A COMPENDIUM OF
NEUROPSYCHOLOGICAL TESTS

A COMPENDIUM OF NEUROPSYCHOLOGICAL TESTS

Administration, Norms, and Commentary

Third Edition

ESTHER STRAUSS
ELISABETH M. S. SHERMAN
OTFRIED SPREEN

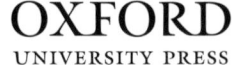

UNIVERSITY PRESS

2006

OXFORD
UNIVERSITY PRESS

Oxford University Press, Inc., publishes works that further
Oxford University's objective of excellence
in research, scholarship, and education.

Oxford   New York
Auckland   Cape Town   Dar es Salaam   Hong Kong   Karachi
Kuala Lumpur   Madrid   Melbourne   Mexico City   Nairobi
New Delhi   Shanghai   Taipei   Toronto

With offices in
Argentina   Austria   Brazil   Chile   Czech Republic   France   Greece
Guatemala   Hungary   Italy   Japan   Poland   Portugal   Singapore
South Korea   Switzerland   Thailand   Turkey   Ukraine   Vietnam

Copyright © 2006 by Oxford University Press

Published by Oxford University Press, Inc.
198 Madison Avenue, New York, New York 10016

www.oup.com

Oxford is a registered trademark of Oxford University Press

Library of Congress Cataloging-in-Publication Data
Strauss, Esther.
A compendium of neuropsychological tests : administration, norms, and commentary /
Esther Strauss, Elisabeth M. S. Sherman, Otfried Spreen.— 3rd ed.
    p.   cm.
Rev. ed. of: A compendium of neuropsychological tests / Otfried Spreen, Esther Strauss.
2nd ed. 1998.
Includes bibliographical references and index.
ISBN-13 978-0-19-515957-8
ISBN 0-19-515957-8
1. Neuropsychological tests—Handbooks, manuals, etc.
[DNLM: 1. Neuropsychological Tests. 2. Reference Values. WL 141 S768c 2006]
I. Sherman, Elisabeth M. S.   II. Spreen, Otfried.   III. Spreen, Otfried. Compendium of
neuropsychological tests.   IV. Title.
RC386.6.N48S67 2006
616.8'0475—dc22   2005020769

9 8 7 6 5 4

Printed in China

We dedicate this volume to Dr. Edgar J. Strauss and Dr. Norman K. Sherman, fathers who gracefully mixed family and work/science and who inspired us with their love of learning, warmth, humor, and intelligence. This book is also dedicated to Dr. Arthur L. Benton, who served as a mentor for generations of neuropsychologists and whose work served as the basis for many of the measures reviewed in this volume.

Preface

RATIONALE: KNOW YOUR TOOLS

How well do you know your tools? While most of us have a working knowledge of the features and limitations of the tests we use, too often our knowledge of the basic psychometrics of our tests, and the research that accompanies their use, appears inadequate. For example, how many neuropsychologists can easily summon test-retest reliability coefficients for all the tests in their battery or relate the sensitivity/specificity of these tests in the clinical population they routinely assess? This is not because the information is lacking (although this is also at times a problem) or difficult to find. Indeed, most of the information one could ever want on psychological tests can be found in test manuals on the office shelves of most practicing neuropsychologists; the rest can be easily obtained via electronic literature searches. Working knowledge of neuropsychological tests is hampered by the most common of modern day afflictions: lack of time, and for want of a better term, "information overload."

Determining whether important information is lacking on any given test requires enough time to survey the literature and scrutinize test manuals for omissions. However, there are simply too many manuals and too many studies for the average neuropsychologist to continually stay up to date on the various strengths and weaknesses of every test he or she uses. The longer the neuropsychological battery, the more time required. The reality is that most of these tests have manuals that are several hundred pages long. Other tests are associated with literally hundreds of research studies. Gaining full familiarity with every aspect of these tests' psychometrics and clinical relevance, in addition to expert competency in administration and scoring, requires hours and hours of time, which for most practicing neuropsychologists is simply an impossible task.

Our own experience bears this out. Prior to commencing the revision, several major tests were released (e.g., D-KEFS, NEPSY, WAIS-III). During the four-year time span spent revising this text, there was a virtual explosion of tests, with several additional major batteries released, including the NAB,

WISC-IV, WPPSI-III, Stanford-Binet-V, WJ III, and WRAML-2, with many more forthcoming (e.g., BSID-III, NEPSY-III, PPVT-IV). As authors of the book and practicing clinicians, we were not sure whether we should have been excited about these new releases or frankly dismayed. The sheer volume of information that we reviewed for this book was indeed staggering, with some test reviews requiring days of effort, and in some cases, weeks. Our offices filled up continually with stacks of studies to review and piles of new test manuals to read. At the very least, we hope that the investment of our time into this book will save readers some of their own time—that most elusive of modern-day commodities.

Our goal was to design a text that would provide, in an easy-to-read, easy-to-reference format, all the major highlights of the most commonly used neuropsychological tests in the form of comprehensive, empirically based critical reviews. In addition, the book was designed to provide an overview of basic and advanced issues germane to neuropsychological assessment, and as such, serves as a guidebook for neuropsychological practice.

"Know Your Tools": this is the driving force behind the newest edition of the *Compendium of Neuropsychological Tests*. We hope that after reading it, users may gain a greater understanding of critical issues relevant to the broader practice of neuropsychological assessment, a strong working knowledge of the specific strengths and weaknesses of the tests in their test portfolio, and most importantly, an enhanced understanding of neuropsychological assessment grounded in empirical evidence and research.

CHANGES

Since its first publication in 1991, the *Compendium of Neuropsychological Tests* has been an essential reference text used both to guide the reader through the maze of published and unpublished literature on tests and to inform clinicians and researchers on the psychometric properties of their instruments so that they can make informed choices and sound interpretations. The goals of the third edition of the *Compendium* remain the same, although admittedly given the huge expansion of the field, our coverage is necessarily selective.

For this edition, we cover most of the tests and topics covered in the previous edition. However, all chapters have been extensively revised and updated. Outdated information has been removed and tests that appear to have met with little use have been deleted. In addition, we have expanded considerably our treatment of topics and tests. New topics include chapters on psychometric issues, normative considerations, and adaptive function. New tests include the Cognitive Assessment System (CAS), Kaplan Baycrest Neurocognitive Assessment (KBNA), Neuropsychological Assessment Battery (NAB), NEPSY, RBANS, TONI-3, SCOLP, WASI, WAIS-III, WISC-IV, WPPSI-III, WTAR, SB5, WJ III COG, GORT-4, CANTAB, D-KEFS, Hayling and Brixton Tests, Comprehensive Trail Making Test, CPT-II, IVA+Plus, Ruff 2 & 7, TEA, TEA-Ch, TOVA, CVLT-II, CVLT-C, Children's Memory Scale (CMS), Doors and People Test, HVLT-R, RBMT-II, RULIT, WMS-III, WRAML-2, BDAE-3, EOWPVT3, EVT, MAE, PPVT-III, Balloons Test, Facial Recognition Test, JLO, VOSP, RASP, Smell Identification Test, Grooved Pegboard, BRIEF, IADL, PAI, SIB-R, Trauma Symptom Inventory (TSI), the b Test, Dot Counting, and the Word Memory Test. We also elected not to cover many of the psychosocial/behavioral scales for children that we had covered in previous editions (e.g., PIC, CBCL) because these were already well-reviewed elsewhere (e.g., Sattler, 2001), and in order to focus our energy on more neuropsychologically based scales such as the BRIEF.

In addition to updating and modifying earlier versions and adding new topics and tests, the presentation format has been altered. For this edition, additional headings have been used, including separate sections for reliability and validity, and more information is provided in tables and figures. We hope that these changes will make it easier for readers to locate critical information and to compare characteristics across measures.

ORGANIZATION OF THE BOOK

The first chapter in this volume presents basic psychometric concepts in neuropsychological assessment and provides an overview of critical issues to consider in evaluating a measure for clinical use. The second chapter considers the basic principles involved in evaluating norms and selecting a normative dataset. Chapters 3 and 4 consider practical aspects of the history-taking interview and the evaluation of the examinee, that is, the assessment process itself. Chapter 5 provides guidelines on report writing and the provision of feedback. Chapters 6 to 16 address specific cognitive domains (intelligence, achievement, executive functions, attention, memory, language, visual perception, somatosensory and olfactory function, mood/personality, response bias), with tests assigned in a rational manner to each of the domains—and the recognition that there is considerable potential for overlap of tests across domains.

To make educated choices regarding the many instruments currently available, the introduction to each domain provides an overview of that area and the various tests covered in that section. A unique feature of each introduction is the inclusion of a table that summarizes salient features (e.g., age ranges covered, tasks included, administration time, key processes thought to be assessed, test-retest reliability, etc.) of each test included in that domain. In this way, readers can quickly determine which test is most appropriate for a particular patient/situation.

To promote clarity, each test review follows a fixed format: purpose, source, age range, description, administration, administration time, scoring, demographic effects, normative data, reliability, validity, and commentary. In each review, we have taken a lifespan perspective so that we could highlight developmental trends and provide a valuable reference text for use with a wide variety of examinees. Thus, many of the measures that we consider pertain to both children and adults, including the elderly; some, however, are geared to one segment of the population. As such, the *Compendium* should be considered a core reference text for adult, geriatric, and pediatric neuropsychological assessment.

CAUTIONS AND CAVEATS

We want to point out that the writing of a book of this scope and complexity will unfortunately—but necessarily—contain some errors. We encourage readers to inform us of any omissions, misinterpretations, typographical errors, or frank gaffes so that we can correct them in the next edition. Despite any test limitations noted here, we also want to highlight that some tests may be useful in clinical or research situations not reviewed in this volume, and that the final decision as to a test's utility and validity rests with the user.

ACKNOWLEDGMENTS

We express our gratitude to the numerous authors whose published work has provided the basis for our work and who frequently provided additional information, clarification, and helpful comments.

In particular, we wish to acknowledge the significant contribution of Daniel Slick to Chapter 1. Special thanks also go to Gordon Chelune, Mike Hunter, Tom Tombaugh, Glenn Larrabee, and Morris Moscovitch, who provided clarifications and insights based on their unique scientific expertise and experience. Over the years, Bob Smith and Travis White at PAR and Aurelio Prifitera at Harcourt Assessment have graciously provided us with test materials for review, and we are indebted to them for their generous support. We also thank the other test authors and publishers who kindly provided us with materials.

We also wish to thank the many individuals who served as ad hoc reviewers for test reviews. These include Nancy Wilde, Stephanie Griffiths, Charmaine Miranda, Ruth Grunau, Diane

Roche, and Laurie Ford. We are indebted to Dr. Ira Bernstein, who graciously offered comments on the *Psychometrics* chapter, and to the graduate students at the University of Victoria, who also provided feedback. Special thanks go to Rob McInerney for his helpful insights on the PASAT. Special thanks also go to Kim Eyrl, who served as a tireless and efficient assistant for aspects of the book. A special note of thanks goes to Joan Bossert, Keith Faivre, Fiona Stevens, and Jeffrey House, our editors at Oxford University Press, for their encouragement and assistance.

Finally, we thank our families for their understanding and support during the many hours it took to write this book. In particular, Esther thanks Josef and their three children (Zeev, Tali, and Tamar), who let her practice tasks on them and who continue to make her life interesting and sweet. Elisabeth wishes to thank Daniel Slick, partner in life, parenthood, and neuropsychology, who was a valued intellectual resource, a tireless supporter for the book, and a dedicated father to their three young children (Madeleine, Tessa, and Lucas)—the last two born during the writing of this book.

Contents

List of Acronyms, xiii

1. **Psychometrics in Neuropsychological Assessment, 1**

2. **Norms Selection in Neuropsychological Assessment, 44**

3. **History Taking, 55**

4. **Test Selection, Test Administration, and Preparation of the Patient, 75**

5. **Report Writing and Feedback Sessions, 86**

6. **General Cognitive Functioning, Neuropsychological Batteries, and Assessment of Premorbid Intelligence, 98**
   Introduction, 98
   Bayley Scales of Infant Development—Second Edition (BSID-II), 114
   Cognitive Assessment System (CAS), 133
   Dementia Rating Scale—2 (DRS-2), 144
   Kaplan Baycrest Neurocognitive Assessment (KBNA), 159
   Kaufman Brief Intelligence Test (K-BIT), 164
   Mini-Mental State Examination (MMSE), 168
   National Adult Reading Test (NART), 189
   NEPSY: A Developmental Neuropsychological Assessment, 201
   Neuropsychological Assessment Battery (NAB), 218
   Raven's Progressive Matrices (RPM), 229
   Repeatable Battery for the Assessment of Neuropsychological Status (RBANS), 237
   Stanford-Binet Intelligence Scales—Fifth Edition (SB5), 258
   The Test of Nonverbal Intelligence—3 (TONI-3), 268
   The Speed and Capacity of Language Processing Test (SCOLP), 272
   Wechsler Abbreviated Scale of Intelligence (WASI), 279
   Wechsler Adult Intelligence Scale—III (WAIS-III), 283
   Wechsler Intelligence Scale for Children—Fourth Edition (WISC-IV), 310

   Wechsler Preschool and Primary Scale of Intelligence—Third Edition (WPPSI-III), 337
   Wechsler Test of Adult Reading (WTAR), 347
   Woodcock-Johnson III Tests of Cognitive Abilities (WJ III COG), 351

7. **Achievement Tests, 363**
   Introduction, 363
   The Gray Oral Reading Test—Fourth Edition (GORT-4), 365
   Wechsler Individual Achievement Test—Second Edition (WIAT-II), 370
   Wide Range Achievement Test—3 (WRAT3), 384
   Woodcock-Johnson III Tests of Achievement (WJ III ACH), 390

8. **Executive Functions, 401**
   Introduction, 401
   Behavioral Assessment of the Dysexecutive Syndrome (BADS), 408
   CANTAB, 415
   Category Test (CT), 424
   Cognitive Estimation Test (CET), 437
   Delis-Kaplan Executive Function System (D-KEFS), 443
   Design Fluency Test, 450
   Five-Point Test, 456
   The Hayling and Brixton Tests, 460
   Ruff Figural Fluency Test (RFFT), 466
   Self-Ordered Pointing Test (SOPT), 471
   Stroop Test, 477
   Verbal Fluency, 499
   Wisconsin Card Sorting Test (WCST), 526

9. **Attention, 546**
   Introduction, 546
   Brief Test of Attention (BTA), 547
   Color Trails Test (CTT) and Children's Color Trails Test (CCTT), 554

Comprehensive Trail Making Test (CTMT), 557
Conners' Continuous Performance Test II
    (CPT-II), 562
Integrated Visual and Auditory Continuous Performance
    Test (IVA + Plus), 575
Paced Auditory Serial Addition Test (PASAT) and
    Children's Paced Auditory Serial Addition Test
    (CHIPASAT), 582
Ruff 2 & 7 Selective Attention Test (2 & 7 Test), 610
Symbol Digit Modalities Test (SDMT), 617
Test of Everyday Attention (TEA), 628
Test of Everyday Attention for Children
    (TEA-Ch), 638
Test of Variables of Attention (T.O.V.A.), 645
Trail Making Test (TMT), 655

10. **Memory, 678**
Introduction, 678
Autobiographical Memory Interview (AMI), 687
Benton Visual Retention Test (BVRT-5), 691
Brief Visuospatial Memory Test—Revised
    (BVMT-R), 701
Brown-Peterson Task, 704
Buschke Selective Reminding Test (SRT), 713
California Verbal Learning Test-II (CVLT-II), 730
California Verbal Learning Test—Children's Version
    (CVLT-C), 735
Children's Memory Scale (CMS), 746
Doors and People Test (DPT), 755
Hopkins Verbal Learning Test—Revised
    (HVLT-R), 760
Recognition Memory Test (RMT), 769
Rey-Osterrieth Auditory Verbal Learning Test
    (RAVLT), 776
Rey Complex Figure Test (ROCF), 811
Rivermead Behavioural Memory Test—Second
    Edition (RBMT-II), 841
Ruff-Light Trail Learning Test (RULIT), 851
Sentence Repetition Test, 854
Wechsler Memory Scale—Third Edition (WMS-III), 860
Wide Range Assessment of Memory and
    Learning—Second Edition (WRAML2), 881

11. **Language Tests, 891**
Introduction, 891
Boston Diagnostic Aphasia Examination—
    Third Edition (BDAE-3), 892
Boston Naming Test—2 (BNT-2), 901
Dichotic Listening—Words, 916
Expressive One-Word Picture Vocabulary Test—
    Third Edition (EOWPVT3), 922
Expressive Vocabulary Test (EVT), 928
Multilingual Aphasia Examination (MAE), 933
Peabody Picture Vocabulary Test—Third Edition
    (PPVT-III), 940
Token Test (TT), 953

12. **Tests of Visual Perception, 963**
Introduction, 963
Balloons Test, 965
Bells Cancellation Test, 968
Clock Drawing Test (CDT), 972
Facial Recognition Test (FRT), 983
Hooper Visual Organization Test (VOT), 990
Judgement of Line Orientation (JLO), 997
Visual Object and Space Perception Battery
    (VOSP), 1006

13. **Tests of Somatosensory Function, Olfactory Function,
    and Body Orientation, 1012**
Introduction, 1012
Finger Localization, 1013
Right-Left Orientation (RLO), 1017
Rivermead Assessment of Somatosensory
    Performance (RASP), 1020
Smell Identification Test (SIT), 1023
Tactual Performance Test (TPT), 1031

14. **Tests of Motor Function, 1042**
Introduction, 1042
Finger Tapping Test (FTT), 1043
Grip Strength, 1052
Grooved Pegboard, 1061
Purdue Pegboard Test, 1068

15. **Assessment of Mood, Personality,
    and Adaptive Functions, 1080**
Introduction, 1080
Beck Depression Inventory—Second Edition
    (BDI-II), 1084
Behavior Rating Inventory of Executive Function
    (BRIEF), 1090
Geriatric Depression Scale (GDS), 1099
Instrumental Activities of Daily Living (IADL), 1107
Minnesota Multiphasic Personality Inventory-2
    (MMPI-2), 1113
Personality Assessment Inventory (PAI), 1126
Scales of Independent Behavior—Revised
    (SIB-R), 1134
Trauma Symptom Inventory (TSI), 1140

16. **Assessment of Response Bias
    and Suboptimal Performance, 1145**
Introduction, 1145
The b Test, 1158
The Dot Counting Test (DCT), 1161
Rey Fifteen-Item Test (FIT), 1166
Test of Memory Malingering (TOMM), 1171
21 Item Test, 1176
Victoria Symptom Validity Test (VSVT), 1179
Word Memory Test (WMT), 1184

Test Index, 1189
Subject Index, 1204

List of Acronyms

3MS	Modified Mini-Mental State Examination
2 & 7 Test	Ruff 2 & 7 test
AAE	African American English
ACI	Attention/ Concentration Index
AcoA	Anterior communicating artery
AD	Alzheimer's disease or absolute deviation
ADHD	Attention Deficit Hyperactivity Disorder
ADL	Activities of daily living
AERA	American Educational Research Association
AIS	Autobiographical Incidents Schedule
ALS	Amyotrophic lateral sclerosis
AMI	Autobiographical Memory Interview or Asocial Maladaptic Index
AMNART	American National Adult Reading Test
A-MSS	Age-corrected MOANS scaled score
A&E-MSS	Age- and education-corrected MOANS scaled score
ANELT-A	Nijmwegen Everyday Language Test
APA	American Psychological Association
APM	Advanced Progressive Matrices
Arith	Arithmetic
ASHA	American Speech and Hearing Association
ASTM	Amsterdam Short Term Memory Test
ATR	Atypical Response
ATT	Attention
Aud. Imm.	Auditory Immediate
Aud. Del.	Auditory Delay
Aud. Recog	Auditory Recognition
AVLT	Auditory Verbal Learning Test
BADS	Behavioral Assessment of the Dysexecutive Syndrome
BAI	Beck Anxiety Inventory
BASC	Behavior Assessment System for Children
BCET	Biber Cognitive Estimation Test
BCT	Booklet Category Test
BD	Block Design
BDAE	Boston Diagnostic Aphasia Examination
BDI	Beck Depression Inventory
BIA	Brief Intellectual Ability
BLC	Big Little Circle
BNT	Boston Naming Test
BQSS	Boston Qualitative Scoring System
BRB-N	Brief Repeatable Battery of Neuropsychological Tests
BRI	Behavior Regulation Index
BRIEF	Behavior Rating Inventory of Executive Function
BRIEF-A	Behavior Rating Inventory of Executive Function—Adult
BRIEF-P	Behavior Rating Inventory of Executive Function-Preschool Version
BRIEF-SR	Behavior Rating Inventory of Executive Function—Self-Report
BRR	Back Random Responding
BRS	Behavior Rating Scale
BSI	Brief Symptom Inventory
BSID	Bayley Scales of Infant Development
B-SIT	Brief Smell Identification Test
BTA	Brief Test of Attention
BVMT-R	Brief Visuospatial Memory Test—Revised
BVRT	Benton Visual Retention Test
CAARS	Conners' Adult ADHD Rating Scale
CANTAB	Cambridge Neuropsychological Test Automated Batteries
CARB	Computerized Assessment of Response Bias
CAS	Cognitive Assessment System
C-AUSNART	Contextual Australian NART
CBCL	Child Behavior Checklist
CCC	Consonant Trigrams
CCF	Cattell Culture Fair Intelligence Test
CCRT	Cambridge Contextual Reading Test
CCTT	Children's Color Trails Test
CCT	Children's Category Test
CDF	Cashel Discriminant Function
CDT	Clock Drawing Test

CELF	Clinical Evaluation of Language Fundamentals	DRS	Dementia Rating Scale
CERAD	Consortium for the Establishment of a Registry for Alzheimer's Disease	DSM-IV	Diagnostic and Statistical Manual of Mental Disorders
CES-D	Center for Epidemiological Studies Depression Scale	DSp	Digit Span
		DSS-ROCF	Developmental Scoring System for the Rey-Osterrieth Complex Figure
CET	Cognitive Estimation Test	DSym	Digit Symbol
CFT	Complex Figure Test	DT	Dual Task
CFQ	Cognitive Failures Questionnaire	Ed	Education
CHC	Carroll-Horn-Cattell	EI	Exaggeration Index
CHI	Closed head injury	ELF	Excluded Letter Fluency
CHIPASAT	Children's Paced Auditory Serial Addition Test	EMI	Externalized Maladaptive Index
		EMQ	Everyday Memory Questionnaire
CI	Confidence interval	EOWPVT	Expressive One-Word Picture Vocabulary Test
CLR	Conceptual Level Responses		
CLTR	Consistent Long-Term Retrieval	ERP	Event-related potential
CMS	Children's Memory Scale	ERR	Errors
CNS	Central nervous system	E-Score	Effort-Index Score
CO	Correlation Score	EVT	Expressive Vocabulary Test
Comp	Comprehension	EXIT25	Executive Interview
CONCEPT	Conceptualization	Fam Pic (Pix)	Family Pictures
Cons	Consistency	FAS	Letters commonly used to assess phonemic fluency (COWA) or Fetal Alcohol Syndrome
CONSRT	Construction		
COWA	Controlled Oral Word Association		
CPM	Colored Progressive Matrices	FBS	Fake Bad Scale
CPT	Continuous Performance Test	FDWT	Fused Dichotic Words Test
CRI	Concussion Resolution Index	FIM	Functional Independence Measures
CSHA	Canadian Study of Health and Aging	FFD	Freedom from Distractibility
CT	Category Test or computed tomography	FIT	Rey Fifteen-Item Test
CTMT	Comprehensive Trail Making Test	FLD	Frontal lobe dementia
CTT	Color Trails Test	FLE	Frontal lobe epilepsy
CV	Consonant Vowel	FMS	Failure to Maintain Set
CVA	Cerebrovascular accident	FP	False Positive
CVLT	California Verbal Learning Test	FRT	Facial Recognition Test
CVLT-C	California Verbal Learning Test—Children's Version	FTD	Frontotemporal dementia
		FTT	Finger Tapping Test
CVLT-SF	California Verbal Learning Test—Short Form	FSIQ	Full Scale IQ
		FWSTM	Four-Word Short-Term Memory Test
CW	Color-Word	GAI	General Ability Index
DAFS	Direct Assessment of Functional Status	*Ga*	Auditory Processing
DAI	Diffuse axonal injury	*Gc*	Crystallized Ability
DAS	Das Assessment System	GCS	Glascow Coma Scale
DCT	Dot Counting Test	GDS	Geriatric Depression Scale or Gordon Diagnostic System
DEF	Defensiveness Index		
DEX	Dysexecutive Questionnaire	GEC	Global Executive Composite
DFR	Delayed Free Recall	*Gf*	Fluid Ability
DFT	Design Fluency Test	GLR	Long-Term Retrieval
DH	Dominant Hand	*GQ*	Quantitative Knowledge
DICA	Diagnostic Interview for Children and Adolescents	*Grw*	Reading-Writing
		GS	Processing Speed
D-KEFS	Delis-Kaplan Executive Function System	*Gsm*	Short-Term Memory
DL	Dichotic Listening	*GV*	Visual Processing
DLB	Dementia with Lewy bodies	GIA	General Intellectual Ability
DMS	Delayed Matching to Sample	GLC	General Language Composite
DPT	Doors and People Test	GMI	General Memory Index or General Maladaptic Index
DR	Delayed Recall or Recognition		
DRI	Delayed Recall Index		

GNDS	General Neuropsychological Deficit Scale
GORT	Gray Oral Reading Test
GRI	General Recognition Index
HD	Huntington's disease
HMGT	Homophone Meaning Generation Test
HRCT	Halstead-Reitan Category Test
HRNES	Halstead-Russell Neuropsychological Evaluation System
HS	High school
HVLT-R	Hopkins Verbal Learning Test—Revised
IADL	Instrumental Activities of Daily Living
ICC	Intraclass correlation
IED	Intra/Extra-Dimensional Shift
IES	Impact of Event Scale
IMC	Information-Memory-Concentration Test
IMI	Immediate Memory Index or Internalized Maladaptive Index
ImPACT	Immediate Post-Concussion Assessment and Cognitive Testing
Info	Information
INS	International Neuropsychological Society
I/P	Initiation/Perseveration
IR	Immediate Recognition
ISI	Inter-Stimulus Interval
IVA	Integrated Visual and Auditory Continuous Performance Test
JOLO(JLO)	Judgement of Line Orientation
K-ABC	Kaufman Assessment Battery for Children
KAIT	Kaufman Adolescent and Adult Intelligence Test
K-BIT	Kaufman Brief Intelligence Test
K-FAST	Kaufman Functional Academic Skills Test
KBNA	Kaplan Baycrest Neurocognitive Assessment
KTEA	Kaufman Test of Educational Achievement
LAMB	Learning and Memory Battery
LD	Learning disability
LDFR	Long Delay Free Recall
LEA	Left ear advantage
LEI	Learning Efficiency Index
Let-Num Seq	Letter Number Sequencing
LH	Left hemisphere
LL	Learning to Learn
LM	Logical Memory
LOC	Loss of consciousness
LOT	Learning Over Trials
LTPR	Long-Term Percent Retention
LTR	Long-Term Retrieval
LTS	Long-Term Storage
MAE	Multilingual Aphasia Examination
MAI	Multilevel Assessment Instrument
MAL	Malingering Index
MAVDRI	Mayo Auditory-Verbal Delayed Recall Index
MAVLEI	Mayo Auditory-Verbal Learning Efficiency Index
MAVPRI	Mayo Auditory-Verbal Percent Retention Index
MBA	Mini-Battery of Achievement
MC	Multiple Choice
MCG	Medical College of Georgia
MCI	Mild Cognitive Impairment or Metacognitive Index
MDI	Mental Development Index
MEM	Memory
MHT	Moray House Test
MMPI	Minnesota Multiphasic Personality Inventory
MMSE	Mini Mental State Examination
MND	Malingered Neurocognitive Dysfunction
MOANS	Mayo's Older Americans Normative Studies
MOAANS	Mayo's African American Normative Studies
MOT	Motor
MR	Matrix Reasoning
MRI	Magnetic resonance imaging
MS	Multiple Sclerosis
MSB	Meyers Short battery
MSI	Memory Screening Index
MSS	MOANS Scaled Score
MTBI	Mild traumatic brain injury
MTCF	Modified Taylor Complex Figure
MTS	Matching to Sample
NAB	Neuropsychological Assessment Battery
NAN	National Academy of Neuropsychology
NART	National Adult Reading Test
NAART	North American Reading Test
NCCEA	Neurosensory Center Comprehensive Examination for Aphasia
NCE	Normal Curve Equivalent
NDH	Non-Dominant Hand
NFT	Neurofibrillary tangles
NIM	Negative Impression Management
NIS	Neuropsychological Impairment Scale
NPA	Negative Predictive Accuracy
NPE	Non-Perseverative errors
NPP	Negative predictive power
NPV	Negative predictive value
NVIQ	Nonverbal IQ
OA	Object Assembly
OARS	Older Americans Resources and Services
ODD	Oppositional Defiant Disorder
OPIE	Oklahoma Premorbid Intelligence Estimate
ORQ	Oral Reading Quotient
PA	Picture Arrangement
PAI	Personality Assessment Inventory
PAL	Paired Associate Learning
PASAT	Paced Auditory Serial Addition Test
PASS	Planning, Attention, Simultaneous, Successive
PC	Picture Completion
PCS	Post-concussive symptoms (or syndrome)
PD	Parkinson's disease
PDD	Pervasive developmental disorder
PDI	Psychomotor Development Index

PDRT	Portland Digit Recognition Test	ROWPVT	Receptive One-Word Picture Vocabulary Test
PE	Perseverative Errors or practice effects	RPC	Recognition Percent Correct
PET	Positron emission tomography	RPI	Relative Proficiency Index
PIM	Positive Impression Management	RPM	Raven's Progressive Matrices
PKU	Phenylketonuria	RT	Reaction Time
POI	Perceptual Organization Index	RULIT	Ruff-Light Trail Learning Test
PICA	Porch Index of Communicative Ability	RVP	Rapid Visual Information Processing
PIQ	Performance IQ	SADI	Self-Awareness of Deficits Interview
PMA	Primary Mental Abilities	SAILS	Structured Assessment of Independent Living Skills
PNES	Psychogenic nonepileptic seizures		
PPA	Positive predictive accuracy	SAS	Standard Age Score
PPP	Positive predictive power	SAT9	Stanford Achievement Test, Ninth Edition
PPV	Positive predictive value	SB	Stanford-Binet
PPVT	Peabody Picture Vocabulary Test	SB-IV	Stanford-Binet Intelligence Scales, Fourth Edition
PR	Perseverative Responses or percentile rank		
PRI	Perceptual Reasoning Index or Percent Retention Index	SBE	Spanish Bilingual Edition
		SBI	Screening Battery Index
PRM	Pattern Recognition Memory	SCID	Structured Clinical Interview for DSM
PSAT	Paced Serial Addition Test	SCL-90	Symptom Checklist-90
PSI	Processing Speed Index	SCOLP	Speed and Capacity of Language Processing Test
PSQ	Processing Speed Quotient	SCT	Short Cateogry Test
PSS	Pernal Semantic Schedule	SD	Standard deviation
PTA	Post-traumatic amnesia	SDMT	Symbol Digit Modalities Test
PTSD	Post-traumatic stress disorder	SEE	Standard error of the estimate
PVSAT	Paced Visual Serial Addition Test	SEM	Standard error of measurement
RASP	Rivermead Assessment of Somatosensory Performance	SEP	Standard error of prediction
		SES	Socioeconomic status
RAVLT	Rey Auditory Verbal Learning Test	SIB-R	Scales of Independent Behavior-Revised
RAVLT-EI	Rey Auditory Verbal Test—Exaggeration Index	SIM	Similarities
RBANS	Repeatable Battery for the Assessment of Neuropsychological Status	SIT	Smell Identification Test
		SOAP	Subject-Relative, Object-Relative, Active, Passive
RBMT	Rivermead Behavioral Memory Test	SOC	Stockings of Cambridge
RBMT-C	Rivermead Behavioral Memory Test for Children	SOP	Sub-Optimal Performance
		SOPT	Self-Ordered Pointing Test
RBMT-E	Rivermead Behavioral Memory Test-Extended Version	SPECT	Single photon emission computed tomography
		SPIE	Australian version of the OPIE
RC	Recognition (hit rate) or Restructured Clinical	SPM	Standard Progressive Matrices
		SPS	Standardized Profile Score
rCBF	Regional cerebral blood flow	SRB	Standardized regression-based
RCI	Reliable Change Index	SRM	Spatial Recognition Memory
RCI-PE	Reliable Change Index with practice effects	SRT	Selective Reminding Test
RD	Reading disorder	SS	Symbol Search or standard score
RDF	Rogers Discriminant Function	SSP	Spatial Span
RDS	Reliable Digit Span	SST	Silly Sentences Test
REA	Right ear advantage	ST	Sub-Test
REC	Recognition	STPR	Short-Term Percent Retention
RFFT	Ruff Figural Fluency Test	STR	Short-Term Recall
RH	Right hemisphere	SVT	Symptom Validity Test
RLO	Right-Left Orientation	SWT	Spot-the-Word Test
RLTR	Random Long-Term Retrieval	SWM	Spatial Working Memory
RMF	Recognition Memory for Faces	TACL-R	Test for Auditory Comprehension of Language- Revised
RMI	Rarely Missed Index or Relative Mastery Index		
RMT	Recognition Memory Test	TBI	Traumatic brain injury
ROC	Receiver Operating Curve	TE	Total Errors
ROCF	Rey-Osterrieth Complex Figure	TEA	Test of Everyday Attention
ROR	Reach Out and Read	TEA-Ch	Test of Everyday Attention for Children

TIA	Transient ischemic attack	VR	Visual Reproduction
TLE	Temporal lobe epilepsy	VST	Victoria Stroop Test
TMT	Trail Making Test	VSVT	Victoria Symptom Validity Test
TOLD-P	Test of Language Development-Primary	WAB	Western Aphasia Battery
TOMAL	Test of Memory and Learning	WAIS	Wechsler Adult Intelligence Scale
TOMM	Test of Memory Malingering	WAIS-R	Wechsler Adult Intelligence Scale, Revised
TONI	Test of Nonverbal Intelligence	WAIS-III	Wechsler Adult Intelligence Scale, Third Edition
T.O.V.A.	Test of Variables of Attention		
TP	True Positive	WASI	Wechsler Abbreviated Scale of Intelligence
TPT	Tactual Performance Test	WCST	Wisconsin Card Sorting Test
TRF	Teacher's Report Form	WIAT	Wechsler Individual Achievement Test
TSI	Trauma Symptom Inventory	WISC	Wechsler Intelligence Scale for Children
TT	Token Test	WISC-III	Wechsler Intelligence Scale for Children, Third Edition
TTF	Trials to Complete First Category		
TVIP	Test de Vocabulario en Imagenes Peabody	WISC-IV	Wechsler Intelligence Scale for Children, Fourth Edition
UCO	Uses for Common Objects		
UH-DRS	Unified Huntington's Disease Rating Scale	WJ III ACH	Woodcock-Johnson Tests of Achievement, Third Edition
UNIT	Universal Nonverbal Intelligence Test		
UPSIT	University of Pennsylvania Smell Identification Test (see also SIT)	WJ III COG	Woodcock-Johnson Tests of Cognitive Abilities, Third Edition
VABS	Vineland Adaptive Behavior Scale	WJ-R	Woodcock-Johnson Revised
VaD	Vascular dementia	WMH	White matter hyperintensities
VCI	Verbal Comprehension Index	WMI	Working Memory Index
VD	Vascular dementia	WMS	Wechsler Memory Scale
VIQ	Verbal IQ	WMT	Word Memory Test
Vis. Imm.	Visual Immediate	WPPSI	Wechsler Preschool and Primary Scale of Intelligence
Vis. Del.	Visual Delay		
VLS	Victoria Longitudinal Study	WPPSI-III	Wechsler Preschool and Primary Scale of Intelligence, Third Edition
VMI	Developmental Test of Visual-Motor Integration		
VOC	Vocabulary	WPPSI-R	Wechsler Preschool and Primary Scale of Intelligence, Revised
VOSP	Visual and Object Space Perception Battery	WRAML	Wide Range Assessment of Memory and Learning
VOT	Hooper Visual Organization Test	WRAT	Wide Range Achievement Test
VPA	Verbal Paired Associates	WTAR	Wechsler Test of Adult Reading

A COMPENDIUM OF
NEUROPSYCHOLOGICAL TESTS

1

Psychometrics in Neuropsychological Assessment
with Daniel J. Slick

OVERVIEW

The process of neuropsychological assessment depends to a large extent on the reliability and validity of neuropsychological tests. Unfortunately, not all neuropsychological tests are created equal, and, like any other product, published tests vary in terms of their "quality," as defined in psychometric terms such as reliability, measurement error, temporal stability, sensitivity, specificity, predictive validity, and with respect to the care with which test items are derived and normative data are obtained. In addition to commercial measures, numerous tests developed primarily for research purposes have found their way into wide clinical usage; these vary considerably with regard to psychometric properties. With few exceptions, when tests originate from clinical research contexts, there is often validity data but little else, which makes estimating measurement precision and stability of test scores a challenge.

Regardless of the origins of neuropsychological tests, their competent use in clinical practice demands a good working knowledge of test standards and of the specific psychometric characteristics of each test used. This includes familiarity with the Standards for Educational and Psychological Testing (American Educational Research Association [AERA] et al., 1999) and a working knowledge of basic psychometrics. Texts such as those by Nunnally and Bernstein (1994) and Anastasi and Urbina (1997) outline some of the fundamental psychometric prerequisites for competent selection of tests and interpretation of obtained scores. Other, neuropsychologically focused texts such as Mitrushina et al. (2005), Lezak et al. (2004), Baron (2004), Franklin (2003a), and Franzen (2000) also provide guidance. The following is intended to provide a broad overview of important psychometric concepts in neuropsychological assessment and coverage of important issues to consider when critically evaluating tests for clinical usage. Much of the information provided also serves as a conceptual framework for the test reviews in this volume.

THE NORMAL CURVE

The frequency distributions of many physical, biological, and psychological attributes, as they occur across individuals in nature, tend to conform, to a greater or lesser degree, to a bell-shaped curve (see Figure 1–1). This *normal curve* or *normal distribution*, so named by Karl Pearson, is also known as the Gaussian or Laplace-Gauss distribution, after the 18th-century mathematicians who first defined it. The normal curve is the basis of many commonly used statistical and psychometric models (e.g., classical test theory) and is the assumed distribution for many psychological variables.[1]

Definition and Characteristics

The normal curve has a number of specific properties. It is unimodal, perfectly symmetrical and asymptotic at the tails. With respect to scores from measures that are normally distributed, the ordinate, or height of the curve at any point along the x (test score) axis, is the proportion of persons within the sample who obtained a given score. The ordinates for a range of scores (i.e., between two points on the x axis) may also be summed to give the proportion of persons that obtained a score within the specified range. If a specified normal curve accurately reflects a population distribution, then ordinate values are also equivalent to the probability of observing a given score or range of scores when randomly sampling from the population. Thus, the normal curve may also be referred to as a probability distribution.

Figure 1–1 The normal curve.

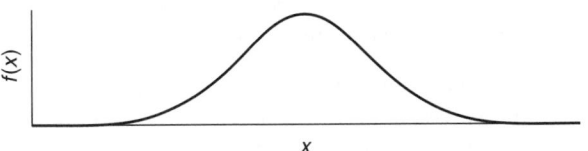

The normal curve is mathematically defined as follows:

$$f(x) = \frac{1}{\sqrt{2\pi\sigma^2}} e - (x - \mu)^2 \qquad [1]$$

Where:

x = measurement values (test scores)
μ = the mean of the test score distribution
σ = the standard deviation of the test score distribution
π = the constant pi (3.14 . . .)
e = the base of natural logarithms (2.71 . . .)
$f(x)$ = the height (ordinate) of the curve for any given test score

Relevance for Assessment

As noted previously, because it is a frequency distribution, the area under any given segment of the normal curve indicates the frequency of observations or cases within that interval. From a practical standpoint, this provides psychologists with an estimate of the "normality" or "abnormality" of any given test score or range of scores (i.e., whether it falls in the center of the bell shape, where the majority of scores lie, or instead, at either of the tail ends, where few scores can be found). The way in which the degree of "normality" or "abnormality" of test scores is quantified varies, but perhaps the most useful and inherently understandable metric is the *percentile*.

Z Scores and Percentiles

A percentile indicates the percentage of scores that fall at or below a given test score. As an example, we will assume that a given test score is plotted on a normal curve. When all of the ordinate values at and below this test score are summed, the resulting value is the percentile associated with that test score (e.g., a score in the 75th percentile indicates that 75% of the reference sample obtained equal or lower scores).

To convert scores to percentiles, raw scores may be linearly transformed or "standardized" in several ways. The simplest and perhaps most commonly calculated standard score is the *z score*, which is obtained by subtracting the sample mean score from an obtained score and dividing the result by the sample *SD*, as show below:

$$z = (x - X)/SD \qquad [2]$$

Where:

x = measurement value (test score)
X = the mean of the test score distribution
SD = the standard deviation of the test score distribution

The resulting distribution of z scores has a mean of 0 and an *SD* of 1, regardless of the metric of raw scores from which they were derived. For example, given a mean of 25 and an *SD* of 5, a raw score of 20 translates into a z score of −1. The percentile

corresponding to any resulting z score can then be easily looked up in tables available in most statistical texts. Z score conversions to percentiles are also shown in Table 1–1.

Interpretation of Percentiles

An important property of the normal curve is that the relationship between raw or z scores (which for purposes of this discussion are equivalent, since they are linear transformations of each other) and percentiles is not linear. That is, a constant difference between raw or z scores will be associated with a variable difference in percentile scores, as a function of the distance of the two scores from the mean. This is due to the fact that there are proportionally more observations (scores) near the mean than there are farther from the mean; otherwise, the distribution would be rectangular, or non-normal. This can readily be seen in Figure 1–2, which shows the normal distribution with demarcation of z scores and corresponding percentile ranges.

The nonlinear relation between z scores and percentiles has important interpretive implications. For example, a one-point difference between two z scores may be interpreted differently, depending on where the two scores fall on the normal curve. As can be seen, the difference between a z score of 0 and a z score of +1 is 34 percentile points, because 34% of scores fall between these two z scores (i.e., the scores being compared are at the 50th and 84th percentiles). However, the difference between a z score of +2 and a z score of +3 is less than 3 percentile points, because only 2.5% of the distribution falls between these two points (i.e., the scores being compared are at the 98th and 99.9th percentiles). On the other hand, interpretation of percentile–score differences is also not straightforward, in that an equivalent "difference" between two percentile rankings may entail different clinical implications if the scores occur at the tail end of the curve than if they occur near the middle of the distribution. For example, a 30-point difference between scores at the 1st percentile versus the 31st percentile may be more clinically meaningful than the same difference between scores at the 35th percentile versus the 65th percentile.

Linear Transformation of Z Scores: T Scores and Other Standard Scores

In addition to the z score, linear transformation can be used to produce other standardized scores that have the same properties with regard to easy conversion via table look-up (see Table 1–1). The most common of these are T scores ($M = 50$, $SD = 10$), scaled scores, and standard scores such as those used in most IQ tests ($M = 10$, $SD = 3$, and $M = 100$, $SD = 15$). It must be remembered that z scores, T scores, standard scores, and percentile equivalents are derived from *samples*; although these are often treated as population values, any limitations of generalizability due to reference sample composition or testing circumstances must be taken into consideration when standardized scores are interpreted.

Table 1–1 Score Conversion Table

IQ[a]	T	SS[b]	Percentile	−z ǀ +z	Percentile	SS[b]	T	IQ[a]
≤55	≤20	≤1	≤0.1	≤3.00≥	≥99.9	≥19	≥80	≥145
56–60	21–23	2	<1	2.67–2.99	>99	18	77–99	140–144
61–67	24–27	3	1	2.20–2.66	99	17	73–76	133–139
68–70	28–30	4	2	1.96–2.19	98	16	70–72	130–132
71–72	31		3	1.82–1.95	97		69	128–129
73–74	32–33		4	1.70–1.81	96		67–68	126–127
75–76	34	5	5	1.60–1.69	95	15	66	124–125
77			6	1.52–1.59	94			123
78	35		7	1.44–1.51	93		65	122
79	36		8	1.38–1.43	92		64	121
80		6	9	1.32–1.37	91	14		120
81	37		10	1.26–1.31	90		63	119
			11	1.21–1.25	89			
82	38		12	1.16–1.20	88		62	118
83			13	1.11–1.15	87			117
84	39		14	1.06–1.10	86		61	116
			15	1.02–1.05	85			
85	40	7	16	.98–1.01	84	13	60	115
			17	.94–.97	83			
86	41		18	.90–.93	82		59	114
87			19	.86–.89	81			113
			20	.83–.85	80			
88	42		21	.79–.82	79		58	112
			22	.76–.78	78			
89			23	.73–.75	77			111
	43		24	.70–.72	76		57	
90		8	25	.66–.69	75	12		110
			26	.63–.65	74			
91	44		27	.60–.62	73		56	109
			28	.57–.59	72			
			29	.54–.56	71			
92			30	.52–.53	70			108
	45		31	.49–.51	69		55	
93			32	.46–.48	68			107
			33	.43–.45	67			
94	46		34	.40–.42	66		54	106
			35	.38–.39	65			
			36	.35–.37	64			
95		9	37	.32–.34	63	11		105
	47		38	.30–.31	62		53	
96			39	.27–.29	61			104
			40	.25–.26	60			
			41	.22–.24	59			
97	48		42	.19–.21	58		52	103
			43	.17–.18	57			
			44	.14–.16	56			
98			45	.12–.13	55			102
	49		46	.09–.11	54		51	
99			47	.07–.08	53			101
			48	.04–.06	52			
			49	.02–.03	51			
100	50	10	50	.00–.01	50	10	50	100

[a]$M = 100$, $SD = 15$; [b]$M = 10$, $SD = 3$.

Note: SS = Scaled

Figure 1–2 The normal curve demarcated by z scores.

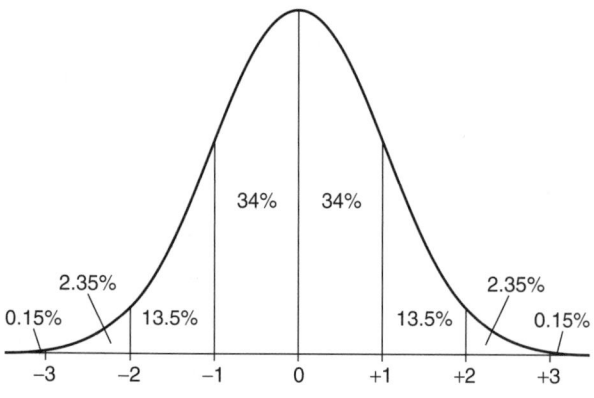

The Meaning of Standardized Test Scores: Score Interpretation

As well as facilitating translation of raw scores to estimated population ranks, standardization of test scores, by virtue of conversion to a common metric, facilitates comparison of scores across measures. However, this is only advisable when the raw score distributions for tests that are being compared are approximately normal in the population. In addition, if standardized scores are to be compared, they should be derived from similar samples, or more ideally, from the same sample. A score at the 50th percentile on a test normed on a population of university students does not have the same meaning as an "equivalent" score on a test normed on a population of elderly individuals. When comparing test scores, one must also take into consideration both the reliability of the two measures and their intercorrelation before determining if a significant difference exists (see Crawford & Garthwaite, 2002). In some cases, relatively large disparities between standard scores may not actually reflect reliable differences, and therefore may not be clinically meaningful. Furthermore, statistically significant or reliable differences between test scores may be common in a reference sample; therefore, the baserate of differences must also be considered, depending on the level of the scores (an IQ of 90 versus 110 as compared to 110 versus 130). One should also keep in mind that when test scores are not normally distributed, standardized scores may not accurately reflect actual population rank. In these circumstances, differences between standard scores may be misleading.

Note also that comparability across tests does not imply equality in meaning and relative importance of scores. For example, one may compare standard scores on measures of pitch discrimination and intelligence, but it will rarely be the case that these scores are of equal clinical or practical meaning or significance.

Interpreting Extreme Scores

A final critical issue with respect to the meaning of standardized scores (e.g., z scores) has to do with extreme observations.

In clinical practice, one may encounter standard scores that are either extremely low or extremely high. The meaning and comparability of such scores will depend critically on the characteristics of the normative sample from which they derive.

For example, consider a hypothetical case in which an examinee obtains a raw score that is below the range of scores found in a normal sample. Suppose further that the SD in the normal sample is very small and thus the examinee's raw score translates to a z score of −5, indicating that the probability of encountering this score in the normal population would be 3 in 10 million (i.e., a percentile ranking of .00003). This represents a considerable extrapolation from the actual normative data, as (1) the normative sample did not include 10 million individuals (2) not a single individual in the normative sample obtained a score anywhere close to the examinee's score. The percentile value is therefore an extrapolation and confers a false sense of precision. While one may be confident that it indicates impairment, there may be no basis to assume that it represents a meaningfully "worse" performance than a z score of −3, or of −4.

The *estimated prevalence value* of an obtained z score (or T score, etc.) can be calculated to determine whether interpretation of extreme scores may be appropriate. This is simply accomplished by inverting the percentile score corresponding to the z score (i.e., dividing 1 by the percentile score). For example, a z score of −4 is associated with an estimated frequency of occurrence or prevalence of approximately 0.00003. Dividing 1 by this value gives a rounded result of 31,560. Thus, the estimated prevalence value of this score in the population is 1 in 31,560. If the normative sample from which a z score is derived is considerably smaller than the denominator of the estimated prevalence value (i.e., 31,560 in the example), then some caution may be warranted in interpreting the percentile. In addition, whenever such extreme scores are being interpreted, examiners should also verify that the examinee's raw score falls within the range of raw scores in the normative sample. If the normative sample size is substantially smaller than the estimated prevalence sample size *and* the examinee's score falls outside the sample range, then considerable caution may be indicated in interpreting the percentile associated with the standardized score. Regardless of the z score value, it must also be kept in mind that interpretation of the associated percentile value may not be justifiable if the normative sample has a significantly non-normal distribution (see later for further discussion of non-normality). In sum, the clinical interpretation of extreme scores depends to a large extent on the properties of the normal samples involved; one can have more confidence that the percentile is reasonably accurate if the normative sample is large and well constructed and the shape of the normative sample distribution is approximately normal, particularly in tail regions where extreme scores are found.

The Normal Curve and Test Construction

Although the normal curve is from many standpoints an ideal or even expected distribution for psychological data, test score

Figure 1–3 Skewed distributions.

Positive Skew   Negative Skew

samples do not always conform to a normal distribution. When a new test is constructed, non-normality can be "corrected" by examining the distribution of scores on the prototype test, adjusting test properties, and resampling until a normal distribution is reached. For example, when a test is first administered during a try-out phase and a positively skewed distribution is obtained (i.e., with most scores clustering at the tail end of the distribution), the test likely has too high a floor, causing most examinees to obtain low scores. Easy items can then be added so that the majority of scores fall in the middle of the distribution rather than at the lower end (Anastasi & Urbina, 1997). When this is successful, the greatest numbers of individuals obtain about 50% of items correct. This level of difficulty usually provides the best differentiation between individuals at all ability levels (Anastasi & Urbina, 1997).

It must be noted that a test with a normal distribution in the general population may show extreme skew or other divergence from normality when administered to a population that differs considerably from the average individual. For example, a vocabulary test that produces normally distributed scores in a general sample of individuals may display a negatively skewed distribution due to a low ceiling when administered to doctoral students in literature, and a positively skewed distribution due to a high floor when administered to preschoolers from recently immigrated, Spanish-speaking families (see Figure 1–3 for examples of positive and negative skew). In this case, the test would be incapable of effectively discriminating between individuals within either group because of ceiling effects and floor effects, respectively, even though it is of considerable utility in the general population. Thus, a test's distribution, including floors and ceilings, must always be considered when assessing individuals who differ from the normative sample in terms of characteristics that affect test scores (e.g., in this example, degree of exposure to English words). In addition, whether a test produces a normal distribution (i.e., without positive or negative skew) is also an important aspect of evaluating tests for bias across different populations (see Chapter 2 for more discussion of bias).

Depending on the characteristics of the construct being measured and the purpose for which a test is being designed, a normal distribution of scores may not be obtainable or even desirable. For example, the population distribution of the construct being measured may not be normally distributed. Alternatively, one may want only to identify and/or discriminate between persons at only one end of a continuum of abilities (e.g., a creativity test for gifted students). In this case, the characteristics of only one side of the sample score distribution (i.e., the upper end) are critical, while the characteristics on the other side of the distribution are of no particular concern. The measure may even be deliberately designed to have floor or ceiling effects. For example, if one is not interested in one tail (or even one-half) of the distribution, items that would provide discrimination in that region may be omitted to save administration time. In this case, a test with a high floor or low ceiling in the general population (and with positive or negative skew) may be more desirable than a test with a normal distribution. In most applications, however, a more normal-looking curve within the targeted subpopulation is usually desirable.

Non-Normality

Although the normal curve is an excellent model for psychological data and many sample distributions of natural processes are approximately normal, it is not unusual for test score distributions to be markedly non-normal, even when samples are large (Miccerti, 1989).[2] For example, neuropsychological tests such as the Boston Naming Test (BNT) and Wisconsin Card Sorting Test (WCST) do not have normal distributions when raw scores are examined, and, even when demographic correction methods are applied, some tests continue to show a non-normal, multimodal distribution in some populations (Fastenau, 1998). (An example of a non-normal distribution is shown in Figure 1–4.)

The degree to which a given distribution approximates the underlying population distribution increases as the number of observations (N) increases and becomes less accurate as N decreases. This has important implications for norms comprised of small samples. Thus, a larger sample will produce a more normal distribution, but only if the underlying population distribution from which the sample is obtained is normal. In other words, a large N does not "correct" for non-normality of an underlying population distribution. However,

Figure 1–4 A non-normal test score distribution.

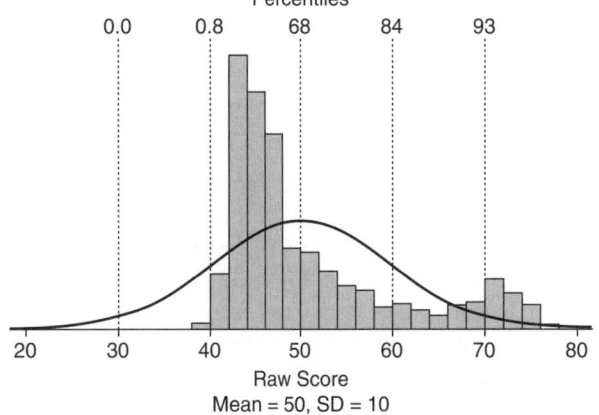

small samples may yield non-normal distribution due to random sampling effects, even though the population from which the sample is drawn has a normal distribution. That is, one may not automatically assume, given a non-normal distribution in a small sample, that the population distribution is in fact non-normal (note that the converse may also be true).

Several factors may lead to non-normal test score distributions: (a) the existence of discrete subpopulations within the general population with differing abilities, (b) ceiling or floor effects, and (c) treatment effects that change the location of means, medians, and modes and affect variability and distribution shape (Miccerti, 1989).

Skew

As with the normal curve, some varieties of non-normality may be characterized mathematically. Skew is a formal measure of asymmetry in a frequency distribution that can be calculated using a specific formula (see Nunnally & Bernstein, 1994). It is also known as the *third moment of a distribution* (the mean and variance are the first and second moments, respectively). A true normal distribution is perfectly symmetrical about the mean and has a skew of zero. A non-normal but symmetric distribution will have a skew value that is near zero. Negative skew values indicate that the left tail of the distribution is heavier (and often more elongated) than the right tail, which may be truncated, while positive skew values indicate that the opposite pattern is present (see Figure 1–3). When distributions are skewed, the mean and median are not identical because the mean will not be at the midpoint in rank and z scores will not accurately translate into sample percentile rank values. The error in mapping of z scores to sample percentile ranks increases as skew increases.

Truncated Distributions

Significant skew often indicates the presence of a truncated distribution. This may occur when the range of scores is restricted on one side but not the other, as is the case, for example, with reaction time measures, which cannot be lower than several hundred milliseconds, but can reach very high positive values in some individuals. In fact, distributions of scores from reaction time measures, whether aggregated across trials on an individual level or across individuals, are often characterized by positive skew and positive outliers. Mean values may therefore be positively biased with respect to the "central tendency" of the distribution as defined by other indices, such as the median. Truncated distributions are also commonly seen on error scores. A good example of this is Failure to Maintain Set (FMS) scores on the WCST (see review in this volume). In the normative sample of 30- to 39-year-old persons, observed raw scores range from 0 to 21, but the majority of persons (84%) obtain scores of 0 or 1, and less than 1% obtain scores greater than 3.

Floor/Ceiling Effects

Floor and ceiling effects may be defined as the presence of truncated tails in the context of limitations in range of item difficulty. For example, a test may be said to have a *high floor* when a large proportion of the examinees obtain raw scores at or near the lowest possible score. This may indicate that the test lacks a sufficient number and range of easier items. Conversely, a test may be said to have a *low ceiling* when the opposite pattern is present (i.e., when a high number of examinees obtain raw scores at or near the highest possible score). Floor and ceiling effects may significantly limit the usefulness of a measure. For example, a measure with a high floor may not be suitable for use with low functioning examinees, particularly if one wishes to delineate level of impairment.

Multimodality and Other Types of Non-Normality

Multimodality is the presence of more than one "peak" in a frequency distribution (see histogram in Figure 1–4 for an example). Another form of significant non-normality is the uniform or near-uniform distribution (a distribution with no or minimal peak and relatively equal frequency across scores). When such distributions are present, linearly transformed scores (z scores, T scores, and other deviation scores) may be totally inaccurate with respect to actual sample/population percentile rank and should not be interpreted in that framework. In these cases, sample-derived rank percentile scores may be more clinically useful.

Non-Normality and Percentile Derivations

Non-normality is not trivial; it has major implications for derivation and interpretation of standard scores and comparison of such scores across tests: standardized scores derived by linear transformation (e.g., z scores) will not correspond to sample percentiles, and the degree of divergence may be quite large.

Consider the histogram in Figure 1–4, which shows the distribution of scores obtained for a hypothetical test. This test, with a sample size of 1000, has a mean raw score of 50 and a standard deviation of 10; therefore (and very conveniently), no linear transformation is required to obtain T scores. An expected normal distribution based on the observed mean and standard deviation has been overlaid on the observed histogram for purposes of comparison.

The histogram in Figure 1–4 shows that the distribution of scores for the hypothetical test is grossly non-normal, with a truncated lower tail and significant positive skew, indicating floor effects and the existence of two distinct subpopulations. If the distribution were normal (i.e., if we follow the normal curve, superimposed on the histogram in Figure 1–4, instead of the histogram itself), a raw score of 40 would correspond to a T score of 40, a score that is 1 *SD* or 10 points from the mean, and translate to the 16th percentile (percentile not shown in the graph). However, when we calculate a percentile for the actual score distribution (i.e., the histogram), a score of 40 is actually below the 1st percentile with respect to the observed sample distribution (percentile = 0.8). Clearly, the difference in percentiles in this example is not trivial and has significant implications for score interpretation.

Normalizing Test Scores

When confronted with problematic score distributions, many test developers employ "normalizing" transformations in an attempt to correct departures from normality (examples of this can be found throughout this volume, in the *Normative Data* section for tests reviewed). Although helpful, these procedures are by no means a panacea, as they often introduce problems of their own with respect to interpretation. Additionally, many test manuals contain only a cursory discussion of normalization of test scores. Anastasi and Urbina (1997) state that scores should only be normalized if: (1) they come from a large and representative sample, or (2) any deviation from normality arises from defects in the test rather than characteristics of the sample. Furthermore, as we have noted above, it is preferable to adjust score distributions prior to normalization by modifying test content (e.g., by adding or modifying items) rather than statistically transforming non-normal scores into a normal distribution. Although a detailed discussion of normalization procedures is beyond the scope of this chapter (interested readers are referred to Anastasi & Urbina, 1997), ideally, test makers should describe in detail the nature of any significant sample non-normality and the procedures used to correct it for derivation of standardized scores. The reasons for correction should also be justified, and direct percentile conversions based on the uncorrected sample distribution should be provided as an option for users. Despite the limitations inherent in correcting for non-normality, Anastasi and Urbina (1997) note that most test developers will probably continue to do so because of the need to use test scores in statistical analyses that assume normality of distributions. From a practical point of view, test users should be aware of the mathematical computations and transformations involved in deriving scores for their instruments. When all other things are equal, test users should choose tests that provide information on score distributions and any procedures that were undertaken to correct non-normality, over those that provide partial or no information.

Extrapolation/Interpolation

Despite all the best efforts, there are times when norms fall short in terms of range or cell size. This includes missing data in some cells, inconsistent age coverage, or inadequate demographic composition of some cells compared to the population. In these cases, data are often extrapolated or interpolated using the existing score distribution and techniques such as multiple regression. For example, Heaton and colleagues have published sets of norms that use multiple regression to correct for demographic characteristics and compensate for few subjects in some cells (Heaton et al., 2003). Although multiple regression is robust to slight violations of assumptions, estimation errors may occur when using normative data that violates the assumptions of homoscedasticity (uniform variance across the range of scores) and normal distribution of scores necessary for multiple regression (Fastenau & Adams, 1996; Heaton et al., 1996).

Age extrapolations beyond the bounds of the actual ages of the individuals in the samples are also sometimes seen in normative data sets, based on projected developmental curves. These norms should be used with caution due to the lack of actual data points in these age ranges. Extrapolation methods, such as those that employ regression techniques, depend on the shape of the distribution of scores. Including only a subset of the distribution of age scores in the regression (e.g., by omitting very young or very old individuals) may change the projected developmental slope of certain tests dramatically. Tests that appear to have linear relationships, when considered only in adulthood, may actually have highly positively skewed binomial functions when the entire age range is considered. One example is vocabulary, which tends to increase exponentially during the preschool years, shows a slower rate of progress during early adulthood, remains relatively stable with continued gradual increase, and then shows a minor decrease with advancing age. If only a subset of the age range (e.g., adults) is used to estimate performance at the tail ends of the distribution (e.g., preschoolers and elderly), the estimation will not fit the shape of the actual distribution.

Thus, normalization may introduce error when the relationship between a test and a demographic variable is nonlinear. In this case, linear correction using multiple regression distorts the true relationship between variables (Fastenau, 1998).

MEASUREMENT PRECISION: RELIABILITY AND STANDARD ERROR

Like all forms of measurement, psychological tests are not perfectly precise; rather, test scores must be seen as *estimates* of abilities or functions, each associated with some degree of measurement error.[3] Each test differs in the precision of the scores that it produces. Of critical importance is the fact that no test has only one specific level of precision. Rather, precision always varies to some degree, and potentially substantially, across different populations and test-use settings. Therefore, estimates of measurement error relevant to specific testing circumstances are a prerequisite for correct interpretation. For example, even the most precise test may produce highly imprecise results if administered in a nonstandard fashion, in a nonoptimal environment, or to an uncooperative examinee. Aside from these obvious caveats, a few basic principles help in determining whether a test generally provides precise measurements in most situations where it will be used. We begin with an overview of the related concepts of *reliability, true scores, obtained scores*, the various estimates of measurement error, and the notion of *confidence intervals*. These are reviewed below.

Definition of Reliability

Reliability refers to the consistency of measurement of a given test and can be defined in several ways, including consistency within itself (internal consistency reliability), consistency over time (test-retest reliability), consistency across alternate forms (alternate form reliability), and consistency across raters (interrater reliability). Indices of reliability indicate the degree to which a test is free from measurement error (or the proportion of variance in observed scores attributable to variance in true scores). The interpretation of such indices is often not so straightforward.

It is important to note that the term "error" in this context does not actually refer to "incorrect" or "wrong" information. Rather, "error" consists of the multiple sources of variability that affect test scores. What may be termed error variance in one application may be considered part of the true score in another, depending on the construct being measured (state or trait), the nature of the test employed, and whether it is deemed relevant or irrelevant to the purpose of the testing (Anastasi & Urbina, 1997). An example relevant to neuropsychology is that internal reliability coefficients tend to be smaller at either end of the age continuum. This finding has been attributed to both limitations of tests (e.g., measurement error) and increased intrinsic performance variability among very young and very old examinees.

Factors Affecting Reliability

Reliability coefficients are influenced by (a) test characteristics (e.g., length, item type, item homogeneity, and influence of guessing) and (b) sample characteristics (e.g., sample size, range, and variability). The extent of a test's "clarity" is intimately related to its reliability: reliable measures typically have (a) clearly written items, (b) easily understood test instructions, (c) standardized administration conditions, (d) explicit scoring rules that minimize subjectivity, and (e) a process for training raters to a performance criterion (Nunnally & Bernstein, 1994). For a list of commonly used reliability coefficients and their associated sources of error variance, see Table 1–2.

Internal Reliability

Internal reliability reflects the extent to which items within a test measure the same cognitive domain or construct. It is a core index in classical test theory. A measure of the intercorrelation of items, internal reliability is an estimate of the correlation between randomly parallel test forms, and by extension,

Table 1–2 Sources of Error Variance in Relation to Reliability Coefficients

Type of Reliability Coefficient	Error Variance
Split-half	Content sampling
Kuder-Richardson	Content sampling
Coefficient alpha	Content sampling
Test-retest	Time sampling
Alternate-form (immediate)	Content sampling
Alternate-form (delayed)	Content sampling and time sampling
Interrater	Interscorer differences

Source: Adapted from Anastasi & Urbina, 1997, with permission.

of the correlation between test scores and true scores. This is why it is used for estimating true scores and associated standard errors (Nunnally & Bernstein, 1994). All things being equal, longer tests will generally yield higher reliability estimates (Sattler, 2001). Internal reliability is usually assessed with some measure of the average correlation among items within a test (Nunnally & Bernstein, 1994). These include the split-half or Spearman-Brown reliability coefficient (obtained by correlating two halves of items from the same test) and coefficient alpha, which provides a general estimate of reliability based on all the possible ways of splitting test items. Alpha is essentially based on the average intercorrelation between test items and any other set of items, and is used for tests with items that yield more than two response types (i.e., possible scores of 0, 1, or 2). For additional useful references concerning alpha, see Chronback (2004) and Streiner (2003a, 2003b). The Kuder-Richardson reliability coefficient is used for items with yes/no answers or heterogeneous tests where split-half methods must be used (i.e., the mean of all the different split-half coefficients if the test were split into all possible ways). Generally, Kuder-Richardson coefficients will be lower than split-half coefficients when tests are heterogeneous in terms of content (Anastasi & Urbina, 1997).

The Special Case of Speed Tests

Tests involving speed, where the score exclusively depends on the number of items completed within a time limit rather than the number correct, will cause spuriously high internal reliability estimates if internal reliability indices such as split-half reliability are used. For example, dividing the items into two halves to calculate a split-half reliability coefficient will yield two half-tests with 100% item completion rates, whether the individual obtained a score of 4 (i.e., yielding two half-tests totaling 2 points each, or perfect agreement) or 44 (i.e., yielding two half-tests both totaling 22 points, also yielding perfect agreement). The result in both cases is a split-half reliability of 1.00 (Anastasi & Urbina, 1997). Some alternatives are to use test-retest reliability or alternate form reliability, ideally with the alternate forms administered in immediate succession to avoid time sampling error. Reliabilities can also be calculated for any test that can be divided into specific time intervals; scores per interval can then be compared in a procedure akin to the split-half method, as long as items are of relatively equivalent difficulty (Anastasi & Urbina, 1997). For most of the speed tests reviewed in this volume, reliability is estimated by using the test-retest reliability coefficient, or else by a generalizability coefficient (see below).

Test-Retest Reliability

Test-retest reliability, also known as temporal stability, provides an estimate of the correlation between two test scores from the same test administered at two different ponts in time. A test with good temporal stability should show little change over time, providing that the trait being measured is stable and there are no differential effects of prior exposure. It is important to note that tests measuring dynamic (i.e., changeable) abilities will by definition produce lower test-retest reliabilities than tests measuring domains that are more trait-like and stable (Nunnally & Bernstein, 1994). See Table 1–3 for common sources of bias and error in test-retest situations.

A test has an infinite number of possible test-retest reliabilities, depending on the length of the time interval between testing. In some cases, reliability estimates are inversely related to the time interval between baseline and retest (Anastasi & Urbina, 1997). In other words, the shorter the time interval between test and retest, the higher the reliability coefficient will be. However, the extent to which the time interval affects the test-retest coefficient will depend on the type of ability evaluated (i.e., stable versus more variable). Reliability may also depend on the type of individual being assessed, as some groups are intrinsically more variable over time than others. For example, the extent to which scores fluctuate over time may depend on subject characteristics, including age (e.g., normal preschoolers will show more variability than adults) and neurological status (e.g., TBI examinees' scores may vary more in the acute state than in the post-acute state). Ideally, reliability estimates should be provided for both normal individuals and the clinical populations in which the test is intended to be used, and the specific demographic characteristics of the samples should be fully specified. Test stability coefficients presented in published test manuals are usually derived from relatively small normal samples tested over much shorter intervals than are typical for retesting in clinical practice and should therefore be considered with due caution when drawing inferences regarding clinical cases. However, there is some evidence that duration of interval has less of an impact on test-retest scores than subject characteristics (Dikmen et al., 1999).

Prior Exposure and Practice Effects

Variability in scores on the same test over time may be related to situational variables such as examinee state, examiner state, examiner identity (same versus different examiner at retest), or environmental conditions that are often unsystematic and

Table 1–3 Common Sources of Bias and Error in Test-Retest Situations

Bias	Intervening variables	Events of interest (e.g., surgery, medical intervention, rehabilitation) Extraneous events
	Practice effects	Memory for content Procedural learning Other factors (a) Familiarity with testing context and examiner (b) Performance anxiety
	Demographic considerations	Age (maturational effects and aging) Education Gender Ethnicity Baseline ability
Error	Statistical errors	Measurement error (*SEM*) Regression to the mean (SE_e)
	Random or uncontrolled events	

Source: From Lineweaver & Chelune, 2003, p. 308. Reprinted with permission from Elsevier.

may or may not be considered sources of measurement error. Apart from these variables, one must consider, and possibly parse out, effects of prior exposure, which are often conceptualized as involving implicit or explicit learning. Hence the term *practice effects* is often used. However, prior exposure to a test does not necessarily lead to increased performance at retest. Note also that the actual nature of the test may sometimes change with exposure. For instance, tests that rely on a "novelty effect" and/or require deduction of a strategy or problem solving (e.g., WCST, Tower of London) may not be conducted in the same way once the examinee has prior familiarity with the testing paradigm.

Like some measures of problem-solving abilities, measures of learning and memory are also highly susceptible to practice effects, though these are less likely to reflect a fundamental change in how examinees approach tasks. In either case, practice effects may lead to low test-retest correlations by effectively lowering the ceiling at retest, resulting in a restriction of range (i.e., many examinees obtain scores at near the maximum possible at retest). Nevertheless, restriction of range should not be assumed when test-retest correlations are low until this has been verified by inspection of data.

The relationship between prior exposure and test stability coefficients is complex, and although test-retest coefficients may be affected by practice or prior exposure, the coefficient does not indicate the magnitude of such effects. That is, retest correlations will be very high when individual retest scores all change by a similar amount, whether the practice effect is nil or very large. When stability coefficients are low, then there may be (1) no systematic effects of prior exposure, (2) the relation of prior exposure may be nonlinear, or (3) ceiling effects/ restriction of range related to prior exposure may be attenuating the coefficient. For example, certain subgroups may benefit more from prior exposure to test material than others (e.g., high-IQ individuals; Rapport et al., 1998), or some subgroups may demonstrate more stable scores or consistent practice effects than do others. This causes the score distribution to change at retest (effectively "shuffling" the individuals' rankings in the distribution), which will attenuate the correlation. In these cases, the test-retest correlation may vary significantly across subgroups and the correlation for the entire sample will not be the best estimate of reliability for any of the subgroups, overestimating reliability for some and underestimating reliability for others. In some cases, practice effects, as long as they are relatively systematic and accurately assessed, will not render a test unusable from a reliability perspective, though they should always be taken into account when retest scores are interpreted. In addition, individual factors must always be considered. For example, while improved performance may usually be expected with a particular measure, an individual examinee may approach tests that he or she had difficulty with previously with heightened anxiety that leads to decreased performance. Lastly, it must be kept in mind that factors other than prior exposure (e.g., changes in environment or examinee state) may affect test-retest reliability.

Alternate Forms Reliability

Some investigators advocate the use of alternate forms to eliminate the confounding effects of practice when a test must be administered more than once (e.g., Anastasi & Urbina, 1997). However, this practice introduces a second form of error variance into the mix (i.e., content sampling error), in addition to the time sampling error inherent in test-retest paradigms (see Table 1–3; see also Lineweaver & Chelune, 2003). Thus, tests with alternate forms must have extremely high correlations between forms in addition to high test-retest reliability to confer any advantage over using the same form administered twice. Moreover, they must demonstrate equivalence in terms of mean scores from test to retest, as well as consistency in score classification within individuals from test to retest. Furthermore, alternate forms do not necessarily eliminate effects of prior exposure, as exposure to stimuli and procedures can confer some positive carry-over effect (e.g., procedural learning) despite the use of a different set of items. These effects may be minimal across some types of well-constructed parallel forms, such as those assessing acquired knowledge. For measures such as the WCST, where specific learning and problem solving are involved, it may be difficult or impossible to produce an equivalent alternate form that will be free of effects of prior exposure to the original form. While it is possible to attain this degree of psychometric sophistication through careful item analysis, reliability studies, and administration to a representative normative group, it is rare for alternate forms to be constructed with the same psychometric rigor as were the original forms from which they were derived. Even well-constructed alternate forms often lack crucial validation evidence such as similar correlations to criterion measures as the original test form. This is especially true for older neuropsychological tests, particularly those with original forms that were never subjected to any item analysis or reliability studies whatsoever (e.g., BVRT). Inadequate test construction and psychometric properties are also found for alternate forms in more general published tests in common usage (e.g., WRAT-3). Because so few alternate forms are available and few of those that are meet these psychometric standards, our tendency is to use reliable change indices or standardized regression-based scores for estimating change from test to retest.

Interrater Reliability

Most test manuals provide specific and detailed instructions on how to administer and score tests according to standard procedures to minimize error variance due to different examiners and scorers. However, some degree of examiner variance remains in individually administered tests, particularly when scores involve a degree of judgment (e.g., multiple-response verbal tests such as the Wechsler Vocabulary Scales, which require the rater to administer a score from 0 to 2). In this case, an estimate of the reliability of administration and scoring across examiners is needed.

Interrater reliability can be evaluated using percentage agreement, kappa, product-moment correlation, and intraclass correlation coefficient (Sattler, 2001). For any given test, Pearson correlations will provide an upper limit for the intraclass correlations, but intraclass correlations are preferred because, unlike the Pearson's r, they take into account paired assessments made by the same set of examiners from those made by different examiners. Thus, the intraclass correlation distinguishes those sets of scores ranked in the same order from those that are ranked in the same order but have low, moderate, or complete agreement with each other, and corrects for interexaminer or test-retest agreement expected by chance alone (Cicchetti & Sparrow, 1981). However, advantages of the Pearson correlation are that it is familiar, is readily interpretable, and can be easily compared using standard statistical techniques; it is best for evaluating consistency in ranking rather than agreement per se (Fastenau et al., 1996).

Generalizability Coefficients

One reliability coefficient type not covered in this list is the generalizability coefficient, which is starting to appear more frequently in test manuals, particularly in the larger test batteries (e.g., Wechsler scales and NEPSY). In generalizability theory, or *G theory*, reliability is evaluated by decomposing test score variance using the general linear model (e.g., variance components analysis). This is a variant of the mathematical methods used to apportion variance in general linear model analyses such as ANOVA. In the case of G theory, the between-groups variance is considered an estimate of a true score variance and within-groups variance is considered an estimate of error variance. The generalizability coefficient is the ratio of estimated true variance to the sum of the estimated true variance and estimated error variance. A discussion of this flexible and powerful model is beyond the scope of this chapter, but detailed discussions can be found in Nunnally and Bernstein (1994) and Shavelson et al. (1989). Nunnally and Bernstein (1994) also discuss related issues pertinent to estimating reliabilities of variables reflecting sums such as composite scores, and the fact that reliabilities of difference scores based on correlated measures can be very low.

Evaluating a Test's Reliability

A test cannot be said to have a single or overall level of reliability. Rather, tests can be said to exhibit different kinds of reliability, the relative importance of which will vary depending on how the test is to be used. Moreover, each kind of reliability may vary across different populations. For instance, a test may be highly reliable in normally functioning adults, but be highly unreliable in young children or in individuals with neurological illness. It is important to note that while high reliability is a prerequisite for high validity, the latter does not follow automatically from the former. For example, height can be measured with great reliability, but it is not a valid index of intelligence. It is usually preferable to choose a test of slightly lesser reliability if it can be demonstrated that the test is associated with a meaningfully higher level of validity (Nunnally & Bernstein, 1994).

Some have argued that internal reliability is more important than other forms of reliability; thus, if alpha is low but test-retest reliability is high, a test should not be considered reliable (Nunnally, 1978, as cited by Cicchetti, 1989). Note that it is possible to have low alpha values and high test-retest reliability (if a measure is made up of heterogeneous items but yields the same responses at retest), or low alpha values but high interrater reliability (if the test is heterogeneous in item content but yields highly consistent scores across trained experts; an example would be a mental status examination). Internal consistency is therefore not necessarily the primary index of reliability, but should be evaluated within the broader context of test-retest and interrater reliability (Cicchetti, 1989).

Some argue that test-retest reliability is not as important as other forms of reliability if the test will only be used once and is not likely to be administered again in future. However, depending on the nature of the test and retest sampling procedures (as discussed previously), stability coefficients may provide valuable insight into the replicability of test results, particularly as these coefficients are a gauge of "real-world" reliability rather than accuracy of measurement of true scores or hypothetical reliability across infinite randomly parallel forms (as is internal reliability). In addition, as was stated previously, clinical decision making will almost always be based on the obtained score. Therefore, it is critically important to know the degree to which scores are replicable at retesting, whether or not the test may be used again in future.

It is our belief that test users should take an informed and pragmatic, rather than dogmatic, approach to evaluating reliability of tests used to inform diagnosis or other clinical decisions. If a test has been designed to measure a single, one-dimensional construct, then high internal consistency reliability should be considered an essential property. High test-retest reliability should also be considered an essential property unless the test is designed to measure state variables that are expected to fluctuate, or if systematic factors such as practice effects attenuate stability coefficients.

What Is an Adequate Reliability Coefficient?

The reliability coefficient can be interpreted directly in terms of the percentage of score variance attributed to different sources (i.e., unlike the correlation coefficient, which must be squared). Thus, with a reliability of .85, 85% of the variance can be attributed to the trait being measured, and 15% can be attributed to error variance (Anastasi & Urbina, 1997). When all sources of variance are known for the same group (i.e., when one knows the reliability coefficients for internal, test-retest, alternate form, and interrater reliability on the same sample), it is possible to calculate the true score variance (for an example, see Anastasi & Urbina, 1997, pp. 101–102). As noted above, although a detailed discussion of this topic is beyond the scope of this volume, the portioning of total score variance into components is the crux of generalizability theory of reliability, which forms the basis for reliability estimates for many well-known speed tests (e.g., Wechsler scale subtests such as Digit Symbol).

Sattler (2001) notes that reliabilities of .80 or higher are needed for tests used in individual assessment. Tests used for decision making should have reliabilities of .90 or above. Nunnally and Bernstein (1994) note that a reliability of .90 is a "bare minimum" for tests used to make important decisions about individuals (e.g., IQ tests), and .95 should be the optimal standard. When important decisions will be based on test scores (e.g., placement into special education), small score differences can make a great difference to outcome, and precision is paramount. They note that even with a reliability of .90, the *SEM* is almost one-third as large as the overall *SD* of test scores.

Given these issues, what is a clinically acceptable level of reliability? According to Sattler (2001), tests with reliabilities below .60 are unreliable; those above .60 are marginally reliable, and those above .70 are relatively reliable. Of note, tests with reliabilities of .70 may be sufficient in the early stages of validation research to determine whether the test correlates with other validation evidence; if so, additional effort can be expended to increase reliabilities to more acceptable levels (e.g., .80) by reducing measurement error (Nunnally & Bernstein, 1994). In outcome studies using psychological tests, internal consistencies of .80 to .90 and test-retest reliabilities of .70 are considered a minimum acceptable standard (Andrews et al., 1994; Burlingame et al., 1995).

Table 1–4 Magnitude of Reliability Coefficients

Magnitude of Coefficient
Very high (.90+)
High (.80–.89)
Adequate (.70–.79)
Marginal (.60–.69)
Low (<.59)

In terms of internal reliability of neuropsychological tests, Cicchetti et al. (1990) have proposed that internal consistency estimates of less than .70 are unacceptable, reliabilities between .70 and .79 are fair, reliabilities between .80 and .89 are good, and reliabilities above .90 are excellent.

For interrater reliabilities, Cicchetti and Sparrow (1981) report that clinical significance is poor for reliability coefficients below .40, fair between .40 and .59, good between .60 and .74, and excellent between .75 and 1.00. Fastenau et al. (1996), in summarizing guidelines on the interpretation of intraclass correlations and kappa coefficients for interrater reliability, consider coefficients larger than .60 as substantial and of .75 or .80 as almost perfect.

These are the general guidelines that we have used throughout the text to evaluate the reliability of neuropsychological tests (see Table 1–4) so that the text can be used as a reference when selecting tests with the highest reliability. Users should note that there is a great deal of variability with regard to the acceptability of reliability coefficients for neuropsychological tests, as perusal of this volume will indicate. In general, for tests involving multiple subtests and multiple scores (e.g., Wechsler scales, NEPSY, D-KEFS), including those derived from qualitative observations of performance (e.g., error analyses), the farther away a score gets from the composite score itself and the more difficult the score is to quantify, the lower the reliability. A quick review of the reliability data presented in this volume also indicates that verbal tests, with few exceptions, tend to have consistently higher reliability than tests measuring other cognitive domains.

Limits of Reliability

Although it is possible to have a reliable test that is not valid for some purposes, the converse is not the case (see later). Further, it is also conceivable that there are some neuropsychological domains that simply cannot be measured reliably. Thus, even though there is the assumption that questionable reliability is always a function of the test, reliability may depend on the nature of the psychological process measured or on the nature of the population evaluated. For example, many of the executive functioning tests reviewed in this volume have relatively modest reliabilities, suggesting that this ability is difficult to assess reliably. Additionally, tests used in populations with high response variability, such as preschoolers, elderly individuals, or individuals with brain disorders, may invariably yield low reliability coefficients despite the best efforts of test developers.

Lastly, as previously discussed, reliability coefficients do not provide complete information on the reproducibility of individual test scores. Thus, with regard to test-retest reliability, it is possible for a test to have high reliability ($r = .80$) but have retest means that are 10 points higher than baseline scores. Reliability coefficients do not provide information on whether individuals retain their relative place in the distribution from baseline to retest. Procedures such as the Bland-Altman method (Altman & Bland, 1983; Bland & Altman, 1986) are one way to determine the limits of agreement between two assessments for individuals in a group.

MEASUREMENT ERROR

A good working understanding of conceptual issues and methods of quantifying measurement error is essential for competent clinical practice. We start our discussion of this topic with concepts arising from classical test theory.

True Scores

A central element of classical test theory is the concept of a *true score*, or the score an examinee would obtain on a measure in the absence of any measurement error (Lord & Novick, 1968). True scores can never be known. Instead, they are estimated, and are conceptually defined as the mean score an examinee would obtain across an infinite number of randomly parallel forms of a test, assuming that the examinee's scores were not systematically affected by test exposure/practice or other time-related factors such as maturation (Lord & Novick, 1968). In contrast to true scores, *obtained scores* are the actual scores yielded by tests. Obtained scores include any measurement error associated with a given test.[4] That is, they are the sum of true scores and error.

In the classical model, the relation between obtained and true scores is expressed in the following formula, where error (*e*) is random and all variables are assumed to be normal in distribution:

$$x = t + e \qquad [3]$$

Where:

x = obtained score
t = true score
e = error

When test reliability is less than perfect, as is always the case, the net effect of measurement error across examinees is to bias obtained scores outward from the population mean. That is, scores above the mean are most likely to be higher than true scores, while those below the mean are most likely to be lower than true scores (Lord & Novick, 1968). *Estimated true scores* correct this bias by regressing obtained scores toward the normative mean, with the amount of regression depending on test reliability and deviation of the obtained score from the mean. The formula for estimated true scores (t') is:

$$t' = X + [r_{xx}(x - X)] \qquad [4]$$

Where:

X = mean test score
r_{xx} = test reliability (internal consistency reliability in classical test theory)
x = obtained score

If working with z scores, the formula is simpler:

$$t' = r_{xx} \times z \qquad [5]$$

Formula 4 shows that an examinee's estimated true score is the sum of the mean score of the group to which he or she belongs (i.e., the normative sample) and the deviation of his or her obtained score from the normative mean weighted by test reliability (as derived from the same normative sample). Further, as test reliability approaches unity (i.e., $r = 1.0$), estimated true scores approach obtained scores (i.e., there is little measurement error, so estimated true scores and obtained scores are nearly equivalent). Conversely, as test reliability approaches zero (i.e., when a test is extremely unreliable and subject to excessive measurement error), estimated true scores approach the mean test score. *That is, when a test is highly reliable, greater weight is given to obtained scores than to the normative mean score, but when a test is very unreliable, greater weight is given to the normative mean score than to obtained scores.* Practically speaking, estimated true scores will always be closer to the mean than obtained scores are (except, of course, where the obtained score is at the mean).

The Use of True Scores in Clinical Practice

Although the true score model is abstract, it has practical utility and important implications for test score interpretation. For example, what may not be immediately obvious from formulas 4 and 5 is readily apparent in Table 1–5: estimated true scores translate test reliability (or lack thereof) into the same metric as actual test scores.

As can be seen in Table 1–5, the degree of regression to the mean of true scores is inversely related to test reliability and directly related to degree of deviation from the reference mean. This means that the more reliable a test is, the closer are obtained scores to true scores and that the further away the obtained score is from the sample mean, the greater the discrep-

ancy between true and obtained scores. For a highly reliable measure such as Test 1 ($r = .95$), true score regression is minimal, even when an obtained score lies a considerable distance from the sample mean; in this example, a standard score of 130, or two SDs above the mean, is associated with an estimated true score of 129. In contrast, for a test with low reliability such as Test 3 ($r = .65$), true score regression is quite substantial. For this test, an obtained score of 130 is associated with an estimated true score of 120; in this case, fully one-third of the observed deviation is "lost" to regression when the estimated true score is calculated.

Such information may have important implications with respect to interpretation of test results. For example, as shown in Table 1–5, as a result of differences in reliability, obtained scores of 120 on Test 1 and 130 on Test 3 are associated with essentially equivalent estimated true scores (i.e., 119 and 120, respectively). If only obtained scores are considered, one might interpret scores from Test 1 and Test 3 as significantly different, even though these "differences" actually disappear when measurement precision is taken into account. It should also be noted that such differences may not be limited to comparisons of scores across different tests within the same individual, but may also apply to comparisons between scores from the same test across different individuals when the individuals come from different groups and the test in question has variable reliability across those groups.

Regression to the mean may also manifest as pronounced asymmetry of confidence intervals centered on true scores, relative to obtained scores, as discussed in more detail later. Although calculation of true scores is encouraged as a means of gauging the limitations of reliability, it is important to consider that any significant difference between characteristics of an examinee and the sample from which a mean sample score and reliability estimate were derived may invalidate the process. For example, in some cases it makes little sense to estimate true scores for severely brain-injured individuals on tests of cognition using test parameters from healthy normative samples, as mean scores within the brain-injured population are likely to be substantially different from those seen in healthy normative samples; reliabilities may differ substantially as well. Instead, one may be justified in deriving estimated true scores using data from a comparable clinical sample if this is available. Overall, these issues underline the complexities inherent in comparing scores from different tests in different populations.

The Standard Error of Measurement

Examiners may wish to quantify the margin of error associated with using obtained scores as estimates of true scores. When the sample SD and the reliability of obtained scores are known, an estimate of the SD of obtained scores about true scores may be calculated. This value is known as the *standard error of measurement*, or *SEM* (Lord & Novick, 1968). More simply, the *SEM* provides an estimate of the amount of error in a person's observed score. It is a function of the reliability

Table 1–5 Estimated True Score Values for Three Observed Scores at Three Levels of Reliability

		Observed Scores ($M = 100$, $SD = 15$)		
	Reliability	110	120	130
Test 1	.95	110	119	129
Test 2	.80	108	116	124
Test 3	.65	107	113	120

Estimated true scores rounded to whole values.

of the test, and of the variability of scores within the sample. The *SEM* is inversely related to the reliability of the test. Thus, the greater the reliability of the test is, the smaller the *SEM* is, and the more confidence the examiner can have in the precision of the score.

The *SEM* is defined by the following formula:

$$SEM = SD\sqrt{1 - r_{xx}}$$ [6]

Where:

SD = the standard deviation of the test, as derived from an appropriate normative sample

r_{xx} = the reliability coefficient of the test (usually internal reliability)

Confidence Intervals

While the *SEM* can be considered on its own as an index of test precision, it is not necessarily intuitively interpretable,[5] and there is often a tendency to focus excessively on test scores as point estimates at the expense of consideration of associated estimation error ranges. Such a tendency to disregard imprecision is particularly inappropriate when interpreting scores from tests of lower reliability. Clinically, it may therefore be very important to report, in a concrete and easily understandable manner, the degree of precision associated with specific test scores. One method of doing this is to use *confidence intervals.*

The *SEM* is used to form a confidence interval (or range of scores), around estimated true scores, within which obtained scores are most likely to fall. The distribution of obtained scores about the true score (the error distribution) is assumed to be normal, with a mean of zero and an *SD* equal to the *SEM*; therefore, the bounds of confidence intervals can be set to include any desired range of probabilities by multiplying by the appropriate *z* value. Thus, if an individual were to take a large number of randomly parallel versions of a test, the resulting obtained scores would fall within an interval of ±1 *SEM* of the estimated true score 68% of the time, and within 1.96 *SEM* 95% of the time (see Table 1–1).

Obviously, confidence intervals for unreliable tests (i.e., with a large *SEM*) will be larger than those for highly reliable tests. For example, we may again use data from Table 1–5. For a highly reliable test such as Test 1, a 95% confidence interval for an obtained score of 110 ranges from 103 to 116. In contrast, the confidence interval for Test 3, a less reliable test, is larger, ranging from 89 to 124.

It is important to bear in mind that confidence intervals for obtained scores that are based on the *SEM* are centered on *estimated true scores.*[6] Such confidence intervals will be symmetric around obtained scores only when obtained scores are at the test mean or when reliability is perfect. Confidence intervals will be asymmetric about obtained scores to the same degree that true scores diverge from obtained scores. Therefore, when a test is highly reliable, the degree of asymmetry will often be trivial, particularly for obtained scores within

one SD of the mean. For tests of lesser reliability, the asymmetry may be marked. For example, in Table 1–5, consider the obtained score of 130 on Test 2. The estimated true score in this case is 124 (see equations 4 and 5). Using equation 5 and a z-multiplier of 1.96, we find that a 95% confidence interval for the obtained scores spans ±13 points, or from 111 to 137. This confidence interval is substantially asymmetric about the obtained score.

It is also important to note that *SEM*-based confidence intervals should not be used for estimating the likelihood of obtaining a given score at retesting with the same measure, as effects of prior exposure are not accounted for. In addition, Nunally and Bernstein (1994) point out that use of *SEM*-based confidence intervals assumes that error distributions are normally distributed and homoscedastic (i.e., equal in spread) across the range of scores obtainable for a given test. However, this assumption may often be violated. A number of alternate error models do not require these assumptions and may thus be more appropriate in some circumstances (see Nunally and Bernstein, 1994, for a detailed discussion).[7]

Lastly, as with the derivation of estimated true scores, when an examinee is known to belong to a group that markedly differs from the normative sample, it may not be appropriate to derive *SEM*s and associated confidence intervals using normative sample parameters (i.e., SD and r_{xx}), as these would likely differ significantly from parameters derived from an applicable clinical sample.

The Standard Error of Estimation

In addition to estimating confidence intervals for obtained scores, one may also be interested in estimating confidence intervals for estimated true scores (i.e., the likely range of true scores about the estimated true score). For this purpose, one may construct confidence intervals using the *standard error of estimation* (SE$_E$; Lord & Novick, 1968). The formula for this is:

$$SE_E = SD\sqrt{r_{xx}(1 - r_{xx})}$$ [7]

Where:

SD = the standard deviation of the variable being estimated

r_{xx} = the test reliability coefficient

The SE$_E$, like the *SEM*, is an indication of test precision. As with the *SEM*, confidence intervals are formed around estimated true scores by multiplying the SE$_E$ by a desired *z* value. That is, one would expect that over a large number of randomly parallel versions of a test, an individual's true score would fall within an interval of ±1 SE$_E$ of the estimated true score 68% of the time, and fall within 1.96 SE$_E$ 95% of the time. As with confidence intervals based on the *SEM*, those based on the SE$_E$ will usually not be symmetric around obtained scores. All of the other caveats detailed previously regarding *SEM*-based confidence intervals also apply.

The choice of constructing confidence intervals based on the *SEM* versus the SE$_E$ will depend on whether one is more interested in true scores or obtained scores. That is, while the *SEM* is a gauge of test accuracy in that it is used to determine the expected range of *obtained* scores about true scores over parallel assessments (the range of error in *measurement* of the true score), the SE_E is a gauge of estimation accuracy in that it is used to determine the likely range within which *true* scores fall (the range of error of *estimation* of the true score). Regardless, both *SEM*-based and SE_E-based confidence intervals are symmetric with respect to estimated true scores rather than the obtained scores, and the boundaries of both will be similar for any given level of confidence interval when a test is highly reliable.

The Standard Error of Prediction

When the standard deviation of obtained scores for an alternate form is known, one may calculate the likely range of obtained scores expected on retesting with an alternate form. For this purpose, the *standard error of prediction* (SE_P; Lord & Novick, 1968) may be used to construct confidence intervals. The formula for this is:

$$SE_P = SD_y \sqrt{1 - r_{xx}^2} \qquad [8]$$

Where:

SD_y = the standard deviation of the parallel form administered at retest

r_{xx} = the reliability of the form used at initial testing

In this case, confidence intervals are formed around estimated true scores (derived from initial obtained scores) by multiplying the SE_P by a desired *z* value. That is, one would expect that when retested over a large number of randomly parallel versions of a test, an individual's obtained score would fall within an interval of ±1 SE_P of the estimated true score 68% of the time, and fall within 1.96 SE_E 95% of the time. As with confidence intervals based on the *SEM*, those based on the SE_P will generally not be symmetric around obtained scores. All of the other caveats detailed previously regarding the *SEM*-based confidence intervals also apply. In addition, while it may be tempting to use SE_P-based confidence intervals for evaluating significance of change at retesting with the same measure, this practice violates the assumptions that a parallel form is used at retest and, particularly, that no prior exposure effects apply.

SEMs and True Scores: Practical Issues

Nunnally and Bernstein (1994) note that most test manuals do "an exceptionally poor job of reporting estimated true scores and confidence intervals for expected obtained scores on alternative forms. For example, intervals are often erroneously centered about obtained scores rather than estimated true scores. Often the topic is not even discussed" (p. 260). Sattler (2001) also notes that test manuals often base confidence intervals on the overall *SEM* for the entire standardization sample, rather than on *SEMs* for each age band. Using the average *SEM* across age is not always appropriate, given that some age groups are inherently more variable than others (e.g., preschoolers versus adults). In general, confidence intervals based on age-specific *SEMs* are preferable to those based on the overall *SEM* (particularly at the extremes of the age distribution, where there is the most variability) and can often be constructed using age-based *SEMs* found in most manuals.

It is important to acknowledge that while estimated true scores and associated confidence intervals have merit, there are practical reasons to focus on obtained scores instead. For example, essentially all validity studies and actuarial prediction methods for most tests are based on obtained scores. Therefore, obtained scores must usually be employed for diagnostic and other purposes to maintain consistency to prior research and test usage. For more discussion regarding the calculation and uses of the *SEM*, SE_E, SE_P, and alternative error models, see Dudek (1979), Lord and Novick (1968), and Nunnally and Bernstein (1994).

VALIDITY

Models of validity are not abstract conceptual frameworks that are only minimally related to neuropsychological practice. The Standards for Educational and Psychological Testing (AERA et al., 1999) state that validation is the joint responsibility of the test developer and the test user (1999). Thus, a working knowledge of validity models and the validity characteristics of specific tests is a central requirement for responsible and competent test use. From a practical perspective, a working knowledge of validity allows users to determine which tests are appropriate for use and which fall below standards for clinical practice or research utility. Thus, neuropsychologists who use tests to detect and diagnose neurocognitive difficulties should be thoroughly familiar with commonly used validity models and how these can be used to evaluate neuropsychological tools. Assuming that a test is valid because it was purchased from a reputable test publisher, appears to have a large normative sample, or came with a large user's manual can be a serious error, as some well-known and commonly used neuropsychological tests are lacking with regard to crucial aspects of validity.

Definition of Validity

Cronbach and Meehl (1955) were some of the first theorists to discuss the concept of construct validity. Since then, the basic definition of validity evolved as testing needs changed over the years. Although construct validity was first introduced as a separate type of validity (e.g., Anastasi & Urbina, 1997), it has moved, in some models, to encompass all types of validity (e.g., Messick, 1993). In other models, the term "construct validity" has been deemed redundant and has simply been replaced by "validity," since all types of validity ultimately inform as to the construct measured by the test. Accordingly, the term "construct validity" has not been used in the Standards for Educational and Psychological Testing since 1974 (AERA et al., 1999). However, whether it is deemed "construct validity" or simply "validity," the concept is central to evaluating the utility of a test in the clinical or research arena.

Test validity may be defined at the most basic level as *the degree to which a test actually measures what it is intended to measure*, or in the words of Nunnally and Bernstein (1994), "how well it measures what it purports to measure in the context in which it is to be applied" (p. 112). As with reliability, an important point to be made here is that a test cannot be said to have one single level of validity. Rather, it can be said to exhibit various types and levels of validity across a spectrum of usage and populations. That is, *validity is not a property of a test*, but rather, *validity is a property of the meaning attached to a test score*; validity can only arise and be defined in the specific context of test usage. Therefore, while it is certainly necessary to understand the validity of tests in particular contexts, ultimate decisions regarding the validity of test score interpretation must take into account any unique factors pertaining to validity at the level of individual assessment, such as deviations from standard administration, unusual testing environments, examinee cooperation, and the like.

In the past, assessment of validity was generally test-centric. That is, test validity was largely indexed by comparison with other tests, especially "standards" in the field. Since Cronbach (1971), there has been a move away from test-based or "measure-centered validity" (Zimiles, 1996) toward the interpretation and external utility of tests. Messick (1989, 1993) expanded the definition of validity to encompass an overall judgment of the extent to which empirical evidence and theoretical rationales support the adequacy and effectiveness of interpretations and actions resulting from test scores. Subsequently, Messick (1995) proposed a comprehensive model of construct validity wherein six different, distinguishable types of evidence contribute to construct validity. These are (1) content related, (2) substantive, (3) structural, (4) generalizability, (5) external, and (6) consequential evidence sources (see Table 1–6), and they form the "evidential basis for score

Table 1–6 Messick's Model of Construct Validity

Type of Evidence	Definition
Content-related	Relevance, representativeness, and technical quality of test content
Substantive	Theoretical rationales for the test and test responses
Structural	Fidelity of scoring structure to the structure of the construct measured by the test
Generalizability	Scores and interpretations generalize across groups, settings, and tasks
External	Convergent and divergent validity, criterion relevance, and applied utility
Consequential	Actual and potential consequences of test use, relating to sources of invalidity related to bias, fairness, and distributive justice[a]

Source: Adapted from Messick, 1995.

[a]See Lees-Haley (1996) for limitations of this component.

interpretation" (Messick, 1995, p. 743). Likewise, the Standards for Educational and Psychological Testing (AERA et al., 1999) follows a model very much like Messick's, where different kinds of evidence are used to bolster test validity based on each of the following sources: (1) evidence based on test content, (2) response processes, (3) internal structure, (4) relations to other variables, and (5) consequences of testing. The most controversial aspect of these models is the requirement for consequential evidence to support validity. Some argue that judging validity according to whether use of a test results in positive or negative social consequences is too far-reaching and may lead to abuses of scientific inquiry, as when a test result does not agree with the overriding social climate of the time (Lees-Haley, 1996). Social and ethical consequences, although crucial, may therefore need to be treated separately from validity (Anastasi & Urbina, 1997).

Validity Models

Since Cronbach and Meehl, various models of validity have been proposed. The most frequently encountered is the tripartite model whereby validity is divided into three components: content validity, criterion-related validity, and construct validity (see Anastasi & Urbina, 1997; Mitrushina et al., 2005; Nunnally & Bernstein, 1994; Sattler, 2001). Other validity subtypes, including convergent, divergent, predictive, treatment, clinical, and face validity, are subsumed within these three domains. For example, convergent and divergent validity are most often treated as subsets of construct validity (Sattler, 2001) and concurrent and predictive validity as subsets of criterion validity (e.g., Mitrushina et al., 2005). Concurrent and predictive validity only differ in terms of a temporal gradient; concurrent validity is relevant for tests used to identify existing diagnoses or conditions, whereas predictive validity applies when determining whether a test predicts future outcomes (Anastasi & Urbana, 1997). Although face validity appears to have fallen out of favor as a type of validity, the extent to which examinees believe a test measures what it appears to measure can affect motivation, self-disclosure, and effort. Consequently, face validity can be seen as a moderator variable affecting concurrent and predictive validity that can be operationalized and measured (Bornstein, 1996; Nevo, 1985). Again, all these labels for distinct categories of validity are ways of providing different types of *evidence for validity* and are not, in and of themselves, different types of validity, as older sources might claim (AERA et al., 1999; Yun & Ulrich, 2002). Lastly, validity is a matter of degree rather than an all-or-none property; validity is therefore never actually "finalized," since tests must be continually reevaluated as populations and testing contexts change over time (Nunnally & Bernstein, 1994).

How to Evaluate the Validity of a Test

Pragmatically speaking, all the theoretical models in the world will be of no utility to the practicing clinician unless they can be translated into specific, step-by-step procedures for evaluating a test's validity. Table 1–7 presents a comprehensive (but not exhaustive) list of specific features users can look for when evaluating a test and reviewing test manuals. Each is organized according to the type of validity evidence provided. For example, construct validity can be assessed via correlations with other tests, factor analysis, internal consistency (e.g., subtest intercorrelations), convergent and discriminant validation (e.g., multitrait-multimethod matrix), experimental interventions (e.g., sensitivity to treatment), structural equation modeling, and response processes (e.g., task decomposition, protocol analysis; Anastasi & Urbina, 1997). Most importantly, users should also remember that even if all other conditions are met, a test cannot be considered valid if it is not reliable (see previous discussion).

It is important to note that not all tests will have sufficient evidence to satisfy all aspects of validity, but test users should have a sufficiently broad knowledge of neuropsychological tools to be able to select one test over another, based on the quality of the validation evidence available. In essence, we

have used this model to critically evaluate all the tests reviewed in this volume.

Note that there is a certain degree of overlap between categories in Table 1–7. For example, correlations between a specific test and another test measuring IQ can simultaneously provide criterion-related evidence and construct-related evidence of validity. Regardless of the terminology, it is important to understand how specific techniques such as factor analysis serve to inform the validity of test interpretation across the range of settings in which neuropsychologists work.

What Is an Adequate Validity Coefficient?

Some investigators have proposed criteria for evaluating evidence related to criterion validity in outcome assessments. For instance, Andrews et al. (1994) and Burlingame et al. (1995) recommend that a minimum level of acceptability for correlations involving criterion validity is .50. However, Nunnally

Table 1–7 Sources of Evidence and Techniques for Critically Evaluating the Validity of Neuropsychological Tests

Type of Evidence	Required Evidence
Content-related	Refers to themes, wording, format, tasks, or questions on a test, and administration and scoring
	Description of theoretical model on which test is based
	Review of literature with supporting evidence
	Definition of domain of interest (e.g., literature review, theoretical reasoning)
	Operationalization of definition through thorough and systematic review of test domain from which items are to be sampled, with listing of sources (e.g., word frequency sources for vocabulary tests)
	Collection of sample of items large enough to be representative of domain and with sufficient range of difficulty for target population
	Selection of panel of judges for expert review, based on specific selection criteria (e.g., academic and practical backgrounds or expertise within specific subdomains)
	Evaluation of items by expert panel based on specific criteria concerning accuracy and relevance
	Resolution of judgment conflicts within panel for items lacking cross-panel agreement (e.g., empirical means such as Index of Item Congruence; Hambleton, 1980)
Construct-related	Formal definition of construct
	Formulation of hypotheses to measure construct
	Gathering empirical evidence of construct validation
	Evaluating psychometric properties of instrument (i.e., reliability)
	Demonstration of test sensitivity to developmental changes, correlation with other tests, group differences studies, factor analysis, internal consistency (e.g., correlations between subtests, or to composites within the same test), convergent and divergent validation (e.g., multitrait-multimethod matrix), sensitivity to experimental manipulation (e.g., treatment sensitivity), structural equation modeling, and analysis of process variables underlying test performance.
Criterion-related	Identification of appropriate criterion
	Identification of relevant sample group reflecting the entire population of interest; if only a subgroup is examined, then generalization must remain within subgroup definition (e.g., keeping in mind potential sources of error such as restriction of range)
	Analysis of test-criterion relationships through empirical means such as contrasting groups, correlations with previously available tests, classification of accuracy statistics (e.g., positive predictive power), outcome studies, and meta-analysis
Response processes	Determining whether performance on the test actually relates to the domain being measured
	Analysis of individual responses to determine the processes underlying performance (e.g., questioning test takers about strategy, analysis of test performance with regard to other variables, determining whether the test measures the same construct in different populations, such as age)

Source: Adapted from Anastasi & Urbina, 1997; American Educational Research Association et al., 1999; Messick, 1995; and Yun and Ulrich, 2002.

and Bernstein (1994) note that validity coefficients rarely exceed .30 or .40 in most circumstances involving psychological tests, given the complexities involved in measuring and predicting human behavior. There are no hard and fast rules when evaluating evidence supportive of validity, and interpretation should consider how the test results will be used. Thus, tests with even quite modest predictive validities ($r = .30$) may be of considerable utility, depending on the circumstances in which they will be used (Anastasi & Urbina, 1997; Nunnally & Bernstein, 1994), particularly if they serve to significantly increase the test's "hit rate" over chance. It is also important to note that in some circumstances, criterion validity may be measured in a categorical rather than continuous fashion, such as when test scores are used to inform binary diagnoses (e.g., demented versus not demented). In these cases, one would likely be more interested in indices such as predictive power than other measures of criterion validity (see below for a discussion of classification accuracy statistics).

USE OF TESTS IN THE CONTEXT OF SCREENING AND DIAGNOSIS: CLASSIFICATION ACCURACY STATISTICS

In some cases, clinicians use tests to measure *how much* of an attribute (e.g., intelligence) an examinee has, while in other cases, tests are used to help determine whether or not an examinee has a specific attribute, condition, or illness that may be either *present or absent* (e.g., Alzheimer's disease). In the latter case, a special distinction in test use may be made. *Screening tests* are those which are broadly or routinely used to detect a specific attribute, often referred to as a *condition of interest,* or COI, among persons who are not "symptomatic" but who may nonetheless have the COI[8] (Streiner, 2003c). *Diagnostic tests* are used to assist in ruling in or out a specific condition in persons who present with "symptoms" that suggest the diagnosis in question. Another related use of tests is for purposes of prediction of outcome. As with screening and diagnostic tests, the outcome of interest may be defined in binary terms—it will either occur or not occur (e.g., return to the same type and level of employment). Thus, in all three cases, clinicians will be interested in the relation of the measure's distribution of scores to an attribute or outcome that is defined in binary terms.

Typically, data concerning screening or diagnostic accuracy are obtained by administering a test to a sample of persons who are also classified, with respect to the COI, by a so-called gold standard. Those who have the condition according to the gold standard are labeled *COI+*, while those who do not have the condition are labeled *COI-*. In medicine, the gold standard is often a highly accurate diagnostic test that is more expensive and/or has a higher level of associated risk of morbidity than some new diagnostic method that is being evaluated for use as a screening measure or as a possible replacement for the existing gold standard. In neuropsychology, the situation is often more complex, as the COI may be a psychological construct (e.g., malingering) for which consensus with respect to fundamental definitions is lacking or diagnostic gold standards may not exist. These issues may be less problematic when tests are used to predict outcome (e.g., return to work), though other problems that may afflict outcome data such as intervening variables and sample attrition may complicate interpretation of predictive accuracy.

The simplest way to relate test results to binary diagnoses or outcomes is to utilize a cutoff score. This is a single point along the continuum of possible scores for a given test. Scores at or above the cutoff classify examinees as belonging to one of two groups; scores below the cutoff classify examinees as belonging to the other group. Those who have the COI according to the test are labeled as *Test Positive* (Test+), while those who do not have the COI are labeled *Test Negative* (Test-).

Table 1–8 shows the relation between examinee classifications based on test results versus classifications based on a gold standard measure. By convention, test classification is denoted by row membership and gold standard classification is denoted by column membership. Cell values represent the total number of persons from the sample falling into each of four possible outcomes with respect to agreement between a test and respective gold standard. By convention, agreements between gold standard and test classifications are referred to as *True Positive* and *True Negative* cases, while disagreements are referred to as *False Positive* and *False Negative* cases, with *positive* and *negative* referring to the presence or absence of a COI as per classification by the gold standard. When considering outcome data, observed outcome is substituted for the gold standard. It is important to keep in mind while reading the following section that while gold standard measures are often implicitly treated as 100% accurate, this may not always be the case. Any limitations in accuracy or applicability of a gold standard or outcome measure need to be accounted for when interpreting classification accuracy statistics.

Table 1–8 Classification/Prediction Accuracy of a Test in Relation to a "Gold Standard" or Actual Outcome

Test Result	Gold Standard		
	COI+	COI-	Row Total
Test+	A (True Positive)	B (False Positive)	A + B
Test-	C (False Negative)	D (True Negative)	C + D
Column total	A + C	B + D	$N = A + B + C + D$

Test Accuracy and Efficiency

The general accuracy of a test with respect to a specific COI is reflected by data in the *columns* of a classification accuracy table (Streiner, 2003c). The column-based indices include *Sensitivity*, *Specificity*, and the *Positive* and *Negative Likelihood Ratios* (LR$^+$ and LR$^-$). The formulas for calculation of the column-based classification accuracy statistics from data in Table 1–9 are given below:

$$\text{Sensitivity} = A/(A + C) \qquad [9]$$

$$\text{Specificity} = D/(D + B) \qquad [10]$$

$$\text{LR}^+ = \text{Sensitivity}/(1 - \text{Specificity}) \qquad [11]$$

$$\text{LR}^- = \text{Specificity}/(1 - \text{Sensitivity}) \qquad [12]$$

Sensitivity is defined as the proportion of COI$^+$ examinees who are correctly classified as such by a test. Specificity is defined as the proportion of COI$^-$ examinees who are correctly classified as such by a test. The Positive Likelihood Ratio (LR$^+$) combines sensitivity and specificity into a single index of overall test accuracy indicating the odds (likelihood) that a positive test result has come from a COI$^+$ examinee. For example, a likelihood ratio of 3.0 may be interpreted as indicating that a positive test result is three times as likely to have come from a COI$^+$ examinee as a COI$^-$ one. The LR$^-$ is interpreted conversely to the LR$^+$. As the LR approaches 1, test classification approximates random assignment of examinees. That is, a person who is Test$^+$ is equally likely to be COI$^+$ or COI$^-$. Given that they are derived from an adequate normative sample, Sensitivity, Specificity and LR$^{+/-}$ are assumed to reflect fixed (i.e., constant) properties of a test that are applicable whenever a test is used within the normative population. For purposes of working examples, Table 1–9 presents hypothetical test and gold standard data.

Using equations 9 to 12 above, the hypothetical test demonstrates moderate Sensitivity (.75) and high Specificity (.95), with a LR$^+$ of 15 and an LR$^-$ of 3.8. Thus, for the hypothetical measure, a positive result is 15 times more likely to be obtained by an examinee who has the COI than one who does not, while a negative result is 3.8 times more likely to be obtained by an examinee who does not have the COI than one who does.

Note that Sensitivity, Specificity, and LR$^{+/-}$ are parameter estimates that have associated errors of estimation that can be quantified. The magnitude of estimation error is inversely related to sample size, and can be quite large when samples size

is small. The formulae for calculating standard errors for Sensitivity, Specificity, and the LR are complex and will not be presented here (see McKenzie et al., 1997). Fortunately, these values may also be easily calculated using a number of readily available computer programs. Using one of these (by Mackinnon, 2000) with data from Table 1–9, the 95% confidence interval for Sensitivity was found to be .59 to .87, while that for Specificity was .83 to .99. LR$^+$ was 3.8 to 58.6, and LR$^-$ was 2.2 to 6.5. Clearly, the range of measurement error is not trivial for this hypothetical study. In addition to appreciating issues relating to estimation error, it is also important to understand that while column-based indices provide useful information about test validity and utility, a test may nevertheless have high sensitivity and specificity but still be of limited clinical value in some situations, as will be detailed below.

Predictive Power

As opposed to being concerned with test accuracy at the *group* level, clinicians are typically more concerned with test accuracy in the context of diagnosis and other decision making at the level of *individual* examinees. That is, clinicians wish to determine whether or not an individual examinee does or does not have a given COI. In this scenario, clinicians must consider indices derived from the data in the *rows* of a classification accuracy table (Streiner, 2003c). These row-based indices are Positive Predictive Power (PPP) and Negative Predictive Power (NPP).[9] The formulas for calculation of these from data in Table 1–8 are given below:

$$\text{PPP} = A/(A + B) \qquad [13]$$

$$\text{NPP} = D/(C + D) \qquad [14]$$

Positive Predictive Power is defined as the probability that an individual with a positive test result has the COI. Conversely, *Negative Predictive Power* is defined as the probability that an individual with a negative test result does *not* have the COI. For example, predictive power estimates derived from the data presented in Table 1–9 indicate that PPP = .94 and NPP = .79; thus, in the hypothetical data set, 94% of persons who obtain a positive test result actually have the COI, while 79% of people who obtain a negative test result do not in fact have the COI. When predictive power is close to .50, examinees are approximately equally likely to be COI$^+$ as COI$^-$, regardless of whether they are Test$^+$ or Test$^-$. When predictive power is less than .50, test-based classifications or diagnoses will be incorrect more often than not.[10]

As with Sensitivity and Specificity, PPP and NPP are parameter estimates that should always be considered in the context of estimation error. Unfortunately, standard errors or confidence intervals for estimates of predictive power are rarely listed when these values are reported; clinicians are thus left to their own devices to calculate them. Fortunately, these values may be easily calculated using a number of computer programs. Using one of these (by Mackinnon, 2000) with data from Table 1–9, the 95% confidence intervals for PPP and NPP were found to be .94 to .99 and .65 to .90, respectively.

Table 1–9 Classification/Prediction Accuracy of a Test in Relation to a "Gold Standard" or Actual Outcome—Hypothetical Data

| Test Result | Gold Standard | | |
	COI$^+$	COI$^-$	Row Total
Test$^+$	30	2	32
Test$^-$	10	38	48
Column total	40	40	$N = 80$

Figure 1–5 Relation of predictive power to prevalence—hypothetical data.

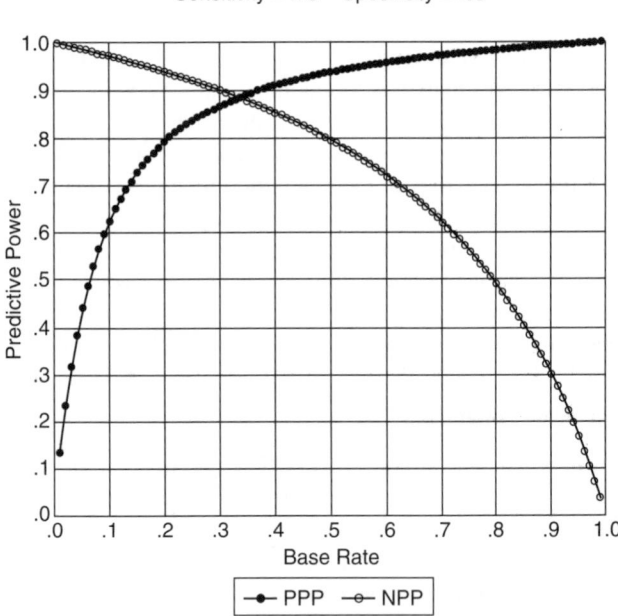

Clearly, the CI range is not trivial for this small data set. Of critical importance to clinical interpretation of test scores, PPP and NPP are *not* fixed properties of a test like row-based indices, but vary with the baserate or prevalence of a COI.

Sample vs. Actual Baserates and Relation to Predictive Power

The prevalence of a COI is defined with respect to Table 1–8 as:

$$(A + C)/N \qquad [15]$$

As should be readily apparent from inspection of Table 1–9, the prevalence of the COI in the sample is 50 percent. Formulas for deriving Predictive Power for any level of sensitivity and specificity and a specified prevalence are given below:

$$PPP = \frac{Prevalence \times Sensitivity}{(Prevalence \times Sensitivity) + [(1 - Prevalence) \times (1 - Specificity)]} \qquad [16]$$

$$NPP = \frac{(1 - Prevalence) \times Specificity}{[(1 - Prevalence) \times Specificity] + [Prevalence \times (1 - Sensitivity)]} \qquad [17]$$

From inspection of these formulas, it should be apparent that regardless of sensitivity and specificity, predictive power will vary between 0 and 1 as a function of prevalence. Application of formulas 16 and 17 to the data presented in Table 1–9 across the range of possible baserates provides the range of possible PPP and NPP values depicted in Figure 1–5.

As can be seen in Figure 1–5, the relation between predictive power and prevalence is curvilinear and asymptotic with

endpoints at 0 and 1. For any given test cutoff score, PPP will always increase with baserate, while NPP will simultaneously decrease. For the hypothetical test being considered, one can see that both PPP and NPP are moderately high (at or above .80) when the COI baserate ranges from 20% to 50%. The tradeoff between PPP and NPP at high and low baserate levels is also readily apparent; as the baserate increases above 50%, PPP exceeds .95, while NPP declines, falling below .50 as the baserate exceeds 80%. Conversely, as the baserate falls below 30%, NPP exceeds .95 while PPP rapidly drops off, falling below 50% as the baserate falls below 7%.

From the forgoing, it is apparent that the predictive power values derived from data presented in Table 1–9 would not be applicable in settings where baserates vary from the 50% value in the hypothetical data set. This is important because in practice, clinicians may often be presented with PPP values based on data where "prevalence" values are near 50%. This is due to the fact that, regardless of the prevalence of a COI in the population, diagnostic validity studies typically employ equal sized samples of COI+ and COI– individuals to facilitate statistical analyses. In contrast, the actual prevalence of COIs in the population is rarely 50%. The actual prevalence of a COI and the PPP in some clinical settings may be substantially lower than that reported in validity studies, particularly when a test is used for screening purposes.

For example, suppose that the data from Table 1–9 were from a validity trial of a neuropsychological measure designed for administration to young children for purposes of predicting later development of schizophrenia. The question then arises: should the measure be used for broad screening given a lifetime schizophrenia prevalence of .008? Using Formula 16, one can determine that for this purpose the measures PPP is only .11 and thus the "positive" test results would be incorrect 89% of the time.[11] Conversely, the prevalence of a COI may in some settings be substantially higher than 50%. As an example of the other extreme, the baserate of head injuries among persons referred to a head-injury rehabilitation service based on documented evidence of a blow to the head leading to loss of consciousness is essentially 100%, in which case the use of neuropsychological tests to determine whether or not examinees had sustained a "head injury" would not only be redundant, but very likely lead to false negative errors (such tests could of course be legitimately used for other purposes, such as grading injury severity). Clearly, clinicians need to carefully consider published data concerning sensitivity, specificity, and predictive power in light of intended test use and, if necessary, calculate PPP and NPP values and COI baserate estimates applicable to specific groups of examinees seen in their own practices.

Difficulties With Estimating and Applying Baserates

Prevalence estimates for some COIs may be based on large-scale epidemiological studies that provide very accurate prevalence estimates for the general population or within specific subpopulations (e.g., the prevalence rates of various psychiatric disorders in inpatient psychiatric settings). However, in some cases, no prevalence data may be available or reported prevalence data may not be applicable to specific settings or subpopulations. In these cases, clinicians who wish to determine predictive power must develop their own baserate estimates. Ideally, these can be derived from data collected within the same setting in which the test will be employed, though this is typically time consuming and many methodological challenges may be faced, including limitations associated with small sample sizes. Methods for estimating baserates in such context are beyond the scope of this chapter; interested readers are directed to Mossmann (2003), Pepe (2003), and Rorer and Dawes (1982).

Why Are Classification Actuary Statistics Not Ubiquitous in Neuropsychological Research and Clinical Practice?

Of note, the mathematical relations between sensitivity, specificity, prevalence, and predictive power were first elucidated by Thomas Bayes and published in 1763; methods for deriving predictive power and other related indices of confidence in decision making are thus often referred to as *Bayesian* statistics.[12] Needless to say, Bayes's work predated the first diagnostic applications of psychological tests as we know them today. However, although neuropsychological tests are routinely used for diagnostic decision making, information on the predictive power of most tests is often absent from both test manuals and applicable research literature. This is so despite the fact that the importance and relevance of Bayesian approaches to the practice of clinical psychology was well described 50 years ago by Meehl and Rosen (1955), and has been periodically addressed since then (Willis, 1984; Elwood, 1993; Ivnik et al., 2001). Bayesian statistics are finally making major inroads into the mainstream of neuropsychology, particularly in the research literature concerning symptom validity measures, in which estimates of predictive power have become de rigueur, although these are still typically presented without associated standard errors, thus greatly reducing utility of the data.

Determining the Optimum Cutoff Score—ROC Analyses and Other Methods

The forgoing discussion has focused on the diagnostic accuracy of tests using specific cutoff points, presumably ones that are optimum cutoffs for given tasks such as diagnosing dementia. A number of methods for determining an optimum cutoff point are available and although they may lead to similar results, the differences between them are not trivial. Many of these methods are mathematically complex and/or computationally demanding, thus requiring computer applications.

The determination of an optimum cutoff score for detection or diagnosis of a COI is often based on simultaneous evaluation of sensitivity and specificity or predictive power across a range of scores. In some cases, this information, in

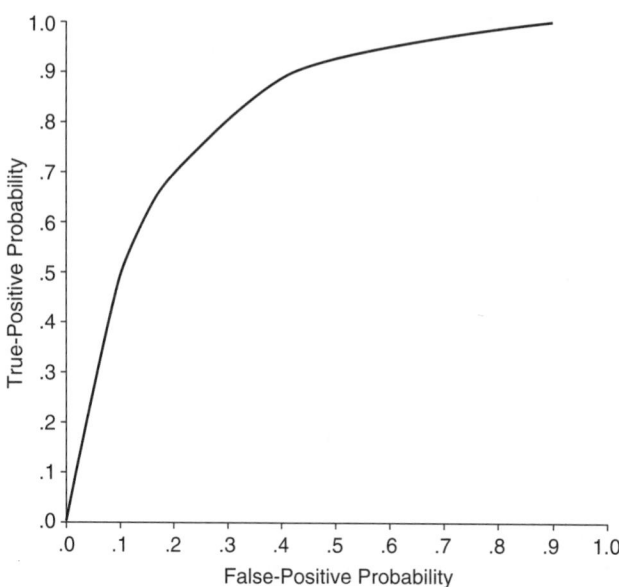

Figure 1–6 An ROC graph.

tabular or graphical form, is simply inspected and a score is chosen based on a researcher or clinician's comfort with a particular error rate. For example, in malingering research, cutoffs that minimize false-positive errors or hold them below a low threshold are often implicitly or explicitly chosen, even when such cutoffs are associated with relatively large false-negative error rates.

A more formal, rigorous and often very useful set of tools for choosing cutoff points and for evaluating and comparing test utility for diagnosis and decision making and for determining optimum cutoff scores falls under the rubric of Receiver Operating Characteristics (ROC) analyses. Clinicians who use tests for diagnostic or other decision-making purposes should be familiar with ROC procedures. The statistical procedures utilized in ROC analyses are closely related to and substantially overlap those of Bayesian analyses. The central graphic element of ROC analyses is the ROC graph, which is a plot of the true positive proportion (Y-axis) against the false positive proportion (X-axis) associated with each specific score in a range of test scores. Figure 1–6 shows an example ROC graph. The area under the curve is equivalent to the overall accuracy of the test (proportion of the entire sample correctly classified), while the slope of the curve at any point is equivalent to the LR^+ associated with a specific test score.

A number of ROC methods have been developed for determining cutoff points that consider not only accuracy, but also allow for factoring in quantifiable or quasi-quantifiable costs and benefits, and the relative importance of specific costs and benefits associated with any given cutoff score. ROC methods may also be used to compare the diagnostic utility of two or more measures, which may be very useful for purposes of test selection. Although ROC methods can be very useful clinically, they have not yet made great inroads in clinical neuropsychological literature. A detailed discussion of ROC methods is beyond the scope of this chapter; interested readers are referred to Mossmann and Somoza (1992), Pepe (2003), Somoza and Mossmann (1992), and Swets, Dawes and Monahan (2000).

Evaluation of Predictive Power Across a Range of Cutoff Scores and Baserates

As noted above, it is important to recognize that positive and negative predictive power are *not* properties of tests, but rather are properties of specific test scores in specific contexts. The forgoing sections describing the calculation and interpretation of predictive power have focused on methods for evaluating the value of a single cutoff point for a given test for purposes of classifying examinees as COI+ or COI−. However, by focusing exclusively on single cutoff points, clinicians are essentially transforming continuous test scores into binary scores, thus discarding much potentially useful information, particularly when scores are considerably above or below a cutoff. Lindeboom (1989) proposed an alternative approach in which predictive power across a range of test scores and baserates can be displayed in a single Bayesian probability table. In this approach, test scores define the rows and baserates define the columns of a table; individual table cells contain the associated PPP and NPP for a specific score and specific baserate. Such tables have rarely been constructed for standardized measures, but examples can be found in some test manuals (e.g., the Victoria Symptom Validity Test; Slick et al., 1997). The advantage of this approach is that it allows clinicians to consider the diagnostic confidence associated with an examinee's specific score, leading to more accurate assessments. A limiting factor for use of Bayesian probability tables is that they can only be constructed when sensitivity and specificity values for an entire range of scores are available, which is rarely the case for most tests. In addition, predictive power values in such tables are subject to any validity limitations of underlying data, and should include associated standard errors or confidence intervals.

Evaluating Predictive Power in the Context of Multiple Tests

Often more than one test that provides data relevant to a specific diagnosis is administered. In these cases, clinicians may wish to integrate predictive power estimates *across* measures. There may be a temptation to use the PPP associated with a score on one measure as the "baserate" when the PPP for a score from a second measure is calculated. For example, suppose that the baserate of a COI is 15%. When a test designed to detect the COI is administered, an examinee's score translates to a PPP of 65%. The examiner then administers a second test designed to detect the COI, but when PPP for the examinee's score on the second test is calculated, a "baserate" of 65% is used rather than 15%, as the former is now the

assumed prior probability that the examinee has the COI, given their score on the first test administered. The resulting PPP for the examinee's score on the second measure is now 99% and the examiner concludes that the examinee has the COI. While this procedure may seem logical, it will produce an inflated PPP estimate for the second test score whenever the two measures are correlated, which will almost always be the case when both measures are designed to screen for or diagnose the same COI. At present, there is no simple mathematical model that can be used to correct for the degree of correlation between measures so that they can be used in such an iterative manner; therefore this practice should be avoided.

A preferred psychometric method for integrating scores from multiple measures, which can only be used when normative data are available, is to construct optimum group membership (i.e., COI+ vs. COI−) prediction equations or classification rules using logistic regression or multiway frequency analyses, which can then be cross-validated, and ideally distributed in an easy-to-use format such as software. More details on methods for combining information across measures may be found in Franklin (2003b) and Pepe (2003).

ASSESSING CHANGE OVER TIME

Neuropsychologists are often interested in and/or confronted with issues of change in function over time. In these contexts three interrelated questions arise:

- To what degree do changes in examinee test scores reflect "real" changes in function as opposed to measurement error?
- To what degree do real changes in examinee test scores reflect clinically significant changes in function as opposed to clinically trivial changes?
- To what degree do changes in examinee test scores conform to expectations, given the application of treatments or the occurrence of other events or processes occurring between test and retest, such as head injury, dementia or brain surgery?

A number of statistical/psychometric methods have been developed for assessing changes observed over repeated administrations of neuropsychological tests; these differ considerably with respect to mathematical models and assumptions regarding the nature of test data. As with most areas of psychometrics, the problems and processes involved in decomposing observed scores (i.e., change scores) into measurement error and "true" scores are often complex. Clinicians are certainly not aided by the lack of agreement about which methods to use for analysing test-retest data, limited retest data for many tests and limited coverage and direction concerning retest procedures in most test manuals. Only a relatively brief discussion of this important area of psychometrics is presented here. Interested readers are referred to other sources (e.g., Chelune, 2003) for a more in-depth review.

Reference Group Change Score Distributions

If a reference or normative sample is administered a test twice, the distribution of observed change scores ("change score" = retest score minus baseline score) can be quantified. When such information is available, individual examinee change scores can be transformed into *standardized* change scores (e.g., percentiles), thus providing information on the degree of unusualness of any observed change in score. Unfortunately, it is rarely possible to use this method of evaluating change due to major limitations in most data available in test manuals. Retest samples tend to be relatively small for many tests, thus limiting generalizability. This is particularly important when change scores vary with demographic variables (e.g., age and level of education) and/or initial test score level (e.g., normal vs. abnormal), because retest samples typically are restricted with respect to both. Second, retest samples are often obtained within a short period of time after initial testing, typically less than two months, whereas in clinical practice typical test-retest intervals are often much longer. Thus any effects of extended test-retest intervals on change score distributions are not reflected in most change-score data presented in test manuals. Lastly, change score information is typically presented in the form of summary statistics (e.g., mean and *SD*) that have limited utility if change scores are not normally distributed (in which case percentile tables would be much preferable). As a result of these limitations, clinicians often must turn to other methods for analyzing change.

The Reliable Change Index (RCI)

Jacobson and Truax (1991; see also Jacobson et al., 1999) proposed a psychometric method for determining if changes in test scores over time are reliable (i.e., not an artefact of imperfect test reliability). This method involves calculation of a *Reliable Change Index* (RCI). The RCI is an indicator of the probability that an observed difference between two scores from the same examinee on the same test can be attributed to measurement error (i.e., to imperfect reliability). When there is a low probability that the observed change is due to measurement error, one may infer that it reflects other factors, such as progression of illness, treatment effects, and/or prior exposure to the test.

The RCI is calculated using the *Standard Error of the Difference* (SE$_D$), an index of measurement error derived from classical test theory. It is the standard deviation of expected test-retest difference scores about a mean of 0 given an assumption that no actual change has occurred.[13] The formula for the SE$_D$ is:

$$SE_D = \sqrt{2 \cdot (SEM)^2} \qquad [18]$$

where *SEM* is the Standard Error of Measurement, as previously defined in Formula 6. Inspection of Formula 18 reveals that tests with a large *SEM* will have a large SE$_D$. The RCI for a specific score is calculated by dividing the observed amount of change by the SE$_D$, transforming observed change scores into SE$_D$ units. The formula is given below:

$$(S_2 - S_1)/SE_D \qquad [19]$$

Where:

S$_1$ = an examinee's initial test score
S$_2$ = an examinee's score at retest on the same measure

The resulting RCI scores can be either negative or positive and can be thought of as a type of *z* score that can be interpreted with reference to upper or lower tails of a normal probability distribution. Therefore, RCI scores falling outside a range of −1.96 to 1.96 would be expected to occur less than 5% of the time as a result of measurement error alone, assuming that an examinee's true retest score had not changed since the first test. The assumption that an examinee's true score has not changed can therefore be rejected at *p* < .05 (two-tailed) when his or her RCI score is above 1.96 or below −1.96.

The RCI is directly derived from classical test theory. Thus internal-consistency reliability (Cronbach's α) is used to estimate measurement error rather than test-retest reliability, as the latter reflects not just test-intrinsic measurement error, but also any additional variation over time arising from real changes in function and the effect of other intervening variables. Thus use of test-retest reliability introduces additional complexity into the meaning of the RCI.

The RCI is often calculated using *SD* (to calculate *SEM*) and reliability estimates obtained from test normative samples. However, as these values may not be applicable to the clinical group to which an examinee belongs, care must be taken in interpretation of the RCI in such circumstances. It may be preferable to use *SD* and reliability estimates from samples similar to an examinee, if these are available. Because the SE$_D$ value is constant for any given combination of test and reference sample, it can be used to construct RCI confidence intervals applicable to any initial test score obtained from a person similar to the reference sample, using the formula below:

$$RCI - CI = S_1 \pm (z \cdot SE_D) \qquad [20]$$

Where:

S$_1$ = Initial test score
z = *z* score associated with a given confidence range (e.g., 1.64 for a 90% C.I.)

Retest scores falling outside the desired confidence interval about initial scores can be considered evidence of a significant change. Note that while a "significant" RCI value may be considered as a prerequisite, it is *not* by itself sufficient evidence that clinically significant change has occurred. Consider RCIs in the context of highly reliable tests: relatively small score changes at retest can produce significant RCIs, but both the initial test score and retest score may remain within the same classification range (e.g., normal) so that the clinical implications of observed change may be minimal. In addition, use of the RCI implicitly assumes that no practice effects pertain. When practice effects are present, significant RCI values may partially or wholly reflect effects of prior test exposure rather than a change in underlying functional level.

To allow RCIs to be used with tests that have practice effects, Chelune et al. (1993) suggest a modification to calculation of the RCI in which the mean change score for a reference group is subtracted from the observed change score of an individual examinee and the result is used as an Adjusted Change Score for purposes of calculating an Adjusted RCI. Alternatively, an RCI confidence interval calculated using Formula 21 could have its endpoints adjusted by addition of the mean change score.

$$\text{Adj. RCI} - \text{CI} = (S_1 + M_C) \pm (z \cdot SE_D) \qquad [21]$$

Where:

S_1 = Initial test score
M_C = Mean change score (Retest – Test)
z = z score associated with a given confidence range
    (e.g., 1.64 for a 90% C.I.)

This approach appears to offer some advantages over the traditional RCI, particularly for tests where large practice effects are expected. However, adjusting for practice in this way is problematic in a number of ways, first and foremost of which is the use of a constant term for the practice effect, which will not reflect any systematic variability in practice effects across individuals. Secondly, neither standard nor adjusted RCIs account for regression toward the mean because the associated estimated measurement error is not adjusted proportionally for the extremity of observed change.

Standardized Regression-Based Change Scores

The RCI may provide useful information regarding the likelihood of a meaningful change in the function being measured by a test, but as noted above, it may have limited validity in some circumstances. Many quantifiable factors not accounted for by RCI may influence or predict retest scores, including test-retest interval, baseline ability level (Time 1 score), scores from other tests, and examinee characteristics such as gender, education, age, acculturation, and neurological or medical conditions. In addition, while RCI scores factor in test reliability, error is operationalized as a constant that does not account for regression to the mean (i.e., the increase in measurement error associated with more extreme scores). One method for evaluating change that does allow clinicians to account for additional predictors and also controls for regression to the mean is the use of linear regression models (Crawford & Howell, 1998; Hermann et al., 1991).[14]

With linear regression models, predicted retest scores are derived and then compared with observed retest scores for purposes of determining if deviations are "significant." In the preferred method, this is accomplished by dividing the difference between obtained retest scores and regression-predicted retest scores by the *Standard Error for Individual Predicted*

Scores ($SE_{\hat{Y}}$). Because score differences are divided by a standard error, the resulting value is considered to be standardized. The resulting standardized score is in fact a *t* statistic that can be translated into a probability value using an appropriate program or table. Small probability values indicate that the observed retest score differs significantly from the predicted value. The $SE_{\hat{Y}}$ is used because, unlike the Standard Error of the Regression, it is not constant across cases, but increases as individual values of independent variables deviate from the mean, thus accounting for regression to the mean on a case-by-case basis (Crawford & Howell, 1998). Thus, persons who are outliers with respect to their scores on predictor variables will have larger margins of error associated with their predicted scores and thus larger changes in raw scores will be required to reach significance for these individuals.

As with other standardized scores (e.g., *z* scores), standardized regression-based change scores (SRB scores) from different measures can be directly compared, regardless of the original test score metric. However, a number of inferential limitations of such comparisons, described in the section on standardized scores earlier in this chapter, still apply. Regression models can also be used when one wishes to consider change scores from multiple tests simultaneously; these are more complex and will not be covered here (see McCleary, et al., 1996).

As an example of the application of SRB scores, consider data on IQ in children with epilepsy reported by Sherman et al. (2003). They found that in samples of children with intractable epilepsy who were not treated surgically, FSIQ scores at retest could be predicted by baseline FSIQ and number of anti-epileptic medications (AEDs) that the children were taking at baseline. The resulting Multiple R^2 value was large (.92), indicating that the equation had acceptable predictive value. The resulting regression equation is given below:

$$\begin{aligned} \text{FSIQ}_{retest} = &(0.965 \times \text{FSIQ}_{baseline}) \\ &+ (-4.519 \times \text{AEDs}_{baseline}) + 7.358 \end{aligned}$$

It can be seen from inspection of this equation that predicted retest FSIQ values were positively related to baseline IQ and inversely related to number of AEDs being taken at baseline. Therefore, for children who were not taking any AEDs at baseline, a modest increase in FSIQ at retest was expected, while for those taking one or more AEDs (a marker of epilepsy severity), IQs tended to decline over time. Given a baseline FSIQ of 100, the predicted FSIQs at retest for children taking 0, 1, 2, and 3 AEDs at baseline were 104, 99, 95, and 90, respectively. Using a program developed by Crawford & Howell (1998), Sherman et al. (2003) were able to determine which children in the surgery sample demonstrated unusual change, relative to expectations for children who did not receive surgery. For example, a child in the sample was taking 2 AEDs and had a FSIQ of 53 at baseline. The predicted retest IQ was thus 49 but the actual retest IQ following right anterior temporal lobectomy was 63. The observed change was 14 points higher than the predicted change; the associated *p* value was .039 and thus the child was classified as obtaining a significantly higher than predicted retest score. The inference in this case was that better than expected FSIQ outcome was a positive effect of epilepsy surgery. Other examples of regression equations developed for specific neuropsychological tests are presented throughout this volume.

Limitations of Regression-Based Change Scores

It is important to understand the limitations of regression methods. Regression equations based on smaller sample sizes will lead to large error terms so that meaningful predicted-obtained differences may be missed. Equations from large-scale studies or from cross-validation efforts are therefore preferred. In order to maximize utility, sample characteristics should match populations seen clinically and predictor variables should be carefully chosen to match data that will likely be available to clinicians. Test users should generally avoid interpolation—that is, they should avoid applying a regression equation to an examinee's data (predictor variables and test-retest scores) when the data values fall outside the ranges for corresponding variables comprising the regression equation. For example, if a regression equation is developed for predicting IQ at retest from a sample with initial IQ scores ranging from 85 to 125, it should not be applied to an examinee whose initial IQ is 65. Finally, SRB scores should only be derived and used when necessary assumptions concerning residuals are met (see Pedhazur, 1997, pp. 33–34).

It is critical to understand that SRB scores do not necessarily indicate whether a clinically significant change from baseline level has occurred—for which use of RCIs may be more appropriate. Instead, SRB scores are an index of the degree to which observed change conforms to established trends in a reference population. These trends may consist of increases or decreases in performance over time in association with combinations of influential predictor variables, such as type and severity of illness, treatment type, baseline cognitive level, gender, age, and test-retest interval. Expected trends may involve increased scores at retest for healthy individuals, but decreased scores for individuals with progressive neurological disease. The following two examples will illustrate this point.

In the first example, consider a hypothetical scenario of a treatment for depression that is associated with improved post-treatment scores on a depression inventory, such that in a clinical reference sample, the test-retest correlation is high and the average improvement in scores at retest exceeds the threshold for clinical significance as established by RCI. In the simplest case (i.e., using only scores from Time 1), regression-predicted retest scores would be equivalent to the mean score change observed in the clinical reference sample. In this case, an examinee who at retest obtained a depression score at or near the post-treatment mean would obtain a *non-significant* SRB score but a *significant* RCI score, indicating that they demonstrated the typically seen clinically significant improvement in response to treatment. Conversely, an examinee who obtained an unchanged depression score following treatment would obtain a *significant* SRB score but a *non-significant* RCI

score, indicating that they did not show the typically seen significant improvement in response to treatment.

In the second example, consider a hypothetical scenario of a memory test that has significant prior-exposure (i.e., learning) effects such that in the normative sample the test-retest correlation is high and the average improvement in scores at retest exceeds the threshold for clinical significance as established by RCI. As with the depression score example, in the simplest case (i.e., using only scores from Time 1), regression-predicted retest scores would be equivalent to the mean score change observed in the reference sample. In this case, an examinee who at retest obtained a memory score at or near the retest mean would obtain a *non-significant* SRBC score but a *significant* RCI score, indicating that they demonstrated the typically seen prior exposure/learning effect (note the difference in interpretation from the previous example—the improvement in score is assumed to reflect treatment effects in the first case and to be artifactual in the second case). Conversely, an examinee who obtained an unchanged memory score following treatment would obtain a *significant* SRB score but a *non-significant* RCI score, indicating that they did not show the typically seen prior exposure/learning effect. Conceivably, in the context of a clinical referral, the latter finding might be interpreted as reflective of memory problems (see Sawrie, et al., 1996, and Temkin et al., 1999, for excellent examples of studies comparing utility of RCIs and SRB scores in clinical samples).

Clinically Significant Change

Once a clinician has determined that an observed test score change is reliable, he or she will usually need to determine whether the amount of change is clinically meaningful. Jacobson and Truax (1991) proposed that clinically significant change occurs, in the context of treatment, when an examinee's score (e.g., on the Beck Depression Inventory) moves from within the clinical "depressed" range into the normal population range. However, this definition of clinically significant change is not always relevant to neuropsychological assessment. There are at present no widely accepted criteria for clinically significant change within the context of neuropsychological assessment. Rather, the determination of clinical significance of any observed change that is reliable will depend greatly on the specific context of the assessment.

NORMAL VARIATION

Ingraham and Aiken (1996) have noted that when clinicians attempt to interpret examinee profiles of scores across multiple tests they "confront the problem of determining how many deviant scores are necessary to diagnose a patient as abnormal or whether the configuration of scores is significantly different from an expected pattern" (p. 120). They further note that the likelihood that a profile of tests scores will exceed criteria for abnormality increases as: (1) the number of tests in a battery *increases*; (2) the *z* score cutoff used to classify a test score as abnormal *decreases*; and (3) the number of abnormal test scores required to reach criteria *decreases*. Ingraham and Aiken (1996) developed a mathematical model that may be used for determining the likelihood of obtaining an abnormal test result from a given number of tests. Implicit in this model is an assumption that some "abnormal" test scores are spurious. As Ingraham and Aiken (1996) note, the problem of determining whether a profile of test scores meets criteria for abnormality is considerably complicated by the fact that most neuropsychological measures are intercorrelated and therefore the probabilities of obtaining abnormal results from each test are not independent. However, they provide some suggested guidelines for adapting their model or using other methods to provide useful approximations.

In a related vein of research, Schretlen et al. (2003), noting that little is known about what constitutes the normal range of intraindividual variation across cognitive domains and, by extension, associated test scores, evaluated normal variation in a sample of 197 healthy adults who were participants in a study on normal aging. For each individual, the Maximum Discrepancy, or MD (the absolute difference between standard scores from two measures expressed in units of standard deviation) across scores from 15 commonly used neuropsychological measures was calculated. The smallest MD value observed was 1.6 *SD*, while the largest was 6.1 *SD*. Two thirds of the sample obtained MD scores in excess of 3 *SD*, and when these were recalculated with highest and lowest scores omitted, 27% of the sample still obtained MD scores exceeding 3 *SD*. Schretlen et al. (2003) concluded from this data that "marked intraindividual variability is very common in normal adults, and underscores the need to base diagnostic inferences on clinically recognizable patterns rather than psychometric variability alone" (p. 864). While the number of "impaired" scores obtained by each healthy participant was not reported, 44% of the sample were found to have at least one test score more than 2 *SD* below their estimated IQ score. Similarly Palmer et al. (1998) and Taylor and Heaton (2001) have reported that it is not uncommon for healthy people to show isolated weakness in one test or area. These data are certainly provocative and strongly suggest that additional large-scale studies of normal variability and prevalence of impaired-range scores among healthy persons are clearly warranted. Clinicians should always consider available data on normal variability (e.g., Index Score discrepancy baserates for Wechsler Scales) when interpreting test scores. When these data are not available, mathematical models and research data suggest that a conservative approach to interpretation is warranted when considering a small number of score discrepancies or abnormal scores from a large test battery.

A Final Word on the Imprecision of Psychological Tests

Though progress has been made, much work remains to be done in developing more psychometrically sound and clinically efficient and useful measures. At times, the technical limitations of many neuropsychological tests currently available with regard to measurement error, reliability, validity, diagnostic accuracy, and other important psychometric characteristics may lead to questions regarding their worth in clinical practice. Indeed, informed consideration may, quite appropriately, lead neuropsychologists to limit or completely curtail their use of some measures. The extreme argument would be to completely exclude any tests that entail measurement error, effectively eliminating all forms of objective measurement of human characteristics. However, it is important to keep in mind the limited and unreliable nature of human judgment, even expert judgment, when left to its own devices.

Dahlstom (1993) provides the following historical example. While in the midst of their groundbreaking work on human intelligence and prior to the use of standardized tests to diagnose conditions affecting cognition, Binet and Simon (1907) carried out a study on the reliability of diagnoses assigned to children with mental retardation by staff psychiatrists in three Paris hospitals. The specific categories included "l'idiotie," "l'imbécilité," and "la debilité mentale" (corresponding to the unfortunate diagnostic categories of idiot, imbecile, and moron, respectively). Binet and Simon reported the following:

> We have made a methodical comparison between the admission certificates filled out for the same children within only a few days' interval by the doctors of Sainte-Anne, Bicêtre, the Salpétrière, and Vaucluse. We have compared several hundreds of these certificates, and we think we may say without exaggeration that they looked as if they had been drawn by chance out of a sack. (p. 76)

Dahlstom (1993) goes on to state that "this fallibility in the judgments made by humans about fellow humans is one of the primary reasons that psychological tests have been developed and applied in ever-increasing numbers over the past century" (p. 393). In this context, neuropsychological tests need not be perfect, or even psychometrically exceptional; they need only meaningfully improve clinical decision making and significantly reduce errors of judgment—those errors stemming from prejudice, personal bias, halo effects, ignorance, and stereotyping—made by people when judging other people (Dahlstom, 1993; see also Meehl, 1973). The judicious selection, appropriate administration, and well-informed interpretation of standardized tests will usually achieve this result.

GRAPHICAL REPRESENTATIONS OF TEST DATA

It is often useful to have a visual representation of test performance in order to facilitate interpretation and cross-test comparison. For this purpose, we include example profile forms (Figures 1–7 and 1–8 on pp. 32–43) which we use to graphically or numerically represent neuropsychological performance in the individual patient. We suggest that these forms be used to draw in confidence intervals for each test rather than point estimates. We also include a sample form that we use for evaluation of children involving repeat assessment, such as epilepsy surgical candidates.

NOTES

1. It should be noted that Pearson later stated that he regretted his choice of "normal" as a descriptor for the normal curve; this "[had] the disadvantage of leading people to believe that all other distributions of frequency are in one sense or another 'abnormal'. That belief is, of course, not justifiable" (Pearson, 1920, p. 25).

2. Micceti analyzed 400 datasets, including 30 from national tests and 131 from regional tests, on 89 different populations administered various psychological and education tests and found that extremes of asymmetry and "lumpiness" (i.e., appearance of distinct subpopulations in the distribution) were the norm rather than the exception. General ability measures tended to fare better than other types of tests such as achievement tests, but the results suggested that the vast majority of groups tested in the real world consist of subgroups that produce non-normal distributions, leading Micceti to state that despite "widespread belief [. . .] in the naïve assumption of normality," there is a "startling" lack of evidence to this effect for achievement tests and psychometric measures (p. 156).

3. Ironically, measurement error cannot be known precisely and must also be estimated.

4. Note that this model focuses on test characteristics and does not explicitly address measurement error arising from particular characteristics of individual examinees or testing circumstances.

5. In most cases, even though it is usually provided in the same metric as test scores (i.e., standard score units), users should note that some test publishers report *SEM*s in raw score units, which further impedes interpretation.

6. When interpreting confidence intervals based on the *SEM*, it is important to bear in mind that while these provide useful information about the expected range of scores, such confidence intervals are based on a model that assumes expected performance across a large number of randomly parallel forms. Ideally, test users would therefore have an understanding of the nature and limitations of classical test models and their applicability to specific tests in order to use estimates such as the *SEM* appropriately.

7. There are quite a number of alternate methods for estimating error intervals and adjusting obtained scores for regression to the mean and other sources of measurement error (Glutting, McDermott & Stanley, 1987) and there is no universally agreed-upon method. Indeed, the most appropriate methods may vary across different types of tests and interpretive uses, though the majority of methods will produce roughly similar results in many cases. A review of alternate methods for estimating and correcting for measurement error is beyond the scope of this book; the methods presented were chosen because they continue to be widely used and accepted and they are relatively easy to grasp conceptually and mathematically. Regardless, in most cases, the choice of *which* specific method is used for estimating and correcting for measurement error is far less important than the issue of whether *any* such estimates and corrections are calculated and incorporated into test score interpretation. That is, test scores should not be interpreted in the absence of consideration of measurement error.

8. COIs and outcomes of interest may also be defined along a continuum from binary (present–absent) to multiple discrete categories (mild, moderate, severe) to fully continuous (percent impairment). This chapter will only consider the binary case.

9. In medical literature, these may be referred to as the *Predictive Value of a Positive Test* (PV+) or *Positive Predictive Value* (PPV) and the *Predictive Value of a Negative Test* (PV−) or *Negative Predictive Value* (NPV).

10. Predictive power values at or below .50 should *not* be automatically interpreted as indicating that a COI is not present or that a test has no utility. For example, if the population prevalence of a COI is .05 and the PPP based on test results is .45, a clinician can rightly conclude that an examinee is much more likely to have the COI than members of the general population, which may be clinically relevant.

11. Recalculating the PPP for this scenario using low and high values of Sensitivity and Specificity as defined by 95% confidence limits derived earlier from the data in Table 1–9 gives a worst-case to best-case PPP range of .03 to .41.

12. In Bayesian terminology, prevalence of a COI is known as the *prior* probability, while PPP and NPP are known as *posterior* probabilities. Conceptually, the difference between the prior and posterior probabilities associated with information added by a test score is an index of the diagnostic utility of a test. There is an entire literature concerning Bayesian methods for statistical analysis of test utility. These will not be covered here and interested readers are referred to Pepe (2003).

13. Compare this approach with use and limitations of the SE_P, as described earlier in this chapter.

14. The basics of linear regression will not be covered here; see Pedhauzer (1997).

REFERENCES

Altman, D. G., & Bland, J. M. (1983). Measurement in medicine: The analysis of method comparison. *Statistician, 32*, 307–317.

American Educational Research Association, American Psychological Association, & National Council on Measurement in Education. (1999). *Standards for educational and psychological testing.* Washington, DC: American Psychological Association.

Anastasi, A., & Urbina, S. (1997). *Psychological testing* (7th ed.). Upper Saddle River, NJ: Prentice Hall.

Andrews, G., Peters, L., & Teesson, M. (1994). *The measurement of consumer outcomes in mental health.* Canberra, Australia: Australian Government Publishing Services.

Axelrod, B. N., & Goldman, R. S. (1996). Use of demographic corrections in neuropsychological interpretation: How standard are standard scores? *The Clinical Neuropsychologist, 10*(2), 159–162.

Baron, I. S. (2004). *Neuropsychological evaluation of the child.* New York: Oxford University Press.

Binet, A., & Simon, T. (1907). *Les enfants anormaux.* Paris: Armond Colin.

Bland, J. M., & Altman, D. G. (1986). Statistical methods for assessing agreement between two methods of clinical measurement. *Lancet, i*, 307–310.

Bornstein, R. F. (1996). Face validity in psychological assessment: Implications for a unified model of validity. *American Psychologist, 51*(9), 983–984.

Burlingame, G. M., Lambert, M. J., Reisinger, C. W., Neff, W. M., & Mosier, J. (1995). Pragmatics of tracking mental health outcomes in a managed care setting. *Journal of Mental Health Administration, 22*, 226–236.

Canadian Psychological Association. (1987). *Guidelines for educational and psychological testing.* Ottawa, Canada: Canadian Psychological Association.

Chelune, G. J. (2003). Assessing reliable neuropsychological change. In R. D. Franklin (Ed.), *Prediction in Forensic and Neuropsychology: Sound Statistical Practices* (pp. 65–88). Mahwah, NJ: Lawrence Erlbaum Associates.

Chronbach, L. (1971). Test validation. In R. Thorndike (Ed.), *Educational measurement* (2nd ed., pp. 443–507). Washington, DC: American Council on Education.

Chronbach, L., & Meehl, P. E. (1955). Construct validity in psychological tests. *Psychological Bulletin, 52*, 167–186.

Cicchetti, D. V. (1994). Guidelines, criteria, and rules of thumb for evaluating normed and standardized assessment instruments in psychology. *Psychological Assessment, 6*(4), 284–290.

Cicchetti, D. V., & Sparrow, S. S. (1981). Developing criteria for establishing interrater reliability of specific items: Applications to assessment of adaptive behavior. *American Journal of Mental Deficiency, 86*, 127–137.

Cicchetti, D. V., Volkmar, F., Sparrow, S. S., Cohen, D., Fermanian, J., & Rourke, B. P. (1992). Assessing reliability of clinical scales when data have both nominal and ordinal features: Proposed guidelines for neuropsychological assessments. *Journal of Clinical and Experimental Neuropsychology, 14*(5), 673–686.

Crawford, J. R., & Garthwaite, P. H. (2002). Investigation of the single case in neuropsychology: Confidence limits on the abnormality of test scores and test score differences. *Neuropsychologia, 40,* 1196–1208.

Crawford, J. R., & Howell, D. C. (1998). Regression equations in clinical neuropsychology: An evaluation of statistical methods for comparing predicted and obtained scores. *Journal of Clinical and Experimental Neuropsychology, 20*(5), 755–762.

Dahlstom, W. G. (1993). Small samples, large consequences. *American Psychologist, 48*(4), 393–399.

Dikmen S. S., Heaton R. K., Grant I., & Temkin N. R. (1999). Test-retest reliability and practice effects of expanded Halstead-Reitan Neuropsychological Test Battery. *Journal of the International Neuropsychological Society, 5*(4):346–56.

Dudek, F. J. (1979). The continuing misinterpretation of the standard error of measurement. *Psychological Bulletin, 86*(2), 335–337.

Elwood, R. W. (1993). Clinical discriminations and neuropsychological tests: An appeal to Bayes' theorem. *The Clinical Neuropsychologist, 7*, 224–233.

Fastenau, P. S. (1998). Validity of regression-based norms: An empirical test of the Comprehensive Norms with older adults. *Journal of Clinical and Experimental Neuropsychology, 20*(6), 906–916.

Fastenau, P. S., & Adams, K. M. (1996). Heaton, Grant, and Matthews' Comprehensive Norms: An overzealous attempt. *Journal of Clinical and Experimental Neuropsychology, 18*(3), 444–448.

Fastenau, P. S., Bennett, J. M., & Denburg, N. L. (1996). Application of psychometric standards to scoring system evaluation: Is "new" necessarily "improved"? *Journal of Clinical and Experimental Neuropsychology, 18*(3), 462–472.

Ferguson, G. A. (1981). *Statistical analysis in psychology and education* (5th ed.). New York: McGraw-Hill.

Franklin, R. D. (Ed.). (2003a). *Prediction in Forensic and Neuropsychology: Sound Statistical Practices.* Mahwah, NJ: Lawrence Erlbaum Associates.

Franklin, R. D., & Krueger, J. (2003b). Bayesian Inference and Belief networks. In R. D. Franklin (Ed.), *Prediction in Forensic and Neuropsychology: Sound Statistical Practices* (pp. 65–88). Mahwah, NJ: Lawrence Erlbaum Associates.

Franzen, M. D. (2000). *Reliability and validity in neuropsychological assessment* (2nd ed.). New York: Kluwer Academic/Plenum Publishers.

Gasquoine, P. G. (1999). Variables moderating cultural and ethnic differences in neuropsychological assessment: The case of Hispanic Americans. *The Clinical Neuropsychologist, 13*(3), 376–383.

Glutting, J. J., McDermott, P. A., & Stanley, J. C. (1987). Resolving differences among methods of establishing confidence limits for test scores. *Educational and Psychological Measurement, 47*(3), 607–614.

Gottfredson, L. S. (1994). The science and politics of race-norming. *American Psychologist, 49*(11), 955–963.

Greenslaw, P. S., & Jensen, S. S. (1996). Race-norming and the Civil Rights Act of 1991. *Public Personnel Management, 25*(1), 13–24.

Hambelton, R. K. (1980). Test score validity and standard-setting methods. In R. A. Berk (Ed.), *Criterion-referenced measurement: The state of the art* (pp. 80–123). Baltimore, MD: Johns Hopkins University Press.

Harris, J. G., & Tulsky, D. S. (2003). Assessment of the non-native English speaker: Assimilating history and research findings to guide clinical practice. In D. S. Tulsky, D. H. Saklofske, G. J. Chelune, R. K. Heaton, R. Ivnik, R. Bornstein, A. Prifitera, & M. F. Ledbetter (Eds.), *Clinical interpretation of the WAIS-III and WMS-III* (pp. 343–390). New York: Academic Press.

Heaton, R. K., Chelune, G. J., Talley, J. L., Kay, G. G., & Curtiss, G. (1993). *Wisconsin Card Sorting Test Manual.* Odessa, FL: PAR.

Heaton, R. K., Taylor, M. J., & Manly, J. (2003). Demographic effects and use of demographically corrected norms with the WAIS-III and WMS-III. In D. S. Tulsky, D. H. Saklofske, G. J. Chelune, R. K. Heaton, R. Ivnik, R. Bornstein, A. Prifitera, & M. F. Ledbetter (Eds.), *Clinical interpretation of the WAIS-III and WMS-III* (pp. 181–210). New York: Academic Press.

Hermann, B. P., Wyler, A. R., VanderZwagg, R., LeBailly, R. K., Whitman, S., Somes, G., & Ward, J. (1991). Predictors of neuropsychological change following anterior temporal lobectomy: Role of regression toward the mean. *Journal of Epilepsy, 4,* 139–148.

Ingraham, L. J., & Aiken, C. B. (1996). An empirical approach to determining criteria for abnormality in test batteries with multiple measures. *Neuropsychology, 10*(1), 120–124.

Ivnik, R. J., Smith, G. E., & Cerhan, J. H. (2001). Understanding the diagnostic capabilities of cognitive tests. *Clinical Neuropsychologist. 15*(1), 114–124.

Jacobson, N. S., Roberts, L. J., Berns, S. B., & McGlinchey, J. B. (1999). Methods for defining and determining the clinical significance of treatment effects description, application, and alternatives. *Journal of Consulting and Clinical Psychology, 67*(3), 300–307.

Jacobson, N. S. & Truax, P. (1991). Clinical significance: A statistical approach to defining meaningful change in psychotherapy research. *Journal of Consulting and Clinical Psychology, 59*, 12–19.

Kalechstein, A. D., van Gorp, W. G., & Rapport, L. J. (1998). Variability in clinical classification of raw test scores across normative data sets. *The Clinical Neuropsychologist, 12*(3), 339–347.

Lees-Haley, P. R. (1996). Alice in validityland, or the dangerous consequences of consequential validity. *American Psychologist, 51*(9), 981–983.

Lezak, M. D., Howieson, D. B., & Loring, D. W. (2004). *Neuropsychological assessment* (4th ed.). New York: Oxford University Press.

Lindeboom, J. (1989). Who needs cutting points? *Journal of Clinical Psychology, 45*(4), 679–683.

Lineweaver, T. T., & Chelune, G. J. (2003). Use of the WAIS-III and WMS-III in the context of serial assessments: Interpreting reliable and meaningful change. In D. S. Tulsky, D. H. Saklofske, G. J. Chelune, R. K. Heaton, R. Ivnik, R. Bornstein, A. Prifitera, & M. F. Ledbetter (Eds.), *Clinical interpretation of the WAIS-III and WMS-III* (pp. 303–337). New York: Academic Press.

Lord, F. M., & Novick, M. R. (1968). *Statistical theories of mental test scores.* Reading, MA: Addison-Wesley.

Makinnon, A. (2000). A spreadsheet for the calculation of comprehensive statistics for the assessment of diagnostic tests and interrater agreement. *Computers in Biology and Medicine, 30,* 127–134.

McCleary, R., Dick, M. B., Buckwalter, G., Henderson, V., & Shankle, W. R. (1996). Full-information models for multiple psychometric tests: Annualized rates of change in normal aging and dementia. *Alzheimer Disease and Associated Disorders, 10*(4), 216–223.

McFadden, T. U. (1996). Creating language impairments in typically achieving children: The pitfalls of "normal" normative sampling. *Language, Speech, and Hearing Services in Schools, 27*, 3–9.

McKenzie, D., Vida, S., Mackinnon, A. J., Onghena, P. and Clarke, D. (1997) Accurate confidence intervals for measures of test performance. *Psychiatry Research, 69*, 207–209.

Meehl, P. E. (1973). Why I do not attend case conferences. In P. E. Meehl (Ed.), *Psychodiagnosis: Selected papers* (pp. 225–302). Minneapolis: University of Minnesota.

Meehl, P. E., & Rosen, A. (1955). Antecedent probability and the efficiency of psychometric signs, patterns, or cutting scores. *Psychological Bulletin. 52*, 194–216.

Messick, S. (1989). Validity. In R. L. Linn (Ed.), *Educational measurement* (3rd ed., p. 13–103). New York: Macmillan.

Messick, S. (1993). Validity. In R. L. Lin (Ed.), *Educational measurement* (3rd ed., pp. 13–103). Phoenix, AZ.: The Oryx Press.

Messick, S. (1995). Validity of psychological assessment: Validation of inferences from persons' responses and performance as scientific inquiry into scoring meaning. *American Psychologist, 9*, 741–749.

Messick, S. (1996). Validity of psychological assessment: Validation of inferences from persons' responses and performances as scientific inquiry into score meaning. *American Psychologist, 50*(9), 741–749.

Micceri, T. (1989). The unicorn, the normal curve, and other improbable creatures. *Psychological Bulletin, 105*(1), 156–166.

Mitrushina, M. N., Boone, K. B., & D'Elia, L. F. (1999). *Handbook of normative data for neuropsychological assessment.* New York: Oxford University Press.

Mitrushina, M. N., Boone, K. B., Razani, J., & D'Elia, L. F. (2005). *Handbook of normative data for neuropsychological assessment* (2nd ed.). New York: Oxford University Press.

Mossman, D. (2003). Daubert, cognitive malingering, and test accuracy. *Law and Human Behavior, 27*(3), 229–249.

Mossman D., & Somoza E. (1992). Balancing risks and benefits: another approach to optimizing diagnostic tests. *Journal of Neuropsychiatry and Clinical Neurosciences, 4*(3), 331–335.

Nevo, B. (1985). Face validity revisited. *Journal of Educational Measurement, 22*, 287–293.

Nunnally, J. C., & Bernstein, I. H. (1994). *Psychometric theory* (3rd ed.). New York: McGraw-Hill, Inc.

Palmer, B. W., Boone, K. B., Lesser, I. R., & Wohl, M. A. (1998). Base rates of "impaired' neuropsychological test performance among healthy older adults. *Archives of Clinical Neuropsychology, 13*, 503–511.

Pavel, D., Sanchez, T., & Machamer, A. (1994). Ethnic fraud, native peoples and higher education. *Thought and Action, 10*, 91–100.

Pearson, K. (1920). Notes on the history of correlation. *Biometrika, 13*, 25–45.

Pedhazur, E. (1997). *Multiple Regression in Behavioral Research.* New York: Harcourt Brace.

Pepe, M. S. (2003). *The Statistical Evaluation of Medical Tests for Classification and Prediction.* New York: Oxford.

Puente, A. E., Mora, M. S., & Munoz-Cespedes, J. M. (1997). Neuropsychological assessment of Spanish-Speaking children and youth. In C. R. Reynolds & E. Fletcher-Janzen (Eds.), *Handbook of clinical child neuropsychology* (2nd ed., pp. 371–383). New York: Plenum Press.

Rapport, L. J., Brines, D. B., & Axelrod, B. N. (1997). Full Scale IQ as mediator of practice effects: The rich get richer. *Clinical Neuropsychologist, 11*(4), 375–380.

Rey, G. J., Feldman, E., & Rivas-Vazquez. (1999). Neuropsychological test development and normative data on Hispanics. *Archives of Clinical Neuropsychology, 14*(7), 593–601.

Rorer, L. G., & Dawes, R. M. (1982). A base-rate bootstrap. *Journal of Consulting and Clinical Psychology, 50*(3), 419–425.

Sacket, P. R., & Wilk, S. L. (1994). Within-group norming and other forms of score adjustment in preemployment testing. *American Psychologist, 49*(11), 929–954.

Sattler, J. M. (2001). *Assessment of children: Cognitive applications* (4th ed.). San Diego: Jerome M. Sattler Publisher, Inc.

Sawrie, S. M., Chelune, G. J., Naugle, R. I., & Luders, H. O. (1996). Empirical methods for assessing meaningful neuropsychological change following epilepsy surgery. *Journal of the International Neuropsychological Society, 2*, 556–564.

Schretlen D. J., Munro C. A., Anthony J. C., & Pearlson G. D. (2003). Examining the range of normal intraindividual variability in neuropsychological test performance. *Journal of the International Neuropsychological Society, 9*(6): 864–70.

Shavelson, R. J., Webb, N. M., & Rowley, G. (1989). Generalizability theory. *American Psychologist, 44*, 922–932.

Sherman, E. M. S., Slick, D. J., Connolly, M. B., Steinbok, P., Martin, R., Strauss, E., Chelune, G. J., & Farrell, K. (2003). Re-examining the effects of epilepsy surgery on IQ in children: An empirically derived method for measuring change. *Journal of the International Neuropsychological Society, 9*, 879–886.

Slick, D. J., Hopp, G., Strauss, E., & Thompson, G. (1997). *The Victoria Symptom Validity Test.* Odessa, FL: Psychological Assessment Resources.

Sokal, R. R., & Rohlf, J. F. (1995). *Biometry.* San Fransisco, CA: W.H. Freeman.

Somoza E., & Mossman D. (1992). Comparing diagnostic tests using information theory: the INFO-ROC technique. *Journal of Neuropsychiatry and Clinical Neurosciences, 4*(2), 214–219.

Streiner, D. L. (2003a). Being inconsistent about consistency: When coefficient alpha does and doesn't matter. *Journal of Personality Assessment, 80*(3), 217–222.

Streiner, D. L. (2003b). Starting at the beginning: An introduction to coefficient alpha and internal consistency. *Journal of Personality Assessment, 80*(1), 99–103.

Streiner, D. L. (2003c). Diagnosing tests: Using and misusing diagnostic and screening tests. *Journal of Personality Assessment, 81*(3), 209–219.

Swets, J. A., Dawes, R. M., & Monahan, J. (2000). Psychological science can improve diagnostic decisions. *Psychological Science in the Public Interest, 1*(1), 1–26.

Taylor, M. J., & Heaton, R. K. (2001). Sensitivity and specificity of WAIS-III/WMS-III demographically corrected factor scores in neuropsychological assessment. *Journal of the International Neuropsychological Society, 7*, 867–874.

Temkin, N. R., Heaton, R. K., Grant, I., & Dikmen, S. S. (1999). Detecting significant change in neuropsychological test performance: A comparison of four models. *Journal of the International Neuropsychological Society, 5*, 357–369.

Tulsky, D. S., Saklofske, D. H., & Zhu, J. (2003). Revising a standard: An evaluation of the origin and development of the WAIS-III. In D. S. Tulsky, D. H. Saklofske, G. J. Chelune, R. K. Heaton, R. Ivnik, R. Bornstein, A. Prifitera, & M. F. Ledbetter (Eds.), *Clinical interpretation of the WAIS-III and WMS-III* (pp. 43–92). New York: Academic Press.

Willis, W. G. (1984). Reanalysis of an actuarial approach to neuropsychological diagnosis in consideration of base rates. *Journal of Consulting and Clinical Psychology, 52*(4), 567–569.

Woods, S. P., Weinborn, M., & Lovejoy, D. W. (2003). Are classification accuracy statistics underused in neuropsychological research? *Journal of Clinical and Experimental Neuropsychology*, 25(3), 431–439.

Yun, J., & Ulrich, D. A. (2002). Estimating measurement validity: A tutorial. *Adapted Physical Activity Quarterly, 19,* 32–47.

Zimiles, H. (1996). Rethinking the validity of psychological assessment. *American Psychologist, 51*(9), 980–981.

Figure 1–7 Profile form—Adult

Name _____ D.O.B. _____ Age _____ Sex _____

Education _____ Handedness _____ Examiner _____

Test Dates _____ Previous Testing _____

COGNITIVE

	Score	Age SS	%ile	10 20 30 40 50 60 70 80 90
WAIS-III				
Vocabulary	_____	_____	_____	
Similarities	_____	_____	_____	
Arithmetic	_____	_____	_____	
Digit Span **F B**	_____	_____	_____	
Information	_____	_____	_____	
Comprehension	_____	_____	_____	
Letter-Number Sequencing	_____	_____	_____	
Picture Completion	_____	_____	_____	
Digit-Symbol-Coding	_____	_____	_____	
Block Design	_____	_____	_____	
Matrix Reasoning	_____	_____	_____	
Picture Arrangement	_____	_____	_____	
Symbol Search	_____	_____	_____	
Object Assembly	_____	_____	_____	
VIQ	_____	_____	_____	
PIQ	_____	_____	_____	
FSIQ	_____	_____	_____	
VCI	_____	_____	_____	
POI	_____	_____	_____	
WMI	_____	_____	_____	
PSI	_____	_____	_____	
NAART				
VIQ	_____	_____	_____	
PIQ	_____	_____	_____	
FSIQ	_____	_____	_____	
Raven's Matrices (_____)	_____	_____	_____	
Other _____	_____	_____	_____	
Other _____	_____	_____	_____	
Other _____	_____	_____	_____	

(continued)

Figure 1–7 (*continued*)

EXECUTIVE FUNCTION

	Score	Z	%ile	10 20 30 40 50 60 70 80 90
WCST				
Categories	_____	_____	_____	
Perseverative Errors	_____	_____	_____	
FMS	_____	_____	_____	
Category Test	_____	_____	_____	
Cognitive Estimation Test	_____	_____	_____	
Stroop (_____)				
I	_____	_____	_____	
II	_____	_____	_____	
III	_____	_____	_____	
Interference	_____	_____	_____	
Verbal Fluency				
FAS	_____	_____	_____	
Animals	_____	_____	_____	
Ruff Figural Fluency				
Total Unique Designs	_____	_____	_____	
Error Ratio	_____	_____	_____	
BADS				
6-Elements	_____	_____	_____	
Key Search	_____	_____	_____	
Other _____	_____	_____	_____	

ATTENTION/CONCENTRATION

	Score	Z	%ile	10 20 30 40 50 60 70 80 90
Trails (_____)				
A	_____	_____	_____	
B	_____	_____	_____	
Interference	_____	_____	_____	
CPT				
Omissions	_____	_____	_____	
Commissions	_____	_____	_____	
BTA	_____	_____	_____	
Symbol-Digit	_____	_____	_____	
PASAT				
2.4	_____	_____	_____	
2.0	_____	_____	_____	
1.6	_____	_____	_____	
1.2	_____	_____	_____	
Other _____	_____	_____	_____	

(*continued*)

Figure 1–7 *(continued)*

MEMORY

	Score	Age SS	%ile	10 20 30 40 50 60 70 80 90

WMS-III

	Score	Age SS	%ile
Logical Memory I	_____	_____	_____
Logical Memory II	_____	_____	_____
Faces I	_____	_____	_____
Faces II	_____	_____	_____
VPA I	_____	_____	_____
VPA II	_____	_____	_____
Family Pictures I	_____	_____	_____
Family Pictures II	_____	_____	_____
Spatial Span	_____	_____	_____
Visual Reprod. I	_____	_____	_____
Visual Reprod. II	_____	_____	_____
Visual Reprod. Recognition	_____	_____	_____
Word Lists I	_____	_____	_____
Word Lists II	_____	_____	_____
Auditory Immediate	_____	_____	_____
Visual Immediate	_____	_____	_____
Immediate Memory	_____	_____	_____
Auditory Delayed	_____	_____	_____
Visual Delayed	_____	_____	_____
Aud. Recogn. Delayed	_____	_____	_____
General Memory	_____	_____	_____
Working Memory	_____	_____	_____

CVLT-II

	Score	Age SS	%ile
List A Total	_____	_____	_____
List A Trial 1	_____	_____	_____
List A Trial 5	_____	_____	_____
List B	_____	_____	_____
List A Short-Delay Free Recall	_____	_____	_____
List A Short-Delay Cued Recall	_____	_____	_____
List A Long-Delay Free Recall	_____	_____	_____
List A Long-Delay Cued Recall	_____	_____	_____
Semantic Cluster Ratio	_____	_____	_____
Serial Cluster Ratio	_____	_____	_____
% Primacy	_____	_____	_____
% Middle	_____	_____	_____
% Recency	_____	_____	_____
Learning Slope	_____	_____	_____
Recall Consistency	_____	_____	_____
Perservations	_____	_____	_____
Free Recall Instrustions	_____	_____	_____
Cued Recall Intrusions	_____	_____	_____
Recognition Hits	_____	_____	_____
False Positives	_____	_____	_____
Response Bias	_____	_____	_____
			_____
B-A1	_____	_____	_____
Short Delay A5	_____	_____	_____
Long Delay - Short Delay Free	_____	_____	_____
Recognition - Long Delay Free	_____	_____	_____

(continued)

Figure 1–7 (*continued*)

MEMORY (Contd.)

	Score	Z	%ile	10 20 30 40 50 60 70 80 90
Rey Complex Figure				
Copy	_____	_____	_____	
3″ Recall	_____	_____	_____	
30″ Recall	_____	_____	_____	
Recognition	_____	_____	_____	
BVMT-R				
Trial 1	_____	_____	_____	
Trial 2	_____	_____	_____	
Trial 3	_____	_____	_____	
Total Recall	_____	_____	_____	
Delayed Recall	_____	_____	_____	
Recognition Hits	_____	_____	_____	
Recog. False Alarms	_____	_____	_____	
RAVLT				
Trial 1	_____	_____	_____	
Trial 2	_____	_____	_____	
Trial 3	_____	_____	_____	
Trial 4	_____	_____	_____	
Trial 5	_____	_____	_____	
Total	_____	_____	_____	
Recognition	_____	_____	_____	
Other _____	_____	_____	_____	
Other _____	_____	_____	_____	
Other _____	_____	_____	_____	

MEMORY/MOTIVATION

	Score			10 20 30 40 50 60 70 80 90
VSVT				
Easy Correct	_____	z =	p =	
Hard Correct	_____	z =	p =	
Easy Time	_____	sd =		
Hard Time	_____	sd =		
TOMM				
Trial 1	_____	_____	_____	
Trial 2	_____	_____	_____	
Retention	_____	_____	_____	
Word Memory Test				
Immediate Recognition	_____	_____	_____	
Delayed Recognition	_____	_____	_____	
Consistency	_____	_____	_____	
Multiple Choice	_____	_____	_____	
Paired Associate	_____	_____	_____	
Delayed Free Recall	_____	_____	_____	
Other _____	_____	_____	_____	

(*continued*)

Figure 1–7 (continued)

LANGUAGE

	Score	Z	%ile	10 20 30 40 50 60 70 80 90
Boston Naming Test	____	____	____	
Dichotic Listening				
R. Ear	____	____	____	
L. Ear	____	____	____	
Total	____	____	____	
Token Test	____	____	____	
PPVT-III	____	____	____	
Other _____	____	____	____	

VISUAL

	Score	Z	%ile	10 20 30 40 50 60 70 80 90
Hooper VOT	____	____	____	
VOSP				
Incomplete Letters	____	____	____	
Silhouettes	____	____	____	
Object Decision	____	____	____	
Progressive Silhouettes	____	____	____	
Dot Counting	____	____	____	
Position Discrimination	____	____	____	
Number Location	____	____	____	
Cube Analysis	____	____	____	
Judgment of Line Orientation	____	____	____	
Right-Left Orientation				
Total Correct	____	____	____	
Reversal Score	____	____	____	
Other _____	____	____	____	

MOTOR

	Score	Z	%ile	10 20 30 40 50 60 70 80 90
Grooved Pegboard				
Right	____	____	____	
Left	____	____	____	
Finger Tapping				
Right	____	____	____	
Left	____	____	____	
Dynamometer				
Right	____	____	____	
Left	____	____	____	
Other _____	____	____	____	

(continued)

Figure 1–7 (*continued*)

SOMATOSENSORY/OLFACTION

	Score	Z	%ile	10 20 30 40 50 60 70 80 90
Smell Identification	_____	_____	_____	
TPT				
Right	_____	_____	_____	
Left	_____	_____	_____	
Both	_____	_____	_____	
Memory	_____	_____	_____	
Location	_____	_____	_____	
Other _____	_____	_____	_____	
Other _____	_____	_____	_____	

ACADEMIC ACHIEVEMENT

	Score	Z	%ile	10 20 30 40 50 60 70 80 90
WRAT-III				
Reading	_____	_____	_____	
Spelling	_____	_____	_____	
Arithmetic	_____	_____	_____	
WJ-III Achievement				
Letter/Word Identification	_____	_____	_____	
Passage Comprehension	_____	_____	_____	
Word Attack	_____	_____	_____	
Reading Vocabulary	_____	_____	_____	
Calculation	_____	_____	_____	
Applied Problems	_____	_____	_____	
Quantitative Concepts	_____	_____	_____	
Dictation	_____	_____	_____	
Writing Samples	_____	_____	_____	
Other _____	_____	_____	_____	

PERSONALITY/MOOD

MMPI-2

_____
_____
_____

PAI

_____
_____
_____

BDI-II

_____
_____
_____

IADL

_____
_____
_____

Other

_____
_____
_____

Figure 1–8 Profile form—Children

CHILDREN'S NEUROPSYCHOLOGICAL TEST PROFILE

Name: _____ **Patient No:** _____ **D.O.B.:** _____ **Sex:** _____

Handedness: _____

Test Date 1: _____ **Test Date 2:** _____ **Test Date 3:** _____

Age: _____ **Grade:** _____ **Age:** _____ **Grade:** _____ **Age:** _____ **Grade:** _____

WISC-IV	Raw	Scaled/Age Eq.	%ile
SI		/ / /	
VC		/ / /	
CO		/ / /	
IN		/ / /	
WR		/ / /	
BD		/ / /	
PCn		/ / /	
MR		/ / /	
PCm		/ / /	
DS		/ / /	
LN		/ / /	
AR		/ / /	
CD		/ / /	
SS		/ / /	
CA		/ / /	

FSIQ		/ / /	
VCI		/ / /	
PRI		/ / /	
WMI		/ / /	
PSI		/ / /	

	Raw	p	%ile
VC–PR			
VC–FD			
VC–PS			
PR–FD			
PR–PS			
FD–PS			

Attention/Executive

	Raw	Scaled	%ile
CAT			
Hits			
FA			
RT			
ADHD-IV—Parent			
HI			
IA			
ADHD-IV—Teacher			
HI			
IA			

(continued)

Figure 1–8 *(continued)*

Attention/Executive (Contd.)

	Raw			Scaled			%ile		

WCST (64 / 128)
- Errors
- PR
- CLR
- Cat
- FMS

D-KEFS
- Letter Fluency
- Category Fluency
- Ca. Switching Correct
- Cat. Switching Accuracy

Color-Word Interference Test
- Naming Time
- Reading Time
- Inhibition Time
- Inhibition Errors
- Inhibition vs. Reading
- Switching Time
- Switching Errors
- Switching vs. Inhibition

MNI Design Fluency
- Perseverations
- Novel Output

NEPSY
- Tower
- Tower Rule Violations

- AA & RS
- Attention
- Response Set

- Visual Attention

BRIEF—Parent
- Inhibit
- Shift
- Emotional Control
- Initiate
- Working Memory
- Plan/Organize
- Organization of Materials
- Monitor
- BRI
- MI
- Composite

(continued)

Figure 1–8 (*continued*)

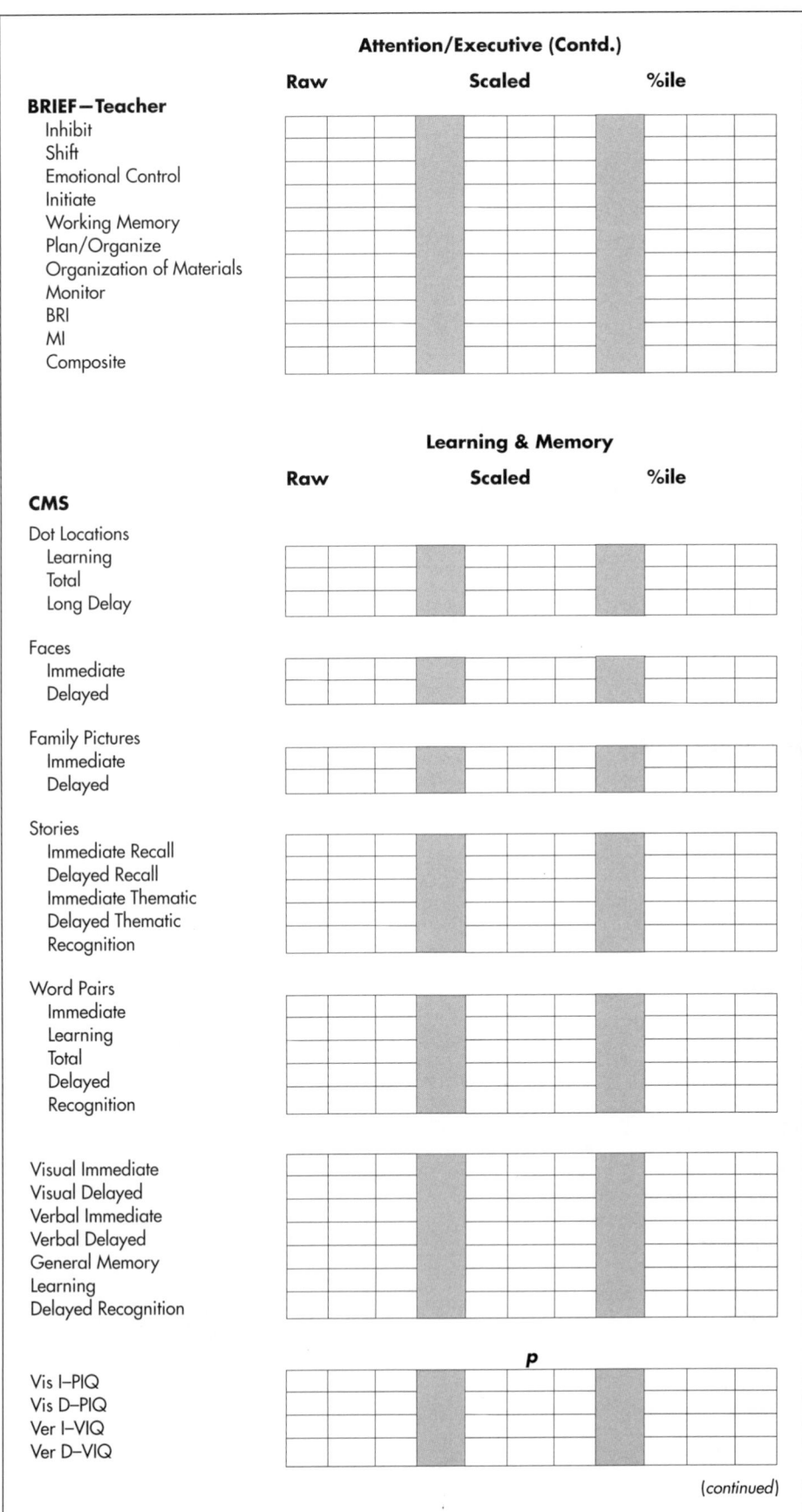

Attention/Executive (Contd.)

BRIEF—Teacher
  Inhibit
  Shift
  Emotional Control
  Initiate
  Working Memory
  Plan/Organize
  Organization of Materials
  Monitor
  BRI
  MI
  Composite

Learning & Memory

CMS
Dot Locations
  Learning
  Total
  Long Delay

Faces
  Immediate
  Delayed

Family Pictures
  Immediate
  Delayed

Stories
  Immediate Recall
  Delayed Recall
  Immediate Thematic
  Delayed Thematic
  Recognition

Word Pairs
  Immediate
  Learning
  Total
  Delayed
  Recognition

Visual Immediate
Visual Delayed
Verbal Immediate
Verbal Delayed
General Memory
Learning
Delayed Recognition

P

Vis I–PIQ
Vis D–PIQ
Ver I–VIQ
Ver D–VIQ

(*continued*)

Figure 1-8 *(continued)*

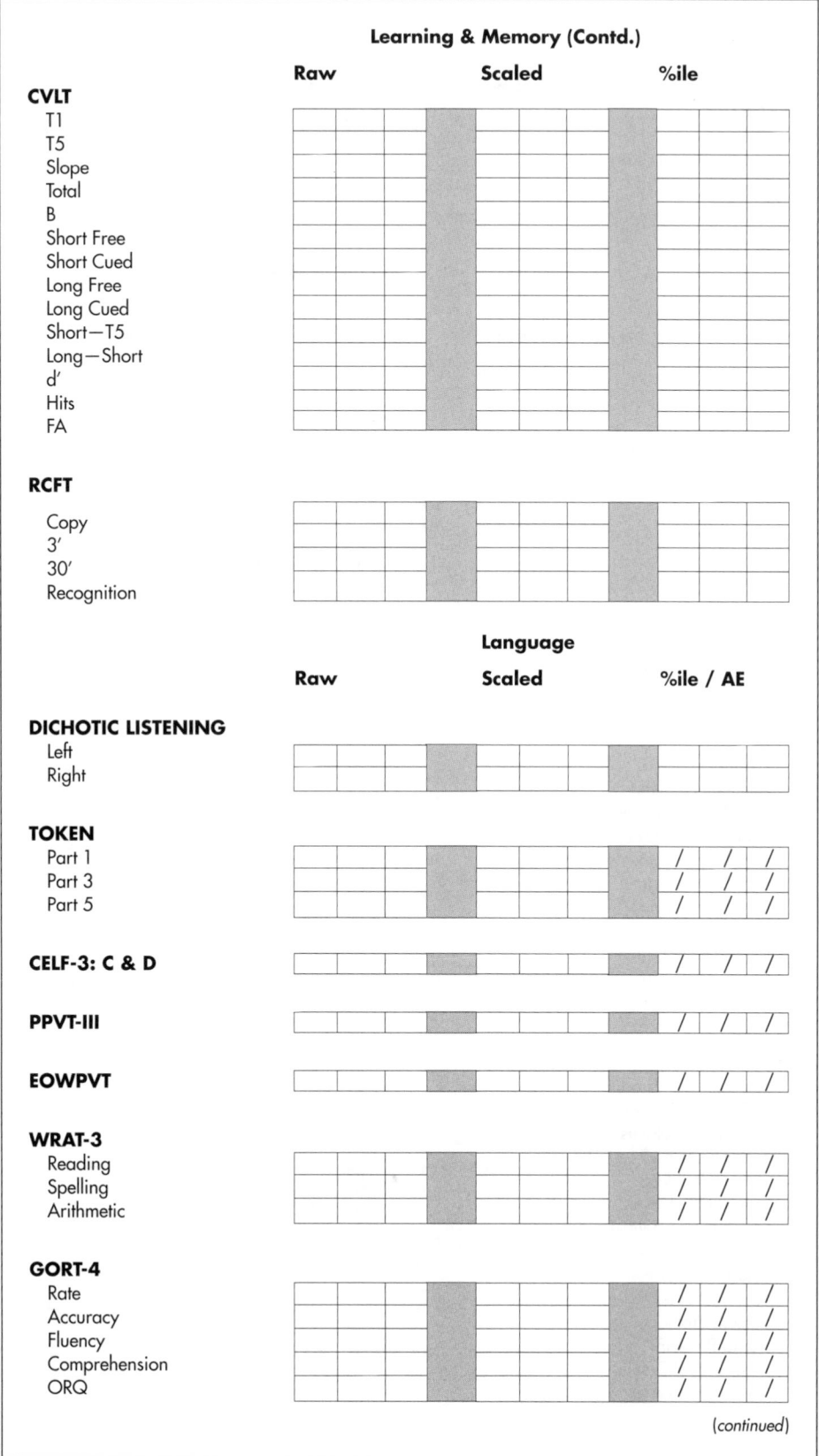

Figure 1–8 *(continued)*

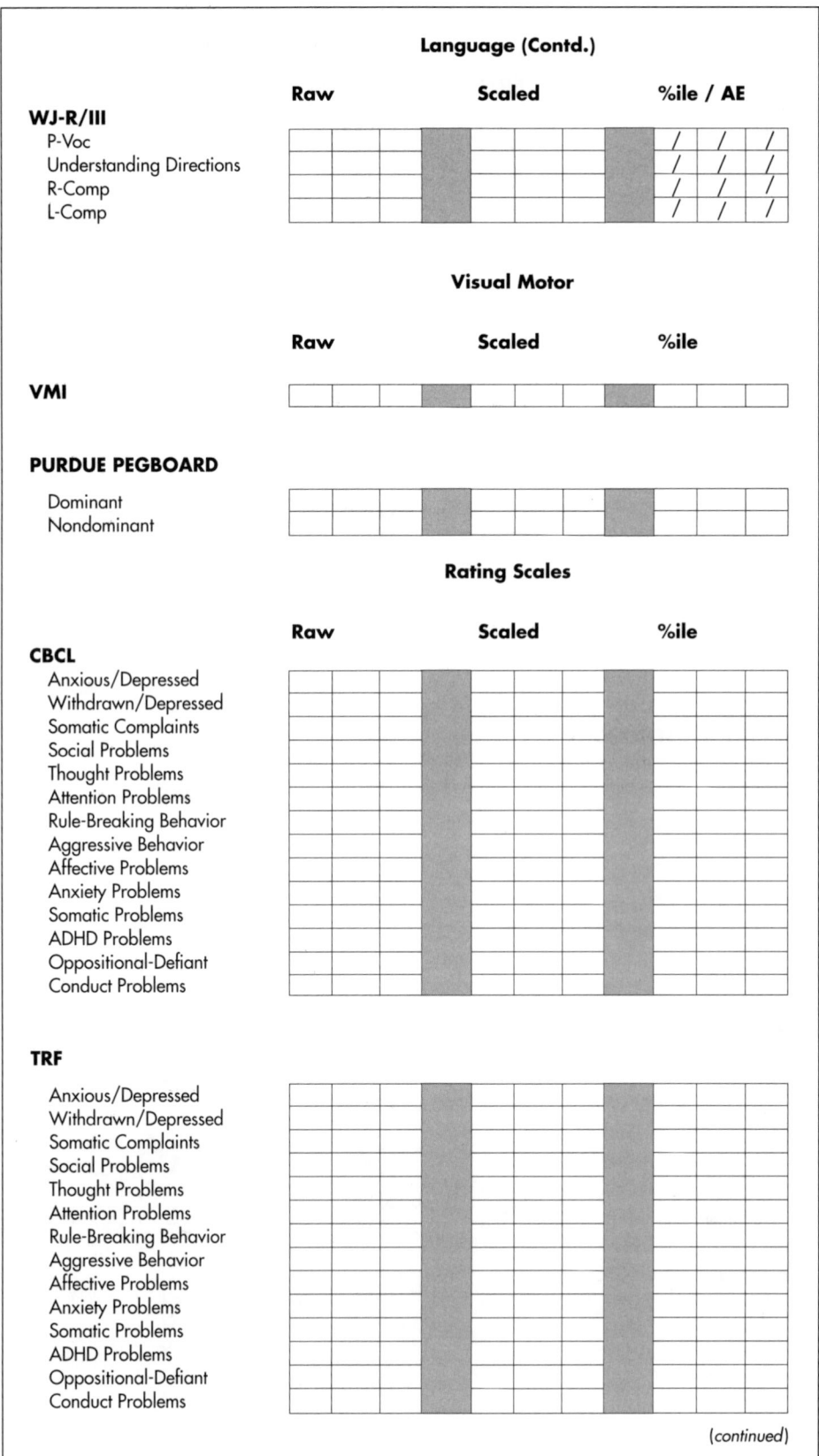

Language (Contd.)

	Raw			Scaled			%ile / AE		
WJ-R/III									
P-Voc							/	/	/
Understanding Directions							/	/	/
R-Comp							/	/	/
L-Comp							/	/	/

Visual Motor

	Raw			Scaled			%ile		
VMI									

PURDUE PEGBOARD

Dominant									
Nondominant									

Rating Scales

	Raw			Scaled			%ile		
CBCL									
Anxious/Depressed									
Withdrawn/Depressed									
Somatic Complaints									
Social Problems									
Thought Problems									
Attention Problems									
Rule-Breaking Behavior									
Aggressive Behavior									
Affective Problems									
Anxiety Problems									
Somatic Problems									
ADHD Problems									
Oppositional-Defiant									
Conduct Problems									
TRF									
Anxious/Depressed									
Withdrawn/Depressed									
Somatic Complaints									
Social Problems									
Thought Problems									
Attention Problems									
Rule-Breaking Behavior									
Aggressive Behavior									
Affective Problems									
Anxiety Problems									
Somatic Problems									
ADHD Problems									
Oppositional-Defiant									
Conduct Problems									

(continued)

Figure 1–8 *(continued)*

Rating Scales (Contd.)

	Raw			Scaled			%ile		

CDI (Long/Short)

Negative Mood
Interpersonal Problems
Ineffectiveness
Anhedonia
Negative Self-Esteem
Total

	Raw			Scaled			%ile / AE		

SIB-R

Broad Independence
Motor Skills
Social & Com. Skills
Personal Living Skills
Community Living Skills

2

Norms Selection in Neuropsychological Assessment

OVERVIEW

In this chapter, we present an overview of factors pertinent to (1) understanding normative data and (2) selecting norms so that they best meet the goals of the assessment and meet the needs of the patient evaluated. The goal of the chapter is to facilitate the user's task in making informed choices about norms.

One of the main considerations in choosing norms is whether a broadly representative sample should be selected, or whether a more specific subgroup is more appropriate, such as one defined by specific gender, education, ethnicity, socioeconomic status (SES), or other variables. Additional considerations are sample size, sample composition, and date of norms collection. All of these factors are discussed in this chapter. Other pertinent psychometric issues such as score transformations, extrapolation/interpolation, and normative adjustments by case weighting are also essential factors to consider when selecting normative datasets for clinical practice or research; these are considered in Chapter 1.

NORMS SELECTION: BASIC PRINCIPLES

Selecting an appropriate normative dataset is a prerequisite for effective and competent neuropsychological practice. Norms selection is as important as test selection; choosing an inadequate normative sample is as disastrous as choosing a test with poor reliability or validity, as considerable variability in obtained scores can occur depending on which normative dataset was the basis of normed-referenced scores (Kalechstein et al., 1998; Mitrushina et al., 2005). Because scores are directly tied to measurable consequences such as diagnoses, treatment recommendations, and funding decisions, neuropsychologists need to be aware of the specific characteristics of the norms they use.

Ideally, norms should be selected a priori in order to avoid confirmatory bias (Kalechstein et al., 1998). From a practical

standpoint, this also avoids wasted time and resources; many clinicians have administered a test to a patient, but only later realized that there existed no appropriate normative data corresponding to the patient's specific demographic characteristics (Mitrushina et al., 2005).

As most clinicians know, the process of norms selection often occurs in tandem with test selection. Subtle administration differences may characterize similar paradigms tied to different normative data sets. Word fluency is a case in point. To administer this test, users may employ the administration protocol described in this volume and derive standardized scores based on a variety of norms from several published studies. Or, one can use a word fluency paradigm as operationalized by the D-KEFS, NEPSY, or RBANS, and use the specific normative dataset tied to each test. Because each normative dataset differs in terms of its demographic composition, deciding which word fluency test to use will rest on an evaluation of the individual patient's demographic characteristics such as age and education. Norms selection is therefore facilitated by a strong working knowledge of the similarities and differences between tests in the field, as well as by the varying characteristics of their respective normative data sets. In addition to our volume, Mitrushina et al. (2005) and Baron (2004) are invaluable sources in this regard.

ARE LARGER NORMATIVE DATASETS
ALWAYS BETTER?

When choosing a test, most clinicians are primarily concerned with the size of the normative sample. The assumption is that the larger the N, the more reliable and representative the scores derived. As we have seen in Chapter 1, norms should be as large as possible to avoid sampling error, and to maximize the representativeness of the sample vis-à-vis the general population. As a rule of thumb, at least 200 subjects are needed to conduct item analysis (Nunnally & Bernstein, 1994), and many sources consider norms of less than 150 cases inadequate.

However, it is important to note that even large normative sets yield small cell sizes when scores are divided into demographically defined subgroups according to variables such as age, gender, and education. For example, for a given patient, a smaller, homogenous normative dataset comprised only of individuals from a similar demographic subgroup (e.g., elderly, white females from Minnesota with 12 years of education) may actually provide a larger N and a better demographic fit than norms from large, commercially produced, nationally representative tests whose cell sizes are the result of minute subdivision according to multiple demographic factors. This is one of the reasons that we provide additional normative datasets for commercially available tests that already have large normative databases.

On the other hand, there are clear advantages to norms derived from large datasets from the general population based on statistical techniques that correct for the irregularities inherent in smaller samples. To maximize clinical validity, users should be fully familiar with the properties of the normative sets they use, including techniques such as case weighting, to increase or adjust the composition of norm subgroups (e.g., by statistically increasing the number of cases defined by a demographic variable such as race or age, when the actual cell size falls short). Users should note that although techniques such as case weighting are relatively common and used in many large-scale tests (e.g., Wechsler scales), this practice means that derived scores are partially based on an estimate rather than on actual, real-world data.

THE FLYNN EFFECT AND THE DATE OF NORMING

New tests and new normative datasets appear with regularity in the neuropsychological assessment field. As a result, users are regularly faced with deciding whether to use existing, well-known normative datasets or the newest, most recently published normative datasets. Some have suggested that when choosing norms, recency of publication is less important than demographic match and cell size (Kalechstein et al., 1998). However, the effect of the passage of time on test scores should not be underestimated. The Flynn effect, which is the general trend for increased IQs over time with each subsequent generation, is estimated to contribute to an increase of 0.3 IQ points per year. Depending on the test, estimates range from 3 to 9 points per decade. A 20-point increase over one generation on some nonverbal tests such as the Raven's has even been recorded (i.e. Flynn, 1984, 2000). Gains have also been noted on neuropsychological tests such as the Halstead-Reitan Battery (Bengston et al., 1996). However, there is some evidence that the Flynn effect is more pronounced in fluid/nonverbal tests than in crystallized/verbal tests (see Kanaya et al., 2003a, 2003b for review). Score increases attributed to the Flynn effect are thought to result from improved nutrition, cultural changes, experience with testing, changes in schooling or child-rearing practices, or other factors as yet unknown (Neisser et al., 1996).

We know that normed tests have a "lifespan" of about 15 to 20 years, assuming that all other factors, such as the relevance of test items, remain constant (Tulsky et al., 2003). After this time, new norms need to be collected; this ensures that scores are reanchored to correct for the Flynn effect and this counteracts the tendency for increased scores over time. With renorming, the older test becomes "easier" and the new test becomes "harder": an individual given both the old and the new versions of the same test would obtain higher scores on the test with older norms. In light of the well-known Flynn effect, one would assume that most normative datasets used by neuropsychologists include only data from the most recent age cohorts. Surprisingly, some normative samples still used by neuropsychologists contain data that are as much as 40 years old. These old datasets, when considered in light of the Flynn effect, introduce the potential for considerable score inflation.

The Flynn effect has not been studied sufficiently in neuropsychology. However, we do know that it has a number of potential effects of major consequence for neuropsychological assessment. The first is that it alters cutoffs used for determination of certain conditions, depending on the recency of the norms used. For example, in the year a new re-standardized normative sample from an IQ test is released, an average child obtains a hypothetical score of 100. If tested with the older instrument, his or her score might be 105. Although this slight shift in scores has minimal consequences in the middle of the score distribution (i.e., within the average range), it may have major consequences for children whose ability lies closer to the tail ends of the distribution. If their scores lie in the vicinity of standard cut-scores used in diagnosing major conditions such as mental retardation or giftedness (e.g., 70 and 130, on IQ tests), these children may obtain scores above or below the cut-score, depending on whether they were given the older test or the re-standardized version. Conceivably, this could also affect factors such as eligibility for the death penalty, in some countries (Kanaya et al., 2003b). Thus, in these cases, the choice of norms has significant impact on whether an obtained score lies above or below a determined cutoff, and greatly alters the proportion of individuals with a specific condition that are detected by a test.

On a group level, the Flynn effect also has far-reaching consequences. For instance, in a large longitudinal study, Kanaya et al. (2003a, 2003b) documented the effects of subsequent re-normings of IQ tests, including cyclical fluctuations in the average score obtained by children consisting of increases up until the year of publication of new norms, followed by an immediate decrease in scores. Score levels were therefore tied to how closely children were tested to the year in which new norms appeared. On a national level, the year in which children were tested affected the reported prevalence of mental retardation, with possible large-scale implications for national policy regarding education financing, social security eligibility, and other issues of national importance. Similar findings have been reported for children with LD tested with new and older versions of the WISC-III (Truscott & Frank,

2001), potentially affecting the reported prevalence of LD. Additional research is needed to determine how the Flynn effect might affect other kinds of cut-scores, such as those used to screen for dementia.

Another reason that the Flynn effect is relevant for neuropsychologists is that single tests are rarely used as the sole basis of the neuropsychological evaluation. Potentially, the Flynn effect could add additional sources of complexity for users of flexible batteries, if a number of different tests normed in different decades are used. Batteries such as the NAB or NEPSY, which provide co-normed subtests in a variety of neuropsychological domains, provide a clear advantage over other test combinations in this regard. Alternatively, existing large-scale batteries from the intelligence, memory, and psychoeducational domain, co-normed contemporaneously on a single sample (i.e., WAIS-III/ WMS-III/ WIAT-II; WJ-III-COG/WJ-III-ACH), can also form much of the core of a neuropsychological battery, when supplemented with additional tests normed during a similar timeframe.

As a result of the Flynn effect, some tests may lose their ability to discriminate among individuals with higher ability levels. This happens because score inflation secondary to the Flynn effect causes more and more higher functioning individuals to reach ceiling on the test. In fact, in some cases (e.g., Raven's or SPM), ceiling effects are now quite noticeable.

OLDER NORMS AND INTERACTIONS WITH SOCIODEMOGRAPHIC FACTORS

Importantly, outdated norms can interact with demographic factors to raise the risk of misinterpretation of test results. Over the last few decades, the demographic composition of the U.S. population has changed dramatically, with increasing numbers of ethnic minority representation, particularly in the younger age ranges (e.g., Llorente et al., 1999). By 2010, Hispanics will comprise 15% of the U.S. population; by 2050, this percentage is projected to reach 25% (Pontón & León-Carrión, 2001). Because these demographic factors impact test scores, use of older norms may differentially penalize individuals from minority groups because of limited minority representation compared with more contemporary norms (see discussion of PPVT-R in *PPVT-III* review, for example).

Cohort effects also raise the risk that older normative datasets may be obsolete. In elderly individuals, educational level may be restricted by a lack of universal access to education; when norms based on these cohorts are applied to later cohorts with better educational opportunities, the result is artificial score inflation and reduced test sensitivity. Additional distortion is introduced to particular subgroups when cohort-specific features such as access to education interact with demographic factors such as gender and ethnicity as a result of institutionalized sexism and racism (e.g., Manly et al., 2003). Special care must therefore be exercised when selecting norms

in these groups. Note that cohort effects have been documented in even the youngest of subjects, in some cases as early as age 3 (Bocérean et al., 2003).

PRACTICAL CONSIDERATIONS REGARDING THE DATE OF NORMING

Practically speaking, consumers of increasingly expensive psychological tests must carefully scrutinize test manuals for the date of normative data collection before assuming that recently released normative sets actually contain recently collected normative data. The reality is that some recently published norms actually include very old data. Several instances of this were noted in tests reviewed for this volume. The year in which normative data were collected should be explicitly stated in test manuals; omitting this information is not appropriate practice (see Standards for Educational and Psychological Testing [AERA] et al., 1999). Consequently, users are urged to contact test publishers when this information is lacking. In this volume, we have attempted to include the date of norming to facilitate the task for users.

TYPES OF NORMS

It was not so long ago that neuropsychologists relied exclusively on raw scores and cut-offs for determining level of performance, and that normative samples consisted solely of "normals" and "brain-damaged" individuals. Over time, the field has shifted toward the notion of general population norms comprised of a large sample of individuals characterized by specific demographic characteristics. Use of these norms then allows the user to better determine whether the individual differs from the general population. While IQ and achievement tests have for many years set the standard and perfected techniques for constructing large, representative normative datasets, neuropsychological datasets have only recently begun to include a variety of individuals reflecting the composition of the general population.

At the same time, demographically corrected normative datasets, which represent only a subset of the general population most similar to the patient under scrutiny, are increasingly used and demanded by practitioners. Demographic corrections have come to be routinely applied to most normative data in neuropsychology, first in the form of age-corrected norms, and in some cases, gender-corrected norms, and later, as education-corrected norms. As more and more neuropsychological tests become commercially produced, some norms specifically include a certain proportion of individuals who represent groups defined by race/ethnicity, in order to make norms as representative of the general population as possible. This has also allowed additional levels of within-group norming. This gradual shift away from raw scores as the basis of interpretation to scores adjusted for multiple demographic factors occurred because of an acknowledgment by clinicians and researchers that demographics are significantly correlated with performance on neuropsychological tests, as they are for most cognitive tests in common usage (see test reviews in this volume for specific references, as well as sources below). The reasons for this shift, and the ways in which general population and demographically corrected normative datasets can be used effectively, will be reviewed in this chapter.

NORMS: POPULATION-BASED VERSUS DEMOGRAPHICALLY ADJUSTED

There are two schools of thought regarding how closely matched the norms must be to the demographic characteristics of the individual being assessed, and these views are diametrically opposed. These are: (1) that norms should be as representative of the general population as possible, and (2) that norms should approximate, as closely as possible, the unique subgroup to which the individual belongs. The latter view is the central tenet of Mitrushina et al.'s text (Mitrushina et al., 2005), which is essentially a guidebook for choosing norms that most closely fit the demographic characteristics of the individual patient being assessed. Although most neuropsychologists assume that the latter is always preferable, this is not necessarily the best choice at all times. Because a test's sensitivity, specificity and impairment cutoffs (see Chapter 1) depend to some extent on the norms selected, choosing norms necessitates a trade-off between the risk of making false negative errors and the risk of making false positive errors. Thus, the use of broadly representative versus demographically specific norms will depend on the purpose of the testing.

At times, it will be paramount to compare the individual to all other persons of the same age in the general population. Determining a diagnosis of mental retardation or learning disability would be one example. At other times, the goal will be to compare the individual to the best-matched demographic subgroup. Here, the goal might involve mapping out an individual's relative strengths and weaknesses in order to inform diagnostic considerations, plan classroom accommodations or return to work, or to obtain a best estimate of premorbid level in a dementia work-up. In many clinical situations, the assessment will involve both approaches because the results serve to address questions at many levels, including diagnosis, individual strengths and weaknesses, and areas in need of treatment/accommodation. For a more complete discussion of these and related issues, see *Ethnicity, Race and Culture.*

STRATIFIED GENERAL POPULATION NORMS

The rationale for stratifying norms according to demographic characteristics is to maximize the likelihood that norms are representative of the general population. Major tests are usually stratified based on age, gender, education, ethnicity/race,

socioeconomic status (SES), the latter defined as either actual SES, occupation, or education/parental education. Additional variables include geographic region and urban versus rural residence. Stratification occurs according to representative proportions such as those provided by U.S. Census data to best approximate the composition of the general population.

Although each of these demographic factors tend to be treated as separate stratification variables, it is important to note there is considerable overlap between supposedly separate demographic characteristics. In most cases, some demographic characteristics (e.g., ethnicity, geographic location) are actually surrogate variables for other more fundamental variables that influence test scores (e.g., SES, education).

When nationally representative norms are considered, the sample should have an even distribution of demographic variables across ages, unless certain demographics are more heavily weighted in some age groups versus others. For example, because of factors related to parity and longevity, there is a larger ethnic minority representation among young children in the United States than in adults, and a higher representation of women in the oldest age bands. Because the demographic composition of nations changes over time, this suggests additional caution in using normative data that are outdated, as the norms may no longer be representative of the population being evaluated.

DEMOGRAPHICALLY CORRECTED NORMS

The second kind of normative dataset is one that includes only individuals from a specific category; these are sometimes known as within-group norms. The utility of these norms rests in the fact that individuals with particular demographic characteristics can be compared with the subgroup that best approximates their unique and specific demographic constellation. Demographically corrected norms will be discussed throughout the following sections, but in particular in the sections devoted to ethnicity, race, and culture.

AGE RANGE, DEVELOPMENTAL GROWTH CURVES, AND AGE BANDS

Most neuropsychological functions exhibit specific developmental growth curves when considered across age. For example, growth curves for different abilities will depend on factors such as the age at which the function displays its greatest growth, the extent to which the function changes during adulthood, and the extent of its vulnerability to age-related decline. Thus, a developmental growth curve for a test of executive function may differ markedly from that of a test of vocabulary in terms of slope during the period from early childhood to adolescence (i.e., a steeper, earlier increase for the vocabulary test), and during old age (i.e., a steeper, earlier decline for the executive function test). Figure 2–1 shows

Figure 2–1 Developmental growth curves for abilities measured by the WJ-III. *Source:* Reprinted with permission from McGrew & Woodcock, 2001.

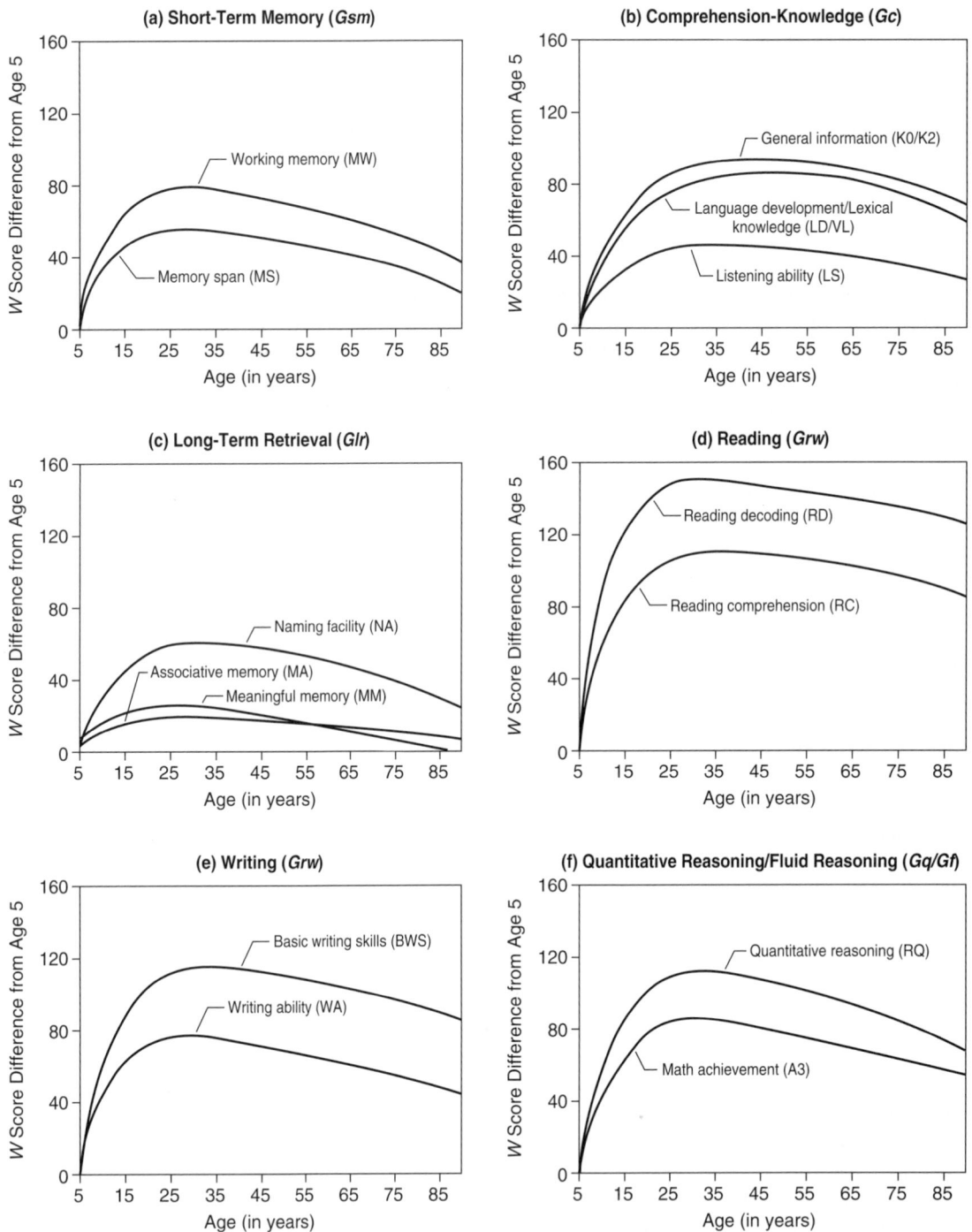

age-related changes in performance in the different WJ-III cognitive and achievement domains.

While age correction has become an almost automatic process in transforming and interpreting scores in neuropsychological assessment, the selection of age range and the range of each age band should not be arbitrarily determined. Rather, the portioning of norms by age and the range of each age band will depend on the shape of the growth curve for each test. Ideally, a well-constructed test will base its age band on growth curves and provide shorter age bands during periods of rapid development/change and longer age bands when the ability under question shows little developmental change. Batteries that use uniform age bands across domains (e.g., the same age bands for each subtest) should demonstrate that this approach is based on empirical evidence of similarity of developmental trajectories across each domain sampled.

A working knowledge of developmental growth curves for functions assessed by neuropsychological tests is useful in order to evaluate norms and their derived test scores. Note that age effects are also often considered evidence of test validity in those functions that display developmental growth curves. Although most manuals for major intelligence, achievement, and language tests tend to include this information, growth curves are not routinely included in manuals for neuropsychological tests. As a result, we have endeavored to provide information on developmental/age effects for each of the tests reviewed in this volume, in the *Normative Data* section of each test.

EDUCATION

Many normative datasets offer education-corrected norms. In the case of children, parental education is often used as a stratification variable. Although some authors provide detailed instructions on how to code educational level in order to minimize error variance, most often this is left to the individual examiner who has to deal with complex educational histories that require considerable judgment. Heaton et al. (2004) offer guidelines for use with their normative data and these are shown in Table 2–1. A discussion of education effects is included in almost all test reviews in this volume.

Table 2–1 Guidelines for Assigning Years of Education

Counted in Years of Education	Not Counted
Only full years of regular academic coursework that are successfully completed are counted	Years in which person obtained failing grades not counted; partial years not counted
	General Equivalency Diploma (GED)
Regular college or university	Vocational training
No matter how much time it takes to complete a diploma or degree, standard numbers of education years are assigned:	
High school 12	
Associate's degree 14	
Bachelor's degree 16	
Master's degree 18	
Doctoral degree 20	

Source: Reproduced by special permission of the publisher, Psychological Assessment Resources, Inc., 16204 North Florida Avenue, Lutz, FL 33549, from the Revised Comprehensive Norms for an Expanded Halstead-Reitan Battery: Demographically adjusted Neuropsychological Norms for African American and Caucasian Adults by Robert K. Heaton, PhD, S. Walden Miller, PhD, Michael J. Taylor, PhD, and Igor Grant, MD, Copyright 1991, 1992, 2004 by PAR, Inc. Further reproduction is prohibited without permission from PAR, Inc.

ETHNICITY, RACE, AND CULTURE

Differences Between Ethnicity, Race, and Culture

The terms "ethnicity," "culture," and "race" are often used interchangeably. However, ethnicity and culture are multidimensional constructs that reflect groups characterized by common language, customs, heritage, or nationality, whereas race carries the implication of genetically based traits (Ardila et al., 1994; see also Gasquoine, 1999; Harris & Tulsky, 2003; and Tulsky et al., 2003, for further discussion). All of these terms, in most instances, are used when referring to minority groups that differ from the majority group. Test manuals that stratify according to ethnicity and/or race, or that provide within-group norms of racial or cultural groups, do not typically provide detailed information on how minority groups are defined, even though the method by which race, culture, or ethnicity is determined may influence the composition of norms. Thus, minority groups defined by self-identification, observed physical differences, or rating scales reflecting degree of acculturation will necessarily differ to some extent. In addition, there is increasing evidence that some of the variance in test scores predicted by "ethnicity" actually relates to level of acculturation, literacy or quality of education (Harris & Tulsky, 2003; Manly et al., 1998, 2002, 2003; Shuttleworth-Edwards et al., 2004).

Rationale for Ethnically Adjusted Norms

There are numerous studies that document lower performance estimates on cognitive tests in minority populations (e.g., Manly & Jacobs, 2001; Manly et al., 1998, 2002; Pontón & Ardila, 1999). When scores are then used to make inferences about brain functioning, the result is an overestimate of deficits and misattribution about neuropsychological dysfunction. For example, when normally functioning African Americans are assessed, a statistically high base rate of impairment has been documented using conventional cutoff scores (e.g., Campbell et al., 2002; Heaton et al., 2004; Patton et al., 2003). Numerous examples can also be found with regard to groups such as Spanish-speaking individuals (e.g., Ardila et al., 1994) and people in southern Africa (Shuttleworth-Edwards et al., 2004). In other words, the specificity (i.e., the extent to which normal individuals are correctly identified) of many neuropsychological tests is inadequate when unadjusted cutoffs are used in minority and/or disadvantaged groups.

In children, the whole issue of ethnicity and neuropsychological assessment is relatively uncharted territory, despite considerable evidence from intelligence and language research that ethnicity significantly impacts test scores in children (Brooks-Gunn et al., 2003; Padilla et al., 2002; Sattler, 2001). Children's neuropsychological norms that take into account additional demographic variables besides age would therefore be of considerable utility.

In addition to ethical issues regarding misdiagnosis, the costs of false positive errors in normal individuals are obvious.

These include adverse psychological effects on the patient, unnecessary treatment, and negative financial repercussions (e.g., Patton et al., 2003). Thus, there is a critical need for representative normative data for minority subgroups, as well as adjusted cutoffs to reflect more clinically acceptable impairment levels within subgroups (e.g., Campbell et al., 2002; Heaton et al., 2004; Heaton et al., 2003; Manly & Jacobs, 2001; Patton et al., 2003). The field has begun to respond to this need, as shown by an ever-increasing pool of demographically corrected normative data, and by the recent publication of several neuropsychological texts devoted to cross-cultural assessment. The reader is highly encouraged to consult these texts for a more complete discussion of the issues (e.g., Ardila et al., 1994; Ferraro, 2002; Fletcher-Janzen et al., 2000; Pontón & León-Carrión, 2001).

Types of Norms for Minority Groups

Norms that take into consideration ethnicity, race, and/or culture typically consist of separate normative datasets that include only specific members such as African Americans or Spanish speakers (e.g., Manly et al., 1998; Ardila et al., 1994; Heaton et al., 2004; Pontón, 2001). There are other methods to adjust scores, including: bonus points (i.e., adding a constant to the score of all members of a subgroup so that the group mean is equivalent to the majority group's), separate cutoffs for each subgroup, and banding (i.e., treating all individuals within a specific score range as having equivalent scores to avoid interpretation of small score differences) (Sacket & Wilk, 1994). With the exception of the use of subgroup-specific cutoffs, these techniques are not commonly used in neuropsychology.

Of historical interest is the fact that neuropsychology's recent shift toward demographically corrected scores based on race/ethnicity and other variables has occurred with surprisingly little fanfare or controversy despite ongoing debate in other domains of psychology. For example, when race-norming was applied to pre-employment screening in the United States to increase the number of minorities chosen as job applicants, the result was the Civil Rights Act of 1991, which outlawed race-norming for applicant selection or referral (see Sackett & Wilk, 1994; Gottfredson, 1994; and Greenlaw & Jensen, 1996, for an interesting historical review of the ill-fated attempt at race-norming the GATB).

Limitations of Demographically Adjusted Norms

There are some cases where adjustment for demographic influences might be questioned. For example, age and education are risk factors for dementia; removing the effects of these demographic variables might therefore remove some of the predictive power of measures of cognitive impairment (Sliwinski et al., 1997, 2003). O'Connell et al. (2004) have recently reported that use of age- and education-corrected normative data failed to improve the diagnostic accuracy of the 3MS, a version of the MMSE, when screening for dementia or cognitive

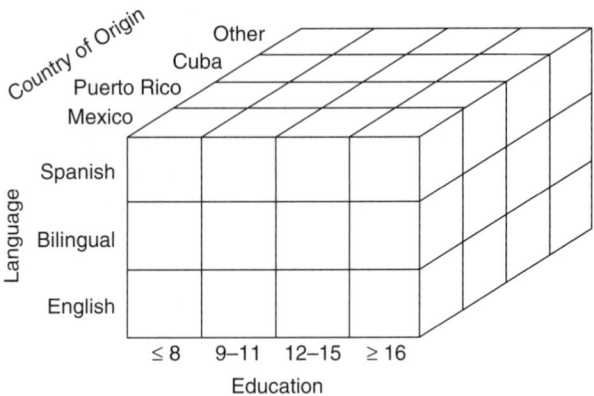

Figure 2–2 Model of Hispanic diversity in neuropsychological assessment. *Source:* Adapted from Pontón & León-Carrión, 2001.

impairment. Instead, they recommended that the unadjusted normative data be used for screening purposes. In a similar vein, Reitan and Wolfson (1995, 1996) have argued that age and education corrections are appropriate for normal, healthy individuals, but that they are not needed for brain-damaged subjects. This view has been disputed, however (e.g., Lezak et al., 2004; also see *Test Selection* in this volume). There is also evidence that when "corrective norms" are applied, some demographic influences remain, and overcorrection may occur, resulting in score distortion for some subgroups and a risk of increased false negatives (e.g., Fastenau, 1998).

Some of the limitations of ethnically adjusted norms are summarized by Sattler (2001), including the fact that they may provide (1) a basis for negative comparisons between groups, (2) lower expectations for children from groups that differ culturally and linguistically from the majority, and (3) have little relevance outside of the specific geographic area in which they were collected. Gasquoine (1999) also argues that within-group norming in neuropsychology has limited merit due to the complexities inherent in measuring ethnicity and culture; subgroups can be divided exponentially, limited only by the number of demographic variables available. Figure 2–2 shows the various subgroups that can be derived from subdividing within the U.S. Hispanic population alone.

One alternative to within-group norming is to directly take into account the influence of specific variables on test scores, since these factors presumably operate across ethnicity and culture. These include factors such as English language fluency, acculturation, length of residence in the United States, education, quality of education, and SES, including quality of the home environment, health/nutritional status, income, and degree and persistence of poverty (Gasquoine, 1999). Therefore, norms that correct for ethnicity may be correcting for the "wrong" variable, particularly if other variables appear to better account for observed differences between groups. For instance, differences between minority groups and the majority culture on cognitive tests may remain even after important variables such as number of years of education are accounted for (e.g., Farias et al., 2004; Shuttleworth-Edwards et al., 2004), but procedures that take into account quality of education by coding for quality directly (e.g., Shuttleworth-Edwards et al., 2004) or using literacy corrections yield few group differences (e.g., Byrd et al., 2004; Manly et al., 1998; 2002).

It is important to note, as well, that variables such as the persistence of poverty and education level/quality within and across minority groups cannot be fully dissociated. For instance, in some Western countries, the prevalence of continuous periods of poverty versus temporary instances of poverty may be much higher in some minority subgroups than in children from the majority culture with similar SES. It is difficult to conceptualize how norms could be made to correct for these multiple factors, but multivariate corrections on large, varied samples, including cross-validation, might be feasible.

Lastly, there are individuals who, despite apparent similarities such as race, differ substantially from the overall characteristics of the target normative subgroup, and who actually may be more closely matched to another group that does not share obvious racial, cultural, or ethnic characteristics. For example, in the United States, the terms "Hispanic" and "African American" are associated with a unique sociopolitical environment related to SES, education, and health status. However, these terms have limited applicability to individuals who may share only superficial characteristics such as race or language (e.g., Shuttleworth-Edwards et al., 2004), but who are recent immigrants to the United States, or who are citizens of other countries. Thus, demographically corrected norms developed in the United States may have limited utility for (1) individuals who differ from the target subgroup in important aspects such as quality of education, or (2) in other countries where ethnic subgroups may have different educational/SES correlates. However, given the state of the field, the provision of normative data for minority groups is a step in the right direction, as is increased awareness on the part of practitioners and researchers that diversity is an inherent characteristic of human populations that needs to be reflected in our neuropsychological tools and practice.

Caveats in the Clinical Use of Demographically Based Norms for Minority Groups

As we have already alluded to, within-group norms significantly affect sensitivity and specificity with regard to tests that employ cutoffs for assigning individuals to specific groups, such as those based on diagnosis (e.g., diagnostic criteria for dementia or language disorder), or for assigning individuals to treatment (e.g., Aricept trial, language intervention). The costs of a false positive may be high in one subgroup (e.g., African American elders undergoing a dementia workup), but false negatives might be of larger consequence in another subgroup (i.e., Hispanic preschoolers in an early screening program). In the former, a false positive is associated with clearly adverse consequences (e.g., false dementia diagnosis). However, in the latter, a false negative might be worse if it means losing access to a service that might have far-reaching benefits

(e.g., a screening program that provides free language intervention, literacy materials, and parent support for at-risk inner-city preschoolers). Ideally, the decision to use adjusted cutoff and within-group norms should be based on a full understanding of the context in which they are destined to be used, including the base rate of the particular disorder within the subgroup, the sensitivity and specificity of the measure, and the costs of false positive and false negative errors.

Importantly, with regard to the WAIS-III/WMS-III, the Psychological Corporation explicitly states that demographically adjusted scores are not intended for use in psychoeducational assessment, determination of intellectual deficiency, vocational assessment, or any other context where the goal is to determine absolute functional level (IQ or memory) in comparison to the general population. Rather, demographically adjusted scores are best used for neurodiagnostic assessment in order to minimize the impact of confounding variables on the diagnosis of cognitive impairment. That is, they should be used to infer strengths and weakness relative to a presumed pre-morbid standard (The Psychological Corporation, 2002). Therefore, neuropsychologists need to balance the risks and benefits of using within-group norms, and use them with a full understanding of their implications and the situations in which they are most appropriate.

Finally, eliminating score differences across demographic groups with demographic corrections or within-group norms will not adjust the current disparities in life circumstances and outcomes that are at times reflected in test scores, nor will it adjust for the relative lack of neuropsychological models that include sociocultural factors (e.g., Campbell et al., 2002; Pérez-Arce, 1999). Above all else, as noted by Ardila et al. (1994), "the clinical neuropsychologist must entertain the notion that human diversity does not translate into human deficiency" (p. 5).

PRACTICAL CONSIDERATIONS IN THE USE OF DEMOGRAPHICALLY CORRECTED NORMS

By necessity, neuropsychologists often adopt a compromise between using population-wide norms and within-group norms. Almost all tests provide age-based scores, but the availability of norms based on education and minority status (ethnicity/race/culture) varies greatly across tests. As a result, practicing clinicians are therefore only able to demographically correct some scores but not others, unless a uniform battery such as the WAIS-III/WMS-III or NAB is employed. The problem is that if only some scores are adjusted for moderator variables (e.g., education), and then compared with non-corrected scores, false attributions of impairment may occur (Kalechstein et al., 1998).

As a practical solution, given equivalent sampling quality, the a priori selection of the normative set should be primarily guided by the particular moderating variable that is most likely to affect the classification of test performance (Kalechstein et al., 1998). For example, on tests of psychomotor speed, it would be preferable to match on the basis of age rather than education, if a choice was required. In contrast, on tests of verbal achievement, education would likely be the primary selection criterion.

In each test review in this volume, we have included information on demographic influences on test performance. With this information, users can determine for themselves whether demographic corrections are necessary, and whether test scores need to be interpreted within a demographically relevant context.

EXCLUSIONARY CRITERIA AND THE PROBLEM OF THE TRUNCATED DISTRIBUTION

Although many test developers make specific efforts to exclude individuals with disabilities or deficits from normative samples, there is a strong argument for including impaired individuals within normative sets, in a proportion that approximates that found in the general population. The reason is that excluding individuals with disabilities from normative sets actually distorts the normal distribution of scores (McFadden, 1996). When the "tail" of the population is truncated by removing the scores of individuals with disabilities or disease, this forces lower-functioning but healthy individuals in the normative group to then represent the lowest performance rankings in the population and to substitute for the missing lower tail. When this distribution is then used to derive a norm-derived score for a healthy but low functioning person, the result is a significant overestimation of deficits (see *PPVT-III* for additional discussion of this issue).

In particular, using exclusionary criteria in older individuals based on health status may disproportionately restrict normative samples because of the increased prevalence of medical or other health conditions in this age range. The result is a "normal" sample that includes only the upper ranges of scores for older individuals, and which will disproportionately render impairment scores for low-functioning but typically aging elders (Kalechstein et al., 1998).

Hebben and Milberg (2002) discuss additional problems specific to constructing appropriate norms for use in the neuropsychological examination of the elderly patient. These include cohort effects, the presence of non-neurological illness in many normal elderly persons, the increased likelihood of persons with early dementia in older age groups, and floor effects. The inclusion of older adults in the terminal stages of decline associated with impending mortality also needs to be evaluated since such individuals are likely to show cognitive dysfunction (Macdonald, 2004).

For individual patient evaluations, there is the potential for erroneous interpretations of strengths and weaknesses and inconsistencies across testing domains if test scores derived from truncated distributions are unknowingly compared with scores derived from full distributions (McFadden, 1996). Thus, a well-constructed normative set would indicate the number of individuals with disabilities in the sample (typically in a proportion that parallels that found in the general population), and indicate how the sample was screened for conditions affecting performance on the test. Users would then need to adjust interpretations when comparing tests with full and truncated distributions. In most cases, we have indicated screening criteria for the tests reviewed in this volume so that neuropsychologists can effectively make these comparisons. However, further research on the comparability of tests with different inclusion and exclusion criteria regarding individuals with disabilities or health conditions is needed.

GEOGRAPHIC LOCATION

Test manuals should always include information on where normative data were collected because of regional variation in demographic factors that can affect test scores, such as SES, education, and cultural background. Most large test batteries developed in the United States sample data from four or five major regions. These include the Northeast, South, West, and North Central, plus or minus the additional category of Southwest. In most cases, both urban and rural individuals are represented in order to represent regional variations in test performance. However, not all tests include this additional stratification variable.

On a much larger scale, norms may also differ to a significant extent depending on the country in which they were collected. Differences occur on two levels: content differences due to different exposure or culturally specific responses to individual items, and ability differences related to socioeconomic, sociodemographic, or other differences between countries. For instance, there are significant demographic differences between English-speaking nations such that people from Britain and individuals from the United States perform differently on common language tests such as the PPVT-III and WTAR, even when words are "translated" to reflect national dialect. Similarly, major IQ tests are typically re-normed in other countries because of cultural and socioeconomic differences that translate into measurable score differences. For example, Canadian individuals tend to have higher IQ scores when U.S.-based IQ test versions are used; this may or may not be related to educational differences, but also likely reflects the different sociodemographic composition of the two countries (e.g., see *WAIS-III, Comment,* in this volume). Similar findings have been reported for Australian children with regard to U.S. norms on Wechsler tests (e.g., Kamieniecki et al., 2002). Regardless of the underlying factors, these differences between countries necessitate re-normings for all the major Wechsler tests, including the WPPSI-III, WISC-IV, WAIS-III and WIAT-II. A detailed review of WAIS-based differences across nations was recently provided by Shuttleworth-Edwards et al. (2004).

Because the vast majority of English-language neuropsychological tests are normed in the United States, additional research on the representativeness of different neuropsychological norms across regions and across nations would be helpful. Caution is therefore warranted in using norms collected in other regions because of variation of important demographic factors (Patton et al., 2003). Local norms are therefore an asset when available. With regard to cross-test comparisons, clinicians need to be aware of the origins of the normative data they use, and keep any possible demographic differences in mind when comparing scores across tests normed in different countries or geographic regions.

A FINAL COMMENT ON SAMPLES OF CONVENIENCE

A well-constructed normative data set should consist of an actual standardization sample rather than a sample of convenience. This means that standard procedures should have been followed in the recruitment of subjects, test administration, scoring, and data collection, including assessing examiners for consistency in administration and scoring, data error checks, and the like. Although this point seems obvious, the number of neuropsychological tests that rely on samples of convenience is surprising. These samples consist of data originally collected for another purpose, such as research, or under non- or semi-standardized conditions, including tests with aggregate normative data collected over several years, control data collected as part of several research projects, pilot data, partial standardization data, and even data collected as part of neuropsychological workshops for practitioners. As much as possible, we have attempted to identify the type and source of the normative data included in this volume so that clinicians can assess the conditions under which norms were collected, and judge the quality of the norming effort for themselves.

REFERENCES

American Educational Research Association, American Psychological Association, & National Council on Measurement in Education. (1999). *Standards for educational and psychological testing.* Washington, DC: American Psychological Association.

Ardila, A., Rosselli, M., & Puente, A. E. (1994). *Neuropsychological evaluation of the Spanish speaker.* New York: Plenum Press.

Baron, I. S. (2004). *Neuropsychological evaluation of the child.* New York: Oxford University Press.

Bengston, M. L., Mittenberg, W., Schneider, B., & Seller, A. (1996). An assessment of Halstead-Reitan test score changes over 20 years. [Abstract]. *Archives of Clinical Neuropsychology, 11,* 386.

Bocéréan, C., Fisher, J.-P., & Fliellier, A. (2003). Long-term comparison (1921-2001) of numerical knowledge in three to five-and-a-half year-old children. *European Journal of Psychology of Education, XVIII, 4,* 403–424.

Brooks-Gunn, J., Klebanov, P. K., Smith, J., Duncan, G. J., & Lee, K. (2003). The Black-White test score gap in young children: Contributions of test and family characteristics. *Applied Developmental Science, 7*(4), 239–252.

Byrd, D. E., Touradji, P., Tang, M.-X., & Manly, J. J. (2004). Cancellation test performance in African American, Hispanic, and White elderly. *Journal of the International Neuropsychological Society, 10,* 401–411.

Campbell, A. L., Ocampo, C., Rorie, K. D., Lewis, S., Combs, S., Ford-Booker, P., Briscoe, J., Lewis-Jack, O., Brown, A., Wood, D., Dennis, G., Weir, R., & Hastings, A. (2002). Caveats in the neuropsychological assessment of African Americans. *Journal of the National Medical Association, 94*(7), 591–601.

Farias, S. T., Mungas, D., Reed, B., Haan, M. N., & Jagust, W. J. (2004). Everyday functioning in relation to cognitive functioning and neuroimaging in community-dwelling Hispanic and non-Hispanic older adults. *Journal of the International Neuropsychological Society, 10,* 342–354.

Fasteneau, P. S. (1998). Validity of regression-based norms: An empirical test of the comprehensive norms with older adults. *Journal of Clinical and Experimental Neuropsychology, 20*(6), 906–916.

Fasteneau, P. S., & Adams, K. M. (1996a). Heaton, Grant, and Matthews' Comprehensive Norms: An overzealous attempt. *Journal of Clinical and Experimental Neuropsychology, 18*(3), 444–448.

Ferraro, F. R. (2002). *Minority and cross-cultural aspects of neuropsychological assessment.* Lisse, Netherlands: Swets & Zeitlinger Publishers.

Fletcher-Janzen, E., Strickland, T. L., & Reynolds, C.R. (2000). *Handbook of cross-cultural neuropsychology.* New York: Springer.

Flynn, J. R. (1984). The mean IQ of Americans: Massive gains 1932 to 1978. *Psychological Bulletin, 95,* 29–51.

Flynn, J. R. (2000). The hidden history of IQ and special education: Can the problems be solved? *Psychology, Public Policy and Law, 6*(1), 191–198.

Gasquoine, P. G. (1999). Variables moderating cultural and ethnic differences in neuropsychological assessment: The case of Hispanic Americans. *The Clinical Neuropsychologist, 13*(3), 376–383.

Gottfredson, L. S. (1994). The science and politics of race-norming. *American Psychologist, 49*(11), 955–963.

Greenslaw, P. S., & Jensen, S. S. (1996). Race-norming and the Civil Rights Act of 1991. *Public Personnel Management, 25*(1), 13–24.

Harris, J. G., & Tulsky, D. S. (2003). Assessment of the non-native English speaker: Assimilating history and research findings to guide clinical practice. In D. S. Tulsky, D. H. Saklofske, G. J. Chelune, R. K. Heaton, R. Ivnik, R. Bornstein, A. Prifitera, & M. F. Ledbetter (Eds.), *Clinical interpretation of the WAIS-III and WMS-III* (pp. 343–390). New York: Academic Press.

Heaton, R. K., Miller, S. W., Taylor, M. J., & Grant, I. (2004). *Revised Comprehensive Norms for an Expanded Halstead-Reitan Battery: Demographically adjusted neuropsychological norms for African American and Caucasian adults.* Lutz, FL: PAR.

Heaton, R. K., Taylor, M. J., & Manly, J. (2003). Demographic effects and use of demographically corrected norms with the WAIS-III and WMS-III. In D. S. Tulsky, D. H. Saklofske, G. J. Chelune, R. K. Heaton, R. Ivnik, R. Bornstein, A. Prifitera, & M. F. Ledbetter (Eds.), *Clinical interpretation of the WAIS-III and WMS-III* (pp. 181–210). New York: Academic Press.

Hebben, N., & Milberg, W. (2002). *Essentials of neuropsychological assessment.* New York: John Wiley & Sons.

Kalechstein, A. D., van Gorp, W. G., & Rapport, L. J. (1998). Variability in clinical classification of raw test scores across normative data sets. *The Clinical Neuropsychologist, 12,* 339–347.

Kamieniecki, G. W., & Lynd-Stevenson, R. M. (2002). Is it appropriate to use United States norms to assess the "intelligence" of Australian children? *Australian Journal of Psychology, 54*(2), 67–78.

Kanaya, T., Ceci, S. J., & Scullin, M. H. (2003a). The rise and fall of IQ in special ed: Historical trends and their implications. *Journal of School Psychology, 41,* 453–465.

Kanaya, T., Scullin, M. H., & Ceci, S. J. (2003b). The Flynn effect and U.S. policies: The impact of rising IQ scores on American society via mental retardation diagnoses. *American Psychologist, 58*(10), 887–890.

Lezak, M. D., Howieson, D. B., Loring, D. W., Hannary, H. J., & Fischer, J. S. (2004). *Neuropsychological assessment* (4th ed.). New York: Oxford University Press.

Llorente, A. M., Ponton, M. O., Taussig, I. M., & Satz, P. (1999). Patterns of American immigration and their influence on the acquisition of neuropsychological norms for Hispanics. *Archives of Clinical Neuropsychology, 14*(7), 603–614.

Macdonald, S. W. S. (2004). Longitudinal profiles of terminal decline: Associations between cognitive decline, age, time to death, and cause of death. PhD dissertation, University of Victoria.

Manly, J. J., & Jacobs, D. M. (2001). Future directions in neuropsychological assessment with African Americans. In F. R. Ferraro (Ed.), *Minority and cross-cultural aspects of neuropsychological assessment* (pp. 79–96). Heereweg, Lisse, The Netherlands: Swets & Zeitlinger.

Manly, J. J., Jacobs, D. M., Touradji, P., Small, S. A., & Stern, Y. (2002). Reading level attenuates differences in neuropsychological test performance between African American and White elders. *Journal of the International Neuropsychological Society, 8,* 341–348.

Manly, J. J., Miller, W., Heaton, R. K., Byrd, D., Reilly, J., Velasquez, R. J., Saccuzzo, D. P., Grant, I., and the HIV Neurobehavioral Research Center (HNRC) Group. (1998). The effect of African-American acculturation on neuropsychological test performance in normal and HIV-positive individuals. *Journal of the International Neuropsychological Society, 4,* 291–302.

Manly, J. J., Touradji, P., Tang, M. X., & Stern, Y. (2003). Literacy and memory decline among ethnically diverse elders. *Journal of Clinical and Experimental Neuropsychology, 25*(5), 680–690.

McFadden, T. U. (1996). Creating language impairments in typically achieving children: The pitfalls of "normal" normative sampling. *Language, Speech, and Hearing Services in Schools, 27,* 3–9.

McGrew, K. S., & Woodcock, R. W. (2001). *Woodcock-Johnson III technical manual.* Itasca, IL: Riverside Publishing.

Mitrushina, M. N., Boone, K. B., Razani, J., & D'Elia, L.F. (2005). *Handbook of normative data for neuropsychological assessment* (2nd ed.). New York: Oxford University Press.

Mitrushina, M. N., Boone, K. B., & D'Elia, L. F. (1999). *Handbook of normative data for neuropsychological assessment.* New York: Oxford University Press.

Neisser, U., Boodoo, G., Bouchards, T. J., Boykin, A. W., Broday, N., Ceci, S. J., Halpersn, D. F., Loehlin, J. C., Perloff, R., Sternberg, R. J., & Urbina, S. (1996). Intelligence: Knowns and unknowns. *American Psychologist, 13*(51), 77–101.

Nunnally, J. C., & Bernstein, I. H. (1994). *Psychometric theory* (3rd ed.). New York: McGraw-Hill.

O'Connell, M. E., Tuokko, H., Graves, R. E., & Kadlec, H. (2004). Correcting the 3MS for bias does not improve accuracy when screening for cognitive impairment or dementia. *Journal of Clinical and Experimental Neuropsychology, 26,* 970–980.

Padilla, Y. C., Boardman, J. D., Hummer, R. A., & Espitia, M. (2002). Is the Mexican American epidemiologic paradox advantage at birth maintained through early childhood? *Social Forces, 80*(3), 1101–1123.

Patton, D. E., Duff, K., Schoenberg, M. R., Mold, J., Scott, J. G., & Adams, R. L. (2003). Performance of cognitively normal African Americans on the RBANS in community dwelling older adults. *The Clinical Neuropsychologist, 17*(4), 515–530.

Pérez-Arce, P. (1999). The influence of culture on cognition. *Archives of Clinical Neuropsychology, 14*(7), 581–592.

Pontón, M. O. (2001). Research and assessment issues with Hispanic populations. In M. O. Pontón & J. León-Carrión (Eds.), *Neuropsychology and the Hispanic patient* (pp. 39–58). Mahwah, NJ: Lawrence Erlbaum Associates.

Pontón, M. O., & Ardila, A. (1999). The future of neuropsychology with Hispanic populations in the United States. *Archives of Clinical Neuropsychology, 14*(7), 565–580.

Pontón, M. O., & León-Carrión, J. (2001). *Neuropsychology and the Hispanic patient.* Mahwah, NJ: Lawrence Erlbaum Associates, Publishers.

The Psychological Corporation. (2002). *WAIS-III/WMS-III Updated Technical Manual.* San Antonio, TX: Author.

Reitan, R. M., & Wolfson, D. (1995). Influence of age and education on neuropsychological test results. *The Clinical Neuropsychologist, 9,* 151–158.

Reitan, R. M., & Wolfson, D. (1996). The influence of age and education on the neuropsychological test performance of older children. *Child Neuropsychology, 1,* 165–169.

Sacket, P. R., & Wilk, S. L. (1994). Within-group norming and other forms of score adjustment in preemployment testing. *American Psychologist, 49*(11), 929–954.

Sattler, J. M. (2001) *Assessment of children: Cognitive applications* (4th ed.). San Diego, CA: J. M. Sattler.

Shuttleworth-Edwards, A. B., Kemp, R. D., Rust, A. L., Muirhead, J. G. L., Hartman, N. P., & Radloff, S. E. (2004). Cross-cultural effects on IQ test performance: A review and preliminary normative indications on WAIS-III test performance. *Journal of Clinical and Educational Neuropsychology, 26*(7), 903–920.

Sliwinski, M., Buschke, H., Stewart, W. F., Masur, D., & Lipton, R.D. (1997). The effect of dementia risk factors on comparative and diagnostic selective reminding norms. *Journal of the International Neuropsychological Society, 3,* 317–326.

Sliwinski, M., Lipton, R., Buschke, H., & Wasylyshyn, C. (2003). Optimizing cognitive test norms for detection. In R. Petersen (Ed.), *Mild cognitive impairment: Aging to Alzheimer's disease.* New York: Oxford University Press.

Truscott, S. D., & Frank, A. J. (2001). Does the Flynn effect affect IQ scores of students classified as LD? *Journal of School Psychology, 39*(4), 319–334.

Tulsky, D. S., Saklofske, D. H., Chelune, G. J., Heaton, R. K., Ivnik, R., Bornstein, R., Prifitera, A., & Ledbetter, M. F. (2003). *Clinical interpretation of the WAIS-III and WMS-III.* New York: Academic Press.

3

History Taking

The interview is one of the four main pillars of the assessment process, along with formal tests, observations, and informal test procedures (Sattler, 2002). The patient's account of his or her prior and present life circumstances, the current problem, and his or her behavior/style during the initial interview can provide a wealth of information regarding the presence, nature, and impact of neuropsychological disturbances. Consequently, taking a detailed history is essential to the evaluation and often invaluable since it helps to guide the test selection process, allows for interpretation of test data within a suitable context, and may yield important clues to a correct diagnosis, to the effects of the disorder on daily life, and to decisions regarding rehabilitative interventions. In fact, the interview and case history will determine whether it is even possible to pursue formal testing (Vanderploeg, 2000). If formal assessment is possible, the history helps to determine the range of processes to be examined, the complexity of tests to be used, the accommodations that may be necessary given the patient's disabilities, and the level of cooperation and insight of the patient. In neuropsychological assessment, test scores take on diagnostic or practical significance only when evaluated in the context of the individual's personal circumstances, academic or vocational accomplishments, and behavior during the interview (Lezak et al., 2004).

Competent history taking is a skill that requires, in addition to a broad knowledge of neuropsychology and a wide experiential base, an awareness of the interactions that may occur in interview situations. Often patients are tense and concerned about their symptoms. They are seeking an evaluation often in spite of their fears about what they will learn about themselves or their family member. The clinician's job is to put the client at ease and convey that the assessment is a collaborative venture to determine the presence, nature, severity, and impact of the problem (see also Chapter 4, *Test Selection, Test Administration, and Preparation of the Patient*). Yet, as Sattler (2002) points out, the clinical interview is not an ordinary conversation; nor is it a psychotherapeutic session. Rather, it involves an interpersonal interaction that has a specific goal, with formal, clearly defined roles and a set of norms governing the interaction. Thus, the interview is typically a formally arranged meeting where the patient is obliged to attend and respond to questions posed by the examiner. The interviewer sets the agenda, which covers specific topics and directs the interaction, using probing questions to obtain detailed and accurate information. Further, the examiner follows guidelines concerning confidentiality and privileged communication.

Although interviews can be structured or unstructured, history taking typically follows a semistructured, flexible format where referring questions are clarified and the following information is obtained (see also Lezak et al., 2004; Stowe, 1998; Vanderploeg, 2000):

1. *basic descriptive data* including age, marital status, place of birth, etc.;
2. *developmental history* including early risk factors and deviations from normal development;
3. *social history* including educational level/achievement, vocational history, family/personal relationships, and confrontations with legal system;
4. *relevant past medical history* including alcohol/drug/medication use, exposure to toxins, and relevant family history;
5. *current medical status* including description of the illness (nature of onset; duration; physical, intellectual, and emotional/behavioral changes), and medication/treatment regimens (including compliance); and
6. *the effect of the disorder* on daily life, aspirations, and personal relations.

In addition, with a view toward future management and rehabilitation, the clinician should obtain information on the coping styles and compensatory techniques that the patient uses to negotiate impairments and reduce or solve problems. Because compensatory strategies rely on functions that are relatively spared, the clinician should also identify the patient's resources and strengths. At the end of the history, the clinician may wish to go over the material with the patient to ensure that the details and chronology are correct and to check for additional information or answer questions/concerns that the patient may have. The examiner should also clarify the circumstances surrounding the examination (e.g., medical-legal context) and what the patient believes may be gained or lost from the examination, since this may affect test performance. Informal test questions about a patient's orientation and memory for current events, TV shows, local politics, or geography may be included in the interview. Ideally, the examiner should proceed in an orderly fashion, finishing one area before going on to the next. However, the examiner must be flexible and prepared to deal with unanticipated findings.

The length of interview varies but often lasts between 30 and 90 minutes. If the clinical focus is a young child, the parent(s) or caregiver is typically interviewed alone since the child's presence may compromise the data to be collected (Sattler, 2002) as the parent/caregiver may feel uncomfortable disclosing concerns. In addition, small children can be distracting.

FRAMING OF QUESTIONS

The way in which questions are framed will determine the information elicited during the assessment. Open-ended questions are useful in discovering the patient's point of view and emotional state. More-focused questions are better at eliciting specific information and help to speed the pace of the assessment. Both have their place in the assessment. There are, however, a number of question types that should be avoided (e.g., yes/no questions; double-barreled questions; long, multiple questions; coercive, accusatory, or embarrassing questions), since they may not elicit the desired information and may create a climate of interrogation and defensiveness (Sattler, 2002).

OBSERVATIONS OF BEHAVIOR

The content of the interview is important; however, the patient's behavior and style are also noteworthy. During the interview, additional, diagnostically valuable information can be gleaned from (a) level of consciousness, (b) general appearance (e.g., eye contact, modulation of face and voice, personal hygiene, habits of dress), (c) motor activity (e.g., hemiplegia, tics, tenseness, hyper- or hypokinesia), (d) mood, (e) degree of cooperation, and (f) abnormalities in language, prosody, thinking, judgment, or memory.

Because memory is unreliable, it is important to take careful notes during the interview. Patients are usually forgiving of examiners' writing rates. However, the note taking should not be so slow as to interfere with rapport. Audiotapes can also be used; however, the examiner must obtain written consent to use an audio recorder, and it should be remembered that audio recording can impact neuropsychological test performance. Constantinou et al. (2002) found that in the presence of an audio recorder the performance of participants on memory tests declined (see Chapter 4 on *Test Selection* for additional discussion of the presence of observers and audio-video recordings). Clinicians who see clients for repeat assessments may also want to obtain consent for a photograph for the file.

REVIEW OF RECORDS

Often, the patient's account will have to be supplemented by information from other sources (e.g., informants, documents), since a patient's statements may prove misleading with regard to the presence/absence of events and symptoms, the gravity of symptoms, and the time course of their evolution. For example, patients with a memory disorder or who lack insight are likely to be poor historians. Similarly, children may not be reliable informants. In forensic matters in particular, it is important to verify the history given by the patient by obtaining and reviewing records. Distortion of past performance may be linked to prospects for compensation, and the clinician runs the risk of setting the normal reference range too high, causing false diagnoses of neurological conditions (Greiffenstein & Baker, 2003; Greiffenstein et al., 2002). Reynolds (1998) provides a listing of various records that the clinician should consider for review, shown in Table 3–1. The relevance of these records varies, depending on the case.

Table 3–1 Records to Consider in the Evaluation of a Patient's History

Educational records	Including primary, secondary, and postsecondary records, results of any standardized testing, and records of special education
Employment records	Including evaluations, workers' compensation claims, and results of any personnel testing
Legal records	Including criminal and civil litigation
Medical records	Both pre- and postmorbid
Mental health records	Including any prior contact with a mental health professional whether psychiatrist, psychologist, social worker, counselor, etc., including therapy notes, history and intake forms, test results, reports, and protocols
Substance abuse treatment records	Such records may be more difficult to obtain because of federal privacy laws
Military records	Including results of ASVAB, GATB, etc.

Source: Adapted from Reynolds, 1998.

SYMPTOM REPORT/RESPONSE STYLES

It should be noted that patients may falsely attribute preexisting symptoms to an accident or insult, report a higher than actual level of premorbid function, catastrophize or over-report current symptoms, or have difficulty reporting symptoms precisely, without intending to deceive (Greiffenstein et al., 2002; Slick et al., 1999). In addition to motivational issues (e.g., Youngjohn et al., 1995), a number of non-neurologic factors have been shown to influence self-report of premorbid status and subjective complaints of physical, cognitive, and psychological functioning. These include emotional status and negative affectivity (e.g., Fox et al., 1995b; Gunstad & Suhr, 2001, 2002; Sawchyn et al., 2000; Seidenberg et al., 1994), chronic pain (Iverson & McCracken, 1997), suggestibility or expectations regarding outcome (Ferguson et al., 1999; Mittenberg et al., 1992; Suhr & Gunstad, 2002, 2005), and response biases shaped by the social context (Greiffenstein et al., 2002). There is also evidence that following any negative life event (be it accident or illness, neurological or not), individuals may attribute all symptoms, both current and preexisting, to that negative event (Gunstad & Suhr, 2001, 2002).

Patients also have certain ways of answering questions, and some of these response styles or sets may affect the accuracy of the information. For example, children with developmental disabilities may be deficient in assertiveness skills and thus may be prone to acquiesce by answering "yes" to yes/no questions (Horton & Kochurka, 1995). Other pitfalls in obtaining information from certain patients include position bias (e.g., the tendency to choose the first answer in a list), misunderstanding negatively worded items (prominent in young children), and difficulty with time sense (that is, relating past symptoms to current health status; Dodson, 1994).

These considerations underscore the fact that self-report of particular symptoms or symptom clusters can suggest but should not be viewed as diagnostic of specific disorders. For example, complaints of headache, fatigue, and irritability may be found in such diverse conditions as head injury, chronic fatigue syndrome, gastrointestinal disorder, and the common cold (Binder, 1997; Gunstad & Suhr, 2002). Further, base rates of reported postconcussive symptoms (PCSs) have been found to be similar in comparisons of injured and noninjured individuals using symptom checklists (e.g., Ferguson et al., 1999; Fox et al., 1995a, 1995b; Gouvier et al., 1988; Gunstad & Suhr, 2001; Paniak et al., 2002), suggesting that self-report of PCSs are not unique to that disorder. In a similar vein, complaints of memory disturbance are a consistent feature of early AD but are also evident in other disorders such as depression (American Psychiatric Association, 1994).

QUESTIONNAIRES

A good interview takes careful planning. It requires that the examiner learn as much as possible about the person and the purpose(s) of the assessment prior to the interview (e.g., by reviewing medical reports). Questionnaires have also been developed to provide documentation of information routinely collected during the interview (e.g., Baron, 2004; Baron et al., 1995; Dougherty & Schinka, 1989a, 1989b; Goldstein & Goldstein, 1999; Sattler, 2002; Schinka, 1989). Clinicians may construct their own forms or refer to ones that we have developed. We use two questionnaires, one designed for adult patients (Figure 3–1) and the other for use with parents when children are clients (Figure 3–2). Note that none of the forms (our own or others) has data on validity or reliability. Accordingly, the questionnaires should be viewed as complementary to and not as substitutes for the interview. We emphasize that they are not diagnostic instruments. The most efficient use of these instruments is to have the client or caregiver complete them prior to the meeting. In this way, the interview can clarify or focus on the major concerns of the individual and need not touch on minor details already provided in the questionnaire. Such a complementary process increases the confidence in the information obtained and ensures that no topics are overlooked.

REFERENCES

American Psychiatric Association. (1994). *Diagnostic and Statistical Manual of Mental Disorders* (4th ed.). Washington, DC: Author.

Baron, I. S. (2004). *Neuropsychological evaluation of the child.* New York: Oxford University Press.

Baron, I. S., Fennell, E. B., & Voeller, K. S. (1995). *Pediatric neuropsychology in the medical setting.* New York: Oxford University Press.

Binder, L. M. (1997). A review of mild head trauma. Part II: Clinical implications. *Journal of Clinical and Experimental Neuropsychology, 19,* 432–457.

Constantinou, M., Ashendorf, L., & McCaffrey, R. J. (2002). When the third party observer of a neuropsychological examination is an audio-recorder. *The Clinical Neuropsychologist, 16,* 407–412.

Dodson, W. E. (1994). Quality of life measurement in children with epilepsy. In M. R. Trimble & W. E. Dodson (Eds.), *Epilepsy and quality of life* (pp. 217–226). New York: Raven Press.

Dougherty, E., & Schinka, J. A. (1989a). *Developmental History Checklist.* Odessa, FL: PAR.

Dougherty, E., & Schinka, J. A. (1989b). *Personal History Checklist—Adolescent.* Odessa, FL: PAR.

Ferguson, R. J., Mittenberg, W., Barone, D. F., & Schneider, B. (1999). Postconcussion syndrome following sports-related head injury: expectation as etiology. *Neuropsychology, 13,* 582–589.

Fox, D. D., Lees-Haley, P. R., Earnest, K., & Dolezal-Wood, S. (1995a). Base rates of postconcussive symptoms in health maintenance organization patients and controls. *Neuropsychology, 9,* 606–611.

Fox, D. D., Lees-Haley, P. R., Earnest, K., & Dolezal-Wood, S. (1995b). Post-concussive symptoms: base rates and etiology in psychiatric patients. *Clinical Neuropsychologist, 9,* 89–92.

Goldstein, A., & Goldstein, M. (1999). *Childhood History Form.* Salt Lake City: Neurology, Learning and Behavior Center.

Gouvier, W. D., Uddo-Crane, M., & Brown, L. M. (1988). Base rates of post-concussional symptoms. *Archives of Clinical Neuropsychology, 3,* 273–278.

Greiffenstein, M. F., & Baker, W. J. (2003). Premorbid clues? Preinjury scholastic performance and present neuropsychological functioning in late postconcussion syndrome. *The Clinical Neuropsychologist, 17,* 561–573.

Greiffenstein, M. F., Baker, W. J., & Johnson-Greene, D. (2002). Actual versus self-reported scholastic achievement of litigating postconcussion and severe closed head injury claimants. *Psychological Assessment, 14,* 202–208.

Gunstad, J., & Suhr, J. A. (2001). Expectation as etiology versus the good old days: Postconcussion syndrome reporting in athletes, headache sufferers, and depressed individuals. *Journal of the International Neuropsychological Society, 7,* 323–333.

Gunstad, J., & Suhr, J. A. (2002). Perception of illness: nonspecificity of postconcussion syndrome symptom expectation. *Journal of the International Neuropsychological Society, 8,* 37–47.

Horton, C. B., & Kochurka, K. A. (1995). The assessment of children with disabilities who report sexual abuse: A special look at those most vulnerable. In T. Ney (Ed.), *True and false allegations of child sexual abuse: Assessment and case management* (pp. 275–289). New York: Brunner/Mazel.

Iverson, G., & McKracken, L. (1997). "Postconcussive" symptoms in persons with chronic pain. *Brain Injury, 10,* 783–790.

Lezak, M. D., Howieson, D. B., & Loring, D. W. (2004). *Neuropsychological assessment* (4th ed.). New York: Oxford University Press.

Mittenberg, W., Diguilio, D. V., Perrin, S., & Bass, A. E. (1992). Symptoms following mild head injury: Expectation as aetiology. *Journal of Neurology, Neurosurgery and Psychiatry, 55,* 200–204.

Paniak, C., Reynolds, S., Phillips, K., Toller-Lobe, G., Melnyk, A., & Nagy, J. (2002). Patient complaints within 1 month of mild traumatic brain injury: A controlled study. *Archives of Clinical Neuropsychology, 17,* 319–334.

Reynolds, C. R. (1998). Common sense, clinicians, and actuarialism in the detection of malingering during head injury litigation. In C. R. Reynolds (Ed.), *Detection of malingering during head injury litigation* (pp. 261–286). New York: Plenum Press.

Sattler, J. (2002). *Assessment of children: behavioral and clinical applications,* (4th ed.) San Diego: Sattler.

Sawchyn, J., Brulot, M., & Strauss, E. (2000). Note on the use of the Postconcussion Symptom Checklist. *Archives of Clinical Neuropsychology, 15,* 1–8.

Schinka, J. A. (1989). *Personal History Checklist—Adult.* Odessa, FL: PAR.

Seidenberg, M., Taylor, M. A., & Haltiner, A. (1994). Personality and self-report of cognitive functioning. *Archives of Clinical Neuropsychology, 9,* 353–361.

Slick, D. J., Sherman, E. M. S., & Iverson, G. L. (1999). Diagnostic criteria for malingered neurocognitive dysfunction: Proposed standards for clinical practice and research. *The Clinical Neuropsychologist, 13,* 545–561.

Stowe, R. M. (1998). Assessment methods in behavioural neurology and neuropsychiatry. In G. Goldstein, P. D. Nussbaum, & S. R. Beers (Eds.), *Neuropsychology* (pp. 439–485). New York: Plenum Press.

Suhr, J. A., & Gunstad, J. (2002). "Diagnosis threat": The effect of negative expectations on cognitive performance in head injury. *Journal of Clinical and Experimental Neuropsychology, 24,* 448–457.

Suhr, J. A., & Gunstad, J. (2005). Further exploration of the effect of "diagnosis threat" on cognitive performance in individuals with mild head injury. *Journal of the International Neuropsychological Society, 11,* 23–29.

Vanderploeg, R. D. (2000). Interview and testing: The data collection phase of neuropsychological evaluations. In R. D. Vanderploeg (Ed.), *Clinican's guide to neuropsychological assessment* (2nd ed., pp. 3–38). New Jersey: Lawrence Erlbaum Associates.

Youngjohn, J. R., Burrows, L., & Erdal, K. (1995). Brain damage or compensation neurosis? The controversial post-concussion syndrome. *The Clinical Neuropsychologist, 9,* 112–123.

Figure 3–1 Background questionnaire—Adult version.

BACKGROUND QUESTIONNAIRE—ADULT

Confidential

The following is a detailed questionnaire on your development, medical history, and current functioning at home and at work. This information will be integrated with the testing results in order to provide a better picture of your abilities as well as any problem areas. Please fill out this questionnaire as completely as you can.

Client's Name: _____ Today's Date: _____
   (If not client, name of person completing this form _____
   Relationship to Client _____)
Home address _____ Work _____
Client's Phone (H) _____ (W) _____
Date of Birth _____ Age _____ Sex _____
Place of Birth _____
Primary Language _____ Secondary Language _____
   Fluent/Nonfluent (circle one)
Hand used for writing (check one)   ☐ Right   ☐ Left

Medical Diagnosis (if any) (1) _____

                  (2) _____

Who referred you for this evaluation? _____
Briefly describe problem: _____
_____
_____

Date of the accident, injury, or onset of illness _____
What specific questions would you like answered by this evaluation?
(1) _____

(2) _____

(3) _____

SYMPTOM SURVEY
For each symptom that applies, place a check mark in the box. Add any comments as needed.

Physical Concerns

Motor	Rt	Lt	Both	Date of Onset
☐ Headaches				_____
☐ Dizziness				_____
☐ Nausea or vomiting				_____
☐ Excessive fatigue				_____
☐ Urinary incontinence				_____
☐ Bowel problems				_____
☐ Weakness on one side of body (Indicate body part)	___	___	___	_____
☐ Problems with fine motor control	___	___	___	_____
☐ Tremor or shakiness	___	___	___	_____
☐ Tics or strange movements	___	___	___	_____
☐ Balance problems				_____
☐ Often bump into things				_____
☐ Blackout spells (fainting)				_____
☐ Other motor problems _____				_____

(continued)

Figure 3–1 (*continued*)

Sensory	Rt	Lt	Both	Date of Onset
❏ Loss of feeling/numbness (Indicate where)	___	___	___	_____
❏ Tingling or strange skin sensations (Indicate where)	___	___	___	_____
❏ Difficulty telling hot from cold	___	___	___	_____
❏ Visual Impairment				_____
❏ Wear glasses ☐ Yes ☐ No				_____
❏ Problems seeing on one side	___	___	___	_____
❏ Sensitivity to bright lights				_____
❏ Blurred vision	___	___	___	_____
❏ See things that are not there	___	___	___	_____
❏ Brief periods of blindness	___	___	___	_____
❏ Need to squint or move closer to see clearly				_____
❏ Hearing loss	___	___	___	_____
❏ Wear hearing aid ☐ Yes ☐ No				_____
❏ Ringing in ears	___	___	___	_____
❏ Hear strange sounds	___	___	___	_____
❏ Unaware of things on one side of my body	___	___	___	_____
❏ Problems with taste				_____
❏ (___ Increased ___ Decreased sensitivity) Problems with smell				_____
❏ (___ Increased ___ Decreased sensitivity)				_____
❏ Pain (describe)				_____
❏ Other sensory problems _____				

Intellectual Concerns
Problem Solving   Date of Onset

❏ Difficulty figuring out how to do new things _____
❏ Difficulty figuring out problems that most others can do _____
❏ Difficulty planning ahead _____
❏ Difficulty changing a plan or activity when necessary _____
❏ Difficulty thinking as quickly as needed _____
❏ Difficulty completing an activity in a reasonable time _____
❏ Difficulty doing things in the right order (sequencing) _____

Language and Math Skills   Date of Onset

❏ Difficulty finding the right word _____
❏ Slurred speech _____
❏ Odd or unusual speech sounds _____
❏ Difficulty expressing thoughts _____
❏ Difficulty understanding what others say _____
❏ Difficulty understanding what I read _____
❏ Difficulty writing letters or words (not due to motor problems) _____
❏ Difficulty with math (e.g., balancing checkbook, making change, etc.) _____
❏ Other language or math problems _____

Nonverbal Skills   Date of Onset

❏ Difficulty telling right from left _____
❏ Difficulty drawing or copying _____
❏ Difficulty dressing (not due to motor problems) _____
❏ Difficulty doing things I should automatically be able to do (e.g., brushing teeth) _____
❏ Problems finding way around familiar places _____
❏ Difficulty recognizing objects or people _____
❏ Parts of my body do not seem as if they belong to me _____
❏ Decline in my musical abilities _____

(*continued*)

Figure 3–1 (*continued*)

❏ Not aware of time (e.g., day, season, year) _____
❏ Slow reaction time _____
❏ Other nonverbal problems _____

_____

Awareness and Concentration   Date of Onset
❏ Highly distractible _____
❏ Lose my train of thought easily _____
❏ My mind goes blank a lot _____
❏ Difficulty doing more than one thing at a time _____
❏ Become easily confused and disoriented _____
❏ Aura (strange feelings) _____
❏ Don't feel very alert or aware of things _____
❏ Tasks require more effort or attention _____

Memory   Date of Onset
❏ Forget where I leave things (e.g., keys, gloves, etc.) _____
❏ Forget names _____
❏ Forget what I should be doing _____
❏ Forget where I am or where I am going _____
❏ Forget recent events (e.g., breakfast) _____
❏ Forget appointments _____
❏ Forget events that happened long ago _____
❏ More reliant on others to remind me of things _____
❏ More reliant on notes to remember things _____
❏ Forget the order of events _____
❏ Forget facts but can remember how to do things _____
❏ Forget faces of people I know (when not present) _____
❏ Other memory problems _____

_____

Mood/Behavior/Personality   Rate Severity   Date of Onset
                              Mild   Moderate   Severe
❏ Sadness or depression   ❏   ❏   ❏   _____
❏ Anxiety or nervousness   ❏   ❏   ❏   _____
❏ Stress   ❏   ❏   ❏   _____
❏ Sleep problems (falling asleep ❏ staying asleep ❏) _____
❏ Experience nightmares on a daily/weekly basis _____
❏ Become angry more easily _____
❏ Euphoria (feeling on top of the world) _____
❏ Much more emotional (e.g., cry more easily) _____
❏ Feel as if I just don't care anymore _____
❏ Easily frustrated _____
❏ Doing things automatically (without awareness) _____
❏ Less inhibited (do things I would not do before) _____
❏ Difficulty being spontaneous _____
❏ Change in energy (❏ loss ❏ increase) _____
❏ Change in appetite (❏ loss ❏ increase) _____
❏ Increase ❏ or loss ❏ of weight _____
❏ Change in sexual interest (increase ❏ decline ❏) _____
❏ Lack of interest in pleasurable activities _____
❏ Increase in irritability _____
❏ Increase in aggression _____
❏ Other changes in mood or personality or in how you deal with people

_____

Have others commented to you about changes in your thinking, behavior, personality, or mood? If yes, who and what have they said? ❏ Yes ❏ No

_____
_____
_____

(continued)

61

Figure 3–1 (*continued*)

Are you experiencing any problems in the following aspects of your life? If so, please explain:

Marital/Family _____

_____

Financial/Legal _____

_____

Housekeeping/Money Management _____

_____

Driving _____

Overall, my symptoms have developed ☐ slowly ☐ quickly

My symptoms occur ☐ occasionally ☐ often

Over the past six months my symptoms have ☐ improved ☐ stayed the same ☐ worsened

Is there anything you can do (or someone does) that gets the problems to stop or be less intense, less frequent, or shorter? _____

_____

What seems to make the problems worse? _____

_____

In summary, there is ☐ definitely something wrong with me
☐ possibly something wrong with me
☐ nothing wrong with me

What are your goals and aspirations for the future? _____

_____

EARLY HISTORY

You were born: ☐ on time ☐ prematurely ☐ late
Your weight at birth: _____

Were there any problems associated with your birth (e.g., oxygen deprivation, unusual birth position, etc.) or the period afterward (e.g., need for oxygen, convulsions, illness, etc.)? ☐ Yes ☐ No
Describe: _____

Check all that applied to your mother while she was pregnant with you:
❑ Accident
❑ Alcohol use
❑ Cigarette smoking
❑ Drug use (marijuana, cocaine, LSD, etc.)
❑ Illness (toxemia, diabetes, high blood pressure, infection, etc.)
❑ Poor nutrition
❑ Psychological problems
❑ Medications (prescribed or over the counter) taken during pregnancy
❑ Other problems _____

List all medications (prescribed or over the counter) that your mother took while pregnant:

_____

Rate your developmental progress as it has been reported to you, by checking one description for each area:

	Early	Average	Late
Walking	☐	☐	☐
Language	☐	☐	☐
Toilet training	☐	☐	☐
Overall development	☐	☐	☐

(*continued*)

Figure 3–1 (*continued*)

As a child, did you have any of these conditions:

- ❏ Attentional problems
- ❏ Clumsiness
- ❏ Developmental delay
- ❏ Hyperactivity
- ❏ Muscle weakness

- ❏ Learning disability
- ❏ Speech problems
- ❏ Hearing problems
- ❏ Frequent ear infections
- ❏ Visual problems

MEDICAL HISTORY

Medical problems **prior** to the onset of current condition

If yes, give date(s) and brief description

- ❏ Head injuries _____
- ❏ Loss of consciousness _____
- ❏ Motor vehicle accidents _____
- ❏ Major falls, sports accidents, or industrial injuries _____
- ❏ Seizures _____
- ❏ Stroke _____
- ❏ Arteriosclerosis _____
- ❏ Dementia _____
- ❏ Other brain infection or disorder (meningitis, encephalitis, oxygen deprivation etc.) _____
- ❏ Diabetes _____
- ❏ Heart disease _____
- ❏ Cancer _____
- ❏ Back or neck injury _____
- ❏ Serious illnesses/disorder (Immune disorder, cerebral palsy, polio, lung, etc.) _____
- ❏ Poisoning _____
- ❏ Exposure toxins (e.g., lead, solvents, chemicals) _____
- ❏ Major surgeries _____
- ❏ Psychiatric problems _____
- ❏ Other _____

Are you currently taking any medication?

Name	Reason for taking	Dosage	Date started

Are you currently in counseling or under psychiatric care? ☐ Yes ☐ No

Please list date therapy initiated and name(s) of professional(s) treating you:

_____

Have you ever been in counseling or under psychiatric care? ☐ Yes ☐ No

If yes, please list dates of therapy and name(s) of professional(s) who treated you:

_____

Please list all inpatient hospitalizations including the name of the hospital, date of hospitalization, duration, and diagnosis:

_____

(*continued*)

Figure 3–1 (*continued*)

SUBSTANCE USE HISTORY

I started drinking at age:
☐ less than 10 years old   ☐ 10–15   ☐ 16–19   ☐ 20–21   ☐ over 21

I drink alcohol: ☐ rarely or never   ☐ 1–2 days/week
                          ☐ 3–5 days/week   ☐ daily

I used to drink alcohol but stopped: ___ Date stopped: _____
Preferred type(s) of drinks: _____

Usual number of drinks I have at one time: _____

My last drink was: ☐ less than 24 hours ago   ☐ 24–48 hours ago
                          ☐ over 48 hours ago

Check all that apply:
☐ I can drink more than most people my age and size before I get drunk.
☐ I sometimes get into trouble (fights, legal difficulty, work problems, conflicts with family, accidents, etc.) after
   drinking (specify): _____
☐ I sometimes black out after drinking.

Please check all the drugs you are now using or have used in the past:

	Presently Using	Used in Past
Amphetamines (including diet pills)	☐	☐
Barbiturates (downers, etc.)	☐	☐
Cocaine or crack	☐	☐
Hallucinogenics (LSD, acid, STP, etc.)	☐	☐
Inhalants (glue, nitrous oxide, etc.)	☐	☐
Marijuana	☐	☐
Opiate narcotics (heroin, morphine, etc.)	☐	☐
PCP (or angel dust)	☐	☐
Others (list)	☐	☐

Do you consider yourself dependent on any of the above drugs?   ☐ Yes   ☐ No
If yes, which one(s): _____

Do you consider yourself dependent on any prescription drugs?   ☐ Yes   ☐ No
If yes, which one(s): _____

Check all that apply:
☐ I have gone through drug withdrawal.
☐ I have used IV drugs.
☐ I have been in drug treatment.

Has use of drugs ever affected your work performance? _____
Has use of drugs or alcohol ever affected your driving ability? _____
Do you smoke?   ☐ Yes   ☐ No
If yes, amount per day: _____
Do you drink coffee: ☐ Yes   ☐ No
If yes, amount per day: _____

FAMILY HISTORY

The following questions deal with your biological mother, father, brothers, and sisters:
Is your mother alive?   ☐ Yes   ☐ No
If deceased, what was the cause of her death?

_____

Mother's highest level of education: _____
Mother's occupation: _____

(*continued*)

Figure 3–1 (*continued*)

Does your mother have a known or suspected learning disability? ☐ Yes ☐ No

If yes, describe: _____

Is your father alive? ☐ Yes ☐ No

If deceased, what was the cause of his death?

_____

Father's highest level of education: _____

Father's occupation: _____

Does your father have a known or suspected learning disability? ☐ Yes ☐ No

If yes, describe: _____

How many brothers and sisters do you have? _____

What are their ages? _____

Are there any unusual problems (physical, academic, psychological) associated with any of your brothers or sisters?

If yes, describe: _____

Please check all problems that exist(ed) in close biological family members (parents, brothers, sisters, grandparents, aunts, uncles). Note who it is (was) and describe the problem where indicated

	Who?	Describe
Neurologic disease		
☐ Alzheimer's disease or senility	_____	
☐ Huntington's disease	_____	
☐ Multiple sclerosis	_____	
☐ Parkinson's disease	_____	
☐ Epilepsy or seizures	_____	
☐ Other neurologic disease	_____	_____
Psychiatric illness		
☐ Depression	_____	
☐ Bipolar illness (manic-depression)	_____	
☐ Schizophrenia	_____	
☐ Other		
Other disorders		
☐ Mental retardation	_____	
☐ Speech or language disorder	_____	_____
☐ Learning problems	_____	_____
☐ Attention problems	_____	_____
☐ Behavior problems	_____	_____
☐ Other major disease or disorder	_____	_____

PERSONAL HISTORY

Marital History

Current marital status: ☐ Single   ☐ Married   ☐ Common-law
                          ☐ Separated   ☐ Divorced   ☐ Widowed

Years married to current spouse: _____

Dates of previous marriages: From _____ to _____
                               From _____ to _____

Spouse's name: _____   Age: _____

Spouse's occupation: _____

Spouse's health: ☐ Excellent   ☐ Good   ☐ Poor

Children (include stepchildren)

Name	Age	Gender	Occupation
_____	_____	_____	_____
_____	_____	_____	_____
_____	_____	_____	_____
_____	_____	_____	_____
_____	_____	_____	_____

Who currently lives at home? _____

Do any family members have any significant health concerns/special needs? _____

_____

(*continued*)

Figure 3–1 *(continued)*

Educational History

	Name of School Attended	Grades and Years Attended	Degree certifications
Elementary	_____	_____	_____
High school	_____	_____	_____
College/university	_____	_____	_____
	_____	_____	_____
Trade school	_____	_____	_____

If a high school diploma was not awarded, did you complete a GED? _____

Were any grades repeated? ☐ Yes ☐ No
Reason: _____

Were there any special problems learning to read, write, or do math? _____
_____

Were you ever in any special class(es) or did you ever receive special services?
☐ Yes ☐ No
If yes, what grade(s) _____ or age? _____
What type of class? _____

How would you describe your usual performance as a student?
☐ A & B   Provide any additional helpful comments about your academic
☐ B & C   performance: _____
☐ C & D   _____
☐ D & F   _____

Military Service
Did you serve in the military? ☐ Yes ☐ No
If yes, what branch? _____ Dates: _____
Certifications/Duties: _____
_____
_____

Did you serve in war time? _____ If so, what arena? _____

Did you receive injuries of were you ever exposed to any dangerous or unusual substances during your service?
☐ Yes ☐ No

If yes, explain: _____

Do you have any continuing problems related to your military service? Describe:
_____

Occupational History
Are you currently working? ☐ Yes ☐ No
Current job title: _____
Name of employer: _____
Current responsibilities: _____
Dates of employment: _____
Are you currently experiencing any problems at work? ☐ Yes ☐ No
If yes, describe: _____
_____
Do you see your current work situation as stable? ☐ Yes ☐ No

(continued)

Figure 3–1 *(continued)*

Approximate annual income: Prior to injury or illness   _____
                              After injury or illness_____

Previous employers:
Name   Dates   Duties/position   Reason for leaving
_____
_____
_____
_____

Recreation
Briefly list the types of recreations (e.g., sports, games, TV, hobbies, etc.) that you enjoy:
_____
_____
Are you still able to do these activities? _____
_____

Recent Tests
Check all tests that recently have been done and report any abnormal findings.

	Check if normal	Abnormal findings
❑ Angiography	_____	_____
❑ Blood work	_____	_____
❑ CT scan	_____	_____
❑ MRI	_____	_____
❑ PET scan	_____	_____
❑ SPECT	_____	_____
❑ Skull x-ray	_____	_____
❑ EEG	_____	_____
❑ Neurological exam	_____	_____
❑ Other_____	_____	_____

Identify the physician who is most familiar with your recent problems: _____
_____

Date of last vision exam: _____
Date of last hearing exam: _____

Have you had a prior psychological or neuropsychological exam?   ☐ Yes   ☐ No
If yes, complete the following:
Name of psychologist: _____
Date: _____
Reason for evaluation: _____
Finding of the evaluation: _____
_____

Please provide any additional information that you feel is relevant to this referral:
_____
_____
_____

Figure 3–2 Background questionnaire—Child version.

BACKGROUND QUESTIONNAIRE—CHILD

Confidential

The following is a detailed questionnaire on your child's development, medical history, and current functioning at home and at school. This information will be integrated with the testing results to provide a better picture of your child's abilities as well as any problem areas. Please fill out this questionnaire as completely as you can.

CHILD'S FAMILY

Child's Name: _____ Today's Date: _____

Birthdate: _____ Age: _____ Grade: _____ Name of School: _____

Birth Country: _____ Age on arrival in country if born elsewhere:_____

Person filling out this form: ☐ Mother ☐ Father ☐ Stepmother ☐ Stepfather ☐ Other: _____

Biological Mother's Name: _____ Age: _____ Highest Grade Completed: _____

Number of Years of Education: _____ Degree/Diploma (if applicable): _____

Occupation: _____

Biological Father's Name: _____ Age: _____ Highest Grade Completed: _____

Number of Years of Education: _____ Degree/Diploma (if applicable): _____

Occupation: _____

Marital status of biological parents: ☐ Married ☐ Separated ☐ Divorced ☐ Widowed ☐ Other: _____

If biological parents are separated or divorced:

   How old was this child when the separation occurred? _____

   Who has legal custody of the child? (Check one) ☐ Mother ☐ Father ☐ Joint/Both ☐ Other:_____

   Stepparent's Name: _____ Age: _____ Occupation: _____

If this child is not living with underline either biological parent:

   Reason: _____

   ☐ Adoptive parents ☐ Foster parents ☐ Other family members ☐ Group home ☐ Other: _____

   Name(s) of legal guardian(s): _____

List all people currently living in your child's household:

Name	Relationship to child	Age

If any brothers or sisters are living outside the home, list their names and ages:

_____

_____

Primary language spoken in the home: _____

Other languages spoken in the home: _____

If your child's first language is not English, please complete the following:

   Child's first language: _____ Age at which your child learned

   English: _____

CURRENT MEDICATIONS

List *all* medications that your child is currently taking:

Medication	Reason taken	Dosage (if known)	Start date

(continued)

68

Figure 3–2 (*continued*)

BEHAVIOR CHECKLIST

Place a check mark (√) next to behaviors that you believe your child exhibits to an excessive or exaggerated degree when compared to other children his or her age.

Sleeping and Eating
- ❏ Nightmares
- ❏ Trouble sleeping
- ❏ Eats poorly
- ❏ Eats excessively

Social Development
- ❏ Prefers to be alone
- ❏ Excessively shy or timid
- ❏ More interested in objects than in people
- ❏ Difficulty making friends
- ❏ Teased by other children
- ❏ Bullies other children
- ❏ Not sought out for friendship by peers
- ❏ Difficulty seeing another person's point of view
- ❏ Doesn't empathize with others
- ❏ Overly trusting of others
- ❏ Doesn't appreciate humor

Behavior
- ❏ Stubborn
- ❏ Irritable, angry, or resentful
- ❏ Frequent tantrums
- ❏ Strikes out at others
- ❏ Throws or destroys things
- ❏ Lying
- ❏ Stealing
- ❏ Argues with adults
- ❏ Low frustration threshold
- ❏ Daredevil behavior
- ❏ Runs away
- ❏ Needs a lot of supervision
- ❏ Impulsive (does things without thinking)
- ❏ Poor sense of danger
- ❏ Skips school

- ❏ Dangerous to self or others (describe):
  _____
  _____
- ❏ Purposely harms or injures self (describe):
  _____
  _____
- ❏ Talks about killing self (describe):
  _____
  _____
- ❏ Unusual fears, habits or mannerisms (describe):
  _____
- ❏ Seems depressed
- ❏ Cries frequently
- ❏ Excessively worried and anxious
- ❏ Overly preoccupied with details
- ❏ Overly attached to certain objects
- ❏ Not affected by negative consequences
- ❏ Drug abuse
- ❏ Alcohol abuse
- ❏ Sexually active

Other Problems
- ❏ Bladder control problems (not during seizure)
- ❏ Poor bowel control (soils self)
- ❏ Motor/vocal tics
- ❏ Overreacts to noises
- ❏ Overreacts to touch
- ❏ Excessive daydreaming and fantasy life
- ❏ Problems with taste or smell

Motor Skills
- ❏ Poor fine motor coordination
- ❏ Poor gross motor coordination

OTHER PROBLEMS:

_____
_____
_____
_____
_____

EDUCATION PROGRAM

Does your child have a modified learning program? ☐ Yes ☐ No

Is there an individual education plan (IEP)? ☐ Yes ☐ No

Are you satisfied with your child's current learning program? If not, please explain: _____
_____

(*continued*)

Figure 3–2 (*continued*)

Has your child been held back a grade?   ☐ No   ☐ Yes (Indicate grade: _____)
Is your child in any special education classes?   ☐ Yes   ☐ No
  If yes, please describe: _____
  _____

Is your child receiving learning assistance at school?   ☐ Yes ☐ No
  If yes, please describe: _____
  _____

Has your child been suspended or expelled from school?   ☐ Yes   ☐ No
  If yes, please describe: _____
  _____

Has your child ever received tutoring?   ☐ Yes   ☐ No
  If yes, please describe: _____
  _____

Briefly describe classroom or school problems if applicable: _____
_____
_____

COGNITIVE SKILLS

Rate your child's cognitive skills relative to other children of the <u>same age</u>.

	Above average	Average	Below average	Severe problem
Speech	☐	☐	☐	☐
Comprehension of speech	☐	☐	☐	☐
Problem solving	☐	☐	☐	☐
Attention span	☐	☐	☐	☐
Organizational skills	☐	☐	☐	☐
Remembering events	☐	☐	☐	☐
Remembering facts	☐	☐	☐	☐
Learning from experience	☐	☐	☐	☐
Understanding concepts	☐	☐	☐	☐
Overall intelligence	☐	☐	☐	☐

Check any specific problems:

☐ Poor articulation
☐ Difficulty finding words to express self
☐ Disorganized speech
☐ Ungrammatical speech
☐ Talks like a younger child
☐ Slow learner
☐ Forgets to do things
☐ Easily distracted
☐ Frequently forgets instructions

☐ Frequently loses belongings
☐ Difficulty planning tasks
☐ Doesn't foresee consequences of actions
☐ Slow thinking
☐ Difficulty with math/handling money
☐ Poor understanding of time

Describe briefly any other cognitive problems that your child may have: _____
_____
_____

Describe any special skills or abilities that your child may have: _____
_____
_____

DEVELOPMENTAL HISTORY

If your child is adopted, please fill in as much of the following information as you are aware of.

During pregnancy, did the mother of this child:

  Take any medication?   ☐ Yes   ☐ No
    If yes, what kind?_____

(*continued*)

Figure 3–2 (*continued*)

Smoke? ☐ Yes ☐ No
   If yes, how many cigarettes each day? _____

Drink alcoholic beverages? ☐ Yes ☐ No
   If yes, what kind? _____
   Approximately how much alcohol was consumed each day? _____

Use drugs? ☐ Yes ☐ No
   If yes, what kind? _____
   How often were drugs used? _____

List any complications during pregnancy (excessive vomiting, excessive staining/blood loss, threatened miscarriage, infections, toxemia, fainting, dizziness, etc.): _____

_____

Duration of pregnancy (weeks): _____ Duration of labor (hours): _____ Apgars: _____ / _____

Were there any indications of fetal distress? ☐ Yes ☐ No
   If yes on any of other above, for what reason? _____

_____

Check any that apply to the birth: ☐ Labor induced ☐ Forceps ☐ Breech ☐ Cesarean
   If yes on any of other above, for what reason? _____

_____

What was your child's birth weight? _____
Check any that apply following birth: ☐ Jaundice ☐ Breathing problems ☐ Incubator ☐ Birth defect
   If any, please describe: _____

_____

_____

Were there any other complications? ☐ Yes ☐ No
   If yes, please describe: _____

_____

Were there any feeding problems? ☐ Yes ☐ No
   If yes, please describe: _____

_____

Were there any sleeping problems? ☐ Yes ☐ No
   If yes, please describe: _____

_____

Were there any growth or development problems during the first few years of life? ☐ Yes ☐ No
   If yes, please describe: _____

_____

Were any of the following present (to a significant degree) during infancy or the first few years of life?

❏ Unusually quiet or inactive   ❏ Colic   ❏ Headbanging

❏ Did not like to be held or cuddled   ❏ Excessive restlessness   ❏ Constantly into everything

❏ Not alert   ❏ Excessive sleep   ❏ Excessive number of accidents compared with other children

❏ Difficult to soothe   ❏ Diminished sleep

(*continued*)

Figure 3–2 (*continued*)

Please indicate the approximate age at which your child first showed the following behaviors by checking the appropriate box. Check "Never" if your child has never shown the listed behavior.

	Early	Average	Late	Never		Early	Average	Late	Never
Smiled	☐	☐	☐	☐	Tied shoelaces	☐	☐	☐	☐
Rolled over	☐	☐	☐	☐	Dressed self	☐	☐	☐	☐
Sat alone	☐	☐	☐	☐	Fed self	☐	☐	☐	☐
Crawled	☐	☐	☐	☐	Bladder trained, day	☐	☐	☐	☐
Walked	☐	☐	☐	☐	Bladder trained, night	☐	☐	☐	☐
Ran	☐	☐	☐	☐	Bowel trained	☐	☐	☐	☐
Babbled	☐	☐	☐	☐	Rode tricycle	☐	☐	☐	☐
First word	☐	☐	☐	☐	Rode bicycle	☐	☐	☐	☐
Sentences	☐	☐	☐	☐					

MEDICAL HISTORY

Vision problems ☐ No ☐ Yes (describe: _____) Date of last vision examination: _____

Hearing problems ☐ No ☐ Yes (describe: _____) Date of last hearing examination: _____

Place a check next to any illness or condition that your child has had. When you check an item, also note the approximate date of the illness (if you prefer, you can simply indicate the child's age at illness).

Illness or condition	Date(s) or age(s)	Illness or condition	Date(s) or age(s)
☐ Measles	_____	☐ Loss of consciousness	_____
☐ German measles	_____	☐ Poisoning	_____
☐ Mumps	_____	☐ Severe headaches	_____
☐ Chicken pox	_____	☐ Rheumatic fever	_____
☐ Whooping cough	_____	☐ Tuberculosis	_____
☐ Diphtheria	_____	☐ Bone or joint disease	_____
☐ Scarlet fever	_____	☐ Sexually transmitted disease	_____
☐ Meningitis	_____	☐ Anemia	_____
☐ Pneumonia	_____	☐ Jaundice/hepatitis	_____
☐ Encephalitis	_____	☐ Diabetes	_____
☐ High fever	_____	☐ Cancer	_____
☐ Seizures	_____	☐ High blood pressure	_____
☐ Allergy	_____	☐ Heart disease	_____
☐ Hay fever	_____	☐ Asthma	_____
☐ Injuries to head	_____	☐ Bleeding problems	_____
☐ Broken bones	_____	☐ Eczema or hives	_____
☐ Hospitalizations	_____	☐ Physical abuse	_____
☐ Operations	_____	☐ Sexual abuse	_____
☐ Ear infections	_____	☐ Other: _____	_____
☐ Paralysis	_____		

FAMILY MEDICAL HISTORY

Place a check next to any illness or condition that any member of the immediate family (i.e., brothers, sisters, aunts, uncles, cousins, grandparents) has had. Please note the family member's relationship to the child.

Condition	Relationship to child		Relationship to child
☐ Seizures or epilepsy	_____	☐ Tics or Tourette's syndrome	_____
☐ Attention deficit	_____	☐ Alcohol abuse	_____
☐ Hyperactivity	_____	☐ Drug abuse	_____
☐ Learning disabilities	_____	☐ Suicide attempt	_____
☐ Mental retardation	_____	☐ Physical abuse	_____

(*continued*)

Figure 3–2 (*continued*)

Condition	**Relationship to child**			**Relationship to child**
☐ Childhood behavior problems	_____	☐ Sexual abuse		_____
☐ Mental illness	_____	☐ Neurological illness or disease		_____
☐ Depression or anxiety	_____	☐ Antisocial behavior (assaults, thefts, etc.)		_____

List any previous assessments that your child has had:

	Dates of testing	Name of examiner
Psychiatric	_____ _____	_____ _____
Psychological	_____	_____
Neuropsychological	_____	_____
Educational	_____	_____
Speech pathology	_____ _____	_____ _____

List any form of psychological/psychiatric treatment that your child has had (e.g., psychotherapy, family therapy, inpatient or residential treatment):

Type of treatment	Dates	Name of therapist

_____
_____
_____
_____

Have there been any recent stressors that you think may be contributing to your child's difficulties (e.g., illness, deaths, operations, accidents, separations, divorce of parents, parent changed job, changed schools, family moved, family financial problems, remarriage, sexual trauma, other losses)? _____
_____
_____
_____
_____

OTHER INFORMATION

What are your child's favorite activities? _____
_____

Has your child ever been in trouble with the law? ☐ Yes ☐ No
  If yes, please describe briefly: _____
_____

On the average, what percentage of the time does your child comply with requests or commands? _____
_____

What have you found to be the most satisfactory ways of helping your child? _____
_____

What are your child's assets or strengths? _____
_____

Is there any other information that you think may help me in assessing your child? _____
_____
_____
_____
_____

(*continued*)

Figure 3–2 (*continued*)

_____

Thank you for filling out this questionnaire.

4

Test Selection, Test Administration, and Preparation of the Patient

TEST SELECTION

Although the terms "psychological testing" and "psychological assessment" are often used synonymously, they do represent different aspects of practice. While "testing" is one aspect, often referring to the administration of a particular scale to obtain a specific score, psychological assessment is the more appropriate term for the evaluation of individual clients and includes the "integration of test results, life history information, collateral data, and clinical observations into a unified description of the individual being assessed" (Hunsley, 2002, p. 139). It is "a complex activity requiring the interplay of knowledge of psychometric concepts with expertise in an area of professional practice or application. Assessment is a conceptual, problem-solving process of gathering dependable, relevant information . . . to make informed decisions" (Turner et al., 2001, p. 1100). As such, it provides a valuable source of clinical information, perhaps as informative as that provided by medical tests (Meyer et al., 2001).

The American Psychological Association (APA; Turner et al., 2001) has developed guidelines to inform test users and the public of the qualifications the APA considers important for the competent and responsible use of psychological tests. The guidelines indicate that psychologists possess (a) core generic psychometric knowledge and skills and (b) specific qualifications for the responsible use of tests in particular settings or for specific purposes. With regard to test selection, the guidelines specify that "test users should select the best test or test version for a specific purpose and should have knowledge of testing practice in the content area and of the most appropriate norms when more than one normative set is available. Knowledge of test characteristics such as psychometric properties, basis in theory and research, and normative data . . . should influence test selection" (Turner et al., 2001, p. 1101).

Thus, test selection should be based on knowledge of the literature and the appropriateness of a particular test for a given individual under a unique set of circumstances and the distinctive set of referral questions. Well-standardized tests should be chosen, as the standardization process minimizes the error variance within a patient's assessment data (Miller & Rohling, 2001).

Norms

The reader is referred to Chapter 2 (*Norms Selection in Neuropsychological Practice*) for a discussion of factors to consider with regard to the adequacy of norms.

Approaches to Assessment

There are three main approaches to assessment. In the *fixed battery approach*, the clinician gives the same tests to every patient regardless of the specific referral question. In the *flexible battery approach*, the unique nature of the patient's deficits guides the choice of tasks, and this selection may vary from one patient to another. An *intermediate position* is the flexible battery approach in which the assessment is tailored so that homogeneous groups of patients are routinely given specific subsets of tests.

In our practice, the selection of tests for a given patient usually starts with a "core battery" based on the information available (or initial hypotheses) about the patient's problem (e.g., epilepsy, traumatic head injury, dementia, etc.) and the specific referral questions (e.g., differential diagnosis, post-treatment reevaluation, routine follow-up). Thus, we may begin with a general screening battery (e.g., RBANS, NAB, DRS-2) designed to be sensitive to various conditions and follow up with more detailed testing. Alternatively, depending on the patient and our understanding of the presenting problem(s), our approach may incorporate a routine grouping of tests that includes an intelligence test appropriate for the age of the patient and several tests in the areas of presumed deficit (e.g., tests of memory, concentration/attention, executive function) to confirm the presence and severity of the deficit. Tests sampling other domains (e.g., language, sensory function, mood) are also included to explore alternative hypotheses, obtain a broad overview of the person's functioning, and provide information useful for a given question or referral source. The remainder of the test selection is often "open-ended" (i.e., not all tests to be given in a particular case are determined in advance). Rather, some tests are selected after a review of the results of the initial testing, of the client's complaints, and of the person's behavior during testing. In this way, we can clarify relevant issues and more precisely characterize the nature of any areas of impairment. Occasionally, it is obvious that the patient fatigues easily or is likely to fail demanding tests. In that case, the selection of additional or alternative tests is critical, and must focus directly on the target problems and the patient's capacity to work with the examiner. When we work exclusively with a particular population, we often use specific "custom" batteries designed with a flexible approach but administered routinely to all patients with similar presenting problems. This facilitates retesting for clinical purposes as well as using data for research and program evaluation.

The conorming of some commonly used tests (e.g., Wechsler intelligence with memory and with achievement tests, MAYO norms, NAB) permits the comparison of one set of test scores directly with another. However, such coordinated norming is relatively uncommon. Thus, in most cases, the flexible battery approach does not allow the use of score comparisons across tests with common metrics. This is a distinct advantage of fixed batteries, or of "impairment indices" resulting from fixed test batteries (e.g., the Halstead Impairment Index, the GNDS: Oestreicher & O'Donnell, 1995; Reitan & Wolfson, 1988; HRNES: Russell, 2000a, 2000b). There are also statistical problems (e.g., the likelihood of obtaining at least one score in the impaired range increases as more tests are administered) and biases (hind-bias, over-reliance on salient data, underutilization of base rates, failure to take into account covariation) inherent in the administration of multiple tests. Miller and Rohling (2001) presented a statistically based method for calculating summary scores and interpreting data within a flexible battery approach. Test scores are converted to a common metric (T scores) and assigned to particular cognitive domains. Overall, domain and individual test battery means are then evaluated with reference to premorbid estimates using various statistical indices. The percentage of tests that fall in the impaired range is also calculated. Rohling et al. (2003) have provided some evidence supporting their claim that their method of analysis for generating summary scores from a flexible battery performs as well as the GNDS, Average Impairment Rating, and the Halstead Impairment Index in determining neuropathology.

Sweet et al. (2000a, 2000b) report that, according to a survey of 422 neuropsychologists in 1999, the flexible battery approach (i.e., variable but routine groupings of tests for different types of patients such as head injury, alcoholism, elderly, etc.) is the favorite, with endorsement rates of about 70%. Fixed (or standard) battery use has dwindled to about 15% as has a totally flexible approach to test selection. Thus, impairment indices have become more obsolete as

neuropsychologists are less and less called upon to determine whether deficits are "organic or not organic," a question that is now better answered by neuroradiological and electrophysiological techniques. Instead, neuropsychological evaluations have moved toward providing a detailed description of the nature of the deficit, its impact on daily living, and its rehabilitation.

A variant of the flexible battery framework is the Boston "*process*" approach, which focuses on a qualitative exploration of how the patient attained the test score and how he or she succeeded or failed at a task (Kaplan, 1988; Lezak et al., 2004). The process approach requires careful observation of the patient's strategy during each task and a follow-up of unusual approaches or errors by questioning or by the readministration of tasks with modified materials or instructions to clarify the nature of the specific deficit underlying poor performance (see Milberg et al., 1986). Thus, to understand how the neuropathological process has impacted response strategy, the examiner may "test the limits" by allowing the person more time to complete the problem or by providing specific structure or cueing not present in the standard administration format (Bauer, 2000). In general, the Boston Process Approach has been criticized for not having sufficient norms or detailed information regarding reliability and validity (e.g., Erickson, 1995; Slick et al., 1996). In addition, the practice of readministering tasks in a modified or nonstandard fashion complicates readministration. Thus, when patients have been evaluated using a process approach in the past, interpretation of results from readministration with the standard instrument should be done with caution. Process-based versions of well-known intelligence tests have been published (e.g., WAIS-R NI, WISC-IV Integrated), and recently, proponents of the Boston Process Approach have published versions of list-learning and executive functioning tasks that are normed and based on advancements in cognitive psychology (e.g., CVLT-2, D-KEFS). Parallel to this trend, researchers have attempted to quantify the process by which patients solve existing tests (e.g., by supplementing traditional memory tests with incidental and recognition tasks, by generating new indices of clustering and switching for fluency tasks; Poreh, 2000). These tests and techniques show promise in their ability to parse neuropsychological processes in a way that might allow a more detailed and thorough detection and characterization of neuropsychological deficits.

TEST ADMINISTRATION

Timing of Assessment

Lezak et al. (2004) recommend that formal assessment typically should not be done during the acute or postacute period. During the first 3 months, changes in the patient's status can be so rapid as to make test results obtained in one week obsolete by the next. In addition, fatigue often has significant deleterious effects during this period, making it difficult to evaluate actual patient competencies. Examiners should also bear in mind that both fatigue and awareness of poor performance can activate symptoms of depression and anxiety, which can further interfere with cognitive functioning and perpetuate and exacerbate symptoms. Accordingly, scheduling an initial assessment typically occurs within about three to six months after the event, unless early baseline testing is needed to document severity of deficits and to track progress over time.

The assessment may be needed for a variety of reasons including to determine if the individual is able to resume previous activities (e.g., employment, schooling); to evaluate competency (e.g., manage financial affairs); to ascertain strengths and weaknesses; to provide information for diagnostic purposes; to help determine the types of adaptations, supports, or remediations that may be needed; and to provide input regarding likely long-term outcome. The course of recovery is frequently prolonged (e.g., following traumatic brain injury), with many patients experiencing dramatic change in outcome from the time of insult to one year postevent (Dikmen et al., 1995). The rate of change tends to slow in subsequent years (Powell & Wilson, 1994). Accordingly, a second assessment may be needed about 6 to 12 months after the first to provide firmer opinions regarding outcome. In evolving conditions (e.g., dementia, MS, Parkinson's), additional assessments at one- or two-year intervals may also be useful (for a more complete discussion, see Lezak et al., 2004).

Amount of Time Required

Not surprisingly, a large amount of time is spent in test administration alone. We include administration times for the measures provided in this volume. A recent survey of U.S. clinical neuropsychologists revealed an average estimate of about five hours, with forensic evaluations taking considerably longer (Sweet et al., 2002). The reader can also refer to a useful survey from Lundin and DeFilippis (1999) pertaining to usual times to complete specific neuropsychological tests (note this refers to time to administer, score, interpret, and report).

Use of Psychometrists

Although many neuropsychologists prefer to administer the tests personally, test administration by a well-trained psychometrician is both accepted and widespread (Brandt & van Gorp, 1999; The NAN Policy and Planning Committee, 2000a). Sweet et al.'s (2000a; 2002) surveys showed that between 42% and 69% of neuropsychologists use a psychometrician. In general, neuropsychologists in private practice are less likely to use an assistant than clinicians employed in institutions. However, most (>75%) conducted the interview personally and most (>75%) observed the patient during some part of the testing. Record review, interpretation and report write-up, patient feedback, and consultation to the referral source are almost always (>80%) conducted by the clinician (Sweet et al., 2002).

Written Notes

Regardless of who does the testing (clinician, technician), it is important to keep detailed written notes about the patient's behaviors and responses during the course of the assessment. This is critical because the examiner may forget salient information or not realize its significance until after the examination is complete. It is also good practice to keep a continuous record of the order in which the tests were administered as well as the time used for each test and rest period. This helps later if the potential effects of interference or fatigue need clarification.

Computer Administration

This is becoming popular, in part because of the advantages offered to the neuropsychologist in terms of presentation format. Thus, extensive training is not required for the tester, and by limiting client/examiner interaction, a potential source of bias is removed and a truly standard administration is achieved. The computer provides precisely the same test each time; responses are automatically recorded and analyzed, also reducing error. The program can also be modified to allow considerable variation in test parameters. Another advantage is the ease with which different indices of performance can be obtained (e.g., accuracy, reaction time, variability). A number of tests have been specially developed for computer administration (e.g., ANAM: Bleiberg et al., 2000; CANTAB: Robbins et al., 1994; CARB: Condor et al., 1992; CPT-II: Connors & MHS staff, 2000; VSVT: Slick et al., 1997). However, close supervision is needed for computer-administered tests to ensure that the patient is able to follow instructions properly to provide valid results.

Computer-administered tests do not necessarily provide identical or even similar results as the same test administered by an examiner in person (Feldstein et al., 1999; Ozonoff, 1995; Van Schijndel & van der Vlugt, 1992). Hence, the existing normative data may not be applicable. For example, a study by Feldstein et al. (1999) compared the distribution properties of central tendency, variability, and shape (e.g., skewedness) between the manual version of the WCST and four computerized versions. None of the computerized versions was found to be equivalent to the manual version on all assessment measures, suggesting that norms provided for the standard version could not be used for the computer versions. Rather, new norms needed to be established for each computer version. A study by French and Beaumont (1987) compared automated and standard forms of 8 tests in 367 subjects: While some tests, including Raven's Progressive Matrices, the Mill Hill Vocabulary Test, and Eysenck's Personality Questionnaire, showed acceptable reliability, others, especially the Digit Span Test and the Differential Aptitude Test, produced quite low reliabilities. The authors concluded that some tests were not amenable to automation. It is also possible that computer administration can mask deficits that would otherwise be apparent in some populations. For example, some individuals (e.g., those with autism) may perform better when faced with a computer than a person, tapping cognitive functions at a level that is rarely demanded in real-life settings (Luciana, 2003). In short, using a computer for administration of standard tests requires demonstrating that meaningful and equivalent results can be obtained with computer testing. Moreover, there is some evidence that as computer-related anxiety increases, performance on computer administered measures tends to decrease (Browndyke et al., 2002).

Order of Administration

In general, test order has little impact on performance. For example, participants in the standardization sample took the WAIS-III and WMS-III in one session, in roughly counterbalanced order. There were few test-order effects noted (Zhu & Tulsky, 2000). When tests (e.g., WCST, Category Test) do show order of administration effects, the clinician should consider which of the instruments will provide the best information regarding the referral question and should use only that test for the patient.

There are a number of issues to consider with regard to ordering the tests. Thus, test administration does require careful planning to avoid interference effects. For example, various memory tests call for the recall of stimuli after a period of 10 to 30 minutes. While the examiner may wish to fill this delay with other tasks, it is important that tests with similar visual or verbal content be avoided because the patient may substitute the content of intervening tests during the delayed recall of the first test.

There are other considerations as well. For example, some measures (e.g., broad-ranging measures such as Wechsler Intelligence Scales) are frequently placed early in the examination to answer initial questions and to generate hypotheses regarding spared and impaired functions. Others (e.g., relatively easy ones) may be saved for last so that the patient leaves with a sense of success. Certain measures of motivational status are best placed at the very beginning of a neuropsychological examination. Some of these tasks (e.g., Rey 15-Item, 21-Item) likely will prove less sensitive to exaggeration if used reactively (i.e., if used midway through the evaluation after suspicions of biased effort have been raised). The patient will have been exposed to a variety of difficult neuropsychological measures so that these tasks will appear relatively simple and straightforward.

NEUROPSYCHOLOGICAL ASSESSMENT

Informed Consent

The 2002 APA Ethics Code, effective June 1, 2003, specifies the need for informed consent for assessments, evaluations, or diagnostic services, albeit with several exceptions in which patient assent represents the appropriate standard of care (Johnson-Greene, 2005). The code states that consent should include (a) an explanation of the nature and purpose of the assessment, (b) fees, (c) involvement of third parties, and (d) limits of confidentiality. The examinee should also be provided with sufficient opportunity to ask questions and receive answers. Johnson-Greene (2005) states that there are also good practical and ethical reasons to provide information concerning the referral source, foreseeable risks, discomforts and benefits, and time commitment, as such elements may well be intrinsic to consent that really is adequately informed.

Informed consent is not required in some instances in which assent, as defined as the absence of objection to assessment procedures, would be considered sufficient. Such situations include the following (Johnson-Greene, 2005): (a) testing is mandated by law or governmental regulations, (b) informed consent is implied because testing is conducted as a routine educational, institutional, or organizational activity, or (c) where the purpose of testing is to evaluate decisional capacity. In such cases, as well as with children, patients should be provided with basic information about the procedures, their preferences should be noted, and their assent should be documented along with the consent of a legally authorized person. Forensic cases are viewed similarly in that a normal doctor-patient relationship does not exist but the basic components of patient assent would be expected (Johnson-Greene, 2005). Persons undergoing forensic evaluations may also be precluded from receiving an explanation of their test results normally afforded to patients, which should be explained in advance of any forensic evaluation (Johnson-Greene, 2005).

The National Academy of Neuropsychology strongly encourages neuropsychologists to provide informed consent to patients seeking services and views its conveyance as a basic professional and ethical responsibility. A flowchart (Johnson-Greene, 2005) is provided in Figure 4–1, which outlines the process of determining consent content and conveyance. A sample informed consent document (Johnson-Greene, 2005) is provided in Figure 4–2.

Additional Considerations

Relatively little attention has been paid to the consumer side of neuropsychological assessments (see also Prigatano, 2000). To be of maximum benefit to the patient, however, the neuropsychologist should be prepared to follow some of the basic rules that emerged from a mail follow-up of 129 outpatients seen in five Australian centers. These rules would seem to apply equally to other geographic locations (adapted from Bennett-Levy et al., 1994):

- *Patient Preparation.* Patients are usually not prepared for what to expect during an assessment. Sixty percent of the patients in the study had no information on what to expect or were unaware that the assessment

Figure 4–1 Flowchart for informed consent. *Source:* Johnson-Greene, 2005. Reprinted with permission from Elsevier.

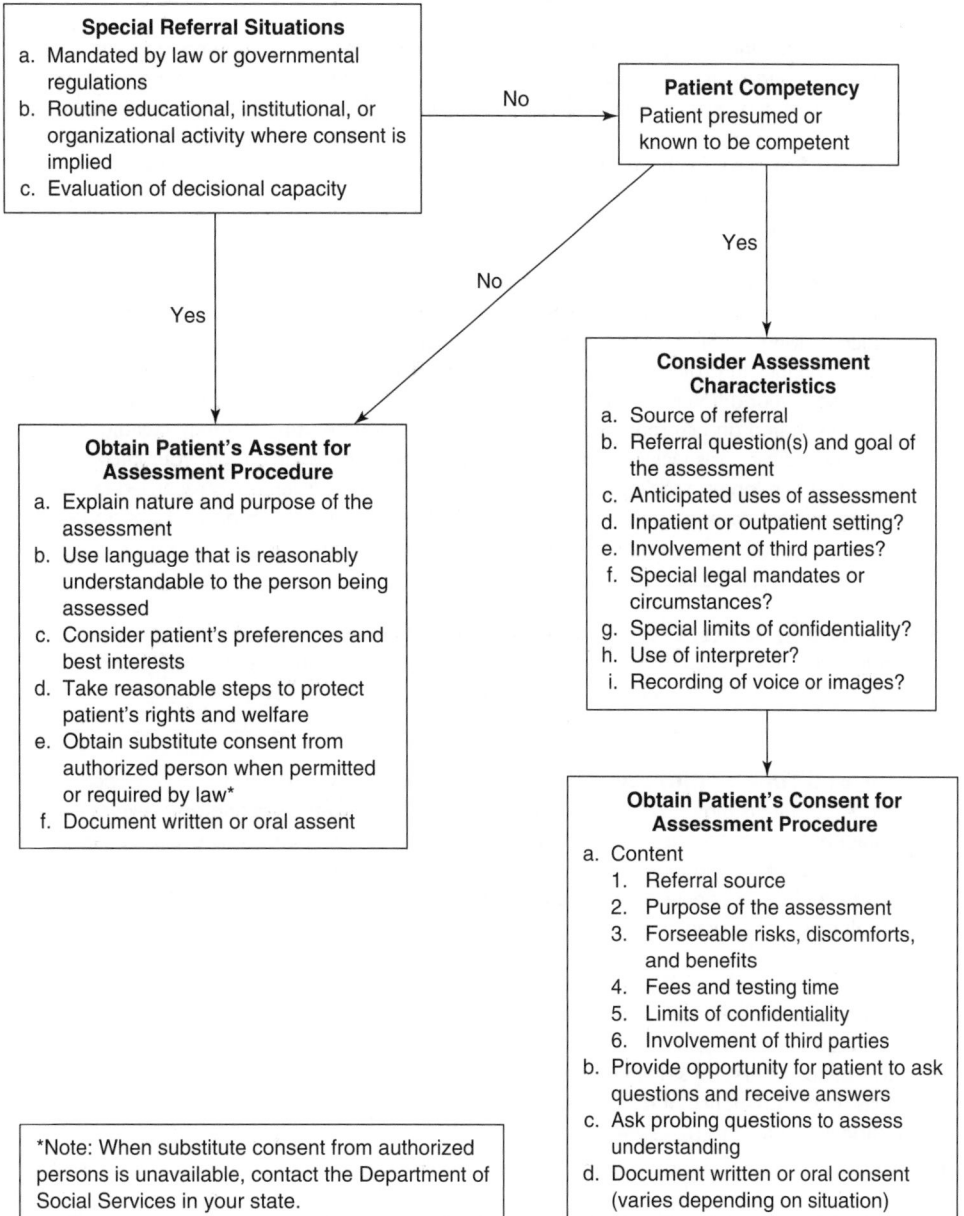

could take up to three hours. This can be remedied by educating referring agents, sending an informative letter before the assessment (e.g., who will be performing the assessment, how long it will last, what to bring), and giving an introduction before the beginning of testing that can be tailored for children and adults (see also Hebben & Milberg, 2002; Sattler, 2001; and Figure 4–2).
- *Provision of feedback.* Feedback on strengths and problem areas with suggestions about how to get around problem areas is recommended.
- *Presence of third parties/recordings.* Inviting a relative to accompany the patient may be beneficial to alleviate

anxiety, but may also help in history taking and in the informing interview. In most cases, the accompanying person should be interviewed separately to avoid embarrassment to both patient and interviewee. Also, the discrepancies between statements made by the informant and the patient may provide clues about the patient's insight or awareness of deficits and about the effects of such deficits on daily functioning. However, the presence of third-party observers in the test situation (or behind one-way mirrors or via electronic recording) is generally discouraged since it creates the potential for distraction and may increase the risk that motivational disturbances may impact

Figure 4–2 Sample informed consent. *Source:* Johnson–Greene (2005). Reprinted with permission from Elsevier.

Please note that this is a general template for informed consent that may not apply to your specific jurisdiction. It is recommended that psychologists seek advice from personal counsel to determine if this consent is appropriate for their specific jurisdictions.

Referral Source: You have been referred for a neuropsychological assessment (i.e., evaluation of your thinking abilities) by _____ (name of referral source).

Nature and Purpose of Assessment: The goal of neuropsychological assessment is to determine if any changes have occurred in your attention, memory, language, problem solving, or other cognitive functions. A neuropsychological assessment may point to changes in brain function and suggest possible methods and treatments for rehabilitation. In addition to an interview where we will be asking you questions about your background and current medical symptoms, we may be using different techniques and standardized tests including but not limited to asking questions about your knowledge of certain topics, reading, drawing figures and shapes, listening to recorded tapes, viewing printed material, and manipulating objects. Other specific goals and anticipated uses of the information we gather today include the following: _____ _____

Foreseeable Risks, Discomforts, and Benefits: For some individuals, assessments can cause fatigue, frustration, and anxiousness. Other anticipated risks, discomforts, and benefits associated with this assessment include the following: _____ _____

Fees and Time Commitment: The hourly fee for this assessment is _____ per hour. Assessments may take several hours or more of face-to-face testing and several additional hours for scoring, interpretation, and report preparation. This evaluation is estimated to take approximately _____ hours of face-to-face assessment time. Though the fees are generally covered by insurance, patients are responsible for any and all fees for the assessment.

Limits of Confidentiality: Information obtained during assessments is confidential and can ordinarily be released only with your written permission. There are some special circumstances that can limit confidentiality, including (a) a statement of intent to harm self or others, (b) statements indicating harm or abuse of children or vulnerable adults, and (c) issuance of a subpoena from a court of law. Other foreseeable limits to confidentiality for this assessment include: _____ _____

I have read and agree with the nature and purpose of this assessment and to each of the points listed above. I have had an opportunity to clarify any questions and discuss any points of concern before signing.

_____   _____

Patient Signature   Date

_____   _____

Parent/Guardian or Authorized Surrogate (if applicable)   Date

_____   _____

Witness Signature   Date

test performance (the NAN Policy and Planning Committee, 2000b). Thus, even audio recording affects neuropsychological test performance. Constantinou et al. (2002) found that in the presence of an audio recorder, the performance of participants on memory (but not motor) tests declined. Also bear in mind that neuropsychological test measures have been standardized under a specific set of highly controlled circumstances that did not include the presence of a third-party observer. Therefore, the presence of a third-party observer may represent a threat to the validity and reliability of the data generated under such circumstances. In addition, exposure of test procedures to nonpsychologists jeopardizes the validity of these methods for future use (The NAN Policy and Planning Committee, 2000c). Note, however, that there are circumstances that support the presence of a neutral party in nonforensic situations (e.g., in the training of students; a parent providing a calming influence during the evaluation of a child).

- *Reduction of stress.* The patient's anxiety should be alleviated as much as possible. The testing experience can have a significant impact on self-confidence. Reassurance that not all items of a test can be completed by most clients or that on some tests (e.g., PAI, MMPI-2) there are no "correct" answers should be provided routinely. Most clients understand that a test contains high-difficulty items to avoid a ceiling effect for very bright subjects.

- *Reduction of discomfort/fatigue.* A comfortable testing environment should be provided, and the patient should be asked how it can be made more comfortable. More than 90% of clients in the Bennett-Levy study mentioned that it was too hot, too cold, or too noisy. Some patients complain of backache; the availability of a back support may alleviate these complaints. Children should be provided with appropriately sized desks and chairs. Adequate rest breaks and hot and cold refreshments should be provided. Usually, a break after 1½ hours of testing is indicated. The patient should be offered the choice of a one-session assessment, or a split one. Seventy-two percent of clients in the Bennett-Levy study stated that, for a 3-hour assessment, they would have preferred two sessions instead of one.

Cooperation/Effort

In situations where the client is a "third party" (i.e., in forensic assessments where the psychologist works for the defendant or insurer, ostensibly "against" the client), the client should be assured that the aim of the assessment is to provide a valid picture of his or her strengths and weaknesses. The client should be encouraged to cooperate fully to avoid misleading results.

Most patients who are referred for neuropsychological examinations try to perform optimally, particularly if they understand the reasons for testing and that their efforts may improve their opportunities with regard to their treatment, job, or school performance. We rarely encounter clients who refuse outright to collaborate. In such cases, a repeated brief discussion of the purpose of the assessment and/or a break is indicated. If a patient refuses to collaborate on a given test, switching to a very different test may be an option. General refusal to cooperate, though extremely rare, should be accepted by the examiner, who then discontinues the session. In such cases, offer the patient a face-saving way out of the situation by assuring him or her that the tests can be scheduled at another time when the patient feels better or if he or she changes his or her mind. Test refusal in children may also indicate poor underlying skills (Mäntynen et al., 2001).

Some patients, however, do not display optimal effort. This may occur for a variety of reasons. For example, the person may be ill, may not understand the reasons for the assessment, or may gain (e.g., financially) from poor performance. A recent survey (Slick et al., 2004) revealed that experts rely on indicators of suboptimal performance from conventional tests and always give at least one symptom validity test, although the precise measure varies from one expert to another. There was no firm consensus on when the tests should be given or whether warnings at the outset of testing should be provided. Once suspicion is aroused, however, experts typically alter test routines. They administer additional symptom validity tests and encourage clients to give good effort. On occasion, they discontinue entirely the testing session.

Testing of Children

When testing children or adolescents, the establishment of a good rapport is especially important. As with adults, an attitude of acceptance, understanding, and respect for the patient is more important than entertaining tricks to establish and maintain rapport. Older children may think of the testing as similar to a school test situation, which may evoke fear of failure and anxiety. The use of reinforcements such as stickers or tokens used in many schools may contribute to better cooperation. However, at present, there is little evidence that scores obtained using tangible or social reinforcement provide better estimates of children's abilities than those obtained under standard administration conditions (Sattler, 2001). It should also be noted that most tests were not standardized with the use of incentives. Therefore, their use should be reserved for exceptional circumstances (e.g., an extremely uncooperative child) and their use should be noted in the test protocol and report. Reassurance and encouragement for the effort may work better than praise for correct responses, because most tests progress from easy to difficult items, where failure is inevitable (Sattler, 2001). Younger children and children with behavior problems may try to manipulate the examiner by asking questions, refusing to answer, getting up, constantly asking for breaks, or even displaying open hostility or leaving the testing room. This can be avoided by changing to tasks with which the examinee is more comfortable. The examiner should keep in mind that the behavior of the child does not reflect on the examiner, but shows a manner of "coping" the child may use in similar situations and that is a clinically relevant piece of information. The examiner should also note whether refusals to cooperate occur only with certain types of tasks (e.g., young children with aphasic disturbances may act out during verbally challenging tasks but show interest in nonverbal tasks). Open confrontation ("Do you want to do this, or should I send you back to your parents?") should be avoided. In cases of outright test refusal, although test scores may not be interpretable (i.e., scores could be poor due to refusal or to inability), the testing behavior itself will still be informative, particularly when taken in the context of other sources of information (e.g., parents' and teachers' questionnaires). It is important to note that it may be better to discontinue testing altogether in an uncooperative child than to obtain test data that may lead to erroneous estimates of cognitive ability. Retesting can be attempted when the child is older or when the testing situation is less stressful for the child (e.g., following discharge from hospital or after family intervention).

Testing Older Adults

When evaluating older adults, it is critical that the examiner determine that the patient's vision and audition are sufficient for adequate task performance, and if not, to assist him or her to compensate for any losses (Lezak et al., 2004). Storandt (1994) discusses characteristics of elderly patients that may affect the progress and the results of the assessment: for the overly loquacious, usually elderly adult who may frequently stray off-target and may relay long personal stories while being tested, Storandt recommends a pleasant but businesslike attitude on the part of the examiner, deferring all discussions to the end of the session, explaining that during testing there is much to be covered. Again, the examiner should be aware that tangential and overly talkative behavior may be clinically significant and be evidence of possible executive or comprehension difficulties. In contrast, the depressed or despondent patient may require considerable encouragement and patience from the examiner (and also more time). In all cases, it is important that the examiner maintains a friendly, neutral attitude and be aware of countertranference issues (e.g., viewing the elderly patient as a parent, showing irritation toward a difficult child).

Circadian arousal may impact performance, at least in older adults (May & Hasher, 1998; Paradee et al., 2005). There is evidence that when older adults are tested at their nonoptimal times (i.e., evening), processing is compromised. Thus, time of testing must be considered in the administration of tasks to allow appropriate assessment of behavior in both single-test and test-retest situations. It is also possible that normative data need to be reevaluated with testing time controlled (May & Hasher, 1998).

Test Modifications and Testing Patients With Special Needs or English as a Second Language

With patients who have significant disabilities (e.g., problems with vision, audition, or the use of upper limbs), it is often necessary to modify standard testing procedures, either by allowing more time or by using modifications of the response mode (e.g., pointing rather than giving a verbal response). Most modifications invalidate the existing norms, although they may lead to valid inferences. Braden (2003) noted that the essential purpose of accommodations is to maintain assessment validity by decreasing (and hopefully eliminating) construct irrelevant variance. He noted that assessments are intended to measure certain constructs; however, the process may capture other, unintended constructs. For example, a low score on the Wechsler Performance Scale in a vision-impaired client confounds visual acuity with the construct intended to be measured (fluid intelligence). However, clinicians may underrepresent the construct of interest when they use methods that fail to capture adequately the intended construct. Thus, omitting the Performance Scale would reduce construct irrelevant variance but may underrepresent the construct of intelligence (limiting it to an assessment of crystallized ability). The clinician might ensure representation of fluid abilities by including an orally administered test of fluid abilities (e.g., a verbal analogies test) along with the standard Wechsler verbal subtests. Accommodations must balance the need to reduce construct irrelevant variance with the simultaneous goal of maintaining construct representation, or they run the risk of invalidating the assessment results (Braden 2003). Any accommodations should be clearly noted on the test protocols as well as stated in the report, and any conclusions (including limitations in representing the construct) should be qualified appropriately (see Braden, 2003, and Sattler, 2001, for suggestions on test administration for visually impaired and other populations).

The bilingual patient with English as a second language deserves specific considerations. Even though the patient's English may appear fully fluent, some first-language habits, such as silent counting and spelling in the first language, frequently persist and may invalidate some test results requiring these skills (e.g., digit repetition, recitation of the alphabet). Language preference and the amount and quality of education received within North America significantly impact cognitive performance, even when traditional demographic variables (e.g., age, level of education) are taken into account (Harris et al., 2003). If the examinee does not indicate a preference for English and is only a recent resident in North America, then his or her scores may be adversely affected, and as the individual diverges from the standardization sample, the norms may become less meaningful (Harris et al., 2003; O'Bryant et al., 2004). If the examination proceeds in English, then this should be noted in the report.

Even more problems are posed by the patient with poor English and different sociocultural experiences; this may invalidate not only verbal tests, but also the so-called nonverbal and culture-free tests with complex instructions. Sociocultural effects have been reported even for seemingly nonverbal tasks, such as the TPT, Seashore Rhythm, Category Test, and Performance portions of the WAIS-III (e.g., Arnold et al., 1994; Harris et al., 2003; Shuttleworth-Edwards et al., 2004b). Of note, recent research suggests that the WAIS-III Digit Symbol-Incidental Learning optional procedure (Pairing and Free Recall) may be a relatively culture-independent task with utility as a neuropsychological screening instrument. Shuttleworth-Edwards et al. (2004a) gave the task to a South African sample stratified for ethnicity in association with language of origin (white English first language versus black African first language), education level (grade 12, graduate), and quality of education (advantaged, disadvantaged). They found no significant differences for ethnicity/language of origin and level or quality of education.

The psychologist may wish to resort to an interpreter, but interpreters are not skilled clinicians and good practice suggests that the patient be referred to a colleague who is fully fluent in that language (Artiola I Fortuny & Mullaney, 1998). In addition to limited clinical skills of interpreters, there is no way for the clinician to assess whether clinician and patient statements are in fact translated accurately, which seriously undermines any conclusions that are made from interview data. Inability to communicate directly makes it difficult to assess not only the patient's statements, but also the quality and fluency of the language produced, the modulations of phrasing, the mood, and the level of cooperation (Artiola I Fortuny & Mullaney, 1998). However, in the event of a highly uncommon language and the unavailability of a colleague from the patient's country or linguistic group, use of an interpreter may be unavoidable. Artiola I Fortuny and Mullaney state that in such cases, a professional interpreter or an individual with advanced fluency should be used. Friends or relatives of the patient should not be used because of the potential to contaminate data collection in ways that the neuropsychologist cannot appreciate. It should be noted that a simple translation of English-language tests may also distort the results. In particular, translated verbal tests may not be equivalent to the original English version in terms of lexical difficulty, lexical frequency, linguistic correctness, and cultural relevance and thus invalidate the available norms. The use of foreign-language versions of existing tests (e.g., the Wechsler Scales are available in a large number of foreign adaptations; see Harris et al., 2003, for a recent listing) may be appropriate, but this approach may also lead to problems: A test adapted and standardized for Spain or France may not contain items appropriate for Spanish-speaking Americans or for Quebec Francophones, nor would the published norms for such tests be valid. Fortunately, some local (e.g., Hispanic, French-Canadian) language versions have been developed, and these are listed together with foreign adaptations in the test descriptions of this book. In addition, a number of authors have published instruments with normative data applicable to Spanish-speaking populations (e.g., Artiola I Fortuny et al., 1999; Ostroski-Solis et al., 1999), although issues of reliability and validity (e.g., impact of racial socialization, sensitivity to neurological insult) require further study. For a more complete discussion of cross-cultural and minority concerns pertaining to assessment, see Artiola I Fortuny et al. (2005), Ferraro (2002), Gasquoine (2001), Manly et al. (2002), Ponton and Leon-Carrion (2001), and Shuttleworth-Edwards et al. (2004a, 2004b), as well as Chapter 2 in this volume.

REFERENCES

Arnold, B. R., Montgomery, G. T., Castaneda, I., & Longoria, R. (1994). Acculturation and performance of Hispanics on selected Halstead-Reitan neuropsychological tests. *Assessment, 1*, 239–248.

Artiola I Fortuny, L., & Mullaney, H. A. (1998). Assessing patients whose language you do not know: Can the absurd be ethical? *The Clinical Neuropsychologist, 12*, 113–126.

Artiola I Fortuny, L., Romo, D. H., Heaton, R. K., & Pardee, R. E. (1999). *Manual de normas y procedimeintos para la bateria neuropsicologica en espanol*. Lisse, the Netherlands: Swets & Zeitlinger.

Artiola I Fortuny, L., Garola, M., Romo, D. H., Feldman, E., Barillas, F., Keefe, R., Lemaitre, M. J., Martin, A. O., Mirsky, A., Monguio, I., Morote, G., Parchment, S., Parchment, L. J., de Pena, E., Politis, D. G., Sedo, M. A., Taussik, I., Valdivia, F., de Valdivia, L. S., & Maestre, K. V. (2005). Research with Spanish-speaking populations in the United States: Lost in translation. A commentary and a plea. *Journal of Clinical and Experimental Neuropsychology, 27*, 555–564.

Bauer, R. M. (2000). The flexible battery approach to neuropsychological assessment. In R. D. Vanderploeg (Ed.), *Clinician's guide to neuropsychological assessment* (2nd ed., pp. 419–448). Mahwah, NJ: LEA.

Bennett-Levy, J., Klein-Boonschate, M. A., Batchelor, J., McCarter, R. & Walton, N. (1994). Encounters with Anna Thompson: The consumer's experience of neuropsychological assessments. *The Clinical Neuropsychologist, 8*, 219–238.

Bleiberg, J., Kane, R. L., Reeves, D. L., Garmoe, W. S., & Halpern, E. (2000). Factor analysis of computerized and traditional tests used in mild brain injury research. *The Clinical Neuropsychologist, 14*, 287–294.

Braden, J. P. (2003). Accommodating clients with disabilities on the WAIS-III and WMS. In D. Tulsky, R. K. Saklofske, G. Heaton, G. Chelune, R. A. Ivnik, R. A. Bornstein, A. Prifitera, & M. Ledbetter, (Eds.), *Clinical interpretation of the WAIS-III and WMS-III*. San Diego, CA: Academic Press.

Brandt, J., & van Gorp, W. G. (1999). American Academy of Clinical Neuropsychology policy on the use of non-doctoral-level personnel in conducting clinical neuropsychological evaluations. *The Clinical Neuropsychologist, 13*, 385.

Browndyke, J. N., Albert, A. L., Malone, W., Schatz, P., Paul, R. H., Cohen, R. A., Tucker, K. A., & Gouvier, W. D. (2002). Computer-related anxiety: Examining the impact of technology-specific affect on the performance of a computerized neuropsychological assessment measure. *Applied Neuropsychology, 4*, 210–218.

Condor, R., Allen, L., & Cox, D. (1992). *Computerized assessment of response bias test manual*. Durham, NC: Cognisyst.

Conners, C. K., & MHS Staff. (2000). *Conners' Continuous Performance Test II (CPT II)*. Toronto, Ontario: Multi-Health Systems, Inc.

Constantinou, M., Ashendorf, L., & McCaffrey, R. J. (2002). When the third party observer of a neuropsychological examination is an audio-recorder. *The Clinical Neuropsychologist, 16*, 407–412.

Dikmen, S. S., Machamer, J. E., Winn, H. R., & Temkin, N. R. (1995). Neuropsychological outcome at 1-year post head injury. *Neuropsychology, 9*, 80–91.

Erickson, R. C. (1995). A review and critique of the process approach in neuropsychological assessment. *Neuropsychology Review, 5*, 223–243.

Feldstein, S. N., Keller, F. R., Portman, R. E., Durham, R. L., Klebe, K. J., & Davis, H. P. (1999). A comparison of computerized and standard versions of the Wisconsin Card Sorting Test. *The Clinical Neuropsychologist, 13*, 303–313.

Ferraro, F. R. (Ed.). (2002). *Minority and cross-cultural aspects of neuropsychological assessment. Studies on neuropsychology, development, and cognition.* Bristol, PA: Swets & Zeitlinger Publishers.

French, C. C., & Beaumont, J. G. (1987). The reaction of psychiatric patients to computerized assessment. *British Journal of Clinical Psychology, 26*, 267–278.

Gasquoine, P. G. (2001). Research in clinical neuropsychology with Hispanic American participants: A review. *The Clinical Neuropsychologist, 15*, 2–12.

Harris, J. G., Tulsky, D. S., & Schultheis, M. T. (2003). Assessment of the non-native English speaker: Assimilating history and research findings to guide clinical practice. In D. S. Tulsky, D. H. Saklofske, G. J. Chelune, R. K. Heaton, R. J. Ivnik, R. Bornstein, A. Prifitera, & M. F. Ledbetter (Eds.), *Clinical Interpretation of the WAIS-III and WMS-III.* New York: Academic Press.

Hebben, N., & Milberg, W. (2002). *Essentials of neuropsychological assessment.* New York: John Wiley & Sons.

Hunsley, J. (2002). Psychological testing and psychological assessment: A closer examination. *American Psychologist, 57*, 139–140.

Kaplan, E. (1988). A process approach to neuropsychological assessment. In T. Boll & B. K. Bryant (Eds.), *Clinical neuropsychology and brain function: Research, measurement, and practice* (pp. 127–167). Washington, DC: American Psychological Association.

Johnson-Greene, D. (2005). Informed consent in clinical neuropsychology practice. Official statement of the National Academy of Neuropsychology. *Archives of Clinical Neuropsychology, 20*, 335–340.

Lezak, M. D., Howieson, D. B., & Loring, D. W. (2004). *Neuropsychological assessment* (4th ed.). New York: Oxford University Press.

Luciana, M. (2003). Practitioner review: Computerized assessment of neuropsychological function in children: Clinical and research applications of the Cambridge Neuropsychological Testing Automated Battery (CANTAB). *Journal of Child Psychology and Psychiatry, 44*, 649–663.

Lundin, K. A., & DeFilippis, N. A. (1999). Proposed schedule of usual and customary test administration times. *The Clinical Neuropsychologist, 13*, 433–436.

Manly, J. L., Jacobs, D. M., Touradji, P., Small, S. A., & Stern, Y. (2002). Reading level attenuates differences in neuropsychological test performance between African American and White elders. *Journal of the International Neuropsychological Society, 8*, 341–348.

Mäntynen, H., Poikkeus, A. M., Ahonen, T., Aro, T., & Korkman, M. (2001). Clinical significance of test refusal among young children. *Child Neurology, 7*, 241–250.

May, C. P., & Hasher, L. (1998). Synchrony effects in inhibitory control over thought and action. *Journal of Experimental Psychology: Human Perception and Performance, 24*, 363–379.

Meyer, G. L., Finn, S. E., Eyde, L. D., Kay, G. G., Moreland, K. L., Dies, R. R., Eisman, E. J., Kubiszyn, T. W., & Reed, G. M. (2001). Psychological testing and psychological assessment: A review of evidence and issues. *American Psychologist, 56*, 128–165.

Milberg, W. P., Hebben, N., & Kaplan, E. (1986). The Boston process approach to neuropsychological assessment. In I. Grant & K. M. Adams (Eds.), *Neuropsychological assessment of neuropsychiatric disorders* (pp. 65–86). New York: Oxford University Press.

Miller, L. S., & Rohling, M. L. (2001). A statistical interpretive method for neuropsychological test data. *Neuropsychology Review, 11*, 143–169.

The NAN Policy and Planning Committee. (2000a). The use of neuropsychology test technicians in clinical practice: Official statement of the National Academy of Neuropsychology. *Archives of Clinical Neuropsychology, 15, 381.*

The NAN Policy and Planning Committee. (2000b). Presence of third party observers during neuropsychological testing: Official statement of the National Academy of Neuropsychology. *Archives of Clinical Neuropsychology, 15, 379.*

The NAN Policy and Planning Committee. (2000c). Test security: Official statement of the National Academy of Neuropsychology. *Archives of Clinical Neuropsychology, 15*, 383–386.

O'Bryant, S. E., O'Jile, J. R., & McCaffrey, R. J. (2004). Reporting of demographic variables in neuropsychological research: Trends in the current literature. *The Clinical Neuropsychologist, 18*, 229–233.

Oestreicher, J. M. & O'Donnell, J. P. (1995) Validation of the General Neuropsychological Deficit Scale with nondisabled, learning-disabled, and head-injured young adults. *Archives of Clinical Neuropsychology, 10*, 185–191.

Ostrosky-Solis, F., Ardila, A., & Rosselli, M. (1999). NEUROPSI: A brief neuropsychological test battery in Spanish with norms by age and educational level. *Journal of the International Neuropsychological Society, 5*, 413–433.

Ozonoff, S. (1995). Reliability and validity of the Wisconsin Card Sorting Test in studies of autism. *Neuropsychologia, 9*, 491–500.

Paradee, C. V., Rapport, L. J., Hanks, R. A., & Levy, J. A. (2005). Circadian preference and cognitive functioning among rehabilitation inpatients. *The Clinical Neuropsychologist, 19*, 55–72.

Ponton, M. O., & Leon-Carrion, J. (2001). *Neuropsychology and the Hispanic patient: A clinical handbook.* Mahwah, NJ: Lawrence Erlbaum Associates.

Poreh, A. M. (2000). The quantified process approach: An emerging methodology to neuropsychological assessment. *The Clinical Neuropsychologist, 14*, 212–222.

Powell, G. E., & Wilson, S. L. (1994). Recovery curves for patients who have suffered very severe brain injury. *Clinical Rehabilitation, 8*, 54–69.

Prigatano, G. P. (2000). Neuropsychology, the patient's experience, and the political forces within our field. *Archives of Clinical Neuropsychology, 15*, 71–82.

Reitan, R. M., & Wolfson, D. (1988). *Traumatic brain injury: Recovery and rehabilitation.* Tucson, AZ: Neuropsychology Press.

Robbins, T., James, M., Owen, A., Sahakian, B., McInnes, L., & Rabbitt, P. (1994). The Cambridge Neuropsychological Test Automated Battery (CANTAB): A factor analytic study in a large number of elderly volunteers. *Dementia, 5*, 266–281.

Rohling, M. L., Williamson, D. J., Miller, L. S., & Adams, R. L. (2003). Using the Halstead-Reitan Battery to diagnose brain damage: A comparison of the predictive power of traditional techniques to Rohling's Interpretive Method. *The Clinical Neuropsychologist, 17*, 531–543.

Russell, E. W. (2000a). The cognitive-metric, fixed battery approach to neuropsychological assessment. In R. D. Vanderploeg (Ed.), *Clinician's guide to neuropsychological assessment* (2nd ed., pp. 449–481). Mahwah, NJ: LEA.

Russell, E. W. (2000b). The application of computerized scoring programs to neuropsychological assessment. In R. D. Vanderploeg (Ed.), *Clinician's guide to neuropsychological assessment* (2nd ed., pp. 483–515). Mahwah, NJ: LEA.

Sattler, J. M. (2001). *Assessment of children: Cognitive applications* (4th ed.). San Diego: J. M. Sattler.

Shuttleworth-Edwards, A. B., Donnelly, M. J. R., Reid, I., & Radloff, S. E. (2004a). A cross-cultural study with culture fair normative indications on WAIS-III Digit Symbol-Incidental Learning. *Journal of Clinical and Experimental Neuropsychology, 26,* 921–932.

Shuttleworth-Edwards, A. B., Kemp, R. D., Rust, A. L., Muirhead, G. G. L., Hartman, N. P., & Radloff, S. E. (2004b). Cross-cultural effects on IQ test performance: A review and preliminary normative indications on WAIS-III test performance. *Journal of Clinical and Experimental Neuropsychology, 26,* 903–920.

Slick, D., Hopp, G., Strauss, E., Fox, D., Pinch, D., & Stickgold, K. (1996). Effects of prior testing with the WAIS-R NI on subsequent retest with the WAIS-R. *Archives of Clinical Neuropsychology, 11,* 123–130.

Slick, D., Hopp, G., Strauss, E., & Thompson, G. B. (1997). *Victoria Symptom Validity Test.* Odessa, FL: PAR.

Slick, D. J., Tan, J. E., Strauss, E. H., & Hultsch, D. F. (2004). Detecting malingering: A survey of Experts' practices. *Archives of Clinical Neuropsychology, 19,* 465–473.

Storandt, M. (1994). General principles of assessment of older adults. In M. Storandt & G. R. Vanden Bos (Eds.), *Neuropsychological assessment of dementia and depression.* Washington, DC: American Psychological Association.

Sweet, J. J., Moberg, P. J., & Sucy, Y. (2000a). Ten-year follow-up survey of clinical neuropsychologists: Part 1. Practices and beliefs. *The Clinical Neuropsychologist, 14,* 18–37.

Sweet, J. J., Moberg, P. J., & Sucy, Y. (2000b). Ten-year follow-up survey of clinical neuropsychologists: Part II. Private practices and economics. *The Clinical Neuropsychologist, 14,* 479–495.

Sweet, J. J., Peck, E. A., Abramowitz, C., & Etzweiler, S. (2002). National Academy of Neuropsychology/Division 40 of the American Psychological Association Practice Survey of clinical neuropsychology, part 1: Practitioner and practice characteristics, professional activities, and time requirements. *The Clinical Neuropsychologist, 16,* 109–127.

Turner, S. M., DeMers, S. T., Fox, H. R., & Reed, G. M. (2001). APA's guidelines for test user qualifications: An executive summary. *American Psychologist, 12,* 1099–1113.

Van Schijndel, F. A. A., & van der Vlugt, H. (1992). Equivalence between classical neuropsychological tests and their computer version: Four neuropsychological tests put to the test. *Journal of Clinical and Experimental Neuropsychology, 14,* 45 (abstract).

Zhu, J., & Tulsky, D. S. (2000). Co-norming the WAIS-III and WMS-III: Is there a test-order effect on IQ and memory scores? *The Clinical Neuropsychologist, 14,* 461–467.

5

Report Writing and Feedback Sessions

THE NEUROPSYCHOLOGICAL REPORT

Ultimately, the purpose of the neuropsychological assessment is to answer the referral question; practically speaking, the assessment serves to meet the needs of the referring party while helping the patient. In all cases, a report is prepared that reflects background, test findings, observations, and recommendations. Neuropsychological assessment reports vary greatly in format, content, and language; no fixed format is appropriate for all purposes. Nevertheless, the steps in preparing the report are often similar across settings; these will be outlined in this chapter. Additional guidelines on report writing for the neuropsychologist can be found in Axelrod (2000), Baron (2004), Hebben and Milberg (2002), and Williams and Boll (2000). Sample neuropsychological reports are presented in these texts as well as in Donders (1999) and other sources. For general guides on report writing, see Ownby (1997), Sattler (2001), and Tallent (1993). This chapter will cover style, content, confidentiality, computer use, and other relevant issues in report writing.

Wording

Wording should be kept as clear and simple as possible regardless of whom the recipient of the report is. In particular, psychological jargon and acronyms should be avoided and technical terms, if necessary, should be explained. When choosing wording, it must be kept in mind that in many cases the patient or family will read the report (see *Feedback Session*). In addition, the report is likely to be read by many other individuals other than the referring party and will likely remain on file for several years to come (e.g., as part of a hospital chart or permanent school record). Consequently, wording must be carefully and deliberately chosen, with an avoidance of unsubstantiated statements, wording that minimizes the individual, and terms with unnecessarily negative connotations (i.e., the patient should not be described as "a 43-year-old hemiplegic," but rather as "a 43-year-old man with

hemiplegia"). The patient should be referred to by name rather than as "the patient" (Hebben & Milberg, 2002). A clinician's thesaurus for wording psychological reports (American Psychological Association [APA], 1997; Zuckerman, 1995) and dictionary of neuropsychological terms (Loring, 1999) may be useful for choosing appropriate, precise, and comprehensible wording.

Style and Length

The report should be problem-oriented and should clearly answer the referral question. Depending on the recipient, the style and length of reports will vary and can be as informal as letters, as brief as a consultation form, or as comprehensive as a narrative report (Axelrod, 2000). The length of a report also depends on the purpose and on the complexity of the findings. However, the report should be kept as brief as possible by avoiding irrelevant or redundant information. Duplication of information readily available from other sources should be avoided. This only adds bulk to the report and wastes both the writer's and the reader's time. The guiding principle for inclusion should be whether the information is relevant to the purposes of the report and whether it contributes to a clearer understanding of the current test findings, interpretations, and recommendations.

Ideally, the report should be written in short sentences to maximize clarity. The report should also "contain enough information so an educated lay person will be able to grasp the major ideas, conclusions, and recommendations" (Axelrod, 2000, p. 247). However, too much information, particularly when paired with excessive verbosity, is aversive to readers. Further, lengthy and wordy reports are less likely to be read in full by the recipient: a busy physician may read no more than the summary statement. Brevity can be maximized by covering normal-range test results in a single sentence (e.g., "All other test results were in the normal range"; "Motor and sensory testing showed average results without significant side differences").

In some settings, a single-page report may be perfectly adequate. A recent survey by Donders (2001) found a mean length of seven pages for neuropsychological reports. Those surveyed included clinicians whose reports routinely were only one page long while others regularly prepared reports of 30 pages or more. Donders (1999) pleaded for brevity in reports dealing with children; he provides an example report that is only one to two pages in length.

Privacy and Confidential Information

Information that is valid but not relevant to the referral question (e.g., dental history) should be omitted, unless it is pertinent to test findings. Omitting irrelevant information throughout the report is also mandated by principle 4.04 of the APA Ethical Principles of Psychologists and Code of Conduct (2002). According to this principle, the psychologist must not include statements that are not germane to the evaluation or that are an undue invasion of privacy. Similarly, caution should be employed when including confidential or negative information that involves a third party (e.g., ex-spouse, parent, sibling). Further, reports with identifiable references to a third party should not be released without that person's consent. Unless the information is absolutely essential to the referral question and has been verified, third-party information should be avoided as much as possible. In cases where references to third parties are important for the referral question, the information should be written in a way that does not identify individuals without their consent (e.g., "There is a family history of bipolar disorder in first-degree relatives," rather than "The client's brother John has bipolar disorder"). In many cases, information on third parties is only marginally relevant to the referral question; in all cases, inclusion of third-party information should be done with caution.

Content

Most neuropsychological assessment reports contain certain basic information. These sections can either be formally identified subheadings or be only briefly touched upon, depending on the format of the report. See Table 5–1 for an example.

Identifying Information

To avoid confusion, the full name, birth date, age, date of testing, date of the report, and referral source should be listed, along with any other crucial identifying information such as chart number. Whether the report is written on a standard form provided by the hospital or agency or in letter form, this information is best listed separately at the beginning of the report.

Reason for Referral

It is essential to state the reason for referral at the beginning of the report. This serves to focus the report and to clarify why

Table 5–1 Organization of Information in the Neuropsychological Report

Report Sections

Identifying information
Reason for referral
Relevant history
Review of relevant previous reports
Current concerns
Report of informant(s)
Observations during history taking and testing
Test results
    General intellectual status
    Achievement
    Executive function
    Attention
    Memory
    Language
    Visual-spatial skills
    Motor function
    Sensory function
    Psychosocial functioning
Summary and opinion
Recommendations
Appendix: Tests administered

the evaluation was conducted and who requested it. Since the reason for referral often guides the selection of tests, citing this information helps clarify why certain tests were given as well as the rationale for the formulation and recommendations. A sentence or two confirms that the neuropsychologist has understood the request and will address relevant questions in the body of the report (e.g., "The patient was referred because of possible cognitive decline"; "The patient was referred because of learning and memory problems"). This does not preclude addressing other important issues in the report.

Some referrals are made without a clear statement of purpose (e.g., "request neuropsychological assessment"; "query organicity"). In some cases, the actual reason for referral is evident after review of pertinent records. In other cases, the referring party may need to clarify the reason for the referral. A referral form that lists several types of evaluations can be used (e.g., "Diagnostic Evaluation"; "Follow-Up Evaluation"; "Postsurgical Evaluation"; "Screening Evaluation"), as this helps to focus the reason for referral and provides referring parties with information on other services provided by the neuropsychologist.

Relevant History

The history section sets the stage for the interpretation of test results and provides the context for conclusions and recommendations. This section is based on history taking as outlined in Chapter 3 and typically includes information regarding the examinee's relevant personal and family medical history (including birth history, developmental milestones), educational attainment and school history, occupational history, alcohol and drug use, legal history, family and living situation, and interpersonal relationships. As noted previously, any information listed here will be relevant and germane to the assessment itself.

The history section contains information that bears directly on the interpretation of results. For example, in dementia evaluations, any genetic contributions can be outlined by a description of family medical history, and the description of cognitive complaints contributes to an understanding of the course of the disorder (e.g., abrupt or insidious onset). This section also provides clues to premorbid functioning by describing highlights of educational and occupational achievement. It also contributes to an understanding of the impact of the disorder on the patient's social and occupational situation. The extent to which particular aspects are emphasized over others will depend on the type of evaluation conducted. For instance, if the assessment was requested to determine whether the client suffered traumatic brain injury, a detailed report of loss of consciousness and posttraumatic amnesia would be crucial since this information will have bearing on the diagnosis and prognosis. However, this information might not be reviewed with the same amount of detail if the same patient were later seen to determine the presence of a specific type of learning disability.

Review of Relevant Previous Reports

Specific sources of information, in addition to information gleaned in the interview, will include medical reports (e.g., neurological reports, MRI, CT, EEG), school reports, and employment records (see also Chapter 3). Treatment information, including current medications and ongoing mental health interventions (e.g., therapy/counseling), should be included, and prior testing, including prior psychological or neuropsychological evaluations, should be summarized. Snyder and Ceravolo (1998) provide steps to efficiently retrieve all the relevant information from medical charts, a task that can be time-consuming unless approached strategically. McConnell (1998) provides assistance for understanding results from laboratory tests commonly found in hospital charts that may have implications for neuropsychologists (e.g., hematologic and endocrinologic tests).

The client's background history is often obtained through a mix of self-report and information gleaned from other records. It is therefore important to differentiate the source of the information. For instance, a sentence such as "Mr. Smith reported that he was depressed as an adolescent" is not as informative for the reader as "Mr. Smith was diagnosed with depression in adolescence by Dr. Jones." Such seemingly minor changes in wording may influence the interpretation of results. The source of the information obtained should be indicated clearly, along with the date. Specifying the source can serve to inform the reader about the accuracy of the information as well as indicate any potential for bias (Hebben & Milberg, 2002). Again, detailed repetition of information already

available to the reader is not helpful. For instance, in some medical settings such as inpatient wards, only the most cursory review of neurological history may be required because the information is already fully available to the treatment team.

Current Concerns

It is important to include a description of the examinee's complaints and concerns (or of those of spouses or parents, in cases of low-functioning adults or children; see below). In addition to physical and cognitive concerns, this section should also include information about the patient's emotional state (e.g., stress, anxiety, depression) and the impact of symptoms or complaints on daily living, since this may affect the interpretation of the test results as well as the recommendations. The history of presenting problems should include a description of current complaints in terms of severity, pervasiveness, duration, and onset (Hebben & Milberg, 2002). In many cases, each area (physical, cognitive, emotional) will be specifically reviewed (e.g., "In terms of physical complaints, the patient reported nausea, dizziness, etc."). Children and patients with limited insight should also be queried about their current concerns, albeit in a briefer and simpler form.

The patient's current concerns may be quite different from those of the referral source. Often, this discrepancy directly affects the interpretation of test results, which underlines the value of conducting a thorough interview with the patient and not relying solely on test scores for interpretation. In some cases, a discrepancy between the referring party and the patient is due to the patient's impaired insight secondary to a neurological condition (e.g., dementia). In others, the discrepancy suggests that the difficulties that prompted the referral are due to other factors altogether (e.g., a patient referred for a dementia workup due to poor work performance denies cognitive difficulties but reveals a complicated grief reaction after a spouse's death). In the case of children, discrepancies between the referring party and parents' concerns are commonplace and differ depending on the age of the child. Awareness and sensitivity about issues important to the child or adolescent, even when these differ markedly from those of the adults involved, ensures better cooperation with any subsequent treatment recommendations. This may also apply to adults who have significant cognitive impairments and whose concerns differ from those of their caregivers.

Report of Informant(s)

This section includes information provided by other informants such as a spouse, relative, teacher, or employer. Although informants such as parents and teachers are routinely polled in evaluations of children, informant information is a valuable component of the evaluation of adults, particularly in cases where adult self-report may not be accurate, either because of neurological disorder affecting insight (e.g., TBI) or because of outside factors such as litigation. In many cases, informant report is essential for diagnosis to determine whether a condition is situation-specific or pervasive (e.g., ADHD). In most cases, information from informants may highlight additional concerns and symptoms as well as uncover examinee statements that are misleading with regard to both the gravity of the symptoms and the time course of their evolution, which is of interest from a clinical standpoint. In children and in adults with limited insight, this section may be greatly expanded compared with the previous section. Specific forms have been developed to document informant and client reports (see Chapter 3).

Observations During History Taking and Testing

Since testing frequently extends over several hours or days, the patient's behavior during that period provides valuable information about day-to-day functioning. Competence as a historian, personal appearance, punctuality, cooperativeness, rapport with the examiner, approach to novel or routine tasks, comprehension of instructions, response to encouragement, reaction to failure, and degree of effort should all be evaluated by the examiner. The behavior at the beginning and toward the end of the session or the effect of breaks during testing on subsequent motivation allows an estimate of persistence, fatigue, speed of response, and emotional control. In fact, substantial changes in behavior during the course of the assessment should be carefully documented because they may affect the validity of the test results. Any concerns that assessment findings may not be reliable or valid indicators of an individual's ability should be stated clearly in this section along with reasons for the concerns (e.g., "*The test results may underestimate the client's abilities because he had a severe cold on the day of testing*" or "*Concern about her motivation to perform well emerged on the tests described below. Accordingly, the test results likely do not provide an accurate indication of her current strengths and weaknesses*"). Again, this section of the report should be kept to a minimum of relevant details. There is no need to overload the report with lengthy observations not pertinent to the purpose of the assessment.

In many cases, the specific behaviors listed will differ depending on the setting. For instance, evaluations of examinees in psychiatric settings may include lengthy observations on reality testing, thought content, and coherence of verbal expression. These would not be addressed in detail in other settings, where the focus may be on distractibility, overactivity, or inattentiveness during testing (e.g., ADHD workup) or on effort, consistency of self-reported complaints versus test performance, and pain behaviors (e.g., medico-legal TBI evaluation).

In some cases, neuropsychology reports include a section on the validity of test findings; in others, this consists of a detailed, stand-alone section (e.g., medico-legal reports). In other cases, the entire report may be prefaced with a qualifying statement that specifies that the results are time-limited and may no longer be applicable after a certain period of time. This is particularly true in pediatric reports due to de-velopmental changes, but may also be the case in settings where patients are seen while in an acute state (e.g., inpatient TBI or in the postoperative period after neurosurgery). Other general caveats can also be detailed, such as the relevance of norms for the particular individual and the degree to which the results likely reflect an adequate reflection of the individual's ability, given the individual's perceived effort and the degree to which testing conditions were optimal.

Test Results

The section on test results is the most technical aspect of the report. While the tendency may be to describe scores test by test, ideally, the information is organized into logical domains, and results are presented in terms of performance (e.g., "Sustained attention skills were significantly below age expectations") rather than in terms of the test (e.g., "The patient's score on a computerized test requiring her to respond to the letter X when presented with multiple letter trials over time was poor").

The domains covered (see Table 5–1) may vary depending on the purpose of the assessment. Noncontributory results may be omitted or summed up briefly. Other formats exist as well. For example, Donders (1999) advocates the use of a brief report that summarizes the entire results in one paragraph (devoid of scores), describing results in a way that is easily interpretable by a lay reader. Other settings also demand a more general summary of results without a domain-by-domain explanation (e.g., inpatient medical chart entries, screening evaluations).

Many outpatient reports include separate sections for each domain (with subtitles). We use a variety of formats, depending on the referral question; in some cases, a one- or two-paragraph summary of results is sufficient to integrate all the neuropsychological data. In longer reports, topic sentences integrate the information from different tests that are relevant to interpreting the examinee's functioning within that domain. This is followed by a listing of the test data that led to the interpretation, with supporting data (usually described in percentile form) and references to the relevant tests. For example:

> Verbal comprehension appeared intact. She was able to follow complex commands (Token Test—within average range). By contrast, expressive functions were poor. Her ability to generate words on command within a fixed time period (Verbal Fluency) was low, below the 10th percentile. She also had considerable difficulty naming pictured objects (Boston Naming Test), her score falling in the impaired range, below the 5th percentile. Some paraphasias [substitution of sounds] were apparent on naming tasks (e.g., acorn—aircorn). The provision of phonemic cues facilitated naming.

It is also useful to keep in mind that most tests provide results for several different domains. For example, the WAIS-III subtest scores need not all be referenced under "Intellectual

Ability." Rather, Digit Span may be considered under "Attention" or "Working Memory," Vocabulary under "Language," Block Design under "Visual-Spatial Ability," etc. Similarly, the Trail Making Test may be considered under "Executive Function," "Attention," and "Visuomotor Ability."

Special mention should be made regarding validity indices. There is growing concern in the medical-legal context that individuals may familiarize themselves with neuropsychological tests to manipulate the test findings for gain (e.g., to evade detection in the case of malingering). Accordingly, names of tests of motivational status can be provided in the list of tests administered, but it should not be stated in the body of the report that these tasks are measures of effort (see also Chapter 16, *Assessment of Response Bias and Suboptimal Performance*). That is, comments on the validity of test data should be made without naming any specific test (Green, 2003). For example:

> The patient obtained very low scores on a number of memory tests that are objectively very easy. While such low scores can occur in severely demented individuals, they rarely if ever occur in normal individuals or from people suffering from mild brain injuries. These findings raise significant concerns regarding the validity of the test results.

Alternatively:

> The patient was given some tasks that are relatively insensitive to severe brain injury, but that can be greatly affected by effort. Her performance was at a level that is rarely seen among non-compensation-seeking patients with documented significant brain damage and indicates suboptimal effort.

It is important to note areas of strength as well as weaknesses. Strengths in certain cognitive or other areas provide the main basis for intervention strategies. Crosson (2000) notes that a deficit-centered approach can have a negative impact when providing feedback to the patient and family. This is also true with regard to report writing. Again, the discussion of strengths and weaknesses refers to functional domains and not to tests. In cases where few strengths can be found on objective testing (i.e., severe developmental delay), the individual's personal assets can be highlighted (e.g., "Despite these cognitive limitations, Sarah is an engaging, sociable girl").

Describing Test Scores

The question of whether to include raw data and standard or other scores within reports is controversial. Naugle and McSweeny (1995) point out that the practice of including raw data and scores such as IQs may lead to misinterpretations and contravenes the Ethical Principles of Psychologists, which state that psychological data should not be released to individuals unqualified to interpret them. By contrast, the routine reporting of raw scores is recommended by authors like Freides

(1993, 1995), Mitrushina et al. (2005), and Tallent (1993). Both Matarazzo (1995) and Freides (1995) argue that it is illogical to restrict access to scores when conclusions and interpretations of these scores, which are equally sensitive, are presented in reports. Others have argued that the practice of deliberately omitting important and detailed information such as IQ scores in reports goes against the accepted practice of all other professionals such as physicians, who freely provide the information gathered during their assessments to other health professionals. For example, Lees-Haley and Courtney (2000) argue that current practice of restricting the disclosure of tests and raw tests to courts undermines psychologists' credibility and is contrary to the best interest of consumers. Routinely omitting scores also makes interpretations impossible to verify. In this vein, Hebben and Milberg (2002) argue that test scores are the only common referent that will be used by future readers of the report and that labels such as "average" or "below average" are not precise and may refer to different score ranges depending on the individual clinician.

The practice of including scores in reports also allows for more precise information to be conveyed to the reader and permits the next examiner to measure change more accurately. Hebben and Milberg recommend providing actual test scores in standard form in the body of the report or a summary table, with specification of the norms used and raw score, if several norms exist for a test (e.g., Boston Naming Test). A similar approach is taken by Donders (1999), who appends a list of test scores in standard or in raw score format to the report, along with the corresponding normative means and standard deviations. Most neuropsychologists include scores in their reports (Donders, 2001). According to a survey of Division 40 members, raw scores are rarely reported in the body of the report, although there are some exceptions (e.g., the number of categories achieved on the WCST). Age and grade equivalents are also rarely mentioned, consistent with the significant psychometric problems associated with such scores (e.g., the lack of equal distances between measurement points and the gross exaggeration of small performance differences) (Donders 2001). Most neuropsychologists express scores in percentile ranks or standard scores (e.g., z or T scores; Donders, 2001), as described in Chapter 1.

Few lay individuals understand the meaning of test scores, including percentiles. Bowman (2002) found that third-year undergraduates in a psychometrics course grossly underestimated below-normal percentile values and overestimated above-average percentile values when asked to interpret them in terms of corresponding IQ values. Thus, the communication of scores is facilitated by the use of descriptors of ranges of ability. Commonly accepted classification systems of ability levels are provided by Wechsler (1997; see Table 5–2) and by Heaton et al. (2004; Table 5–3).

Unless the recipient of the report can be expected to be fully familiar with the system used, we recommend that the test results section be prefaced with an explanation of the metric used. For example:

Table 5–2 Classification/Descriptors of Test Scores Using the Wechsler System

Classification	IQ	z Score	T Score	Percent Included	Lower Limit of Percentile Range
Very superior	130 and above	+2 and above	70+	2.2	98
Superior	120–129	1.3 to 2	63–69	6.7	91
High average	110–129	0.6 to 1.3	56–62	16.1	75
Average	90–109	±0.6	44–55	50.0	25
Low average	80–89	−0.6 to −1.3	43–37	16.1	9
Borderline	70–79	−1.3 to −2.0	36–30	6.7	2
Extremely low	69 and below	−2.0 and below	29 and below	2.2	—

Source: Based on WAIS-III (Wechsler, 1997) description system.

The following description of Ms. A's abilities is based on her performance in comparison to same-aged peers. A percentile ranking refers to the percentage of people in her age group who would be expected to score equal to or below her on that particular measure. Thus, a score of 50, falling at the 60th percentile, would mean that 40% of her peers obtained higher scores while 60% obtained lower scores. Test scores that are better than 75% to 84% of individuals with the same background are considered to be above average. Scores that fall within the 25th to 74th percentile are considered to be within the average range. Scores that are within the 9th to 24th percentile are termed low average. Scores that fall within the 2nd to 8th percentile are borderline or mildly impaired, while scores below this range are considered to be extremely low or moderately/severely impaired.

One drawback of percentile-rank reporting is the pseudoaccuracy implied in such scores. Basically, percentile ranks represent the number of people covered by the normal distribution curve as expressed in standard deviations. One-half of a standard deviation from the mean changes the percentile ranks from 50 to 69, a seemingly large difference that is in most cases clinically insignificant. With computer calculations, scores that differ by even small fractions of a standard deviation can be translated into percentile points that may seem to reflect real differences to the reader unfamiliar with basic psychometrics.

Lezak et al. (2004) provide an illustrative example of this phenomenon. Lay individuals who see a Wechsler report of a Similarities score at the 37th percentile (scaled score of 9) and an Arithmetic score at the 63rd percentile (scaled score of 11) are likely to conclude erroneously that the client performs better in Arithmetic than in verbal reasoning. However, score differences of this magnitude are chance variations, and the individual's performance in these two areas is best viewed as equivalent.

Some test scores are not normally distributed, and norms for these tests allow only a very limited range of scores (see Chapter 1). When most individuals succeed on the majority of items (e.g., Boston Naming Test, Hooper, Rey Complex Figure, RBANS, some WMS-III subtests), the distribution is negatively skewed and variability of scores falling within the normal or above-normal range is highly limited. The test has its highest discriminative power at the lower end of ability levels (Mitrushina et al., 2005). In the case where test items present difficulty for most of the subjects (e.g., Raven's Advanced Progressive Matrices), the score distribution is positively skewed and variability within the lower ranges is highly limited. Such a task would be most appropriate for the selection of a few outstanding individuals from a larger sample (Mitrushina et al., 2005). In either case, the use of standard scores (e.g., z scores, T scores) is not advised. In such cases, it is more appropriate to describe the test results in terms of a cutoff of frequency of occurrence (e.g., at the 5th percentile; Lezak et al., 2004).

The interpretation of scores described according to impairment classifications must consider the premorbid abilities of the examinee. "Average" or "normal range" scores in a previously gifted individual may very well indicate considerable loss of abilities. On the other hand, for a person with borderline premorbid intelligence, impairment may only be inferred from scores two or three standard deviations below the mean. Reference to indicators of premorbid functioning and to demographically corrected scores are required for the interpretation of scores for people with nonaverage premorbid abilities

Table 5–3 Classification/Descriptors of Test Scores Using the Heaton et al. System

Performance Range	Classification	T-Score Range	Lower Limit of Percentile Range
Normal	Above average	55+	68
	Average	45–54	31
	Below average	40–44	16
Impaired	Mild	35–39	7
	Mild to moderate	30–34	2
	Moderate	25–29	<1
	Moderate to severe	20–24	—
	Severe	0–19	—

Source: Heaton et al., 2004.

(Bell & Roper, 1998; Heaton et al., 2003, 2004; Larrabee, 2000a; Tremont, 1998).

It is also important to bear in mind that there are relationships among tests due to shared common factors (Larrabee, 2000a). Each score must be interpreted in the context of scores on other tests of related abilities. Further, the findings must make neuropsychological sense; that is, they must be meaningful in terms of the patient's history and the suspected disorder (Lezak et al., 2004). Note, too, that a single "deviant" score may be the result of one of several error sources: misunderstanding of instructions, inattention, distraction, momentary lapse of effort, etc. Thus, it is not at all uncommon for healthy people to show isolated impairment on one or two tests in the course of an assessment (Heaton et al., 2004; Ingraham & Aiken, 1996; Taylor & Heaton, 2001). However, consistent impairment within specific cognitive domains is relatively unusual (Palmer et al., 1998).

Norms

When different norms are available for a test, the clinician may want to specify the norm set that was used to derive scores (either in parentheses in the body of the report or in an appendix of test scores). This information can be particularly helpful given that patients are often assessed multiple times. See Chapter 2 for an extended discussion of norms selection in neuropsychological assessment.

Test Adaptations and Deviations from Standard Administration

Test adaptations for the client with visual, auditory, or motor impairments, and any test modifications used for testing clients for whom English is a second language as discussed in Chapter 4, should be clearly stated, and restrictions on the use of published norms and consequent limitations in interpretation should be explained in the report.

Summary, Opinion, and Recommendations

A summary is often provided in point form. It includes a brief restatement of the client's history, the major neuropsychological findings, and a diagnostic statement that includes the presumed origin of the deficit. A prognostic statement is also expected. For example:

1. This is a 54-year-old right-handed accountant with no previous history of neurological disorder.
2. She was in a motor vehicle accident on Dec. 12, 2000, and suffered a severe head injury; she was comatose for two weeks and had significantly abnormal findings on neurological examination and imaging.
3. Neuropsychological findings reveal significant deficits in memory and slowed processing speed.
4. There are no concurrent conditions to account for these cognitive difficulties (i.e., she does not have significant depression, pain, or PTSD). In addition, she appeared to put forth maximum effort on the tests administered.
5. It is therefore likely that she suffered significant neuropsychological compromise as a result of her accident.
6. Given the time since her injury, further significant improvement is unlikely.

Alternatively, this part of the report can be divided into relevant sections of interest to different readers. For example, the report can include a "Neurological Implications" or "Medical Implications" section written primarily for medical staff including likely etiology, chronicity, diffuse or focal nature of deficits, and need for medical follow-up. Often, the summary will include major recommendations. For example:

The pattern of neuropsychological test results was consistent with dementia. Given the neurological results and history provided by his wife, it is likely that this represents dementia of the Alzheimer's type. Consultation with his neurologist or treating physician is recommended to ensure neurological follow-up.

Or:

Neuropsychological testing suggests preserved language skills in this left-handed boy with intractable seizures and a history of perinatal stroke in the left frontal lobe in areas presumed to subserve language functioning. Consequently, the possibility of atypical language dominance (i.e., bilateral or right hemisphere language) should be confirmed with Wada testing prior to epilepsy surgery. Language mapping is also recommended prior to any surgery involving the left frontal lobe.

The interpretation, based on quantitative and qualitative information, must respect what is known about brain-behavior relations (i.e., it must make sense from a neurological and neuropsychological point of view) and must also take into account information regarding test reliability and validity. Hebben and Milberg (2002) stress that if neuropsychological data do not fit with the other information such as neurological data or prior history, this should be stated. Further, they caution that there are few single test scores that are valid predictors of lesions in specific areas of the brain. Even though conclusions about impaired function can be made, predictions about abnormal brain areas should be made with caution. They provide a list of questions to follow when interpreting neuropsychological data, including considering base rates, premorbid levels, confounding factors, and specific points to consider when making inferences about brain damage or dysfunction based on neuropsychological data. Cimino (2000) also notes that conceptualization and interpretation needs to take into account the influence of subject-specific variables, effects of interaction between different cognitive domains, and consistency/inconsistency within cognitive domains, and should avoid erroneous assumptions (e.g., overinterpretation of test scores) and other issues central to making appropriate interpretations of neuropsychological data. For a full discussion of these and related issues, the reader is urged to consult comprehensive texts on neuropsychological assessment such as Baron (2004), Groth-Marnat (2000), Lezak et al. (2004), McCaffrey et al. (1997), Mitrushina et al. (2005), and Vanderploeg (2000).

Diagnostic information and recommendations relevant for follow-up by other professionals are also highlighted in this section. This often includes implications for daily living and education (e.g., Baron et al., 1995, 2004). For example:

Neuropsychological results show a clear discrepancy between measured intelligence and achievement levels in the area of reading. As a result, John meets criteria for a reading disability and will require a modified program and designation as a student with special educational needs.

Or:

Mr. Jones's pattern of test results and history suggest that his post-injury course has been complicated by PTSD. Referral to a therapist or counselor with expertise in this area is highly recommended. Referral has been discussed with Mr. Jones and names of local providers have been suggested.

Unfortunately, in many settings, recommendations remain the most overlooked aspect of the neuropsychological evaluation (Hebben & Milberg, 2002). Recommendations should be both practical and realistic. The neuropsychologist preparing the assessment report should be familiar with remedial techniques, therapies, and basic management procedures in his or her field of expertise as well as with the available local resources that provide such assistance. Names and phone numbers for specific treatment, training, or support facilities may need to be included or provided as separate attachments during the feedback session.

Other recommendations include practical hints for the patient and the caregiver for the management of particular problems in daily living, educational and occupational implications, and, in some cases, an estimate of when reassessment should be scheduled to measure future progress or decline. Examples of recommendations can be found in many sources (e.g., Eslinger, 2002; Ylvisaker, 1997).

Driving deserves special mention. The ability to drive a motor vehicle is often an issue of concern for the patient, the caregiver, and the referring psychologist or physician. In many jurisdictions, psychologists must, by law, report any patient they suspect is not competent to drive. Neuropsychological tests do not provide direct information about the ability to drive safely, although they can provide some relevant information (e.g., Brown et al., 2005), and in instances of severe impairment it is obvious that the driver's license should be suspended. Brouwer and Withaar (1997) provide a framework for determining fitness to drive after brain injury. For further discussion of driving and neuropsychological assessment, see Dobbs (1997) and Lemsky (2000).

Appendix: Tests Administered

The need for appendices varies depending on the report type. Some neuropsychologists include a full listing of all tests administered in the course of the assessment, while others supplement the list with actual test scores. Others include the test list in the body of the report. Briefer reports may not include any mention of the tests administered. When brevity is required, we favor the practice of including test names for the more important findings and describing other findings in general terms in the body of the report (e.g., "The patient showed severe executive functioning deficits [<1st percentile, WCST]. However, attention, memory and language were all within normal limits").

RECIPIENTS

The contents of a neuropsychological report are confidential and not to be shared with others not specifically designated by the patient or referring party. Even if the report is not directly shared with the patient, in most cases, he or she has the right to see the report. Although this is not always feasible in medical settings, it is good practice to allow the patient to read the report before it is distributed (see *Feedback Session*) and to clarify with the patient in writing who should receive a copy. This practice is followed, at least on an occasional basis, by a majority of neuropsychologists in a recent survey (Donders, 2001). Neuropsychologists whose clientele is predominantly pediatric may defer report distribution until after review with the patient or family (e.g., see Baron, 2004; Baron et al., 1995).

The distribution list should be indicated at the end of the report. Most neuropsychologists do not vary the content of the report depending on the distribution list. However, some clinicians working with children may draft an abbreviated version of the report or a letter for distribution to the school when the full report contains sensitive material that parents may not want disclosed to the school system.

FORENSIC ASSESSMENT REPORTS

Forensic assessment is a specialty in itself (McCaffrey et al., 1997; Otto & Heilbrun, 2002). Typically, forensic reports are longer, more detailed, and more comprehensive than those used in routine clinical practice (Donders, 2001). However, it is important to remember that any report written for clinical purposes may be scrutinized in court at a later time. Forensic assessment reports are written for lawyers on both sides of the case and should be couched in clear language that cannot be misinterpreted. Most often the report will address questions regarding the existence of brain injury, cause of brain injury, degree of impairment, and prognosis. Reports may also focus on child custody, diminished criminal responsibility, and competency. Competency can be assessed in terms of specific questions such as the competency to stand trial, make a will, manage one's affairs (e.g., contracts, estate), determine residence (commitment to an institution or hospital), or give informed consent (Grisso & Appelbaum, 1998). In addition to neuropsychological tests, specific instruments have been developed for assessing competency (e.g., the MacArthur Competency Assessment Tool–Criminal Adjudication; Appelbaum & Grisso, 1995).

In reports written for forensic purposes, the qualifications of the psychologist (registration or license, board certification, area of specialization, years of experience) are required and usually form the first sentence of the report ("*I am a psychologist registered to practice in ___ . Attached is my curriculum vitae outlining some of my qualifications*"). The section detailing informant reports may also be quite detailed in medico-legal evaluations when corroboration of subjective complaints is necessary. The section on observations will also frequently be expanded to include a detailed opinion about the validity of the test findings (see later, and Chapter 16, *Assessment of Response Bias and Suboptimal Effort*, in this volume). Additionally, the report should include specifics regarding norms (Williams, 1997a) because the neuropsychologist should be able to justify why a particular normative set was used. Some neuropsychologists also divide the interpretation section into "preexisting" (e.g., prior head injury), "concurrent" (e.g., medication use), and "intervening factors" (e.g., PTSD) to fully discuss all the possible factors that may account for the obtained pattern of test results (Williams, 1997b).

The question of admissibility of testimony by neuropsychologists in various states is guided by two standards. The Frye rule holds that the evidence should be conditioned on having been sufficiently established that it is generally accepted in the particular field in which it belongs. The standards for admissibility changed in 1993 with the U.S. Supreme Court's decision in *Daubert v. Merrell Dow Pharmaceuticals*. It rejected the Frye standard on the ground that it focused too narrowly on a single criterion, general acceptance; rather, the court must decide whether the reasoning and methodology underlying the testimony is scientifically valid and can properly be applied to the facts at issue. Criteria for deciding acceptability include testability of the theoretical basis, error rates of the methods used, peer review and publication, and general acceptance.

Due to the adversarial nature of court proceedings, the testifying neuropsychologist can expect extremely critical analysis of his or her report. Well-prepared lawyers are familiar with many of the tests and their weaknesses, based on books specifically written for that purpose (e.g., Doerr & Carlin, 1991; Faust et al., 1991; Hall & Pritchard, 1996; Melton et al., 1997; Sbordone, 1995; Ziskin & Faust, 1988). Additionally, expert neuropsychologists are frequently hired by the opposing side to critically review the neuropsychological report. Attacks may be expected, particularly regarding results based on personality tests like the MMPI or the Rorschach Test and on results based on experimental or nonstandard measures of

neuropsychological functioning (see also McCaffrey et al., 1997, and Mitrushina et al., 2005, for a discussion of guidelines for determining whether a neuropsychological test is considered standard). The report writer may also consider the ecological validity of neuropsychological tests, which may be dubious unless supported by sound studies. Authors like Larrabee (2000b), Lees-Haley and Cohen (1999), and Sweet (1999) provide guidance for the neuropsychologist, while Pope et al. (1993) focus their book primarily on the MMPI, the MMPI-2, and the MMPI-A. Neuropsychologists specializing in forensic assessment should also refer to the Specialty Guidelines for Forensic Psychologists (Committee on Ethical Guidelines for Forensic Psychologists, 1991).

A particularly important aspect of forensic reports is the question of symptom validity: Was the patient cooperating fully? Are some or all of the symptoms valid or are they influenced by a tendency to exaggerate or even to malinger? Many tests, especially the MMPI-2 and other personality tests, have developed scales or indices that can assist in the detection of response bias (see Chapter 15, *Assessment of Mood, Personality, and Adaptive Functions*). In addition, special testing for symptom validity has been developed (described in Chapter 16, *Assessment of Response Bias and Suboptimal Performance*). Such information is crucial for the interpretation of test results. However, the problem is complicated by the fact that these tests can at best only indicate that motivational and/or emotional factors (e.g., depression, anxiety, lack of effort) may be influencing task performance. Even in cases where financial or other incentives exist and the patient's performance is suspect, the patient may be impaired and/or acting without conscious intent. Accurate diagnosis requires examination of both test and extra-test behavior as well as a thorough evaluation of the patient's history and pertinent reports, including injury characteristics (Slick et al., 1999). Communication of findings can be problematic, given the difficulty in diagnosing malingering and the complexity of an individual's motivations. The report should be written in a factual manner, providing a detailed description of the patient's behavior, and should acknowledge any limitations in the assessment. In some cases, the clinician may merely comment that the invalidity of the testing precludes firm conclusions. A recent survey of experts in the area (Slick et al., 2004) suggests that the term "malingering" is rarely used. Rather, most experts typically state that the test results are invalid, inconsistent with the severity of the injury, or indicative of exaggeration (for a further discussion, see Chapter 16, *Assessment of Response Bias and Suboptimal Performance*).

COMPUTER-GENERATED SCORES AND REPORTS

Computer scoring programs are fairly common, and the sophistication of interpretative programs has increased over time. Several data management and storage, "report building," and report writing computer programs are available, with options ranging from organizing inputted test scores to providing outlines and fully written reports. The clinician, however, remains responsible for what goes into the report. For this reason, he or she should be thoroughly familiar with all material used in such programs as well as with the standards for educational and psychological testing that pertain to computer testing and interpretation (American Educational Research Association et al., 1999).

Clinicians may be tempted to use the computer as a "cheap consultant" and take the validity of the computer-generated report for granted. It is important to bear in mind that computer-generated reports, by their very nature, use a shotgun rather than a problem-oriented approach, and they address a hypothetical, "typical" individual based on averages of certain test scores, not the particular examinee who is the subject of the report. It follows, then, that a computer-generated report can only be used selectively and with modifications required by the referral questions and the specific circumstances of the examinee.

Computer scoring can save time and often avoids computation errors. However, the translation of raw scores into standardized scores must be scrutinized by the psychologist to check which normative database is used and to ensure that proper corrections for age, education, and other factors are applied.

FEEDBACK SESSION

Psychological assessment results are of direct interest to the patient, who is usually concerned about his or her mental or emotional problems. Informing interviews serve three purposes: (1) to review and clarify test results, (2) to acquire additional information of relevance to the assessment process, and (3) to educate the patient and family about their condition (Baron, 2004; Baron et al., 1995). A step-by-step guide to communicating results to patients and treatment teams is provided by Ryan et al. (1998). Crosson (2000) also discusses pitfalls and principles of giving feedback to patients and families.

It is good practice to schedule an informing interview with the examinee soon after the assessment. Spouses and primary caregivers are typically invited to attend. In many cases (especially with children), teachers, employers, case workers, or other persons directly involved may also be included at the discretion of the family. The informing interview usually starts with a review of the purpose of the assessment. The clinician may also ask the examinee and/or family about their expectations and what they hope to learn from the assessment, which helps clarify misinformation about the purpose and limits of the evaluation (Baron 2004; Baron et al., 1995). Test results can be summarized briefly and should be explained in easily understood terms. It is good practice to be explicit and use examples. To prevent the impression that test results are kept "secret" from the client, it may be appropriate to explain why the psychologist came to a certain conclusion ("You remember that list of words that you had to repeat? You had a lot of trouble remembering words compared to other people your age"). While it is true that few examinees have the training and sophistication to fully understand test scores (Lezak et al., 2004), terms like "average" or "seriously below average for your age" do make sense to most people.

The most important parts of the informing interview, however, are the conclusions reached and the recommendations. The patient wants to know whether he or she has a serious problem, whether it is progressive, and what can be done about it. This should be discussed at some length and repeated as necessary. Most clients retain only a small portion of the information given during a single feedback session. It is helpful to provide the examinee and/or family with additional written materials in some cases (i.e., phone and address of therapist, training group, or rehabilitation facility).

At times, the psychologist may gain additional information during the informing interview that necessitates modifying the report in some way or leads to additional recommendations. For this reason, some psychologists typically send out reports only after the informing interview is concluded (Baron, 2004; Baron et al., 1995). However, we find that this practice can cause unnecessary delays in the distribution of the report to the referring party in settings where results are needed quickly (i.e., inpatient settings). Additional, pertinent information may always be sent out in a letter or as an addendum to the report.

As noted previously with regard to the report itself, focusing primarily on deficits during the feedback session may make patients (and their families) feel devastated; insensitive delivery of negative findings can also injure self-esteem and increase the risk of significant depression (Crosson, 2000); in the case of children, parents may feel hopeless and responsible for their children's limitations. When extreme, these reactions may interfere with adjustment and rehabilitation processes. Such considerations underscore the importance of emphasizing strengths as well as weaknesses. Baron (2004; Baron et al. 1995) provides guidelines useful to pediatric neuropsychologists on how to gain parental acceptance, communicate results simply and define terminology, use restatement, provide examples, encourage questions and participation, and decide when to include children in feedback sessions.

As noted above, it may be appropriate to allow patients to read the report at the end of the session and to take a copy home. Providing written as well as oral feedback is one of the recommendations resulting from a study of consumers of neuropsychological assessment (Bennett-Levy et al., 1994; Gass & Brown, 1992).

REFERENCES

American Educational Research Association, American Psychological Association, & National Council on Measurement in Education. (1999). *Standards for educational and psychological testing.* Washington, DC: American Educational Research Association.

American Psychological Association. (1996). Statement on the disclosure of test data. *American Psychologist, 51,* 644–648.

American Psychological Association. (1997). *Thesaurus of psychological index terms* (8th ed.). Washington, DC: Author.

American Psychological Association. (2002). Ethical principles of psychologists and code of conduct. *American Psychologist, 57,* 1060–1073.

Appelbaum, P. S., & Grisso, T. (1995). The MacArthur treatment competency study. I: Mental illness and competency to consent to treatment. *Law and Human Behavior, 19,* 105–126.

Axelrod, B. N. (2000). Neuropsychological report writing. In R. D. Vanderploeg (Ed.), *Clinician's guide to neuropsychological assessment* (2nd ed., pp. 245–273). Mahwah, NJ: Lawrence Erlbaum Associates.

Baron, I. S. (2004). *Neuropsychological evaluation of the child.* New York: Oxford University Press.

Baron, I. S., Fennell, E. B., & Voeller, K. K. S. (1995). *Pediatric neuropsychology in the medical setting.* New York: Oxford University Press.

Bau, C., Edwards, D., Yonan, C., & Storandt, M. (1996). The relationship of neuropsychological test performance to performance on functional tasks in dementia of the Alzheimer type. *Archives of Clinical Neuropsychology, 11,* 69–75.

Bell, B. D., & Roper, B. L. (1998). "Myths of neuropsychology": Another view. *The Clinical Neuropsychologist, 12,* 237–244.

Bennett-Levy, J., Klein-Boonschate, M. A., Batchelor, J., et al. (1994). Encounters with Anna Thompson: The consumer's experience of neuropsychological assessment. *The Clinical Neuropsychologist, 8,* 219–238.

Bowman, M. L. (2002). The perfidy of percentiles. *Archives of Clinical Neuropsychology, 17,* 295–303.

Brouwer, H. W., & Withaar, F. K. (1997). Fitness to drive after traumatic brain injury. *Neuropsychological Rehabilitation, 3,* 177–193.

Brown, L. B., Stern, R. A., Cahn-Weiner, D. A., Rogers, B., Messer, M. A., Lannon, M. C., Maxwell, C., Souza, T., White, T., & Ott, B. R. (2005). Driving scenes test of the Neuropsychological Assessment Battery (NAB) and on-road driving performance in aging and very mild dementia. *Archives of Clinical Neuropsychology, 20,* 209–216.

Cimino, C. (2000). Principles of neuropsychological interpretation. In R. D. Vanderploeg (Ed.), *Clinician's guide to neuropsychological assessment* (2nd ed., pp. 69–109). Mahwah, NJ: LEA Publishers.

Committee on Ethical Guidelines for Forensic Psychologists (1991). Specialty guidelines for forensic psychologists. *Law and Human Behavior, 6,* 655–665.

Crosson, B. (2000). Application of neuropsychological assessment results. In R. D. Vanderploeg (Ed.), *Clinician's guide to neuropsychological assessment* (2nd ed., pp. 195–244). Mahwah, NJ: LEA Publishers.

Dobbs, A. R. (1997). Evaluating the driving competence of dementia patients. *Alzheimers Disease and Related Disorders, 11*(Suppl. 1), 8–12.

Donders, J. (1999). Pediatric neuropsychological reports: Do they really have to be so long? *Child Neuropsychology, 5,* 70–78.

Donders, J. (2001). A survey of report writing by neuropsychologists. II: Test data, report format, and document length. *Clinical Neuropsychologist, 15,* 150–161.

Doerr, H. O., & Carlin, A. S. (Eds.). (1991). *Forensic neuropsychology: Legal and scientific bases.* Odessa, FL: Psychological Assessment Resources.

Dougherty, E., & Bortnick, D. M. (1990). *Report writer: Adult's Intellectual Achievement and Neuropsychological Screening Test.* Toronto, Ontario: Multi-Health Systems.

Erickson, R. C., Eimon, P., & Hebben, N. (1992). A bibliography of normative articles on cognition tests for older adults. *The Clinical Neuropsychologist, 6,* 98–102.

Eslinger, P. (2002). *Neuropsychological interventions: Clinical research and practice.* New York: Guilford Press.

Faust, D., Ziskin, J., & Hiers, J. B. (1991). *Brain damage claims: Coping with neuropsychological evidence* (Vol. 2). Odessa, FL: Psychological Assessment Resources.

Freides, D. (1993). Proposed standard of professional practice: Neuropsychological reports display all quantitative data. *The Clinical Neuropsychologist, 7,* 234–235.

Freides, D. (1995). Interpretations are more benign than data? *The Clinical Neuropsychologist, 9,* 248.

Gass, C. S., & Brown, M. C. (1992). Neuropsychological test feedback to patients with brain dysfunction. *Psychological Assessment, 4,* 272–277.

Green, P. (2003). *Green's Word Memory Test.* Edmonton: Green's Publishing Inc.

Grisso, T., & Appelbaum, P. (1998). *Assessing competence to consent to treatment: A guide for physicians and other health professionals.* New York: Oxford University Press.

Groth-Marnat, G. (2000). *Neuropsychological assessment in clinical practice.* New York: John Wiley & Sons.

Hall, H. V., & Pritchard, D. A. (1996). *Detecting malingering and deception. Forensic decision analysis.* Delray Beach, FL: St. Lucie Press.

Heaton, R. K., Miller, S. W., Taylor, M. J., & Grant, I. (2004). *Revised comprehensive norms for an Expanded Halstead-Reitan Battery: Demographically adjusted neuropsychological norms for African American and Caucasian adults.* Lutz, FL: Psychological Assessment Resources.

Heaton, R. K., Taylor, M. J., & Manly, J. J. (2003). Demographic effects and use of demographically corrected norms with the WAIS-III and WMS-III. In Tulsky, D., Saklofske, R. K., Heaton, G., Chelune G., Ivnik, R. A., Bornstein, R. A., Prifitera, A., & Ledbetter, M. (Eds.), *Clinical interpretation of the WAIS-III and WMS-III* (pp. 183–210). San Diego, CA: Academic Press.

Hebben, N., & Millberg, W. (2002). *Essentials of neuropsychological assessment.* New York: John Wiley and Sons.

Ingraham, L. J., & Aiken, C. B. (1996). An empirical approach to determining criteria for abnormality in test batteries with multiple measures. *Neuropsychology, 10,* 120–124.

Larrabee, G. J. (2000a). Association between IQ and neuropsychological test performance: Commentary on Tremont, Hoffman, Scott and Adams (1998). *The Clinical Neuropsychologist, 14,* 139–145.

Larrabee, G. J. (2000b). Forensic neuropsychological assessment. In R. D. Vanderploeg (Ed.), *Clinician's guide to neuropsychological assessment,* (2nd ed.). Mahwah, NJ: LEA.

Lees-Haley, P. R., & Cohen, L. J. (1999). The neuropsychologist as expert witness: Toward credible science in the courtroom. In J. J. Sweet (Ed.), *Forensic neuropsychology: Fundamentals and practice.* Lisse, the Netherlands: Swetts & Zeitlinger.

Lees-Haley, P. R., & Courtney, J. C. (2000). Disclosure of tests and raw test data to the courts: A need for reform. *Neuropsychology Review, 10*(3), 169–182.

Lemsky, C. M. (2000). Neuropsychological assessment and treatment planning. In G. Groth-Marnat (Ed.), *Neuropsychological assessment in clinical practice: A guide to test interpretation and integration* (pp. 535–574). New York: John Wiley & Sons, Inc.

Lezak, M. D., Howieson, D. B., & Loring, D. W. (2004). *Neuropsychological assessment* (4th ed.). New York: Oxford University Press.

Loring, D. W. (Ed.). (1999). *INS dictionary of neuropsychology.* New York: Oxford University Press.

Matarazzo, J. D. (1995). Psychological report standards in neuropsychology. *The Clinical Neuropsychologist, 9,* 249–250.

McCaffrey, R. J., Williams, A. D., Fisher, J. M., & Laing, L. C. (1997). *The practice of forensic neuropsychology: Meeting challenges in the courtroom.* New York: Plenum Press.

McConnell, H. W. (1998). Laboratory testing in neuropsychology. In P. J. Snyder & P. D. Nussbaum (Eds.), *Clinical neuropsychology: A pocket handbook for assessment* (pp. 29–53). New York: American Psychological Association.

Melton, G. B., Petrila, J., Poythress, N. G., & Slobogin, C. (1997). *Psychological evaluations for the courts* (2nd ed.). New York: Guilford.

Mitrushina, M. N., Boone, K. B., Razani, J., & D'Elia, L. F. (2005). *Handbook of normative data for neuropsychological assessment* (2nd ed.). New York: Oxford University Press.

Naugle, R. I., & McSweeny, A. J. (1995). On the practice of routinely appending neuropsychological data to reports. *The Clinical Neuropsychologist, 9,* 245–247.

Otto, R. K., & Heilbrun, K. (2002). The practice of forensic psychology. *American Psychologist, 57,* 5–18.

Ownby, R. L. (1997). *Psychological reports* (3rd ed.). New York: Wiley.

Palmer, B. W., Boone, K. B., Lesser, J. M., & Wohl, M. A. (1998). Base rates of "impaired" neuropsychological test performance among healthy older adults. *Archives of Clinical Neuropsychology, 13,* 503–511.

Pope, K. S., Butcher, J. N., & Seelen, J. (1993). *The MMPI, MMPI-2, and MMPI-A in court: A practical guide for expert witnesses and attorneys.* Washington, D.C.: American Psychological Association.

Reynolds, C. R., & Fletcher-Janzen, E. (1997). *Handbook of clinical child neuropsychology* (2nd ed.). New York: Plenum Press.

Ryan, C. M., Hammond, K., & Beers, S. R. (1998). General assessment issues for a pediatric population. In P. J. Snyder & P. D. Nussbaum (Eds.), *Clinical neuropsychology: A pocket handbook for assessment* (pp. 105–123). Washington, D.C.: American Psychological Association.

Sattler, J. (2001). *Assessment of children: Cognitive applications* (4th ed.). San Diego, CA: Jerome M. Sattler.

Sbordone, R. J. (1995). *Neuropsychology for the attorney.* Delray Beach, FL: St. Lucie Press.

Slick, D. J., Sherman, E. M. S., & Iverson, G. L. (1999). Diagnostic criteria for malingered neurocognitive dysfunction: Proposed standards for clinical practice and research. *Clinical Neuropsychologist, 13,* 545–561.

Slick, D. J., Tan, J. E., Strauss, E. H., & Hultsch, D. F. (2004). Detecting malingering: A survey of experts' practices. *Archives of Clinical Neuropsychology, 19,* 465–473.

Snyder, P. J., & Ceravolo, N. A. (1998). The medical chart: Efficient information-gathering strategies and proper chart noting. In P. J. Snyder & P. D. Nussbaum (Eds.), *Clinical neuropsychology: A pocket handbook for assessment* (pp. 3–10). New York: American Psychological Association.

Sweet, J. J. (1999). *Forensic neuropsychology: Fundamentals and practice.* Lisse, the Netherlands: Swets & Zeitlinger.

Sweet, J. J., Newman, P., & Bell, B. (1992). Significance of depression in clinical neuropsychological assessment. *Clinical Psychology Review, 12,* 21–45.

Tallent, N. (1993). *Psychological report writing* (4th ed.). Englewood Cliffs, NJ: Prentice Hall.

Taylor, M. J., & Heaton, R. K. (2001). Sensitivity and specificity of WAIS-III/WMS-III demographically corrected factor scores in neuropsychological assessment. *Journal of the International Neuropsychological Society, 7,* 867–874.

Tremont, G. (1998). Effect of intellectual level on neuropsychological test performance: A response to Dodrill (1997). *The Clinical Neuropsychologist, 12,* 560–567.

Vanderploeg, R. D. (2000). *Clinician's guide to neuropsychological assessment* (2nd ed.). Mahwah, NJ: Lawrence Erlbaum Associates.

Wechsler, D. (1997). *Wechsler Adult Intelligence Scale—III.* San Antonio, TX: The Psychological Corporation.

Williams, A. D. (1997a). Fixed versus flexible battery. In R. J. McCaffrey, A. D. Williams, J. M. Fisher, & L. C. Laing (Eds.), *The practice of forensic neuropsychology: Meeting challenges in the courtroom* (pp. 57–70). New York: Plenum Press.

Williams, A. D. (1997b). The forensic evaluation of adult traumatic brain injury. In R. J. McCaffrey, A. D. Williams, J. M. Fisher, & L. C. Laing (Eds.), *The practice of forensic neuropsychology: Meeting challenges in the courtroom* (pp. 37–56). New York: Plenum Press.

Williams, M. A., & Boll, T. J. (2000). Report writing in clinical neuropsychology. In G. Groth-Marnat (Ed.), *Neuropsychological assessment in clinical practice: A guide to test interpretation and integration* (pp. 575–602). New York: John Wiley & Sons, Inc.

Ylvisaker, M. (1997). *Traumatic brain injury rehabilitation: Children and adolescents* (2nd ed.). New York: Butterworth-Heinemann.

Ziskin, J., & Faust, D. (1988). *Coping with psychiatric and psychological testimony* (4th ed., Vol. 1–3). Marina Del Rey, CA: Law & Psychologys Press.

Zuckerman, E. L. (1995). *The clinician's thesaurus: A guidebook for wording psychological reports and other evaluations* (4th ed.). Toronto, Ontario: Mental Health Systems.

6

General Cognitive Functioning, Neuropsychological Batteries, and Assessment of Premorbid Intelligence

GENERAL COGNITIVE FUNCTIONING

IQ Tests

Models of Intelligence

There are diverse conceptions of intelligence and how it should be measured (e.g., Neisser et al., 1996; Sattler, 2001). Some theorists (e.g., Spearman, 1927) have emphasized the importance of a general factor, g, which represents what all the tests (or subtests) have in common and determines how one would perform on the variety of tasks tapping intelligence; others (e.g., Thurstone, 1938) have theorized that there are actually multiple intelligences, each reflecting a specific dimension of cognitive ability, such as memory, verbal comprehension, or number facility. One of the most important theories in contemporary intelligence research is based on the factor-analytic work of Carroll (1993, 1997) and Horn and Noll (1997). The Carroll-Horn-Cattell (CHC) framework (Flanagan & McGrew, 1997) is a model that synthesizes Carroll and Horn-Cattell's models and stresses several broad classes of abilities at the higher level (e.g., fluid ability [Gf], crystallized intelligence [Gc], short-term memory, long-term storage and retrieval, processing speed), and a number of primary factors at the lower level (e.g., quantitative reasoning, spelling ability, free recall, simple reaction time). The CHC factor-analytic theory of cognitive abilities is shown in Figure 6–1. Because contemporary theories of the structure of cognitive functioning emphasize multiple, somewhat independent factors of intelligence (e.g., Carroll, 1997; Flanagan et al., 2000; Larrabee, 2004; McGrew, 1997; Tulsky et al., 2003a, 2003b), intelligence is best evaluated with multifaceted instruments and techniques.

While modern models of intelligence such as the CHC model derive from an empirical framework (i.e., factor analysis), they are a relatively recent development in the history of applied intelligence testing. From the time of the very first standardized tests, intelligence tests were used by clinicians not because of empirically demonstrated rigor, but because of practical concerns and clinical utility. For instance, part of the impetus for the development of the Binet-Simon Scale (1905) was the French government's request that Binet and Simon find a way to examine school-aged children who had mental retardation (Sattler, 2001; Tulsky et al., 2003b). The goals of the Army Alpha and Beta forms developed by Robert M. Yerkes (1921) and his colleagues were to guide military selection, that is, to screen intellectually incompetent individuals to exempt them from military service and to identify those capable of more responsibility and greater duties (Tulsky et al., 2003b). David Wechsler developed the first version of his famous test to detect impairments in psychiatric inpatients in New York's Bellevue Hospital. Thus, the main criterion for selecting and constructing these early IQ tests was clinical relevance, not congruence with empirically derived theories of cognitive functioning.

While they were revered and almost universally accepted by practicing clinicians, traditional IQ tests were not well received by contemporary theorists, particularly in the light of hindsight afforded by statistical techniques. As a result, tests grounded in clinical tradition, such as the Wechsler scales, have been criticized for spawning simplistic models of human intelligence such as the dichotomy of verbal versus nonverbal intelligence (Flanagan & McGrew, 1997), or more recently, the four-factor model of intelligence composed of verbal, nonverbal, working memory, and processing speed components (Flanagan & McGrew, 1997). However, regardless of empirically based criticisms, traditional tests, including the many descendents of the first Binet and Wechsler scales, are some of the most important milestones in the history of psychological assessment, and as such, have contributed extensively to our knowledge of cognitive function in abnormal and normal populations. What is most intriguing is that there appears to be a rapprochement between traditional clinically based tests and those based on factor-analytic models of intelligence. For example, tests derived from different traditions are becoming increasingly similar in content, as a review of several of the major intelligence batteries in this volume will indicate, as test

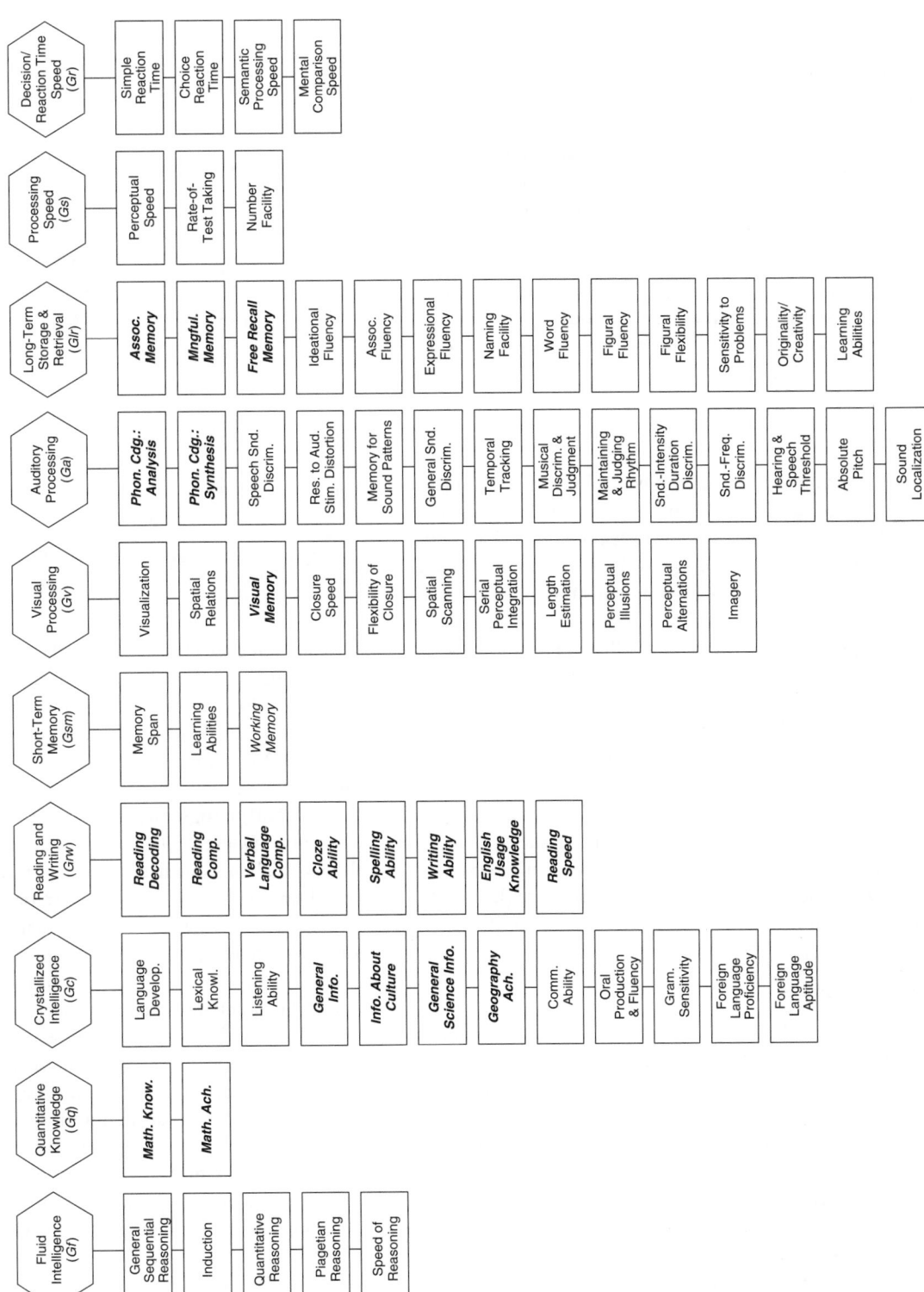

Figure 6–1 An integrated Cattell-Horn-Carroll *Gf-Gc* model of the structure of cognitive abilities. *Note:* Italic font indicates abilities that were not included in Carroll's three-stratum model but were included by Carroll in the domains of knowledge and achievement. Bold font indicates abilities that are placed under different *Gf-Gc* broad abilities than in Carroll's model. These changes are based on the Cattell-Horn model and/or recent research (see McGrew, 1997, and McGrew & Flanagan, 1998). *Source:* Reprinted with permission from Flanagan et al., 2000.

developers adapt traditional tests to fit models such as the CHC model (e.g., SB-5, WJ III, WPPSI-III, WISC-IV). Another example is the use of factor-analytic techniques to parse traditional measures into more contemporary models of cognitive functioning (e.g., Tulsky's six-factor model of the WAIS-III/WMS-III). Still another is the combination of subtests from traditional and nontraditional batteries, including the Stanford-Binet, the Wechsler, and factor-analysis-based scales such as the WJ III, into combined batteries that assess all the different dimensions of cognitive ability posited by factor-analytic approaches (i.e., Cross-Battery Approach) (Flanagan & McGrew, 1997; Flanagan et al., 2000). Overall, new tests based on empirical models such as factor analysis (e.g., Woodcock-Johnson-III, CAS) and new conceptualizations of existing tests (e.g., WAIS-III, WISC-IV) tend to assess a broader spectrum of abilities than previously represented and tend to be more consonant with factor-based theories of cognitive functioning.

Content

The more common measures of general intellectual function (e.g., the Wechsler Tests, WJ III, CAS, and the Stanford-Binet) include many different types of items, both verbal and nonverbal. Examinees may be asked to give the meaning of words, to complete a series of pictures, to construct block patterns, etc. Performance can then be scored to yield several subscores and composite scores. Although intelligence tests usually correlate highly with each other (e.g., .50 to .70), each test provides a significant amount of unique variance such that intelligence tests are not necessarily interchangeable. Thus, because the various intelligence tests sample different combinations of abilities, an individual's IQ is likely to vary from one test to another. It is also worth bearing in mind that a wide range of human abilities are outside the domain of standard intelligence tests (e.g., Neisser et al., 1996; Tulsky et al., 2003a). Obvious facets include wisdom, creativity, practical knowledge, and social skills.

Utility of IQ scores

There has been dispute over the utility of IQ scores. Some argue that these scores are exceedingly reliable and therefore worthy of attention. Indeed, IQ tests are unique in that their reliabilities commonly exceed .95, a level that few other tests are able to achieve (e.g., Kaufman & Lichtenberger, 1999). Others (e.g., Lezak et al., 2004) contend that because of the multiplicity of cognitive functions assessed in these batteries, composites such as IQ scores are not useful in describing cognitive test performance and only serve to obscure important information obtainable only by examining discrete scores. In addition to more traditional summary or IQ scores, most contemporary tests (e.g., Wechsler, WJ III, CAS, Stanford-Binet) typically include measures of more discrete factors and domains. Such an approach is also consistent with current views of cognitive functioning outlined previously.

Table 6–1 Percentile Ranks by Educational Level

Percentile	Years of Education					
	0–7	8	9–11	12	13–15	16+
VIQ						
95th	105	108	119	120	126	135
75th	91	98	105	108	115	123
50th	82	90	96	100	108	116
25th	73	83	87	92	100	108
5th	60	72	73	80	90	97
PIQ						
95th	109	117	122	122	125	132
75th	95	103	108	109	113	120
50th	84	93	98	100	105	111
25th	74	83	88	91	97	102
5th	60	69	73	78	86	90
FSIQ						
95th	106	111	120	121	126	135
75th	92	99	106	108	115	123
50th	82	91	96	100	107	115
25th	73	83	87	92	100	107
5th	59	71	73	79	89	95

Source: Adapted from Ryan et al., 1991. Copyright by the American Psychological Association. Reprinted with permission.

While some are critical of IQ tests, they do not dispute the fact that IQ scores predict certain forms of achievement—especially school achievement—quite effectively. Table 6–1 presents estimated percentile ranks for WAIS-R VIQ, PIQ, and FSIQ at six different educational levels (Ryan et al., 1991). Similar findings are obtained for the WAIS-III (see *WTAR Manual*, 2001; also, see WAIS-III in this volume). This table shows how IQ levels differ across education levels. For example, one might assume that following a traumatic brain injury, a child who obtains an FSIQ of 90 or lower would be unlikely to complete college since fewer than 5% of university-educated individuals have IQ scores in this range.

Because IQ scores predict educational achievement, they also predict occupational and financial outcome (Neisser et al., 1996). The correlation between IQ scores and grades is about .50; correlations with achievement test results are higher (the Psychological Corporation, 2002). Note, however, that correlations of this magnitude account for only about 25% of the overall variance. Other individual characteristics (e.g., persistence, interest) are probably of equal or greater importance in achieving academically. However, we may not have equally reliable ways of measuring these traits. With these reservations in mind, IQ scores are clearly relevant to the neuropsychological context and need to be considered.

Comprehensive IQ Batteries

Choosing the appropriate IQ test is an integral part of the assessment process. The breadth of abilities that are tapped by various measures is obviously a critical concern. For example, with the exception of the WAIS-III Matrix Reasoning subtest, the scale does not contain any strong indicators of fluid reasoning (see Flanagan et al., 2000, for a more complete discussion of the limitations of most current batteries in containing measures that sufficiently approximate the full range of abilities that define current views of intelligence). Further, while many clinicians routinely administer the same IQ test to all examinees, there are instances where a different IQ battery may be more appropriate. For instance, individuals who will require longitudinal assessment may be better suited to an IQ test that spans all the age ranges (e.g., WJ III), whereas others may require a test with a major nonverbal component (e.g., SB5). Considerations about conorming should also inform battery selection (e.g., depending on whether a memory workup or learning disability assessment will be conducted), since not all IQ tests are conormed with major memory or achievement tests. In Table 6–2, we list the major assessment batteries, with respective age ranges, domains assessed, typical administration times, and conormed tests. We tend to give the IQ test early in the course of the assessment because it allows the examiner to observe how the client behaves on a wide array of tasks. In this way, the examiner can develop hypotheses about the patient's spared and impaired abilities that can then be tested more thoroughly during the course of the assessment.

In this chapter, we present the Wechsler Intelligence Scales (WPPSI-III, WISC-IV, WAIS-III), which have played a central role in neuropsychological thinking about intelligence and psychological testing. For example, the WAIS-III (and its previous versions) is one of the most frequently used measures in neuropsychological batteries (e.g., Camara et al., 2000; Rabin et al., 2005) and is often considered "the gold standard" in intelligence testing (e.g., Ivnik et al., 1992). The same can be said for the WISC-IV, and to a lesser extent, for the WPPSI-III.

A number of authors (e.g., Flanagan et al., 2000; Larrabee, 2004; Tulsky et al., 2003b) argue that a more complete evaluation of intellectual functioning necessitates supplementing the traditional Wechsler scales with other instruments to measure facets of g that are either not covered or insufficiently covered by the Wechsler tests. Thus, Tulsky et al. (2003b) have developed a six-factor model from the WAIS-III and WMS-III (see *WAIS-III* and *WMS-III*) that includes verbal, perceptual, processing speed, working memory, auditory memory, and visual memory constructs. Whether the model increases clinical sensitivity and specificity remains to be determined. Another technique is to use the Cross-Battery Approach, which adds on specific subtests from other major IQ tests to supplement areas not fully assessed by the Wechsler scales (e.g., Flanagan et al., 2000).

We include a number of other measures of general intellectual functioning that have taken advantage of recent theoretical advances in the field. The structure of the WJ III COG is closely modeled after the CHC theory of intelligence. It has a three-level hierarchical structure consisting of (a) psycho-metric g (i.e., the General Intellectual Ability score [GIA]), (b) Stratum II level abilities (represented by seven factors), and (c) Stratum III abilities (represented by 20 subtests measuring narrow abilities). In addition, it yields five Clinical Clusters that measure abilities important for clinical evaluation, including executive functioning, working memory, and attention.

The SB5 also measures a range of abilities in the CHC framework. The nonverbal domain includes a broad range of subtests that may prove useful in the neuropsychological setting. However, the omission of measures of speed of processing likely limits the test's sensitivity to impairment.

The Cognitive Assessment Scale (CAS; Naglieri & Das, 1997) is a theory-based measure of intelligence, deriving from the work of A. Luria. It is based on the notions that "cognitive processes" should replace the term "intelligence" and that a test of cognitive processing should rely as little as possible on acquired knowledge such as vocabulary or arithmetic. The authors propose that cognition depends on four interrelated essential elements: planning, attention, simultaneous processes, and successive processes. These are thought to interact with the individual's knowledge base and skills.

The Bayley Scales (BSID-II; Bayley, 1993) are the most widely used measures for infants and very young children. The BSID-II is a developmental assessment test that measures cognitive, motor, and physical development with an item content that is theoretically eclectic and broad. Despite the considerable challenges of assessing infants and toddlers, the test has a strong psychometric base.

IQ Screening Methods

For screening purposes, when a global IQ estimate is sufficient or when time constraints are an issue, examiners might consider giving a test such as the K-BIT (Kaufman & Kaufman, 1990). It has the advantage of being motor-free, is brief to administer, and provides measures of both verbal and nonverbal functioning.

However, tests such as the WASI (the Psychological Corporation, 2001), with its four subtests (Vocabulary, Similarities, Block Design, Matrix Reasoning), show lower correlations among subtests and therefore may provide the clinician with more meaningful information by tapping a broader array of cognitive functions (Hays et al., 2002). The WASI also has the advantage that it was developed using linking samples with the WISC-III and WAIS-III. Wechsler short forms (see *WAIS-III* in this volume), however, are somewhat better at predicting WAIS-III summary scores and some (e.g., Kaufman's tetrad of Arithmetic, Similarities, Picture Completion, and Digit Symbol) require less time to administer. In addition, the short forms have the advantage that, should there be a need for a complete Wechsler profile, the nonadministered subtests can be administered at a later date (Eisenstein & Engelhart, 1997). Many other established batteries (e.g., CAS, WJ III) provide a short-form IQ estimate based on a smaller number of subtests than the standard form.

Table 6-2 Characteristics of Tests of General Intellectual Functioning

Test	Age Range	Administration Time	Domains Purported to Assess	Normative Linking Samples
Bayley	1 month–3 years, 5 months	Depends on age: 25–60 min	Mental Development Motor Development Behavioral Rating Scale	
CAS	5–17 years, 11 months	Basic: 40 min Standard: 60 min	Planning Processes Attention Processes Simultaneous Processes Successive Processes	
DRS-2	55+ years	Depends on mental status: Healthy elderly: 10–15 min Impaired: 30–45 min	Attention Initiation/Perseveration Construction Conceptualization Memory and Attention	
K-BIT	4–90 years	15–30 min	Verbal Knowledge/Reasoning Nonverbal Reasoning	
KBNA	20–89 years	120 min	Attention/Concentration Memory—Immediate, Delayed, Recognition Spatial Processing Verbal Fluency Reasoning/Conceptual Shifting	
NAB	18–97 years	Depends on which modules are given: Screening: 45 min Individual modules: 25–45 min All modules except screening: 3 hr All modules: ~4 hr	Screening Attention Language Memory Spatial Executive Functions	
NEPSY	3–12 years	Depends on age: Age 3–4: 45 min Core; 1 hr full Ages 5+: 65 min Core; 2 hr full	Attention/Executive Language Sensorimotor Functions Visuospatial Processing Memory and Learning	
MMSE	18–85+ years with some limited data available for children	10–15 min	Orientation Registration Attention/ Calculation Recall Language	
Raven's	5 years 5 months+	SPM: 40 min CPM: 25 min APM: 40–60 min	Nonverbal Reasoning	
RBANS	20–89 years	20–30 min	Immediate Memory Visuospatial/Constructional Language Attention Delayed Memory	
SB5	2–85+ years	Abbreviated: 15–20 min Full: 45–75 min	Fluid Reasoning Knowledge Quantitative Reasoning Visual-Spatial Reasoning Working Memory	WJ III ACH
TONI-3	6–89 years, 11 months	15–20 min	Nonverbal Reasoning	

(continued)

Table 6–2 Characteristics of Tests of General Intellectual Functioning (*continued*)

Test	Age Range	Administration Time	Domains Purported to Assess	Normative Linking Samples
WAIS-III	16–89	45–90 min	Verbal Knowledge/Reasoning Working Memory Nonverbal Reasoning Speed of Processing	WMS-III WIAT-II WASI WTAR
WISC-IV	6–16 years, 11 months	~90 min	Verbal Knowledge/Reasoning Perceptual Reasoning Working Memory Speed of Processing	
WPPSI-III	2 years, 6 months–7 years, 3 months	Young children: ~40 min Older children: 40–85 min, depending on which subtests are given	Verbal Knowledge/Reasoning Nonverbal Reasoning Speed of Processing Language Ability	WIAT-II
WASI	6–89 years	15–30 min, depending on whether two or four subtests are given	Verbal Reasoning Nonverbal Reasoning	WAIS-III WISC-III
WJ III COG	2–90+ years	Standard: 25–35 min Extended: 90–120 min Brief: 15 min	Comprehension-Knowledge Long-Term Retrieval Visual-Spatial Thinking Auditory Processing Fluid Reasoning Processing Speed Short-Term/Working Memory Attention Cognitive Fluency Executive Processes Delayed Recall	WJ III ACH

Overall, screening forms should not be used to categorize an individual's intelligence for diagnostic purposes or disability determination. Rather, they should be reserved for situations where gross estimates will suffice or when patient stamina is an issue. The choice of test should be guided by a number of considerations, including the test's clinical utility, psychometric characteristics, and time constraints.

Nonverbal IQ Tests

The TONI-3 (Brown et al., 1997) and Raven's Progressive Matrices (Raven, 1938, 1947, 1965) may be considered in patients whose test performance may be confounded by language, hearing, or motor impairments, or who lack proficiency with English and/or come from diverse ethnic and racial backgrounds. The Raven's tests are older and better researched. While not culture-free, they are more culture-fair than traditional IQ tests such as the Wechsler. New versions of the Raven's tests have also been developed to overcome the erosion of discriminative power as a result of the worldwide increase in intellectual ability over the years (i.e., Flynn effect).

It is important to bear in mind that the one-dimensional nature of tasks such as the Raven's and the TONI-3 provide little information about an individual's strengths or weak-

nesses, and both suffer from psychometric limitations. The motor-reduced component and untimed nature of these tasks may also make them relatively insensitive to various forms of impairment. Lastly, comprehensive nonverbal batteries such as the UNIT, C-TONI, or Leiter-R are more appropriate for diagnostic assessment than the one-dimensional tests such as the TONI-3 or Raven's (these are reviewed in Essentials of Nonverbal Assessment: McCallum et al., 2001).

Neuropsychological Batteries

Broad-based neuropsychological test batteries, such as the Halstead-Reitan Neuropsychological Battery (HRNB; Reitan & Wolfson, 1993) and the Luria-Nebraska Neuropsychological Battery (LNNB; Golden et al., 1985) have been used in the past to assess the presence, location, and extent of cerebral damage. With the advent of sophisticated neuroimaging procedures, the role of neuropsychology has shifted, with clinicians being asked to address other issues (e.g., nature of the cognitive deficit, potential for cognitive compensation/retraining and functional impact). In addition, the economics of health care has shifted focus toward brief assessment. In response to these changes, a number of authors have developed new tools for the assessment of a wide array of cognitive skills. Thus, the KBNA

(Leach et al., 2000) consists of 25 subtests, some of which can be combined into indices that represent higher-order domains of functioning. The KBNA also measures behaviors commonly overlooked by neuropsychologists and behavioral neurologists (e.g., praxis, emotion expression).

The Neuropsychology Assessment Battery (NAB; Stern & White, 2003) is a "new-generation" battery that provides a fairly comprehensive evaluation of functions in about 3.5 to 4 hours (White & Stern, 2003). It offers a separate screening module to determine the presence/absence of impaired performance and the need for additional follow-up testing with any of the main NAB modules. Table 6–2 shows the six NAB modules. Each NAB module has two equivalent/parallel forms (Form 1 and 2) and each form consists of 33 individual tests. Of note, each module contains one daily living task that is designed to be congruent with an analogous real-world behavior. Because each test was normed on the same standardization sample, the examiner can use a single set (rather than several different sets) of normative tables including appropriate age, sex, and education corrections. These coordinated norms allow for within- and between-patient score comparisons across the NAB tests.

For children, the NEPSY (Korkman et al., 1998) is the first instrument designed exclusively and a priori as a neuropsychological battery for children. Although there are other neuropsychological batteries for children, they are based on modifications and downward extensions of existing adult batteries.

Screening Tools

Comprehensive batteries provide considerable data but can be time consuming. Another approach involves brief screening instruments such as the MMSE (Folstein et al., 1975), DRS (Jurica et al., 2001; Mattis, 1976), and RBANS (Randolph, 1998).

The MMSE is very popular. Most studies report that the MMSE summary score is sensitive to the presence of dementia, particularly in those with moderate to severe forms of cognitive impairment. However, it is less than ideal in those with mild cognitive deficits.

The DRS is more comprehensive than the MMSE. It more accurately tracks progression of decline and is better able to discriminate among patients with dementia. Nonetheless, the clinician may prefer the MMSE, particularly with those individuals who have difficulty concentrating longer than five to 10 minutes. Further, although sensitive to differences at the lower end of functioning, the DRS may not detect impairment in the higher ranges of intelligence, since it was developed to avoid floor effects in clinically impaired populations rather than ceiling effects in high-functioning individuals.

The RBANS appears to be more sensitive to impairment than either the MMSE or the DRS. However, it too was designed for use with healthy adults as well as people with moderate/severe dementia, suggesting that it may have limited utility at the higher end of the intellectual continuum.

PREMORBID ESTIMATION

In neuropsychological assessment, the diagnosis of impairment requires some standard against which to compare current performance. Effectively comparing a person's performance to some population average score will depend on how closely the individual matches the population in terms of demographics and past experiences. However, the predictions are to a hypothetical average rather than to the specific individual under consideration (Franzen et al., 1997). The same test score can represent an entirely normal level of functioning for one individual and yet a serious decline for another (Crawford et al., 2001). Therefore, it is necessary to compare performance against an individualized comparison standard. Since premorbid neuropsychological test data are rarely available, it becomes necessary to estimate an individual's premorbid level of functioning.

Self-report is not a reliable basis for the estimation of premorbid ability. Even individuals with no external incentives to misrepresent their past achievements tend to inflate their recall of their high school grades and past achievements. Studies of college students (Bahrick et al., 1996) and of psychiatric patients (Johnson-Greene et al., 1997) reveal that accuracy of grade recall declines with actual letter grade; namely, worse actual achievement is associated with more inflated reports. There are probably a variety of reasons that patients, and nonpatients, overestimate their achievements. Some may inflate their preinjury ability or deny premorbid difficulties as a response to an adversarial context (Greiffenstein & Baker, 2001; Greiffenstein et al., 2002); others may misrepresent their abilities because of cognitive compromise. If a clinician interprets test scores in the context of exaggerated reports of past performance, he or she may overestimate the extent of a patient's decline and may infer deterioration when none exists (Gladsjo et al., 1999).

Past school, employment or military records may provide clues regarding premorbid ability. Relying on school records avoids the pitfalls of accepting unsubstantiated self-report. Grades in school records or performance reports on the job are confounded by the subjectivity in judgment of the various raters. Nonetheless, there is evidence that grade point average (GPA) is related to subsequent neuropsychological test performance in well-motivated neurologically intact individuals, suggesting that grade markings can provide an important context for interpretation of such measures (Greiffenstein & Baker, 2003).

Standardized test scores from school records can be invaluable as indicators of preinsult ability. In addition, it is known that achievement tests show moderate/strong correlations with measures of intelligence (e.g., Baade & Schoenberg, 2004; the Psychological Corporation, 2002). Spelling scores correlate less with Wechsler FSIQ than do reading and mathematics scores. Recently, Baade and Schoenberg (2004) suggested a procedure to predict WAIS-R FSIQ using group-administered achievement test scores. However, additional studies that examine the relations between achievement tests (e.g., American College Test, Scholastic Achievement Test) given during school years and measures such as the WAIS-III given many years later are needed to ensure the adequacy of this method. Further, historical data are often difficult to acquire or may not even exist. Therefore, other approaches to estimating premorbid cognitive functioning are necessary.

Premorbid Estimation in Adults

The most investigated procedures to estimate premorbid ability are based on (a) demographics alone, (b) current performance on tasks thought to be fairly resistant to neurological insult, and (c) combinations of demographics and current performance. We consider each of these methods in the following sections. It should be noted that much of the work conducted in this area has focused on premorbid estimation of IQ (and typically as measured by the Wechsler scale); however, increasingly efforts are being directed to other functions as well.

Interestingly, while methods to predict premorbid ability receive considerable study in the literature, practitioners tend not to use these measures in clinical practice (Smith-Seemiller et al., 1997). The extent to which this may reflect a lack of awareness of these measures, as opposed to the perception that they are unnecessary or ineffective, is unclear (Smith-Seemiller et al., 1997). Some of the limitations of these methods are that they may not detect patients with clinically significant impairment, either (a) because of inadequate sensitivity (e.g., error band is too wide) or (b) because of inadequate resistance of the predictor to withstand the effects of the disease. However, our view is that it is worthwhile to use one of these methods. If the discrepancy between estimated and obtained performance does not exceed the cutoff, then the technique has failed to show evidence of abnormality and the patient may still have clinically significant decline; however, if the obtained discrepancy does exceed the cutoff, then the result may have clinical value (Graves et al., 1999). Although the various methods reviewed have limited sensitivity, it is important to bear in mind that clinicians' informal estimates are even less accurate (Crawford et al., 2001; Williams, 1997).

Demographic Prediction

In this approach, premorbid ability is estimated on the basis of demographic variables, such as age, education, occupation, sex, and ethnicity. In the case of IQ, education, race, and occupation are the strongest predictors and these variables are combined in multiple regression equations to predict the various IQ scores. The power of demographics in predicting Wechsler IQ scores is highest for FSIQ and VIQ (and VCI). Thus, Wilson et al. (1978) evaluated the ability of five demographic variables (age, sex, race, education, and occupation) to predict WAIS IQs and obtained moderately favorable results. The equations were able to predict 54%, 53%, and 42% of the variance in FSIQ, VIQ, and PIQ, respectively. The original WAIS was revised in 1981 and Barona et al. (1984) updated the formulas for use with the revision, the WAIS-R (see Spreen & Strauss, 1998, for the formulas and worksheet). These indices were able to account for only 36%, 38%, and 24% of FSIQ, VIQ, and PIQ scores, respectively. In addition, the standard errors of estimate for the regression equations were rather large (e.g., 12.14 for WAIS-R FSIQ). The smaller proportion of variance explained in nonverbal ability has also been noted by Crawford and Allen (1997). They used the demographic approach to predict the WAIS-R IQ in the United Kingdom. Their regression equations predicted 53%, 53%, and 32% of the variance in FSIQ, VIQ, and PIQ, respectively.

Methods for predicting premorbid IQ involving demographic factors alone have also been developed for the most recent version of the WAIS (WAIS-III) based on a subsample of the Wechsler standardization sample (see Table 6–3). The *WTAR Manual* (2001; see review in this volume) provides regression-based indices and tables (separately for ages 16–19 and 20–89 years) that allow the examiner to predict WAIS-III VIQ, PIQ, FSIQ, and VCI from a combination of educational level, race/ethnicity, and sex. The strongest predictor is education, followed by ethnicity. The contribution of sex is larger for minority groups than for Caucasians. As was the case with earlier Wechsler versions, prediction is better for VIQ, VCI, and FSIQ than for PIQ.

Demographic methods (formal regression equations) have the advantage of being applicable to a wide variety of clients and, unlike performance on cognitive tests, they are not subject to decline in clinical conditions (e.g., dementia). They are also not compromised by suboptimal effort—a problem that may plague performance-based measures, particularly in medical-legal contexts. In fact, large discrepancies between expected and obtained scores may even prove helpful in identifying insufficient effort (Demakis et al., 2001). In addition, regression equations are more accurate than clinicians' informal estimates based on the same information (Crawford et al., 2001). Actuarial methods apply the optimal weights to the demographic predictor variables, thereby maximizing accuracy, whereas clinical estimates are often based on vague or distorted impressions of cognition-demographic relationships (Crawford et al., 2001). Actuarial methods also have higher rates of interrater reliability than clinical judgment because they limit subjective estimates (Barona et al., 1984).

There are however, a number of concerns associated with demographic methods. First, the band of error associated with these various demographic equations is considerable (see also Basso et al., 2000). For example, the predicted WAIS-III FSIQ for a white male aged 20 to 89 years with 12 years of education is 102; however, the 90% confidence interval has a range of almost 40 points (83–121). As such, we may be 90% confident that the individual may have had a premorbid intelligence that was either low average, average, above average, or superior! Unless a very large decline has occurred, it may be very difficult to decide whether a patient's obtained IQ is genuinely less than expected. Further, given that 68% of the Wechsler normative sample obtained IQs between 85 and

Table 6–3 Examples of Methods to Predict Premorbid Ability in Adults

Method	Tool	Prediction
Demographics only	WTAR Manual (age, educational level, race/ethnicity, and gender)	WAIS-III VIQ, PIQ, FSIQ, VCI
Current performance	NART/NAART/AMNART	WAIS-R VIQ, PIQ, FSIQ FAS PASAT Raven's Progressive Matrices Doors and People Test
	WTAR	WAIS-III VIQ, PIQ, FSIQ, VCI, POI, WMI, PSI WMS-III Immediate Memory, General Memory, Working Memory
	SCOLP—Spot-the-Word	IQ Boston Naming Test FAS
	WRAT-R/3 Reading	IQ
	Word Accentuation Test	WAIS Raven's Progressive Matrices
Combined method	WTAR and Demographics	WAIS-III VIQ, PIQ, FSIQ, VCI, POI, WMI, PSI WMS-III Immediate Memory, General Memory, Working Memory
	NART/NAART/AMNART and Demographics	WAIS-R FSIQ WAIS-R Vocabulary Raven's SPM
	SCOLP—Spot-the-Word and demographics	FAS
	OPIE-3 (Demographics and WAIS-III Vocabulary, Matrix Reasoning, Information, Picture Completion)	WAIS-III FSIQ, VIQ, PIQ

Note: The relevant prediction equations are located in the chapters on the WAIS-III (OPIE), NART, SCOLP, Raven's, PASAT, FAS, and BNT.

115, the demographic prediction renders minimal improvement over an estimate based on base-rate information alone (Basso et al., 2000). In addition, the demographic method yields severely restricted IQ ranges and is affected by regression to the mean, resulting in serious overestimation of premorbid IQ at the lower end and underestimation at the higher end of ability (e.g., Barona et al., 1984; Basso et al., 2000; Langeluddecke & Lucas, 2004; Sweet et al., 1990). As a consequence, those at the higher end of the IQ continuum who have suffered a decline may go undetected, while those at the lower end of the IQ distribution risk being diagnosed with impairment when none has occurred.

Accordingly, the demographic indices should be used with considerable caution in the individual case since much prediction error may be expected. While they may be of use with individuals whose premorbid IQ is likely to have been in the average range, they should not be used to estimate the premorbid ability of exceptional individuals such as the gifted, mentally handicapped, or even slow learners (e.g., Basso et al., 2000; Langeluddecke & Lucas, 2004; Ryan & Prifitera, 1990). Performance-based methods (e.g., OPIE, NART, WTAR), considered below, tend to provide better predictors of IQ than de-

mographic indices (e.g., Basso et al., 2000; Blair & Spreen, 1989; Crawford, 1992; Langeluddecke & Lucas, 2004).

Demographic indices alone may be preferred for estimating premorbid IQ in patients for whom reliance on cognitive performance (e.g., NART, WRAT-3, WTAR) would be inappropriate (e.g., patients with moderate or advanced dementia or aphasia, with severe brain injury, or who are suspected of insufficient effort). It is worth noting, however, that the deficits in cases of moderate/severe dysfunction are often clinically obvious and establishing a patient's premorbid IQ may be less critical in such cases. Caution should also be exercised when using demographic-based estimates with patients suffering from disorders that may have a lengthy prodromal phase. In such cases, the prodromal phase may have resulted in a failure to achieve patients' educational and occupational potential. Of course, a similar degree of caution must be exercised with performance-based estimates of premorbid ability (Crawford et al., 2001).

The power of demographics to predict functions other than IQ appears limited. For example, low levels of association have been reported between demographic variables (age, education, race/ethnicity, sex, geographic region) and performance on measures of memory (Gladsjo et al., 1999; Williams, 1997), including the WMS-III indices (correlations ranging from .02 to .31 in the U.S. standardization sample; the Psychological Corporation, 2001).

Current Performance

Assumptions that overall premorbid functioning can be reliably predicted from a single "spared" cognitive domain ("best performance" method) have been criticized by research showing that normal individuals demonstrate significant variability in functioning across different cognitive domains (e.g., Taylor & Heaton, 2001). As a consequence, the final result will be a systematic overestimation of intellectual impairment or deficits (Mortensen et al., 1991; but see Hoofien et al., 2000). Lezak et al. (2004) caution that an estimate of premorbid ability should never be based on a single test score but should take into account as much information as possible about the patient.

An alternative approach relies on the assessment of current abilities that are considered to be relatively resistant to the effects of cerebral insult (i.e., "hold" tests). This method uses test scores obtained during the formal test session to estimate premorbid ability. These are reviewed below.

Wechsler Subtests. Wechsler (1958) suggested that tests such as Vocabulary, Information, and Picture Completion were minimally affected by the effects of aging and brain impairment in adults and could therefore serve to estimate overall levels of premorbid cognitive function. However, this method has significant limitations. Although Vocabulary is among the most resistant of the Wechsler subtests, performance is markedly impaired in a range of clinical conditions. Vocabulary scores are therefore likely to seriously underestimate premorbid intelligence (Crawford, 1989; Lezak et al., 2004). The Information subtest reflects a person's general fund of knowledge. However, this score may be misleading in examinees with poor educational opportunities. In addition, there is evidence that tests such as Information and Picture Completion demonstrate decline following neurologic injury (e.g., Russell, 1972).

Word Reading Tests. Nelson and O'Connell (Nelson, 1982; Nelson & O'Connell, 1978) proposed that a reading test for irregularly spelled words would be a better indicator of premorbid ability based on the rationale that (a) reading skills are fairly resistant to brain insult, and (b) that irregularly spelled words cannot be decoded phonologically and hence rely on previously acquired skills. They developed in Britain a test called the National Adult Reading Test (NART), which consists of 50 irregular words (e.g., debt, naïve; see review in this volume). Subsequently, the NART was standardized against the WAIS-R (Crawford, 1992; Ryan & Paolo, 1992). Blair and Spreen (1989) adapted the NART for use with a North American population (North American Adult Reading Test or NAART or NART-R). Similar versions (AMNART:

Grober & Sliwinski, 1991; ANART: Schwartz & Saffran, 1987, cited in Grober & Sliwinski, 1991) have been developed for use in the United States.

NART scores correlate well with measures of IQ given concurrently. In addition, the NART has been validated against an actual premorbid criterion. Crawford et al. (2001) followed up 177 people who were given an IQ test at age 11. They found a correlation of .77 between these scores and NART scores at age 77.

NART (NAART/AMNART) scores correlate highly with FSIQ and VIQ and less with PIQ, a not surprising finding since it is a verbal test. Although much of the research on the NART has focussed on the estimation of premorbid Wechsler IQ, prediction equations have also been developed for use with tests such as the FAS, Raven's, PASAT, and Doors and People Test (see Table 6–3).

Prediction of IQ tends to be more accurate with equations based on NART (and its various adaptations) scores than with the Wechsler Vocabulary subtest (Crawford et al., 1989; Sharpe & O'Carroll, 1991) or with demographic variables (Blair & Spreen, 1989; Bright et al., 2002; Grober & Sliwinski, 1991; Ryan & Paolo, 1992). Further, while a fairly large decline in cognitive ability (about 15–20 points) may need to occur before the reading test can reliably identify abnormality, other methods (e.g., demographic estimates) require larger declines (about 20–25 points) (e.g., Graves et al., 1999).

The NART is not insensitive to decline; deterioration in NART performance does occur in patients with a variety of neurological conditions, for example, in cases of moderate to severe dementia (Patterson et al., 1994; Stebbins, Wilson, et al., 1988, 1990) and in those with mild dementia who have accompanying linguistic deficits (Stebbins, Gilley, et al., 1990). However, the NART appears less sensitive to neurological compromise than other measures (e.g., Wechsler Vocabulary). In short, it may prove useful in providing a lower limit to the estimate of premorbid IQ (Stebbins, Gilley, et al., 1990, Stebbins, Wilson, et al. 1990).

One should also note that the NART cannot be used with aphasic or dyslexic patients, nor in patients with significant articulatory or visual acuity problems (Crawford, 1989, 1992). Further, like any regression-based procedure, the NART overestimates FSIQ at the lower end of the IQ range and underestimates it at the higher end (Ryan & Paolo, 1992; Wiens et al., 1993).

Nelson, the NART's author, selected English words with an irregular pronunciation whose proper reading would depend on the previous knowledge of the subject rather than on phonological decoding skills. In the Spanish language, this cannot be done because every word is read in a regular way (with phonological decoding). Del Ser et al. (1997) therefore developed a reading task (Word Accentuation Test, WAT) with an ambiguous graphic clue for the Spanish reader: the accentuation of 30 infrequent words written in capital letters without accent marks. Its correlations with the WAIS (.84) and the Raven's Progressive Matrices (.63) are high, and the task appears fairly resistant to mild cognitive deterioration.

The test was developed in Spain, and since Spanish has marked geographical differences, a version has also been developed for use in Argentina (Burin et al., 2000). The reliability and validity of the WAT among Spanish speakers in other regions (e.g., the United States) has not yet been determined.

The WTAR (the Psychological Corporation, 2001; see also description in this volume) is a relatively new tool that is similar to the NART in that it requires reading of irregularly spelled words. Although its validity is less researched, only the WTAR, not the NART (or its variants), has been validated against the WAIS-III. Like the NART, WTAR scores correlate highly with FSIQ and the verbal composites (VIQ and Verbal Comprehension Index) and only moderately well with other Wechsler scores.

While the WTAR appears to provide a reasonable estimate of intellectual functioning, its utility in other domains (e.g., memory) appears more modest. Nonetheless, it displays a better prediction of WAIS-III and WMS-III scores than demographic variables. For example, the amount of variance accounted for by WTAR-predicted FSIQ (56%) is higher than that based on demographics alone (36%; the Psychological Corporation, 2001). Like the NART, it is relatively but not completely resistant to cerebral insult; also like the NART, it should not be used in those with a preexisting learning disorder or in those who suffer language or perceptual disorders.

The SCOLP (Baddeley et al., 1992) Spot-the-Word test (STW) is a brief lexical decision task consisting of 60 word-nonword pairs. Individuals have to identify the real word in each pair. Scores on the task correlate moderately well with crystallized ability. However, other tests (e.g., NART) prove more resistant to neurological impairment and correlate higher with Wechsler IQ (e.g., Watt & O'Carroll, 1999). Of note, equations based on the STW test have been developed for a variety of functions (see Table 6–3 and test descriptions elsewhere in this volume). In addition, because it does not involve a spoken response, the STW may be particularly useful for aphasic or dysarthric people. It can even be administered in a group setting to provide a gross estimate of ability.

The reading subtest of the Wide Range Achievement Test (WRAT, WRAT-R, WRAT-3) is used more frequently than other reading tests (e.g., NART) as an indicator of premorbid intellectual status (Smith-Seemiller et al., 1997). WRAT Reading shows a moderate relation with WAIS-R/WAIS-III IQ ($r = .45–.63$; Griffin et al., 2002; Johnstone et al., 1996; Wiens et al., 1993), although the relation is somewhat lower than that observed for the NART (Griffin et al., 2002) or the STW test (Lucas et al., 2003).

WRAT Reading scores do not remain stable in patients with a history of neurological insult, suggesting that this measure can be affected by CNS disease (Johnstone & Wilhelm, 1996) and other factors (e.g., motivational status). In addition, the task tends to underestimate Wechsler IQ, particularly in the high IQ ranges, to an even greater degree than the NART/NAART (Griffin et al., 2002; Weins et al., 1993). At the lower end of the IQ range (e.g., below 89), the WRAT-R/WRAT-3 may, however, be more appropriate than the NART/NAART or

demographic indicators (Griffin et al., 2002; Johnstone et al., 1996; Weins et al., 1993). In the average range, WRAT-3 and NAART scores provide equivalent and adequate classification (Griffin et al., 2002). In short, no one estimation method appears uniformly accurate, and different estimation methods are relatively better within specific IQ categories (see also Basso et al., 2000).

Accordingly, clinicians have to consider using multiple methods to derive estimates of premorbid ability rather than rely on a single estimate. In the event of differing classifications, clinicians are forced to rely on clinical judgement with regard to weighing the particular methodology that most accurately reflects premorbid functioning. Hybrid methods of premorbid estimation tend to provide for more accurate estimates.

Combinations of Demographics and Current Performance

Pairing test behavior with data from demographic variables appears to increase the power of prediction, producing less range restriction and less over- or underestimation of premorbid ability. The addition of demographics serves to buffer some of the effects of clinical status impacting cognitive performance (the Psychological Corporation, 2001); the inclusion of current performance indicators (e.g., reading test scores) can improve predictive accuracy particularly in those with unusual combinations (e.g., lower than expected reading ability given their educational achievement; Gladsjo et al., 1999).

Demographic variables (education level, race/ethnicity, and gender) and WTAR performance have been combined to predict intellectual (WAIS-III) and memory (WMS-III) functioning. The addition of demographic data to WTAR performance resulted in an increase of 4% to 7% over WTAR performance alone in the prediction of intellectual and memory performance (the Psychological Corporation, 2001). In addition, the ranges of possible scores are increased modestly (the Psychological Corporation, 2001). Others have reported similar gains when combining demographics with scores on reading tests such as the NART (e.g., Grober & Sliwinski, 1991; Watt & O'Carroll, 1999; Willshire et al., 1991).

Another method (OPIE, or Oklahoma Premorbid Intelligence Estimate formulas) combines select WAIS-III subtests that are relatively insensitive to neurological dysfunction (Vocabulary, Matrix Reasoning, Information, and Picture Completion) and demographic information (i.e., age, education, ethnicity, region of country, and gender) in prediction algorithms. Such formulas were initially developed by Krull et al. (1995) and Vanderploeg et al. (1996) for use with the WAIS-R and have been shown to correlate highly with premorbid ability (premorbid military data) (Hoofien et al., 2000). Formulas have recently been generated by Schoenberg et al. (2002) for the WAIS-III. Six OPIE-3 algorithms were developed from the WAIS-III standardization sample to predict FSIQ (other formulas are available to predict VIQ and PIQ; see Premorbid Estimation in our review of the *WAIS-III* in this volume). The subtests comprising the formulas are as follows (note that ST refers to subtest):

- OPIE-3 (4 ST): Vocabulary, Information, Matrix Reasoning, and Picture Completion
- OPIE-3 (2 ST): Vocabulary and Matrix Reasoning
- OPIE-3V: Vocabulary only
- OPIE-3P: Matrix Reasoning and Picture Completion
- OPIE-3MR: Matrix Reasoning only
- OPIE-3 (Best): OPIE-3V used if Vocabulary age-scaled score is higher, OPIE-3MR used if Matrix Reasoning age-scaled score is higher, and OPIE-3 (2ST) used if the age-scaled scores are equivalent

The OPIE-3 algorithms yield estimates of FSIQ that closely match the general population mean (Langeluddecke & Lucas, 2004; Schoenberg et al., 2002). They show a better range of scores in comparison with demographically based indices (Langeluddecke & Lucas, 2004) as well as NART-based estimates (see *NART* chapter in this volume), and while susceptible to relatively large errors of prediction (standard errors of estimation, SE_Es), other methods (i.e., demographic indexes) may yield larger prediction errors (Basso et al., 2000). The OPIE-3V, OPIE-3MR, and OPIE-3 (2ST) appear to be fairly robust where intellectual impairment is mild/moderate; the OPIE-3 (Best) is suitable for cases of severe brain injury (Langelluddecke & Lucas, 2004; Schoenberg et al., 2003). However, OPIE estimates, particularly those including two nonverbal subtests, are susceptible to neurological impairment (Langeluddecke & Lucas, 2004).

The differential clinical utility of the OPIE-3 and reading test-demographics (e.g.,WTAR-Demographics) approaches is not known. The OPIE-3 correlations with WAIS-III IQ are likely inflated due to the lack of independence (WAIS-III subtests are used in the computation of IQ scores), which also inflates the overlap in score distributions (Schoenberg et al., 2002); the OPIE-3 algorithms provide a greater range of IQ estimates (depending on the equation, range: 72–112 IQ score points; Schoenberg et al., 2002) than the WTAR used alone (depending on the IQ index, range: 30–49; the Psychological Corporation, 2001, p. 45) or when combined with demographic variables (range: 38–50; the Psychological Corporation, 2001, p. 57). Similarly, the proportion of OPIE-3 FSIQ estimates that fall within ±10 points of actual IQ (75%–93%; Schoenberg et al., 2002) is greater than the WTAR alone (70.4%), demographics alone (60.9%), or the combined WTAR-demographics approach (73.4%; the Psychological Corporation, 2001, p. 59).

Despite the potential theoretical and psychometric problems of the OPIE estimates (regression to the mean, high correlations between predictors and criterion), the available data suggest that the OPIE-3 is useful in predicting premorbid ability in neurologically impaired populations (Langelluddecke & Lucas, 2004; Schoenberg et al., 2003). An advantage of the OPIE-3 is that an estimate can be obtained when the WTAR (or NART) is not administered. Nonetheless, both methods (OPIE-3 and WTAR-demographics) require additional validation studies, including against an actual premorbid criterion.

Table 6–4 Examples of Methods to Predict Premorbid Ability in Children

Method	Tool	Prediction
Demographics only	Parental education, ethnicity	WISC-III VIQ, PIQ, and FSIQ
Performance of family members	IQ of parents or siblings	IQ
Combined methods	Parent ratings, maternal ethnicity, SES, word recognition	CVLT VMI WISC-III PIQ

Premorbid Estimation in Children

Methods to estimate premorbid cognitive functioning in adults have been well researched. In contrast, researchers have directed little attention to the development of prediction methods for children. The issue is also more complicated in children as their skills are not fully developed, and unlike adults, children often do not achieve stable levels of functioning prior to trauma or disease onset (Redfield, 2001). Table 6–4 shows that a number of methods have been used to predict premorbid ability in children. These include (a) demographic information, (b) familial intellect, and (c) a combination of sociodemographic information and current performance. Overall, attempts to develop measures of premorbid or expected ability for children have generally been less successful than for adults, typically producing estimates with inadequate precision for clinical use (Klesges & Sanchez, 1981; Yeates & Taylor, 1997).

Table 6–5 Regression Equations to Predict WISC-III IQ Scores

Outcome Measure	Regression Equation	SE_E	R^2
FSIQ	5.44 (mean education) + 2.80 (white/non-white) − 9.01 (black/non-black) + 81.68	12.56	.28
VIQ	5.71 (mean education) + 4.64 (white/non-white) − 5.04 (black/non-black) + 79.06	12.79	.27
PIQ	4.18 (mean education) + 0.26 (white/non-white) − 11.85 (black/non-black) + 88.09	13.35	.20

Ethnicity is composed of two coded variables, white/non-white (white = 1, non-white = 0) and black/non-black (black = 1, non-black = 0). Hispanic people would be uniquely identified with 0 on both white/non-white and black/ non-black. The regression equations had information for only three categories: white, black, and Hispanic; therefore, the regression equations should not be used with other ethnic groups. For parental education, the mean of the codings for the mother's and father's level of education is used in the regression formulas or the single parent's educational code if data from only one parent is available (parental education: 0–8 years = 1, 9–11 years = 2, 12 years (or GED) = 3, 13–15 years = 4, 16+ years = 5).

Source: From Vanderploeg et al., 1998. Reprinted with permission of APA.

Reynolds and Gutkin (1979) used demographic variables (father's occupational status, child's gender, ethnicity, urban versus rural residence, and geographic region) from the WISC-R to predict IQ scores. The equations had multiple correlations of .44, .44, and .37 with FSIQ, VIQ, and PIQ, respectively. Similar equations have been developed on the basis of the WISC-III standardization data. Vanderploeg et al. (1998) used mean parental education and ethnicity to predict IQ scores. The equations had correlations with FSIQ, VIQ, and PIQ of .53, .52, and .45, respectively, accounting for slightly more variance in actual IQ scores than the formulas developed by Reynolds and Gutkin (1979) from the WISC-R standardization data. Equations that relied on demographics alone proved just as effective as combining demographic variables with a WISC-III subtest scaled scores in a best-performance fashion (i.e., including Vocabulary or Picture Completion, whichever produced the higher estimated score), both of which were significantly more effective than using Vocabulary plus demographics or Picture Completion plus demographics individual formulas. Given that a purely demographic approach proved just as effective as the more complicated best-performance approach, it may be a better choice for premorbid estimation in children (Vanderploeg et al., 1998). The equations are provided in Table 6–5. Note that the equations refer to the WISC-III, not the more up-to-date WISC-IV, and that the demographic variables account for less

Table 6–6 Cumulative Percentages of Expected Discrepancies (Regardless of Sign) Between Obtained and Predicted IQ for Several Estimation Methods

Amount of Discrepancy (IQ points)	Discrepancy from IQ Estimated by				
	One Parent's IQ[a]	One Sibling's IQ[a]	Two Parents' Mean IQ[a]	Demographic Variables[b]	Previous IQ[a]
30	3	2	2	2	0
29	3	3	3	2	0
28	4	3	3	3	0
27	5	4	4	3	0
26	6	5	5	4	0
25	7	6	5	5	0.01
24	8	7	6	6	0.01
23	9	8	8	7	0.02
22	11	10	9	8	0.04
21	12	11	11	9	0.1
20	14	13	12	11	0.1
19	16	15	14	13	0.2
18	19	17	17	15	0.4
17	21	20	19	18	0.6
16	24	23	22	20	1
15	27	26	25	23	2
14	30	29	28	27	2
13	34	33	32	30	4
12	38	36	36	34	5
11	42	41	40	38	8
10	46	45	44	43	11
9	51	50	49	47	15
8	56	55	54	52	20
7	61	60	59	58	26
6	66	65	64	63	33
5	71	71	70	69	42
4	77	76	76	75	52
3	83	82	82	81	63
2	88	88	88	87	75
1	94	94	94	94	87

Note: All values refer to discrepancies between obtained and estimated Full-Scale IQ; discrepancies between obtained IQs of family members may be larger. For directional comparisons (e.g., the cumulative frequency with which an obtained IQ is below predicted IQ by a specified amount), divide the entries by 2.

[a]Estimated IQ is calculated by the equation $IQ_{est} = r(x - 100) + 100$, where IQ_{est} is estimated IQ score, r is the correlation coefficient with IQ for a particular estimation method (.42 for one parent's IQ, .47 for one sibling's IQ, .50 for two parents' mean IQ, .91 for a previous IQ) and x is the familial or previous IQ used as an estimator.

[b]Equation for estimating IQ using demographic variables from Vanderploeg et al., 1998.

Source: From Redfield, 2001. Reprinted by kind permission of Psychology Press.

than 30% of the variance in IQ scores. Note, too, the large standard errors of estimation suggesting that a very large discrepancy between observed and expected values will be needed to infer decline. In addition, bear in mind that any regression-based approach predicts scores toward the population mean, overestimating scores of persons with low ability and underestimating scores of those with high ability.

Some have suggested using parental or sibling intelligence as an index of expected intellectual ability of children (e.g., Baron, 2000; Reynolds, 1997)—a recommendation based on the well-known finding that IQs among biological relatives are correlated. However, IQ is significantly correlated within families (*r* values ranging from .42–.50), but at a level that limits the precision of IQ estimates based on measures of other family members' abilities (Redfield, 2001). The confidence limits around an IQ estimate based on familial intelligence, with or without the addition of demographic variables, span a wide range of values. To assist clinicians wishing to compare a child's IQ with estimates based on familial IQ or demographic variables, Table 6–6 lists cumulative percentages of expected discrepancies between obtained and predicted IQ for several estimation methods. Reference to Table 6–6 shows that sizeable discrepancies from familial IQ are required to infer abnormality, thus reducing their sensitivity (Redfield, 2001). Thus, while a significant discrepancy may be meaningful, the absence of one is often inconclusive. Redfield (2001) notes that estimates based on family members' IQ are not substantially more accurate than discrepancies derived from demographic indices. In short, there appears to be little justification to actually test family members' IQ, because an equally accurate measure can be obtained from the less costly procedure of ascertaining selected demographic characteristics (Redfield, 2001).

Attempts have also been made to predict premorbid ability using sociodemographic variables and measures of skills such as word recognition. Yeates and Taylor (1997) derived prediction equations from 80 children with orthopedic injuries between the ages of 6 and 12 years. A combination of parent ratings of premorbid school performance (Child Behavior Checklist, CBCL), maternal ethnicity, family socioeconomic status, and children's word recognition skill (WJ-R) predicted 13%, 36%, and 45% of the variance in three measures (respectively, a shortened version of the CVLT, Developmental Test of Visual-Motor Integration [VMI], and WISC-III prorated PIQ). Although prediction was statistically significant for all three outcomes, the regression equations were not especially accurate for individual children, especially those with the lowest and highest scores. Less than two-thirds of the group had a predicted score within 10 points of their actual scores regardless of the outcome considered.

In short, while clinicians can refer to multiple sources of information (i.e., demographics, family members' IQ, parent ratings, concurrent word reading skills) to predict premorbid functioning in children, the resulting estimates are not likely to be sufficiently accurate for individual cases, particularly those with milder forms of cerebral dysfunction. The various

equations, however, may be of greater use in research contexts (e.g., to show that a group with TBI were similar to a group of noninjured counterparts premorbidly).

REFERENCES

Baade, L. E., & Schoenberg, M. R. (2004). A proposed method to estimate premorbid intelligence utilising group achievement measures from school records. *Archives of Clinical Neuropsychology, 19,* 227–243.

Baddeley, A., Emslie, H., & Nimmo Smith, I. (1992). *The Speed and Capacity of Language-Processing Test.* Suffolk, England: Thames Valley Test Company.

Bahrick, H. P., Hall, L. K., & Berger, S. A. (1996). Accuracy and distortion in memory for high school grades. *Psychological Science, 7,* 265–271.

Baron, I. S. (2000). Clinical implications and practical applications of child neuropsychological evaluations. In K. O. Yeates, M. D., Ris, & H. G. Taylor (Eds.), *Pediatric neuropsychology: Research, theory, and practice* (pp. 439–456). New York: Guilford Press.

Barona, A., Reynolds, C. R., & Chastain, R. (1984). A demographically based index of pre-morbid intelligence for the WAIS-R. *Journal of Consulting and Clinical Psychology, 52,* 885–887.

Basso, M. R., Bornstein, R. A., Roper, B. L., & McCoy, V. L. (2000). Limited accuracy of premorbid intelligence estimators: A demonstration of regression to the mean. *The Clinical Neuropsychologist, 14,* 325–340.

Bayley, N. (1993). *Bayley Scales of Infant Development* (2nd ed.; Bayley-II). San Antonio, TX: Psychological Corporation.

Blair, J. R., & Spreen, O. (1989). Predicting premorbid IQ: A revision of the National Adult Reading Test. *The Clinical Neuropsychologist, 3,* 129–136.

Bright, P., Jadlow, E., & Kopelman, M. D. (2002). The National Adult Reading Test as a measure of premorbid intelligence: A comparison with estimates derived from premorbid levels. *Journal of the International Neuropsychological Society, 8,* 847–854.

Brown, L., Sherbenou, R. J., & Johnson, S. K. (1997). *Test of Nonverbal Intelligence: A language-free measure of cognitive ability* (3rd ed.). Austin, TX: Pro-Ed.

Burin, D. I., Jorge, R. E., Aizaga, R. A., & Paulsen, J. S. (2000). Estimation of premorbid intelligence: The word accentuation test—Buenos Aires version. *Journal of Clinical and Experimental Neuropsychology, 22,* 677–685.

Camara, W. J., Nathan, J. S., & Puente, A. E. (2000). Psychological test usage: Implications in professional psychology. *Professional Psychology: Research and Practice, 31,* 141–154.

Carroll, J. B. (1993). *Human cognitive abilities: A survey of factor analytic studies.* Cambridge: MA: Cambridge University Press.

Carroll, J. B. (1997). The three-stratum theory of cognitive abilities. In D. P. Flanagan, J. L. Genshaft, & P. L. Harrison (Eds.), *Contemporary intellectual assessment: Theories, tests and issues* (pp. 122–130). New York: Guilford.

Crawford, J. R. (1989). Estimation of premorbid intelligence: A review of recent developments. In J. R. Crawford & D. M. Parker (Eds.), *Developments in clinical and experimental neuropsychology.* London: Plenum.

Crawford, J. R. (1992). Current and premorbid intelligence measures in neuropsychological assessment. In J. R. Crawford, D. M. Parker, & W. M. McKinlay (Eds.), *A handbook of neuropsychological assessment.* West Sussex: LEA.

Crawford, J. R., & Allan, K. M. (1997). Estimating premorbid WAIS-R IQ with demographic variables: Regression equation derived from a U.K. sample. *The Clinical Neuropsychologist, 11,* 192–197.

Crawford, J. R., Millar, J., & Milne, A. B. (2001). Estimating premorbid IQ from demographic variables: A comparison of a regression equation vs. clinical judgement. *British Journal of Clinical Psychology, 40,* 97–105.

Del Ser, T., Gonzalez-Montalvo, J-I., Martinez-Espinosa, S., Delgado-Villapalos, C., & Bermejo, F. (1997). Estimation of premorbid intelligence in Spanish people with the Word Accentuation Test and its application to the diagnosis of dementia. *Brain and Cognition, 33,* 343–356.

Demakis, G. J., Sweet, J. J., Sawyer, T. P., Moulthrop, M., Nies, K., & Clingerman, S. (2001). Discrepancy between predicted and obtained WAIS-R IQ scores discriminates between traumatic brain injury and insufficient effort. *Psychological Assessment, 13,* 240–248.

Eisenstein, N., & Engelhart, C. I. (1997). Comparison of the K-BIT with short forms of the WAIS-R in a neuropsychological population. *Psychological Assessment, 9,* 57–62.

Flanagan, D. P., & McGrew, K. S. (1997). A cross-battery approach in assessing and interpreting cognitive abilities: Narrowing the gap between practice and cognitive science. In D. P. Flanagan & J. L. Genschaft (Eds.), *Contemporary intellectual assessment: Theories, tests, and issues.* New York: Guilford Press.

Flanagan, D. P., McGrew, K. S., & Ortiz, S.O. (2000). *The Wechsler Intelligence Scales and Gf-Gc theory: A contemporary approach to interpretation.* Boston: McGraw-Hill.

Folstein, M. F., Folstein, S. E., & McHugh, P. R. (1975). "Mini-mental state": A practical method for grading the cognitive state of outpatients for the clinician. *The Journal of Psychiatric Research, 12,* 189–198.

Franzen, M. D., Burgess, E. J., & Smith-Seemiller, L. (1997). Methods of estimating premorbid functioning. *Archives of General Neuropsychology, 12,* 711–738.

Gladsjo, J. A., Heaton, R. K., Palmer, B. W., Taylor, M. J., & Jeste, D. V. (1999). Use of oral reading to estimate premorbid intellectual and neuropsychological functioning. *Journal of the International Neuropsychological Society, 5,* 247–254.

Golden, C. J., Purisch, A. D., & Hammeke, T. A. (1985). *Luria-Nebraska Neuropsychological Battery: Forms I and II.* Los Angeles: Western Psychological Services.

Graves, R. E., Carswell, L. M. N., & Snow, W. G. (1999). An evaluation of the sensitivity of premorbid IQ estimators for detecting cognitive decline. *Psychological Assessment, 11,* 29–38.

Greiffenstein, M. F. & Baker, W. J. (2001). Comparison of premorbid and postinjury MMPI-2 profiles in late postconcussion claimants. *The Clinical Neuropsychologist, 15,* 162–170.

Greiffenstein, M. F., & Baker, W. J. (2003). Premorbid clues? Preinjury scholastic performance and present neuropsychological functioning in late postconcussion syndrome. *The Clinical Neuropsychologist, 17,* 561–573.

Greiffenstein, M. F., Baker, W. J., & Johnson-Greene, D. (2002). Actual versus self-reported scholastic achievement of litigating postconcussion and severe closed head injury claimants. *Psychological Assessment, 14,* 202–208.

Griffin, S. L., Mindt, M. R., Rankin, E. J., Ritchie, A. J., & Scott, J. G. (2002). Estimating premorbid intelligence: Comparison of traditional and contemporary methods across the intelligence continuum. *Archives of Clinical Neuropsychology, 17,* 497–507.

Grober, E., & Sliwinski, M. (1991). Development and validation of a model for estimating premorbid verbal intelligence in the elderly. *Journal of Clinical and Experimental Neuropsychology, 13,* 933–949.

Hays, J. R., Reas, D. L., & Shaw, J. B. (2002). Concurrent validity of the Wechsler Abbreviated Scale of Intelligence and the Kaufman Brief Intelligence Test among psychiatric patients. *Psychological Reports, 90,* 355–359.

Hoofien, D., Vakil, E., & Gilboa, A. (2000). Criterion validation of premorbid intelligence estimation in persons with traumatic brain injury: "Hold/don't hold" versus "best performance" procedures. *Journal of Clinical and Experimental Neuropsychology, 22,* 305–315.

Horn, J. L. & Noll, J. (1997). Human cognitive capabilities. In D. P. Flanagan, J. L. Genshaft (Eds.), *Contemporary intellectual assessment: Theories, tests, and issues* (pp. 53–91). New York: Guilford Press.

Ivnik, R. J., Malec, J. F., Smith, G. E., Tangalos, E. G., Peterson, R. C., Kokmen, E., & Kurland, L. T. (1992). Mayo's Older American Normative Studies: WAIS-R norms for ages 56 to 97. *The Clinical Neuropsychologist, 6*(Supplement), 1–30.

Johnson-Greene, D., Dehring, M., Adams, K. M., Miller, T., Arora, S., Beylin, A., & Brandon, R. (1997). Accuracy of self-reported educational attainment among diverse patient populations: A preliminary investigation. *Archives of Clinical Neuropsychology, 12,* 635–643.

Johnstone, B., Callahan, C. D., Kapila, C. J., & Bouman, D. E. (1996). The comparability of the WRAT-R reading test and NAART as estimates of premorbid intelligence in neurologically impaired patients. *Archives of Clinical Neuropsychology, 11,* 513–519.

Johnstone, B., & Wilhelm, K. L. (1996). The longitudinal stability of the WRAT-reading subtest: Is it an appropriate estimate of premorbid intelligence? *Journal of the International Neuropsychological Society, 2,* 282–285.

Jurica, P. J., Leitten, C. L., & Mattis, S. (2001). *Dementia Rating Scale-2.* Odessa, FL: Psychological Assessment Resources.

Kaufman, A. S., & Kaufman, N. L. (1990). *Kaufman Brief Intelligence Test.* Circle Pines, MN: American Guidance Service.

Kaufman, A. S., & Lichtenberger, E. O. (1999). *Essentials of WAIS-III assessment.* New York: John Wiley & Sons, Inc.

Klesges, R. C., & Sanchez, V. C. (1981). Cross-validation of an index of premorbid intellectual functioning in children. *Journal of Consulting and Clinical Psychology, 49,* 141.

Korkman, M., Kirk, U., & Kemp, S. (1998). *NEPSY: A developmental neuropsychological assessment manual.* San Antonio, TX: The Psychological Corporation.

Krull, K. R., Scott, J. G., & Sherer, M. (1995). Estimation of premorbid intelligence from combined performance and demographic variables. *The Clinical Neuropsychologist, 9,* 83–88.

Langeluddecke, P. M., & Lucas, S. K. (2004). Evaluation of two methods for estimating premorbid intelligence on the WAIS-III in a clinical sample. *The Clinical Neuropsychologist, 18,* 423–432.

Larrabee, G. J. (2004). A review of clinical interpretation of the WAIS-III and WMS-III: Where do we go from here and what should we do with WAIS-IV and WMS-IV? *Journal of Clinical and Experimental Neuropsychology, 24,* 707–717.

Leach, L., Kaplan, E., Rewilak, D., Richards, B., & Proulx, B-B. (2000). *Kaplan Baycrest Neurocognitive Assessment.* San Antonio, TX: The Psychological Corporation.

Lezak, M. D., Howieson, D. B., & Loring, D. W. (2004). *Neuropsychological assessment* (4th ed.). New York: Oxford University Press

Lucas, S. K., Carstairs, J. R., & Shores, E. A. (2003). A comparison of methods to estimate premorbid intelligence in an Australian sample: Data from the Macquarie University neuropsychological normative study (MUNNS). *Australian Neuropsychologist, 38,* 227–237.

Mattis, S. (1976). Mental status examination for organic mental syndrome in the elderly patient. In L. Bellak & T. B. Karasu (Eds.), *Geriatric psychiatry.* New York: Grune & Stratton.

McCallum, R. S., Bracken, B. A., & Wassermna, J. D. (2001). *Essentials of nonverbal assessment.* New York: John Wiley & Sons.

McGrew, K. S. (1997). Analysis of the major intelligence batteries according to a proposed comprehensive GF-Gc framework. In D. F. Flanagan, J. L. Genshaft, & P. L. Harrison (Eds.), *Contemporary intellectual assessment: Theories, tests, and issues* (pp. 151–182). New York: Guilford Press.

Mortensen, E. L., Gade, A., & Reinisch, J. M. (1991). A critical note on Lezak's "best performance method" in clinical neuropsychology. *Journal of Clinical and Experimental Neuropsychology, 13,* 361–371.

Naglieri, J. A., & Das, J. P. (1997). *Cognitive Assessment System interpretive handbook.* Itasca, IL: Riverside Publishing.

Neisser, U., Boodoo, G., Bouchard, T. J., Boykin, A. W., Brody, N., Ceci, S. J., Halpern, D. F., Loehlin, J. C., Perloff, R., Sternberg, R. J., & Urbina, S. (1996). Intelligence: Knowns and unknowns. *American Psychologist, 51,* 77–101.

Nelson, H. E. (1982). *National Adult Reading Test (NART): Test manual.* Windsor, England: NFER Nelson.

Nelson, H. E., & O'Connell, A. (1978). Dementia: The estimation of pre-morbid intelligence levels using the New Adult Reading Test. *Cortex, 14,* 234–244.

Patterson, K., Graham, N., & Hodges, J. R. (1994). Reading in dementia of the Alzheimer type: A preserved ability? *Neuropsychology, 8,* 395–407.

The Psychological Corporation. (2001). *Wechsler Test of Adult Reading manual.* San Antonio, TX: Author.

The Psychological Corporation. (2002). *WAIS-III/WMS-III technical manual: Updated.* San Antonio, TX: Author.

Rabin, L. A., Barr, W. B., & Burton, L. A. (2005). Assessment practices of clinical neuropsychologists in the United States and Canada: A survey of INS, NAN, and APA Division 40 members. *Archives of Clinical Neuropsychology, 20,* 33–66.

Randolph, C. (1998). *RBANS manual.* San Antonio, TX: The Psychological Corporation.

Raven, J. C. (1938). *Progressive Matrices: A perceptual test of intelligence.* London: H.K. Lewis.

Raven, J. C. (1947). *Colored Progressive Matrices sets A, Ab, B.* London: H.K. Lewis.

Raven, J. C. (1965). *Advanced Progressive Matrices sets I and II.* London: H.K. Lewis.

Redfield, J. (2001). Familial intelligence as an estimate of expected ability in children. *The Clinical Neuropsychologist, 15,* 446–460.

Reitan, R. M., & Wolfson, D. (1993). *The Halstead-Reitan neuropsychological test battery: Theory and clinical interpretation* (2nd ed.). Tucson, AZ: Neuropsychology Press.

Reynolds, C. R. (1997). Postscripts on premorbid ability estimation: Conceptual addenda and a few words on alternative and conditional approaches. *Archives of Clinical Neuropsychology, 12,* 769–778.

Reynolds, C. R., & Gutkin, T. B. (1979). Predicting the premorbid intellectual status of children using demographic data. *Clinical Neuropsychology, 1,* 36–38.

Russell, E. (1972). WAIS factor analysis with brain damaged subjects using criterion measures. *Journal of Consulting and Clinical Psychology, 39,* 133–139.

Ryan, J. J., & Paolo, A. M. (1992). A screening procedure for estimating premorbid intelligence in the elderly. *The Clinical Neuropsychologist, 6,* 53–62.

Ryan, J. J., Paolo, A. M., & Findley, G. (1991). Percentile rank conversion tables for WAIS-R IQs at six educational levels. *Journal of Clinical Psychology, 47,* 104–107.

Ryan, J. J., & Prifitera, A. (1990). The WAIS-R index for estimating premorbid intelligence: Accuracy in predicting short form IQ. *International Journal of Clinical Neuropsychology, 12,* 20–23.

Sattler, J. M. (2001). *Assessment of children: Cognitive applications* (4th ed.). San Diego: Jerome M. Sattler, Publishers, Inc.

Schoenberg, M. R., Duff, K., Scott, J. G., & Adams, R. L. (2003). An evaluation of the clinical utility of the OPIE-3 as an estimate of premorbid WAIS-III FSIQ. *The Clinical Neuropsychologist, 17,* 308–321.

Schoenberg, M. R., Scott, J. G., Duff, K., & Adams, R. L. (2002). Estimation of WAIS-III intelligence from combined performance and demographic variables: Development of the OPIE-3. *The Clinical Neuropsychologist, 16,* 426–438.

Sharpe, K., & O'Carroll, R. (1991). Estimating premorbid intellectual level in dementia using the National Adult Reading Test: A Canadian study. *British Journal of Clinical Psychology, 30,* 381–384.

Smith-Seemiller, L., Franzen, M. D., Burgess, E. J., & Prieto, L. R. (1997). Neuropsychologists' practice patterns in assessing premorbid intelligence. *Archives of Clinical Neuropsychology, 12,* 739–744.

Spearman, C. (1927). *The abilities of man.* New York: MacMillan.

Spreen, O., & Strauss, E. (1998). *A compendium of neuropsychological tests: Administration, norms and commentary.* New York: Oxford University Press.

Stebbins, G. T., Gilley, D. W., Wilson, R. S., Bernard, B. A., & Fox, J. H. (1990). Effects of language disturbances on premorbid estimates of IQ in mild dementia. *The Clinical Neuropsychologist, 4,* 64–68.

Stebbins, G. T., Wilson, R. S., Gilley, D. W., Bernard, B. A., & Fox, J. H. (1988). Estimation of premorbid intelligence in dementia. *Journal of Clinical and Experimental Neuropsychology, 10,* 63–64.

Stebbins, G. T., Wilson, R. S., Gilley, D. W., Bernard, B. A., & Fox, J. H. (1990). Use of the National Adult Reading Test to estimate premorbid IQ in dementia. *The Clinical Neuropsychologist, 4,* 18–24.

Stern, R. A., & White, T. (2003). *Neuropsychological Assessment Battery.* Lutz, FL: PAR.

Sweet, J., Moberg, P., & Tovian, S. (1990). Evaluation of Wechsler adult intelligence scale—revised premorbid IQ clinical formulas in clinical populations. *Psychological Assessment, 2,* 41–44.

Taylor, M. J., & Heaton, R. K. (2001). Sensitivity and specificity of WAIS-III/WMS-III demographically corrected factor scores in neuropsychological assessment. *Journal of the International Neuropsychological Society, 7,* 867–874.

Thurstone, L. L. (1938). *Primary mental abilities.* Chicago: University of Chicago Press.

Tulsky, D. S., Ivnik, R. J., Price, L. R., & Wilkins, C. (2003). Assessment of cognitive functioning with the WAIS-III and WMS-III: Development of a six-factor model. In D. S. Tulsky, D. H. Saklofske, G. J. Chelune, R. K. Heaton, R. J. Ivnik, R. Bornstein, A. Prifitera, & M. F. Ledbetter (Eds.), *Clinical interpretation of the WAIS-III and WMS-III* (pp. 149–182). San Diego: Academic Press.

Tulsky, D. S., Saklofske, D. S., & Ricker, J. (2003). Historical overview of intelligence and memory: Factors influencing the Wechsler Scales. In D. S. Tulsky, D. H. Saklofske, G. J. Chelune, R. K. Heaton, R. J. Ivnik, R. Bornstein, A. Prifitera, & M. F. Ledbetter (Eds.), *Clinical interpretation of the WAIS-III and WMS-III* (pp. 7–41). San Diego: Academic Press.

Vanderploeg, R. D., Schinka, J. A., & Axelrod, B. N. (1996). Estimation of WAIS-R premorbid intelligence: Current ability and demographic data used in a best-performance fashion. *Psychological Assessment, 8,* 404–411.

Vanderploeg, R. D., Schinka, J. A., Baum, K. M., Tremont, G., & Mittenberg, W. (1998). WISC-III premorbid prediction strategies: Demographic and best performance approaches. *Psychological Assessment, 10,* 277–284.

Watt, K. J., & O'Carroll, R. E. (1999). Evaluating methods for estimating premorbid intellectual ability in closed head injury. *Journal of Neurology, Neurosurgery, and Psychiatry, 66,* 474–479.

Wechsler, D. (1958). *The measurement and appraisal of adult intelligence* (4th ed.). Baltimore, MD: Williams and Wilkins.

White, T., & Stern, R. A. (2003). *Neuropsychological Assessment Battery: Psychometric and technical manual.* Lutz, FL: PAR.

Wiens, A. N., Bryan, J. E., & Crossen, J. R. (1993). Estimating WAIS-R FSIQ from the National Adult Reading Test—Revised in normal subjects. *The Clinical Neuropsychologist, 8,* 70–84.

Wilson, R. S., Rosenbaum, G., Brown, G., Rourke, D., Whitman, D., & Grisell, J. (1978). An index of premorbid intelligence. *Journal of Consulting and Clinical Psychology, 46,* 1554–1555.

Williams, J. M. (1997). The prediction of premorbid memory ability. *Archives of Clinical Neuropsychology, 12,* 745–756.

Willshire, D., Kinsella, G., & Prior, M. (1991). Estimating WAIS-R IQ from the national adult reading test: A cross-validation. *Journal of Clinical and Experimental Neuropsychology, 13,* 204–216.

Yeates, K. O., & Taylor, H. G. (1997). Predicting premorbid neuropsychological functioning following pediatric traumatic brain injury. *Journal of Clinical and Experimental Neuropsychology, 19,* 825–837.

Bayley Scales of Infant Development—Second Edition (BSID-II)

PURPOSE

The Bayley Scales of Infant Development, Second Edition (BSID-II) are designed to assess mental, motor, and behavioral development of infants and preschoolers.

SOURCE

The BSID-II (Bayley, 1993) can be ordered from the Psychological Corporation, P.O. Box 9954, San Antonio, TX 78204-0354 (www.harcourtassessment.com). A complete kit with manual, 25 Record Forms, Motor Scale Forms, Behavior Rating Scale Forms, Stimulus Cards, and other necessary materials costs $995 US. A Dutch version normed in the Netherlands, the BOS-II, will also soon be available.

AGE RANGE

The test can be administered to children between the ages of 1 month and 3 1/2 years (i.e., 42 months).

DESCRIPTION

Overview

The Bayley is the most important and most widely used developmental assessment test. The original Bayley Scales of Infant Development were published in 1969 (Bayley, 1969); a second edition appeared in 1993 (BSID-II; Bayley, 1993). A new edition is forthcoming (BSID-III). Items from the Bayley tests have as origins some of the earliest tests of infant development (e.g., Bayley, 1933, 1936; Gesell, 1925; Jaffa, 1934; see Bendersky & Lewis, 2001; Bracken & Walker, 1997; and Brooks-Gunn & Weintraub, 1983, for reviews of the early history of infant assessment).

The BSID-II is designed to assess cognitive, physical, language, and psychosocial development of infants, toddlers, and preschoolers (Bayley, 1993). Although it arose out of the study of normal infant development, one of its primary uses is to evaluate infants suspected of delay or atypical development to determine eligibility for services and to track progress over time. Often, these are young children who were born premature or of low birth weight or who have a major congenital anomaly, delayed milestones, or other risk factors for developmental disability. In addition, it is a preferred tool for developmental research: hundreds of studies on clinical and nonclinical populations have been published involving the original BSID (see Black & Matula, 2000), and many more appear each year using the BSID-II.

The BSID-II is a *developmental* test, not an intelligence test (Bayley, 1993). Unlike intelligence tests that assume a curvilinear function between age and ability, the manual specifies that a developmental test assesses different abilities present at different ages. The BSID-II is therefore "designed to sample a wide array of emergent developmental abilities and to inventory the attainment of developmental milestones" (Bayley, 1993, p. 8).

According to the manual, the Bayley Scales were designed to provide a set of standard situations and tasks that would allow the child to display an observable set of behavioral responses. One of its primary goals is to provide a method for standardized assessment that nevertheless allows considerable flexibility in administration. For example, the examiner can vary the order of item administration depending on the child's temperament, interest level, and the level of rapport established with the child (e.g., an item can be administered later, once an initially shy child becomes more sociable; Bayley, 1993). Incidentally observed behaviors are also scorable, even if they occur before or after the actual test administration; testing can also occur over more than one session if required.

Test Structure

The BSID-II consists of three parts (see Table 6–7). According to the manual, each is designed to be complementary and to contribute unique information. The first two scales consist of structured assessment batteries designed to assess general

Table 6–7 BSID-II Scales and Scores

Scale	Score	Overview
Mental Scale	Mental Development Index (MDI)	Measures general cognitive development, including items that tap memory, habituation, problem solving, early number concepts, generalization, classification, vocalizations, language, and social skills; facet scores can also be derived using specific item clusters
Motor Scale	Psychomotor Development Index (PDI)	Measures overall motor development, including items assessing gross and fine motor skills (e.g., rolling, crawling, creeping, sitting, standing, walking, running, jumping, prehension, use of writing implements, imitation of hand movements)
Behavior Rating Scale (BRS)	Total Score Attention/Arousal (up to 6 months) Orientation/Engagement (6 months +) Emotional Regulation (6 months +) Motor Quality (all ages)	A rating scale completed by the examiner that provides a qualitative assessment in percentile form that reflects two or three factors, depending on age

Adapted from Bayley, 1993.

cognitive and motor development (Mental and Motor Scales), and the third component is a rating scale (Behavior Rating Scale [BRS]). The Mental Scale provides an index score for general cognitive development (i.e., the Mental Development Index [MDI]). The Motor Scale provides an index of overall motor development (i.e., Psychomotor Development Index [PDI]). From these two scales, four "facet" scores can be derived: Cognitive, Language, Motor, and Personal/Social. Although the manual does not provide additional information on the development or psychometric characteristics of the facet subscales, it notes that the facet scores are not intended for identifying impairment in specific subdomains, but rather for identifying relative strengths and weaknesses. The facet scores were derived on rational and semi-empirical grounds (i.e., item placement into facets by expert review and based on correlation between each item and the final scales; Bayley, 1993).

The BRS provides a qualitative assessment of behavior reflecting three main factors: Orientation/Engagement, Emotional Regulation, and Motor Quality (infants under 6 months of age are assessed for Motor Quality and Attention/Arousal only). Items are rated on a five-point Likert scale by the examiner, based in part on information provided by the caregiver. Unlike tests for older children that primarily assess test performance (e.g., Wechsler scales), the BRS is considered a critical aspect of the BSID-II because an infant's state (including engagement, arousal level, and motivation at the time of testing) may substantially influence the Mental and Motor Scale scores (Black & Matula, 2000). In other words, the BRS is designed to supplement the Mental and Motor Scales by providing information on the validity of the evaluation, as well as on the child's relations with others and how the child adapts to the testing situation.

Item Sets and Test Content

One of the major features of the BSID-II is the organization of the test into a series of separate item sets of increasing difficulty that correspond to developmental ages. This arrangement makes sense theoretically because the test is designed to measure attainment of developmental milestones rather than specific cognitive domains. Developmental progression is reflected in the relative domain content of item sets across age, in addition to the difficulty level of each item set. The result is a Mental Scale that primarily measures sensory and perceptual development in infancy and language skills and other cognitive abilities after 12 months (Fugate, 1998). Likewise, the Motor Scale assesses primarily gross motor skills in infancy and fine motor skills, along with other aspects of gross motor abilities, after 12 months (Fugate, 1998). The manual notes that this results in less predictability from one testing to the next compared to intelligence tests (Bayley, 1993) because different item types are tested at different ages. However, items reflecting abilities that predict later functioning were specifically added to the BSID-II, and items for the older age bands are similar to those of intelligence tests for preschoolers such as the WPPSI-R (Bayley, 1993), which should afford some predictive validity.

Item content for the BSID-II, according to the manual, is "theoretically eclectic," with items gleaned from a broad cross-section of developmental research and developmental testing (Bayley, 1993). New items were selected based on careful review of developmental research; these include items tapping recognition memory, habituation of attention, problem solving, number concepts, language, personal/social development, and motor abilities (see pp. 12–14 of manual).

BSID-II Versus BSID

The BSID-II differs from the original BSID in several ways. It has extended age bands (1–42 months compared with 2–30 months of age) and a newer normative sample. Many original items were dropped and many new items were added; older items were also rewritten and modified (Black & Matula, 2000). About 76% of the Mental Scale items and 84% of the Motor Scale items were retained. Stimulus materials were also redesigned and updated (Bayley, 1993). In the original BSID, items were arranged in order of increasing difficulty, and basals and ceilings were established by passing or failing

10 consecutive items. Because this technique was thought to be too time-consuming and frustrating for children, the BSID-II was revised to include item sets that correspond to specific age levels. As a result of the newer normative sample, altered format, and changed content, children retested with the BSID-II obtain significantly lower scores than when tested with the original BSID. Caution is therefore recommended when comparing scores from different versions of the test, particularly when retest scores suggest a decline in functioning (DeWitt et al., 1998; see also *Validity* for details).

BSID-II Translations

The *BSID-II Manual* does not provide information on how to use the test with children whose first language is not English, and, to our knowledge, there currently exist no official versions of the BSID-II normed in other languages apart from the BOS-II. It has nevertheless been used within the United States to assess Spanish-speaking children (e.g., Leslie et al., 2002) and in Canada to assess Francophone children from Quebec (e.g., Pomerleau et al., 2003). The test has also been used in Norway (Moe & Slinning, 2001), Finland (Lyytinen et al., 1999; Sajaniemi et al., 2001a, 2001b), Germany (e.g., Walkowiak et al., 2001), Malaysia (Ong et al., 2001), and Bangladesh (Hamadani et al., 2002). The original BSID was adapted for use in Nigeria; the modified version appears to show higher predictive ability than the original scale (Ogunnaike & Houser, 2002). Similar adaptations have been employed in Kenya (Sigman et al., 1988).

ADMINISTRATION

For details, see manual. Testing is conducted under optimal conditions (i.e., when the infant is fully alert and in the presence of the primary caregiver. Other aspects of testing infants, such as an appropriate testing environment, reinforcement, providing feedback, and dealing with tantrums and fatigue are discussed in Black and Matula (2000) and in the manual. Above all else, examiners should ensure that examinees are well-fed and well-rested prior to attempting administration (Bendersky & Lewis, 2001).

Because the examiner alters test administration in response to the child's performance, examiners should be knowledgeable about infant behavior and be experienced in test administration. Black and Matula (2000) state that testing infants with the Bayley is a difficult skill that requires mastery of administration rules, thorough knowledge of normal and atypical infant development, and careful attention to the infant and caregiver during test administration. Both novice and experienced test users should attend at least one workshop in its use prior to administering the BSID-II (Nellis & Gridley, 1994). Training should include lectures, demonstrations, practice testing of infants, and evaluation of videotaped administrations, as well as training to a criterion of greater than 90% agreement between experienced examiners (Black & Matula, 2000). Special care should be given to learning specific items, given the low agreement between raters. Chandlee

et al. (2002) provide detailed administration/scoring guidelines for specific items that tend to have low interrater agreement even in experienced, trained examiners. These are reproduced in Table 6–8. Familiarity with Black and Matula's text (2000) is also highly recommended.

Materials and Setting

Manipulatives are an integral part of the Bayley. The test kit therefore contains numerous small items (e.g., toys, cups, blocks, etc.). These are appealing and child-friendly, and maintain the interest of most infants and toddlers (Nellis & Gridley, 1994). Other items needed for administration but not included in the testing kit are plain paper, small plastic bags, tissues, and a stopwatch. Following each testing session, testing materials should be washed. Note that testing needs to occur in a location that allows administration of all the motor items, which includes access to three steps and to at least 9 feet of floor space to allow the child to stop from a full run. Because of practicality and safety issues related to using stairs in public settings (C. Miranda, personal communication, January 2005), many examiners build a set of stairs according to the height/width specifications detailed in the manual.

Although the test is designed to be portable, the kit itself is quite large and heavy, and contains many small parts that can be difficult to pack away quickly (Black & Matula, 2000). The testing manual includes both administration instructions and technical information. Record booklets are well designed and contain much helpful information on administration.

Start Points, Basals, and Ceilings

Start points for item sets are based on chronological age. However, start points can be altered depending on the examiner's judgment of the child's actual ability levels. For example, earlier start points can be selected for low-functioning children or those with atypical development, based on the examiner's estimation of the child's developmental level as determined by behavioral observation, caregiver report, or other test scores (but see *Comments* for further discussion of this issue)

Testing proceeds by item set until the child has met basal and ceiling criteria. On the Mental Scale, the basal is five or more correct items anywhere within the item set. A ceiling is attained when a child fails three or more items anywhere within the item set. On the Motor Scale, these values are four and two, respectively.

BRS

The BRS is filled out by the examiner following completion of the test, combined with information provided by the caregiver (e.g., whether the session was typical of the child's behavior and reflective of his or her skills). Items are rated on a five-point Likert-type scale.

Table 6–8 Recommended Administration and Scoring Guidelines for BSID-II Items With Low Interscorer Agreement

BSID-II Mental Scale Item	Possible Problems Encountered During Administration or Scoring	Recommended Administration and Scoring Practices
111.	Incidental scoring issue Vague scoring criteria—minimal examples provided as to what constitutes a pass	Examiner must closely monitor and record each vocalization produced Examiner must carefully determine whether word and gesture occur *simultaneously* Scoring criteria need clarification in manual (e.g., further exemplars) As stated in manual, caregiver's interpretation or report is not sufficient for credit
113.	Incidental scoring issue Vague scoring criteria—examiners may differ on acceptance of "poorly articulated words" and "word approximations" as well as degree of temporal delay necessary for words to be considered nonimitative	Examiner must closely monitor and record each vocalization produced Examiner must carefully note whether the child's "intent is clear" for poorly articulated words or word approximations to be credited Examiner must carefully determine whether words occur *spontaneously* rather than in imitation Scoring criteria need clarification in manual (e.g., degree of temporal delay necessary for words to be considered nonimitative) As stated in manual, caregiver's interpretation or report is not sufficient for credit
114.	Incidental scoring issue Vague scoring criteria—examiners may differ on multiple criteria, including word articulation, interpretation of one or more concepts, and pauses between words	Examiner must closely monitor and record each vocalization produced Examiner must carefully note whether words signify "different concepts," are not separated by "distinct pause," and are used "appropriately" Scoring criteria need clarification in manual (e.g., further specification of above concepts) As stated in manual, caregiver's interpretation or report is not sufficient for credit
116.	Vague scoring criteria—difficult to differentiate between a "scribble" and a stroke Child may make definitive stroke on Item 91, then scribble definitively on Item 116, but does not make another stroke	Scoring criteria need clarification in manual (e.g., whether imitation or discrimination of different fine-motor movements is critically variable) According to manual, if child does not make another stroke on Item 116 after making scribble, child does not receive pass (temporal delay from Item 91 negates pass)
117.	Vague scoring criteria—examiners may differ on acceptance of "poorly"	Scoring criteria need clarification in manual
119.	Inaccurate timing—child may pick up first peg before examiner completes directions, delaying start of timing Child may place and remove pegs	Critically important for examiner to time *accurately* (e.g., begin timing as soon as child picks up first peg; stop timing immediately when six pegs are in board; time allotted 70 seconds) All six pegs must be "standing" in pegboard at end of 25 seconds to score a pass As stated in manual, this item may be administered up to three times
121.	May be incidental scoring issue Vague scoring criteria—examiners may differ on acceptability of pronouns that are not used in a "grammatically correct" manner	Examiner must closely monitor and record each vocalization produced Examiner should note specific directions in the manual for eliciting a response if none occurs spontaneously Scoring criteria need clarification in manual (e.g., exemplars of pronouns not used in grammatically correct manner, but credited) As stated in manual, use of pronouns need not be grammatically correct

(continued)

Table 6–8 Recommended Administration and Scoring Guidelines for BSID-II Items With Low Interscorer Agreement (*continued*)

BSID-II Mental Scale Item	Possible Problems Encountered During Administration or Scoring	Recommended Administration and Scoring Practices
127.	Incidental scoring issue Vague scoring criteria—examiners may differ on acceptability of multiple-word utterances that are not "grammatically correct"	Examiner must closely monitor and record each vocalization produced Unclear whether examiner must note whether words are not separated by "distinct pause," and are used "appropriately" (see Item 114) Scoring criteria need clarification in manual (e.g., clarify above concepts) As stated in manual, caregiver's interpretation or report is not sufficient for credit
129.	Incidental scoring issue Vague scoring criteria— requires judgment as to whether "new information" is included	Examiner must closely monitor and record each vocalization produced Critical for examiner to accurately record each vocalization to determine if multiple-word utterances include topics of prior utterances Also critical for examiner to make judgment as to whether "new information" is included in multiple-word utterances Scoring criteria need clarification in manual (e.g., further exemplars of utterances including "new information")
136.	Incidental scoring issue Vague scoring criteria—examiners may differ on degree of temporal delay necessary for question to be nonimitative	Examiner must closely monitor and record each vocalization produced Examiner should note specific directions in the manual for evoking a response if none occurs spontaneously Scoring criteria need clarification in manual (e.g., how much temporal delay necessary for question to be considered nonimitative)
142.	Vague scoring criteria—multiple-word utterances may not be different Child may make utterances during reading of the story (Item 131)	Two identical multiple-word utterances may be scored as pass if temporal delay between them Utterances during reading of story scored as pass Scoring criteria need clarification in manual (e.g., further exemplars and nonexemplars)
148.	May be incidental scoring issue Vague scoring criteria—examiners may differ on acceptability of past tense verbs that are not "correctly formed"	Examiner must closely monitor and record each vocalization produced Scoring criteria need clarification in manual (e.g., further exemplars)
159.	Vague scoring criteria—child may state numbers in same order (Items 146 and 164), but not stop at same endpoint	Even if child does not stop at same endpoint, if numbers stated in same order (Items 146 and 164), score as pass Scoring criteria need clarification in manual (e.g., inclusion of exemplars and nonexemplars)
165.	Inaccurate timing—child may pick up first shape before examiner completes directions, delaying start of timing Child may place and remove shapes	Critically important for examiner to time *accurately* (e.g., begin timing as soon as child picks up first shape; stop timing immediately when all nine shapes are in board; time allotted 150 seconds) All nine shapes must be completely inserted in board at end of 30 seconds to score a pass As stated in manual, only one trial permitted

Source: From Chandlee et al., 2002. Reprinted with permission.

ADMINISTRATION TIME

Testing time for children less than 15 months of age is 25 to 35 minutes; for older children, it is up to 60 minutes. Actual testing time varies depending on the experience of the examiner, the choice of an appropriate basal level, the child's level of cooperation, variability of responses, and level of competence.

SCORING

Scores

There is no computerized scoring system available as of this writing, but one is anticipated for the third edition. Raw scores are converted into standard scores (MDI and PDI) based on

Table 6–9 BSID-II Developmental Index Scores Classification and Frequencies

Score Range	Classification	Theoretical Normal Curve %	Mental Scale (Actual Sample %)	Motor Scale (Actual Sample %)
115 and above	Accelerated Performance	16.0	14.8	16.5
85–114	Within Normal Limits	68.0	72.6	68.7
70–84	Mildly Delayed Performance	13.5	11.1	12.5
69 and below	Significantly Delayed Performance	2.5	1.5	2.3

Source: From Bayley, 1993. Reprinted with permission.

the child's chronological age by using the appropriate tables in the manual ($M = 100$, $SD = 15$, range 50–150). Corrected age (i.e., gestational as opposed to chronological) is used for premature infants (see *Comment* for further discussion of this issue). Significance levels and cumulative percentages of the standardization sample obtaining various MDI-PDI discrepancies can be obtained in the manual (Bayley, 1993).

Facet scores reflecting age-equivalent performance in four areas of development can also be derived (Cognitive, Language, Motor, and Social). However, only developmental ages can be derived, based on the number of items passed at each age level; these are shown on the Record Form. Percentile ranks only are provided for the BRS.

Classification of Developmental Index Scores and BRS Scores

BSID-II scores can be interpreted using the four recommended classifications shown in the manual (e.g., Accelerated Performance, Within Normal Limits, Mildly Delayed Performance, or Significantly Delayed Performance). These are presented in Table 6–9, along with corresponding score ranges. For the BRS, scores are described in terms of three classification levels (i.e., Within Normal Limits, Questionable, and Nonoptimal). Corresponding ranges are shown in Table 6–10.

Additional Domain Scores

Although not expressly designed for this purpose, researchers have attempted to organize the items into subscales assessing specific domains of ability. For instance, Seigel et al. (1995) formed language subtests from BSID

Table 6–10 BSID-II Behavior Rating Scale (BRS) Cutoff Scores

Score	Percentile Range
Within Normal Limits	At or above the 26th percentile
Questionable	Between 11th and 25th percentile
Nonoptimal	At or below the 10th percentile

Source: From Bayley, 1993. Reprinted with permission.

items that were useful in the identification of children with delayed language. From the BSID-II, Choudhury and Gorman (2000) developed a scale of items measuring cognitive ability with reported sensitivity to attentional functioning (COG scale). For a list of items, see Table 6–11. Although they show promise in providing additional information on strengths and weaknesses, these scales need further refinement before they can be used in the diagnostic evaluation of individual children.

Table 6–11 BSID-II Mental Scale Items Used for the COG Scale

Item Number	Description
97	Builds tower of two cubes
98	Places pegs in 70 seconds
102	Retrieves toy (visible displacement)
103	Imitates crayon stroke
104	Retrieves toy (clear box II)
105	Uses rod to attain toy
112	Places four pieces in 150 seconds
115	Completes pink board in 180 seconds
116	Differentiates scribble from stroke
118	Identifies objects in photograph
119	Places pegs in 25 seconds
120	Completes reversed pink board
123	Builds tower of six cubes
125	Matches pictures
128	Matches colors
130	Completes blue board in 75 seconds
132	Attends to story
135	Places beads in tube in 120 seconds
137	Builds tower of eight cubes
138	Matches four colors
139	Builds train of cubes
143	Imitates horizontal stroke
144	Recalls geometric form
144	Discriminates picture I
147	Compares masses

Notes: Items excluded from the COG composite score were predominantly language-related items that assessed preexisting skills (semantics and conceptual labels). It is important to note that although attention is required to correctly respond to these language-based items, they do not necessarily require children to sustain attention to the items to correctly respond and receive credit.

Source: From Choudhury & Gorman, 2000. Reprinted with permission.

DEMOGRAPHIC EFFECTS

Age

As noted above, items for the BSID-II were specifically included if they showed sensitivity to age.

Gender

There is some evidence, using the previous test version, that girls' scores are more predictive of later IQ than boys' (Andersson et al., 1998). However, most studies report little or no effect of gender on test scores (e.g., $r = -.16$; Lyttinen et al., 1999), apart from interactions between developmental insult and gender suggesting that boys are more vulnerable to cognitive delays (e.g., Moe & Slinning, 2001; Sajaniemi et al., 2001a).

Education/Socioeconomic Status

Parental education, often used as a marker for socioeconomic status (SES), tends to be positively associated with scores on cognitive tests in children. Evidence for an effect of parental education on BSID-II scores is mixed, due to the use of different samples across studies. For example, correlations between BSID-II scores and parental education were moderate to high in one study of normal 27-month-olds, with both mothers' and fathers' education appearing to have about the same association with the MDI ($r = .45–.50$; Roberts et al., 1999). In contrast, modest correlations have been reported in other samples for maternal education (e.g., $r = .21$) but not paternal education (Lyytinen et al., 1999, 2001). In other studies involving low SES samples with diverse ethnic backgrounds, no association between demographic variables such as maternal/paternal education, ethnicity, and BSID-II MDI scores are found (Shannon et al., 2002), possibly due to restricted range. However, scores of children from high parental education/SES backgrounds are typically higher than those of low education/SES backgrounds. For example, in one sample of highly educated, affluent parents, children obtained mean BSID-II MDI scores of 108.2 ($SD = 11.9$; range 84–134). In comparison, MDI scores of 6-month-old infants of at-risk mothers characterized by young age, low education, and low income were slightly lower, though still within normal limits ($M = 93.8$, $SD = 5.0$; Pomerleau et al., 2003). Note that several studies have found that for children of low SES/low parental education, BSID-II scores exhibit a relative decrease or lag over time as children develop (e.g., Mayes et al., 2003) (see also *Ethnicity/SES*).

Ethnicity/SES

Empirical and rational methods for the elimination of bias were employed in the development of the BSID-II, which should minimize differences based on ethnicity/culture (see *Validity, Content*). Additionally, the widespread use of the test across cultures and languages suggests that the test is largely unbiased (see *Translations*), nor does the test appear to differentially penalize ethnic subgroups within the larger U.S. population. For instance, African American preschoolers attending community-based childcare centers obtain scores that are generally within the average range at 18 months of age (i.e., 95.7, $SD = 10.1$, range 79–122), despite a low-income background (Burchinal et al., 2000). Similarly, the proportion of children identified as significantly delayed, mildly delayed, or within normal limits does not differ proportionally by ethnicity in children apprehended for neglect or abuse (Leslie et al., 2002), suggesting that children of minority status are not differentially penalized on the test. Even children living in extreme poverty in the slums of Bangladesh typically achieve scores that are within normal limits, at least on the MDI (i.e., MDI = 102.6, $SD = 10$; PDI = 95.7, $SD = 15$; Hamadani et al., 2002).

Nevertheless, it is important to note that the attainment of developmental milestones may differ depending on cultural beliefs and caregiving practices; therefore, some groups may obtain lower scores on some items, reflecting alternative practices rather than developmental deviance (Leslie et al., 2002). For example, normally developing Brazilian infants obtain lower scores than U.S. infants on the Motor Scale at 3, 4, and 5 months of age. After this time, scores are equivalent to U.S. norms (Santos et al., 2000, 2001). Items exhibiting possible bias (i.e., passed by 15% or less of Brazilian infants) measured sitting, grasping, and hand posture (see Table 6–12 for specific items). However, items tapping motor behavior characteristics of older infants, such as crawling, cruising, and walking, were not different between groups. This is attributed to different child rearing practices, possibly mediated in part by parental education, such that Brazilian infants are held and carried most of the time, are rarely placed on the floor or seated without support, and have fewer opportunities to manipulate toys compared with U.S. infants (Santos et al., 2000, 2001). Other research within the United States indicates that performance on some BSID-II motor items are mediated in part by caregiving practices involving sleep position (Ratliff-Shaub et al., 2001; see *Normative Data* for more details).

Table 6–12 Items Failed by 85% or More of Normally Developing Brazilian Infants (Ages 3 to 5 Months)

Item	Movement Group
Rotates wrist	Ungrouped
Sits alone momentarily	Sitting
Uses whole hand to grasp rod	Grasping
Uses partial thumb opposition to grasp cube	Grasping
Attempts to secure pellets	Grasping
Sits alone for 30 seconds	Sitting
Sits alone while playing with toys	Sitting
Sits alone steadily	Sitting
Uses whole hand to grasp pellets	Grasping

Source: From Santos et al., 2000. Reprinted with permission.

When scoring BSID-II items from cultural groups with caregiving practices that differ from North American practices, adjusting scores on these items may be appropriate to avoid underestimating ability.

It is important to note that research shows that children from at-risk backgrounds, including those of poor, primarily minority, single-parent families with significant familial chaos, have decreasing BSID-II scores over time when multiple assessments are compared, despite normal-range scores in infancy (e.g., DeWitt et al., 1998; Mayes et al., 2003). The oft-cited explanation for this decline is that environmental factors become more important in determining skills as children grow, which maximizes the adverse impact of inadequate environments on development over time. An additional explanation is that the change in BSID-II item type from infancy to toddlerhood interacts with cultural factors. Thus, familiarity with situations similar to item sets for older toddlers (e.g., compliance and table-top activities) may differ across ethnic groups because of cultural factors. Lower scores in older children may therefore signify that that the BSID-II does not capture relevant competence as defined in these cultural subgroups, which explains the decrease in scores over time for some low SES, primarily minority groups (Black et al., 2001; Leslie et al., 2002). It is important to note that, regardless of the reason for the decrease in scores over time, the result is that a larger proportion of at-risk children may be identified as requiring intervention services with increasing age.

NORMATIVE DATA

Standardization Sample

The BSID-II standardization sample consists of a national, stratified, random sample of 1700 children, stratified according to data from the 1988 U.S. Census. Table 6–13 shows sample characteristics with regard to stratification variables (e.g., parental education, ethnicity). One hundred children in 17 separate age bands corresponding to specific ages were tested (i.e., 1, 2, 3, 4, 5, 6, 8, 10, 12, 15, 18, 21, 24, 27, 30, 36, and 42 months). Note that not all age intervals are represented. Therefore, to derive standard scores for the Mental and Motor Scales across age, raw score distributions for each age group from the standardization sample were normalized. Irregularities within and across ages were eliminated by smoothing, and raw to index score conversions for age groups not included in the sampled age bands were interpolated (Bayley, 1993).

To derive percentiles for the BRS, data from the standardization sample, in addition to data from 370 children with clinical diagnoses, were analyzed for three age groups (1–5 months, 6–12 months, and 13–42 months). Frequency distributions were constructed, and cutoffs were derived to reflect three categories: (1) Within Normal Limits, (2) Questionable, and (3) Nonoptimal (see Table 6–10 for actual score ranges).

Table 6–13 Characteristics of the BSID-II Normative Sample

Number	1700[a]
Age	1 to 42 months
Geographic location	
Northeast	18.7%
South	33.4%
North Central	23.9%
West	24.0%
Sample type	National, stratified, random sample[b]
Parental education	
0–11 years	16.5%
12 years	36.5%
13–15 years	26.0%
16 years or more	21.2%
SES	Not specified
Gender	
Males	50%
Females	50%
Race/ethnicity	
African American	15.0%
Hispanic	11.6%
White	69.7%
Other	3.7%
Screening	Only healthy children were included, defined as any child born without significant medical complications, without history of medical complications, and not currently diagnosed with or receiving treatment for mental, physical, or behavioral problems, based on parent report

[a]Based on 17 age groupings of 100 cases each; more age groupings appear in the younger children (1–12 months) because of more rapid development compared to the older children (13–42 months); actual ages included are 1, 2, 3, 4, 5, 6, 8, 10, 12, 15, 18, 21, 24, 27, 30, 36, and 42 months.
[b]Based on 1988 U.S. Census data.

Source: Adapted from Bayley, 1993.

Demographically Adjusted Norms

Given an apparent effect of caregiving practices on the emergence of certain motor milestones (see *Ethnicity*), score adjustment may be considered for infants with cultural backgrounds that differ from that of the normative group. Raw score ranges and confidence intervals for Brazilian infants are shown in Table 6–14, given the temporary delay in the emergence of some motor skills in this group compared with the standardization sample.

Note that even within North American samples, caregiving practices may influence performance on certain motor items. For example, healthy infants who sleep supine (i.e., on their back) fail more motor items than infants who sleep prone,

Table 6–14 Raw Score Ranges for Brazilian Infants on the BSID-II PDI (Modal Maternal Education Level = 8 Years or Less)

Age in Months	N	Mean Score	95% Confidence Interval
1	47	11.0	10.4–11.7
2	40	16.2	15.6–16.9
3	42	21.1	20.5–21.8
4	36	25.1	24.4–25.9
5	38	31.0	30.1–32.1
6	39	38.7	37.7–39.7

Note: Raw scores represent the same children retested over time.

Source: From Santos et al., 2000. Reprinted with permission.

particularly those items assessing head control tested prone. In addition, infants are more likely to fail items that are administered in the position opposite to their usual sleeping position (Ratliff-Schaub et al., 2001). The authors note that the BSID-II was normed during a time when the majority of young infants slept prone, a practice that is no longer recommended because of an associated increased risk of Sudden Infant Death Syndrome (SIDS), but which may have been associated with better head control in the standardization sample. Sleep practices may therefore need to be queried closely, particularly in infants with suspected motor delays.

Estimation of Ability Levels Beyond Available Standard Score Range

For very high or very low functioning infants (e.g., a standard score above 150 or below 50), the raw scores do not allow the calculation of a precise standard score. Because the test is intended for assessment of children with atypical and delayed development, scores below 50 are often needed. Age equivalents provided in the manual are one alternative (p. 325 of the manual). Derived (i.e., extrapolated) scores are another. Lindsay and Brouwers (1999) provide alternate age equivalents based on a linear derivation method for evaluating longitudinal development in very low or very high functioning infants. These are presented in Table 6–15.

Robinson and Mervis (1996) also derived a regression equation to provide extrapolated standard scores for the MDI and PDI for very low scorers obtaining standard scores below 50. Extrapolated standard scores are provided in Tables 6–16a and 6–16b. Because these scores are extrapolated and not based on actual data points, the authors note that they should be considered estimates only and used for research purposes.

RELIABILITY

Internal Reliability

Internal consistency of the scales as measured by average coefficient alpha across age is high (i.e., .88 for the MDI, .84 for the PDI, and .88 for the BRS; Bayley, 1993). Within age bands,

coefficients are also generally high, except for some of the younger age bands on the BRS (i.e., BRS alpha coefficient at age 2 months = .64, and falls between .71 and .77 for ages 3–5 months; see manual for details).

In the standardization sample, the *SEM* is 5.21 for the Mental Scale and 6.01 for the Motor Scale. Knowledge of these *SEM*s therefore provides a basis for constructing confidence intervals around the obtained score. However, the manual provides 90% and 95% confidence intervals for index scores based on the SE_E, which is a more precise estimation method (see manual for details).

Test-Retest Reliability

Reliability is high for the Mental Scale and adequate for the Motor Scale, across age (i.e., $r = .87$ and .78, respectively, after a median interval of 4 days). Although adequate given the nature of the sample, test-retest reliability of some BSID-II scales, in some age groups, falls short in terms of standards for diagnostic evaluation of individual children. Overall, Mental Scale reliability is impressive at 2 to 3 years, and certainly meets criteria for clinical decision making. BRS total score reliabilities are variable (i.e., quite low in the youngest group tested, but acceptable in 12-month olds; range of .55–.90, depending on age). BRS factors, on average, are low to marginal except for Motor Quality, which demonstrates acceptable to high reliability across age. Stability by age is shown in Table 6–17 based on test-retest stability estimates reported in the manual for 175 children from the standardization sample, drawn from four age groups (1, 12, 24, and 36 months) and retested after a median interval of four days.

Because reliability coefficients do not inform on whether actual score ranges are maintained over time, percentage agreement for classification categories of the BRS are also presented in the manual, based on dichotomous classification (e.g., Within Normal Limits vs. Nonoptimal/Questionable). Classification accuracy ranged from 73% (i.e., total score at 1 month) to almost 97% (i.e., Motor Quality at 24–36 months), depending on age. Overall, Motor Quality ratings were highly consistent across age (all over 90% correctly classified), with all other factor scores showing at least 80% classification accuracy (Bayley, 1993). Classification accuracy information over time, to our knowledge, is not available for other BSID-II scores.

Long-term stability of the BSID-II has not been thoroughly investigated. One study reports a one-year test-retest reliability of .67, based on testing at 12 months and 24 months in normally developing toddlers (Markus et al., 2000). Pomerleau et al. (2003) report low test-retest reliability from a one-month visit to six-month visit in a small mixed sample of infants of high-risk, moderate-risk, and low-risk mothers, with scores actually decreasing at 6 months (i.e., $r = .30$ for MDI; $N = 68$). Thus, as noted by Bayley (1993), the test is not designed for long-term prediction of developmental level.

It is important to note that test-retest reliability coefficients may be misleading (i.e., a low r may reflect sample

Table 6–15 Extrapolated Age Equivalents for the BSID-II for High- and Low-Functioning Infants

Raw Score	Developmental Age (Months)			Raw Score	Developmental Age (Months)			Raw Score	Developmental Age (Months)		
	Loess	Manual	Linear		Loess	Manual	Linear		Loess	Manual	Linear
0		<1	0.3	60	6.2	5	5.6	120	19.8	20	20.0
1		<1	0.4	61	6.3	6	5.7	121	20.1	20	20.3
2		<1	0.4	62	6.5	6	5.9	122	20.4	20	20.5
3		<1	0.5	63	6.7	6	6.0	123	20.7	21	20.8
4		<1	0.5	64	6.9	6	6.3	124	20.9	21	21.0
5		<1	0.6	65	7.1	6	6.5	125	21.2	21	21.3
6		<1	0.6	66	7.3	7	6.8	126	21.5	22	21.7
7		<1	0.7	67	7.4	7	7.0	127	21.8	22	22.0
8		<1	0.7	68	7.6	7	7.2	128	22.1	22	22.3
9		<1	0.8	69	7.8	7	7.4	129	22.4	23	22.7
10		<1	0.8	70	8.0	7	7.6	130	22.8	23	23.0
11		<1	0.9	71	8.2	8	7.8	131	23.1	23	23.3
12		<1	0.9	72	8.4	8	8.0	132	23.5	24	23.7
13		<1	1.0	73	8.6	8	8.3	133	23.9	24	24.0
14	1.0	1	1.0	74	8.8	8	8.7	134	24.3	24	24.3
15	1.1	1	1.1	75	9.0	9	9.0	135	24.8	25	24.7
16	1.1	1	1.1	76	9.3	9	9.3	136	25.2	25	25.0
17	1.2	1	1.2	77	9.5	9	9.5	137	25.6	25	25.3
18	1.3	1	1.3	78	9.7	10	9.8	138	26.1	26	25.7
19	1.3	1	1.4	79	9.9	10	10.0	139	26.5	26	26.0
20	1.4	1	1.4	80	10.1	10	10.3	140	27.0	26	26.3
21	1.5	1	1.5	81	10.3	11	10.5	141	27.5	27	26.7
22	1.5	2	1.6	82	10.6	11	10.8	142	28.0	27	27.0
23	1.6	2	1.6	83	10.8	11	11.0	143	28.5	27	28.0
24	1.7	2	1.7	84	11.0	11	11.2	144	29.0	29	28.5
25	1.8	2	1.8	85	11.3	11	11.4	145	29.5	29	29.0
26	1.9	2	1.9	86	11.5	11	11.6	146	30.1	30	29.5
27	1.9	2	1.9	87	11.7	12	11.8	147	30.6	30	30.0
28	2.0	2	2.0	88	12.0	12	12.0	148	31.2	31	31.0
29	2.1	2	2.2	89	12.2	12	12.3	149	31.8	32	31.5
30	2.2	2	2.3	90	12.5	12	12.7	150	32.3	32	32.0
31	2.3	2	2.5	91	12.7	13	13.0	151	32.9	33	33.0
32	2.4	3	2.7	92	13.0	13	13.3	152	33.5	34	34.0
33	2.5	3	2.8	93	13.2	13	13.5	153	34.1	35	34.5
34	2.6	3	3.0	94	13.5	14	13.8	154	34.8	35	35.0
35	2.7	3	3.1	95	13.7	14	14.0	155	35.4	36	36.0
36	2.8	3	3.2	96	14.0	14	14.3	156	36.1	36	36.8
37	2.9	3	3.3	97	14.3	14	14.5	157	36.7	36	37.5
38	3.0	3	3.4	98	14.5	15	14.8	158	37.4	37–39	38.3
39	3.2	3	3.5	99	14.8	15	15.0	159	38.1	37–39	39.0
40	3.3	3	3.5	100	15.0	15	15.3	160	38.8	37–39	39.5
41	3.4	4	3.6	101	15.2	15	15.5	161	39.5	37–39	40.0
42	3.5	4	3.7	102	15.5	16	15.8	162	40.2	37–39	40.5
43	3.6	4	3.8	103	15.7	16	16.0	163	40.9	40–42	41.0
44	3.8	4	3.9	104	15.9	16	16.2	164	41.7	40–42	41.5
45	3.9	4	4.0	105	16.1	16	16.4	165	42.4	40–42	42.0
46	4.0	4	4.1	106	16.4	16	16.6	166		42+	42.9
47	4.2	4	4.2	107	16.6	17	16.8	167		42+	43.8
48	4.3	4	4.3	108	16.8	17	17.0	168		42+	44.7
49	4.5	4	4.4	109	17.0	17	17.2	169		42+	45.6
50	4.6	4	4.5	110	17.3	17	17.4	170		42+	46.5
51	4.7	4	4.5	111	17.5	17	17.6	171		42+	47.4
52	4.9	5	4.6	112	17.7	18	17.8	172		42+	48.2
53	5.0	5	4.7	113	18.0	18	18.0	173		42+	49.1
54	5.2	5	4.8	114	18.2	18	18.3	174		42+	50.0
55	5.4	5	4.9	115	18.5	18	18.5	175		42+	50.9
56	5.5	5	5.0	116	18.7	19	18.8	176		42+	51.8
57	5.7	5	5.1	117	19.0	19	19.0	177		42+	52.7
58	5.8	5	5.3	118	19.3	19	19.3	178		42+	53.6
59	6.0	5	5.4	119	19.6	19	19.7				

Source: From Lindsay & Brouwers, 1999. Reprinted with permission.

Table 6–16a Extrapolated Scores for the BSID-II Mental Developmental Index (MDI)

MDI	2	3	4	5	6	8	10	12	15	18	21	24	27	30	36	42
								Age in Months								
50	3	—	—	—	38	47	55	—	74	—	99	108	117	—	130	140
49	—	8	19	30	—	—	—	65	73	87	—	—	—	122	—	—
48	2	—	—	—	37	46	—	—	—	—	98	107	116	—	129	139
47	—	7	18	29	—	—	54	64	72	86	—	—	—	121	—	—
46	1	—	—	—	36	45	—	—	—	—	97	106	115	—	128	138
45	—	6	17	28	—	—	53	63	71	85	—	—	—	120	—	—
44	—	—	—	—	35	44	—	—	—	—	96	105	114	—	127	137
43	—	5	16	27	—	—	52	62	70	84	—	—	—	119	—	—
42	—	—	—	—	34	43	—	—	—	—	95	104	113	—	126	136
41	—	4	15	26	—	—	51	61	69	83	—	—	—	118	—	
40	—	—	—	—	33	42	—	—	—	—	94	103	112	—	125	135
39	—	3	14	25	—	—	50	60	68	82	—	—	—	117	—	
38	—		—	—	32	41	—	—	—	—	93	102	111	—	124	134
37	—	2	13	24	—	—	49	—	67	81	—	—	—	116	—	
36			—	—	31	40	—	59	—	—	92	101	110	—	123	133
35	—	1	12	23	—	—	48	—	66	80	—	—	—	115	—	
34	—	—	—	—	30	39	—	58	—	—	91	100	109	—	122	132
33	—	—	11	22	—	—	47	—	65	79	—	—	—	114	—	
32	—		—	—	29	38	—	57	—	—	90	99	108	—	121	131
31	—		10	21	—	—	—	—	64	78	—	—	—	113	—	
30	—	—	—	—	28	37	46	56	—	—	89	98	107	—	120	130

Note: To use the table, find the appropriate age column and move down the rows until you reach the obtained raw score; the number in the far left column of that row represents the estimated index score. Researchers using these tables should be aware that both the accuracy and the interval nature of the index scores may not be retained in the estimated tables.

Source: Adapted from Robinson & Mervis, 1996. Reprinted with permission.

Table 6–16b Extrapolated Scores for the Psychomotor Developmental Index (PDI)

PDI	2	3	4	5	6	8	10	12	15	18	21	24	27	30	36	42
								Age in Months								
50	—	—	—	—	—	—	—	—	—	—	—	—	—	—	—	—
49	—	8	—	—	23	—	—	52	57	—	66	71	77	—	84	—
48	—	—	—	17	—	—	—	—	—	—	—	—	—	—	—	92
47	—	—	11	—	—	35	41	—	—	62	—	—	—	80	—	—
46	—	7	—	—	22	—	—	51	—	—	—	—	—	—	83	—
45	—	—	—	16	—	—	—	—	56	—	65	70	76	—	—	—
44	—	—	10	—	—	34	40	—	—	—	—	—	—	—	—	91
43	—	6	—	—	21	—	—	—	—	61	—	—	—	79	82	—
42	—	—	9	15	—	—	—	50	—	—	64	69	—	—	—	—
41	—	—	—	—	—	33	39	—	55	—	—	—	75	—	—	90
40	—	5	—	—	20	—	—	—	—	—	—	—	—	—	81	—
39	—	—	—	14	—	—	—	—	—	60	—	—	—	78	—	
38	—	—	8	—	—	32	38	49	—	—	—	68	—	—	—	
37	—	4	—	—	19	—	—	—	54	—	63	—	74	—	80	—
36	—	—	—	13	—	—	—	—	—	—	—	—	—	—	—	89
35	—	—	7	—	—	31	37	—	—	59	—	—	—	77	—	—
34	—	3	—	—	18	—	—	48	—	—	—	67	—	—	79	
33	—	—	6	12	—	—	36	—	53	—	62	—	73	—	—	—
32	—	—	—	—	—	30	—	—	—	—	—	—	—	—	—	88
31	—	2	—	—	17	—	—	—	—	58	—	—	—	76	78	—
30	—	—	5	11	—	29	35	47	—	—	—	66	—	—	—	—

Note: To use the table, find the appropriate age column and move down the rows until you reach the obtained raw score; the number in the far left column of that row represents the estimated index score. Researchers using these tables should be aware that both the accuracy and the interval nature of the index scores may not be retained in the estimated tables.

Source: Adapted from Robinson & Mervis, 1996. Reprinted with permission.

Table 6–17 Test-Retest Reliability Coefficients for the BSID-II, by Age

Magnitude of Coefficient	Age 1 Month	Age 12 Months	Ages 24 and 36 Months
Very high (.90+)		BRS Total Score	Mental Scale
High (.80–.89)	Mental Scale[a]	Mental Scale[a] BRS Motor Quality	
Adequate (.70–.79)	Motor Scale[a] BRS Motor Quality	Motor Scale	Motor Scale BRS Motor Quality
Marginal (.60–.69)		BRS Emotional Regulation	BRS Total Score BRS Orientation/ Engagement BRS Emotional Regulation
Low (<.59)	BRS Total Score BRS Attention/ Arousal	BRS Orientation/ Engagement	

Note: Scores for Mental and Motor Scales are standard scores; scores for BRS are raw scores.
[a]Based on combined 1- and 12-month data.

Source: Adapted from Bayley, 1993.

characteristics rather than test characteristics). Stability estimates may therefore differ significantly across conditions, depending on expected developmental trajectory, as well as on the age at which children are tested. For example, Niccols and Latchman (2002) reported that one-year BSID-II stability coefficients for children with Down syndrome were higher than those for medically fragile infants (i.e., .65 and .37, respectively). However, when actual developmental quotient scores were examined, on average, scores of children with Down syndrome dropped after one year, but scores of medically fragile infants increased in the same time span, consistent with their expected developmental trajectories. Additionally, BSID-II classifications (i.e., Normal/Borderline vs. Abnormal) in infancy, compared with those obtained one year later, showed low agreement for Down syndrome children but moderate agreement for medically fragile infants (kappa = .04 vs. .41). As noted above (see *Ethnicity/SES*), research shows that children from at-risk backgrounds, including those with high rates of poverty, single-parent families, and familial chaos, have decreasing BSID-II scores with time when multiple assessments are compared (e.g., Mayes et al., 2003). Lower test-retest stability estimates may occur in these subgroups. Additionally, these studies underline the need to examine other indices of test-retest stability (including expected developmental trajectories and actual score ranges) in addition to reliability coefficients when evaluating test characteristics in clinical groups.

Practice Effects

The manual reports that scores increased an average of two points on both the Mental and Motor Scales across all ages, indicating a minimal practice effect in the standardization sample after a median interval of four days (Bayley, 1993).

Practice effects have not been found in all studies (e.g., Markus et al., 2000). Again, practice effects would not be expected in populations whose developmental trajectory includes a decrease from infancy to toddlerhood.

Assessing Change

A new way of modeling change using developmental trajectories based on Rossavik modeling shows promise in determining whether individual infants deviate from their projected developmental growth curve. These are estimates of change modeled on BSID-II raw scores for normally and atypically developing infants tested serially over time. Using these models, Deter et al. (2001) found that differences of ± 10% raw score points between two assessment points in time were beyond the bounds expected by measurement or prediction error, and were thus indicative of probable alternation of normal development in the individual infant between 4 and 26 months of age.

Interrater Reliability

Interscorer reliability is reported as .96 for the Mental Scale and .75 for the Motor Scale. BRS interscorer reliability is generally high (over .90 for total and factor scores for 1–5-month-olds level, and over 87% for 13–42-month-olds; Bayley, 1993). Good interobserver agreement has also been found in other studies, in samples differing significantly from the standardization sample (e.g., Hamadani et al., 2002). However, when interscorer reliability of experienced Bayley examiners is assessed at the item level, considerable variability may occur on certain items. Chandlee et al. (2002) reported that although agreement was generally high for the majority of items, there were certain items that were not scored consistently across raters (i.e., 23% of items sampled). This inconsistency yielded underestimations or overestimations of as much as −16 to +14 standard score points on the MDI, even though the mean difference across raters was small (i.e., −1.7 points). They also found greater scoring variability in younger children and for items requiring incidental observation of language or involving timing. As noted above, Chandlee et al. (2002) provide recommendations for administering and scoring these items to improve interrater agreement (see Table 6–8).

VALIDITY

Content

Items for the BSID-II were selected with considerable care to ensure appropriate item content and absence of bias. Techniques included a survey of BSID users, literature review, panel review including experts in child development who were provided with specific guidelines on how to evaluate items, new item generation (based on literature review and generation of items from 25 experts), three pilot testings, testing using a tryout version, and bias analyses (including empirical analysis such as Rasch techniques, and expert panel bias review). After completion of standardization testing, items were re-reviewed, and only those demonstrating strong age trends, appropriate difficulty level, statistical relationship to other scale items, lack of bias, and no administration/scoring problems were retained in the final test version (Bayley, 1993).

Comparison With the Original BSID

Correlations between the two versions are high in the standardization sample for the Mental and Motor Scales (i.e., $r = .62$ and .63, respectively). However, the size of the correlations indicates that the two tests nevertheless have a significant amount of unique variance (Bayley, 1993). Similar correlations have been reported in other samples, including children from low SES and African American mothers ($r = .78$ and .70, respectively; Black et al., 2001). Raw scores and age equivalents of profoundly delayed individuals whose ages fall outside the test norms are very highly intercorrelated between test versions ($r = .90–.97$; DeWitt et al., 1998).

BSID scores are, on average, 10 to 12 points higher than BSID-II scores when both tests are administered (Bayley, 1993; Black & Matula, 2000). For example, mean standard score differences in MDI between the two scales have ranged from 9.2 to 18.2 points in normally developing infants (Bayley, 1993; Glenn et al., 2001; Tasbihsazan et al., 1997) and 9 to 11 raw score points in profoundly delayed individuals outside the age range (DeWitt et al., 1998). Similar results have been reported in children with Down syndrome (8.4 standard score points; Glenn et al., 2001) and preterm infants (7.3 points; Goldstein et al., 1995). Additionally, children who obtain BSID scores that differ significantly from the norm (i.e., at the extremes of the distribution such as developmental delay or

above average), tend to have larger BSID-BSID-II differences (i.e., 13 to 18 points; Bayley, 1993; Gagnon & Nagle, 2000; Glenn et al., 2001; Tasbihsazan et al., 1997), although this is not always found (e.g., DeWitt et al., 1998).

Subscale Intercorrelations

According to the manual, the Mental and Motor Scales are moderately intercorrelated across age (average $r = .44$, range .24 to .72; Bayley, 1993). One study on normal 6-month-old infants reported a high correlation between scales ($r = .66$; Porter et al., 2003). The manual also reports that the BRS's correlation to the Mental and Motor Scales is low to moderate across age (i.e., .27 to .45 for the BRS total score). Porter et al. (2003) reported negligible correlations between the BRS Emotional Regulation factor and MDI/PDI in 6-month-old infants ($r = .11$). Overall, these findings suggest that each of the three BSID-II components tap different sources of variance not necessarily covered by the other two BSID-II scales.

Factor Structure

The manual does not provide information on whether the three BSID-II components actually emerge as separate factors (Flanagan & Alfonso, 1995), or whether facet scores are replicable in factor solutions. Factor analyses of clinical groups are also needed (Fugate, 1998).

With regard to the BRS, the manual reports factor solutions corresponding to the factor scores in the scale. These include two factors, Motor Quality and Attention/Arousal, in the youngest age group (1–5 months), and three factors in the two older age groups, representing Orientation/Engagement, Motor Quality, and Emotional Regulation. Of note, the factor solutions only accounted for moderate amounts of variance (i.e., 46%, 54%, and 44%, respectively), which suggests that other ways of portioning variance may provide a better fit. In particular, one study suggests that Motor Quality appeared to dominate factor solutions generated using standardization and clinical samples in both first-order and second-order factor solutions, either because motor behavior is easily observed by raters, or because motor quality mediates all other aspects of performance on the BRS (Thompson et al., 1996). Of note, factor solutions became increasingly complex as samples became more heterogeneous, with the simplest factor solution occurring in the youngest, normally developing infants (Thompson et al., 1996).

Correlations With IQ

Even though the manual is careful to explain that the test is a developmental scale and not an IQ test, the BSID-II shows substantial associations with IQ. For example, the BSID-II Mental Scale correlates highly with composite measures of general intelligence, including scores from the McCarthy

Scales ($r = .79$), WPPSI-R ($r = .73$), and DAS ($r = .49$; Bayley, 1993). As expected, correlations between the Motor Scale and composites from these measures are not as high. For example, the manual reports moderate correlations between the Motor Scale and McCarthy Scales ($r = .45$), WPPSI-R ($r = .41$), and DAS ($r = .35$; Bayley, 1993).

Substantial correlations between tests do not necessarily inform on whether scores obtained from different instruments are similar, particularly in children whose development may be uneven or atypical. For example, in preschoolers with autism, Magiati and Howlin (2001) found that BSID-II scores were significantly lower than those yielded by the Merrill-Palmer, despite high correlations between the two tests ($r = .82$). In contrast, BSID-II and Vineland Scales appeared to show higher agreement; intercorrelations were high, and scores were comparable (55.6 versus 55.1). Correlations to other measures are discussed in further detail in the manual (Bayley, 1993), and validity studies are also discussed in Black and Matula (2000). There is currently limited empirical evidence on the validity of the facet scores in terms of correlations to other measures.

Scores on the BSID-II are usually predictive of subsequent IQ, but this may depend on the sample assessed and the timeframe evaluated. Overall, BSID-II scores of infants with significant delays or atypical development are more predictive of later IQ than those with scores in the average range (Bracken & Walker, 1997). For example, in one study of extremely low birth weight infants, BSID-II scores at the age of 2 were highly related to WPPSI-R IQ at 4 years, especially in girls ($r = . 73$; Sajaniemi et al., 2001b). BSID-II scores of children under age 2 may be less predictive of later IQ because perceptual motor skills, rather than mental skills, are mostly assessed by earlier items on the Mental Scale (Roberts et al., 1999).

Correlations With Other Cognitive Tests

Research has also examined whether the BSID-II is a good predictor of more specific cognitive domains such as language or attention. Some studies report that BSID-II MDI scores are significantly correlated with language measures, with increasingly large associations with increasing age (e.g., .26–.33 in 14-month-olds versus .50–.53 in 18-month-olds; Lyytinen et al., 1999). However, this has not been found in all studies. For example, in toddlers with developmental delay, prelinguistic vocalizations (e.g., rate, extent of consonant use, and rate of interactive vocalizations), but not BSID-MDI or Mental Age scores, predict expressive language scores assessed one year later (McCathren et al., 1999). Similarly, children with a positive family history of dyslexia perform similarly to controls (i.e., both groups within normal limits) on the BSID-II MDI, despite group differences on expressive language tests (Lyytinen et al., 2001). Lack of group differences were also found for the BSID-II expressive score, a subset of items thought to be a more precise estimate of language competence compared to the entire scale (but see Seigel et al., 1995). This raises questions about the test's sensitivity to language deficits.

Other research has examined the association between BSID-II and attention. For example, the MDI is highly related to the ability to respond to joint attention (Markus et al., 2000), an early precursor of focused and sustained attention (Bono & Stifter, 2003). Further, a composite score comprised of specific MDI items measuring cognitive ability (COG) appears to be more predictive of the duration of attention in 17- to 24-month olds than the standard MDI (see Table 6–11 for specific items). This may be because the MDI reflects broader aspects of ability tapping general cognitive and perceptual skill development rather than specific cognitive skills such as attention (Choudhury & Gorman, 2000).

Clinical Studies

The manual provides preliminary data on BSID-II performance in specific clinical samples such as children with prematurity, HIV infection, prenatal drug exposure, birth asphyxia, development delay, chronic otitis media, autism, and Down syndrome. Many of the clinical groups performed below normal limits on the MDI and the PDI, with the Down syndrome group having the lowest scores and the otitis media group the highest scores. Although the manual recommends that these data be interpreted with caution, it is difficult to determine their clinical significance in the absence of information on score differences compared to matched normal samples, as well as diagnostic classification statistics such as sensitivity, specificity, and positive/negative predictive power. Note that other studies on children with Down syndrome (Niccols & Latchman, 2002) and drug exposure (Schuler et al., 2003) report significantly lower mean scores than those presented in the manual.

The BSID-II has been used in a large number of studies on various clinical populations. For instance, in infants with extremely low birth weight, each additional pre-/perinatal risk factor (e.g., low maternal education, neonatal ultrasound abnormalities, intraventricular hemorrhage, respiratory intervention, etc.) is associated with a 3.5-point decrease in BSID-II MDI scores (Sajaniemi et al., 2001b). Similarly, periventricular leukomalacia in premature infants is found to be a strong risk factor for low BSID-II scores (Nelson et al., 2001). The test has shown sensitivity to the effects of prenatal exposure to polysubstance abuse, where boys show increased vulnerability to delay (Moe et al., 2001). The BSID-II has also demonstrated sensitivity to developmental trajectories in Down syndrome such that scores typically drop from the first to the second year of life (Niccols & Latchman, 2002). In contrast, BSID-II scores of medically fragile children tested in the first year of life may underestimate cognitive potential, as seen by the increase in scores with age (Niccols & Latchman, 2002). The BSID-II has also been used in studies assessing developmental delay in adoptees from Eastern European countries, where the rate of developmental delay detected by the test may be as high as 55% (Boone et al., 2003). The test has also been used in large-scale studies on vulnerable children, including those managed by child welfare and foster care (Leslie et al., 2002).

Variability in BSID-II scores within groups, as evidenced by large standard deviations or large score ranges, may also be a feature of at-risk children. This has been documented in children with early risk factors such as neurological abnormality or prematurity (e.g., MDIs ranging from <50 to +110; Nelson et al., 2001), in children of families with extreme poverty and environmental instability (Mayes et al., 2003), and in prenatally drug-exposed children (Moe & Slinning, 2001).

The BSID-II has also been used in treatment studies, including multisensory intervention administered in the neonatal intensive care unit to infants with neurological injury or extreme prematurity (Nelson et al., 2001; Sajaniemi et al., 2001b). In children with PKU, the test has shown sensitivity to mild delay and has provided evidence for the beneficial effect of breastfeeding on neurodevelopment via intake of long-chain polyunsaturated fatty acids, thought to be involved in the development of frontal regions in the developing brain (Agostoni et al., 2003). In healthy infants, supplementation of formula with docosahexaenoic acid (DHA) during the first four months of life is reported to be associated with a seven-point increase in MDI but not PDI or BRS, supporting the hypotheses that this nutritional component is selectively related to cognitive development (Birch et al., 2000).

In typically developing children, the BSID-II has contributed to our understanding of normal development. For instance, BSID-II MDI scores are significantly related to symbolic play in preschoolers (Lyytinen et al., 1999); symbolic play is thought to represent prelinguistic skills that are a foundation for later language ability (Lyytinen et al., 2001). The BSID-II has also been used in research showing the importance of family environment on early cognitive development. BSID-II scores are moderately correlated to measures of the home environment reflecting the quality of parenting in medically fragile infants ($r = .41$–.42; Holditch-Davis et al., 2000). Similarly, in research on developmental neurotoxicity examining the effect of PCB in breast milk, increased concentrations are associated with poorer BSID-II scores; however, a good home environment appears to be a significant protective factor that may offset adverse cognitive effects of exposure (Walkowiak et al., 2001). BSID-II scores also appear to be related to parenting characteristics, which provides evidence for the association between rearing practices and cognitive development. For instance, maternal vocalizations and maternal contingency (i.e., contingent responding to infant needs) are moderately associated with MDI and BRS scores, but not PDI (Pomerleau et al., 2003). Specific parenting behaviors that inhibit toddlers' competence (e.g., forceful redirection, ignoring/reinforcing misbehavior) are moderately and inversely related to MDI scores (Coleman et al., 2002). Similarly, parental beliefs about parenting competence are moderately related to MDI scores in easy toddlers, but not in difficult tod-

dlers (Coleman & Karraker, 2003). Extent of marital conflict appears to be inversely related to scores on the BRS Emotional Regulation factor in infants (Porter et al., 2003), suggesting that conflict in the home may adversely affect developing regulatory abilities in infants. The BSID-II has also been used in research demonstrating the role of fathers' parenting style in cognitive development. For example, a responsive-didactic parenting style in fathers is predictive of risk of delay in low-income fathers of varied ethnicity (Shannon et al., 2002). When other factors are controlled, the MDI is also related to the quality of daycare centers (i.e., operationalized as adult to child ratio and group size) in low-income African American preschoolers (Burchinal et al., 2000), again providing evidence for the impact of early environmental influences on cognitive development.

COMMENT

The BSID-II is a well-designed, psychometrically sound test that is probably the most frequently used infant development assessment test in North America and, like its predecessor, is considered the best available assessment tool for infants (Sattler, 2001). It is also a preferred test for research. Especially compelling is the fact that, despite the considerable challenges of assessing infants and preschoolers, including inherent variability in behavior, limited attention, distractibility, and susceptibility to interference (Chandlee et al., 2002), the test boasts impressive psychometrics (Dunst, 1998; Flanagan & Alfonso, 1995). Additionally, the manual is well written and comprehensive (including historical overview), and test content was developed with substantial care, including literature review and bias review.

However, as with any test, users need to be aware of its limitations. First, there are a few psychometric issues. Although the test has impressive reliabilities, particularly with regard to the MDI and BRS Motor Quality Scales, there are still concerns about stability of some scores over time (e.g., Bradley-Johnson, 2001; Flanagan & Alfonso, 1995). Some BRS factor scores also have questionable reliability at some ages (i.e., Attention/Arousal). The test may also have steep item gradients in the younger age bands (Nellis & Gridley, 1994). Facet scores have limited empirical evidence of validity, have a potential for misuse (Schock & Buck, 1995), and should be used, if at all, "with extreme caution" (Fugate, 1998; see also *Interpretation*). Information on sensitivity, specificity, and other classification statistics such as positive predictive power are lacking for the MDI, PDI, and BRS, as well as for facet scores and BRS factor scores.

The norms are based on 1988 Census data, which makes them outdated in terms of demographic composition and potentially vulnerable to the Flynn effect. Healthy children only are included in the sample, which is problematic because the test is commonly used to assess children with developmental delay (see McFadden, 1996, for the limitations of "truncated" norm distributions). On the other hand, other tests are hampered by floor effects, so that standard scores for low-functioning children are based on a flat profile consisting of few or no raw score points, which provides no information on what a child can actually accomplish (Flanagan & Alfonso, 1995). Unlike these, the BSID-II has a range of items that are appropriate for even low-functioning preschoolers. As a result, most children pass several items, which provides substantial information on their capabilities—not just their limitations—and is of considerable utility in planning interventions and remedial programs (Flanagan & Alfonso, 1995). Others disagree (Dunst, 1998), and note that the test was not designed for this purpose, nor is it capable of identifying behavioral goals for intervention, particularly when the same MDI score can be obtained by different children passing and failing completely different combinations of item types and levels (Bendersky & Lewis, 2001). Note, too, that the BSID-II has limited utility in discriminating ability level below mild to moderate delay (i.e., minimum standard score = 50), and has been criticized as an assessment tool for children with disabilities (Dunst, 1998). Use of developmental age equivalents for quantifying deficit in extremely low-functioning individuals instead is an inadequate substitute.

There is also the issue of cutoff points for adjacent norms tables for children whose ages are close to the next oldest or youngest age classification. Bradley-Johnson (2001) provides the following example: on a given day, a child aged 4 months, 15 days obtains a raw score of 40, which yields an MDI of 91. If the child had been tested the next day instead, when she was aged 4 months, 16 days, her MDI score would be 69. Note that this problem with age cutoffs only occurs between 1 and 5 months of age (Bradley-Johnson, 2001). As a possible solution, users are urged to consider adjacent age-norms tables when calculating scores for infants whose ages are at the top or the bottom of an age band. However, this appears a rather inadequate solution, especially when scores can result in such divergent classifications.

Because toddlers and preschoolers are known to either (a) not be able to express themselves verbally, (b) not choose to express themselves verbally, or (c) be difficult to understand when they actually do express themselves verbally, a nonverbal score would be a significant asset (Bradley-Johnson, 2001). In addition, lack of a nonverbal score limits the utility of the test in children with language or speech impairments given the large number of items that are language-based, particularly in the older age bands (Bradley-Johnson, 2001). In assessing young children with developmental delay, the BSID-II is probably not sufficient to accurately predict future language scores (McCathren et al., 1999); the test should therefore be supplemented by other language measures. Likewise, the test is heavily loaded with motor items, and therefore may not be appropriate for children with physical impairments such as cerebral palsy (Mayes, 1999).

Given the outdated norms that inflate test scores, use of the original BSID for clinical or research purposes is not recommended (Tasbihsazan et al., 1997). Alternatively, researchers who have been using the BSID for longitudinal studies may consider reporting raw scores (Black & Matula, 2000).

Start Points

Competent administration of the BSID-II demands a thorough understanding of the practical limits and benefits of using estimated starting points, whether based on estimated level or corrected age (i.e., gestational versus chronological). Specifically, BSID-II scores may vary depending on which item set was chosen as the starting point of the child's assessment. Minor changes to the administration of the Bayley, such as those based on the examiner's assumptions of a child's levels, can significantly affect test scores and lead to underestimation or overestimation of levels (Gauthier et al., 1999; Washington et al., 1998). Note that one major contributor to poor replicability of MDI scores across raters is the use of different start points by different examiners (Chandlee et al., 2002).

Ross and Lawson (1997) conducted an informal survey and found that most psychologists use the corrected age as a basis for selecting the starting point in premature infants. However, when the authors compared MDI and PDI scores of premature children using both corrected and chronological ages, equivalent scores were obtained only for children with major developmental delays. Children with average scores when chronological age was used as a starting point had lower levels when corrected age was used to determine the initial item set. In another study (Glenn et al., 2001), infants could pass items in higher item sets despite reaching ceiling criteria on lower ranked items. The authors noted that some children with atypical development tend to have scattered or variable performance, which could exacerbate any inaccuracies related to the starting point. To avoid this problem, they recommend preceding the BSID-II administration by the administration of other nonverbal tests/materials covering a wide range of age levels to identify an appropriate BSID-II starting point. This may be time-consuming in some contexts. A practical alternative is simply to use item types that span several start points, such as items involving cubes, pegs, or picture naming/pointing (C. Miranda, personal communication, January 2005).

Users should keep in mind that delay in one area might not necessarily mean delay in other areas of functioning (Matula et al., 1997). For example, selecting a starting point based on a child's language deficits may result in item sets that are inappropriately low for their motor strengths, and vice versa. Black and Matula (2000) recommend that designated starting points therefore only be altered when definitive information exists on a child's levels. Alternatively, the simplest approach is simply to use chronological age in all cases (Gauthier et al., 1999).

Scoring: Corrected Age Versus Chronological Age

The second issue concerns the selection of age level for conversion of raw scores to standard scores. The manual recommends that corrected age be used for children with prematurity when deriving standard scores. However, it is unclear whether a correction should be applied at all ages or only to younger infants. In Ross and Lawson's (1997) survey, most psychologists corrected for age until 2 years of age, after which chronological age was used in score conversions. They noted that this was based on convention, not on empirical evidence. The authors review some of the research on age correction, which indicates that the need to correct for age is more complex than it appears (e.g., it may relate to such factors as birth weight and functional domain assessed, given cross-domain variability in children with uneven development). For more information on this issue, see Black and Matula (2000).

Interpretation

It is important to note that BSID-II scores should be used as general indicators of functioning, not as definitive predictors of future ability or potential (Nellis & Gridley, 1994). The BSID-II was not designed to provide information on specific subdomains of infant ability, and the test does not measure specific, well-defined cognitive processes, but is rather "a standardized, developmentally ordered checklist of complex criterion behaviors" (Bendersky & Lewis, 2001, p. 443). The manual explicitly indicates that the test should *not* be used to measure deficit in a specific skill area such as language, nor to obtain a norm-referenced score for a severely physically or sensorially impaired child.

As noted above, there are psychometric issues and limited validity evidence for the facet scores, including unequal item representation across ages. Black and Matula (2000) recommend that these be used with caution, keeping in mind that the scores may provide a general description of functioning within domains but that a precise evaluation of particular abilities should be obtained via other instruments designed for this purpose. The manual stresses that only the MDI and PDI summary scores should be used in interpreting test results, and that failure on a particular cluster of items (e.g., language) "should not be used as a measure of deficit in a specific skill area" (p. 4).

Lastly, the test is also at times used to characterize the developmental level of severely or profoundly impaired children and adults who are outside the actual BSID-II age range by deriving developmental age equivalents of raw scores. Although this technique can yield useful clinical information, use of the test in this way should be done with caution, keeping in mind the practical and psychometric limitations of age equivalents (Bayley, 1993; DeWitt et al., 1998).

REFERENCES

Agostoni, C., Verduci, E., Massetto, N., Radaelli, G., Riva, E., & Giovannini, M. (2003). Plasma long-chain polyunsaturated fatty acids and neurodevelopment through the first 12 months of life in phenylketonuria. *Developmental Medicine & Child Neurology, 45*, 257–261.

Andersson, H. W., Sonnander, K., & Sommerfelt, K. (1998). Gender and its contribution to the prediction of cognitive abilities at 5 years. *Scandinavian Journal of Psychology, 39*, 267–274.

Atkinson, L. (1990). Intellectual and adaptive functioning: Some tables for interpreting the Vineland in combination with intelligence tests. *American Journal of Mental Retardation, 95*, 198–203.

Bayley, N. (1933). *The California First-Year Mental Scale.* Berkeley: University of California Press.

Bayley, N. (1936). *The California Infant Scale of Motor Development.* Berkeley: University of California Press.

Bayley, N. (1969). *Bayley Scales of Infant Development.* Manual. New York: Psychological Corporation.

Bayley, N. (1970). Development of mental abilities. In P. H. Mussen (Ed.), *Carmichael's manual of child psychology* (3rd ed.). New York: Wiley.

Bayley, N. (1993). *Bayley Scales of Infant Development* (2nd ed.; Bayley-II). San Antonio, TX: Psychological Corporation.

Bendersky, M., & Lewis, M. (2001). The Bayley Scales of Infant Development: Is there a role in biobehavioral assessment? In L. T. Singer & P. S. Zeskind (Eds.), *Biobehavioral assessment of the infant* (pp. 443–462). New York: Guilford Press.

Birch, E. E., Garfield, S., Hoffman, D. R., Uauy, E., & Birch, D. G. (2000). A randomized controlled trial of early dietary supply of long-chain polyunsaturated fatty acids and mental development in term infants. *Developmental Medicine & Child Neurology, 42*, 174–181.

Black, M. M., Hess, C., & Berenson-Howard, J. (2001). Toddlers from low-income families have below normal mental, motor and behavior scores on the revised Bayley scales. *Journal of Applied Developmental Psychology, 21*, 655–666.

Black, M. M., & Matula, K. (2000). *Essentials of Bayley Scales of Infant Development-II assessment.* New York: John Wiley and Sons, Inc.

Bono, M. A., & Stifter, C. A. (2003). Maternal attention-directing strategies and infant focused attention during problem solving. *Infancy, 4*(2), 235–250.

Boone, J. L., Hostetter, M. K., & Weitzman, C. C. (2003). The predictive accuracy of pre-adoption video review in adoptees from Russian and Eastern European orphanages. *Clinical Pediatrics, 42*, 585–590.

Bracken, B. A. (1987). Limitations of preschool instruments and standards for minimal levels of technical adequacy. *Journal of Psychoeducational Assessment, 4*, 313–326.

Bracken, B. A., & Walker, K. C. (1997). The utility of intelligence tests for preschool children. In D. P. Flanagan, J. L. Genshaft, & P. L. Harrison (Eds.), *Contemporary intellectual assessment: Theories, tests and issues* (pp. 484–502). New York: Guilford Press.

Bradley-Johnson, S. (2001). Cognitive assessment for the youngest children: A critical review of tests. *Journal of Psychoeducational Assessment, 19*, 19–44.

Braungart, J. M., Plomin, R., DeFries, J. C., & Fulker, D. W. (1992). Genetic influence on tester-rated infant temperament as assessed by Bayley's Infant Behavior Record: Nonadoptive and adoptive siblings and twins. *Developmental Psychology, 28*, 40–47.

Brooks-Gunn, J., & Weinraub, M. (1983). Origins of infant intelligence testing. In M. Lewis (Ed.), *Origins of intelligence: Infancy and early childhood* (2nd ed., pp. 25–66). New York: Plenum Press.

Burchinal, M. R., Roberts, J. E., Riggins, R., Zeisel, S. A., Neebe, E., & Bryant, D. (2000). Relating quality of center-based child care to early cognitive and language development longitudinally. *Child Development, 71*(2), 339–357.

Campbell, S. K., Siegel, E., & Parr, C. A. (1986). Evidence for the need to renorm the Bayley Scales of Infant Development based on the performance of a population-based sample of 12-month-old infants. *Topics in Early Childhood Special Education, 6,* 83–96.

Cattell, P. (1940). *Cattell Infant Intelligence Scale.* San Antonio, TX: Psychological Corporation.

Chandlee, J., Heathfield, L. T., Selganik, M., Damokosh, A., & Radcliffe, J. (2002). Are we consistent in administering and scoring the Bayley Scales of Infant Development–II? *Journal of Psychoeducational Assessment, 20,* 183–200.

Choudhury, N., & Gorman, K. S. (2000). The relationship between sustained attention and cognitive performance in 17–24-month old toddlers. *Infant and Child Development, 9,* 127–146.

Coleman, P. K., & Karraker, K. H. (2003). Maternal self-efficacy beliefs, competence in parenting, and toddler's behavior and development status. *Infant Mental Health Journal, 24*(2), 126–148.

Coleman, P. K., Trent, A., Bryan, S., King, B., Rogers, N., & Nazir, M. (2002). Parenting behavior, mother's self-efficacy beliefs, and toddler performance on the Bayley Scales of Infant Development. *Early Child Development and Care, 172*(2), 123–140.

Cook, M. J., Holder-Brown, L., Johnson, L. J., & Kilgo, J. L. (1989). An examination of the stability of the Bayley Scales of Infant Development with high-risk infants. *Journal of Early Intervention, 13,* 45–49.

Damarin, F. (1978). Bayley Scales of Infant Development. In O. K. Buros (Ed.), *The eighth mental measurement yearbook* (Vol. 1, pp. 290–293). Highland Park, NJ: Gryphon.

Deter, R. L., Karmel, B., Gardner, J. M., & Flory, M. J. (2001). Predicting 2nd year Bayley raw scores in normal infants: Individualized assessment of early developmental trajectories using Rossavik modeling. *Infant Behavior & Development, 24,* 57–82.

DeWitt, M. B., Schreck, K. A., & Mulick, J. A. (1998). Use of Bayley Scales in individuals with profound mental retardation: Comparison of the first and second editions. *Journal of Developmental and Physical Disabilities, 10,* 307–313.

DiLalla, L. F., Thompson, L. A., Plomin, R., Phillips, K., Fagan, J. F., Haith, M. M., Cyphers, L. H., & Fulker, D. W. (1990). Infant predictors of preschool and adult IQ: A study of infant twins and their parents. *Developmental Psychology, 26,* 759–769.

Dunst, C. (1998). Review of the Bayley Scales of Infant Development—Second edition. In J. C. Impara & B. S. Plake (Eds.), *The thirteenth mental measurements yearbook* (pp. 92–93). Lincoln, NE: The University of Nebraska-Lincoln.

Flanagan, D. P., & Alfonso, V. C. (1995). A critical review of the technical characteristics of new and recently revised intelligence tests for preschool children. *Journal of Psychoeducational Assessment, 13,* 66–90.

Fugate, M. H. (1998). Review of the Bayley Scales of Infant Development—Second Edition. In J. C. Impara & B. S. Plake (Eds.), *The thirteenth mental measurements yearbook* (pp. 93–96). Lincoln, NE: The University of Nebraska-Lincoln.

Gagnon, S. G., & Nagle, R. J. (2000). Comparison of the revised and original versions of the Bayley Scales of Infant Development. *School Psychology International, 21,* 293–305.

Gauthier, S. M., Bauer, C. R., Messinger, D. S., & Closius, J. M. (1999). The Bayley Scales of Infant Development-II: Where to start? *Journal of Developmental and Behavioral Pediatrics, 20,* 75–79.

Gesell, A. (1925). *The mental growth of the preschool child.* New York: MacMillan.

Glenn, S. M., Cunningham, C. C., & Dayus, B. (2001). Comparison of 1969 and 1993 standardizations of the Bayley Mental Scales of Infant Development for infants with Down syndrome. *Journal of Intellectual Disability Research, 45,* 56–62.

Goldstein, D. J., Fogle, E. E., Wieber, J. L., & O'Shea, T. M. (1995). Comparison of the Bayley Scales of Infant Development, Second Edition, and the Bayley Scales of Infant Development with premature infants. *Journal of Psychosocial Assessment, 13,* 391–396.

Hamadani, J. D., Fuchs, G. J., Osendarp, S. J. M., Huda, S. N., & Grantham-McGregor, S. M. (2002). Zinc supplementation during pregnancy and effects on mental development and behaviour of infants: A follow-up study. *The Lancet, 360,* 290–294.

Holditch-Davis, D., Tesh, E. M., Goldman, B. D., Miles, M. S., & D'Auria, J. (2000). Use of the HOME inventory with medically fragile infants. *Children's Health Care, 29*(4), 257–278.

Jaffa, A. S. (1934). *The California Preschool Mental Scale.* Berkeley: University of California Press.

Kaplan, M. G., Jacobson, S. W., & Jacobson, J. L. (1991). *Alternative approaches to clustering and scoring the Bayley Infant Behavior Record at 13 months.* Paper presented at the meeting of the Society for Research in Child Development, Seattle, WA.

Kohen-Raz, R. (1967). Scalogram analysis of some developmental sequences of infant behavior as measured by the Bayley Infant Scales of Mental Development. *Genetic Psychology Monographs, 76,* 3–21.

Lehr, C. A., Ysseldyke, J. E., & Thurlow, M. L. (1987). Assessment practices in model early childhood special education programs. *Psychology in the Schools, 24,* 390–399.

Leslie, L. K., Gordon, J. N., Ganger, W., & Gist, K. (2002). Developmental delay in young children in child welfare by initial placement type. *Infant Mental Health Journal, 23*(5), 496–516.

LeTendre, D., Spiker, D., Scott, D. T., & Constantine, N. A. (1992). Establishing the "ceiling" on the Bayley Scales of Infant Development at 25 months. *Advances in Infancy Research, 7,* 187–198.

Lindsay, J. C., & Brouwers, P. (1999). Intrapolation and extrapolation of age-equivalent scores for the Bayley II: A comparison of two methods of estimation. *Clinical Neuropharmacology, 22,* 44–53.

Lyytinen, P., Laasko, M.-L., Poikkeus, A.-M., & Rita, N. (1999). The development and predictive relations of play and language across the second year. *Scandinavian Journal of Psychology, 40,* 177–186.

Lyytinen, P., Poikkeus, A.-M., Laasko, M.-L., Eklund, K., & Lyytinen, H. (2001). Language development and symbolic play in children with and without familial risk for dyslexia. *Journal of Speech, Language, and Hearing Research, 44,* 873–885.

Magiati, I., & Howlin, P. (2001). Monitoring the progress of preschool children with autism enrolled in early intervention programmes. *Autism, 5*(4), 399–406.

Markus, J., Mundy, P., Morales, M., Delgado, C. E. F., & Yale, M. (2000). Individual differences in infant skills as predictors of child-caregiver joint attention and language. *Social Development, 9*(3), 302–315.

Matula, K., Gyurke, J. S., & Aylward, G. P. (1997). Bayley Scales II. *Journal of Developmental and Behavioral Pediatrics, 18,* 112–113.

Mayes, S. D. (1999). Mayes Motor-Free Compilation (MMFC) for assessing mental ability in children with physical impairments. *International Journal of Disability, Development and Education, 46*(4), 475–482.

Mayes, L. C., Cicchetti, D., Acharyya, S., & Zhang, H. (2003). Developmental trajectories of cocaine-and-other-drug-exposed and non-cocaine-exposed children. *Developmental and Behavioral Pediatrics, 24*(5), 323–335.

McCathren, R. B., Yoder, P. J., & Warren, S. F. (1999). The relationship between prelinguistic vocalization and later expressive vocabulary in young children with developmental delay. *Journal of Speech, Language and Hearing Research, 42,* 915–924.

McFadden, T. U. (1996). Creating language impairments in typically achieving children: The pitfalls of "normal" normative sampling. *Language, Speech, and Hearing in the Schools, 27,* 3–9.

Moe, V., & Slinning, K. (2001). Children prenatally exposed to substances: Gender-related differences in outcome from infancy to 3 years of age. *Infant Mental Health Journal, 22*(3), 334–350.

Nellis, L., & Gridley, B. E. (1994). Review of the Bayley Scales of Infant Development, Second Edition. *Journal of School Psychology, 32*(2), 201–209.

Nelson, M. N., White-Traut, R. C., Vasan, U., Silvestri, J., Comiskey, E., Meleedy-Rey, P., Littau, S., Gu, G., & Patel, M. (2001). One-year outcome of auditory-tactile-visual-vestibular intervention in the neonatal intensive care unit: Effects of severe prematurity and central nervous system injury. *Journal of Child Neurology, 16,* 493–498.

Niccols, A., & Latchman, A. (2002). Stability of the Bayley Mental Scale of Infant Development with high-risk infants. *British Journal of Developmental Disabilities, 48,* 3–13.

Ogunnaike, O. A., & Houser, R. F. (2002). Yoruba toddler's engagement in errands and cognitive performance on the Yoruda Mental Subscale. *International Journal of Behavioral Development, 26*(2), 145–153.

Ong, L., Boo, N., & Chandran, V. (2001). Predictors of neurodevelopmental outcome of Malaysian very low birthweight children at 4 years of age. *Journal of Paediatric Child Health, 37,* 363–368.

Pomerleau, A., Scuccimarri, C., & Malcuit, G. (2003). Mother-infant behavioral interactions in teenage and adult mothers during the first six months postpartum: Relations with infant development. *Infant Mental Health Journal, 24*(5), 495–509.

Porter, C. L., Wouden-Miller, M., Silva, S. S., & Porter, A. E. (2003). Marital harmony and conflict: Links to infants' emotional regulation and cardiac vagal tone. *Infancy, 4*(2), 297–307.

Ramey, C. T., Campbell, F. A., & Nicholson, J. E. (1973). The predictive power of the Bayley Scales of Infant Development and the Stanford-Binet Intelligence Test in a relatively constant environment. *Child Development, 44,* 790–795.

Ratliff-Schaub, K., Hunt, C. E., Crowell, D., Golub, H., Smok-Pearsall, S., Palmer, P., Schafer, S., Bak, S., Cantey-Kiser, J., O'Bell, R., & the CHIME Study Group. (2001). Relationship between infant sleep position and motor development in preterm infants. *Developmental and Behavioral Pediatrics, 22*(5), 293–299.

Roberts, E., Bornstein, M. H., Slater, A. M., & Barrett, J. (1999). Early cognitive development and parental education. *Infant and Child Development, 8,* 49–62.

Robinson, B. F., & Mervis, C. B. (1996). Extrapolated raw scores for the second edition of the Bayley Scales of Infant Development. *American Journal on Mental Retardation, 100*(6), 666–670.

Ross, G., & Lawson, K. (1997). Using the Bayley-II: Unresolved issues in assessing the development of prematurely born children. *Journal of Developmental and Behavioral Pediatrics, 18,* 109–111.

Sajaniemi, N., Hakamies-Blomqvist, L., Katainen, S., & von Wendt, L. (2001a). Early cognitive and behavioral predictors of later performance: A follow-up study of ELBW children from ages 2 to 4. *Early Childhood Research Quarterly, 16,* 343–361.

Sajaniemi, N., Mäkelä, J., Salokorpi, T., von Wendt, L., Hämäläinen, T., & Hakamies-Blomqvist, L. (2001b). Cognitive performance and attachment patterns at four years of age in extremely low birth weight infants after early intervention. *European Child & Adolescent Psychiatry, 10,* 122–129.

Samson, J. F., & de Groot, L. (2001). Study of a group of extremely preterm infants (25–27 weeks): How do they function at 1 year of age? *Journal of Child Neurology, 16,* 832–837.

Santos, D. C. C., Gabbard, C., & Goncalves, V. M. G. (2000). Motor development during the first 6 months: The case of Brazilian infants. *Infant and Child Development, 9*(3), 161–166.

Santos, D. C. C., Gabbard, C., & Goncalves, V. M. G. (2001). Motor development during the first year: A comparative study. *The Journal of Genetic Psychology, 162*(2), 143–153.

Sattler, J. M. (2001). Assessment of children: Cognitive applications (4th ed.). San Diego, CA: Jerome M. Sattler Publisher, Inc.

Schock, H. H., & Buck, K. (1995). Review of Bayley Scales of Infant Development—Second Edition. *Child Assessment News, 5*(2), 1, 12.

Schuler, M. E., Nair, P., & Harrington, D. (2003). Developmental outcome of drug-exposed children through 30 months: A comparison of Bayley and Bayley-II. *Psychological Assessment, 15*(3), 435–438.

Seigel, L. S., Cooper, D. C., Fitzhardinge, P. M., & Ash, A. J. (1995). The use of the Mental Development Index of the Bayley Scale to diagnose language delay in 2-year-old high risk infants. *Infant Behavior and Development, 18,* 483–486.

Shannon, J. D., Tamis-LeMonda, C. S., London, K., & Cabrera, N. (2002). Beyond rough and tumble: Low-income fathers' interactions and children's cognitive development at 24 months. *Parenting: Science and practice, 2*(2), 77–104.

Shapiro, B. K., Palmer, F. B., Antell, S. E., Bilker, S., Ross, A., & Capute, A. J. (1989). Giftedness: Can it be predicted in infancy? *Clinical Pediatrics, 28,* 205–209.

Sigman, M., Neumann, C., Carter, E., Cattle, D. J., D'Souza, N., & Bwibo, N. (1988). Home interactions and the development of Embu toddlers in Kenya. *Child Development, 59,* 1251–1261.

Tasbihsazan, R., Nettelbeck, T., & Kirby, N. (1997). Increasing mental development index in Australian children: A comparative study of two versions of the Bayley Mental Scale. *Australian Psychologist, 32,* 120–125.

Thompson, B., Wasserman, J. D., & Matula, K. (1996). The factor structure of the Behavioral Rating Scale of the Bayley Scales of Infant Development-II. *Educational and Psychological Measurement, 56,* 460–474.

Walkowiak, J., Wiener, J.-A., Fastabend, A., Heinzow, B., Kramer, U., Schmidt, E., Steingruber, H. J., Wundram, S., & Winneke, G. (2001). Environmental exposure to polychlorinated biphenyls and quality of the home environment: Effects on psychodevelopment in early childhood. *Lancet, 358,* 1602–1607.

Washington, K., Scott, D. T., & Wendel, S. (1998). The Bayley Scales of Infant Development-II and children with developmental delays: A clinical perspective. *Developmental and Behavioral Pediatrics, 19*(5), 346–349.

Yarrow, L. J., Morgan, G. A., Jennings, K. D., Harmon, R., & Gaiter, J. (1982). Infants' persistence at tasks: Relationship to cognitive functioning and early experience. *Infant Behavior and Development, 5,* 131–141.

PURPOSE

The Cognitive Assessment System (CAS) is designed to assess cognitive processes in children and adolescents.

SOURCE

The CAS (Naglieri & Das, 1997) can be ordered from Riverside Publishing Company, 425 Spring Lake Drive, Itasca, IL 60143-2079 (1-800-323-9540; fax: 630-467-7192; http://www.riverpub.com). The complete test kit price is $629 US. Computer scoring (CAS Rapid Score) is $165 US. There is also a Dutch translation of the test (Kroesbergen et al., 2003).

AGE RANGE

The test is designed for ages 5 years to 17 years, 11 months.

DESCRIPTION

Theoretical Underpinnings

The CAS is based on the PASS theory of cognitive processing, which posits that cognition depends on four interrelated functions (i.e., Planning, Attention, Simultaneous, and Successive) that interact with the individual's knowledge base and skills (Das et al., 1994; see Figure 6–2). Like other nontraditional IQ tests such as the WJ III and the Kaufman tests (e.g., K-ABC, KAI), its theoretical underpinnings include cognitive psychology and factor analysis (Naglieri, 1996). The CAS is based on the theory that PASS processes are the essential elements of human cognition (Naglieri & Das, 1997). This differs from traditional IQ tests such as the Wechsler scales and the Stanford-Binet, which posit a general ability score ("*g*") and whose content derives from clinical applications rather

Figure 6–2 Model of PASS processes. *Source:* Reprinted with permission from Naglieri, 1999a.

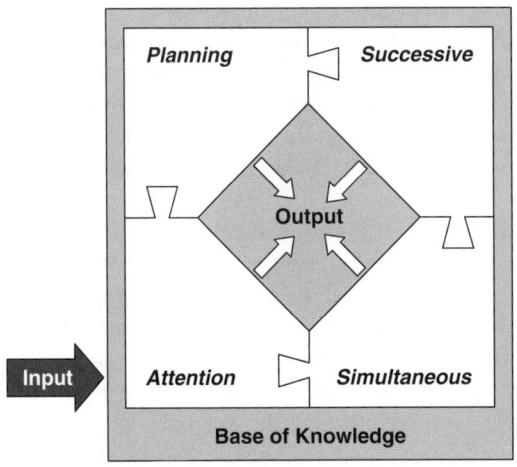

than specific models of intelligence (note that the newest versions of these instruments are also based, to some extent, on factor-analytic theories of intelligence). The CAS model assumes that the term "cognitive processes" should replace the term "intelligence" and that a test of cognitive processing should rely as little as possible on acquired knowledge such as vocabulary or arithmetic. The CAS is conceived by its author to be a technological improvement over its more traditional predecessors (Naglieri, 1999a).

The CAS consists of four main scales assessing each of the four PASS processes. Table 6–18 shows the functions measured by each scale. Briefly, the CAS Planning subtest measures self-control, self-monitoring, and plan development; the Attention subtest measures the various attentional processes as well as inhibition (e.g., sustained, focused, selective attention, resistance to distraction). Simultaneous subtests measure the ability to integrate information into a whole (e.g., integration of words into ideas), and Successive subtests measure the ability to integrate information into a specific progression involving strong serial or syntactic components (e.g., the linking of separate sounds into speech).

According to the test authors, the four PASS processes correspond to Luria's three functional units, which Luria associated with specific brain systems. Attention is posited to reflect Luria's first functional unit (brainstem, diencephalon, medial regions). Simultaneous and Successive processes reflect the second functional unit (occipital, parietal, and temporal lobes posterior to the central sulcus), and Planning reflects the third functional unit (frontal lobes, particularly prefrontal cortex). Like Luria's model, the four PASS processes are thought to be interrelated, not independent. Although more than one PASS process might be involved in each CAS subtest, the PASS scale to which each subtest belongs reflects the PASS process with the most influence on subtest performance (Naglieri, 1999a).

The CAS is of particular interest to neuropsychologists because it is based on Lurian theory and contains several subtests that approximate well-known neuropsychological testing paradigms such as the Trail Making Test and Stroop. In addition, it contains scales of potential use in the neuropsychological assessment of children (i.e., Planning and Attention) and a method for tracking strategy use during test administration that may be of utility in assessing executive functions (i.e., Strategy Assessment; see Figure 6–3).

Uses

According to the authors, the CAS allows examiners to determine (a) intraindividual strengths and weaknesses, (b) competence relative to peers, and (c) the relationship between cognitive functioning and achievement. This means that the CAS, like other intelligence tests, is intended to be used for diagnosis (i.e., learning disability, mental retardation,

Table 6–18 Descriptive Characteristics of PASS Processes

Planning Scale	Simultaneous Scale
Generation of strategies	Integration of words into ideas
Execution of plans	Seeing parts as a whole or group
Anticipation of consequences	Seeing several things at one time
Impulse control	Comprehension of word relationships
Organization of action	Understanding of inflection
Planful responses to new situations	Understanding verbal relationships and concepts
Self-control	Working with spatial information
Self-evaluation	
Self-monitoring	
Strategy use	
Use of feedback	

Attention Scale	Successive Scale
Directed concentration	Articulation of separate sounds into a consecutive series
Focus on essential details	Comprehension when word order drives meaning
Focus on important information	Execution of movements in order
Resistance to distraction	Perception of stimuli in sequence
Selective attention	Serial organization of spoken speech
Sustained attention over time	Working with sounds in a specific order
Sustained effort	

Source: Adapted from Naglieri & Das, 1997.

Figure 6–3 Example protocol for a CAS Planning subtest (i.e., Planned Codes). *Source:* Reprinted with permission from Naglieri, 1999a.

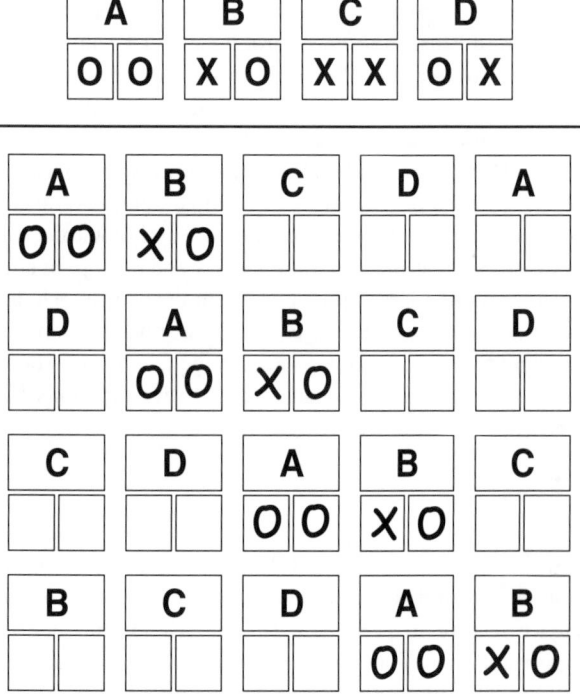

giftedness) and eligibility for services (e.g., state- or province-mandated special education criteria). However, because it is purported by its authors to be broader in scope than other more traditional IQ tests, the CAS is intended to be sensitive to conditions that typically elude other intelligence tests. These include ADHD, learning disability, traumatic brain injury, and giftedness (Gutentag et al., 1998; Naglieri, 1999a, 2001; Naglieri & Das, 1997; Naglieri & Edwards, 2004; Naglieri et al., 2003).

The way in which particular diagnoses are detected also differs. For example, in the traditional model, IQ tests are presumed to be insensitive to learning disability. Consequently, a discrepancy between IQ and achievement is required for diagnosis in most cases. This differs from the CAS, which is presumed to detect specific scale weaknesses in learning disabled children. A discrepancy/consistency analysis is therefore required, presuming both discrepancies and similarities between the CAS and the achievement measure used in diagnosis (Naglieri, 1999a; Naglieri & Edwards, 2004).

Unlike other intelligence tests, the CAS is also designed for use in planning specific interventions. To this end, it can be used in conjunction with a related training program, the PASS Remedial Program. Interested readers can consult the interpretive manual as well as the following publications for more information on this program: Das et al. (1994, 1995, 1997). This approach includes specific programs for training "planful" approaches to completing schoolwork, which may be of

Table 6–19 CAS Subtests by PASS Domain

PASS Domain	Standard Battery
Planning	*Matching Numbers*
	Planned Codes
	Planned Connections
Simultaneous	*Nonverbal Matrices*
	Verbal-Spatial Relations
	Figure Memory
Attention	*Expressive Attention*
	Number Detection
	Receptive Attention
Successive	*Word Series*
	Sentence Repetition
	Speech Rate
	Sentence Questions

Note: Subtests included in the Basic Battery are shown in italics; all subtests are included in the Standard Battery.

particular interest to neuropsychologists involved in rehabilitation of children with attention or executive deficits. Examples of interventions that can be used to facilitate learning for children with specific PASS weaknesses are also outlined in Naglieri (1999b).

Test Structure

The CAS has two forms: the Standard Battery, and a shorter version, the Basic Battery. The Standard Battery includes three subtests for each of the four PASS domains, for a total of 12 subtests. The Basic Battery involves two subtests per domain, for a total of eight subtests. See Table 6–19 for a summary of the subtests in the Standard and Basic Batteries (Basic Battery subtests are shown in italics). A detailed description of each subtest is provided in Table 6–20.

The CAS is organized into three levels: the Full-Scale score, the four separate PASS scales, and the 12 separate subtests making up the PASS scales. However, it is not intended to have a hierarchical structure (Naglieri, 1999b). PASS scales are derived from multiple subtests that are each thought to measure that particular PASS process. When these are combined, the result is a PASS scale with higher reliability than the individual subtests themselves. In other words, the different subtests of the Attention scale were not designed to measure different components of attention, but rather were chosen because they were presumed to be good measures of the broader construct of attention. Interpretation is therefore at the PASS scale level. Naglieri (1999a) recommends that subtest-level interpretation occur only if there is a specific reason to do so (e.g., inconsistent strategy use associated with variable Planning subtests). The authors note that the CAS Full-Scale score, which is a composite score based on the four PASS scales, is only provided for convenience to allow designations consistent with state regulations for special education, not because it is based on a hierarchical model of intelligence.

ADMINISTRATION TIME

The Basic Battery takes about 40 minutes; the Standard Battery takes about 60 minutes.

ADMINISTRATION

Materials

The CAS comes in an easily portable carrying case. It contains fewer materials than other intelligence batteries for children, which is an advantage when portability is an issue. Test materials are well designed. The manual is split-back, which allows it to stand independently to facilitate test administration, similar to the Wechsler scales manuals. The test also includes a tabbed, spiral-bound stimulus book. Scoring templates are bound separately in a tabbed, spiral-bound booklet, which makes them easy to use and less likely to get damaged or lost (note that there are 19 different scoring templates in all). A separate Interpretive Handbook provides information on test development, standardization, psychometric properties, and interpretation. Test protocols are well designed and easy to use. There are three Response Books (one for each age group and a separate booklet for responses to the Figure Memory subtest). There is also a Record Form for use by the examiner for entering scores and recording responses, including a space to record strategy use during Planning subtests (i.e., the Strategy Assessment Checklist). Two red pencils are also included for use in some of the paper-and-pencil subtests.

General Administration

See manual and Naglieri (1999a) for additional administration guidelines. Items are administered according to two age classifications (5–7 years and 8–17 years). With few exceptions, this simply means using different start-points for different ages. Each subtest is administered until the time limit runs out or the discontinue criterion is met (i.e., four consecutive failed responses).

Unlike other tests that require strict adherence to instructions, the CAS allows the examiner to provide a brief explanation if the child does not understand what is required after standard sample items and demonstration. The additional instructions can include gestures or verbal explanations in any language.

Strategy Assessment

In addition to providing subtest scores, the Planning subtests allow the examiner to conduct a Strategy Assessment. This allows the examiner to record the strategy used by the child and to determine whether it was similar to that used by the standardization sample. Strategies are recorded in two ways. The "Observed Strategies" are recorded by the examiner during the test, and "Reported Strategies" are

Table 6–20 Description of CAS Subtests

Planning

Matching Numbers
This is similar to a paper-and-pencil cancellation task. The child is instructed to find two matching numbers among a line of numbers, under time constraints. Although this subtest is purported to measure Planning, it does require that the child employ visual scanning, visual attention, and processing speed. The total score is a ratio of number correct and time.

Planned Codes
The child must fill in codes (Xs or Os) that correspond to letters presented at the top of the page, under time constraints. The basic paradigm is similar to the Wechsler Digit Symbol and Coding tasks, but uses a less involved motor response (X or O only), is more complex (requires a code pair instead of a single symbol), and does not require that items be completed in a prescribed order. Instead, the child is explicitly told to "do it any way you want," which is presumed to elicit strategy use that would maximize the number of items completed before the time limit. The total score is a ratio of number correct and time.

Planned Connections
This subtest follows the basic Trail Making Test paradigm. Numbers are initially presented on a page in random array. The child is instructed to connect the numbers as quickly as possible, under time constraints. Longer number series are presented until ceiling is reached. As in Trails, the child is corrected when an error is made. For younger children (5–7 years), this is the extent of the test. Older children are given two additional items that require switching between number and letters (similar to part B of the Trail Making Test). The total score is the sum of the time taken (one score reflects both serial order and switching items).

Attention

Expressive Attention
This is a Stroop task analog. For ages 5 to 7, the interference paradigm involves naming the size of pictured animals according to two features: relative size of the animal on the page or absolute size of the animal itself in real life. The interference trial shows conflict between the relative and absolute size (e.g., small picture of a dinosaur, big picture of a butterfly). Items are presented in rows, so that the child can "read" across the page. For older children (8–17 years), the subtest closely follows the Stroop paradigm (i.e., word reading, color reading, color-word interference trial). The subtest score is a ratio score of time and accuracy for the interference trial only.

Number Detection
This is a classic cancellation task. The child is shown specified targets (three to six numbers, depending on age), and then must cross out these targets among an array of numbers, working row by row from left to right under time constraints. Older children are also presented targets in two different fonts to make the task more difficult. The total score is the number of hits (corrected for errors of commission), which is then transformed to a ratio score involving time taken. Errors of commission and hits cannot be scored separately.

Receptive Attention
This is another paper-and-pencil task that requires the child to underline pairs of like objects or letters, working row by row from left to right under time constraints. Targets are those pairs that "have the same name" (i.e., may differ on appearance, but are from the same category, such as two kinds of trees, or upper- and lowercase letters). A ratio score of time and hits (corrected for errors of commission) is then computed; hits and errors of commission cannot be scored separately.

Simultaneous

Nonverbal Matrices
This is a classic nonverbal pattern-matching task similar to Raven's Progressive Matrices. The total score is the number correct.

Visual-Spatial Relations
This is a multiple-choice receptive language test that requires the examinee to pick out a specific picture corresponding to a sentence read aloud by the examiner. Sentences get increasingly grammatically and syntactically complex.

Figure Memory
The child is instructed to remember a geometric figure presented for 5 seconds; the figure must then be identified and traced from memory within a larger, more complicated geometric figure presented in the record book. Given the task requirements, this subtest likely involves aspects of visual-spatial pattern matching and visual memory.

Successive

Word Series
The child must repeat words in series of increasing length, to a maximum of nine words (e.g., "Cat—Boy—Book"). The words are all of equal difficulty and not linked semantically or logically. Given these task requirements, this subtest appears to measure aspects of verbal memory span.

Sentence Repetition
Unlike other sentence repetition subtests from other children's batteries (e.g., WPPSI-R, NEPSY, WRAML), this involves novel sentences that cannot be easily recalled based on prior knowledge or on filling in missing words based on logic. All sentences are constructed of color words only (e.g., "The white greened the yellow").

(continued)

Table 6–20 Description of CAS Subtests (*continued*)

Speech Rate	Administered only to 5 to 7-year-olds, this subtest involves the rapid repetition of short word series under time constraints. The child is instructed to repeat a word sequence 10 times (e.g., "wall, car, girl"), with a time limit of 30 seconds. Errors are alterations in the word sequence, but not mispronunciations, distortions, or other articulation difficulties. If the child has not completed 10 correct sequences in the 30-second time limit, he or she is given a time of 31 for that item. The total score is the time taken, summed across items. This subtest requires oralmotor speed as well as verbal memory span.
Sentence Questions	Administered only to 8 to 17-year-olds, this subtest involves the auditory comprehension of novel spoken sentences (e.g., "The green is yellowing. Who is yellowing?"). As such, it requires an understanding of grammar and semantic relationships independent of vocabulary level, and would be an interesting measure of auditory comprehension when vocabulary skills are suspected to be weak.

Adapted from Naglieri & Das, 1997.

queried by the examiner using prompts (e.g., "Tell me how you did these"). During each of the Planning subtests, the examiner may complete the Strategy Assessment Checklist, which allows a quantification of strategy use. See Figure 6–4 for an example.

In theory, the examiner is instructed to observe and record strategy use during the test. In practice, this is sometimes difficult to do, given the nature of the task and the speed with which it is executed (e.g., cancellation-type tasks such as *Matching Numbers*). Practically speaking, although this should be possible for all Planning subtests, only Planned Codes allows the examiner to objectively record strategy use without depending to some extent on self-report (Haddad, 2004).

SCORING

Scores

See manual, as well as additional scoring guidelines provided in Naglieri (1999a). Raw subtest scores are converted to scaled scores ($M = 10$, $SD = 3$), which are then summed to derive PASS domain standard scores and the Full-Scale standard score. The four PASS scales are equally weighted to form the Full-Scale score, as are each group of three subtests making up each PASS scale score. Percentile ranks and confidence intervals (90% and 95%) are provided in the manual for both the Standard and Basic Battery. Tables in the manual also provide confidence intervals based on the estimated true score. Age equivalents are also provided, as are cumulative percentages

of differences between PASS scores and Full-Scale score, and differences between subtest scaled scores required for statistical significance. Several tables are also provided to compare CAS scores to predicted WJ-R scores. These may be of limited utility now that a newer version of the WJ has been published (WJ III).

Strategy Use

Strategy use is coded on the response forms according to a checklist (see Figure 6–5). Higher scores reflect better strategy use. However, the manual provides limited information on how to score observed strategies and does not provide information on the relative accuracy of observed versus reported strategy use for different ages.

Figure 6–5 Sample CAS Strategy Assessment Checklist. *Source:* Reprinted with permission from Naglieri, 1999a.

Strategy Assessment Checklist

Obs	Rep	Description of Strategy
		1. Looked at first then last digits
		2. Looked at first then last digit
		3. Looked at first two digits
✔	✔	4. Looked at the last number
		5. Looked at the first digit
		6. Put finger on the number
✔		7. Verbalized the number
		8. Scanned the row for a match
		9. No strategy

Other:
Observed _____

_____

Reported _____

_____

Figure 6–4 Example protocol for a CAS Attention subtest (i.e., Number Detection). *Source:* Reprinted with permission from Naglieri, 1999a.

Find the numbers that look like this: **1 2** 4 5

4	2	6	4	2	1	3	2	5
2	3	2	4	1	2	5	5	3
1	6	2	5	6	3	4	2	4

Repeat Testing

The manual allows standard score comparisons for use with repeat testing (i.e., the score range expected, given a specific baseline score). The ranges are based on a method that accounts for regression to the mean and internal reliability. Specifics are outlined in Anderson (1991, as cited in Naglieri & Das, 1997). Tables in the manual can be used to determine whether a change in CAS performance pre- and postintervention is statistically significant. These scores are based on calculation of the standard error of prediction (SE_p; see Chapter 1), and are not based on test-retest data per se.

DEMOGRAPHIC EFFECTS

Age

The CAS's sensitivity to age-related changes is supported by raw score increases with increasing age for all subtests, as shown in the manual (p. 51, Naglieri & Das, 1997). Age-related changes in the percentage of children using strategies on the Planning subtests are also shown in the manual (p. 82, Naglieri & Das, 1997). However, the authors note that not all strategies are of equivalent utility across age (e.g., saying codes aloud might be effective in the younger age group, but not in older children). Further, while only 25% of younger children use strategies on the CAS, almost all adolescents do so (e.g., Planned Connections). In terms of predictive validity, the amount of variance in achievement accounted for by the CAS increases with age (Naglieri & Rojahn, 2004).

Gender

Gender differences have been found on PASS scales, with girls obtaining slightly higher scores than boys on Planning and Attention subtests.

Ethnicity

The CAS is purported to be less culturally biased than other traditional IQ tests due to its lack of heavily language- or achievement-based subtests and its flexible instructions. During construction of the CAS, detailed bias analysis was conducted, including differential item functioning analysis to determine whether any subgroups performed differently on certain items of the test. In addition, the test was evaluated for predictive bias (i.e., whether the relationship of the test to a criterion measure—in this case, achievement—would differ by subgroup). There were no significant differences across groups defined by gender, race, or Hispanic status with regard to regression slopes predicting WJ-R performance (Naglieri & Das, 1997).

In a comparison of the CAS and WISC-III in a group of children in special education placement, the WISC-III identified disproportionately more African American children as having mental retardation, consistent with criticisms that the use of the WISC-III is partly responsible for the overrepresentation of African American children in special education programs (Naglieri & Rojahn, 2001). Compared with Caucasian children, African American children had lower scores on the "achievement-loaded" WISC-III Verbal scales (Naglieri & Rojahn, 2001, p. 365). In contrast, African American children had higher scores on the Planning and Attention scales of the CAS. Importantly, use of the CAS would have led to a 30% decrease in the identification of children with mental retardation within this group, which has significant implications for using this measure in diagnosis in minority groups. Based on these and other results, Naglieri (2001) notes that minority children are more likely to be fairly evaluated using the CAS than with other intelligence tests that rely more on English language or academic skills.

NORMATIVE DATA

Standardization Sample

The standardization sample consists of 2200 children stratified according to age, gender, race, Hispanic origin, region, community setting, and parental education level based on 1990 U.S. Census data. See Table 6–21 for sample characteristics. To allow ability-achievement comparisons, 1600 children were administered the CAS and the WJ-R, with sampling again closely matching the 1990 U.S. Census. An additional 872 children were recruited for validity/reliability studies.

Derivation of Scaled and Standard Scores

To construct norms for the CAS, cumulative frequency distributions from the raw score distributions from each 1-year age interval from the standardization sample were normalized to produce scaled scores. Scaled score progression both within and across age bands were examined, and smoothing was used to correct for any irregularities (Naglieri & Das, 1997).

RELIABILITY

Internal Reliability

CAS Full-Scale reliability coefficients provided in the manual are high, ranging from .95 to .97 across age. Reliabilities for the PASS scales are also high (i.e., with average reliabilities of $r = .88$ for Planning, .88 for Attention, .93 for Simultaneous, and .93 for Successive). Additionally, reliability coefficients were adequate to high for all CAS subtests, averaged across age (see Table 6–22). Of note, internal reliability estimates are based on split-half reliability (Spearman-Brown; Simultaneous and Successive subtests except Speech Rate), test-retest reliability (timed tests such as Planning and Attention subtests, and Speech Rate), or on a formula for estimating the reliability of linear combinations (composite scores). Reliability information on the Strategy Assessment is lacking.

Table 6–21 Normative Sample Characteristics for the CAS

Number	2200[a]
Age	5 to 17 years, 11 months
Geographic location	
Midwest	25%
Northeast	19%
South	34%
West	23%
Sample type	National, stratified, random sample[b]
Parental education	
Less than high school	20%
High school	29%
Some college	29%
Four or more years of college	23%
Community setting	
Urban	75%
Rural	25%
Gender	
Males	50%
Females	50%
Race	
Black	14%
White	77%
Other	10%
Hispanic origin	
Hispanic	11%
Non-Hispanic	89%
Screening	None indicated; sample includes special populations such as learning disabled (5%), speech/language impaired (1%), seriously emotionally disturbed (0.8%), mentally retarded (1%), and gifted (4%) children

[a]Based on nine age groupings representing one-year intervals for age 5 to 10 years, 11 months, two-year intervals for age 11 to 14 years, 11 months, and three-year interval for age 15 to 17 years, 11 months; 100 to 150 cases are represented in each age band.
[b]Based on 1990 U.S. Census data and collected between 1993 and 1996.

Source: Adapted from Naglieri & Das, 1997.

Standard Error of Measurement

Average *SEM*s across age for the Full Scale and four composites are within acceptable limits (i.e., 5.4 for the Full Scale and between 4.8 and 6.2 for the four composites). Average subtest *SEM*s across age range from 1.0 to 1.5 (Naglieri & Das, 1997).

Test-Retest Reliability

Test-retest stability was assessed in 215 children tested twice over a median interval of 21 days (Naglieri & Das, 1997). For the standard battery, PASS scales demonstrated adequate to high reliability ($r = .77$ to .86 for individual PASS scales, and .89 for the Full-Scale score). At the subtest level, most CAS subtests showed adequate to high test-retest stability (Table 6–23). Verbal-Spatial Relations showed marginal stability in every age range assessed, as did Figure Memory in the two younger age groups. There is no information on the stability of the Strategy Assessment in the manual.

Practice Effects

The test-retest scores differed by approximately four standard score points on the Planning and Successive scales, by five points on the Simultaneous scale, and by six points on the Attention scale and Full-Scale score (Naglieri & Das, 1997). This suggests a small practice effect on the Standard Battery, based on data presented in the manual for test-retest stability. For the Basic Battery, these values were three, two, four, and five points, respectively.

VALIDITY

Content

As noted in *Description*, the test is based on a detailed theoretical foundation. Significant effort also went into the creation of the CAS subtests, including item selection, data analysis,

Table 6–22 Internal Reliability Coefficients for CAS Subtests, Averaged Across Age

Magnitude of Coefficient	Subtest
Very high (.90+)	—
High (.80–.89)	Planned Codes
	Nonverbal Matrices
	Verbal-Spatial Relations
	Figure Memory
	Expressive Attention
	Word Series
	Sentence Repetition
	Speech Rate
	Sentence Questions
Adequate (.70–.79)	Matching Numbers
	Planned Comparisons
	Number Detection
	Receptive Attention
Marginal (.60–.69)	—
Low (<.59)	—

Source: Adapted from Naglieri and Das, 1997.

test revision, pilot testing, national tryout, and standardization (Naglieri, 1999a). See also *Demographic Effects, Ethnicity* for information on bias analyses conducted in the development of the test.

Subtest Intercorrelations

As reported in the *Interpretive Manual*, subtest intercorrelations within each PASS scale are high in the standardization sample (Naglieri & Das, 1997). For instance, on average, subtests for the Simultaneous domain are moderately to highly intercorrelated ($r = .45–.53$), as are the Successive subtests ($r = .48–.65$). Planning and Attention also have moderate to high subtest intercorrelations within each scale ($r = .39–57$, Planning; $r = .39–.44$, Attention), but also appear to be related to subtests from other scales. In fact, in some cases, correlations between Attention and Planning subtests were higher than those within each scale (e.g., $r = .51$, Matching Numbers and Receptive Attention; $r = .50$, Planned Connections and Expressive Attention). This is not entirely surprising, given the similarities between some of the subtests between these two domains and the interrelated nature of planning/executive and attention skills in the real world. This is also supported by some factor-analytic studies (see later discussion).

Factor Structure and Scale Specificity

Factor-analytic studies provided in the manual support the four-factor PASS model, along with a three-factor solution that combines the Planning and Attention scales. The authors report that their decision to retain the four-factor model rather than the three-factor solution was based on clinical, empirical, and theoretical grounds. Other authors have reported

Table 6–23 Test-Retest Stability Coefficients for CAS Subtests Across Age Groups

Magnitude of Coefficient	Ages 5–7	Ages 8–11	Ages 12–17
Very high (.90+)	—	—	—
High (.80–.89)	Planned Codes	Planned Codes	Planned Codes
	Sentence Repetition	Planned Connections	Sentence Repetition
		Nonverbal Matrices	
		Sentence Questions	
Adequate (.70–.79)	Matching Numbers	Expressive Attention	Matching Numbers
	Planned Connections	Number Detection	Planned Connections
	Nonverbal Matrices	Word Series	Nonverbal Matrices
	Number Detection	Sentence Repetition	Figure Memory
	Receptive Attention		Expressive Attention
	Word Series		Number Detection
	Speech Rate		Receptive Attention
			Word Series
			Sentence Questions
Marginal (.60–.69)	Verbal-Spatial Relations	Matching Numbers	Verbal-Spatial Relations
	Figure Memory	Verbal-Spatial Relations	
	Expressive Attention	Figure Memory	
		Receptive Attention	
Low (≤ .59)	—	—	—

Note: Correlations were corrected for restriction in range.

Source: Adapted from Naglieri and Das, 1997.

different findings. In a confirmatory factor analysis of the standardization data, Kranzler and Keith (1999) and Keith et al. (2001) found only marginal fit for the four-factor model, and Planning and Attention were virtually indistinguishable in the factor solution. The best fit was a hierarchical solution with four first-order factors corresponding to the PASS processes, a second-order Attention-Planning factor, and a large third-order "g" factor. Kranzler and Keith (1999) also found better fit statistics for other ability tests such as the WISC-III and WJ-R. Overall, the CAS was felt to lack structural fidelity (i.e., correspondence between theory and test structure), a necessary but not sufficient condition for construct validity (Keith & Kranzler, 1999). Naglieri (1999a) countered that these authors overinterpreted a minor difference in factor-analytic results, overemphasized the role of factor analysis in determining the structure of human abilities, and undervalued the need to measure validity in a broad manner. Interestingly, although Naglieri (1999a) asserts that the CAS does not have a hierarchical structure, which Keith et al. dispute on the basis of factor analysis, Luria's theory was hierarchical in nature. Primary, secondary, and tertiary zones were found within each functional unit, and the tertiary zones of the frontal lobes were considered a "superstructure" above all other parts of the cortex (Luria, 1973, p. 89).

Keith et al. also conducted a joint confirmatory factor analysis of the CAS and WJ III (Keith et al., 2001; Kranzler et al., 2000), which led them to conclude that PASS scales actually measure other abilities than those specified by Naglieri—namely, processing speed for Attention and Planning, verbal memory span for the Successive scale, and fluid intelligence and broad visualization for the Successive scale. Note that Haddad (2004) concluded that one of the Planning subtests (Planned Codes) was not a simple speed measure; over 50% of children performed better on Planned Codes when they were not told to complete the test items in sequential (i.e., nonstrategic) order.

Keith et al. (2001) concluded that only the Successive scale measured g, and that it was the only scale with enough unique variance to be interpreted separately from the rest of the test. They concluded that, contrary to the authors' claims, the CAS measures the same psychometric g as other tests of intelligence and that the PASS theory was likely an inadequate model of human cognitive abilities. In contrast, Naglieri (1999a) stressed that the CAS has ample validity based on predictive validity and relevance to treatment and that when specificity was calculated for the PASS scales, all four scales were found to have sufficient unique variance to be interpreted on their own.

Correlations With Other Neuropsychological Tests

CAS subtests have moderate criterion validity when compared with other neuropsychological tests. In a small sample of children with TBI described in the manual ($N = 22$), the Planning scale was related to Trail Making A ($r = -.40$) but not Trail Making B, or to the Tower of London, a test measuring planning, in-

hibition, and working memory. The implication is that the Planning scale is more a measure of speed than of planning (see later discussion). The authors explain the latter finding by stating that the Tower test has a stronger successive than planning aspect, consistent with the sequential nature of the task (Das & Naglieri, 1997). In this same group, the Simultaneous scale was related to the Token Test and Embedded Figures ($r = .45$ and .39, respectively). The Attention scale was related to Trail Making A and Stroop, and the Successive scale was related to Trail Making A, the Tower of London, and the Sentence Repetition Test. In another study, Simultaneous and Successive scales were related to facial recognition (Kroeger et al., 2001).

Correlations With IQ

Based on data presented in the manual, correlations between CAS and Wechsler IQ tests are for the most part high, particularly between the CAS Full-Scale score and FSIQ scores from Wechsler scales ($r = .66–.71$, WISC-III; $r = .60$, WPPSI-R). Of the four PASS scales, Simultaneous and Successive appear to measure an aspect of cognitive ability most related to the traditional notion of FSIQ, with average correlations between WISC-III FSIQ and Simultaneous/Successive scales in the moderate to high range (i.e., $.36–.64$, with most $\geq .59$). In contrast, correlations between WISC-III FSIQ and Planning/Attention domains are moderate (i.e., $.30–.48$). Similar effects occur with the WPPSI-R, with high correlations between WPPSI-R FSIQ and CAS Simultaneous/Successive scores ($r = .73$ and .67, respectively) but only modest correlations between WPPSI-R FSIQ and CAS Planning/Attention ($r = .12$ and .22; Naglieri & Das, 1997).

At the PASS or factor index level, Planning correlates most highly with WISC-III Processing Speed ($r = .70$), PIQ ($r = .53$), and Perceptual Organization ($r = .45$, in a small sample of regular education students described in the manual; $N = 54$). The Simultaneous scale correlates moderately to highly with all the WISC-III factor scores ($r = .35–.69$). Successive processing also appears to correlate strongly with all WISC-III index scores ($r = .58–.64$), except Processing Speed, where the correlation fails to reach significance ($r = .32$). CAS Attention correlates most highly with Processing Speed ($r = .54$) and PIQ ($r = .35$). These results seem to support the view of a substantial processing speed component to the CAS Planning and Attention scales (but see Haddad, 2004).

In comparisons using the WPPSI-R in a small sample of 5- to 7-year-olds ($N = 33$; see manual), Simultaneous processing was most related to PIQ ($r = .76$) and FSIQ ($r = .73$), but the correlation with VIQ was also substantial ($r = .53$). Successive processing was related to both VIQ ($r = .57$) and PIQ ($r = .52$). Neither Attention nor Planning was related to any WPPSI-R indices, as would be expected based on the theories underlying the CAS.

When children are administered the CAS and other tests of intelligence, there are slight Full-Score differences (see test manual). In general, CAS scores are higher. For instance, there is a one-point difference between CAS and WISC-III Full-Scale scores in normal children ($N = 54$), a two-point difference in children with learning disabilities ($N = 81$), and a five-point difference in children with mental handicap ($N = 84$; CAS = 65.9, WISC-III = 60.7). The CAS Full-Scale score was seven points higher in younger children administered the WPPSI-R ($N = 33$). In a separate study, children in special education placements obtained Full-Scale CAS scores that were approximately six points higher than WISC-III Full-Scale scores (Naglieri & Rojahn, 2001). Score differences using the WISC-IV and WPPSI-III are likely to be smaller, given the more recent standardization samples for these measures.

Correlations With Achievement

Like all IQ tests, the CAS is moderately to highly related to achievement. In fact, in a recent review, Naglieri and Bornstein (2003) noted that CAS correlations with achievement were some of the highest of all the intelligence batteries, along with the K-ABC and WJ III (i.e., $r = .70–.74$). CAS associations with achievement are reviewed in the *Interpretive Manual* and in Naglieri and Edwards (2004).

Unlike other IQ tests that are minimally sensitive to learning difficulties (hence the need for ability-achievement discrepancy analyses), specific patterns of CAS performance across PASS subtests are claimed to be related to certain kinds of academic difficulties. Specific profile differences on the CAS are also reported for different subgroups of children with academic difficulties. For instance, children with reading difficulties have lower Successive scores than children in regular education and children with ADHD, and lower Simultaneous scores than children in regular education (Naglieri & Edwards, 2004). The manual also indicates that PASS scales are associated with specific weaknesses on the WJ-R (e.g., low Planning scores are associated with low Calculation, Dictation, and Basic Writing on the WJ-R). The CAS authors also compared the sensitivity of the CAS to that of the WISC-III in detecting learning disability using the WJ-R. Both scales were moderately correlated with the Skills cluster of the WJ-R in regular students. The authors note that this occurred despite the fact that the CAS contains no items relating to achievement (i.e., learned information such as Vocabulary, Information, and Arithmetic), as does the WISC-III.

Clinical Studies

The manual provides CAS data on several clinical groups as evidence of further construct validity (Naglieri & Das, 1997). Children with ADHD ($N = 66$) were found to have relative weaknesses on the Planning and Attention scales ($M = 88.4$, $SD = .10.0$; and $M = 92.1$, $SD = .11.9$, respectively), which the authors argued was consistent with the conceptualization of ADHD as a disorder of inhibition processes. In a subsequent study, lower Planning scores were also found for ADHD children compared with both normal children and children with anxiety/depression (Naglieri et al., 2003). The manual also indicates that children with reading disability identified using WISC-III/WJ-R discrepancies have relative weaknesses in the Successive scale ($N = 24$), which the authors interpreted as consistent with the view of reading disability as being related to phonological processing deficits. This has also been shown in a subsequent study, along with differences in Simultaneous scores (Naglieri & Edwards, 2004). The manual also reports that children with intellectual deficits ($N = 86$) had consistently depressed PASS scale scores consistent with presumed global deficits, whereas gifted children had Full-Scale scores that were, on average, one standard deviation above the mean, with slightly different elevations across domains (Das & Naglieri, 1997). In published studies, head-injured children have shown a relative weakness in Planning compared with non-head-injured children (Gutentag et al., 1998). Children with written expression disabilities also show specific CAS profiles (Johnson et al., 2003).

In the educational setting, children with low Planning scores benefit from intervention to increase planning skills, while untreated controls show no improvement in math computation (Naglieri & Johnson, 2000). In another study, children with a selective Planning weakness benefited from a cognitive strategy instruction program in increasing their posttest reading comprehension scores (Haddad et al., 2003). However, not all studies have found a positive association between CAS profiles and responsivity to intervention. Kroesbergen et al. (2003) found that an intervention to increase math skills did not differentially improve scores of children with mathematical learning difficulties, despite evidence that children with mathematically based learning difficulties could be grouped into three subgroups based on CAS performance.

Children with higher strategy use during Planning tasks appear to earn higher Planning scores than those who do not use strategies (Naglieri & Das, 1997). This serves as some evidence of the tests' construct validity. Planning subtests, which may tap creativity, may also be useful in the assessment of giftedness (Naglieri, 2001). There is also some indication that the CAS may have some utility in training environments and that its predictive validity may extend beyond achievement, based on research involving aviation simulations (Fein & Day, 2004). This may be because the CAS is more highly loaded with attention and executive tasks than most standard IQ tests.

COMMENT

From a test development perspective, the CAS appears to be a well-designed, psychometrically sound instrument with a large standardization sample and good reliability. The manual is well written, thorough, and comprehensive, and contains detailed information on the psychometric properties of the test that are sometimes not available in many test manuals (e.g., psychometrics of the short form or Basic Battery). The test is also based on modern theories of ability and on over 20 years of research and development by the test authors. Other features may make it more useable across populations and cultures (i.e., limited reliance on language- or achievement-type content, flexible instructions to facilitate comprehension, and evidence of lack of bias in minorities). It also includes interesting and novel subtests, including a number of executive and attention subtests, as well as subtests modeled after classic neuropsychological tests such as the Stroop and Trail Making Test. Although these deserve further study, the test is also associated with intervention programs based on CAS strengths and weaknesses. A small number of research studies have shown that PASS profiles may be used to determine responsivity to training in cognitive strategies to improve planning skills, which should be of considerable practical and clinical utility in making recommendations for individual children, as well as in designing interventions to improve executive skills.

On the other hand, there continue to be significant concerns about its factor structure and the meaning of the factors. Tables to enable CAS-achievement comparisons are also outdated because of the arrival of the WJ III. Some subtests demonstrate marginal test-retest reliabilities (see Table 6–23). The psychometric properties of the Strategy Assessment are mostly unknown; these scores should therefore not be used in diagnostic decision making. Users should also note that Planned Codes is the only Planning subtest where strategy can be objectively observed by the examiner rather than relied upon via verbal report (Haddad, 2004).

In addition, some of the features do not allow a process-based analysis of performance, despite the test's foundation in Lurian theories. For instance, there is no differentiation between accuracy (pass/fail) and speed (time) on several Planning and Attention subtests, and Attention subtests do not allow the differentiation of inattention (missed targets) from response inhibition (errors of commission). Although allowing this level of analysis was never a goal of the CAS, in the neuropsychological context, knowledge of the patient's ability on these separate processes is helpful in diagnosis and treatment planning. Granted, many other intelligence tests such as the Wechsler scales also use similar omnibus scores, and the reality is that parsing performance in this way sometimes leads to less-than-stellar reliabilities for some scores (e.g., see *CPT-II; D-KEFS*). However, because some CAS subtests model themselves after neuropsychological tests that commonly allow these distinctions (e.g., Stroop), the clinician must therefore find alternate means to assess these processes in detail. In this way, the CAS suffers somewhat from the difficulties inherent in translating Luria's methods to a clinically applied instrument (e.g., omnibus scores that reflect multiple neuropsychological processes are not consistent with Lurian principles), as have other instruments based on Lurian theory (e.g., Adams, 1980; Spiers, 1981). However, it is important to state that, overall, the CAS is a well-constructed, well-researched,

theory-based measure of intelligence with several features of particular interest to neuropsychologists.

REFERENCES

Adams, K. M. (1980). In search of Luria's battery: A false start. *Journal of Consulting and Clinical Psychology, 48*, 511–516.

Atkinson, L. (1991). Three standard errors of measurement and the Wechsler Memory Scale-Revised. *Psychological Assessment, 3*(1), 136–138.

Das, J. P., Carlson, J., Davidon, M. B., & Longe, K. (1997). *PREP: PASS remedial program.* Seattle, WA: Hogrefe.

Das, J. P., Mishra, R. K., & Pool, J. (1995). An experiment on cognitive remediation of word-reading difficulty. *Journal of Learning Disabilities, 28*, 66–79.

Das, J. P., Naglieri, J. A., & Kirby, J.R. (1994). *Assessment of cognitive processes: The PASS theory of intelligence.* Boston: Allyn & Bacon.

Fein, E. C., & Day, E. A. (2004). The PASS theory of intelligence and the acquisition of a complex skill: A criterion-related validation study of Cognitive Assessment System scores. *Personality and Individual Differences, 37*, 1123–1136.

Gutentag, S., Naglieri, J. A., & Yeates, K. O. (1998). Performance on children with traumatic brain injury on the Cognitive Assessment System. *Assessment, 5*, 263–272.

Haddad, F. A. (2004). Planning versus speed: An experimental examination of what planned codes of the Cognitive Assessment System measures. *Archives of Clinical Neuropsychology, 19*, 313–317.

Haddad, F. A., Garcia, Y. E., Naglieri, J. A., Grimditch, M., McAndrews, A., & Eubanks, J. (2003). Planning facilitation and reading comprehension: Instructional relevance and the PASS theory. *Journal of Psychoeducational Assessment, 21*, 282–289.

Johnson, J. A., Bardos, A. N., & Tayebi, K.A. (2003). Discriminant validity of the Cognitive Assessment System for students with written expression disabilities. *Journal of Psychoeducational Assessment, 21*, 180–195.

Keith, T. Z., & Kranzler, J. H. (1999). The absence of structural fidelity precludes construct validity: Rejoinder to Naglieri on what the Cognitive Assessment System does and does not measure. *School Psychology Review, 28*(2), 303–321.

Keith, T. Z., Kranzler, J. H., & Flanagan, D. P. (2001). What does the Cognitive Assessment System (CAS) measure? Joint confirmatory factor analysis of the CAS and the Woodcock-Johnson Tests of Cognitive Ability (3rd Edition). *School Psychology Review, 30*(1), 89–119.

Kranzler, J. H., & Keith, T. Z. (1999). Independent confirmatory factor analysis of the Cognitive Assessment System (CAS): What does the CAS measure? *School Psychology Review, 28*(1), 117–144.

Kranzler, J. H., Keith, T. Z., & Flanagan, D. P. (2000). Independent examination of the factor structure of the Cognitive Assessment System (CAS): Further evidence challenging the construct validity of the CAS. *Journal of Psychoeducational Assessment, 18*(2), 143–159.

Kroeger, T. L., Rojahn, J., & Naglieri, J. A. (2001). Role of planning, attention, and simultaneous and successive cognitive processing in facial recognition in adults with mental retardation. *American Journal on Mental Retardation, 106*(2), 151–161.

Kroesbergen, E. H., Van Luit, J. E. H., & Naglieri, J. A. (2003). Mathematical learning difficulties and PASS cognitive processes. *Journal of Learning Disabilities, 36*(6), 574–582.

Luria, A. R. (1973). *The working brain: An introduction to neuropsychology.* New York: Basic Books.

Naglieri, J. A. (1996). Cognitive assessment: Nontraditional intelligence tests. In T. Fagan & P. Warden (Eds.), *Encyclopedia of school psychology* (pp. 69–70). Westport, CT: Greenwood Press.

Naglieri, J. A. (1997). IQ: Knowns and unknowns, hits and misses. *American Psychologist, 52*(1), 75–76.

Naglieri, J. A. (1999a). *Essentials of CAS assessment.* New York: John Wiley & Sons.

Naglieri, J. A. (1999b). How valid is PASS theory and CAS? *School Psychology Review, 28*(1), 145–162.

Naglieri, J. A. (2001). Understanding intelligence, giftedness and creativity using the PASS theory. *Roeper Review, 23*(3), 151–157.

Naglieri, J. A., & Bornstein, B. T. (2003). Intelligence and achievement: Just how correlated are they? *Journal of Psychoeducational Assessment, 21*(3), 244–260.

Naglieri, J. A., & Das, J. P. (1997). *Cognitive Assessment System interpretive handbook.* Itasca, IL: Riverside Publishing.

Naglieri, J. A., & Edwards, G. H. (2004). Assessment of children with attention and reading difficulties using the PASS theory and Cognitive Assessment System. *Journal of Psychoeducational Assessment, 22*, 93–105.

Naglieri, J. A., Goldstein, S., Iseman, J. S., & Schwebach, A. (2003). Performance of children with attention deficit hyperactivity disorder and anxiety/depression on the WISC-III and Cognitive Assessment System (CAS). *Journal of Psychoeducational Assessment, 21*, 32–42.

Naglieri, J. A., & Gottling, S. H. (1997). Mathematics instruction and PASS cognitive processes: An intervention study. *Journal of Learning Disabilities, 30*(5), 513–520.

Naglieri, J. A., & Johnson, D. (2000). Effectiveness of a cognitive strategy intervention in improving arithmetic computation based on the PASS theory. *Journal of Learning Disabilities, 33*(6), 591–597.

Naglieri, J. A., & Rojahn, J. (2001). Gender differences in planning, attention, simultaneous and successive (PASS) cognitive processes and achievement. *Journal of Educational Psychology, 93*(2), 430–437.

Naglieri, J. A., & Rojahn, J. (2004). Construct validity of the PASS theory and CAS: Correlations with achievement. *Journal of Educational Psychology, 96*(1), 174–181.

Nunnally, J. C., & Bernstein, I. H. (1994). *Psychometric theory* (3rd ed.). New York: McGraw-Hill, Inc.

Spiers, P. A. (1981). Have they come to praise Luria or to bury him? The Luria-Nebraska neuropsychological battery controversy. *Journal of Consulting and Clinical Psychology, 49*, 331–341.

Dementia Rating Scale-2 (DRS-2)

PURPOSE

The purpose of this scale is to provide an index of cognitive function in people with known or suspected dementia.

SOURCE

The test (including Professional Manual, 50 scoring booklets and profile forms, and one set of stimulus cards) can be ordered from Psychological Assessment Resources, Inc., P.O. Box 998, Odessa, FL (www.parinc.com), at a cost of $229 US. An alternate form is also available.

AGE RANGE

The test is intended for individuals aged 55 years and older.

DESCRIPTION

Some patients, such as the elderly with profound cognitive impairments, may generate very few responses on such standard tests as the Wechsler Adult Intelligence Scale or the Wechsler Memory Scale, making it difficult to assess the magnitude of their mental impairments. The Dementia Rating Scale (DRS) was developed to quantify the mental status of such patients (Coblentz et al., 1973; Mattis, 1976, 1988). A new version, the Dementia Rating Scale-2 (DRS-2), has recently been published (Jurica et al., 2001). Although the manual has been updated, the scoring booklet improved, and new norms provided, the test is the same. In addition, an alternate form (DRS-2: Alternate Form), consisting of new item content, has been provided (Schmidt & Mattis, 2004).

The items on the test are similar to those employed by neurologists in bedside mental status examinations. They are arranged hierarchically, from difficult to easier items, so that adequate performance on an initial item allows the examiner to discontinue testing within that section and to assume that credit can be given for adequate performance on the subsequent tasks. A global measure of dementia severity is derived from subscales of specific cognitive capacities. The subscales include measures of attention (e.g., digit span, detecting 'As'), initiation and perseveration (e.g., performing alternating movements, copying repeated patterns, semantic fluency), construction (e.g., copying designs, writing name), conceptualization (e.g., similarities), and verbal and nonverbal short-term memory (e.g., sentence recall, design recognition; see Table 6–24).

ADMINISTRATION

See *Source.* Briefly, the examiner asks questions or gives instructions (e.g. "In what way are an apple and a banana alike?") and records responses. The DRS subtests are presented in a fixed order generally corresponding to the Attention (ATT), Initiation/Perseveration (I/P), Construction (CONST), Conceptualization (CONCEPT), and Memory (MEM) subscales; however, not all Attention tasks are presented in a sequence because some also serve as time-filling distracters between presentations of memory tasks.

Generally, if the first one or two tasks in a subscale are performed well, subsequent (easier) tasks are credited with a correct performance, and the examiner proceeds to the next subscale.

Table 6–24 Subscales and Subtests of the DRS-2

Subscale	Subtests	Maximum Points
Attention	Digit Span Two Successive Commands Single Command Imitation Counting Distraction 1 and 2 Verbal Recognition—Presentation Visual Matching	37
Initiation/Perseveration	Complex Verbal Initiation/Perseveration Consonant Perseveration Vowel Perseveration Double Alternating Movements Alternate Tapping Graphomotor Design	37
Construction	Construction Designs	6
Conceptualization	Identities and Oddities Similarities Priming Inductive Reasoning Differences Similarities-Multiple Choice	39
Memory and Attention	Orientation Verbal Recall—Reading Verbal Recall—Sentence Initiation Verbal Recognition Visual Recognition	25

ADMINISTRATION TIME

The time required is approximately 10 to 15 minutes for normal elderly subjects. With a demented patient, administration may take 30 to 45 minutes to complete.

SCORING

See *Source*. One point is given for each item performed correctly. Maximum score is 144.

DEMOGRAPHIC EFFECTS

Age

Age affects performance, with younger adults obtaining higher scores than older ones (e.g., Bank et al., 2000; Lucas et al., 1998; Rilling et al., 2005; Smith et al., 1994).

Education/IQ

Numerous authors (Bank et al., 2000; Chan et al., 2001, 2003; Freidl et al., 1996, 1997; Kantarci et al., 2002; Lucas et al., 1998; Marcopulos & McLain, 2003; Marcopulos et al., 1997; Monsch et al., 1995; Rilling et al., 2005; Schmidt et al., 1994, Smith et al., 1994) have reported that performance varies not only by age, but also by education and IQ. Accordingly, normative data broken down by age and education are preferred.

Gender/Race and Culture

Gender (Bank et al., 2000; Chan et al., 2001; Lucas et al., 1998; Monsch et al., 1995; Rilling et al., 2005; Schmidt et al., 1994) has little impact on test scores. African Americans tend to obtain lower scores than Caucasians (Rilling et al., 2005), suggesting the need for ethnicity-specific norms. Cultural factors also appear to have an impact (see *Validity*).

NORMATIVE DATA

Mattis (1976; cited in Montgomery, 1982) initially recommended a cutoff score of 137 for identifying impairment. However, this cutoff is of limited value since the sample sizes on which the score is based (Coblentz et al., 1973) were extremely small (i.e., 20 brain-damaged subjects, 11 normals). Different cutoff scores (e.g., DRS < 123) have been provided by others (e.g., Montgomery, 1982); however, the clinical utility of these scores is also limited, because sample sizes were small and the subjects were relatively well educated. Because studies have demonstrated significant relationships between age as well as education and DRS performance (see previous discussion as well as DRS-2 manual), simple cutoff scores are considered inappropriate. Recent studies have provided data stratified by both age and education.

Schmidt et al. (1994) collected data from 1001 Austrian subjects, aged 50 to 80 years, who were free of neuropsychiatric or severe general diseases. The mean age of participants was 66.3 years (range 50–80), with a mean education of 10.8 years $(SD = 2.3)$. Although the sample size is superior, the data may not be suitable for use with North American samples, given the cultural and language differences and the lack of participants over the age of 80 years.

Lucas et al. (1998; see also DRS-2 manual) present norms for 623 community-dwelling adults over the age of 55 years (age, $M = 79.2$ years, $SD = 7.6$). The participants were predominantly Caucasian with a relatively high level of education ($M = 13.1$ years, $SD = 7.6$) and were reported by their physician to have no active medical disorder with potential to affect cognition. These data were collected as part of Mayo's Older Americans Normative Studies (MOANS) and afford the clinician the advantage of being able to compare DRS scores to patient performance on other tests having the MOANS norms (e.g., WAIS-R, WMS-R, RAVLT) (Lucas et al., 1998). The DRS data are shown in Tables 6–25 through 6–33. Age-corrected MOANS scaled scores ($M = 10$, $SD = 3$) are presented in the left-hand column of the table while corresponding percentile ranks are given in the right-hand column. To further adjust for the effects of education, a standard linear regression was used to derive age- and education corrected MOANS Total scaled scores. This formula is

presented in Table 6–34. Efforts to provide adjustment for education at the subtest level resulted in scaling problems due to the highly skewed nature of some subtests. Therefore, education corrections are applied only to the total score. Note, however, that the underrepresentation of participants with limited educational backgrounds (i.e., <8 years) cautions against the application of this formula in such individuals.

Although the MOANS (Lucas et al. 1998) data represent a very important contribution to the normative base, the sample consists largely of Caucasian adults living in economically stable regions of the United States. As a result, their norms will likely overestimate cognitive impairment in those with limited education and different cultural or health-related experiences (Bank et al., 2000; Yochim et al., 2003). A number of authors (Bank et al., 2000; Vangel & Lichtenberg, 1995) have attempted to address the issue by increasing African American representation in the normative samples. Recently, Rilling et al. (2005) provided age- and education-adjusted normative data based on 307 African American community-dwelling participants from the MOAANS (Mayo African American Normative Studies) project in Jacksonville, Florida. Participants were predominantly female (75%), ranged in age from 56 to 94 years ($M = 69.6$ years, $SD = 6.87$), and varied in education from 0 to 20 years of formal education ($M = 12.2$ years, $SD = 3.48$). They were screened to exclude those with active neurological, psychiatric, or other conditions that might affect cognition. Age-corrected MOAANS scaled scores and percentile ranks for the DRS total and subtest scores are presented in Tables 6–35 through 6–41. The computational formula to calculate age- and education-corrected MOAANS

Table 6–25 MOANS Scaled Scores for Persons Under Age 69 Years

Scaled Scores	Dementia Rating Scale Subtests					Total	Percentile Ranges
	Attention	Initiation/Perseveration	Construction	Conceptualization	Memory		
2	<27	<24	0–2	<25	<17	<115	<1
3	27–28	24–26	3	25–26	17	115–119	1
4	29–30	27–28	—	27	18–19	120–121	2
5	31	29–30	4	28–29	20	122–127	3–5
6	32	31–33	—	30–32	21	128–130	6–10
7	33	34	5	33	22	131–132	11–18
8	34	35	—	34–35	—	133–134	19–28
9	—	—	—	36	23	135–136	29–40
10	35	36	6	37	24	137–139	41–59
11	36	37	—	38	—	140	60–71
12	—	—	—	39	—	141	72–81
13	37	—	—	—	25	142	82–89
14	—	—	—	—	—	143	90–94
15	—	—	—	—	—	144	95–97
16	—	—	—	—	—	—	98
17	—	—	—	—	—	—	99
18	—	—	—	—	—	—	>99

Source: From Lucas et al., 1998. Reprinted with the kind permission of Psychology Press.

Table 6–26 MOANS Scaled Scores for Persons Aged 69–71 Years

Scaled Scores	Dementia Rating Scale Subtests					Total	Percentile Ranges
	Attention	Initiation/Perseveration	Construction	Conceptualization	Memory		
2	<27	<24	0–2	<25	<17	<110	<1
3	27–28	24–26	3	25–26	17	110–119	1
4	29–30	27–28	—	27	18–19	120–121	2
5	31	29–30	4	28–29	20	122–126	3–5
6	32	31–32	—	30–31	21	127–129	6–10
7	33	33–34	5	32–33	22	130–132	11–18
8	34	35	—	34	—	133–134	19–28
9	—	—	—	35	23	135–136	29–40
10	35	36	6	36–37	24	137–139	41–59
11	36	37	—	38	—	140	60–71
12	—	—	—	—	—	141	72–81
13	37	—	—	39	25	142	82–89
14	—	—	—	—	—	143	90–94
15	—	—	—	—	—	144	95–97
16	—	—	—	—	—	—	98
17	—	—	—	—	—	—	99
18	—	—	—	—	—	—	>99

Source: From Lucas et al., 1998. Reprinted with the kind permission of Psychology Press.

scaled scores ($MSS_{A\&E}$) for the DRS total score is shown in Table 6–42.

The MOAANS normative data are similar to normative estimates provided by others (Banks et al., 2000; Marcopulos & McLain, 2003), based on mixed-ethnic samples with significant proportions of older African American partici-pants. Of note, norms for the DRS were developed in conjunction with norms for other tests (e.g., BNT, RAVLT, JLO, verbal fluency, MAE Token Test; see descriptions elsewhere in this volume), allowing the clinician to compare an individual's performance across tasks included in the MOANS/ MOAANS battery.

Table 6–27 MOANS Scaled Scores for Persons Aged 72–74 Years

Scaled Scores	Dementia Rating Scale Subtests					Total	Percentile Ranges
	Attention	Initiation/Perseveration	Construction	Conceptualization	Memory		
2	<27	<24	0–2	<25	<17	<110	<1
3	27–28	24–26	3	25–26	17	110–119	1
4	29	27–28	—	27	18–19	120–121	2
5	30	29–30	4	28–29	20	122–126	3–5
6	31	31	—	30–31	21	127–129	6–10
7	32	32–33	5	32–33	—	130–131	11–18
8	33–34	34–35	—	34	22	132–133	19–28
9	—	—	—	35	—	134–135	29–40
10	35	36	6	36–37	23–24	136–138	41–59
11	36	—	—	38	—	139	60–71
12	—	37	—	—	—	140–141	72–81
13	37	—	—	39	25	142	82–89
14	—	—	—	—	—	—	90–94
15	—	—	—	—	—	143–144	95–97
16	—	—	—	—	—	—	98
17	—	—	—	—	—	—	99
18	—	—	—	—	—	—	>99

Source: From Lucas et al., 1998. Reprinted with the kind permission of Psychology Press.

Table 6–28 MOANS Scaled Scores for Persons Aged 75–77 Years

| Scaled Scores | Dementia Rating Scale Subtests | | | | | Total | Percentile Ranges |
	Attention	Initiation/Perseveration	Construction	Conceptualization	Memory		
2	<27	<24	0–2	<23	<17	<109	<1
3	27–28	24–26	3	23–26	17	109–119	1
4	29	27–28	—	27	18	120–121	2
5	30	29–30	4	28–29	19–20	122–125	3–5
6	31	31	—	30–31	—	126–128	6–10
7	32	32–33	5	32	21	129–130	11–18
8	33–34	34	—	33–34	22	131–132	19–28
9	—	35	—	35		133–134	29–40
10	35	36	6	36–37	23	135–137	41–59
11	—	—	—	—	24	138–139	60–71
12	36	37	—	38	—	140	72–81
13	37	—	—	39	25	141–142	82–89
14	—	—	—	—	—	—	90–94
15	—	—	—	—	—	143	95–97
16	—	—	—	—	—	144	98
17	—	—	—	—	—	—	99
18	—	—	—	—	—	—	>99

Source: From Lucas et al., 1998. Reprinted with the kind permission of Psychology Press.

RELIABILITY

Internal Consistency

Gardner et al. (1981) reported a split-half reliability of .90 for the total scale in a sample of nursing home patients with neurological disorders. Vitaliano, Breen, Russo, et al. (1984) examined internal consistency of the DRS in a small sample of individuals with probable AD. The alpha coefficients were adequate to high for the subscales: Attention (.95), Initiation/Perseveration (.87), Conceptualization (.95), and Memory (.75). Smith et al. (1994) found mixed support for the reliability of DRS scales in a sample of 274

Table 6–29 MOANS Scaled Scores for Persons Aged 78–80 Years

| Scaled Scores | Dementia Rating Scale Subtests | | | | | Total | Percentile Ranges |
	Attention	Initiation/Perseveration	Construction	Conceptualization	Memory		
2	<26	<24	0–2	<19	<17	<108	<1
3	26–28	24–26	3	19–25	17	108–115	1
4	29	27–28	—	26	18	116–119	2
5	30	29–30	4	27–28	19–20	120–122	3–5
6	31	31	—	29–30	—	123–126	6–10
7	32	32	5	31–32	21	127–129	11–18
8	33	33–34	—	33–34	22	130–131	19–28
9	34	—	—	35	—	132–134	29–40
10	35	35–36	6	36	23	135–136	41–59
11	—	—	—	37	24	137–138	60–71
12	36	37	—	38	—	139–140	72–81
13	—	—	—	—	25	141	82–89
14	37	—	—	39	—	142	90–94
15	—	—	—	—	—	143	95–97
16	—	—	—	—	—	144	98
17	—	—	—	—	—	—	99
18	—	—	—	—	—	—	>99

Source: From Lucas et al., 1998. Reprinted with the kind permission of Psychology Press.

Table 6–30 MOANS Scaled Scores for Persons Aged 81–83 Years

| Scaled Scores | Dementia Rating Scale Subtests | | | | | Total | Percentile Ranges |
	Attention	Initiation/Perseveration	Construction	Conceptualization	Memory		
2	<26	<24	0–2	<19	<16	<108	<1
3	26–28	24–25	3	19–24	16	108–114	1
4	29	26–27	—	25	17–18	115–117	2
5	30	28–29	4	26–27	19	118–121	3–5
6	31	30	—	28–30	20	122–126	6–10
7	32	31–32	5	31–32	21	127–128	11–18
8	33	33–34	—	33	22	129–130	19–28
9	34	—	—	34	—	131–133	29–40
10	35	35	6	35–36	23	134–136	41–59
11	—	36	—	37	—	137	60–71
12	36	—	—	38	24	138–139	72–81
13	—	37	—	—	—	140–141	82–89
14	37	—	—	39	25	—	90–94
15	—	—	—	—	—	142	95–97
16	—	—	—	—	—	143	98
17	—	—	—	—	—	144	99
18	—	—	—	—	—	—	>99

Source: From Lucas et al., 1998. Reprinted with the kind permission of Psychology Press.

older patients with cognitive impairment. Internal consistency (Cronbach's alpha) was greater than .70 for Construction, Conceptualization, Memory, and total score, greater than .65 for Attention, and only about .45 for Initiation and Perseveration. Interpretation of the Initiation and Perseveration scale as measuring a single construct is, therefore, hazardous.

Test-Retest Reliability and Practice Effects

When 30 patients with provisional diagnoses of AD were retested following a one-week interval, the correlation for the DRS total score was .97, whereas subscale correlations ranged from .61 to .94 (Coblentz et al., 1973). The means and standard deviations for the total score and subtest scores at test

Table 6–31 MOANS Scaled Scores for Persons Aged 84–86 Years

| Scaled Scores | Dementia Rating Scale Subtests | | | | | Total | Percentile Ranges |
	Attention	Initiation/Perseveration	Construction	Conceptualization	Memory		
2	<26	<24	0–2	<19	<15	<107	<1
3	26–28	24–25	3	19–23	15	107–112	1
4	29	26	—	24	16	113	2
5	30	27–28	4	25–26	17–19	114–120	3–5
6	31	29–30	—	27–29	20	121–124	6–10
7	32	31	—	30–31	—	125–127	11–18
8	33	32–33	5	32–33	21	128–129	19–28
9	—	34	—	34	22	130–132	29–40
10	34–35	35	6	35–36	23	133–135	41–59
11	—	36	—	37	—	136–137	60–71
12	36	—	—	38	24	138	72–81
13	—	37	—	—	—	139–140	82–89
14	37	—	—	39	25	141	90–94
15	—	—	—	—	—	142	95–97
16	—	—	—	—	—	—	98
17	—	—	—	—	—	143–144	99
18	—	—	—	—	—	—	>99

Source: From Lucas et al., 1998. Reprinted with the kind permission of Psychology Press.

Table 6-32 MOANS Scaled Scores for Persons Aged 87–89 Years

| Scaled Scores | Dementia Rating Scale Subtests | | | | | Total | Percentile Ranges |
	Attention	Initiation/Perseveration	Construction	Conceptualization	Memory		
2	<26	<19	0–1	<19	<14	<104	<1
3	26–28	19–21	2	19–22	14–15	104–109	1
4	29	22–23	3	23–24	—	110–112	2
5	30	24–26	—	25–26	16	113–115	3–5
6	31	27–29	4	27–28	17–19	116–122	6–10
7	32	30–31	—	29–30	20	123–126	11–18
8	—	32–33	5	31–32	21	127–129	19–28
9	33	34	—	33–34	22	130–131	29–40
10	34–35	35	6	35–36	23	132–134	41–59
11	—	36	—	37	—	135–136	60–71
12	36	—	—	—	24	137–138	72–81
13	—	37	—	38	—	139	82–89
14	37	—	—	39	25	140–141	90–94
15	—	—	—	—	—	142	95–97
16	—	—	—	—	—	—	98
17	—	—	—	—	—	143	99
18	—	—	—	—	—	144	>99

Source: From Lucas et al., 1998. Reprinted with the kind permission of Psychology Press.

and retest, as well as the retest correlations, are shown in Table 6–43 and reveal minimal effects of practice in this population. Smith et al. (1994) retested a sample of 154 older normal individuals following an interval of about one year and found that DRS total score declines of 10 points or greater occurred in less than 5% of normals. Not surprisingly, over this comparable interval, 61% of 110 dementia patients displayed a decline in DRS total scores of 10 or more points.

Alternate Form Reliability

This is reported to be high in community-dwelling elderly individuals, with a correlation coefficient of .82 for the total score and correlations ranging from .66 (Initiation/Perseveration) to .80 (Memory) for the subscales. In addition, no significant differences were found between total scale and subscale scores of the two forms (Schmidt et al., 2005).

Table 6-33 MOANS Scaled Scores for Persons Over Age 89 Years

| Scaled Scores | Dementia Rating Scale Subtests | | | | | Total | Percentile Ranges |
	Attention	Initiation/Perseveration	Construction	Conceptualization	Memory		
2	<26	<19	0–1	<19	<14	<104	<1
3	26–28	19–20	2	19–21	14	104–108	1
4	29	21	3	22	15	109–112	2
5	30	22–25	—	23–25	16	113–114	3–5
6	31	26–27	4	26–27	17	115–118	6–10
7	32	28–29	—	28–30	18–19	119–123	11–18
8	—	30–32	5	31	20	124–126	19–28
9	33	33	—	32–33	21	127–129	29–40
10	34–35	34	6	34–36	22	130–133	41–59
11	—	35	—	37	23	134–135	60–71
12	36	36	—	—	—	136–137	72–81
13	—	—	—	38	24	138–139	82–89
14	37	37	—	—	—	140–141	90–94
15	—	—	—	39	25	142	95–97
16	—	—	—	—	—	—	98
17	—	—	—	—	—	143	99
18	—	—	—	—	—	144	>99

Source: From Lucas et al., 1998. Reprinted with the kind permission of Psychology Press.

Table 6–34 Regression Formula for Age- and Education-Corrected MOANS Scaled Scores for DRS Total

Age- and education-corrected MOANS scaled scores (AEMSS) can be calculated for DRS Total scores by using age-corrected MOANS scaled scores (AMSS) and education (expressed in years completed) in the following formula:

$$AEMSS = 2.56 + (1.11 \times AMSS) - (0.30 \times EDUC).$$

Source: From Lucas et al., 1998. Reprinted with the kind permission of Psychology Press.

VALIDITY

Construct Validity

The test correlates well with the Wechsler Memory Scale Memory Quotient (.70), the WAIS Full-Scale IQ (.67), cortical metabolism (.59) as determined by positron emission tomography (PET) (Chase et al., 1984), and composite scores derived from standard neuropsychological tests (Knox et al., 2003), supporting its use as a global assessment measure. Smith et al. (1994) found that in older adults who were cognitively impaired, DRS total score shared 54% of its variance with MAYO FSIQ and 57% with MAYO VIQ. In individuals with mental deficiency, the test loaded on the same factor as the Peabody Picture Vocabulary Test-Revised (Das et al., 1995). Moreover, the test correlates highly (about r .70–.80) with other commonly used standardized mental status examinations, such as the Mini-Mental-State-Exam (MMSE) and the Information-Memory-Concentration test (IMC), suggesting that they evaluate overlapping mental abilities (e.g., Bob-

holz & Brandt, 1993; Salmon et al., 1990). Freidl et al. (1996; 2002), however, found only a weak relationship between the DRS and MMSE ($r = .29$) and low agreement with regard to cognitive impairment in a community sample. Conversion formulas are available (see *Comparing Scores on Different Tests*) but given their lack of precision should be used with considerable caution.

In designing the test, Mattis grouped the tasks according to their face validity into five subsets: Memory, Construction, Initiation and Perseveration, Conceptualization, and Attention. Although there are generally high correlations between DRS and MMSE total scores, subscales of the DRS do not always show the expected relationships with items of the MMSE. For example, Bobholz and Brandt (1993) reported that the Attention item of the MMSE (serial sevens) was not significantly correlated with the Attention subscale of the DRS. Smith et al. (1994) provided evidence of convergent validity for some of the DRS scales. In a sample of 234 elderly patients with cognitive impairment, DRS subscale scores for Memory, Attention, and Conceptualization were significantly correlated with appropriate indices (GMI, ACI, and VIQ, respectively) from the WAIS-R and Wechsler Memory Scale-Revised, as assessed in the Mayo Older Americans Normative Studies. Support for the convergent validity of the Construction scale was more problematic. Smith et al. found that this scale correlated more highly with VIQ and ACI scales than with PIQ, raising the concern that it may provide a better index of attention and general cognitive status than of visual-perceptual/visual-constructional skills per se. Marson et al. (1997) reported that in a sample of 50 patients with mild to moderate AD, four of the five DRS subscales correlated most strongly with their assigned criterion

Table 6–35 MOAANS Scaled Scores for Persons Aged 56–62 Years (Midpoint Age = 61, Age Range for Norms = 56–66, N = 108)

Scaled Scores	Dementia Rating Scale Subtests					Total	Percentile Range
	Attention	Initiation/Perseveration	Construction	Conceptualization	Memory		
2	0–23	0–27	0–1	0–23	0–15	0–110	<1
3	24–29	28–29	2	24–25	16–17	111–115	1
4	—	30	—	26	18	116	2
5	30	31	—	27–28	—	117–121	3–5
6	31	32	3	29	19–20	122–123	6–10
7	32	33–34	—	30–31	21	124–126	11–18
8	33	35	4	32	22	127–129	19–28
9	34	36	5	33–34	23	130–132	29–40
10	35	—	—	35	24	133–135	41–59
11	36	—	—	36	—	136–137	60–71
12	—	37	6	37	25	138	72–81
13	—	—	—	38	—	139–141	82–89
14	37	—	—	—	—	142	90–94
15	—	—	—	39	—	143	95–97
16	—	—	—	—	—	—	98
17	—	—	—	—	—	144	99
18	—	—	—	—	—	—	>99

Source: From Rilling et al., 2005. Reprinted by permission of the Mayo Foundation for Medical Education and Research.

Table 6-36 MOAANS Scaled Scores for Persons Aged 63–65 Years (Midpoint Age = 64, Age Range for Norms = 59–69, N = 130)

Scaled Scores	Dementia Rating Scale Subtests					Total	Percentile Range
	Attention	Initiation/Perseveration	Construction	Conceptualization	Memory		
2	0–23	0–27	0–1	0–21	0–15	0–102	<1
3	24–27	28–29	2	22–23	16–17	103–107	1
4	28–29	30	—	24	—	108–114	2
5	—	31	—	25–27	18	115–118	3–5
6	30–31	32	3	28–29	19	119–122	6–10
7	32	33–34	—	30	20	123–125	11–18
8	33	35	4	31–32	21–22	126–129	19–28
9	34	36	5	33	23	130–131	29–40
10	35	—	—	34–35	—	132–134	41–59
11	—	—	—	36	24	135–136	60–71
12	36	37	6	—	—	137–138	72–81
13	—	—	—	37–38	25	139–140	82–89
14	37	—	—	—	—	141	90–94
15	—	—	—	39	—	142–143	95–97
16	—	—	—	—	—	—	98
17	—	—	—	—	—	144	99
18	—	—	—	—	—	—	>99

Source: From Rilling et al., 2005. Reprinted by permission of the Mayo Foundation for Medical Education and Research.

variables (Attention with WMS-R Attention, Initiation/Perseveration with COWA, Conceptualization with WAIS-R Similarities, Memory with WMS-R Verbal Memory). However, the Construction scale correlated as highly with Block Design as with WMS-R Attention. Brown et al. (1999) found that in a sample of patients with Parkinson's disease, some DRS subscales correlated significantly with conceptually related measures from other tests (Attention with WAIS-R Digit Span Forward, Initiation/Perseveration with WCST perseverative responses, Conceptualization with WAIS-R Similarities, Memory with WMS Immediate Logical Memory). No signification correlation was observed between the Construction subscale and other tests. Thus, the available literature suggests that the DRS does not assess aspects of visual-constructional/visual-spatial functioning and that additional measures will need to be supplemented to adequately examine this domain.

Table 6-37 MOAANS Scaled Scores for Persons Aged 66–68 Years (Midpoint Age = 67, Age Range for Norms = 62–72, N = 167)

Scaled Scores	Dementia Rating Scale Subtests					Total	Percentile Range
	Attention	Initiation/Perseveration	Construction	Conceptualization	Memory		
2	0–23	0–27	0–1	0–21	0–15	0–102	<1
3	24–27	28	2	22–23	16	103–107	1
4	28–29	29	—	24	17	108–113	2
5	—	30	—	25–26	18	114–117	3–5
6	30–31	31–32	3	27–28	19	118–121	6–10
7	32	33–34	—	29	20	122–125	11–18
8	33	35	4	30–31	21	126–128	19–28
9	34	36	—	32–33	22	129–130	29–40
10	35	—	5	34–35	23	131–133	41–59
11	—	—	—	—	24	134–135	60–71
12	36	37	6	36	—	136–137	72–81
13	—	—	—	37	25	138–139	82–89
14	37	—	—	38	—	140	90–94
15	—	—	—	39	—	141–142	95–97
16	—	—	—	—	—	143	98
17	—	—	—	—	—	144	99
18	—	—	—	—	—	—	>99

Source: From Rilling et al., 2005. Reprinted by permission of the Mayo Foundation for Medical Education and Research.

Table 6–38 MOAANS Scaled Scores for Persons Aged 69–71 Years (Midpoint Age = 70, Age Range for Norms = 65–75, N = 182)

Scaled Scores	Dementia Rating Scale Subtests					Total	Percentile Ranges
	Attention	Initiation/Perseveration	Construction	Conceptualization	Memory		
2	0–23	0–24	0–1	0–21	0–15	0–100	<1
3	24–27	25–28	2	22–23	16	101–106	1
4	28–29	29	—	24	—	107	2
5	30	30	—	25	17–18	108–116	3–5
6	31	31	3	26–27	19	117–119	6–10
7	32	32–33	—	28–29	20	120–123	11–18
8	33	34–35	4	30	21	124–127	19–28
9	34	36	—	31–32	22	128–130	29–40
10	35	—	5	33–35	23	131–133	41–59
11	—	—	—	—	24	134–135	60–71
12	36	37	6	36	—	136–137	72–81
13	—	—	—	37	25	138	82–89
14	37	—	—	38	—	139–140	90–94
15	—	—	—	—	—	141	95–97
16	—	—	—	39	—	142	98
17	—	—	—	—	—	143	99
18	—	—	—	—	—	144	>99

Source: From Rilling et al., 2005. Reprinted by permission of the Mayo Foundation for Medical Education and Research.

Factor-analytic studies suggest that the five subscales do not reflect exclusively the constructs with which they are labeled (Colantonio et al., 1993; Kessler et al., 1994; Woodard et al., 1996). Kessler et al. (1994) found that a two-factor model, specifying separate verbal and nonverbal functions, provided the best fit for the data in a heterogeneous sample, approximately two-thirds of which carried psychiatric (depression) or dementia (AD-type) diagnoses. Similar results were reported by Das et al. (1995) in a sample of individuals with mental retardation of moderate to severe degree. In a study by Colantonio et al. (1993) with a sample of patients with probable AD, three factors emerged, which they labeled: (1) Conceptualization/Organization, containing tasks of priming inductive reasoning, similarities, differences, identities and oddities, and sentence generation; (2) Visuospatial, containing subtests of graphomotor, construction, attention, alternating movements,

Table 6–39 MOAANS Scaled Scores for Persons Aged 72–74 Years (Midpoint Age = 73, Age Range for Norms = 68–78, N = 157)

Scaled Scores	Dementia Rating Scale Subtests					Total	Percentile Range
	Attention	Initiation/Perseveration	Construction	Conceptualization	Memory		
2	0–23	0–22	—	0–21	0–15	0–100	>1
3	24–27	23–25	0–1	22–23	16	101–106	1
4	28	26–27	2	24	—	107	2
5	29	28–30	—	25	17–18	108–114	3–5
6	30–31	31	3	26	19	115–118	6–10
7	32	32	—	27–28	20	119–121	11–18
8	33	33–34	4	29	21	122–126	19–28
9	34	35	—	30–32	22	127–129	29–40
10	—	36	5	33–34	23	130–133	41–59
11	35	—	—	35	24	134–135	60–71
12	36	37	6	36	—	136–137	72–81
13	—	—	—	37	25	138	82–89
14	37	—	—	38	—	139–140	90–94
15	—	—	—	—	—	141	95–97
16	—	—	—	39	—	142	98
17	—	—	—	—	—	143	99
18	—	—	—	—	—	144	>99

Source: From Rilling et al., 2005. Reprinted by permission of the Mayo Foundation for Medical Education and Research.

Table 6-40 MOAANS Scaled Scores for Persons Aged 75–77 Years (Midpoint Age = 76, Age Range for Norms = 71–81, N = 119)

Scaled Scores	Dementia Rating Scale Subtests					Total	Percentile Range
	Attention	Initiation/Perseveration	Construction	Conceptualization	Memory		
2	0–23	0–22	—	0–21	0–15	0–100	<1
3	24–27	23–24	0–1	22–23	16	101–106	1
4	28	25–26	—	—	—	107	2
5	29	27–29	2	24	17	108–111	3–5
6	30–31	30	3	25–26	18	112–117	6–10
7	32	31–32	—	27	19–20	118–121	11–18
8	33	33–34	4	28–29	21	122–125	19–28
9	34	35	—	30–31	22	126–128	29–40
10	—	36	5	32–34	23	129–132	41–59
11	35	—	—	35	24	133–134	60–71
12	36	37	6	36	—	135–137	72–81
13	—	—	—	37	25	138	82–89
14	—	—	—	38	—	139–140	90–94
15	37	—	—	—	—	141	95–97
16	—	—	—	39	—	142	98
17	—	—	—	—	—	143	99
18	—	—	—	—	—	144	>99

Source: From Rilling et al., 2005. Reprinted by permission of the Mayo Foundation for Medical Education and Research.

and word and design recognition memory; and (3) Memory, consisting of sentence recall and orientation. Similar results have been reported by Woodard et al. (1996) in a sample of patients with probable AD. Moderate correlations were also found between these factors and supplementary neuropsychological measures, supporting the validity of these factors. On the other hand, Hofer et al. (1996) examined the factor structure of the test in patients with dementia and healthy elderly controls grouped together. They found five factors, which they labeled Long-term Memory (Recall)/Verbal Fluency, Construction, Memory (Short-term), Initiation/Perseveration, and Simple Commands. The contrasting results (Hofer et al., 1996; Kessler et al., 1994 versus Colantonio et al., 1993; Woodard et al., 1996) highlight the fact that the resulting factor structure

Table 6-41 MOAANS Scaled Scores for Persons Aged 78 + (Midpoint Age = 79, Age Range for Norms = 74–94, N = 79)

Scaled Scores	Dementia Rating Scale Subtests					Total	Percentile Range
	Attention	Initiation/Perseveration	Construction	Conceptualization	Memory		
2	0–23	0–17	—	0–17	0–3	0–78	<1
3	24–27	18–23	0–1	18–22	4–12	79–103	1
4	28	24	—	23	13–16	104–106	2
5	29	25–27	2	24	17	107–110	3–5
6	30	28–30	3	25–26	18	111–115	6–10
7	31	31	—	27	19	116–118	11–18
8	32	32	4	28	20	119–121	19–28
9	33	33–34	—	29–30	21	122–126	29–40
10	34	35–36	5	31–33	22–23	127–130	41–59
11	35	—	—	34–35	—	131–133	60–71
12	36	—	6	36	24	134–135	72–81
13	—	37	—	37	25	136–138	82–89
14	—	—	—	38	—	139	90–94
15	37	—	—	—	—	140	95–97
16	—	—	—	39	—	141	98
17	—	—	—	—	—	142–143	99
18	—	—	—	—	—	144	>99

Source: From Rilling et al., 2005. Reprinted by permission of the Mayo Foundation for Medical Education and Research.

Table 6–42 Regression Formula for Age- and Education-Corrected MOAANS Scaled Scores for DRS Total

Age- and education-corrected MOAANS scaled scores ($MSS_{A\&E}$) can be calculated for DRS Total scores by using aged-corrected MOAANS scaled scores (MSS_A) and education (expressed in years completed) in the following formula:

$$MSS_{A\&E} = 3.01 + (1.19 \times MSS_A) - (0.41 \times EDUC)$$

Source: From Rilling et al., 2005. Reprinted by permission of the Mayo Foundation for Medical Education and Research.

depends critically on the characteristics of the population studied including the severity of their impairment.

Clinical Studies

The DRS is useful in detecting cognitive impairment in older adults (e.g., Yochim et al., 2003). It can differentiate patients with dementia of the Alzheimer's type from normal elderly subjects (Chan et al., 2003; Monsch et al., 1995; Salmon et al., 2002); is sensitive to early stages of dementia (Knox et al., 2003; Monsch et al., 1995; Salmon et al., 2002; Vitaliano, Breen, Albert, et al., 1984), even in individuals with mental retardation (Das et al., 1995); and is useful in identifying stages (severity) of impairment (Chan et al., 2003; Shay et al., 1991; Vitaliano, Breen, Albert, et al., 1984). Further, the DRS has demonstrated the ability to accurately track progression of cognitive decline, even in the later stages of AD (Salmon et al., 1990). Although the DRS tends to be highly correlated with other mental status exams, such as the Information Memory Concentration (IMC) and MMSE, and shows equal sensitivity to dementia (Chan et al., 2003; van Gorp et al., 1999), it provides more precise estimates of change than these tests, likely due to its wider sampling of item difficulty (Gould et al. 2001; Salmon et al., 1990). Therefore, to follow progression in severely demented patients, the DRS is clearly the instrument of choice.

Unlike other standardized mental status examinations that were developed as screening instruments (e.g., MMSE), the DRS was designed with the intention of discriminating among patients with dementia. There is evidence that pattern analysis of the DRS can distinguish the dementias associated with AD from those associated with Huntington's disease (HD), Parkinson's disease (PD), or vascular dementia (VaD) (e.g., Cahn-Weiner et al., 2002; Kertesz & Clydesdale, 1994; Lukatela et al., 2000; Paolo et al., 1994; Paulsen et al., 1995; Salmon et al., 1989). Patients with AD display more severe memory impairment; patients with HD are more severely impaired on items that involve the programming of motor sequences (Initiation/Perseveration subtest), while patients with PD or VaD display more severe constructional problems. Patients with PD may also show memory impairment on the DRS, although this might reflect the effects of depression (Norman et al., 2002). Further, patients with frontotemporal dementia are less impaired on the Memory subscale than AD patients (Rascovsky et al., 2002). It is worth noting that these various distinctions among patient groups emerge even when patients are similar in terms of overall level of cognitive impairment.

These findings are generally consistent with neuroimaging findings suggesting relationships between particular brain regions and specific cognitive functions assessed by the DRS. For example, Fama et al. (1997) found that Memory subscale scores in patients with AD were related to MRI-derived hippocampal volumes, while Initiation/Perseveration scores were related to prefrontal sulcal widening. Others have also observed that scores on select subscales are related to the integrity of specific brain regions. In patients with vascular dementia, performance on the Memory subscale is associated with whole brain volume, whereas the Initiation and Construction subscales are related to subcortical hyperintensities (Paul et al., 2001). Even in the absence of dementia, subcortical ischemic vascular disease is associated with subtle declines in executive functioning, as measured by the Initiation/Perseveration subscale (Kramer et al., 2002).

There is evidence that depression impairs DRS performance, at least to some extent (Harrell et al., 1991; van Reekum et al., 2000). For example, one group of investigators (Butters et al., 2000) studied 45 nondemented, elderly depressed patients before and after successful treatment with pharmacotherapy. Among depressed patients with concomitant cognitive impairment at baseline, successful treatment of

Table 6–43 DRS Test-Retest Reliability in People With Presumed AD

	Initial Test		Retest		Test-Retest Correlation
	M	SD	M	SD	r
Total Score	79.55	33.98	83.18	30.60	.97
Attention	23.55	9.91	24.16	6.80	.61
Initiation/Perseveration	21.36	9.78	22.00	7.34	.89
Construction	2.55	1.81	2.91	1.70	.83
Conceptualization	21.18	10.58	21.91	9.28	.94
Memory	10.91	6.58	12.20	6.00	.92

Source: From Coblentz et al., 1973. Reprinted with permission from the AMA.

depression was associated with gains on the DRS measures of Conceptualization and Initiation/Perseveration. Nonetheless, the overall level of cognitive functioning in these patients remained mildly impaired, especially in the Memory and Initiation/Perseveration domains.

Although the DRS is typically used with older adults, it has found use in other groups as well. Thus, it has been given to adolescents and adults with mental retardation (spanning the spectrum from mild to severe; Das et al., 1995; McDaniel & McLaughlin, 2000). However, it should not be used to diagnose mental retardation.

Ecological Validity

DRS scores show modest correlations with measures of functional competence (the ability to perform activities of daily living as well as engage in complex recreational activities; e.g., Cahn et al., 1998; LaBuda & Lichtenberg, 1999; Lemsky et al., 1996; Loewenstein et al., 1992; Smith et al., 1994; Vitaliano, Breen, Albert, et al., 1984, Vitaliano, Breen, Russo, et al., 1984). In particular, the Initiation/Perseveration and Memory subtests have proved valuable indicators of functional status in the elderly (Nadler et al., 1993; Plehn et al., 2004).

In addition, the DRS may be useful in predicting functional decline (Hochberg et al., 1989) and survival (Smith et al., 1994). Smith et al. (1994) reported that in sample of 274 persons over age 55 with cognitive impairment, DRS total scores supplemented age information and provided a better basis for estimating survival than did gender or duration of disease. Median survival for those with DRS total scores below 100 was 3.7 years.

Other DRS Versions and Item Bias

Attempts to develop other language versions of the DRS have met with varying success, perhaps because of cultural bias inherent in the subscales or individual subscale items. For example, Hohl et al. (1999) found that Hispanic AD patients performed significantly worse than non-Hispanics in terms of total DRS score (on a translated version), despite being matched by MMSE score. This difference was accounted for primarily by poorer performance of the Hispanic patients, relative to the non-Hispanic patients, on the Memory and Conceptualization subtests. A Chinese version (Chan et al., 2001, 2003) has also been developed that shows similar sensitivity and specificity as the English version. Comparison of age- and education-matched groups in Hong Kong and San Diego revealed differences in the pattern of subtest performance, even though groups did not differ in total DRS scores. Individuals in Hong Kong scored significantly higher than the San Diego participants on the Construction scale, whereas the opposite pattern was observed on the Initiation/Perseveration and Memory subscales.

Woodard et al. (1998) investigated possible racial bias in the test by comparing 40 pairs of African American and Caucasian dementia patients matched for age, years of education, and gender. Principal component analysis revealed similar patterns and magnitudes across component loadings for each racial group, suggesting no evidence of test bias. In addition, they identified only 4 of the 36 items of the DRS that showed differential item functioning: "palm up/palm down, fist clenched/fist extended, point out and count the As, and visual recognition." The implication is that the DRS may be used in both African American and Caucasian populations to assess dementia severity. Another study, by Teresi et al. (2000), found that most items of the Attention subscale of the DRS performed in an education-fair manner.

Comparing Scores on Different Tests

If a patient has been given a different mental status test (e.g., MMSE), one can translate the score on the test into scale-free units such as a z score or percentile score, or one can use a conversion formula. Equations have been developed to convert total scores from one test to the other (Bobholz & Brandt, 1993; Meiran et al., 1996; Salmon et al., 1990), but given the mixed results in the literature (see *Construct Validity*), these should be used with caution. The equations are shown in Table 6–44. The formulas should be applied to similar patients.

Table 6–44 Conversion Formulas to Derive DRS Scores From the MMSE

Test	Formula	Reference
DRS	41.53 + 3.26 (MMSE)	Salmon et al., 1990 Based on a sample of 92 patients with probable AD
DRS	33.86 + 3.39 (MMSE)	Bobholz & Brandt, 1993 Based on a sample of 50 patients with suspected cognitive impairment
DRS	45.5 + 3.01 (MMSE)	Meiran et al., 1996 Based on a sample of 466 patients in a memory disorders clinic; the expected error associated with this formula is ±11.1

COMMENT

The DRS is a fairly comprehensive screening test, evaluating aspects of cognition (e.g., verbal conceptualization, verbal fluency) not well assessed by tests such as MMSE. It also appears to be more useful than other measures (e.g., the MMSE) in tracking change. On the other hand, the DRS takes about four times longer to administer (Bobholz & Brandt, 1993) and may be more susceptible to cultural or educational factors in some populations (e.g., Hispanics) (Hohl et al., 1999).

The summary score appears to have relatively good concurrent and predictive validity. Given that the DRS may also be helpful in distinguishing among dementing disorders even in later stages of disease, the focus should also be on specific cognitive dimensions that the test offers. In this context, it is worth bearing in mind that the Conceptualization and Memory subscales appear fairly reliable and seem to represent discrete constructs. Construction, Attention, and Initiation/Perseveration items should also be administered, but given concerns regarding reliability and validity, their interpretation is more problematic.

It is also important to note that the test is a screening device and the clinician may need to follow up with a more in-depth investigation. Thus, individuals identified as cognitively impaired on the test should undergo additional assessment to determine the presence or absence of dementia. Further, although sensitive to differences at the lower end of functioning, the DRS may not detect impairment in the higher ranges of intelligence (Jurica et al., 2001; Teresi et al., 2001). This is because the DRS was developed to avoid floor effects in clinically impaired populations rather than ceiling effects in high-functioning individuals (Jurica et al., 2001).

Some (Chan et al., 2002; Monsch et al., 1995) have suggested that an abbreviated version composed only of the Memory and Initiation/Perseveration subscales may be useful as a quick screening for individuals suspected of AD. This focus is consistent with literature suggesting that deterioration of memory is an early, prominent symptom of the disease. However, with use of such a shortened procedure, the comprehensive data on different aspects of cognitive functioning will be lost (Chan et al., 2003).

REFERENCES

Bank, A. L., Yochim, B. P., MacNeill, S. E., & Lichtenberg, P. A. (2000). Expanded normative data for the Mattis dementia rating scale for use with urban, elderly medical patients. *The Clinical Neuropsychologist, 14*, 149–156.

Bobholz, J. H., & Brandt, J. (1993). Assessment of cognitive impairment: Relationship of the Dementia Rating Scale to the Mini-Mental State Examination. *Journal of Geriatric Psychiatry and Neurology, 6*, 210–213.

Brown, G. G., Rahill, A. A., Gorell, J. M., McDonald, C., Brown, S. J., Sillanpaa, M., & Shults, C. (1999). Validity of the Dementia Rating Scale in assessing cognitive function in Parkinson's disease. *Journal of Geriatric Psychiatry and Neurology, 12*, 180–188.

Butters, M. A., Becker, J. T., Nebes, R. D., Zmuda, M. D., Mulsant, B. H., Pollock, B. G., & Reynolds, C. F., III. (2000). Changes in cognitive functioning following treatment of late-life depression. *American Journal of Psychiatry, 157*, 1949–1954.

Cahn, D. A., Sullivan, E. V., Shear, P. K., Pfefferbaum, A., Heit, G., & Silverberg, G. (1998). Differential contributions of cognitive and motor component processes to physical and instrumental activities of daily living in Parkinson's disease. *Archives of Clinical Neuropsychology, 13*, 575–583.

Cahn-Weiner, D. A., Grace, J., Ott, B. R., Fernandez, H. H., & Friedman, J. H. (2002). Cognitive and behavioural features discriminate between Alzheimer's and Parkinson's disease. *Neuropsychiatry, Neuropsychology, & Behavioural Neurology, 15*, 79–87.

Chan, A. S., Choi, A., Chiu, H., & Liu, L. (2003). Clinical validity of the Chinese version of Mattis Dementia Rating Scale in differentiating dementia of Alzheimer's type in Hong Kong. *Journal of the International Neuropsychological Society, 9*, 45–55.

Chan, A. S., Salmon, D. P., & Choi, M-K. (2001). The effects of age, education, and gender on the Mattis Dementia Rating Scale performance of elderly Chinese and American individuals. *Journal of Gerontology: Series B: Psychological Sciences & Social Sciences, 56B*, 356–363.

Chase, T. N., Foster, N. L., Fedio, P., Brooks, R., Mansi, L., & Di Chiro, G. (1984). Regional cortical dysfunction in Alzheimer's disease as determined by positron emission tomography. *Annals of Neurology, 15*, S170–S174.

Coblentz, J. M., Mattis, S., Zingesser, L. H., Kasoff, S. S., Wisniewski, H. M., & Katzman, R. (1973). Presenile dementia. *Archives of Neurology, 29*, 299–308.

Colantonio, A., Becker, J. T., & Huff, F. J. (1993). Factor structure of the Mattis Dementia Rating Scale among patients with probable Alzheimer's disease. *The Clinical Neuropsychologist 7*, 313–318.

Das, J. P., Mishra, R. K., Davison, M., & Naglieri, J. A. (1995). Measurement of dementia in individuals with mental retardation: Comparison based on PPVT and Dementia Rating Scale. *The Clinical Neuropsychologist, 9*, 32–37.

Fama, R., Sullivan, E. V., Shear, P. K., Marsh, L., Yesavage, J., Tinklenberg, J. R., Lim, K. O., & Pfefferbaum, A. (1997). Selective cortical and hippocampal volume correlates of Mattis Dementia Rating Scale in Alzheimer disease. *Archives of Neurology, 54*, 719–728.

Freidl, W., Schmidt, R., Stronegger, W. J., Fazekas, F., & Reinhart, B. (1996). Sociodemographic predictors and concurrent validity of the Mini Mental State Examination and the Mattis Dementia Rating Scale. *European Archives of Psychiatry and Clinical Neuroscience, 246*, 317–319.

Freidl, W., Schmidt, R., Stronegger, W. J., & Reinhart, B. (1997). The impact of sociodemographic, environmental, and behavioural factors, and cerebrovascular risk factors as potential predictors on the Mattis Dementia Rating Scale. *Journal of Gerontology, 52A*, M111–M116.

Freidl, W., Stronegger, W.-J., Berghold, A., Reinhart, B., Petrovic, K., & Schmidt, R. (2002). The agreement of the Mattis Dementia Rating Scale with the Mini-Mental State Examination. *International Journal of Psychiatry, 17*, 685–686.

Gardner, R., Oliver-Munoz, S., Fisher, L., & Empting, L. (1981). Mattis Dementia Rating Scale: Internal reliability study using a diffusely impaired population. *Journal of Clinical Neuropsychology, 3*, 271–275.

Gould, R., Abramson, I., Galasko, D., & Salmon, D. (2001). Rate of cognitive change in Alzheimer's disease: Methodological approaches using random effects models. *Journal of the International Neuropsychological Society, 7,* 813–824.

Harrell, L. E., Duvall, E., Folks, D. G., Duke, L., Bartolucci, A., Conboy, T., Callaway, R., & Kerns, D. (1991). The relationship of high-intensity signals on magnetic resonance images to cognitive and psychiatric state in Alzheimer's disease. *Archives of Neurology, 48,* 1136–1140.

Hochberg, M. G., Russo, J., Vitaliano, P. P., Prinz, P. N., Vitiello, M. V., & Yi, S. (1989). Initiation and perseveration as a subscale of the Dementia Rating Scale. *Clinical Gerontologist, 8,* 27–41.

Hofer, S. M., Piccinin, A. M., & Hershey, D. (1996). Analysis of structure and discriminative power of the Mattis Dementia Rating Scale. *Journal of Clinical Psychology, 52,* 395–409.

Hohl, U., Grundman, M., Salmon, D. P., Thomas, R. G., & Thal, L. J. (1999). Mini-Mental State Examination and Mattis Dementia Rating Scale performance differs in Hispanic and non-Hispanic Alzheimer's disease patients. *Journal of the International Neuropsychological Society, 5,* 301–307.

Jurica, P. J., Leitten, C. L., & Mattis, S. (2001). *Dementia Rating Scale-2.* Odessa, FL: Psychological Assessment Resources.

Kantarci, K., Smith, G. E., Ivnik, R. J., Petersen, R. C., Boeve, B. F., Knopman, D. S., Tangalos, E. G., & Jack, C. R. (2002). H magnetic resonance spectroscopy, cognitive function, and apolipoprotein E genotype in normal aging, mild cognitive impairment and Alzheimer's disease. *Journal of the International Neuropsychological Society, 8,* 934–942.

Kertesz, A., & Clydesdale, S. (1994). Neuropsychological deficits in vascular dementia vs Alzheimer's disease. *Archives of Neurology, 51,* 1226–1231.

Kessler, H. R., Roth, D. L., Kaplan, R. F., & Goode, K. T. (1994). Confirmatory factor analysis of the Mattis Dementia Rating Scale. *The Clinical Neuropsychologist, 8,* 451–461.

Knox, M. R., Lacritz, L. H., Chandler, M. J., & Cullum, C. M. (2003). Association between Dementia Rating Scale performance and neurocognitive domains in Alzheimer's disease. *The Clinical Neuropsychologist, 17,* 216–219.

Kramer, J. H., Reed, B. R., Mungas, D., Weiner, N. W., & Chui, H. C. (2002). Executive dysfunction in subcortical ischaemic vascular disease. *Journal of Neurology, Neurosurgery and Psychiatry, 72,* 217–220.

LaBuda, J., & Lichtenberg, P. (1999). The role of cognition, depression, and awareness of deficit in predicting geriatric rehabilitation patients' IADL performance. *The Clinical Neuropsychologist, 13,* 258–267.

Lemsky, C. M., Smith, G., Malec, J. F., & Ivnik, R. J. (1996). Identifying risk for functional impairment using cognitive measures: An application of CART modeling. *Neuropsychology, 10,* 368–375.

Loewenstein, D. A., Rupert, M. P., Berkowitz-Zimmer, N., Guterman, A., Morgan, R., Hayden, S. (1992) Neuropsychological test performance and prediction of functional capacities in dementia. *Behavior, Health, and Aging, 2,* 149–158.

Lucas, J. A., Ivnick, R. J., Smith, G. E., Bohac, D. L., Tangalos, E. G., Kokmen, E., Graff-Radford, N. R., & Petersen, R. C. (1998). Normative data for the Mattis Dementia Rating Scale. *Journal of Clinical and Experimental Neuropsychology, 20,* 536–547.

Lukatela, K., Cohen, R. A., Kessler, H., Jenkins, M. A., Moser, D. J., Stone, W. F., Gordon, N., & Kaplan, R. F. (2000). Dementia Rating Scale performance: A comparison of vascular and Alzheimer's dementia. *Journal of Clinical and Experimental Neuropsychology, 22,* 445–454.

Marcopulos, B. A., & McLain, C. A. (2003). Are our norms "normal"? A 4-year follow-up study of a biracial sample of rural elders with low education. *The Clinical Neuropsychologist, 17,* 19–33.

Marcopulos, B. A., McLain, C. A., & Giuliano, A. J. (1997). Cognitive impairment or inadequate norms? A study of healthy, rural, older adults with limited education. *The Clinical Neuropsychologist, 11,* 111–113.

Marson, D. C., Dymek, M. P., Duke, L. W., & Harrell, L. E. (1997). Subscale validity of the Mattis Dementia Rating Scale. *Archives of Clinical Neuropsychology, 12,* 269–275.

Mattis, S. (1976). Mental status examination for organic mental syndrome in the elderly patient. In L. Bellak & T. B. Karasu (Eds.), *Geriatric psychiatry.* New York: Grune and Stratton.

Mattis, S. (1988). *Dementia Rating Scale: Professional manual.* Odessa, FL: Psychological Assessment Resources.

McDaniel, W. F., & McLaughlin, T. (2000). Further support for using the Dementia Rating Scale in the assessment of neuro-cognitive functions of individuals with mental retardation. *The Clinical Neuropsychologist, 14,* 72–75.

Meiran, N., Stuss, D. T., Guzman, D. A., Lafleche, G., & Willmer, J. (1996). Diagnosis of dementia: Methods for interpretation of scores of 5 neuropsychological tests. *Archives of Neurology, 53,* 1043–1054.

Monsch, A. U., Bondi, M. W., Salmon, D. P., Butters, N., Thal, L. J., Hansen, L. A., Wiederholt, W. C., Cahn, D. A., & Klauber, M. R. (1995). Clinical validity of the Mattis Dementia Rating Scale in detecting dementia of the Alzheimer type. *Archives of Neurology, 52,* 899–904.

Montgomery, K. M. (1982). *A normative study of neuropsychological test performance of a normal elderly sample* (unpublished Master's thesis). University of Victoria, Victoria, British Columbia.

Nadler, J. D., Richardson, E. D., Malloy, P. F., Marran, M. E., & Hostetler Brinson, M. E. (1993). The ability of the Dementia Rating Scale to predict everyday functioning. *Archives of Clinical Neuropsychology, 8,* 449–460.

Norman, S., Troster, A. I., Fields, J. A., & Brooks, R. (2002). Effects of depression and Parkinson's disease on cognitive functioning. *Journal of Neuropsychiatry and Clinical Neurosciences, 14,* 31–36.

Paolo, A. M., Troster, A. I., Glatt, S. L., Hubble, J. P., & Koller, W. C. (1994). *Utility of the Dementia Rating Scale to differentiate the dementias of Alzheimer's and Parkinson's disease.* Paper presented to the International Neuropsychological Society, Cincinnati, OH.

Paul, R. H., Cohen, R. A., Moser, D., Ott, B. R., Zawacki, T., Gordon, N., Bell, S., & Stone, W. (2001). Performance on the Mattis Dementia Rating Scale in patients with vascular dementia: Relationships to neuroimaging findings. *Journal of Geriatric Psychiatry & Neurology, 14,* 33–36.

Paulsen, J. S., Butters, N., Sadek, B. S., Johnson, B. S., Salmon, D. P., Swerdlow, N. R., & Swenson. M. R. (1995). Distinct cognitive profiles of cortical and subcortical dementia in advanced illness. *Neurology, 45,* 951–956.

Plehn, K., Marcopulos, B. A., & McLain, C. A. (2004). The relationship between neuropsychological test performance, social functioning, and instrumental activities of daily living in a sample of rural older adults. *The Clinical Neuropsychologist, 18,* 101–113.

Rascovsky, K., Salmon, D. P., Hi, G. J., Galasko, D., Peavy, G. M., Hansen, L. A., & Thal, L. J. (2002). Cognitive profiles differ in autopsy-confirmed frontotemporal dementia and AD. *Neurology,* 1801–1807.

Rilling, L. M., Lucas, J. A., Ivnik, R. J., Smith, G. E., Willis, F. B., Ferman, T. J., Petersen, R. C., & Graff-Radford, N. R. (2005). Mayo's Older African American Normative Studies: Norms for the Mattis Dementia Rating Scale. *The Clinical Neuropsychologist, 19,* 229–242.

Salmon, D. P., Kwo-on-Yuen, P. F., Heindel, W. C., Butters, N., & Thal, L. J. (1989). Differentiation of Alzheiner's disease and Huntington's disease with the Dementia Rating Scale. *Archives of Neurology, 46,* 1204–1208.

Salmon, D. P., Thal, L. J., Butters, N., & Heindel, W. C. (1990). Longitudinal evaluation of dementia of the Alzheimer's type: A comparison of 3 standardized mental status examinations. *Neurology, 40,* 1225–1230.

Salmon, D. P., Thomas, R. G., Pay, M. M., Booth, A., Hofstetter, C. R., Thal, L. J., & Katzman, R. (2002). Alzheimer's disease can be accurately diagnosed in very mildly impaired individuals. *Neurology, 59,* 1022–1028.

Schmidt, R., Freidl, W., Fazekas, F., Reinhart, P., Greishofer, P., Koch, M., Eber, B., Smith, G. E., Ivnik, R. J., Malec, J. F., Kokmen, E., Tangalos, E., & Petersen, R. C. (1994). Psychometric properties of the Mattis Dementia Rating Scale. *Assessment, 1,* 123–131.

Schmidt, K., & Mattis, S. (2004). *Dementia Rating Scale-2: Alternate form.* Lutz, FL: PAR.

Schmidt, K. S., Mattis, P. J., Adams, J., & Nestor, P. (2005). Alternate-form reliability of the Dementia Rating Scale-2. *Archives of Clinical Neuropsychology, 20,* 435–441.

Shay, K. A., Duke, L. W., Conboy, T., Harrell, L. E., Callaway, R., & Folks, D. G. (1991). The clinical validity of the Mattis Dementia Rating Scale in staging Alzheimer's dementia. *Journal of Geriatric Psychiatry and Neurology, 4,* 18–25.

Smith, G. E., Ivnik, R. J., Malec, J. F., Kokmen, E., Tangalos, E. G., & Petersen, R. C. (1994). Psychometric properties of the Mattis Dementia Rating Scale. *Assessment, 1,* 123–131.

Teresi, J. A., Holmes, D., Ramirez, M., Gurland, B. J., & Lantigua, R. (2001). Performance of cognitive tests among different racial/ethnic and education groups: Findings of differential item functioning and possible item bias. *Journal of Mental Health and Aging, 17,* 79–89.

Teresi, J. A., Kleinman, M., & Ocepek-Welikson, K. (2000). Modern psychometric methods for detection of differential item functioning: Application to cognitive assessment measures. *Statistics in Medicine, 19,* 1651–1683.

Van Gorp, W. G., Marcotte, T. D., Sultzer, D., Hinkin, C., Mahler, M., & Cummings, J. L. (1999). Screening for dementia: Comparison of three commonly used instruments. *Journal of Clinical and Experimental Neuropsychology, 21,* 29–38.

Van Reekum, R., Simard, M., Clarke, D., Conn, D., Cohen, T., & Wong, J. (2000). The role of depression severity in the cognitive functioning of elderly subjects with central nervous system disease. *Journal of Psychiatry and Neuroscience, 25,* 262–268.

Vangel Jr., S. J., & Lichtenberg, P. A. (1995) Mattis Dementia Rating Scale: Clinical utility and relationship with demographic variables. *The Clinical Neuropsychologist, 9,* 209–213.

Vitaliano, P. P., Breen, A. R., Albert, M. S., Russo, J., & Prinz, P. N. (1984). Memory, attention, and functional status in community-residing Alzheimer type dementia patients and optimally healthy aged individuals. *Journal of Gerontology, 39,* 58–64.

Vitaliano, P. P., Breen, A. R., Russo, J., Albert, M., Vitiello, M., & Prinz, P. N. (1984). The clinical utility of the Dementia Rating Scale for assessing Alzheimer's patients. *Journal of Chronic Disabilities, 37*(9/10), 743–753.

Woodard, J. L., Auchus, A. P., Godsall, R. E., & Green, R. C. (1998). An analysis of test bias and differential item functioning due to race on the Mattis Dementia Rating Scale. *Journal of Gerontology: Psychological Sciences, 53B,* 370–374.

Woodard, J. L., Salthouse, T. A., Godsall, R. E., & Green, R. C. (1996). Confirmatory factor analysis of the Mattis Dementia Rating Scale in patients with Alzheimer's disease. *Psychological Assessment, 8,* 85–91.

Yochim, B. P., Bank, A. L., Mast, B. T., MacNeill, S. E., & Lichtenberg, P. A. (2003). Clinical utility of the Mattis Dementia Rating Scale in older, urban medical patients: An expanded study. *Aging, Neuropsychology and Cognition, 10,* 230–237.

Kaplan Baycrest Neurocognitive Assessment (KBNA)

PURPOSE

The purpose of this test is to provide a comprehensive evaluation of cognitive abilities in individuals aged 20 to 89 years.

SOURCE

The test (including Test Manual, Stimulus Book, Response Chips, cassette, Response Grid, 25 Response Booklets, and Record Forms) can be ordered from the Psychological Corporation, 19500 Bulverde Road, San Antonio, TX 78259 (www.harcourtassessment.com). The kit costs $264 US.

AGE RANGE

The test can be given to individuals aged 20 to 89 years.

DESCRIPTION

The KBNA (Leach et al., 2000) was designed as a comprehensive test to identify and characterize mild as well as severe forms of cognitive dysfunction in adults, including the elderly. The KBNA is intended to capture within a reasonable time period (less than two hours) the full range of neuropsychological functioning using tasks that derive from both behavioral neurology and psychometric approaches. Thus, the KBNA consists of 25 subtests similar in format to those found in widespread clinical use (Orientation, Sequences, Numbers, Word Lists 1 and 2, Complex Figure 1 and 2, Motor Programming, Auditory Signal Detection, Symbol Cancellation, Clocks, Picture Naming, Sentence Reading—Arithmetic, Reading Single Words, Spatial Location, Verbal Fluency, Praxis, Picture Recognition, Expression of Emotion, Practical Problem Solving, Conceptual Shifting, Picture Description—Oral, Auditory Comprehension, Repetition, Picture Description—Written; see Table 6–45 for descriptions).

The subtests were designed to measure specific aspects of functioning and to yield multiple scores (including error analyses) so that the clinician can evaluate the process or processes by which the person completed the tasks. Some of the subtest scores can also be combined to represent higher order

Table 6–45 Description of KBNA Subtests

	Subtest	Description
1	Orientation	Declarative memory for personally relevant information (e.g., date of birth, age)
2	Sequences	Mental control tasks (e.g., recite months of year in normal and reverse sequence, name letters that rhyme with word key)
3	Numbers	Recall set of telephone numbers in two oral-response trials and one written-response trial
4	Word Lists 1	Learn and remember a list of 12 words on four list-learning trials; the list is categorized with four words representing each of three categories
5	Complex Figure 1	Copy of a complex figure
6	Motor Programming	Examinee performs five alternating movements with hands
7	Auditory Signal Detection	Examinee listens to a tape of alphabet letters and signals, by tapping, each time the letter A appears; subtest last for 195 seconds
8	Symbol Cancellation	Examinee is presented with a page containing over 200 geometric figures and asked to circle the figures that match a designated target; time limit is 2 minutes
9	Clocks	Consists of five components: free drawing (with hands set at 10 after 11), predrawn, copy, reading without numbers, and reading with numbers
10	Word List 2	Free recall, cued recall, and recognition of target words from Word List 1
11	Complex Figure 2	Recall and recognition of Complex Figure 1
12	Picture Naming	Naming of 20 black-and-white line drawings; semantic and phonemic cues are provided if patient cannot name item
13	Sentence Reading—Arithmetic	One task requires examinee to read two word problems out loud and calculate the answers, using paper and pencil. The second task requires solving nine calculations involving addition, subtraction, or multiplication
14	Reading Single Words	Examinee reads aloud a set of 10 words and five nonsense words
15	Spatial Location	Examinee is shown a series of figures, each consisting of a rectangle in which are arrayed three to seven dots. The design is hidden and the examinee is asked to place response chips on a response grid in the corresponding locations
16	Verbal Fluency	Consists of three components: "c" words, animals, and first names; 1 minute for each
17	Praxis	Tests of ideomotor praxis for intransitive (e.g., waving), transitive (e.g., turning a key), and buccofacial (e.g., blowing out a candle) movements. If patient fails to perform any movement, the patient is asked to imitate the examiner's performance
18	Picture Recognition	Patient is presented with a series of 40 pictures including those from the Picture Naming task and is asked to indicate if each picture was presented before
19	Expression of Emotion	Examinee must demonstrate a series of facial expressions (angry, happy, surprised, sad); if patient fails, he or she is asked to imitate the examiner's expression
20	Practical Problem Solving	Examiner reads aloud scenarios representing situations of urgency (e.g., if smelled smoke) and examinee has to indicate how he or she would respond
21	Conceptual Shifting	Examinee is presented with a set of four line drawings that can be variously grouped and must indicate the three drawings that are alike and in what way. The examinee must then select three of the same four designs according to another shared attribute and state or describe the attribute
22	Picture Description—Oral	Examinee must describe orally events depicted in a line drawing
23	Auditory Comprehension	Examinee is read five questions (e.g., "Do you put on your shoes after your socks?") and must respond with yes or no
24	Repetition	Examinee is asked to repeat five orally presented items, ranging from single words (e.g., *president*) to complete sentences (e.g., "If he comes, I will go")
25	Picture Description—Written	Examinee is asked to describe events depicted in a line-drawn scene

Table 6–46 KBNA Indices and Contributing Scores

Index	Scores
Attention/Concentration	Sequences total score Spatial Location adjusted score
Memory—Immediate Recall	Word Lists 1—Recall Total score Complex Figure 1—Recall Total score
Memory—Delayed Recall	Word Lists 2—Recall Total score Complex Figure 2—Recall Total score
Memory—Delayed Recognition	Word Lists 2—Recognition Total score Complex Figure 2—Recognition Total score
Spatial Processing	Complex Figure 1—Copy/Clocks combined score
Verbal Fluency	Verbal Fluency—Phonemic score Verbal Fluency—Semantic score
Reasoning/Conceptual Shifting	Practical Problem Solving/Conceptual shifting combined score
Total	Attention/Concentration Index Memory—Immediate Recall Index Memory—Delayed Recall Index Memory—Delayed Recognition Index Spatial Processing Index Verbal Fluency Index Reasoning/Conceptual Shifting Index

domains of functioning that are represented by eight indices. The indices and their contributing subtests (or components of subtests) are shown in Table 6–46. Note that only half of the subtests contribute to the indices. Subtests with acceptable score distributions are included in the indices; the other tests, not in the indices, represent those with highly skewed distributions.

ADMINISTRATION

Directions for administering the items, time limits, and correct responses appear in the test manual. Instructions for recording information for each subtest are also provided on the record form. The subtests should be given in the numbered order in which they appear in the subtest instructions because the durations of the delay intervals are determined by the administration of the intervening tasks. The authors recommend that the test be given in one test session. However, not all subtests need be given to each client (L. Leach, personal

communication, November 7, 2002); the choice depends on whether specific problems need more elaborate testing. In addition, the authors caution that circumstances may warrant deviations from the order and time frame. For example, in cases of suspected aphasia, it is suggested that the examiner begin with the Picture Naming subtest since doing so may allow the examiner to assess the impact of language disturbance on tests of memory and comprehension.

ADMINISTRATION TIME

The test can be administered in about two hours.

SCORING

Most of the subtests require little interpretation of scoring criteria. However, detailed scoring criteria are provided (see Appendix A of the test manual) for Complex Figure 1, Picture Description—Oral, Picture Description—Written, and the Free Drawing Component of Clocks.

The record form provides space to note responses, to convert raw scores to age-based scaled scores (1–19, $M = 10$, $SD = 3$), and to index scores (T score, $M = 50$, $SD = 10$) using tables in Appendices B and C of the Examiner's Manual. Percentile-rank equivalents and confidence intervals at the 90% and 95% levels are also provided for the index scores (Appendix C of the manual). A graph is also available to plot the index scores. The various process scores can also be converted to percentile ranges (<2, 2–16, >16) using age-based tables in Appendix D of the manual. These bands correspond to below average, equivocal, and average, respectively. Subtest and index discrepancy criteria are also provided (Appendix E). The difference between pairs of subtest or index scores required for statistical significance (.05 level) ranges from about four to six points. Discrepancies between indices of about 20 points or more would be considered rare, although this varies considerably depending upon the particular indices selected.

DEMOGRAPHIC EFFECTS

Age

The test authors noted that age impacts performance, with scores declining with advancing age. Accordingly, performance is evaluated relative to age-based norms.

Education

The authors report that level of education may also impact performance, and they provide some data (Table 5.2 in the test manual) showing that performance across the various indices increases with increasing education. However, the various subtest and index scores are not broken down by age as well as education.

Ethnicity

No information is available.

NORMATIVE DATA

Standardization Sample

Norms presented in the KBNA Manual are based on a sample of 700 healthy individuals, aged 20 to 89 years, considered representative of the U.S. population (See Table 6–47).

RELIABILITY

Internal Consistency

Split-half reliability coefficients for the subtests vary depending upon the age group. Considering the average reliability coefficients, they range from marginal (Sequences, $r = .67$) to high (Word Lists 2-Recall, $r = .90$) (see Table 6–48). The average reliability coefficients for the index scores are reported by the authors to be in the .70s to .80s. The average reliability for the total scale score is .81.

Test-Retest Reliability and Practice Effects

The stability of KBNA scores was evaluated in 94 adults (from the normative sample; L. Leach personal communication, November 15, 2004) who were retested following an interval ranging from two to eight weeks. Reliability coefficients were high for the total scale (.85), but lower for the individual sub-

Table 6–47 Characteristics of the KBNA Normative Sample

Number	700
Age	20–89 years[a]
Geographic location	Proportional representation from northeast, north central, south, and west regions of the United States
Sample type	Stratified sample according to 1999 U.S. Census data
Education	≤8 to ≥16 years
Gender	Approximate census proportions of males and females in each age group. About 53% female overall
Race/ethnicity	For each age group, based on racial/ethnic proportions of individuals in those age bands in the U.S. population according to Census data. About 78% Caucasian
Screening	Screened by self-report for medical and psychiatric conditions that could affect cognitive functioning

[a]Broken down into seven age groups: 20–29, 30–39, 40–49, 50–59, 60–69, 70–79, and 80–89, each consisting of 100 participants.

tests (see Table 6–48). Many of these stability coefficients are low due to truncated distributions. Classification as to extent of impairment (below average, equivocal, average) for many of the subtests was, however, relatively consistent from test to retest (see KBNA Manual).

Mean retest scores were generally higher than initial scores (particularly in the areas of memory and spatial processing where gains of about 8 to 10 standard score points were evident); however, on two of the indices (Memory—Delayed Recognition, Verbal Fluency), scores declined by about one point on retest.

Interrater Reliability

Interscorer agreement for some of the subtests that require interpretation (e.g, Complex Figure; Picture Description—Oral, Written; and the Free Drawing Component of Clocks) is not provided, raising concern about the interpretation of these scores.

VALIDITY

Construct Validity

The authors report correlational data suggesting that the KBNA is broadly consistent with the results of other global measures of cognitive status. Thus, the authors report that the KBNA total index score correlated .67 with the WASI FSIQ in about 500 nonimpaired people who participated in the standardization sample. In a small ($N = 14$) mixed clinical sample, the KBNA total index score correlated fairly strongly (.82) with the total score on the Dementia Rating Scale (DRS).

The subtests comprising each index were determined by the authors in part on theoretical grounds. However, intercorrelations between subtests comprising an index are low (see Table 6–49), raising questions regarding the meaning of these indices in individual patients. The manual provides some evidence of construct validity by examining the pattern of intercorrelations among the various indices. The authors note that that the correlations between related KBNA indices (i.e., Immediate, Delayed, and Recognition Memory) are relatively high (.6–.8), while correlations with other indices are relatively lower. However in light of the low correlations between subtests, further research is needed to determine whether these index scores are measuring distinct cognitive constructs.

The authors provide some evidence of convergent validity for some of the KBNA indices in small, clinically mixed samples. Thus, correlations between the KBNA Attention/Concentration Index and various measures of attention on the WAIS-R (Digit Symbol, $r = .64$; Digit Span, $r = .76$) and WMS-III (Spatial Span, $r = .71$) were high, with one exception (WMS-III Mental Control, $r = .24$). With regard to the memory indices, verbal memory (CVLT) scores showed a moderate to high degree of association with the relevant memory indices of the KBNA (.48–.77); however, correlations were low between the Rey-O Delayed Recall measure and the delayed measures of

Table 6–48 Magnitude of Reliability Coefficients of KBNA Subtests and Indices

Magnitude of Coefficient	Internal Consistency	Test-Retest
Very high (.90+)	Word List 2—Recall	

High (.80–.89)	Word Lists 1
	Word List 2—Recognition
	Complex Figure 1—Recall
	Complex Figure 2—Recognition
	Attention/Concentration Index
	Memory—Immediate
	    Recall Index
	Memory—Delayed
	    Recall Index
	Spatial Processing Index
	Total Index
		Sequences
		Attention/Concentration Index
		Total Index

Adequate (.70–.79)	Complex Figure 2—Recall
	Complex Figure 1—Copy/Clocks
	Spatial Location
	Practical Problem Solving/
	    Conceptual Shifting
	Memory—Delayed
	    Recognition Index
	Verbal Fluency Index
	Reasoning/Conceptual
	    Shifting Index
		Word Lists 1
		Word Lists 2—Recall
		Verbal Fluency—Semantic
		Memory-Immediate Recall Index
		Memory—Delayed Recall Index
		Memory—Delayed Recognition
		    Index

Marginal (.60–.69)	Sequences Verbal Fluency—Phonemic Verbal Fluency—Semantic	Complex Figure 1—Recall Complex Figure 2—Recognition Spatial Location Spatial Processing Index

Low (≤.59)		Word Lists 2—Recognition
		Complex Figure 2—Recall
		Complex Figure 1—Copy/Clocks
		Practical Problem Solving/
		    Conceptual Shifting
		Verbal Fluency Index
		Reasoning/Conceptual Shifting
		    Index

the KBNA (−.03 to −.12). As might be expected, the KBNA spatial processing index correlated most strongly with the Rey-O copy score, and the KBNA Reasoning/Conceptual Shifting Index showed a strong relation to WAIS-R measures of crystallized (Vocabulary, $r = .80$) and fluid (Block Design, $r = .81$) ability. While FAS verbal fluency correlated highly with the KBNA Verbal Fluency-Phonemic score ($r = .91$), associations between KBNA Verbal Fluency and the Boston Naming Test were moderate ($r = .49$).

It should also be noted that no information is provided in the manual regarding the construct validity of subtests/process scores not included in the indices.

Clinical Studies

The authors compared a mixed sample, consisting mostly of patients (size of sample not reported) with dementia or head injury, with a matched group of controls and found that the

patients scored significantly below the nonimpaired individuals on all indices except the Reasoning/Conceptual Shifting Index. Unfortunately, no information is provided regarding the severity of impairments in the clinical sample. Therefore, it is not clear if the KBNA is sensitive to mild forms of cognitive disturbance.

COMMENT

The KBNA is not intended as a brief screening tool. Rather, the goal of the authors was to design a measure that could identify domain-specific disorders while maintaining a reasonable administration time. Thus, it has the potential to provide considerable information regarding an individual's functioning in an efficient manner. In addition to assessing a wide array of traditional areas (e.g., memory, attention, naming), it measures behaviors commonly overlooked by neuropsychologists (e.g., praxis, emotion expression). Further, the battery

Table 6–49 Intercorrelations Between Subtests Comprising Indices for Ages 20–89

Index	Correlation Between Subtests
Attention/Concentration	.42
Memory—Immediate Recall	.20
Memory—Delayed Recall	.24
Memory—Delayed Recognition	.22
Verbal Fluency	.57

Note that the Spatial Processing and Reasoning/Conceptual Shifting Index scores are direct linear transformations of their respective contributing scaled scores.

approach facilitates cross-subtest comparisons afforded by a common normative sample. The quantification of process scores (e.g., intrusions, repetitions, perseverations, semantic errors) is also an asset.

However, the KBNA is a new tool, and some of its psychometric properties are less than optimal. Although age-based normative data are provided, users cannot evaluate test performance in the context of both age and education. Further, information on the impact of other demographic variables (e.g., sex, ethnicity/culture) is not reported. The lack of data on the impact of ethnicity suggests considerable caution in the use of the test with members of minority groups.

Many subtests (except Word Lists 1 and Phonemic and Semantic Fluency) have truncated floors and ceilings. For example, an 80-year-old who recalls nothing of the complex figure following the delay obtains a scaled score of 5. Similarly, a 20-year-old who recognizes all of the items from the Complex

Figure only achieves a scaled score of 12. Accordingly, scores from the various subtests must be interpreted with care.

Information needs to be provided regarding interrater reliability. Another consideration is that some of the subtests have reliabilities necessitating considerable caution in interpretation—particularly when the issue of change is of concern. Users are encouraged to refer to tables in the test manual (Tables 3.7–3.12) to determine the confidence that can be had in the accuracy of a particular score.

In addition, the meaning of many of the subtests is unclear and the evidence supporting interpretation of the indices is rather weak. How effective the test is at identifying and characterizing different disorders is also not known, and whether it is more sensitive to impairment than other tests (e.g., DRS, RBANS) remains to be determined. Its sensitivity to change/progression of disorder and relation to functional capacity also needs study.

The KBNA yields a variety of scores, including index scores, subtest scaled scores, process scores, and discrepancy scores. Given the large number of scores that are evaluated in this battery, the process of score conversion/recording is cumbersome. A computerized scoring program would be beneficial. A scoring template for the Symbol Cancellation task would also be helpful.

REFERENCE

Leach, L., Kaplan, E., Rewilak, D., Richards, B., & Proulx, B-B. (2000). *Kaplan Baycrest Neurocognitive Assessment*. San Antonio, TX: The Psychological Corporation.

Kaufman Brief Intelligence Test (K-BIT)

PURPOSE

The aim of this individually administered test is to provide a brief estimate of intelligence for screening and related purposes.

SOURCE

The kit (including Manual, easel, 25 Record Forms, and carry bag) can be ordered from the American Guidance Service, 4201 Woodland Road, Circle Pines, MN 55014-1796 (www.agsnet.com). A new version, the K-BIT-2, has been recently released but is not yet available to us. The cost is $199.99 US for the new version.

AGE RANGE

The test can be given to individuals aged 4 through 90 years.

DESCRIPTION

The test (Kaufman & Kaufman, 1990) is based on the measurement of both verbal and nonverbal abilities. It consists of

two subtests, Vocabulary and Matrices, that are presented in an easel format. The Vocabulary subtest provides an estimated Verbal IQ, the Matrices subtest provides an estimated Nonverbal IQ, and the scores from both measures provide a Composite IQ.

Subtest 1, Vocabulary, is an 82-item measure of verbal ability that demands oral responses for all items. Part A, Expressive Vocabulary (45 items), administered to individuals of all ages, requires the person to provide the name of a pictured object such as a lamp or calendar. Part B, Definitions (37 items), administered to individuals 8 years and older, requires the person to provide the word that best fits two clues (a phrase description and a partial spelling of the word). For example, a dark color: BR__W__. The Vocabulary subtest measures word knowledge and verbal concept formation and is thought to assess crystallized intelligence.

Subtest 2, Matrices, is a 48-item nonverbal measure composed of several types of items involving visual stimuli, both meaningful (people and objects) and abstract (designs and symbols). All items require understanding of relations among stimuli, and all are multiple choice, requiring the patient either to point to the correct response or to say the letter corresponding to the position of the item. For the easiest items, the patient selects which one of five items goes best with a stimulus picture (e.g., a car goes with a truck). For the next set of items, the patient must choose which one of six or eight pictures completes a 2 × 2 or 3 × 3 matrix. Abstract matrices were popularized by Raven (1956, 1960) as a method of assessing intelligence in a more "culture-fair" manner. The ability to solve visual analogies, especially those with abstract stimuli, is considered an excellent measure of fluid reasoning (i.e., the ability to be flexible when encountering novel problem-solving situations).

ADMINISTRATION

Directions for administering the items, the correct responses, and examples of typical responses that should be queried appear on the easel facing the examiner. The only task that requires timing is Definitions. Clients are allowed 30 seconds to respond to each item. Starting points for each task are tailored to the patient's age. Items are organized in units, and the examiner discontinues the task if the patient fails every item in one unit. The order of K-BIT tasks (Vocabulary, Matrices) is fixed but not inviolable. The inclusion of both verbal and nonverbal subtests in the K-BIT allows the examiner flexibility when testing a patient with special needs (e.g., patients with aphasic disorders can be given only the Matrices subtest).

ADMINISTRATION TIME

The test can be administered in about 15 to 30 minutes, depending in part on the age of the patient.

SCORING

The examiner records scores on each task and converts, by means of tables provided in the K-BIT Manual, raw scores to age-based standard scores ($M = 100$, $SD = 15$) for the separate subtests (Vocabulary and Matrices) and the total scale (the K-BIT IQ Composite). Space is also provided on the record form to record confidence intervals (a 90% confidence interval is recommended), percentile ranks, descriptive categories (e.g., average, below average, etc.), normal curve equivalents, and stanines, using tables provided in the K-BIT Manual. Examiners can also compare the patient's performance on the two K-BIT subtests to determine if the difference is significant and unusual by referring to tables in the manual.

DEMOGRAPHIC EFFECTS

Age

Age affects performance. Raw scores on the Expressive Vocabulary task increase steadily from ages 4 to 15 years, begin to peak at about age 16, and maintain that same high level through age 74 before declining in the oldest age group (see

Source). Mean raw scores on the Definitions task increase steadily from ages 6 to 44 years before declining gradually from ages 45 to 69 years; a large decrease is evident for ages 70 and above (see *Source*). Average raw scores on the Matrices subtest increase steadily from ages 4 to 17, peak at ages 17 to 19, and decline steadily across the rest of the adult age range (see *Source*).

Education

In clinical populations, K-BIT scores show a moderate relation with educational attainment (r = about .40) (Hays et al., 2002; Naugle et al., 1993).

Gender

Item analysis suggests no consistent gender differences (Webber & McGillivray, 1998); that is, no single item appears easier for one gender.

Ethnicity

No information is available.

NORMATIVE DATA

Standardization Sample

The K-BIT was normed on a nationwide standardization sample of 2022 people, ages 4 to 92 years (age 4–6: $N = 327$; age 7–19: $N = 1195$; age 20–44: $N = 320$; age 45–92: $N = 180$), stratified according to 1985 and 1990 U.S. Census data on four background variables: gender, geographic region, socioeconomic status, and race or ethnic group (see Table 6–50). Educational attainment of subjects ages 20 to 90 and of the parents of subjects ages 4 to 19 was used to estimate socioeconomic status.

RELIABILITY

Internal Consistency

Split-half reliability coefficients for Vocabulary are excellent, ranging from .89 to .98 ($M = .92$) depending upon the age range. Matrices split-half coefficients range from .74 to .95 ($M = .87$). Matrices coefficients for very young children, ages 4 to 6 years, are acceptable ($M = .78$) but improve with older age groups. The split-half reliability of the K-BIT IQ composite is excellent, with values ranging from .88 to .98 ($M = .93$) (see *Source*; Webber & McGillivray, 1998).

Standard Errors of Measurement

The K-BIT IQ Composite and Vocabulary standard scores have an average standard error of measurement (*SEM*) of about four points across the entire age range, whereas the Matrices standard scores have an average *SEM* of about 5.5

Table 6–50   Characteristics of the K-BIT Normative Sample

Number	2022
Age	4–90 years[a]
Geographic location	Proportional representation from northeast, north central, south, and west regions of the United States
Sample type	Stratified sample so that equal numbers of males and females tested and the sample had same proportional distribution as the U.S. population across dimensions of geographic region, SES, and race or ethnic group according to 1985 and 1990 U.S. Census data
Education	≤4 to ≥16 years[b]
Gender	
Male	50.4%
Females	49.6%
Race/ethnicity	
Caucasian	72%
African American	14.8%
Hispanic	9.4%
Other	3.8%
Screening	Not reported

[a]The oldest person was actually 92 years old.
[b]For ages 4–19 parental education used; ages 20–90 rely on examinee's educational level.

points. A slightly higher standard error was found for the Matrices subtest (about 8.0) in Australian adolescents with an intellectual disability (Webber & McGillivray, 1998).

Test-Retest Reliability and Practice Effects

Test-retest reliability was evaluated by administering the K-BIT twice to 232 normal children and adults ages 5 to 89. The interval between tests ranged from 12 to 145 days, with a mean of 21 days. Reliability coefficients are high (>.90) for all age groups (see *Source*; see also Webber & McGillivray, 1998). Slight practice effects emerge following such short retest periods. One can expect increases of about three standard score points on the K-BIT IQ Composite and about two to four standard score points on the Vocabulary and Matrices subtests on retest. These small increases caused by practice apply equally to all age groups. Thompson et al. (1997) reported similar findings.

VALIDITY

Age Differentiation

As evidence of construct validity, a test that purports to measure intelligence must demonstrate age differentiation. Consistent with expectation (Horn, 1985), average raw scores on

the Expressive Vocabulary task increase steadily during childhood, peak at about age 16, and maintain that same high level through age 74 before declining for the oldest age group. Raw scores on the Definitions task increase steadily to 44 years and then decline gradually. Average raw scores on the Matrices subtest increase up to 17 years and decline steadily with advancing age (see *Demographic Effects* and *Source*).

Correlations to IQ Tests

K-BIT verbal and nonverbal IQ scores correlate moderately well (*r* = about .59) with one another (see *Source*). K-BIT IQ scores also correlate well with other measures of intelligence such as the Wechsler (WISC-R, WISC-III, WAIS-R, WASI), the Stanford-Binet, the Kaufman Assessment Battery for Children, the Peabody Picture Vocabulary Test–3, the Shipley Institute for Living Scale, the Slosson, the Raven's Colored Progressive Matrices and the Test of Nonverbal Intelligence (see *Source*; Bowers & Pantle, 1998; Chin et al., 2001; Donders, 1995; Eisenstein & Engelhart, 1997; Grados & Russo-Garcia, 1999; Lafavor & Brundage, 2000; Naugle et al., 1993; Powell et al., 2002; Prewett, 1992a, 1992b, 1995; Prewett & McCaffery, 1993; Thompson et al., 1997; Webber & McGillivray, 1998). Correlations ranging from .61 to .89 have been reported between K-BIT Composite and Wechsler Full-Scale IQ scores. Correlations tend to be higher for the Vocabulary/VIQ and Composite/Full-Scale IQ indices than for Matrices and Performance IQ scores. For example, in a heterogeneous group of 200 patients referred for neuropsychological assessment, Naugle et al. (1993) reported that correlations between the Verbal, Nonverbal, and Composite scales of the two measures were .83, .77, and .88, respectively. K-BIT scores tend to be about five points higher than their Wechsler counterparts (Chin et al., 2001; Eisenstein & Engelhart, 1997; Grados & Russo-Garcia, 1999; Hays et al., 2002; Naugle et al., 1993; Prewett, 1995; Thompson et al., 1997; Webber & McGillivray, 1998). However, standard errors of estimation between corresponding indices tend to be large (6–12 points), and in a significant proportion of individuals (more than 20%), K-BIT scores under- or overestimate Wechsler scores by 10 points or more (Axelrod & Naugle, 1998; Chin et al., 2001; Donders, 1995; Thompson et al., 1997). For example, Naugle et al. (1993) reported that K-BIT composite scores ranged from 12 points lower to 22 points higher than WAIS-R FSIQ; 5% of the differences between tests exceeded 15 points, or one standard deviation. In short, in individual cases, K-BIT scores can differ markedly from their corresponding Wechsler scores. If the aim is to predict Wechsler IQ indices, then a more accurate estimate can be obtained by using a Wechsler short form (Axelrod & Naugle, 1998; Thompson et al., 1997). Thus, Axelrod and Naugle (1998) noted that on a seven-subtest short form, 92% of the cases fell within 5% of their full WAIS-R score, while on the K-BIT only 50% fell within five points. Even two- and four-subtest short forms of the Wechsler test do better than the K-BIT in predicting Wechsler IQ scores (Axelrod & Naugle,

1998; Eisenstein and Engelhart, 1997). K-BIT IQ composite scores are on average about five points lower than the mean Stanford-Binet Test Composite (Prewett & McCaffery, 1993).

Like longer tests of intelligence (e.g., the Wechsler tests), the K-BIT includes measures of both verbal and nonverbal intelligence. For this reason, the K-BIT has an advantage over alternative screening measures such as the Peabody Picture Vocabulary Test-3, the Test of Nonverbal Intelligence, or the Raven Progressive Matrices, which tap primarily one type of ability (Naugle et al., 1993). However, tests such as the WASI (with its four subtests: Vocabulary, Similarities, Block Design, Matrix Reasoning) show lower correlations among subtests and therefore may provide the clinician with more clinically meaningful information by tapping a broader array of cognitive functions than the K-BIT (Hays et al., 2002). Wechsler short forms may also be appropriate in some situations (see review in this volume).

Although the verbal-nonverbal dichotomy invites the user to contrast the two, the discrepancy derived from the K-BIT tends to correlate only modestly (.23–.59) with that of the WAIS-R (Naugle et al., 1993). Structural equation analysis of the K-BIT and the WAIS-R in a sample of neurologically impaired adults revealed that the K-BIT Vocabulary subtest had a significant visual-spatial component (Burton et al., 1995). That is, the K-BIT appears to provide less of a differentiation between verbal and nonverbal intellectual functions than the WAIS-R. Given this substantial visual-spatial component on the Vocabulary subtest, the K-BIT Verbal IQ may give a spuriously low estimate of verbal intelligence in persons with visual-spatial difficulties and consequently may obscure performance discrepancies between K-BIT Verbal and Matrices IQs (Burton et al., 1995).

Correlations With Other Cognitive Tests

Additional evidence of validity comes from using achievement tests as the criteria. K-BIT Composite scores correlate moderately well (.3–.8) with measures of achievement, such as the WRAT-R/3, the Kaufman Test of Educational Achievement, and the K-FAST (see *Source*; Bowers & Pantle, 1998; Klimczak et al., 2000; Powell et al., 2002; Prewett & McCaffery, 1993). Correlations with measures of memory (CVLT) appear high (.57–.68) (Powell et al., 2002).

Clinical Studies

There is evidence that the test is sensitive to severe forms of central nervous system disturbance. Donovick et al. (1996) reported that neurosurgical patients in the acute stages of recovery and psychiatric patients performed more poorly than healthy college students, individuals with closed head injuries, and children with learning disabilities. However, the test appears to be relatively insensitive to deficits that may occur in those with mild or moderate head injury (Donovick et al., 1996). Donders (1995) reported that in children with loss of consciousness greater than 30 minutes (mean length of coma

about six days), severity of traumatic brain injury (as measured by length of coma) was not related to K-BIT indices, whereas correlations were statistically significant for several WISC-III indices. The K-BIT does not emphasize speed of performance, and this fact may explain the reason why it showed little sensitivity to sequelae associated with traumatic brain injury.

COMMENT

The K-BIT is a useful screening measure of verbal, nonverbal, and general intellectual ability when global estimates are sufficient (e.g., for research purposes or when a subtest profile is not needed), when the examiner wishes to avoid speeded tasks, when time constraints or functional abilities of the patient preclude the use of a longer measure, or when the patient is familiar with standard tests such as the Wechsler. It is also relatively simple to administer, does not require manual or rapid responses, and covers a wide age range. Psychometric properties (reliability, validity) are very good, and the test was normed as a brief test, not as an extrapolation from a comprehensive test—a problem with many of the Wechsler short forms (Kaufman & Kaufman, 2001).

K-BIT scores, however, should be considered tentatively when making clinical decisions, particularly with regard to the presence of impairment and differences between verbal and nonverbal performance. That is, when clinicians need to characterize a person's IQ for possible diagnosis or placement, or will be making inferences about the person's ability profile, then test results need to be supported by a more comprehensive assessment (Kaufman & Kaufman, 2001). Despite the finding that K-BIT scores are highly correlated with IQ scores from other standardized tests, K-BIT scores can differ markedly from their counterparts. Thus, the K-BIT and Wechsler test are not interchangeable. If the goal is to predict Wechsler IQ scores, then Wechsler short forms are the tools of choice. Further, the limited response alternatives (e.g., no manual or rapid responses) that make the K-BIT easy to administer and score preclude an assessment of the diversity of behavior often required in a clinical setting (Naugle et al., 1993). Tests such as the WASI may tap more diverse functions and provide more clinically useful information; however, this issue requires further study. It is also important to bear in mind that the K-BIT does require reading and spelling. The K-BIT-2 does not require these skills and therefore may be more appropriate for individuals with written language disorders.

Users should also bear in mind that the norms for the K-BIT were collected about 20 years ago and some inflation in scores is expected due to the Flynn effect. Therefore, use of the newer version (K-BIT-2) is recommended.

Finally, it should be noted that the K-BIT does not allow the examiner to make meaningful discriminations among individuals with very low levels of functioning (Powell et al., 2002). For example, individuals aged 25 to 34 years who obtain raw scores of 25 or below on the Vocabulary subtest receive a standard score of 40. In patients with severe deficits, tests that have a lower floor (e.g., the Stanford-Binet) may be preferred.

REFERENCES

Axelrod, B. N., & Naugle, R. I. (1998). Evaluation of two brief and reliable estimates of the WAIS-R. *International Journal of Neuroscience, 94,* 85–91.

Bowers, T. L. & Pantle, M. L. (1998). Shipley Institute for Living Scale and the Kaufman Brief Intelligence Test as screening instruments for intelligence. *Assessment, 5,* 187–195.

Burton, D. B., Naugle, R. I., & Schuster, J. M. (1995). A structural equation analysis of the Kaufman Brief Intelligence Test and the Wechsler Intelligence Scale—Revised. *Psychological Assessment, 7,* 538–540.

Chin, C. E., Ledesma, H. M., & Cirino, P. T. (2001). Relation between Kaufman Brief Intelligence Test and WISC-III scores of children with RD. *Journal of Learning Disabilities, 34,* 2–8.

Donders, J. (1995). Validity of the Kaufman Brief Intelligence Test (K-BIT) in children with traumatic brain injury. *Assessment, 2,* 219–224.

Donovick, P. J., Burright, R. G., Burg, J. S., Gronendyke, S. J., Klimczak, N., Mathews, A., & Sardo, J. (1996). The K-BIT: A screen for IQ in six diverse populations. *Journal of Clinical Psychology in Medical Settings, 3,* 131–139.

Eisenstein, N., & Engelhart, C. I. (1997). Comparison of the K-BIT with short forms of the WAIS-R in a neuropsychological population. *Psychological Assessment, 9,* 57–62.

Grados, J. J., & Russo-Garcia, K. A. (1999). Comparison of the Kaufman Brief Intelligence Test and the Wechsler Intelligence Scale for Children-third edition in economically disadvantaged African American youth. *Journal of Clinical Psychology, 59,* 1063–1071.

Hays, J. R., Reas, D. L., & Shaw, J. B. (2002). Concurrent validity of the Wechsler Abbreviated Scale of Intelligence and the Kaufman Brief Intelligence Test among psychiatric patients. *Psychological Reports, 90,* 355–359.

Horn, J. L. (1985). Remodeling old models of intelligence. In B. B. Wolman (Ed.), *Handbook of intelligence.* New York: Wiley.

Kaufman, A. S., & Kaufman, N. L. (1990). *Kaufman Brief Intelligence Test manual.* Circle Pines, MN: American Guidance Service.

Kaufman, J. C., & Kaufman, A. S. (2001). Time for changing of the guard: A farewell to short forms of intelligence. *Journal of Psychoeducational Assessment, 19,* 245–267.

Klimczak, N. C., Bradford, K. A., Burright, R. G., & Donovick, P. J. (2000). K-FAST and WRAT-3: Are they really different? *The Clinical Neuropsychologist, 14,* 135–138.

Lafavor, J. M., & Brundage, S. B. (2000). Correlation among demographic estimates of intellectual abilities, performance IQ scores, and verbal IQ scores in non-brain-damaged and aphasic adults. *Aphasiology, 14,* 1091–1103.

Naugle, R. I., Chelune, G. J., & Tucker, G. D. (1993). Validity of the Kaufman Brief Intelligence Test. *Psychological Assessment, 5,* 182–186.

Powell, S., Plamondon, R., & Retzlaff, P. (2002). Screening cognitive abilities in adults with developmental disabilities: Correlations of the K-BIT, PPVT-3, WRAT-3, and CVLT. *Journal of Developmental and Physical Disabilities, 14,* 239–246.

Prewett, P. N. (1992a). The relationship between the K-BIT and the Wechsler Intelligence Scale for Children—Revised (WISC-R). *Psychology in the Schools, 29,* 25–27.

Prewett, P. N. (1992b). The relationship between the Kaufman Brief Intelligence Test (K-BIT) and the WISC-R with incarcerated juvenile delinquents. *Educational and Psychological Measurement, 52,* 977–982.

Prewett, P. N. (1995). A comparison of two screening tests (the Matrix Analogies Test—short form and the Kaufman Brief Intelligence Test) with the WISC-III. *Psychological Assessment, 7,* 69–72.

Prewett, P. N., & McCaffery, L. K. (1993). A comparison of the Kaufman Brief Intelligence Test (K-BIT) with the Stanford-Binet, a two subtest short form, and the Kaufman Test of Educational Achievement (K-TEA brief form). *Psychology in the Schools, 30,* 299–304.

Raven, J. C. (1956). *Guide to using the Coloured Progressive Matrices* (rev. ed.). London: H.K. Lewis.

Raven, J. C. (1960). *Guide to using the Standard Progressive Matrices* (rev. ed.). London: H.K. Lewis.

Thompson, A., Browne, J., Schmidt, F., & Boer, M. (1997). Validity of the Kaufman Brief Intelligence Test and a four-subtest WISC-III short form with adolescent offenders. *Assessment, 4,* 385–394.

Webber, L. S., & McGillivray, J. A. (1998). An Australian validation of the Kaufman Brief Intelligence Test (K-BIT) with adolescents with an intellectual disability. *The Australian Psychologist, 33,* 234–237.

Mini-Mental State Examination (MMSE)

PURPOSE

The purpose of this test is to screen for mental impairment, particularly in the elderly.

SOURCE

The test (MMSE User's Guide and 50 Test Forms) can be obtained from Psychological Assessment Resources, Inc., P.O. Box 998, Odessa, FL (www.parinc.com), at a cost of $63 US.

AGE RANGE

The test can be given to individuals aged 18 to 85+, although some limited data are available for children aged 10 and older for the MMSE and aged 4 and older for the 3MS.

DESCRIPTION

The MMSE is a popular measure to screen for cognitive impairment, to track cognitive changes that occur with time, and to assess the effects of potential therapeutic agents on cognitive functioning. It is attractive because it is brief, easily administered, and easily scored.

Many of the items were used routinely by neurologists to screen mental ability informally. The items were formalized by Folstein et al. (1975) to distinguish neurological from psychiatric patients. The items were designed to assess orientation to time and place, attention and calculation (serial 7s, spell "world" backward), language (naming, repetition, comprehension, reading, writing, copying), and immediate and delayed recall (three words; see Figure 6–6). Over 100 translations of the MMSE have also been developed, although most

Figure 6–6 Mini-Mental State Examination. Note that the choice of words used to test a person's ability to learn and retain three words was left originally to the discretion of the examiner. Most studies, however, have adopted the words *apple*, *penny*, and *table*. For the pur-pose of testing Canadian patients, the orientation item is modified by replacing state and county with country and province (Lamarre & Patten, 1991). *Source:* Reprinted from Tombaugh & McIntyre, 1992. Copyright Blackwell Publishing.

Item	Max. points
1. What is the: Year? Season? Date? Day? Month?	5
2. Where are we: State (Country)? County (Province)? Town or City? Hospital (Place)? Floor (Street)?	5
3. Name three objects (apple, penny, table), taking one second to say each. Then ask the patient to tell you the three words. Repeat the answers until the patient learns all three, up to six trials. The score is based on the first trial.	3
4. Serial 7s: Subtract 7 from 100. Then subtract 7 from that number, etc. Stop after five subtractions (93, 86, 79, 72, 65).	5
Score the total number of correct answers.	
Alternate: Spell "world" backwards. The score is the number of letters in correct order (e.g., dlrow = 5, dlorw = 3).	
5. Ask for the names of the three objects learned in #3.	3
6. Point to a pencil and watch. Have the patient name them as you point.	2
7. Have the patient repeat "No ifs, ands, or buts" (only one trial).	1
8. Have the patient follow a three-stage command: "Take the paper in your right hand. Fold the paper in half. Put the paper on the floor."	3
9. Have the patient read and obey the following: "Close your eyes." (Write in large letters.)	1
10. Have the patient write a sentence of his or her own choice.	1
11. Have the patient copy the following design (overlapping pentagons).	1

have not been extensively validated (Auer et al., 2000). The interested reader can contact PAR (MMSE Permissions) for one of the available translations.

An expanded version of the MMSE, the Modified Mini-Mental State Examination (3MS), has been developed (Teng & Chui, 1987) to increase the test's sensitivity. Four additional questions that assess temporal and spatial orientation, the ability to see relations between objects, and verbal fluency (i.e., date and place of birth, word fluency, similarities, and delayed recall of words) were added (Figure 6–7). In addition, the 3MS includes items that assess different aspects of memory including cued recall, recognition memory, delayed free and cued recall, and delayed recognition memory. The maximum score was increased from 30 to 100 points, and a modified scoring procedure was introduced that allows partial credit for some items. One of the advantages of the 3MS is that both a 3MS and an MMSE score can be derived from a single administration.

The 3MS has been studied in a pediatric sample (Besson & Labbe, 1997) and the MMSE has been adapted for use in pediatric settings (Ouvrier et al., 1993). The items are shown in Figure 6–8.

ADMINISTRATION

The examiner asks questions and records responses. Questions are asked in the order listed (see Figures 6–6 through 6–8) and are scored immediately. In addition, the following suggestions are offered:

1. The version for adults should not be given unless the person has at least an eighth-grade education level and is fluent in English (Tombaugh & McIntyre, 1992).
2. A written version of the test may be preferable for hearing-impaired individuals (Uhlmann et al., 1989).

Figure 6–7 Modified Mini-Mental State (3MS) Examination. *Source:* Reprinted from Teng & Chui, 1987. Copyright 1987 by the Physicians Postgraduate Press. Reprinted with permission.

Name: _____   Date: _____   Age: _____

Education: _____   Gender: _____

Total Score: _____ **/100**

Administered by: _____

Date & Place of Birth

- "What is your date of birth?"   Year _____ (1)   Month _____ (1)   Day_____ (1)

- "What is your place of birth?"   Town/City _____ (1)   Province/State _____ (1)

Total Score ___ /5

Registration

- "I shall say three words for you to remember. Repeat them after I have said all 3 words":

  ☐ SHIRT . . . ☐ BROWN . . . ☐ HONESTY   (or: SHOES . . . BLACK . . . MODESTY, or: SOCKS . . . BLUE . . . CHARITY)

- "Remember what they are because I am going to ask you to name them again in a few minutes." Accurate repetition (1 point each) Score _____ (3) # of trials needed to repeat all three words _____ (no score)

Total Score ___ /3

Mental Reversal

- "Can you count from 1 to 10? Like this, 1,2,3, all the way to 10. Go." Answer _____

  If correct say:

- "Now, can you to count backwards from 5? Go."

  Answer _____ Accurate repetition (2); 1 or 2 misses (1)   Score_____ (2)

- "Now I am going to spell a word forwards and I want you to spell it backwards. The word is 'world,' W-O-R-L-D. Spell 'world' backwards."

  (Print letters) _____ (D L R O W)

  Accurate repetition (1) each correctly placed letter Score _____ (5)

Total Score ___ /7

First Recall

- "What are the 3 words that I asked you to remember?" (If not recalled, provide a category prompt; if not recalled ask them to choose one of the three multiple-choice options; if correct answer not given, score 0 and provide the correct answer.)

Spontaneous Recall	*Category Prompt*	*Multiple Choice*
☐ Shirt (3)	☐ Something to wear (2)	☐ Shoes, Shirt, Socks (1)
☐ Brown (3)	☐ A color (2)	☐ Blue, Black, Brown (1)
☐ Honesty (3)	☐ A good personal quality (2)	☐ Honesty, Charity, Modesty (1)

Total Score ___ /9

(continued)

Figure 6–7 (*continued*)

Temporal Orientation

- "What is the year?" _____ Accurate (8); miss by 1 year (4); miss by 2–5 years (2)   Score _____ (8)

- "What is the season?" _____ Accurate or within 1 month (1)   Score _____ (1)

- "What is the month?" _____ Accurate within 5 days (2); miss by 1 month (1)   Score _____ (2)

- "What is the date?" _____ Accurate (3); miss by 1–2 days (2); miss by 3–5 days (1)   Score _____ (3)

- "What is the day of the week?" _____ Accurate (1)   Score _____ (1)

Total Score ___ /15

Spatial Orientation

- "Can you tell me where we are right now? For instance, what state/province are we in?" _____ (2)

- "What city are we in?" _____ (1)

- "Are we in a hospital or office building or home?" _____ (1)

- "What is the name of this place?" _____ (1)

- "What floor of the building are we on?" (no score) _____ (0)

Total Score ___ /5

Naming

- "What is this called?" (show wristwatch) ☐ (no score)

- "What is this called?" (show pencil) ☐ (no score)

- "What is this called?" (point to a part of your own body; score 0 if subject cannot readily name)

  Shoulder ☐ (1) Chin ☐ (1) Forehead ☐ (1) Elbow ☐ (1) Knuckle ☐ (1)

Total Score ___ /5

Four-Legged Animals

- "What animals have four legs?" ***Allow 30 seconds*** (record responses). If no response after 10 seconds repeat the question once. Prompt after only the first incorrect answer by saying: "I want four-legged animals."

_____ (1) _____ (1) _____ (1) _____ (1)

_____ (1) _____ (1) _____ (1) _____ (1)

_____ (1) _____ (1)

Total Score ___ /10

Similarities

- "In what way are an arm and a leg alike?"

_____

If incorrect, this time only, prompt with: "An arm and leg are both limbs or parts of the body."

Score _____ Both are body parts; limbs; etc. (2)

Score _____ Less accurate answer (0 or 1)

(*continued*)

Figure 6–7 *(continued)*

- "In what way are laughing and crying alike?"

  _____

  Score _____ Both are feelings, emotions (2)

  Score _____ Less accurate answer (0 or 1)

- "In what way are eating and sleeping alike?"

  _____

  Score _____ Both are essential for life (2)

  Score _____ Less accurate answer (0 or 1)

  Total Score ___ /6

Repetition

- "Repeat what I say: 'I would like to go home/out.'"   Accurate   Score _____ (2)

                                                    1–2 missed/wrong words   Score _____ (0 or 1)

- "Now repeat: No ifs □, ands □, or buts □."   Accurate   Score _____ (3)

  (no credit if "s" is left off a word)   One point each   Score _____ (1 or 2)

  Total Score ___ /5

Read & Obey   Hold up piece of paper on which the command is printed "Close your eyes."

- "Please do this." (wait 5 seconds, if no response provide next prompt)

- "Read and do what this says." (if already said or reads the sentence only provide next prompt)

- "Do what this says."

  Obeys without prompting   Score _____ (3)

  Obeys after prompting   Score _____ (2)

  Reads aloud only (no eye closure) Score _____ (0 or 1)

  Total Score ___ /3

Writing

  Provide subject with a pencil with eraser and say:

- "Please write this down, 'I would like to go home/out.'" Repeat sentence word by word, if necessary.

  Allow one minute.

  Do not penalize self-corrections. (1) point for each word, except "I"   Score _____ (5)

  Total Score ___ /5

  (continued)

Figure 6–7 (*continued*)

Copying Two Pentagons

- "Here is a drawing. Please copy the drawing on the same paper." **Allow one minute**. If subject needs longer, document how much of design was completed in one minute and allow him or her to finish.

	Pentagon 1	*Pentagon 2*	
5 approximately equal sides	Score _____ (4)	Score _____ (4)	Intersection
5 unequal sides (>2:1)	Score _____ (3)	Score _____ (3)	4 corners _____ (2)
Other enclosed figure	Score _____ (2)	Score _____ (2)	Not-4-corner enclosure _____ (1)
2 or more lines	Score _____ (1)	Score _____ (1)	No enclosure (0)
Less than 2 lines	Score _____ (0)	Score _____ (0)	

Total Score ___ /10

Three-Stage Command

Hold up a sheet of plain paper and say:

- "Take this paper with your left hand ☐, fold it in half ☐, and hand it back to me ☐."

(Note: use right hand for left-handed patients; *do not* repeat any part of the command or give visual cues to return the paper, such as keeping hand in ready to receive posture. Score (1) point for each step.)

Total Score ___ /3

Second Recall

- "What are the 3 words that I asked you to remember?" (If not recalled, provide a category prompt; if not recalled ask them to choose one of the three multiple-choice options; if correct answer not given, score 0)

Spontaneous Recall	*Category Prompt*	*Multiple Choice*
☐ Shirt (3)	☐ Something to wear (2)	☐ Shoes, shirt, socks (1)
☐ Brown (3)	☐ A color (2)	☐ Blue, black, brown (1)
☐ Honesty (3)	☐ A good personal quality (2)	☐ Honesty, charity, modesty (1)

Total Score ___ /9

Total Score: _____ /100

(*continued*)

Figure 6–7 *(continued)*

CLOSE YOUR EYES

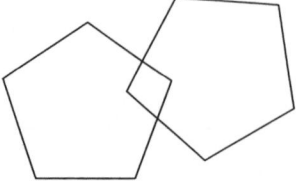

Figure 6–8 MMSE for children. *Source:* From Ouvrier et al., 1993. Reprinted with permission of BC Decker.

Orientation		Score	Points
1. What is the	Year?		1
	Season?		1
	Date?		1
	Day?		1
	Month?		1
2. Where are we?	Country		1
	State or territory		1
	Town or city		1
	Hospital or suburb		1
	Floor or address		1

Registration

3. Name three objects, taking one second to say each. Then ask the patient all three after you have said them twice (tree, clock, boat). Give one point for each correct answer. Repeat the items until patient learns all three. **3**

Attention and Calculation

4. Serial 7s. Give one point for each correct answer.
   Stop after five answers. **5**

5. Spell "world" backwards.
   The practice word "cat" can be used for younger or children suspected of significant intellectual deficits.
   Older children are first asked to spell "world" forward and then backward. **5**

Recall

6. Ask for names of three objects learned in Q3. Give one point for each correct answer. **3**

Language

7. Point to a pencil and a watch. Have the patient name them as you point. **2**

8. Have the patient repeat "No ifs, ands, or buts."
   Say the sentence twice before asking the patient to repeat. **1**

9. Have the patient follow a three-stage command. "Take a piece of paper in your right hand.
   Fold the paper in half.
   Put the paper on the floor." **3**

10. Have the patient read and obey the following: "Close your eyes." (Write in large letters.) **1**

11. Have the patient write a sentence of his or her choice. (The sentence should contain a subject and an object, and should make sense. Ignore spelling errors when scoring.) **1**

12. Have the patient copy the design printed below. (Give one point if all sides and angles are preserved and if the intersecting sides form diamond shape.) **1**

Total **35**

3. Serial 7s and "world" should not be considered equivalent items. Tombaugh and McIntyre (1992) recommend that both items should be given and the higher of the two used, although Espino et al. (2004) recommend giving serial 7s alone to increase reliability and discriminative ability. Folstein et al. (2001) indicate that "world" should only be given if the examinee refuses to perform the serial 7s task. Further, "world" should be spelled forward (and corrected) prior to spelling it backward (Folstein et al., 2001; Tombaugh & McIntyre, 1992).

4. Item 2 of the MMSE (i.e., "where are we" orientation-to-place questions) should be modified. The name of the county (province) where the person lives should be asked rather than the name of the county where the test is given. The name of the street where the individual lives should be asked rather than the name of the floor where the testing takes place (Tombaugh & McIntyre, 1992).

5. The words *apple, penny,* and *table* should be used for registration and recall. If necessary, the words may be administered up to three times to obtain perfect registration, but the score is based on the first trial (Tombaugh & McIntyre, 1992).

6. Alternative word sets (e.g., *pony, quarter, orange*) can be substituted (Folstein et al., 2001; Teng & Chui, 1987) when retesting an examinee. Note, however, that the equivalence of the various sets has not been established.

7. If any physical limitations prevent the individual from using the right hand on the Comprehension task or for placing the paper on the floor, it is acceptable to instruct the individual to use his or her left hand or to place the paper on a table.

ADMINISTRATION TIME

The task can be administered in 5 to 10 minutes.

SCORING

The score is the total number of correct answers. The maximum score for the MMSE is 30 points for the adult version and 35 points for the children's version. See Folstein et al. (2001) for detailed scoring criteria. For the 3MS, the maximum score is 100. Failures to respond should be scored as errors (Fillenbaum, Hughes, et al., 1988).

Scoring criteria are fairly explicit for the 3MS. However, the following is recommended:

1. Registration/recall: Accept only the correct suffix. For example, do not accept "shoe" for "shoes" or "honest" for "honesty."

2. Repetition: Give no credit if the "s" is omitted.

3. Writing: Assign one point for each correct word, but give no credit for "I." Do not penalize self-corrected errors.

DEMOGRAPHIC EFFECTS

Age

MMSE/3MS scores increase with age in children (Ouvrier et al., 1993) and decrease with advancing age in adults (Antsey et al., 2000; Bleeker et al., 1988; Bravo & Hebert, 1997a; Brown et al., 2003; Crum et al., 1993; Dufouil et al., 2000; Freidl et al., 1996; Jorm et al., 1988; O'Connell et al., 2004; O'Connor et al., 1989; Olin & Zelinski, 1991; Starr et al., 1992; Tombaugh & McIntyre, 1992; Tombaugh et al., 1996). In children, scores for both the MMSE and 3MS reach a plateau at about 9 or 10 years of age (Besson & Labbe, 1997; Ouvrier et al., 1993). Most of the age-related change in adults begins at about age 55 to 60 and then dramatically accelerates at the age of 75 to 80. These age effects persist even when individuals are stratified by educational level.

IQ/Education

MMSE/3MS scores are related to premorbid intelligence and educational attainment: Individuals with higher premorbid ability and/or more education tend to score higher than those with lower IQs and/or few years of schooling (Anthony et al., 1982; Antsey et al., 2000; Bravo & Hebert, 1997a; Brown et al., 2003; Christensen & Jorm, 1992; Crum et al., 1993; Dufouil et al., 2000; Fountoulakis et al., 2000; Freidl et al., 1996; Ishizaki et al., 1998; Jorm et al., 1988; Marcopulos et al., 1997; O'Connell et al., 2004; O'Connor et al., 1989; Olin & Zelinski, 1991; Ouvrier et al., 1993; Starr et al., 1992; Taussig et al., 1996; Tombaugh et al., 1996; Van Der Cammen et al., 1992). IQ has a stronger relationship to MMSE scores than education (Bieliauskas et al., 2000). There is evidence that low educational or intelligence levels increase the likelihood of misclassifying normal people as cognitively impaired while higher ability and educational levels may mask mild impairment. Education and premorbid ability, however, may also reflect etiological factors (e.g., hypertension, obesity) critical in the process that eventually results in some form of dementia (e.g., ischemic vascular dementia). In short, education may represent a psychometric bias and/or a risk factor (for further discussion, see Crum et al., 1993; Jorm et al., 1988; Tombaugh & McIntyre, 1992).

Gender

Gender has little impact on the total score (e.g., Antsey et al., 2000; Besson & Labbe, 1997; Bleecker et al., 1988; Bravo & Hebert, 1997a; O'Connor et al., 1989; but see Brown et al., 2003). Some (Bleecker et al., 1988; Jones & Gallo, 2002; O'Connor et al., 1989) have reported that gender influences performance on some items. For example, Jones and Gallo (2002) reported that women are more likely to err on serial subtractions and men on spelling and other language tasks; however, the magnitude of the effect tends to be quite small.

Race/Ethnicity/Language

There is some evidence that MMSE scores are affected by race/ethnicity and social class (e.g., Espino et al., 2004; Mulgrew et al., 1999; Taussig et al., 1996). MMSE scores tend to be decreased in individuals of nonwhite ethnicity (Espino et al., 2001; Espino et al., 2004; Shadlen et al., 1999; but see Ford et al., 1996; Marcopulos et al., 1997; Marcopulos & McLain, 2003) and lower social class. Ethnic differences, at least in the case of Mexican Americans, appear related to educational differences and location of residence (neighbourhood) with barrio residents scoring considerably lower than Mexican Americans living in transitional neighbourhoods and the suburbs (Espino et al., 2001). Espino and colleagues (2001) have speculated that the regional differences reflect cultural and/or social factors (e.g., differences in familiarity with the kinds of skills measured by the MMSE, daily stress, assimilation).

Some of the items appear to be biased with respect to race/ethnicity and education (Jones & Gallo, 2002; Mulgrew et al., 1999; Teresi et al., 2001). For example, the sentence production item appears easier for Caucasians than for African Americans. The items "close your eyes" and serial 7s are also problematic, having different results for various ethnic and education groups.

There is also some evidence that language of testing may impact performance. For example, Bravo and Hebert (1997a) noted that English-speaking older adults performed slightly better than their French-speaking counterparts, although the effect was very small (less than one point for the MMSE and about two points for the 3MS).

Other

Health status (e.g., history of heart disease) impacts performance (Antsey et al., 2000). There is also evidence that impending mortality lowers performance. The mortality-related effects appear most pronounced within three years before death; however, the magnitude of the effect is relatively small (Tan, 2004).

NORMATIVE DATA—ADULTS

MMSE

Extensive norms by age (18 to approximately 85 years) and education (no formal schooling to one or more college degrees) have been reported (Crum et al., 1993), based on probability sampling of more than 18,000 community-dwelling adults. The sample includes individuals, regardless of their physical or mental health status, from five metropolitan areas: New Haven, Baltimore, Durham, St. Louis, and Los Angeles. The data are presented in Table 6–51. Iverson (1998) derived age- and education-corrected cutoff scores for individuals aged 60 and above in this dataset. The cutoffs, also shown in Table 6–51, are greater than 1.64 standard deviations below the sample mean (if normally distributed, 90% of all scores

should fall within ± 1.64 z score units from the mean). Note that the MMSE scores were based on either the response to serial 7s or spelling "world" backwards, whichever yielded the higher score. Also note the wider range of scores in the lowest educational groups and at the oldest ages. MMSE scores ranged from a median of 29 for those aged 18 to 24 years to 25 for individuals aged 80 years and older. The median MMSE score was 29 for individuals with at least 9 years of schooling, 26 for those with 5 to 8 years of schooling, and 22 for those with 0 to 4 years of schooling.

Similar data have been reported for rural U.S. elderly (ages 55+) with low education (Marcopulos & McLain, 2003), older adults (aged 62–95) living in retirement villages and institutions in Australia (Antsey et al., 2000), and participants (ages 65+) drawn from various geographical regions in Canada, who were classified as cognitively intact on the basis of an extensive battery of neuropsychological and medical tests (Bravo & Hebert, 1997a; Tombaugh et al., 1996). About 95% of nondemented older adults score over 23 on the MMSE (Bravo and Hebert, 1997a; Meiran et al., 1996).

3MS

Bravo and Hebert (1997a) provide data based on 7,754 adults, aged 65+, randomly chosen to take part in the Canadian Study of Health and Aging (CSHA). Individuals classed as cognitively impaired or demented following a clinical and neuropsychological examination were excluded. The reference values, stratified by age and education, are shown in Table 6–52. About 95% of the sample obtained a score over 76.

Other smaller normative sets have also been provided. Thus, Tombaugh et al. (1996) report percentile scores derived from a select subsample of the CSHA, judged to be cognitively intact on the basis of an extensive clinical examination. The normative data were stratified across two age groups (65–79 and 80–89) and two educational levels (0–8 and 9+ years). Jones et al. (2002) present normative data on the 3MS for a sample of 393 U.S. community-dwelling, primarily Caucasian, older adults. Their sample of individuals aged 80+ or with less than 12 years of education is relatively small ($N = 44$).

Brown et al. (2003) have recently reported normative data based on a sample of 238 African American, community-dwelling older adults, aged 60 to 84. Tables 6–53 and 6–54 provide these data along with the score adjustments for education and gender. Brown et al. (2003) caution that the quality of education varies greatly within the population of African Americans and that matching on years of education does not necessarily mean that the quality of education is comparable.

NORMATIVE DATA—CHILDREN

MMSE

For the children's version of the MMSE, Ouvrier et al. (1993) tested a heterogeneous sample of 117 children who attended

Table 6–51 Mini-Mental State Examination Score by Age and Education Level, Number of Participants, Mean, *SD*, and Selected Percentiles

Educational Level	Age (Years)							
	18–24	25–29	30–34	35–39	40–44	45–49	50–54	55–59
0–4 years *N*	17	23	41	33	36	28	34	49
Mean	22	25	25	23	23	23	23	22
SD	2.9	2.0	2.4	2.5	2.6	3.7	2.6	2.7
Lower quartile	21	23	23	20	20	20	20	20
Median	23	25	26	24	23	23	22	22
Upper quartile	25	27	28	27	27	26	25	26
5–8 years *N*	94	83	74	101	100	121	154	208
Mean	27	27	26	26	27	26	27	26
SD	2.7	2.5	1.8	2.8	1.8	2.5	2.4	2.9
Lower quartile	24	25	24	23	25	24	25	25
Median	28	27	26	27	27	27	27	27
Upper quartile	29	29	28	29	29	29	29	29
9–12 years or high school diploma *N*	1326	958	822	668	489	423	462	525
Mean	29	29	29	28	28	28	28	28
SD	2.2	1.3	1.3	1.8	1.9	2.4	2.2	2.2
Lower quartile	28	28	28	28	28	27	27	27
Median	29	29	29	29	29	29	29	29
Upper quartile	30	30	30	30	30	30	30	30
College experience or higher degree *N*	783	1012	989	641	354	259	220	231
Mean	29	29	29	29	29	29	29	29
SD	1.3	0.9	1.0	1.0	1.7	1.6	1.9	1.5
Lower quartile	29	29	29	29	29	29	28	28
Median	30	30	30	30	30	30	30	29
Upper quartile	30	30	30	30	30	30	30	30
Total *N*	2220	2076	1926	1443	979	831	870	1013
Mean	29	29	29	29	28	28	28	28
SD	2.0	1.3	1.3	1.8	2.0	2.5	2.4	2.5
Lower quartile	28	28	28	28	27	27	27	26
Median	29	29	29	29	29	29	29	29
Upper quartile	30	30	30	30	30	30	30	30

Educational Level	Age (Years)						Total
	60–64	65–69	70–74	75–79	80–84	≥85	
0–4 years *N*	88	126	139	112	105	61	892
Mean	23	22	22	21	20	19	22
SD	1.9	1.9	1.7	2.0	2.2	2.9	2.3
Lower quartile	19	19	19	18	16	15	19
Median	22	22	21	21	19	20	22
Upper quartile	26	25	24	24	23	23	25
Abnormal cutoff	19	18	19	17	16	14	
5–8 years *N*	310	633	533	437	241	134	3223
Mean	26	26	26	25	25	23	26
SD	2.3	1.7	1.8	2.1	1.9	3.3	2.2
Lower quartile	24	24	24	22	22	21	23
Median	27	27	26	26	25	24	26
Upper quartile	29	29	28	28	27	27	28
Abnormal cutoff	22	23	23	21	21	17	
9–12 years or high school diploma *N*	626	814	550	315	163	99	8240
Mean	28	28	27	27	25	26	28
SD	1.7	1.4	1.6	1.5	2.3	2.0	1.9

(continued)

Table 6-51 Mini-Mental State Examination Score by Age and Education Level, Number of Participants, Mean, *SD*, and Selected Percentiles (*continued*)

Educational Level	Age (Years)						
	60–64	65–69	70–74	75–79	80–84	≥85	Total
Lower quartile	27	27	26	25	23	23	27
Median	28	28	28	27	26	26	29
Upper quartile	30	29	29	29	28	28	30
Abnormal cutoff	25	25	24	24	21	22	
College experience or higher degree *N*	270	358	255	181	96	52	5701
Mean	29	29	28	28	27	27	29
SD	1.3	1.0	1.6	1.6	0.9	1.3	1.3
Lower quartile	28	28	27	27	26	25	29
Median	29	29	29	28	28	28	29
Upper quartile	30	30	29	29	29	29	30
Abnormal cutoff	26	27	25	25	25	24	
Total *N*	1294	1931	1477	1045	605	346	18,056
Mean	28	27	27	26	25	24	28
SD	2.0	1.6	1.8	2.1	2.2	2.9	2.0
Lower quartile	26	26	24	23	21	21	27
Median	28	28	27	26	25	25	29
Upper quartile	29	29	29	28	28	28	30
Abnormal cutoff	24	24	24	22	21	19	

Data from the Epidemiologic Catchment Area household surveys in New Haven, CT; Baltimore, MD; St. Louis, MO; Durham, NC; and Los Angeles, CA, between 1980 and 1984. The data are weighted based on the 1980 U.S. population Census by age, gender, and race.

Source: From Crum et al., 1993. Copyright, American Medical Association. Iverson (1998) provides the abnormal cutoff scores, which are greater than 1.64 standard deviations below the sample means for participants aged 60 and above.

private or outpatient clinics. They suggest that values below 27/35 are abnormal in children over the age of 10 years; however, definition of lower limits of normal at various ages remains to be determined.

3MS

Besson and Labbe (1997) gathered preliminary data on the 3MS in a sample of 79 children, free of neurological impairment as reported by parents and medical history. Means and stan-

Table 6-52 Age- and Education-Specific Reference Values for the 3MS Based on a Sample 7754 Normal Elderly Across Canada

Education	Age (Years)				
	65–69	70–74	75–79	80–84	85+
0–4 years	*N* = 78	*N* = 85	*N* = 93	*N* = 78	*N* = 65
	82.0 (8.7)	82.6 (7.5)	81.0 (5.4)	79.6 (8.1)	77.0 (8.8)
	(70, 79, 82)	(71, 78, 83)	(70, 77, 83)	(65, 76, 81)	(50, 74, 80)
5–8 years	*N* = 495	*N* = 422	*N* = 556	*N* = 277	*N* = 239
	87.1 (7.7)	87.1 (8.1)	85.7 (5.8)	84.0 (6.0)	82.6 (5.1)
	(76, 83, 88)	(78, 83, 87)	(75, 81, 86)	(70, 79, 85)	(66, 78, 83)
9–12 years	*N* = 942	*N* = 752	*N* = 921	*N* = 455	*N* = 332
	91.7 (6.5)	90.7 (6.3)	89.8 (4.7)	87.5 (5.1)	85.6 (4.3)
	(81, 89, 93)	(80, 87, 92)	(79, 86, 90)	(76, 83, 88)	(72, 81, 86)
13 years and over	*N* = 581	*N* = 375	*N* = 535	*N* = 236	*N* = 208
	93.9 (5.7)	92.9 (6.4)	91.3 (5.2)	89.8 (5.3)	88.0 (4.2)
	(85, 92, 95)	(82, 91, 94)	(80, 88, 92)	(79, 86, 91)	(75, 84, 89)

Data reported as sample size, mean (standard deviation), and (5th, 25th, 50th) percentiles.

Source: From Bravo & Hebert, 1997a. Reproduced with permission, John Wiley & Sons.

Table 6–53 Percentile Scores for 3MS Raw Scores Based on a Sample of Elderly African American Adults

Raw Score	Age Group	
	60–71	72–84
100		
99	97	99
98	94	98
97	89	98
96	87	94
95	84	92
94	80	89
93	75	81
92	69	78
91	60	76
90	54	73
89	48	69
88	46	63
87	41	60
86	38	58
85	34	52
84	28	50
83	23	47
82	20	43
81	16	38
80	13	36
79	12	33
78	10	32
77	8	32
76	8	29
75	7	26
74	6	26
73	5	25
72	4	23
71	3	21
70	3	21
69	2	18
68	2	17
67	1	15
66	1	15
65	1	14
64	1	13
63	<1	10
62	<1	9
61	<1	7
60	<1	6
59	<1	6
58	<1	6
57	<1	3
56	<1	2
55	<1	2
54	<1	1

Based on a sample of 238 African Americans who reported no history of neurological disorder. The sample was not screened for psychiatric disorder.

Source: From Brown et al., 2003. Reproduced with the kind permission of Psychology Press.

Table 6–54 Adjustments for 3MS Raw Scores for Elderly African Americans

Years of Education	Age Group			
	60–71		72–84	
	Male	Female	Male	Female
<12	+4	0	+7	−3
12	0	−2	−1	−11
>12	−4	−7	−13	−12

Source: From Brown et al., 2003. Reproduced with the kind permission of Psychology Press.

dard deviations of scores are shown in Table 6–55. Note that cell sizes are very small.

RELIABILITY

MMSE

Internal Consistency. With regard to the standard version, estimates of internal consistency range from .31 for community-based samples to .96 for a mixed group of medical patients (Espino et al., 2004; Foreman, 1987; Hopp et al., 1997; Jorm et al., 1988; Lopez et al., 2005; Tombaugh et al., 1996). The lower reliability in some samples likely reflects the reduced variability in healthy and better-educated samples. Lopez et al. (2005) suggest that reliabilities may be sufficiently high for clinical use if examiners use true score confidence intervals.

The MMSE can be scored using three strategies: serial 7s or spelling (using the greater number of correct responses from either item), serial 7s only, and spelling only. The serial 7s-only method maximized variability and yielded the highest alpha coefficient ($r = .81$) in a community-based sample. The serial 7s or spelling method yielded a marginally adequate level ($r = .68$), while the alpha coefficient for the spelling only method was less than optimal ($r = .59$; Espino et al., 2004).

Table 6–55 Children's Norms for the 3MS

Age	Mean	SD	N
4	26.9	11.6	11
5	46.6	11.2	16
6	59.7	9.5	11
7	78.1	12.9	9
8	84.5	4.3	11
9	85.3	6.2	7
10	89.6	2.4	4
11	92.0	2.9	5
12	90.6	6.5	5

Based on a sample of 79 children, aged 4–12 years, with no history of neurological disorder.

Source: From Besson & Labbe, 1997. Reprinted with permission of BC Decker.

Table 6–56 Regression Formula for Detecting Reliable Change on the MMSE and 3MS

	Percent of Variance Explained by all Variables (R^2) Total	Formula for Obtaining Predicted Score	Value Needed for Detecting Reliable Change
MMSE Short Interval	.41	.38 (test 1)−.07 (age) + .10 (educ) + 21.65	±2.73
3MS Short Interval	.60	.53 (test 1)−.27 (age) + .20 (educ) + 62.60	±7.41
MMSE Long Interval	.37	.45 (test 1)−.09 (age) + 1.06 (sex) + 19.12	±3.60
3MS Long Interval	.53	.52 (test 1)−.23 (age) + .30 (educ) + 1.93 (sex) + 53.86	±9.82

Based on a sample of 232 older adults who were retested following three-month and five-year intervals and who received consensus diagnoses of no cognitive impairment on both examinations. RCI-Reg-Reliable Change Index—Regression: After the predicted retest score is obtained, it is subtracted from the observed retest score. If this change score exceeds the Value Needed for Dectecting Reliable Change, it is considered to represent a significant change at .05 (one tailed). Age and education are expressed in years. Sex was coded as male = 1 and female = 2.

Source: Reprinted from Tombaugh (2005). Reprinted with permission from Elsevier.

Test-Retest Reliability and Practice Effects. Test-retest reliability estimates for intervals of less than two months generally fall between .80 and .95 (see Clark et al., 1999; Folstein et al., 1975; O'Connor et al., 1989; Tombaugh & McIntyre, 1992, for a review). In patients with probable AD retested within a two-week period, slight improvement is noted (.2 to ± 2.1 points), with most patients (95%) showing a short-term change of four points or less (Doraiswamy & Kaiser, 2000). Following retest intervals of about three months, nondemented individuals tend to show slight improvement (less than one point) (Tombaugh, 2005), while individuals with dementia or mild cognitive impairment tend not to benefit from prior exposure to the test (Helkala et al., 2002).

With lengthier retest intervals (e.g., 1–2 years), normal subjects typically show a small amount of change (less than two points), and retest correlations are lower (<.80) (Hopp et al., 1997; Mitrushina & Satz, 1991; Olin & Zelinski, 1991), perhaps due in part to the inclusion at one time of individuals with mild cognitive impairment (Tombaugh, in press). Recall and Attention subtests tend to be the least reliable (Olin & Zelinski, 1991).

In patients with probable AD, the average annual change in MMSE score is about four points, although there is high measurement error (which almost equals the average annual score change) and there is striking variability among individuals (Clark et al., 1999; Doody et al., 2001). It is not uncommon for patients to have a stable or even an improved score during a one-year interval (Chan et al., 1999). The implication of these findings is that clinicians monitoring change in older adults should be cautious in interpreting small changes in scores. Iverson (1998) has reported that depending upon the age and education of the patient, changes of about two points may be statistically reliable. However, Clark et al. (1999) have suggested that to be clinically meaningful (rather than merely reflecting testing imprecision), a change in MMSE score must exceed three points. Doody et al. (2001) recommend a drop of five or more points to reflect clinically meaningful decline.

Over intervals of five years, test-retest correlations are limited for older adults (65–99 years) classed as intact on both test occasions (.55) as well as for individuals who were reclassified as

showing mild cognitive impairment on the second test session (.59) (Tombaugh, 2005). In part, the modest correlation for intact individuals is due to regression to the mean (high scores tend to decline whereas low scores tend to increase on subsequent testing). However, there is also considerable variability among older individuals over the five-year period. On average, MMSE scores remain relatively stable among intact older adults, changing less than one point (+.08) over the five-year interval, but declining (−1.38) in those with mild cognitive impairment.

Tombaugh (2005) used reliable change methodology to provide a better estimate of whether an individual's retest score has changed significantly from the initial test score over both short (<3 months) and long (five years) retest intervals. Table 6–56 shows the regression formulas, the percent of variance explained by all variables (e.g., test one score, age, education, gender), and the amount of change needed to exceed the .05 level (one-tailed). Note that most of the variance is accounted for by the score on the first test occasion. A normative table containing the percentile equivalents for various change scores is also provided (see Table 6–57). The data are based on a sample of 232 older adults who were retested following both short and long intervals and who received consensus diagnoses of no cognitive impairment on both examinations. The values needed for clinically meaningful change agree fairly well with those suggested by Clark et al. (1999), Doody et al. (2001), and Eslinger et al. (2003).

Interrater Reliability. Scoring of some items (e.g., overlapping polygons) is somewhat subjective, and there is no suggested time limit for any item. Interrater reliability is marginal (above .65) (Folstein et al., 1975; Foster et al., 1988) and could be enhanced with more precise administration and scoring criteria (Molloy et al., 1991; Olin & Zelinski, 1991).

Pediatric Adaptations

No information regarding reliability is yet available for the pediatric adaptation of the MMSE by Ouvrier et al. (1993).

Table 6–57 Percentiles for the Difference Between Obtained Retest Scores and Retest Scores Predicted on the Basis of Regression Equations Using Baseline Scores and Demographic Information as Regressors for the MMSE and 3MS

Percentiles	MMSE Short Interval (<3 months)	MMSE Long Interval (5 years)	3MS Short Interval (<3 months)	3MS Long Interval (5 years)
98 (+2 SD)	3.08	4.26	11.27	12.06
95	2.53	3.79	7.48	8.90
90	2.05	3.44	4.90	7.05
84 (+1 SD)	1.43	3.16	3.99	4.62
75	1.06	2.55	2.66	3.45
50 (0 SD)	0.13	1.18	0.21	0.47
25	−0.78	0.01	−1.54	−3.12
16 (−1 SD)	−1.50	−0.84	−2.96	−5.47
10	−2.16	−1.67	−5.40	−7.79
05	−3.20	−2.99	−8.47	−10.15
02 (−2 SD)	−4.22	−4.67	−10.28	−17.31

Based on a sample of 232 older adults who were retested following three-month and five-year intervals and who received consensus diagnoses of no cognitive impairment on both examinations.

Source: From Tombaugh, 2005. Reprinted with permission from Elsevier.

3MS

The reliability (internal consistency, test-retest) of the 3MS tends to be higher than that of the MMSE (e.g., Besson & Labbe, 1997; Bravo & Hebert, 1997b; Tombaugh et al., 1996; Tombaugh, in press). For example, Tombaugh et al. (1996) reported that in normal individuals, Cronbach's alpha was .82 for the 3MS and .62 for the MMSE. For patients with AD, Cronbach's alpha was .88 for the 3MS and .81 for the MMSE. The consistently higher alphas for the 3MS reflect, at least in part, its larger number of items.

Test-retest reliability is reported to be high for intervals of one to four weeks in children (.85–.99; Besson & Labbe, 1997) and for intervals of about three months in individuals diagnosed with dementia (intraclass correlation of .85; Correa et al., 2001).

A recent study (Correa et al., 2001) showed that, under conditions of repeat testing (<90 days but >14 days) with two different assessors in a setting compatible with no change in cognitive status, the discrepancy between repeat 3MS scores of people with dementia can be as large as ± 16 points. This suggests that the smallest individual change in score that can be reliably detected must exceed 16 points. With lengthier retest intervals (five years), declines of about seven points are unusual in normal older adults (Tombaugh, in press; see Table 6–57).

Interrater reliability is reported to be high ($r = .98$) for the overlapping figures (Teng & Chui, 1987). The interrater reliability of the 3MS was moderate when measured by agreement of clinician categorization of cognitive impairment versus no cognitive impairment based on 3MS scores (kappa = 0.67; Lamarre & Patten, 1991).

VALIDITY

Construct Validity—MMSE

The MMSE shows modest to high correlations with other brief screening tests such as the Blessed Test, the DRS, Spanish versions of the Mental Status Questionnaire, the Information-Memory-Concentration Test, the Orientation-Memory-Concentration Test, and the Clock Drawing Task (e.g., Adunsky et al., 2002; Fillenbaum et al., 1987; Foreman, 1987; Freidl et al., 1996; Salmon et al., 1990; Taussig et al., 1996), suggesting that the various tests tap similar, though not necessarily identical, cognitive domains. For example, 9 of 30 (40%) points on the MMSE relate to memory and attention. By contrast, only 25 of 144 points (17%) on the DRS are for memory items. Not surprisingly, agreement between tests (e.g., MMSE and DRS) regarding cognitive impairment can be low (Freidl et al., 1996, 2002). Thus, in a large sample of healthy adults ($N = 1957$), Freidl et al. reported a correlation of .29 between the total scores of the MMSE and DRS. Using recommended cutoff scores for each test, the DRS classified 4.2% of study participants as cognitively impaired in comparison to 1.6% for the MMSE. Equations have been developed to convert total scores from one test to the other (e.g., MMSE and DRS), but given the mixed results in the literature, they should be used with caution (see also *DRS-2* in this volume). The equations are provided in Table 6–58.

Modest to high correlations have also been reported between total MMSE scores and a variety of other cognitive measures, including tests of intelligence, memory, attention/concentration, constructional ability, and executive function (e.g., Axelrod et al., 1992; Bieliauskas et al., 2000; Feher et al.,

Table 6–58 Conversion Formulas From DRS to MMSE

Test	Formula	Reference
MMSE	−12.72 + 0.31 (DRS)	Salmon et al., 1990 Based on a sample of 92 patients with probable AD
MMSE	−10.0 + 0.29 (DRS)	Bobholz & Brandt, 1993 Based on a sample of 50 patients with suspected cognitive impairment
MMSE	−3.1 + 0.23 (DRS)	Meiran et al., 1996 Based on a sample of 466 patients in a memory disorders clinic. The expected error associated with this formula is ±3

1992; Folstein et al., 1975; Giordani et al., 1990; Jefferson et al., 2002; Mitrushina & Satz, 1991; Perna et al., 2001; Tombaugh & McIntyre, 1992). Thus, the total score seems to measure some general cognitive ability.

Folstein et al. (1975) grouped the items into discrete subsections (e.g., orientation, registration, attention and calculation, recall, language); however, these categories were derived without empirical justification and it is not clear whether the MMSE subsections and individual items can be viewed as measures of specific aspects of cognition (Giordani et al., 1990; Mitrushina & Satz, 1994). Concordance rates between individual MMSE tasks and neuropsychological tests addressing corresponding cognitive domains can be quite low (Benedict & Brandt, 1992; Giordani et al., 1990; Jefferson et al., 2002; Mitrushina & Satz, 1994).

Factor-analytic studies of the MMSE often yield a two-factor solution (Braekhus et al., 1992; Giordani et al., 1990; Tombaugh & McIntyre, 1992), although other solutions have also been found. For example, a study with a large ($N = 8556$) sample of community-dwelling older adults suggested the presence of five separate dimensions (concentration, language and praxis, orientation, memory, and attention), although the MMSE also satisfied criteria of unidimensionality (Jones & Gallo, 2000). Similar findings have been reported by Banos and Franklin (2002) in 339 adult inpatients at a nonforensic state psychiatric hospital. It is difficult to compare the various studies due to differences in variable construction, sample composition, and statistical method. The two most recent studies (Banos & Franklin, 2002; Jones & Gallo, 2000) provide empirical support for some of the traditional categories, such as orientation (time and place), attention (serial 7s), and memory (recall of three words). There is less empirical support for the categories of registration, language, and construction.

Clinical Findings

MMSE. Most studies report that the MMSE summary score is sensitive to the presence of dementia, particularly in those with moderate to severe forms of cognitive impairment; however, the MMSE appears less than ideal when those with mild cognitive impairment are evaluated, when focal neurological deficits are present (e.g., poststroke), or when psychiatric patients are included (Benedict & Brandt, 1992; Feher et al., 1992; Grut et al., 1993; Kupke et al., 1993; Kuslansky et al., 2004; Meyer et al., 2001; Nys et al., 2005; O'Connor et al., 1989; Shah et al., 1992; Tombaugh & McIntyre, 1992; Van Der Cammen et al., 1992; Wells et al., 1992). There are a number of possible explanations for this decreased sensitivity and specificity. One possibility rests on the fact that the MMSE is biased toward verbal items and does not adequately measure other functions such as ability to attend to relevant input, ability to solve abstract problems, ability to retain information over prolonged time intervals, visual-spatial ability, constructional praxis, and mood. Accordingly, it may overestimate dementia in aphasic patients. At the same time, it may be relatively insensitive to various dysexecutive and amnestic syndromes as well as disturbances of the right hemisphere, resulting in an increase in false negatives. In addition, the language items are very simple, and mild impairments may go undetected.

The results from the factor-analytic studies reported previously (*Construct Validity*) imply that the individual subsection scores of the MMSE should not be used in lieu of more comprehensive assessments if a detailed diagnostic profile is desired (Banos & Franklin, 2002; Giordani et al., 1990). This does not mean that the MMSE cannot provide useful information in differentiating among patients with dementia. For example, Brandt et al. (1988) showed different profiles on the MMSE in patients with AD and patients with Huntington's disease. The differences between the groups rested on different scores on the memory and attention/concentration items. Patients with AD did worse on the memory items, whereas patients with Huntington's disease did worse on the attention/concentration items. Similarly, Jefferson et al. (2002) found that patients with AD scored lower than patients with ischemic vascular dementia (VaD) or Parkinson's disease (PD) on temporal orientation and recall tasks, while those with VaD obtained lower scores than patients with AD on motor/constructional tasks (copying, writing) and an index comprising items requiring working memory (spelling "world" backward, carrying out three-step commands). The VaD and PD groups also made more errors in writing a sentence and copying intersecting polygons.

The MMSE may also be useful in predicting who will develop AD or VaD (e.g., Small, Herlitz, et al., 1997; Jones et al., 2004). For example, Jones et al. (2004) found that lower baseline scores on the MMSE in nondemented persons were associated with an increased risk of AD or VaD after a three-year follow-up period. Delayed memory was the best predictor in both preclinical VaD and preclinical AD. It is worth bearing in mind, however, that although a large proportion (more than two-thirds) of cognitively impaired individuals (one or more *SD* below their age and education mean) become demented or die in three years, a substantial proportion improve over the same period without a higher risk of later progressing to dementia (Palmer et al., 2002).

The MMSE is also sensitive to cognitive decline; however, as the disorder becomes more severe, the test loses its sensitivity to change (Salmon et al., 1990; Tombaugh & McIntyre, 1992). In such cases, other tests are preferred, such as the DRS, which includes more easy items. For example, the DRS contains a number of simple items that assess attentional processes. Severely demented patients can complete these items since attention is often preserved until late in the course of the disease. Thus, severely demented patients who can make few, if any, correct responses on the MMSE can still respond adequately on the DRS.

A number of investigators report an *average* annual rate of decline of about two to four points on the MMSE for patients with probable dementia of the Alzheimer type (Becker et al., 1988; Clark et al., 1999; Doody et al., 2001; Salmon et al., 1990; Small, Viitanen, et al., 1997). However, progression rates of AD are nonlinear and quite variable between persons (Clark et al., 1999; Doody et al., 2001). Nonetheless, there is some consistency in that patients who begin with progression rates that are more rapid than average (≥5 MMSE points per year) continue to decline sooner than patients who begin at slow (≤1.9 points per year) or average rates (2–4.9 points per year; Doody et al., 2001). Further, individuals with AD decline at a faster rate than patients with VaD (Nyenhuis et al., 2002) or frontotemporal dementia (Pasquier et al., 2004).

MMSE scores correlate with histopathological findings in in vivo brain images and event-related potentials (Aylward et al., 1996; Bigler et al., 2002; Colohan et al., 1989; DeKoskey et al., 1990; Finley et al., 1985; Martin et al., 1987; Pearlson & Tune, 1986; Stout et al., 1996; Tsai & Tsuang, 1979). For instance, a number of authors (e.g., Bigler et al., 2002; Stout et al. 1996) have reported an association between white matter lesions, noted on MRI, and impaired cognitive function as measured by the MMSE. Clinical-pathological study of patients with AD reveal that the best predictors of MMSE scores are the total counts of neurofibrillary tangles (NFT) in the entorhinal cortex and area 9 as well as degree of neuronal loss in the CA1 field of the hippocampus (Ginnakapoulos et al., 2003).

Sensitivity of Items

Analyses of individual items reveal that errors rarely occur on questions related to orientation to place and language; for both normal and demented individuals, most errors occur for the recall of three words, serial 7s/"world," pentagon, and orientation to time. In short, these latter items are the most sensitive to normal aging and a variety of diseases (e.g., diabetes, cardiovascular disease) including dementing processes (Hill & Backman, 1995; Nilsson et al., 2002; Tombaugh & McIntyre, 1992; Tombaugh et al., 1996; Wells et al., 1992). Sensitivity of specific items to cognitive impairment in children has not yet been established.

Serial 7s/"World"

There is evidence that serial 7s and reverse spelling of "world" represent different tasks. Spelling "world" backward consistently produces higher scores than does counting backward by sevens (Tombaugh & McIntyre, 1992). Serial 7s maximizes variability, increases internal consistency, and reduces measurement error, thus increasing the likelihood of discriminating between individuals in their level of cognitive ability (Espino et al., 2004). In fact, Espino et al. (2004) have argued that only serial 7s should be given. However, users should bear in mind that performance on the serial 7s task appears heavily influenced by basic arithmetic skills and therefore should be used with caution as a measure of concentration (Karzmark, 2000).

Ecological Validity

MMSE. MMSE scores show modest relations with measures of functional capacity (e.g., driving, cooking, caring for finances, consent to participate in studies), functional outcome after stroke, and time to nursing home care and death (e.g., Adunsky et al., 2002; Bigler et al., 2002; Burns et al., 1991; Fillenbaum et al., 1988a, 1988b; Kim & Caine, 2002; Lemsky et al., 1996; Marcopulos et al., 1997; Stern et al., 1997; Taussig et al., 1996; see also Ruchinskas & Curyto, 2003, for a recent review). For example, Gallo et al. (1998) reported that poor performance on the copy polygons task is associated with an increase in motor vehicle crashes. In addition, the test is somewhat sensitive to mortality-related effects with declines in scores evident about three to five years prior to death (e.g., Nguyen et al., 2003; Tan, 2004). The greatest risk is for those with moderate to severe cognitive impairment, although mild impairment (e.g., MMSE scores 18–23) is also associated with increased risk (Nguyen et al., 2003). A decline of at least four points over two years is also predictive of an increased risk of mortality, perhaps reflecting symptoms of medical diseases that carry with them long-term risk of mortality (Nguyen et al., 2003). Stern et al. (1997) have developed an equation to predict the estimated time to nursing home care and death in people with AD. The prediction equation is available at the following site: cpmcnet.columbia.edu/dept/sergievsky/predictor.html.

Because cognitive deficits can render self-report (e.g., including responses on the Geriatric Depression Scale, Beck Depression Inventory) invalid, interpretation is considered hazardous once MMSE scores decline below 20 (Bedard et al., 2003). In such cases, reports from informants and observations are critical. A threshold of 20 may also apply to patient involvement in medical decision making (Hirschman et al., 2003). However, Kim and Caine (2002) noted that in a sample of patients with mild to moderate Alzheimer's disease, a fairly wide range of MMSE scores (21–25, which includes an often used cutoff for normal) did not discriminate consent capacity status well. They recommend that if there are strong ethical reasons to select only patients who are clearly capable of providing consent, then the researcher/practitioner is advised to use a higher MMSE cutoff score (e.g., 26).

The 3MS and Other Versions

Several attempts have been made to improve the utility of the MMSE by omitting items of limited diagnostic utility and/or adding items or tests known to be sensitive to cognitive impairment. For example, Loewenstein et al. (2000) incorporated three extended-delay recall trials (for the recall items) at five-minute intervals. The modification showed increased sensitivity and specificity in differentiating cognitively normal older adults from those with mild cognitive impairment.

As noted earlier (see *Description*), the 3MS by Teng et al. (1987) added four additional items (date and place of birth, word fluency, similarities, and delayed recall of words), included items that assess different aspects of memory, and increased the maximum score to permit greater differentiation among individuals. A factor analysis of the 3MS yielded the following five domains: psychomotor skills, memory, identification and association, orientation, and concentration and calculation (Abraham et al., 1993). In addition, the 3MS has moderate to high correlations with neuropsychological tests that assess similar domains (Grace et al., 1995), providing evidence for its concurrent validity.

Although some studies have found the sensitivity and specificity of the 3MS and MMSE to be similar (Nadler et al., 1995; Tombaugh et al., 1996), others have found the 3MS to be more sensitive in detecting cognitive deficits and to be a better predictor of functional outcome (Grace et al., 1995). In all studies, the criterion validity of the 3MS is high. For example, Tombaugh et al. (1996) reported that the sensitivity of the 3MS was 92.6% when screening for AD versus no cognitive impairment at a cutoff score of 77/78 (i.e., those who scored 77 or below were classed as impaired whereas those who scored 78 or above were classed as normal).

Recently, the 3MS has been modified (3MS-R; Tschantz et al., 2002). The modifications are primarily in the area of assessing remote memory where the authors substituted the recall of personal demographic information (date and place of birth) with the recall of current and past prominent politicians to make the information easier to verify. They also changed some of the item scaling in the orientation section and shortened the time allotted for the verbal fluency item (from 30 to 20 seconds). As might be expected, the test is sensitive to dementia. Lower age, higher education, and female gender were linked to higher 3MS-R scores. Normative data, stratified by age, education, and gender, are available based on a sample of over 2000 cognitively intact older people.

COMMENT

The MMSE has been used widely to detect dementia for over 25 years. Part of its popularity can be attributed to its ease of administration, its brevity, and the large volume of literature that has accumulated.

The choice of screening measure for identifying dementia will depend on the goals of the examination and on the sample studied. In geriatric or neurological samples with a high prevalence of patients with illiteracy or language or motoric disorders, the MMSE may not be ideal and may lead to an overestimation of dementia (e.g., Kuslansky et al., 2004; Tombaugh & McIntyre, 1992). At the same time, it may miss a significant proportion of individuals who have mild memory or other cognitive losses. Nonetheless, it may offer equally effective detection of dementia as lengthier tests (e.g., DRS, Neurobehavioral Cognitive Status Examination, Hopkins Verbal Learning Test), at least in some populations (Chan et al., 2003; Kuslansky et al., 2004; van Gorp et al., 1999; but see Meyer et al., 2001). However, it is important to bear in mind that agreement between tests is not assured.

Further, the MMSE lacks diagnostic specificity: Low scores signal that there *may* be important changes in cognition and health. Analysis of some of the items (particularly those related to orientation, attention, and memory) may generate more targeted questions and/or offer clues with regard to the type of disorder. In short, the presence and nature of cognitive impairment should not be diagnosed on the basis of MMSE scores alone. The examiner needs to follow up suspicions of impairment with a more in-depth evaluation.

The use of age- and education-stratified normative variables when screening for dementia or cognitive impairment has recently been questioned. O'Connell et al. (2004) reported that correcting for demographic influences (age, education, gender) failed to improve the accuracy of the 3MS. Similar findings have been reported with regard to the MMSE (Kraemer et al., 1998). Because age and education are in themselves apparent risk factors for dementia, removal of the effects of these demographic variables (i.e., age or education, or both) might remove some of the predictive power of the screening measure (Sliwinski et al., 1997). Additional research is needed to determine whether correction is important to improve diagnostic accuracy and whether it is critical in some contexts but not others.

It should also be noted that the use of simple cutoffs, while widely used, oversimplifies the situation by ignoring the prevalence of dementia in a given setting. In other words, the sensitivity and specificity of specific cutoffs will vary with the base rates of dementia in each setting. Meiran et al. (1996) show that a score of 26 is unlikely to be associated with dementia in an environment where most individuals do not have dementia (e.g., 20% prevalence). In that setting (i.e., low base rate), a score of 26 probably indicates dementia with a 52% probability. However, a score of 26 in a nursing home setting is likely to be associated with dementia since many of the patients (e.g., 50%) have dementia (i.e., high base rate). In this case, the chances are 81% that the patient has dementia. On the other hand, in ambulatory memory disorder clinics, the presence of dementia is about 75%. In that setting, a score of 26 indicates dementia with a 93% probability.

While the test may be a useful screening instrument to assess level of performance, it has limited value in measuring progression of disease in individual patients. This is because of a large measurement error and substantial variation in change in annual scores (Clark et al., 1999).

Finally, a number of revisions of the MMSE have been proposed, including the 3MS—a modification that has promising psychometric characteristics. The various revisions, however, have not yet gained widespread use.

REFERENCES

Abraham, I. L., Manning, C. A., Boyd, M. R., Neese, J. B., Newman, M. C., Plowfield, L. A., et al. (1993). Cognitive screening of nursing home residents: Factor analytic structure of the modified Mini-Mental State (3MS) examination. *International Journal of Geriatric Psychiatry, 8*, 133–138.

Adunsky, A., Fleissig, Y., Levenkrohn, S., Arad, M., & Noy, S. (2002). Clock drawing task, Mini-Mental State Examination and cognitive-functional independence measure: Relation to functional outcome of stroke patients. *Archives of Gerontology and Geriatrics, 35*, 153–160.

Anthony, J. C., LeResche, L., Niaz, U., Von Korff, M. R., & Folstein, M. F. (1982). Limits of the "Mini-Mental State" as a screening test for dementia and delirium among hospital patients. *Psychological Medicine, 12*, 397–408.

Antsey, K. J., Matters, B., Brown, A. K., & Lord, S. R. (2000). Normative data on neuropsychological tests for very old adults living in retirement villages and hostels. *The Clinical Neuropsychologist, 14*, 309–317.

Auer, S., Hampel, H., Moller, H-J., & Reisberg, B. (2000). Translations of measurements and scales: Opportunities and diversities. *International Geriatrics, 12*, 391–394.

Axelrod, B. N., Goldman, R. S., & Henry, R. R. (1992). Sensitivity of the Mini-Mental State Examination to frontal lobe dysfunction in normal aging. *Journal of Clinical Psychology, 48*, 68–71.

Aylward, E. H., Rasmussen, D. X., Brandt, J., Raimundo, L., Folstein, M., & Pearlson, G. D. (1996). CT measurement of supracellar cistern predicts rate of cognitive decline in Alzheimer's disease. *Journal of the International Neuropsychological Society, 2*, 89–95.

Banos, J. H., & Franklin, L. M. (2002). Factor structure of the Mini-Mental State Examination in adult psychiatric inpatients. *Psychological Assessment, 14*, 397–400.

Becker, J. T., Huff, F. J., Nebes, R. D., Holland, A., & Boller, F. (1988). Neuropsychological function in Alzheimer's disease: Pattern of impairment and rate of progression. *Archives of Neurology, 45*, 263–268.

Bedard, M., Molloy, D. W., Squire, L., Minthorn-Biggs, M-B., Dubois, S., Lever, J. A., & O'Donnell, M. (2003). Validity of self-reports in dementia research: The Geriatric Depression Scale. *Clinical Gerontologist, 26*, 155–163.

Benedict, R. H. B., & Brandt, J. (1992). Limitation of the Mini-Mental State Examination for the detection of amnesia. *Journal of Geriatric Psychiatry and Neurology, 5233–5237*.

Besson, P. S., & Labbe, E. E. (1997). Use of the modified Mini-Mental State Examination with children. *Journal of Child Neurology, 12*, 455–460.

Bieliauskas, L. A., Depp, C., Kauszler, M. L., Steinberg, B. A., & Lacy, M. (2000). IQ and scores on the Mini-Mental State Examination (MMSE). *Aging, Neuropsychology, and Cognition, 7*, 227–229.

Bigler, E. D., Kerr, B., Victoroff, J., Tate, D. F., & Breitmner, J. C. S. (2002). White matter lesions, quantitative magnetic resonance imaging and dementia. *Alzheimer Disease and Associated Disorders, 16*, 161–170.

Bleecker, M. L., Bolla-Wilson, K., Kawas, C., & Agnew, J. (1988). Age-specific norms for the Mini-Mental State Exam. *Neurology, 33*, 1565–1568.

Bobholz, J. H., & Brandt, J. (1993). Assessment of cognitive impairment: Relationship of the Dementia Rating Scale to the Mini-Mental State Examination. *Journal of Geriatric Psychiatry and Neurology, 12*, 180–188.

Braekhus, A., Laake, K., & Engedal, K. (1992). The Mini-Mental State Examination: Identifying the most efficient variables for detecting cognitive impairment in the elderly. *Journal of the American Geriatrics Society, 40*, 1139–1145.

Brandt, J., Folstein, S. E., & Folstein, M. F. (1988). Differential cognitive impairment in Alzheimer's disease and Huntington's disease. *Annals of Neurology, 23*, 555–561.

Bravo, G., & Hebert, R. (1997a). Age- and education-specific references values for the Mini-Mental and Modified Mini-Mental State Examinations derived from a non-demented elderly population. *International Journal of Geriatric Psychiatry, 12*, 1008–1018.

Bravo, G., & Hebert, R. (1997b). Reliability of the modified Mini-Mental State Examination in the context of a two-phase community prevalence study. *Neuroepidemiology, 16*, 141–148.

Brown, L. M., Schinka, J. A., Mortimer, J. A., & Graves, A. B. (2003). 3MS normative data for elderly African Americans. *Journal of Clinical and Experimental Neuropsychology, 25*, 234–241.

Burns, A., Jacoby, R., & Levy, R. (1991). Progression of cognitive impairment in Alzheimer's disease. *Journal of the American Geriatric Society, 39*, 39–45.

Chan, A. S., Choi, A., Chiu, H., & Liu, L. (2003). Clinical validity of the Chinese version of Mattis dementia rating scale in differentiating dementia of Alzheimer's type in Hong Kong. *Journal of the International Neuropsychological Society, 9*, 45–55.

Christensen, H., & Jorm, A. F. (1992). Effect of premorbid intelligence on the Mini-Mental State and IQCODE. *International Journal of Geriatric Psychiatry, 7*, 159–160.

Clark, C. M., Sheppard, L., Fillenbaum, G. G., Galasko, D., Morris, J. C., Koss, E., Mohs, R., Heyman, A., & the Cerad Investigators. (1999). Variability in annual Mini-Mental State Examination score in patients with probable Alzheimer disease. *Archives of Neurology, 56*, 857–862.

Colohan, H., O'Callaghan, E., Larkin, C., Waddington, J. L. (1989). An evaluation of cranial CT scanning in clinical psychiatry. *Irish Journal of Medical Science, 158*, 178–181.

Correa, J. A., Perrault, H., & Wolfson, C. (2001). Reliable individual change scores on the 3MS in older persons with dementia: Results from the Canadian study of health and aging. *International Psychogeriatrics, 13*, 71–78.

Crum, R. M., Anthony, J. C., Bassett, S. S., & Folstein, M. F. (1993). Population-based norms for the Mini-Mental State Examination by age and educational level. *Journal of the American Medical Association, 269*, 2386–2391.

DeKosky, S. T., Shih, W. J., Schmitt, F. A., Coupal, J., & Kirkpatrick, C. (1990). Assessing utility of single photon emission computed tomography (SPECT) scan in Alzheimer disease: Correlation with cognitive severity. *Alzheimer Disease and Associated Disorders, 4*, 14–23.

Doody, R. S., Massman, P., & Dunn, J. K. (2001). A method for estimating progression rates in Alzheimer disease. *Archives of Neurology, 58*, 449–454.

Doraiswamy, P. M., & Kaiser, L. (2000). Variability of the Mini-Mental State Examination in dementia. *Neurology, 54,* 1538–1539.

Dufouil, C., Clayton, D., Brayne, C., Chi, L. Y., Dening, T. R., Paykel, E. S., O'Connor, D. W., Ahmed, A., McGee, M. A., & Huppert, F. A. (2000). Population norms for the MMSE in the very old. *Neurology, 55,* 1609–1612.

Eslinger, P. J., Swan, G. E., & Carmelli, D. (2003). Changes in the mini-mental state exam in community-dwelling older persons over 6 years: Relationships to health and neuropsychological measures. *Neuroepidemiology, 22,* 23–30.

Espino, D. V., Lichtenstein, M. J., Palmer, R. F., & Hazuda, H. P. (2001). Ethnic differences in Mini-Mental State Examination (MMSE) scores: Where you live makes a difference. *Journal of the American Geriatric Society, 49,* 538–548.

Espino, D. V., Lichtenstein, M. J., Palmer, R. F., & Hazuda, H. P. (2004). Evaluation of the Mini-Mental State Examination's internal consistency in a community-based sample of Mexican-American and European-American elders: Results from the San Antonio longitudinal study of aging. *Journal of the American Geriatrics Society, 52,* 822–827.

Feher, E. P., Mahurin, R. K., Doody, R. S., Cooke, N., Sims, J., & Pirozzolo, F. J. (1992). Establishing the limits of the Mini-Mental State. *Archives of Neurology, 49,* 87–92.

Fillenbaum, G. G., George, L. K., & Blazer, D. G. (1988a). Scoring nonresponse on the Mini-Mental State Examination. *Psychological Medicine, 18,* 1021–1025.

Fillenbaum, G. G., Heyman, A., Wilkinson, W. E., & Haynes, C. S. (1987). Comparison of two screening tests in Alzheimer's disease. *Archives of Neurology, 44,* 924–927.

Fillenbaum, G. G., Hughes, D. C., Heyman, A., George, L. K., et al. (1988b). Relationship of health and demographic characteristics to Mini-Mental State Examination scores among community residents. *Psychological Medicine, 18,* 719–726.

Finley, W. W., Faux, S. F., Hutcheson, J., & Amstutz, L. (1985). Long-latency event-related potentials in the evaluation of cognitive function in children. *Neurology, 35,* 323–327.

Folstein, M. F., Folstein, S. E., & McHugh, P. R. (1975). "Mini-Mental State." A practical method for grading the cognitive state of patients for the clinician. *Journal of Psychiatric Research, 12,* 189–198.

Folstein, M. F., Folstein, S. E., McHugh, P. R., & Fanjiang, G. (2001). *Mini-Mental State Examination: User's guide.* Odessa, FL: PAR.

Ford, G. R., Haley, W. E., Thrower, S. L., West, C. A. C., & Harrell, L. E. (1996). Utility of Mini-Mental State Exam scores in predicting functional impairment among White and African American dementia patients. *Journal of Gerontology: Medical Sciences, 51A,* M185–M188.

Foreman, M. D. (1987). Reliability and validity of mental status questionnaires in elderly hospitalized patients. *Nursing Research, 36,* 216–220.

Foster, J. R., Sclan, S., Welkowitz, J., Boksay, I., & Seeland, I. (1988). Psychiatric assessment in medical long-term care facilities: Reliability of commonly used rating scales. *International Journal of Geriatric Psychiatry, 3,* 229–233.

Fountoulakis, K. N., Tsolaki, M., Chantzi, H., & Kazis, A. (2000). Mini Mental State Examination (MMSE): A validation study in Greece. *American Journal of Alzheimer's Disease and Other Dementias, 15,* 342–345.

Freidl, W., Schmidt, R., Stronegger, W. J., Fazekas, F., & Reinhart, B. (1996). Sociodemographic predictors and concurrent validity of the Mini Mental State Examination and the Mattis Dementia Rating Scale. *European Archives of Psychiatry and Clinical Neuroscience, 246,* 317–319.

Freidl, W., Stronegger, W.-J., Berghold, A., Reinhart, B., Petrovic, K., & Schmidt, R. (2002). The agreement of the Mattis Dementia Rating Scale with the Mini-Mental State Examination. *International Journal of Psychiatry, 17,* 685–686.

Gallo, J. J., Rebok, G., & Lesikar, S. (1998). The driving habits of adults aged 60 years and older. *Journal of the American Geriatrics Society, 47,* 335–341.

Giannakopoulos, P., Herrmann, F. R., Bussiere, T., Bouras, C., Kovari, E., Perl, D. P., Morrison, J. H., Gold, G., & Hof, P. R. (2003). Tangle and neuron numbers, but not amyloid load, predict cognitive status in Alzheimer's disease. *Neurology, 60,* 1495–1500.

Giordani, B., Boivin, M. J., Hall, A. L., Foster, N. L., Lehtinen, S. J., Bluemlein, M. S., & Berent, S. (1990). The utility and generality of Mini-Mental State Examination scores in Alzheimer's disease. *Neurology, 40,* 1894–1896.

Grace, J., Nadler, J. D., White, D. A., Guilmette, T. J., et al. (1995). Folstein vs modified Mini-Mental State Examination in geriatric stroke: Stability, validity, and screening utility. *Archives of Neurology, 52,* 477–484.

Grut, M., Fraiglioni, L., Viitanen, M., & Winblad, B. (1993). Accuracy of the Mini-Mental Status Examination as a screening test for dementia in a Swedish elderly population. *Acta Neurologica Scandinavica, 87,* 312–317.

Helkala, E.-L., Kivipelto, M., Hallikainen, M., Alhainen, K., Heinonen, H., Tuomilehto, J., Soininen, H., & Nissines, A. (2002). Usefulness of repeated presentation of Mini-Mental State Examination as a diagnostic procedure—a population-based study. *Acta Neurologica Scandinavica, 106,* 341–346.

Hill, R. D., & Backman, L. (1995). The relationships between the Mini-Mental State Examination and cognitive functioning in normal elderly adults: A componential analysis. *Age Aging, 24,* 440–446.

Hirschman, K. B., Xie, S. X., Feudtner, C., & Karlawish, J. H. T. (2003). How does Alzheimer's disease patient's role in medical decision making change over time? *Journal of Geriatric Psychiatry & Neurology, 17,* 55–60.

Hopp, G. A., Dixon, R. A., Backman, I., & Grut, M. (1997). Stability of two measures of cognitive functioning in nondemented old-old adults. *Journal of Clinical Psychology, 53,* 673–686.

Ishizaki, J., Meguro, K., Ambo, H., Shimada, M., Yamaguchi, S., Hayasaka, C., Komatsu, H., Sekita, Y., & Yamadori, A. (1998). A normative, community-based study of Mini-Mental State in elderly adults: The effect of age and educational level. *Journal of Gerontology: Psychological Sciences, 53B,* P359–P363.

Iverson, G. L. (1998). Interpretation of Mini-Mental State Examination scores in community-dwelling elderly and geriatric neuropsychiatry patients. *International Journal of Geriatric Psychiatry, 13,* 661–666.

Jefferson, A. L., Consentino, S. A., Ball, S. K., Bogdanoff, B., Kaplan, E., & Libon, D. J. (2002). Errors produced on the Mini-Mental State Examination and neuropsychological test performance in Alzheimer's disease, ischemic vascular dementia, and Parkinson's disease. *Journal of Neuropsychiatry and Clinical Neurosciences, 14,* 311–320.

Jones, R. N., & Gallo, J. J. (2000). Dimensions of the Mini-Mental State Examination among community dwelling older adults. *Psychological Medicine, 30,* 605–618.

Jones, R. N., & Gallo, J. J. (2002). Education and sex differences in the Mini-Mental State Examination: Effects of differential item functioning. *Journals of Gerontology: Series B: Psychological Sciences & Social Sciences, 57B,* P548–P558.

Jones, S., Laukka, E. J., Small, B. J., Fratiglioni, L., & Backman, L. (2004). A preclinical phase in vascular dementia: Cognitive impairment three years before diagnosis. *Dementia & Geriatric Cognitive Disorders, 18,* 233–239.

Jones, T. G., Schinka, J. A., Vanderploeg, R. D., Small, B. J., Graves, A. B., & Mortimer, J. A. (2002). 3MS normative data for the elderly. *Archives of Clinical Neuropsychology, 17,* 171–177.

Jorm, A. F., Scott, R., Henderson, A. S., & Kay, D. W. (1988). Educational level differences on the Mini-Mental State. *Psychological Medicine, 18,* 727–788.

Karzmark, P. (2000). Validity of the serial seven procedure. *International Journal of Geriatric Psychiatry, 15,* 677–679.

Kim, S. Y. K., & Caine, E. D. (2002). Utility and limits of the Mini Mental State Examination in evaluating consent capacity in Alzheimer's disease. *Psychiatric Services, 53,* 1322–1324.

Kraemer, H. C., Moritz, D. J., & Yesavage, J. (1998). Adjusting Mini-Mental State Examination scores for age and education level to screen for dementia: Correcting bias or reducing variability. *International Psychogeriatrics, 10,* 43–51.

Kupke, T., Revis, E. S., & Gantner, A. B. (1993). Hemispheric bias of the Mini-Mental State Examination in elderly males. *The Clinical Neuropsychologist, 7,* 210–214.

Kuslansky, G., Katz, M., Verhese, J., Hall, C. B., Lapuerta, P., LaRuffa, G., & Lipton, R. B. (2004). Detecting dementia with the Hopkins learning test and the Mini-Mental State Examination. *Archives of Clinical Neuropsychology, 19,* 89–104.

Lamarre, C. J., & Patten, S. B. (1991). Evaluation of the modified Mini-Mental State Examination in a general psychiatric population. *Canadian Journal of Psychiatry, 36,* 507–511.

Lemsky, C. M., Smith, G., Malec, J. R., & Ivnik, R. J. (1996). Identifying risk for functional impairment using cognitive measures: An application of CART modeling. *Neuropsychology, 10,* 368–375.

Loewenstein, D. A., Barker, W. W., Harwood, D. G., Luis, C., Acevedo, A., Rodriguez, I., & Duara, R. (2000). Utility of a modified Mini-Mental State Examination with extended delayed recall in screening for mild cognitive impairment and dementia among community dwelling elders. *International Journal of Geriatric Psychiatry, 15,* 434–440.

Lopez, M. N., Charter, R. A., Mostafavi, B., Nibut, L. P., & Smith, W. E. (2005). Psychometric properties of the Folstein Mini-Mental State Examination. *Assessment, 12,* 137–144.

Marcopulos, B. A., & McLain, C. A. (2003). Are our norms "normal"? A 4-year follow-up study of a biracial sample of rural elders with low education. *The Clinical Neuropsychologist, 17,* 19–33.

Marcopulos, B. A., McLain, C. A., & Giuliano, A. J. (1997). Cognitive impairment or inadequate norms? A study of healthy, rural, older adults with limited education. *The Clinical Neuropsychologist, 11,* 111–131.

Martin, E. M., Wilson, R. S., & Penn, R. D., Penn, R. D., Fox, J. H., et al. (1987). Cortical biopsy results in Alzheimer's disease: Correlation with cognitive deficits. *Neurology, 37,* 1201–1204.

Meiran, N., Stuss, D. T., Guzman, A., Lafleche, G., & Willmer, J. (1996). Diagnosis of dementia: Methods for interpretation of scores of 5 neuropsychological tests. *Archives of Neurology, 53,* 1043–1054.

Meyer, J. S., Li, Y-S., & Thornby, J. (2001). Validating Mini-Mental Status, cognitive capacity screening and Hamilton Depression scales utilizing subjects with vascular headaches. *International Journal of Geriatric Psychiatry, 16,* 430–435.

Mitrushina, M., & Satz, P. (1991). Reliability and validity of the Mini-Mental State Exam in neurologically intact elderly. *Journal of Clinical Psychology, 47,* 537–543.

Mitrushina, M., & Satz, P. (1994). Utility of Mini-Mental State Examination in assessing cognition in the elderly. Paper presented to the International Neuropsychological Society, Cincinnati, OH.

Molloy, D. W., Alemayehu, E., & Roberts, R. (1991). Reliability of a standardized Mini-Mental State Examination compared with the traditional Mini-Mental State Examination. *American Journal of Psychiatry, 148,* 102–105.

Mulgrew, C. L., Morgenstern, N., Shtterly, S. M., Baxter, J., Baron, A. E., & Hamman, R. F. (1999). Cognitive functioning and impairment among rural elderly Hispanics and non-Hispanic Whites as assessed by the Mini-Mental State Examination. *Journal of Gerontology: Psychological Sciences, 54B,* P223–230.

Nadler, J. D., Relkin, N. R., Cohen, M. S., Hodder, R. A., Reingold, J., & Plum, F. (1995). Mental status testing in the elderly nursing home populations. *Journal of Geriatric Neurology, 8,* 177–183.

Nilsson, E., Fastbom, J., & Wahlin, A. (2002). Cognitive functioning in a population-based sample of very old non-demented and non-depressed persons: The impact of diabetes. *Archives of Gerontology and Geriatrics, 35,* 95–105.

Nguyen, H. T., Black, S. A., Ray, L., Espino, D. V., & Markides, K. S. (2003). Cognitive impairment and mortality in older Mexican Americans. *Journal of the American Geriatrics Society, 51,* 178–183.

Nyenhuis, D. L., Gorelick, P. B., Freels, S., & Garron, D. C. (2002). Cognitive and functional decline in African Americans with VaD, AD, and stroke without dementia. *Neurology, 58,* 56–61.

Nys, G. M. S., van Zandvoort, M. J. E., de Kort, P. L. M., Jansen, B. P. W., Kappelle, L. J., & de Haan, E. H. F. (2005). Restrictions of the Mini-Mental State Examination in acute stroke. *Archives of Clinical Neuropsychology, 20,* 623–629.

O'Connell, M. E., Tuokko, H., Graves, R. E., & Kadlec, H. (2004). Correcting the 3MS for bias does not improve accuracy when screening for cognitive impairment or dementia. *Journal of Clinical and Experimental Neuropsychology, 26,* 970–980.

O'Connor, D. W., Pollitt, P. A., Treasure, F. P., Brook, C. P. B., & Reiss, B. B. (1989). The influence of education, social class and sex on Mini-Mental State scores. *Psychological Medicine, 19,* 771–776.

Olin, J. T., & Zelinski, E. M. (1991). The 12-month stability of the Mini-Mental State Examination. *Psychological Assessment, 3,* 427–432.

Ouvrier, R. A., Goldsmith, R. F., Ouvrier, S., & Williams, I. C. (1993). The value of the Mini-Mental State Examination in childhood: A preliminary study. *Journal of Child Neurology, 8,* 145–149.

Palmer, K., Wang, H-X., Backman, L., Winblad, B., & Fratiglioni, L. (2002). Differential evolution of cognitive impairment in nondemented older persons: Results from the Kungholmen project. *American Journal of Psychiatry, 159,* 436–442.

Pasquier, F., Richard, F., & Lebert, F. (2004). Natural history of frontotemporal dementia: Comparison with Alzheimer's disease. *Dementia & Geriatric Cognitive Disorders, 17,* 253–257.

Pearlson, G. D., & Tune, L. E. (1986). Cerebral ventricular size and cerebrospinal fluid acetylcholinesterase levels in senile dementia of the Alzheimer type. *Psychiatry Research, 17,* 23–29.

Perna, R. B., Bordini, E. J., & Boozer, R. H. (2001). Mini-Mental Status Exam: Concurrent validity with the Rey Complex Figure Test in a geriatric population with depression. *The Journal of Cognitive Rehabilitation, 19,* 24–29.

Ruchinskas, R. A., & Curyto, K. J. (2003). Cognitive screening in geriatric rehabilitation. *Rehabilitation Psychology, 48,* 14–22.

Salmon, D. P., Thal, L. J., Butters, N., & Heindel, W. C. (1990). Longitudinal evaluation of dementia of the Alzheimer type: A comparison of 3 standardized mental status examinations. *Neurology, 40,* 1225–1230.

Shadlen, M-F., Larson, E. B., Gibbons, L., McCormick, W. C., & Teri, L. (1999). Alzheimer's disease symptom severity in blacks and whites. *Journal of the American Geriatrics Society, 47,* 482–486.

Shah, A., Phongsathorn, V., George, C., Bielawska, C., & Katona, C. (1992). Psychiatric morbidity among continuing care geriatric inpatients. *International Journal of Geriatric Psychiatry, 7,* 517–525.

Sliwinski, M., Buschke, H., Stewart, W. F., Masur, D., & Lipton, R. D. (1997). The effect of dementia risk factors on comparative and diagnostic selective reminding norms. *Journal of the International Neuropsychological Society, 3,* 317–326.

Small, B. J., Herlitz, A., Fratiglioni, L., Almkvist, O., & Bäckman, L. (1997a). Cognitive predictors of incident Alzheimer's disease: A prospective longitudinal study. *Neuropsychology, 11,* 413–420.

Small, B. J., Viitanen, M., Winblad, B., & Bäckman, L. (1997b). Cognitive changes in very old persons with dementia: The influence of demographic, psychometric, and biological variables. *Journal of Clinical and Experimental Neuropsychology, 19,* 245–260.

Starr, J. M., Whalley, L. J., Inch, S., & Shering, P. A. (1992). The quantification of the relative effects of age and NART-predicted IQ on cognitive function in healthy old people. *International Journal of Geriatric Psychiatry, 7,* 153–157.

Stern, Y., Tang, M-X., Albert, M. S., Brandt, J., Jacobs, D. M., Bell, K., Marder, K., Sano, M., Devanand, D., Slbert, S. M., Blysma, F., & Tsai, W-Y. Predicting time to nursing home care and death in individuals with Alzheimer disease. *Journal of the American Medical Association, 277,* 806–812.

Stout, J. C., Jernigan, T. L., Archibald, S. L., & Salmon, D. P. (1996). Association of dementia severity with cortical gray matter and abnormal white matter volumes in dementia of the Alzheimer type. *Archives of Neurology, 53,* 742–749.

Tan, J. (2004). *Influence of impending death on the MMSE.* MSc Thesis, University of Victoria.

Taussig, I. M., Mack, W. J., & Henderson, V. W. (1996). Concurrent validity of Spanish-language versions of the Mini-Mental State Examination, Mental Status Questionnaire, Information-Concentration Test, and Orientation-Memory-Concentration Test: Alzheimer's disease patients and non-demented elderly comparison subjects. *Journal of the International Neuropsychological Society, 2,* 286–298.

Teng, E. L., & Chui, H. C. (1987). The modified Mini-Mental State (3MS) Examination. *Journal of Clinical Psychiatry, 48,* 314–318.

Teng, E. L., Chiu, H. C., Schneider, L. S., & Metzger, L. E. (1987). Alzheimer's dementia: Performance on the Mini-Mental State Examination. *Journal of Consulting and Clinical Psychology, 55,* 96–100.

Teresi, J. A., Holmes, D., Ramirez, M., Gurland, B. J., & Lantigua, R. (2001). Performance of cognitive tests among different racial/ethnic and education groups: Findings of differential item functioning and possible item bias. *Journal of Mental Health and Aging, 7,* 79–89.

Tombaugh, T. N. (2005). Test-retest reliable coefficients and 5-year change scores for the MMSE and the 3MS. *Archives of Clinical Neuropsychology, 20,* 485–503.

Tombaugh, T. N. (in press). How much change in the MMSE and 3MS is a significant change? *Psychological Assessment.*

Tombaugh, T. N., McDowell, I., Krisjansson, B., & Hubley, A. M. (1996). Mini-Mental State Examination (MMSE) and the modified MMSE (3MS): A psychometric comparison and normative data. *Psychological Assessment, 8,* 48–59.

Tombaugh, T. N., & McIntyre, N. J. (1992). The Mini-Mental State Examination: A comprehensive review. *Journal of American Geriatric Society, 40,* 922–935.

Tsai, L., & Tsuang, M. T. (1979). The Mini-Mental State Test and computerized tomography. *American Journal of Psychiatry, 136,* 436–439.

Tschanz, J. T., Welsh-Bohmer, K. A., Plassman, B. L., Norton, M. C., Wyse, B. W., & Breitner, J. C. S. (2002). An adaptation of the modified Mini-Mental State Examination: Analysis of demographic influences and normative data. *Neuropsychiatry, Neuropsychology, and Behavioral Neurology, 15,* 28–38.

Uhlmann, R. F., Teri, L., Rees, T. S., Mozlowski, K. J., & Larson, E. B. (1989). Impact of mild to moderate hearing loss on mental status testing. *Journal of the American Geriatrics Society, 37,* 223–228.

Van Der Cammen, T. J. M., Van Harskamp, F., Stronks, D. L., Passchier, J., & Schudel, W. J. (1992). Value of the Mini-Mental State Examination and informants' data for the detection of dementia in geriatric outpatients. *Psychological Reports, 71,* 1003–1009.

Van Gorp, W. G., Marcotte, T. D., Sultzer, D., Hinkin, C., Mahler, M., & Cummings, J. L. (1999). Screening for dementia: Comparison of three commonly used instruments. *Journal of Clinical and Experimental Neuropsychology, 21,* 29–38.

Wells, J. C., Keyl, P. M., Aboraya, A., Folstein, M. F., & Anthony, J. C. (1992). Discriminant validity of a reduced set of Mini-Mental State Examination items for dementia and Alzheimer's disease. *Acta Psychiatrica Scandinavica, 86,* 23–31.

National Adult Reading Test (NART)

OTHER TEST NAMES

There are three main versions of this test (see Table 6–59). Nelson (1982) developed the NART using a British sample and the original WAIS. For the second edition (NART-2), the test was restandardized for use with the WAIS-R (Nelson & Willison, 1991). The test has also been adapted for use in the United States (American National Adult Reading Test, AMNART: Grober & Sliwinski, 1991) and in the United States and Canada (North American Adult Reading Test, NAART: Blair & Spreen, 1989).

PURPOSE

The purpose of the test is to provide an estimate of premorbid intellectual ability.

SOURCE

The NART-2 (word card and booklet, manual including pronunciation guide, and scoring forms) can be purchased from NFER-Nelson, Unit 28, Bramble Road, Techno Trading Centre, Swindon, Wiltshire, SNZ 8E2, at a cost of £74.25 sterling + vat.

Table 6–59 NART Versions

Test	Test Predicted	Number of Items
NART-2	WAIS-R	50
	FAS	
	PASAT	
	Raven's SPM	
NAART	WAIS-R	61
	Vocabulary	
AMNART	WAIS-R	45

There is no commercial source for the NAART or the AM-NART. Users may refer to the following text to design their own material (Figures 6–10 and 6–11).

AGE RANGE

The test can be used with individuals aged 18 and older.

DESCRIPTION

There are a number of clinical, medico-legal, or research situations where knowledge of premorbid cognitive ability (e.g., IQ) is essential. Since premorbid test data are rarely available, methods of estimation are needed. The National Adult Reading Test or NART-2 (Nelson, 1982; Nelson & O'Connell, 1978; Nelson & Willison, 1991), a reading test of 50 irregularly spelled words (e.g., ache, naive, thyme), has promise as an assessment tool for the determination of premorbid intellectual function (Figure 6–9). Assuming that the patient is familiar with the word, accuracy of pronunciation is used to predict IQ. As the words are short, patients do not have to analyze a complex visual stimulus, and because they are irregular, phonological decoding or intelligent guesswork will not provide the correct pronunciation. Therefore, it has been argued that performance depends more on previous knowledge than on current cognitive capacity (Nelson & O'-Connell, 1978). The value of the test lies in (a) the high correlation between reading ability and intelligence in the normal population (Crawford, Stewart, Cochrane, et al., 1989), (b) the fact that word reading tends to produce a fairly accurate estimate of preinjury IQ (Crawford et al., 2001; Moss & Dowd, 1991), and (c) the fact that the ability to pronounce irregular words is generally retained in mildly demented individuals (Crawford, Parker, et al., 1988; Fromm et al., 1991; Sharpe & O'Carroll, 1991; Stebbins, Gilley, et al., 1990; see *Validity*). It is important to note that the NART and its various versions (see Table 6–59), as of this writing, can only be used to predict WAIS-R IQ. To predict WAIS-III scores, the reader is referred to the reviews of the WTAR and WAIS III and the introduction to Chapter 6, which also considers methods for premorbid estimation (*General Cognitive Functioning, Neuropsychological Batteries and Assessment of Premorbid Intelligence*).

Figure 6–9 The New Adult Reading Test-2. *Source:* Extract from the National Adult Reading Test. Hazel S. Nelson, 1991, by permission of the publishers, NFER-Nelson.

Ache	Procreate	Leviathan
Debt	Quadruped	Aeon
Psalm	Catacomb	Detente
Depot	Superfluous	Gauche
Chord	Radix	Drachm
Bouquet	Assignate	Idyll
Deny	Gist	Beatify
Capon	Hiatus	Banal
Heir	Simile	Sidereal
Aisle	Rarefy	Puerperal
Subtle	Cellist	Topiary
Nausea	Zealot	Demesne
Equivocal	Abstemious	Campanile
Naive	Gouge	Labile
Thyme	Placebo	Syncope
Courteous	Facade	Prelate
Gaoled	Aver	

Nelson (1982) developed the test in England for use with the WAIS. Nelson and Willison (1991) restandardized the NART (NART-2) on a British sample so that it is possible to convert NART-2 scores directly to WAIS-R scores. Ryan and Paolo (1992) also standardized the NART for the WAIS-R, using an American sample of people 75 years and older. Blair and Spreen (1989) modified the test for use with North American populations (NAART) and validated it against the WAIS-R. The NAART consists of a list of 61 words printed in two columns on both sides of an 8 ½" × 11" card, which is given to the subject to read. The examiner records errors on a NAART scoring sheet. A sample scoring sheet along with the correct pronunciations is given in Figure 6–10. A short version, the NAART35, has recently been developed by Uttl (2002) and appears to provide a reliable and valid measure of verbal intelligence. The 35 items comprising this version are highlighted in Figure 6–10. Grober and Sliwinski (1991) also developed their own North American version, the AM-NART, which consists of 45 items. The items are shown in Figure 6–11.

In addition to these three main versions, other modifications have also appeared in the literature. An abbreviated NART (Short NART) is described later, which is based on the first half of the test (Beardsall & Brayne, 1990). Another useful modification is to place the words into sentences (e.g., the Cambridge Contextual Reading Test or CCRT: Beardsall & Huppert, 1994; C-AUSNART: Lucas et al., 2003), since the

Figure 6–10 NAART and NAART35 sample scoring sheet. Pronunciation symbols follow Webster's. Single asterisk indicates correct U.S. pronunciation only. Double asterisks indicate correct Canadian pronunciation only. Items in bold comprise the NAART35.

NAART
Sample Scoring Sheet

Page 1

DEBT det	SUBPOENA se·pē'·nə
DEBRIS də·brē, dā·brē', dā'·brē	PLACEBO plə·sē'·bō
AISLE īl	PROCREATE prō'·krē·āt
REIGN rān	PSALM säm, sälm*
DEPOT dē·,pō, de'·pō	BANAL bə·nál', bā·nal', bān'·əl
SIMILE sim'·ə·lē	**RAREFY** rãr'·ə·fī
LINGERIE lan'·zhə·rē', lon'·zhə·rā'	**GIST** jist
RECIPE res'·ə·pē	**CORPS** kor, korz
GOUGE gauj	**HORS D'OEUVRE** ȯr' dərv(r)'
HEIR ãr	**SIEVE** siv
SUBTLE sət'·əl	**HIATUS** hī·ā·təs
CATACOMB kaṯ'·ə·kōm	**GAUCHE** gōsh
BOUQUET bō·kā', bü·kā'	**ZEALOT** zel'·ət
GAUGE gāj	**PARADIGM** par'·ə·dīm, par'·ə·dim
COLONEL kərn'·əl	**FACADE** fə·säd'

Page 2

CELLIST chel'·əst	**LEVIATHAN** li·vī'·ə·thən
INDICT in·dīt'	PRELATE prel'·ət, prē'·lāt*
DETENTE dā·tä(n)t	**QUADRUPED** kwäd'·rə·ped
IMPUGN im·pyün'	**SIDEREAL** sī·dir'·ē·al, sə·dir'·ē·al
CAPON kā'·pən, kā'·pon	**ABSTEMIOUS** ab·stē'·mē·əs
RADIX rād'·iks	**BEATIFY** bē·aṯ'·ə·fī
AEON ē'·ən, e'·an	**GAOLED** jāld
EPITOME i·piṯ'·ə·mē	**DEMESNE** di·mān', di·mēn'
EQUIVOCAL i·kwiv'·ə·kəl	**SYNCOPE** sing'·kə·pē, sin'·k'rrn·pē
REIFY rā'·ə·fī, rē'·ə·fi	**ENNUI** an·wē'
INDICES in'·də·sēz	DRACHM dram
ASSIGNATE as'·ig·nāt'	CIDEVANT sēd·ə·vä(n)'
TOPIARY tō·pē·er'·ē	EPERGNE i·pərn', ā·pərn'
CAVEAT kav'·ē·at, kāv'·ē·at, kā·vē·aṯ'**	VIVACE vē·väch'·ā, vē·väch'·ē
SUPERFLUOUS sụ·pẻr'·flü·əs	TALIPES tal'·ə·pēz
	SYNECDOCHE sə·nek'·də·kē

provision of semantic and syntactic cues (context) results in a larger number of words being read correctly and, hence, in a higher estimate of IQ, particularly among demented people and poor-to-average readers (Beardsall & Huppert, 1994; Conway & O'Carroll, 1997; Watt & O'Carroll, 1999). Beardsall (1998) has developed an equation to convert CCRT errors to WAIS-R Verbal IQ scores based on a relatively small sample (73) of healthy British individuals aged 70 years and older. The inclusion of demographic information (education, gender) improved prediction. The CCRT as well as a conversion table (to convert CCRT errors to Verbal IQ) is available upon request from the author (L. Beardsall, School of Psychology, University of Birmingham, Edgbaston, Birmingham, B15 2TT, UK). The test has not yet been adjusted for use in North America.

ADMINISTRATION

NART-2

See *Source*. Briefly, the patient is presented with the word card and is instructed to read each word. Because the reading of words in a list format may be confusing for some subjects, the NART-2 is available in booklet format with each word

Figure 6–11 AMNART list of words. *Source:* From Grober & Sliwinski, 1991. Reprinted with permission of the authors and Psychology Press.

ACHE	CHASSIS
AISLE	CELLIST
CAPON	ALGAE
DEBT	SUPERFLUOUS
CHORD	CHAMOIS
HEIR	THYME
DENY	APROPOS
BOUQUET	VIRULENT
CAPRICE	ZEALOT
GAUGE	FACADE
WORSTED	CABAL
DEPOT	ABSTEMIOUS
NAUSEA	DETENTE
NAÏVE	SCION
SUBTLE	PAPYRUS
PUGILIST	QUADRUPED
FETAL	PRELATE
BLATANT	EPITOME
PLACEBO	BEATIFY
HIATUS	HYPERBOLE
SIMILE	IMBROGLIO
MERINGUE	SYNCOPE
SIEVE	

displayed in large print on a separate card. The reading of words is paced by requiring the patient to pause between words until the examiner calls, "next."

Short NART

An optional criterion for discontinuation of the NART-2 (14 incorrect in 15 consecutive responses) is presented in the test manual. However, Beardsall and Brayne (1990) have reported that, in a sample of elderly subjects, this criterion was rarely met. To reduce anxiety or distress in people with poor reading skills, they developed an equation that estimates a person's score on the second half of the NART (items 26–50) from the first half (the Short NART). If a patient scores less than 12 correct on the Short NART, this is taken as the total correct score, since Beardsall and Brayne (1990) showed that people who score 0 to 11 correct are unlikely to add to their score by completing the second half of the test. For those scoring between 12 and 20, a conversion table (Table 6–60) is used to predict the full error score. For people scoring more than 20 correct, the complete NART is administered. The accuracy of the Short NART in estimating premorbid IQ has been found to be virtually equivalent to the full NART in a cross-validation study (Crawford et al., 1991).

Table 6–60 Conversion Table for Predicted Full NART Error Score From Short NART Score

Correct Score	Conversion to Full NART Error Score
0–11	As in Full NART (50 minus correct)
12	38
13	36
14	34
15	33
16	31
17	30
18	28
19	26
20	24
21+	As in Full NART (50 minus correct)

Compute the number of correct words in the Short NART. If 0 to 20 are correct, then do not continue to the Full NART. If 21 to 25 are correct, then continue to the Full NART. These scores can then be converted to predicted IQ scores using appropriate equations.

Source: From Beardsall & Brayne, 1990. Copyright British Psychological Society. Reprinted with permission.

NAART/NAART35

The instructions are shown in Figure 6–12.

AMNART

For the AMNART, the person is asked to read each word aloud. If the individual changes a response, the last response is scored as correct or not correct. Boekamp et al. (1995) reported that no discontinuation rule could be established for the AMNART because word difficulty order was not invariant across different samples.

ADMINISTRATION TIME

The approximate time required is 10 minutes.

SCORING

The use of a pronunciation guide and a tape recorder is recommended to facilitate scoring. Each incorrectly pronounced word counts as one error. Slight variations in pronunciation are acceptable when they are due to regional accents. The total number of errors is tabulated.

NART-2 and Short NART

These scores can be converted to WAIS-R VIQ, PIQ, and FSIQ using a table provided in the manual (Nelson & Willison, 1991). Note that Short NART scores must be converted to full NART-2 scores. An additional table is provided in the test

Figure 6–12 Instructions for NAART and NAART35.

"I want you to read slowly down this list of words starting here (indicate 'debt') and continuing down this column and on to the next. When you have finished reading the words on the page, turn the page over and begin here" (indicate top of second page).

"After each word please wait until I say 'Next' before reading the next word."

"I must warn you that there are many words that you probably won't recognize; in fact, *most* people don't know them, so just guess at these, OK? Go ahead."

The examinee should be encouraged to guess, and all responses should be reinforced ("good," "that's fine," etc.). The examinee may change a response if he or she wishes to do so but if more than one version is given, the examinee must decide on the final choice. No time limit is imposed.

manual to evaluate whether the predicted minus obtained discrepancy is unusual. Alternatively, examiners working with American patients can use Ryan and Paolo's (1992) equations to predict WAIS-R IQ:

$$\text{Estimated VIQ} = 132.3893 + (\text{NART-2 errors})(-1.164)$$

$$\text{Estimated PIQ} = 123.0684 + (\text{NART-2 errors})(-0.823)$$

$$\text{Estimated FSIQ} = 131.3845 + (\text{NART-2 errors})(-1.124)$$

The standard errors of estimate (SE_Es) are 7.70, 12.08, and 8.83 for WAIS-R VIQ, PIQ, and FSIQ, respectively. Note that the regression equations were developed on a sample of normal, community-dwelling subjects, 75 years and older. The inclusion of education (plus NART errors) in the equation did not significantly improve prediction. Carswell et al. (1997) cross-validated the equation for VIQ and also noted that demographic variables (age and education) failed to significantly improve the accuracy of postdiction.

Willshire et al. (1991), however, included demographic variables with the NART and provided a substantially better estimate of premorbid cognitive functioning than that given by the NART or by demographic information alone. The equation (appropriate for subjects between the ages of 55 and 69 years) is as follows:

$$\text{Estimated IQ} = 123.7 - 0.8 \, (\text{NART errors})$$
$$+ 3.8 \, \text{education} - 7.4 \, \text{gender}$$

To use this equation, note that educational level comprised the following five categories: (1) some primary school, (2) some secondary school, (3) some secondary school plus trade qualifications, (4) secondary school completed, and (5) tertiary education begun. Gender was assigned as males = 1 and females = 2.

NAART/NAART35

NAART equations (Blair & Spreen, 1989) to predict WAIS-R VIQ, PIQ, and FSIQ are as follows:

$$\text{Estimated VIQ} = 128.7 - .89(\text{NAART errors})$$

$$\text{Estimated PIQ} = 119.4 - .42(\text{NAART errors})$$

$$\text{Estimated FSIQ} = 127.8 - .78(\text{NAART errors})$$

The SE_Es for VIQ, PIQ, and FSIQ are 6.56, 10.67, and 7.63, respectively.

NAART equations (Uttl, 2002) to predict WAIS-R Vocabulary are:

Estimated Vocabulary (raw score)
$$= 31.30 + 0.622(\text{NAART correct}) \, (SE_E = 5.14)$$

Estimated Vocabulary (raw score)
$$= 25.71 + 0.566(\text{NAART correct}) + 0.508$$
$$(\text{Education}) \, (SE_E = 5.02)$$

Estimated Vocabulary Scaled Score
$$= 5.383 + 0.179(\text{NAART}) \, (SE_E = 1.71)$$

Estimated Vocabulary Scaled Score
$$= 4.112 + 0.167(\text{NAART}) + 0.115$$
$$(\text{Education}) \, (SE_E = 1.69)$$

For the NAART35, Uttl (2002) provides the following equations to predict WAIS-R Vocabulary:

Estimated Vocabulary (raw score)
$$= 38.67 + 0.811(\text{NAART35 correct}) \, (SE_E = 5.11)$$

Estimated Vocabulary (raw score)
$$= 32.50 + 0.740(\text{NAART35 correct}) + 0.500$$
$$(\text{Education}) \, (SE_E = 5.00)$$

Estimated Vocabulary Scaled Score
$$= 7.52 + 0.233(\text{NAART35}) \, (SE_E = 1.71)$$

Estimated Vocabulary Scaled Score
$$= 6.12 + 0.217(\text{NAART35}) + 0.114(\text{Education})$$
$$(SE_E = 1.69)$$

The equation to predict NAART from the NAART35 is:

$$\text{NAART correct} = 12.39 + 1.282(\text{NAART35}) \, (SE_E = 1.54)$$

AMNART

For the AMNART (Grober & Sliwinski, 1991), the equation to estimate WAIS-R VIQ is:

Estimated VIQ
= 118.2 – .89 (AMNART errors)
+ .64 (years of education). The SE_E is 7.94.

DEMOGRAPHIC EFFECTS

As might be expected, NART (NART-2, NAART) errors systematically decrease with increasing FSIQ (Wiens et al., 1993). NART (NAART, AMNART) performance is correlated with years of education and social class. Age, gender, and ethnicity (Caucasian versus African American) have little effect on performance (Antsey et al., 2000; Beardsall, 1998; Boekamp et al., 1995; Cockburn et al., 2000; Crawford, Stewart, et al., 1988; Freeman & Godfrey, 2000; Graf & Uttl, 1995; Grober & Sliwinski, 1991; Ivnik et al., 1996: Nelson, 1982; Nelson & Willison, 1991; Starr et al., 1992; Storandt et al., 1995; Wiens et al., 1993), although when a wide age range is studied (well-educated healthy individuals aged 16–84 years), an age-related increase in "correct" NAART scores appears to emerge (see Table 6–61) (Graf & Uttl, 1995; Parkin & Java, 1999; Uttl 2002; Uttl & Graf, 1997) due largely to the relatively weak performance of young adults.

While cross-sectional studies do not suggest significant decline in NART (all versions) scores in older adults, a recent longitudinal study (Deary et al., 1998) showed evidence of decline with aging. In that study, 387 healthy elderly people were tested with the NART-2 at baseline and followed up four years later. NART-estimated IQ fell by a mean of 2.1 points over four years. Further, the amount of decline was differentially related to initial cognitive status, social class, and education. Those with higher baseline ability, in higher social groups, with more education, and who were younger were relatively protected from decline.

INTERPRETIVE GUIDELINES

Prediction of Wechsler Intelligence Scores

NART-2. Nelson and Willison (1991) have provided a discrepancy table to determine the probability of a chance oc-

currence of a discrepancy in favor of NART-2-estimated IQ over observed WAIS-R IQ. The equations are based on a British sample. For North American samples, Ryan and Paolo (1992) developed regression equations to predict WAIS-R IQs from NART error scores (see *Scoring*), but they did not provide corresponding discrepancy tables.

Willshire et al. (1991) have developed regression equations to predict WAIS-R IQs for use with adults, aged 55 to 69 years, based on a combination of NART errors and demographic variables. The equation (see *Scoring*) is based on an Australian sample. However, standard errors of estimate and discrepancy tables are not provided.

Crawford, Stewart, Parker, et al. (1989) have also developed regression equations that combine NART errors and demographic variables to predict premorbid IQ. Unfortunately, these equations are based on the WAIS, not the newer versions (WAIS-R, WAIS-III).

Because there are limitations in estimating premorbid ability from NART scores (e.g., regression to the mean, limited range of scores, vulnerability of performance to disease), Crawford et al. (1990) have developed a regression equation to predict NART scores from demographic variables (years of education, social class, age, and gender).[1] The equation is as follows:

Predicted NART error score
= 37.9 – 1.77 (education) + 2.7 (class) – .07 (age)
– 0.03 (gender); Se_{est} = 6.93

The equation can also be downloaded from Dr. Crawford's site www.psyc.abdn.ac.uk. The equation allows the clinician to compare a current NART score against a predicted score. A large discrepancy between the predicted and obtained scores (obtained error score more than 11.4 points over the predicted score) suggests impaired NART performance and alerts the clinician to the fact that the NART will not provide an accurate estimate of premorbid ability.

NAART. Blair and Spreen (1989) recommended that for PIQ, a positive discrepancy of at least 21 points between estimated and actual IQs indicates the possibility of deterioration. For VIQ and FSIQ, a positive discrepancy of 15 or more points between estimated and actual IQ scores indicates the

Table 6–61 NAART and NAART35 Mean Number Correct by Age Group

Performance on NAART and NAART35 by Midpoint Overlapping Age Groups

Midpoint	20	25	30	35	40	45	50	55	60	65	70	75	80
Range	18–25	20–30	25–35	30–40	35–45	40–50	45–55	50–60	55–65	60–70	65–75	70–80	75–91
N	52	63	55	51	51	59	68	62	59	56	57	52	48
NAART M	38.46	39.90	39.44	38.58	40.05	40.20	41.57	42.88	44.38	42.28	43.15	43.55	43.82
SD	9.29	8.30	8.57	9.33	10.87	10.79	9.16	8.33	8.26	9.31	9.42	8.84	8.09
NAART35 M	20.60	21.76	21.39	20.59	21.80	21.72	22.75	23.76	24.84	22.90	23.70	24.18	24.51
SD	6.63	6.04	6.32	7.11	8.48	8.29	7.27	6.66	6.32	7.31	7.59	7.08	6.59

Source: Adapted from Uttl, 2002.

possibility of intellectual deterioration or impairment (based on the calculation of 95% confidence levels). Wiens et al. (1993) reported that only about 10% of normal individuals have predicted-obtained FSIQ differences as large as 15 points. Thus, a difference of this size is infrequent enough among healthy people to merit clinical attention (see also Berry et al., 1994).

To evaluate whether the obtained NAART score is within the expected range, Uttl (2002) has developed NAART prediction equations based on age as well as age and education. The equations are as follows:

$$\text{NAART correct} = 36.60 + 0.0925(\text{Age}) \ (SE_E = 9.15)$$

$$\text{NAART correct} = 14.07 + 1.518(\text{Education}) + 0.071$$
$$(\text{Age}) \ (SE_E = 8.38)$$

AMNART.   Grober and Sliwinski (1991) recommend a discrepancy of 10 or more points between estimated and obtained VIQ values to suggest the possibility of intellectual decline. However, Boekamp et al. (1995) suggest caution in applying this rule; in their study, such a heuristic resulted in considerable overlap between participants who were demented and those who were not. Ivnik et al. (1996) have provided age- and education-based normative information derived from a sample of older adults (aged 55+), almost exclusively Caucasian, living in an economically stable region of the United States (as part of the MOANS project). Their data are shown in Table 6–62 and may help the examiner to determine whether the obtained score provides a reasonable estimate of premorbid ability (see also *Comment*).

Caveat.   It is important to note the ranges of possible predicted WAIS-R scores. The range of possible NAART-predicted IQs is 129 to 74 for the Verbal Scale, 119 to 94 for the Performance Scale, and 128 to 80 for the Full Scale (Wiens et al., 1993). The range of possible NART-predicted IQs is 132 to 74 for the Verbal Scale, 123 to 82 for the Performance Scale, and 131 to 75 for the Full Scale (Ryan & Paolo, 1992). The range of possible VIQ estimates for the AMNART is about 131 to 83 (Grober & Sliwinski, 1991). Thus, there is truncation of the spread of predicted IQs on either end of the distribution, leading to unreliable estimates for individuals at other than average levels of ability (Ryan & Paolo, 1992; Wiens et al., 1993).

Prediction of Other Cognitive Tests

The majority of research on the NART has focussed on estimating premorbid intelligence and has employed the Wechsler intelligence scales as the criterion variable. NART equations are, however, also available for estimating premorbid performance on other cognitive tasks (see Table 6–59), including the FAS verbal fluency task (Crawford et al., 1992), the PASAT (Crawford et al., 1998), and the Raven's Standard Progressive Matrices (Freeman & Godfrey, 2000; Van den Broek & Bradshaw, 1994). The equations are provided below (see also reviews of *Verbal Fluency*, *PASAT*, and *Raven's* in this book):

Estimated FAS
$$= 57.5 - (0.76 \times \text{NART errors}), \ SE_{est} = 9.09;$$
also see www.abdn.ac.uk

Table 6–62 AMNART (Correct Count) MOANS Norms for Persons Aged 56–97 Years

Percentile Ranges	Scaled Score	Age										
		56–62	63–65	66–68	69–71	72–74	75–77	78–80	81–83	84–86	87–89	90–97
<1	2	>34	>34	>34	>34	>34	>35	>35	>35	>35	>35	>35
1	3	34	34	34	34	34	35	35	35	35	35	35
2	4	33	33	33	33	33	34	34	34	34	34	34
3–5	5	30–32	30–32	30–32	30–32	30–32	30–33	32–33	32–33	32–33	32–33	32–33
6–10	6	28–29	28–29	28–29	28–29	28–29	28–29	28–31	28–31	28–31	28–31	28–31
11–18	7	25–27	25–27	25–27	25–27	25–27	25–27	25–27	25–27	25–27	25–27	25–27
19–28	8	23–24	23–24	23–24	23–24	23–24	23–24	23–24	23–24	23–24	23–24	23–24
29–40	9	20–22	20–22	20–22	20–22	20–22	20–22	20–22	20–22	20–22	20–22	20–22
41–50	10	14–19	15–19	15–19	17–19	17–19	17–19	17–19	17–19	17–19	17–19	17–19
60–71	11	11–13	12–14	12–14	13–16	13–16	13–16	13–16	13–16	13–16	13–16	13–16
72–81	12	9–10	9–11	9–11	9–12	9–12	9–12	10–12	10–12	10–12	10–12	10–12
82–89	13	7–8	7–8	7–8	7–8	7–8	7–8	7–9	7–9	7–9	7–9	7–9
90–94	14	6	6	6	6	6	6	6	6	6	6	6
95–97	15	5	5	5	5	5	5	5	5	5	5	5
98	16	3–4	4	4	4	4	4	4	4	4	4	4
99	17	1–2	1–3	1–3	2–3	3	3	3	3	3	3	3
>99	18	0	0	0	0–1	0–2	0–2	0–2	0–2	0–2	0–2	0–2
N		160	169	152	134	125	112	91	83	83	83	83

Note: Age- and education-corrected MOANS scales scores ($MSS_{A\&E}$) are calculated from a person's age-corrected MOANS scaled score (MSS_A) and that person's education expressed in years of formal schooling completed as follows: $MSS_{A\&E} = 6.77 + (1.25 \times \text{A-MSS}) - (0.73 \times \text{Education})$.

Source: Adapted from Ivnik et al., 1996, based on Mayo's Older Normative Studies (MOANS). Reprinted with the kind permission of Psychology Press.

Estimated PASAT Total
   $= 215.74 - (1.85 \times \text{NART errors}) - (.77 \times \text{Age})$
   $\text{SE}_{est} = 34.87$; also see www.abdn.ac.uk

Estimated RSPM
   $= 66.65 + (-.462 \times \text{NART errors}) + (-.254 \times \text{age})$

RELIABILITY

The NART/NART-2/NAART/AMNART is among the most reliable tests in clinical use.

Internal Consistency

Reliability estimates are above .90 for the various versions, including the NAART35 (Blair & Spreen, 1989; Crawford, Stewart, et al., 1988; Grober & Sliwinski, 1991; Uttl, 2002).

Test-Retest Reliability and Practice Effects

A test-retest reliability of .98 has been reported for the NART, with practice effects emerging over the short term (10 days; Crawford, Stewart, Besson, et al., 1989). However, the mean decrease is less than one NART error, suggesting that practice effects are of little clinical significance. One-year test-retest coefficients are high (.89) (Deary et al., 2004). With longer retest intervals (e.g., four years), reliability is lower, though still respectable (.67–.72; Deary et al., 1998; Kondel et al., 2003).

Raguet et al. (1996) gave the NAART to 51 normal adults on two separate occasions, separated by about one year. NAART estimates were highly reliable, with a coefficient of .92. Practice effects were minimal.

Interrater Reliability

The NART also has high interrater reliability (above .88; Crawford, Stewart, Besson, et al., 1989; O'Carroll, 1987; Riley & Simmonds, 2003; Sharpe & O'Carroll, 1991). Some NART words, however, have a disproportionately high rate of interrater disagreement (*aeon*, *puerperal*, *aver*, *sidereal*, and *prelate*) and particular care should be taken when scoring these words (Crawford, Stewart, Besson, et al., 1989). Training by an experienced examiner and use of the pronunciation guide appears to improve accuracy for these items (Alcott et al., 1999). Blair and Spreen (1989) report that a measure of interscorer reliability for the NAART was .99 ($p < .001$).

VALIDITY

Construct Validity

Researchers generally report moderate to high correlations (.40–.80) between NART (NAART, AMNART) performance and concurrently given measures of general intellectual status (Blair & Spreen, 1989; Carswell et al., 1997; Cockburn et al.,

2000; Crawford, Stewart, Besson, et al., 1989, 2001; Freeman & Godfrey, 2000; Grober & Sliwinski, 1991; Johnstone et al., 1996; Nelson & O'Connell, 1978; Paolo et al., 1997; Raguet et al., 1996; Sharpe & O'Carroll, 1991; Uttl, 2002; Wiens et al., 1993; Willshire et al., 1991), WRAT-R Reading (Johnstone et al., 1993; Wiens et al., 1993), and education (Maddrey et al., 1996). In the standardization sample, the NART predicted 55%, 60%, and 30% of the variance in prorated WAIS Full Scale, Verbal, and Performance IQ, respectively (Nelson, 1982). Similar results have been reported by others for the various versions (e.g., Blair & Spreen, 1989; Crawford, Stewart, Besson, et al., 1989; Ryan & Paolo, 1992; Wiens et al., 1993). In short, the test is a good predictor of VIQ and FSIQ, but is relatively poor at predicting PIQ. Among verbal subtests, NART (NAART) errors correlate most highly with Vocabulary and Information (Wiens et al., 1993). Combined factor analysis of the NART and WAIS (Crawford, Stewart, Cochrane, et al., 1989) has revealed that the NART has a very high loading (.85) on the first unrotated principal component, which is regarded as representing general intelligence (*g*). Further, the NAART appears to measure verbal intelligence with the same degree of accuracy in various age groups (Uttl, 2002).

The test has good accuracy in the retrospective estimation of IQ (Berry et al., 1994; Carswell et al., 1997; Moss & Dowd, 1991; Raguet et al., 1996). A recent study by Crawford et al. (2001) followed up 177 individuals who had been administered an IQ test (Moray House Test, MHT) at age 11. They found a correlation of .73 between these scores and NART scores at age 77. The NART also had a significant correlation with the MMSE ($r = .25$), but this correlation fell near zero after controlling for the influence of childhood IQ. These results provide strong support for the claim that NART scores estimate premorbid, rather than current, intelligence.

There is also evidence that an estimate of cognitive change (as indexed by the discrepancy between current performance on the NART and Raven's Standard Progressive Matrices) reflects lifetime cognitive change. Deary et al. (2004) followed up 80 nondemented people who took the MHT at age 11 and retested them at age 77, on the NART, Raven's, and two WAIS-R subtests (Digit Symbol, Object Assembly). The NART-Raven difference correlated highly with the MHT-Raven difference ($r = .64$) and with MHT-WAIS difference ($r = .66$). That is, the estimate of cognitive change based on the NART-Raven's difference correlated highly with actual cognitive change that took place over a course of 67 years.

Prediction of IQ tends to be more accurate with equations based on NART (or NAART/AMNART) scores than with the Wechsler Vocabulary subtest (Crawford, Parker, & Besson, 1988; Sharpe & O'Carroll, 1991) or with demographic variables (Blair & Spreen, 1989; Bright et al., 2002; Grober & Sliwinski, 1991; Ryan & Paolo, 1992). However, Paolo et al. (1997) reported that both the NART and Barona demographic procedures demonstrated adequate ability to detect intellectual decline in persons with mild dementia.

Whether combining demographic and NART (or NAART/AMNART) estimates increases predictive accuracy is of some debate. Bright et al. (2002) found that an equation combining NART scores with demographic variables did not significantly increase the amount of variance in WAIS/WAIS-R IQ explained by NART only, either in patients (e.g., with AD, Korsakoff's) or healthy controls. By contrast, other authors have concluded that the addition of NART to demographic information improves prediction. For example, Willshire et al. (1991) reported that in a sample of residents in Melbourne, Australia, 56% of the variance in WAIS-R IQ scores could be predicted on the basis of a formula that included NART error score, education, and gender. This was 24% more than could be predicted on the basis of education alone and 18% more than on the basis of NART error score alone (see *Scoring*). Similarly, Watt and O'Carroll (1999) reported that in healthy participants, the addition of demographic variables improved the amount of explained variance in current WAIS-R Verbal IQ when using the NART. Carswell et al. (1997) found that a regression equation that combined NART errors and WAIS-R Vocabulary age-scaled scores provided a better estimate of VIQ scores obtained three years previously than did NART errors or Vocabulary scores alone. Grober and Sliwinski (1991) found that inclusion of both AMNART errors and education permitted a larger range of possible VIQ estimates and was slightly more accurate in estimating VIQ than the equation using only AMNART errors. Finally, Gladsjo et al. (1999) found that in normal individuals (aged 20–81 years), addition of the ANART (a 50-item American variant of the NART) improved prediction of WAIS-R VIQ, FSIQ, and learning score (based on CVLT, Story and Figure Learning Tests) beyond that achieved by demographics alone. The use of the ANART with demographic information appeared particularly useful in those examinees who have unusual combinations of lower than expected reading ability given their educational achievement. Of note, the ANART did not improve estimates of other premorbid abilities (general cognitive impairment as indexed by the Average Impairment Rating, which is a summary of 12 measures from the Halstead-Reitan Battery, Delayed Memory) beyond that accomplished by demographic correction.

The test is generally resistant to neurological insults such as closed head injury (Crawford, Parker, et al., 1988; Watt & O'Carroll, 1999) and is one of the few cognitive measures that is relatively robust against the effects of disease and decline in old age (Anstey et al., 2001). However, the test is not insensitive to cerebral damage, and deterioration in reading test performance does occur in some patients with cerebral dysfunction, for example, in patients with a severe TBI tested within 12 months of injury (Riley & Simmonds, 2003); in patients with moderate to severe levels of dementia (Boekamp et al., 1995; Fromm et al., 1991; Grober & Sliwinski, 1991; Paolo et al., 1997; Stebbins et al., 1988; Stebbins, Gilley, et al., 1990), even when obviously aphasic or alexic patients are excluded (Taylor, 1999); in patients with mild dementia who have accompanying linguistic or semantic memory deficits (Grober & Sliwinski, 1991; Stebbins, Wilson, et al., 1990; Storandt et al., 1995); and in some other specific conditions

(e.g., patients with multiple sclerosis (MS), particularly those with a chronic-progressive course; Friend & Grattan, 1998). Although some (O'Carroll et al., 1992) have reported that NART scores are low in patients with Korsakoff's syndrome or frontal disturbance, others (Bright et al., 2002; Crawford & Warrington, 2002) have not found that NART performance is affected in these patients.

There are other reports of deterioration in NART performance in the later stages of dementia. Patterson et al. (1994) found a dramatic decrease in NART performance as a function of AD severity and reported a correlation of .56 between MMSE and NART scores. They attributed the specific reading deficit manifested on the NART to the deterioration of semantic memory in AD and to an impaired ability to perform specific phonological manipulations. Paque and Warrington (1995) compared the performance of 57 dementing patients on the NART and the WAIS-R. Patients were examined on two occasions spaced at least 10 months apart. Although NART performance declined over time, the deterioration on VIQ and PIQ was more rapid and severe. Patients whose reading declined tended to have a lower VIQ than PIQ, raising the concern that verbal skills may have already been compromised by disease. Taylor et al. (1996) tested a sample of AD patients on three or four occasions each separated by about one year. AMNART performance declined with increasing dementia severity as measured by the MMSE. Cockburn et al. (2000) assessed patients with AD on four yearly occasions. They also found that NART scores declined over time, particularly if the initial MMSE score was low. Whereas initial NART scores were associated with educational level, the extent of change depended more on initial MMSE performance. However, they also noted individual differences in the rate of decline, suggesting that reliance on group data may be quite misleading. Cockburn et al. also found that lower frequency words disappear faster from the lexicon than higher frequency words. However, there were widespread individual differences and also wide variability in word recognition over time. That is, words might be recognized at one visit, not a year later, but then correctly recognized in later visits.

The influence of psychiatric disorder is not clear. Some have reported that NART performance is not affected by depression (Crawford et al., 1987). However, others (Watt & O'-Carroll, 1999) have found that NART scores are influenced by depression, at least in patients who have suffered head injuries. Findings by Kondel et al. (2003) in people with schizophrenia suggest that the NART may provide a reasonable estimate of premorbid IQ in younger patients (20–51 years), but not necessarily in older ones (52–85 years). Russell et al. (2000) gave the NART and WAIS-R to a sample of adults with schizophrenia who had a measure of IQ (WISC/WISC-R) taken during childhood (i.e., about 23 years earlier). There were no significant differences between childhood and adult measures of IQ; however, there were significant differences between these two indices and NART-estimated IQ, particularly when IQ did not fall in the average range. The NART overestimated IQ by an average of 15 IQ points. The authors recommended the use of more than one index of premorbid functioning.

COMMENT

Administration of this measure is relatively straightforward and takes little time. The test has high levels of internal, test-retest, and interrater reliability. It correlates moderately well with measures of intelligence (particularly VIQ and FSIQ) and is less related to demographic variables than various measures of cognitive functioning (e.g., Wechsler test; Bright et al., 2002). Although the reading ability assessed by the NART/NAART/AMNART may not be entirely insensitive to cerebral damage, the available evidence suggests that it may be less vulnerable than many other cognitive measures, such as the MMSE and Wechsler tests (Berry et al., 1994; Christensen et al., 1991; Cockburn et al., 2000; Maddrey et al., 1996). Thus, although far from perfect, tests like the NART may be the instruments of choice for assessing premorbid IQ.

The test, however, should not be used with patients who have compromised language or reading ability, with those who have VIQs less than PIQs, or with those who have significant articulatory or visual acuity problems. Use of the NART (or its variants) within 12 months of a severe head injury is also not recommended since doing so runs the risk of significantly underestimating premorbid IQ (Riley & Simmonds, 2003). Further, while the test may provide an acceptable premorbid index in the early stages of a dementing disorder, it is susceptible to changes that occur with disease progression. The potential confounding effect of depression requires additional study.

It is also important to bear in mind that use of regression procedures has some limitations, including regression toward the mean and limited range of scores. These limitations suggest that two types of errors may occur when the equations are applied to individuals with suspected dementia (Boekamp et al., 1995; Ryan & Paolo, 1992; Wiens et al., 1993). In the case of superior premorbid ability, the predicted IQ will represent an underestimate of the amount of cognitive deterioration present. However, since patients with dementia are rarely referred for psychological assessment when their intelligence levels remain in the superior range, this ceiling effect should not necessarily invalidate the clinical utility of the test (Ryan & Paolo, 1992). On the other hand, in individuals whose premorbid abilities are relatively low, the estimated IQ might suggest cognitive deterioration when, in actuality, it has not occurred. Note, too, that a fairly large loss in cognitive ability (about 15–21 IQ points) may need to occur before the NART (NAART) can reliably identify potential abnormality. Accordingly, the clinician needs to be cautious in inferring an absence of decline when cutoff discrepancies are not met.

These limitations underscore the need to supplement NART (NAART/AMNART) estimates of premorbid functioning with clinical observations and information about a patient's educational and occupational accomplishments as well as other performance-based data (e.g., MMSE, Vocabulary). Raguet et al. (1996) recommend averaging estimates from the Barona formula and NAART. Crawford et al. (1990) and Uttl (2002) have attempted to address the problem by developing regression equations to predict NART/NAART scores from demographic variables (see *Interpretive Guidelines*). A similar procedure has been developed for use with the new WTAR.

The majority of research on the NART has focussed on estimating premorbid intelligence. NART equations are, however, also available for estimating premorbid performance on other cognitive tasks (see Table 6–59 and *Interpretive Guidelines*). Some (Schlosser & Ivison, 1989) have speculated that NART equations based on memory test performance may be capable of assessing dementia earlier than the NART/WAIS-R combination. However, findings by Gladsjo et al. (1999) and Issella et al. (2005) suggest that the NART (or its variants) does not improve accuracy of prediction of premorbid memory abilities beyond that accomplished by demographic correction.

Although the rationale for developing various versions of the NART (NAART, AMNART, CCRT) appears sound, there is no empirical comparison of their relative efficacy (Franzen et al., 1997). The various forms and equations should not be used interchangeably, and the exact version should be specified in clinical or research reports (Franzen et al., 1997). Note, too, that the equations developed for the NAART35 remain to be cross-validated in other samples.

One other limitation deserves attention. The various NART versions have been developed for use with the WAIS and WAIS-R. To date, only the WTAR, not the NART (NAART, AMNART), has been validated against the updated WAIS-III, the version currently used in most research and clinical settings.

NOTE

1. Social class coding: 1: professional (e.g., architect, church minister); 2: intermediate (e.g., computer programmer, teacher); 3: skilled (e.g., carpenter, salesperson); 4: semiskilled (e.g., assembly-line worker, waiter); 5: unskilled (e.g., cleaner, laborer). Gender coding: male = 1, female = 2.

REFERENCES

Alcott, D., Swann, R., & Grafhan, A. (1999). The effect of training on rater reliability on the scoring of the NART. *British Journal of Clinical Psychology, 38,* 431–434.

Anstey, K. J., Luszcz, M. A., Giles, L. C., & Andrews, G. R. (2001). Demographic, health, cognitive, and sensory variables as predictors of mortality in very old adults. *Psychology and Aging, 16,* 3–11.

Beardsall, L. (1998). Development of the Cambridge Contextual Reading Test for improving the estimation of premorbid verbal intelligence in older persons with dementia. *British Journal of Clinical Psychology, 37,* 229–240.

Beardsall, L., & Brayne, C. (1990). Estimation of verbal intelligence in an elderly community: A prediction analysis using a shortened NART. *British Journal of Clinical Psychology, 29*, 83–90.

Beardsall, L., & Huppert, F. A. (1994). Improvement in NART word reading in demented and normal older persons using the Cambridge Contextual Reading Test. *Journal of Clinical and Experimental Neuropsychology, 16*, 232–242.

Berry, D. T. R., Carpenter, G. S., Campbell, D. A., Schmitt, F. A., Helton, K., & Lipke-Molby, T. (1994). The new adult reading test-revised: Accuracy in estimating WAIS-R IQ scores obtained 3.5 years earlier from normal older persons. *Archives of Clinical Neuropsychology, 9*, 239–250.

Blair, J. R., & Spreen, O. (1989). Predicting premorbid IQ: A revision of the National Adult Reading Test. *The Clinical Neuropsychologist, 3*, 129–136.

Boekamp, J. R., Strauss, M. E., & Adams, N. (1995). Estimating premorbid intelligence in African-American and white elderly veterans using the American version of the National Adult Reading Test. *Journal of Clinical and Experimental Neuropsychology, 17*, 645–653.

Bright, P., Jadlow, E., & Kopelman, M. D. (2002). The National Adult Reading Test as a measure of premorbid intelligence: A comparison with estimates derived from premorbid levels. *Journal of the International Neuropsychological Society, 8*, 847–854.

Carswell, L. M., Graves, R. E., Snow, W. G., & Tierney, M. C. (1997). Postdicting verbal IQ of elderly individuals. *Journal of Clinical and Experimental Neuropsychology, 19*, 914–921.

Christensen, H., Hadzi-Pavlovic, D., & Jacomb, P. (1991). The psychometric differentiation of dementia from normal aging: A meta-analysis. *Psychological Assessment, 3*, 147–155.

Cockburn, J., Keene, J., Hope, T., & Smith, P. (2000). Progressive decline in NART scores with increasing dementia severity. *Journal of Clinical and Experimental Neuropsychology, 22*, 508–517.

Conway, S. C., & O'Carroll, R. E. (1997). An evaluation of the Cambridge Contextual Reading Test (CCRT) in Alzheimer's disease. *British Journal of Clinical Psychology, 36*, 623–625.

Crawford, J. R., Allan, K. M., Cochrane, R. H. B., & Parker, D. M. (1990). Assessing the validity of NART-estimated premorbid IQs in the individual case. *British Journal of Clinical Psychology, 29*, 435–436.

Crawford, J. R., Besson, J. A. O., Parker, D. M., Sutherland, K. M., & Keen, P. L. (1987). Estimation of premorbid intellectual status in depression. *British Journal of Clinical Psychology, 26*, 313–314.

Crawford, J. R., Deary, I. J., Starr, J., & Whalley, L. J. (2001). The NART as an index of prior intellectual functioning: A retrospective validity study covering a 66-year interval. *Psychological Medicine, 31*, 451–458.

Crawford, J. R., Moore, J. W., & Cameron, I. M. (1992). Verbal fluency: A NART-based equation for the estimation of premorbid performance. *British Journal of Clinical Psychology, 31*, 327–329.

Crawford, J. R., Parker, D. M., Allan, K. M., Jack, A. M., & Morrison, F. M. (1991). The Short NART: Cross-validation, relationship to IQ and some practical considerations. *British Journal of Clinical Psychology, 30*, 223–229.

Crawford, J. R., Obansawin, M. C., & Allan, K. M. (1998). PASAT and components of WAIS-R performance: Convergent and discriminant validity. *Neuropsychological Rehabilitation, 8*, 255–272.

Crawford, J. R., Parker, D. M., & Besson, J. A. O. (1988). Estimation of premorbid intelligence in organic conditions. *British Journal of Psychiatry, 153*, 178–181.

Crawford, J. R., Stewart, L. E., Garthwaite, P. H., Parker, D. M., and Besson, J. A. O. (1988). The relationship between demographic variables and NART performance in normal subjects. *British Journal of Clinical Psychology, 27*, 181–182.

Crawford, J. R., Stewart, L. E., Besson, J. A. O., Parker, D. M., & De Lacey, G. (1989). Prediction of WAIS IQ with the National Adult Reading Test: Cross-validation and extension. *British Journal of Clinical Psychology, 28*, 267–273.

Crawford, J. R., Stewart, L. E., Cochrane, R. H. B., Parker, D. M., & Besson, J. A. O. (1989). Construct validity of the National Adult Reading Test: A factor analytic study. *Personality and Individual Differences, 10*, 585–587.

Crawford, J. R., Stewart, L. E., Parker, D. M., Besson, J. A. O., & Cochrane, R. H. B. (1989). Estimation of premorbid intelligence: Combining psychometric and demographic approaches improves predictive accuracy. *Personality and Individual Differences, 10*, 793–796.

Crawford, J. R., & Warrington, E. K. (2002). The Homophone Meaning Generation Test: Psychometric properties and a method for estimating premorbid performance. *Journal of the International Neuropsychological Society, 8*, 547–554.

Deary, I. J., MacLennan, W. J., & Starr, J. M. (1998). Is age kinder to the initially more able?: Differential ageing of a verbal ability in the healthy old people in Edinburgh study. *Intelligence, 26*, 357–375.

Deary, I. J., Whalley, L. J., & Crawford, J. R. (2004). An "instantaneous" estimate of a lifetime's cognitive change. *Intelligence, 32*, 113–119.

Franzen, M. D., Burgess, E. J., & Smith-See-Miller, L. (1997). Methods of estimating premorbid functioning. *Archives of Clinical Neuropsychology, 12*, 711–738.

Freeman, J., & Godfrey, H. (2000). The validity of the NART-RSPM index in detecting intellectual declines following traumatic brain injury: A controlled study. *British Journal of Clinical Psychology, 39*, 95–103.

Friend, K. B., & Grattan, L. (1998). Use of the North American Adult Reading Test to estimate premorbid intellectual function in patients with multiple sclerosis. *Journal of Clinical and Experimental Neuropsychology, 20*, 846, 851.

Fromm, D., Holland, A. L., Nebes, R. D., & Oakley, M. A. (1991). A longitudinal study of word-reading ability in Alzheimer's disease: Evidence from the National Adult Reading Test. *Cortex, 27*, 367–376.

Gladsjo, J. A., Heaton, R. K., Palmer, B. W. M. Taylor, M. J., & Jeste, D. V. (1999). Use of oral reading to estimate premorbid intellectual and neuropsychological functioning. *Journal of the International Neuropsychological Society, 5*, 247–254.

Graf, P., & Uttl, B. (1995). Component processes of memory: Changes across the adult lifespan. *Swiss Journal of Psychology, 54*, 113–130.

Grober, E., & Sliwinski, M. (1991). Development and validation of a model for estimating premorbid verbal intelligence in the elderly. *Journal of Clinical and Experimental Neuropsychology, 13*, 933–949.

Isella, V., Villa, M. L., Forapani, F., Piamarta, A., Russo, I. M., & Appolonio, I. M. (2005). Ineffectiveness of an Italian NART-equivalent for the estimation of verbal learning ability in normal elderly. *Journal of Clinical and Experimental Neuropsychology, 27*, 618–623.

Ivnik, R. J., Malec, J. F., Smith, G. E., Tangalos, E. G., & Petersen, R. C. (1996). Neuropsychological tests norms above age 55: COWAT, BNT, token, WRAT-R reading, AMNART, Stroop, TMT, JLO. *The Clinical Neuropsychologist, 10*, 262–278.

Johnstone, B., Callahan, C. D., Kapila, C. J., & Bouman, D. E. (1996). The comparability of the WRAT-R reading test and NAART as estimates of premorbid intelligence in neurologically impaired patients. *Archives of Clinical Neuropsychology, 11*, 513–519.

Kondel, T. K., Mortimer, A. M., Leeson, M. C., Laws, K. R., & Hirsch, S. R. (2003). Intellectual differences between schizophrenic patients and normal controls across the adult lifespan. *Journal of Clinical and Experimental Neuropsychology, 25*, 1045–1056.

Lucas, S. K., Carstairs, J. R., & Shores, E. A. (2003). A comparison of methods to estimate premorbid intelligence in an Australian sample: Data from the Macquarie University Neuropsychological Normative Study (MUNNS). *Australian Psychologist, 38*, 227–237.

Maddrey, A. M., Cullum, C. M., Weiner, M. F., & Filley, C. M. (1996). Premorbid intelligence estimation and level of dementia in Alzheimer's disease. *Journal of the International Neuropsychological Society, 2*, 551–555.

Moss, A. R., & Dowd, T. (1991). Does the NART hold after head injury: A case report. *British Journal of Clinical Psychology, 30*, 179–180.

Nelson, H. E. (1982). *National Adult Reading Test (NART): Test manual*. Windsor, UK: NFER Nelson.

Nelson, H. E., & O'Connell, A. (1978). Dementia: The estimation of pre-morbid intelligence levels using the new adult reading test. *Cortex, 14*, 234–244.

Nelson, H. E., & Willison, J. (1991). *National Adult Reading Test (NART): Test manual* (2nd ed.). Windsor, UK: NFER Nelson.

O'Carroll, R. E. (1987). The inter-rater reliability of the National Adult Reading Test (NART): A pilot study. *British Journal of Clinical Psychology, 26*, 229–230.

O'Carroll, R. E., Moffoot, A., Ebmeier, K. P., & Goodwin, G. M. (1992). Estimating pre-morbid intellectual ability in the alcoholic Korsakoff syndrome. *Psychological Medicine, 22*, 903–909.

Paque, L., & Warrington, E. K. (1995). A longitudinal study of reading ability in patients suffering from dementia. *Journal of the International Neuropsychological Society, 1*, 517–524.

Paolo, A. M., Troster, A. I., Ryan, J. J., & Koller, W. C. (1997). Comparison of NART and Barona demographic equation premorbid IQ estimates in Alzheimer's disease. *Journal of Clinical Psychology, 53*, 713–722.

Parkin, A. J., & Java, R. I. (1999). Deterioration of frontal lobe function in normal aging: Influences of fluid intelligence versus perceptual speed. *Neuropsychology, 13*, 539–545.

Patterson, K., Graham, N., & Hodges, J. R. (1994). Reading in dementia of the Alzheimer type: A preserved ability? *Neuropsychology, 8*, 395–407.

Raguet, M. L., Campbell, D. A., Berry, D. T. R., Schmitt, F. A., & Smith, G. T. (1996). Stability of intelligence and intellectual predictors in older persons. *Psychological Assessment, 8*, 154–160.

Riley, G. A., & Simmonds, L. V. (2003). How robust is performance on the National Adult Reading Test following traumatic brain injury? *British Journal of Clinical Psychology, 42*, 319–328.

Russell, A. J., Munro, J., Jones, P. B., Hayward, P., Hemsley, D. R., & Murray, R. M. (2000). The National Adult Reading Test as a measure of premorbid IQ in schizophrenia. *British Journal of Clinical Psychology, 39*, 297–305.

Ryan, J. J., & Paolo, A. M. (1992). A screening procedure for estimating premorbid intelligence in the elderly. *The Clinical Neuropsychologist, 6*, 53–62.

Schlosser, D., & Ivison, D. (1989). Assessing memory deterioration with the Wechsler Memory Scale, the National Adult Reading Test, and the Schonell Graded Word Reading Test. *Journal of Clinical and Experimental Neuropsychology, 11*, 785–792.

Sharpe, K., & O'Carroll, R. (1991). Estimating premorbid intellectual level in dementia using the National Adult Reading Test: A Canadian study. *British Journal of Clinical Psychology, 30*, 381–384.

Starr, J. M., Whalley, L. J., Inch, S., & Shering, P. A. (1992). The quantification of the relative effects of age and NART-predicted IQ on cognitive function in healthy old people. *International Journal of Geriatric Psychiatry, 7*, 153–157.

Stebbins, G. T., Gilley, D. W., Wilson, R. S., Bernard, B. A., & Fox, J. H. (1990). Effects of language disturbances on premorbid estimates of IQ in mild dementia. *The Clinical Neuropsychologist, 4*, 64–68.

Stebbins, G. T., Wilson, R. S., Gilley, D. W., Bernard, B. A., & Fox, J. H. (1988). Estimation of premorbid intelligence in dementia. *Journal of Clinical and Experimental Neuropsychology, 10*, 63–64.

Stebbins, G. T., Wilson, R. S., Gilley, D. W., Bernard, B. A., & Fox, J. H. (1990). Use of the National Adult Reading Test to estimate premorbid IQ in dementia. *The Clinical Neuropsychologist, 4*, 18–24.

Storandt, M., Stone, K., & LaBarge, E. (1995). Deficits in reading performance in very mild dementia of the Alzheimer type. *Neuropsychology, 9*, 174–176.

Taylor, R. (1999). National Adult Reading Test performance in established dementia. *Archives of Gerontology and Geriatrics, 29*, 291–296.

Taylor, K. I., Salmon, D. P., Rice, V. A., Bondi, M. W., Hill, L. R., Ernesto, C. R., & Butters, N. (1996). A longitudinal examination of American National Adult Reading Test (AMNART) performance in dementia of the Alzheimer type (DAT): Validation and correction based on rate of cognitive decline. *Journal of Clinical and Experimental Neuropsychology, 18*, 883–891.

Uttl, B. (2002). North American Reading Test: Age norms, reliability, and validity. *Journal of Clinical and Experimental Neuropsychology, 24*, 1123–1137.

Uttl, B., & Graf, P. (1997). Color Word Stroop test performance across the life span. *Journal of Clinical and Experimental Neuropsychology, 19*, 405–420.

Van den Broek, M. D., & Bradshaw, C. M. (1994). Detection of acquired deficits in general intelligence using the National Adult Reading Test and Raven's Standard Progressive Matrices. *British Journal of Clinical Psychology, 33*, 509–515.

Watt, K. J., & O'Carroll, R. E. (1999). Evaluating methods for estimating premorbid intellectual ability in closed head injury. *Journal of Neurology, Neurosurgery, and Psychiatry, 66*, 474–479.

Wiens, A. N., Bryan, J. E., & Crossen, J. R. (1993). Estimating WAIS-R FSIQ from the National Adult Reading Test-Revised in normal subjects. *The Clinical Neuropsychologist, 7*, 70–84.

Willshire, D., Kinsella, G., & Prior, M. (1991). Estimating WAIS-R from the National Adult Reading Test: A cross-validation. *Journal of Clinical and Experimental Neuropsychology, 13*, 204–216.

NEPSY: A Developmental Neuropsychological Assessment

PURPOSE

The NEPSY was designed to assess neuropsychological development in preschoolers and children.

SOURCE

The NEPSY (Korkman et al., 1998) can be obtained from the Psychological Corporation, 19500 Bulverde Rd, San Antonio, TX 78259 (www.harcourtassessment.com). American and Finnish versions are available from this publisher. The complete NEPSY testing kit costs approximately $600 US. The NEPSY Scoring Assistant for computer scoring costs approximately $150 US.

A French version of the test is available from Les Éditions du Centre de Psychologie Appliquée (ECPA; www.ecpa.fr), and French-Canadian norms from Quebec have also reportedly been collected. A revised Swedish version was also published in 2000 (www.psykologiforlaget.se). The test has also been used in German-speaking children from Austria (Perner et al., 2002).

AGE RANGE

The test can be administered to children aged 3 to 12 years.

TEST DESCRIPTION

Background

The NEPSY is the American adaptation of the NEPS, a Finnish instrument that first appeared over 25 years ago (Korkman, 1980). As noted by Korkman (1999), the test originally consisted of only two to five tasks for 5- and 6-year-olds, designed along traditional Lurian approaches, scored in a simple pass/fail manner, and calibrated so that items were passed by the vast majority of children. The NEPS was revised and expanded in 1988 and 1990 to include more tasks (including the VMI and Token Test as complements) and a wider age range (NEPS-U; Korkman, 1988a; 1988b). A Swedish version was also developed (Korkman, 1990). The most recent version of the NEPSY, again revised and expanded to an even broader age range, was standardized in Finland (Korkman et al., 1997) and in the United States (Korkman et al., 1998). Specific differences between the 1988 Finnish version and the most recent American and Finnish versions are listed in several sources (Korkman, 1999; Korkman et al., 1998; Mäntynen et al., 2001).

Overview and Theoretical Orientation

The NEPSY is the first instrument designed exclusively and a priori as a neuropsychological battery for children. Although there are other neuropsychological batteries for children, these are based on modifications and downward extensions of existing adult batteries (e.g., Luria-Nebraska Neuropsychological Battery—Children's Version: Golden, 1987; Reitan-Indiana Neuropsychological Test Battery for Children and Halstead-Reitan Neuropsychological Test Battery for Older Children: Reitan & Davidson, 1974; Reitan & Wolfson, 1985, 1992). The NEPSY was created as an instrument with four main functions: (1) sensitivity to subtle deficits that interfere with learning in children, (2) detection and clarification of the effects of brain damage or dysfunction in young children, (3) utility for long-term follow-up of children with brain damage and dysfunction, and (4) provision of reliable and valid results for studying normal and atypical neuropsychological development in children (Korkman et al., 1998).

The test's theoretical orientation is a melding of Lurian principles with developmental neuropsychological assessment. Although the precise way in which these two orientations interact is not fully described in the manual, further detail is provided by Korkman (1999). The most important similarity to Luria's method is the approach of analyzing neurocognitive disorders through an evaluation of component processes, using systematic component-by-component assessment. Cognitive processes are viewed as complex capacities mediated by interacting functional systems. Some subtests were therefore designed to assess basic components within functional domains, whereas others were designed to assess cognitive functions that require integration of several functional domains. Level of performance and qualitative aspects of performance are both measured within and across functional domains (Korkman et al., 1998). The pattern of errors and qualitative behaviors is expected to change with age, which the authors indicate would provide information on normal and atypical development (Korkman et al., 1998).

There are also significant differences compared to Luria's approach. Whereas Luria used a hypothesis-driven approach to assessment that included forming and revising hypotheses as the evaluation unfolded, the NEPSY approach is to screen across all Core domains first (using the Core battery), followed by a more in-depth analysis within domains where deficits are suspected (i.e., Expanded or Selective assessment; Korkman, 1999). Another obvious difference is that the NEPSY comprises standardized subtests that are relatively homogenous for content and that provide norm-based comparisons, an approach that is more in line with traditional psychological assessment of cognitive ability (e.g., Wechsler scales) than to Luria's methods.

To interpret the test, the authors recommend the use of Core domains to identify impairments and subtest-level analysis to analyze the nature of impairments, followed by verification with corroborating information (Korkman et al., 1998). The authors stress that without appropriate training in pediatric neuropsychology, interpretation must be limited to a description of neurocognitive strengths and weaknesses.

Test Structure

The NEPSY was designed as a flexible testing instrument. It includes five Core domains, along with additional Expanded and Supplemental subtests that can be administered selectively, depending on the type of assessment and characteristics of the examinee. Interestingly, unlike other cognitive batteries such as the Wechsler scales and WJ III, or neuropsychological batteries such as the Halstead-Reitan, the NEPSY does not yield an overall score. This is consistent with a conceptualization of neuropsychological functioning as reflecting independent but related functional systems.

The five Core domains, shown in Table 6–63 with their associated subtests, include: (1) Attention/Executive Functions, (2) Language, (3) Sensorimotor Functions, (4) Visuospatial Processing, and (5) Memory and Learning. There are two versions of the test depending on the age range of the child (i.e.,

Table 6–63 NEPSY Core and Expanded Subtests Across Age

	Ages 3–4	Ages 5–12
Attention/Executive		
Tower		✓
Auditory Attention and Response Set		✓
Visual Attention	✓	✓
Statue	✓	
Design Fluency		*
Knock and Tap		*
Language		
Body Part Naming	✓	
Phonological Processing	✓	✓
Speeded Naming		✓
Comprehension of Instructions	✓	✓
Repetition of Nonwords		*
Verbal Fluency	*	*
Oromotor Sequencing	*	*
Sensorimotor Functions		
Fingertip Tapping		✓
Imitating Hand Movements	✓	✓
Visuomotor Precision	✓	✓
Manual Motor Sequences	*	*
Finger Discrimination		*
Visuospatial Processing		
Design Copy	✓	✓
Arrows		✓
Block Construction	✓	*
Route Finding		*
Memory and Learning		
Memory for Faces		✓
Memory for Names		✓
Narrative Memory	✓	✓
Sentence Repetition	✓	*
List Learning		*

✓ Core Subtest. * Expanded Subtest.

Source: Adapted from Korkman et al., 1998.

3–4 years, and 5–12 years). Core and Expanded subtests differ somewhat for the two age ranges (see Table 6-63). Subtests are described in Table 6-64.

An Expanded or Selective Assessment, with additional subtests not included in the Core domains, can also be administered when specific neuropsychological aspects need to be evaluated in more depth. Additionally, "Supplemental Scores" allow a more fine-grained analysis of performance on Core domain subtests; these are conceptually separate from the two "Supplemental Subtests" that assess basic skills such as orientation and handedness. Qualitative Observations, taken by the examiner during the administration of the NEPSY subtests, can also be quantified and compared with expected levels in the standardization sample to provide a process-approach component to the assessment. See Table 6–65 for a listing of specific Qualitative Observation scores. A schematic representation of NEPSY domains, subtests, and scores is shown in Figure 6-13.

Because it allows broad and specific analyses of test performance along with qualitative analysis of testing behavior, the NEPSY allows the examiner to design a multidimensional assessment that can be customized to suit the needs of the individual child (Kemp et al., 2001).

ADMINISTRATION TIME

Administration time depends on the type of assessment performed and the age of the child. The Core Assessment takes approximately 45 minutes in children ages 3 to 4 years and 65 minutes in children age 5 and older. The full NEPSY takes about one hour in younger children and two hours in children 5 and older.

ADMINISTRATION

See manual for specific instructions. Different subtests are administered depending on the age of the child (see Table 6–63). Consequently, different forms are used for younger (ages 3–4) and older children (ages 5–12). Specific administration procedures for children with special needs, including those with attention problems, language disorder, or hearing, visual, or motor impairments, are outlined in Kemp et al. (2001).

Test refusal is common for some NEPSY subtests in 3½-year-olds, especially in subtests requiring verbal expression or that have no manipulatives (e.g., Sentence Repetition, Finger Discrimination), with the best cooperation rate obtained for Visuomotor Precision (Mäntynen et al., 2001). Users who test recalcitrant preschoolers may therefore wish to begin the evaluation with tests that yield the best cooperation rates, such as Visuomotor Precision, Visual Closure, Phonological Processing, and Comprehension of Instructions (see Mäntynen et al., 2001, for specific refusal rates per subtest).

Materials

NEPSY testing materials are bright, child-friendly, and easy to administer. Test protocols are attractively designed and easy to

Table 6–64 Descriptions of NEPSY Subtests

Attention/Executive Domain

Tower	Designed to assess planning, monitoring, self-regulation, and problem solving; similar to other tower paradigms (e.g., Tower of Hanoi). The child must move three colored balls to specific positions on three pegs in a specific number of moves and under time constraints.
Auditory Attention and Response Set	Continuous performance task purported to measure vigilance, selective auditory attention, and set shifting. The first condition is an auditory attention task during which the child must respond to specific words on a tape and resist responding to distracters. The second condition introduces conflicting demands between the actual stimuli and the response required (i.e., when the child hears "red," he or she must pick up a yellow square), which demands set shifting and response inhibition
Visual Attention	Two-part visual cancellation task that assesses both speed and accuracy at detecting targets among distracters
Design Fluency	A nonverbal fluency task during which the child must draw as many novel designs as possible in a given time limit from both structured and unstructured dot arrays
Statue	Assesses response inhibition and motor persistence. During this subtest, the child is asked to stand still over a 75-second interval during which the examiner produces distracting stimuli.
Knock and Tap	A motor task that measures self-regulation and response inhibition. The child is required to learn simple hand gestures in response to specific hand gestures from the examiner, and then learn a conflicting set of responses that requires the child to inhibit the previously learned gestures as well as the tendency to imitate the examiner's gestures

Language Domain

Body Part Naming	Simple naming task for younger children that involves naming body parts on a picture of a child or on the child's own body
Phonological Processing	A two-part test that requires the child to identify words based on presented word segments, and then to create a new word by omitting or substituting word segments or phonemes
Speeded Naming	Requires the child to name the size, shape, and color of familiar stimuli as rapidly as possible
Comprehension of Instructions	Auditory comprehension task that requires the child to point to the correct picture in response to examiner commands of increasing syntactic complexity
Repetition of Nonsense Words	Assesses the child's phonological encoding and decoding skills with regard to novel sound patterns by requiring the child to repeat nonsense words presented on audiotape
Verbal Fluency	A standard verbal fluency paradigm. The child must produce as many words as possible from semantic and/or phonological categories (in younger children, animals and foods; children ages 7+ also must provide as many words as possible beginning with the letters "F" and "S")
Oromotor Sequencing	Involves the repetition of tongue twisters to assess oromotor coordination

Sensorimotor Domain

Fingertip Tapping	Tapping test that assesses speeded finger dexterity
Imitating Hand Movements	Involves the child copying complex hand positions demonstrated by the examiner
Visuomotor Precision	A paper-and-pencil task involving timed eye-hand coordination in which the child is asked to rapidly trace the path of a vehicle on paper without crossing any lines
Manual Motor Sequences	Involves the imitation of rhythmic hand movement sequences
Finger Discrimination	A finger agnosia test in which the examiner touches the child's fingers, who then must identify the fingers without visual input

Visuospatial Processing Domain

Design Copy	Similar to the Beery Visuomotor Integration Test in that the child must copy two-dimensional designs of increasing difficulty on paper
Arrows	Subtest is similar to the Judgment of Line Orientation test in that the child must select the arrow that points to a target from a number of arrows with different orientations
Block Construction	Requires the child to reproduce three-dimensional block constructions using actual models and pictures, using unicolored blocks
Route Finding	Visual-spatial task involving finding the correct route leading to a target on a map

(continued)

Table 6–64 Descriptions of NEPSY Subtests (*continued*)

Memory and Learning Domain	
Memory for Faces	A face recall task involving recalling a series of photographs of children's faces
Memory for Names	Involves repeated exposure trials to a set of cards on which are drawn children's faces; the child is required to learn the name associated with each face
Narrative Memory	A story recall task; the examiner reads a story to the child, who then must recite it from memory; if trials are failed, multiple-choice items are administered
Sentence Repetition	Sentences are aurally presented to the child, who must then recite the sentences to the examiner

Note: The NEPSY also includes additional Supplementary subtests assessing Orientation and Handedness.

Source: Adapted from Korkman et al., 1998.

use during test administration and hand scoring. Instructions for administering the NEPSY are included on an easel for some tests and in the manual for others. Because the manual is a small paperback, accessing and using the instructions in the manual while engaged in testing is somewhat cumbersome. However, the entire test is easily portable in a carrying case, which facilitates test administration at the bedside.

SCORING

Index scores for the five Core domains are provided in standard score format ($M = 100$, $SD = 15$), with corresponding percentile ranks and confidence intervals. All of the Core and most of the Expanded subtest scores are derived in scaled score format ($M = 10$, $SD = 3$). For Core domain subtests that have either non-normal distributions or significant ceiling or floor effects in the standardization sample, percentile ranges are provided instead. This includes Knock and Tap, Finger Discrimination, Route Finding, Manual Motor Sequences, and Oromotor Sequences. Percentages of children in the normative sample with specific scores are provided for the optional Handedness and Orientation subtests. The NEPSY Manual provides tables to evaluate the significance of Core domain and subtest scores as well as frequencies of discrepancy scores.

Supplemental Scores (see Table 6–65) are all derived as cumulative percentages of the standardization sample. Qualitative Observations are derived as either cumulative percentages of the standardization sample or as base rates reflecting the percentage of children in the standardization sample showing the particular behavior. The authors note that the Supplemental and Qualitative Observation scores are not equivalent to the percentiles obtained for the Expanded subtests described previously. While the former reflect actual base rates of occurrence of specific behaviors, the latter represent percentile ranks that underwent smoothing to adjust for sampling irregularities (Korkman et al., 1998).

The NEPSY computer-scoring program greatly facilitates derivation of scores and is a significant time saver. It is well designed and easy to use, and printouts are easy to read and interpret.

DEMOGRAPHIC EFFECTS

Age

Significant age effects are found on all NEPSY subtests. These are strongest from 5 to 8 years of age and moderate from 9 to 12 years (Korkman et al., 2001). From 10 to 12 years, only fluency subtests and Sentence Repetition show age-related increases, which may relate to either psychometric limitations of the tasks or to an actual developmental plateau. Memory for Faces does not improve significantly after age 8, and ceiling effects may curtail age-related increases on Imitating Hand Positions. Overall, the subtests that show the greatest sensitivity to age, with continued, steady improvements over the age span, are Design Fluency, Verbal Fluency, Speeded Naming, and Sentence Repetition (Korkman et al., 2001). Significant age effects, graphically illustrated by growth curves, have also been published for Phonological Processing, Speeded Naming, and Sentence Repetition for the NEPSY's Finnish standardization sample (Korkman et al., 1999), with the most significant increments occurring before age 9.

Gender

Overall, gender effects are minimal. However, there is a small but significant, temporary advantage for girls on language subtests assessing Phonological Processing and Sentence Repetition (Korkman et al., 1999), at least at the start of reading instruction. A small gender effect favoring boys on the Arrows subtest in Zambian schoolchildren has also been reported (Mulenga et al., 2001). An interaction between gender and prenatal drug exposure favoring girls over boys has also been reported for the NEPSY Language domain (Bandstra et al., 2002), with boys scoring about one-fifth of an *SD* below girls.

Ethnicity

There are few studies on cultural influences and performance on the NEPSY. A study in urban Zambian children found that most scores were within one SD of U.S. norms. However, lower scores were found on the NEPSY Attention/Executive and

Table 6–65 Supplemental Scores and Qualitative Observations for Each NEPSY Subtest

Domain	Subtest	Supplemental Scores	Qualitative Observations
Attention/Executive	Tower		Rule violations Motor difficulty Off-task behavior
	Auditory Attention and Response Set	Attention task score Response Set task score Omission Errors (by task) Commission Errors (by task)	
	Visual Attention	Time to Completion (by task) Omission Errors (by task) Commission Errors (by task)	Off-task behavior
	Design Fluency	Structured Array score Random Array score	
Language	Body Part Naming		Poor articulation
	Phonological Processing		Asks for repetition
	Speeded Naming	Time to Completion Accuracy	Increasing voice volume Reversed sequences Body movement
	Comprehension of Instructions		Asks for repetition
	Repetition of Nonsense Words		Stable misarticulation
	Verbal Fluency	Animals Trial score Food/Drink Trial score Semantic score Phonemic score	Increasing voice volume Body movement
	Oromotor Sequences		Stable misarticulation Oromotor hypotonia Rate change
Sensorimotor	Fingertip Tapping	Repetitions score Sequences score Preferred Hand score Nonpreferred Hand score	Visual guidance Incorrect positioning Posturing Mirroring Overflow Rate change
	Imitating Hand Positions	Preferred Hand score Nonpreferred Hand score	Mirror hand Other hand helps
	Visuomotor Precision	Time to Completion (by item) Errors (by item)	Pencil grip
	Manual Motor Sequences		Recruitment Overflow Perseveration Loss of asymmetry Body movement Forceful tapping Rate change
Visuospatial	Design Copying		Pencil grip Hand tremor
	Arrows		Rotation
Learning and Memory	Sentence Repetition		Asks for repetition Off-task behavior
	Memory for Faces	Immediate Memory score Delayed Memory score	
	Memory for Names	Learning Trials score Delayed Memory score	
	Narrative Memory	Free Recall points Cued Recall points	
	List Learning	Learning effect Interference effect Delay effect Learning curve	Repetitions Novel intrusions Interference intrusions

Note: Supplemental scores are in addition to Total scores for each subtest.

Source: Adapted from Korkman et al., 1998.

Figure 6–13 Schematic representation of NEPSY structure. *Source:* Reprinted with permission from Korkman et al., 1998.

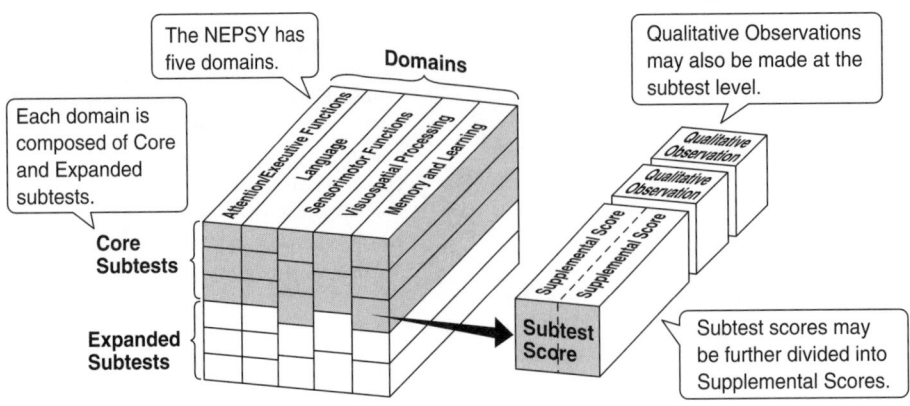

Language domains, and higher scores were found on the Visuospatial domain compared with U.S. norms (Mulenga et al., 2001). Interestingly, Mulenga et al. (2001) observed that Zambian schoolchildren tended to work slowly on NEPSY tests involving speed, despite explicit instructions to work quickly. In British preschoolers, scores are marginally higher than U.S. norms and show lower variability on subtest scores, particularly on language subtests. This suggests that the NEPSY may be less sensitive to underachievement in England if U.S. norms are used (Dixon & Kelly, 2001). In studies involving African American, inner-city children, mean scores on the Language Core domain are somewhat lower than average (Bandstra et al., 2002, 2004), but generally within the broad range typically obtained for language tests in this group (see *PPVT-III*).

IQ

As expected, IQ is related to NEPSY performance. Correlations of NEPSY Domain scores to WISC-III FSIQ in the standardization sample are highest for Language ($r = .59$), in the moderate range for Visuospatial, Memory and Learning, and Attention/Executive ($r = .45, .41,$ and $.37,$ respectively), and modest for the Sensorimotor domain ($r = .25$). Correlations to WPPSI-R follow the same general pattern, with the highest association between IQ and NEPSY Language ($r = .57$) and the lowest occurring between NEPSY Sensorimotor and Attention/Executive ($r = .31$ and $.26,$ respectively). See also *Validity* for further discussion.

NORMATIVE DATA

Standardization Sample

Table 6–66 shows detailed sample characteristics. The NEPSY normative sample is a national, stratified random sample of 1000 children, aged 3 to 12 years, with data collected between 1994 and 1996. There were 100 children (50 boys, 50 girls) in each of 10 age groups. Stratification by age, race/ethnicity,

geographic location, and parental education was based on 1995 U.S. Census data (Korkman et al., 1998). Children with neurological or other conditions were excluded (Kemp et al., 2001).

Table 6–66 Characteristics of the NEPSY Normative Sample

Number	1000[a]
Age	3 to 12 years, 11 months
Geographic location	
Northeast	20%
South	35%
North Central	24%
West	23%
Sample type	National, stratified, random sample[b]
Parental education	
0–11 years	10%
12–15 years	60%
16 years or more	30%
SES	Reflected by parental education
Gender	
Males	50% (overall, and in each age band)
Females	50%
Race/ethnicity	
African American	16%
Hispanic	12%
White	69%
Other	4%
Screening	Children with diagnosed neurological, psychological, developmental, or learning disabilities were excluded

[a]Based on 10 age groupings of 100 cases each. [b]Based on 1995 U.S. Census data, stratified according to age, gender, geographic location, race/ethnicity, and parental education.

Source: Adapted from Korkman et al., 1998, and Kemp et al., 2001.

Table 6–67 NEPSY Domain Scores and Subtest Scores for Zambian Schoolchildren

Domains and Subtests	9-Year-Olds		11-Year-Olds	
	M	SD	M	SD
Attention and Executive Functioning	93.56	10.30	89.60	15.50
Tower	9.80	1.85	11.10	3.65
Auditory Attention and Response Set	11.28	2.05	10.45	2.35
Visual Attention	6.40	3.73	4.25	3.31
Design Fluency	7.88	3.19	7.05	3.36
Language	85.64	11.32	87.05	13.37
Phonological Processing	8.84	2.85	10.15	2.70
Speeded Naming	6.28	3.60	5.95	2.87
Comprehension of Instructions	8.12	3.72	7.65	3.96
Repetition of Nonsense Words	7.48	2.68	6.45	4.85
Verbal Fluency	8.48	3.12	8.55	2.74
Sensorimotor Functioning	94.16	19.71	99.45	10.00
Fingertip Tapping	9.52	4.56	10.80	2.14
Imitating Hand Positions	9.80	2.57	10.25	2.24
Visuomotor Precision	8.28	4.46	8.90	1.52
Visuospatial Processing	111.80	16.14	113.70	20.38
Design Copying	15.44	3.15	15.30	3.66
Arrows	8.72	4.60	9.55	5.35
Block Construction	9.36	2.91	8.25	3.68
Memory and Learning	100.76	14.32	97.25	14.45
Memory for Faces	12.28	2.94	10.20	2.86
Memory for Names	9.72	2.113	8.20	3.68
Narrative Memory	8.24	3.33	10.45	2.83
Sentence Repetition	9.44	4.02	9.25	3.70
List Learning	9.92	2.50	8.95	2.21

Source: Mulenga et al., 2001. Reprinted with permission from Lawrence Erlbaum.

Other Normative Data

Mulenga et al. (2001) reported that there is an overall lack of normative data for children in the developing world. As a result, these investigators administered the NEPSY to 45 Zambian schoolchildren tested in English. Means and standard deviations are presented in Table 6–67. Note that children were schooled in English and spoke English as a second language, in addition to local dialects. Attention/Executive and Language domain scores are lower than those in the U.S. norms, but scores for the Visuospatial Processing domain are higher. In comparison, the mean score for 7-year-old, African American, low SES, inner-city children on the Language Core domain is approximately 87 points ($M = 86.8$, $SD = 13.3$; $N = 176$; Bandstra et al., 2002; $M = 87.3$, $SD = 13.3$, $N = 192$; Bandstra et al., 2004).

Score Conversion Procedures

To form the NEPSY normative tables, scale score conversions were derived through conversion of raw scores to normalized z-scores through direct lookup tables corresponding to normal curve values (Korkman et al., 1998). Comparisons of resulting distributions across age were evaluated, and irregularities were eliminated by smoothing and polynomial curve fitting. The process was repeated for sums of scaled scores to derive index scores. Six-month interval values for subtests were interpolated from the whole-year norms (Korkman et al., 1998).

Five subtests had highly skewed raw score distributions. These were Finger Discrimination, Route Finding, Manual Motor Sequences, Oromotor Sequences, and Knock and Tap. Percentile rankings were derived for these subtests instead of scaled scores after elimination of minor sampling irregularities by smoothing (Korkman et al., 1998). As noted in Korkman et al. (2001), as a general rule, subtests with skewness of ±2.5 were converted to percentiles. A table containing information on raw score ranges, means, SDs, standard error, and degree of skewness and kurtosis is provided in Korkman et al. (2001). Because percentile rankings can be misleading when they are derived from non-normal samples, the authors made a decision to include only general percentile ranking classifications for these subtests. These are shown in Table 6–68.

Some subtests require consideration of both speed and accuracy to adequately describe performance (i.e., Visual Attention, Visuomotor Precision). However, in most cases, accuracy scores were highly skewed in the standardization sample. Weights were therefore assigned to accuracy and speed scores to normalize the distribution, and to enable assessment of the combined effect of speed and accuracy on performance. The

Table 6–68 Percentile Ranking Classifications for NEPSY Subtests* With Non-Normal Raw Score Distributions

Percentile Ranking	Classification
≤ 2nd percentile	Well below expected level
3rd–10th percentile	Below expected level
11th–25th percentile	Borderline
26th to 75th percentile	At expected level
>75th percentile	Above expected level

*Finger Discrimination, Route Finding, Manual Motor Sequences, Oromotor Sequences, and Knock and Tap.

Source: Adapted from Korkman et al., 1998.

total score for these subtests takes into account weighted accuracy and speed scores and is normally distributed (see p. 39 of the manual for further details; Korkman et al., 1998). Tables are provided in the manual to calculate these combined scores; this is done automatically by the scoring program.

RELIABILITY

Internal Consistency

The manual presents detailed information on internal reliability based on the standardization sample (Korkman et al., 1998). With regard to Core domain scores, reliability was adequate to high across age (Table 6–69). The authors note that the lower coefficient for the Attention/Executive domain in 3- to 4-year-olds, which is marginally adequate ($r = .70$), may be a result of developmental variability in this age range. The lowest domain score reliability in the 5 to 12 age group was for the Sensorimotor domain ($r = .79$). All other domain scores for this age group showed high reliability, but none were over .90, a minimal level recommended for clinical decision making (see Chapter 1).

With regard to subtests, reliability coefficients were for the most part adequate to high. Reliabilities for ages 3 to 4 and 5 to 12 are presented in Table 6–70. Reliabilities were marginal for Verbal Fluency in the 3 to 4 age group and for Visuomotor Precision in the 5 to 12 age group. Coefficients for Statue, Design Fluency, and Immediate Memory for Faces were low.

Standard Error of Measurement

For the Core domain scores, standard error of measurement (SEM) is largest for the Attention/Executive domain for ages 3 to 4 (i.e., 8.22). Other SEMs range between four and seven standard score points. In the case of NEPSY subtests, the SEM for Statue at age 3 to 4 was 2.12; all other SEMs were less than two scaled score points (Korkman et al., 1998). Overall, these values are comparable to those obtained by other major assessment measures for children such as the WISC-III.

Test-Retest Stability

Because one of the NEPSY's goals is to facilitate assessment of children over time (Korkman et al., 1998), evidence of its temporal stability is particularly important. Test-retest stability coefficients in the manual are based on 168 normal children tested twice over a mean testing interval of 38 days (range 2–10 weeks). Coefficients were calculated separately for each of five age groups consisting of 30 to 41 children and consist of Pearson's correlations corrected for variability. For those subtests with normative scores based on percentiles due to skewed distribution, consistency of percentile range classifications from test to retest was used instead (e.g., Knock and Tap, Finger Discrimination, Route Finding, Manual Motor Sequences, and Oromotor Sequences).

A number of NEPSY subtests had less than optimal test-retest stability. Table 6-71 shows the NEPSY subtests classified according to the magnitude of their test-retest coefficients for different age groups. Over half of the NEPSY subtests had test-retest reliabilities that were marginal or low, even at this relatively short testing interval. This was the case for both age groups. Some reliabilities were adequate to high in the younger age group, but marginal or low in the older children

Table 6–69 Internal Reliability of NEPSY Core Domain Scores

Magnitude of Coefficient	Core Domain Score Ages 3–4	Core Domain Score Ages 5–12
Very High (.90+)	Language Memory and Learning	
High (.80–.89)	Sensorimotor Visuospatial	Attention/Executive Language Visuospatial Memory and Learning
Adequate (.70–.79)	Attention/Executive	Sensorimotor
Marginal (.60–.69)		
Low (<.59)		

Source: Adapted from Korkman et al., 1998.

Table 6–70 Internal Reliability of NEPSY Subtests

Magnitude of Coefficient	Ages 3–4	Ages 5–12
Very high (.90+)	Sentence Repetition	Phonological Processing List Learning
High (.80–.89)	Phonological Processing Comprehension of Instructions Imitating Hand Positions Visuomotor Precision[a] Design Copying Block Construction Narrative Memory	Tower Repetition of Nonsense Words Imitating Hand Positions Memory for Names Sentence Repetition Auditory Attention and Response Set[a] *Immediate Memory for Names*
Adequate (.70–.79)	Body Part Naming Visual Attention[a]	Comprehension of Instructions Design Copying Arrows Block Construction Memory for Faces Narrative Memory Verbal Fluency[b] Fingertip Tapping[b] Visual Attention[a] Speeded Naming[a] *Auditory Attention*[b] *Auditory Response Set*[b]
Marginal (.60–.69)		Visuomotor Precision[a] *Delayed Memory for Faces* *Delayed Memory for Names*
Low (<.59)	Statue[b] Verbal Fluency[b]	Design Fluency[b] *Immediate Memory for Faces*

Note: Supplemental scores are shown in italics.
[a]Generalizability coefficient. [b]Test-retest reliability coefficient.

Source: Adapted from Korkman et al., 1998.

(e.g., Narrative Memory, Imitating Hand Positions). The reverse was also true (e.g., Verbal Fluency).

Many subtests that base scores on percentile rankings had poor test-retest classification accuracy (see Table 6–72). At age 3 to 4, subtest classifications were at chance levels. Although consistency from test to retest is better in older children, almost half of the sample was misclassified at retest on some subtests (e.g., Manual Motor Sequences). The highest accuracy was obtained for Statue at age 5, which correctly classified 69% of children at retest. While this is clearly an improvement over chance, about 30% of children would be misclassified at retest, which is problematic if the test is to be used in clinical evaluation. Note that classification accuracy may be affected by practice effects, if children are classified in a higher category at retest because of improved performance. Whether practice effects actually affected classification accuracy is not detailed in the manual.

Practice Effects

Both practice effects and test-retest ability are important in assessing an instrument's ability to produce valid measurements over time. Practice effects, defined as improvements in performance at retest, were largest for the Core Memory domain score and the Memory and Learning subtests, based on tables provided in the NEPSY Manual (Korkman et al., 1998).

Specifically, in the 3 to 4 age group, all Core domain scores increased on average three to four points from test to retest. In the 5 to 6 age group, the Attention/Executive and Memory and Learning Core domain scores increased approximately 15 points, with the remainder of domain scores increasing six to seven standard score points. In the 9 to 10 age group, all changes were less than five points except for Memory and Learning, which increased 15 points from test to retest. In the 11 to 12 age group, all changes were less than six points, with the exception of Memory and Learning, which increased 11 points (Korkman et al., 1998). It is unclear whether lower gains seen in older children may be due to ceiling effects.

Overall, the magnitude of standard score changes from test to retest was considerable for some scores (e.g., Memory and Learning, and Attention/Executive domain in the 5-to-6-year group). These large test-retest differences must be taken into account when interpreting test-retest scores of individual children, as only very large increases are likely to be due to actual improvement over and above the effects of practice. Interestingly, the NEPSY Visuospatial Domain showed less of

Table 6–71 Test-Retest Stability Coefficients for NEPSY Subtests

Magnitude of Coefficient	Ages 3–4	Ages 5–12
Very high (.90+)		
High (.80–.89)	Narrative Memory Sentence Repetition	Auditory Attention and Response Set
Adequate (.70–.79)	Imitating Hand Positions Design Copying	Repetition of Nonsense Words Verbal Fluency Fingertip Tapping Design Copying Memory for Names Sentence Repetition *Auditory Attention* *Auditory Response Set* *Immediate Memory for Names* *Delayed Memory for Names*
Marginal (.60–.69)	Visual Attention Body Part Naming Comprehension of Instructions Visuomotor Precision	Visual Attention Phonological Processing Block Construction Narrative Memory List Learning
Low (≤.59)	Statue Phonological Processing Verbal Fluency Block Construction	Tower Design Fluency Speeded Naming Comprehension of Instructions Imitating Hand Positions Visuomotor Precision Arrows Memory for Faces *Immediate Memory for Faces* *Delayed Memory for Faces*

Note: Correlations denote Pearson's coefficients corrected for variability; Supplemental scores are shown in italics.

Source: Adapted from Korkman et al., 1988.

a practice effect (i.e., about 0–6 points, depending on age) than the conceptually similar Perceptual Organization Index from the WISC-III, which shows a 10-to-11-point increase from test to retest in its standardization sample (Wechsler, 1991). Again, it is unclear whether ceiling effects may be confounding results in the older age range.

Interrater Reliability

According to the manual, for tests requiring examiner judgment/interpretation for scoring (i.e., Design Copying, Visuomotor Precision, Repetition of Nonsense Words), a high degree of interrater reliability was obtained in a subsample of 50 children in the standardization sample (.97–.99; Korkman et al., 1998).

For Qualitative Observations, two trained raters independently rated a mixed sample of 21 children (Nash, 1995, as cited in Korkman et al., 1998). Interrater reliability of Qualitative Observations varied dramatically across domains (e.g., from as high as 1.00 for Tower Motor Difficulty to as low as 0.34 for Fingertip Tapping Mirroring; see Korkman et al., 1998, p. 188, or Kemp et al., 2001, p. 222, for specific

values). Kappas were below .50 for four Qualitative Observation scores. These were Misarticulations During the Repetition of Nonsense Words, Mirroring and Rate Change During Fingertip Tapping, and Pencil Grip During Visuomotor Precision (Korkman et al., 1998). Due to their poor

Table 6–72 Classification Accuracy of Test-Retest Rankings for NEPSY Subtests

Subtest	Ages 3–4	Ages 5–12
Statue		69%
Knock and Tap		65%
Route Finding		65%
Oromotor Sequences	50%	62%
Finger Discrimination—Preferred		61%
Finger Discrimination—Nonpreferred		56%
Manual Motor Sequences	47%	54%

Note: Values reflect the percentage of children correctly classified in the same percentile rankings at retest (i.e., decision consistency of classification).

Source: Adapted from Korkman et al., 1998. The test-retest correlation for Statue at age 3–4 is presented in Table 6–71.

interrater reliability, interpretation of these specific scores is not recommended.

VALIDITY

Content

The subtests comprising each Core domain were selected by the authors a priori, based on theoretical grounds and on prior research with the NEPSY. The test itself was developed in several phases. Based on experience with the previous Finnish and Swedish versions, the test was adapted for use in the United States following additional literature reviews, a pilot phase, bias review, a tryout version (comprised of 52 subtests), second bias review, second tryout version, and national standardization and further validation.

Subtest Intercorrelations

In some cases, intercorrelations of subtests within each Core domain are low, and some subtests are more highly correlated with subtests outside their assigned Core domain than with subtests within their Core domain (see pp. 361–363 in Korkman et al., 1998, for subtest correlation matrix). Only the Language and Visuospatial subtests are moderately intercorrelated within their respective Core domains (see Table 6–73 for actual correlation ranges in the standardization sample). Strong intercorrelations of similar magnitude are also reported in a clinical study for these two domains (Till et al., 2001).

Subtest intercorrelations for the Attention/Executive domain are especially weak in the standardization sample. For example, in the 3 to 4 age group, the two subtests making up the Attention/Executive Core domain are only modestly correlated ($r = .24$). Intercorrelations for the 5 to 12 age group are even lower (see Table 6–73). However, higher values are reported by Till et al. (2004), with moderate intercorrelations between some subtests (i.e., $r = .42$, NEPSY Visual Attention and NEPSY Statue) but not others ($r = .17$, NEPSY Visual Attention and NEPSY Tower). See *Comment* for further discussion of this issue.

Factor Structure and Subtest Specificity

Only one study to date has examined whether the NEPSY's five-domain structure can be replicated empirically. Stinnett et al. (2002) conducted a principal axis factor analysis on standardization data for ages 5 to 12 and found little evidence for a five-factor model. Instead, they found a robust one-factor solution on which language-based subtests loaded most highly. This omnibus factor included Phonological Processing, Comprehension of Instructions, Memory for Names, and Speeded Naming. Stinnett et al. noted that further research using confirmatory factor analysis and factor analyses using clinical samples are needed. However, these results, in conjunction with the low correlations between some Core domain subtests, raise questions about the valid-

Table 6–73 Intercorrelations Between Core Subtests Within NEPSY Core Domains

Domain	Ages 3–4	Ages 5–12
Attention/Executive	.24	.07–.18
Language	.40–.59	.32–.38
Sensorimotor	.25	.14–.18
Visuospatial	.40	.34
Memory and Learning	.40	.14–.34

Source: Adapted from Korkman et al., 1998.

ity of interpreting Core domain scores in the evaluation of individual children.

Stinnett et al. (2002) also examined the subtest specificity of NEPSY subtests (i.e., comparing unique variance contributed by each factor to common variance with the test as a whole, while taking into account each subtest's error variance). To be considered as having ample specificity, a subtest should have unique variance that exceeds 25% of the total variance and have a total variance that is larger than error variance (Kaufman, 1994). Stinnett et al. concluded that only Phonological Processing and Memory for Names had enough unique variance and low enough error variance to be interpreted separately from the main factor underlying the NEPSY. The remainder of subtests with sufficient unique variance had as much error variance as common variance, making individual interpretation of subtests dubious at best. The authors also noted that nine subtests were judged to be too unreliable to be used individually in the interpretation of performance. These included Comprehension of Instructions, Speeded Naming, Design Copying, Narrative Memory, Arrows, Visual Attention, Visuomotor Precision, Finger Tapping, and Memory for Faces. Whether these conclusions also apply to clinical samples remains an open question.

Correlations With IQ

Correlations between the NEPSY and WISC-III/WPPSI-R are shown in Table 6–74 for nonclinical data provided in the manual (Korkman et al., 1998). Overall, these indicate that the NEPSY clearly measures abilities that overlap with, but are distinct from, measures of general intelligence. Correlations to WISC-III FSIQ for NEPSY domain scores in the standardization sample are highest for Language ($r = .59$), in the moderate range for Visuospatial, Memory and Learning, and Attention/Executive ($r = .45$, .41, and .37, respectively), and modest for Sensorimotor ($r = .25$; Korkman et al., 1998). Correlations to WPPSI-R FSIQ follow the same general pattern, with the highest association between IQ and NEPSY Language ($r = .57$) and the lowest for NEPSY Sensorimotor and Attention/Executive ($r = .31$ and .26, respectively).

In particular, correlations between IQ tests and NEPSY provide particular support for the convergent validity of the NEPSY Language and NEPSY Visuospatial Index scores,

Table 6–74 Correlations Between the NEPSY and Tests of IQ/Mental Development

NEPSY Index	WISC-III FSIQ	WISC-III VCI	WISC-III POI	WISC-III FFD	WISC-III PSI	WPPSI-R FSIQ	BSID-II MDI	BSID-II PSI
Attention/Executive	.37	.33	.25	.35	.26	.26	−.31	−.37
Language	.59	.58	.36	.57	.29	.57	.61	−.11
Sensorimotor	.25	.17	.18	.24	.32	.31	.31	.22
Visuospatial	.45	.36	.45	.30	.19	.47	−.04	−.09
Memory and Learning	.41	.43	.22	.35	.26	.51	.05	−.56

Note: WISC-III data represents 127 nonclinical cases (mean age of 9), WPPSI-R data represents 45 nonclinical cases (mean age of 4), and BSID-II data represents data on 20 3-year-olds. WISC-III = Wechsler Intelligence Scale for Children—Third Edition; FSIQ = Full-Scale Intelligence Quotient; VCI = Verbal Comprehension Index; POI = Perceptual Organization Index; FFD = Freedom from Distractibility; PSI = Processing Speed Index; WPPSI-R = Wechsler Preschool and Primary Scale of Intelligence—Revised; BSID-II = Bayley Scales of Infant Development—Second Edition; MDI = Mental Development Index; PSI = Psychomotor Development Index.

Source: Adapted from Korkman et al., 1998.

which correlate moderately to highly with similar scores from IQ tests (e.g., $r = .57$ between NEPSY Language and WISC-III VCI, and $r = .45$ between NEPSY Visuospatial and WISC-III POI). Less convergent support is found for other NEPSY domains. However, the NEPSY Attention/Executive domain score is modestly related to WISC-III FFD to about the same extent as it is to the FSIQ ($r = .35$ and .37, respectively; Korkman et al., 1998).

Note that the mean index scores for the WISC-III presented in the manual are slightly higher than NEPSY scores (i.e., about three points), which may relate to the older WISC-III norms. However, NEPSY and WPPSI-R scores were generally equivalent (see data in Korkman et al., 1998). Correlations to newer versions of these Wechsler scales (WISC-IV, WPPSI-III) are not yet available.

The manual also presents NEPSY and BSID-II data for a small group of normal 3-year-olds. Unexpectedly, negative correlations are found between some scores (see Table 6–74), despite the strong association between NEPSY Language domain and developmental level as measured by the MDI (i.e., $r = .61$; Korkman et al., 1998). Differences in mean scores were also relatively large; the most pronounced was between the NEPSY Attention/Executive score and the MDI, which showed a mean difference of over 16 points. While these discrepancies may reflect the limitations of a small sample size, caution is recommended in comparing test scores in this age range until further research is conducted comparing the two measures.

Correlations With Achievement Tests and School Grades

One of the main uses of testing children is predicting how deficits impact school functioning. As a result, measures that are sensitive to school performance are of considerable utility for clinical assessment. The NEPSY Manual presents data on correlations between NEPSY scores and school grades for a large sample of children ($N = 445$; Korkman et al., 1998). As is the case for most test batteries, the language-based score (i.e., NEPSY Language domain) was most predictive of school grades and showed the highest correlations with language-based school grades ($r = .40$). The NEPSY Language domain also predicted school grades in nonlanguage areas such as mathematics and science ($r = .37$ and .34, respectively). All other correlations were modest (range .10–.32), with some of the lowest correlations to school grades occurring for the NEPSY Attention/Executive domain ($r = .10–.17$) and Sensorimotor domain (.13–.17).

Similar relationships occur when the NEPSY is compared to standardized achievement tests such as the WIAT. In a small sample of children with LD presented in the manual ($N = 39$), NEPSY Language is highly related to almost all WIAT test composites, including Reading, Mathematics, and Writing ($r = .26–.41$; Korkman et al., 1998). One exception is NEPSY Attention/Executive, which demonstrates an impressive correlation with WIAT Language but not WIAT Reading ($r = .57$ versus $r = .08$). Although the NEPSY Visuospatial Index is moderately related to the Mathematics Composite, NEPSY Language is equally related to success in this area ($r = .44$ versus $r = .41$). The NEPSY Memory and Learning Index is virtually unrelated to WIAT scores ($r = .06–.15$), except for a modest correlation with WIAT Language ($r = .24$). Correlations between the newer WIAT-II are not available. Correlations with other achievement tests are also shown in the manual; these generally show similar findings (i.e., that NEPSY Language is most associated with academic achievement).

Correlations With Other Neuropsychological Tests

Certain NEPSY subtests are very similar to classic neuropsychological paradigms. The manual presents correlations between conceptually similar NEPSY subtests and other, well-known neuropsychological tests (Korkman et al., 1998). For the most part, these provide some criterion-based evidence of the validity of NEPSY subtests.

For example, there is a very high correlation between NEPSY Arrows and the conceptually similar Judgement of Line Orientation ($r = .77$) in a small mixed sample in the manual ($N = 18$; Korkman et al., 1998). Other correlations with conceptually similar tests are moderate (NEPSY Statue and Benton Motor Impersistence; NEPSY Design Copying and BVRT-Copy) or minimal (NEPSY Finger Discrimination and Benton Finger Localization; NEPSY Immediate Memory For Faces and Benton Facial Recognition; see manual for more details). Correlations between NEPSY Comprehension of Instructions and the MAE are moderate ($r = .48$, MAE Token test) to high ($r = .76$, MAE Aural Comprehension of Words and Phrases). Sentence Repetition subtests from the NEPSY and MAE are uncorrelated ($r = .01$), whereas word fluency tests from both measures exhibit a moderate degree of overlap ($r = .44$, NEPSY Verbal Fluency and MAE Controlled Word Association).

With regard to memory, correlations between NEPSY memory subtests and conceptually similar CMS subtests are in the moderate to high range in a group of 27 nonclinical children presented in the manual ($r = .36–.56$; p. 210 of Korkman et al., 1998). CMS correlations with other NEPSY nonmemory subtests are not shown, which complicates interpretation of discriminant validity. However, index score intercorrelations are presented, which indicate that although NEPSY Memory and Learning is highly related to CMS General Memory ($r = .57$), NEPSY Memory and Learning is actually more highly related to CMS Attention/Concentration ($r = .74$) than to any other memory-related CMS index. Whether this is due to a large attentional component in the NEPSY Memory and Learning score or to sample characteristics is unknown, but does suggest care in comparing index scores from the two scales in individual children, as they may measure different cognitive domains despite similar nomenclature.

With regard to attention, the NEPSY Attention/Executive domain score correlates moderately with the CMS Attention/Concentration Index ($r = .31$). However, this NEPSY Index is not selectively associated with CMS-based attention, since moderate to high correlations are also found across CMS index scores purported to measure aspects of memory functioning (see manual for details, p. 211). In children with ADHD, the NEPSY Attention/Executive Index is moderately related to performance on the Auditory Continuous Performance Test ($r = -.27$ to $-.28$; Keith, 1994) but not to performance on the Conners' CPT ($r = -.06$ to $-.09$). This holds true even when only NEPSY Attention/Executive subtests specifically related to attention are examined, such as Visual Attention ($r = -.05$ to $-.11$). Instead, Conners' CPT scores appear to be more closely related to performance on the NEPSY Sensorimotor and Visuospatial domains (see manual for details). In other studies, the NEPSY Attention/Executive domain subtests appear to correlate with some tests of theory of mind in preschoolers (Perner et al., 2002), even after partialing out IQ ($N = 22$).

Examples of criterion-based evidence of the validity of the NEPSY Language domain are provided by studies involving the EOWPVT-R, PPVT-III, and CELF-P, well-known and well-validated language measures for children. For instance, NEPSY Body Part Naming and EOWPVT-R are highly correlated in children with sleep-disordered breathing and matched con-

trols ($r = .52$; Till et al., 2001). Likewise, NEPSY Phonological Processing and NEPSY Comprehension of Instructions are both moderately to highly associated with PPVT-III scores ($r = .53$ and $.42$, respectively; Till et al., 2001). In a longitudinal study on the effects of cocaine on language development, both the CELF-P at ages 3 and 5 and the NEPSY Language score at age 7 showed the same magnitude of cocaine-related performance decrement (i.e., approximately one-fifth of an SD). This provides some evidence for the fact that the CELF-P and the NEPSY Language domain measure a similar dimension of functioning in preschoolers (Bandstra et al., 2002).

With regard to visual-spatial abilities, NEPSY Block Construction and NEPSY Hand Positions are both moderately correlated to the Wide Range Assessment of Visual-Motor Abilities (WRAVMA; Adams & Sheslow, 1995).

Clinical Studies

The manual provides NEPSY data on a number of small clinical groups compared with matched controls, including children with ADHD, LD/ADHD, LD-reading, language disorder, autism, FAS, TBI, and hearing impairment ($N = 8–51$; Korkman et al., 1998). The manual concludes that these studies support the clinical validity of the test, and can be used as a guide for determining which NEPSY components to use in the diagnostic workup for conditions such as ADHD (see Kemp et al., 2001). However, the data are not compelling for three main reasons: (1) the actual number of children with clinical-level impairments in each group is sometimes quite low, (2) some group means are actually in the broadly normal range, despite statistically significantly lower scores compared with matched controls, and (3) no data showing that the NEPSY can discriminate between clinical groups are provided, given that demonstration of group differences versus controls is an inadequate metric of the clinical utility of neuropsychological tests. A higher standard is the percent of children with impairments who are actually detected by the test, and an even higher standard is whether the test can discriminate *between* clinical groups. Overall, the percentage of children in the clinical groups with impaired performance on the NEPSY raises serious questions about the test's sensitivity to neurocognitive impairment in the context of these specific disorders. Table 6–75 shows the percentage of children identified as "impaired" (i.e., with scores <2 SD below the mean) for each of the clinical groups presented in the manual.

Previous test reviews of the NEPSY have noted the paucity of validity information on the test (e.g., Ahmad & Warriner, 2001). Nevertheless, composites comprised of NEPSY Language domain subtests, PPVT-III, and EOWPVT-R appear sensitive to the effects of prenatal organic solvent exposure based on group comparisons (Till et al., 2001), along with NEPSY subtests measuring graphomotor ability (Visuomotor Precision, Design Copying), but not Attention/Executive subtests or a composite comprised of NEPSY Visuospatial subtests and WRAVMA (Till et al., 2001). However, the NEPSY

Table 6–75 Percent of Clinical Groups With Impaired Performance on the NEPSY

NEPSY Core Domain	ADHD $N = 51$	LD/ADHD $N = 20$	LD-Reading $N = 36$	Language Disorder $N = 19$	Autism $N = 23$	FAS $N = 10$	TBI $N = 8$	Hearing Impairment $N = 32$
Attention/Executive	2.0	25.0	2.8	37.5	17.6	77.8	62.5	20.0
Language	2.0	20.0	2.8	7.7	11.1	33.3	50.0	—
Sensorimotor	9.8	0.0	16.7	11.8	17.6	22.2	62.5	4.0
Visuospatial	2.0	10.0	13.9	5.6	8.7	30.0	28.6	12.5
Memory and Learning	3.9	15.0	11.1	31.6	27.3	40.0	25.0	9.4

Note: Impairment = scores less than two *SD*s below the mean.

Source: Adapted from Korkman et al., 1998.

Attention/Executive Index score appears to be sensitive to the neurocognitive effects of sleep-disordered breathing in 5-year olds, at least as measured by group differences (Gottlieb et al., 2004; O'Brien et al., 2004), as is the NEPSY Memory domain (Gottlieb et al., 2004). In particular, an index measuring the total number of arousals per hour of sleep time was negatively associated with performance on the Tower subtest ($r = -.43$; O'Brien et al., 2004). Preschoolers at risk for ADHD also appear to have lower scores on Attention/Executive domain scores compared with controls (Perner et al., 2002). NEPSY Language domain scores are reportedly sensitive to the effects of prenatal cocaine exposure (Brandstra et al., 2002, 2004).

A study by Schmitt and Wodrich (2004) examined whether the NEPSY domain scores provide additional information not already accounted for by IQ tests. They compared three groups of children (neurological, scholastic concerns, and standardization controls) and found that, after controlling for IQ, only the NEPSY Language and NEPSY Sensorimotor domain scores differed between groups. They concluded that although the test passes preliminary evidence of validity (i.e., group differences without controlling for IQ), other more rigorous evidence supportive of the sensitivity of index scores to group differences is lacking. Specifically, differences between children with neurological conditions and controls disappeared when IQ was controlled for on the Attention/Executive and Memory and Learning domains. Even when IQ was not controlled for, there were no group differences on the Visuospatial domain. The authors note that the main practical implication of these findings is that there is empirical evidence for the practice of supplementing IQ tests with NEPSY Language and Sensorimotor domains (i.e., Phonological Processing, Speeded Naming, and all the Sensorimotor subtests), but not for the other NEPSY subtests. We would temper these group-based conclusions by adding that only those Sensorimotor subtests with adequate reliabilities should be considered for differential diagnosis of individual children (e.g., Imitating Hand Movements in younger children and Fingertip Tapping in older children).

Other group studies on the Finnish NEPSY, or on prior versions of the NEPSY in Finnish and Swedish samples, are reviewed in Korkman et al. (1998), Korkman (1999), and Kemp et al. (2001). These include outcome studies on congenital hypothyroidism (Song, 2001), early-onset hemiparesis (Kolk & Talvik, 2000), congenital brain lesions and epilepsy (Kolk et al., 2001), juvenile neuronal ceroid lipofuscinosis (Lamminranta et al., 2001), fetal alcohol (Korkman et al., 1998), and low birth weight and asphyxia (Korkman et al., 1996; Sajaniemi et al., 2001; see also Korkman, 1988; Korkman & Haekkinen-Rihu, 1994; and Korkman et al., 1996). Although of interest, these studies provide little information on the test's sensitivity/specificity to clinical conditions, other than group comparisons. Further, given considerable changes compared with the 1988 Finnish edition, some results based on earlier test versions may not necessarily be applicable to the newer American version.

COMMENT

When one considers some of the limitations of existing neuropsychological tests for children, the NEPSY is a major technological advancement in pediatric neuropsychology. It is the only neuropsychological battery for children that is not simply a downward extension of an adult battery, and it is the only existing comprehensive neuropsychological battery for children normed on a single, large, randomized, stratified normative sample. As such, it allows users to compare performance across domains, unencumbered by the psychometric and methodological limitations inherent in cross-test comparisons of tests normed on different samples. In addition, it is a test that is modeled, to some extent, on Luria's approach to assessment, and many of its subtests are adaptations of classic neuropsychological testing paradigms (e.g., Word Fluency, Tower of London/Hanoi, Design Fluency, Finger Agnosia, Judgment of Line Orientation, etc.). It therefore has a respectable theoretical foundation, and from a practical standpoint, it provides users with a wide array of subtests that were previously unavailable for children or that had inadequate norms. In addition, even though it is well normed and employs standardized administration procedures, it allows a process-oriented approach by measuring how children arrive at a certain level of performance (i.e., through the Qualitative Observation scores). It has brightly colored, child-friendly stimuli, is a relatively simple battery to learn and administer, and maintains the interests of most young children. Additionally, its age range extends to preschoolers (i.e., 3–5 years), an age band overlooked by many tests. Lastly, although many North Americans see it as a new test, it is actually one of the oldest instruments in pediatric neuropsychology, used in Finland for over 25 years. It is a test with a distinguished past and is hardly a newcomer in the field.

Despite its many assets, the NEPSY has some significant limitations, and could benefit greatly from additional validation research and psychometric refinement. Although it remains a major milestone in the evolution of pediatric neuropsychological assessment, it may have been overly ambitious in its attempts to cover the whole breadth and depth of neuropsychological functioning in children and may have been better served by including fewer subtests with better psychometric properties.

Psychometric Properties

Some NEPSY subtests, and their related Core domains, have poor psychometric properties and should probably rarely be administered in a diagnostic clinical context. These include Verbal Fluency, Statue, Phonological Processing, and Block Construction at ages 3 to 4, and Visuomotor Precision, Design Fluency, Tower, Speeded Naming, Comprehension of Instructions, Imitating Hand Positions, Arrows, and Memory for Faces at ages 5 to 12. It is possible that in some cases (i.e., older children), poor reliabilities may be due to ceiling effects. Note that almost all the subtests that use percentile classifications rather than scaled scores show poor reproducibility (e.g., Knock and Tap, Finger Discrimination, Route Finding, Manual Motor Sequences, Oromotor Sequences). Due to poor reliabilities for some Qualitative Observation scores and a lack of corroborative clinical evidence overall, these scores should be used with caution in the clinical assessment of individual children. Reliability and validity information are entirely lacking for a number of Supplemental Scores. Given that these are based on even fewer items than the total scores from which they derive, it is doubtful that their reliabilities would attain those of the Core domain scores shown in Tables 6–70 and 6–71.

Although this seems like a long list of subtests and scores with psychometric limitations, it should be remembered that the NEPSY includes 27 subtests, a number of which demonstrate at least adequate reliability. It should nevertheless be noted that only two subtests have both high internal reliability and high test-retest reliability defined as r greater than .80 (i.e., Sentence Repetition at ages 3–4, and Auditory Attention and Response Set at ages 5–12). No NEPSY subtest demonstrates both types of reliability above .90, a level recommended for clinical decision making. See Tables 6–70 to 6–72 for specific subtests.

Substantial practice effects must also be taken into account when assessing children for change over time with certain subtests such as those from the Memory and Learning domain.

Clinical Utility and Differential Diagnosis

The sensitivity of a test (i.e., its ability to detect impairment) is one of the main prerequisites for using it in a clinical context. As noted above in *Validity*, data from the manual on the proportion of children with impairments in specific domains within various neurocognitive conditions of childhood (e.g., ADHD, LD/ADHD, language disorder, autism, etc.) suggest poor sensitivity to impairment for NEPSY domain scores (see Table 6–75). It is difficult, for example, to see how the test would be of any utility in the evaluation of children with ADHD, since almost the entire group performed well on the test (e.g., only 2% had Attention/Executive scores in the impaired range). Similarly, excluding conditions with excessively small samples sizes (i.e., TBI, FAS), the proportion of children identified was at best 38%, which again suggests that the test "missed" more children than it actually identified.

While low test sensitivity may be the norm in certain conditions (e.g., see discussion of diagnosis of ADHD in reviews of CPTs in this volume), a minimally acceptable level of sensitivity—at the very least exceeding chance—should be demonstrated as evidence of a test's clinical utility and predictive validity (i.e., sensitivity >50%, or more than 50% of a clinical group identified by the test). Although the manual points out that the NEPSY was not designed to yield specific diagnoses such as ADHD or LD, it indicates that the test may be useful in determining whether a child fulfills diagnostic criteria for certain conditions, including ADHD, LD, autism, and other neurological conditions of childhood (Korkman et al., 1998, p. 237; see also Kemp et al., 2001). To date, there does not appear to be enough evidence to support this practice.

Overall, more research needs to be conducted to support the diagnostic utility of the NEPSY in conditions with known cognitive impairments. Until such time, the NEPSY should be used with caution for clinical diagnosis (i.e., absence of impaired scores may not allow one to rule out cognitive impairments), particularly given other limitations reviewed here.

Interpretation of NEPSY Scores

Evidence supporting the interpretability of the Core domain scores as reflecting five separate dimensions of neuropsychological functioning is limited. According to Stinnett et al., the interpretation of Core domain scores as measuring separate neuropsychological domains could lead to "very faulty decision making about a child's neuropsychological status" (Stinnett et al., 2002, p. 78).

Kemp et al. (2001) note that in the development of the NEPSY, domains were specified a priori based on neuropsychological theory/tradition rather than on factor analysis. Each subtest within a given domain assesses a diverse aspect within that functional area, and subtest-level interpretation is most important. Thus, Kemp et al. (2001) note that domain subtests are for the most part heterogeneous; they reflect a "comprehensive variety of measures" rather than "convergent measures of some underlying factors" (p. 335). Domains are therefore presumably constructed to be maximally sensitive for screening different types of disorders, which presumably may differ with regard to performance on domain subcomponents.

Overall, weak intercorrelations within certain NEPSY domains seriously undermine the validity and utility of some of the Core domain scores (excluding the Language and Visuospatial domains). Despite Kemp et al.'s (2001) argument that NEPSY domains measure diverse functions that are of clinical relevance, subtests comprising Core Index scores should measure a broadly similar construct if individual composite scores are to be used in differential diagnosis, or as major components in the interpretive process. A high degree of predictive validity for these domain scores may obviate the need for domain homogeneity, but this has yet to be demonstrated.

Subtest Specificity

In terms of subtest specificity, while all subtests meet criteria for "ample" specificity, only Phonological Processing and Memory for Names can really be interpreted as measuring something distinct from the rest of the test (Stinnett et al., 2002). Other subtests, while possibly assessing unique dimensions, are associated with too much error variance to allow reliable measurement for clinical purposes. Stinnett et al. (2002) conclude that the NEPSY "does not appear to measure much besides language function" (p. 79), and is not likely to detect subtle neuropsychological deficits. They also suspect that it is language-based deficits that fuel group differences in clinical groups reported in the manual as evidence of validity. We must concur with these conclusions.

Given weak subtest specificity for some subtests but lack of evidence for five separate Core domains, it is difficult to determine how exactly NEPSY performance should be interpreted in a clinical context. At the very least, clinicians would be well advised to make a careful test selection based on reliability coefficients, paying particular attention to subtests with adequate to high reliabilities for the specific age band needed. Specific subtests can then be selected among those with good psychometric properties. On the other hand, given the evidence that subtest specificity may be inadequate in some cases (Stinnett et al., 2002), clinicians may want to continue interpreting those index scores with good reliability/validity and relatively homogenous content domains (e.g., Language and Visuospatial).

Ceilings, Floors, and Item Gradients

Ceiling and floor effects on the NEPSY are defined as scores falling within one *SD* of minimum/maximum levels on each subtest (Korkman et al., 2001). Thus defined, only Imitating Hand Positions demonstrates possible ceiling effects in older children (Korkman et al., 2001). However, other authors suggest that ceilings and floors be at least two *SD*s from the mean, with a distance of three to four *SD*s preferred (Bracken & Walker, 1997). This is especially important for tests designed for use in clinical groups, where floor effects must be

eliminated to properly detect impairments. Floor effects are certainly present on some NEPSY subtests; for example, a 3-year-old who obtains a raw score of 0 on Narrative Memory will receive a scaled score of 7, and it is impossible to obtain a scaled score lower than 5 on Statue. Comprehension of Instructions, Imitating Hand Positions, and Memory for Names—Delayed also show ceiling effects in the older age groups (e.g., the maximum possible scaled score for 12-year-olds on Comprehension of Instructions is 13, and the maximum for Memory for Names—Delayed is 12). This limits utility for assessing high functioning children (e.g., gifted older children). Overall, most NEPSY subtests are not significantly affected by inadequate floors and ceilings. However, it is not clear that the NEPSY would be sensitive to changes over time in the older age groups (i.e., 10- to 12-year-olds), given plateauing of abilities in this age group (Korkman et al., 2001).

Item gradients for Memory for Names are too steep in some age groups. For example, at age 5, a score of 0 on Memory for Names—Delayed yields a scaled score of 4, but a score of 1 yields a scaled score of 7.

Is the NEPSY Truly More Flexible Than Other Batteries?

The NEPSY's flexibility as a testing instrument has yet to be supported by empirical evidence. Although this is presented as a major asset of the test, no evidence has been provided that the test is any more flexible than any other battery composed of various subtests. Evidence that the test is not hampered by subtest order effects, carry-over effects, or other confounds should be provided to support its "flexibility." For instance, because the standardization sample was presumably administered to the entire battery in a fixed order, it is possible that scores from subtests administered later in the battery would be more affected by fatigue or carry-over effects than those administered earlier on, which would be reflected in the norms. As well, carry-over effects, secondary to administering several subtests within a single domain in sequential order versus interspersed with subtests measuring different domains should also be evaluated.

Other Considerations

With 27 subtests to choose from and countless related possible scores and Qualitative Observations, subtest selection and interpretation can be a daunting task and elicit confusion in novice users. A major time commitment is required to learn to administer and understand the psychometric strengths and weaknesses of all the subtests. As a result, our impression is that many clinicians administer only a small subtest of the battery.

The test also has norms that exclude all children with impairments; this may be an issue if scores are compared with other tests based on nontruncated distributions (see McFadden, 1996, for a discussion of this issue). Norms for adolescents are also lacking, which may be an issue when longitudinal assessment is required.

Visual assessment is restricted to Memory for Faces, due to poor reliability of other visual memory subtests in the standardization sample and cost considerations during test development (Korkman et al., 1998). Therefore, in populations where a thorough memory evaluation is needed, supplementation with other memory tests is advisable. Note that for Narrative Memory, a story-recall task, full points are obtained for spontaneous recall, with partial points awarded for recognition. However, recall and recognition trials cannot be scored separately, which is a limitation when memory needs to be assessed in detail. For all the other Memory and Learning subtests, an Immediate and Delayed Supplemental Score can be derived separately. Some of the specific differences between NEPSY subtests and conceptually similar subtests available on their own or as part of other batteries are discussed by Baron (2004).

REFERENCES

Adams, D., & Sheslow, D. (1995). *Wide Range Assessment of Visual Motor Abilities.* Wilmington, DE: Wide Range.

Ahmad, S. A., & Warriner, E. M. (2001). Review of the NEPSY: A Developmental Neuropsychological Assessment. *Clinical Neuropsychologist, 15*(2), 240–249.

Bandstra, E. S., Morrow, C. E., Vogel, A. L., Fifer, R. C., Ofir, A. Y., Dausa, A. T., Xue, L., & Anthony, J. C. (2002). Longitudinal influence of prenatal cocaine exposure on child language functioning. *Neurotoxicology and Teratology, 24,* 297–308.

Bandstra, E. S., Vogel, A. L., Morrow, C. E., Xue, L., & Anthony, J. C. (2004). Severity of prenatal cocaine exposure and child language functioning through age seven years: A longitudinal latent growth curve analysis. *Substance Use & Misuse, 39*(1), 25–59.

Baron, I. S. (2004). *Neuropsychological evaluation of the child.* New York: Oxford University Press.

Bracken, B. A., & Walker, K. C. (1997). The utility of intelligence tests for preschool children. In D. P. Flanagan, J. L. Genshaft, & P. L. Harrison (Eds.), *Contemporary intellectual assessment: Theories, tests and issues* (pp. 484–502). New York: Guilford Press.

Dixon, L. A., & Kelly, T. P. (2001). A comparison of the performance of preschool children from England and USA on the NEPSY: Developmental Neuropsychological Assessment. *Clinical Neuropsychological Assessment: An International Journal for Research and Clinical Practice, 2*(1).

Gottlieb, D. J., Chase, C., Vezina, R. M., Heeren, T. C., Corwin, M. J., Auerbach, S. H., Weese-Mayer, D. E., & Lesko, S. M. (2004). Sleep-disordered breathing symptoms are associated with poorer cognitive function in 5-year-old children. *Journal of Pediatrics, 145,* 458–464.

Kaufman, A. S. (1994). *Intelligent testing with the WISC-III.* New York: John Wiley & Sons.

Keith, R. W. (1994). *Auditory Continuous Performance Test.* San Antonio, TX: The Psychological Corporation.

Kemp, S. L., Kirk, U., & Korkman, M. (2001). *Essentials of NEPSY assessment.* New York: John Wiley & Sons, Inc.

Kolk, A., Beilmann, A., Tomberg, T., Napa, A., & Talvik, T. (2001). Neurocognitive development of children with congenital unilateral brain lesion and epilepsy. *Brain and Development, 23*(2), 88–96.

Kolk, A., & Talvik, T. (2001). Cognitive outcome of children with early-onset hemiparesis. *Journal of Child Neurology, 15*(9), 581–587.

Korkman, M. (1980). *NEPS. Lasten neuropsykologinen tutkimus. Käsikirja* [NEPS. neuropsychological assessment of children manual]. Helsinki, Finland: Psykologien kustannus.

Korkman, M. (1988a). *NEPS-U. Lasten neuropsykologinen tutkimus. Uudistettu laitos* [NEPSY. neuropsychological assessment of children—revised edition]. Helsinki, Finland: Psykologien kustannus.

Korkman, M. (1988b). NEPSY: An application of Luria's investigation for young children. *Clinical Neuropsychologist, 2*(4), 375–392.

Korkman, M. (1990). *NEPSY. Neuropsykologisk undersökning: 4-7 år. Svensk version* [NEPSY. Neuropsychological assessment: 4–7 years. Swedish version]. Stockholm: Psykologiförlaget, Stockholm.

Korkman, M. (1999). Applying Luria's diagnostic principles in the neuropsychological assessment of children. *Neuropsychology Review, 9*(2), 89–105.

Korkman, M., Barron-Linnankoski, S., & Lahti-Nuuttila, P. (1999). Effects of age and duration of reading instruction on the development of phonological awareness, rapid naming, and verbal memory span. *Developmental Neuropsychology, 16*(3), 415–431.

Korkman, M., & Haekkinen-Rihu, P. (1994). A new classification of developmental language disorders. *Brain and Language, 47*(1), 96–116.

Korkman, M., Likanen, A., & Fellman, V. (1996). Neuropsychological consequences of very low birth weight and asphyxia at term: Follow-up until school age. *Journal of Clinical Neuropsychology, 18*(2), 220–233.

Korkman, M., Kemp, S. L., & Kirk, U. (2001). Effects of age on neurocognitive measures of children ages 5 to 12: A cross-sectional study on 800 children from the United States. *Developmental Neuropsychology, 20*(1), 331–354.

Korkman, M., Kirk, U., & Kemp, S. (1997). *NEPSY. Lasten neuropsykologinen tutkimus* [NEPSY. A Developmental Neuropsychological Assessment. In Finnish]. San Antonio, TX: The Psychological Corporation.

Korkman, M., Kirk, U., & Kemp, S. (1998). *NEPSY: A Developmental Neuropsychological Assessment manual.* San Antonio, TX: The Psychological Corporation.

Korkman, M., Renvaktar, A., & Sjostrom, P. (2001). Verbal and comorbid impairments in Finnish children with specific reading disorder. *Clinical Neuropsychological Assessment: An International Journal for Research and Practice, 2*(1).

Lamminranta, S., Aberg, L. E., Autti, T., Moren, R., Laine, T., Kaukoranta, J., & Santavuori, P. (2001). Neuropsychological test battery in the follow-up of patients with juvenile neuronal ceroid lipofuscinosis. *Journal of Intellectual Disability Research, 45*(1), 8–17.

Mäntynen, H., Poikkeu, A.-M., Ahonen, T., Aro, T., & Korkman, M. (2001). Clinical significance of test refusal among young children. *Child Neuropsychology, 7*(4), 241–250.

McFadden, T. U. (1996). Creating language impairments in typically achieving children: The pitfalls of "normal" normative sampling. *Language, Speech, and Hearing in the Schools, 27,* 3–9.

Mulenga, K., Ahonen, T., & Aro, M. (2001). Performance of Zambian children on the NEPSY: A pilot study. *Developmental Neuropsychology, 20*(1), 375–383.

O'Brien, L. M., Mervis, C. B., Holbrook, C. R., Bruner, J. L., Smith, N. H., McNally, N., McClimment, M. C., & Gozal, D. (2004). Neurobehavioral correlates of sleep-disordered breathing in children. *Journal of Sleep Research, 13,* 165–172.

Perner, J., Kain, W., & Barchfeld, P. (2002). Executive control and higher-order theory of mind in children at risk of ADHD. *Infant and Child Development, 11,* 141–158.

Schmitt, A. J., & Wodrich, D. L. (2004). Validation of a Developmental Neuropsychological Assessment (NEPSY) through comparison of neurological, scholastic concerns, and control groups. *Archives of Clinical Neuropsychology, 19,* 1077–1093.

Song, S. I. (2001). The influence of etiology and treatment factors on intellectual outcome in congenital hypothyroidism. *Journal of Developmental and Behavioral Pediatrics, 22,* 376–384.

Stinnett, T. A., Oehler-Stinnett, J., Fuqua, D. R., & Palmer, L. S. (2002). Examination of the underlying structure of the NEPSY, A Developmental Neuropsychological Assessment. *Journal of Psychoeducational Assessment, 20,* 66–82.

Till, C., Koren, G., & Rovet, J. F. (2001). Prenatal exposure to organic solvents and child neurobehavioral performance. *Neurotoxicology and Teratology, 23,* 235–245.

Wechsler, D. (1991). *The Wechsler Intelligence Scale for Children—Third Edition.* San Antonio, TX: The Psychological Corporation.

Neuropsychological Assessment Battery (NAB)

PURPOSE

The NAB is a modular battery of neuropsychological tests covering the areas of Attention, Language, Memory, Spatial, and Executive Functioning. A Screening Module is also available to examine these same five cognitive domains.

SOURCE

The NAB is published by PAR (www.parinc.com). The Complete Kit (33 tests) includes two alternate forms (Form 1 and Form 2) and costs $2995 US. The Screening Kit comprises 12 tests and costs $795 US, while the NAB Form 1 Kit (33 tests—Form 1) costs $1995 US. A training video and unlimited scoring software (NAB-SP) are included in the various kits.

AGE RANGE

The NAB was designed for use with individuals aged 18 to 97 years.

DESCRIPTION

The choice of functional domains and properties of the NAB (Stern & White, 2003) were guided by a survey of neuropsychologists' assessment practices in the United States and by consultations with an advisory council. Thus, the NAB was designed as an integrated yet modular battery of tests to assess the major functional domains of attention, language, memory, spatial, and executive functions. The NAB provides coordinated norms for all of the modules along with a recently published screening measure of intelligence (Reynolds Intellectual Screening Test, RIST; Reynolds & Kamphaus, 2003). That is, the examiner can use a single set of normative tables that allow for within-patient and between-patient score comparisons across the NAB and between these measures and estimated IQ level. Additional positive features include the provision of demographically corrected norms, the availability of two equivalent parallel forms, and the inclusion in each module of tasks that tap activities of daily living. The authors note that some areas (e.g., IQ, motor functioning, mood/personality) are not included in the NAB, and the examiner can expand upon the NAB assessment depending upon the specific clinical needs.

The organization of the NAB is shown in Table 6–76 and descriptions of the individual tests are provided in Table 6–77. The battery focuses on five major domains that are measured by five main NAB modules: Attention, Language, Memory, Spatial, and Executive Functions. A Screening Module is also provided that measures the same functional domains that are assessed by the main NAB modules. The Screening Module can be given alone or to indicate the need to administer one or more of the main NAB modules. For example, those who perform very poorly or very well on sections of the Screening Module may be judged not to need additional examination with the corresponding main module(s). Alternatively, the examiner can forego the Screening Module and administer any or all of the five main modules (or individual tests) to a patient.

By definition, the NAB Screening Module is based on a limited range of items. So that Screening domain scores can predict performance on the corresponding module within the same functional domain, Screening Module tests are either (a) similar to main module tests but with different stimuli and tasks parameters (e.g., Shape Learning, Story Learning), (b) shorter versions of the same tests included in the main modules (e.g., Numbers & Letters, Mazes), or (c) identical to the main module tests (e.g., Orientation, Digits Forward).

The types of testing paradigms found on the NAB will be familiar to most neuropsychologists. For example, the Attention Module includes measures of forward and backward digit span. The Language Module includes measures of picture naming and comprehension of commands of increasing complexity. The Memory Module incorporates measures of list, story, and shape learning. The Spatial Module includes tests of design construction and complex figure drawing. The Executive Functions Module contains tasks such as mazes, categorization, and word generation. A novel feature is that each NAB module (except Screening) also includes one Daily Living test that is designed to be highly congruent with real-life behavior.

The NAB yields a variety of scores. Each NAB test (with the exception of the Screening Attention Module Orientation test and the Language Module Reading Comprehension test) results in one or more primary scores and, in some cases,

Table 6–76 NAB Modules, Tests, and Administration Time

Module	Tests	Administration Time (min)	Index Scores
Screening		45	
Attention	Orientation Digits Forward Digits Backward Numbers & Letters		Screening Attention Domain (S-ATT)
Language	Auditory Comprehension Naming		Screening Language Domain (S-LAN)
Memory	Shape Learning Story Learning		Screening Memory Domain (S-MEM)
Spatial	Visual Discrimination Design Construction		Screening Spatial Domain (S-SPT)
Executive	Mazes Word Generation		Screening Executive Function Domain (S-EXE) Total Screening Index (S-NAB)
Main			
Attention	Orientation Digits Forward Digits Backward Dots Numbers & Letters *Driving Scenes*	45	Attention Index (ATT)
Language	Oral Production Auditory Comprehension Naming Reading Comprehension Writing *Bill Payment*	35	Language Index (LAN)
Memory	List Learning Shape Learning Story Learning *Daily Living Memory: medication instructions, name, address, phone number*	45	Memory Index (MEM)
Spatial	Visual Discrimination Design Construction Figure Drawing *Map Reading*	45	Spatial Index (SPT)
Executive	Mazes *Judgment* Categories Word Generation	30	Executive Functions Index (EXE)
			Total NAB Index (T-NAB)

Note: Italicized subtests refer to Daily Living tests designed to be congruent with analogous real-world behavior.

additional secondary and/or descriptive test scores. The secondary and descriptive scores provide an assessment of "process" variables. For example, on the Memory Module List Learning task, there are four primary scores that indicate the total correct across the three List A learning trials, the total correct on the List B free recall trial, the total List A correct following a short delay, and the total List A correct following a long delay. Secondary and descriptive scores provide an indication of how much information is retained from the short to the long delay (providing a measure of forgetting), the ability to discriminate hits from false alarms on the recognition test (discriminability), the extent to which an examinee uses a semantic encoding strategy when learning the list, and the presence of perseverations and intrusions. Similarly, the copy and

Table 6–77 Description of NAB Tasks

Module	Test	Description
Attention/Screening	Orientation	Questions about orientation to self, time, place, and situation (e.g., name, year, city, why here)
Attention/Screening	Digits Forward	Examinee must repeat digits spoken by the examiner (span length is three to nine)
Attention/Screening	Digits Backward	Examinee must orally reverse digits spoken by the examiner (span length is three to nine)
Attention	Dots	An array of dots is briefly exposed, followed by a blank interference page, followed by a new array with one additional dot that the examinee is asked to identify.
Attention; similar, abbreviated versions of Parts A and D are included in the Screening Module	Numbers & Letters	Part A: a letter-cancellation task requiring the examinee to mark target X's in 24 rows of numbers and letters
		Part B: examinee must count the number of X's in each row and write the total at the end of each row.
		Part C: examinee must add the numbers in each row and write the sum at the end of each row.
		Part D: examinee must mark a slash through each X and simultaneously add the numbers and write the sum at the end of each row.
Attention	Driving Scenes	Examinee is presented with a base stimulus depicting a driving scene as viewed from behind the steering wheel of a car. Examinee is presented with additional scenes and must identify modifications.
Language	Oral Production	Examinee must orally describe a scene in a picture.
Language; identical Colors, Shapes, and Color/Shapes/Numbers subtests are included in the Screening Module	Auditory Comprehension	Six separate subtests that require the patient to listen to orally presented commands and to respond by pointing to stimuli such as (a) colored rectangles, (b) geometric shapes, and (c) colored geometric shapes with numbers printed on them; or to respond (d) by pointing to body parts or places in the room; (e) by answering orally presented pairs of yes/no questions; or (f) by folding paper according to one- to four-step commands.
Language; Screening Module contains shorter version	Naming	The examinee is asked to name pictured items.
Language	Reading Comprehension	The examinee must select the target word or sentence from a set of foils that best matches a photograph of an object or a scene.
Language	Writing	A narrative writing sample depicted in a stimulus picture
Language	Bill Payment	The examinee is presented with a bill statement, a blank check, a check ledger, and an envelope and is required to respond to questions based on the available information.
Memory	List Learning	Three learning trials of a 12-word list, followed by an interference list, then short-delay free recall, long-delay free recall, and long-delay forced-choice recognition task. The word list includes three semantic categories with four words in each category.
Memory; Screening Module contains a similar, shorter version	Shape Learning	Three learning trials of nine target nonsense shapes, each learning trial followed by nine, four-stimulus, multiple-choice recognition items (target and three foils). After a 15-minute delay, there is another multiple-choice recognition trial, followed by an 18-item forced-choice, yes/no recognition trial composed of nine targets and nine foils.
Memory; Screening Module contains a single trial, shorter version	Story Learning	Includes two learning trials of a passage, separate measures of verbatim and gist recall, and both immediate and delayed recall trials
Memory	Daily Living Memory	The examinee is required to learn a name, address, and phone number as well as medication dosing instructions; involves immediate free recall, delayed free recall, and delayed multiple-choice recognition trials
Spatial; Screening Module contains a shorter version	Visual Discrimination	Requires matching of nonsense shapes to one of four choices (target and three foils)

(continued)

Table 6–77 Description of NAB Tasks (*continued*)

Module	Test	Description
Spatial; Screening Module contains a shorter version	Design Construction	Examinee uses shapes (tans) to reproduce designs of increasing difficulty.
Spatial	Figure Drawing	Requires copying and immediate free recall of a complex figure; the scoring system includes an overall summary score (based on presence, accuracy, and placement of elements) as well an evaluation of qualitative features: fragmentation, planning, and organization. A pen-switching procedure is used.
Spatial	Map Reading	Examinee must respond to a number of questions regarding map locations/directions
Executive; Screening Module contains a shorter version	Mazes	Examinee must trace a route through mazes of increasing difficulty.
Executive	Judgment	Examinee answers a series of questions about home safety, health, and medical issues.
Executive	Concept Formation	Two panels of photographs of six adults with identifying information are presented. For each panel, the examinee must indicate as many ways as possible to sort the photos into two categories.
Executive; Screening Module contains a similar version	Word Generation	Examinee is presented with a set of letters from which to generate as many three-letter words as possible within a specific time limit.

recall productions of the figure on the Spatial Module Figure Drawing task are scored not only for the overall presence, accuracy, and placement of elements, but also with regard to the extent of fragmentation, planning, and overall organization (similar to scores available for the Rey Figure). In addition to the quantitative primary, secondary, and descriptive scores for individual tests, many tests provide space for recording various qualitative features of performance such as confabulation, micrographia, and neglect.

For the Screening Module, selected primary T scores are summed to obtain each Screening domain score, and the five Screening domain scores are summed to obtain the Total Screening Index (S-NAB). Similarly, for each of the main domain-specific modules, a module index score is calculated as the sum of selected primary T scores in that module. The Total NAB Index (T-NAB) is based on the sum of the five module index scores and represents the examinee's overall performance.

ADMINISTRATION

Record forms are color coded according to module. Instructions for administration are given in the record form. The recording, discontinue rules, and time limits are clearly displayed to examiners in the record form, eliminating the need for the manual during administration.

Depending upon the individual's performance on the screening module, a judgment can be made, based on recommended cutoffs provided on the record form, as to whether the corresponding main module should be given. Thus, individuals who achieve very low (e.g., standard scores below 74 or 75) or very high (e.g., standard scores above 115) scores on a Screening Module may be judged not to require administration of the corresponding main module (see *Validity* below).

Whenever the Screening Module is given, it should be administered before any other NAB modules or tests. There is a suggested order of domain-specific module administration: Attention, Language, Memory, Spatial, and Executive Functions.

ADMINISTRATION TIME

According to the test authors, the entire battery (including the Screening Module) can be given in about four hours. The administration times for the various modules are shown in Table 6–76.

SCORING

Scoring guidelines for each test are found on the record form. There are three types of NAB scores: primary, secondary, and descriptive (see Table 6–78). Primary scores represent the most important ones for interpreting performance and are also used to compute composite scores (Module index scores, Screening domain/index scores), which contribute equally to the overall composites: T-NAB and S-NAB indices. Primary scores tend to have a relatively large range of possible raw scores and approximately normal score distributions. Secondary scores

Table 6–78 Types of NAB Test Scores

Score Type	Description	Normative Metric
Primary	Most important; in most cases, there is only one primary score per test; but some tests yield multiple primary scores	Primary test scores are converted to T scores ($M = 50$, $SD = 10$)
	Select primary scores contribute to composites: Module Index, Screening Domain/Index scores	Module Indices, Screening Domain scores, S-NAB and T-NAB indices have a mean of 100 and SD of 15
Secondary	Less important but can provide significant information; have lower reliability and nonparametric distributions; do not contribute to Module Index and Total NAB Index scores	Percentiles by nine age groups
Descriptive	Have poor reliability and/or highly skewed distributions in healthy people; provide qualitative indicators of performance; do not contribute to Module Index and Total NAB Index scores	Cumulative percentages for the overall sample

have skewed distributions and/or limited score ranges. All secondary scores are scaled so that higher percentiles reflect better performance. Descriptive scores also have highly skewed score distributions and/or limited score ranges but to an even greater degree. Higher cumulative percentages reflect better performance for all scores except List Learning Perseverations and List Learning Intrusions; for these two scores, higher cumulative percentages reflect poorer performance. Secondary and descriptive scores are viewed as useful sources of qualitative information.

DEMOGRAPHIC EFFECTS

Age

Age affects performance (White & Stern, 2003b).

Education/IQ

Education/IQ also impacts test scores, although typically less so than age (White & Stern, 2003a).

Gender

Gender tends to have a small effect on performance (White & Stern, 2003a).

Ethnicity

The impact of ethnicity is not reported, although the authors indicate that the advisory counsel reviewed all items for ethnicity/racial/cultural bias and those items with the highest biases were eliminated.

NORMATIVE DATA

Standardization Sample

The NAB standardization data were collected in 2001–2002 at five sites selected to provide representation in each of four geographic regions of the United States: Rhode Island, Florida, Indiana, and California (Los Angeles). The NAB provides both demographically corrected norms ($N = 1448$) and age-based, U.S. Census-matched norms ($N = 950$), consisting of a subsample of the overall NAB standardization sample selected to closely match the current U.S. population with respect to education, gender, race/ethnicity, and geographic region. However, the demographically corrected norms are the primary normative standard and facilitate interpretation of an individual's NAB performance relative to neurologically healthy individuals of the same age, gender, and educational level. The characteristics of the demographically corrected standardization sample are shown in Table 6–79. Of the 1448 participants, 711 received Form 1 and 737 received Form 2 as part of the standardization study; no participant completed both forms.

Normative data are provided in two separate manuals: the NAB Demographically Corrected Norms Manual (White & Stern, 2003a) and the NAB U.S. Census-Matched Norms Manual (White & Stern, 2003c). The user selects the most appropriate normative group (typically demographically corrected norms). Raw primary scores for each test are converted to z scores, which are then converted to T scores (e.g., by gender, age group, and education level) and percentiles. In general, T scores less than 40 are classed as impaired. Secondary raw scores are converted to percentiles while descriptive raw scores are converted to cumulative percentiles. Secondary

Table 6–79 Characteristics of the NAB Demographically Corrected Normative Sample

Number	1,448
Age	18–97 years[a]
Geographic location	
Northeast	21.3%
Midwest	23.0%
South	33.1%
West	22.6%
Sample type	Community-dwelling individuals
Education	
≤11 years	20.9%[b]
12 years	22.7%
13–15 years	27.1%
≥16 years	29.4%
Gender	
Female	53.5%
Male	46.5%
Race/ethnicity	
Caucasian	84.8%
African American	6.9%
Hispanic	4.8%
Other	3.5%
Screening	Screened for substance abuse and medical, psychiatric, motor, or sensory condition that could potentially affect performance; in addition, 14 subjects judged to be disoriented on the basis of their Orientation scores were removed

[a]The sample was divided into the following age groups: 18–29, 30–39, 40–49, 50–59, 60–64, 65–69, 70–74, 75–79, and 80–97. Note that a majority of the subjects in the oldest age group were less than 90 years of age. [b]A graduate equivalency degree (GED) was coded as 11 years.

score percentiles less than the 16th percentile are categorized as impaired.

Selected primary T scores are used to obtain module domain/index scores, and the latter are used to obtain total index scores. These summary scores are converted to standard scores with a mean of 100 and a standard deviation of 15. The Total NAB Index represents the sum of the five module indices, with each module contributing equally to the Total NAB Index. Similarly, the Total Screening Index reflects the sum of the five Screening domain scores. The NAB uses the interpretive ranges suggested by Heaton et al. (2004; See Chapter 5, *Report Writing and Feedback Sessions*, Table 5–3). Index scores below 85 are classed as impaired.

Tables are also provided in the manuals to determine the significance and rarity between scores. For example, depending upon the combination of Screening domain and Total Screening Index comparison, a difference of about 14 to 25 points is required to be statistically significant at the p .05 level. Discrepancies for combinations of the module indices and Total NAB Index scores range from about 10 to 16 points at the p .05 level.

The frequencies of score differences are also provided in the test manuals. These tables present the cumulative percentages

of the absolute differences (i.e., regardless of the direction of the score difference) between each possible pair of scores. In general, fairly large discrepancies are needed to confirm their rarity. For example, a discrepancy of about 30 points between the Screening Attention and Language domain/index scores occurred in about 13% of the demographically corrected standardization sample. Unfortunately, directional prevalence rates of discrepancy scores are not provided.

Participants in the standardization sample also completed a measure of intelligence, the RIST. Tables are provided in the NAB Psychometric and Technical Manual to evaluate an individual's raw score by level of estimated intelligence.

RELIABILITY

Internal Consistency

Many of the NAB primary subtests were excluded from internal consistency analyses for a variety of reasons, including the use of unique item presentation formats, interitem dependency issues that would artificially inflate the reliability estimate, and the use of speed of performance formats for a number of test measures (White & Stern , 2003b). The range of alpha coefficients in the normative sample is quite diverse for selected primary scores for the six modules, when averaged for both forms across the age groups (Psychometric and Technical Manual). As shown in Table 6–80, coefficients range from high (e.g., Oral Production; Story Learning Phrase Unit, Immediate and Delayed Recall) to inadequate, likely in part a reflection of the limited range of scores on some tests (e.g., Auditory Comprehension, Screening Naming) and construct heterogeneity (e.g., Judgment).

Generalizability coefficients were used to calculate the reliability estimates of Screening domain, Total Screening Index, module index, and Total NAB Index scores. The reliabilities for the Screening domain scores ranged from .55 for the Screening Language domain score to .91 for the Screening Attention domain score, and the Total Screening Index reliability coefficient was .80. The module index scores reliabilities were higher, ranging from .79 for the Language index score to .93 for both the Attention and Memory index scores. The reliability coefficient of the Total NAB Index score was .96.

Test-Retest Reliability

The authors (White & Stern, 2003b) indicate that the stability of both NAB forms was assessed with an average test-retest interval of more than six months ($M = 193.1$ days, $SD = 20.3$) and sampling across a wide age range (20–97 years). Thus, 45 healthy individuals were given Form 1 on two occasions and 50 healthy people were administered Form 2 on two occasions. As Table 6–80 shows, test-retest correlations of the primary scores tend to be marginal or low.

As might be expected, composite scores (Screening domain, domain, Total Screening, and Total NAB) tend to be more stable than the individual test scores (Table 6–80). However,

Table 6–80 Magnitude of Reliability Coefficients for NAB Primary Scores and Domains and Total Index Scores for the Demographically Corrected Standardization Sample for All Age Groups

	Internal Consistency*	Test-Retest Primary Scores	Test-Retest Domain and Total Index Scores
Very high (.90+)			
High (.80–.89)	Oral Production Story Learning Phrase Unit IR Story Learning Phrase Unit DR	Numbers & Letters Part A Speed Numbers & Letters Part A Efficiency	Attention Index Total NAB Index
Adequate (.70–.79)	Screening Digits Forward Screening Digits Backward Screening Story Learning DR Naming Mazes	Screening Numbers & Letters Part A Efficiency Naming	Screening Attention Domain Total Screening Index Spatial Index
Marginal (.60–.69)	Screening Story Learning IR Bill Payment Shape Learning IR Visual Discrimination Design Construction Map Reading	Screening Digits Forward Screening Digits Backward Screening Numbers & Letters Part A Speed Screening Mazes Screening Word Generation Numbers & Letters Part D Efficiency Driving Scenes Story Learning Phrase Unit DR Design Construction Word Generation	Screening Language Domain Screening Executive Functions Domain Memory Index Executive Functions Index
Low (≤.59)	Screening Auditory Comprehension Screening Naming Screening Visual Discrimination Screening Design Construction Screening Mazes Auditory Comprehension Shape Learning DR Judgment	Screening Numbers & Letters Part A Errors Screening Numbers & Letters Part B Efficiency Screening Auditory Comprehension Screening Naming Screening Shape Learning IR & DR Screening Story Learning IR & DR Screening Visual Discrimination Screening Design Construction Dots Number & Letters Part A Errors Numbers & Letters Part B Efficiency Numbers & Letters Part C Efficiency Numbers & Letters Part D Disruption Oral Production Auditory Comprehension Writing Bill Payment List Learning List A IR List Learning List B IR List Learning List A Short DR List Learning List A Long DR Shape Learning IR Shape Learning DR Story Learning Phrase Unit IR Daily Living Memory IR Daily Living Memory DR Visual Discrimination Figure Drawing Copy Figure Drawing Copy Organization Figure Drawing IR Map Reading Mazes Judgment Categories	Screening Memory Domain Screening Spatial Domain Language Index

*Internal reliability estimates were not computed for all subtests.

Table 6–81 Median Percentage Agreement Coefficients for Correct Classifications for Secondary and Descriptive Scores

Module	Secondary Scores	Descriptive
Screening	86.4%	99.2%
Attention	90.3%	100%
Language	99.2%	98.3%
Memory	91.6%	83.3%
Spatial	84.8%	—
Executive	82.4%	—

Note: Test and retest scores were divided into three categories ($\leq$−2.0 SD, −1.9 SD to +1.9 SD, $\geq$2.0 SD) and the test and retest ranges were then evaluated to determine the percentage agreement of each category from test to retest.

reliabilities of some of the domains (e.g., Language, Screening Spatial, Executive Functions) are less than adequate.

To examine the temporal stability of the secondary and descriptive scores, a percentage agreement coefficient was calculated with test and retest scores divided into three categories based on standard deviation units ($\leq$−2.0 *SD*, −1.9 to +1.9 *SD*, $\geq$2.0 *SD*). The test and retest ranges were then evaluated to determine the percentage agreement of each category from test to retest. Using this coarse scheme, the authors report high classification agreement (based on the average correct classification performance for all ages; see Table 6–81).

Reliability coefficients for Form 2 tend to be somewhat higher than those for Form 1. For example, the reliability coefficient (corrected for restriction of range using the initial test) for the Total Screening Index for Form 1 is .66, but .85 for Form 2. Similarly, the reliability coefficient for the Total NAB Index for Form 1 is .74 and .89 for Form 2. Currently, no information is available on test-retest reliability in clinical groups.

Practice Effects

Practice effects are evident for most of the NAB tasks; however, gains are small (about 1–2 T-score points) across a six-month interval (White & Stern, 2003b). With the exception of the Screening Memory domain score, the NAB Screening domain scores demonstrate relatively small practice effects (less than half of a standard deviation). A similar pattern of practice effects is seen for the module index scores and the Total NAB Index score.

Equivalent Form Reliability

The authors (White & Stern, 2003b) conducted a generalizability study in which 100 participants (aged 18–84 years, *M* = 57.9 years, *SD* = 19.5) were given NAB Forms 1 and 2 in a counterbalanced design. The mean interval between administrations was 25 days (*SD* = 6.3). Median generalizability coefficients for the Screening Module and for the module primary scores tend to exceed .60, suggesting adequate reliability. The mean difference between versions is not reported.

Interrater Reliability

Thirty Form 1 and thirty Form 2 standardization protocols were independently scored by two raters (White & Stern, 2003b) with interrater reliability evaluated for the following subtests that require some subjectivity: Writing, Story Learning, Figure Drawing, Judgment, and Categories. Scoring reliability was high for all subtests.

Standard Errors of Measurement

Tables are provided in the Psychometric and Technical Manual (White & Stern, 2003b) that summarize the various estimates of reliability (e.g., alpha coefficients, test-retest reliability, generalizability coefficients) as well as the standard error of measurement (*SEM*) corresponding to the relevant reliability coefficient. The Screening domain, Total Screening Index, module index, and Total NAB Index scores are considered the main focus of interpretation, and 90% and 95% confidence intervals are presented in the tables of the norms manuals. Note, however, that the *SEM*s are quite large. Standard errors or measurement, reported in T-score units, for the Screening domain/index scores range from 4.5 (Screening Attention) to 10.06 (Screening Language). For the main module scores, *SEM*s (reported in T-score units) range from 3.00 (T-NAB Index) to 6.87 (Language index). Because *SEM*s are large, confidence intervals are also sizeable. For example, if an individual obtains a Total Screening Index (S-NAB) score of 100, the examiner can be 95% confident that the individual's true score falls in the low-average to above-average range; that is, 87 to 113. Similarly, if an individual obtains a standard score of 90 on the Executive Functions module, the examiner can be 95% confident that the individual's true score is between 80 and 100.

Users should note that traditional Pearson correlations and associated *SEM*s are presented to evaluate the stability of primary scores and module indexes for each form separately. By contrast, generalizability coefficients (and associated *SEM*s) are provided with regard to equivalent forms reliability. Why different metrics (Pearson correlations, generalizability coefficients) were chosen to evaluate the various aspects of reliability is not reported. Standard errors or measurement based on generalizability coefficients appear smaller than those based on Pearson correlations. It is not clear whether this reflects increased reliability when two alternate forms are given (as opposed to the same form given on both occasions—a surprising finding) or characteristics of the methods used to derive the reliability estimates.

VALIDITY

Content Validity

The test authors (White & Stern, 2003b) report that reviews of the neuropsychological literature and results of the publisher's survey of neuropsychological needs and practices (Stern &

White, 2000) led to decisions regarding the content of the NAB. An expert panel of consultants provided guidance regarding the appropriateness of each item and/or test. Coverage of content extends to ecologically relevant tasks. In addition, pilot testing was used to empirically determine the difficulty level of items and to equate items between forms. A variety of quality assurance procedures (e.g., examiner training, rescoring of protocols, random selection of protocols to check for accuracy) were employed to reduce errors and enhance the accuracy of the data collected.

Task Intercorrelations

The intercorrelations among the primary scores of tasks within a module domain tend to be positive and of modest to moderate strength. In general, the module primary scores correlate most highly with the module index score that subsumes them. Further, Screening domain scores generally have the highest correlations with their respective main module index score counterparts. The correlations range from .35 (between the Screening Language domain score and the Language index score) to .78 (the Screening Attention domain score and the Attention index score). The Total Screening Index score and the Total NAB Index score are highly correlated ($r = .79$) (White & Stern, 2003b).

Relations Between Screening Domain and Module Index Scores

One of the primary goals of the NAB was to construct Screening Module domain score ranges that could reliably predict performance on the corresponding full NAB module at both the severely impaired and above-average ends of the ability spectrum. In this way, one could use the Screening domain scores to identify individuals who are so impaired (or intact) that they would be expected to obtain similarly impaired (or intact) scores on the corresponding domain-specific module, thus obviating the need to administer the main module (Stern & White, 2003).

The ability of the Screening domain scores to predict performance on the corresponding module index scores was evaluated in the standardization sample as well as a number of clinical groups (White & Stern, 2003b). Each of the five module index scores was classed into one of three groups: moderate to severely impaired (index score of 45–61), with the goal of identifying these individuals and recommending against testing them with the corresponding main NAB module; moderately impaired to average (index score of 62–106), with the goal of identifying such individuals and recommending that they be tested with the corresponding main NAB module; and above average and better (index score of 107–155), with the goal of identifying individuals in this range and recommending against testing them with the corresponding NAB module. For each module, the cumulative score distribution of the Screening domain score was computed for each of the three index score ranges and a conservative criterion was selected to identify at least 95% of the individuals who are recommended to receive the full module. This criterion was based on the belief that it is more desirable to give the main module unnecessarily than to screen out an individual who may, in fact, require the main module. As Table 6–82 shows, only 5% of the individuals who obtained index scores in the 62 to 106 range (i.e., who are judged to require administration of the main module) were missed by the

Table 6–82 Recommendations for Administering NAB Modules Based on Screening Domain Scores: Decision Accuracy Rates

Screening Domain	Cutoff	False-Positive Rate	False-Negative Rate
Attention	Moderate-severely impaired (≤74)	.41	.05
	Above average (≥114)	.57	.05
Language	Moderate-severely impaired (≤75)	.25	.05
	Above average (≥126)	.97	.04
Memory	Moderate-severely impaired (≤75)	.29	.05
	Above average (≥119)	.79	.05
Spatial	Moderate-severely impaired (≤74)	.56	.05
	Above average (≥120)	.78	.05
Executive	Moderate-severely impaired (≤73)	.33	.05
	Above average (≥115)	.62	.05

Source: From White & Stern, 2003b. Reproduced by special permission of the publisher, Psychological Assessment Resources, Inc., 16204 North Florida Avenue, Lutz, Florida 33549, from the Neuropsychological Assessment Battery by Robert A. Stern, PhD, and Travis White, PhD. Copyright 2001, 2003 by PAR, Inc. Further reproduction is prohibited without permission from PAR, Inc.

respective cutoff scores. However, the false-positive rates are high, with many intact individuals falsely flagged for main module administration. For example, the above-average and higher cutoff scores correctly identify only between 3% (Language domain) and 43% (Attention domain) of individuals who obtained index scores in the 107 to 155 range (i.e., who were judged not to require administration of the main module). Overall, the cutoffs appear more useful for lower, as opposed to higher, functioning patients. The above-average and higher cutoffs are not very useful for identifying fully intact individuals who do not require administration of the full module.

Factor-Analytic Findings

Exploratory and confirmatory factor-analytic studies are presented in the Psychometric and Technical Manual (White & Stern, 2003b). The models that were derived are somewhat different than the models originally hypothesized (e.g., psychomotor speed tended to emerge as a separate factor with loadings from Mazes and Numbers & Letters Efficiency). These models should be considered as hypotheses that need to be evaluated further in other samples, including clinical ones.

Correlations With Other Measures

A subset of 50 unimpaired individuals (aged 20–85 years, $M = 59.5$, $SD = 17.5$ years) who participated in the NAB standardization study also completed a number of standard cognitive measures (White & Stern, 2003b). Positive relations were found between NAB scores and scores on other brief measures of general cognitive ability such as the MMSE, 3MS, RBANS, and Reynolds Intellectual Screening Test (RIST). Thus, the Total NAB Index correlates with the 3MS, MMSE, RBANS, and RIST scores in the .40 to .65 range, suggesting that this composite has a substantial overlap with overall intellectual ability while still measuring something unique.

The authors also compared NAB scores with other measures of specific cognitive functions (e.g., with WMS-III, CVLT-II, TMT, RBANS, Ruff 2 & 7, Boston Naming Test, Token Test, COWA, ROCF, JOLO, WCST, Porteus Mazes) to examine both the convergent and divergent validity of the NAB scores (White & Stern, 2003b). Correlational analyses based on unimpaired and impaired samples (e.g., patients with dementia, patients with aphasia) tend to show the expected pattern of relations, with criterion measures correlating more highly with those NAB scores that tap similar, as opposed to different, cognitive processes.

Clinical Studies

Data are presented in the test manual (White & Stern, 2003b) on NAB performance in various clinical groups, including individuals with dementia, aphasia, traumatic brain injury, HIV/AIDS, multiple sclerosis, conditions requiring inpatient rehabilitation, and adult ADHD. Overall, the findings con-

form to expectation. For example, almost 90% of the patients with dementia score in the impaired range on the Memory index. Similarly, a sizeable percentage of mild to moderate TBI patients (screened for suboptimal effort) show impairments in the Attention, Memory, and Executive Function areas. Although these findings provide preliminary information regarding the validity of the NAB, additional studies are needed regarding the test's diagnostic utility.

Ecological Validity

There is some evidence of ecological validity of NAB scores. Thus, Screening domain Memory scores correlate moderately well with therapists' ratings of memory functioning of inpatients in a rehabilitation hospital (White & Stern, 2003b). Further, the Driving Scenes test appears relevant to everyday driving ability. Brown et al. (2005) found that healthy persons performed better than very mildly demented individuals on the test. The correlation between the Driving Scenes test and on-road performance was .55, and those rated as safe by the driving instructor performed better on the NAB Driving Scenes test than those rated as marginal or unsafe.

Malingering

The authors (White & Stern, 2003b) used a simulation paradigm to examine the impact of feigned or exaggerated impairment of head injury on NAB performance. Simulators performed significantly worse than controls on most NAB primary scores and module indices. In addition, simulators could be distinguished from controls as well as patients with TBI by their pattern of very poor scores on 11 NAB indicators: Driving Scenes, Auditory Comprehension, Visual Discrimination, Figure Drawing Immediate Recall, Daily Living Immediate and Delayed Recall, Judgment, Categories, Attention index, Language index, and Memory index. Low to moderately high correlations were obtained between these 11 NAB scores and three criterion measures of motivational status: the TOMM, WMT, and VSVT.

COMMENT

The authors of the NAB should be commended for developing a battery of tests that can be given in a reasonably brief period of time that includes quantitative summary scores along with numerous qualitative indices (e.g., extent of fragmentation and planning in drawing a complex figure) and that provides coordinated norming of tests. The provision of equivalent, parallel forms that were separately normed is also useful. The inclusion of measures that tap daily living skills is another unique feature of the battery. Other strengths include its portability, the fact that manipulatives are kept to a minimum, and its ease of administration and scoring. Like any new, complex measure, there are also some limitations/ reservations, but these do not diminish the overall value of the test.

The Technical Manual is thorough and well written. Normative data are extensive, although it should be noted that about 85% of the standardization sample is Caucasian and norms are not corrected for ethnicity. Additional research is necessary in this regard.

The availability of a single comprehensive set of demographically corrected normative data is a key asset. As a consequence, standardized scores on these tasks can be compared directly and different profiles of strengths and weaknesses can be identified. Data are provided to determine whether discrepancies are significant and unusual. Unfortunately, the manuals do not provide the frequencies with which discrepancies occurred in either direction.

Users should note that internal reliabilities are low for many scores (see Table 6–81), and even for composite scores, SEMs and corresponding confidence intervals can be quite large. A positive feature of the NAB compared with many other batteries (e.g., WAIS-III) is that test-retest reliability was evaluated over an interval more commonly used in clinical situations (six months). However, reliabilities of the primary scores tend to be less than optimal, especially for the Spatial, Memory, and Executive Functions domains. Greater confidence can be had in the composite scores, although even the reliabilities of some of these (e.g., Executive Functions, Memory, Language) are not sufficiently high for clinical decision making and suggest that some tasks may have limited utility for longitudinal assessment. There is also a lack of clarity regarding the use of different metrics (Pearson correlations, generalizability coefficients) that were chosen to evaluate various aspects of reliability (test-retest, alternate form).

Screening scores may also yield different results than the full modules (e.g., Language). The NAB screening recommendations for follow-up administration of a module were developed to ensure that at least 95% of individuals who would be expected to require administration of a NAB module are in fact recommended for that module; that is, the goal was to maximize the hit rate and minimize the false-negative rate (Stern & White, 2003). In practice, use of this conservative screening criterion means that for most patients (particularly higher functioning ones), the recommendation will be to administer all five main modules, increasing perhaps unnecessarily the administration time. Accordingly, the desire for increased sensitivity will need to be balanced with the need to limit the length of the testing.

The authors provide considerable evidence of test validity, including content, construct, and criterion-related validity. The inclusion of clinical samples is also a strength, as users can have access to some preliminary information even though independent research has not yet been published. Preliminary evidence of ecological utility is also included, along with information potentially useful in the interpretation of NAB scores in forensic situations. Users should note, however, that support for the five main module/index scores is mixed at present and additional studies are needed to evaluate the structure of the NAB, particularly in clinical populations.

Although the NAB was developed with the goal of providing a common set of core tests that could serve as a reasonably comprehensive neuropsychological test battery for most clinical applications, users should bear in mind that a comprehensive neuropsychological evaluation will require additional tests of important domains not assessed by the NAB such as IQ, motor functioning, and personality. The selection of these additional tests may be informed by the individual patient's performance on the NAB.

Finally, users should note that the NAB was developed by attending to feedback from users and experts, and in an attempt to cater to the consensus opinion, the NAB does not represent a fundamental shift in neuropsychological thinking. The NAB tests will be familiar to most neuropsychologists as the tasks incorporate existing methods of assessment. For example, the Memory tests have the capacity to measure various aspects of episodic memory, including visual and verbal memory, recognition memory, discriminability, and susceptibility to interference, as well as the extent to which the examinee gains from repetition and uses a semantic encoding strategy. This familiarity may prove an asset, encouraging its use among clinicians and researchers, and it may replace existing tests that are not conormed. However, the NAB is not clearly theory driven and the authors admit that development was guided by both empiricism and cognitivism. However, because it employs standard testing paradigms, it does not contribute new approaches or new conceptualizations of neuropsychological functioning. Accordingly, examiners will have to choose other techniques for coverage of additional domains (e.g., implicit memory) and for identification of the particular component processes (e.g., familiarity versus recollection) that may be affected in a given patient. Finally, it is not yet clear whether NAB subtests, designed after familiar neuropsychological paradigms (e.g., Rey Complex Figure, CVLT, Word Fluency), confer added sensitivity over existing, well-established tests.

REFERENCES

Brown, L. B., Stern, R. A., Cahn-Weiner, D. A., Rogers, B., Messer, M. A., Lannon, M. C., Maxwell, C., Souza, T., White, T., & Ott, B. R. (2005). Driving Scenes test of the Neuropsychological Assessment Battery (NAB) and on-road driving performance in aging and very mild dementia. *Archives of Clinical Neuropsychology, 20,* 209–216.

Heaton, R. K., Miller, S. W., Taylor, M. J., & Grant, I. (2004). *Revised comprehensive norms for an expanded Halstead-Reitan Battery: Demographically adjusted neuropsychological norms for African American and Caucasian adults.* Lutz, FL: Psychological Assessment Resources.

Reynolds, C. R., & Kamphaus, R. W. (2003). *Reynolds Intellectual Screening Test.* Lutz, FL: Psychological Assessment Resources.

Stern, R. A., & White, T. (2000). Survey of neuropsychological assessment practices [Abstract]. *Journal of the International Neuropsychological Society, 6,* 137.

Stern, R. A., & White, T. (2003). *Neuropsychological Assessment Battery: Administration, Scoring, and Interpretation manual.* Lutz, FL: Psychological Assessment Resources.

White, T., & Stern, R.A. (2003a). *Neuropsychological Assessment Battery: Demographically corrected norms manual.* Lutz, FL: Psychological Assessment Resources.

White, T., & Stern, R.A. (2003b). *Neuropsychological Assessment Battery: Psychometric and Technical manual.* Lutz, FL: Psychological Assessment Resources.

White, T., & Stern, R. A. (2003c). *U.S. census-matched norms manual.* Lutz, FL: Psychological Assessment Resources.

Raven's Progressive Matrices (RPM)

PURPOSE

The purpose of Raven's Progressive Matrices (RPM) is to assess reasoning in the visual modality.

SOURCE

The test can be ordered from Harcourt Assessment (www.harcourtassessment.com). The complete kit includes two each of the Colored, Standard, and Advanced (I and II) test booklets, 50 hand-scorable answer documents and keys for each level, the Comprehensive Technical Manual (1998), and the Research Supplement 3 (2000), which contains American normative data. The kit costs $725 US. The various components (booklets, answer documents, manuals) can also be purchased individually.

AGE RANGE

Norms begin at age 6.5 for the Standard PM (SPM), age 5.5 for the Colored PM (CPM), and age 12 for the Advanced RM (APM).

DESCRIPTION

The RPM is consensually accepted as the quintessential test of inductive reasoning (Alderton & Larson, 1990). Test items require the examinee to infer a rule relating to a collection of elements, and then to use the rule to generate the next items in a series or to verify that a presented element is legitimate relative to the rule (Alderton & Larson, 1990). Problems become progressively more difficult, the easier items serving as a learning experience for later and more difficult items. Thus, the test has been used to assess intellectual efficiency or the ability to become more efficient by learning from immediate experience with the problems (Mills et al., 1993). The test is a popular measure of conceptual ability because responses require neither verbalization, skilled manipulative ability, nor subtle differentiation of visual-spatial information. In addition, verbal instruction is kept to a minimum (Zaidel et al., 1981).

Three forms of this test have been developed. The Standard Progressive Matrices (also known as the classic SPM or SPM-C) was originally published in 1938 (Raven, 1938). Normative studies, a linkage to a measure of word knowledge (the Mill Hill Vocabulary Scale), and the development of the Colored Progressive Matrices (CPM) and Advanced Progressive Matrices (APM) followed in the 1940s. In 1956, the SPM items were resequenced and the CPM and APM were revised (McCallum et al., 2000). In 1998, several new versions (Parallel CPM, Parallel SPM, and SPM+) were introduced.

SPM

The SPM consists of 60 items grouped into five sets (A to E), each set containing 12 items. Each item contains a pattern problem with one part removed and six to eight pictured inserts, one of which contains the correct pattern (see Figure 6–14). Each set involves different principles of matrix transformation, and within each set the items become increasingly more difficult. The scale is intended for the entire range of intellectual development starting with the time a child is able to grasp the idea of finding a missing piece to complete a pattern. All individuals, regardless of their age, are given the same series of problems in the same order and asked to work at their own speed, without interruption from the beginning to the end. It can be given individually or as a group test. Young children, intellectually impaired people, and very old individuals, however, are not expected to solve more than the problems in Sets

Figure 6–14 Simulated example of the SPM. *Source:* Courtesy of Harcourt Assessment.

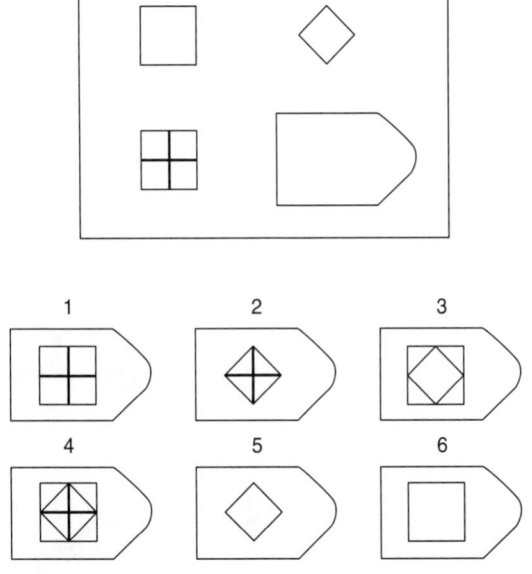

A and B of the scale and the easier problems of Sets C and D, where reasoning by analogy is not essential. A parallel version has also been developed (SPM-P; Raven et al., 2000a). The original version (1938) had, at the time it was developed, enough difficult problems to discriminate between adults of different ability levels. However, this discriminative power eroded as a result of the worldwide increase in intellectual ability over the years (Raven et al., 2000a). In fact, ceiling effects are quite noticeable in adolescence (Pind et al., 2003). The new Extended Plus version (SPM+) has been developed, which contains more difficult items but retains the 60-item format (Raven et al., 2000a).

CPM

The CPM (classic CPM or CPM-C; Raven, 1947; Raven et al., 1998b) provide a shorter and simpler form of the test. The test consists of 36 items, grouped into three sets (A, Ab, B) of 12 items each. That is, Sets C, D, and E of the Standard series have been omitted and an additional set of 12 problems (Ab) has been interpolated between Sets A and B. The last few problems in Set B are printed in the Colored version exactly as they appear in the Standard Test. In this way, a person who succeeds in solving these problems can proceed without interruption to Sets C, D, and E of the SPM so that intellectual capacity can be more accurately assessed (Raven et al., 1998a). By omitting a person's score on Set Ab, the total score on Sets A, B, C, D, and E can be used to determine the percentile grade on the SPM. Set A consists of problems in the form of a continuous pattern (or gestalt continuation; see Figure 6–15). As one progresses in the set, the items are of increasing perceptual difficulty. Items in the Ab and B series are made up of four elements or parts, three of which are given and one to be selected among the response alternatives (see Figure 6–14). There is a gradual shift through the Ab and B sets from four parts, which form a coherent whole or gestalt to problems in which each part is a symbol in an analogies test and there is no perceptual gestalt per se (Costa, 1976).

The CPM was developed for use with children (age 5.5+) and older people, for anthropological studies, and for clinical work. The test can be used with people who, for any reason, cannot understand English; people who suffer from physical disabilities, aphasias, cerebral palsy, or deafness; and people who are intellectually below normal. The problems are printed on colored backgrounds to attract the patient's attention. The scale is arranged so that it can be presented in the form of illustrations in a book or as boards with movable pieces. The board form makes the nature of the task even clearer to the patient. The CPM can be given individually, or after about age 8 in group format. The test covers the cognitive processes of which children under the age of 11 years are usually capable. Once the intellectual capacity to reason by analogy has developed, the SPM is the more suitable scale to use. A parallel form (CPM-P) has also been developed (Raven et al., 1998b).

APM

The Advanced Progressive Matrices (APM) (Raven, 1965, 1994; Raven et al., 1998c) were constructed as a test of intellectual efficiency that could be used with people of more than average intellectual ability and that could differentiate clearly between people of even superior ability (see Figure 6–16). It is intended for those for whom the SPM is too easy (i.e., for

Figure 6–15 Simulated example of the CPM. *Source:* Courtesy of Harcourt Assessment.

Figure 6–16 Simulated example of the APM. *Source:* Courtesy of Harcourt Assessment.

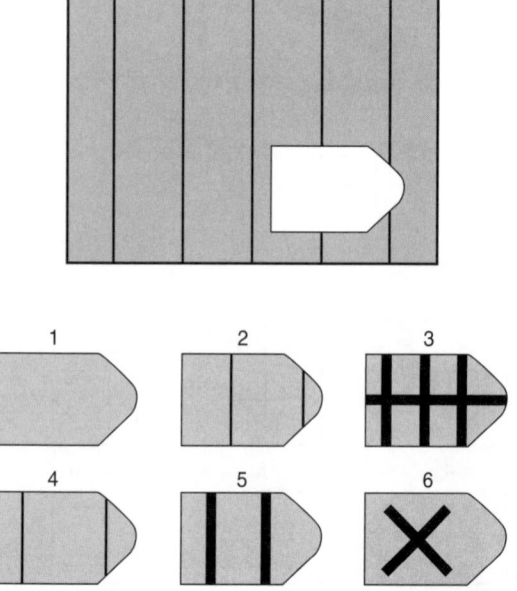

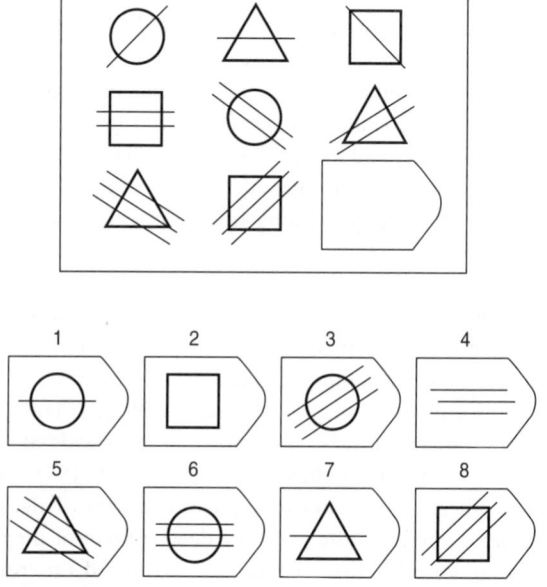

persons obtaining a raw score above about 50 on the SPM). With highly able children beyond the age of 10 years, the APM may be the most appropriate level to ensure an adequate ceiling (Mills et al., 1993). It consists of two sets of items. In Set I, there are 12 problems designed to introduce a person to the method of working and to cover the intellectual processes assessed by the SPM. It can be used as a short 10-minute test or as a practice test before starting Set II. The 36 items in Set II are identical in presentation and reasoning with those in Set I. They increase in difficulty more steadily and become considerably more complex.

ADMINISTRATION

See *Source*. Briefly, the examinee points to the pattern piece he or she selects as correct or writes its number on an answer sheet. There is some evidence that computerized forms can produce the same results as paper-and-pencil forms (Raven, 1996; Raven et al., 2000a). Raven cautions that, in order to obtain equivalence with the printed version, the answer selected by respondents should be shown on the screen and be alterable and that the respondents should be required to make a second, separate response to move the display to the next item.

ADMINISTRATION TIME

Both the SPM and CPM are untimed tests. The SPM takes about 40 minutes and the CPM requires about 25 minutes. Some give the APM under time constraints while others do not. Set II of the APM can be used without a time limit to assess a person's total reasoning capacity. In that case, the examinee should be shown the problems of Set I as examples to explain the principles of the test. About one hour should be allowed to complete the task. To assess a person's intellectual efficiency, Set I can be given as a short practice test followed by Set II as a speed test. The most common time limit for Set II is 40 minutes.

SCORING

The total number correct is recorded. Score conversion is to percentiles. The parallel versions of the CPM and SPM were developed to foil respondents who have memorized the correct answers (Raven et al., 1998b). Accordingly, the correct answer on each item differs from that in the classic versions of the tests. This is also the case for the SPM+. The authors warn that it is essential that the answer sheets and/or scoring keys correspond to the test used.

Using estimates of relative item difficulties, the authors constructed tables to convert scores on one test version to another. Thus, it is possible to transform CPM to SPM scores (and vice versa) using a table provided in the test manual (Raven et al., 1998b, 2000a). One can also convert SPM-C/SPM-P to SPM+ scores (Raven et al., 2000a) as well as to APM scores (Raven et al., 1998c).

DEMOGRAPHIC EFFECTS

Age

Scores on the Raven are correlated with the examinee's age (Locascio et al., 2003; Marcopulos & McLain, 2003; Raven et al., 2000b; Salthouse, 1993). There is an increase of ability through childhood, a period of maximum ability from adolescence to adulthood, and then a decline with advancing age.

Gender

According to Raven (Raven et al., 1998c), gender has little impact on SPM and CPM performance. However, others have reported gender-related differences at least in various age groups (e.g., Lynn et al., 2004). For Set II of the APM, the performance of men tends to be slightly superior to that of women (Bors & Stokes, 1998). The male advantage may reflect the test's visual-spatial nature (Abad et al., 2004).

Education/SES/Ethnicity

Raven scores show a significant increase with increasing years of education and socioeconomic status (Burke, 1985; Freeman & Godfrey, 2000; Marcopulos et al., 1997; Measso et al., 1993; O'Leary et al., 1991; Smits et al., 1997; also see *Source*). Ethnicity can also impact performance (Raven et al., 2000b; see *Validity*).

NORMATIVE DATA

Numerous reports of normative data have appeared in the literature (see *Source*). Many norms are derived from studies conducted in the 1930s and 1940s. Since that time, there has been an upward shift in levels of performance (Daley et al., 2003; Raven et al., 1998b, 1998a, 2000b). Consequently, more recent normative data are preferred. International and local norms are available from the source. Given the evidence of some cultural bias, the use of local norms may be desirable. In general, norms for high socioeconomic status districts are higher than others. Those for rural areas are lower (Raven et al., 1998b, 2000a). Local norms appear preferable for clinical use but are problematic when used to make comparative judgments across populations (Mills et al., 1993). Tables giving detailed percentages of test scores are also available (see *Source*) but should be used with caution given that the test may not be sufficiently precise to support such fine discrimination. Although conversion of percentages to IQ scores is possible (see Table 6–83 and Table 1–1), the practice is discouraged. Progressive Matrices scores are not interchangeable with those obtained from intelligence tests, which sample a wider range of abilities.

SPM

Summary North American norms for ages 6.5 to 19.5 are given by Raven et al. (2000a, 2000b). These data are derived

Table 6–83 Conversion of Percentile Ranks to Wechsler-type IQs

IQ	Percentile	IQ	Percentile	IQ	Percentile	IQ	Percentile
155	99.9	117	87	101	53	85	16
144	99.8	116	86	100	50	84	14
142	99.7	115	84	99	47	83	13
140	99.6	114	82	98	45	82	12
139	99.5	113	81	97	42	81	10
138	99	112	79	96	39	80	9
132	98	111	77	95	37	79	8
129	97	110	75	94	34	78	7
127	96	109	73	93	32	77	6
125	96	108	70	92	30	76	5
123	94	107	68	91	27	74	4
122	93	106	66	90	25	71	3
121	92	105	61	89	23	70	2
120	91	104	61	89	21	67	1
119	90	103	58	87	19	61	<1
118	88	102	55	86	18		

from a series of systematic random samples of schoolchildren (N not provided). American norms for ages 18+ have been developed by Raven et al. (2000a, 2000b) (N not provided). By early adolescence, ceiling effects begin to emerge, suggesting that it is not a suitable measure of mental ability for all age groups, not even among school-age children (see also Pind et al., 2003). Because the SPM+ does not yet have independent norms, it can only be interpreted by converting its scores to Classic SPM scores (SPM-C; Raven et al., 2000a), and this conversion effectively minimizes many of the benefits of its increased ceiling (McCallum et al., 2000).

Regression equations to predict premorbid SPM scores have been developed (Freeman & Godfrey, 2000; Van den Broek & Bradshaw, 1994). Both equations appear equally sensitive to neurological impairment (Freeman & Godfrey, 2000). The Van den Broek and Bradshaw equation (see also *NART* section) is somewhat easier to compute and is as follows:

$$SPM = (-0.462 \times NART\ errors) + (-0.254 \times age)$$
$$+ 66.65, r^2 = .548, SE_{est} = 5.556$$

CPM

Summary North American norms for ages 5.5 to 11.5 are presented by Raven et al. (1998b, 2000b). These data are derived from a series of norming studies with schoolchildren (N not provided). By about age 9 years, a nearly perfect score (35 out of 36) is obtained by the upper 5% of the normative sample, suggesting that a ceiling has probably been reached.

Yeudall et al. (1986) tested 225 normal Canadian men and women, ages 15 to 40, with the CPM. At each age-group interval (e.g., 15–20, 21–25, etc.), there were few, if any, errors. The mean number correct for the combined group (aged 15–40) was 34.9 ($SD = 1.25$). Norms for the elderly, ages 55 to 85, are provided by Smits et al. (1997). Note that in this study, only Sets A and B were given (Ab was omitted). Because section Ab

correlated strongly (>.90) with the sum of sections A and B, estimated total scores have been derived (Raven et al., 1998b).

Marcopulos et al. (1997) report a mean of 17.5 ($SD = 6.0$) for 110 community-dwelling older adults (age, $M = 76.48$ years, $SD = 7.87$) with an average educational level of 6.65 years ($SD = 2.14$). Marcopulos and McLain (2003) retested this sample four years later and the data are shown in Table 6–84. In this way, those who dropped out or who demonstrated significant decline (at least one SD) over the four-year period on the MMSE, DRS, and Fuld Object Memory Evaluation could be excluded to leave 73 "robust" participants. Note that some of the cell sizes are very small (<20). These data are included to illustrate trends and should not be considered normative estimates.

APM

Raven et al. (1998c) provide North American norms for adolescents (aged 12–16.5; Set II) and adults (18–68+; Sets I and II) for untimed (ages 12–70+) and timed (ages 17–28) versions.

Table 6–84 CPM Normative Data Stratified by Age and Education ($N = 73$)

	Education Level					
	0–6 years			7–10 years		
Age	N	M	SD	N	M	SD
55–74	8	15.3	4.0	25	20.5	6.3
75+	15	15.3	4.2	25	18.6	6.3

Total sample: $M = 18.2$, $SD = 6.1$.

Source: From Marcopulos & McLain, 2003. Reprinted with the kind permission of Psychology Press.

RELIABILITY

SPM

Raven et al. (2000a) summarize numerous studies and report that split-half reliability is high (>.80). Test-retest reliability is also high (>.80) with retest intervals less than a year. With longer intervals (years), values tend to be lower. Practice effects are not reported in the manual. The two forms appear to be interchangeable based on Rasch analysis (Raven et al., 2000a).

CPM

Raven et al. (1998b) summarize a number of studies with children which suggest that split-half reliability is high (typically above .80). Test-retest reliability is reported to be high (>.80) following intervals of days or weeks. Over longer intervals (6 months–1 year), however, values decline (.59–.79) (Raven et al., 1998b). Practice effects are not reported in the manual.

Raven et al. (1998b) report that more than 1000 respondents were used to calculate the difficulty levels of the original and parallel items in Sets A and B and about 500 for the old and new items in Set Ab. At an overall level, scores on the Parallel Form closely matched those obtained on the Classic Form of the test; at an individual level, the item difficulties of both forms expressed in Rasch logits were also very similar.

APM

APM Set II has high internal consistency, with split-half reliability coefficients varying between .83 and .87 (Bors & Stokes, 1998; Raven et al., 1998c). Set I, which has only 12 items, naturally yields lower figures. Data on retest reliability were originally collected for a 48-item version of the test that was in use from 1947–1962. There were 109 children and 243 adults who took the test (with a 40-minute time limit), and they were retested after six to eight weeks. The test was highly reliable for adults and children aged 11½ + (>.80), but only reasonably reliable for 10½-year-olds (.76). Overall, Set II scores increased by about three points on retest (Raven et al., 1998c). Scores on Set I correlate moderately well with those of Set II (.53; Bors & Stokes, 1998).

VALIDITY

Construct Validity

According to the authors, the RPM was constructed to measure the educative component of *g* as defined in Spearman's theory of cognitive ability. They define educative ability as "the ability to forge new insights, the ability to discern meaning in confusion, the ability to perceive, and the ability to identify relationships" (Raven et al., 2000a, p. 1). Although not strictly a pure measure of Spearman's *g*, the RPM comes as close as many consider possible (Llabre, 1984; Neisser, 1998). The RPM is also regarded by some theorists who endorse Cattell's (1957) decomposition of *g* into fluid intelligence (ability to solve novel problems) and crystallized intelligence (domain-specific knowledge acquired over time) as a quintessential measure of fluid intelligence.

While the RPM is largely a pure measure of *g*, a number of authors have contended that it also contains small spatial ability and verbal reasoning factors. For example, Lynn et al. (2004) examined 12- to 18-year-olds on the SPM. Exploratory and confirmatory factor analyses showed loadings of the items on three factors, which were identified as gestalt continuation (present in the early items), verbal analytical reasoning (includes arithmetical addition and subtraction problems), and visual-spatial ability (items where solution can be found perceptually). Further, the three factors showed a higher order factor identifiable as *g*.

It has been suggested that the core abilities tapped by the RPM include an incremental, reiterative strategy for encoding and inducing the regularities in each problem, the ability to induce abstract relations, and the ability to dynamically manage a large set of problem-solving goals in working memory (Carpenter et al., 1990). Indeed, a number of studies have found strong correlations between working memory and RPM performance in aging and Parkinson's disease. For example, statistically controlling for age-related decline in working memory accounts for much of the age-related decline in RPM performance (Gabrieli, 1996; Salthouse, 1993). Similarly, statistical control for reduced working memory in Parkinson's patients virtually eliminates their deficit on the RPM relative to age-matched healthy people (Gabrieli, 1996). Speed of processing (e.g., inspection time) also correlates with test performance, with high scores on the RPM associated with more rapid processing (Bates & Rock, 2004).

Concurrent Validity

Studies show moderately strong correlations (about .5–.7) between Raven tests and conventional tests of intelligence such as the Wechsler and Stanford-Binet scales, the NART, and the TONI-2 (Bostantjopoulou et al., 2001; Burke, 1985; Deary et al., 2004; Jensen et al., 1988; O'Leary et al., 1991; also see *Source*). When the Wechsler subtests are considered, the strongest relationship is found with Block Design, which involves visual-spatial skills and is considered a good measure of fluid intelligence (Mills et al., 1993).

Culture Fairness

The RPM is considered more culture fair than the Wechsler test for measuring reasoning ability (O'Leary et al., 1991). One approach to demonstrating test fairness is to compare the item difficulty calibrations across independent racial and ethnic groups. Overall, such studies reveal that the test has similar psychometric properties across various groups (e.g., African American, Caucasian, Hispanic, Asian, African, East

Indian; McCallum et al., 2000; Rushton et al., 2004). It has relatively low correlations with tests of academic achievement (Esquivel, 1984; Llabre, 1984; see *Source*), consistent with the notion that it is a fairer (but not necessarily more valid) measure than most intelligence tests or specific ability measures (Mills et al., 1993; Raven et al., 1990). Matrices (SPM) show the highest correlation with mathematics, with lower correlations being found for language subjects (Pind et al., 2003). The RPM, however, is not culture blind (Owen, 1992). Research on the ability of the RPM (SPM, in particular) to predict scholastic achievement or occupational success has produced conflicting results (Raven et al., 2000a). This appears particularly the case in certain cultural contexts.

Clinical Findings

The bulk of the evidence suggests that RPM performance (CPM and SPM) is impaired in various neurological and neuropsychiatric conditions. For example, patients with dementia tend to show impairment on the RPM (see Court et al. in Raven et al., 2000b, for a recent review of the RPM in various neurological populations). Similarly, patients with schizophrenia show lower performance on the RPM (CPM) (Parnas et al., 2001) as do individuals who suffer from severe depression (Naismith et al., 2003). Like the Wechsler IQ, it is somewhat sensitive to the consequences of traumatic brain injury (Freeman & Godfrey, 2000; Hiscock et al., 2002).

Gainotti et al. (1992) found that qualitative analysis of responses on the CPM can increase the diagnostic accuracy with regard to AD. The tendency to give globalistic (reproducing on a reduced scale the whole shape of the model instead of completing it) and odd (completely different from the missing part and from the general form of the model) responses are good markers of dementia and point more to AD than to a vascular form of dementia. Nondemented patients with PD show impairment on the CPM; however, the impairment appears to be accounted for at least in part by a visual-spatial deficit. In such patients, performance on subtest A of the CPM (with most items assessing gestalt continuation or visual closure) is predicted by other visual-spatial tasks but not by scores on tests of verbal memory or executive function (Cronin-Golomb & Braun, 1997).

Visual field defects and visual neglect impact performance (Court et al., in Raven et al., 2000b). Costa et al. (1969) developed criteria for assessing the presence of unilateral spatial inattention from CPM protocols. The number of answers chosen from the right side of the page (alternatives 3 and 6) is subtracted from the number of answers from the left side of the page (alternatives 1 and 4). The probability of this score, called the *position preference score* (PP), being 7 or greater or −7 or less is less than .01 in a normal population. A positive score of 7 or greater suggests right-sided neglect, whereas a negative score of 7 or less suggests left-sided neglect. The measure appears more sensitive than copying and drawing tasks to unilateral spatial inattention (Campbell & Oxbury, 1976). To reduce the influence that neglect for left-sided alternatives

may have on the performance of right-brain-damaged patients, the response array for each item on the CPM can be arranged vertically (Caltagirone et al., 1977; Villardita, 1985).

The RPM is often described as a measure of nonverbal reasoning ability. The question arises whether language plays a central role in mediating performance on the task. While the literature suggests that aphasic patients perform worse than normal controls on the RPM, findings are less consistent when aphasic patients are compared with other nonaphasic patients with left-hemisphere damage (Court et al., in Raven et al., 2000b). Unlike the findings with respect to aphasia, the findings with regard to RPM performance in the presence of constructional apraxia are quite consistent. Constructional apraxia is associated with lower RPM scores (Court et al., in Raven et al., 2000b).

The literature suggests that there is no significant difference between average scores of right- and left-brain-damaged individuals (e.g., Costa et al., 1969; Denes et al., 1978; Villardita, 1985). This may reflect a lack of homogeneity of items composing the CPM (e.g., Burke, 1958; Costa, 1976). There is some evidence that left-right hemispheric differences emerge when the items of the CPM are categorized on the basis of the cognitive ability presumed to underlie their solution (Denes et al., 1978; Villardita, 1985; Zaidel et al., 1981). Some have suggested that subtest A performance (with most items tapping gestalt continuation; see Figure 6–15) tends to be associated with the functions of the right (visual-spatial) hemisphere and subtest B performance (items requiring analogical reasoning; see Figure 6–14) with the functions of the left hemisphere (Costa 1976; Cronin-Golomb & Braun, 1997; Denes et al., 1978; Zaidel, 1981).

Activation studies suggest that an extensive network in both posterior and frontal regions is involved in RPM performance. For example, studies using cerebral blood flow or positron emission tomography (PET) reveal that performance on the RPM is associated with increased blood flow or glucose metabolism in the posterior part of the brain (parietal-temporal-occipital), that is, in regions important for visual cognition (Abe et al., 2003; Esposito et al., 1999; Haier et al., 1988; Risberg et al., 1977). Results of an fMRI study by Prabhakaran et al. (1997) in young, healthy participants suggested RPM performance activates an extensive network of working memory systems, consistent with behavioral studies suggesting a link between working memory and RPM performance (see previous discussion).

Malingering

A formula (Gudjonsson & Shackleton, 1986; McKinzey et al., 1999) to detect malingering has been developed for use with the SPM. The formula compares the number of correct answers for the first 24 items against the number of correct answers for the last 24 items (the "rate of decay"), using a set of cutoff numbers derived from the expected, theoretical rate of decay (see Table 6–85). In 46 simulators and 381 people from the adult standardization sample (Raven et al., 2000a), the

Table 6–85 Cutoff Values for Each Total SPM Score

Total Score	Cutoff	Total Score	Cutoff
2	1	32	12
3	2	33	10
4	3	34	10
5	4	35	10
6	5	36	10
7	6	37	10
8	7	38	8
9	7	39	8
10	7	40	8
11	7	41	8
12	7	42	8
13	9	43	7
14	9	44	7
15	9	45	7
16	9	46	7
17	9	47	7
18	10	48	6
19	10	49	6
20	10	50	6
21	10	51	6
22	10	52	6
23	11	53	2
24	11	54	2
25	11	55	2
26	11	56	2
27	11	57	0
28	12	58	0
29	12	59	−1
30	12	60	−1
31	12		

Note: The rate of decay is calculated by comparing the number of correct answers in each subset according to the formula $([2A + B] − [D + 2E])$. The cutoff is determined by the total score. The SPM is considered invalid if the rate of decay is below the cutoff listed for each total score.

From McKinzey et al., 1999. Reprinted with the permission of the British Psychological Society.

formula yielded a 26% false-negative rate and 5% false-positive rate (McKinzey et al., 1999). However, in children and adolescents (ages 7–17) instructed first to take the SPM according to standard instructions and then to malinger, the formula proved highly inaccurate, with a false-positive rate of 7% and a false-negative rate of 64%. By contrast, missing any of items A3, A4, or B1 (all extremely easy items) produced a 95% hit rate, with equal false-positive and false-negative rates of 5%. The indices remain to be cross-validated in neurologically impaired and forensic samples.

COMMENT

The RPM is the most well researched of all the nonverbal measures, with over 1500 published studies involving its use (McCallum et al., 2000). The simplicity, the nonverbal nature of the RPM, and the culture fairness of the task are distinct advantages for certain patients, particularly those from diverse ethnic and racial groups. For these reasons, the test is particularly valuable in the evaluation of people whose test performance may be confounded by language, hearing, or motor impairments or who lack proficiency with English and/or familiarity with the dominant North American culture. However, the test provides little information about an individual's strengths or weaknesses. The motor-reduced component and its untimed nature may also make it relatively insensitive to various forms of impairment. It also provides only a unidimensional estimate of cognitive functioning, which may limit its predictive validity. That is, multidimensional measures may have a better chance of accurately predicting multidimensional abilities such as school achievement or job success than measures that tap only a single ability. Thus, the RPM may provide additional information, but alternative measures are needed to gain a true picture of an individual's abilities (Court et al., in Ravens et al., 2000b; Mills et al., 1993). It is also important to note that performance is affected by factors such as visual field defects, unilateral neglect, and aphasia. Accordingly, interpretation may be difficult in the presence of these factors. Results should not be interpreted with respect to level of intellectual functioning when there is a significant position preference score (Court et al., in Raven et al., 2000b). In such cases, the test may provide important information regarding the presence of specific disorders (e.g., neglect).

The different formats of the test (CPM, SPM, SPM+, APM) provide the examiner with various choices. For example, adolescents can be given the SPM or SPM+, and high-ability adolescents and adults can be given the SPM+ or the APM. However, there is little guidance provided as to which version should be administered. One recommendation might be to select the version that has the most rigorous norms for that particular person (McCallum et al., 2000). Bear in mind that ceiling effects tend to emerge by about age 9 years on the CPM and by about age 12 to 13 years on SPM. Because the SPM+ has not yet been normed, it should be considered experimental until norms and percentile ranks are available (McCallum et al., 2000).

Like other cognitive tests (e.g., Wechsler), scores have been increasing over time (Raven et al., 2000a). The magnitude of the increase for the RPM is about 6 IQ points or 0.4 z units per decade (Hiscock et al., 2002). For example, on the classic SPM, people born in 1877 and tested in 1942 averaged 24 raw score points on the test, while people born in 1947 and tested in 1992 averaged 54 raw score points. Accordingly, newer normative data are preferred since use of older norms will diminish the test's ability to detect impairment (Hiscock et al., 2002).

The manuals offer the user a wide array of international norms; however, insufficient information is provided regarding the representativeness of each sample (McCallum et al., 2000). In this context, questions can also be raised about the most recent 1993 standardization involving adults in the United States in Des Moines, Iowa (McCallum et al., 2000). Although the test authors concluded that the data were representative of the

United States as a whole, one minority group (African American) appears to be significantly underrepresented in the sample.

REFERENCES

Abad, F. J., Colom, R., Rebollo, I., & Escorial, S. (2004). Sex differential item functioning in the Raven's Advanced Progressive Matrices: Evidence for bias. *Personality and Individual Differences, 36,* 1459–1470.

Abe, Y., Kachi, T., Kato, T., Arahata, Y., Vamada, T., Washimi, Y., Iwai, K., Ito, K., Yanagisawa, N., & Sobue, G. (2003). Occipital hypoperfusion in Parkinson's disease without dementia: Correlation to impaired cortical visual processing. *Journal of Neurology, Neurosurgery & Psychiatry, 74,* 419–422.

Alderton, D. L., & Larson, G. E. (1990). Dimensionality of Raven's Advanced Progressive Matrices items. *Educational and Psychological Measurement, 50,* 887–900.

Bates, T. C., & Rock, A. (2004). Personality and information processing speed: Independent influences on intelligent performance. *Intelligence, 32,* 33–46.

Bors, D. A., & Stokes, T. L. (1998). Raven's Advanced Progressive Matrices: Norms for first-year university students and the development of a short form. *Educational and Psychological Measurement, 58,* 382–398.

Bostantjopoulou, S., Kiosseoglou, G., Katsarou, Z., & Alevriadou, A. (2001). Concurrent validity of the Test of Nonverbal Intelligence in Parkinson's disease patients. *Journal of Psychology, 135,* 205–212.

Burke, H. R. (1958). Raven's Progressive Matrices: Validity, reliability, and norms. *Journal of Psychology, 22,* 252–257.

Burke, H. R. (1985). Raven's Progressive Matrices: More on norms, reliability, and validity. *Journal of Clinical Psychology, 41,* 231–235.

Caltagirone, C., Gainotti, G., & Miceli, G. (1977). A new version of Raven's Colored Matrices designed for patients with focal hemispherical lesion. *Minerva Psichiatrica, 18,* 9–16.

Campbell, D., & Oxbury, J. (1976). Recovery from unilateral visuospatial neglect? *Cortex, 12,* 303–312.

Carpenter, P. A., Just, M. A., & Shell, P. (1990). What one intelligence test measures: A theoretical account of the processing in the Raven Progressive Matrices test. *Psychological Review, 97,* 404–431.

Cattell, R. B. (1957). *Personality and motivation structure and measurement.* New York: Harcourt, Brace & World.

Costa, L. D. (1976). Interset variability on the Raven Colored Progressive Matrices as an indicator of specific ability deficit in brain-lesioned patients. *Cortex, 12,* 31–40.

Costa, L. D., Vaughan, H. G., Horwitz, M., & Ritter, W. (1969). Patterns of behavioral deficit associated with visual spatial neglect. *Cortex, 5,* 242–263.

Cronin-Golomb, A., & Braun, A. E. (1997). Visuospatial dysfunction and problem-solving in Parkinson's disease. *Neuropsychology, 11,* 44–52.

Daley, T. C., Whaley, S. E., Sigman, M. D., Espinosa, M. P., & Neumann, C. (2003). IQ on the rise: The Flynn effect in rural Kenyan children. *Psychological Science, 14,* 215–219.

Deary, I. J., Whalley, L. J., & Crawford, J. R. (2004). An "instantaneous" estimate of a lifetime's cognitive change. *Intelligence, 32,* 113–119.

Denes, F., Semenza, C., & Stoppa, E. (1978). Selective improvement by unilateral brain-damaged patients on Raven Coloured Matrices. *Neuropsychologia, 16,* 749–752.

Esposito, G., Kirkby, B. S., Van Horn, J. D., Ellmore, T. M., & Berman, K. F. (1999). Context-dependent, neural system-specific neurophysiological concomitants of ageing: Mapping PET correlates during cognitive activation. *Brain, 122,* 963–979.

Esquivel, G. B. (1984). Coloured Progressive Matrices. In D. J. Keyser & R. C. Sweetland (Eds.), *Test critiques* (Vol. 1, pp. 206–213). Kansas City, MO: Test Corporation of America.

Freeman, J., & Godfrey, H. (2000). The validity of the NART-RSPM index in detecting intellectual decline following traumatic brain injury: A controlled study. *British Journal of Clinical Psychology, 39,* 95–103.

Gabrieli, J. D. E. (1996). Memory systems analyses of mnemonic disorders in aging and age-related disease. *Proceedings of the New York Academy of Sciences of the United States of America, 93,* 13534–13540.

Gainotti, G., Parlato, V., Monteleone, D., & Carlomagno, S. (1992). Neuropsychological markers of dementia on visual-spatial tasks: A comparison between Alzheimer's type and vascular forms of dementia. *Journal of Clinical and Experimental Neuropsychology, 14,* 239–252.

Gudjonsson, G., & Schackleton, H. (1986). The pattern of scores on Raven's Matrices during "faking bad" and "non-faking" performance. *British Journal of Clinical Psychology, 25,* 35–41.

Haier, R., Seigel, B., Nuechterlein, K., & Hazlett, E. (1988). Cortical glucose metabolic rate correlates of abstract reasoning and attention studied with positron emission tomography. *Intelligence, 12,* 199–217.

Hiscock, M., Inch, R., & Gleason, A. (2002). Raven's Progressive Matrices performance in adults with traumatic brain injury. *Applied Neuropsychology, 9,* 129–138.

Jensen, A. R., Saccuzzo, D. P., & Larsen, G. E. (1988). Equating the Standard and Advanced forms of the Raven Progressive Matrices. *Educational and Psychological Measurement, 48,* 1091–1095.

Llabre, M. M. (1984). Standard Progressive Matrices. In D. J. Keyser & R. C. Sweetland (Eds.), *Test critiques* (Vol. 1, pp. 595–602). Missouri: Test Corporation of America.

Locascio, J. J., Corkin, S., & Growde, J. H. (2003). Relation between clinical characteristics of Parkinson's disease and cognitive decline. *Journal of Clinical and Experimental Neuropsychology, 25,* 94–109.

Lynn, R., Allik, J., & Irwing, P. (2004). Sex differences on three factors identified in Raven's Standard Progressive Matrices. *Intelligence, 32,* 411–424.

Marcopulos, B. A., & McLain, C. A. (2003). Are our norms "normal"? A 4-year follow-up study of a biracial sample of rural elders with low education. *The Clinical Neuropsychologist, 17,* 19–33.

Marcopulos, B. A., McLain, C. A., & Giuliano, A. J. (1997). Cognitive impairment or inadequate norms? A study of healthy, rural, older adults with limited education. *The Clinical Neuropsychologist, 11,* 111–131.

McCallum, S., Bracken, B., & Wasserman, J. (2000). *Essentials of nonverbal assessment.* New York: John Wiley & Sons.

McKinzey, R. M., Podd, M. H., Krehbiel, M. A., & Raven, J. (1999). Detection of malingering on Raven's Standard Progressive Matrices: A cross-validation. *British Journal of Clinical Psychology, 38,* 435–439.

Measso, G., Zaooala, G., Cavarzeran, F., Crook, T. H., Romani, L., Pirozzolo, F. J., Grigoletto, F., Amaducci, L., Massari, D., & Lebowitz, B. D. (1993). Raven's Colored Progressive Matrices: A normative study of a random sample of healthy adults. *Acta Neurologica Scandinavia, 88,* 70–74.

Mills, C. J., Ablard, K. E., & Brody, L. E. (1993). The Raven's Progressive Matrices: Its usefulness for identifying gifted/talented students. *Roeper Review, 15,* 183–186.

Naismith, S. L., Hickie, I. B., Turner, K., Little, C. L., Winter, V., Ward, P. B., Wilhelm, K., Mitchell, P., & Parker, G. (2003). Neuropsychological performance in patients with depression is associated with clinical, etiological and genetic risk factors. *Journal of Clinical and Experimental Neuropsychology, 25,* 866–877.

Neisser, U. (1998). Introduction: Rising test scores and what they mean. In U. Neisser (Ed.), *The rising curve: Long-term gains in IQ and related measures* (pp. 3–22). Washington, DC: American Psychological Association.

O'Leary, U-M., Rusch, K. M., & Guastello, S. J. (1991). Estimating age-stratified WAIS-R IQs from scores on the Raven's Standard Progressive Matrices. *Journal of Clinical Psychology, 47,* 277–284.

Owen, K. (1992). The suitability of Raven's Standard Progressive Matrices for various groups in South Africa. *Personality and Individual Differences, 13,* 149–159.

Parnas, J., Vianin, P., Saebye, D., Jansson, L., Volmer-Larsen, A., & Bovet, P. (2001). Visual binding abilities in the initial and advanced stages of schizophrenia. *Acta Psychiatrica Scandinavia, 103,* 171–189.

Pind, J., Gunnarsdottir, E. K., & Johannesson, H. S. (2003). Raven's Standard Progressive Matrices: New school age norms and a study of the test's validity. *Personality and Individual Differences, 34,* 375–386.

Prabhakaran, V., Smith, J. A. L., Desmond, J. E., Glover, G. H., & Gabrieli, J. D. E. (1997). Neural substrates of fluid reasoning: An fMRI study of neocortical activation during performance of the Raven's Progressive Matrices. *Cognitive Psychology, 33,* 43–63.

Raven, J. C. (1938, 1996). *Progressive Matrices: A perceptual test of intelligence. Individual Form.* Oxford: Oxford Psychologists Press Ltd.

Raven, J. C. (1947). *Colored Progressive Matrices Sets A, Ab, B.* Oxford: Oxford Psychologists Press Ltd.

Raven, J. C. (1965, 1994). *Advanced Progressive Matrices Sets I and II.* Oxford: Oxford Psychologists Press Ltd.

Raven, J., Raven, J. C., & Court, J. H. (1998a). *Raven manual: Section 1. General overview.* Oxford: Oxford Psychologists Press Ltd.

Raven, J., Raven, J. C., & Court, J. H. (1998b). *Raven manual: Section 2. Colored Progressive Matrices.* Oxford: Oxford Psychologists Press Ltd.

Raven, J., Raven, J. C., & Court, J. H. (1998c). *Raven manual: Section 4. Advanced Progressive Matrices.* Oxford: Oxford Psychologists Press Ltd.

Raven, J., Raven, J. C., & Court, H. H. (2000a). *Raven manual: Section 3. Standard Progressive Matrices.* Oxford: Oxford Psychologists Press Ltd.

Raven, J., et al. (2000b). *Raven manual research supplement 3: American norms, neuropsychological applications.* Oxford: Oxford Psychologists Press Ltd.

Raven, J., Summers, B., Birchfield, M., et al. (1990). *Manual for Raven's Progressive Matrices and Vocabulary scales. Research Supplement No. 3: A Compendium of North American Normative and Validity Studies.* Oxford: Oxford Psychologists Press Ltd.

Risberg, J., Maximilian, A., & Prohovnik, I. (1977). Changes of cortical activity patterns during habituation to a reasoning test. *Neuropsychologia, 15,* 793–798.

Rushton, J. P., Skuy, M., & Bon, T. A. (2004). Construct validity of Raven's Advanced Progressive Matrices for African and non-African engineering students in South Africa. *International Journal of Selection & Assessment, 12,* 220–229.

Salthouse, T. A. (1993). Influence of working memory on adult age differences in matrix reasoning. *British Journal of Psychology, 84,* 171–179.

Smits, C. H. M., Smit, J. H., van den Heuvel, N., & Jonker, C. (1997). Norms for an abbreviated Raven's Coloured Progressive Matrices in an older sample. *Journal of Clinical Psychology, 53,* 687–697.

Van den Broek, M. D., & Bradshaw, C. M. (1994). Detection of acquired deficits in general intelligence using the National Adult Reading Test and Raven's Standard Progressive Matrices. *British Journal of Clinical Psychology, 33,* 509–515.

Villardita, C. (1985). Raven's Colored Progressive Matrices and intellectual impairment in patients with focal brain damage. *Cortex, 21,* 627–634.

Yeudall, L. T., Fromm, D., Reddon, J. R., & Stefanyuk, W. O. (1986). Normative data stratified by age and sex for 12 neuropsychological tests. *Journal of Clinical Psychology, 42,* 920–946.

Zaidel, E., Zaidel, D. W., & Sperry, R. W. (1981). Left and right intelligence: Case studies of Raven's Progressive Matrices following brain bisection and hemidecortication. *Cortex, 17,* 167–186.

Repeatable Battery for the Assessment of Neuropsychological Status (RBANS)

PURPOSE

The purpose of this scale is to provide a brief evaluation of cognitive function in adults with neurological disturbance such as dementia, head injury, and stroke.

SOURCE

The test can be ordered from Harcourt Assessment (www.harcourtassessment.com). The Primary Form kit costs $169 US while the Alternate Form kit costs $149 US. A Spanish version is forthcoming.

AGE RANGE

Norms are available for ages 20 through 89 years.

DESCRIPTION

The RBANS (Randolph, 1998) was designed as a brief test to identify and characterize mild as well as severe forms of dementia in older adults. As its potential utility for screening cognitive status in younger individuals became apparent, the normative base was modified to include younger adults. The test comprises 12 subtests, similar to measures in widespread clinical use, that contribute to one of five domains/indices: Immediate Memory (List learning, Story memory), Visuospatial/Constructional (Figure Copy, Line Orientation), Language (Picture Naming, Semantic Fluency—Fruits & Vegetables), Attention (Digit Span, Coding), and Delayed Memory (List Recall, List Recognition, Story Memory, Figure Recall). In addition, a total scale score can be computed and is formed by combining the five domain scores. The descriptions of the subtests and indices are shown in Table 6–86.

Table 6-86 Description of RBANS Indices and Subtests

Index	Subtest	Description
Immediate Memory	List Learning	10 semantically unrelated items presented orally and patient asked to recall words; four learning trials are provided.
	Story Memory	Short story is orally presented and patient must retell the story; two learning trials.
Visuospatial/Constructional	Figure Copy	Patient must draw a complex figure.
	Line Orientation	Patient presented with pattern of 13 equal lines radiating from a single point. Below are two lines and patient must identify which two lines they match in the pattern.
Language	Picture Naming	Patient must name line drawings; a semantic cue is provided if an object is obviously misperceived.
	Semantic Fluency	Patient is given one minute to generate fruits and vegetables (Form A) and animals found in a zoo (Form B).
Attention	Digit Span	Forward Span
	Coding	Patient must code numbers to symbols in 90 sec.
Delayed Memory	List Recall	Patient must recall the list of 10 words from the List Learning subtest.
	List Recognition	Examinee is read 20 words and asked to indicate the 10 from the word list.
	Story Memory	Examinee is asked to recall story learned earlier.
	Figure Recall	Patient redraws the figure shown earlier.
Total Scale		Sum of Indices: Immediate Memory Visuospatial/Constructional Language Attention Delayed Memory

The stimuli are contained in a wire-bound, easel-backed booklet, making the test portable and allowing for bedside administration. One alternate form is available so that the test can be repeated on another occasion. This may allow the examiner to track disease progression or to assess the effects of therapeutic intervention.

ADMINISTRATION

Directions for administering the items, discontinue rules, correct responses, time limits, and prompts appear on the record form. Instructions for recording information for each subtest are also provided on the record form. The subtests should be given in the numbered order in which they appear on the record form, because the duration of the delay interval is determined by the administration of the intervening tasks.

ADMINISTRATION TIME

The test can be administered in about 20 to 30 minutes.

SCORING

Subtest raw scores are converted to age-based index scores by means of tables included in the Stimulus Booklet. Index scores ($M = 100$, $SD = 15$) range from 40 to 160. The RBANS Manual also provides the index means and standard deviations broken down by age groups (20–49, 50–69, and 70–89) and educational level (<HS, HS, >HS; see pp. 63–64 in test manual). Note that the raw total scores from two subtests are needed for the conversion to an index score for the domains of Immediate Memory, Visuospatial/Constructional, Language, and Attention. The List Recall, List Recognition, Story Recall, and Figure Recall total scores are summed for the Delayed Memory Index. That sum, along with the List Recognition total score, is used for the conversion to an index score. Thus, the focus is on the index scores, not the individual subtests. Percentile equivalents, confidence intervals (90% and 95%), and index discrepancy criteria are also provided.

There are two errors in the test publication. In Appendix 1 of both stimulus booklets, the scoring criteria for the drawing of the horizontal line should read: "It should not exceed ½ the length of the rectangle." In Appendix 2 of both stimulus booklets, in calculating the Immediate Memory index score for ages 70 to 79, at the intersection of Story Memory = 21 and List Learning = 20, the index score should be *100*, not 103.

DEMOGRAPHIC EFFECTS

Age

Age impacts performance (Duff et al., 2003; Gontkovsky et al., 2002; Randolph, 1998), with scores tending to decline with advancing age. However, in psychiatric samples, age has little relation to performance (Gold et al., 1999; Hobart et al., 1999; Wilk et al., 2004). However, these samples did not include elderly individuals, limiting their ability to detect age-related effects.

Education

As might be expected, cognitive performance on all indices improves with educational achievement (Duff et al., 2003; Gold et al., 1999; Gontkovsky et al., 2002; Hobart et al., 1999; Randolph, 1998; Wilk et al., 2004). Thus, it is important to adjust for education.

Gender

Modest effects have been reported with regard to gender. Men tend to perform better on the visual-spatial/constructional index (Gold et al., 1999; Wilk et al., 2004) and Attention Index (Wilk et al., 2004; but see Beatty, Mold, et al., 2003). Females perform slightly better on the Delayed Memory Index (Beatty, Mold, et al., 2003; Wilk et al., 2004) and the Language Index (Beatty, Mold, et al., 2003).

Ethnicity/Race

Gold et al. (1999) reported that in persons with schizophrenia, the RBANS total score of Caucasian patients was higher than that of African American patients; however, this difference disappeared when groups were statistically equated on WRAT-3 reading scores. By contrast, Patton et al. (2003) reported that racial discrepancies exist in older adults matched for age, education (years of education), and gender, with Caucasians performing higher than African Americans. These

Table 6–87 Characteristics of the RBANS Normative Sample

Number	540
Age	20–89 years[a]
Geographic location[b]	
Northeast	7%
South	23.7%
North Central	62.4%
West	6.9%
Sample type	Standardization sample considered representative of U.S. adult population in terms of gender, educational level, and race/ethnicity based on 1995 U.S. Census data
Education	
<HS	109
= HS	187
>HS	244
Gender	
Males	Not provided
Females	Not provided
Race/ethnicity	
White	~81%
African American	~13%
Hispanic	~7%
Screening	Screened to exclude participants with medical and psychiatric disorders

[a]Based on several age groupings: 20–39, 40–49, 50–59, 60–69, 70–79, 80–89. $N = 90$ per age group. [b]Sample is overrepresented by individuals in the North Central regions and underrepresented by individuals in the West and Northeast. However, subsequent analysis did not suggest any significant regional differences with regard to the total scale index score.

findings highlight the fact that years of education and quality of education may well yield discrepant results and that race may be a proxy for other variables.

NORMATIVE DATA

Standardization Sample

Norms are presented in the RBANS stimulus booklet and are based on a sample of 540 individuals, aged 20 to 89 years, considered representative of the U.S. population. Table 6–87 shows characteristics of the sample. RBANS subtest scores by age group are shown in Table 6–88.

Other Normative Data

Recently, Duff et al. (2003) extended the normative information on the RBANS by calculating age- and education-corrected scaled scores for the individual subtests. Age-corrected and education-corrected index and total scores are also provided.

Table 6–88 RBANS Subtest Means (*SD*), by Age Group

Subtest	Age Group					
	20–39	40–49	50–59	60–69	70–79	80–89
List Learning	30.7 (4.3)	27.6 (4.4)	27.5 (4.7)	28.0 (4.5)	26.6 (5.0)	23.2 (4.5)
Story Memory	19.1 (3.3)	16.9 (3.2)	17.5 (3.7)	18.4 (3.5)	17.4 (3.6)	15.3 (3.9)
Figure Copy	19.1 (1.3)	18.3 (1.4)	18.2 (1.4)	18.1 (1.7)	17.8 (1.8)	17.3 (2.0)
Line Orientation	16.8 (3.0)	15.4 (3.0)	16.4 (2.9)	16.6 (2.9)	16.4 (2.8)	15.7 (2.6)
Picture Naming	9.6 (0.7)	9.4 (1.1)	9.4 (0.9)	9.7 (0.5)	9.6 (0.7)	9.1 (1.0)
Semantic Fluency	21.6 (3.7)	20.8 (5.0)	21.0 (5.0)	21.0 (4.6)	19.8 (5.2)	17.4 (3.7)
Digit Span	11.7 (2.5)	10.6 (2.2)	10.5 (2.4)	10.2 (2.1)	10.4 (2.5)	9.2 (2.2)
Coding	56.5 (8.8)	49.8 (8.1)	46.3 (8.9)	46.1 (7.9)	41.3 (9.0)	34.0 (6.8)
List Recall	7.5 (1.8)	6.3 (1.9)	6.0 (2.1)	6.0 (2.2)	4.9 (2.5)	3.9 (2.3)
List Recognition	19.8 (0.7)	19.7 (0.6)	19.5 (1.0)	19.4 (1.2)	19.2 (1.2)	18.8 (1.4)
Story Recall	10.1 (2.1)	8.9 (1.8)	9.1 (2.2)	9.3 (2.1)	9.0 (2.2)	7.4 (2.8)
Figure Recall	16.1 (2.9)	13.5 (3.3)	13.5 (3.3)	13.6 (4.0)	12.5 (4.2)	11.4 (4.1)

The table contains subtest information from the standardization sample (*N* = 540). The data are from Form A.

Source: From C. Randolph, personal communication, October 18, 2002.

The data are based on a group of 718 community-dwelling older adults (65 years or older), predominantly Caucasians, recruited from an outpatient primary care setting in Oklahoma. Participants were excluded due to a variety of medical conditions (e.g., stroke or TIA, head injury, seizures, Parkinson's disease, macular degeneration) that clearly impact cognitive functioning. Tables 6–89 to 6–92 provide conversions of subtest raw scores to age-corrected scaled scores based on four midpoint age groups (70, 75, 80, 85). The age scaled scores have a mean of 10 and an *SD* of three. Tables 6–93 to 6–96 provide conversions of subtest age-corrected scaled scores to age- and education-corrected scaled scores based on four education groups (i.e., ≤11 years, 12 years, 13–15 years, ≥ 16 years). The age- and education-corrected scaled scores also have a mean of 10 and an *SD* of three. Table 6–97 provides conversions of age-corrected scaled scores to age-

Table 6–89 RBANS Raw Score Conversions to Age-Corrected Scaled Score for Midpoint Age = 70 (Age Range = 65–75, *N* = 495)

Scaled Score Range	List Learn	Story Mem	Figure Copy	Line Orient	Pict Nam	Sem Fluen	Digit Span	Cod	List Recall	List Recog	Score Recall	Figure Recall	%ile
2	0–7	0–3	0–10	0	0–4	0–4	0–4	0–3	—	0–11	—	—	<1
3	8–13	4	11	1–5	5–6	5–8	5	4–14	—	12–13	0	0–1	1
4	14	5–6	12	6	7	9	6	15–18	—	14	1	2–3	2
5	15	7–8	13–14	7–8	—	10	7	19–22	0	15	2	4–5	3–5
6	16–17	9–10	15	9–10	8	11	—	23–26	1	16	3–4	6–7	6–10
7	18–19	11	16	11–12	—	12–13	8	27–29	2	17	5	8–9	11–18
8	20–21	12–13	17	13–14	9	14	9	30–32	3	18	6	10	19–28
9	22–23	14–15	18	15	—	15–16	10	33–35	4	—	7	11–12	29–40
10	24–26	16–17	—	16–17	10	17–18	11	36–40	5	19	8–9	13–14	41–59
11	27–28	18	19	18	—	19–20	12	41–43	6	20	—	15	60–71
12	29	19	20	—	—	21	13	44–46	7	—	10	16	72–81
13	30–31	20	—	19	—	22–23	14	47–50	8	—	—	17	82–89
14	32–33	21	—	20	—	24–25	15	51–52	—	—	11	18	90–94
15	34–35	22	—	—	—	26	16	53–58	9	—	12	19	95–97
16	36–38	23	—	—	—	27	—	59–60	10	—	—	20	98
17	39	24	—	—	—	28–30	—	61–65	—	—	—	—	99
18	40	—	—	—	—	≥31	—	≥66	—	—	—	—	>99

Note: RBANS = Repeatable Battery for the Assessment of Neuropsychological Status, Learn = Learning, Mem = Memory, Orient = Orientation, Pict Nam = Picture Naming, Sem Fluen = Semantic Fluency, Cod = Coding, Recog = Recognition.

Source: From Duff et al., 2003. Reprinted with the kind permission of Psychology Press.

Table 6–90 RBANS Raw Score Conversions to Age-Corrected Scaled Score for Midpoint Age = 75 (Age Range = 70–80, N = 396)

Scaled Score	List Learn	Story Mem	Figure Copy	Line Orient	Pict Nam	Sem Fluen	Digit Span	Cod	List Recall	List Recog	Story Recall	Figure Recall	%ile Range
2	0–7	0–2	0–6	0	0–3	0–5	0–4	0–3	—	0–11	—	0–1	< 1
3	8–11	3–5	7–11	1–5	4–6	6	5	4–6	—	12	—	2	1
4	12	—	12	6	7	—	—	7–13	—	13	0	—	2
5	13–14	6–7	13	7–8	—	7–9	6	14–18	—	14	1–2	3–4	3–5
6	15–16	8–9	14–15	9–10	8	10–11	7	19–20	0	15	3	5–6	6–10
7	17–18	10–11	16	11–12	—	12	8	21–25	1	16–17	4	7–8	11–18
8	19–20	12	17	13	—	13	9	26–28	2	—	5–6	9	19–28
9	21–22	13–14	—	14–15	9	14–15	—	29–32	3	18	7	10–11	29–40
10	23–25	15–17	18	16	10	16–17	10–11	33–37	4–5	19	8	12–13	41–59
11	26–27	18	19	17–18	—	18–19	12	38–40	—	20	9	14	60–71
12	28–29	19	20	—	—	20	13	41–43	6–7	—	10	15–16	72–81
13	30	20	—	19	—	21–22	14–15	44–46	—	—	—	17	82–89
14	31–33	21	—	20	—	23–25	16	47–51	8	—	11	18	90–94
15	34	22	—	—	—	26	—	52–54	9	—	12	19	95–97
16	35	23	—	—	—	27–28	—	55–56	10	—	—	20	98
17	36	24	—	—	—	29–31	—	57–59	—	—	—	—	99
18	37–40	—	—	—	—	≥ 32	—	≥60	—	—	—	—	>99

Note: RBANS = Repeatable Battery for the Assessment of Neuropsychological Status, Learn = Learning, Mem = Memory, Orient = Orientation, Pict Nam = Picture Naming, Sem Fluen = Semantic Fluency, Cod = Coding, Recog = Recognition.

Source: From Duff et al., 2003. Reprinted with the kind permission of Psychology Press.

corrected index scores and total scores, and Table 6–98 provides conversions of age- and education-corrected index and total scores. Index and total scores have a mean of 100 and an *SD* of 15. Of note, scoring criteria of Figure Copy and Figure Recall were relaxed (e.g., discouraging the use of a ruler or protractor measuring elements), since it was noted that when the original scoring criteria were applied, the resulting data were significantly below expectation.

The sample studied by Duff et al. (2003) performed slightly lower than the original RBANS standardization sample and demonstrated greater variability in their scores. The sample studied by Duff et al. (2003) may be considered more

Table 6–91 RBANS Raw Score Conversions to Age-Corrected Scaled Score for Midpoint Age = 80 (Age Range = 75–85, N = 239)

Scaled Score	List Learn	Story Mem	Figure Copy	Line Orient	Pict Nam	Sem Fluen	Digit Span	Cod	List Recall	List Recog	Story Recall	Figure Recall	%ile Range
2	0–7	0–1	0–6	0–1	0–5	0–5	—	0–5	—	0–11	—	—	< 1
3	8–9	2–4	7–10	2–5	6	6–7	0–3	6–7	—	12	—	0–1	1
4	10–12	5	11–12	6	—	—	4	8–11	—	13	—	2	2
5	13–14	—	13	7–8	7	8	5–6	12–15	—	14	0	3	3–5
6	15	6–7	14	9–10	8	9–10	7	16–18	0	15	1–2	4–6	6–10
7	16–17	8–10	15	11	—	11–12	8	19–21	1	16	3	7	11–18
8	18–19	11	16	12–13	—	13	9	22–25	2	17	4	8–9	19–28
9	20–21	12–13	17	14	9	14	—	26–29	—	18	5–6	10	29–40
10	22–23	14–16	18	15–16	10	15–17	10–11	30–33	3–4	19	7–8	11–13	41–59
11	24–25	17	—	17	—	18	12–13	34–37	5	20	—	14	60–71
12	26–28	18–19	19	18	—	19	—	38–39	6	—	9	15	72–81
13	29	20	20	19	—	20–21	14–15	40–42	7	—	10	16	82–89
14	30–31	21	—	20	—	22–24	16	43–44	8	—	—	17	90–94
15	32–34	22	—	—	—	25–26	—	45–48	—	—	11	18–19	95–97
16	35	—	—	—	—	27–28	—	49–50	9	—	12	20	98
17	36–37	23	—	—	—	29–31	—	51–53	10	—	—	—	99
18	38–40	24	—	—	—	≥32	—	≥54	—	—	—	—	>99

Note: RBANS = Repeatable Battery for the Assessment of Neuropsychological Status, Learn = Learning, Mem = Memory, Orient = Orientation, Pict Nam = Picture Naming, Sem Fluen = Semantic Fluency, Cod = Coding, Recog = Recognition.

Source: From Duff et al., 2003. Reprinted with the kind permission of Psychology Press.

Table 6–92 RBANS Raw Score Conversions to Age-Corrected Scaled Score for Midpoint Age = 85 (Age Range = 80–94, N = 116)

Scaled Score	List Learn	Story Mem	Figure Copy	Line Orient	Pict Nam	Sem Fluen	Digit Span	Cod	List Recall	List Recog	Story Recall	Figure Recall	%ile Range
2	0–8	0–3	0–7	0	—	0–3	—	0–5	—	0–12	—	—	<1
3	9	4	8	1	0–4	4	—	6	—	13	—	—	1
4	10	—	9–11	2–5	5	5–6	0–3	7	—	—	—	—	2
5	11–12	5	12–13	6	6	7–8	4	8–10	—	14	—	0	3–5
6	13	—	14	7–10	7	9	5–6	11–15	—	15	0	1–4	6–10
7	14–15	6–8	—	11	8	10	7	16–18	0–1	16	1	5–6	11–18
8	16–17	9–10	15–16	12	—	11–12	8–9	19–21	2	17	2–4	7–8	19–28
9	18–20	11–12	17	13–14	—	13	—	22–25	—	18	5	9	29–40
10	21–22	13–15	—	15–16	9	14–16	10–11	26–30	3–4	—	6–7	10–12	41–59
11	23–24	16	18	17	10	17–18	—	31–32	—	19	8	13	60–71
12	25–27	17–18	19	18	—	19	12–13	33–36	5	20	9	14	72–81
13	28–29	19	20	—	—	20	14	37–39	6	—	—	15	82–89
14	30	20	—	19	—	21	15	40–41	7	—	10	16	90–94
15	31–37	21	—	20	—	22–24	16	42–44	8	—	11	17–18	95–97
16	38–40	22	—	—	—	25	—	45	—	—	12	—	98
17	—	23–24	—	—	—	26–27	—	46–50	9	—	—	19	99
18	—	—	—	—	—	≥28	—	≥51	10	—	—	20	>99

Note: RBANS = Repeatable Battery for the Assessment of Neuropsychological Status, Learn = Learning, Mem = Memory, Orient = Orientation, Pict Nam = Picture Naming, Sem Fluen = Semantic Fluency, Cod = Coding, Recog = Recognition.

Source: From Duff et al., 2003. Reprinted with the kind permission of Psychology Press.

representative of a population of older adults living in the Midwest who regularly visit their primary care physicians.

Others have also provided demographic adjustments based on the OKLAHOMA project. Gontkovsky et al. (2002) have provided regression-based adjustments for education and

Beatty, Mold, et al. (2003) have reported corrections for gender. The corrections are given only for the index scores, not the individual subtests. As noted previously (*Demographic Effects*), gender is not as powerful an influence on RBANS performance as is education. It accounts for 1% or less of the

Table 6–93 RBANS Age-Corrected Scaled Score Conversions to Age- and Education-Corrected Scaled Score for ≤ 11 Years of Education (N = 100)

Scaled Score	List Learn	Story Mem	Figure Copy	Line Orient	Pict Nam	Sem Fluen	Digit Span	Cod	List Recall	List Recog	Story Recall	Figure Recall	%ile Range
2	—	—	2	—	—	—	—	—	—	—	—	—	<1
3	2	2	3	2	2	2	2	2	—	2	—	3	1
4	3	3	—	3	—	3	—	—	2–4	3	2–3	—	2
5	4–5	—	4	4	3	4–5	3–4	3	5	4–5	4	—	3–5
6	—	4	5	5	4–5	6	5	4	6	6	—	4–5	6–10
7	6	5	6	—	—	—	6	5	7	—	5–6	6	11–18
8	7	6	7	6–7	6	7–8	7	6	—	7	7	7	19–28
9	8	7	8	—	7	—	8	7	8	8	8	8	29–40
10	9	8	9–10	8–9	8	9	9	8	9	9	9	9	41–59
11	—	9	—	—	9	10	—	9	10	10	—	10	60–71
12	10–11	10	11	10	—	11	10	—	—	—	10–11	11	72–81
13	12	11	—	11	10	12	11–12	10	11–12	11	—	12	82–89
14	13–14	12	12	12	11	13	13	11–12	13	12	12–13	13–14	90–94
15	15–17	—	13	13	12–18	14–16	14	—	—	13–18	14	—	95–97
16	18	13	14–18	14	—	17	15	13	14	—	15	15	98
17	—	14	—	15–18	—	18	16–18	14	15	—	16–18	16–18	99
18	—	15–18	—	—	—	—	—	15–18	16–18	—	—	—	> 99

Note: Age scaled scores were taken from Tables 6–89 to 6–92. RBANS = Repeatable Battery for the Assessment of Neuropsychological Status, Learn = Learning, Mem = Memory, Orient = Orientation, Pict Nam = Picture Naming, Sem Fluen = Semantic Fluency, Cod = Coding, Recog = Recognition.

Source: From Duff et al., 2003. Reprinted with the kind permission of Psychology Press.

Table 6–94 RBANS Age-Corrected Scaled Score Conversions to Age- and Education-Corrected Scaled Score for 12 Years of Education (N = 188)

Scaled Score	List Learn	Story Mem	Figure Copy	Line Orient	Pict Nam	Sem Fluen	Digit Span	Cod	List Recall	List Recog	Story Recall	Figure Recall	%ile Range
2	—	2	2	2–3	—	2–3	—	2–4	—	2	2	2–3	<1
3	2–3	3	3	—	—	—	—	—	—	3	3	—	1
4	4	4	—	4	—	4	2–3	—	2–4	—	4	—	2
5	5	5	4	5	2–5	5	4–5	5	5	4–5	5	4–5	3–5
6	6	6	5–6	6	6	6	6	6	6	6	—	6	6–10
7	7	7	7	7	—	7	7	—	7	7	6	7	11–18
8	8	8	8	—	7–8	8	8	7–8	8	8–9	7	8	19–28
9	9	—	9	8–9	9	9	9	—	9	—	8–9	9	29–40
10	10	9	10	—	—	10	10	9	10	10	—	10	41–59
11	—	10–11	11	10	10	11	11	10	11	—	10–11	11	60–71
12	11–12	12	—	11–12	11	12	12	11	12	11	12	12	72–81
13	—	13	12	—	12–18	—	13	12	13	12	13	13	82–89
14	13	—	13	13	—	13	14	13	14	13–18	14	—	90–94
15	14	14	14–18	—	—	14	15	14	15	—	—	14–15	95–97
16	15	15	—	14	—	15	16	15	—	—	15	16–18	98
17	16	16–17	—	15–18	—	16–17	17–18	16	16	—	16–18	—	99
18	17–18	18	—	—	—	18	—	17–18	17–18	—	—	—	>99

Note: Age scaled scores were taken from Tables 6–89 to 6–92. RBANS = Repeatable Battery for the Assessment of Neuropsychological Status, Learn = Learning, Mem = Memory, Orient = Orientation, Pict Nam = Picture Naming, Sem Fluen = Semantic Fluency, Cod = Coding, Recog = Recognition.

Source: From Duff et al., 2003. Reprinted with the kind permission of Psychology Press.

variance in the various index scores. Nonetheless, users may find the adjustments useful and the corrections are shown in Table 6–99.

Demographically adjusted normative data based on a sub-sample of 61 African Americans (39 males, 22 females, ages 65–94) from the OKLAHOMA project are also available (Patton et al., 2003). As with the larger sample, participants were recruited from their primary care physicians and screened to exclude medical conditions likely to affect cognitive functioning. All were living independently and two-thirds had completed high school (62%). Data are grouped into overlapping midpoint ranges at five-year intervals for midpoint

Table 6–95 RBANS Age-Corrected Scaled Score Conversions to Age- and Education-Corrected Scaled Score for 13–15 Years of Education (N = 230)

Scaled Score	List Learn	Story Mem	Figure Copy	Line Orient	Pict Nam	Sem Fluen	Digit Span	Cod	List Recall	List Recog	Story Recall	Figure Recall	%ile Range
2	—	—	2	2	2	—	2–3	2	—	2	2–3	2	<1
3	2	2–3	3–4	—	3–4	2	4	—	2–4	3–4	4	3	1
4	3	—	5	3–4	—	3	5	3–5	5	—	5	4	2
5	4–5	5	6	5	6–7	5–6	6	6	—	5	—	5–6	3–5
6	6	6	7	6	—	—	—	—	6	6	6	—	6–10
7	7	7	8	7	8	7	7	7	7	7	7–8	7	11–18
8	8	8	—	8	9	8	8	8	8	8–9	9	8	19–28
9	9	9	9–10	9	—	9	9	9	9	—	—	9	29–40
10	10	10	—	10	10	10	10	10	10–11	10	10–11	10	41–59
11	11	11	11	11–12	11	11–12	11–12	11	—	—	—	11	60–71
12	12	12	—	—	12–18	—	—	12	12	11	12–13	12	72–81
13	13	13	12	13	—	13	13	13	13–14	12	—	13	82–89
14	14	14	13	14	—	14	14	14	15	13–18	14–16	14	90–94
15	—	15	14–18	15	—	15–16	15	15	—	—	—	15	95–97
16	15	16	—	16–18	—	—	16–18	16	16	—	—	16	98
17	16–17	17	—	—	—	17	—	17	17–18	—	17	17–18	99
18	18	18	—	—	—	18	—	18	—	—	18	—	>99

Note: Age scaled scores were taken from Tables 6–89 to 6–92. RBANS = Repeatable Battery for the Assessment of Neuropsychological Status, Learn = Learning, Mem = Memory, Orient = Orientation, Pict Nam = Picture Naming, Sem Fluen = Semantic Fluency, Cod = Coding, Recog = Recognition.

Source: From Duff et al., 2003. Reprinted with the kind permission of Psychology Press.

Table 6–96 RBANS Age-Corrected Scaled Score Conversions to Age- and Education-Corrected Scaled Score for ≥16 Years of Education (N = 200)

Scaled Score	List Learn	Story Mem	Figure Copy	Line Orient	Pict Nam	Sem Fluen	Digit Span	Cod	List Recall	List Recog	Story Recall	Figure Recall	%ile Range
2	2	2	2	2	2–4	—	—	2	—	2–3	2–3	2	<1
3	3	3	—	3	—	2–4	2	3	2–4	4	4	—	1
4	—	—	3	—	—	5	3	4	5	—	—	3	2
5	4–6	4–6	4–6	4–6	5–6	—	4–6	5	—	5–6	—	4–5	3–5
6	—	7	7	7	7	6	—	6–7	6	7	6–7	6	6–10
7	7	8	8	8	8–9	7–8	7–8	8	7	8	8	7–8	11–18
8	8	9	9	9	—	—	9	9	8	9	9	—	19–28
9	9	—	10	—	10	9	—	—	9	10	—	9	29–40
10	10–11	10–11	11	10–12	11	10	10–11	10	10–11	—	10–11	10–11	41–59
11	12	12	—	—	12–18	11	12	11	—	11	12–13	—	60–71
12	13	13	12	13	—	12	13	12	12–13	12	—	12	72–81
13	14	14	13	—	—	13	—	13	14	13–18	14	13–14	82–89
14	—	15	14–18	14	—	14	14	14	15	—	—	15	90–94
15	15	16	—	15	—	15	15	15	—	—	15	—	95–97
16	16	17	—	16–18	—	16	16–18	16	16	—	16	16	98
17	17	18	—	—	—	17	—	17	17–18	—	17–18	17–18	99
18	18	—	—	—	—	18	—	18	—	—	—	—	>99

Note: Age scaled scores were taken from Tables 6–89 to 6–92. RBANS = Repeatable Battery for the Assessment of Neuropsychological Status, Learn = Learning, Mem = Memory, Orient = Orientation, Pict Nam = Picture Naming, Sem Fluen = Semantic Fluency, Cod = Coding, Recog = Recognition.

Source: From Duff et al., 2003. Reprinted with the kind permission of Psychology Press.

ages of 70 to 80. Because sample sizes tapered for participants over age 75, data are presented for individuals 75 to 94 (N = 24). Tables 6–100 to 6–102 provide raw score to scaled score conversions for the RBANS subtests, while Table 6–103 provides the age-corrected scaled score to index score conversions. It is important to bear in mind that scoring of the figure reflects the less stringent adherence to the manual's scoring criteria. Note, too, that there are restrictions in the range of scores for a number of the subtests.

Wilk et al. (2004) have recently provided normative data for a large sample (N = 575, ages 18–59 years) of patients with schizophrenia or schizoaffective disorder. Such data are of use when the clinician wishes to determine whether the pattern or severity of impairment is unusual relative to expectations based on the diagnosis. In this way, the clinician can determine whether more extensive investigation is warranted. The interested reader is referred to normative tables provided in their article.

RELIABILITY

Internal Consistency

Reliability for the individual subtests is not provided in the test manual. Split-half reliability coefficients of RBANS indices are reported to be in the .80s (Randolph, 1998). The average reliability for the Total Scale score is also high (.86–.94) in adults (Gontkovsky et al., 2004; Hobart et al., 1999; Randolph, 1998).

Standard Errors of Measurement (SEM)

The RBANS index scores have average SEMs that are relatively large, about five to six points across the entire age range. The difference between pairs of index scores required for statistical significance (.05 level) ranges from about 11 to 19 points. Discrepancies between indices of about 30 points or more would be considered rare.

Test-Retest Reliability and Assessment of Change

The stability of Form A RBANS index scores was evaluated in 40 older adults (age, M = 70.7 years) who were retested following an interval of about 39 weeks (Randolph, 1998). Reliability coefficients were high for the total scale (.88), but lower for the individual indices (Language, .55; Immediate Memory, .78). Mean retest scores were generally higher than initial scores (by about five points); however, on the Language Index, scores declined by about two points on retest.

In "typically aging" older adults, aged 65 and above, who were retested with Form A following a one-year interval, stability coefficients ranged from .58 (Language) to .83 (Total Score) for the index scores, and from .51 (Figure Copy) to .83 (Coding) for the subtests (Duff, Beglinger, et al., 2005). Practice effects were largely absent, with most scores slightly decreasing at retest.

Duff et al. (2004; Duff, Schoenberg, et al., 2005) have recently provided regression-based equations to assess change across time based on these older adults. The equations were

Table 6–97 RBANS Age-Corrected Scaled Score Conversions to Age-Corrected Index Scores

Index Score	IM	VC	Lang	Attn	DM	Total	%ile	Index Score	IM	VC	Lang	Attn	DM	Total	%ile
≤62	≤6	≤6	≤7	≤9	≤14	≤74	<1	100				20		124	50
65	7–9	7–10	8–10	10–11	15–21	75–78	1	101					42	125	53
70	10	11	11		22–23	79–85	2	102	21	21				126	55
71	11		12	12	24–25	86	3	103			20	21	43	127–128	58
72		12	13		26	87	3	104						129	61
73				13	27	88	4	105	22				44	130	63
74						89	4	106				22		131–132	66
75	12		14		28	90	5	107		22			45	133	68
76		13				91–92	5	108	23					134	70
77						93	6	109			21	23	46	135	73
78	13				29	94–95	7	110		23				136	75
79		14		14		96	8	111	24					137	77
80					30	97	9	112			22		47	138	79
81			15			98	10	113		24			48	139	81
82	14	15		15	31	99–100	12	114	25						82
83						101	13	115						140	84
84			16		32	102	14	116					49	141–142	86
85	15	16		16	33	103	16	117	26			25			87
86						104–105	18	118					50	143–144	88
87					34	106	19	119	27		23		51	145	90
88	16					107	21	120		25		26		146	91
89		17		17	35	108	23	121					52	147	92
90	17		17		36	109–110	25	122						148	93
91						111	27	123	28		24	27		149	94
92		18		18		112–113	30	124					53	150–151	95
93	18		18		37	114	32	126	29		25		54	152–154	96
94					38	115–116	34	128				28		155	97
95		19				117	37	130	30		26		55	156	98
96	19			19	39	118	39	132		26		29	56	157–158	98
97					40	119–120	42	134	31			30		159–161	99
98			19			121–122	45	137	32	27	27	31	57–58	162–164	99
99	20	20			41	123	47	≥138	≥33	≥28	≥28	≥32	≥59	≥165	>99

Note: IM = Immediate Memory; VC = Visuospatial/Constructional; Lang = Language; Attn = Attention; DM = Delayed Memory. To determine the Index (Standard) Scores, add up the age-corrected scaled scores of the subtests that comprise the Index (i.e., IM = List Learning + Story Memory; VC = Figure Copy + Line Orientation; Lang = Picture Naming + Semantic Fluency; Attn = Digit Span + Coding; DM = List Recall + List Recognition + Story Recall + Figure Recall), and refer to the appropriate column in the table above. To determine the Total Score, add up the age-corrected scaled scores of all the subtests of the RBANS, and refer to the appropriate column in the table above.

Source: From Duff et al., 2003. Reprinted with the kind permission of Psychology Press.

developed on a sample of 223 adults and cross-validated in a separate sample of 222 adults. All subtests were administered and scored as defined in the manual, with the exception of Figure Copy and Recall, which were scored with the revised scoring criteria of Duff et al. (2003). Prediction equations for each of the indices and the Total Scale score are shown in Table 6–104. Algorithms for the 12 subtests are shown in Table 6–105.

Not surprisingly, initial performance was the best predictor of follow-up performance, although demographic variables also added to the predictive value of the formulas. The authors caution that like most regression-based prediction equations, these are likely to provide the best estimates of time 2 performances for individuals who do not fall at the extremes of functioning at time 1 (e.g., <2nd percentile or >98th

percentile). That is, they are susceptible to regression to the mean effects and will likely over- or underestimate time 2 scores in those at the extremes. Similarly, use of these formulas outside the demographic and situational parameters (e.g., <64 or >90 years old, relatively brief or extended retest intervals) may increase error.

One alternative to reliable change algorithms is the use of base rate data for discrepancy scores across a clinically meaningful period of time. If a discrepancy between two scores (time 1 and time 2) exceeds a predetermined threshold (<10th percentile), this change in performance is interpreted to be clinically significant. Recently, Patton et al. (2005) provided base rate data of RBANS scores using a cognitively intact community-dwelling sample of older adults for one- and two-year retest intervals. Base rates of discrepancies were calculated

Table 6–98 RBANS Age- and Education-Corrected Scaled Score Conversions to Age- and Education-Corrected Index Scores

Index Score	IM	VC	Lang	Attn	DM	Total	%ile	Index Score	IM	VC	Lang	Attn	DM	Total	%ile
≤62	≤8	≤9	≤8	≤10	≤18	≤77	<1	100			24		44	132	50
65	9–10	10	9–11	11	20–21	78–84	1	101				21		133	53
70	11	11	12	12	22–23	85–89	2	102	21	22			45	134	55
71		12	13	13	24–25	90–91	3	103					46	135	58
72	12					92	3	104	22	23	25			136–137	61
73					26	93	4	105				22	47	138–139	63
74						94	4	106						140	66
75		13		14	27	95	5	107					48	141	68
76			14		28	96	5	108	23	24	26	23	49	142	70
77	13				29	97–98	6	109						143	73
78		14	15			99–101	7	110					50	144	75
79					30	102	8	111	24	25		24		145	77
80				15		103	9	112						146	79
81	14				31	104	10	113					51	147–148	81
82		15	16		32	105–107	12	114	25		27			149	82
83				16		108	13	115		26	28		52	150	84
84	15		17				14	116	26			25		151	86
85		16			33	109	16	117					53	152	87
86	16		18		34	110–111	18	118		27			54	153	88
87				17			19	119	27			26		154–155	90
88		17	19		35	112–113	21	120					55	156	91
89	17					114	23	121			29				92
90			20		36	115–116	25	122	28	28			56	157–158	93
91	18	18		18	37	117–118	27	123		29			57	159–160	94
92			21		38	119–120	30	124						161	95
93					39	121	32	126	29		30	28	58	162	96
94	19	19	22	19	40	122	34	128	30					163–165	97
95						123–124	37	130		30		29	59	166	98
96					41	125	39	132	31		31		60–61	167–168	98
97		20	23	20	42	126–127	42	134		31	32	30	62	169–170	99
98	20					128–129	45	137		32	33	31	63–64	171–174	99
99		21			43	130–131	47	≥138	≥32	≥33	≥34	≥32	≥65	≥175	>99

Note: IM = Immediate Memory; VC = Visuospatial/Constructional; Lang = Language; Attn = Attention; DM = Delayed Memory. To determine the Index (Standard) Scores, add up the age- and education-corrected scaled scores of the subtests that comprise the Index (i.e., IM = List Learning + Story Memory; VC = Figure Copy + Line Orientation; Lang = Picture Naming + Semantic Fluency; Attn = Digit Span + Coding; DM = List Recall + List Recognition + Story Recall + Figure Recall), and refer to the appropriate column in the table above. To determine the Total Score, add up the age- and education-corrected scaled scores of all the subtests of the RBANS, and refer to the appropriate column in the table above.

Source: From Duff et al., 2003. Reprinted with the kind permission of Psychology Press.

and organized into three groups (i.e., below average, average, and above average) with respect to their age- and education-corrected RBANS Total Scale score (see Table 6–98) in an attempt to reduce the influence of regression to the mean and practice effects that are associated with varying levels of cognitive ability. The below-average group was composed of participants who obtained age- and education-corrected total scale scores less than 90 at Time 1, the average group scored between 90 and 109 at Time 1; and the above-average groups scored 110 or above. These data are shown in Tables 6–106 to 6–108 with base rates drawn from three sources: OKLAHOMA age-corrected index scores, OKLAHOMA age- and educated-corrected index scores, and age-corrected index scores based on the original RBANS normative sample (Randolph, 1998).

Form A was used in at each assessment. The data show that relatively large differences across time are common in many cases. Note that discrepancy data for the two-year interval include interim testing at one year while one-year discrepancies from Time 3 minus Time 2 are predicated on the fact that testing occurred at Time 1. Therefore, these data should only be used when evaluating cases where similar serial testing occurred.

Alternate Forms

Randolph (1998) reported that a test-retest study, Form A—Form B, was performed using 100 participants (mean age not reported) who were tested twice following an interval of one to

Table 6–99 Adjustment for Education and Gender for RBANS Indexes

Index	Education Adjustment							Sex	
	≤8 Grade	Some HS	GED	HS	Some College	College Grad	Some Grad School	Male	Female
Immediate Memory	+8	+5	+3	0	−3	−5	−8	+1	−1
Visuospatial/ Construction	+8	+5	+3	0	−3	−5	−8	−3	+3
Language	+3	+2	+1	0	−1	−2	−3	+2	−2
Attention	+8	+5	+3	0	−3	−5	−8	0	0
Delayed Memory	+5	+4	+2	0	−2	−4	−5	+2/0	−2/0
Total	+8	+6	+3	0	−3	−6	−8	0	0

Compute index from RBANS Manual and add education or gender correction.

Source: Adapted from Gonkovsky et al., 2002 and Beatty et al., 2003a.

seven days using a counterbalanced design. Stability coefficients were high for the Total Scale (.82) but variable for the index scores (Language, .46; Attention, .80). Gold et al. (1999) gave the different forms of the RBANS to 53 patients with schizophrenia on two occasions with a mean retest interval of 12 weeks. The Total score ($r = .84$) and the Attention Index ($r = .91$) demonstrated excellent reliability. The other four indices had lower reliability (Language, .56; Immediate Memory, .73).

A follow-up study (Wilk et al., 2002) examined the test-retest stability of the RBANS in 181 patients with schizophrenia or schizoaffective disorder (aged 18–64) and 99 healthy subjects (aged 24–86) recruited as part of the RBANS stan-

dardization. Participants were administered one form of the RBANS on one occasion and another form at a later date, with intervals ranging from 1 to 134 days. Despite having a markedly longer interval between test occasions, patients tended to display slightly higher alternate form test stability than the healthy comparison group. Overall, the Total Scale demonstrated the highest capacity for stable measurement across testing sessions (schizophrenic patients ICC = .84, normal controls ICC = .77). The other four indices had lower reliability (normal controls: Language ICC = .36; Attention ICC = .76). About 75% of individuals had differences in scores within ± 10 points. A decline of greater than 10 points

Table 6–100 RBANS Raw Score to Age-Corrected Scaled Score Conversions for Midpoint Age = 70 (Age Range = 65–75; N = 45)

Scale Score	List Learn	Story Mem	Figure Copy	Line Orient	Pict Naming	Sem Fluency	Digit Span	Coding	List Recall	List Recog	Story Recall	Figure Recall	Percentile Range
2	—	—	—	—	—	—	—	—	—	—	—	—	<1
3	—	0–2	—	0–4	0–5	—	0–6	0–10	—	0–11	—	—	1
4	0–14	3–5	—	5	6	0–7	7	11–12	—	12	0–1	0–4	2
5	15	6–7	0–12	6	—	8	—	13–17	—	13–14	2	5	3–5
6	16–17	8–9	13	8	—	9–11	—	18	0	15	—	6	6–10
7	18	10	—	9	7	—	—	19–23	1	16	3	—	11–18
8	19–20	11	14–15	10–11	8	12–13	8–9	24	—	—	4	7–8	19–28
9	21–22	12–13	16–17	12–13	—	14	10	25–30	2	17	5–6	9	29–40
10	23	14–16	—	14–15	9	15	11	31–34	3	18	7–8	10–11	41–59
11	24–26	17	18	16	10	16–17	12	35–36	4	19	—	12–14	60–71
12	27–28	18	19	17	—	18	—	37–43	5	20	9	15	72–81
13	29–31	19	20	18	—	19–21	13	44–49	6	—	10	16–17	82–89
14	32–33	20–21	—	19	—	22	14–15	—	7	—	—	—	90–94
15	34	—	—	20	—	—	16	—	8	—	11	18	95–97
16	35	22	—	—	—	23	—	50	9–10	—	12	19–20	98
17	—	—	—	—	—	—	—	—	—	—	—	—	99
18	40	23–24	—	—	—	24–44	—	51–89	—	—	—	—	<99

Note: The OKLAHOMA normative sample consists of individuals who reside in the southern Midwest. Caution is advised in utilizing the current data for individuals who differ from the OKLAHOMA sample with respect to important demographic factors such as age, education, and cultural background. The sample size (N = 61) of the OKLAHOMA norms for African Americans should also be taken into consideration, as pertaining to its influence on clinical interpretation, when utilizing these data. RBANS = Repeatable Battery for the Assessment of Neuropsychological Status, Learn = Learning, Mem = Memory, Orient = Orientation, Pict Naming = Picture Naming, Recog = Recognition.

Source: From Patton et al., 2003. Reprinted with the kind permission of Psychology Press.

Table 6–101 RBANS Raw Score to Age-Corrected Scaled Score Conversions for Midpoint Age = 75 (Age Range = 70–80; N = 33)

Scale Score	List Learn	Story Mem	Figure Copy	Line Orient	Pict Naming	Sem Fluency	Digit Span	Coding	List Recall	List Recog	Story Recall	Figure Recall	Percentile Range
2	—	—	—	—	—	—	—	—	—	—	—	—	<1
3	—	—	—	—	—	—	0–6	0–5	—	0–11	—	—	1
4	0–14	0–6	0–12	0–4	0–5	0–7	7	6–10	—	12	0	0	2
5	15	7	13	5	6	8	—	11	—	13–14	1–2	1–3	3–5
6	16	8–9	14	6–7	7	9–10	—	13–14	0	15	—	4–5	6–10
7	17	10	15	8	—	11	—	15–17	1	—	3	6	11–18
8	18	11	16	9	8	12	8–9	18	—	16	4	—	19–28
9	19–20	—	—	10–12	9	13–14	10	19–22	2	—	5	7–9	29–40
10	21–22	12–13	17	13–14	—	15	11	23–31	—	17–18	6	10–11	41–59
11	23	14	18	15	10	16	12	34–32	3–4	—	7–8	12–13	60–71
12	24–26	15	19	16	—	17–18	—	33–35	5	19	9	14–15	72–81
13	27–29	16–17	20	17–18	—	19–20	13	36–39	—	20	10	16–17	82–89
14	30–32	—	—	19	—	21	—	40–45	6	—	11–12	—	90–94
15	33–34	18	—	—	—	22–25	14–15	46–47	7–8	—	—	18	95–97
16	—	19–20	—	20	—	26	16	48–89	9	—	—	19	98
17	35–39	21	—	—	—	27	—	—	10	—	—	20	99
18	40	22–24	—	—	—	29–44	—	—	—	—	—	—	<99

Note: RBANS = Repeatable Battery for the Assessment of Neuropsychological Status, Learn = Learning, Mem = Memory, Orient = Orientation, Pict Naming = Picture Naming, Recog = Recognition.

Source: Patton et al., 2003. Reprinted with the kind permission of Psychology Press.

occurred in fewer than 10% of the healthy participants. About 16% of the participants showed an increase of greater than 10 points on retest. Confidence limits for the Total Scale change in scores for the healthy comparison group are shown in Table 6–109. Overall, the confidence intervals tend to be large, requiring about a 15-point change in either direction to establish even a 90% confidence interval.

Interrater Reliability

Interscorer agreement for the Figure Copy subtest was determined by using three trained scorers who each blindly scored 20 Copy/Recall tests. The intraclass correlation was .85, indicating that relatively consistent results were obtained across different scorers (Randolph, 1998).

Table 6–102 RBANS Raw Score to Age-Corrected Scaled Score Conversions for Age Range = 75–94 (N = 24)

Scale Score	List Learn	Story Mem	Figure Copy	Line Orient	Pict Naming	Sem Fluency	Digit Span	Coding	List Recall	List Recog	Story Recall	Figure Recall	Percentile Range
2	—	—	—	—	—	—	—	—	—	—	—	—	< 1
3	—	—	—	—	—	—	—	—	—	—	—	—	1
4	0–9	0–4	0–11	0–4	0–4	0–3	0–5	0–5	—	—	—	—	2
5	10–15	5–6	12	5	5	4–8	6	6–7	—	—	—	—	3–5
6	16	7–8	—	6	6	9	7	8	—	0–12	—	—	6–10
7	17	9	13	7	7	10–11	8	9–10	0	13–14	0–1	0–3	11–18
8	18	10	14	8	—	12	9	11–14	—	15	2–3	4–5	19–28
9	—	11	15	9–10	8	13	10	15–18	1	16–17	4	6	29–40
10	19–20	12	16–17	11–14	9	14–18	11	19–25	2	—	5	7–9	41–59
11	21	13–14	18	15	10	19	12	26–30	—	18	6	10–11	60–71
12	22	15	19	16	—	20	—	31	—	—	—	—	72–81
13	23	16	20	17	—	21–23	13	32–36	—	—	7–8	12–15	82–89
14	24–26	17	—	18	—	24–25	—	—	3	19	9–10	16	90–94
15	27–33	18–24	—	19	—	26	14	37	5	20	—	17	95–97
16	34–40	—	—	20	—	27–29	15–16	38–89	6–10	—	—	18–20	98
17	—	—	—	—	—	30–44	—	—	—	—	—	—	99
18	—	—	—	—	—	—	—	—	—	—	—	—	< 99

Note: RBANS = Repeatable Battery for the Assessment of Neuropsychological Status, Learn = Learning, Mem = Memory, Orient = Orientation, Pict Naming = Picture Naming, Recog = Recognition.

Source: Patton et al., 2003. Reprinted with the kind permission of Psychology Press.

Table 6–103 RBANS Age-Corrected Scaled Score to Age-Corrected Index Score Conversions

Index Score	IM	VC	Lang	Attn	DM	Total	%ile
≤62	≤6	≤6	≤8	≤10	≤20	≤80	≤1
65	7	7–10	9	11	21	81	1
70	8	11	10	12	22–24	82	2
71	9		11	13	25	83	3
72					26	84	3
73	10	12				86	4
74					27	87	4
75			12			88–89	5
76						90–93	5
77		13		14	28	94	6
78			13		29	95	7
79	11		14		30	96	8
80	12	14			31	97	9
81	13			15	32	98–100	10
82	14	15				101	12
83	15		15	16		102	13
84						103–104	14
85	16	16	16	17	33	105	16
86						106	18
87	17				34	107	19
88			17			108–109	21
89					35	110	23
90		17			36		25
91	18		18		37	111	27
92				18	38	112	30
93		18				113–114	32
94						115–116	34
95				19			37
96		19	19			117–118	39
97	19				39	119–121	42
98					40	122–123	45
99	20				41	124	47
100		20		20	42	125–126	50
101	21	21	20			127	53
102						128–129	55
103	22	22		21	43	130	58
104			21			131–132	61
105	23				44	133	63
106						134	66
107					45	135	68
108			22		46	136	70
109				22	47	137	73
110		23	23			138	75
111					48	139–140	77
112				23		141–142	79
113				24		143	81
114	24	24	24			144	82
115					49		84
116	25					145	86
117		25		25			87
118	26		25		50	146	88
119				26			90
120	27						91
121	28	26	26	27	51	147–149	92
122	29			28	52	150	93
123		27		29	53	151	94
124	30		27		54	152–153	95
126				30	55	154–155	96
128		28	28			156–157	97
130	31				56	158	98
132						159–163	98
134	32				57	164–167	99
137						168–169	99
≤138	≤33	≤29	≤29	≤31	≤58	≤170	≤99

Note: To determine the Index (Standard) scores, add up the age-corrected scaled scores of the subtests that comprise the Index (i.e., IM = List Learning + Story Memory; VC = Figure Copy + Line Orientation; Lang = Picture Naming + Semantic Fluency; Attn = Digit Span + Coding; DM = List Recall + List Recognition + Story Recall + Figure Recall), and refer to the appropriate column in the table above. To determine the Total score, add up the age-corrected scaled scores of all the subtests of the RBANS, and refer to the appropriate column in the table above. IM = Immediate Memory; VC = Visuospatial/Constructional; Lang = Language; Attn = Attention; DM = Delayed Memory.

Source: Patton et al., 2003. Reprinted with the kind permission of Psychology Press.

VALIDITY

Correlations With Other Measures

RBANS scores are strongly correlated with more extensive assessments. Thus, Randolph (1998) reported that in a mixed clinical sample (most with dementia), the RBANS total scale score correlated fairly strongly (.78) with the FSIQ of a WAIS-R short form (Arithmetic, Similarities, Picture Completion, Digit Symbol). Similarly, Gold et al. (1999) found that in patients with schizophrenia, the Total score on the RBANS demonstrated moderately high correlations with WAIS-III FSIQ (.77) and WMS-III indices (.67–.69). Hobart et al. (1999) also found that RBANS Total score correlated highly (.79) with a composite *z* score derived from 22 standard measures of IQ, memory,

language, motor, attention, and executive function in a diagnostically heterogeneous sample drawn from a public mental health system. The RBANS index scores correlated most highly with a general ability factor and had limited correlations with measures of motor performance, vigilance, and executive function. Of note, mean Wechsler FSIQ or memory index scores tend to be substantially above the mean RBANS Total Scale index score, suggesting that the RBANS may be more sensitive to impairment than the Wechsler tests.

Unfortunately, the RBANS Manual does not provide factor-analytic data supporting the subscale structure. It also does not report how well the subtests comprising specific indices intercorrelate. Some evidence of construct validity is provided by the pattern of intercorrelations for the five content indices

Table 6–104 Algorithms to Predict Time 2 RBANS Index Scores in Older Adults Who Are Given Form A

Index	R^2	SE_{est}^a	C^b	B^c	B^d	B^e	B^f
Immediate Memory	.56	11.08	53.76	.63	−.37	2.58	
Visuospatial/ Construction	.43	12.50	35.89	.57		2.81	
Language	.39	8.79	35.28	.63			
Attention	.60	9.65	37.04	.75	−.30		.03
Delayed Memory	.51	11.46	30.60	.71			
Total Score	.72	7.81	37.65	.75	−.23	1.47	

To calculate the Predicted Time 2 score based on the formulas above, use the age-corrected scaled score from the RBANS Manual for the Time 1 score; use age in years; use the education coding listed below; and use the number of days for the retest interval.

Education Coding:
11 years or less = 1
12 years = 2
13–15 years = 3
16 years or more = 4

Change indices can be calculated as follows:
Observed Time 2 score–Predicted Time 2 score = Predicted Difference score
Predicted Difference score/Standard error of the estimate = z score of difference
If z score of difference >±1.64, then significant change at 90% confidence.

[a]Standard error of the estimate. [b]Constant. [c]Unstandardized beta weight for Time 1 Index score. [d]Unstandardized beta weight for age. [e]Unstandardized beta weight for education. [f]Unstandardized beta weight for retest interval.

Source: From Duff et al., 2004. Based on older adults, aged 65+, retested following about one year. Reprinted with the permission of Cambridge University Press.

(i.e., Immediate Memory, Visuospatial/Constructional, Language, Attention, and Delayed Memory). Randolph (1998) reported that in the standardization sample, the highest correlation is between the Immediate and Delayed Memory Indices (.63), while the correlations between other indices are lower and range from .28 to .41, suggesting that the different index scores are measuring relatively distinct cognitive constructs. Similar findings have been reported by Gontkovsky et al. (2004) in a sample of normal geriatric patients with no documented or reported history of central nervous system dysfunction. Correlations between individual RBANS indices with corresponding functions assessed on tests such as the WAIS-R, WMS-R, Rey Complex Figure, Judgment of Line Orientation, Boston Naming Test, WRAT-3, and COWAT tended to show modest to moderately high (.21–.82) correlations (Randolph, 1998).

Gold et al. (1999) provided evidence of convergent validity for some of the RBANS scales in a sample of patients with schizophrenia. Three of the five indices (Immediate Memory, Attention, Delayed Memory) correlated most closely with their assigned criterion variables (Immediate Memory with WMS-III Immediate and Delayed Memory indices, Attention with WAIS-III Working Memory Index, Delayed Memory with WMS Delayed Memory Index). However, the Language Index correlated as highly with the WAIS-III Verbal Comprehension Index as with the WAIS-III Processing Speed and

Table 6–105 Algorithms to Predict Time 2 RBANS Subtests in Older Adults Who Were Given Form A

Subtest	R^2	SE_{est}^a	C^b	B^c	Other Variables in Equation[d]
List Learning	.52	3.74	19.34	.55	(ed × 1.18) − (age × .16)
Story Memory	.43	3.48	18.25	.61	− (age × .17)
Figure Copy	.25	1.65	8.50	.53	
Line Orientation	.46	2.28	11.23	.45	(gender × .69) − (age × .07) + (ed × .56) + (race × 1.73)
Picture Naming	.42	0.59	3.45	.62	(gender × .21)
Semantic Fluency	.35	3.60	6.48	.53	(ed × .59)
Digit Span	.39	1.90	8.25	.51	−(age × .07) + (interval × .01)
Coding	.75	5.45	18.86	.86	−(age × 19)
List Recall	.47	1.96	6.78	.64	−(age × .07)
List Recognition	.33	1.22	11.88	.51	−(age × .04)
Story Recall	.45	2.10	2.03	.63	(ed × .34)
Figure Recall	.39	3.16	10.31	.57	−(age × .08) + (ed × .59)

[a]Standard error of the estimate. [b]Constant. [c]Unstandardized beta weight for the same Time 1 subtest. [d]Unstandardized beta weights for other variables in the equation. To calculate the Predicted Time 2 score, use the subtest raw scores; use age in years; use the education, gender, and race codings listed below; use the number of days for the retest interval. Use the following formula: (Constant value for the subtest) + (Unstandardized beta weight for the subtest at Time 1 × raw score for the subtest at Time 1) + (Other variables in equation as noted in the table).

Education Coding:	Gender Coding:	Race Coding:
11 years or less = 1	Female = 0	Non-white/Non-Caucasian = 0
12 years = 2	Male = 1	White/Caucasian = 1
13–15 years = 3		
16 years or more = 4		

Change indices can be calculated as follows:
Observed Time 2 score − Predicted Time 2 score = Predicted Difference score
Predicted Difference score/Standard error of the estimate = z score of difference
If z of difference > ±1.64, then significant change at 90% confidence. A copy of the computer program used to calculate the predicted scores, differences scores, and the test of the differences' significance can be obtained from K. Duff (Kevin-duff@ uiowa.edu).

Source: Duff et al., 2005. Based on older adults, aged 65+, retested following about one year. Reprinted with permission from Elsevier.

Table 6–106 Frequencies (Cumulative Percentages) of Discrepancies Between RBANS (Form A) Age- and Age- and Education-Corrected Index Scores at one- and two- year Intervals: Age- and Education-Corrected Total Scale Score at Time 1 <90 (*N* = 50)

	Cumulative Percentages										
	Decline in Scores Over Time						Increase in Scores Over Time				
	≤1%	2%	5%	10%	20%	50%	20%	10%	5%	2%	≤1%
Total Scale											
Age-Corrected (OKLAHOMA)[a]											
One-year Interval (T2–T1)	−17.0	−17.0	−14.4	−7.7	−1.8	5.0	9.0	12.8	15.9	18.0	18.0
Two-year Interval (T3–T1)	−22.0	−21.9	−17.9	−10.9	−4.6	4.5	12.0	16.0	18.4	22.0	22.0
One-year Interval (T3–T2)	−10.0	−10.0	−10.0	−9.0	−6.8	0.0	6.0	8.0	9.9	13.9	14.0
Age- and Education-Corrected[a]											
One-year Interval (T2-T1)	−16.0	−15.9	−12.0	−6.7	−2.8	3.0	10.0	12.8	16.9	20.0	20.0
Two-year Interval (T3–T1)	−21.0	−20.9	−16.4	−10.9	−4.8	3.5	10.0	14.8	19.3	23.0	23.0
One-year Interval (T3–T2)	−12.0	−12.0	−9.9	−8.0	−6.8	0.0	4.0	8.0	9.5	16.9	17.0
Age-Corrected (Randolph, 1998)[b]											
One-year Interval (T2–T1)	−19.0	−18.9	−12.8	−7.0	−2.8	3.5	11.6	14.9	17.9	20.0	20.0
Two-year Interval (T3–T1)	−29.0	−28.8	−19.9	−7.9	−4.0	4.0	11.8	17.6	23.9	26.0	26.0
One-year Interval (T3–T2)	−15.0	−15.0	−12.9	−11.0	−9.0	−1.0	6.8	10.9	13.9	20.9	21.0
Immediate Memory Index											
Age-Corrected (OKLAHOMA)[a]											
One-year Interval (T2–T1)	−17.0	−17.0	−17.0	−11.6	−4.8	4.0	11.0	16.7	18.9	26.9	27.0
Two-year Interval (T3–T1)	−30.0	−29.7	−15.5	−12.6	−7.0	3.5	13.6	17.9	23.5	26.9	27.0
One-year Interval (T3–T2)	−15.0	−15.0	−13.0	−10.8	−8.0	0.0	7.6	10.8	15.4	18.0	18.0
Age- and Education-Corrected[a]											
One-year Interval (T2–T1)	−18.0	−18.0	−17.5	−8.9	−4.8	3.5	12.0	17.0	21.3	29.9	30.0
Two-year Interval (T3–T1)	−27.0	−26.8	−15.5	−13.9	−7.8	4.5	14.0	17.9	21.9	29.9	30.0
One-year Interval (T3–T2)	−17.0	−17.0	−13.4	−11.9	−8.0	0.0	7.8	12.8	15.4	19.9	20.0
Age-Corrected (Randolph, 1998)[b]											
One-year Interval (T2–T1)	−28.0	−28.0	−25.9	−10.8	−3.8	5.0	15.4	21.0	29.4	39.8	40.0
Two-year Interval (T3–T1)	−37.0	−36.8	−22.3	−13.7	−7.4	5.5	18.8	22.9	28.2	39.8	40.0
One-year Interval (T3–T2)	−29.0	−28.9	−17.0	−12.0	−9.0	0.0	9.8	17.5	21.8	25.0	25.0
Visuospatial/Constructional Index											
Age-Corrected (OKLAHOMA)[a]											
One-year Interval (T2–T1)	−34.0	−33.8	−20.9	−16.9	−7.0	1.5	10.0	16.7	29.1	36.9	37.0
Two-year Interval (T3–T1)	−35.0	−34.9	−28.9	−19.8	−15.0	0.0	10.0	18.9	21.8	49.5	50.0
One-year Interval (T3–T2)	−33.0	−32.8	−21.3	−16.8	−14.8	−4.0	7.8	13.9	22.3	32.8	33.0
Age- and Education-Corrected[a]											
One-year Interval (T2–T1)	−29.0	−28.9	−21.8	−12.7	−5.8	0.0	9.8	18.7	24.0	26.9	27.0
Two-year Interval (T3–T1)	−26.0	−26.0	−23.5	−18.8	−13.8	0.0	12.4	16.9	20.9	39.6	40.0
One-year Interval (T3–T2)	−26.0	−25.9	−18.8	−17.0	−13.8	−6.0	8.0	11.9	19.9	23.9	24.0
Age-Corrected (Randolph, 1998)[b]											
One-year Interval (T2-T1)	−40.0	−39.8	−26.2	−13.0	−9.0	3.0	12.0	21.8	34.5	39.9	40.0
Two-year Interval (T3–T1)	−34.0	−34.0	−31.5	−26.5	−18.8	0.0	15.8	21.0	28.4	52.5	53.0
One-year Interval (T3–T2)	−31.0	−31.0	−28.8	−22.0	−18.0	−6.0	10.2	16.0	21.8	30.9	31.0
Language Index											
Age-Corrected (OKLAHOMA)[a]											
One-year Interval (T2–T1)	−31.0	−30.9	−23.1	−16.9	−9.0	−0.5	9.8	24.3	32.8	43.8	44.0
Two-year Interval (T3–T1)	−28.0	−27.8	−17.4	−11.8	−9.0	0.0	12.6	20.8	29.3	45.8	46.0
One-year Interval (T3–T2)	−25.0	−24.9	−19.9	−13.9	−9.8	3.0	11.8	15.9	21.5	32.8	33.0
Age- and Education-Corrected[a]											
One-year Interval (T2–T1)	−19.0	−18.9	−14.4	−8.0	−6.0	0.0	6.0	11.8	17.8	22.9	23.0
Two-year Interval (T3–T1)	−14.0	−13.9	−11.0	−8.0	−4.0	0.0	7.8	12.0	18.3	30.8	31.0
One-year Interval (T3–T2)	−11.0	−11.0	−10.0	−6.0	−4.0	0.0	6.0	12.7	15.9	20.9	21.0

(continued)

Table 6–106 Frequencies (Cumulative Percentages) of Discrepancies Between RBANS (Form A) Age- and Age- and Education-Corrected Index Scores at one- and two- year Intervals: Age- and Education-Corrected Total Scale Score at Time 1 <90 (*N* = 50) (*continued*)

	Cumulative Percentages										
	Decline in Scores Over Time						Increase in Scores Over Time				
	≤1%	2%	5%	10%	20%	50%	20%	10%	5%	2%	≤1%
Age-Corrected (Randolph, 1998)[b]											
One-year Interval (T2–T1)	−32.0	−31.7	−16.3	−10.7	−6.0	0.0	8.6	14.9	27.8	31.0	31.0
Two-year Interval (T3–T1)	−28.0	−27.7	−13.5	−10.8	−8.0	0.0	6.8	16.8	21.4	31.8	32.0
One-year Interval (T3–T2)	−28.0	−27.8	−16.7	−8.9	−7.0	0.0	6.8	11.9	20.7	27.9	28.0
Attention Index											
Age-Corrected (OKLAHOMA)[a]											
One-year Interval (T2–T1)	−14.0	−13.9	−10.5	−6.9	−3.8	3.0	8.0	14.8	17.5	18.0	18.0
Two-year Interval (T3-T1)	−21.0	−21.0	−18.3	−11.0	−5.6	3.0	10.8	15.0	21.0	24.9	25.0
One-year Interval (T3–T2)	−20.0	−20.0	−17.5	−15.6	−7.0	0.0	7.0	9.8	13.5	16.9	17.0
Age- and Education-Corrected[a]											
One-year Interval (T2–T1)	−14.0	−14.0	−11.9	−9.9	−4.0	3.0	7.8	14.0	14.5	20.9	21.0
Two-year Interval (T3–T1)	−24.0	−23.9	−17.2	−12.8	−6.6	3.0	13.4	17.0	22.0	24.0	24.0
One-year Interval (T3–T2)	−18.0	−18.0	−17.5	−10.9	−7.0	0.0	8.0	11.0	14.0	16.9	17.0
Age-Corrected (Randolph, 1998)[b]											
One-year Interval (T2–T1)	−19.0	−18.9	−10.4	−6.0	−6.0	3.0	12.0	15.0	18.0	21.9	22.0
Two-year Interval (T3–T1)	−22.0	−22.0	−18.3	−13.7	−3.8	3.0	14.4	18.0	21.5	24.0	24.0
One-year Interval (T3–T2)	−22.0	−22.0	−18.8	−11.9	−8.4	0.0	6.0	11.8	13.4	17.9	18.0
Delayed Memory Index											
Age-Corrected (OKLAHOMA)[a]											
One-year Interval (T2–T1)	−19.0	−18.8	−9.5	−6.0	−4.8	4.0	11.8	16.9	24.5	32.9	33.0
Two-year Interval (T3–T1)	−19.0	−19.0	−15.9	−9.9	−3.6	7.0	13.8	16.0	26.3	33.9	34.0
One-year Interval (T3–T2)	−14.0	−14.0	−13.0	−8.9	−4.8	0.5	6.8	9.8	12.5	13.0	13.0
Age- and Education-Corrected[a]											
One-year Interval (T2–T1)	−62.0	−61.0	−9.5	−6.0	−4.0	3.5	8.8	13.9	20.3	28.9	29.0
Two-year Interval (T3–T1)	−19.0	−19.0	−15.4	−9.0	−2.8	4.5	11.8	14.0	18.4	28.8	29.0
One-year Interval (T3–T2)	−13.0	−13.0	−11.5	−6.9	−4.0	0.5	6.0	9.0	12.4	42.4	43.0
Age-Corrected (Randolph, 1998)[b]											
One-year Interval (T2–T1)	−38.0	−37.7	−20.5	−16.0	−8.8	3.5	13.8	23.3	25.9	33.9	34.0
Two-year Interval (T3–T1)	−38.0	−37.8	−22.5	−16.9	−10.6	3.5	17.8	23.9	26.0	37.8	38.0
One-year Interval (T3–T2)	−28.0	−28.0	−23.7	−18.1	−5.8	0.0	14.4	17.0	19.0	24.9	25.0

Note: T1 = testing at year 1 score; T2 = testing at year 2 score; T3 = testing at year 3 score. In determining which table to use, calculate the T1 age- and education-corrected Total scale score based on Duff et al. (2003) normative data. For Scores <90 use Table 6–106; for scores from 90–109, use Table 6–107; and for scores ≥110, use Table 6–108.
[a]Age-corrected Index discrepancy scores designated "(OKLAHOMA)" and age- and education-corrected Index discrepancy scores are based on the OKLAHOMA normative studies (Duff et al., 2003).
[b]Age-corrected Index discrepancy scores designated "(Randolph, 1998)" are based on the original RBANS normative data.

Source: Patton et al., 2005. Reprinted with the kind permission of Psychology Press.

WMS-III Immediate and General Memory Indices. Similarly, the Visuospatial/Constructional Index correlated at similar levels with the WAIS-III Verbal Comprehension, Perceptual Organization, and Working Memory Index scores, raising concerns about the meaning of the Language and Visuospatial/Constructional Indices.

By contrast, Larson et al. (2005) examined relations between the RBANS and a variety of other measures (e.g., TMT, line cancellation, EXIT, BDAE repetition and commands, WAIS-R Vocabulary, Raven's CPM, Benton Faces, Rivermead BMT, and CES-D 10) in stroke patients and reported that convergent and discriminant validity were adequate for most RBANS indices, with the exception of the Attention Index. They also noted that all RBANS indices correlated moderately with measures of language function, reflecting the heavy reliance of verbal response in the RBANS and raising questions about its utility in aphasic patients.

Clinical Studies

The RBANS is sensitive to a number of disorders, including concussion (Killam et al., 2005; Moser & Schaatz, 2002) and

Table 6–107 Frequencies (Cumulative Percentages) of Discrepancies Between RBANS (Form A) Age- and Age- and Education-Corrected Index Scores at one- and two-year Intervals: Age- and Education-Corrected Total Scale Score at Time 1 = 90–109 (N = 172)

	Cumulative Percentages										
	Decline in Scores Over Time						Increase in Scores Over Time				
	≤1%	2%	5%	10%	20%	50%	20%	10%	5%	2%	≤1%
Total Scale											
Age-Corrected (OKLAHOMA)[a]											
One-year Interval (T2-T1)	−21.5	−18.2	−12.0	−9.0	−6.0	0.0	7.0	10.0	12.0	16.1	18.1
Two-year Interval (T3-T1)	−21.0	−16.5	−14.0	−8.7	−5.0	0.5	8.0	12.7	18.0	22.5	25.9
One-year Interval (T3-T2)	−20.3	−15.5	−10.4	−8.0	−5.0	1.0	8.0	12.0	16.0	20.5	24.0
Age- and Education-Corrected[a]											
One-year Interval (T2-T1)	−19.6	−14.5	−10.0	−8.0	−6.0	0.0	6.0	9.0	11.0	13.5	16.6
Two-year Interval (T3-T1)	−17.0	−15.5	−12.0	−8.0	−5.0	1.0	7.4	12.0	15.4	19.5	24.5
One-year Interval (T3-T2)	−18.1	−16.5	−10.4	−8.0	−4.0	0.5	7.0	11.0	15.0	19.1	22.8
Age-Corrected (Randolph, 1998)[b]											
One-year Interval (T2-T1)	−20.3	−16.5	−14.0	−12.0	−8.0	0.0	8.4	12.7	16.0	20.0	21.4
Two-year Interval (T3-T1)	−17.5	−16.0	−13.0	−11.0	−5.4	1.0	9.4	13.7	21.0	27.5	28.3
One-year Interval (T3-T2)	−24.6	−17.0	−12.0	−8.0	−5.0	1.0	8.0	13.0	16.0	19.5	21.3
Immediate Memory Index											
Age-Corrected (OKLAHOMA)[a]											
One-year Interval (T2-T1)	−29.3	−27.0	−19.4	−15.0	−9.8	0.0	6.0	11.7	15.0	20.5	21.0
Two-year Interval (T3-T1)	−33.3	−26.5	−18.0	−13.4	−9.0	0.0	11.4	18.0	22.1	27.0	33.0
One-year Interval (T3-T2)	−21.5	−19.6	−12.0	−11.0	−6.0	3.0	11.4	15.0	19.4	24.0	30.9
Age- and Education-Corrected[a]											
One-year Interval (T2-T1)	−28.0	−28.0	−20.0	−17.0	−11.0	0.0	8.0	12.0	14.4	19.1	20.3
Two-year Interval (T3-T1)	−30.2	−27.5	−18.7	−14.0	−9.0	0.0	13.0	18.0	25.0	29.1	35.9
One-year Interval (T3-T2)	−22.8	−21.0	−12.0	−11.0	−5.4	4.0	12.0	16.0	20.0	26.1	33.5
Age-Corrected (Randolph, 1998)[b]											
One-year Interval (T2-T1)	−40.4	−32.3	−25.0	−18.7	−13.0	0.0	9.0	16.7	21.4	25.5	27.0
Two-year Interval (T3-T1)	−41.3	−34.1	−22.7	−15.7	−9.0	3.0	15.0	20.0	27.0	34.6	40.6
One-year Interval (T3-T2)	−25.5	−22.0	−17.0	−12.0	−6.4	6.0	14.0	19.7	22.4	29.5	37.1
Visuospatial/Constructional Index											
Age-Corrected (OKLAHOMA)[a]											
One-year Interval (T2-T1)	−34.1	−28.2	−23.7	−18.0	−11.0	0.0	12.0	18.0	22.0	29.6	33.5
Two-year Interval (T3-T1)	−43.0	−35.2	−22.7	−19.0	−13.0	0.0	8.0	13.0	21.0	25.0	36.8
One-year Interval (T3-T2)	−37.3	−32.7	−25.0	−19.0	−10.4	0.0	7.0	12.0	20.1	27.7	30.0
Age- and Education-Corrected[a]											
One-year Interval (T2-T1)	−27.1	−25.1	−16.4	−12.0	−8.4	0.0	7.4	13.7	16.4	22.6	27.8
Two-year Interval (T3-T1)	−33.0	−25.6	−18.0	−15.7	−10.4	0.0	6.0	11.0	14.4	20.5	26.4
One-year Interval (T3-T2)	−31.2	−26.5	−20.4	−14.0	−9.0	0.0	6.0	11.0	14.4	18.0	18.8
Age-Corrected (Randolph, 1998)[b]											
One-year Interval (T2-T1)	−33.4	−28.2	−21.4	−18.4	−12.0	0.0	14.4	20.0	24.0	31.7	39.2
Two-year Interval (T3-T1)	−47.0	−31.0	−24.4	−19.0	−14.4	0.0	10.0	18.0	22.0	29.0	36.9
One-year Interval (T3-T2)	−42.2	−33.1	−26.7	−22.4	−13.0	0.0	8.0	14.7	19.0	25.1	29.5
Language Index											
Age-Corrected (OKLAHOMA)[a]											
One-year Interval (T2-T1)	−31.5	−30.0	−22.4	−16.7	−11.0	0.0	9.4	13.0	16.7	24.7	31.7
Two-year Interval (T3-T1)	−35.5	−29.5	−25.0	−14.0	−10.0	0.0	10.0	14.0	17.7	29.5	36.1
One-year Interval (T3-T2)	−34.0	−29.6	−20.4	−14.0	−10.4	0.0	10.0	16.7	21.0	27.5	28.3
Age- and Education-Corrected[a]											
One-year Interval (T2-T1)	−22.0	−18.5	−13.4	−9.7	−6.0	0.0	4.0	6.0	11.4	15.1	16.5
Two-year Interval (T3-T1)	−18.4	−14.0	−12.0	−8.7	−6.0	0.0	4.0	7.0	14.0	20.5	24.5
One-year Interval (T3-T2)	−20.8	−18.5	−12.0	−8.0	−4.4	0.0	6.0	11.0	14.0	20.0	22.3

(continued)

Table 6–107 Frequencies (Cumulative Percentages) of Discrepancies Between RBANS (Form A) Age- and Age- and Education-Corrected Index Scores at one- and two-year Intervals: Age- and Education-Corrected Total Scale Score at Time 1 = 90–109 (N = 172) (continued)

	Cumulative Percentages										
	Decline in Scores Over Time						Increase in Scores Over Time				
	≤1%	2%	5%	10%	20%	50%	20%	10%	5%	2%	≤1%
Age-Corrected (Randolph, 1998)[b]											
One-year Interval (T2-T1)	−24.0	−21.0	−14.4	−11.0	−7.0	0.0	7.0	9.0	16.0	20.5	25.9
Two-year Interval (T3-T1)	−25.3	−22.6	−14.7	−9.7	−6.0	0.0	8.0	12.0	18.0	24.2	29.5
One-year Interval (T3-T2)	−36.2	−23.2	−14.0	−10.4	−7.0	0.0	7.0	12.0	16.0	21.0	24.6
Attention Index											
Age-Corrected (OKLAHOMA)[a]											
One-year Interval (T2-T1)	−23.4	−20.5	−14.7	−11.0	−7.0	0.0	7.0	11.0	14.0	20.5	22.8
Two-year Interval (T3-T1)	−19.3	−16.1	−14.0	−13.0	−9.0	0.0	7.0	11.0	17.0	20.1	24.0
One-year Interval (T3-T2)	−21.0	−16.6	−14.0	−10.0	−6.4	0.0	9.0	14.0	17.0	23.2	26.3
Age- and Education-Corrected[a]											
One-year Interval (T2-T1)	−25.8	−23.6	−15.4	−11.7	−8.0	0.0	7.4	11.0	14.0	21.0	22.5
Two-year Interval (T3-T1)	−18.5	−17.5	−14.4	−14.0	−10.0	0.0	8.0	13.1	18.0	20.5	25.8
One-year Interval (T3-T2)	−21.6	−17.5	−14.0	−11.0	−7.0	0.0	10.0	14.0	18.4	25.0	28.8
Age-Corrected (Randolph, 1998)[b]											
One-year Interval (T2-T1)	−18.3	−15.0	−15.0	−13.0	−9.0	0.0	9.0	15.0	21.0	23.1	27.0
Two-year Interval (T3-T1)	−21.8	−18.0	−15.0	−12.0	−9.0	3.0	10.0	15.0	19.0	24.5	28.1
One-year Interval (T3-T2)	−21.8	−18.5	−15.0	−12.0	−6.0	0.0	9.0	14.4	19.0	22.5	25.5
Delayed Memory Index											
Age-Corrected (OKLAHOMA)[a]											
One-year Interval (T2-T1)	−25.0	−19.0	−16.4	−11.0	−6.0	1.0	10.0	13.7	17.0	23.0	25.5
Two-year Interval (T3-T1)	−20.3	−19.0	−14.4	−9.7	−4.0	4.0	12.0	15.0	18.7	23.0	26.2
One-year Interval (T3-T2)	−20.8	−17.5	−15.4	−11.0	−5.0	2.0	10.4	14.0	17.4	22.5	25.5
Age- and Education-Corrected[a]											
One-year Interval (T2-T1)	−20.5	−16.1	−14.4	−10.0	−6.0	1.0	8.0	11.0	14.0	19.1	20.3
Two-year Interval (T3-T1)	−19.4	−15.5	−11.7	−8.0	−4.0	3.0	10.0	13.0	16.0	20.7	24.1
One-year Interval (T3-T2)	−19.4	−14.5	−12.0	−9.0	−5.0	1.5	9.0	13.0	16.0	20.5	24.1
Age-Corrected (Randolph, 1998)[b]											
One-year Interval (T2-T1)	−29.0	−26.5	−21.4	−16.0	−9.0	2.5	10.0	18.1	21.0	23.5	28.5
Two-year Interval (T3-T1)	−26.3	−22.2	−19.0	−11.7	−4.0	3.5	13.0	20.0	24.0	29.0	32.8
One-year Interval (T3-T2)	−29.8	−24.6	−16.0	−11.4	−6.4	2.5	13.0	17.0	22.4	26.5	28.8

Note: T1 = testing at year 1 score; T2 = testing at year 2 score; T3 = testing at year 3 score. In determining which table to use, calculate the T1 age- and education-corrected Total scale score based on Duff et al. (2003) normative data. For scores <90 use Table 6–106; for scores from 90–109, use Table 6–107; and for scores ≥110, use Table 6–108.

[a]Age-corrected Index discrepancy scores designated "(OKLAHOMA)" and age- and education-corrected Index discrepancy scores are based on the OKLAHOMA normative studies (Duff et al., 2003).

[b]Age-corrected Index discrepancy scores designated "(Randolph, 1998)" are based on the original RBANS normative data.

Source: Patton et al., 2005. Reprinted with the kind permission of Psychology Press.

dementia, and is useful in differentiating among dementing disorders (Beatty, Ryder, et al., 2003; Randolph, 1998). For example, Randolph et al. (1998) reported that patients with probable AD performed most poorly on Language and Delayed Memory subsections, while patients with Huntington's disease (HD) obtained their lowest scaled scores on the Attention and Visuospatial/Constructional subsections. In addition, even those patients who performed above the suggested cutoff points on the MMSE and DRS scored significantly below their controls on the RBANS, suggesting that the RBANS is effective in both detecting and characterizing these different

dementing disorders. Similar findings distinguishing patients with primarily cortical versus subcortical disorders have been reported by Beatty, Ryder, et al. (2003). They found that patients with AD showed more severe impairment on the Language and Delayed Memory indices (like patients with HD), while patients with Parkinson's disease (PD) showed a greater deficit on the Attention Index. Classification accuracy using an algorithm suggested by Randolph et al. (1998) ([Visuospatial/Construction + Attention]/2)] − ([Language + Delayed Memory]/2) was good, provided patients were already classed as demented. Classification was poor among patients with PD

Table 6–108 Frequencies (Cumulative Percentages) of Discrepancies Between RBANS (Form A) Age- and Age- and Education-Corrected Index Scores at 1- and 2-year Intervals: Age- & Education-Corrected Total Scale Score at Time 1 ≥ 110 (N = 61)

| | Cumulative Percentages | | | | | | | | | | |
| | Decline in Scores Over Time | | | | | | Increase in Scores Over Time | | | | |
	≤1%	2%	5%	10%	20%	50%	20%	10%	5%	2%	≤1%
Total Scale											
Age-Corrected (OKLAHOMA)[a]											
One-year Interval (T2–T1)	−25.0	−24.0	−17.8	−14.4	−9.0	−6.0	4.0	6.0	8.0	14.0	15.0
Two-year Interval (T3–T1)	−16.0	−15.8	−13.9	−12.8	−11.0	−4.0	2.0	4.8	6.9	14.0	14.0
One-year Interval (T3–T2)	−15.0	−14.3	−11.0	−9.8	−8.0	0.0	7.6	9.8	13.0	20.6	22.0
Age- and Education-Corrected[a]											
One-year Interval (T2–T1)	−20.0	−19.0	−16.0	−14.0	−10.6	−5.0	2.0	7.8	9.8	15.0	16.0
Two-year Interval (T3–T1)	−19.0	−18.0	−12.9	−11.0	−10.0	−4.0	2.0	5.8	8.8	12.8	13.0
One-year Interval (T3–T2)	−18.0	−17.3	−12.8	−9.0	−8.0	0.0	7.6	10.8	14.8	15.0	15.0
Age-Corrected (Randolph, 1998)[b]											
One-year Interval (T2–T1)	−23.0	−22.3	−19.9	−16.0	−11.6	−3.0	3.6	7.0	13.0	22.0	22.0
Two-year Interval (T3–T1)	−21.0	−21.0	−19.9	−13.8	−10.6	−4.0	6.0	9.8	12.8	26.4	30.0
One-year Interval (T3–T2)	−15.0	−14.8	−13.9	−11.8	−7.0	−1.0	8.6	14.8	21.3	36.1	39.0
Immediate Memory Index											
Age-Corrected (OKLAHOMA)[a]											
One-year Interval (T2–T1)	−32.0	−30.8	−25.9	−21.0	−18.6	−4.0	4.0	11.4	15.9	21.0	22.0
Two-year Interval (T3–T1)	−24.0	−23.5	−21.6	−17.0	−11.6	−3.0	7.6	11.8	17.7	20.3	21.0
One-year Interval (T3–T2)	−21.0	−20.3	−17.8	−15.0	−9.0	3.0	12.0	18.0	21.0	22.5	23.0
Age- and Education-Corrected[a]											
One-year Interval (T2–T1)	−30.0	−29.5	−28.0	−22.0	−17.0	−5.0	4.6	10.8	17.8	22.8	24.0
Two-year Interval (T3–T1)	−26.0	−25.5	−21.7	−17.6	−12.0	0.0	7.6	13.0	17.8	21.0	22.0
One-year Interval (T3–T2)	−21.0	−20.3	−16.9	−16.0	−7.2	3.0	13.6	18.0	20.7	24.0	24.0
Age-Corrected (Randolph, 1998)[b]											
One-year Interval (T2–T1)	−35.0	−34.0	−23.9	−23.0	−15.0	−6.0	6.0	14.8	17.0	23.0	24.0
Two-year Interval (T3–T1)	−27.0	−27.0	−25.6	−17.0	−9.0	0.0	9.6	17.0	20.0	25.3	26.0
One-year Interval (T3–T2)	−24.0	−22.8	−16.9	−12.0	−8.0	3.0	15.2	19.6	25.9	32.0	33.0
Visuospatial/Constructional Index											
Age-Corrected (OKLAHOMA)[a]											
One-year Interval (T2–T1)	−30.0	−29.5	−25.0	−24.8	−13.0	0.0	11.2	17.8	23.8	28.8	30.0
Two-year Interval (T3–T1)	−33.0	−33.0	−30.7	−25.0	−15.0	0.0	10.6	13.0	18.6	23.6	25.0
One-year Interval (T3–T2)	−33.0	−33.0	−26.8	−21.0	−13.0	0.0	12.0	18.0	22.0	24.8	25.0
Age- and Education-Corrected[a]											
One-year Interval (T2–T1)	−27.0	−26.3	−20.9	−15.8	−10.6	0.0	9.6	12.6	19.9	20.8	21.0
Two-year Interval (T3–T1)	−30.0	−28.6	−22.8	−18.6	−13.0	0.0	7.0	9.8	12.8	14.0	14.0
One-year Interval (T3–T2)	−28.0	−27.0	−20.9	−15.4	−10.0	0.0	7.0	13.0	16.7	19.8	20.0
Age-Corrected (Randolph, 1998)[b]											
One-year Interval (T2–T1)	−34.0	−32.8	−28.7	−22.0	−14.6	0.0	6.2	19.0	22.8	31.3	32.0
Two-year Interval (T3–T1)	−37.0	−36.5	−31.8	−20.8	−15.2	0.0	7.0	14.8	18.7	23.8	25.0
One-year Interval (T3–T2)	−31.0	−29.8	−21.0	−18.4	−12.6	0.0	11.2	15.8	18.8	21.8	22.0
Language Index											
Age-Corrected (OKLAHOMA)[a]											
One-year Interval (T2–T1)	−38.0	−37.3	−34.2	−24.2	−14.0	0.0	10.0	15.6	21.7	25.3	26.0
Two-year Interval (T3–T1)	−30.0	−27.6	−19.9	−17.0	−11.0	−4.0	9.6	14.0	21.8	24.3	25.0
One-year Interval (T3–T2)	−28.0	−26.6	−20.8	−16.0	−8.8	0.0	12.8	18.0	24.6	28.0	28.0
Age- and Education-Corrected[a]											
One-year Interval (T2–T1)	−21.0	−20.8	−18.9	−15.6	−10.6	0.0	6.0	10.8	13.7	20.8	22.0
Two-year Interval (T3–T1)	−18.0	−17.5	−11.8	−10.0	−7.0	0.0	6.0	9.8	14.6	16.8	17.0
One-year Interval (T3–T2)	−18.0	−18.0	−16.6	−11.0	−6.2	0.0	7.0	11.8	15.8	17.0	17.0

(*continued*)

Table 6–108 Frequencies (Cumulative Percentages) of Discrepancies Between RBANS (Form A) Age- and Age- and Education-Corrected Index Scores at 1- and 2-year Intervals: Age- & Education-Corrected Total Scale Score at Time 1 ≥ 110 (N = 61) (continued)

| | Cumulative Percentages | | | | | | | | | | |
| | Decline in Scores Over Time | | | | | | Increase in Scores Over Time | | | | |
	≤1%	2%	5%	10%	20%	50%	20%	10%	5%	2%	≤1%
Age-Corrected (Randolph, 1998)[b]											
One-year Interval (T2–T1)	−29.0	−26.8	−19.9	−17.6	−12.0	0.0	8.2	13.8	16.9	25.0	26.0
Two-year Interval (T3–T1)	−26.0	−25.3	−22.9	−14.4	−7.6	0.0	9.6	13.0	19.7	29.0	30.0
One-year Interval (T3–T2)	−30.0	−26.4	−11.9	−9.0	−4.0	0.0	9.0	15.2	19.9	21.8	22.0
Attention Index											
Age-Corrected (OKLAHOMA)[a]											
One-year Interval (T2–T1)	−20.0	−19.8	−17.0	−14.0	−11.0	−5.0	5.2	10.6	14.9	19.6	21.0
Two-year Interval (T3–T1)	−23.0	−22.5	−20.9	−14.8	−12.8	−3.0	5.6	10.8	16.8	17.0	17.0
One-year Interval (T3–T2)	−28.0	−26.3	−20.8	−15.0	−8.0	−0.0	11.0	14.0	19.8	24.0	25.0
Age- and Education-Corrected[a]											
One-year Interval (T2–T1)	−21.0	−20.5	−18.0	−17.6	−14.0	−4.0	4.0	10.4	14.0	16.3	17.0
Two-year Interval (T3–T1)	−25.0	−24.3	−21.0	−18.0	−11.0	−3.0	5.8	10.8	17.9	18.0	18.0
One-year Interval (T3–T2)	−29.0	−27.1	−19.8	−14.0	−9.8	0.0	11.6	15.0	20.6	26.0	27.0
Age-Corrected (Randolph, 1998)[b]											
One-year Interval (T2–T1)	−21.0	−21.0	−18.4	−13.0	−12.0	−3.0	7.0	10.8	16.6	26.8	27.0
Two-year Interval (T3–T1)	−24.0	−23.3	−20.9	−16.0	−12.6	0.0	10.0	17.0	22.5	30.3	32.0
One-year Interval (T3–T2)	−37.0	−33.6	−21.9	−12.4	−9.0	0.0	11.8	19.0	23.8	38.8	39.0
Delayed Memory Index											
Age-Corrected (OKLAHOMA)[a]											
One-year Interval (T2–T1)	−21.0	−20.5	−18.0	−14.8	−11.6	−4.0	6.0	11.4	13.8	24.8	27.0
Two-year Interval (T3–T1)	−32.0	−30.3	−24.6	−19.8	−12.2	−3.0	6.0	11.6	17.7	19.5	20.0
One-year Interval (T3–T2)	−27.0	−26.5	−20.6	−14.0	−11.0	0.0	7.6	12.6	16.0	17.8	18.0
Age- and Education-Corrected[a]											
One-year Interval (T2–T1)	−16.0	−16.0	−15.9	−13.0	−9.2	−2.0	7.0	10.4	14.7	21.8	23.0
Two-year Interval (T3–T1)	−21.0	−20.5	−17.9	−15.0	−12.0	−1.0	5.0	10.4	17.7	20.3	21.0
One-year Interval (T3–T2)	−23.0	−22.3	−18.0	−12.8	−9.6	0.0	5.6	10.8	15.7	20.6	22.0
Age-Corrected (Randolph, 1998)[b]											
One-year Interval (T2–T1)	−24.0	−22.8	−14.0	−13.0	−9.0	0.0	6.6	10.0	14.9	29.4	32.0
Two-year Interval (T3–T1)	−38.0	−35.4	−24.8	−18.4	−12.0	0.0	5.6	13.6	16.9	20.5	21.0
One-year Interval (T3–T2)	−33.0	−30.8	−18.7	−15.0	−10.0	0.0	5.0	9.8	14.0	17.8	19.0

Note: T1 = testing at year 1 score; T2 = testing at year 2 score; T3 = testing at year 3 score. In determining which table to use, calculate the T1 age- and education-corrected Total scale score based on Duff et al. (2003) normative data. For scores <90 use Table 6–106; for scores from 90–109, use Table 6–107; and for scores ≥110, use Table 6–108.
[a]Age-corrected Index discrepancy scores designated "(OKLAHOMA)" and age- and education-corrected Index discrepancy scores are based on the OKLAHOMA normative studies (Duff et al., 2003).
[b]Age-corrected Index discrepancy scores designated "(Randolph, 1998)" are based on the original RBANS normative data.

Source: Patton et al., 2005. Reprinted with the kind permission of Psychology Press.

who were of normal mental status. Cognitive slowing was evident in all groups.

There is also evidence that the memory disturbances that accompany Parkinson's disease (PD) and multiple sclerosis (MS) can be differentiated using the RBANS. Patients with PD did not learn or remember stories better than unrelated word lists and they also did not perform better on recognition than on recall tests for memory for word lists, raising questions about the validity of the retrieval failure explanation of impaired memory in PD (Beatty, Ryder, et al., 2003). By contrast, the patients with MS exhibited better recall of stories than of lists and better list recognition than recall (Beatty, 2004).

The RBANS also appears to be a useful screening instrument in psychiatric patients (Gold et al., 1999; Hobart et al., 1999; Wilk et al., 2002, 2004). Patients with schizophrenia demonstrate marked impairment on the test, despite showing relatively adequate performance on a measure of premorbid competence (WRAT-3 Reading; e.g., Gold et al., 1999; Wilk et al., 2002, 2004). Index scores suggest that patients have relatively less impairment of language and visual functions than of memory and attention. RBANS performance is minimally related to symptoms of the illness but strongly related to employment status. The Immediate Memory Index is the most discriminating with regard to employment status (Gold et al.,

Table 6–109 Confidence Intervals for Test-Retest Change in RBANS Total Scores for Healthy People Given Alternate Forms

Level of Confidence	Lower Limit	Upper Limit
99%	−25.1	22.1
95%	−19.1	16.3
90%	−16.4	13.4
85%	−14.5	10.4
80%	−13.1	10.1
70%	−7.9	10.8

Note: This group consisted of 99 healthy participants (28 men, 71 women) between the ages of 24 and 86 years with a mean education of 15.43 years (*SD* = 14.76). Difference scores outside these intervals indicate significant change.

Source: From Wilk et al., 2002. Reprinted with permission from the American Journal of Psychiatry, copyright © 2002. American Psychiatric Association.

1999). A study by Hobart et al. (1999) found that patients with schizophrenia demonstrated greater deficits on the RBANS than did patients with bipolar disorder.

With regard to predictive validity, Larson et al. (2005) reported that for stroke patients, the RBANS predicted well self-report of cognitive disability as well as instrumental activities of daily living 12 months later.

Finally, there is some evidence that time of testing can impact story memory performance in older adults. Older individuals obtained slightly lower recall scores when tested at their nonpreferred, rather than at their preferred, time of day (Paradee et al., 2005).

COMMENT

The RBANS is a useful screening tool to measure general performance level. The test is brief and appears well tolerated by patients who might not be able to cooperate with a lengthier examination (Hobart et al., 1999). It also may be more sensitive to impairment than other standard tests (e.g., MMSE, DRS, WMS-III).

The RBANS does not, however, take the place of a more comprehensive examination. Thus, depending upon the diagnostic question, data from the RBANS will have to be supplemented by measures of vigilance and executive and motor function (Hobart et al., 1999). Estimates of premorbid function, orientation, and mood also should be obtained. In addition, evidence supporting the interpretability of the five indices, and of the Language, Visuospatial/Constructional, and Attention indices in particular, appears weak. Thus, to confirm diagnostic impressions and to derive a detailed profile of cognitive strengths and weaknesses, the restricted assessment offered by the RBANS may be inadequate. Further, the lack of information on the individual subtests limits its utility.

Some of the subtests have a restricted range in the normal population (e.g., Figure Copy, Line Orientation, Picture Naming, List Recognition); that is, most healthy individuals obtain raw scores that approach the maximum possible for the subtest, with few individuals scoring below a perfect score. Thus, comparisons to other, more evenly distributed subtests should be avoided (e.g., comparing a "superior" performance [SS = 16] on Semantic Fluency to an "average" performance [SS = 10] on Picture Naming; Duff et al., 2003).

It is also worth bearing in mind that the test was designed to be used with healthy adults as well as individuals who may have moderately severe dementia. As a consequence, it may have limited utility in detecting impairment at the higher end of the intellectual distribution. It also appears to place a heavy demand on verbal responses and therefore is likely not appropriate for use with aphasic patients (Larson et al., 2005).

Finally, the test-retest stability appears adequate/high for the Total score; however, reliabilities of most of the indices appear low. The Total score, and possibly the Attention Index, should be the primary scores to consider in assessing change over time. Nonetheless, even for these indices, fairly large differences are needed to confirm reliable change. Thus, the ability of the RBANS to monitor change/progression of disorders may be limited in conditions where progress or decline is relatively subtle.

REFERENCES

Beatty, W. W. (2004). RBANS analysis of verbal memory in multiple sclerosis. *Archives of Clinical Neuropsychology, 19,* 825–834.

Beatty, W. W., Mold, J. W., & Gontkovsky, S. T. (2003a). RBANS performance: Influences of sex and education. *Journal of Clinical and Experimental Neuropsychology, 25,* 1065–1069.

Beatty, W. W., Ryder, K. A., Gontkovsky, S. T., Scott, J. G., McSwan, K. L., & Bharucha, K. J. (2003b). Analyzing the subcortical dementia syndrome of Parkinson's disease using the RBANS. *Archives of Clinical Neuropsychology, 18,* 509–520.

Duff, K., Beglinger, L. J., Schoenberg, M. R., Patton, D. E., Mold, J., Scott, J. G., & Adams, R. L. (2005). Test-retest stability and practice effects of the RBANS in a community dwelling elderly sample. *Journal of Clinical and Experimental Neuropsychology, 27,* 565–575.

Duff, K., Patton, D., Schoenberg, M. R., Mold, J., Scott, J. G., & Adams, R. L. (2003). Age- and education-corrected independent normative data for the RBANS in a community dwelling elderly sample. *The Clinical Neuropsychologist, 17,* 351–366.

Duff, K., Schoenberg, M. R., Patton, D., Mold, J., Scott, J. G., & Adams, R. L. (2004). Predicting change with the RBANS in an elderly sample. *Journal of the International Neuropsychological Society, 10,* 828–834.

Duff, K., Schoenberg, M. R., Patton, D., Paulsen, J. S., Bayless, J. D., Mold, J., Scott, J. G., & Adams, R. L. (2005). Regression-based formulas for predicting change in RBANS subtests with older adults. *Archives of Clinical Neuropsychology, 20,* 281–290.

Gold, J. M., Queern, C., Iannone, V. N., & Buchanan, R. B. (1999). Repeatable Battery for the Assessment of Neuropsychological Status as a screening test in schizophrenia, I: Sensitivity, reliability, and validity. *American Journal of Psychiatry, 158,* 1944–1950.

Gontkovsky, S. T., Beatty, W. W., & Mold, J. W. (2004). Repeatable Battery for the Assessment of Neurological Status in a normal, geriatric sample. *Clinical Gerontology, 27,* 79–86.

Gontkovsky, S. T., Mold, J. W., & Beatty, E. E. (2002). Age and educational influences on RBANS index scores in a nondemented geriatric sample. *The Clinical Neuropsychologist, 16,* 258–263.

Hobart, M. P., Goldberg, R., Bartko, J. J., & Gold, J. M. (1999). Repeatable Battery for the Assessment of Neuropsychological Status as a screening test in schizophrenia, II: Convergent/discriminant validity and diagnostic group comparisons. *American Journal of Psychiatry, 156,* 1951–1957.

Killam, C., Cautin, R. L., & Santucci, A.C. (2005). Assessing the enduring residual neuropsychological effects of head trauma in college athletes who participate in contact sports. *Archives of Clinical Neuropsychology, 20,* 599–611.

Larson, E. B., Kirschner, K., Bode, R., Heinemann, A., & Goodman, R. (2005). Construct and predictive validity of the Repeatable Battery for the Assessment of Neuropsychological Status in the evaluation of stroke patients. *Journal of Clinical and Experimental Neuropsychology, 27,* 16–32.

Moser, R. S., & Schatz, P. (2002). Enduring effects of concussion in youth athletes. *Archives of Clinical Neuropsychology, 17,* 91–100.

Paradee, C. V., Rapport, L. J., Hanks, R. A., & Levy, J. A. (2005). Circadian preference and cognitive functioning among rehabilitation inpatients. *The Clinical Neuropsychologist, 19,* 55–72.

Patton, D. E., Duff, K., Schoenberg, M. R., Mold, J., Scott, J. G., & Adams, R. L. (2003). Performance of cognitively normal African Americans on the RBANS in community dwelling older adults. *The Clinical Neuropsychologist, 17,* 515–530.

Patton, D. E., Duff, K., Schoenberg, M. R., Mold, J., Scott, J. G., & Adams, R. L. (2005). Base rates of longitudinal RBANS discrepancies at one- and two-year intervals in community-dwelling older adults. *The Clinical Neuropsychologist, 19,* 27–44.

Randolph, C. (1998). *RBANS manual.* San Antonio, TX: The Psychological Corporation.

Randolph, C., Tierney, M. C., Mohr, E., & Chase, T. N. (1998). The Repeatable Battery for the Assessment of Neuropsychological Status (RBANS): Preliminary clinical validity. *Journal of Clinical and Experimental Neuropsychology, 20,* 310–319.

Wilk, C. M., Gold, J. M., Bartko, J. J., Dickerson, F., Fenton, W. S., Knable, M., Randolph, C., & Buchanaan, R. W. (2002). Test-retest stability of the Repeatable Battery for the Assessment of Neuropsychological Status in schizophrenia. *American Journal of Psychiatry, 159,* 838–844.

Wilk, C. M., Gold, J. M., Humber, K., Dickerson, F., Fenton, W. S., & Buchanan, R. W. (2004). Brief cognitive assessment in schizophrenia: Normative data for the Repeatable Battery for the Assessment of Neuropsychological Status. *Schizophrenia Research, 70,* 175–186.

Stanford-Binet Intelligence Scales—Fifth Edition (SB5)

PURPOSE

The Stanford-Binet Intelligence Scales—Fifth Edition (SB5) is a standardized intelligence battery for children and adults.

SOURCE

The SB5 can be obtained from Riverside Publishing, 425 Spring Lake Drive, Itasca, IL 60143-2079, USA (www.riverpub.com; general: 1-800-323-9540; outside the United States: 1-630-467-7000; fax: 1-630-467-7192). The Complete Kit costs $825 US (3 Item Books, Examiner's Manual, Technical Manual, 25 Test Records, and a plastic case containing all manipulatives and carrying case). Scoring software (SB5 Scoring Pro) is available for $195 US.

AGE RANGE

The SB5 can be administered to people aged 2 to 85+ years.

DESCRIPTION

Overview

The SB5 (Roid, 2003a) is the latest revision of the Stanford-Binet scales. The Stanford-Binet is a direct descendent of the very first test of intelligence, the 1905 Binet scale (Binet & Simon, 1905), a test that determined to a large extent how intelligence came to be conceptualized and measured (Ittenbach, 1997). Beginning with Terman's American revision of the original Binet-Simon Intelligence Scale (Terman, 1916), the test was revised in 1937 (Terman & Merrill, 1937), renormed in 1960

(Terman & Merrill, 1960), and revised again in 1986 (Stanford-Binet Intelligence Scale—Fourth Edition or SB-IV; Thorndike et al., 1986; see Figure 6–17).

The earlier editions of the test used item groupings to assess functional ability, arranged by levels into order of difficulty. The 1986 revision shifted to a subtest-based point system based on items of increasing difficulty, similar to those of other intelligence tests such as the Wechsler scales. It also based itself on modern theories of a hierarchical *g* measuring crystallized and fluid abilities.

The main goals of the fifth revision included (a) expanding the range of the test to allow assessment of very low and very high levels of cognitive ability, (b) restoring the original toys and manipulatives for assessing preschoolers that had been removed in recent versions, (c) increasing clinical utility,

Figure 6–17 History of the Stanford-Binet. *Source:* Reprinted with permission from Roid & Barram, 2004.

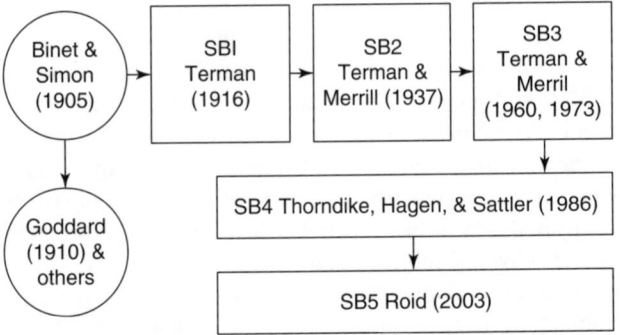

(d) updating materials, (e) increasing the nonverbal items, and (f) increasing the range of domains measured by the test (Roid, 2003b). Accordingly, a number of new subtests have been added, while many of the classic Stanford-Binet subtests were retained. The SB5 retains the routing subtest technique of the 1986 revision (i.e., where the examiner first administers a subtest to get an idea of the examinee's level of ability, then uses this estimation to choose starting points on subsequent subtests). In addition, the SB5 presents items according to functional levels. The presentation of a variety of items that each measure a different domain of ability but that are grouped together by level of difficulty was a feature of even earlier versions. Both routing subtests and functional levels were redesigned using modern psychometric methods such as item response theory.

According to Flanagan and Ortiz (2001), the previous version (SB-IV) had several strengths. First, it measured a broader range of abilities in the Cattell-Horn-Cattell (CHC) framework (see section introduction for a definition of this model, as well as Figure 6–18) than most other intelligence tests except the WJ III. Second, it did not oversample certain abilities, as did other tests such as the WISC-III (e.g., visual processing). Third, it allowed practitioners flexibility in choosing specific subtests contributing to the total composite score.

These features appear to have been retained in the newer SB5. While the earlier version measured four factors (Verbal, Quantitative, Abstract/Visual Reasoning, and Short-Term Memory), the new SB5 measures five factors (Fluid Reasoning, Knowledge, Quantitative Reasoning, Visual-Spatial Processing, and Working Memory) that are based on modern factor-analytic CHC theories of intelligence. These factors correspond to *Gf* (Fluid Intelligence), *Gc* (Crystallized Knowledge), *Gq* (Quantitative Knowledge), *Gv* (Visual Processing), and *Gsm* (Short-Term Memory) in the CHC model (see Figures 6–18 and 6–19). Factors not measured by the SB5, excluded because of difficulties with usability, testing time, or priority (Roid, 2003c), are *Ga* (Auditory Processing), *Glr* (Long-Term Retrieval), and *Gs* (Processing Speed). The latter

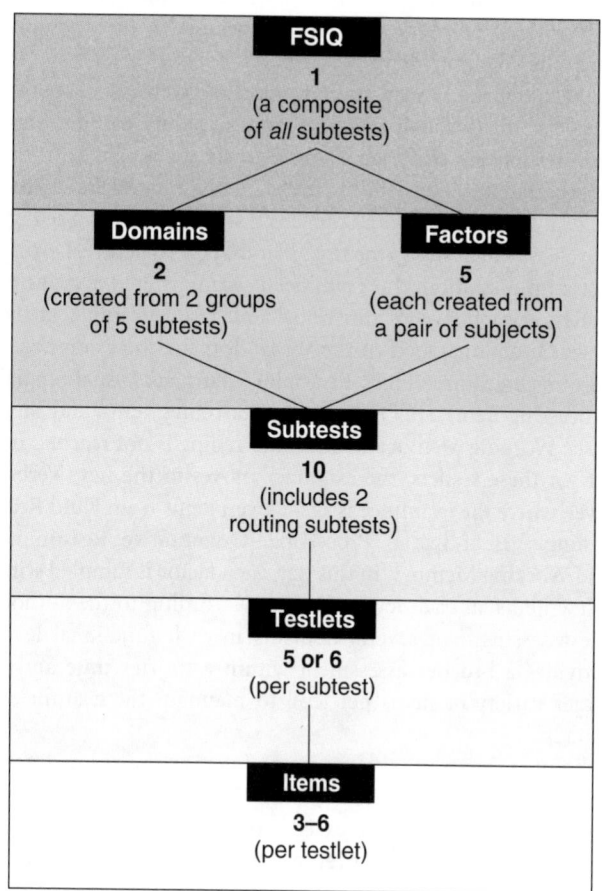

Figure 6–19 Hierarchy of SB5 Components. *Source:* Reprinted with permission from Roid, 2003b.

omission is likely a significant drawback in neuropsychological contexts. See Table 6–110 for the list of factors included in the test.

Test Structure

The Full-Scale IQ is based on 10 subtests forming five factors. Each of the five factors is made up of two subtests—one from the Nonverbal domain and the other from the Verbal domain. The name of each subtest reflects both the factor on which it

Figure 6–18 Test Structure of the SB5. *Note:* FSIQ = Full Scale IQ; *g* = general ability; NVIQ = Nonverbal IQ; VIQ = Verbal IQ; FR = Fluid Reasoning; KN = Knowledge; QR = Quantitative Reasoning; VS = Visual-Spatial Processing; WM = Working Memory. *Source:* Reprinted with permission from Roid & Barram, 2004.

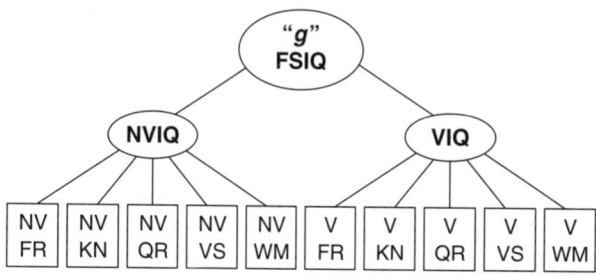

Table 6–110 CHC Factor Coverage of the SB5

CHC Factors Included in the SB5	CHC Factors Not Included in the SB5
Gf (Fluid Intelligence)	*Ga* (Auditory Processing)
Gc (Crystallized Knowledge)	*Glr* (Long-Term Retrieval)
Gq (Quantitative Knowledge)	*Gs* (Processing Speed)
Gv (Visual Processing)	
Gsm (Short-Term Memory)	

loads and its "domain" (i.e., whether it is Nonverbal or Verbal in nature). For example, the Nonverbal Knowledge and Verbal Knowledge subtests form the Knowledge factor; the Nonverbal Working Memory and Verbal Working Memory subtests form the Working Memory factor.

Each subtest is in turn comprised of five or six separate "testlets" that measure different levels of ability within a subtest. Testlets are made up of three to six items that have the same difficulty level (Roid, 2003b). Levels range from 1 to 6 (except for the Verbal domain, which starts at level 2). See Figure 6–19, which shows the test's hierarchical structure. During test administration, the examinee is administered a series of testlets at each level of functional ability. For example, at the lowest functional level of the Verbal domain, the examinee is administered three Fluid Reasoning items, six Visual-Spatial Processing items, six Quantitative Reasoning items, and then three Working Memory items. If the ceiling is not reached on any of these testlets, the examiner moves to the next Verbal level, where the examinee is again given items from Fluid Reasoning, Visual-Spatial Processing, Quantitative Reasoning, and Working Memory. In this way, each factor is sampled with a few items, at each level of ability. According to the author, the assessment of several domains in each functional level provides a broader assessment within a shorter time and a larger variety of items per level to maintain the examinee's interest.

Some subtests are also made up of items comprising different types of "activities" (see Table 6–111 for specific activities by subtest), which do not exactly conform to testlets (e.g., an activity may be extended over several testlets of increasing difficulty).

Two of the 10 SB5 subtests are designated as Routing Subtests; these are Nonverbal Fluid Reasoning and Verbal Knowledge. Scores on these subtests determine the entry point for each subtest (i.e., the particular testlet that corresponds to the examinee's level; see Figure 6–20). According to the author, testlets are therefore a modern equivalent of age levels designed to simulate modern computerized adaptive testing (Roid, 2003c). A mix of factors at each level of ability is also similar to the earlier Stanford-Binet version.

An Abbreviated Battery IQ is based on the two Routing subtests (Object Series/Matrices and Vocabulary). The Nonverbal IQ, based on the five nonverbal subtests, can be administered to individuals with limited linguistic ability. The Verbal IQ, based on the five verbal subtests, can be used in individuals with motor or visual impairments.

ADMINISTRATION TIME

The full battery takes approximately 45 to 75 minutes. The Abbreviated Battery can be administered in 15 to 20 minutes.

ADMINISTRATION

See manual. The test is divided into three major components that are presented in three different Item Books. Book 1 contains the two routing subtests (Object Series/Matrices and Vocabulary), used to determine an estimate of ability for determining starting points in Book 2 (i.e., functional ability level). Appropriate entry points are printed on the record form after the Routing subtests. Book 2 contains all the nonverbal subtests and Book 3 contains all the verbal subtests.

For ease of administration, a plastic case with compartments is provided to store manipulatives (e.g., small toys, blocks, etc.). Although instructions are printed in the Stimulus books for ease of administration, new users should refer to the Examiner's Manual for additional instructions for administering each subtest. Subtests in Books 2 and 3 are organized into "testlets" arranged into levels of difficulty. Each subtest includes five or six of these testlets, each of which generally contains six items or yields six points. The Record Form is arranged so that each page reflects a functional level of difficulty, with four testlets reflecting each of the separate factors (note that the fifth factor is assessed via routing subtests). Each testlet begins with teaching items. Basals and ceilings are indicated for each testlet on the record form.

The author provides specific instructions on how to administer the test using accommodations and adaptations for special populations, including deaf/hard of hearing, blind/visually impaired, and physically impaired individuals (see Interpretive Manual; Roid, in press).

SCORING

Scores

SB5 standard scores ($M = 100$) have an SD of 15, not 16 as in previous editions. The Full-Scale IQ ranges from 40 to 160. Tables for conducting discrepancy analyses and frequency analyses (e.g., between IQ and factor indices, between single subtest and average subtest, and scatter) are presented in the Technical Manual. Age equivalents were derived using change-sensitive score methodology, an improvement over standard age equivalents, based on item response theory scaling (see p. 127 of the Examiner's Manual for details, and Roid, in press). These scores are reportedly useful in the evaluation of examinees who obtain extreme scores (i.e., low functioning and gifted individuals), but cautions about interpreting age-equivalent-based scores also apply (see p. 129 of Examiner's Manual).

Scoring can be done by hand or by using computer scoring software (SB5 Scoring Pro; Roid, 2003d); computer scoring is recommended given the number and complexity of scores.

Ability-Achievement Discrepancies

Tables for calculating ability-achievement discrepancies based on a linking sample between the SB5 and the WJ III ACH are provided in the Technical Manual for the predicted-achievement method and simple-difference method. Tables are provided for the three IQ composites (FSIQ, VIQ, and NVIQ) and for 19 WJ III ACH scores, including the five cluster scores for each of the separate achievement domains on the WJ III.

Table 6–111 Factors, Subtests, and Activities of the SB5

Factors and Subtests	Activities	Description
Fluid Reasoning (FR)		
Nonverbal Fluid Reasoning	Object Series Matrices	This is a matrices task that uses manipulatives in young children, pictured objects in older children, and standard abstract matrices in older age groups.
Verbal Fluid Reasoning	Early Reasoning Verbal Absurdities Verbal Analogies	Early items (Early Reasoning) require the child to sort picture chips into categories; later items involve Verbal Absurdities; the examiner says a sentence with an impossible or incongruous element, which the child must explain; Verbal Analogies is a standard analogies task (e.g., "North is to South as East is to") requiring the examinee to provide missing words.
Knowledge (KN)		
Nonverbal Knowledge	Procedural Knowledge Picture Absurdities	Early items require the child to pantomime common actions in response to examiner commands; later items involve the classic "Absurdities" paradigm of earlier test versions, which requires the examinee to verbally explain how a series of pictured scenes is incongruous or impossible.
Verbal Knowledge	Vocabulary	Simpler items involve body part naming and providing verbal descriptions of common scenes; in older children and adults, the examinee must provide word definitions.
Quantitative Reasoning (QR)		
Nonverbal Quantitative Reasoning	Quantitative Reasoning	Early items employ blocks and pictures to assess knowledge of simple math concepts (e.g., bigger/smaller); later items assess counting, number recognition, and mathematical reasoning skills; responses are largely nonverbal.
Verbal Quantitative Reasoning	Quantitative Reasoning	Items are similar to the Nonverbal Quantitative Reasoning, but require a verbal response; items also contain a number of word problems that the examiner reads aloud.
Visual-Spatial Processing (VS)		
Nonverbal Visual-Spatial Processing	Form Board Form Patterns	Early items employ the classic Stanford-Binet form board of earlier test versions; later items require the examinee to assemble form board pieces into semirepresentational objects, people, or animals from a pictured model.
Verbal Visual-Spatial Processing	Position and Direction	The examinee must demonstrate understanding of verbal instructions involving spatial directions, using either manipulatives or pointing (early items); on later items, the examinee must use directional terms (e.g., north, south) to give directions, or solve word problems involving spatial information.
Working Memory (WM)		
Nonverbal Working Memory	Delayed Response Block Span	The first three items consist of a simple Delayed Response paradigm involving a cup and a hidden toy; all other items involve a visual span task similar to the classic Knox Cubes paradigm, with additional complexity in the later items.
Verbal Working Memory	Memory for Sentences Last Word	Early items involve sentence repetition; later items from the "Last Word" task are similar to a sustained attention task under interference conditions; the examinee is asked a series of yes/no questions; following the series, the examinee must recite the last word of each question posed.

Note: Factors are in bold; subtests are in italics.

Adapted from Roid, 2003a, 2003b, and 2003c.

Figure 6–20 Administration Procedure for the SB5. *Source:* Reprinted with permission from Roid, 2003b.

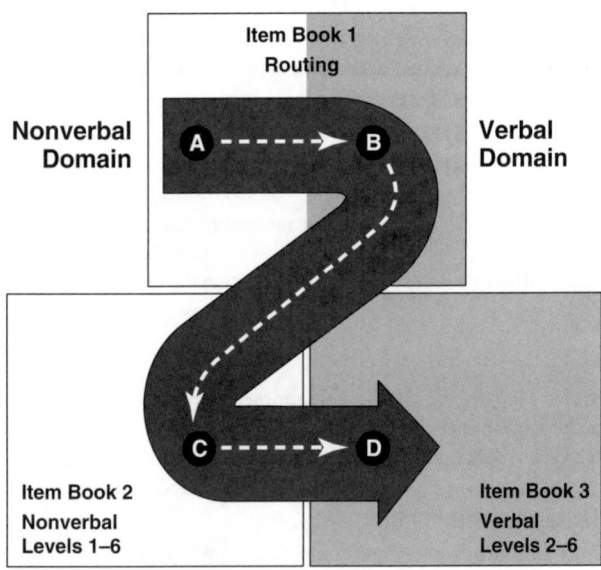

A Administer the Nonverbal Fluid Reasoning routing subtest (Object Series/Matrices).

B Administer the Verbal Knowledge routing subtest (Vocabulary).

C Begin at the appropriate Nonverbal level based on the Object Series/Matrices score. Continue testing until the examinee reaches a ceiling on all four subtests.

D Proceed to the appropriate Verbal level based on the Vocabulary score. Continue testing until the examinee reaches a ceiling on all four subtests.

DEMOGRAPHIC EFFECTS

Age

SB5 performance typically increases until late adolescence or middle adulthood, depending on the function, and gradually declines later in adulthood (Roid, 2003c). This supports the test's sensitivity to age-related changes in cognitive ability. For a full discussion of age trends for the SB5, see pp. 103 to 105 of the Technical Manual. Growth curves based on cross-sectional data for the Knowledge, Working Memory, Fluid Reasoning, Quantitative Reasoning, and Visual-Spatial factors for the SB5 are shown in Figure 6–21. According to these curves, the Knowledge factor reaches its peak latest in life (ages 50–60), and the Working Memory factor reaches its peak earliest (at approximately age 20).

Education

Information on education effects, particularly in adults, is lacking.

Figure 6–21 Growth Curves for the Five SB5 Factors. *Note:* FR = Fluid Reasoning; WM = Working Memory; VS = Visual-Spatial; QR = Quantitative Reasoning; and KN = Knowledge. *Source:* Reprinted with permission from Roid, 2003c.

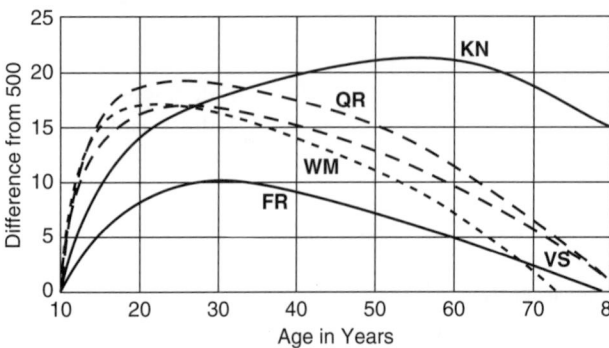

Ethnicity

Considerable care went into ensuring that SB5 content was fair in terms of bias against subgroups defined by ethnicity and race (see *Validity, Content*). However, there are as yet no independent studies on the test's usage in minorities or subgroups defined by ethnicity.

NORMATIVE DATA

Standardization Sample

As shown in Table 6–112, the normative sample consists of 4800 subjects aged 2 to 85+. Norms were collected from 2001 to 2002, and were stratified according to age, gender, race/ethnicity, geographic region, and socioeconomic level (based on years of education in adults and parental years of education in children). There were 400 children in each one-year age band at the younger age levels (2–4 years), 400 per one-year age band in older children (5–16 years), and 100 to 200 cases in each 10-year age band in adults. Note that there is a higher percentage of women in the older age levels due to differential life expectancy. Normative data were smoothed with polynomial regression (see p. 61 of the Technical Manual for details).

In addition to the standardization sample, the SB5 was administered to 1365 individuals with clinical diagnoses (e.g., ADHD, autism, developmental disability, limited English, gifted, learning disability, motor impaired, mental retardation, speech/language impairment, deafness/hard of hearing, and emotional disturbance).

Note that the standardization edition upon which normative data are based contained more items than the final published version and used a mixture of verbal and nonverbal items in each functional level (see p. 46 of Technical Manual for details). A study of 136 subjects administered both

Table 6–112 SB5 Normative Sample Characteristics

Number	4800[a]
Age	2 to 85+ years
Geographic location	
Northeast	19%
South	35%
Midwest	23%
West	23%
Sample type	National, stratified random sample[b]
Parental education/education	
<12 years	18%
12 years	33%
>12 years	49%
SES	Designated by educational level
Gender	
Males	49%
Females	51%
Race/ethnicity	
White/Anglo American	69%
Black/African American	12%
Hispanic	12%
Asian	4%
Other	3%
Screening	Persons with severe medical conditions, limited English language proficiency, severe sensory or communication deficit (i.e., speech, hearing, visual, orthopedic, or TBI), severe behavioral/emotional disturbance (e.g., autism), or enrollment in special education for the majority of the school day[c]

[a]Based on 30 separate age bands. [b]Based on 2001 U.S. Census data, stratified by age, gender, race/ethnicity, geographic region, and SES (i.e., education). [c]The standardization sample includes students who were enrolled in special education but were in regular classrooms for more than 50% of their day (i.e., 5% of the school-age sample).

Source: Adapted from Roid, 2003c.

versions reportedly supports the equivalence of the standardization and published versions.

The SB5 and WJ III ACH linking sample consists of 472 children aged 6 to 19; data from this sample form the basis of the ability-achievement discrepancy analysis.

RELIABILITY

Internal Consistency

Internal reliability is very high for the Full-Scale IQ at all ages ($r = .97–.98$; see *Source*). Reliabilities for the Nonverbal IQ and Verbal IQ are also high (mean $r = .95$ and .96, respectively). The Abbreviated Battery IQ reliabilities are somewhat lower (mean $r = .91$, range .85–.96), but are still quite respectable for

a two-subtest composite. Average reliabilities for the five factor index scores are very high ($r = .90–.92$); average subtest internal consistencies are also good, with average subtest coefficients ranging from $r = .84$ to .89.

Standard Errors of Measurement

According to the Technical Manual, SB5 *SEM*s are generally small, as would be expected given the test's high internal reliability. *SEM*s for the Full-Scale IQ are about two standard score points across all ages ($M = 2.30$). Nonverbal IQ *SEM*s range from three to almost four points ($M = 3.26$), and those for the Verbal IQ range from two to three points ($M = 3.05$). Abbreviated Battery IQ *SEM*s range from three to five points across age ($M = 4.55$). Factor index score *SEM*s are generally similar (about four points, on average). At the subtest level, average *SEM*s across age are small (about one point).

Test-Retest Reliability

Test-retest reliability is for the most part also excellent. Temporal stability was evaluated in four groups retested after a test interval of five to eight days: 96 preschoolers (aged 2–5), 87 children and young adults (aged 6–20), 81 adults (aged 21–59), and 92 older adults (aged 60 and over; see Technical Manual). Full-Scale IQ and Verbal IQ stability was very high for all ages ($r = .93–.95$). Reliability for the Nonverbal IQ, although also quite high ($r = .89–.93$), was slightly lower. As expected due to its significantly shorter length, Abbreviated Battery IQ stability was high, but lower than that of the other IQ composites and lower than would be optimal (e.g., >.95) for diagnostic decision making (i.e., $r = .84–.87$).

Subtest and factor index stability was generally high to very high (>.80; see Table 6–113), but there were some exceptions. Notably, the Working Memory Index attained only adequate reliability in adults, and Working Memory—Nonverbal subtest reliability was only marginal. The Knowledge factor index had very high test-retest reliability in all age groups.

Practice Effects

Practice effects are minimal with the SB5 after a five- to eight-day interval (Technical Manual). Specifically, the Full-Scale IQ increased two to four points. The author notes that this is a notable improvement over the SB-IV (six to eight points), WISC-III (seven to eight points), and WAIS-III (three to six points); this is despite a shorter testing interval, which they state tends to maximize practice effects (although others might disagree; see Chapter 1). SB5 Verbal IQs increased on average two to three points, whereas Nonverbal IQs increased by two to five points. As noted by the author, the Nonverbal IQ increase is considerably smaller than that of corresponding indices on most of the other major IQ batteries (e.g., PIQ increases 11 to 13 points on the WISC-III). The Abbreviated Battery IQs increased 2.5 to 3.9 points across age

Table 6–113 Magnitude of Test-Retest Reliability Coefficients for the SB5 Factor Indices and Subtests

Magnitude of Coefficient	Ages 2 to 5	Ages 6 to 20	Ages 21 to 59	Ages 60+
Very high (.90+)	Knowledge—V Working Memory—V *Knowledge* *Working Memory*	Knowledge—NV Quantitative Reasoning—V *Knowledge* *Quantitative Reasoning*	Knowledge—NV Knowledge—V Quantitative Reasoning—V *Knowledge*	Knowledge—NV Knowledge—V Quantitative Reasoning—V *Knowledge* *Quantitative Reasoning*
High (.80–.89)	Knowledge—NV Quantitative Reasoning—NV Fluid Reasoning—V *Fluid Reasoning* *Quantitative Reasoning* *Visual-Spatial Processing*	Quantitative Reasoning—NV Visual-Spatial Processing—NV Working Memory—NV Fluid Reasoning—V Knowledge—V Working Memory—V *Fluid Reasoning* *Visual-Spatial Processing* *Working Memory*	Fluid Reasoning—V *Fluid Reasoning* *Quantitative Reasoning* *Visual-Spatial Processing*	Quantitative Reasoning—NV Visual-Spatial Processing—NV Working Memory—NV Fluid Reasoning—V Visual-Spatial Processing—V Working Memory—V *Fluid Reasoning* *Visual-Spatial Processing* *Working Memory*
Adequate (.70–.79)	Fluid Reasoning—NV Visual-Spatial Processing—NV Working Memory—NV Quantitative Reasoning—V Visual-Spatial Processing—V	Fluid Reasoning—NV Visual-Spatial Processing—V	Fluid Reasoning—NV Quantitative Reasoning—NV Visual-Spatial Processing—NV Visual-Spatial Processing—V Working Memory—V *Working Memory*	Fluid Reasoning—NV
Marginal (.60–.69)	—	—	Working Memory—NV	—
Low (< .59)	—	—	—	—

Note: Composites scores are shown in italics. NV denotes Nonverbal subtests and V denotes Verbal subtests.

Adapted from Roid, 2003c.

groups. Factor index scores increased by one to four points, on average.

Interrater Reliability

Interrater agreement is generally high for the subtests with more than one scoring option (i.e., 0, 1, or 2), with a median *r* of .90. For more detailed information, see p. 75 of the Technical Manual.

VALIDITY

Content Validity

The SB5 was published after seven years of development, including literature review, expert advice (including that of intelligence theorists such as John B. Carroll and John L. Horn),

user surveys, factor analyses of previous versions, pilot studies, item response theory modeling, and tryout editions. For details on item development in each of the factor domains and detailed procedures on item analysis, see Roid (2003c, pp. 41–44 and 78–81).

The SB5 items were evaluated for fairness along gender, ethnic, racial, cultural, linguistic, and exceptional group status and, unlike many tests, along religious group status (e.g., Buddhist, Christian, Jewish, Hindu, and Muslim). Techniques for evaluating fairness included logical analyses and "offensiveness review" (p. 134) by expert bias reviewers from each group, and a number of empirical techniques including conventional item analysis, IRT studies using the Rasch model, studies of differential item functioning, construct-related studies (i.e., consistency of reliability and subtest correlations across groups), studies of fairness of prediction (i.e., equivalence of correlations to achievement across groups), and other studies including fairness of interscorer reliability across groups. The authors report that these studies support the SB5 as a fair test across groups. (For additional information on these studies, see Roid, in press.)

SB5 Loadings With *g*

As additional evidence of validity, the authors present *g* loadings for all the SB5 subtests, and review literature indicating that the SB5, with *g* loadings ranging from 56% to 61%, is a better measure of *g* than the WAIS-III (50%), WISC-III (39%), WPPSI-R (40%), and SB-IV (49%; see p. 108 in the Technical Manual for specific references).

The Abbreviated Battery IQ

The Abbreviated Battery IQ is highly related to the Full-Scale IQ. Correlations between Full-Scale and Abbreviated Battery IQs in the standardization sample are very high (i.e., $r = .81$ in younger children aged 2–5, and $r = .87$ in groups aged 6 and up). In a special sample of individuals with mental retardation, this correlation was also very high ($r = .87$). The Technical Manual describes the consistency of the Abbreviated and Full-Scale SB5 IQs in detecting mental retardation. Overall agreement between the two scores was 92% in detecting scores above and below a cutoff of 70. False positives on the Abbreviated Battery IQ (i.e., ABIQ <70, FSIQ ≥ 70) were rare (2 cases out of 4800), and false negatives (i.e., ABIQ ≥ 70, FSIQ <70) were low (8%).

Factor Structure

Confirmatory factor analysis using structural equation modeling and split-half subtest scores (i.e., with two scores for every subtest) is described in detail in the Technical Manual. The authors caution that using the conventional subtest standard scores may not reproduce the same factor solutions. They found support for a two-factor verbal-nonverbal solution, with some of the highest loadings in the older age groups and some of the lowest in the youngest age group. In additional analyses, the five-factor SB5 model provided the best fit compared with single- and other multifactor combinations. The lowest loadings were found in the youngest age group and for some Nonverbal subtests (Fluid Reasoning and Visual-Spatial subtests).

In a "cross-battery" confirmatory factor analysis with subtests from the WJ III corresponding to SB5 factors, a five-factor solution again had the best fit compared with other single- and multifactor solutions, though the difference between models was not large.

Correlations With the SB-IV

In 104 subjects administered both measures in a counterbalanced order, the scales were highly correlated ($r = .90$ between SB5 Full-Scale IQ and SB-IV Composite SAS). Factor scores were also highly correlated ($r = .64$–.77). Due to the Flynn effect, the SB-IV composite score, normed in 1985, was higher than the SB5 Full-Scale IQ by 3.5 points. The Technical Manual presents tables for estimating SB5 scores from SB-IV scores (Table 4.2, p. 83) and Form L-M scores (Table 4.4., p. 85). The correlation between the SB5 Abbreviated IQ and SB-IV CAS score is reportedly high ($r = .71$).

Correlations With Other Intelligence Tests

WPPSI-R. According to the Technical Manual, Full-Scale IQ scores in 71 preschoolers were highly correlated ($r = .83$). Verbal IQ scores were also highly related ($r = .82$), as were the SB5 Nonverbal IQ and WPPSI-R PIQ ($r = .72$). However, mean WPPSI-R scores were six points lower than SB5 scores, which the authors attributed to the increased length and less usage of toys and manipulatives in the WPPSI-R versus the SB5 in this age group (see Technical Manual for further details).

WISC-III. Sixty-six children (aged 6–16) were administered the SB5 and WISC-III (see Technical Manual). Full-Scale IQs were very highly correlated, as were Verbal IQs ($r = .84$ and .85, respectively). The Nonverbal IQ and the PIQ were highly correlated, but to a lesser degree than the other composites ($r = .66$). The WISC-III Full-Scale IQ was five points higher, which the authors attributed to the Flynn Effect. Correlations between the SB5 Working Memory Index and WISC-III FFD were not reported. Correlations between the Abbreviated IQ and the WISC-III Full-Scale IQ were somewhat lower ($r = .69$).

WAIS-III. As with other Wechsler versions, Full-Scale IQ and Verbal IQ were highly correlated between the two batteries ($r = .82$ and .81, respectively) in 87 adults, as reported in the Technical Manual. SB5 Nonverbal IQ and WAIS-III PIQ were also highly correlated, though slightly less so than the other composites ($r = .76$). The WAIS-III Full-Scale IQ was 5.5 points higher than that of the SB5, a difference that is slightly larger than what would be predicted by the Flynn effect. Correlations between the Abbreviated IQ and the WAIS-III Full-Scale IQ were also high ($r = .81$).

WJ III Cognitive. Like the SB5, the WJ III COG is based on the CHC theory of intelligence (see review in this volume). As such, a higher concordance between factors would be expected than with tests not based on this theory, such as the Wechsler test editions listed previously. This was examined by the authors in a sample of 145 children (aged 4–11; Technical Manual). Using only the WJ III COG factors that matched the five factors included in the SB5, the correlation between scales was .90, which is extremely high for separately normed, separately constructed test batteries containing different items. Indeed, with correlations this high, one could argue that these components of the tests are virtually interchangeable.

Correlations between the SB5 Full-Scale IQ and the WJ III COG GIA, which includes factors not measured by the SB5, produced a lower correlation ($r = .76$). Verbal factors were highly correlated ($r = .75$), and correlations between working memory factors were also relatively strong ($r = .61$). Means on the two tests were much closer in magnitude than those involving the Wechsler tests (i.e., within 1.4 points).

Correlations Between the Nonverbal IQ and Other Nonverbal Scales

Correlations between the SB5 Nonverbal IQ and the Universal Nonverbal Intelligence Test (UNIT; Bracken & McCallum, 1998) were .57 in a small sample of children with deafness or who were hard of hearing ($N = 29$; Technical Manual), an acceptable level of association for nonverbal measures.

Correlations With Achievement

Correlations with achievement are within the range expected between IQ and achievement tests. For example, correlations between the Full-Scale and Verbal IQ composites for the SB5 and WJ III ACH Academic Applications score were equally high ($r = .84$ and .82, respectively, in 472 children aged 6–19; Technical Manual). Overall, correlations between the two tests are strong ($r = .50$–.84), and mean scores between the two measures are very close (approximately three points between the Academic Applications and SB5 Full-Scale score). This would be expected in two tests designed to be used in ability/achievement discrepancy analyses.

WIAT-II total composite and SB5 Full-Scale and Verbal IQ scores are also highly related ($r = .80$, in 80 children aged 6–15; Technical Manual). The median correlation across all factors between the two tests is also high ($r = .60$). WIAT-II scores are almost five points higher than SB5 scores, however, despite a relatively similar timing of standardization.

Clinical Studies

Detailed information on SB5 profiles of several clinical groups are outlined in the Technical Manual. As expected, gifted individuals had above-average IQ, individuals with mental retardation showed a flat profile across domains and low overall score, and preschoolers with developmental delay had relatively low scores (i.e., IQ = 124, 57, and 75, respectively).

In another sample of children with developmental delay/mental retardation, correlations between the total composite scores for the SB5 and an adaptive behavior scale (i.e., SIB-R) were moderately high ($r = .59$); both means were below 70, which was expected for this particular sample. Children and adolescents who were not proficient in English (English language learners) had their lowest scores on language-based composites (Knowledge factor = 89.3, VIQ = 88.6), and the Nonverbal IQ was one of their higher scores (95.3). A speech and language delay sample did not show strong evidence of decreased scores on language-based composites; instead, they

had a somewhat flat profile with relatively weaker Verbal than Nonverbal IQ (89 versus 95). No notable differences in NVIQ, VIQ, and FSIQ for children with different types of learning disabilities were found (i.e., math, reading, or writing).

Although the authors state that the various composite scores show evidence of criterion validity for the SB5 in detecting learning disabilities, score differences were very small across composites. For example, the lowest score for children with math disabilities, Quantitative Reasoning, is within approximately one to two points of the NVIQ, VIQ, and FSIQ. Working Memory was the lowest index score in a group of children with ADHD ($M = 90.2$; see Technical Manual); however, from a clinical standpoint, this was not far below the IQ composites (NVIQ, VIQ, and FSIQ), which were about 92 to 93. Groups with severe emotional disturbance or orthopedic/motor delay were about one standard deviation below the standardization mean.

COMMENT

The SB5 appears to be an excellent test that is grounded on strong theoretical foundations, rigorous test development methods, and a respected tradition of psychological assessment. Psychometrically, it is an impressive test. It has excellent reliability and appears to have smaller practice effects than other major intelligence batteries, although additional information on test stability over longer intervals would be informative. The range of difficulty of items is extensive, without restriction by floor or ceiling effects, which make the scale ideal for testing very young children, low-functioning individuals, and gifted examinees. The use of toys and manipulatives, which the author indicates was included in the new version due to users' requests, make it child-friendly, and the testing format (i.e., use of testlets) may indeed maintain the interest of examinees, though this needs to be adequately studied. The SB5 developers also appear to have made every effort to deliver a fair test that is relatively free of cultural or other biases. The manuals are extensive, and in addition to SB5-specific information, contain detailed discussions on several general topics germane to assessment (e.g., history of intelligence testing, review of CHC theory, assessment of special populations).

The SB5 contains a number of novel tasks (e.g., Verbal Working Memory) that have norms for a large range of age groups, which makes them suitable for longitudinal testing (e.g., at-risk preschoolers or other groups where long-term follow-up will be needed).

Testing Format and Administration

Because of its use of routing subtests, testlets, and administration of a cross-section of factors at each level of difficulty (rather than consecutively administering each subtest in its entirety), the SB5 is designed in a way that differs significantly from most other intelligence batteries. This new structure and administration technique takes some getting used to, even for experienced examiners. New users must spend considerable time reviewing the test structure and familiarizing themselves with the administration rules. For example, examiners must keep track of multiple basals and ceilings simultaneously, and rules for ceilings and basals differ depending on the nature of the subtest (routing or standard) and on testlet level. However, this may be an improvement over the previous Stanford-Binet, which itself had subtests that were fairly complex to administer, particularly in examinees who required dropping back to attain a lower-than-expected basal. Future research should be informative in determining whether the newer technique is truly an improvement over more traditional methods that do not employ adaptive testing methods.

Some subtests contain a number of different activities (e.g., Verbal Fluid Reasoning), whereas others contain similar items that only differ in level of difficulty. Users should be aware of this in interpreting scores at different ages or levels of ability.

The Nonverbal IQ

The Nonverbal scale measures five distinct CHC factors, which make it unique compared with all other intelligence batteries (Roid, 2003c). Note that each factor is only represented by a single subtest at the domain level, which some authors consider inadequate for factor interpretation (e.g., Flanagan & Ortiz, 2001). Regardless, because the Nonverbal domain includes a broad range of subtest types and activities, it provides a composite that is not restricted to a narrow aspect of nonverbal functioning (e.g., such as visual-constructional skills, a criticism of some Wechsler versions).

The SB5 Technical and Examiner's Manuals state that individuals with speech problems should be administered the Nonverbal subtests in preference to the other composites. However, the extent to which the Nonverbal IQ is truly "nonverbal" is open to debate. Instructions are generally given verbally, and although verbal responses are for the most part minimal, tasks such as Picture Absurdities require a fairly complex verbal response. (Although the manual states that the answers could be given nonverbally, this would be near impossible in the case of the more complex items.) Further, activities such as Procedural Knowledge demand considerable auditory comprehension. This differs substantially from the recommended requirements for nonverbal tests (see Jensen, 1980, and our review of the *TONI-3*).

To clarify this, the manual indicates that the terms "Nonverbal" and "Verbal" are used in "relative, comparative terms" in the SB5 (Roid, 2003b, p. 134). According to the authors, a more precise description for the Nonverbal domain is that it has lesser language demands, while the Verbal domain requires expressive language or reading skills. The term "Nonverbal IQ" should therefore not be seen as signifying that the Nonverbal IQ score is equivalent to scores from tests such as the Raven's, UNIT, or TONI-3, which eliminate all need for examiner or examinee language. Rather, it should be seen as equivalent to other composites measuring primarily visual-spatial, fluid reasoning, non-language abilities from other major IQ tests (e.g., PIQ, POI, or PRI from Wechsler batteries). In addition,

more evidence for the utility of Nonverbal IQ would be helpful, as correlations with other multifactorial tests such as the UNIT reported in the Technical Manual were only moderately high. Further evidence in clinical samples with limited receptive and/or expressive language deficits is also needed, given that the Nonverbal/Verbal discrepancies in clinical samples in the Technical Manual were not very large (see *Validity*).

Ability-Achievement Discrepancies

The authors recommend the use of the five factor scores for diagnosing LD instead of a single subtest score, because of their higher reliability and concordance with the separate achievement domains identified in IDEA legislation.

Users should employ the WJ III ACH when calculating ability-achievement discrepancies with the SB5. The two tests are linked through a sample of about 500 children who were administered both measures, and tables are provided in the SB5 Manual for determining discrepancies. In addition to this, the WJ III ACH is the recommended achievement measure because of the similarities between the mean scores on both tests, likely due to the contemporaneous standardization of the two batteries. In contrast, WIAT-II scores appear to be slightly higher than SB5 scores, which would complicate comparisons between the tests. Users should note that the WJ III ACH is actually conormed with its own intelligence test battery, the WJ III COG, which provides a broader assessment of CHC factors than does the SB5. Note also that the linking sample between SB5 and WJ III ACH contains only school-aged children and adolescents up to age 19. Other instruments should therefore be used for diagnosing learning disabilities in college-aged students and adults (e.g., WAIS-III/WIAT-II, WJ III COG/WJ III ACH).

Utility in Neuropsychological Populations

Because the SB5 does not measure processing speed, a function important in the differential diagnosis of several important neuropsychological conditions, the test may find less favor among neuropsychologists than among psychoeducational specialists. Additionally, clinical data on groups typically seen by neuropsychologists (e.g., TBI, AD) is lacking at present.

REFERENCES

Binet, A., & Simon, T. (1905). Méthodes nouvelles pour le diagnostic du niveau intellectuel des anormaux. *L'année psychologique, 11,* 191–244.

Bracken, B. A., & McCallum, R. S. (1998). *The Universal Nonverbal Intelligence Test.* Itasca, IL: Riverside Publishing.

Flanagan, D. P., & Ortiz, S. O. (2001). *Essentials of cross-battery assessment.* New York: John Wiley & Sons.

Ittenbach, R. F. (1997). The history of test development. In D. P. Flanagan, J. L. Genshaft, & P. L. Harrison (Eds.), *Contemporary intellectual assessment: Theories, tests and issues* (pp. 17–31). New York: The Guilford Press.

Roid, G. H. (2003a). *Stanford-Binet Intelligence Scales, Fifth Edition.* Itasca, IL: Riverside Publishing.

Roid, G. H. (2003b). *Stanford-Binet Intelligence Scales, Fifth Edition, examiner's manual.* Itasca, IL: Riverside Publishing.

Roid, G. H. (2003c). *Stanford-Binet Intelligence Scales, Fifth Edition, technical manual.* Itasca, IL: Riverside Publishing.

Roid, G. H. (2003d). *SB5 Scoring Pro [Computer Software].* Stanford-Binet Intelligence Scales, Fifth Edition. Itasca, IL: Riverside Publishing.

Roid, G. H. (in press). *Stanford-Binet Intelligence Scales, Fifth Edition, interpretative manual.* Itasca, IL: Riverside Publishing.

Roid, G. H., & Barram, R. A. (2004). *Essentials of Stanford-Binet Intelligence Scales, Fifth Edition (SB5) assessment.* Hoboken, NJ: John Wiley & Sons.

Terman, L. M. (1916). *The measurement of intelligence.* Boston: Houghton Mifflin.

Terman, L. M., & Merrill, M. A. (1937). *Measuring intelligence: A guide to the administration of the new Revised Stanford-Binet Tests of Intelligence.* Boston: Houghton Mifflin.

Terman, L. M., & Merrill, M. A. (1960). *Stanford-Binet Intelligence Scale, Form L-M.* Boston: Houghton Mifflin.

Terman, L. M., & Merrill, M. A. (1973). *Stanford-Binet Intelligence Scale: Manual for the Third Revision Form L-M (1972 norms tables by R.L. Thorndike).* Boston: Houghton Mifflin.

Thorndike, R. L., Hagen, E. P., & Sattler, J. M. (1986). *Stanford-Binet Intelligence Scale—Fourth Edition guide for administering and scoring.* Itasca, IL: Riverside Publishing.

The Test of Nonverbal Intelligence—3 (TONI-3)

PURPOSE

The TONI-3 is a measure of nonverbal intelligence.

SOURCE

The test can be obtained from PRO-ED (www.proedinc.com). The Complete Kit costs $256 US.

AGE RANGE

The test can be administered from ages 6 to 89 years, 11 months.

DESCRIPTION

The TONI-3 (Brown et al., 1997) is the third revision of the TONI, first published in 1982 (Brown et al., 1982) and revised in 1990 (TONI-2; Brown et al., 1990). The TONI-3 is somewhat briefer (10 fewer items) than the TONI-2 and has a newer, larger standardization sample.

The TONI-3 is a test of intelligence that does not involve language in its administration, item content, or response modality (Brown et al., 1997). According to the authors, this makes it well suited for assessing patients with aphasia, dyslexia, language disabilities, learning disabilities, and speech problems as a result of developmental disability or neurological impairment. It is also reportedly useful in assessing persons who have difficulty reading or writing because of limited exposure to English. The lack of words, symbols, numbers, or pictures is supposed to reduce the cultural loading of the test.

The test is comprised of five training items and 45 test items of progressively increasing difficulty. Items resemble matrix analogy-type tests; each page depicts a stimulus figure and a set of possible responses (four or six choices). See Figure 6–22 for a sample item. The examiner pantomimes instructions, and the subject may point, nod, or gesture in response. Individuals with profound motor impairments can respond with eye blink, head stick, light beam, or other method (Brown et al., 1997).

According to its authors, the TONI-3 is not based on any particular theory of intelligence. However, it is intended to be a strong measure of general intelligence (g) and to measure fluid intelligence (Gf) rather than crystallized intelligence (Gc). Instead of other nonverbal skills, abstract reasoning and problem solving were chosen as the basis of the TONI-3 because (a) they are thought to be a major component of general intelligence, (b) they are called upon in everyday life, (c) they allow a language-free, motor-reduced testing format, and (d) they allow items to be novel and culture-free. Item content covers seven different abstract reasoning and problem-solving skills: generalization/classification, discrimination, analogous reasoning, seriation, induction, deduction, and detail recognition (Brown et al., 1997).

Jensen (1980) suggests that language- and culture-free tests should follow seven guidelines: (1) assess performance rather than paper-and-pencil skills, (2) provide pantomimed instructions, not verbal or written, (3) include practice items, (4) be untimed, (5) have abstract content, (6) assess reasoning/problem solving rather than acquired information, and (7) use novel problem solving, not previously learned information. According to the test authors, the TONI-3 meets all these guidelines.

Figure 6–22 TONI-3 Sample Item. *Source:* Reprinted with permission from Brown et al., 1997.

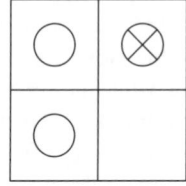

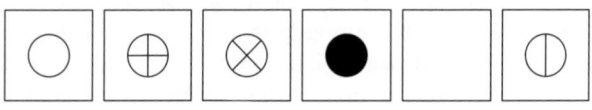

ADMINISTRATION TIME

The test takes 15 to 20 minutes.

ADMINISTRATION

See manual. All examinees start with number 1; a ceiling is attained when the subject fails three out of five items. Test items are presented in a spiral-bound stimulus book. Responses are recorded by the examiner on a separate response sheet and are untimed. There are two equivalent forms (A and B).

SCORING

Raw scores are converted to Deviation Quotients (i.e., standard score format with mean of 100 and *SD* of 15) and to percentile ranks. Only one conversion table is used for both forms because the two forms are "psychometrically equivalent" (Brown et al., 1997, p. 43). Age equivalents can also be derived. However, the authors note that these should be used with extreme caution, both because of the commonly known psychometric limitations of age equivalents and because TONI-3 age equivalents involved smoothing, interpolation, and extrapolation from the original raw score distributions.

DEMOGRAPHIC EFFECTS

Age

TONI-3 scores are strongly related to age up until age 17; they then plateau and begin to decline around age 60 (Brown et al., 1997).

Gender

The manual indicates that females obtain an average score of 101 on Form A of the TONI-3, whereas males have an average score of 99. However, no significant gender effects are reported in the manual.

Education

No information on the impact of education and TONI-3 scores is available.

Ethnicity

The manual indicates that speakers of English as a second language, African American persons, and individuals of Hispanic origin obtain average scores of 93, 95, and 96, respectively, on the TONI-3. This is taken as evidence of the test's suitability across culture and ethnicity (Brown et al., 1997). However, as DeMauro (2001) points out, this means that African American individuals score about a third of a standard deviation below the total sample mean. This indicates that the test may not be as culture-free as claimed by the authors and may be subject to cultural influences, as are most of the so-called nonverbal and culture-free tests in existence.

NORMATIVE DATA

Standardization Data

Norms are based on 3451 subjects tested in 1995 and 1996. The demographics correspond to the 1990 U.S. Census, stratified according to age, gender, race, ethnicity, location, community size, and other SES factors. Table 6–114 shows the characteristics of the normative sample. Overall, the TONI-3 has a comprehensive, inclusive, and well-constructed normative sample.

RELIABILITY

Internal Reliability

Internal reliability is excellent. The manual reports internal reliability both for the normative sample as well as for selected subgroups defined by gender, race, and disability. For these, coefficient alpha values ranged from .89 to .97.

Standard Error of Measurement (*SEM*)

Average *SEM*s range from three to five points for both test forms.

Test-Retest Reliability

Test-retest reliability is also excellent. Information on stability over time is provided for 170 subjects, tested after a one-week interval (see manual). Coefficients range from .89 to .94 for three age groups (13, 15, and 19 to 40 years). However, information on stability in subjects younger than age 13 or in those over age 40 is lacking.

Practice Effects

Information on practice effects (i.e., test-retest means) is not provided in the manual. However, one study found that although TONI-3 scores increased when solutions were attained by students collaboratively, there was no carry-over effect when students were retested with a subset of items and asked to work on solutions independently (Samaha & De Lisi, 2000).

Alternate Form Reliability

The manual reports that reliability of Forms A and B was tested with an immediate administration paradigm (i.e., both forms administered during one testing session). Means differed by less than two raw score points at all ages, with an actual mean difference between forms of one-half of a raw score point. The average correlation between forms across age was .84; however, correlations between forms were not

Table 6–114 Characteristics of the TONI-3 Normative Sample

Normative Sample	School-Age Sample	Adult Sample
Number	3451 subjects in total	
Age	6–18 years[a]	19–89 years[a]
Geographic location[b]		
Northeast	20%	20%
Midwest	24%	25%
South	36%	36%
West	20%	19%
Sample Type	Stratified, national random sample[c]	
Parental Education/Education		
<Bachelor's Degree	75%	73%
Bachelor's Degree	19%	20%
Master's, Professional, Doctoral Degrees	6%	7%
SES	Data on family income presented in the manual (p. 73–74)	
Gender		
Males	51%	47%
Females	49%	53%
Race/Ethnicity		
White	79%	82%
Black	13%	12%
Other	8%	6%
Ethnicity		
Native American	2%	1%
Hispanic	12%	10%
Asian	2%	1%
African American	13%	12%
Other	71%	76%
Disability Status		
No Disability	89%	92%
Learning Disability	6%	3%
Speech-Language Disorder	1%	2%
Mental Retardation	1%	1%
Other Disability	3%	2%
Screening	None noted; individuals with disabilities are included in Census-consistent proportions	

[a]Based on 23 age groupings represented by six-month age bands (6 to 10 years, 11 months), one-year age bands (11 to 16 years, 11 months), and five-year age bands (55 to 79 years, 11 months), as well as an age band from 80 to 89 years, 11 months. [b]Norms were also stratified based on rural versus urban residence. [c]Based on 1990 U.S. Census data.

Source: Adapted from Brown et al., 1997.

uniformly high across all age groups (range .74–.95; see manual for further details). This suggests that the two forms may not necessarily be interchangeable at all age levels. As noted above, a single set of norms is designed to be used with both forms.

Interrater Reliability

Interscorer reliability is high ($r = .99$), according to information presented in the manual.

VALIDITY

Content Validity

In constructing the test, TONI-3 items were selected with care and with regard to theories of nonverbal intellectual functioning, and were evaluated with classical item analysis and differential functioning analysis, the latter to eliminate bias (see pp. 87–94 of test manual for more details).

Factor Structure

Factor analysis, described in the manual, supports the presence of a general factor.

Correlations With Previous Versions

The manual does not provide correlations between the TONI-3 and previous test versions, nor is there information on mean score differences between versions. Presumably, the TONI-3 yields lower standard scores than its predecessor because it is anchored to a newer standardization sample. This information would be of utility for clinicians who may reevaluate patients who were originally tested with an older version.

Correlations With Other Nonverbal IQ tests

Correlations with other nonverbal IQ tests are high and of a magnitude typically observed between standard IQ tests. For example, in a sample of 550 adults reported in the manual, correlations with a test of nonverbal ability, the CTONI (Hammill et al., 1996) were .76 with the Full-Scale IQ score, and .74 and .64 with the Pictorial and Geometric Nonverbal IQ subscales (Brown et al., 1997). One recent study with Greek individuals with Parkinson's disease reported a correlation of .73 between the TONI-2 and Raven's Progressive Matrices (Bostantjopoulou et al., 2001).

Correlations With Standard IQ Tests

Correlations with standard IQ tests are high (Brown et al., 1997). Based on information presented in the manual on a small group of students with learning disabilities, correlation with the WISC-III FSIQ is high ($r = .63$), with no major differences between correlations to VIQ and PIQ ($r = .59$ and .56, respectively). Correlation with the WAIS-R is also high in those with LD ($r = .73$), with slightly higher correlation with PIQ than VIQ ($r = .75$ and .57, respectively). Note that these correlations are based on very small samples (i.e., $N = 34$ and 19, respectively). In addition, no information on mean performance differences between these scales and the TONI-3 is provided in the manual. Information on typically developing individuals, other clinical groups, or on the TONI-3's relationship to other, more recent Wechsler scales (i.e., WAIS-III, WISC-IV) is also lacking.

Fifteen studies on prior research with the TONI-2 and TONI are presented in the manual as further evidence of test validity. Of these, only three have samples of over 50 individuals and are published in peer-reviewed journals. They indicate a moderate correlation between TONI and WISC-R VIQ and a moderate to high correlation with the WISC-R PIQ ($r = .44–.64$) in learning disabled and/or mentally handicapped children.

Correlations With Achievement

Correlations with achievement are high. For example, correlations to the WJ-R Broad Reading and Broad Math are strong ($r = .73$ and .76, respectively), as reported in the manual for a group of 20 students with LD. Notably, despite the assumption that the TONI-3 should assess novel problem solving and not acquired knowledge, correlation with the WJ-R Broad Knowledge is also strong ($r = .56$). Correlations summarized from two studies involving the WRAT and WRAT-R indicate small to moderate correlations between TONI scores and reading, math, and spelling ($r = .28–.38$; see manual for details and correlations with other achievement tests involving previous TONI versions).

Clinical Studies

The manual presents mean scores for several clinical groups (i.e., gifted, dyslexic, deaf, ADHD, RD, LD, emotionally disturbed, and mentally handicapped). According to the information on clinical groups provided, individuals with mental handicaps obtain the lowest mean score (i.e., 71), with other groups obtaining broadly average scores (i.e., 93–111). However, the information shown has only limited clinical relevance because only average group scores are reported, with no associated *SDs*, or percentages within each group attaining clinical cut-offs. Other clinically relevant information such as statistical comparison between clinical groups or comparison with matched controls is not provided. Groups are also not described with regard to demographic characteristics or diagnostic criteria.

Based on the mean performance of a group of gifted children presented in the manual, Sattler (2001) points out that the TONI-3 is limited in its ability to identify gifted individuals (mean score of 110). As noted, the mean TONI-3 score for the mentally handicapped subgroup borders the diagnostic cutoff of 70 and suggests that a number of individuals had scores above the cutoff for intellectual deficit (see *Comment* for discussion of TONI-3 limitations in mental retardation diagnosis).

COMMENT

Some assets of the TONI-3 are its brevity, its lack of reliance on verbal instructions or responses, and its largely motor-free format suitable for most clinical populations. Its manual is well written, includes a comprehensive overview of intelligence testing and nonverbal assessment, and covers several topics of interest, including the use of special norms (i.e., for demographically defined subpopulations) and a detailed discussion of test bias. Unlike many tests, it includes information on internal reliability in different subgroups (e.g., defined by demographic characteristics or clinical condition). Lastly, its forced-choice format may make it useful when suboptimal effort is a concern. However, this has not been formally studied.

The TONI-3 also has a number of limitations. According to McCallum and Bracken (1997), authors of the UNIT, the TONI-2 has a weak theoretical foundation and one-dimensional assessment focus. Although Athanasiou (2000) reported that the TONI-3 was a generally sound instrument, she noted that information on test-retest reliability for upper ages and on predictive validity was scant. Sattler (2001) lists other limitations of the TONI-3, including its reliance on figural reasoning as a measure of intelligence and limited applicability in the assessment of giftedness.

We are most concerned with its limited sensitivity to intellectual impairment. Specifically, the test suffers from significant floor effects. For example, the lowest score possible for a 6-year-old is a standard score of 70, which is the cutoff for diagnosing intellectual impairment. The same problem applies to 80-year-olds, whose lowest possible standard score is 68. The lowest possible standard score across age is only 60, if the subject obtains a score of 0. Consequently, the test should not be used to diagnose intellectual impairments in children or in older adults, and should definitely not be used to yield estimates of the severity of intellectual impairments (i.e., mild, moderate, or severe) in any age group. This significantly limits its clinical utility. Also of concern are its inadequate coverage and analysis of the clinical group data presented in the manual as evidence of validity. Validity information involving populations of interest to neuropsychologists is also quite limited.

There exist surprisingly few studies on the TONI-3 in minorities or ethnic/cultural subgroups to support the view that it is culturally fair, or that it is an accurate assessment method for those whose primary language is not English. Although the manual includes a lengthy discussion of bias and a convincing rationale as to why the TONI-3 would be useful in the assessment of individuals from different cultures, there are few empirical data presented on the test's use in this regard. While it may be "as free of bias as possible" (Brown et al., 1997, p. 123) based on item analysis and psychometric criteria such as internal reliability across groups, criterion validity is limited, particularly in the form of published studies on the TONI-3. Overall, there is an inadequate research basis for supporting the authors' claim that "the TONI-3 is an equally reliable and valid measure for . . . racial and ethnic subgroups, for people who speak English fluently and people who do not, and for people with various sensory and intellectual exceptionalities" (Brown et al., 1997, p. 124).

Some aspects of the psychometric properties of the TONI-3 are also weak. Although internal reliability and test-retest reliability are excellent, alternate form reliability is less than adequate for some age ranges, and correlations between forms presented in the manual are not overly strong at some ages. Concurrent validity data on the test's relationship to standard IQ tests such as the Wechsler scales are inadequate (e.g., derived from small, atypical samples). Further, because the manual restricts itself to correlations, it is difficult to determine how standard scores from the TONI-3 compare with scores from other IQ tests. As a result, it is virtually impossible, in a clinical context, to evaluate change in individual patients whose prior IQ scores were based on other IQ tests or on previous versions of the TONI-3. Sizeable correlations with tests of verbal ability and acquired knowledge are not well explained. Information on practice effects is lacking, as is test-retest reliability information in clinical samples and in children.

Although it might be of use as a screening measure, Sattler recommends using Wechsler tests, SB-IV, or DAS instead, or supplementing the TONI-3 with a verbal test for screening purposes. Although the test authors state that the test is intended to identify subjects with intellectual impairments (Brown et al., 1997), we do not recommend this test when intellectual impairment is suspected, or when comparisons with other IQ tests will be needed to monitor patients over time.

REFERENCES

Athanasiou, M. S. (2000). Current nonverbal assessment instruments: A comparison of psychometric integrity. *Journal of Psychoeducational Assessment, 18,* 211–229.

Bostantjopoulou, S., Kiosseoglou, G., Katsarou, Z., & Alevriadou, A. (2001). Concurrent validity of the Test of Nonverbal Intelligence in Parkinson's disease patients. *The Journal of Psychology, 135*(2), 205–212.

Brown, J., Sherbenou, R. J., & Johnsen, S. (1982). *Test of Nonverbal Intelligence.* Austin, TX: Pro-Ed.

Brown, J., Sherbenou, R. J., & Johnsen, S. (1990). *Test of Nonverbal Intelligence—Second Edition.* Austin, TX: Pro-Ed.

Brown, L., Sherbenou, R. J., & Johnson, S. K. (1997). *Test of Nonverbal Intelligence: A language-free measure of cognitive ability—Third Edition.* Austin, TX: Pro-Ed.

D'Amato, R. K., Lidtak, S. P., & Lassiter, K. S. (1994). Comparing verbal and nonverbal intellectual functioning with the TONI and WISC-R. *Perceptual and Motor Skills, 78,* 701–702.

DeMauro, G. E. (2001). Review of the Test of Nonverbal Intelligence, Third Edition. In B. S. Plake & J. C. Impara (Eds.), *Buros Mental Measurements Yearbook* (14th ed.), pp. 1260–1262. Lincoln, NE: Buros Institute of Mental Measurements.

Hammill, D. D., Pearson, N. A., & Wiederholt, J. L. (1996). *Comprehensive Test of Nonverbal Intelligence.* Austin, TX: Pro-Ed.

Jensen, A. R. (1980). *Bias in mental testing.* New York: Free Press.

Kowall, M. A., Watson, G. M., & Madak, P. R. (1990). Concurrent validity of the Test of Nonverbal Intelligence with referred suburban and Canadian native children. *Journal of Clinical Psychology, 46,* 632–636.

Lopez, E. (1997). Cognitive assessment of LEP and bilingual children. In D. P. Flanagan, J. L. Genshaft, & P. L. Harrison (Eds.), *Contemporary intellectual assessment: Theories, tests, and issues* (pp. 503–516). New York: The Guilford Press.

McCallum, R. S., & Bracken, B. A. (1997). The Universal Nonverbal Intelligence Test. In D. P. Flanagan, J. L. Genshaft, & P. L. Harrison (Eds.), *Contemporary intellectual assessment: Theories, tests, and issues* (pp. 268–280). New York: The Guilford Press.

Salvia, J., & Ysseldyke, J. E. (1995). *Assessment* (6th ed.). Boston: Houghton Mifflin.

Samaha, N. V., & De Lisi, R. (2000). Peer collaboration on nonverbal reasoning task by urban minority students. *Journal of Experimental Education, 69*(1), 5–17.

Sattler, J. M. (2001). *Assessment of children: Cognitive applications* (4th ed.). San Diego: Jerome M. Sattler, Publisher, Inc.

The Speed and Capacity of Language Processing Test (SCOLP)

PURPOSE

The SCOLP consists of two tasks. The first, the Speed of Comprehension Test (Silly Sentences or SST) measures rate of information processing. The second, the Spot-the-Word Test (STW), estimates premorbid verbal ability and provides a framework for interpreting the results of the first test.

SOURCE

The SCOLP (manual, parallel versions, and test forms) can be ordered from Harcourt Assessment (www.harcourt-uk.com), at a cost of about $190 US (£99.87 pounds).

AGE RANGE

Normative data are available for ages 16 and above.

DESCRIPTION

Neurological damage tends to result in a slowing in the rate of information processing. The SCOLP (Baddeley et al., 1992) was designed to provide a measure of this slowing, particularly with regard to language comprehension. This brief, easily administered measure comprises two subtests. The SST requires individuals to verify simple sentences, half of which are true (e.g., "Rats have teeth") and half of which are false (e.g., "Nuns are sold in pairs"). The false statements were produced by mismatching the subject and predicate from two true statements. The individual is given two minutes to evaluate as many of the 100 sentences as possible. Four parallel versions of the test (versions A, B, C, D) are available for the purpose of repeat testing. Each set of 100 sentences has an instruction page with a brief explanation of the test together with six practice items.

The authors note that the speed of verifying statements is related to verbal intelligence. Thus, poor performance may reflect the effect of neurological disturbance or intact performance in an individual with low verbal skills. Accordingly, the authors recommend that the SST be given in conjunction with the STW, which provides an estimate of crystallized verbal intelligence that is much less likely to be influenced by brain damage.

The STW is a brief lexical decision task that consists of 60 pairs of letter strings, each pair comprising one genuine word and one pseudo-word (e.g., kitchen–harrick). Participants work at their own rate, ticking the item they regard as the genuine word. Two parallel versions, A and B, are available. Each set of 60 item pairs has an instruction page with a brief explanation of the test together with six practice items.

The extent to which a person's speed of comprehension on the SST falls below that anticipated by their STW performance allows the clinician to determine whether poor performance on the SST represents a genuine decrement secondary to brain damage or the intact performance of an individual with low verbal functioning. Baddeley et al. (1992) indicate that the STW may also be useful as a broad estimate of premorbid ability. They caution, however, that it was designed principally to aid in the interpretation of the SST.

ADMINISTRATION

See *Source*. For the SST, the patient is presented with one of the parallel versions and the examiner instructs the patient to put a check mark if the sentence is true or sensible and put a cross if the sentence is false or silly. The person must complete as many sentences as possible within two minutes. The authors (Baddeley et al., 1992) suggest that if it is necessary to test people on more than four separate occasions, the examiner can require the person to complete just one page (i.e., 50 sentences) on each occasion, record the time to complete that page as a measure, and estimate the number that would have been completed in two minutes on the basis of the calculated mean time per sentence.

For the STW, the examiner instructs the patient to place a check mark beside the real word in each pair. Guessing is encouraged when the person is uncertain about a word pair. The test is untimed.

ADMINISTRATION TIME

The approximate time required for each task is about five minutes.

SCORING

Scoring templates are provided for each task. For the SST, the total number of sentences completed in the two-minute period is recorded on the test form along with the number of errors. Provided the error rate is small (<10%), the examiner converts the number completed into an age-based scaled score (1–19) or percentile score by means of tables provided in the test manual.

For the STW, the number correct is entered on the test form. Tables in the test manual allow the examiner to obtain age-scaled or percentile scores. The scaled score on the SST is subtracted from the scaled score on the STW. If the scaled score on the SST is lower than the scaled score on the STW, the examiner then refers to a table in the manual that reveals the likelihood of such a discrepancy given that particular vocabulary level. If the difference between the SST and STW is significant and large, then verbal information processing problems may be inferred.

DEMOGRAPHIC EFFECTS

SST

Age. Performance decreases with advancing age (Baddeley et al., 1992; Saxton et al., 2001).

Gender. Although Baddeley et al. (1992) reported a gender difference (with advancing age, males were worse than females), others have not (Saxton et al., 2001).

Education/SES. Education and social class impact performance (Baddeley et al., 1992; Saxton et al., 2001), with the mean number of items correct showing increases with higher social status or education.

STW

Age. The influence of age appears slight. Some have reported that scores improve with increasing age (Baddeley et al., 1992, 1993; Crowell et al., 2002), while others have found no impact of age on test scores (Saxton et al., 2001; Yuspeh & Vanderploeg, 2000).

Gender. Gender does not affect performance (Baddeley et al., 1992, 1993; Crowell et al., 2002; Jorm et al., 2004; Saxton et al., 2001; Yuspeh & Vanderploeg, 2000).

Education/SES. Performance is higher with increases in education and social level (Baddeley et al., 1992; Crowell et al., 2002; Saxton et al., 2001; Watt & O'Carroll, 1999; Yuspeh & Vanderploeg, 2000).

NORMATIVE DATA

Standardization Sample

Baddeley et al. (1992) compiled data for the SCOLP from a stratified sample of 224 volunteers, with approximately equal numbers from each of six social class bands and from four age bands (16–31, 32–47, 48–64, 65–80; Table 6–115). However, the norms provided in the test manual reach to only age 64 and are based on a U.K. sample.

Table 6–115 Characteristics of the SCOLP Normative Sample

Number	224
Age	16–64 years
Geographic location	UK
Sample type	Stratified sample of volunteers with approximately equal numbers sampled from each of six social class bands and from four age bands 16–31, 32–47, 48–64, and 65–80
Education	Not reported
Gender	Not reported
Race/ethnicity	Not reported
Screening	Not reported

Other Normative Data

Saxton et al. (2001) presented normative data for both tasks derived from 424 older adults between 75 and 94 years of age ($M = 81.6$ years) residing in a rural, nonfarming American community (Southwestern Pennsylvania) in economic decline (race not reported). Individuals with evidence of moderate cognitive impairment (e.g., MMSE scores below 24) were excluded, as were people with error rates greater than 12.5% on the SST. Normative data were constructed as described in the SCOLP Manual (Baddeley et al., 1992). Raw scores for both subtests were z-score transformed to a 19-point scale with a mean of 10 and standard deviations of 3. These data are shown in Tables 6–116 and 6–117. If the scaled score on the SST is lower than the scaled score on the STW test, then reference to Table 6–118 will reveal the frequency of such a discrepancy occurring for a given STW score in a participant of a given age. In calculating the discrepancy score, it is expected that an individual's STW score will be higher than the SST score. Although this is the typical finding, some normal individuals may well have a lower STW scaled score. Saxton et al. (2001) noted that among the elderly, many people ended their formal education quite young because of financial and/or family needs and not necessarily because of intellectual difficulty.

Crowell et al. (2002) have recently provided data for the STW test based on 394 healthy, American older adults, aged 60 to 85, dwelling in communities in Florida. The racial composition was largely Caucasian (98.25%). The data are somewhat higher than those reported by Saxton et al. (2001), perhaps reflecting differences in cultural experiences or health status between the samples. Table 6–119 provides the normative frequency distributions for the STW scores in the Crowell et al. sample as well as IQ equivalent scores that are associated with each given cumulative percentile rank. Because significant and moderate effects were found for education ($r = .43$), normative adjustments are provided for education. The study by Crowell et al. (2002) complements the data that focuses on less-educated people (e.g., Saxton et al., 2001) and may be preferred for use with Caucasian adults living in economically stable regions of North America.

Prediction of Premorbid Ability Other Than IQ. Senior et al. (2001) reported moderate relations between the STW and the Boston Naming Test ($r = .45$) and the Controlled Oral Word Association (FAS; $r = .38$) scores in a normal sample of individuals living in Australia. Accordingly, using multiple regression techniques, they suggested that STW raw scores could be used to predict expected raw scores on naming and verbal fluency tasks. The equations are as follows:

Boston Naming Test predicted
$= 36.865 + .355$ (STW raw), $SE_E = 3.30$

FAS predicted
$= .757$ (STW raw) $+ .77$ (years of education) $- 4.747$,
$SE_E = 10.8$

Tables 6–120 (Boston Naming Test-STW) and 6–121 (FAS-STW) can be consulted to determine whether the discrepancy between obtained and expected scores is unusual. Thus, the clinician should (a) use the regression equation to generate the predicted score, (b) subtract the obtained score from the predicted score, ensuring that the subtraction is in the correct direction (i.e., predicted-observed score), (c) using the tables, determine the level of performance using the criterion and ranking for the test to generate the predicted score (this is necessary to compensate for differing restrictions in range of difference scores characteristic of high versus low performance levels), and (d) consult the difference table and determine the frequency of the discrepancy in the normative sample. Note that the direction that cognitive deterioration is most likely to manifest itself is with abnormally large positive difference scores that correspond to the 90th, 95th, and 99th percentiles.

Graves and Carswell (2003) have also developed a regression equation to predict Boston Naming Test scores using scores from the STW. The equation is based on 98 community-dwelling, healthy older adults and is similar to the one provided by Senior et al. (see also *BNT*). The equation is given below:

Predicted BNT score
$= 33.668 + 0.423$(STW raw score); $SE_E = 2.72$ items

RELIABILITY

SST

Internal Consistency. Baddeley et al (1992) report that a sample of 25 people (demographics not provided) was tested with the SST on two occasions separated by a mean of about 19 days, performing version A of the test on one occasion and version B on the other. Participants were separately timed over the first 25 and second 25 sentences on each occasion. The correlation between performance on these two halves was .84 for the first session and .87 for second, suggesting good split-half reliability for these abbreviated versions.

Test-Retest Reliability, Alternate-Form Reliability, and Practice Effects. Baddeley et al. (1992) reported that parallel form

Table 6–116 Speed of Comprehension Test (SST) Scaled Scores by Age Group

Number Completed in 2 min	Age Group (Years)			Number Completed in 2 min	Age Group (Years)		
	75–79	80–84	85+		75–79	80–84	85+
6			1[a]	40	9	11	12
7			1[a]	41	9	11	13[a]
8			2[a]	42	10	11	13
9		1[a]	2[a]	43	10	12	13[a]
10		1[a]	2[a]	44	10	12	14[a]
11		1[a]	3[a]	45	11	12	14[a]
12	1[a]	2[a]	3[a]	46	11	12	14
13	1[a]	2[a]	3[a]	47	11	13	15[a]
14	1[a]	2[a]	4[a]	48	12	13[a]	15
15	1	2[a]	4[a]	49	12	13	15
16	2[a]	3[a]	4[a]	50	12	14	16[a]
17	2[a]	3[a]	5[a]	51	13	14	16[a]
18	2[a]	3	5[a]	52	13	14	16
19	3[a]	4	5	53	13	15	17[a]
20	3	4	6	54	13[a]	15	17[a]
21	3[a]	4	6	55	14	15	17[a]
22	4[a]	5	6[a]	56	14	16	18[a]
23	4[a]	5[a]	7	57	14	16	18[a]
24	4	5	7	58	15	16[a]	18[a]
25	4[a]	6	7[a]	59	15	17[a]	19[a]
26	5	6	8[a]	60	15	17	19[a]
27	5	6	8	61	16[a]	17[a]	19[a]
28	5	7	8	62	16[a]	18[a]	19
29	6	7	9	63	16[a]	18	19[a]
30	6[a]	7	9	64	17[a]	18[a]	19[a]
31	6	8	9	65	17[a]	19[a]	19[a]
32	7	8	10[a]	66	17[a]	19[a]	
33	7	8	10	67	17	19[a]	
34	7	9	10	68	18[a]		
35	8	9	11	69	18[a]		
36	8	9	11	70	18		
37	8	10	11	71	19		
38	8	10	12	72	19[a]		
39	9	10	12	73	19[a]		
				74	19[a]		

N = 424 community-dwelling people, aged 74–95 years, in Southwestern Pennsylvania.
[a]Extrapolations.

Source: From Saxton et al., 2001. Reprinted with the permission of Lawrence Erlbaum Associates, Inc.

reliability (versions A and B) was high (.93). In a larger sample of volunteers, parallel form reliability was also high (.88), although the versions used for these analyses are not indicated (Baddeley et al., 1992). Hinton-Bayre et al. (1997) gave the four alternate forms of the test to rugby players and found the forms to be equivalent in terms of difficulty. Players were tested twice, with a one- to two-week retesting interval. Test-retest reliability of the alternate forms was moderately high (.78), although players improved by an average of 11 sentences on the second exposure, suggesting significant practice effects. Wilson et al. (2000) studied the performance of normal and head-injured people across 20 successive test sessions. They created 10 different forms and used each twice.

Both the normal and brain-injured groups showed an improvement (about 11 seconds) over the 20 occasions, with the control group learning at a faster rate and both groups tending to plateau over the last few occasions.

STW

Internal Consistency.　The authors (Baddeley et al. 1992, 1993) had 50 subjects (aged 20–85 years, M = 38 years; no other information provided) complete versions A and B of the STW. Internal reliability was reported to be good (.78 for version A and .83 for version B).

Table 6–117 Spot-the-Word Test (STW) Scaled Scores by Age Group

Number Correct	Age Group (Years)			Number Correct	Age Group (Years)		
	75–79	80–84	85+		75–79	80–84	85+
30	1[a]	1[a]	1[a]	46	10	10	10
31	1[a]	1[a]	2[a]	47	10	11	10
32	1	1[a]	2[a]	48	11	11	11
33	2[a]	1[a]	3[a]	49	12	12	11
34	3[a]	2[a]	3[a]	50	12	13	12
35	3[a]	3	4	51	13	13	12[a]
36	4	3	4	52	13	14	13
37	4	4	5	53	14	14	14[a]
38	5	5	6	54	15	15	14
39	6	5	6	55	15	16[a]	15
40	6	6	7	56	16[a]	16[a]	15
41	7	7	7	57	17	17	16
42	7	7	8	58	17[a]	18	16
43	8	8	8	59	18[a]	18	17[a]
44	9	9	9	60	18	19[a]	17[a]
45	9	9	9				

N = 424 community-dwelling people, aged 74–95 years, in Southwestern Pennsylvania.

Source: From Saxton et al., 2001. Reprinted with the permission of Lawrence Erlbaum Associates, Inc.

Test-Retest Reliability, Alternate Form Reliability, and Practice Effects. Baddeley et al. (1992, 1993) reported that the correlation between performance on versions A and B was reasonable (.78). In a larger study with healthy volunteers, parallel form reliability yielded a correlation of .88. Hinton-Bayre et al. (1997) constructed abbreviated alternate versions of the task and retested rugby players after a one- to two-week interval. Test-retest reliability was modest (.64). There was no effect of practice on the number of words correctly identified.

VALIDITY

SST

Construct Validity. The SST correlates highly with measures of general language processing capacity (category generation: .52, rapid color naming: .56, semantic categorization: .55, grammatical reasoning: .60, vocabulary: .51, NART: .60, and the STW: .57; Baddeley et al., 1992). Correlations with nonsemantic speeded tasks (e.g., Digit Symbol: .44; Symbol Digit: .44; Letter-Matching: .34–.39) and fluid reasoning (Raven's Matrices: .20) were lower (Baddeley et al., 1992; Hinton-Bayre et al., 1997) .

Clinical Findings. The SST appears sensitive to information-processing deficits associated with mild TBI in the early postinjury phase (Comerford et al., 2002; Hinton-Bayre et al., 1997; Ponsford et al., 2000). Deficits tended to resolve three months postinjury (Ponsford et al., 2000). Impairment has also been reported in patients with schizophrenia

(Tamlyn et al., 1992). No significant impairments, however, were found in patients following repair of a ruptured aneurysm of the anterior communicating artery (Papagno et al., 2003).

Other SST Versions. The paper-and-pencil version is dependent upon literacy and since it was designed for British adults, the items assume a certain cultural familiarity (May et al., 2001). Baddeley et al. (1995) produced an oral version of the task, with simpler materials suitable for children. The items were changed to 40 questions (e.g., "Do cows live under water?"). The whole administration was timed and divided by 40 to obtain a score. In a sample of children, test-retest reliability was reported to be relatively high (.72) after a three-month interval. A computerized version of the oral task has been developed that allows for accuracy as well as decision latencies to be recorded (May et al., 2001). Participants, including children, make few errors on the test and like the standard version, the test does not correlate significantly with scores on the Raven's Matrices (*r* = .09). Preliminary evidence suggests that this oral version appears suitable for use with non-English-speaking preliterate people in developing countries.

STW

Construct Validity. The STW has generally shown adequate convergent validity with other measures of crystallized intelligence and premorbid function. Thus, moderately high correlations have been reported between the STW and the Mill Hill Vocabulary Scale (.60–.71) (Baddeley et al., 1992,

Table 6-118 Comprehension Speed-Vocabulary Discrepancy: Percentile Norms, Overall and by Age Group, for the Spot-the-Word (STW) and Speed of Comprehension (SST) Tests

Scaled STW Score	N	Scaled Score Discrepancy (STW-SST) Percentile			
		25%	10%	5%	1%
Overall					
1–7	99	−1	1	2	3
8–12	244	2	3	4	6
13–19	81	4	6	7	12
Age group: 75–79 years					
1–7	49	0	2	2	2
8–12	95	3	3	4	8
13–19	41	4	5	6	8
Age group: 80–84 years					
1–7	36	−1	0	1	3
8–12	103	2	3	4	7
13–19	36	4	5	7	10
Age group: 85+ years					
1–7	13	0	1	2	2
8–12	40	1	3	3	4
13–19	11	4	8	10	10

N = 424 community-dwelling people, aged 74–95 years, in Southwestern Pennsylvania.

Source: From Saxton et al., 2001. Reprinted with the permission of Lawrence Erlbaum Associates, Inc.

1993) and Wechsler VIQ ($r = .61$) and FSIQ ($r = .58$; Lucas et al., 2003). In a sample of elderly volunteers, Baddeley et al. reported that the STW correlated more strongly with a measure of crystallized (Mill Hill Vocabulary: $r = .86$) than fluid intelligence (AH4: $r = .60$). STW scores correlate highly with NART scores (.58–.86; Baddeley et al., 1992, 1993; Hinton-Bayre et al., 1997) and WRAT-3 Reading scores ($r = .65$; Lucas et al., 2003), suggesting that the STW, NART, and WRAT-3 are measuring a very similar capacity.

There is additional evidence that the STW has good convergent and divergent validity. Yuspeh and Vanderploeg (2000) studied a group of community-dwelling older adults and found that correlations with "nonhold"-type tasks (e.g., Cerad List-Learning, $r = .19$; Symbol Digit Modalities Test, $r = .11$) were low while correlations with other measures used to estimate premorbid IQ were higher (AMNART, $r = .56$; WAIS-R Vocabulary, $r = .58$; note that correlations were higher when corrected for attenuation due to restriction of range in age). The implication is that the STW should be at least relatively stable in the face of neuropsychological impairment, and is therefore a reasonably good measure of premorbid ability.

In fact, Baddeley et al. (1993) hypothesized that the STW would be more resistant to the effects of brain damage than other measures of premorbid ability because it is a fairly basic task with low cognitive demands and relies on a number of parallel processing routes for correct performance (e.g., orthographic appearance, physical appearance, semantic meaning,

and feeling of familiarity of a word) rather than a single factor (Baddeley et al., 1993).

While the STW test appears more resistant than the SST to the effects of brain damage, the literature suggests that it is not immune to such disturbance and that other tests may be preferable. Hinton-Bayre et al. (1997) and Watt and O'Carroll (1999) found that the test is not sensitive to the effects of head trauma. On the other hand, Beardsall and Huppert (1997) reported that performance is grossly impaired in people with mild/moderate dementia. Both the NART and the CCRT (the Cambridge Contextual Reading Test in which NART words are placed in semantic and syntactic context in sentences) proved more resistant to cognitive impairment of mild/moderate severity than did the STW. In addition, the authors noted that demented participants made perseverative errors on the STW, suggesting that it may be unsuitable for patients

Table 6-119 Normative Data for STW Performance for Individuals 60–84 Years of Age

STW Score	Cumulative Percentile	IQ Equivalent[a]
< 34	<1.0	<65
34	1.5	65
35	1.8	67
36	2.8	69
37	3.3	71
38	4.1	73
39	5.1	75
40	7.4	78
41	8.4	79
42	9.4	80
43	13.2	83
44	16.8	86
45	19.3	87
46	25.1	90
47	28.9	92
48	36.0	95
49	42.6	97
50	50.5	100
51	59.6	103
52	68.3	107
53	74.6	110
54	82.0	113
55	85.8	116
56	90.1	119
57	93.7	123
58	97.0	128
59	99.0	135
60	100.0	>135

The above scores provide normative performance data for elderly individuals aged 60–84. To obtain an education-adjusted performance comparison, from the obtained score add or subtract the following adjustments for education prior to looking up level of performance information: years of completed formal education: <12 years, add 5; 12–15 years, add 1; 16+ years, subtract 2.

[a]"IQ equivalent" is meant as the IQ score associated with each given cumulative percentile score.

Source: From Crowell et al., 2002. Reprinted with permission from Elsevier.

Table 6–120 BNT Predicted From STW Raw Score

Ranking	Criterion
Low	STW raw score <46
Average	STW raw score 46–53
High	STW raw score >53

STW	n	BNT Pred—BNT									Descriptives		
		1%	5%	10%	25%	50%	75%	90%	95%	99%	M	SD	SE$_E$
Low	68	−10.8	−9.5	−5.9	−1.8	0.9	3.2	4.5	6.1	8.6	0.22	4.14	0.50
Average	207	−9.3	−6.6	−4.4	−2.3	0.3	2.1	3.7	4.4	5.4	−0.20	3.2	0.22
High	59	−6.7	−4.4	−2.4	−0.7	0.9	2.5	3.0	3.6	4.0	0.45	2.3	0.30
Total	334	−9.9	−6.6	−4.3	−1.9	0.45	2.4	3.7	4.5	6.4	0.0	3.3	0.18

Source: From Senior et al., 2001. Based on a sample of 334 Australian adults (134 males, 200 females), mean age = 33.2 (*SD* = 13.0); mean education = 12.6 (*SD* = 2.2). Reprinted with permission of the authors.

with frontal lobe dysfunction. Papagno and Baddeley (1997), however, described a confabulating patient with evidence of frontal/executive dysfunction who performed without error on an Italian version of the test.

There are additional concerns about the utility of the STW. Watt and O'Carroll (1999) found in a sample of normal healthy people correlations of only moderate degree between the STW and the NART (.69) and the WAIS-R Verbal IQ (.54). The NART and CCRT accounted for about 50% of the variance in Verbal IQ, whereas the STW accounted for only 29%. The more modest relation with what many consider as the "gold standard" of current verbal intelligence, the Wechsler test, is somewhat disappointing and suggests that there is considerable opportunity for error in estimating premorbid Verbal IQ from the STW. Note that to date, studies have evaluated the STW in relation to the WAIS-R. It would be worthwhile to consider the WAIS-III IQ and index scores.

COMMENT

The STW is a brief, easy to administer measure of premorbid functioning in individuals who have had a lengthy exposure to English reading material (Graves et al., 1999). Because it does not involve a spoken response, it can be given to people with aphasic or articulatory problems. It can even be administered as a group test (Baddeley et al., 1993). It can also be presented auditorily, although normative data are only available for the visual presentation format. Computer administration is also possible, facilitating analysis of mean reaction time and variability (Comerford et al., 2002). The availability of algorithms to predict premorbid abilities other than IQ (word generation, naming) is also an asset.

However, correlations with Wechsler test results tend to be disappointing, and some studies have reported better results using other tests of premorbid ability. Further, although the test appears relatively robust in the face of neurological insult, it is not resistant to cognitive decline. It should also be noted that performance on the STW, like other tests of premorbid functioning (e.g., NART), is affected by depression (Watt & O'Carroll, 1999). The fact that depression can increase errors on the test raises the concern of underestimation of premorbid ability and, as a result, false negatives (that is, failing to interpret decline when it has in fact occurred). Finally, the limited sensitivity of the STW means that any dis-

Table 6–121 FAS Predicted From STW Raw Score

Ranking	Criterion
Low	STW raw score <46
Average	STW raw score 46–53
High	STW raw score >53

STW	N	FAS Pred—FAS									Descriptives		
		1%	5%	10%	25%	50%	75%	90%	95%	99%	M	SD	SE$_M$
Low	82	−28.0	−14.0	−12.6	−6.9	−1.4	5.2	10.9	18.0	31.1	−0.9	9.9	1.0
Average	240	−24.6	−16.5	−12.8	−6.8	−0.2	7.9	13.8	18.2	33.3	0.5	11.2	0.72
High	75	−21.6	−19.2	−15.3	−8.7	−0.1	8.5	13.7	15.7	19.8	−0.7	10.4	1.20
Total	397	−24.6	−16.7	−12.8	−6.9	−0.3	7.3	13.7	17.6	31.2	0.0	10.8	0.54

Source: From Senior et al., 2001. Based on a sample of 397 Australian adults (164 males, 233 females), mean age = 33.5 (*SD* = 13.1); mean education = 12.6 (*SD* = 2.2). Reprinted with permission of the authors.

crepancy between it and the SST that falls in the normal range should not be construed as evidence that the patient is normal. The technique may have failed to show evidence of abnormality and the patient may still have a clinically significant degree of cognitive impairment (Graves et al., 1999). Thus, we suggest that clinicians treat the STW results as an initial estimate of premorbid IQ and follow up with evaluation of additional information (e.g., NART, WTAR, demographic).

REFERENCES

Baddeley, A., Emslie, H., & Nimmo Smith, I. (1992). *The Speed and Capacity of Language-Processing test.* Suffolk, England: Thames Valley Test Company.

Baddeley, A., Emslie, H., & Nimmo Smith, I. (1993). The Spot-the-Word test: A robust estimate of verbal intelligence based on lexical decision. *British Journal of Clinical Psychology, 32,* 55–65.

Baddeley, A. D., Gardner, J. M., & Grantham-McGregor, S. (1995). Cross-cultural cognition—developing tests for developing countries. *Applied Cognitive Psychology, 9,* S173–S195.

Beardsall, L., & Huppert, F. (1997). Short NART, CCRT and Spot-the-Word: Comparisons in older and demented persons. *British Journal of Clinical Psychology, 36,* 619–622.

Comerford, V. E., Geffen, G. M., May, C., Medland, S. E., & Geffen, L. B. (2002). A rapid screen of the severity of mild traumatic brain injury. *Journal of Clinical and Experimental Neuropsychology, 24,* 409–419.

Crowell, T. A., Vanderploeg, R. D., Small, B. J., Graves, A. B., & Mortimer, J. A. (2002). Elderly norms for the Spot-the-Word test. *Archives of Clinical Neuropsychology, 17,* 123–130.

Graves, R. E., & Carswell, L. (2003). *Prediction of premorbid Boston Naming and California Verbal Learning Test scores.* Paper presented to the International Neuropsychological Society, Honolulu, HI.

Graves, R. E., Carswell, L. M., & Snow, W. G. (1999). An evaluation of the sensitivity of premorbid IQ estimators for detecting cognitive decline. *Psychological Assessment, 11,* 29–38.

Hinton-Bayre, A. D., Geffen, G., & McFarland, K. (1997). Mild head injury and speed of information processing: A prospective study of professional rugby league players. *Journal of Clinical and Experimental Neuropsychology, 19,* 275–289.

Jorm, A. F., Anstey, K. J., Christensen, H., & Rodgers, B. (2004). Gender differences in cognitive abilities: The mediating role of health state and health habits. *Intelligence, 32,* 7–23.

Lucas, S. K., Carstairs, J. R., & Shores, E. A. (2003). A comparison of methods to estimate premorbid intelligence in an Australian sample: Data from the Macquarie University Neuropsychological Normative Study (MUNNS). *Australian Psychologist, 38,* 227–237.

May, J., Alcock, K. J., Robinson, L., & Mwita, C. (2001). A computerized test of speed of language comprehension unconfounded by literacy. *Applied Cognitive Psychology, 15,* 433–443.

Papagno, C., & Baddelely, A. (1997). Confabulation in a dysexecutive patient: Implication of models of retrieval. *Cortex, 33,* 743–752.

Papagno, C., Rizzo, S., Ligori, L., Lima, J., & Riggio, A. (2003). Memory and executive functions in aneurysms of the anterior communicating artery. *Journal of Clinical and Experimental Neuropsychology, 25,* 24–35.

Ponsford, J., Willmott, C., Rothwell, A., Cameron, P., Kelly, A-M., Nelms, R., Curran, C., & Ng, K. (2000). Factors influencing outcome following mild traumatic brain injury in adults. *Journal of the International Neuropsychological Society, 6,* 568–579.

Saxton, J. A., Ratcliff, G., Dodge, H., Pandav, R., Baddeley, A., & Ganguli, M. (2001). Speed and Capacity of Language Processing Test: Normative data from an older American community-dwelling sample. *Applied Neuropsychology, 8,* 193–203.

Senior, G., Douglas, L., & Dawes, S. (2001). *Discrepancy analysis: A new/old approach to psychological test data interpretation.* Presentation at the 21st annual conference of the National Academy of Neuropsychology, San Francisco, CA.

Tamlyn, D., McKenna, P. J., Mortimer, A. M., Lund, C. E., Hammond, S., & Baddeley, A. D. (1992). Memory impairment in schizophrenia: Its extent, affiliations, and neuropsychological character. *Psychological Medicine, 22,* 101–115.

Watt, K. J. & O'Carroll, R. E. (1999). Evaluating methods for estimating premorbid intellectual ability in closed head injury. *Journal of Neurology, Neurosurgery and Psychiatry, 66,* 474–479.

Wilson, B. A., Watson, P. C., Baddeley, A. D., Emslie, H., & Evans, J. J. (2000). Improvement or simply practice? The effects of twenty repeated assessments on people with and without brain injury. *Journal of the International Neuropsychological Society, 6,* 469–479.

Yuspeh, R. L., & Vanderploeg, R. D. (2000). Spot-the-Word: A measure for estimating premorbid intellectual functioning. *Archives of Clinical Neuropsychology, 15,* 319–326.

Wechsler Abbreviated Scale of Intelligence (WASI)

PURPOSE

The aim of this individually administered test is to provide a brief estimate of intelligence.

SOURCE

The kit (including manual, set of nine blocks, Stimulus Booklet, 25 Record Forms, and carry bag) can be ordered from Harcourt Assessment (www.harcourtassessment.com), at a cost of $250 US.

AGE RANGE

The test can be given to individuals aged 6 to 89 years.

DESCRIPTION

The WASI (The Psychological Corporation, 1999) was developed for use as a screening instrument when a more complete assessment of IQ is not necessary (e.g., for research or vocational purposes), when time constraints are an issue, when screening is needed to determine if a more extensive evaluation

Table 6–122 Composition of the WASI

Indices		Subtests
FSIQ-4	VIQ	Vocabulary
		Similarities
	PIQ	Block Design
		Matrix Reasoning
FSIQ-2		Vocabulary
		Matrix Reasoning

is needed, or for a reassessment of someone who has previously had a more comprehensive evaluation. The WASI has the advantage over similar brief tests (e.g., K-BIT) in that it was developed using linking samples with the WISC-III and WAIS-III, allowing the examiner to estimate full WISC-III and WAIS-III FSIQ score ranges from WASI results (but not WISC-IV ranges).

The test is based on the measurement of both verbal and nonverbal abilities. It consists of four subtests: Vocabulary, Block Design, Similarities, and Matrix Reasoning. The selection of tasks was based in part on previous research that these subtests have high loadings on a general intellectual ability factor (g) and tap both verbal/crystallized and nonverbal/fluid functioning.

There are two options for administration (see Table 6–122). The four-subtest form yields a Full-Scale IQ (FSIQ-4). Vocabulary and Similarities subtests compose the Verbal scale and yield the Verbal IQ (VIQ), and the Block Design and Matrix Reasoning subtests compose the Performance scale and yield the Performance IQ (PIQ). The two-subtest form of the WASI consists of Vocabulary and Matrix Reasoning and also provides a FSIQ (FSIQ-2). Although the subtests are similar in format to their counterparts in the WISC-III and the WAIS-III, none of the items is the same (note that Matrix Reasoning has no counterpart in the WISC-III). The WASI verbal subtests also include some low-end items that require the examinee to name pictures (Vocabulary) or point to one of four pictures that is most similar to three target items (Similarities).

ADMINISTRATION

Directions for administering the items, the correct responses, and examples of typical responses that should be queried appear in the manual. The only task that requires timing is Block Design, and the time limits are provided both in the manual and on the record form. Starting points for each task are tailored to the patient's age. The start points, reverse rules, discontinue rules, and stop points are provided in the manual and record form. The order of tasks (Vocabulary, Block Design, Similarities, Matrix Reasoning) is fixed but not inviolable.

ADMINISTRATION TIME

According to the manual, the four-subtest form takes about 30 minutes, while the two-subtest form takes about 15 min-

utes. WASI subtests tend to contain slightly more items than their WAIS-III counterparts. Both Vocabulary and Similarities require significantly more time to administer with the WASI than with the WAIS-III (Axelrod, 2002), although the difference (about two minutes) is likely not clinically significant.

SCORING

Scoring criteria are provided in the test manual. The WASI differs from other Wechsler scales in that subtest total raw scores are converted to age-corrected T scores instead of subtest scaled scores. A Table in the manual (A.2) provides WISC/WAIS-III subtest scaled score equivalents of WASI T scores. The test age equivalents of subtest raw scores can also be recorded (Table A.7 in the manual). The test age equivalents represent the average performance of each age group on each subtest.

For the four-subtest form, the Verbal IQ is the sum of the T scores on Vocabulary and Similarities. The Performance score is the sum of the T scores on Block Design and Matrix Reasoning and the Full Scale score is the sum of the T scores on all four subtests. For the two-subtest form, the Full Scale score is the sum of T scores on Vocabulary and Matrix Reasoning. The distribution of T scores ranges from 20 to 80 and has a mean of 50 and an SD of 10.

Tables (B.1 and B.2) are provided in the manual so that WISC-III and WAIS-III prediction intervals (90%, 68% levels of confidence) can be determined. Examiners can also compare the patient's Verbal and Performance IQ scores to determine if the difference between these components is significant and unusual by referring to tables in the manual (B.3 and B.4). The frequencies are presented by five ability levels and are given for both VIQ > PIQ and PIQ > VIQ differences. Discrepancy tables for intersubtest differences are not provided.

DEMOGRAPHIC EFFECTS

Age

Age affects performance, and age-based norm tables are provided for the subtests in the WASI Manual (see *Source*).

Gender

No information is provided.

Education

Education is also modestly related to WASI performance (Hays et al., 2002).

Ethnicity

No information is provided.

Table 6–123 Characteristics of the WASI Normative Sample

Number	2245
	1100: Ages 6–16
	1145: Ages 17–89
Age	6–89 years[a]
Geographic location	Proportionate to U.S. population in four major geographic regions: Northeast, North Central, South, and West
Sample type	Standardization sample considered representative of U.S. adult population in terms of gender, educational level, and race/ethnicity based on 1997 Census data
Education[b]	
≤8	32%
9–11	16%
12	26.7%
13–15	14.7%
≥16	10.7%
Gender	
Males	36%
Females	64%
Race/ethnicity	
White	84%
African American	12%
Hispanic	4%
Screening	Screened to exclude participants with insufficient English-language proficiency, uncorrected hearing or visual impairment, or drug or alcohol abuse; taking antidepressant, antianxiety, or antipsychotic medication; or with medical and psychiatric disorders likely to affect cognitive functioning

[a]Divided into 13 age groupings: yearly age groupings from 6–16, 17–19, 20–24, 25–29, 30–34, 35–44, 45–54, 55–64, 65–69, 70–74, 75–79, 80–84, and 85–89; $N = 100$ in each age group from 6–74, $N = 85$ for ages 75–79 and 80–84, and $N = 75$ for ages 85–89.
[b]For participants aged 6–19 years, parent education was used; for participants aged 20–89 years, participant education was used.

NORMATIVE DATA

Standardization Sample

In contrast to previous Wechsler short forms, the WASI was normed on a nationally representative sample of 2245 people, divided into 23 age groups ranging from age 6 to 89 years (Ns of 75–100 in each age group), and stratified according to recent U.S. Census data on three background variables: gender, race/ethnicity, and educational level (see Table 6–123).

RELIABILITY

Internal Consistency

Split-half reliability coefficients for the subtests and IQ scales are excellent (.8–.9; see *Source*; Axelrod, 2002), with slightly higher reliability coefficients for adults than for children. In children, the average reliability coefficients of the subtests range from .87 to .92. For the IQ scales, coefficients are .93, .94, and .86 for the VIQ, PIQ, and FSIQ-4, respectively. The average reliability of the FSIQ-2 is .93. The average coefficients for the adult sample for the subtests range from .92 to .94. Reliability coefficients are .96, .96, and .98 for the VIQ, PIQ, and FSIQ, respectively. The average reliability coefficient of the FSIQ-2 is .96 (see *Source*).

Standard Error of Measurement

The subtest and scale scores of the WASI have average standard errors of measurement of about four points in children and three points in adults.

Test-Retest Reliability and Practice Effects

Test-retest reliability was evaluated by administering the WASI twice to 222 normal children and adults aged 6 to 89. The interval between tests ranged from 2 to 12 weeks, with a mean of 31 days. Stability coefficients for the FSIQ-2 were .85 for children and .88 for adults. Coefficients for the FSIQ-4 were .93 for children and .92 for adults. Practice effects emerge following such short retest periods. The subtest T scores of the second testing are about 0.8 to 4.6 points higher for the children's sample and about 0.6 to 2.8 points higher for the adult sample. The score increases are the highest for Block Design and the lowest for Vocabulary, regardless of age group. Similarly, the IQ scores from the second testing increased about 2.6 to 5.8 points for the children's sample and about 1.8 to 3.9 points for the adult sample, with the increases in PIQ higher than the increases in VIQ. Similar findings occur with the full-form versions.

Axelrod (2002) gave the WAIS-III and WASI to a mixed clinical sample of 72 patients. Despite the fact that the tests were given on the same day, there were no effects of practice.

Interrater Reliability

Interscorer agreement is reported to be high (>.9) for both the verbal and nonverbal subtests (see *Source*).

VALIDITY

Construct Validity

According to the test manual, the WASI measures constructs similar to its WISC-III and WAIS-III counterparts. The WASI and WISC-III were administered in counterbalanced order to a sample of 176 children and adolescents aged 6 to 16 years. The interval between test administrations ranged from 2 to 12 weeks ($M = 23$ days). Correlations between corresponding subtests ranged from .69 (Similarities) to .74 (Block Design). Coefficients for the corresponding VIQ (.82) and PIQ (.76) scales were also high. WISC-III FSIQ correlated .87 with the

WASI FSIQ-4 and .81 with the WASI FSIQ-2. Mean subtest and IQ scores were noted to be slightly higher for the WISC-III. The difference may reflect a Flynn effect, with older tests yielding somewhat higher scores than newer versions.

Validity coefficients were slightly higher in adults (see *Source*). In 248 adults aged 16 to 89 years, correlations between the WASI and WAIS-III subtests ranged from .66 (Matrix Reasoning) to .88 (Vocabulary). For the IQ scores, the coefficients were .84 for PIQ and .88 for VIQ. WAIS-III FSIQ correlated .92 with the WASI FSIQ-4 and .87 with the WASI FSIQ-2. Mean scores between corresponding subtests/IQ scales were nearly equivalent.

A similar study by Axelrod (2002) provided less convincing evidence of the WASI's concurrent validity. In a heterogeneous clinical sample of 72 patients, correlations with WAIS-III summary IQ scores were more modest and ranged from .71 to .82. The WASI VIQ summary score underestimated WAIS-III VIQ scores by about two points, whereas WASI PIQ and FSIQ-4 overestimated the comparable WAIS-III scores (by about eight and three points, respectively). Even more problematic was the finding that only 66% of the WASI FSIQ-4 scores fell within a margin of error of six points. The WASI FSIQ-2 proved even less accurate, with only 50% of the cases falling within the six-point error margin. Better estimates of WAIS-III summary scores were obtained by using WAIS-III (same two or four subtests) or Kaufman (Arithmetic, Similarities, Picture Completion, Digit Symbol) short forms.

Additional evidence of validity comes from using other ability or achievement tests as criteria. Hays et al. (2002) reported that in a sample of 85 psychiatric inpatients, the correlation between the WASI and K-BIT was high (.89). K-BIT Composite and Vocabulary scores were slightly higher than their WASI counterparts (by about two and four points, respectively). Equivalent scores were obtained for the nonverbal subtests. Saklofske et al. (2000) reported that in 64 grade 4 children, the WASI composite scores (FSIQ-2 and particularly FSIQ-4) showed moderate relations with scores from the Canadian Achievement Test/2 and the Canadian Test of Cognitive Skills.

The test authors (see *Source*) gave another ability test, the WIAT, concurrently with the WASI to a group of 210 healthy participants aged 6 to 19 years. WASI scores correlated moderately well (.41–.72) with WIAT subtest and composite scores. The pattern of correlations was similar to those obtained between the WIAT and the WISC/WAIS.

Evidence of convergent and divergent validity is based in part on the intercorrelations of the WASI subtests. For the entire sample, the authors (see *Source*) reported that Vocabulary correlated highest with Similarities (.75). Matrix Reasoning correlated equally with the verbal subtests (Vocabulary: .56, Similarities: .54) and Block Design (.59). The study by Hays et al. (2002) referred to previously also provided evidence of convergent and discriminant validity. In their comparison between the K-BIT and the WASI, they found that subtests tapping similar functions correlated more highly than did dissimilar subtests. For example, the WASI Vocabulary subtest correlated highest with the WASI Similarities (.82) and the K-BIT Vocabulary (.83). Conversely, lower correlations were obtained between verbal and nonverbal subtests.

The test authors (see *Source*) report the results of a joint factor analysis substituting WASI subtests for corresponding WISC-III subtests and the remaining WISC-III subtests. They found that WASI Vocabulary and Similarities subtests load on the Verbal Comprehension factor, along with Information and Comprehension of the full battery. WASI Block Design and Matrix Reasoning load on the Perceptual Organization factor, along with Picture Completion, Picture Arrangement, and Object Assembly of the full battery. Similar results were obtained with exploratory factor analysis of the WASI/WAIS-III (see *Source*). Confirmatory factor analysis provided support for the two-factor model of the WASI (see *Source*). Recently, Ryan et al. (2003) conducted exploratory factor analyses on the WASI adult standardization sample ($N = 1145$) and a diagnostically heterogeneous adult clinical sample ($N = 201$). Two factors (Verbal Comprehension and Perceptual Organization) were identified in each sample. Coefficients of congruence were high and suggested factorial equivalence across the standardization and clinical samples.

Clinical Findings

The authors provide some preliminary evidence showing that the test is sensitive to a variety of clinical conditions, including mental retardation and moderate/severe traumatic brain injury. However, the WASI appears not to have sufficient specificity for distinguishing the severity (e.g., mild, moderate) of disturbance (see *Source*).

COMMENT

The WASI is relatively easy to administer and score. The availability of the four-subtest form or even the briefer two-subtest form provides the examiner with increased flexibility when time constraints are an issue. It has excellent reliability and stability, covers a wide age span, and assesses both verbal and nonverbal domains. An additional benefit is the lack of significant practice effects when either the WASI or WAIS-III is given first. Further, the test has its own separate standardization, and norms are not an extrapolation from a comprehensive test—a problem with many of the Wechsler short forms (Kaufman & Kaufman, 2001). However, other short forms (e.g., same two- or four-subtest forms from the WAIS-III) appear to yield more valid estimates of WAIS-III summary scores, and some (e.g., Kaufman's tetrad of Arithmetic, Similarities, Picture Completion, and Digit Symbol) require less time to administer (Axelrod, 2002). Given concerns about concurrent validity between the WAIS-III and the WASI, the examiner should not use these measures interchangeably (e.g., in serial assessment or to measure change over time). Users should also note that the WASI is linked to the WISC-III, not to the new WISC-IV.

Caution is also recommended when making clinical inferences between verbal and nonverbal ability based on WASI VIQ and PIQ scores. Axelrod (2002) found that less than one-half of the patients obtained WASI scores within six points of their

WAIS-III VIQ and PIQ scores. In addition, in settings where it may be necessary to administer the whole version of the IQ test (e.g., when there is a possibility of mental retardation), it may be more convenient to administer one of the many Wechsler short forms derived from the full-form versions of the WISC-III and WAIS-III (reviewed extensively in Sattler, 2001), and then supplement with additional full-form subtests if need be. It should also be noted that age corrections are provided for WASI scores, but not for other demographic factors such as education and ethnicity. Finally, the WASI should not take the place of a comprehensive examination. Rather, its use should be reserved for screening, for research projects, when a global estimate of intelligence is needed, or when time constraints are an issue.

REFERENCES

Axelrod, B. N. (2002). Validity of the Wechsler Abbreviated Scale of Intelligence and other very short forms of estimating intellectual functioning. *Assessment, 9,* 17–23.

Hays, J. R., Reas, D. L., & Shaw, J. B. (2002). Concurrent validity of the Wechsler Abbreviated Scale of Intelligence and the Kaufman Brief Intelligence Test among psychiatric patients. *Psychological Reports, 90,* 355–359.

Kaufman, J. C., & Kaufman, A. S. (2001). Time for changing of the guard: A farewell to short forms of intelligence. *Journal of Psychoeducational Assessment, 19,* 245–267.

Psychological Corporation (The) (1999). *Wechsler Abbreviated Scale of Intelligence (WASI) manual.* San Antonio, TX: Author.

Ryan, J. J., Carruthers, C. A., Miller, L. J., Souheaver, G. T., Gontkovsky, S. T., & Zehr, M. D. (2003). Exploratory factor analysis of the Wechsler Abbreviated Scale of Intelligence (WASI) in adult standardization and clinical samples. *Applied Neuropsychology, 10,* 252–256.

Saklofske, D. H., Caravan, G., & Schwartz, C. (2000). Concurrent validity of the Wechsler Abbreviated Scale of Intelligence (WASI) with a sample of Canadian children. *Canadian Journal of School Psychology, 16,* 87–94.

Sattler, J. M. (2001). *Assessment of children: Cognitive applications* (4th ed.). San Diego: Jerome M. Sattler, Publisher, Inc.

Wechsler Adult Intelligence Scale—III (WAIS-III)

PURPOSE

The purpose of the WAIS-III is to provide a measure of general intellectual function in older adolescents and adults.

SOURCE

The WAIS-III (materials, Administration and Norms Manual, Technical Manual, Stimulus Booklet, 25 Record Forms, and 25 Response Booklets) can be obtained from Harcourt Assessment, 19500 Bulverde Rd, San Antonio, TX, 78259 (www.harcourtassessment.com). The scale costs about $825 US. Canadian normative data are also available for the WAIS-III. The Psychological Corporation (Harcourt Assessment) provides a computer scoring system (WAIS-III/WMS-III/WIAT-II Scoring Assistant) that gives demographically corrected norms (U.S. normative data only) and costs $225 US. The 6-Factor Model (Tulsky, Ivnik, et al., 2003) is an alternative model for creating composites. Examiners can download the WAIS-III/WMS-III Demographically Adjusted Norms 6-Factor Model Analysis Tool from the Harcourt Assessment web page at http://harcourtassessment.com/haiweb/Cultures/en-US/dotCom/6factormodel/6+Factor+Model.htm. The tool calculates demographically adjusted T scores and base rate discrepancies.

AGE RANGE

The WAIS-III can be given to individuals aged 16 to 89 years.

DESCRIPTION

The Wechsler test has played a critical role in our thinking about intelligence and psychological testing. The interested reader is referred to the excellent reviews of its history by Boake (2002) and Tulsky, Saklofske et al. (2003). It is one of the most frequently used measures in neuropsychological batteries (Butler et al., 1991; Camara et al., 2000; Lees-Haley et al., 1996; Rabin et al., 2005) and is often considered "the gold standard" in intelligence testing (Ivnik et al., 1992). It is a core instrument, giving information about the overall level of intellectual functioning and the presence or absence of significant intellectual disability, and providing clues to altered functions (Lezak et al., 2004).

The WAIS-III (The Psychological Corporation, 1997) is a revision of the WAIS-R (Wechsler, 1981) and differs from its predecessors in several important ways (Tulsky, Ivnik, et al., 2003). First, the structure of the test was altered to make it more compatible with contemporary research and theory on intelligence. The WAIS-III therefore measures new constructs outside of the domain of previous versions (e.g., Working Memory, Processing Speed) and measures some constructs in different ways. For example, the Perceptual Organization Index (POI) includes a new subtest (Matrix Reasoning), developed to enhance the measurement of fluid reasoning. Other subtests (Letter-Number Sequencing, Symbol Search) were developed to assess working memory and processing speed, thereby broadening the scope of the test to include more than just Full-Scale IQ (FSIQ), Verbal IQ (VIQ), and Performance IQ (PIQ). In addition, a contemporary normative reference group has been included. The age range has been extended to cover individuals aged 16 to 89 years. Some changes have been made at the item level, removing or modifying problematic items and adding some new items so that subtests would have more adequate floors and ceilings. Only about 50% to 60% of the WAIS-R items have been retained in either original or slightly modified form. Finally, the test was conormed or linked

Table 6–124 WAIS-III Structure[a]

IQ	IQ	Factor-Based Index	Subtest	Description
FSIQ	Verbal IQ	Verbal Comprehension	Vocabulary	Examinee gives oral definitions for words.
			Similarities	Examinee must state in what way two objects or concepts are alike.
			Information	Examinee responds orally to questions about factual information.
		Working Memory	Arithmetic	Examinee must mentally solve arithmetic word problems presented orally within a time limit.
			Digit Span	Digits Backward—examinee repeats number sequence in same order as presented. Digit Backward—examinee repeats the number sequence in reverse order.
			Letter-Number Sequencing[b]	Examinee is read a combination of numbers and letters and is asked to recall the numbers first in ascending order and then the letters in alphabetic order.
—		—	(Comprehension)	Examinee responds to questions that require understanding of concepts and social practices.
	Performance IQ	Perceptual Organization	Picture Completion	Examinee views a picture and points to or names the important part that is missing.
			Block Design	Examinee is asked to replicate models or pictures of two-color designs with blocks.
			Matrix Reasoning	Examinee looks at a matrix with a section missing and identifies by pointing or by number one of five response options.
		Processing Speed	Digit Symbol	Coding—examinee copies symbols paired with numbers in a 120-sec. limit.
				Incidental Learning: Pairing—examinee is given numbers and must recall associated symbols. Free Recall—examinee writes down as many symbols as can recall.
			Symbol Search[c]	Examinee must determine whether either of two target symbols match any of the symbols in a search group. Examinee responds to as many items as possible in a 120-sec. time limit.
			(Picture Arrangement)	Examinee arranges mixed-up cards to create a logical story.
			(Object Assembly)	Examinee is presented with puzzle pieces that must be put together to depict a common object.

[a]Object Assembly can substitute for a Performance subtest for ages 16–74. [b]Letter-Number Sequencing is an optional subtest that can substitute for Digit Span when that subtest has been spoiled. [c]Symbol Search is an optional supplementary subtest that can substitute for Digit Symbol-Coding. Supplementary subtests are shown in parentheses.

with other measures (e.g., WMS-III, WIAT-II), allowing direct comparison across domains.

In addition to the new subtests (Matrix Reasoning, Letter-Number Sequencing, Symbol Search), optional procedures have been added to the Digit Symbol-Coding subtest to assist the examiner in determining the factors that may be impacting the examinee's performance on the subtest. These optional procedures involve recalling shapes from memory (Pairing and Free Recall) and graphomotor speed (Digit Symbol-Copy).

Thus, the WAIS-III contains a total of 14 subtests, 11 retained from the older version, the WAIS-R, and the three new subtests (see Table 6–124). Although the traditional groupings of FSIQ, VIQ, and PIQ have been retained, a major structural change is that the WAIS-III has incorporated another grouping based on a four-factor model of the test: Verbal Comprehension, Perceptual Organization, Working Memory, and Processing Speed. As shown in Table 6–124, 11 of the 14 subtests are used to create the four-factor indices. Comprehension, Picture Arrangement, and Object Assembly are not included in the calculation of any of the index scores. Like the traditional IQ scores, each index score has a mean of 100 and a standard deviation of 15. The floor of the WAIS-III FSIQ is 45, while the ceiling is 155.

On all three tests (WAIS-III, WISC-IV, WPPSI-III), IQ scores compare the performance of an individual with the average scores attained by members of that person's age group. Identical IQ scores obtained by a 60-year-old and a 20-year-old reflect the same relative standing among people of the subject's age group. In one sense, however, IQ scores at different ages are not identical because test scores change with age, typically rising to a peak during young adulthood, then falling off later on. Consequently, a lower level of test performance is needed to obtain a given IQ at 60 than at 20 years of age.

ADMINISTRATION

See *Source*. Briefly, the examiner asks test questions, displays pictures or puzzles to the patient, and records the patient's responses in an individual response booklet. Start points and reverse, discontinue, and scoring rules as well as time limits are noted in the test manual as well as on the record form. There is a suggested order of subtest administration; however, the examiner can depart from the standard order if there are compelling reasons (e.g., patient is extremely frustrated). Completion of all subtests in one session is preferable, but not obligatory. The examiner can call a recess at the end of a subtest. Rescheduling of the second testing session should be less than one week later. If a subtest must be stopped in the middle, the test can sometimes be resumed where it had been stopped. However, the easy items on some of the subtests (Similarities, Block Design, Matrix Reasoning, Picture Arrangement, Letter-Number Sequencing) provide subjects with the practice they need to succeed at more difficult items. Accordingly, if the examination must be stopped in the middle of any of these subtests, the first few items should be repeated at the next session so that the patient can reestablish the skills necessary to pass the harder items.

The Letter-Number Sequencing task is included in both the WAIS-III and WMS-III; however, in the standardization sample, the task was given only once, during the WMS-III. Even though there is not a very large practice effect on this subtest (see WAIS-/WMS-III Technical Manual), it should be given only once in the testing session (Tulsky & Ledbetter, 2000). There is no significant difference in Letter-Number Sequencing test scores if given as part of the WAIS-III or the WMS-III (Tulsky & Ledbetter, 2000).

The WISC-IV overlaps with the WAIS-III for the age period 16 years to 16 years 11 months. Preliminary data provided in the WISC-IV Technical Manual (Wechsler, 2003) suggest that the WAIS-III composite scores are slightly higher than those of the WISC-IV (about two to five points), with the exception of the WMI. In general, the WAIS-III is preferred because if retesting is necessary after the 17th birthday, then the appropriate comparison is available.

The Wechsler test should be given early in the course of the assessment because it allows the examiner to observe how the patient negotiates a wide array of tasks. In this way, the examiner can begin to develop hypotheses about the patient's spared and impaired functions that can then be tested more thoroughly in the course of the examination.

Short Forms

There are two methods of abbreviating the WAIS-III. One is to reduce the number of items within individual subtests (e.g., Satz-Mogel short form), while the other is to reduce the number of subtests and transform results by referring to special tables (e.g., Jeyakumar et al., 2004; Sattler, 2001) to obtain estimated IQ results.

Reducing the number of items within subtests (Satz-Mogel short form) may result in high correlations with the full form (Wymer et al., 2003) but exacts a price in terms of reliability (Kulas & Axelrod, 2002; Ryan et al., 1999). Moreover, the alternate item approach virtually precludes subsequent administration of the full test should the more precise information be required (Ehrenreich, 1996). Further, it represents a dramatic departure from the standard administration. Because half of the items are excluded, the difficulty slope of the items increases much more rapidly than under standard conditions, while the opportunity for practice decreases equally rapidly (Sattler, 2001). Accordingly, such short forms are not recommended.

With regard to select subtest forms, we often omit Comprehension and Picture Arrangement as well as Object Assembly. Axelrod and Ryan (2000) demonstrated that their omission results in accurate estimates of the traditional IQ scores while retaining all the information needed for the index scores. It also reduces administration time by about 20%. Prorated VIQ scores are obtained by multiplying the sum of Vocabulary, Similarities, Arithmetic, Digit Span, and Information by 6/5. For the PIQ estimate, scaled scores of Picture Completion, Digit Symbol-Coding, Block Design, and Matrix Reasoning are summed and multiplied by 5/4. FSIQ is the total of prorated Verbal and Performance scaled scores.

A number of other short forms have been developed for the WAIS-III (e.g., Wymer et al., 2003; see also Sattler & Ryan, 1999 for an extensive listing). The most time-consuming estimate of FSIQ is given by the seven-subtest combination (40–46 minutes), whereas the most time-efficient combination is Information plus Picture Completion (12 minutes; Ryan et al., 1998).

A popular two-subtest form is Vocabulary and Block Design. It has high reliability (.93 for the average of the 13 age groups in the standardization sample), correlates well (.88–.89) with the Full Scale, and has an administration time of about 26 minutes (Jeyakumar et al., 2004; Sattler & Ryan, 2001). Table 6–125 can be used to convert the sum of scaled scores into an estimated FSIQ (Sattler & Ryan, 2001). Note, however, that despite high correlations, the various two-subtest short forms do not yield sufficiently close estimates of actual FSIQ for precise determination and classification (i.e., average, high average, etc.). Ringe et al. (2002) evaluated various two-subtest short forms (including the dyad Vocabulary and Block Design) in a heterogeneous clinical

Table 6–125 Estimated WAIS-III FSIQ for the Sum
of Vocabulary and Block Design

Sum of Scaled Scores	Est. FSIQ	Sum of Scaled Scores	Est. FSIQ
2	48	21	103
3	51	22	106
4	54	23	109
5	57	24	112
6	60	25	114
7	62	26	117
8	65	27	120
9	68	28	123
10	71	29	126
11	74	30	129
12	77	31	132
13	80	32	135
14	83	33	138
15	86	34	140
16	88	35	143
17	91	36	146
18	94	37	149
19	97	38	152
20	100		

Source: From Sattler & Ryan, 2001. Reprinted with permission.

neurological/neuropsychiatric sample and found that estimated FSIQ scores fell within five points of actual FSIQ in 49% to 74% of the cases (65% for the Vocabulary/Block Design combination).

Longer short forms tend to produce better classification rates. Popular combinations are two seven-subtest forms consisting of Information, Arithmetic, Digit Span, Similarities, Picture Completion, Digit Symbol-Coding, and Block Design or Matrix Reasoning (Ryan & Ward, 1999) that average about 40 to 45 minutes in administration time (Ryan et al., 1998). Sattler and Ryan (1999, 2001) have provided tables (1999: Tables 0-8, 0-9, 0-11; 2001: Tables C-22, C-23, C-25) for converting sums of scaled scores on the seven-subtest short forms into FSIQ, VIQ, and PIQ estimates. Alternatively, prorated sums of scaled scores can be obtained by multiplying the verbal sum of scaled scores by 6/4 and the performance sum by 5/3. The Full Scale sum of scores is the total of prorated verbal and performance sum of scaled scores. These short forms have produced reasonable estimates of FSIQ and VIQ, but not PIQ or the other index scores (Axelrod et al., 2000, 2001; Kulas & Axelrod, 2002; Schopp et al., 2001). For example, Schopp et al. (2001) found that for VIQ and FSIQ, WAIS-III estimates fell within five points of actual scores in 92% of cases with TBI for both the Block Design and Matrix Reasoning seven-subtest versions. For PIQ, the Block Design version gave estimates within five points of actual PIQ scores in 70% of the cases and in 76% of the cases for the Matrix Reasoning version. The Matrix Reasoning version may be preferable when motor limitations or penalties for speed are of concern or when qualitative performance data from Block Design are not

desired. Matrix Reasoning also requires less time to administer than Block Design (see later discussion).

Short form estimations of respective factor scores are not recommended for clinical use (Axelrod et al., 2000; Donders & Axelrod, 2002). Thus, Donders and Axelrod (2002) evaluated the reliability and validity of various two-subtest short forms in a sample of 100 patients with traumatic brain injury and in a demographically matched subgroup from the standardization sample. Although acceptable estimates could be obtained from all short forms for Verbal Comprehension (VC) and for most short forms of Working Memory (WM; Arithmetic and Digit Span, Digit Span and Letter-Number Sequencing), none of the possible short forms for Perceptual Organization (PO) consistently met the minimum criterion regarding the percentage of cases (81%) that fell within the 90% confidence interval of the full-length index (five points for VC, six points for PO and WM). This raises the possibility that the three component subtests (Picture Completion, Block Design, Matrix Reasoning) do not share sufficient variance. Donders and Axelrod (2002) recommend that to obtain the four index scores, clinicians give all 11 subtests (omitting Comprehension, Picture Arrangement, and Object Assembly).

General Ability Index

The FSIQ is one means of generating a global composite IQ score. An alternative global score is the General Ability Index, which is based on subtests from the VCI and POI (Matrix Reasoning, Block Design, Vocabulary, Similarities, Information, and Picture Completion). Tulsky et al. (2001) have argued that the GAI is a better index of general ability, because it excludes Comprehension and Picture Arrangement, subtests that are redundant to those in the VCI and POI, as well as Digit Span and Symbol Search, which have lower loadings on *g*. In addition to a reduction in administration time, the subtests that compose the GAI are fairly resistant to neurological insult. Our own view is that measures of working memory (Digit Span, Letter-Number Sequencing) and processing speed (Symbol Search, Digit Symbol) have the potential to provide very meaningful information within the neuropsychological context (see *Validity*; see also Donders, Tulsky, et al., 2001; Strong et al., 2005), and these subtests should be administered routinely. However, derivation of the GAI might be useful in situations where VCI and POI differ markedly from WMI and PSI, as the best estimate of *g*. From a practical standpoint, the examiner can administer just the 11 subtests that define the four index scores yet still obtain an overall composite score without having to administer the more lengthy Picture Arrangement and Comprehension subtests. Table 6–126 presents information to convert the sum of scaled scores to GAI scores. Tulsky et al. (2001) report that the correlation between the GAI and the FSIQ is .96. The extent of misclassification in comparison with FSIQ based on a complete administration of the scale is not reported.

Table 6–126 General Ability Index (GAI) for the WAIS-III

Sum of Scaled Scores	GAI	90% CI Lower	90% CI Upper	95% CI Lower	95% CI Upper	Sum of Scaled Scores	GAI	90% CI Lower	90% CI Upper	95% CI Lower	95% CI Upper
6	47	44	53	44	54	61	99	95	103	94	104
7	49	46	55	46	56	62	100	96	104	95	105
8	51	48	57	47	58	63	101	97	105	96	106
9	52	49	58	48	59	64	102	98	106	97	107
10	53	50	59	49	60	65	104	100	108	99	109
11	54	51	60	50	60	66	105	101	109	100	110
12	55	52	61	51	61	67	106	102	110	101	111
13	56	53	62	52	62	68	107	103	111	102	112
14	57	54	63	53	63	69	109	105	113	104	114
15	58	55	64	54	64	70	110	105	114	105	115
16	59	56	64	55	65	71	111	106	115	106	116
17	60	57	65	56	66	72	112	107	116	107	117
18	61	58	66	57	67	73	114	109	118	109	119
19	62	59	67	58	68	74	115	110	119	109	120
20	63	60	68	59	69	75	116	111	120	110	121
21	64	61	69	60	70	76	118	113	122	112	122
22	65	62	70	61	71	77	119	114	123	113	123
23	66	63	71	62	72	78	120	115	124	114	124
24	67	64	72	63	73	79	122	117	126	116	126
25	68	65	73	64	74	80	123	118	126	117	127
26	69	66	74	65	75	81	124	119	127	118	128
27	70	67	75	66	76	82	126	121	129	120	130
28	71	68	76	67	77	83	127	122	130	121	131
29	72	69	77	68	78	84	128	123	131	122	132
30	73	70	78	69	79	85	130	125	133	124	134
31	74	71	79	70	80	86	131	126	134	125	135
32	75	72	80	71	81	87	132	127	135	126	136
33	75	72	80	71	81	88	134	129	137	128	138
34	76	73	81	72	82	89	135	130	138	129	139
35	77	74	82	73	83	90	136	131	139	130	140
36	78	74	83	74	84	91	138	133	141	132	142
37	78	74	83	74	84	92	139	134	142	133	143
38	79	75	84	75	85	93	140	135	143	134	144
39	80	76	85	76	86	94	141	136	144	135	145
40	81	77	86	77	87	95	142	136	145	136	146
41	82	78	87	78	88	96	144	138	147	138	148
42	82	78	87	78	88	97	145	139	148	139	149
43	83	79	88	78	89	98	146	140	149	140	150
44	84	80	89	79	90	99	147	141	150	140	151
45	85	81	90	80	91	100	148	142	151	141	152
46	85	81	90	80	91	101	149	143	152	142	153
47	86	82	91	81	91	102	150	144	153	143	153
48	87	83	92	82	92	103	151	145	154	144	154
49	88	84	93	83	93	104	151	145	154	144	154
50	89	85	94	84	94	105	152	146	155	145	155
51	89	85	94	84	94	106	152	146	155	145	155
52	90	86	95	85	95	107	153	147	156	146	156
53	91	87	95	86	96	108	153	147	156	146	156
54	92	88	96	87	97	109	154	148	157	147	157
55	93	89	97	88	98	110	154	148	157	147	157
56	94	90	98	89	99	111	154	148	157	147	157
57	95	91	99	90	100	112	155	149	157	148	158
58	96	92	100	91	101	113	155	149	157	148	158
59	97	93	101	92	102	114	155	149	157	148	158
60	98	94	102	93	103						

Note: CI = confidence interval.

Source: From Tulsky et al., 2001. Reprinted with permission of the authors. Wechsler Adult Intelligence Scale–Third Edition. Copyright © 1997 by Harcourt Assessment, Inc. Reproduced with permission. All rights reserved.

ADMINISTRATION TIME

According to the test publishers, administration of the 11 subtests that yield the three IQ scores averaged 75 minutes (range 60–90 minutes) in the standardization sample. The 11 subtests that comprise the index scores required about 60 minutes (range 45–75 minutes) to administer. The time needed to administer the 13 subtests (Object Assembly omitted) required to generate all summary and index scores is 80 minutes (range 65–95 minutes). However, these times may not generalize to clinical populations.

Ryan et al. (1998) reported somewhat longer administration times (an average of 100 minutes for 13 subtests) in a patient sample with a mean FSIQ of 94.3 (SD = 11.7). By contrast, Axelrod (2001) found shorter times in a clinical sample with a mean FSIQ of 85.9 (SD = 12.8; an average of 65 minutes for 13 subtests). In both studies, however, Block Design, Picture Arrangement, and Comprehension were most time-consuming. Whereas Ryan et al. (1998) reported that level of intelligence influenced administration times, Axelrod (2001) found little relationship between test performance and administration length. The exceptions to this pattern were that Matrix Reasoning took longer for patients who performed better, and longer Digit Span administration was related to higher overall performance on a number of measures in which it is included. As in the study by Ryan et al. (1998), Matrix Reasoning took about one-half the time that was required to administer Block Design.

Note that time estimates reported previously pertain only to the administration of the various WAIS-III measures. This did not include the time requirements associated with scoring, breaks during testing, or interpretation.

SCORING

See *Source*. The Record Form provides space to record and score the subject's responses, to draw a profile of subtest scores, and to summarize information about the patient's behavior in the test situation. Much of the scoring is straightforward, but there are a few subtests (e.g., Vocabulary, Comprehension, Similarities) where subjectivity intrudes (see *Reliability*). So that scoring and qualitative features of the performance can be reviewed later, examiners should record responses to verbal subtests verbatim, or at least record each significant idea expressed by the subject. Atypical solutions on the Performance subtests should also be documented.

The raw scores of subtests are converted to age scaled scores using tables (A1–A2) in the WAIS-III Administration and Scoring Manual. The updated WAIS-III/WMS-III Technical Manual includes a new table of scaled scores for Digit Span Backward (Appendix E). The scaled scores range from 1 to 19 for most subtests and have a mean of 10 and a standard deviation of 3. Thus, scores of 7 and 13 correspond to one *SD* below and above the mean, respectively, and scaled scores of 4 and 16 deviate two *SD*s from the mean. Sums of scaled scores are then converted via tables (A3–A9) to IQ and factor index

scores. The IQs and factor indices range from about 45 to 155 for IQs and from 50 to 150 for indices. They have a mean of 100 and a standard deviation of 15. Tables are provided in the Administration and Scoring Manual to evaluate strengths and weaknesses at the subtest level (i.e., the significance and frequency of differences between the subtest score and the mean of the scale, the differences between subtest scaled scores required for statistical significance, the frequency of intersubtest scatter within various scales) and at the index level (the significance and frequency of differences between indices). The examiner can also evaluate the longest Digit Span Forward and Backward. Tables (B6–B7) are also included in the Administration and Scoring Manual that provide the frequencies of individuals in the standardization sample who obtained these spans as well as the differences between these spans. Normative data (frequencies) for the Digit Symbol optional procedures (Digit Symbol—Incidental Learning, Digit Symbol—Copy) are also provided in the WAIS-III Administration and Scoring Manual (Table A11).

Computer software is available from the test publisher so that raw scores can be automatically converted to appropriate scaled scores, index scores, percentiles, confidence intervals, and corresponding graphs (see *Source*). In addition, it calculates the cumulative percentage of individuals obtaining certain Digits Forward versus Digits Backward discrepancies, and the cumulative percentage of individuals scoring at certain levels on the optional Digit Symbol procedures. The discrepancies among scores (e.g., VIQ-PIQ, VCI-POI) are also computed and evaluated with regard to statistical significance and frequency of occurrence. A table (see also Table B.2 of the WAIS-III Administration and Scoring Manual) provides the percentage of examinees whose scores differed by the given amount or more, regardless of the direction of the difference. Until recently, the manual did not provide the frequencies with which differences between scales occurred in the standardization sample in either direction alone. Tables showing such frequencies have recently been provided by Tulsky et al. (2000; also see Table D6, The Psychological Corporation, 2002). For example, about 3.1% of the standardization sample obtained VIQ and PIQ scores that differed by 24 points or more. Examination of the tables provided by Tulsky et al. (2000) shows that a VIQ > PIQ discrepancy of 24 or more points was obtained by 2.1% of the standardization sample, whereas such a discrepancy favoring PIQ was obtained by 1.0% of the sample. Alternatively, Tulsky et al. (2000) suggest that the examiner can divide the frequencies shown in Table B.2 of the Administration and Scoring Manual by 2 to obtain the approximate base rate information in one direction. Both methods produce similar results, and either one can be used when the examiner has a hypothesis about which score should be greater.

It is important to bear in mind that the discrepancies vary as a function of ability level (see also Hawkins & Tulsky, 2003). The software provides frequencies of various differences based on an average level of performance. However, because IQ and index discrepancies vary as a function of ability level, supplemental tables included in Appendix D (D.1–D.5) of the updated 2002 WAIS-III/WMS-III Technical Manual need to be consulted to ascertain the actual frequency of differences. In general, people with lower IQs tend to have smaller index discrepancies than do those with higher IQs.

These tables (Technical Manual D.1–D.5) reflect the base rates of absolute (bidirectional) discrepancy scores. A separate table (D.6) is provided for directional WAIS-III discrepancies, but these are not stratified by FSIQ. Dori and Chelune (2004) present educationally stratified, directional prevalence rates of discrepancy scores for the WAIS-III, the WMS-III, and between the WAIS-III and WMS-III. In addition, they provide unidirectional cut scores that define simple difference prevalence rates at various decision points (i.e., 5%, 10%, and 15%). Table 6–127 presents within-test base-rate information for the WAIS-III. Tables are also provided in the description of the WMS-III (elsewhere in this book) for within- and between-test discrepancy scores. To illustrate how these tables can be used, assume a patient with 12 years of education obtains a VCI score 13 points greater than PSI. Although the difference is statistically reliable (Table B.1 of the WAIS-III Administration and Scoring Manual), examination of the unidirectional base-rate data for VCI-PSI presented in Table 6–127, where VCI (V1) is greater than PSI (V2), shows that that this discrepancy is not particularly rare in the general population. More than 15% of the standardization sample with 12 years of education had discrepancies greater than or equal to 14 points.

Determination of clinically meaningful differences in the Wechsler profile is guided by rates of discrepancies in the normative sample. Rates of such differences have recently been provided by Axelrod et al. (2002) for a moderate-severe traumatic brain injury sample. Tables 6–128 and 6–129 present directional difference scores for the summary/index and subtest scores, respectively, in this sample. As an example, 33% of the sample had VIQ-PIQ difference scores of greater than or equal to 10, while only 10% had a PIQ-VIQ of greater than or equal to 10. In a similar fashion, a three-point difference in Vocabulary minus Digit Span is relatively rare in this sample, occurring in only about 10% of the cases.

Basals and Ceilings

The WAIS-III Administration and Scoring Manual does not provide guidance on how to credit items that may have been given unnecessarily below the basal level. Sattler and Ryan (2001) recommend that the patient should be given full credit for those items even if the examinee earned partial or no credit. In this way, the patient is not penalized for failing items that should not have been administered in the first place.

Problem With Response Booklet for Digit Symbol Copy

In the second row (Item 14) of the Response Booklet, the symbol to be copied is a three-sided U-shaped figure open to the left. However, the scoring template for this item presents a figure that is open at the top. If examiners use the template, a correctly copied symbol will be scored as an error. Sattler and Ryan (2001) noted this problem and recommended that when scoring Item 14, examiners disregard what is shown on the scoring template and give credit for a drawing that matches the model.

DEMOGRAPHIC EFFECTS

Age

In general, there were few differences between younger and older people in verbal ability (except for Letter-Number Sequencing), but large differences in nonverbal ability. Within the Performance Scale, ability begins to decline with the 45-to-54-year age group. Subtests that measure speed of information processing showed the greatest difference with increasing age (Heaton et al., 2003; Ryan, Sattler, et al., 2000).

Education/SES

Education also impacts WAIS-III scores (Heaton et al., 2003; Schoenberg et al., 2002). Specificity (the likelihood of being correctly classed as normal) of age-corrected scores varies greatly with educational level. Heaton et al. (2003) point out that highly educated individuals would need to show a much greater decrement in test performance to be correctly classified as "impaired" using norms that are corrected only for age. Table 6–130 shows WAIS-III scores for Caucasian males, aged 20 to 89, predicted by education (adapted from the WTAR Manual, 2001). Scores are somewhat lower for African Americans and Hispanics (The Psychological Corporation, 2001).

Education also impacts performance (on Letter-Number Sequencing, Matrix Reasoning, Symbol Search) in a clinical sample. It accounts for a significant amount of variance, above and beyond that accounted for by injury severity (Donders, Tulsky et al., 2001; Strong et al., 2005).

A number of authors (Manly et al., 1998, 2000; Shuttleworth-Edwards, Kemp, et al., 2004) have suggested that while education measured in terms of level of attainment makes a large contribution to test performance, it does not entirely explain different performances, which may be better explained when quality of education is considered. For example, Shuttleworth-Edwards, Kemp, et al. (2004) examined WAIS-III performance (English administration) for a South African sample stratified for white English first language and black African first language, level, and quality of education. The effect of level of education was evident across both the white English and black African first language groups in the direction of poorer performance for lower versus higher levels of education. Further, an even more extensive effect was demonstrated within the black African first language group in the direction of profoundly depressed scores (for both Verbal and Performance tasks) for poor versus good quality of education. These authors recommend

Table 6–127 Unidirectional Base-Rate Information for WAIS-III Discrepancy

WAIS-III Indices	Education <12[a]						Education = 12[b]						Education = 13–15[c]						Education ≥ 16[d]					
	V1 > V2			V1 < V2			V1 > V2			V1 < V2			V1 > V2			V1 < V2			V1 > V2			V1 < V2		
(V1)–(V2)	5%	10%	15%	15%	10%	5%	5%	10%	15%	15%	10%	5%	5%	10%	15%	15%	10%	5%	5%	10%	15%	15%	10%	5%
VIQ-PIQ	16	12	10	13	15	18	17	13	10	13	16	19	21	17	12	12	15	19	23	18	15	9	11	15
VCI-POI	17	12	11	14	17	23	20	15	12	15	19	22	24	18	14	14	18	22	26	20	18	8	12	17
VCI-WMI	17	14	12	12	16	21	20	16	13	14	18	23	23	18	15	15	20	23	29	22	19	9	13	18
VCI-PSI	20	14	11	16	20	25	23	18	14	18	21	28	27	21	17	17	21	26	30	25	22	12	14	21
POI-WMI	25	18	14	13	15	18	25	18	15	15	18	23	21	16	12	13	16	21	23	16	13	14	17	21
POI-PSI	20	15	12	13	16	20	24	19	15	15	20	24	24	19	18	18	21	26	26	21	18	14	18	22
WMI-PSI	22	16	12	14	17	25	26	19	15	15	20	25	29	17	18	18	22	27	25	22	17	15	17	22

Note: WAIS-III = Wechsler Adult Intelligence Scale—Third Edition; V1 = first variable listed; V2 = second variable listed; VIQ = Verbal IQ; PIQ = Performance IQ; VCI = Verbal Comprehension Index; POI = Perceptual Organization Index; WMI = Working Memory Index; PSI = Processing Speed Index. [a] N = 570 for comparisons without WMI; N = 310 for comparisons with WMI. [b] N = 855 for comparisons without WMI; N = 459 for comparisons with WMI. [c] N = 584 for comparisons without WMI; N = 289 for comparisons with WMI. [d] N = 441 for comparisons without WMI; N = 241 for comparisons with WMI.

Source: From Dori & Chelune 2004. Reprinted with permission of the authors. Wechsler Adult Intelligence Scale—Third Edition. Copyright © 1997 by Harcourt Assessment, Inc. Reproduced with permission. All rights reserved.

Table 6-128 Percentages of Postacute TBI Rehabilitation Patients Obtaining Directional Differences Between WAIS-III Index Scores Equal to or Greater Than Specified Values (N = 51)

Magnitude of difference	Percentages of TBI patients	
	VIQ (minus) PIQ	PIQ (minus) VIQ
5	41	26
10	33	10
15	20	6
20	12	–
25	4	–

	VCI (minus)		
	POI	WMI	PSI
5	39	41	65
10	26	24	49
15	16	16	29
20	6	6	22
25	4	–	16

	POI (minus)		
	VCI	WMI	PSI
5	31	39	69
10	20	16	49
15	12	10	31
20	8	6	14
25	4	4	8

	WMI (minus)		
	VCI	POI	PSI
5	37	41	69
10	28	24	45
15	20	18	29
20	12	6	22
25	–	2	10

	PSI (minus)		
	VCI	POI	WMI
5	8	14	8
10	4	4	4
15	2	4	4
20	2	2	2
25	2	–	–

VCI = Verbal Comprehension Index; POI = Perceptual Organization Index; WMI = Working Memory Index; PSI = Processing Speed Index.

Source: From Axelrod et al., 2002. Reproduced with the permission of the Taylor and Francis Group.

that stratification is necessary with regard to both level and quality of education.

Higher income is also associated with better overall WAIS-III performance. This likely relates to the fact that income may serve as a proxy for other more fundamental variables such as quality of education, health status, and the like.

Gender

Gender effects are for the most part trivial (Heaton et al., 2003). The largest differences favor women on Processing Speed, but this translates into specificity differences of only about 5%.

Ethnicity

Ethnicity has an impact on test scores (Heaton et al., 2003; Shuttleworth-Edwards, Kemp, et al., 2004). In the United States, Caucasians score highest, African Americans lowest, and Hispanics intermediate. On most factors, failure to correct for ethnicity results in African Americans being three times likelier than whites to be misclassified as impaired.

Ethnicity, however, may lose its relevance when variables such as level of language ability and/or reading ability and/or quality of education are equivalent (Manly et al., 1998, 2000; Shuttleworth-Edwards, Kemp, et al., 2004). Conversely, when these variables are not equivalent across groups, race groups are unlikely to be homogeneous with respect to psychometric test performance. For example, in a South African black sample, scores for white English and black African first language groups with advantaged education appear comparable with the U.S. standardization, whereas scores for black African first language individuals with disadvantaged education were significantly lower (by about 20–25 points for those with a high school leaving qualification as well as for those with a tertiary graduate level education).

NORMATIVE DATA

Standardization Sample

The WAIS-III is based on a standardization sample of 2450 people, aged 16 to 89 years (see Table 6–131). Data gathered according to 1995 U.S. Census data were used to stratify the sample according to age, gender, race/ethnicity, education level, and geographic region. The sample was divided into 13 age groups, with 100 to 200 in each age group.

Demographic prediction (based on age, education, gender, ethnicity) of WAIS-III scores (VIQ, PIQ, FSIQ, and VCI) is provided in the WTAR Manual. The predicted scores as well as the 90% and 95% confidence intervals are given (Appendix C, WTAR Manual).

Heaton et al. have developed regression-based demographic corrections that adjust for the influences of age, education, gender, and certain ethnicities (Non-Hispanic white, African American, and Hispanic). The corrected norms are available through the Psychological Corporation (see *Source:* WAIS-III/WMS-III/WIAT-II Scoring Assistant) and are described in detail by Heaton et al. (2003) and Taylor and Heaton (2001). The demographically adjusted norms provide the clinician with an estimate of the individual's current performance relative to peers similar in age, education level, gender, and race/ethnicity. Thus, these norms allow the clinician to

Table 6–129 Percentage of Postacute TBI Rehabilitation Patients Obtaining Directional Differences Between WAIS-III Subtests Equal to or Greater Than Specified Values ($N = 51$)

Magnitude of difference	Percentages of TBI patients									
	Vocabulary (VOC) (minus)									
	SIM	ARIT	DSP	INFO	LNS	PC	DSY	BD	MR	SYS
1	35	33	37	31	47	49	67	43	28	59
2	22	26	22	16	29	29	55	31	18	47
3	22	14	10	4	22	22	41	22	12	35
4	8	12	8	2	16	18	29	12	10	26
5	4	4	8	–	8	14	22	10	6	14
6	2	2	6	–	4	10	14	6	2	2

	Similarities (SIM) (minus)									
	VOC	ARIT	DSP	INFO	LNS	PC	DSY	BD	MR	SYS
1	53	37	39	41	37	45	78	55	26	67
2	24	29	24	20	28	31	57	39	14	51
3	14	14	12	14	20	22	41	18	10	35
4	4	8	8	6	12	14	33	12	6	22
5	2	2	4	6	10	10	18	4	2	8
6	2	–	2	–	8	8	12	4	2	6

	Arithmetic (ARIT) (minus)									
	VOC	SIM	DSP	INFO	LNS	PC	DSY	BD	MR	SYS
1	53	43	37	45	49	49	75	49	33	69
2	26	33	26	33	37	41	61	41	22	55
3	22	26	12	29	26	31	47	26	12	45
4	18	14	12	14	14	28	31	14	8	24
5	16	4	6	4	6	20	24	4	6	14
6	2	–	–	2	2	10	18	2	–	6

	Digit Span (DS) (minus)									
	VOC	SIM	ARIT	INFO	LNS	PC	DSY	BD	MR	SYS
1	55	49	45	47	53	53	80	57	35	73
2	31	31	33	31	35	39	71	47	28	67
3	28	26	22	24	26	29	61	31	18	51
4	22	16	8	20	10	26	37	24	14	35
5	16	10	6	12	4	22	28	14	8	16
6	8	8	4	8	4	14	14	4	4	8

	Information (INFO) (minus)									
	VOC	SIM	ARIT	DSP	LNS	PC	DSY	BD	MR	SYS
1	49	37	35	43	53	53	75	51	29	61
2	22	24	28	18	37	33	59	33	18	55
3	6	16	22	12	28	26	45	26	14	43
4	4	10	18	8	16	22	31	20	12	28
5	2	6	8	8	8	16	22	12	6	14
6	–	2	–	4	2	12	16	6	–	8

	Letter-Number Sequencing (LNS) (minus)									
	VOC	SIM	ARIT	DSP	INFO	PC	DSY	BD	MR	SYS
1	47	45	35	24	39	47	73	49	29	67
2	37	24	26	16	28	37	63	35	22	51
3	24	16	14	8	20	26	45	18	10	29
4	12	8	4	4	16	16	26	10	6	22
5	6	6	2	2	6	10	14	8	2	12
6	–	4	–	–	–	2	6	2	–	2

(continued)

Table 6–129 Percentage of Postacute TBI Rehabilitation Patients Obtaining Directional Differences Between WAIS-III Subtests Equal to or Greater Than Specified Values (*N* = 51) (*continued*)

	VOC	SIM	ARIT	DSP	INFO	LNS	DSY	BD	MR	SYS
					Picture Completion (PC) (minus)					
1	39	37	39	31	33	35	59	39	18	59
2	28	20	26	22	26	28	47	29	10	49
3	18	16	20	14	20	14	35	14	8	31
4	14	8	6	8	12	6	28	10	6	16
5	10	2	6	6	6	6	26	8	2	8
6	4	2	2	2	4	6	14	–	2	4

	VOC	SIM	ARIT	DSP	INFO	LNS	PC	BD	MR	SYS
					Digital Symbol (DSY) (minus)					
1	18	14	16	10	16	20	29	20	12	31
2	12	10	8	6	6	14	22	12	6	26
3	4	8	4	6	6	6	12	6	4	10
4	4	4	–	6	4	4	8	4	2	–
5	2	2	–	6	4	2	8	2	–	–
6	–	2		–	4	2	–	2	–	–

	VOC	SIM	ARIT	DSP	INFO	LNS	PC	DSY	MR	SYS
					Block Design (BD) (minus)					
1	39	31	24	26	35	33	41	67	12	55
2	20	16	12	16	24	24	24	51	12	43
3	10	14	6	10	12	10	14	33	10	22
4	6	8	4	6	4	8	10	20	2	8
5	6	2	2	2	2	6	6	12	2	2
6	–	–	–	2	–	2	2	8	–	2

	VOC	SIM	ARIT	DSP	INFO	LNS	PC	DSY	BD	SYS
					Matrix Reasoning (MR) (minus)					
1	65	61	61	55	53	63	65	84	77	77
2	53	43	43	45	43	55	47	73	49	67
3	39	33	33	33	33	37	37	63	35	55
4	24	24	18	20	26	26	28	49	31	41
5	16	10	10	16	16	14	22	35	18	26
6	6	6	4	4	10	10	16	24	6	18

	VOC	SIM	ARIT	DSP	INFO	LNS	PC	DSY	BD	MR
					Sysmbol Search (SYS) (minus)					
1	29	20	24	24	22	18	33	47	26	12
2	16	12	8	14	12	12	24	33	8	6
3	6	4	6	8	8	10	12	22	6	2
4	2	4	2	4	4	6	4	14	2	2
5	–	–	2	2	4	4	4	6	2	–
6	–	–	–	2	2	4	–	4	–	–

Source: Axelrod et al., 2002. Reproduced with the permission of the Taylor and Francis Group.

determine if the patient's current performance is below expectations, given specific background variables (the Psychological Corporation, 2002). They propose a one *SD* cutoff of demographically corrected factor scores (T scores < 40) to define cognitive impairment. This results in an 85% specificity rate (percentage of normals correctly classed as normals) that is constant for the three ethnicity groups and is not affected by differences in age, education, or gender. Note that demographically adjusted norms are not intended to make judgments about intellectual capacity, expected functional capacity, or predicted academic abilities (the Psychological Corporation, 2002). The 6-Factor Model Analysis Tool (that can be downloaded from the Harcourt web site) also provides demographically adjusted norms (based on the 6-Factor Model of Tulsky,

Table 6–130 Education-Predicted WAIS-III Scores for Caucasian Males, ages 20–89

Level of Education	≤8	9–11	12	13–15	16	≥18
FSIQ	90	96	102	107	113	118
VIQ	90	96	102	107	113	118
PIQ	92	96	101	105	110	114

Source: Adapted from The Psychological Corporation, 2001.

Ivnik, et al., 2003) as well as base rates of discrepancies between index scores.

One of the criticisms of the WAIS-R was that the norms for ages 16 to 19 were suspect, likely due to some unknown sampling bias (Kaufman, 1990). With regard to the WAIS-III, Kaufman (in Kaufman & Lichtenberger, 1999) observed expected increases in test scores from ages 16 to 17 to ages 18 to 19. However, from ages 18 to 19 to ages 20 to 24, there was no increase at all, despite the fact that many more individuals in the older age group had attended university. Although he again raised concerns about the norms for the youngest age groups in the standardization sample, Kaufman concluded that the norms for 16- to 19-year-olds are probably valid, especially for ages 16 to 17 years.

In the normative sample, participants took the WAIS-III and WMS-III in one session, in roughly counterbalanced order. There were few test-order effects, suggesting that test order was not a threat to the internal validity of the normative data (Zhu & Tulsky, 2000).

Canadian Norms

The Canadian Technical Manual includes normative data for 1105 individuals aged 16 to 89 years (although because of insufficient N, norms only extend to age 84). Not only do the samples differ, but the Canadian norms also were generated using a different statistical technique (continuous norming) than that used for developing the American norms (based on the cumulative frequency of raw score distributions for samples defined by age cohorts; Lange et al., 2004). Comparison of the scores derived from Canadian and American norms in a forensic psychiatry sample revealed high correlations (>.80) between the two normative systems for all IQ, index, and subtest scores. However, scores were lower for the Canadian versus the American norms, and only 57% to 64% of the sample had IQ scores than fell within ±5 points, and only 54% to 71% of the sample had IQ scores that fell within the same ability classification range. The Processing Speed index had the highest rate of agreement between the two normative systems, with 81.8% falling within the same classification category. The most discordant subtests were Arithmetic, Matrix Reasoning, Picture Arrangement, and Comprehension. In short, interpretation of the WAIS-III performance may well vary when applying Canadian versus American norms.

RELIABILITY

Internal Reliability

The WAIS-III FSIQ score is the most reliable score, with an average split-half reliability coefficient across the 13 age groups of .98 (see Table 6–132). Accordingly, the clinician can have great confidence in the precision of this score. The average split-half reliability coefficients for the other IQ and index scores are also high (VIQ: .97, PIQ: .94, VCI: .96, POI: .93, WMI: .94, PSI: .88). In general, reliability coefficients are higher for the verbal than for the nonverbal scales. They are also higher for the IQ than the index scales, a not surprising finding since the IQ scores are based on a broader range of

Table 6–131 Characteristics of the WAIS-III Normative Sample

Number	2450 adults were tested. This sample was weighted to match 1995 U.S. Census data and each age group was required to have an average FSIQ of 100. This weighting method yielded a sample of 1250.
Age	16–89 years[a]
Geographic location	From geographic regions in proportions consistent with U.S. Census data
Sample type	Based on a representative sample of the U.S. population stratified on the basis of age, gender, race/ethnicity, educational level, and geographic region with concurrent collection of memory ability
Education	<8 to >16 years and consistent with U.S. Census proportions; for examinees aged 16–19 years, parent education was used
Gender	An equal number of males and females in each age group from 16–64; the older age groups included more women than men, in proportions consistent with 1995 U.S. Census data
Race/ethnicity	The proportions of whites, African Americans, Hispanics and other racial/ethnic groups were based on racial/ethnic proportions within each age band according to 1995 U.S. Census data
Screening	Screened via self-report for sensory, substance abuse, medical, psychiatric, or motor condition that could potentially affect performance

[a]Broken down into 13 age groups (16–17, 18–19, 20–24, 25–29, 30–34, 35–44, 45–54, 55–64, 65–69, 70–74, 75–79, 80–84, and 85–89 years); 200 subjects were included in each age group except the two oldest groups. The 80–84 age group consisted of 150 participants and the 85–89 age group included 100 participants.

Table 6–132 Type and Magnitude of Reliability Coefficient of the WAIS-III

	Internal Consistency	Test-Retest
Very high (.90+)	FSIQ	FSIQ
	VIQ	VIQ
	PIQ	PIQ
	VCI	VCI
	POI	Voc
	WMI	Info
	Voc	
	DSp	
	Info	
	MR	
High (.80–.89)	PSI	POI
	Sim	WMI
	Arith	PSI
	Comp	Sim
	Let-Num	Arith
	PC	DSp
	BD	Comp
		DSym
		BD
Adequate (.70–.79)	PA	Let-Num
	OA	PC
		MR
		SS
		OA
Marginal (.60–.69)		PA

For Digit Symbol, Symbol Search, and the Processing Speed Index, only test-retest coefficients are reported because of the timed nature of the subtests.

tasks. Average reliability coefficients are high for most of the individual subtests and range from .93 (Vocabulary) to .70 (Object Assembly). Reliability coefficients of Object Assembly are quite low for older adults (.50 for 85- to 89-year-olds) and contributed to the decision to exclude this subtest from the computation of IQ and index scores.

Split-half reliability coefficients are also high for most clinical samples (e.g., TBI, temporal lobe epilepsy, dementia) recruited as part of the WAIS-III clinical validity studies (Zhu et al., 2001). Internal consistencies were relatively lower for samples with ADHD/ADD and learning disabilities, although not statistically different from the standardization sample. Split-half reliability coefficients have been reported to be high in other populations as well (e.g., substance abusers; Ryan, Arb, et al., 2000).

Standard Error of Measurement (SEM)

According to the test manual, average standard errors of measurement (SEMs) across age groups are smallest for FSIQ (2.33). The remainder of SEMs ranged between 2.55 (VIQ) and 5.13 (PSI) standard score points for the IQ/index

scores. In the case of the subtests, average SEMs were less than two points and ranged from .79 (Vocabulary) to 1.66 (Object Assembly). The 90% and 95% confidence intervals are based on the estimated true score and the standard error of estimation (SE_E). This method results in an asymmetrical interval around the observed score because the estimated true score will always be closer to the mean of the scale than the observed score. Therefore, a confidence interval based on the estimated true score and the SE_E is a correction for regression to the mean. Sattler and Ryan (2001) recommend using confidence intervals (see their text) based on the obtained score and the standard error of measurement. They recommend these confidence intervals because the true score is unknown and they are based on the individual's specific age.

Test-Retest Reliability

A subset of the standardization sample (394 participants) was retested with the WAIS-III following an interval of about 35 days. For the four subgroups (16–29, 30–54, 55–74, and 75–89 years), reliability coefficients are very high, ranging from .94 to .97 for VIQ, .88 to .92 for PIQ, and .95 to .97 for FSIQ. Average stability coefficients for Vocabulary and Information are excellent (in the .90s); those of Similarities, Arithmetic, Digit Span, Comprehension, Digit Symbol, and Block Design are very good (in the .80s), and those of most of the other subtests marginal/adequate (.69–.79; see Table 6–132). Test-retest reliability following an interval of about 60 days tends to be lower (.58–.78) in adolescents (Barr, 2003, see Table 6–134).

When interpreting WAIS-III subtest profiles, clinicians assume that the profiles provide relatively stable patterns of cognitive strengths and weaknesses. Some (e.g., Glutting et al., 1997) have challenged this assumption; for example, by noting that the difference scores across time for individual subtests of the Wechsler scales are unreliable. By contrast, others (Livingston et al., 2003) have suggested that profiles composed of IQ and index scores demonstrate acceptable stability. However, subtest score profiles appear to be inherently less stable.

Practice Effects

Practice effects are evident on the WAIS-III, with FSIQ scores increasing by about three to six points on average (Basso et al., 2002; the Psychological Corporation, 1997). Practice effects tend to be greater for the Performance Scale (about 4 to 11 points) than the Verbal Scale (about two to three points). In addition, there is a trend for the retest gains on the FSIQ and Performance Scale to diminish with increasing age (Lineweaver & Chelune, 2003; the Psychological Corporation, 1997). With regard to changes in factor scores, the largest changes are for Perceptual Organization (increases of about three to eight points), while the smallest are for Working Memory (increases of one to three points; Basso et al., 2002; the Psychological Corporation,

Table 6–133 Confidence Intervals for True Scores for Evaluating Change on the WAIS-III

WAIS-III Score	T1 Mean (SD)	T2 Mean (SD)	r	SEP	90% CI (+/−)
VIQ	111.0 (11.5)	114.8 (11.5)	.87	5.68	9
PIQ	105.4 (12.5)	116.0 (14.4)	.89	6.58	11
FSIQ	109.4 (11.6)	115.0 (12.1)	.90	5.29	9
VCI	111.5 (11.9)	115.8 (12.3)	.85	6.48	11
POI	106.1 (14.1)	114.4 (14.1)	.86	7.74	13
WMI	106.9 (12.4)	108.6 (13.1)	.84	7.11	12
PSI	109.3 (13.0)	116.4 (14.5)	.80	8.66	14

Note: Participants were largely Caucasian, young, well educated (mean 14.5 years), and of average to above average IQ ($M = 109.3$).

Source: Adapted from Basso et al., 2002.

1997). Interestingly, similar increments emerge regardless of whether the intertest interval is one month, three months, or six months (Basso et al., 2002). All age groups show significant gains on retest, with the exception of the 75-to-89-year age group on Working Memory and Processing Speed where the increases (each about one point) are not significant (Sattler & Ryan, 2001). At the subtest level, the largest changes are for Picture Completion (increases of about one to two scaled score points), and the smallest are for Matrix Reasoning (less than one scaled score point). Further, as has been true with previous versions (Rapport et al., 1997), individuals of higher baseline ability tend to demonstrate greater practice effects than those of lower baseline intelligence (Lineweaver & Chelune, 2003). In fact, baseline levels appear to be the major determinants of retest scores (Lineweaver & Chelune, 2003).

Detecting Change

Practice effects are common on the WAIS-III, making detection of clinical change difficult. Reliable change methodology may hold some utility. Basso et al. (2002) tested healthy young adults twice following an intertest interval of three or six months and provide reliable change estimates based on the 90% and 50% confidence intervals. However, this latter interval is too large, as it leaves a 25% interval at both tails of the sampling distribution. Examination of the data in Table 6–133 demonstrates that a relatively wide range of retest scores may

fall within the 90% confidence interval. To utilize the confidence interval for an individual, the estimated true retest score is computed ($Y_{TRUE} = M + r [Y_{obs} - M]$) where M is the sample mean of the test, Y_{obs} is the actual score obtained by an individual, and r is the reliability coefficient. The relevant confidence interval is then applied to the resulting true score. If the observed retest score exceeds the upper or lower limits of the desired confidence interval, then meaningful change is presumed to have occurred. Note that participants were largely Caucasian, young, well educated ($M = 14.5$ years), and of average to above average IQ ($M = 109.3$).

Barr (2003) administered Digit Span (forward, backward), Digit Symbol, and Symbol Search from the WAIS-III to 100 high school athletes (mean age 15.9 years, $SD = 0.98$) at the beginning of the athletic season and retested 48 of them about two months later. Reliable change indices (RCIs; (e.g., Chelune et al., 1993) were computed on the test-retest data and are shown in Table 6–134. The RCIs are followed by the percentage of controls from the test-retest sample with change scores exceeding the lower limit. This is the value of interest in the evaluation of injured individuals. It represents the level of raw score decline that is required to exceed what might be expected on the basis of normal error variance and the effects of practice. Upper limits are also listed to examine the range of improvement that might occur in other contexts. In addition to the traditional 90% level, Barr provides values for less conservative 80% and 70% CIs as well. Examination of Table 6–134

Table 6–134 WAIS-III Confidence Interval (90%) for Reliable Change in High School Athletes

	T1 Mean (SD)	T2 (SD)	r	90% CI	80% CI	70% CI
DS–F Raw	10.8 (1.8)	11.0 (2.1)	.60	−2, +3 (14.5)	−2, +2 (14.6)	−1, +2 (31.3)
DS–B Raw	7.2 (2.2)	7.7 (2.4)	.63	−3, +4 (6.3)	−2, +3 (14.6)	−1, +2 (27.1)
Total–Raw	17.9 (3.2)	18.6 (4.1)	.70	−3, +5 (4.2)	−2, +4 (14.6)	−2, +3 (14.6)
WAIS-III PSI	106.7 (14.8)	114.6 (13.6)	.78	−8, +24 (6.3)	−5, +20 (10.4)	−2, +18 (16.7)
D Sym Raw	84.2 (14.6)	89.4 (16.1)	.73	−12, +23 (4.2)	−9, +19 (8.3)	−6, +16 (10.4)
S Search Raw	39.1 (6.6)	43.1 (6.4)	.58	−6, +14 (4.2)	−4, +12 (4.2)	−2, +10 (10.4)

Based on a largely Caucasian sample of 48 adolescents retested following an interval of about 60 days. All RCI values are followed by the percentage of controls (in parentheses) from the test-retest sample with change scores exceeding the lower limit.

Source: Adapted from Barr, 2003.

Table 6-135 WAIS-III Confidence Interval (90%) for Reliable
Change in Four Clinical Groups

WAIS-III	Alzheimer's	Chronic Alcohol	Schizophrenia	TBI
VIQ	5.17	6.46	7.74	8.63
PIQ	9.18	11.78	10.48	13.12
FSIQ	6.07	6.26	8.23	7.58
VCI	5.56	5.82	8.36	9.73
POI	9.48	12.02	11.92	16.01
WMI	12.84	9.13	11.20	12.76
PSI	11.02	10.43	9.86	10.18

Source: Adapted from Iverson, 1999, 2001.

Table 6-136 WAIS-III Reliable Change Index Values
in Epilepsy Patients

Variable	RC (90%) CI	RC (90%) CI
FSIQ	≤−6	≥+8
VIQ	≤−8	≥+8
PIQ	≤−7	≥+13
VCI	≤−7	≥+9
POI	≤−8	≥+14
WMI	≤−17	≥+13
Information	≤−1	≥+1
Digit Span	≤−3	≥+3
Vocabulary	≤−2	≥+2
Arithmetic	≤−2	≥+2
Comprehension	≤−3	≥+3
Similarities	≤−3	≥+3
Picture Completion	≤−3	≥+5
Picture Arrangement	≤−2	≥+4
Block Design	≤−3	≥+3
Digit Symbol	≤−3	≥+3
Matrix Reasoning	≤−3	≥+5

Note: RCI values have been corrected for practice.

Source: Adapted from Martin et al., 2002.

shows that a drop of 15 points on the Digit Symbol subtest exceeds the lower limit (−12). This level of decline was observed in less than 5% of the retest sample.

Iverson (1999, 2001) provided preliminary data, based on reliable change methodology (e.g., Chelune et al., 1993; Jacobson & Truax, 1991), to assist with determinations of improvement or decline on the WAIS-III in various clinical samples: AD, chronic alcohol use, schizophrenia, and individuals 6 to 18 months post-moderate/severe traumatic brain injury. Table 6–135 shows the 90% confidence intervals for measurement error in these groups. Thus, change scores outside of these intervals are likely not due to measurement error. Note, however, that these data are crude estimates since the clinical subjects were not tested twice and no adjustments were made for practice effects. Rather, the reliability coefficients from the normal population with the *SD*s from the clinical populations were used to calculate *SEM*s and the *SEM* from time 1 was used twice in the formula for the standard error of the difference.

Martin et al. (2002) calculated RCI scores and standardized regression-based (SRB) change scores for WAIS-III subtests and indices (except Symbol Search, Object Assembly, and PSI) in patients with complex partial seizures. Test-retest reliabilities (using a retest interval of about 7.5 months) were within acceptable ranges (.72–.96), although considerable individual subtest variability was found. Preoperative performance was the single largest contributor to each of the predictive regression equations. Age, gender, education, seizure onset, and seizure duration contributed modest variance. Measurement of meaningful cognitive change in the context of epilepsy treatment may provide clinically relevant information regarding effects of epilepsy surgery, drug trials, and repeated seizures or episodes of status. Table 6–136 presents RCI values across the subtest and index scores, corrected for practice. If an individual's change score falls outside the confidence interval, then the change is deemed uncommon, occurring in less than 10% of the patients (i.e., 5% on each end of the change scores distribution).

Standardized regression-based equations predicting postoperative scores are shown in table 6–137. Once the predicted score is determined, a difference score can be transformed

into a standardized z score (SRB change scores) by using the following equation: z score $= (Y_{observed} − Y_{predicted})/SE_{est}$. The z score of change can then be evaluated to determine whether the SRB change score exceeds a value of ±1.64 SRB change score units (90% confidence interval). Scores within the interval are viewed as a relatively frequent occurrence within the overall distribution of change scores and, therefore, do not reflect clinically relevant change. An example of a z-score SRB change calculation is provided for illustration: A woman of 25 years of age obtains a preoperative FSIQ of 86 and a postoperative FSIQ of 80. The predicted postoperative FSIQ (Y_p) becomes (Y_p) = (constant of 3.90) + (0.97 × [baseline score of 86]) + (0.13 × [age of 25]) = 90.57. Using the values from Table 6–137, the z-score change value becomes ($Y_{observed} − Y_{predicted})/SE_{est} = −2.26$. This is outside the ±1.64 90% confidence interval and is therefore considered a clinically relevant

Table 6-137 Regression Equations for Predicting WAIS-III Re-Test
Performance in Epilepsy Patients

Variable	SE$_{est}$	Constant	Unstandardized β for Baseline Measure	Unstandardized β for Age
FSIQ	4.67	3.90	0.97	0.13
VIQ	4.85	1.76	0.98	
PIQ	5.88	10.57	0.91	
VCI	4.67	.21	1.00	
POI	6.31	15.89	0.85	
WMI	8.73	18.13	0.78	
DSYM	1.74	2.01	0.77	

Source: Adapted from Martin et al., 2002.

decline in IQ since it extends beyond the lower 5% of the control sample change scores.

Interrater Reliability

According to the Technical Manual, interscorer agreement is reported to be high (>.90), even for the three subtests (Vocabulary, Similarities, and Comprehension) that require some subjectivity in scoring. However, Ryan and Schnakenberg-Ott (2003) recently asked psychologists and graduate students to score two patient protocols and found that both groups (especially students) made numerous errors despite the fact that they were confident about their scoring. Every protocol contained one or more errors. Vocabulary, Comprehension, Similarities, Picture Completion and Digit-Symbol—Coding subtests were the most difficult to score for both students and practitioners. The authors suggest that in addition to simple carelessness, examiners may not fully understand the scoring criteria. As a consequence, use of a computerized scoring system will reduce but not eliminate errors.

VALIDITY

Comparison With WAIS-R/WISC-III/WISC-IV

There is substantial correlation (.80 and above) between the WAIS-III and its predecessor, the WAIS-R (WAIS-III /WMS-III Technical Manual, 1997). The WAIS-III is somewhat more difficult than the WAIS-R, consistent with previous findings that individuals tend to score lower on newer tests than on older ones (Flynn, 1984, 1987). A sample of 192 people, aged 16 to 74 years, was given the WAIS-III and WAIS-R in counterbalanced order (WAIS-III/WMS-III Technical Manual, 1997) within a 2- to 12-week period. WAIS-III FSIQ was about 2.9 points less than WAIS-R FSIQ; WAIS-III VIQ and PIQ scores were 1.2 and 4.8 points less than corresponding WAIS-R scores. The WAIS-III/WMS-III Technical Manual includes tables (Tables 4.1 and 4.2) that allow the examiner to estimate WAIS-III IQ scores for select WAIS-R IQs. Note that the sample on which this table is based is limited to individuals younger than 75 years and typically of average ability.

The WAIS-III and WISC-III were given in counterbalanced order to a sample of 186 16-year-olds. The interval between test administrations ranged from 2 to 12 weeks. The correlations between the two measures are high (.88, .78, and .88 for VIQ, PIQ, and FSIQ, respectively) and appear to yield comparable IQs (WAIS-III/WMS-III Technical Manual, 1997). However, the WAIS-III is reported to sample a broader range of abilities than the WISC-III (Flanagan & Ortiz, 2001). The WAIS-III /WMS-III Technical Manual includes tables (Tables 4.3 and 4.4) to estimate WISC-III IQ scores for select WAIS-III IQs. As is the case for the WAIS-R, additional research is needed to evaluate the comparability of the measures in clinical groups.

The WAIS-III and WISC-IV also appear to measure similar constructs (Wechsler, 2003). The WAIS-III and WISC-IV were given to 198 children, aged 16, in counterbalanced order, with a testing interval of 10 to 67 days ($M = 22$ days). The correlations between index scores of the two measures are relatively high, ranging from .73 for PRI-POI to .89 for FSIQ-FSIQ and from .56 (Symbol Search) to .83 (Vocabulary) for subtests. With the exception of the WMI, WAIS-III composite scores are about two to five points higher than are those of the WISC-IV. A table is provided in the WISC-IV Technical and Interpretive Manual (Table 5.13) that shows the expected WAIS-III composite scores for selected WISC-IV composite scores.

Correlation With Other Measures

There is also substantial correlation (.6–.92) between the WAIS-III FSIQ and other measures of intelligence, including the Standard Progressive Matrices, the Stanford-Binet-IV (the Psychological Corporation, 1997), the GAMA (Martin et al., 2000), the Dementia Rating Scale (the Psychological Corporation, 2002), and the WASI (Axelrod, 2002; the Psychological Corporation, 1999). However, even strong correlations (e.g., between the WAIS-III and WASI) do not necessarily translate into equivalent test scores (Axelrod, 2002). The WAIS-III FSIQ also correlates moderately well (.36–.86) with measures of academic achievement (the WIAT, WIAT-II, WTAR) and memory (WMS-III) (the Psychological Corporation, 1997, 1999, 2002). This provides some support for the methodology of computing ability-achievement/memory discrepancy scores. The correlation between years of education and WAIS-III IQ scores is moderately high (.46–.55).

Convergent and Divergent Validity

Intercorrelations among the subtests are moderate to high, supporting the notion that a general factor, g, is present (the Psychological Corporation, 2002). Examination of the pattern of intercorrelations between WAIS-III subtests and scales (the Psychological Corporation, 1997) provides some evidence of convergent and discriminant validity of indexes. The Verbal Scale subtests have more in common with each other than do the Performance subtests. The pattern is less distinct for the Performance subtests. Subtests within the various domains (Working Memory, Processing Speed) intercorrelate more highly with each other than with other measures, providing some evidence in favor of the factor-derived scores. Overall, the Verbal Scale subtests have higher correlations with the Full Scale than do Performance Scale subtests (Sattler & Ryan, 2001).

The authors (the Psychological Corporation, 2002) provide some evidence of convergent and discriminant validity for some of the WAIS-III indices in small, clinically mixed samples. Thus, external measures of attention (e.g., the Attention/Concentration index of the WMS-R, Trails B) generally correlate higher with the WAIS-III Working Memory index than with the other IQ and index scores. Language (e.g., Boston Naming Test, FAS, Animal Fluency, Token Test) and verbal memory measures (e.g., WMS-R, CVLT) correlate highest (.38–.71) with the WAIS-III VCI, while nonverbal memory measures (Rey-O) show negligible/small relations with the WAIS-III IQ and factor scores. However, the direct Copy component of the Rey-O correlates moderately well (.51) with the optional procedure, Digit Symbol Copy. As might be expected, speeded tasks (e.g., Finger Tapping, Grooved Pegboard) show moderate relations (.41–.63) with the Processing Speed index. Measures of spatial processing (e.g., JOLO; MicroCog Spatial Processing Index), however, show moderate relations (.41–.67) with all IQ and index scores. As tasks become more constructional (Rey-O copy), correlations with VCI and WMI decrease (.28 and .27, respectively).

Recently, Kennedy et al. (2003) provided support for the interpretation of the Processing Speed index as a measure of central processing speed, although the influence of Working Memory on the Processing Speed index was substantial. In a sample of patients (predominantly male) who sustained traumatic brain injuries, performance on the Trail Making Test—B proved to be the largest independent predictor of the Processing Speed index, accounting for 25.5% of the variance. The WAIS-III Working Memory index scores correlated moderately well with the Processing Speed index scores at .51, a finding similar to that found in the normative sample (.55; the Psychological Corporation, 1997), and uniquely accounted for 10% of the variance in Processing Speed index scores. Psychomotor speed (Finger Tapping) did not account for an appreciable amount of variance in Processing Speed index scores in this population.

Factor-Analytic Findings

The WAIS-III/WMS-III Technical Manual (the Psychological Corporation, 1997) reports a series of factor analyses on about half the standardization sample. The results (with Object Assembly excluded) suggested that a four-factor model best fits the data for the total sample and for all but the oldest age group. They labeled the factors Verbal Comprehension, Perceptual Organization, Working Memory, and Processing Speed. Sattler and Ryan (2001) conducted additional factor analyses on the standardization sample and confirmed that a four-factor model characterizes the WAIS-III, although they noted that the subtests that load on each factor vary somewhat with age. They concluded that their findings provided empirical support for the use of the four summary indices. The four-factor model has also been shown to fit in other healthy (Saklofske et al., 2000) and clinical samples (e.g., Dickinson et al., 2002; van der Heijden & Donders, 2003a), although Ryan and Paolo (2001) found that Arithmetic could not be allocated to any factor in their heterogeneous sample. Similar findings have also been reported for the French version of the WAIS-III (Gregoire, 2004).

Two-factor and three-factor solutions have also appeared in the literature (Caruso & Cliff, 1999; Kaufman et al., 2001; Ward et al., 2000) and others have tested different models. For example, Arnau and Thompson (2000) used the standardization sample and found evidence for a hierarchical factor of general intelligence and four first-order factors of Verbal Comprehension, Perceptual Organization, Working

Memory, and Processing Speed. This factor structure appears to hold across all age groups, implying that the practitioner can be confident that the four factors are measuring the same latent constructs from age 16 to 89 (Taub et al., 2004). Burton et al. (2002) tested more complex models of intelligence in addition to the ones evaluated by the test publishers, crossvalidating results obtained with a mixed clinical sample in the standardization sample. A six-factor model including Semantic Memory (Vocabulary, Information), Verbal Reasoning (Similarities, Arithmetic, Comprehension), Constructional Praxis (Picture Completion, Block Design), Visual Reasoning (Matrix Reasoning, Picture Arrangement), Working Memory (Arithmetic, Digit Span, Letter-Number Sequencing), and Processing Speed (Coding, Symbol Search) had the best fit to the data. The model represents an expansion of Horn's *Gf-Gc* theory. Burton et al. suggest that when evaluating the results for an individual, it might be appropriate, depending upon the specific profile, to combine the subtests in a manner consistent with the six-factor model. Whether the six factors differentiate distinct clinical samples remains to be determined.

Based on an analysis of loadings on the unrotated first factor in principal components analysis, the verbal subtests tend to provide the best measures of *g* (general mental ability; Kaufman & Lichtenberger, 1999; Sattler & Ryan, 2001). Matrix Reasoning and Block Design also show relatively strong loadings (.70 or greater) on the general factor. The weakest measures of *g* include Digit Span, Digit Symbol—Coding, Object Assembly, and Picture Completion, but all of these still are categorized as "fair" measures of *g*, with loadings between .50 and .69. Thus, the variety of tasks that constitute the WAIS-III make the FSIQ a valid measure of *g*. However, some authors (Flanagan & Ortiz, 2001; Flanagan et al., 2000) suggest that a full evaluation of intelligence necessitates supplementing with other instruments to measure facets of *g* that are either not covered or insufficiently covered by the WAIS-III, including auditory processing, long-term storage and retrieval (including naming), and fluid reasoning. Tulsky, Ivnik, et al. (2003) believe that David Wechsler felt that there were more aspects to intelligence than were measured in the WAIS, and they developed a six-factor model from the WAIS-III/WMS-III that may be relevant for practitioners (Tulsky & Price, 2003; Tulsky, Saklofske, et al., 2003). The model includes Verbal, Perceptual, Processing Speed, Working Memory, Auditory Memory, and Visual Memory constructs (see Table 6–138). Based on these factor-analytic findings, new index scores have been developed (Tulsky, Saklofski, et al., 2003) as well as demographically corrected T scores (Heaton et al., 2003; see also *Source*).

Donders, Zhu, et al. (2001) examined whether there were common profile subtypes based on factor index scores in the standardization sample of the WAIS-III. Five reliable subtypes were identified. Three clusters were identified primarily by level of performance across all factor index scores (ranging from below average to average to above average). The other two clusters were characterized by distinct patterns of performance, with

Table 6–138 Composition of WAIS-III–WMS-III Factor Scores in the Six-Factor Model

Verbal Comprehension
  Information
  Vocabulary
  Similarities

Working Memory
  Spatial Span
  Letter-Number Sequencing

Perceptual Organization
  Block Design
  Picture Completion
  Matrix Reasoning

Processing Speed
  Digit Symbol
  Symbol Search

Auditory Memory
  Logical Memory I and II
  Verbal Paired Associates I and II

Visual Memory
  Family Pictures I and II
  Visual Reproductions I and II

Source: Adapted from Tulsky et al., 2003. Reprinted with permission from Elsevier.

relative efficacy on the Processing Speed index being the most prominent distinction (ranging from a relative weakness to a relative strength). The clusters did not differ significantly in age, but ethnicity and income covaried directly with level of performance (Caucasians and those with higher income had higher levels of performance), whereas gender affected differential patterns of performance (predominance of women in subtype with a relative strength on PSI, predominance of men in subtype with relative weakness on PSI).

Subtest Specificity

Subtest specificity refers to the proportion of a subtest's variance that is both reliable (i.e., not due to errors of measurement) and distinctive to the subtest. Subtest specificity is important to determine how feasible it is to interpret the unique abilities or traits attributed to a subtest. To be considered as having ample specificity, a subtest should have unique variance that exceeds 25% or more of the total variance and exceeds the error variance. Kaufman and Lichtenberger (1999) concluded that most subtests had reliable and interpretable unique characteristics. Only Symbol Search and Object Assembly had more error than unique variance, making interpretation of subtests problematic (but see also Sattler and Ryan, 2001, who note that some of the other subtests have inadequate specificity at some ages). They also caution that when unique abilities are interpreted, it is best to have other supportive data (e.g., from an examination of abilities shared with other subtests, background data, behavioral observa-

tions, or supplemental testing). Subtests with inadequate specificity should not be interpreted as measuring specific functions. These subtests, however, can be interpreted as good measures of *g*, and when appropriate, as representing a specific factor (e.g., PSI).

Clinical Findings

With regard to criterion validity, all of the index scores demonstrate some sensitivity to brain disorders (Taylor & Heaton, 2001). Consistent with the notion that the subtests comprising the Verbal Comprehension factor are "hold" tests (Matarazzo & Herman, 1984), this factor is the least sensitive to impairment (Taylor & Heaton, 2001), while the Processing Speed index is most affected (Fisher et al., 2000; Hawkins, 1998; Taylor & Heaton, 2001). With regard to base rate of impairment, most normal individuals (more than 50%) show no impairment (using one *SD* cutoff) on any factor scores, although it is not uncommon for normal individuals to be classed as "impaired" on at least one factor. It is less common for normals to be impaired on more than two factors (Taylor & Heaton, 2001).

Of the WAIS-III factor index scores, a relative strength on the PSI is uncommon following traumatic brain injury (van der Heijden & Donders, 2003b). A relative weakness on PSI appears more likely with increasing severity of TBI (Langeluddecke & Lucas, 2003; Martin et al., 2000; Strong et al., 2005; van der Heijden & Donders, 2003b). Not surprisingly, Digit Symbol is affected by increased injury severity (Donders, Tulsky, et al., 2001). Similarities also are sensitive to severity of brain trauma (Langeluddecke & Lucas, 2003). Letter-Number Sequencing and Symbol Search also demonstrate meaningful relationships with measures of severity of TBI such as length of coma or the presence of intracranial lesions (Donders, Tulsky, et al., 2001), indicating that these tasks should be routinely administered. However, the positive and negative predictive power of depressed scores on these subtests or on the associated factor index, PSI, were somewhat limited, suggesting that clinicians must supplement their assessment with other measures (Donders, Tulsky, et al., 2001). Of note, while Letter-Number Sequencing was sensitive to the sequelae of TBI, other subtests in the WMI (Arithmetic, Digit Span) were not, raising concerns about the diagnostic utility of this index in the context of TBI. Donders et al. also reported that Matrix Reasoning failed to differentiate patients with moderate to severe TBI from matched controls. The fact that this subtest does not involve time constraints may be an important reason for its lack of sensitivity to the effects of TBI. Dugbarty et al. (1999) have also suggested that this subtest correlates as strongly with measures of verbal skills (e.g., verbal fluency) as with measures of nonverbal problem solving (C-TONI). These findings raise the question of whether Matrix Reasoning actually enhances measurement of fluid reasoning on the WAIS-III. Information also holds up relatively well to neurological insult, even severe ones (Langeluddecke & Lucas, 2003).

Digit Symbol

Digit Symbol is a multifaceted task. The WAIS-III Digit Symbol-Coding subtest includes supplementary procedures that assess perceptual-motor speed (Symbol Copy) and incidental learning (Free Recall and Pairing) as a way of determining what might have caused a low Digit Symbol-Coding score. The literature suggests that speed plays a key role. Across the various age groups in the WAIS-III standardization sample, the correlation between Symbol Copy (indexing speed) and Digit Symbol is $r = .70$, indicating that the tests share about 50% of their variance (Joy et al., 2004). The literature (Joy et al., 2004; Kreiner & Ryan, 2001) suggests that Digit Symbol-Coding performance is more related to speed (Symbol Copy) than to the memory requirements of the test (memory accounting for only 5–7% of Digit Symbol variance using the incidental learning tests or at most 14–15% using WMS-III indexes). Joy et al. (2004) note that the contribution of memory to Digit Symbol performance, while relatively small, is nonetheless real.

The Incidental Learning scores (Free Recall and Pairing) measure memory. Thus, in the WAIS-III/WMS-III standardization sample, Free Recall and Pairing scores show moderate correlations ($r =$ about .37) with WMS-III memory index scores; the mean correlation between Symbol Copy and memory was less (.28; Joy et al., 2003). Further, there is evidence that the incidental learning task has diagnostic utility in the evaluation of a variety of conditions that affect memory including Alzheimer's, Huntington's, and sport-related head injury (Joy et al., 2003; Shuttleworth-Edwards, 2002). Based on analyses from the WAIS-III/WMS-III standardization data and a smaller clinical sample, Joy et al. (2003) recommend that on Pairing, scores of 6 or below (i.e., three or fewer pairs mastered) on the part of younger adults (16–49 years) or scores of 4 or below (i.e., two or fewer pairs) on the part of older adults (50–89 years) raise the concern of memory impairment. On Free Recall, scores of 5 or below are sufficiently suggestive of memory impairment to warrant further investigation. Similar findings have recently been reported in South Africa for black African first language individuals (ages 19–30) from a disadvantaged educational setting, suggesting that the task may be relatively culture independent with utility as a screening instrument (Shuttleworth-Edwards, Donnelly, et al., 2004).

Joy et al. (2003) caution, however, that incidental learning scores in the average range by no means rule out memory impairment; only when scores are very high do memory problems become less likely (i.e., specificity is high but sensitivity is low). Thus, only perfect or nearly perfect incidental learning test scores should induce clinicians to abandon previously planned memory testing.

Interpretive Guidelines

Kaufman & Lichtenberger (1999) outline a sequence of steps to aid in the interpretation of WAIS-III profiles. The sequence begins with a look at the most global score (FSIQ), since it is the most reliable score on the measure and moves through multiple steps that deal first with the separate IQs (steps 2 to 4: are IQ scores significantly different, are the IQ differences abnormally large, is the IQ discrepancy interpretable?), and then the factor indices (steps 5 to 7: if the factor scores are interpretable, a variety of interpretive hypotheses are considered), before addressing strengths and weakness in the subtest profile (steps 8 to 9: evaluation of each subtest relative to the person's own average subtest score, generation of hypotheses by considering how different abilities overlap various subtests). Kaufman and Lichtenberger (1999) recommend that the IQs are not interpretable if there is variability between the factors making up the IQs or if there is significant scatter within the Verbal or Performance IQ scale (i.e., if the difference between the highest and lowest subtest on the scale exceeds eight or more points). In a similar vein, they suggest that the factor scores may not provide adequate estimates of the construct being measured if there is significant scatter in the subtest scores comprising the index. For the VCI, they suggest the range is five or more points; for the POI and WMI, the range is six or more points; and for the PSI, the range is four or more points. They determined these latter values by conducting pair-wise comparisons among the subtests making up an index and selecting the smallest scaled score range that ensured significant discrepancies.

The Kaufman and Lichtenberger approach appears reasonable. However, there is insufficient evidence that indices based on widely divergent components are less valid than indices based on subtests of similar magnitude. As Ryan and Paolo (2001) point out, the WAIS-III indices reported in the test manual are based on the entire standardization sample, and it is likely that IQ/factor scores based on widely divergent subtests were not excluded from the scaling of indices during test development. Thus, strict adherence to the method may be premature. There is a recent attempt to determine whether marked intersubtest scatter reduces predictive validity. Ryan et al. (2002) examined WAIS-III/WMS-III data in a sample of patients, half with high intersubtest scatter (scatter range of nine or more) and half with low scatter. The two groups were matched on FSIQ. They found that the accuracy of memory performance estimates based on the WAIS-III were not influenced by the amount of intersubtest scatter in the profiles. Thus, estimates of WMS-III indices based on FSIQ may be done with a reasonable degree of confidence, when the amount of intersubtest scatter in the profile is fairly large. Whether the same holds true for estimation of scores from other instruments (e.g., WIAT) remains to be determined.

Profile Analysis

The advent of demographically adjusted scores does not eliminate interpretive difficulties since they estimate scores of individuals imperfectly. One way to enhance inferential capacity is to interpret the score of interest against the patient's index profile. There are two different types of measures that assist in profile analysis: statistically reliable differences and empirically observed base rates. According to the WAIS-III Technical Manual (the Psychological Corporation, 2002), a discrepancy that is statistically significant yet frequent in the standardization sample likely reflects normal variations in an individual's abilities. On the other hand, discrepancy scores that are statistically significant and rare in the standardization sample are thought to represent both a meaningful and substantial deficit in at least one of the abilities being compared. Whether an occurrence is unusual depends on one's definition of abnormality. Some suggest that to be unusual or rare, the difference should occur in 15% or less (in one direction) of the standardization sample (e.g., Sattler & Ryan, 2001).

There are two methods provided to determine whether a discrepancy is abnormal: simple and predicted difference methods. The predicted difference method is preferred since it takes into account score reliability, the correlation between the two measures and regression to the mean (The Psychological Corporation, 1997). By definition, the stronger the correlation is, the closer two scores are expected to covary, and so the smaller the expected discrepancy is. This implies that for highly correlated variables, even a relatively small discrepancy may be rare in the general population and could reflect a clinically meaningful finding. For moderately correlated variables, a discrepancy of similar magnitude may be relatively common (Dori & Chelune, 2004).

Patterns of discrepancy base rates may also covary as a function of cognitive level (Dori & Chelune, 2004; Hawkins & Tulsky, 2003). Hawkins and Tulsky (2003) note that larger discrepancies are more commonly seen at high IQ levels, although FSIQ does not correlate strongly with discrepancy magnitude. More important are the effects of rising IQ (and any strong correlate such as VCI or education) on the direction of discrepancy, the tendency for one index score to exceed the other at low FSIQ levels, with the situation reversed at higher IQ level. These effects reflect the modest correlation between the contrasted indices, combined with the fact that one of the contrasted pair usually correlates more strongly with FSIQ than the other. They explain that when two indices do not correlate perfectly, a regression to the mean type of effect occurs; that is, if someone has a higher than average score on one index (e.g., FSIQ, VCI), chances are that the second score (e.g., PSI, or memory index) will be lower, as there is more room beneath the first score than above it. Conversely, if the first score is lower than average, chances are the second (contrasted) score will be higher. Further, in any pairing, the index that correlates to the greater extent with general ability tends to be the superior score at higher ability levels and the inferior score at lower ability levels. Thus, the clinician must recognize that when contrasting one score (e.g., PSI) against an index used to set

an expectation for that score (e.g., VCI), a sizeable inferiority of the second score (PSI) is expected on psychometric grounds alone.

As noted earlier (see *Scoring*), Dori and Chelune (2004) provide information on education-stratified, directional prevalence rates (i.e., base rates) of discrepancy scores between the major index scores for the WAIS-III. Hawkins and Tulsky (2003) provide discrepancy base rates for indices derived from the six-factor model to determine whether a discrepancy between demographically adjusted T scores is abnormal. Adjusted score discrepancies still exhibit direction effects. Thus, individuals who perform better on the intellectual indices (VCI, POI) than is typical for their demographic characteristics will typically display lower PSI, WMI, and memory scores, with the converse being true for those with low intellectual index scores. T scores and discrepancy base-rate data based on the six-factor model are available by downloading the analysis tool on the Harcourt Assessment web site (see *Source*). Note that the WMI is derived from the WMS-III.

Premorbid Estimation of Ability

A number of procedures have been developed to estimate premorbid level of intellectual ability. These include methods based on (a) demographics alone, (b) current performance on tasks thought to be fairly resistant to neurological insult, and (c) demographics and current performance.

The WAIS-III is linked to the WTAR, a task requiring reading of irregular words, and allows for comparison between predicted and actual functioning. Tables are provided in the WTAR Manual to predict WAIS-III scores from the WTAR reading score, from demographic information alone (age, gender, education, and ethnicity), or from WTAR reading plus demographic information (see *WTAR*). The combined WTAR demographic estimated FSIQ, VIQ, and PIQ scores correlate .79, .81, and .66 with the standardization samples' actual FSIQ, VIQ, and PIQ scores, respectively. The WTAR may be a particularly useful supplement to the WAIS-III when estimating premorbid status, especially in light of recent research suggesting that reliance only on years of education may not be sufficient in accounting for quality of educational experience (Manly et al., 2002).

Another method to estimate premorbid functioning is to derive algorithms by combining current Wechsler subtest scores with demographic variables (Oklahoma Premorbid Intelligence Estimate; OPIE-3). Recently, Schoenberg et al. (2002) used the Wechsler standardization sample to generate a set of algorithms:

- Four subtest—OPIE-3 (4ST): Vocabulary, Information, Matrix Reasoning, Picture Completion raw scores with demographic variables
- Two subtest—OPIE-3 (2ST): Vocabulary and Matrix Reasoning raw scores and demographic variables

- Single verbal subtest—OPIE-3V: Vocabulary and demographic variables
- Two performance subtests—OPIE-3P: Matrix Reasoning and Picture Completion and demographic variables
- Single performance subtest—OPIE-3MR: Matrix Reasoning and demographic variables
- OPIE-3 Best: a procedure that employs either the OPIE-3V, the OPIE-3MR, or OPIE (2ST) algorithms in a best performance method. To derive the OPIE-3 (Best) estimate, individuals' predicted FSIQ is obtained from the OPIE-3V algorithm if their VOC age-corrected scaled score is one or more points above their MR score. If the MR age-corrected scaled score is greater than VOC, individuals' premorbid IQ is estimated using the OPIE-3MR method. In cases in which VOC and MR age-corrected scaled scores are equivalent, their IQ score is predicted using the OPIE-3 (2ST) equation.

Examination of these algorithms within samples of patients with known brain injury (Schoenberg et al., 2003) indicated that the OPIE-3 (2ST), OPIE-3V, and OPIE-3MR algorithms did not systematically over- or underestimate FSIQ in patients with brain injury or among depressed individuals without brain injury. The OPIE-3 (Best) procedure appeared to slightly overestimate FSIQ in a nonneurologically compromised sample (i.e., the depressed group). Based on these findings, Schoenberg et al. (2003) recommend the OPIE-3 (2ST), OPIE-3V, or OPIE-3MR for general clinical use. The OPIE-3 (Best) procedure is suitable for cases of moderate to severe brain injury. Clinicians might also wish to compare the FSIQ estimate using the OPIE-3 (Best) procedure to the predicted IQs yielded by the OPIE-3 (2ST), OPIE-3V, and OPIE-3MR algorithms. Following recommendations of Veiel and Koopman (2001) regarding estimates derived from regression, a worksheet for computing corrected FSIQ estimates is included in Table 6–139.

Schoenberg et al. (2004) have extended their work and provided algorithms to estimate premorbid VIQ and PIQ scores. These formulas may prove particularly useful in individuals with large natural differences (e.g., 15 points or more) between their verbal and nonverbal abilities. The VIQ OPIE-3 model combines Vocabulary raw scores with demographic variables. The PIQ estimation algorithm uses Matrix Reasoning scores with demographic variables. The formulas are also shown in Table 6–139.

Reliance on demographics alone is of limited clinical utility in individual cases. Recently, Langeluddecke and Lucas (2004) assessed demographic (from the WTAR) and OPIE-3 methods for estimating premorbid intellectual ability. They evaluated three TBI groups that varied in terms of injury severity (moderate, severe, extremely severe) as well as a group of normal controls. The demographic method yielded average scores in keeping with the general population; however, the range was severely restricted. The implication is that

demographic prediction may be of use with individuals whose premorbid IQ is likely to have been in the average range but is inappropriate in individuals at either end of the spectrum of intellectual ability (see also Griffin et al., 2002). The OPIE-3 IQ scores were not subject to severe range restriction. However, they found OPIE estimates (particularly those including two nonverbal subtests) to be susceptible to the effects of neurological impairment. The OPIE-3 (Best) proved particularly robust in more severely injured patients, consistent with the findings of Schoenberg et al. (2003) noted above. There was less support for its use in relation to an injury of mild/moderate severity as it tended to overestimate FSIQ by an average of about six points.

Thus, the available literature suggests that methods that combine demographics and current performance (e.g., OPIE-3, combined WTAR) offer a reasonable approach to premorbid estimation of IQ. The differential utility of the OPIE-3 and other methods such as the WTAR (combined demographics and reading) requires investigation (see Chapter 6, *General Cognitive Functioning, Neuropsychological Batteries, and Assessment of Premorbid Intelligence*, earlier in this volume for comparison of these methods).

Malingering

Qualitative analyses related to poor effort on the Wechsler scales have focused on scatter (excessive failures on easy items), absurd or grossly illogical responses, and approximate answers (e.g., Rawling & Brooks, 1990). The sensitivity and specificity of such qualitative indices are, however, somewhat disappointing (Milanovitch et al., 1996). Suppressed Digit Span performance has been proposed as a potential marker for suboptimal performance since potential malingerers may not realize that Digit Span is often relatively preserved in patients with neurological impairment. Iverson and Tulsky (2003) examined the WAIS-III standardization sample and select clinical groups. They generated base-rate tables for the Digit Span scaled score, longest span forward, longest span backward, and the Vocabulary-Digit Span difference score. They suggested the following guidelines with regard to suspect performance: (a) scaled score of 5 or less, (b) longest span forward score of 4 or less (for persons under age 55), (c) longest span backward score of 2 or less, or (d) Vocabulary-Digit Span difference score of 5 or greater. These suspicion indices are based on base rates in the general population and in clinical groups that generally occur in 5% or less of the subjects. Based on a study of TBI patients with low and high probability of malingering, Axelrod et al. (in press) found that the Digit Span scaled score is more efficient than the other Digit Span indices for detecting incomplete effort. They recommend a cutoff score of 7 or less for purposes of preliminary screening. Such a cutoff accurately classified 75% of persons in the incomplete effort group and 69–77% in good effort groups.

Miller et al. (2004) examined the specificity of a Vocabulary minus Digit Span scaled score of ≥6 points in a sample of

Table 6–139 OPIE-3 Calculation Worksheet

1. OPIE-3 (2ST) estimation formula using Vocabulary and Matrix Reasoning; $SE_E = 6.63$:

FSIQ = 45.997 + .652 (VOC raw score) + 1.287 (MR raw score) + .157 (Age in years)
        + 1.034 (Education) + 0.652 (Ethnicity) − 1.015 (Gender).

Predicted FSIQ = _____ (95% CI = ±1.96 SE_E) _____ − _____

Veiel & Koopman (2001) adjustment:
Adjusted Predicted FSIQ = 100 + (Predicted IQ–100) (1.21) = _____
        Adjusted SE_E = 6.85(95% CI = ±1.96 SE_E) = _____ − _____

2. OPIE-3V estimation formula using Vocabulary; $SE_E = 8.35$:

FSIQ = 57.220 + 0.874 (VOC raw score) + 1.766 (Education) + 1.081 (Ethnicity)
        + 0.674 (Region of the country) − 1.508 (Gender)

Predicted FSIQ = _____ (95% CI = ±1.96 SE_E) _____ − _____

Veiel & Koopman (2001) adjustment:
Adjusted Predicted FSIQ = 100 + (Predicted IQ–100) (1.39) = _____
        Adjusted SE_E = 9.26 (95% CI = ±1.96 SE_E) = _____ − _____

3. OPIE-3MR estimation formula using Matrix Reasoning; $SE_E = 9.06$:

FSIQ = 43.678 + 1.943 (MR raw score) + 0.297 (Age) + 3.564 (Education) + 1.541 (Ethnicity)
        + 0.543 (Region of the country) − 1.137 (Gender)

Predicted FSIQ = _____ (95% CI = ±1.96 SE_E) _____ − _____

Veiel & Koopman (2001) adjustment:
Adjusted Predicted FSIQ = 100 + (Predicted IQ–100) (1.56) = _____
        Adjusted SE_E = 11.14 (95% CI = ±1.96 SE_E) = _____ − _____

For OPIE (Best) FSIQ estimate, administer the WAIS-III. Compare the age-corrected scaled scores. If
    Vocabulary and Matrix Reasoning scores are the same, use Equation 1. If Vocabulary is one or more
    scaled score points greater than Matrix Reasoning, use Equation 2. If MR subtest scaled score is
    greater than Vocabulary, use Equation 3; $SE_E = 7.93$.

Predicted FSIQ = _____ (95% CI = ±1.96 SE_E) _____ − _____.

4. OPIE-3 VIQ = 59.516 + .930 (Vocabulary raw score) + 1.573 (Education) − 2.588 (Gender)
        + .592 (Region of the country) + .521 (Ethnicity). $R^2 = .773$, $SE_E = 7.306$

5. OPIE-3PIQ = 44.435 + 2.232 (Matrix Reasoning raw score) + .301 (Age in years)
        + 1.955 (Education) + 1.452 (Ethnicity). $R^2 = .65$, $SE_E = 9.053$

Coding Variables

Age:	In years
Ethnicity:	1 = African American, 2 = Hispanic, 3 = Other, 4 = Caucasian
Education:	1 = 0–8 years, 2 = 9–11 years, 3 = 12 years, 4 = 13–15 years, 5 = 16+years
Gender:	1 = male, 2 = female
Region:	1 = South, 2 = North Central, 3 = Northeast, 4 = West

Source: Adapted from Schoenberg et al., 2003; Schoenberg et al., 2004.

patients (alcohol abuse, polysubstance abuse) with low base rates for malingering. The overall correct classification rate was 99%. In short, large Vocabulary-Digit Span discrepancies are rare in individuals with these disorders, provided they are not in litigation or seeking compensation/gain.

Another promising technique is to calculate the Reliable Digit Span score (RDS; Greiffenstein et al., 1994) by summing the longest forward and backward digit strings (both trials must be completed without error) from the Digit Span task. For example, a patient who passes both trials of four digits forward and three digits backward attains an RDS score of 7. In TBI samples, the RDS cutoff score of 7 yields sensitivity ranging from about 45–90% with specificity of 57–95% (e.g., Etherton et al., 2005; Larrabee, 2003; Mathias et al., 2002; Strauss, Hultsch, et al., 2000, 2002). Of note, Etherton et al. (2005) have recently shown that laboratory-induced moderate to very severe pain has no impact on RDS scores. Similarly, chronic pain does not negatively impact performance (Etherton et al., 2005). Thus, the presence of moderate to severe pain alone likely cannot account for low RDS scores (<7). Note that these data also support the use of the RDS in detecting response bias in patients complaining of pain as well as in the assessment of pain-related cognitive impairment in patients whose primary complaint is pain (Etherton et al., 2005).

It would be a mistake to rely on Digit Span as the primary method for identifying biased responding. While specificity can be high, sensitivity tends to be modest (Greve et al., 2003; Iverson & Tulsky, 2003). Special symptom validity tasks (e.g., VSVT, PDRT) tend to be more effective than the techniques that rely on Digit Span performance (RDS, Voc-DSp; Mathias et al., 2002; Strauss, Hultsch, et al., 2000, 2002). Nonetheless, abnormal Digit Span or RDS should raise concerns about the validity of the WAIS scores and the evaluation in general.

COMMENT

Significant strengths of the WAIS-III include its excellent standardization, generally high reliability (except in adolescents; Barr, 2003; also see Ryan & Schnakenberg-Ott, 2003, with regard to scoring imprecision), the stability of the IQ and index scores, the inclusion of Working Memory and Processing Speed indices, and the extension of the floor (Kaufman & Lichtenberger, 1999). The co-linking of the WAIS-III with other tests (WTAR, WMS-III, WIAT-II) enables the examiner to evaluate more clearly an individual's conceptual, memory, and achievement level. The availability of demographic estimates of select WAIS-III scores (see WTAR Manual) also facilitates interpretation. However, it is important to bear in mind that the WAIS-III does not evaluate all aspects of intelligence. There are also other considerations.

The range of WAIS-III FSIQs has been extended (45–155); however, the test does not sample a sufficient range of cognitive abilities for individuals with moderate to severe mental retardation and for those who are very gifted. Thus, for individuals who either fail or pass most items on the WAIS-III,

the examiner should consider a different intelligence test (e.g., SB5, WJ-III COG).

The norms for the three IQs are based on administration of 11 standard subtests. Norms for the IQ scores may be difficult to interpret when one of the supplementary subtests (e.g., Letter-Number Sequencing, Symbol Search) or the optional subtest (Object Assembly) is substituted (Ryan & Sattler, 2001). However, clinicians should routinely administer Letter-Number Sequencing and Symbol Search, because otherwise they will not be able to calculate the Working Memory and Processing Speed indices. While administration of these subtests is not necessary for calculation of conventional IQ scores, interpretation of factor scores is more clearly supported by factor-analytic findings (Donders, Zhu, et al., 2001). In addition, the PSI in particular may provide potentially meaningful information that is not otherwise captured by the other indices (which tend to vary more by overall level of performance; Donders, Zhu, et al., 2001). Clinicians should note that a relative strength or weakness on the PSI is moderated to a substantial degree by gender. Thus, a profound decrement on PS may be especially meaningful when the patient is a woman (Donders, Zhu, et al., 2001).

Larrabee (2004), in his recent excellent review, has questioned the advisability of dropping Object Assembly and replacing it with Matrix Reasoning. He noted that prior research with the WAIS and WAIS-R has shown that OA and BD are the highest loading subtests on the Perceptual Organization factor. He also reported that OA has reasonable reliability, appears to measure more than just Processing Speed (despite its timed nature), and likely has greater criterion validity in comparison with Matrix Reasoning and Picture Completion. He argues that OA but not Matrix Reasoning or PC is sensitive to the severity of traumatic brain injury (see also Donders, Zhu, et al., 2001).

Short forms should not be used to categorize an individual's intelligence for diagnostic purposes or disability determination. Rather, they should be reserved for situations where gross estimates will suffice (e.g., as screening measures or within research studies) or when patient stamina is a significant concern. Short-form selection should be based on a number of considerations including clinical utility, psychometric characteristics, and the amount of time saved by the administration of the shortened version (Ryan et al., 1998). Whenever one of the short forms is used, it is recommended that the examiner append the abbreviation "Est." next to the value (Ryan & Ward, 1999). Short forms of PIQ and factor scores are not recommended for clinical use but may be viable when the goal is to obtain group, rather than individual, estimates (Axelrod et al., 2000).

Substantial efforts have been made to examine the effect of ethnicity on the WAIS-III (see WAIS-III/WMS-III Technical Manual). A particular focus has been on reducing bias in items for African American and Hispanic individuals and the provision of normative data for these groups. These steps allow for better interpretation of the test results in these groups.

Studies of additional groups (e.g., Asian Americans) are also needed (Okazaki & Sue, 2000).

When one employs scores that are corrected for age alone, as has been standard practice in the past, normal individuals who have lower education levels or are ethnic minorities have substantially increased probabilities of being incorrectly classified as cognitively impaired. Accordingly, Heaton et al. (2003) have argued for the use of demographically corrected norms. However, there is some recent evidence (Strong et al., 2005) that demographically corrected norms do not offer a clear advantage or disadvantage compared with traditional age-corrected norms, at least among Caucasians who have suffered moderate-severe traumatic head injuries and who have at least a middle-school level of education (grade 8 and above). The authors note that it is possible that the demographically corrected norms may be more convincingly advantageous with other clinical conditions and with other ethnic groups.

The test authors emphasize that the demographically adjusted scores allow the examiner to minimize the impact of psychosocial variables on the diagnosis of cognitive impairment (e.g., to estimate the degree of cognitive impairment following TBI). However, they should not be used in psychoeducational evaluations, determination of intellectual deficiency, vocational assessment, or in any context in which the purpose of the evaluation is to determine the absolute level (IQ or Memory) of the patient relative to a representative sample of the U.S. population. Accordingly, to avoid confusion with traditional IQ and Memory scores, the demographically adjusted scores are reported in a T-score metric.

As was true for previous versions, practice effects tend to be larger for Performance than for Verbal scores. Thus, a trivial advantage favoring performance scales on initial testing may become large on retest simply because of practice effects. Similarly, an advantage favoring the verbal subtests on initial testing may become trivial on retest. Clinicians examining discrepancies for repeat assessments should take into account predictable practice effects. Further, although stability coefficients are high for the WAIS-III, studies are needed to evaluate the stability with particular samples and over longer time periods.

The four-factor solution has good statistical and clinical support. However, when evaluating the results for an individual, it might be appropriate, depending upon the specific profile, to combine the subtests in an alternate manner (e.g., six dimensions). It is important to bear in mind that the VIQ and PIQ groupings are poor representations of *Gc* and *Gf* (Burton et al., 2002; Caruso & Cliff, 1999). Further, users should note that interpretation of the PSI is limited because is consists of only two tasks (Digit Symbol, Symbol Search). In cases where subtest scores comprising the index are highly discrepant, the patient may (a) have a weakness in the factor that is masked by the high score in the narrow area covered by the subtest or (b) have a weakness in the narrow area measured by the subtest but not a broad PS weakness (Taub et al.,

2004). Administration of additional measures of PS may provide clarification.

Evaluation of scatter is important for clinical interpretation. Note that statistically significant differences between specific factor indices are fairly common, and mild fluctuations do not necessarily imply clinical significance (the Psychological Corporation, 1997). Further, there is evidence that the amount of scatter depends on the IQ/education level, with scatter increasing substantially as IQ/education level increases. Base-rate approaches should be used to determine what is truly rare and abnormal or common and normal (Dori & Chelune, 2004).

Revisions

The periodic revisions of the Wechsler scales present problems for investigators and clinicians since every Wechsler standardization sample from 1932 to the present has established norms of a higher standard than its predecessor (Flynn, 1984, 1987). As a result, the Wechsler tests get successively harder to compensate for the increased performance of individuals over time. This means that the older the test is, the greater the overestimation of the participant's IQ is (Parker, 1986). IQ increases of about three points have been reported for the WAIS-III compared with the WAIS-R (WAIS-III/ WMS-III Technical Manual). As was evident with previous versions, the larger differences are in the Performance Scale norms (about five points), with less change in the Verbal Scale norms (about one point; Flynn, 1998). However, Flynn et al. (1998) noted that additional subjects at low IQ levels were added, perhaps making the norms of the new version somewhat less demanding. In addition to differences in difficulty level necessitated by the gain in IQ over time (Flynn, 1984, 1987), there are substantial differences in subtest content. Only about 50–60% of the WAIS-R items have been retained in either original or slightly modified form. Further, the factor structure has changed, measuring new constructs outside of the domain of previous versions and measuring some constructs in different ways (e.g., POI includes Matrix Reasoning; WMI includes Letter-Number Sequencing; Strauss, Spreen, et al., 2000).

These modifications raise significant problems with regard to equating scores on the new WAIS-III with earlier versions and suggest that different versions of the scale may produce different IQ classifications (Kanaya et al., 2003) as well as different subtest patterns for a given individual (Chelune et al., 1987; Reitan & Wolfson, 1990). There is evidence, based on the WISC, that when IQ tests age and are renormed, the impact of mental retardation diagnoses can be significant. Kanaya et al. (2003) reported that in longitudinal IQ records, students in the borderline and mild mental retardation range lost an average of 5.6 points when retested on the renormed version and were more likely to be classed as mentally retarded compared with peers retested on the same test. Kanaya et al. (2003) note that the magnitude of the effect is large and has enormous social implications because of its impact on national policies, including special education financing, eligibility for social security benefits, the death penalty, and military service.

Canadian Version

The WAIS-III norms for the Canadian population are different from those for the U.S. population. With the exception of Processing Speed, clinically different conclusions might be derived on a significant number (more than one-quarter) of individual IQ or index scores depending on whether the Canadian or U.S. normative system is applied. An assessment protocol that follows best practice guidelines recognizes that using U.S. norms may not provide the most appropriate representation of individual performance. It is important to note, however, that in certain circumstances, the U.S. norms may be preferred. For example, American norms extend to age 89 years in contrast to 84 for the Canadian norms. Further, although Canadian linking studies are available with the WIAT-II, similar linking studies have not been done with the WMS-III. Thus, where examiners wish to make use of such data (e.g., predicted-obtained memory discrepancy), the U.S. norms must be used. Clinicians should never substitute Canadian WAIS-III norm-based scores into a discrepancy calculation and apply the U.S. WAIS-III/WMS-III tables (see Canadian Technical Manual). In addition, users should also note that there are no linking studies between the WAIS-R and the Canadian WAIS-III. Thus, to compare current with previous assessment, clinicians need to refer to data contained in the U.S. WAIS-III/WMS-III Technical Manual.

Reporting Data

In terms of reporting IQ test results, it is important to emphasize that there is some variability in all testing and that it is highly unlikely that a person would obtain exactly the same score if retested. Rather, IQ is best thought of as falling within a range of ±2 standard errors of measurement. This defines the interval within which the true score will fall 95% of the time. If one prefers the 90% confidence interval (corresponding to 1.64 SE_M), these are provided in the WAIS-III Administration and Scoring Manual. One way to communicate such information in a psychological report is as follows: "The patient's Full-Scale IQ score on the WAIS-III falls at about the ___ percentile. There is some variability in all testing and it is highly unlikely that a person would obtain exactly the same score on retest. Rather, the IQ score is best thought of as falling within a range. The chances that the range of scores from the ___ to the ___ percentile includes her/his true score are about 95 (or 90) out of 100."

REFERENCES

Arnau, R. C., & Thompson, B. (2000). Second-order confirmatory factor analysis of the WAIS-III. *Assessment, 7,* 237–246.

Axelrod, B. N. (2001). Administration duration for the Wechsler Adult Intelligence Scale-III and Wechsler Memory Scale-III. *Archives of Clinical Neuropsychology, 16,* 293–301.

Axelrod, B. N. (2002). Validity of the Wechsler Abbreviated Scale of Intelligence and other very short forms of estimating intellectual functioning. *Assessment, 9,* 17–23.

Axelrod, B. N., Dingell, J. D., Ryan, J. J., & Ward, L. C. (2000). Estimation of Wechsler Adult Intelligence Scale-III scores with the 7-subtest short form in a clinical sample. *Assessment, 7,* 157–161.

Axelrod, B. N., Fichtenberg, N. L., Liethen, P. C., Czarnota, M. A., & Stucky, K. (2002). Index, summary, and subtest discrepancy scores on the WAIS-III in postacute traumatic brain injury patients. *International Journal of Neuroscience, 112,* 1479–1487.

Axelrod, B. N., Fichtenberg, N. L., Millis, S. R., & Wertheimer, J. C. (in press). Detecting incomplete effort with Digit Span from the Wechsler Adult Intelligence Scale-Third Edition. *The Clinical Neuropsychologist.*

Axelrod, B. N., & Ryan, J. J. (2000). Prorating Wechsler Adult Intelligence Scale-III summary scores. *Journal of Clinical Psychology, 56,* 807–811.

Axelrod, B. N., Ryan, J. J., & Ward, L. C. (2001). Evaluation of seven-subtest short forms of the Wechsler Adult Intelligence Scale-III in a referred sample. *Archives of Clinical Neuropsychology, 16,* 1–8.

Barr, W. B. (2003). Neuropsychological testing of high school athletes. Preliminary norms and test-retest indices. *Archives of Clinical Neuropsychology, 18,* 91–101.

Basso, M. R., Carona, F. D., Lowery, N., & Axelrod, B. N. (2002). Practice effects on the WAIS-III across 3- and 6-month intervals. *The Clinical Neuropsychologist, 16,* 57–63.

Boake, C. (2002). From the Binet-Simon to the Wechsler-Bellevue: Tracing the history of intelligence testing. *Journal of Clinical and Experimental Neuropsychology, 24,* 383–405.

Burton, D. B., Ryan, J. J., Axelrod, B. N., Schellenberger, T. (2002). A confirmatory factor analysis of the WAIS-III in a clinical sample with cross-validation in the standardization sample. *Archives of Clinical Neuropsychology, 17,* 371–387.

Butler, M., Retzlaff, P., & Vanderploeg, R. (1991). Neuropsychological test usage. *Professional Psychology: Research and Practice, 22,* 510–512.

Camara, W. J., Nathan, J. S., & Puente, A. E. (2000). Psychological test usage: Implications in professional psychology. *Professional Psychology: Research and Practice, 31,* 141–154.

Caruso, J. C., & Cliff, N. (1999). The properties of equally and differentially weighted WAIS-III factor scores. *Psychological Assessment, 11,* 198–206.

Chelune, G. J., Eversole, C., Kane, M., & Talbott, R. (1987). WAIS versus WAIS-R subtest patterns: A problem of generalization. *The Clinical Neuropsychologist, 1,* 235–242.

Chelune, G. J., Naugle, R. I., Luders, H., Sedlak, J., & Awad, I. A. (1993). Individual change after epilepsy surgery: Practice effects and base rate information. *Neuropsychology, 7,* 41–52.

Dickinson, D., Iannone, V. N., & Gold, J. M. (2002). Factor structure of the Wechsler Adult Intelligence Scale–III in schizophrenia. *Assessment, 9,* 171–180.

Donders, J., & Axelrod, B. N. (2002). Two-subtest estimations of WAIS-III factor index scores. *Psychological Assessment, 14,* 360–364.

Donders, J., Tulsky, D. S., & Zhu, J. (2001). Criterion validity of new WAIS-III subtest scores after traumatic brain injury. *Journal of the International Neuropsychological Society, 7,* 892–898.

Donders, J., Zhu, J., Tulsky, D. (2001). Factor index score patterns in the WAIS-III standardization sample. *Assessment, 8,* 193–203.

Dori, G. A., & Chelune, G. J. (2004). Education-stratified base-rate information on discrepancy scores within and between the Wechsler Adult Intelligence Scale-Third Edition and the Wechsler Memory Scale-Third Edition. *Psychological Assessment, 16,* 146–154.

Dugbarty, A. T., Sanchez, P. N., Rosenbaum, J. G., Mahurin, R. K., Davis, J. M., & Townes, B. D. (1999). WAIS-III Matrix Reasoning test performance in a mixed clinical sample. *The Clinical Neuropsychologist, 13,* 396–404.

Ehrenreich, J. H. (1996). Clinical use of short forms of the WAIS-R. *Assessment, 3,* 193–200.

Etherton, J. L., Bianchini, K. J., Ciota, M. A., & Greve, K. W. (2005). Reliable Digit Span is unaffected by laboratory-induced pain: Implications for clinical use. *Assessment, 12,* 101–106.

Fisher, D. C., Ledbetter, M. F., Cohen, N. J., Marmor, D., & Tulsky, D. S. (2000). WAIS-III and WMS-III profiles of mildly to severely brain-injured patients. *Applied Neuropsychology, 7,* 126–132.

Flanagan, D. P., McGrew, K. S., & Ortiz, S. O. (2000). *The Wechsler Intelligence Scales and Gf-Gc theory: A contemporary approach to interpretation.* Boston: Allyn and Bacon.

Flanagan, D.P., & Ortiz, S.O. (2001). *Essentials of cross-battery assessment.* New York: John Wiley & Sons.

Flynn, J. R. (1984). The mean IQ of Americans: Massive gains 1932–1978. *Psychological Bulletin, 95,* 29–51.

Flynn, J. R. (1987). Massive IQ gains in 14 nations: What IQ tests really measure. *Psychological Bulletin, 101,* 171–191.

Flynn, J. R. (1998). WAIS-III and WISC-III IQ gains in the United States from 1972 to 1995: How to compensate for obsolete norms. *Perceptual and Motor Skills, 86,* 1231–1239.

Glutting, J., McDermott, P., Watkins, M., Kush, J., & Konold, T. (1997). The base rate problem and its consequences for interpreting children's ability profiles. *School Psychology Review, 26,* 176–188.

Greiffenstein, M. F., Baker, W. J., & Gola, T. (1994). Validation of malingered amnesia measures with a large clinical sample. *Psychological Assessment, 6,* 218–224.

Gregoire, J. (2004). Factor structure of the French version of the Wechsler Adult Intelligence Scale-III. *Educational & Psychological Measurement, 64,* 463–474.

Greve, K. W., Bianchini, K. J., Mathias, C. W., Houston, R. J., & Crouch, J. A. (2003). Detecting malingered performance on the Wechsler Adult Intelligence Scale: Validation of Mittenberg's approach to traumatic brain injury. *Archives of Clinical Neuropsychology, 18,* 245–260.

Griffin, S. L., Mindt, M. R., Rankin, E. J., Ritchie, A. J., & Scott, J. G. (2002). Estimating premorbid intelligence: Comparison of traditional and contemporary methods across the intelligence continuum. *Archives of Clinical Neuropsychology, 17,* 497–507.

Hawkins, K. A. (1998). Indicators of brain dysfunction derived from graphic representations of the WAIS-III/WMS-III technical manual samples: A preliminary approach to clinical utility. *The Clinical Neuropsychologist, 12,* 535–551.

Hawkins, K. A., & Tulsky, D. S. (2003). WAIS-III WMS-III discrepancy analysis: Six factor model index discrepancy base rates, implications, and a preliminary consideration of utility. In D. Tulsky, R. K. Saklofske, G. Heaton, G. Chelune, R. A. Ivnik, R. A. Bornstein, A. Prifitera, & M. Ledbetter (Eds.), *Clinical interpretation of the WAIS-III and WMS-III* (pp. 211–272) San Diego, CA: Academic Press.

Heaton, R. K., Taylor, M. J., & Manly, J. J. (2003). Demographic effects and use of demographically corrected norms with the WAIS-III and WMS-III. In D. Tulsky, R. K. Saklofske, G. Heaton, G.

Chelune, R. A. Ivnik, R. A. Bornstein, A. Prifitera, & M. Ledbetter (Eds.), *Clinical interpretation of the WAIS-III and WMS-III* (pp. 183–210). San Diego, CA: Academic Press.

Iverson, G. (1999). Interpreting change on the WAIS-III/WMS-III following traumatic brain injury. *The Journal of Cognitive Rehabilitation, 17,* 16–20.

Iverson, G. L. (2001). Interpreting change on the WAIS-III-WMS-III in clinical samples. *Archives of Clinical Neuropsychology, 16,* 183–191.

Iverson, G. L., & Tulsky, D. S. (2003). Detecting malingering on the WAIS-III: Unusual Digit Span performance patterns in the normal population and in clinical groups. *Archives of Clinical Neuropsychology, 18,* 1–9.

Ivnik, R. J., Malec, J. F., Smith, G. E., Tangalos, E. G., Peterson, R. C., Kokmen, E., & Kurland, L. T. (1992). Mayo's Older American Normative Studies: WAIS-R norms for ages 56 to 97. *The Clinical Neuropsychologist, 6*(Supplement), 1–30.

Jacobson, N. S., & Truax, P. (1991). Clinical significance: A statistical approach to defining meaningful change in psychotherapy research. *Journal of Consulting and Clinical Psychology, 59,* 12–19.

Jeyakumar, S. L. E., Warriner, E. M., Raval, V. V., & Ahmad, S. A. (2004). Balancing the need for reliability and time efficiency: Short forms of the Wechsler Adult Intelligence Scale-III. *Educational and Psychological Measurement, 64,* 71–87.

Joy, S., Kaplan, E., & Fein, D. (2003). Digit symbol—Incidental Learning in the WAIS-III: Construct validity and clinical significance. *The Clinical Neuropsychologist, 17,* 182–194.

Joy, S. J., Kaplan, E., & Fein, D. (2004). Speed and memory in the WAIS-III Digit Symbol-Coding subtest across the lifespan. *Archives of Clinical Neuropsychology, 19,* 759–767.

Kanaya, T., Scullin, M. H., & Ceci, S. J. (2003). The Flynn effect and U.S. policies: The impact of rising IQ scores on American society via mental retardation diagnoses. *The American Psychologist, 58,* 778–790.

Kaufman, A. S. (1990). *Assessing adolescent and adult intelligence.* Boston: Allyn and Bacon.

Kaufman, A. S., & Lichtenberger, E. O. (1999). *Essentials of WAIS-III assessment.* New York: John Wiley & Sons, Inc.

Kaufman, A. S., Lichtenberger, E. O., & McLean, J. E. (2001). Two- and three-factor solutions of the WAIS-III. *Assessment, 8,* 267–280.

Kennedy, J. E., Clement, P. F., & Curtiss, G. (2003). WAIS-III Processing Speed Index scores after TBI: The influence of working memory, psychomotor speed and perceptual processing. *The Clinical Neuropsychologist, 17,* 303–307.

Kreiner, D. S., & Ryan, J. J. (2001). Memory and motor skill components of the WAIS-III Digit Symbol-Coding subtest. *The Clinical Neuropsychologist, 15,* 109–113.

Kulas, J. F., & Axelrod, B. N. (2002). Comparison of seven-subtest and Satz-Mogel short forms of the WAIS-III. *Journal of Clinical Psychology, 58,* 773–782.

Lange, R., Iverson, G., Viljoen, H., Brickell, T., & Brink, J. (2004). *Interpretive effects of using Canadian versus American WAIS-III normative systems.* Paper presented at the INS, Baltimore, MD.

Langeluddecke, P. M., & Lucas, S. K. (2003). Wechsler Adult Intelligence Scale-Third Edition findings in relation to severity of brain injury in litigants. *The Clinical Neuropsychologist, 17,* 273–284.

Langeluddecke, P. M., & Lucas, S. K. (2004). Evaluation of two methods for estimating premorbid intelligence on the WAIS-III in a clinical sample. *The Clinical Neuropsychologist, 18,* 423–432.

Larrabee, G. J. (2003). Detection of malingering using atypical performance patterns on standard neuropsychological tests. *The Clinical Neuropsychologist, 17,* 410–425.

Larrabee, G. J. (2004). A review of clinical interpretation of the WAIS-III and WMS-III: Where do we go from here and what should we do with WAIS-IV and WMS-IV? *Journal of Clinical and Experimental Neuropsychology, 24,* 707–717.

Lees-Haley, P. R., Smith, H. H., Williams, C. W., & Dunn, J. T. (1996). Forensic neuropsychological test usage: An empirical survey. *Archives of Clinical Neuropsychology, 11,* 45–51.

Lezak, M. D., Howieson, D. B., & Loring, D. W. (2004). *Neuropsychological assessment* (4th ed.). New York: Oxford University Press.

Lineweaver, T. T., & Chelune, G. J. (2003). Use of the WAIS-III and WMS-III in the context of serial assessments: Interpreting reliable and meaningful change. In D. Tulsky, R. K. Saklofske, G. Heaton, G. Chelune, R. A. Ivnik, R. A. Bornstein, A. Prifitera, & M. Ledbetter (Eds.), *Clinical interpretation of the WAIS-III and WMS-III* (pp. 303–337). San Diego, CA: Academic Press.

Livingston, R. B., Jennings, E., Reynolds, C. R., & Gray, R. M. (2003). Multivariate analyses of the profile stability of intelligence tests: High for IQs, low to very low for subtest analyses. *Archives of Clinical Neuropsychology, 18,* 487–507.

Manly, J. J., Jacobes, D. M., Sano, M., Bell, K., Merchant, C. A., Small, S. A., & Stern, Y. (1998). Cognitive test performance among nondemented elderly African Americans and whites. *Neurology, 50,* 1238–1245.

Manly, J., Jacobs, D., Touradji, P., Small, S., Merchant, C., Bell, K., & Stern, Y. (2000). Are ethnic group differences in neuropsychological test performance explained by reading level? A preliminary analysis. *Journal of the International Neuropsychological Society, 6,* 245.

Manly, J. J., Jacobs, D. M., Touradji, P., Small, S. A., & Stern, Y. (2002). Reading level attenuates differences in neuropsychological test performance between African American and White elders. *Journal of the International Neuropsychological Society, 8,* 341–348.

Martin, T. A., Donders, J., & Thompson, E. (2000). Potential of and problems with new measures of psychometric intelligence after traumatic brain injury. *Rehabilitation Psychology, 45,* 402–408.

Martin, R., Sawrie, S., Gilliam, F., MacKey, M., Faught, E., Knowlton, R., & Kuzniekcy, R. (2002). Determining reliable cognitive change after epilepsy surgery: Development of reliable changes indices and standardized regression-based change norms for the WMS-III and the WAIS-III. *Epilepsia, 43,* 1551–1558.

Matarazzo, J. D., & Herman, D. O. (1984). Relationship of education and IQ in the WAIS-R standardization sample. *Journal of Consulting and Clinical Psychology, 52,* 631–634.

Mathias, C. W., Greve, K. W., Bianchini, K. J. (2002). Detecting malingered neurocognitive dysfunction using the Reliable Digit Span in traumatic brain injury. *Assessment, 9,* 254–269.

Milanovitch, J. R., Axelrod, B. N., & Goldberg, J. O. (1996). Validation of the simulations index-revised with a mixed clinical population. *Archives of Clinical Neuropsychology, 11,* 53–59.

Miller, L. J., Ryan, J. J., Carruthers, C. A., & Cluff, R. B. (2004). Brief screening indexes for malingering: A confirmation of Vocabulary minus Digit Span from the WAIS-III and the Rarely Missed Index from the WMS-III. *The Clinical Neuropsychologist, 18,* 327–333.

Okazaki, S., & Sue, S. (2000). Implications of test revisions for assessment with Asian Americans. *Psychological Assessment, 12,* 272–280.

Parker, K. C. H. (1986). Changes with age, year-of-birth cohort interaction, and the standardization of the Wechsler Intelligence tests. *Human Development, 29,* 209–222.

The Psychological Corporation. (1997). *WAIS-III-WMS-II technical manual.* San Antonio: Author.

The Psychological Corporation (1999). *Wechsler Abbreviated Scale of Intelligence.* San Antonio: Author.

The Psychological Corporation (2001). *Wechsler Test of Adult Reading Manual.* San Antonio: Author.

The Psychological Corporation (2002).*WAIS-III/WMS-III: Updated Technical Manual.* San Antonio: Author.

Rabin, L. A., Barr, W. B., & Burton, L. A. (2005). Assessment practices of clinical neuropsychologists in the United States and Canada: A survey of INS, NAN, and APA Division 40 members. *Archives of Clinical Neuropsychology, 20,* 33–66.

Rapport, L. J., Brines, D. B., Axelrod, B. N. (1997). Full scale IQ as mediator of practice effects: The rich get richer. *The Clinical Neuropsychologist, 11,* 375–380.

Rawling, P. J., & Brooks, D. N. (1990). Simulation index: A method for detecting factitious errors on the WAIS-R and WMS. *Neuropsychology, 4,* 223–238.

Reitan, R. M., & Wolfson, D. (1990). A consideration of the comparability of the WAIS and WAIS-R. *The Clinical Neuropsychologist, 4,* 80–85.

Ringe, W. K., Saine, K. C., Lacritz, L. H., Hynan, L. S., & Cullum, C. M. (2002). Dyadic short forms of the Wechsler Adult Intelligence Scale-III. *Assessment, 9,* 254–260.

Ryan, J. J., Arb, J. D., Paul, C. A., & Kreiner, D. S. (2000a). Reliability of the WAIS-III subtests, indexes, and IQs in individuals with substance abuse disorders. *Assessment, 7,* 151–156.

Ryan, J. J., Kreiner, D. S., & Burton, D. B. (2002). Does high scatter affect the predictive validity of WAIS-III IQs? *Applied Neuropsychology, 9,* 173–178.

Ryan, J. J., Lopez, S. J., & Werth, T. R. (1998). Administration time estimates for WAIS-III subtests, scales, and short forms. *Journal of Psychoeducational Assessment, 16,* 315–323.

Ryan, J. J., Lopez, S. J., & Werth, T. (1999). Development and preliminary validation of a Satz-Mogel short form of the WAIS-III in a sample of persons with substance abuse disorders. *International Journal of Neuroscience, 98,* 131–140.

Ryan, J. J., & Paolo, A. M. (2001). Exploratory factor analysis of the WAIS-III in a mixed patient sample. *Archives of Clinical Neuropsychology, 16,* 151–156.

Ryan, J. J., Sattler, J. M., & Lopez, S. J. (2000). Age effects on Wechsler Adult Intelligence Scale-III subtests. *Archives of Clinical Neuropsychology, 15,* 311–317.

Ryan, J. J., & Schnakenberg-Ott, S. D. (2003). Scoring reliability on the Wechsler Adult Intelligence Scale-Third Edition (WAIS-III). *Assessment, 10,* 151–159.

Ryan, J. J., & Ward, L. C. (1999). Validity, reliability, and standard errors of measurement for two 7-subtest forms of the Wechsler Adult Intelligence Scale-III. *Psychological Assessment, 11,* 207–211.

Saklofske, D. H., Hildebrand, D. K., & Gorsuch, R. L. (2000). Replication of the factor structure of the Wechsler Adult Intelligence Scale-Third Edition with a Canadian sample. *Psychological Assessment, 12,* 436–439.

Sattler, J. M. (2001). *Assessment of children: Cognitive applications* (4th ed.). San Diego: Sattler.

Sattler, J. M., & Ryan, J. J. (1999). *Assessment of children revised and updated third edition: WAIS-III supplement.* San Diego: Sattler.

Sattler, J. M., & Ryan, J. J. (2001). Wechsler Adult Intelligence Scale-III (WAIS-III): Description. In J. M. Sattler (Ed.), *Assessment of children: Cognitive applications* (4th ed.). San Diego: Sattler.

Schoenberg, M. R., Duff, K., Scott, J. G., & Adams, R. L. (2003). An evaluation of the clinical utility of the OPIE-3 as an estimate of premorbid WAIS-III FSIQ. *The Clinical Neuropsychologist, 17,* 308–321.

Schoenberg, M. R., Duff, K., Dorfman, K., & Adams, R. L. (2004). Differential estimation of verbal intelligence and performance intelligence scores from combined performance and demographic variables: The OPIE-3 verbal and performance algorithms. *The Clinical Neuropsychologist, 18*, 266–276.

Schoenberg, M. R., Scott, J. G., Duff, K., & Adams, R. L. (2002). Estimation of WAIS-III intelligence from combined performance and demographic variables: Development of the OPIE-3. *The Clinical Neuropsychologist, 16*, 426–438.

Schopp, L. H., Hermann, T. D., Johnstone, B., Callahan, C. D., Roudebush, I. S. (2001). Two abbreviated versions of the Wechsler Adult Intelligence Scale-III: Validation among persons with traumatic brain injury. *Rehabilitation Psychology, 46*, 279–287.

Shuttleworth-Edwards, A. B. (2002). Fine tuning of the Digit Symbol Paired Associate recall test for practitioner purposes in clinical and research settings. *The Clinical Neuropsychologist, 16*, 232–241.

Shuttleworth-Edwards, A. B., Donnelly, M. J. R., Reid, I., & Radloff, S. E. (2004). A cross-cultural study with culture fair normative indications on WAIS-III Digit Symbol-Incidental Learning. *Journal of Clinical and Experimental Neuropsychology, 26*, 921–932.

Shuttleworth-Edwards, A. B., Kemp, R. D., Rust, A. L., Muirhead, G. G. L., Hartman, N. P., & Radloff, S. E. (2004). Cross-cultural effects on IQ test performance: A review and preliminary normative indications on WAIS-III test performance. *Journal of Clinical and Experimental Neuropsychology, 26*, 903–920.

Strauss, E., Hultsch, D. F., Hunter, M., Slick, D. J., Patry, B., & Levy-Bencheton, J. (2000). Using intraindividual variability to detect malingering in cognitive performance. *The Clinical Neuropsychologist, 14*, 420–432.

Strauss, E., Slick, D. J., Levy-Bencheton, J., Hunter, M., Macdonald, S. W. S., & Hultsch, D. F. (2002). Intraindividual variability as an indicator of malingering in head injury. *Archives of Clinical Neuropsychology, 17*, 423–444.

Strauss, E., Spreen, O., & Hunter, M. (2000). Implications of test revisions for research. *Psychological Assessment, 12*, 237–244.

Strong, A-A. H., Donders, J., & Van dyke, S. (2005). Validity of demographically corrected norms for the WAIS-III. *Journal of Clinical and Experimental Neuropsychology, 27*, 746–758.

Taub, G. E., McGrew, K. S., & Witta, E. L. (2004). A confirmatory analysis of the factor structure and cross-age invariance of the Wechsler Adult Intelligence Scale-Third Edition. *Psychological Assessment, 16*, 85–89.

Taylor, M. J., & Heaton, R. K. (2001). Sensitivity and specificity of WAIS-III/WMS-III demographically corrected factor scores in neuropsychological assessment. *Journal of the International Neuropsychological Society, 7*, 867–874.

Tulsky, D. S., Ivnik, R. J., Price, L. R., & Wilkins, C. (2003). Assessment of cognitive functioning with the WAIS-III and WMS-III: Development of a six-factor model. In D. S. Tulsky, D. H. Saklofske, G. J. Chelune, R. K. Heaton, R. J. Ivnik, R. Bornstein, A. Prifitera, & M. F. Ledbetter (Eds.), *Clinical interpretation of the WAIS-III and WMS-III* (pp. 149–182). San Diego: Academic Press.

Tulsky, D. S., & Ledbetter, M. F. (2000). Updating to the WAIS-III and WMS-III: Considerations for research and clinical practice. *Psychological Assessment, 12*, 253–262.

Tulsky, D. S., & Price, L. R. (2003). The joint WAIS-III and WMS-III factor structure: Development and cross-validation of a six-factor model of cognitive functioning. *Psychological Assessment, 15*, 149–162.

Tulsky, D. S., Rolhus, E. L., & Shu, J. (2000). Two-tailed versus one-tailed base rates of discrepancy scores in the WAIS-III. *The Clinical Neuropsychologist, 14*, 451–460.

Tulsky, D. S., Saklofske, D. H., Cheluen, G. J., Heaton, R. K., Ivnik, R. J., Bornstein, R., Prifitera, A., & Ledbetter, M. F. (2003). *Clinical interpretation of the WAIS-III and WMS-III.* San Diego: Academic Press.

Tulsky, D. S., Saklofske, D. H., Wilkins, C., & Weiss, L. G. (2001). Development of a General Ability Index for the Wechsler Adult Intelligence Scale-Third Edition. *Psychological Assessment, 13*, 566–571.

Van der Heijden, P., & Donders, J. (2003a). A confirmatory factor analysis of the WAIS-III in patients with traumatic brain injury. *Journal of Clinical and Experimental Neuropsychology, 25*, 59–65.

Van der Heijden, P., & Donders, J. (2003b). WAIS-III factor index score patterns after traumatic brain injury. *Assessment, 10*, 115–122.

Veiel, H. O., & Koopman, R. F. (2001). The bias in regression-based indices of premorbid IQ. *Psychological Assessment, 13*, 356–368.

Ward, L. C., Ryan, J. J., & Axelrod, B. N. (2000). Confirmatory factor analyses of the WAIS-III standardization data. *Psychological Assessment, 12*, 341–345.

Wechsler, D. (1981). *Wechsler Adult Intelligence Scale—Revised.* New York: The Psychological Corporation.

Wechsler, D. (2003). *Wechsler Intelligence Scale for Children—Fourth Edition.* San Antonio, TX: The Psychological Corporation.

Wymer, J. H., Rayls, K., & Wagner, M. T. (2003). Utility of a clinically derived abbreviated short form of the WAIS-III. *Archives of Clinical Neuropsychology, 18*, 917–927.

Zhu, J., & Tulsky, D. S. (2000). Co-norming the WAIS-III and WMS-III: Is there a test-order effect on IQ and memory scores? *The Clinical Neuropsychologist, 14*, 461–467.

Zhu, J., Tulsky, D. S., Price, L., & Chen, H-Y. (2001). WAIS-III reliability data for clinical groups. *Journal of the International Neuropsychological Society, 7*, 862–866.

Wechsler Intelligence Scale for Children—Fourth Edition (WISC-IV)

PURPOSE

The WISC-IV is intended to assess intelligence in children and adolescents.

SOURCE

The WISC-IV (test materials, Administration and Norms Manual, Technical and Interpretive Manual, Stimulus Booklets, 25 Record Forms, 25 Response Booklets) can be obtained from Harcourt Assessment (www.WISC-IV.com). The scale costs about $825 US. Scoring software comes in two forms: the WISC-IV Scoring Assistant ($199 US), which provides scoring only, or the WISC-IV Writer ($399 US), an interpretive report program. Additional manuals with norms for other countries such as Canada and the United Kingdom can be obtained from the publisher, as can editions in other languages. This includes the WISC-IV Spanish, designed for use in assessing Spanish-speaking children in the United States.

Figure 6–23 History of Wechsler Intelligence Scales. *Note:* WPPSI = Wechsler Preschool and Primary Scale of Intelligence; WISC = Wechsler Intelligence Scale for Children; WAIS = Wechsler Adult Intelligence Scale. *Source:* Reprinted with permission from Flanagan & Kaufman, 2004.

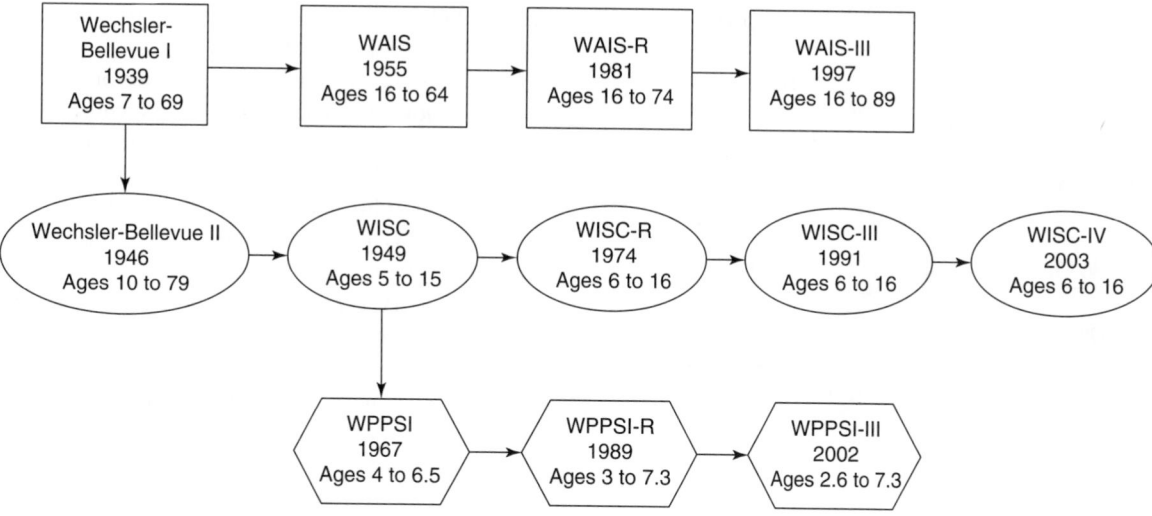

AGE RANGE

The WISC-IV can be administered to children ages 6 to 16 years, 11 months.

DESCRIPTION

The WISC-IV (Wechsler, 2003a) is the fourth edition of the WISC, an intelligence battery for children that originally appeared in 1949 and in two subsequent revisions (i.e., WISC-R, Wechsler, 1974; WISC-III, Wechsler, 1991). Figure 6–23 illustrates the development and evolution of the WISC-IV and other Wechsler scales over time.

The WISC-IV embodies a fundamental shift from previous editions. The test's theoretical underpinnings now reflect current factor analytic theories of intelligence collectively termed CHC theory (e.g., Carroll, 1993; Horn & Noll, 1997; see also *Chapter Introduction*). This represents a major rapprochement among the current three major children's intelligence scales. The Stanford-Binet underwent an analogous shift in its latest incarnation (see *SB5*), and the CHC has for some time been the model for the WJ III Cognitive (also see review in this volume). However, because the WISC-IV dominates the field and is used by so many psychologists, the adoption of this model represents a major historical paradigm shift for the assessment of intelligence in children. While many see this as a major improvement over prior versions, the test has been criticized both by Wechsler traditionalists accustomed to the standard Wechsler model and broad verbal/nonverbal dichotomies (e.g., VIQ-PIQ), and by CHC proponents for not providing coverage of all CHC domains and for an a posteriori adherence to the model (Flanagan & Kaufman, 2004). In many ways, the test is a first-generation hybrid that combines the traditional, clinically derived Wechsler approach and CHC

theory. In so doing, the test belongs to neither model exclusively. In the end, this may prove to be an asset, as there are as yet comparatively few studies on the validity of CHC theory with regard to diagnosis, eligibility, intervention, and instructional planning in clinical populations (Kaufman, 2000), but considerable data on the clinical validity and diagnostic utility of Wechsler scales.

One of the most obvious and drastic deviations from the traditional Wechsler model is the complete elimination of the VIQ and PIQ in favor of four index scores (see Table 6–140). These are the Verbal Comprehension Index (VCI), Perceptual Reasoning Index (PRI), Working Memory Index (WMI), and Processing Speed Index (PSI). Thus, in what has been termed a "scientifically bold move" (Saklofske et al., 2005), the FSIQ remains, but the VCI and PRI supplant the VIQ and PIQ.

Table 6–140 Domains Assessed by WISC-IV Index Scores

Index	Domains Measured
Verbal Comprehension Index (VCI)	Verbal knowledge, verbal reasoning, and verbal conceptualization
Perceptual Reasoning Index (PRI)	Interpretation, reasoning, and organization of visually presented nonverbal information
Working Memory Index (WMI)	Attention, concentration, and working memory for verbal material
Processing Speed Index (PSI)	Speed of mental and graphomotor processing

Source: Adapted from Wechsler, 2003b, and Sattler and Dumont, 2004.

Figure 6–24 WISC-IV Test Framework. *Note:* Supplement subtests are shown in italics. *Source:* Reprinted with permission from Wechsler, 2003b.

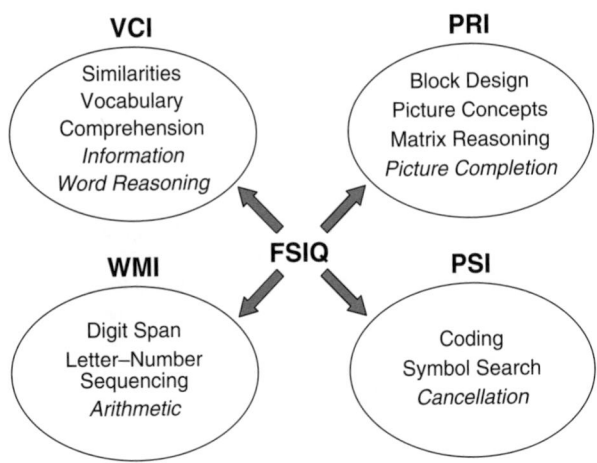

The test's new structure is shown in Figure 6–24. The PRI replaces the WISC-III POI; the WISC-III FFD has been revised as the WMI, with subtests more consistent with those of other Wechsler tests such as the WAIS-III. There are also fewer subtests comprising the VCI and PRI (i.e., three subtests each) compared with the WISC-III. This serves to increase the relative contribution of the WMI and PSI subtests to the WISC-IV FSIQ. In the WISC-III, VIQ and PIQ clearly contribute the greatest number of subtests to the FSIQ. In the WISC-IV, the PSI and WMI contribute more to FSIQ than did the PSI and FFD in the WISC-III (i.e., a 40% versus 20% contribution; Prifitera et al., 2005).

The WISC-IV includes 10 Core subtests and five Supplemental subtests. The Core subtests are the basis for the FSIQ and are used to derive composite scores (see Figure 6–24). Supplemental subtests can be used to extend the evaluation or to substitute for Core subtests (but see *Administration and Scoring*). In the revision, several subtests were removed from the Core index scores (i.e., Information, Arithmetic, Picture Completion, Picture Arrangement, Object Assembly); some were redefined as Supplemental subtests, and others were removed altogether (see later discussion). Five subtests are entirely new (i.e., Picture Concepts, Word Reasoning, Matrix Analogies, Letter-Number Sequencing, Cancellation). A complete list of subtests and definitions is provided in Table 6–141.

The VCI includes two Supplemental tasks: Word Reasoning, a verbally based fluid reasoning task, and Information, a subtest measuring primarily crystallized verbal knowledge that originally contributed to the VIQ in the WISC-III. The PRI emphasizes fluid reasoning through the addition of two new subtests (i.e., Matrix Reasoning, Picture Concepts) while retaining Block Design. To reduce the emphasis on speed, subtests with significant speed elements were either removed (i.e., Picture Arrangement, Object Assembly and Mazes), or redesigned to eliminate or minimize time bonuses (i.e., Arithmetic and Block Design). The measurement of working memory in the WMI is enhanced with the addition of Letter-Number Sequencing, a familiar subtest from the WAIS-III. PSI remains essentially unchanged from the WISC-III, with the addition of a Supplemental PSI subtest, Cancellation. See Table 6–142 for a summary of changes from the WISC-III to WISC-IV (Wechsler, 2003b).

The WISC-IV also includes a number of Process Scores. These are shown in Table 6–143. Process scores provide additional information on performance but are not used to derive index scores. Additional changes to the test were made to improve clinical utility and psychometric properties. Sattler and Dumont (2004) provide sample items similar to WISC-IV items; these are shown in Figure 6–25.

The WISC-IV contains about 56% of the items from the WISC-III (either in the same or updated form; Sattler & Dumont, 2004). Floors and ceilings were extended to improve sensitivity when testing those in the extremes of the population with regard to intellectual ability. Thus, according to the manual, the test should be appropriate for both a 6-year-old with moderate mental retardation and a gifted 16-year-old. Other changes were made to improve user-friendliness of testing materials and to clarify instructions. The number of teaching items, queries, and prompts are also increased relative to the WISC-III. (Interestingly, in revising instructions, in some cases "improper grammar was used to maintain developmental appropriateness and avoid unnecessary verbiage" [Wechsler, 2003b, p. 10].) Lastly, additional scoring samples are provided in the manual to facilitate scoring. Sattler and Dumont (2004), Flanagan and Kaufman (2004), and Prifitera et al. (2005) provide excellent reviews and advice on how to administer and interpret the test; these books should be considered companion volumes for the WISC-IV manuals.

Representing an alternative to the FSIQ, the General Ability Index (GAI) is a constellation of WISC-IV subtests that, when combined, is considered to be theoretically closest to *g* (see Saklofske et al., 2005, for more details). From a practical standpoint, the GAI eliminates any influences of the PSI and WMI on FSIQ because it is based only on the VCI and PRI subtests. The GAI may therefore be appropriate in populations with significant discrepancies between their estimated *g* (as estimated by the VCI/PRI) and attention/processing speed (as estimated by the WMI/PSI). Such groups include children with mental retardation (relative strength in the WMI/PSI), giftedness (relative strength in the VCI/PRI), or head injury (relative weakness in PSI; see Prifitera et al., 2005, for more information). Note that, depending on the discrepancy between *g* (as estimated by the VCI/PRI) and attention/processing speed (as estimated by WMI/PSI), the GAI may yield a slightly lower or higher general ability estimate than the FSIQ, with concomitant implications with regard to diagnosis and eligibility (see Table 6–144).

Like its predecessor, the WISC-IV is linked (but not conormed) with the WIAT-II through a sample of 550 children administered both tests. This allows for the calculation of ability/achievement discrepancies, as described in the Technical Manual (see Yeates & Donders, 2005, for a discussion of

Table 6–141 WISC-IV Subtest Descriptions

Subtest	Description
1. Block Design (BD)	The examinee is required to replicate a set of modeled or printed two-dimensional geometric patterns using red-and-white blocks within a specified time limit.
2. Similarities (SI)	The examinee is required to describe how two words that represent common objects or concepts are similar.
3. Digit Span (DS)	On Digit Span Forward, the examinee is required to repeat numbers verbatim as stated by the examiner. On Digit Span Backward, the examinee is required to repeat numbers in the reverse order as stated by the examiner.
4. Picture Concepts (PCn)	The examinee is required to choose one picture, from among two or three rows of pictures presented, to form a group with a common characteristic.
5. Coding (CD)	The examinee is required to copy symbols that are paired with either geometric shapes or numbers using a key within a specified time limit.
6. Vocabulary (VC)	The examinee is required to name pictures or provide definitions for words.
7. Letter-Number Sequencing (LN)	The examinee is read a number and letter sequence and is required to recall numbers in ascending order and letters in alphabetical order.
8. Matrix Reasoning (MR)	The examinee is required to complete the missing portion of a picture matrix by selecting one of five response options.
9. Comprehension (CO)	The examinee is required to answer a series of questions based on his or her understanding of general principles and social situations.
10. Symbol Search (SS)	The examinee is required to scan a search group and indicate the presence or absence of a target symbol(s) within a specified time limit.
11. *Picture Completion (PCm)*	The examinee is required to view a picture and name the essential missing part of the picture within a specified time limit.
12. *Cancellation (CA)*	The examinee is required to scan both a random and a nonrandom arrangement of pictures and mark target pictures within a specified time limit.
13. *Information (IN)*	The examinee is required to answer questions that address a wide range of general-knowledge topics.
14. *Arithmetic (AR)*	The examinee is required to mentally solve a variety of orally presented arithmetic problems within a specified time limit.
15. *Word Reasoning (WR)*	The examinee is required to identify a common concept being described by a series of clues.

Note: Subtests printed in italics are Supplemental.

Source: From Flanagan & Kaufman, 2004. Reprinted with permission.

Table 6–142 WISC-IV Subtest Modifications Compared with WISC-III

	New Subtest	Administration	Recording & Scoring	New Items
Block Design		✓	✓	✓
Similarities		✓	✓	✓
Digit Span		✓	✓	✓
Picture Concepts	✓			
Coding		✓	✓	
Vocabulary		✓	✓	✓
Letter–Number Sequencing	✓			
Matrix Reasoning	✓			
Comprehension		✓	✓	✓
Symbol Search		✓	✓	✓
Picture Completion		✓	✓	✓
Cancellation	✓			
Information			✓	✓
Arithmetic		✓	✓	✓
Word Reasoning	✓			

Source: From Wechsler, 2003b. Reprinted with permission.

Table 6–143 Process Scores for WISC-IV Subtests

Subtest	Process Score
Block Design	Block Design No Time Bonus
Digit Span	Digit Span Forward
	Digit Span Backward
	Longest Digit Span Forward
	Longest Digit Span Backward
Cancellation	Cancellation Random
	Cancellation Structured

Note: Process scores are not used in index scores or for deriving composites.

limitations of this approach). There is also a process instrument (WISC-IV Integrated; Wechsler, 2004b), which will not be reviewed here (see Chapter 4, *Test Selection, Test Administration, and Preparation of the Patient,* for a discussion of the process approach). The WISC-IV is also linked to the CMS (see review in this volume) to facilitate ability-memory comparisons (see below).

ADMINISTRATION TIME

According to data presented in the Administration Manual, almost all normally developing children complete the test in about an hour and a half (i.e., 90% complete the Core subtests within 94 minutes; Wechsler, 2003a), with about 50% completing the test in little over one hour (i.e., 50% complete the core subtests in 67 minutes or less). As expected, testing time is slightly shorter for children with mental retardation, and slightly longer for gifted children.

The WISC-III technically required administration of additional subtests to yield both the four index scores and the FSIQ (without prorating). In the WISC-IV, the same scores can be obtained by administering 10 subtests. The manual therefore concludes that testing time is reduced by about 15 minutes (Wechsler, 2003b).

ADMINISTRATION

Administration Instructions

See Administration Manual. The test includes one Stimulus Book, blocks, and a split-back, spiral-bound administration manual. Overall, materials are colorful and child-friendly, and are likely to elicit and maintain the attention of children.

Subtest Substitutions

At least one Supplemental subtest is available per index, should substitution of a subtest score be needed because of clinical need or subtest invalidation. Substitutions should only be made when necessary. No more than two substitutions can be made in the derivation of the FSIQ (Wechsler, 2003b; see also *Prorating*).

Queries and Timing

These are outlined in the manual, provided on the record form, and reviewed in Sattler and Dumont (2004) and Flanagan and Kaufman (2004).

SCORING

Scores

Index standard scores range from 40 to 160. Despite this range, Sattler and Dumont (2004) conclude that the test is still insufficiently sensitive for extremely low functioning children in the youngest age ranges. One of the major problems is that scaled scores can be obtained based on nonperformance (i.e., raw scores of 0). See the Administration Manual for rules to follow when children obtain scores of 0 on one or more subtests.

Subtests have a mean of 10 and *SD* of 3. Longest Digits Forward/Backward scores are presented as base rates corresponding to raw scores due to restricted range in the standardization sample. Although not recommended for describing performance, age equivalents can also be derived (see Administration and Scoring Manual).

Confidence intervals based on SE_E and true scores are provided in the manual; alternatively, Sattler and Dumont (2004) recommend calculating confidence intervals based on *SEMs* and obtained scores. These are provided in their text for each age range.

Index Discrepancies and the FSIQ and GAI

Statistical significance of composite score differences and frequencies for composite scale differences are presented in the Administration Manual. Note that frequencies are provided for both positive and negative discrepancies, as these are not symmetrical. Information for calculating the significance and frequency of discrepancies at the subtest level for differences relative to the average subtest score is also provided, as are discrepancy tables for every possible pair of WISC-IV subtests. The significance of intersubtest scatter (i.e., the variability of scores across all subtests) within each composite score can also be analyzed for significance and frequency (see Technical and Interpretive Manual).

WISC-III users were familiar with the fact that the FSIQ could not be interpreted meaningfully if there was a large, significant, and sufficiently rare difference between VIQ and PIQ scores. However, deciding whether the FSIQ should be interpreted in the WISC-IV can be fairly complex. Rather than the single VIQ-PIQ comparison used to evaluate discrepancies on the WISC-III, the WISC-IV requires simultaneous comparison of all four index scores to determine whether significant differences across indices are large enough to invalidate meaningful interpretation of the FSIQ. Although the manual presents dyad-based comparisons (i.e., comparison of a single index score with another single index score),

Similarities (23 items)
In what way are a pencil and a piece of chalk alike?
In what way are tea and coffee alike?
In what way are an inch and a mile alike?
In what way are binoculars and a microscope alike?

Vocabulary (36 items)
What is a ball?
What does *running* mean?
What is a poem?
What does *obstreperous* mean?

Comprehension (21 items)
Why do we wear shoes?
What is the thing to do if you see someone dropping a package?
In what two ways is a lamp better than a candle?
In the United States, why are we tried by a jury of our peers?

Information (33 items)
How many legs do you have?
What must you do to make water freeze?
Who developed the theory of relativity?
What is the capital of France?

Word Reasoning (24 items)
The task is to identify the common concept being described with a series of clues.
Clue 1: This has a motor . . .
Clue 2: . . . and it is used to cut grass.

Block Design (14 items)
The task is to reproduce stimulus designs using four or nine blocks (see below).

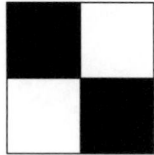

Picture Concepts (28 items)
The task is to choose one picture from each of two or three rows of pictures in such a way that all the pictures selected have a characteristic in common (see below).

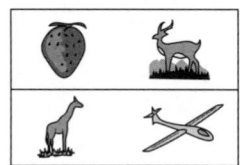

Coding (59 items in Coding A and 119 items in Coding B)
The task is to copy symbols from a key (see below).

1	2	3	4	5	6
x	o	=	L	/	V

2	4	1	5	6	3	5	2	1	6	4	3

Symbol Search (45 items in Part A and 60 items in Part B)
The task is to decide whether a stimulus figure (a symbol) appears in an array (see below).

⌂ ◇	☼ □ ◇ ± △ = □	YES	NO
☼ ±	◇ △ ± □ = □ ⌂	YES	NO
= □	△ ⌂ ☼ □ ± x ◇	YES	NO

Matrix Reasoning (35 items)
The task is to examine an incomplete matrix and select whichever of the five choices best completes the matrix (see below).

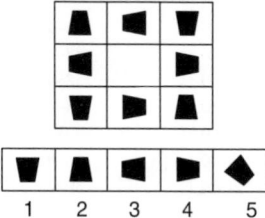

Picture Completion (38 items)
The task is to look at a picture—such as that of a car without a wheel, a scissors without a handle, or a telephone without numbers on the dial—and identify the essential missing part (see below).

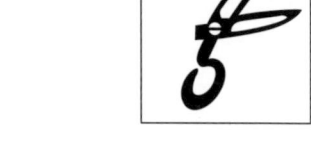

Digit Span (16 items; 8 in Digit Span Forward, 8 in Digit Span Backward)
In the first part, the task is to repeat a string of numbers, ranging from 2 to 9 digits, in a forward direction (example: 1-8). In the second part, the task is to repeat a string of numbers, ranging from 2 to 8 digits, in reverse order (example: 6-4-9).

Letter–Number Sequencing (10 items, each with 3 trials)
The task is to listen to a combination of from 2 to 8 letters and digits (example: 1-b) and repeat the combination back with the numbers acsending order followed by the letters in alphabetical order (example: e-6-d-9 would be repeated back as 6-9-d-e).

Arithmetic (34 items)
If I have one piece of candy and get another one, how many pieces will I have?
At 12 cents each, how much will 4 bars of soap cost?
If suits sell for $1/2$ of the regular price, what is the cost of a $120 suit?

Cancellation (2 items, one Random and one Sequenced)
The task is to scan, within a specific time limit, both a random arrangement and a sequenced arrangement of pictures and mark target pictures (animals; see below).

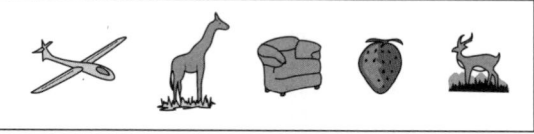

Table 6–144 Generalized Ability Index (GAI) Equivalents for Sums of Scaled Scores for the WISC-IV

Sum of Scaled Scores	GAI	Percentile Rank	Confidence Level 90%	95%	Sum of Scaled Scores	GAI	Percentile Rank	Confidence Level 90%	95%
6	40	<0.1	38–47	37–48	60	100	50	95–105	94–106
7	40	<0.1	38–47	37–48	61	101	53	96–106	95–107
8	40	<0.1	38–47	37–48	62	102	55	97–107	96–108
9	40	<0.1	38–47	37–48	63	103	58	98–108	97–109
10	40	<0.1	38–47	37–48	64	104	61	99–109	98–109
11	40	<0.1	38–47	37–48	65	105	63	100–110	99–110
12	41	<0.1	39–48	38–49	66	106	66	101–110	100–111
13	42	<0.1	40–49	39–50	67	107	68	102–111	101–112
14	43	<0.1	41–50	40–51	68	108	70	103–112	102–113
15	44	<0.1	42–51	41–52	69	110	75	105–114	104–115
16	45	<0.1	42–52	42–53	70	111	77	106–115	105–116
17	46	<0.1	43–53	43–54	71	112	79	107–116	106–117
18	47	<0.1	44–54	43–55	72	113	81	108–117	107–118
19	49	<0.1	46–56	45–57	73	115	84	110–119	109–120
20	51	0.1	48–58	47–59	74	116	86	111–120	110–121
21	52	0.1	49–59	48–60	75	117	87	112–121	111–122
22	53	0.1	50–60	49–61	76	119	90	114–123	113–124
23	55	0.1	52–62	51–62	77	120	91	114–124	114–125
24	57	0.2	54–63	53–64	78	121	92	115–125	115–126
25	58	0.3	55–64	54–65	79	122	93	116–126	115–127
26	59	0.3	56–65	55–66	80	123	94	117–127	116–128
27	61	0.5	58–67	57–68	81	124	95	118–128	117–129
28	63	1	60–69	59–70	82	126	96	120–130	119–131
29	64	1	61–70	60–71	83	127	96	121–131	120–132
30	65	1	62–71	61–72	84	128	97	122–132	121–133
31	67	1	64–73	63–74	85	129	97	123–133	122–133
32	69	2	66–75	65–76	86	130	98	124–134	123–134
33	70	2	66–76	66–77	87	132	98	126–135	125–136
34	71	3	67–77	67–78	88	133	99	127–136	126–137
35	73	4	69–79	68–80	89	135	99	129–138	128–139
36	74	4	70–80	69–81	90	136	99	130–139	129–140
37	75	5	71–81	70–82	91	138	99	132–141	131–142
38	77	6	73–83	72–84	92	139	99.5	133–142	132–143
39	78	7	74–84	73–85	93	140	99.6	134–143	133–144
40	79	8	75–85	74–85	94	142	99.7	136–145	135–146
41	81	10	77–86	76–87	95	143	99.8	137–146	136–147
42	82	12	78–87	77–88	96	144	99.8	138–147	137–148
43	83	13	79–88	78–89	97	146	99.9	139–149	139–150
44	84	14	80–89	79–90	98	147	99.9	140–150	139–151
45	85	16	81–90	80–91	99	148	99.9	141–151	140–152
46	86	18	82–91	81–92	100	150	>99.9	143–153	142–154
47	87	19	83–92	82–93	101	151	>99.9	144–154	143–155
48	88	21	84–93	83–94	102	153	>99.9	146–156	145–157
49	89	23	85–94	84–95	103	154	>99.9	147–157	146–157
50	90	25	86–95	85–96	104	155	>99.9	148–158	147–158
51	91	27	87–96	86–97	105	156	>99.9	149–158	148–159
52	92	30	88–97	87–98	106	157	>99.9	150–159	149–160
53	93	32	89–98	88–99	107	158	>99.9	151–160	150–161
54	94	34	90–99	89–100	108	159	>99.9	152–161	151–162
55	95	37	90–100	90–101	109	160	>99.9	153–162	152–163
56	96	39	91–101	91–102	110	160	>99.9	153–162	152–163
57	97	42	92–102	91–103	111	160	>99.9	153–162	152–163
58	98	45	93–103	92–104	112	160	>99.9	153–162	152–163
59	99	47	94–104	93–105	113	160	>99.9	153–162	152–163
					114	160	>99.9	153–162	152–163

To use the tables, add the scaled scores for Vocabulary, Comprehension, Similarities, Block Design, Matrix Reasoning, and Picture Concepts. Find this value in Column 1, and read across for the corresponding GAI.

Source: From Saklofske et al., 2005. Reprinted with permission.

it is also useful, and potentially more conceptually defensible (given the multiple comparisons required to make such an analysis), to determine whether a given index score deviates from the general pattern of index scores. Longman (2005) therefore provides tables to determine whether a given index score deviates significantly from the mean overall index score on the WISC-IV, and whether that discrepancy is rare or common in the standardization sample (see Tables 6–145 and 6–146).

In cases where the PSI and WMI deviate considerably from the VCI and PRI, the GAI provides an alternative FSIQ estimate. However, users should be wary of the tendency to engage in "cherry picking" in determining whether the FSIQ or the GAI is more appropriate for the particular child (i.e., choosing the index that provides the best outcome with regard to funding category or other desired outcome for the patient, rather than on an a priori, conceptual/rational basis). An important consideration in the use of the GAI is the assumption that the underlying VCI and PRI are not widely divergent from each other (Saklofske et al., 2005).

Prorating

The WISC-IV Administration Manual states that prorating should be used with extreme caution in situations involving diagnostic or placement decisions (Wechsler, 2003a, p. 49). Likewise, Sattler and Dumont (2004) clearly state that prorating is not recommended because it introduces unknown measure-

Table 6–145 Discrepancy Analysis: Required Difference Between an Index Score and the Mean Index Score for the WISC-IV

Ages 6–7	Pooled SEM	Significance Level		
		.15	.05	.01
Verbal Comprehension	4.37	8.25	9.92	11.98
Perceptual Reasoning	4.37	8.25	9.92	11.98
Working Memory	4.50	8.40	10.10	12.19
Processing Speed	6.36	10.69	12.85	15.52

Ages 8–13	Pooled SEM	Significance Level		
		.15	.05	.01
Verbal Comprehension	3.77	7.10	8.53	10.31
Perceptual Reasoning	3.97	7.33	8.81	10.64
Working Memory	4.29	7.71	9.27	11.20
Processing Speed	4.93	8.50	10.21	12.34

Ages 14–16	Pooled SEM	Significance Level		
		.15	.05	.01
Verbal Comprehension	3.35	6.58	7.91	9.55
Perceptual Reasoning	4.33	7.72	9.28	11.21
Working Memory	4.06	7.39	8.89	10.74
Processing Speed	4.89	8.41	10.11	12.21

Source: From Longman, 2005. Reprinted with permission.

ment error and violates standard administration procedures; they note that the procedure is akin to using a short form. If prorating must be used, procedures outlined in the Administration Manual must be followed. Note that the FSIQ cannot be derived if one of the two subtests contributing to either the WMI or PSI is spoiled. Consequently, the manual recommends that Arithmetic and Cancellation also be administered, which may lengthen administration time. The GAI is an alternative when administration yields an invalid or uninterpretable WMI or PSI index.

Ability-Achievement Comparisons

Ability-achievement discrepancies with regard to the WIAT-II can be derived using data presented in the Technical Manual. Although the simple-difference method is also provided, the predicted-difference method is recommended because it accounts for test reliabilities and intercorrelations. Further details on this can be found in the WISC-IV Technical Manual. Saklofske et al. (2005) provide GAI-WIAT-II data for calculating ability-achievement discrepancies when the GAI is determined to be the best general ability estimate. These are reproduced in Tables 6–147 to 6–149.

Ability-Memory Comparisons

WISC-IV scores can be compared to CMS scores to compute ability-memory discrepancies. Using the predicted-actual method, tables for calculating discrepancies involving FSIQ, GAI, VCI, and PRI are shown in Tables 6–150 to 6–153, along with base rates (Table 6–154).

Interpretation

Some qualitative descriptors of composite scores differ compared with the WISC-III (i.e., performance in the lowest range is described as "extremely low" rather than as evidence of "intellectual deficiency"). As is the case for most tests, the manual recommends using confidence intervals in test score descriptions for individual children rather than absolute scores.

DEMOGRAPHIC EFFECTS

Gender

According to Sattler and Dumont (2004), girls and boys obtain similar FSIQs on the WISC-IV. However, boys obtain PSI scores that are about five points higher than girls. It is not yet clear how gender differences might affect scores in clinical groups.

Ethnicity

White American children obtain WISC-IV IQs that are 11.5 points higher than those of African American children and 10 points higher than Hispanic children (Sattler & Dumont,

Table 6–146 Frequency of Differences Between a WISC-IV Index Score and the Overall Mean Index Score for the WISC-IV

Difference	Cumulative Percentile							
	VCI < M[a]	VCI > M	PRI < M	PRI > M	WMI < M	WMI > M	PSI < M	PSI > M
30	0.0	0.1	0.0	0.0	0.2	0.2	0.2	0.0
29	0.0	0.1	0.0	0.0	0.2	0.2	0.3	0.2
28	0.1	0.1	0.0	0.0	0.3	0.3	0.4	0.3
27	0.2	0.1	0.1	0.0	0.4	0.4	0.4	0.4
26	0.3	0.1	0.1	0.0	0.5	0.4	0.6	0.5
25	0.3	0.2	0.1	0.1	0.6	0.5	0.7	0.6
24	0.4	0.2	0.1	0.3	0.7	0.7	0.9	0.9
23	0.6	0.3	0.2	0.4	1.0	1.0	1.1	1.3
22	0.9	0.5	0.3	0.5	1.5	1.3	1.5	1.6
21	1.2	0.9	0.4	0.8	2.0	1.6	2.1	2.0
20	1.5	1.2	0.7	1.0	2.4	2.0	2.7	2.7
19	1.9	1.6	1.2	1.4	2.8	2.5	3.1	3.6
18	2.2	2.1	1.5	2.0	3.6	3.1	4.0	4.5
17	2.8	2.8	2.2	2.5	4.3	3.5	5.2	5.8
16	3.8	3.5	2.9	3.1	5.0	4.4	6.1	7.0
15	5.2	4.1	3.5	4.2	6.0	5.0	7.7	8.0
14	6.3	4.9	4.6	5.4	7.7	6.1	9.1	9.2
13	7.7	6.0	5.7	6.8	8.8	7.4	10.7	11.3
12	9.3	8.0	7.5	8.4	10.8	9.5	12.5	13.4
11	11.7	9.7	9.1	10.3	12.5	11.0	14.6	16.3
10	14.6	12.3	11.5	13.0	15.4	13.4	17.2	19.0
9	17.2	15.0	13.9	15.2	18.0	15.8	19.6	21.8
8	20.0	18.0	17.0	18.3	21.0	18.5	22.1	24.0
7	23.6	21.1	20.5	21.8	25.5	21.9	25.4	27.0
6	27.7	24.9	24.7	26.4	29.3	25.6	28.4	30.1
5	31.7	28.1	29.4	30.2	33.2	29.2	31.0	33.5
4	36.0	31.1	33.2	34.5	37.0	33.6	35.2	37.0
3	40.2	35.0	37.5	39.0	40.7	37.6	39.6	40.0
2	44.7	39.5	42.0	44.0	45.3	41.5	44.1	43.7
1	50.5	44.0	46.8	48.4	49.7	46.1	47.9	47.5
Mean	7.2	7.2	6.8	7.0	7.8	7.5	8.3	8.7
SD	5.2	5.1	4.7	4.9	5.7	5.6	6.1	6.0
Median	6.0	6.0	6.0	6.0	7.0	6.0	7.0	8.0

[a]M stands for the overall mean of four WISC-IV index scores.

Source: From Longman, 2005. Reprinted with permission.

2004). When children are matched for parental education, as was done by Prifitera et al. (2005), White, African American, and Hispanic children obtain FSIQ scores of 103.2, 91.7, and 93.1, respectively. However, the magnitude of differences between groups varies when individual index scores are examined, with the smallest between-group difference found for PSI and WMI. The authors suggest that the FSIQ is somewhat limited in detecting relative strengths and weaknesses within these minority groups.

Ethnicity-based group differences are smallest in the youngest age groups, which provides some evidence of the increasing effect of adverse environmental influences on children's cognitive development in minority groups where disadvantaged children are overrepresented, as has been

suggested in the case of other measures (see *PPVT-III*). Sattler and Dumont (2004) also summarize the existing data on ethnicity and WISC-IV performance. Ethnicity, culture, and test interpretation are also discussed in Harris et al. (2005).

Education

Like those of most IQ tests, WISC-IV scores are related to parental education. For example, the mean FSIQ of children with parents who completed college is about 20 points higher than that of children whose parents have less than nine years of education (Sattler & Dumont, 2004).

Table 6–147 Differences Between WISC-IV GAI and WIAT-II Subtests Required for Statistical
Significance: Predicted-Difference Methods by Age Band

Subtest/Composite	Significance Level	Ages 6–11 Predicted-Difference GAI	Ages 12–16 Predicted-Difference GAI
Word Reading	.05	4.87	6.92
	.01	6.41	9.11
Numerical Operations	.05	12.01	8.59
	.01	15.81	11.31
Reading Comprehension	.05	6.52	7.52
	.01	8.59	9.90
Spelling	.05	8.24	8.38
	.01	10.85	11.03
Pseudoword Decoding	.05	5.42	5.91
	.01	7.14	7.78
Math Reasoning	.05	8.91	8.80
	.01	11.72	11.58
Written Expression	.05	11.18	11.59
	.01	14.72	15.25
Listening Comprehension	.05	12.77	13.41
	.01	16.81	17.65
Oral Expression	.05	10.21	11.73
	.01	13.44	15.44
Reading	.05	5.03	5.65
	.01	6.62	7.43
Math	.05	8.91	7.18
	.01	11.72	9.45
Written Language	.05	8.24	10.82
	.01	10.85	14.24
Oral Language	.05	9.66	8.72
	.01	12.72	11.48
Total	.05	6.25	5.93
	.01	8.23	7.81

Source: From Saklofske et al., 2005. Reprinted with permission.

NORMATIVE DATA

Standardization Sample

American norms are based on 2200 children in 11 age groups from ages 6 years to 16 years 11 months. Specific characteristics of the sample are shown in Table 6–155. Norms were stratified according to 2000 U.S. Census data by age, gender, race, parental education, and geographic region. Specific exclusionary criteria were used in subject selection for the standardization (see Table 6–155). However, after screening, a representative proportion of children from the special group studies (i.e., 5.7%) were then added to the normative sample "to accurately represent the population of children attending school" (Wechsler, 2003b, p. 23). Unlike other subtests, standardization for the Supplemental Arithmetic subtest only included 1100 children.

Canadian norms are also available, based on the fact that Canadian children score higher on the test than the American standardization sample, which may relate to differences with regard to geographic region and SES (PsychCorp, 2003). Other normative versions are available (e.g., WISC-IV[UK]).

Score Conversions

To derive scaled and standard scores for the test from standardization data, raw scores from the normative sample were normalized for each age group. Scaled scores were then derived from these distributions, and minor irregularities in the progression of scaled scores within and across age groups were eliminated by smoothing. Because of a restriction in range, Longest Digits Forward/Backward scores were not converted

Table 6–148 Differences Between WISC-IV GAI Scores and WIAT-II Subtests and Composite Scores Required for Statistical Significance

	WIAT-II														WISC-IV GAI
WISC-IV GAI	Subtest Scores									Composite Scores					
	WR	NO	RC	SP	PD	MR	WE	LC	OE	RD	MA	WL	OL	TA	
40	56	60	55	59	64	54	60	52	66	54	55	57	54	49	40
41	56	60	56	59	65	55	61	53	67	55	56	58	55	50	41
42	57	61	57	60	65	56	62	54	68	55	57	58	55	51	42
43	58	62	57	61	66	57	62	54	68	56	57	59	56	52	43
44	59	62	58	61	66	57	63	55	69	57	58	60	57	52	44
45	59	63	59	62	67	58	64	56	69	58	59	60	58	53	45
46	60	64	60	63	68	59	64	57	70	58	60	61	58	54	46
47	61	64	60	63	68	60	65	58	70	59	60	62	59	55	47
48	62	65	61	64	69	60	66	58	71	60	61	63	60	56	48
49	62	66	62	65	69	61	66	59	71	61	62	63	61	57	49
50	63	67	63	66	70	62	67	60	72	62	63	64	62	58	50
51	64	67	63	66	71	63	68	61	73	62	63	65	62	58	51
52	64	68	64	67	71	64	68	62	73	63	64	65	63	59	52
53	65	69	65	68	72	64	69	62	74	64	65	66	64	60	53
54	66	69	66	68	72	65	70	63	74	65	66	67	65	61	54
55	67	70	66	69	73	66	70	64	75	65	66	68	65	62	55
56	67	71	67	70	74	67	71	65	75	66	67	68	66	63	56
57	68	71	68	70	74	67	72	66	76	67	68	69	67	63	57
58	69	72	69	71	75	68	72	66	76	68	69	70	68	64	58
59	70	73	69	72	75	69	73	67	77	68	69	70	68	65	59
60	70	73	70	72	76	70	74	68	78	69	70	71	69	66	60
61	71	74	71	73	77	70	74	69	78	70	71	72	70	67	61
62	72	75	72	74	77	71	75	70	79	71	72	73	71	68	62
63	73	75	72	74	78	72	76	70	79	72	72	73	72	69	63
64	73	76	73	75	78	73	76	71	80	72	73	74	72	69	64
65	74	77	74	76	79	73	77	72	80	73	74	75	73	70	65
66	75	77	75	77	80	74	78	73	81	74	75	76	74	71	66
67	76	78	75	77	80	75	78	74	82	75	75	76	75	72	67
68	76	79	76	78	81	76	79	74	82	75	76	77	75	73	68
69	77	79	77	79	81	76	80	75	83	76	77	78	76	74	69
70	78	80	78	79	82	77	80	76	83	77	78	78	77	75	70
71	79	81	78	80	83	78	81	77	84	78	78	79	78	75	71
72	79	81	79	81	83	79	82	78	84	78	79	80	78	76	72
73	80	82	80	81	84	79	82	78	85	79	80	81	79	77	73
74	81	83	81	82	84	80	83	79	85	80	81	81	80	78	74
75	82	83	81	83	85	81	84	80	86	81	81	82	81	79	75
76	82	84	82	83	86	82	84	81	87	82	82	83	82	80	76
77	83	85	83	84	86	83	85	82	87	82	83	83	82	80	77
78	84	85	84	85	87	83	85	82	88	83	84	84	83	81	78
79	84	86	84	86	87	84	86	83	88	84	84	85	84	82	79
80	85	87	85	86	88	85	87	84	89	85	85	86	85	83	80
81	86	87	86	87	89	86	87	85	89	85	86	86	85	84	81
82	87	88	87	88	89	86	88	86	90	86	87	87	86	85	82
83	87	89	87	88	90	87	89	86	90	87	87	88	87	86	83
84	88	89	88	89	90	88	89	87	91	88	88	88	88	86	84
85	89	90	89	90	91	89	90	88	92	88	89	89	88	87	85
86	90	91	90	90	92	89	91	89	92	89	90	90	89	88	86
87	90	91	90	91	92	90	91	90	93	90	90	91	90	89	87
88	91	92	91	92	93	91	92	90	93	91	91	91	91	90	88
89	92	93	92	92	93	92	93	91	94	92	92	92	92	91	89
90	93	93	93	93	94	92	93	92	94	92	93	93	92	92	90
91	93	94	93	94	95	93	94	93	95	93	93	94	93	92	91
92	94	95	94	94	95	94	95	94	96	94	94	94	94	93	92

(continued)

320

Table 6–148 Differences Between WISC-IV GAI Scores and WIAT-II Subtests and Composite Scores Required for Statistical Significance
(*continued*)

WISC-IV GAI	WIAT-II														WISC-IV GAI
	Subtest Scores									Composite Scores					
	WR	NO	RC	SP	PD	MR	WE	LC	OE	RD	MA	WL	OL	TA	
93	95	95	95	95	96	95	95	94	96	95	95	95	95	94	93
94	96	96	96	96	96	95	96	95	97	95	96	96	95	95	94
95	96	97	96	97	97	96	97	96	97	96	96	96	96	96	95
96	97	97	97	97	98	97	97	97	98	97	97	97	97	97	96
97	98	98	98	98	98	98	98	98	98	98	98	98	98	97	97
98	99	99	99	99	99	98	99	98	99	98	99	99	98	98	98
99	99	99	99	99	99	99	99	99	99	99	99	99	99	99	99
100	100	100	100	100	100	100	100	100	100	100	100	100	100	100	100
101	101	101	101	101	101	101	101	101	101	101	101	101	101	101	101
102	101	101	102	101	101	102	101	102	101	102	102	101	102	102	102
103	102	102	102	102	102	102	102	102	102	102	102	102	102	103	103
104	103	103	103	103	102	103	103	103	102	103	103	103	103	103	104
105	104	103	104	103	103	104	103	104	103	104	104	104	104	104	105
106	104	104	105	104	104	105	104	105	103	105	105	104	105	105	106
107	105	105	105	105	104	105	105	106	104	105	105	105	105	106	107
108	106	105	106	106	105	106	105	106	104	106	106	106	106	107	108
109	107	106	107	106	105	107	106	107	105	107	107	106	107	108	109
110	107	107	108	107	106	108	107	108	106	108	108	107	108	109	110
111	108	107	108	108	107	108	107	109	106	108	108	108	108	109	111
112	109	108	109	108	107	109	108	110	107	109	109	109	109	110	112
113	110	109	110	109	108	110	109	110	107	110	110	109	110	111	113
114	110	109	111	110	108	111	109	111	108	111	111	110	111	112	114
115	111	110	111	110	109	111	110	112	108	112	111	111	112	113	115
116	112	111	112	111	110	112	111	113	109	112	112	112	112	114	116
117	113	111	113	112	110	113	111	114	110	113	113	112	113	114	117
118	113	112	114	112	111	114	112	114	110	114	114	113	114	115	118
119	114	113	114	113	111	114	113	115	111	115	114	114	115	116	119
120	115	113	115	114	112	115	113	116	111	115	115	114	115	117	120
121	116	114	116	114	113	116	114	117	112	116	116	115	116	118	121
122	116	115	117	115	113	117	115	118	112	117	117	116	117	119	122
123	117	115	117	116	114	117	115	118	113	118	117	117	118	120	123
124	118	116	118	117	114	118	116	119	113	118	118	117	118	120	124
125	119	117	119	117	115	119	117	120	114	119	119	118	119	121	125
126	119	117	120	118	116	120	117	121	115	120	120	119	120	122	126
127	120	118	120	119	116	121	118	122	115	121	120	119	121	123	127
128	121	119	121	119	117	121	118	122	116	122	121	120	122	124	128
129	121	119	122	120	117	122	119	123	116	122	122	121	122	125	129
130	122	120	123	121	118	123	120	124	117	123	123	122	123	126	130
131	123	121	123	121	119	124	120	125	117	124	123	122	124	126	131
132	124	121	124	122	119	124	121	126	118	125	124	123	125	127	132
133	124	122	125	123	120	125	122	126	118	125	125	124	125	128	133
134	125	123	126	123	120	126	122	127	119	126	126	124	126	129	134
135	126	123	126	124	121	127	123	128	120	127	126	125	127	130	135
136	127	124	127	125	122	127	124	129	120	128	127	126	128	131	136
137	127	125	128	126	122	128	124	130	121	128	128	127	128	131	137
138	128	125	129	126	123	129	125	130	121	129	129	127	129	132	138
139	129	126	129	127	123	130	126	131	122	130	129	128	130	133	139
140	130	127	130	128	124	130	126	132	122	131	130	129	131	134	140
141	130	127	131	128	125	131	127	133	123	132	131	130	132	135	141
142	131	128	132	129	125	132	128	134	124	132	132	130	132	136	142
143	132	129	132	130	126	133	128	134	124	133	132	131	133	137	143
144	133	129	133	130	126	133	129	135	125	134	133	132	134	137	144
145	133	130	134	131	127	134	130	136	125	135	134	132	135	138	145

(*continued*)

Table 6–148 Differences Between WISC-IV GAI Scores and WIAT-II Subtests and Composite Scores Required for Statistical Significance (*continued*)

WISC-IV GAI	WIAT-II														WISC-IV GAI
	Subtest Scores									Composite Scores					
	WR	NO	RC	SP	PD	MR	WE	LC	OE	RD	MA	WL	OL	TA	
146	134	131	135	132	128	135	130	137	126	135	135	133	135	139	146
147	135	131	135	132	128	136	131	138	126	136	135	134	136	140	147
148	136	132	136	133	129	136	132	138	127	137	136	135	137	141	148
149	136	133	137	134	129	137	132	139	127	138	137	135	138	142	149
150	137	134	138	135	130	138	133	140	128	139	138	136	139	143	150
151	138	134	138	135	131	139	134	141	129	139	138	137	139	143	151
152	138	135	139	136	131	140	134	142	129	140	139	137	140	144	152
153	139	136	140	137	132	140	135	142	130	141	140	138	141	145	153
154	140	136	141	137	132	141	136	143	130	142	141	139	142	146	154
155	141	137	141	138	133	142	136	144	131	142	141	140	142	147	155
156	141	138	142	139	134	143	137	145	131	143	142	140	143	148	156
157	142	138	143	139	134	143	138	146	132	144	143	141	144	148	157
158	143	139	144	140	135	144	138	146	132	145	144	142	145	149	158
159	144	140	144	141	135	145	139	147	133	145	144	142	145	150	159
160	144	140	145	141	136	146	140	148	134	146	145	143	146	151	160

WR = Word Reading; NO = Numerical Operations; RC = Reading Comp; SP = Spelling; PD = Pseudoword Decoding; MR = Mathematics Reasoning; WE = Written Expression; LC = Listening Comp; OE = Oral Expression; RD = Reading; MA = Mathematics; WL = Written Language; OL = Oral Language; TA = Total Achievement.

Source: From Saklofske et al., 2005. Reprinted with permission.

to scaled scores and are presented as base rates corresponding to raw scores. For composites, the distributions of sums of scaled scores were also normalized, followed by further smoothing.

Linear interpolation methods were used to derive 33 normative age groups from the 11 age groups in the standardization sample. This resulted in 33 four-month age bands ranging from 6 years, 0 months, 0 days, to 16 years, 11 months, 30 days, with scaled scores ranging from 1 to 19 for each age group (Wechsler, 2003b).

Table 6–149 WISC-IV GAI-based Differences Between Predicted and Obtained WIAT-II Subtest and Composite Scores for Various Percentages of the Theoretical Normal Distribution (Base Rates): Predicted-Difference Method

Subtest/Composite	Percentage of Theoretical Normal Distribution (Base Rates)								
	25	20	15	10	5	4	3	2	1
Word Reading	7	9	11	13	17	18	19	21	24
Numerical Operations	8	10	12	15	19	20	21	23	26
Reading Comprehension	7	9	11	13	17	18	19	21	24
Spelling	8	10	12	14	18	20	21	23	26
Pseudoword Decoding	9	11	13	16	20	22	23	25	28
Math Reasoning	7	9	11	13	17	18	19	21	23
Written Expression	8	10	12	15	19	20	22	24	27
Listening Comprehension	7	8	10	12	15	16	17	19	21
Oral Expression	9	11	13	16	21	22	24	26	29
Reading	7	9	10	13	16	17	19	20	23
Mathematics	7	9	11	13	17	18	19	21	24
Written Language	8	9	11	14	18	19	20	22	25
Oral Language	7	9	10	13	16	17	19	20	23
Total	6	7	9	11	13	14	15	17	19

Note: Percentages in table represent the proportions of the sample who obtained WIAT-II scores lower than their WISC-IV GAI scores by the specified amount or more. Reprinted with permission.

Table 6–150 CMS Composite Scores Predicted from WISC-IV FSIQ Scores

WISC-IV FSIQ	Verbal Immediate	Verbal Delayed	General Memory	Attention/ Concentration	Learning	Delayed Recognition
40	66	62	63	57	69	71
41	67	63	64	58	70	72
42	68	63	65	58	70	72
43	68	64	65	59	71	73
44	69	65	66	60	71	73
45	69	65	66	60	72	74
46	70	66	67	61	72	74
47	70	67	68	62	73	75
48	71	67	68	63	73	75
49	71	68	69	63	74	76
50	72	69	70	64	75	76
51	73	69	70	65	75	76
52	73	70	71	65	76	77
53	74	70	71	66	76	77
54	74	71	72	67	77	78
55	75	72	73	68	77	78
56	75	72	73	68	78	79
57	76	73	74	69	78	79
58	76	74	74	70	79	80
59	77	74	75	70	79	80
60	78	75	76	71	80	81
61	78	75	76	72	80	81
62	79	76	77	73	81	82
63	79	77	77	73	81	82
64	80	77	78	74	82	83
65	80	78	79	75	82	83
66	81	79	79	76	83	84
67	82	79	80	76	83	84
68	82	80	80	77	84	85
69	83	80	81	78	84	85
70	83	81	82	78	85	86
71	84	82	82	79	85	86
72	84	82	83	80	86	87
73	85	83	84	81	86	87
74	85	84	84	81	87	88
75	86	84	85	82	87	88
76	87	85	85	83	88	88
77	87	86	86	83	88	89
78	88	86	87	84	89	89
79	88	87	87	85	89	90
80	89	87	88	86	90	90
81	89	88	88	86	90	91
82	90	89	89	87	91	91
83	90	89	90	88	91	92
84	91	90	90	88	92	92
85	92	91	91	89	92	93
86	92	91	91	90	93	93
87	93	92	92	91	93	94
88	93	92	93	91	94	94
89	94	93	93	92	94	95
90	94	94	94	93	95	95
91	95	94	95	94	95	96
92	96	95	95	94	96	96
93	96	96	96	95	96	97
94	97	96	96	96	97	97
95	97	97	97	96	97	98
96	98	97	98	97	98	98
97	98	98	98	98	98	99
98	99	99	99	99	99	99
99	99	99	99	99	99	100
100	100	100	100	100	100	100

(continued)

Table 6-150 CMS Composite Scores Predicted from WISC-IV FSIQ Scores (continued)

WISC-IV FSIQ	Verbal Immediate	Verbal Delayed	General Memory	Attention/ Concentration	Learning	Delayed Recognition
101	101	101	101	101	101	100
102	101	101	101	101	101	101
103	102	102	102	102	102	101
104	102	103	102	103	102	102
105	103	103	103	104	103	102
106	103	104	104	104	103	103
107	104	104	104	105	104	103
108	104	105	105	106	104	104
109	105	106	105	106	105	104
110	106	106	106	107	105	105
111	106	107	107	108	106	105
112	107	108	107	109	106	106
113	107	108	108	109	107	106
114	108	109	109	110	107	107
115	108	109	109	111	108	107
116	109	110	110	112	108	108
117	110	111	110	112	109	108
118	110	111	111	113	109	109
119	111	112	112	114	110	109
120	111	113	112	114	110	110
121	112	113	113	115	111	110
122	112	114	113	116	111	111
123	113	114	114	117	112	111
124	113	115	115	117	112	112
125	114	116	115	118	113	112
126	115	116	116	119	113	112
127	115	117	116	119	114	113
128	116	118	117	120	114	113
129	116	118	118	121	115	114
130	117	119	118	122	115	114
131	117	120	119	122	116	115
132	118	120	120	123	116	115
133	118	121	120	124	117	116
134	119	121	121	124	117	116
135	120	122	121	125	118	117
136	120	123	122	126	118	117
137	121	123	123	127	119	118
138	121	124	123	127	119	118
139	122	125	124	128	120	119
140	122	125	124	129	120	119
141	123	126	125	130	121	120
142	124	126	126	130	121	120
143	124	127	126	131	122	121
144	125	128	127	132	122	121
145	125	128	127	132	123	122
146	126	129	128	133	123	122
147	126	130	129	134	124	123
148	127	130	129	135	124	123
149	127	131	130	135	125	124
150	128	132	131	136	126	124
151	129	132	131	137	126	124
152	129	133	132	137	127	125
153	130	133	132	138	127	125
154	130	134	133	139	128	126
155	131	135	134	140	128	126
156	131	135	134	140	129	127
157	132	136	135	141	129	127
158	132	137	135	142	130	128
159	133	137	136	142	130	128
160	134	138	137	143	131	129

Table 6–151 CMS Composite Scores Predicted from WISC-IV GAI Scores

WISC-IV GAI	Verbal Immediate	Verbal Delayed	General Memory	Attention/ Concentration	Learning	Delayed Recognition
40	71	66	68	63	75	73
41	71	66	68	63	75	73
42	72	67	69	64	76	74
43	72	68	69	65	76	74
44	73	68	70	65	76	75
45	73	69	70	66	77	75
46	74	69	71	67	77	76
47	74	70	71	67	78	76
48	75	70	72	68	78	77
49	75	71	72	68	79	77
50	76	72	73	69	79	78
51	76	72	74	70	79	78
52	76	73	74	70	80	78
53	77	73	75	71	80	79
54	77	74	75	71	81	79
55	78	74	76	72	81	80
56	78	75	76	73	82	80
57	79	75	77	73	82	81
58	79	76	77	74	82	81
59	80	77	78	75	83	82
60	80	77	78	75	83	82
61	81	78	79	76	84	82
62	81	78	79	76	84	83
63	82	79	80	77	84	83
64	82	79	81	78	85	84
65	83	80	81	78	85	84
66	83	81	82	79	86	85
67	84	81	82	80	86	85
68	84	82	83	80	87	86
69	85	82	83	81	87	86
70	85	83	84	81	87	87
71	86	83	84	82	88	87
72	86	84	85	83	88	87
73	87	85	85	83	89	88
74	87	85	86	84	89	88
75	88	86	87	85	90	89
76	88	86	87	85	90	89
77	89	87	88	86	90	90
78	89	87	88	86	91	90
79	90	88	89	87	91	91
80	90	89	89	88	92	91
81	91	89	90	88	92	91
82	91	90	90	89	92	92
83	92	90	91	89	93	92
84	92	91	91	90	93	93
85	93	91	92	91	94	93
86	93	92	92	91	94	94
87	94	93	93	92	95	94
88	94	93	94	93	95	95
89	95	94	94	93	95	95
90	95	94	95	94	96	96
91	96	95	95	94	96	96
92	96	95	96	95	97	96
93	97	96	96	96	97	97
94	97	97	97	96	97	97
95	98	97	97	97	98	98
96	98	98	98	98	98	98
97	99	98	98	98	99	99
98	99	99	99	99	99	99
99	100	99	99	99	100	100
100	100	100	100	100	100	100

(*continued*)

Table 6–151 CMS Composite Scores Predicted from WISC-IV GAI Scores (*continued*)

WISC-IV GAI	Verbal Immediate	Verbal Delayed	General Memory	Attention/ Concentration	Learning	Delayed Recognition
101	100	101	101	101	100	100
102	101	101	101	101	101	101
103	101	102	102	102	101	101
104	102	102	102	102	102	102
105	102	103	103	103	102	102
106	103	103	103	104	103	103
107	103	104	104	104	103	103
108	104	105	104	105	103	104
109	104	105	105	106	104	104
110	105	106	105	106	104	105
111	105	106	106	107	105	105
112	106	107	106	107	105	105
113	106	107	107	108	105	106
114	107	108	108	109	106	106
115	107	109	108	109	106	107
116	108	109	109	110	107	107
117	108	110	109	111	107	108
118	109	110	110	111	108	108
119	109	111	110	112	108	109
120	110	111	111	112	108	109
121	110	112	111	113	109	109
122	111	113	112	114	109	110
123	111	113	112	114	110	110
124	112	114	113	115	110	111
125	112	114	114	116	111	111
126	113	115	114	116	111	112
127	113	115	115	117	111	112
128	114	116	115	117	112	113
129	114	117	116	118	112	113
130	115	117	116	119	113	114
131	115	118	117	119	113	114
132	116	118	117	120	113	114
133	116	119	118	120	114	115
134	117	119	118	121	114	115
135	117	120	119	122	115	116
136	118	121	119	122	115	116
137	118	121	120	123	116	117
138	119	122	121	124	116	117
139	119	122	121	124	116	118
140	120	123	122	125	117	118
141	120	123	122	125	117	118
142	121	124	123	126	118	119
143	121	125	123	127	118	119
144	122	125	124	127	118	120
145	122	126	124	128	119	120
146	123	126	125	129	119	121
147	123	127	125	129	120	121
148	124	127	126	130	120	122
149	124	128	126	130	121	122
150	125	129	127	131	121	123
151	125	129	128	132	121	123
152	125	130	128	132	122	123
153	126	130	129	133	122	124
154	126	131	129	133	123	124
155	127	131	130	134	123	125
156	127	132	130	135	124	125
157	128	132	131	135	124	126
158	128	133	131	136	124	126
159	129	134	132	137	125	127
160	129	134	132	137	125	127

Table 6-152 CMS Composite Scores Predicted from WISC-IV VCI Scores

WISC-IV VCI	Verbal Immediate	Verbal Delayed	General Memory	Attention/ Concentration	Learning	Delayed Recognition
45	70	67	70	68	77	72
46	70	68	71	69	77	72
47	71	68	71	69	78	73
48	71	69	72	70	78	73
49	72	69	72	70	79	74
50	73	70	73	71	79	75
51	73	71	74	72	79	75
52	74	71	74	72	80	76
53	74	72	75	73	80	76
54	75	72	75	73	81	77
55	75	73	76	74	81	77
56	76	74	76	74	82	78
57	76	74	77	75	82	78
58	77	75	77	76	82	79
59	77	75	78	76	83	79
60	78	76	78	77	83	80
61	79	77	79	77	84	80
62	79	77	79	78	84	81
63	80	78	80	79	84	81
64	80	78	81	79	85	82
65	81	79	81	80	85	82
66	81	80	82	80	86	83
67	82	80	82	81	86	83
68	82	81	83	81	87	84
69	83	81	83	82	87	84
70	84	82	84	83	87	85
71	84	83	84	83	88	85
72	85	83	85	84	88	86
73	85	84	85	84	89	86
74	86	84	86	85	89	87
75	86	85	87	86	90	87
76	87	86	87	86	90	88
77	87	86	88	87	90	88
78	88	87	88	87	91	89
79	88	87	89	88	91	89
80	89	88	89	88	92	90
81	90	89	90	89	92	90
82	90	89	90	90	92	91
83	91	90	91	90	93	91
84	91	90	91	91	93	92
85	92	91	92	91	94	92
86	92	92	92	92	94	93
87	93	92	93	92	95	93
88	93	93	94	93	95	94
89	94	93	94	94	95	94
90	95	94	95	94	96	95
91	95	95	95	95	96	95
92	96	95	96	95	97	96
93	96	96	96	96	97	96
94	97	96	97	97	97	97
95	97	97	97	97	98	97
96	98	98	98	98	98	98
97	98	98	98	98	99	98
98	99	99	99	99	99	99
99	99	99	99	99	100	99
100	100	100	100	100	100	100

(continued)

Table 6–152 CMS Composite Scores Predicted from WISC-IV VCI Scores *(continued)*

WISC-IV VCI	Verbal Immediate	Verbal Delayed	General Memory	Attention/ Concentration	Learning	Delayed Recognition
101	101	101	101	101	100	101
102	101	101	101	101	101	101
103	102	102	102	102	101	102
104	102	102	102	102	102	102
105	103	103	103	103	102	103
106	103	104	103	103	103	103
107	104	104	104	104	103	104
108	104	105	104	105	103	104
109	105	105	105	105	104	105
110	106	106	105	106	104	105
111	106	107	106	106	105	106
112	107	107	106	107	105	106
113	107	108	107	108	105	107
114	108	108	108	108	106	107
115	108	109	108	109	106	108
116	109	110	109	109	107	108
117	109	110	109	110	107	109
118	110	111	110	110	108	109
119	110	111	110	111	108	110
120	111	112	111	112	108	110
121	112	113	111	112	109	111
122	112	113	112	113	109	111
123	113	114	112	113	110	112
124	113	114	113	114	110	112
125	114	115	114	115	111	113
126	114	116	114	115	111	113
127	115	116	115	116	111	114
128	115	117	115	116	112	114
129	116	117	116	117	112	115
130	117	118	116	117	113	115
131	117	119	117	118	113	116
132	118	119	117	119	113	116
133	118	120	118	119	114	117
134	119	120	118	120	114	117
135	119	121	119	120	115	118
136	120	122	119	121	115	118
137	120	122	120	121	116	119
138	121	123	121	122	116	119
139	121	123	121	123	116	120
140	122	124	122	123	117	120
141	123	125	122	124	117	121
142	123	125	123	124	118	121
143	124	126	123	125	118	122
144	124	126	124	126	118	122
145	125	127	124	126	119	123
146	125	128	125	127	119	123
147	126	128	125	127	120	124
148	126	129	126	128	120	124
149	127	129	126	128	121	125
150	128	130	127	129	121	126
151	128	131	128	130	121	126
152	129	131	128	130	122	127
153	129	132	129	131	122	127
154	130	132	129	131	123	128
155	130	133	130	132	123	128

Table 6–153 CMS Composite Scores Predicted from WISC-IV PRI Scores

WISC-IV PRI	Verbal Immediate[a]	Verbal Delayed	General Memory	Attention/ Concentration	Learning[a]	Delayed Recognition[a]
45		75	75	70		
46		75	75	70		
47		76	76	71		
48		76	76	71		
49		77	77	72		
50		77	77	73		
51		77	77	73		
52		78	78	74		
53		78	78	74		
54		79	79	75		
55		79	79	75		
56		80	80	76		
57		80	80	76		
58		81	81	77		
59		81	81	77		
60		82	82	78		
61		82	82	79		
62		83	83	79		
63		83	83	80		
64		83	83	80		
65		84	84	81		
66		84	84	81		
67		85	85	82		
68		85	85	82		
69		86	86	83		
70		86	86	84		
71		87	87	84		
72		87	87	85		
73		88	88	85		
74		88	88	86		
75		89	89	86		
76		89	89	87		
77		89	89	87		
78		90	90	88		
79		90	90	88		
80		91	91	89		
81		91	91	90		
82		92	92	90		
83		92	92	91		
84		93	93	91		
85		93	93	92		
86		94	94	92		
87		94	94	93		
88		94	94	93		
89		95	95	94		
90		95	95	95		
91		96	96	95		
92		96	96	96		
93		97	97	96		
94		97	97	97		
95		98	98	97		
96		98	98	98		
97		99	99	98		
98		99	99	99		
99		100	100	99		
100		100	100	100		

(continued)

Table 6-153 CMS Composite Scores Predicted from WISC-IV PRI Scores (continued)

WISC-IV PRI	Verbal Immediate[a]	Verbal Delayed	General Memory	Attention/ Concentration	Learning[a]	Delayed Recognition[a]
101		100	100	101		
102		101	101	101		
103		101	101	102		
104		102	102	102		
105		102	102	103		
106		103	103	103		
107		103	103	104		
108		104	104	104		
109		104	104	105		
110		105	105	106		
111		105	105	106		
112		106	106	107		
113		106	106	107		
114		106	106	108		
115		107	107	108		
116		107	107	109		
117		108	108	109		
118		108	108	110		
119		109	109	110		
120		109	109	111		
121		110	110	112		
122		110	110	112		
123		111	111	113		
124		111	111	113		
125		112	112	114		
126		112	112	114		
127		112	112	115		
128		113	113	115		
129		113	113	116		
130		114	114	117		
131		114	114	117		
132		115	115	118		
133		115	115	118		
134		116	116	119		
135		116	116	119		
136		117	117	120		
137		117	117	120		
138		117	117	121		
139		118	118	121		
140		118	118	122		
141		119	119	123		
142		119	119	123		
143		120	120	124		
144		120	120	124		
145		121	121	125		
146		121	121	125		
147		122	122	126		
148		122	122	126		
149		123	123	127		
150		123	123	128		
151		123	123	128		
152		124	124	129		
153		124	124	129		
154		125	125	130		
155		125	125	130		

[a]Predicted scores were not reported due to correlations with PRI below 0.40.

Table 6–154 Differences Between Predicted and Obtained CMS Subtest and Composite Scores for Various Percentages of the Theoretical Normal Distribution (Base Rates): Predicted-Difference Method Using Various WISC-IV Composite Scores

WISC-IV Composite	CMS Composite	Percentage of Theoretical Normal Distribution (Base Rate)								
		25	20	15	10	5	4	3	2	1
FSIQ	Verbal Immediate	9	11	13	16	21	22	24	26	29
	Verbal Delayed	8	10	13	15	20	21	22	24	28
	General Memory	9	11	13	16	20	21	23	25	28
	Attention/Concentration	8	9	11	14	18	19	20	22	25
	Learning	9	11	14	17	22	23	25	27	31
	Delayed Recognition	9	12	14	17	22	24	25	28	31
GAI	Verbal Immediate	9	12	14	17	22	23	25	27	31
	Verbal Delayed	9	11	13	16	21	22	24	26	29
	General Memory	9	11	14	17	21	23	24	26	30
	Attention/Concentration	8	10	13	16	20	21	23	25	28
	Learning	10	12	15	18	23	24	26	28	32
	Delayed Recognition	10	12	14	18	23	24	26	28	32
VCI	Verbal Immediate	9	11	13	17	21	22	24	26	30
	Verbal Delayed	9	11	13	16	20	22	23	25	28
	General Memory	9	11	14	17	21	23	24	26	30
	Attention/Concentration	9	11	13	16	21	22	23	26	29
	Learning	10	12	15	18	23	24	26	28	32
	Delayed Recognition	9	11	14	17	22	23	25	27	31
PRI	Verbal Immediate	10	12	15	18	24	25	27	29	33
	Verbal Delayed	9	12	14	18	22	24	26	28	31
	General Memory	9	12	14	18	22	24	26	28	31
	Attention/Concentration	9	11	13	17	21	22	24	26	30
	Learning	10	12	15	19	24	25	27	30	33
	Delayed Recognition	10	13	15	19	24	25	27	30	34

Note: Percentages represent the theoretical proportion of CMS scores lower than various WISC-IV composite scores by the specified amount or more.

Short Forms

See Sattler and Dumont (2004) for an extensive review and compilation of WISC-IV short forms.

RELIABILITY

Internal Reliability

The internal reliability of the WISC-IV is excellent, and in many cases, surpasses that of the WISC-III. Split-half reliabilities for subtests, averaged across age, are presented in Table 6–156, along with subtest coefficients for a large group of children with a variety of clinical conditions (i.e., "Special Groups," N = 661). In many cases, subtest reliabilities for children with clinical conditions surpassed those obtained with the standardization sample. Also of note are the lower reliabilities for speeded subtests, as these estimates represent test-retest coefficients. Reliability coefficients are not provided for Longest Digit Span Forward/Backward.

Standard Error of Measurement

*SEM*s are fairly small, as would be expected given the high reliabilities of WISC-IV subtests and index scores. The average SEM across age for the FSIQ is 2.68; others range from 3.78 to 5.21 (index scores) and from .97 to 1.38 (subtests). See the Technical Manual for further details and for *SEM*s by age. Confidence intervals, based on the estimated true score and standard error of estimation, are provided in the manual. Confidence intervals derived using the *SEM* centered around the obtained score will be similar to those presented in the manual because of the high reliability of the test (Wechsler, 2003b). Alternatively, Sattler and Dumont (2004) recommend calculating confidence intervals based on *SEM*s and obtained scores. These are provided in their text for each age range.

Test-Retest Reliability

Test-retest stability is high to excellent for index scores, as reported in the manual (i.e., all index scores in the high .80s or above .90; see Table 6–156). As is typical of most IQ tests, the FSIQ and VCI have the highest reliabilities (>.90). Most subtests also have high reliability (>.80), though some fall only in the "adequate" range (see Table 6–156). Index-level interpretation is therefore preferable when using the WISC-IV in a diagnostic evaluation. Test-retest reliability data are based on a sample of 243 children with 18 to 27 individuals per age group (reliabilities by age are presented in Wechsler, 2003b).

Table 6–155 WISC-IV Normative Sample Characteristics: American Sample

Sample type	National, stratified random sample[a]
Number	2200[b]
Age	6 to 16 years, 11 months
Geographic location	
Northeast	Proportions per region for the sample as a whole presented only
South	in graphical form in the manual
North Central	
West	
Parental education[c]	
≤8 years	5%
9–11years	9%
12 years	28%
13–15 years	33.5%
≥16 years	24.5%
SES	Based on parental education
Gender	
Males	50%
Females	50%
Race/ethnicity[c]	
White	63.5%
African American	15.5%
Hispanic	15%
Asian	4.5%
Other	1.5%
Screening	Individuals were excluded if they were tested on an IQ test in previous six months, had uncorrected visual impairment or hearing loss, were not fluent in English, were nonverbal or noncommunicative, had an upper extremity disability affecting motor performance, were currently admitted to a hospital or mental/psychiatric facility, were currently taking medications that affect test performance, or had been previously diagnosed with a condition that might affect test performance (e.g., stroke, epilepsy, brain tumor, TBI, brain surgery, encephalitis, meningitis)[d]

[a]Based on 11 separate age bands, each representing 12 months (i.e., 6 years, 11 months–7 years, 11 months), with 200 participants in each group. [b]Based on 2000 U.S. Census data, and collected between 2001 and 2002. [c]Proportions reflect data for age 11 only; other age groups differ slightly from these data; proportions presented only graphically for the sample as a whole in the manual. [d]Note that children from the special group studies were then added to the normative sample to reflect the proportion of special needs children in the school-age population (i.e., 5.7%).

Source: Adapted from Wechsler, 2003b.

Mean test interval was 32 days. Currently, there is no information on test-retest reliability in clinical groups.

Practice Effects

A summary of expected practice effects is shown in Table 6–157, as reproduced from Flanagan and Kaufman (2004). These range from small (Comprehension, 0.2 scaled score points) to substantial (Picture Completion, 1.9 scaled score points). As noted by Sattler and Dumont (2004), practice effects are more evident on the PRI and PSI than on the VCI and WMI.

Interscorer Reliability

Interscorer reliability is very high for those subtests requiring judgment on the part of the examiner for scoring (i.e., $r \geq .95$, for Comprehension, Information, Word Reasoning, Similarities, and Vocabulary; Wechsler, 2003b).

VALIDITY

Content Validity

WISC-IV development followed five comprehensive stages: conceptual development (including extensive literature

Table 6–156 Magnitude of Reliability Coefficients for WISC-IV Subtests and Index Scores for the Standardization Sample and Special Groups

Magnitude of Coefficient	Internal Reliability Normative Sample	Internal Reliability Special Groups	Test-Retest Reliability Normative Sample
Very high (.90+)	*Verbal Comprehension Index* *Perceptual Reasoning Index* *Working Memory Index* *FSIQ* Letter-Number Sequencing	Block Design Similarities Vocabulary Letter-Number Sequencing Matrix Reasoning Arithmetic	*Verbal Comprehension Index* *FSIQ* Vocabulary
High (.80–.89)	*Processing Speed Index* Block Design Block Design No Time Bonus Similarities Digit Span Digit Span Forward Digit Span Backward Picture Concepts Coding Vocabulary Matrix Reasoning Comprehension Picture Completion Information Arithmetic	Block Design No Time Bonus Digit Span Picture Concepts Comprehension Picture Completion Information Word Reasoning Digit Span Forward Digit Span Backward	*Perceptual Reasoning Index* *Working Memory Index* *Processing Speed Index* Block Design Similarities Digit Span Coding Letter-Number Sequencing Matrix Reasoning Comprehension Symbol Search Picture Completion Information Word Reasoning
Adequate (.70–.79)	Word Reasoning Symbol Search[a] Cancellation[a] Cancellation Random[a] Cancellation Structured[a]		Block Design No Time Bonus Picture Concepts Cancellation Arithmetic Digit Span Forward Digit Span Backward Cancellation Random Cancellation Structured
Marginal (.60–.69)			
Low (< .59)			

Note: Internal reliability coefficients for subtests represent split-half coefficients averaged across age. The special groups included children with intellectual giftedness, mental retardation, reading disability, reading and written expression disorder, mathematics disorder, learning disorder and ADHD, ADHD, expressive/receptive language disorder, head injury, autistic disorder, and motor impairment. Estimated reliabilities for speeded subtests (e.g., Cancellation) and internal reliability coefficients for Index scores not available in this group.

[a]Represents test-retest coefficient, corrected for sample variability (see Technical Manual).

Source: Adapted from Wechsler, 2003b.

review, professional feedback), pilot, national tryout, standardization, and final assembly and evaluation (Wechsler, 2003b). Bias analyses were conducted on items, including formal expert review and empirical analyses of a bias oversample during the tryout phase and after the standardization. Quality assurance procedures for scoring and data entry were followed in data collection, as was training of examiners. Note that the standardization version included more items than the final version; an average of three items per subtest were dropped after standardization. In addition, changes to the subtest order were made after standardization; these changes were reportedly "minor." According to the Technical Manual, a study comparing performance of 60

children on the final version versus 60 randomly selected children from the standardization indicated no significant mean differences between subtest and composite scores (Wechsler, 2003b).

Subtest Intercorrelations

Intercorrelations among WISC-IV composites and subtests in the standardization sample are extensively reviewed in the Technical and Interpretive Manual (see Tables 6–158 and 6–159). Overall, verbal subtests from the VCI are highly intercorrelated, supporting the construct validity of this index. Correlations for subtests belonging to the PRI are more difficult to

Table 6–157 One-Month Practice Effects for the WISC-IV Indices and Full-Scale IQ (Total $N = 243$)

Scale	Ages 6–7	Ages 8–11	Ages 12–16	All Ages
VCI	+3.4 (.31 SD)	+2.2 (.20 SD)	+1.7 (.14 SD)	+2.1 (.18 SD)
PRI	+6.4 (.46 SD)	+4.2 (.34 SD)	+5.4 (.38 SD)	+5.2 (.39 SD)
WMI	+4.7 (.33 SD)	+2.8 (.22 SD)	+1.6 (.12 SD)	+2.6 (.20 SD)
PSI	+10.9 (.72 SD)	+8.2 (.60 SD)	+4.7 (.35 SD)	+7.1 (.51 SD)
FSIQ	+8.3 (.62 SD)	+5.8 (.53 SD)	+4.3 (.34 SD)	+5.6 (.46 SD)

Note: Intervals ranged from 13 to 63 days with a mean of 32 days.

Source: From Flanagan & Kaufman, 2004. Reprinted with permission.

Table 6–158 Correlations Between WISC-IV Index Scores and Core Subtests

	VCI	PRI	WMI	PSI
Similarities	.89 (.74)	.59	.50	.38
Vocabulary	.91 (.79)	.58	.53	.39
Comprehension	.86 (.70)	.49	.46	.37
Block Design	.50	.81 (.56)	.42	.45
Picture Concepts	.47	.77 (.50)	.39	.36
Matrix Reasoning	.52	.84 (.61)	.46	.44
Digit Span	.44	.42	.86 (.49)	.30
Letter Number	.52	.48	.86 (.49)	.40
Coding	.34	.40	.30	.88 (.53)
Symbol Search	.42	.50	.40	.87 (.53)

Note: Numbers in italics represent subtests belonging to each index; numbers in parentheses represent corrected correlations.
Adapted from Wechsler, 2003b.

interpret, as these subtests demonstrate substantial correlations to the VCI as well as to the PRI itself. Although the manual indicates that this is because of the common *g* loading for VCI and PRI subtests, an alternate interpretation is that the PRI shows more overlap with verbal intelligence than did the PIQ. Likewise, some VCI and PRI subtests show substantial correlations to WMI subtests, underlining the Working Memory requirements of both domains. On the whole, WMI subtests are fairly intercorrelated, as are PSI subtests. The former demonstrate substantial correlations with VCI subtests, likely as a result of the common auditory comprehension demands of both sets of subtests (Wechsler, 2003b). The manual also notes that Cancellation shows the least overlap with other tests, suggesting that it is the least *g*-loaded test in the WISC-IV. Information on subtest and index intercorrelations is needed for clinical groups.

Subtest Specificity

Several WISC-IV subtests have ample specificity, and thus can be interpreted as providing unique information not provided by other subtests or by the test as a whole. The following subtests have ample specificity at all ages: Block Design, Picture Concepts, Matrix Reasoning, Digit Span, Letter-Number Sequencing, Coding, Symbol Search, and Cancellation (Sattler & Dumont, 2004).

Factor Structure

Exploratory and confirmatory factor-analytic studies, with and without the supplemental and optional tests, are presented in detail in the Technical Manual (see Wechsler, 2003b, pp. 52–60). Overall, Sattler and Dumont (2004) found generally good support for the factor-analytic structure of the WISC-IV as reported in the manual. Thus, the four-factor solution composed of the four separate index scores appears to well describe the underlying structure of the test, at least in normal children. Further studies are needed to determine the factor structure of the WISC-IV in clinical populations. Of note, the Picture Concepts subtests appear to load equally on the VCI and PRI in younger children (ages 6 to 7), and had

Table 6–159 Correlations Between WISC-IV Subtests

	SI	VC	CO	BD	PCn	MR	DS	LN	CD	SS
SI	1.00									
VC	.74	1.00								
CO	.62	.68	1.00							
BD	.50	.48	.36	1.00						
PCn	.45	.42	.40	.41	1.00					
MR	.49	.49	.42	.55	.47	1.00				
DS	.39	.42	.36	.35	.30	.38	1.00			
LN	.47	.50	.43	.38	.36	.42	.49	1.00		
CD	.28	.31	.30	.34	.29	.34	.23	.30	1.00	
SS	.39	.38	.34	.45	.34	.42	.30	.40	.53	1.00

Note: Correlations between subtests belonging to the same index are shown in bold. SI = Similarities; VC = Vocabulary; CO = Comprehension; BD = Block Design; PCn = Picture Completion; MR = Matrix Reasoning; DS = Digit Span; LN = Letter-Number; CD = Coding; SS = Symbol Search. Adapted from Wechsler, 2003b.

secondary loadings on the VCI in some factor solutions in older children, suggesting that this subtest has a significant verbal component. For an in-depth discussion of factor analytic-results by age, see Sattler and Dumont (2004).

Correlations With WISC-III and WAIS-III

WISC-IV/WISC-III FSIQ-corrected correlations in normal children are high ($r = .89$). WISC-IV FSIQ scores are about 2.5 points lower than WISC-III scores in normal children (Saklofske et al., 2005). This information is based on 244 children administered both measures in counterbalanced order over a mean test-retest interval of 28 days (Wechsler, 2003b). At the index level, scores are about two to five points higher, on average, than on the WISC-III. Indices are fairly highly correlated (e.g., $r = .88$ for the VCI from both versions); the lowest correlation between versions is for the WISC-IV PRI and WISC-III POI ($r = .72$), reflecting the substantial change in content from the POI to PRI. At the subtest level, the subtests with the largest differences in scores between versions are Block Design, Similarities, Coding, Symbol Search, and Picture Completion, with little over 1 standard score point as the maximum average score difference between versions (i.e., WISC-III subtests slightly higher).

See Wechsler (2003b) for detailed information on the correlation between the WISC-IV and WAIS-III in the overlapping age band of 16-year-olds. As expected, WAIS-III scores are slightly higher than WISC-IV scores. WASI results are also shown in the Technical Manual.

Correlations With WPPSI-III and Other IQ/Developmental Tests

WISC-IV and WPPSI-III group means are practically identical within their overlapping age band (i.e., 6:0 to 7:3), and their respective FSIQs are highly intercorrelated (i.e., $r = .89$; Wechsler, 2003b). At the subtest level, only Coding exhibits a small mean score difference at the group level. However, some subtests exhibit relatively modest overlap between test versions (i.e., Symbol Search, Picture Concepts, Word Reasoning; Wechsler, 2003b). Sattler and Dumont (2004) note that the WISC-IV and WPPSI-III are not completely independent; there is overlap of items on Block Design, Picture Completion, and Information, which complicates interpretation and increases the probability of practice effects in a retesting situation. However, this has yet to be demonstrated empirically. There is also a small amount of item overlap with the WAIS-III in the older age band, which may introduce similar complications (see Sattler & Dumont, 2004, for details).

Correlations With Achievement and Other Cognitive Domains

Correlations with achievement using the WIAT-II are reported in the Technical Manual, based on the administration of both measures to 550 normal children in the linking sample. FSIQ and WIAT-II Total Achievement are highly correlated ($r = .87$)—a level that rivals WISC-IV/WISC-III correlations. At the index level, correlations to Total Achievement are highest for the VCI and lowest for PSI ($r = .80$ and .58, respectively). Predictably, the VCI is most highly related to all aspects of achievement as measured by WIAT-II composites, including reading, mathematics, writing, and oral language ($r = .68–.75$). Notably, the PRI also has substantial correlations with these domains ($r = .61–.67$), as do the WMI and PSI (all r's > .50). Although the manual states that correlations between WISC-IV and WIAT-II demonstrate that specific WISC-IV subtests and composites relate differentially to achievement, most WISC-IV index scores are related at least moderately to most WIAT-II composites. The only exception is that verbal subtests appear to be the most consistent and strong predictors of most achievement domains. Unlike most other subtests, Cancellation demonstrates minimal relationship to achievement ($r \leq .20$).

See Wechsler (2003b) for a detailed discussion of the WISC-IV's relationship to several other PsychCorp measures including the GRS-S (a scale for giftedness), the Bar-On EQ (an emotional intelligence measure), and ABAS-II (see also *Comment*).

Correlations With Memory and Executive Function

The Technical Manual presents data on a group of 126 children administered the WISC-IV and CMS. Yeates and Donders (2005) performed additional analyses on these data and concluded that (a) WISC-IV and CMS measure different constructs despite considerable correlations between the two measures, (b) WISC-IV correlations to CMS Visual memory composites are consistently lower than those involving CMS Verbal memory composites, (c) CMS Visual memory index scores appear to tap working memory, (d) the VCI and WMI appear to overlap more strongly with CMS Verbal memory than other WISC-IV domains, (e) the PSI has the lowest overlap with CMS composites and thus reflects a relatively unique dimension, and (f) WMI and CMS Attention/Concentration are highly related, as would be expected given common subtest content, but all WISC-IV index scores are related to some degree to the latter. Subtest-specific findings are also discussed in detail by these authors, as are correlations between WISC-IV and D-KEFS subtests in a small sample of children with TBI assessed as part of the standardization process. Note that these conclusions are limited by the sample size and the psychometric limitations of the D-KEFS (discussed in this volume).

Clinical Studies

Although additional studies on special groups are needed given small sample sizes, considerable data are presented on WISC-IV performance in various clinical groups in the Technical Manual (e.g., giftedness, mental retardation, autism, ADHD, etc.). Results are supportive of the validity and clinical utility of the test, and are generally consistent with prior research on the WISC-III. These results, along with interpretive guidelines, are discussed in detail in Prifitera et al. (2005), along with useful chapters devoted to the diagnosis of ADHD (Schwean & Saklofske, 2005), giftedness (Sparrow et al., 2005), mental retardation (Spruill et al., 2005), language disabilities (Wigg, 2005), and TBI (Yeates & Donders, 2005). Although an impressive start, these preliminary clinical data need to be supplemented by peer-reviewed research, including results on the test's predictive validity and diagnostic utility.

COMMENT

It is difficult to overstate the WISC's influence on the practice and theoretical understanding of intelligence testing in children. In the words of Flanagan and Kaufman (2004), the "Wechsler scales have had a monumental impact [. . .] on scientific inquiry into the nature of human intelligence and the structure of cognitive abilities" (p. 2). This sentiment is acknowledged by even the harshest critics. The WISC-III, more so than any other Wechsler battery, was the single most commonly used intelligence test in the whole of psychology. Like the WISC-III, the WISC-IV is poised to become the most widely used IQ test in the world. Attesting to this fact are three entire volumes already devoted to the test (e.g., Flanagan & Kaufman, 2004; Prifitera et al., 2005; Sattler & Dumont, 2004); all are excellent references and should be reviewed by WISC-IV users.

Overall, the WISC-IV is an excellent test. It is evident that the revision was undertaken with major feedback from users and substantial attention to detail in terms of theoretical underpinnings, clinical utility, and psychometrics. The standardization has been described as "exemplary" (Flanagan & Kaufman, 2004). The Technical Manual is thorough and well written. The use of a large clinical sample (N of approximately 700) for internal reliability and validity studies is a major technical asset. Because of these features, clinicians already have access to vital information on the WISC-IV in clinical groups even though no independent research has yet been published on the test, as of this writing.

Although it will surely take the place of the WISC-III in this regard, the WISC-IV's exact role in a neuropsychological assessment remains to be defined empirically. Yeates and Donders (2005) predict that the PRI may show less sensitivity to brain dysfunction than did the POI or PIQ, possibly because of the reduced reliance on motor skills and speed, two areas of deficit commonly seen in children with neurological conditions. Similarly, they predict that the PSI may show the greatest sensitivity to acute brain impairment in children, as was the case for the WISC-III. In particular, they note that Cancellation may be useful for neuropsychologists as a substitute for Coding because of its high loading on the PSI factor, its reduced motor demands compared with Coding, and the traditional utility of similar tasks in neuropsychological assessment.

Like all complex test batteries, the WISC-IV has some limitations, which on the whole, do not detract from the value and importance of the test. Information regarding test-retest stability in clinical groups is needed. As well, although reliabilities are impressive for the majority of subtests, test-retest correlations are only adequate for some subtests (e.g., Cancellation). The Working Memory Index does not sample visual working memory, but is instead composed exclusively of auditory/verbal working memory tests. Additional tests are therefore required for a truly comprehensive evaluation of working memory. The Process Variables also need empirical validation. Interestingly, Weiss et al. (2005) report that differences in scores between Block Design with and without time bonuses were extremely rare in the standardization sample (<10%). Future studies will determine whether this score and others demonstrate utility in clinical samples. Lastly, the validity information presented in the Technical Manual is based almost exclusively on other Psychological Corporation products, a practice Sattler and Dumont (2004) find to be less than optimal.

Caution should be employed in comparing WISC-IV and WISC-III scores. First, much of the content underlying the FSIQs differ between versions. For instance, 50% of Core subtests in the WISC-IV are not Core subtests in the WISC-III (Sattler & Dumont, 2004). The WISC-IV is therefore more than just a simple revision of the WISC-III; it is in many ways a different test, even though a good proportion of the test will be familiar to habitual Wechsler test users. Second, the PSI and WMI contribute more highly to the FSIQ than they did in the WISC-III (i.e., 40% versus 20% contribution; Prifitera et al., 2005). Thus, children with strengths in auditory attention and processing speed may obtain higher FSIQs than if they were tested with the WISC-III (particularly if these strengths exceed the expected drop of three points due to the normative reanchoring of the scale). Generally speaking, WISC-IV IQs should be expected to differ to some extent, both in absolute value and in terms of pattern of strengths and weaknesses, in children tested previously with the WISC-III. Ongoing and future research will inform on the degree to which these differences manifest in clinical groups.

Sattler and Dumont (2004) conclude that the test is still insufficiently sensitive for extremely low functioning children in the youngest age ranges, largely because scaled scores can be obtained based on nonperformance (i.e., raw scores of 0). The WPPSI-III or other tests with lower floors (e.g., WJ III COG) may therefore be a better choice for assessing young, very low functioning children with expected IQs in the moderate to severe range of mental handicap.

REFERENCES

Braden, J. P. (2005). Hard-of-hearing and deaf clients: Using the WISC-IV with clients who are hard-of-hearing or deaf. In A. Prifitera, D. H.

Saklofske, & L. G. Weiss (Eds.), *WISC-IV clinical use and interpretation: Scientist-practitioner perspectives.* New York: Elsevier Academic Press.

Carroll, J. B. (1993). *Human cognitive abilities: A survey of factor analytic studies.* New York: Cambridge University Press.

Flanagan, D. P., & Kaufman, A. S. (2004). *Essentials of WISC-IV assessment.* Hoboken, NJ: John Wiley & Sons.

Harris, J. G., & Llorente, A. M. (2005). Cultural considerations in the use of the Wechsler Intelligence Scale for Children—Fourth Edition (WISC-IV). In A. Prifitera, D. H. Saklofske, & L. G. Weiss (Eds.), *WISC-IV clinical use and interpretation: Scientist-practitioner perspectives.* New York: Elsevier Academic Press.

Horn, J. L., & Noll, J. (1997). Human cognitive capabilities: Gf–Gc theory. In D. P. Flanagan, J. L. Genshaft, & P. L. Harrison (Eds.), *Contemporary intellectual assessment: Theories, tests and issues* (pp. 53–91). New York: Guilford.

Kaufman, A. S. (1994). *Intelligent testing with the WISC-III.* New York: John Wiley & Sons, Inc.

Kaufman, A. S. (2000). Seven questions about WAIS-III regarding difference in abilities across the 16 to 89 year life span. *School Psychology Quarterly, 15,* 3–29.

Longman, R. S. (2005). Tables to compare WISC-IV index scores against overall means. In A. Prifitera, D. H. Saklofske, & L. G. Weiss (Eds.), *WISC-IV clinical use and interpretation: Scientist-practitioner perspectives.* New York: Elsevier Academic Press.

Prifitera, A., Saklofske, D. H., Weiss, L. G., & Rolfhus, E. (2005). The WISC-IV in the clinical assessment context. In A. Prifitera, D. H. Saklofske, & L. G. Weiss (Eds.), *WISC-IV clinical use and interpretation: Scientist-practitioner perspectives.* New York: Elsevier Academic Press.

PsycCorp. (2003). *WISC-IV^CDN Canadian manual.* Toronto, Ontario: Harcourt Assessment, Harcourt Canada Ltd.

Saklofske, D. H., Prifitera, A., Weiss, L. G., Rolfhus, E., & Zhu, J. (2005). Clinical interpretation of the WISC-IV FSIQ and GAI. In A. Prifitera, D. H. Saklofske, & L. G. Weiss (Eds.), *WISC-IV clinical use and interpretation: Scientist-practitioner perspectives.* New York: Elsevier Academic Press.

Sattler, J. M., & Dumont, R. (2004). *Assessment of children: WISC-IV and WPPSI-III supplement.* San Diego: Jerome M. Sattler, Publisher, Inc.

Schwean, V. L., & Saklofske, D. H. (2005). Assessment of attention deficit hyperactivity disorder with the WISC-IV. In A. Prifitera, D. H. Saklofske, & L. G. Weiss (Eds.), *WISC-IV clinical use and interpretation: Scientist-practitioner perspectives.* New York: Elsevier Academic Press.

Sparrow, S. S., Pfeiffer, S. I., & Newman, T. M. (2005). Assessment of children who are gifted with the WISC-IV. In A. Prifitera, D. H. Saklofske, & L. G. Weiss (Eds.), *WISC-IV clinical use and interpretation: Scientist-practitioner perspectives.* New York: Elsevier Academic Press.

Spruill, J., Oakland, T., & Harrison, P. (2005). Assessment of mental retardation. In A. Prifitera, D. H. Saklofske, & L. G. Weiss (Eds.), *WISC-IV clinical use and interpretation: Scientist-practitioner perspectives.* New York: Elsevier Academic Press.

Wechsler, D. (1974). *Wechsler Intelligence Scale for Children–Revised.* San Antonio, TX: The Psychological Corporation.

Wechsler, D. (1991). *Wechsler Intelligence Scale for Children–Third Edition.* San Antonio, TX: The Psychological Corporation.

Wechsler, D. (2003a). *WISC-IV administration manual.* San Antonio, TX: The Psychological Corporation.

Wechsler, D. (2003b). *WISC-IV technical and interpretive manual.* San Antonio, TX: The Psychological Corporation.

Wechsler, D. (2004b). *WISC-IV integrated.* San Antonio, TX: The Psychological Corporation.

Weiss, L. G., Saklofske, D. H., & Prifitera, A. (2005). Interpreting the WISC-IV index scores. In A. Prifitera, D. H. Saklofske, & L. G. Weiss (Eds.), *WISC-IV clinical use and interpretation: Scientist-practitioner perspectives.* New York: Elsevier Academic Press.

Wigg, E. H. (2005). Language disabilities. In A. Prifitera, D. H. Saklofske, & L. G. Weiss (Eds.), *WISC-IV clinical use and interpretation: Scientist-practitioner perspectives.* New York: Elsevier Academic Press.

Yeates, K. O., & Donders, J. (2005). The WISC-IV and neuropsychological assessment. In A. Prifitera, D. H. Saklofske, & L. G. Weiss (Eds.), *WISC-IV clinical use and interpretation: Scientist-practitioner perspectives.* New York: Elsevier Academic Press.

Wechsler Preschool and Primary Scale of Intelligence—Third Edition (WPPSI-III)

PURPOSE

The WPPSI-III is intended to assess intelligence in preschoolers and young children.

SOURCE

The WPPSI-III (test materials, Administration and Norms Manual, Technical and Interpretive Manual, Stimulus Booklets, 25 Record Forms, 25 Response Booklets) can be obtained from The Psychological Corporation, 19500 Bulverde Road, San Antonio, TX, 78259 (www.wppsi-iii.com). The scale costs about $725 US ($840 with basic scoring software). Scoring software comes in two forms: the WPPSI-III Scoring Assistant ($165 US), which provides scoring only, and the WPPSI-III Writer ($350 US), an interpretive report program. Additional manuals, such as the Canadian Norms Manual, can also be obtained from the publisher.

AGE RANGE

The WPPSI-III can be administered to children ages 2 years, 6 months, to 7 years, 3 months.

DESCRIPTION

The WPPSI-III (Wechsler, 2002a; 2002b) is the third version of the WPPSI, an intelligence battery for young children that first appeared in 1967 and was later revised in 1989 (Wechsler, 1967, 1989). The WPPSI-R was criticized by test reviewers and users on several fronts, including its limited range of measured abilities, low reliability of some subtests, limited floors and ceilings, nonuniformity of subtest score ranges, long administration time, and complex scoring criteria for some subtests (e.g., Geometric Design). It was also criticized for overemphasizing speed (which may have put some children at a disadvantage), and because of significant item

Table 6–160 WPPSI-III Subtest Changes Compared with WPPSI-R

Subtest	New Subtest	Administration	Recording and Scoring	New Items
		Modifications		
Block Design		✓	✓	✓
Information		✓	✓	✓
Matrix Reasoning	✓			
Vocabulary		✓	✓	✓
Picture Concepts	✓			
Symbol Search	✓			
Word Reasoning	✓			
Coding	✓			
Comprehension			✓	✓
Picture Completion		✓	✓	✓
Similarities		✓	✓	✓
Receptive Vocabulary	✓			
Object Assembly		✓	✓	✓
Picture Naming	✓			

Source: Reprinted with permission from Wechsler, 2002b.

overlap between the WPPSI-R and WISC-III, which complicated interpretation when children were subsequently administered the WISC-III (Flanagan & Ortiz, 2001; Kaufman, 1994; Sattler, 2001).

These limitations have been addressed in the current version, which has been substantially improved compared with its predecessor. First, the test is more consistent with current factor-analytic theories of intelligence and cognitive functioning collectively known as CHC theory (see chapter introduction). This means that the structure of the test is different, and several new subtests have been added (see Table 6–160). The age range has also been extended down from 2 years, 11 months, to 2 years, 6 months. There are now two distinct age groups (2:6 to 3:11, and 4:0 to 7:3), which differ in their score structure, administration time, item difficulty, and reliance on verbal expression. In all, five WPPSI-R subtests were deleted (Arithmetic, Animal Pegs, Geometric Design, Mazes, and Sentences). Two new subtests were added in the younger age band (Receptive Vocabulary, Picture Naming) and five were added in the older age band (Word Reasoning, Matrix Reasoning, Picture Concepts, Coding, and Symbol Search).

The test's overall structure is shown in Figure 6–26. The test yields the traditional FSIQ, VIQ, and PIQ scores in addition to new composite scores. In younger children, the addition of a supplemental subtest provides a General Language Composite (GLC). In older children, supplemental subtests yield a Processing Speed Quotient (PSQ) and a GLC.

There are three different kinds of WPPSI-III subtests. Core subtests are administered when FSIQ, VIQ, and PIQ are needed. Supplemental subtests yield additional scores (GLC in younger children, PSQ in older children), or can be used to substitute for core subtests when needed. Optional subtests yield optional scores; these cannot be used in substitutions for core subtests. These include Receptive Vocabulary and Picture

Naming in older children. A subtest's designation as core, supplemental, or optional may change depending on age (e.g., Receptive Vocabulary). For the younger age band, there are four core subtests (Receptive Vocabulary, Information, Block Design, and Object Assembly) that yield FSIQ, VIQ, and PIQ

Figure 6–26 WPPSI-III structure.

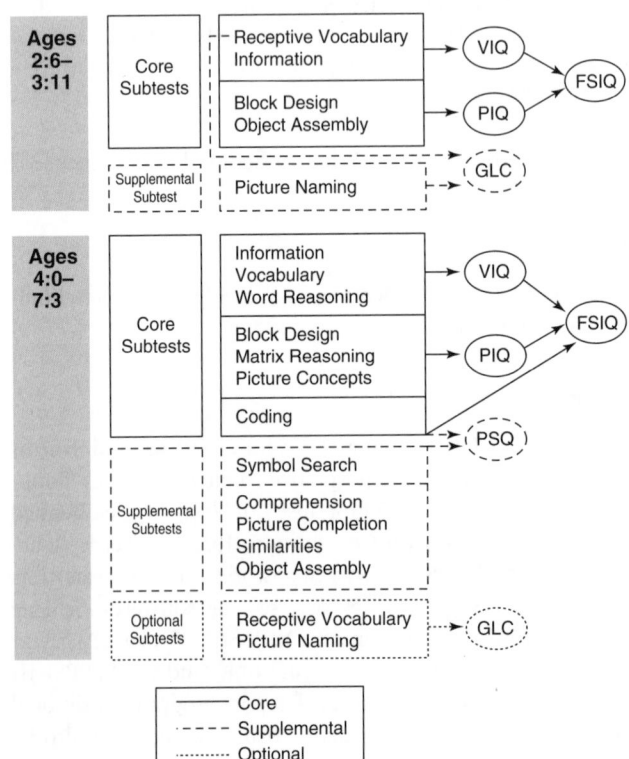

(see Figure 6–26). The GLC is obtained by administering the core subtest of Receptive Vocabulary with the supplemental subtest of Picture Naming. This subtest can also be substituted for Receptive Vocabulary to obtain composite scores. There is no PSQ at this age. WPPSI-III subtests are described in Table 6–161.

To construct the WPPSI-III, floors and ceilings of WPPSI-R subtests were extended with the addition of several new items to improve assessment of delayed and gifted children. In addition, the test's ability to measure fluid reasoning and processing speed was enhanced with new subtests measuring these abilities. The influence of processing speed was somewhat lessened in Performance subtests (e.g., Block Design) with the elimination of bonus points for rapid performance. In the verbal domain, instructions were simplified, and expressive language demands were substantially lessened.

Throughout the test, instructions are simpler, testing materials have been improved, and the manual has been reorganized for ease of use. In addition, norms have been updated and testing time is significantly reduced, particularly at the lower age range where only four subtests need be administered. Although not technically conormed, the WPPSI-III is now statistically linked to achievement through a linkage sample with the WIAT-II. See Sattler and Dumont (2004) and Lichtenberger and Kaufman (2004) for an extensive review and guidelines for administering and interpreting the WPPSI-III.

ADMINISTRATION TIME

Administration of core subtests necessary for deriving the main composite scores takes 30 to 35 minutes in the younger age band, with an additional five to seven minutes for the supplemental Picture Naming subtest. In the older age band, testing takes 40 to 50 minutes for the core subtests, with an additional three to four minutes for the Symbol Search if the PSQ is desired. In older children, total time to administer all the subtests necessary to derive composite scores and required for discrepancy analyses takes approximately 70 to 85 minutes. Additional time is needed if the supplemental tests of Comprehension and Picture Completion are also administered.

ADMINISTRATION

Administration Instructions

See Administration Manual.

Materials

The test includes two Stimulus Books and a split-back, spiral-bound manual. Response booklets are now on special paper meant to discourage unauthorized copying. There are separate record forms for the two age bands. Coding and Symbol Search are presented together in a separate response booklet. The thin Block Design blocks from the WPPSI-R have been replaced with standard Wechsler-type cubes to facilitate manipulation by young children. Overall, materials are colorful and child-friendly, and are likely to elicit and maintain the attention of young children.

Subtest Substitutions

Subtest substitution is recommended only in special circumstances dictated by clinical need (e.g., motor impairment, a spoiled subtest). The Technical Manual states that substitution introduces measurement error; however, substitution should be chosen over prorating. In both cases, results should be interpreted with caution. A supplemental subtest can thus be substituted for a core subtest in the derivation of composite scores, but certain rules apply. Test order may change because all subtests must be administered in standard order as per the manual (e.g., Picture Naming is always administered last in young children), and, in older children, no more than two subtests can be substituted for core subtests when deriving the FSIQ. In young children, only one subtest is available for substitution (Picture Naming), and it must always substitute for Receptive Vocabulary. In the older age band, Comprehension or Similarities can be substituted for core VIQ subtests, and Object Assembly or Picture Completion can be substituted for core PIQ subtests. Allowable substitutions are summarized on p. 25 of the Administration Manual.

Queries and Timing

WPPSI-III verbal tests allow a much more liberal approach regarding querying than those from the WPPSI-R (see Administration Manual). More importantly, there has been a major change to the Performance/Nonverbal tests. Although items are not timed per se (i.e., in the sense of allotting bonus points for rapid performance, as in the WISC-III), items must be completed within a time limit. The time limit depends on the test and the item type (e.g., 30 seconds for Matrix Analogy, 30 to 90 seconds for Block Design, 90 seconds for Object Assembly).

SCORING

Scores

The range of FSIQ for the younger age band is 41 to 155; for the older age band, it is 40 to 160. Slightly different values are found for other editions such as the Canadian standardization (i.e., 45 to 156, and 40 to 160, respectively; Wechsler, 2004). Although not recommended for describing performance, age equivalents can also be derived (see Administration and Scoring Manual). Statistical significance of composite score differences and frequencies for composite scale differences are presented in the Technical and Interpretive Manual. Note that

Table 6–161 WPPSI-III Subtest Description

Subtest	Description
Information	This is a test of general knowledge, organized into two parts. Younger children begin by choosing a picture from a set of four choices in response to an examiner question; older children answer examiner questions orally.
Receptive Vocabulary	This test measures knowledge of vocabulary independent of verbal expression, and follows the format of tests such as the PPVT-III. The examiner says a word and the child must choose the corresponding picture from among a set of four pictures presented in a 2×2 array.
Vocabulary	This test measures word knowledge and verbal expression. Early items involve simple naming (five items); the remaining items require the child to provide definitions for words spoken by the examiner. Responses are rated from zero to two points.
Word Reasoning	This is a test of verbal reasoning that involves verbally presented clues that the child uses to deduce a specific object or concept. Simple items require one clue (e.g., "This is an animal with a trunk. What is it?"), while more complex items involve two or three increasingly specific clues (e.g., "This is something that you eat. And people make it for a party. And it usually has candles on it. What is it?")
Picture Naming	This is a naming task that assesses word knowledge in standard expressive naming task format. The child is simply required to name pictured objects.
Block Design	This is a test of visual-spatial skills and of the ability to analyze and synthesize abstract visual information. The child is asked to arrange blocks to copy a model, under time constraints. Single-color blocks are introduced first; in the last part of the test, the standard Wechsler two-color, red-and-white blocks are used. For early items, the examiner completes all models in full view of the child using real blocks; later items involve reconstructing designs from a pictured model in the stimulus book. Rotations are not penalized. Although not a timed test per se, items must be completed within a specific time limit for credit.
Matrix Reasoning	This is a standard matrix analogy task designed to measure fluid intelligence and abstract reasoning. Four types of items are used requiring either pattern completion, classification, analogical reasoning, or serial reasoning. The child must choose the right response from a set of four or five choices. Items represent both real objects and abstract designs.
Picture Concepts	This test is designed to measure abstract categorical reasoning. It is somewhat analogous to a nonverbal Similarities test. The child is shown two sets of pictured objects and must choose two or three items that go together. Correct answers are typically related by function or by categorical type.
Coding	This is a test of processing speed and visual attention. Test format follows that of Part A of the WISC-IV Coding. The child must draw a simple symbol such as a line or circle within the appropriate geometric shape, based on a key and under timed conditions. Bonus points are awarded for perfect performance within the time limit. The total score is the number correct.
Symbol Search	This is a test of processing speed and visual attention. It is a cancellation task requiring the child to cross out a target symbol appearing among a group of distractor symbols, under time constraints. If it is not found, the child must cross out a question mark that appears on the right of the symbol array. The total score is the number of correct responses minus the number of incorrect responses.
Comprehension	This test measures verbal expression and reasoning. The child is asked to answer questions requiring practical and logical reasoning based on common knowledge and everyday experiences (e.g., "Why do people go to the doctor?"). Responses are rated from zero to two points.
Picture Completion	This test measures visual perception and identification of visual detail. The child is asked to identify, by pointing or naming, an important missing detail from pictures.
Similarities	This test measures verbal reasoning and concept formation. All items are in a sentence completion format. Specifically, the child must complete a sentence by providing the specific concept that links two objects or ideas (e.g., "Carrots and potatoes are both _____"). Responses are rated from zero to two points.
Object Assembly	This test measures visual-spatial skills and visual-constructional ability. The child is required to assemble puzzles in order of increasing complexity. All items represent real objects. Although not a timed test per se, puzzles must be assembled within a time limit of 90 seconds.

frequencies are provided for both positive and negative discrepancies, as these are not symmetrical. Information for calculating the significance and frequency of discrepancies at the subtest level for differences relative to the average subtest score is also provided, as are discrepancy tables for every possible pair of WPPSI-III subtests. The significance of intersubtest scatter (i.e., the variability of scores across all subtests) within each composite score can also be analyzed for significance and frequency (see Technical and Interpretive Manual). Confidence intervals based on SE$_E$ and true scores are provided in the manual; however, Sattler and Dumont (2004) recommend calculating confidence intervals based on *SEM*s

Table 6–162 Suggested Major Abilities and Background Factors Associated With WPPSI-III Composites

Verbal (V)	Performance (P)	Processing Speed (PS)	General Language (GL)	Full Scale (FS)	Major Abilities and Background Factors
V	P	PS		FS	Attention
V				FS	Auditory-vocal processing
	P	PS		FS	Concentration
V			GL	FS	Crystallized knowledge
V			GL	FS	Cultural opportunity
V			GL	FS	Extent of outside reading
	P			FS	Fluid reasoning ability
	P			FS	Immediate problem solving
V			GL	FS	Interest and reading patterns
V			GL	FS	Language development
V			GL	FS	Lexical knowledge
V				FS	Long-term verbal memory
	P			FS	Nonverbal reasoning
	P			FS	Perceptual reasoning
		PS		FS	Processing speed
V			GL	FS	Retrieval of material from long-term memory
		PS		FS	Scanning ability
		PS		FS	Short-term memory
		PS		FS	Short-term visual memory
	P			FS	Spatial perception
		PS		FS	Speed of mental operation
V			GL	FS	Verbal comprehension
V				FS	Verbal processing
	P	PS		FS	Visual acuity and discrimination
		PS		FS	Visual-motor coordination
	P			FS	Visual-motor discrimination
	P	PS		FS	Visual-perceptual processing
	P			FS	Visual-perceptual reasoning
	P			FS	Visual-spatial processing
V			GL	FS	Vocabulary

Source: From Sattler & Dumont, 2004. Reprinted with permission.

and obtained scores. These are provided in their text for each age range.

Prorating

Prorating is not recommended because it introduces unknown measurement error and violates standard administration procedures (Sattler & Dumont, 2004). However, if prorating must be used, procedures outlined in the Administration Manual must be followed (see *Administration*).

Ability-Achievement Comparisons

Ability-achievement discrepancies with regard to the WIAT-II can be derived using Appendix C in the Technical Manual. Although the simple-difference method is provided, the predicted-difference method is recommended because it accounts for test reliabilities and intercorrelations. Further details on this can also be found in the WIAT-II Technical Manual.

Interpretation

Qualitative descriptors of composite scores are reproduced in Table 5–2. Note that descriptors differ compared with previous WPPSI versions. Sattler and Dumont's (2004) suggested content domains are also shown in Table 6–162.

DEMOGRAPHIC EFFECTS

Gender

According to Sattler and Dumont (2004), girls' FSIQ scores are 3.22 points higher than boys', with the most pronounced gender difference on Processing Speed, where girls outperform boys by 6.38 points.

Ethnicity

Sattler and Dumont (2004) summarize the existing data on ethnicity and WPPSI-III performance, based on information provided in the manual. They note that Asian American children obtain the highest FSIQ scores (1.86 points higher than Euro-American children). African American children obtain, on average, scores that are 10.3 points lower than Euro-American children (i.e., 93.8 versus 104.4), whereas those of Hispanic American children are about 11.7 points lower. Hamilton and Burns (2003) note that WPPSI-IIII Processing Speed is based solely on two paper-and-pencil tasks, which may disadvantage children from ethnic groups that do not emphasize speed or writing/drawing skills.

Education

Like those of most IQ tests, WPPSI-III scores are related to parental education. For example, the mean FSIQ of children of parents who completed college is about 22 points higher than that of children whose parents have less than nine years of education (Sattler & Dumont, 2004).

NORMATIVE DATA

Standardization Sample

American norms are based on 1700 children (600 in the younger age band, 1100 in the older age band). In all, nine age bands with 200 individuals per group (100 in the oldest age band) were included. Using these data, linear interpolation was used to produce 18 normative age groups comprised of three-month intervals (2:6 to 5:11) or four-month intervals (6:0 to 7:3). Norms were collected from 2001 to 2002, and stratified according to 2000 U.S. Census data by age, gender, parental education, and geographic region. For purposes of comparing ability to achievement, 200 participants over age 4 were administered the WPPSI-III and WIAT-II. Additional details concerning sample characteristics can be found in the manual; however, overall group composition for certain factors such as ethnicity are presented in graphical form only.

Score Conversions

To derive the scaled scores in the manual from the raw score standardization data, a fairly extensive process was followed; this is detailed in the manual. Polynomial regression was used to determine fit for each age group from raw data, from which percentiles, and then scaled scores, were derived; minor irregularities within and across age groups were eliminated by smoothing. Linear interpolation was used to produce 18 normative groups from the nine sampled age groups. Composite score distributions were also smoothed.

Short Forms

See Sattler and Dumont (2004) for an extensive review and list of subtest combinations that can be used as WPPSI-III short forms.

RELIABILITY

Internal Reliability

Split-half reliabilities of the VIQ, PIQ, GLC, and FSIQ composite scores in the normative sample are very high (.93–.96). Internal reliability is high to very high for all the nonspeeded subtests (.84–.95). This is significantly improved compared with the WPPSI-R. Reliability coefficients in approximately 700 children with clinical diagnoses, including children classified as having giftedness, mental retardation, developmental delay, autism, language disorders, and ADHD, are also high when averaged across groups (i.e., ≥ .90; see Technical Manual). Although most were high to very high, within clinical groups, some subtest reliabilities are lower; however, only the Object Assembly reliability coefficient in the gifted group is in the marginal range (i.e., $r = .61$). Reliability estimates in the Canadian standardization sample are very similar (Wechsler, 2004).

Standard Error of Measurement

Average SEMs across the two age bands were all less than five for the composite scores (ranging from a low of 2.92 for the FSIQ to a high of 4.94 for the PSQ). Subtest SEMs all approximate 1.00.

Test-Retest Reliability

In the manual, stability was assessed using a sample of 157 healthy children in three age groups, tested twice over a mean testing interval of 26 days. Overall, composite score stability was excellent in all three age groups, particularly for FSIQ, VIQ, and PSQ (all with coefficients equal to or above .90). PIQ stability coefficients were in the .84 to .87 range. Test-retest stability of the WPPSI-III in Canadian children ($N = 104$) is quite similar (Wechsler, 2004).

Similarly, the majority of subtests demonstrated adequate to high stability across age (Table 6–163). However, coefficients for Block Design varied substantially across age; stability was only marginal in children aged 4 years to 5 years, 5 months. Across age, Picture Concepts and Object Assembly had the lowest coefficients ($r = .72–.75$).

Practice Effects

Practice effects were least pronounced on verbal tests and for the youngest subjects, based on the data reviewed above. Test-retest gains for the VIQ, PIQ, PSQ, FSIQ, and GLC were 2.8, 5.0, 6.2, 5.2, and 2.7, respectively (Technical and Interpretive Manual).

Interscorer reliability

Interscorer reliability for the verbal tests requiring subjective scoring is high (Technical and Interpretive Manual).

Table 6–163 Magnitude of Reliability Coefficients for WPPSI-III Subtests

Magnitude of Coefficient	Ages 2 Years, 6 Months to 3 Years, 11 Months	Ages 4 to 5 Years, 5 Months	Ages 5 Years, 6 Months to 7 Years, 3 Months
Very high (.90+)	Information Picture Naming	Similarities	
High (.80–.89)	Receptive Vocabulary Block Design	Information Vocabulary Symbol Search Word Reasoning Coding Comprehension Picture Completion Receptive Vocabulary Picture Naming	Information Matrix Reasoning Vocabulary Symbol Search Word Reasoning Comprehension Picture Completion Similarities Receptive Vocabulary Picture Naming
Adequate (.70–.79)	Object Assembly	Matrix Reasoning Picture Concepts Object Assembly	Block Design Picture Concepts Coding Object Assembly
Marginal (.60–.69)	—	Block Design	—
Low (<.59)	—	—	—

Note: Coefficients are corrected for sample variability (see Technical Manual).

VALIDITY

Content Validity

WPPSI-III development followed five comprehensive stages: conceptual development (including extensive literature review, professional feedback), pilot, national tryout, standardization, and final assembly and evaluation (Wechsler, 2002b). Quality assurance procedures for scoring and data entry were followed, as was training of examiners.

Correlations With WPPSI-R

WPPSI-III/WPPSI-R correlations in healthy children are high for FSIQ, VIQ, and PIQ ($r = .85$, .86, and .70, respectively). Score differences were surprisingly small in a group of 176 children administered both measures, with FSIQ differences of 1.2 points only (Technical and Interpretive Manual). VIQ and PIQ differences were 0.4 and 3.1. Object Assembly, Block Design, and Similarities were the least correlated between WPPSI-III and WPPSI-R. This suggests caution in interpreting score changes on these subtests in children tested with both measures.

Subtest Intercorrelations

Intercorrelations among WPPSI-III composites and subtests are extensively reviewed in the Technical and Interpretive Manual. In the younger age band, verbal subtests were more correlated with each other than with performance subtests, but performance subtests were correlated with both verbal and performance subtests. The test publishers interpret this as due to the high g loadings of all the subtests in this age group and the less differentiated cognitive abilities of younger children. In the older age band, verbal subtests were highly intercorrelated, as were processing speed subtests. Performance subtests differed in that some subtests, though highly correlated with PIQ, also correlated with VIQ (i.e., Matrix Reasoning, Block Design), as well as with Symbol Search, a PSQ subtest with a reportedly high g loading. In the older age band, Picture Completion and Picture Concepts were highly correlated with both verbal and performance subtests, which the authors interpreted as evidence for verbal mediation in both these subtests.

In the WPPSI-III, subtests can be substituted for each other to derive composite scores. Correlational evidence in favor of substitution is stronger for the VIQ subtests; some PIQ subtests were only moderately correlated with the PIQ subtests for which they can substitute. Specifically, in younger children, Picture Naming can be substituted for Receptive Vocabulary; their intercorrelation is .71. In older children, Symbol Search can be substituted for Coding ($r = .59$). In the VIQ, Similarities can be substituted for Information, Vocabulary, or Word Reasoning ($r = .67–.69$), as can Comprehension ($r = .66–.70$). In the PIQ, Object Assembly can substitute for Block Design, Matrices, and Picture Concepts ($r = .39–.53$), as can Picture Completion ($r = .46–.50$).

Subtest Specificity

Several WPPSI-III subtests have ample specificity, and thus can be interpreted as providing unique information not provided by other subtests or by the test as a whole. These include Matrix Reasoning, Picture Concepts, Picture Completion, Symbol Search, Receptive Vocabulary, and Object Assembly (Sattler & Dumont, 2004). Block Design, Coding, Comprehension, and Picture Naming have ample subtest specificity at most but not all ages; the specificity of the remaining subtests depends on age (see Sattler & Dumont, 2004, for a detailed listing).

Factor Structure

Exploratory and confirmatory factor-analytic studies, with and without the supplemental and optional tests, are presented in detail in the Technical Manual. In the younger age band, factor-analytic studies support the VIQ/PIQ subtest structure. In the older age band, factor-analytic studies support the validity of the VIQ and PSQ subtest composition. Results are less clear with regard to PIQ. Although generally supportive of the PIQ subtest structure, in some cases, Picture Concepts loads on the Verbal factor and Matrix Reasoning loads on the Processing Speed factor. The test authors note that the cognitive demands of Matrix Reasoning and Picture Concepts might vary depending on the age of the child. Overall, Sattler and Dumont (2004) found generally good agreement with their factor-analytic studies and those reported in the manual.

Correlations With WISC-III, WISC-IV, and Other IQ/Developmental Tests

In older children, correlations with the WISC-III are high ($r = .89$, .82, .79, and .69, for FSIQ, VIQ, PIQ, and PSQ/PSI, respectively), based on 96 normally developing children administered both measures. However, WISC-III composite scores are consistently higher than those of the WPPSI-III, reflecting the older date of publication of the WISC-III and consequent Flynn effect. The FSIQ difference between both measures was 4.9 (3.1 and 7.9 for VIQ and PIQ, respectively). Verbal scores from both measures were in general more highly intercorrelated than performance measures; Object Assembly was only moderately correlated between measures ($r = .46$). Table 5.10 of the Technical Manual presents expected WPPSI-III composite score ranges for given WISC-III scores.

Notably, WISC-IV and WPPSI-III group means are practically identical within their overlapping age band (i.e., 6:0–7:3), and their respective FSIQs are highly intercorrelated (i.e., $r = .89$; Wechsler, 2003). At the subtest level, only Coding exhibits a small mean score difference at the group level. However, some subtests exhibit relatively modest overlap between test versions (i.e., Symbol Search, Picture Concepts, Word Reasoning; Wechsler, 2003). Sattler and Dumont (2004) note that the two tests are not completely independent; there is overlap of items on Block Design, Picture Completion, and Information, which complicates interpretation and increases the probability of practice effects in a retesting situation.

In younger children, the correlation between the WPPSI-III FSIQ and the BSID-II Mental Scale is also high ($r = .80$;

$N = 84$). As might be expected given its cognitive demands, correlation with the Motor Scale is only moderate ($r = .47$). BSID-II composite scores are only slightly higher than WPPSI-III scores (e.g., 0.9-point difference between BSID-II Mental Scale and WPPSI-III FSIQ). Table 5.12 of the Technical Manual presents expected WPPSI-III composite score ranges for given BSID-II scores. Given the near equivalence of scores, both measures can therefore be used with confidence in younger children. Use of the WPPSI-III over the BSID-II would likely yield a more comprehensive assessment of cognitive skills, while use of the BSID-II would yield a better evaluation of motor skills.

Correlations With Achievement

Correlations with achievement using the WIAT-II are also reported in the Technical Manual, based on the administration of both measures to 208 healthy children. FSIQ and WIAT-II Total Achievement were highly correlated ($r = .78$). The VIQ was most related to Total Achievement and Oral Language from the WIAT-II ($r = .77$ and .72, respectively) and least related to the Mathematics composite ($r = .56$), to which the PIQ was most related ($r = .60$). PSQ was also most related to Mathematics ($r = .55$). The GLC was most related to Total Achievement ($r = .76$), Oral Language ($r = .67$), and Reading ($r = .65$) composites from the WIAT-II. Interestingly, Matrix Reasoning and Picture Concepts were only minimally related to achievement, with the largest correlations to achievement subtests or composites attaining only a moderate level of agreement ($r = .35$, Total Achievement, both subtests).

Clinical Studies

Although further studies on special groups are needed, considerable data are presented on WPPSI-III performance in various clinical groups in the Technical Manual (e.g., giftedness, mental retardation, autism, ADHD, etc.). Results are supportive of the validity and clinical utility of the WPPSI-III in clinical groups. Several findings were consistent with prior research, including a relatively lower PSQ in gifted children compared with the other composite scores, less variability across scores in children with mental handicap than in normally developing children, and relative elevations in PIQ compared with other composite scores in children with autism. In children with limited English proficiency, FSIQ, VIQ, and GLC were significantly lower than in a matched control group; there were no group differences in PIQ and PSQ. Therefore, the Technical Manual notes that PIQ may be an appropriate way to estimate intellectual level in children with limited English proficiency. However, Braden (2003) argues that omitting verbal ability from a standardized IQ test does not provide an adequate characterization of general intellectual level because there is not sufficient representation of intellectual abilities in the assessment (e.g., Gf may be represented, but not Gc). Other tests may therefore be more appropriate (e.g., UNIT, Leiter-R).

In contrast, children with motor impairments did not show relative weaknesses in VIQ compared to matched controls despite lower scores on FSIQ, PIQ, and PSQ, indicating that VIQ might provide the best estimate of intellectual abilities for these children. Again, Braden (2003) would argue that this would represent a limited assessment of intellectual ability and, ideally, a nonmotor way of assessing PIQ and PSQ would be needed to ensure adequate representation of fluid abilities in the assessment of general intellectual functioning. Of note, Coding scores were significantly higher in the matched controls, but Symbol Search was not significantly different between groups, demonstrating the differential role of motor skills in these two subtests. Children with ADHD did not show relative weaknesses in PSQ; the significance of this finding is unclear, however, as over half the group was taking medication at the time of testing. Although an impressive start, these clinical studies need to be supplemented by peer-reviewed research, including results on the test's predictive utility.

COMMENT

The WPPSI-III is by and large an excellent test. Almost all aspects of the WPPSI-R were improved. It is evident that the revision was undertaken with major feedback from users and a substantial amount of attention to detail in terms of theoretical underpinnings, clinical utility, and psychometrics. The Technical Manual is also quite thorough and well written. The use of a large clinical sample ($N = 700$) for internal reliability and validity studies is a major technical asset compared with many other intelligence batteries. Because of it, clinicians already have access to vital information on the WPPSI-III in clinical groups even though no independent research has yet been published on the test, as of this writing. Among this information is the fact that the PIQ appears to be minimally affected by limited English proficiency and that the VIQ appears to be minimally affected by motor impairments.

Of note is the fact that the manual recommends using confidence intervals in test score descriptions for individual children (provided in Tables A.2 to A.10 in the Administration and Scoring Manual; but see Sattler & Dumont, 2004). Clinicians should also note that the term "Intellectually Deficient" has been replaced by "Extremely Low" in this revision of the test.

Like all complex test batteries, the WPPSI-III has some limitations. Information on test-retest reliability in clinical groups would have been beneficial. As well, test-retest correlations are not adequate for all subtests (particularly PIQ subtests). Moderate PIQ subtest intercorrelations suggest that this composite may reflect a heterogeneous domain. Factor-analytic studies in older children are also not always supportive of the PIQ as a cohesive dimension of ability. This suggests that the VIQ might be a more stable and unitary measure than the PIQ in older children. Subtest specificity is not covered in the Technical Manual, which would be helpful to determine whether subtests can be interpreted as measuring distinct abilities. Fortunately, Sattler and Dumont provide this information (see above).

In addition, there is the issue of retesting across age bands: IQs derived for younger children are not based on the same subtest clusters as those for older subjects. This raises questions about the comparability of IQs across age, both cross-sectionally (i.e., across individuals of different ages) and longitudinally (i.e., within individuals over time). In older children, a method for deriving a composite IQ estimate based on the same four subtests corresponding to the IQ in the younger age band might be helpful when comparisons are required.

Breadth

In many intelligence batteries, a four-subtest IQ test would be considered a screener or an abbreviated estimate. Although the test is well constructed and its reliability excellent, the use of only four subtests to evaluate IQ in the younger age band requires more study, particularly in terms of predictive validity. Understandably, it is difficult to design IQ tests for young preschoolers, given the two opposing goals of brevity and breadth. That is, a test must be short enough to sustain the interest of young children, but must also be comprehensive enough to adequately measure intelligence and have enough items to ensure adequate reliability. In the case of the WPPSI-III, the four subtests needed to derive the FSIQ have excellent internal and test-retest reliability. However, it is not clear that these four subtests assess a sufficiently broad range of abilities. Flanagan and Ortiz (2001) argue that intellectual assessment of preschool children should cover at least five broad abilities defined by the CHC model: for example, crystallized intelligence (Gc), fluid reasoning (Gf), visual processing (Gv), quantitative ability (Gq), and long-term storage and retrieval (Glr). At most, the four-subtest WPPSI-III covers two broad abilities. Specifically, the VIQ subtests (Information and Receptive Vocabulary) measure Gc, and the PIQ subtests (Block Design and Object Assembly) primarily measure Gv (visual processing).

The test does appear to measure a broad range of abilities in the older age band, particularly when the PSQ and GLC subtests are also administered. The addition of Gf measures in the older children is also a definite asset to the test. However, it is important to note that the two Gf measures (Matrix Reasoning and Picture Concepts) behave somewhat differently than the other PIQ subtests in factor-analytic studies, and their correlations with other PIQ subtests are not always large. They also are minimally related to achievement, which has implications for using these subtests when calculating ability-achievement discrepancies. It is likely that these measures tap a somewhat different set of abilities than the other PIQ subtests, which primarily assess visual processing rather than fluid reasoning. As well, although there is an advantage to administering the optional GLC language subtests because they are conormed with the rest of the battery, clinicians might prefer to administer other, similar language tests that have a more extensive age coverage instead (e.g., PPVT-III). This ensures that changes in performance over time can be more adequately evaluated in children who will require retesting at a later date.

WPPSI-III Versus WPPSI-R

Table 5.8 of the Technical Manual presents expected WPPSI-III composite score ranges for given WPPSI-R scores. However, for children who were administered the WPPSI-R previously, caution should be used in interpreting apparent changes, particularly at the subtest level. Although composite scores may not differ greatly between versions, some subtests were not highly correlated between versions and they assess constructs (e.g., VIQ) in different ways. Given the major content and structural changes to the WPPSI-III, including the use of an up-to-date normative sample and the known limitations of its predecessor, further use of the WPPSI-R for clinical or research purposes is not recommended.

Ceilings and Floors

Most subtests provide a range of scaled scores from 1 to 19 (Sattler & Dumont, 2004). However, some subtests do have floor effects. For example, on Symbol Search, a 4-year-old obtaining a score of 0 would be assigned a scaled score of 6. Floor effects are also apparent for Similarities in this age group. Object Assembly also has a mild ceiling effect in the oldest age band, where a 7-year-old's maximum possible score is 14.

Despite many of its strengths, Sattler and Dumont (2004) conclude that the test is not adequately sensitive to very low intellectual functioning. For example, the lowest possible IQ for a 2½- year-old, if the procedure for calculating IQs of low functioning children is followed (i.e., an IQ cannot be derived using only raw scores of 0), is 52. For the older age band, the lowest possible IQ is 50. Thus, the test will be inappropriate for estimating IQ in children whose levels fall three or more standard deviations below the normative mean. If within the age range, it may therefore be better to administer another measure with lower floors in children suspected of significant intellectual delays (i.e., BSID-II).

Subtest Substitution

The issue of substituting subtests for core subtests in deriving the FSIQ also deserves more study. Although substitutions are discouraged generally, it is an allowable practice if the clinician feels there is sufficient reason to do so. However, this complicates interpretation of IQs that are based on substitutions. For instance, in young children who are given the standard four-subtest IQ, if a supplemental test is used to obtain the VIQ when deriving a FSIQ, fully 25% of the test content will differ from that of children who were administered the standard core subtests. In older children, where two of seven subtests can be substituted, this means that almost 30% of content could potentially differ. Given that correlations between substituted and standard core subtests are only moderate in some cases (e.g., PIQ subtests), the FSIQ could differ substantially depending on the subtests selected for substitution. It is also important to note that in neuropsychological populations, motor and language impairments might differentially affect certain subtests and yield fairly discrepant results, depending on which subtests were used in substitutions.

In addition, the Administration and Scoring Manual states that supplemental subtests should be substituted for core subtests in the case of retests. However, there is no information on how subtest substitutions might affect practice effects or test-retest reliabilities of composite scores, as stability information is only provided in the Technical Manual for children who received identical measures at both evaluations. Given the potential complication in interpreting results when a child was given a standard IQ at one time and a substituted IQ in a subsequent testing, it is recommended that substitutions not be used unless absolutely necessary, particularly in the case of substitutions involving PIQ subtests. Substitutions should be clearly indicated in the assessment report to inform clinicians who might see the child later on for reevaluation.

Test Selection and Age

The WPPSI-III overlaps with the BSID-II at the lower age range (2½–3½) and with the WISC-IV at the upper age range (6–7 years). The manual states that younger children suspected of intellectual delay should therefore be administered the BSID-II, while older children suspected of delay should be administered the WPPSI-III. However, excluding cases with moderate to severe intellectual impairments, when monitoring of cognitive functioning is needed over time in older children who are approaching the age limit of the WPPSI-III, it may be best to simply administer the WISC-IV to avoid having to interpret retesting results that involve two different measures.

REFERENCES

Braden, J. P. (2003). Accommodating clients with disabilities on the WAIS-III and WMS-III. In D. S. Tulsky, D. H. Saklofske, G. J. Chelune, R. K. Heaton, R. Ivnik, R. Bornstein, A. Prifitera, & M. F. Ledbetter (Eds.), *Clinical interpretation of the WAIS-III and WMS-III* (pp. 451–486). New York: Academic Press.

Flanagan, D. P., McGrew, K. S., & Ortiz, S. O. (2000). *The Wechsler intelligence scales and Gf-Gc theory: A contemporary approach to interpretation.* Boston: Allyn & Bacon.

Flanagan, D. P., & Ortiz, S. O. (2001). *Essentials of cross-battery assessment.* New York: John Wiley & Sons.

Hamilton, W., & Burns, T. G. (2003). Review of the Wechsler Preschool and Primary Scale of Intelligence (3rd ed.). *Applied Neuropsychology, 10*(3), 182–190.

Kaufman, A. S. (1994). *Intelligent testing with the WISC-III.* New York: John Wiley & Sons, Inc.

Lichtenberger, E. O., & Kaufman, A. S. (2004). *Essentials of WPPSI-III assessment.* New York: John Wiley & Sons.

Sattler, J. M. (2001). *Assessment of children: Cognitive applications* (4th ed.). San Diego: Jerome M. Sattler, Publisher, Inc.

Sattler, J. M., & Dumont, R. (2004). *Assessment of children: WISC-IV and WPPSI-III supplement.* San Diego: Jerome M. Sattler, Publisher, Inc.

Wechsler, D. (1967). *Wechsler Preschool and Primary Scale of Intelligence.* San Antonio, TX: The Psychological Corporation.

Wechsler, D. (1989). *Wechsler Preschool and Primary Scale of Intelligence—Revised.* San Antonio, TX: The Psychological Corporation.

Wechsler, D. (2002a). *WPPSI-III administration and scoring manual.* San Antonio, TX: The Psychological Corporation.

Wechsler, D. (2002b). *WPPSI-III technical and interpretive manual.* San Antonio, TX: The Psychological Corporation.

Wechsler, D. (2003). *WISC-IV technical and interpretive manual.* San Antonio, TX: The Psychological Corporation.

Wechsler, D. (2004). *Wechsler Preschool and Primary Scale of Intelligence—Third Edition: Canadian manual.* Toronto, Ontario: Harcourt Assessment.

Wechsler Test of Adult Reading (WTAR)

PURPOSE

The WTAR was developed to help clinicians assess premorbid functioning in adults.

SOURCE

The WTAR (Manual, Word Card, 25 Record Forms, and audiotape) can be purchased from Harcourt Assessment, Inc., 19500 Bulverde Road, San Antonio, TX 78259 (www.harcourtassessment.com) at a cost of $115 US.

AGE RANGE

The test can be used with individuals aged 16 to 89 years.

DESCRIPTION

The WTAR (The Psychological Corporation, 2001) is similar to the NART (NAART) in that it requires reading of irregularly spelled words (e.g., *cough*). Use of irregular words minimizes the assessment of the person's current ability to apply standard pronunciation rules and maximizes the assessment of the individual's prior learning of the word. The utility of the method relies on (a) the relatively strong correlation between reading ability and intellectual functioning in normal people and (b) the fact that reading recognition is relatively resistant to the cognitive declines associated with normal aging and brain insult. As a consequence, word reading tends to result in a fairly reasonable estimate of premorbid ability.

The 50-item WTAR was developed for use in the United States and the United Kingdom. It has the advantage over other similar reading tests (e.g., NART) in that it was co-normed with the WAIS-III (Wechsler, 1997a) and the WMS-III (Wechsler, 1997b) in both these countries. This co-norming allows for direct comparison between predicted and actual functioning with regard to general intellectual status and memory. Further, the norms cover a wide age range, from adolescence to late adulthood (16–89 years). It is important to note that the WTAR is not appropriate for the assessment of developmental disorders. Rather, the purpose is the estimation of premorbid abilities, that is, abilities that presumably attained an adult-like status prior to the insult.

The test manual provides tables for predicting WAIS-III (VIQ, PIQ, FSIQ, and VCI) and WTAR scores from the examinee's demographic characteristics (age, gender, education, ethnicity). Such information is useful in determining whether the current performance has been compromised and also allows the clinician to determine which method (e.g., reading and/or demographics) is most appropriate for evaluating an individual client. Tables for converting the WTAR score, and WTAR plus demographic information, to predicted WAIS-III (VIQ, PIQ, FSIQ, VCI, POI, WMI, and PSI) and WMS-III (Immediate Memory, General Memory, Working Memory) scores are also provided. Unless WTAR performance is severely compromised as determined by a comparison of predicted and actual scores, the preferred methodology is the combined WTAR-demographics prediction of functioning.

Statistically significant differences between WTAR-predicted and actual WAIS-III and WMS-III scores and between WTAR-demographics-predicted and actual WAIS-III and WMS-III scores are provided by age group separately for the U.S. and U.K. samples. The frequency of observed differences between predicted and actual WAIS-III and WMS-III scores is provided for all prediction methodologies (demographics only, WTAR only, and combined WTAR-demographics) separately for the U.S. and U.K. samples.

ADMINISTRATION

See *Source.* Briefly, the examiner presents the word card and asks the patient to pronounce each word. The criterion for discontinuation is 12 consecutive scores of 0.

ADMINISTRATION TIME

The approximate time required is 10 minutes.

SCORING

The examinee is required to give only one pronunciation of a word. Acceptable pronunciations are provided on the record form and pronunciation tape. The maximum raw score is 50.

Scoring would be facilitated by the provision of a computer-scoring system. The current method, in which the examiner must refer to many tables in the manual, is rather cumbersome and prone to error. Briefly, the individual's age is needed to locate the correct norms table. The WTAR raw score is then converted to a standard score (Appendix A), and the demographics-predicted WTAR score (Appendix B) is also entered. The predicted WTAR score is subtracted from the actual score and the magnitude of the difference score is evaluated with reference to the cumulative percentages. Assuming the current WTAR score is not unusually below expected levels (20 points or more), tables in the manual allow WAIS-III/WMS-III scores to be predicted by WTAR performance only (Appendix D) and by a combination of WTAR performance and demographics (Appendices E, F, and G). Additional tables allow the examiner to evaluate the significance and rarity of the discrepancy between predicted and obtained values (Appendices H, I, J). Tables also are provided in the manual that allow the examiner to determine whether test-retest differences are significant and rare (Appendix H). Tables are also provided in the WTAR Manual to derive demographic-predicted WAIS-III scores (Appendix C).

DEMOGRAPHIC EFFECTS

Age

For the U.S. standardization sample, the effect of age on performance was relatively small. The distribution of mean scores revealed a curvilinear pattern with gradual performance increases from the 16-to-17-year age group to the 45-to-54-year age group (The Psychological Corporation, 2001). Performance gradually declined from the 45-to-54-year age group to the oldest group (80–89). A similar pattern of age effects was also observed for the U.K. sample.

Gender

Gender has little effect on WTAR scores (The Psychological Corporation, 2001).

Education

Education is moderately correlated with WTAR scores (The Psychological Corporation, 2001).

Ethnicity/Geographic Region

Race/ethnicity is significantly associated with WTAR performance (The Psychological Corporation, 2001). Also of note, the U.K. sample outperformed the U.S. sample across education levels and particularly with increasing age. Accordingly, norms are provided separately for U.S.- and U.K.-based samples.

NORMATIVE DATA AND PREDICTION OF WAIS-III/WMS-III SCORES

Standardization Sample

The WTAR was administered concurrently with the WAIS-III and WMS-III during standardization to 1134 participants in the United States and 331 participants in the United Kingdom, aged 16 to 89 years (note that in the United Kingdom the sample was aged 16–80 years while the prediction equations are for individuals aged 20–89 years). The characteristics of the samples are shown in Table 6–164.

Two sets of normative scores are presented for the WTAR. The age-adjusted scores are based on the score distributions for a particular age group (e.g., in the United States: 16–17, 18–19, 20–24). They are used to predict WAIS-III and WMS-III scores as those tests use age-adjusted norms for IQ and index score derivation. An additional set of normative scores, based on a reference group aged 20 to 34 years, is also provided but should not be used to predict WAIS-III or WMS-III scores.

While demographic variables (age, education, gender, ethnicity) showed little association with WMS-III performance, associations emerged with WAIS-III performance in some race/ethnic and gender groups in the United States. Accordingly, separate prediction equations were developed for white, African American, and Hispanic males and females (except in the 16–19-years age range for Hispanics where demographic data did not predict WAIS-III/WMS-III performance). The U.K. sample was not sufficiently diverse in terms of race/ethnicity, and prediction equations in this sample were developed taking into account only gender and educational level.

The frequency of differences between predicted and actual WAIS-III/WMS-III scores is presented as collapsed, cumulative percentage distributions. Because the accuracy of prediction fluctuates at the upper and lower ends of the IQ distribution, frequencies of differences are also provided separately for the U.S. and U.K. samples according to ranges of intellectual functioning based on FSIQ scores.

RELIABILITY

Internal Consistency

According to the test manual, the WTAR shows excellent internal consistency for the various age groups, with coefficients ranging from .90 to .97 for the U.S. standardization sample and from .87 to .95 for the U.K. sample. Standard errors of measurement derived from the internal consistency coefficient are about four points.

Test-Retest Reliability and Practice Effects

Performance tends to be fairly stable over time. According to the test manual, 319 participants completed the test on two separate occasions, spaced 2 to 12 weeks apart with an average

Table 6-164 Characteristics of the WTAR Normative Sample

Number	
U. S.	1,134
U. K.	331
Age	16–89 years[a]
Geographic location	U.S.: From geographic regions in proportions consistent with U.S. Census data
Sample type	In both the United States and the United Kingdom, the WTAR was normed on nationally representative samples, stratified like the WAIS-III
Education	
U. S.	≤ 8, 9–11, 12, 13–15, ≥ 16 years and consistent with U.S. Census proportions; for examinees aged 16–19 years, parent education was used
U. K.	Stratified according to six education levels: None, Other, GSCE, A-Level, Diploma, Degree
Gender	
U. S.	An equal number of males and females in each age group from ages 16–64; the older age groups included more women than men, in proportions consistent with 1995 U.S. Census data
U. K.	More females than males
Race/ethnicity	
U. S.	The proportions of whites, African Americans, Hispanics, and other racial/ethnic groups were based on racial/ethnic proportions within each age band according to 1995 U.S. Census data
U. K.	Sample is predominantly Caucasian
Screening	Screened via self-report for sensory, substance abuse, medical, psychiatric, or motor condition that could potentially affect performance

[a]U.S.: Broken down into 13 age groups (16–17, 18–19, 20–24, 25–29, 30–34, 35–44, 45–54, 55–64, 65–69, 70–74, 75–79, 80–84, and 85–89 years); 90 subjects were included in each age group except the two oldest groups. The 80–84 age group and the 85–89 age group each consisted of 72 participants. U.K.: Broken down into four age bands: 16–24 ($N = 88$), 25–44 ($N = 97$), 45–64, ($N = 82$), and 65–80 ($N = 64$).

interval of about 35 days. Test-retest correlations were very good (>.90) and practice effects were minimal. Across all age groups in the test-retest sample, the average difference between time 1 and time 2 scores was −0.8, with a standard deviation of 5.4.

VALIDITY

Correlations With Measures of Reading

The WTAR shows high correlations with other measures of reading (e.g, AMNART, $r = .90$; WRATR, $r = .73$; WTAR, 2001). Mean performances were generally consistent across tasks with the exception of relatively high AMNART scores in comparison with WTAR scores.

Correlations to Measures of Intelligence and Memory

Like the NART (NAART), WTAR scores correlate highly with WAIS-III VIQ ($r = .75$), VC ($r = .74$), and FSIQ ($r = .73$) and only moderately well with other Wechsler intelligence scores (WMI, $r = .62$; PIQ, $r = .59$; POI, $r = .56$; PSI, $r = .47$) in the U.S. standardization sample. Similar correlations were found for the U.K. sample. Correlations were weaker in clinical samples (.34–.66), perhaps because WAIS-III scores are more affected by CNS disease than are WTAR scores.

In the standardization samples, moderate correlations emerged between WTAR and WMS-III memory performance (U.S. sample: Working Memory, $r = .51$; General Memory, $r = .49$; Immediate Memory, $r = .47$). Again in a clinical sample, correlations were smaller (.32–.33).

With regard to accuracy of classification based on the WTAR alone, in about 70.4% of the cases, predicted FSIQ was within ±10 points (38.7% were within ±5 points); however, estimates for WMS-III memory performance were poor (about 55% within ±10 points). In short, WTAR performance appears to be a reasonable predictor of premorbid intellectual functioning (particularly verbal IQ) but should only be considered a modest predictor of premorbid memory ability.

Correlations With Language Measures

While the WTAR can be used to predict intellectual and, to a lesser extent, memory functioning, its utility in other cognitive domains appears more limited. According to the manual, the WTAR had low to moderate correlations with measures of language production (BNT, $r = .29$; COWAT, $r = .37$) and comprehension (Token Test, $r = .51$) at least in neurologically impaired samples.

Prediction of Intellectual and Memory Functioning

The WTAR displays better prediction of WAIS-III/WMS-III scores than demographic variables, with a larger range of scores and smaller standard errors of prediction (The Psychological Corporation, 2001). For example, for a Caucasian male aged 20 to 89 years living in the United States, the predicted FSIQ can range from 90 to 118 depending upon the educational achievement. WTAR-predicted FSIQ scores can range from 64 to 124.

The addition of demographic data to WTAR performance in the regression equations resulted in a modest increase of 4% to 7% over WTAR performance alone in the prediction of intellectual and memory functioning. The most accurate assessment of premorbid abilities is based on WAIS-III FSIQ and VIQ scores predicted with the combined WTAR-demographics methodology. These scores have the smallest prediction error, although they are still quite large. For example, for an 85-year-old male patient with 12 years of education, a WTAR standard score of 100 yields a predicted VIQ of 103. The 95% prediction interval indicates that the individual's actual score likely falls between 86 and 120 (i.e., 103 ± 17). Note, too, that the lowest prediction accuracy occurs for the WMS-III indices.

It is also important to bear in mind that use of regression techniques has limitations, including regression to the mean and limited range of scores. Accordingly, for patients with high premorbid functioning, WTAR-predicted scores will underestimate the amount of cognitive deterioration that has occurred. For people at the lower end of the distribution, the equation overpredicts ability and may suggest cognitive deterioration when, in reality, it has not occurred. The differences between predicted and actual scores vary across IQ levels, and this factor also must be considered in the evaluation of difference scores. The user is referred to tables in Appendix J of the manual, which provide cumulative percentages of differences by IQ ranges.

Clinical Findings

WTAR performance appears relatively resistant to cerebral damage; however, it is not insensitive to such impairment. WTAR performance was evaluated in patients with AD (mild and moderate), PD, Huntington's disease, Korsakoff's syndrome, traumatic brain injury, and neuropsychiatric disorders, as well as matched groups of controls (The Psychological Corporation, 2001). WTAR performance was not significantly below that of controls, except in the group with moderate AD. Further, in patients with AD, WTAR performance was related to overall intellectual impairment as determined by the Mattis DRS. That is, the more cognitively impaired performed more poorly on the WTAR, although even these individuals generally functioned in the average range on the WTAR. Finally, across diagnostic groups, WTAR scores "held" better than VIQ scores.

The authors provide some evidence indicating that differences between predicted and obtained measures may be helpful in discriminating clinical groups from one another (The Psychological Corporation, 2001). In general, differentiation tended to be better for dementia (e.g., AD, Huntington's disease, Parkinson's disease) than for nondementia (e.g., TBI, chronic alcoholism, schizophrenia) disorders. However, further research is needed with larger samples to verify these findings and determine whether such discrepancy analysis

yields useful diagnostic information beyond that provided by examination of obtained WAIS-III/WMS-III test scores alone.

The test should not be used to predict premorbid ability in those with preexisting learning disorders. The authors report that reading-disabled individuals performed more poorly than did controls on the WTAR and that for this clinical group, WTAR scores were significantly below most WAIS-III measures.

COMMENT

The WTAR appears to provide a reasonable estimate of intellectual functioning (particularly verbal ability); however, its ability to predict other domains of functioning (including memory) appears limited. Nonetheless, it displays a better prediction of WAIS-III and WMS-III scores than demographic variables (See Chapter 6, *General Cognitive Functioning, Neuropsychological Batteries, and Assessment of Premorbid Intelligence*).

The WTAR may prove particularly valuable in detecting cognitive decline since recent research suggests that reliance only on years of schooling to predict premorbid status may not be sufficient in accounting for the quality of the educational experience (Manly et al., 2002). However, the task should not be used to diagnose learning disorders, nor should it be employed in those with a preexisting learning disorder, in those who suffer language and perceptual disorders (e.g., aphasia and alexia), or in those who have not had lengthy exposure to English reading material. Like other performance-based methods (e.g., NART, WRAT-3), it is also not impervious to the effects of cerebral dysfunction (e.g., moderate dementia).

Although the provision of demographic variables in addition to WTAR scores provides only a modest improvement in prediction of performance in healthy people, the use of demographic variables is recommended to buffer the effects of clinical conditions with regard to prediction of premorbid status. If WTAR performance is severely compromised as determined by a comparison of actual and predicted scores, then the examiner should use demographics-predicted scores only. Note, however, that memory scores are poorly predicted by demographic data alone and therefore should not be used to predict premorbid memory functioning. In addition, prediction of IQ by WTAR demographics alone is subject to severe restriction of range, suggesting that this technique is appropriate for use with individuals whose premorbid IQ is likely to have been within the average range (Langeluddecke & Lucas, 2004; The Psychological Corporation, 2001). It is not suitable for use with exceptional individuals at either end of the ability spectrum.

The authors suggest that the WTAR-demographics methodology is useful in detecting impairment and may prove effective in classifying and discriminating among clinical disorders. The tool, however, is relatively new and in need of further study (e.g., large-scale studies of diverse patient samples).

REFERENCES

Langeluddecke, P. M., & Lucas, S. K. (2004). Evaluation of two methods for estimating premorbid intelligence on the WAIS-III in a clinical sample. *The Clinical Neuropsychologist, 18,* 423–432.

Manly, J. J., Jacobs, D. M., Touradji, P., Small, S. A., & Stern, Y. (2002). Reading level attenuates differences in neuropsychological test performance between African American and White elders. *Journal of the International Neuropsychological Society, 8,* 341–348.

The Psychological Corporation (2001). *Wechsler Test of Adult Reading.* San Antonio, TX: Harcourt Assessment.

Wechsler, D. (1997a). *Wechsler Adult Intelligence Scale—Third Edition.* San Antonio, TX: The Psychological Corporation.

Wechsler, D. (1997b). *Wechsler Memory Scale—Third Edition.* San Antonio, TX: The Psychological Corporation.

Woodcock-Johnson III Tests of Cognitive Abilities (WJ III COG)

PURPOSE

The Woodcock-Johnson III Tests of Cognitive Abilities (WJ III COG) are designed to assess cognitive processes in children and adults.

SOURCE

The WJ III COG (Woodcock et al., 2001b) can be ordered from Riverside Publishing Company (www.riverpub.com). The complete test kit price is $619 US. Computer scoring is included in the test kit (WJ III Compuscore and Profiles Program). Additional report-writing software is also available (WJ III Report Writer). Several training options for learning WJ III administration and scoring are available through the web site, including self-study materials (training manuals, CD-ROMs, and training videos), group training sessions, and workshops offered throughout the United States and Canada. An online Resource Center also provides regular updates on the WJ III in the form of newsletters and research bulletins; these can be downloaded in Adobe format (www.riverpub.com/products/clinical/wj3).

AGE RANGE

The age range is from 2 to 90+ years.

DESCRIPTION

Background

The WJ III, a theory-based measure of intelligence, is the third revision of the original Woodcock-Johnson Psycho-Educational Battery first published in 1977 (Woodcock & Johnson, 1977). The original WJ was not theory-based (Schrank et al., 2002). The WJ-R (Woodcock & Johnson, 1989a, 1989b) was based on *Gf-Gc* theory, whereas the Cattell-Horn-Carroll (CHC) theory of intelligence provided the "blueprint" for the WJ-III (McGrew & Woodcock, 2001; see Figure 6–27). Cattell-Horn-Carroll theory postulates that cognitive abilities can be divided into three main levels: general intellectual ability (Stratum III level), CHC factors representing broad cognitive subdomains (Stratum II level), and specific abilities representing narrow cognitive subdomains (Stratum I level; see chapter introduction for a description of CHC theory). The WJ III consists of two components: the WJ III COG and the WJ III ACH (Woodcock et al., 2001a; see review of the *WJ III ACH* in this volume).

Test Structure and Theoretical Underpinnings

The structure of the WJ III COG is closely modeled after CHC theory. It has a three-level hierarchical system consisting of (1) psychometric *g* (i.e., the General Intellectual Ability [GIA] score, (2) Stratum II level abilities (represented by seven Factors), and (3) Stratum I abilities (represented by 20 subtests measuring narrow abilities). The test provides Standard, Extended, and Brief batteries (based on 7, 14, and 3 subtests, respectively; see Table 6–165). In addition, it yields five Clinical Clusters that measure abilities important for clinical evaluation, including Executive Processes, Working Memory, and Broad Attention (see Table 6–166). Scores can be derived at several levels of interpretation (i.e., overall performance, factor scores, clinical cluster scores, and subtest scores). Most tasks can be given to all ages, except for a few exceptions in the youngest age bands (see Table 6–167 for a list of subtests for preschoolers).

The WJ III differs from other tests of intelligence in that its full-scale score, the GIA, is not the arithmetic mean of all the contributing subcomposites or subtests but is weighted to provide the best estimate of *g* (see *Scoring* for details). However, unlike other tests that are designed primarily as measures of *g*, the WJ III is conceptualized as a strong measure of broad factors/Stratum II abilities (Schrank et al., 2002). Subtests comprising each CHC factor were therefore chosen not because they measured a similar ability but because they were "qualitatively different" from each other, while still measuring the broader CHC factor (McGrew & Woodcock, 2001). For example, Sound Blending and Auditory Attention, both Stratum I subtests, load together on the broad ability or factor of Auditory Processing (a Stratum II level of analysis). This differs from other intelligence tests where subtests may (a) measure a common factor rather than individual abilities (e.g., CAS) or (b) provide a mix of different CHC factors within each composite (e.g., older Wechsler tests). The multifaceted nature of WJ III factors is intended to increase validity and generalizability of scores (Schrank

Figure 6–27 Relationship of the WJ III to CHC Theory. *Source:* Reprinted with permission from McGrew & Woodcock, 2001.

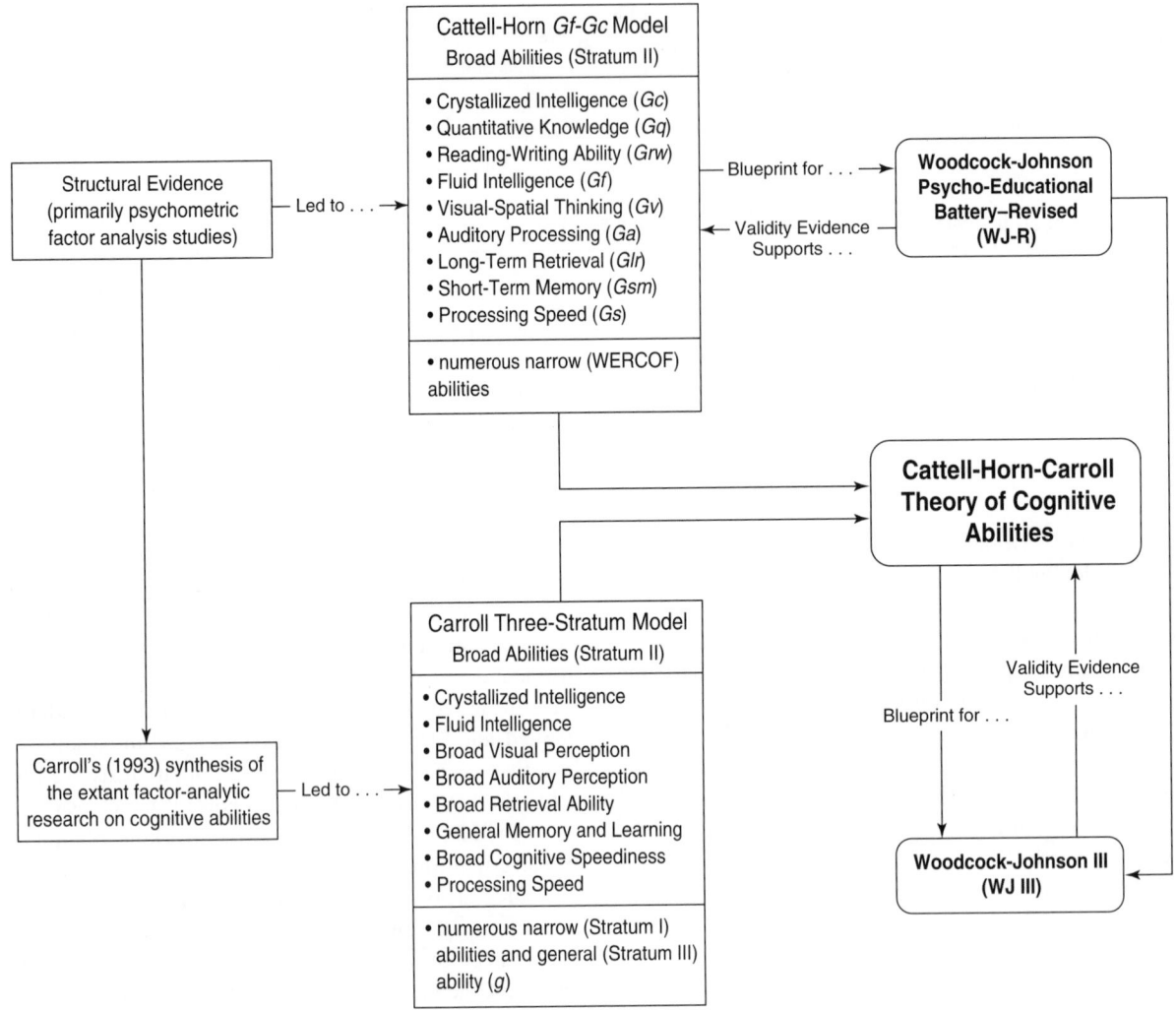

Table 6–165 WJ III COG Categories and Factors Measured by Each Subtest

Category	CHC Factors	Standard Battery Subtests	Extended Battery Subtests
Verbal Ability	*Comprehension-Knowledge (Gc)*	Verbal Comprehension*	General Information
Thinking Ability	*Long-Term Retrieval (Glr)*	Visual-Auditory Learning	Retrieval Fluency
	Visual-Spatial Thinking (Gv)	Spatial Relations	Picture Recognition
	Auditory Processing (Ga)	Sound Blending	Auditory Attention
	Fluid Reasoning (Gf)	Concept Formation*	Analysis-Synthesis
Cognitive Efficiency	*Processing Speed (Gs)*	Visual Matching*	Decision Speed
	Short-Term Memory (Gsm)	Number Reversed	Memory for Words
Supplemental Tests[a]		Auditory Working Memory	Rapid Picture Naming
			Planning
			Pair Cancellation

Note: Factor scores are based on administration of both the Standard and Extended subtest corresponding to that factor. Brief Intellectual Assessment (BIA) subtests are denoted by an asterisk.

[a]Supplemental Tests are used to assess specific Clinical Clusters (see Table 6–166).

Table 6–166 WJ III Clinical Clusters (Obtained by Combining Standard/Extended Subtests and Supplemental Subtests)

Clinical Cluster	WJ III Subtest
Phonemic Awareness	Sound Blending
	Incomplete Words
Working Memory	Numbers Reversed
	Auditory Working Memory
Broad Attention	Number Reversed
	Auditory Working Memory
	Auditory Attention
	Pair Cancellation
Cognitive Fluency	Retrieval Fluency
	Decision Speed
	Rapid Picture Naming
Executive Processes	Concept Formation
	Planning
	Pair Cancellation
Delayed Recall	Visual-Auditory Learning Delayed[a]
Knowledge	General Information[b]

Note: Tests in italics are from the Extended Battery.
[a]Includes Story Recall Delayed from the WJ III Tests of Achievement.
[b]Includes Academic Knowledge from the WJ III Tests of Achievement.

et al., 2002) and to reduce the risk inherent to generalizing from a single narrow aspect of ability to a multifaceted ability (McGrew & Woodcock, 2001). Table 6–168 describes the WJ III COG subtests.

Like other intelligence tests, the WJ III is intended to be used to (a) diagnose learning disabilities, (b) determine discrepancies, (c) plan educational programs, and (d) assess change over time. The Examiner's Manual states that the WJ III can be used in neuropsychological settings to "substantiate the type and extent of a specific impairment in functioning" (p. 6). Its predecessor, the WJ-R, can also be used in combination with the Dean-Woodcock Sensory Motor Battery (D-WSMB) to form a comprehensive neuropsychological assessment battery (i.e., the Dean-Woodcock Neuropsycholog-

Table 6–167 WJ III Subtests for Preschoolers

WJ III COG	WJ III ACH
Verbal Comprehension	Letter-Word Identification
Visual/Auditory Learning	Story Recall
Spatial Relations	Understanding Directions
Sound Blending	Passage Comprehension
Concept Formation	Applied Problems
Visual Matching	Word Attack
Memory for Words	Picture Vocabulary
	Oral Comprehension
	Academic Knowledge
	Sound Awareness

Note: COG = Cognitive battery; ACH = Achievement battery.

ical Assessment System; Dean & Woodcock, 1999). A newer edition of the former is anticipated.

The WJ III is designed to be administered following the principle of selective testing (i.e., matching the tests selected to the specific referral question). Thus, test selection may be based on the need for a full-scale score (GIA) screener (Brief Intellectual Assessment or BIA), or on those specific clusters or factors that require evaluation (Schrank et al., 2002).

WJ III Versus WJ-R

Several improvements were made in the revision of the WJ. The WJ-R measured seven broad abilities (Long-Term Retrieval, Short-Term Memory, Processing Speed, Auditory Processing, Visual-Spatial Thinking, Comprehension-Knowledge, Fluid Reasoning), with an additional eighth ability (i.e., Quantitative Ability) measured by its companion scale, the WJ-R Tests of Achievement (Woodcock & Johnson, 1989a). Although it still measures seven broad abilities (factors), the WJ III has been revised to include a number of new subtests and five new interpretive clusters. Oral language tests, originally in the cognitive battery of the WJ-R, have been moved to the Achievement battery in the WJ III. In addition, ability-achievement comparisons using the conormed WJ III ACH have been expanded to include comparisons of oral language and academic performance, among other features. Test materials have also been redesigned (see *Administration*).

ADMINISTRATION TIME

Each subtest takes 5 to 10 minutes to administer. The Standard battery takes 35 to 45 minutes. The Extended battery takes 90 minutes to almost 2 hours. The Brief Intellectual Assessment (BIA) takes approximately 15 minutes.

ADMINISTRATION

See manual. Additional administration guidelines are also provided in Schrank et al. (2002), including a checklist of common examiner errors that would be useful as a learning aid.

The WJ III was expressly designed for convenience in test administration. Accordingly, it consists of only two folding easels, with no associated manipulatives. Easel size has also been reduced from the previous edition to further facilitate portability. Test items are colorful and of interest to young test takers. Administration is straightforward, requiring simple entry-level guidelines based on age, and, in general, a six-item basal and ceiling rule. All instructions are presented on the easel on the examiner's side, which eliminates the need for a separate examiner's manual. A cassette tape is provided for standardized administration of auditory subtests. There is only one test form for the WJ III COG battery; only the WJ ACH test has alternate forms (A and B).

Table 6-168 Description of WJ III Cognitive Subtests, Grouped by CHC Factor

Subtests	Description
Comprehension-Knowledge (Gc)	
Verbal Comprehension	This subtest is actually made up of four different tasks, each measuring a different aspect of acquired language. All four tasks are required for the total score: (1) Picture Vocabulary (a simple naming task with picture stimuli); (2) Synonyms (the subject provides a synonym for a word printed on the page); (4) Antonyms (the subject provides antonyms); and (4) Verbal Analogies (the subject must provide a fourth word to complete a three-word analogy). All verbal tests require only a one-word answer.
General Information	This test measures verbal knowledge. The subtest has two parts; first, the subject is asked to describe where one would find common objects (e.g., "Where would you find a ladle?"); then the subject is asked to describe the use of common objects (e.g., "What do people usually do with an escalator?").
Long-Term Retrieval (Glr)	
Visual-Auditory Learning	This subtest measures long-term storage and retrieval. The subject must remember picture-sound associations learned over several trials. The stimuli are rebuses (pictorial representations of words), which are eventually arranged in sentence-like sequences and "read" by the subject.
Retrieval Fluency	This is a semantic fluency test. The subject must provide, within a one-minute time interval, as many exemplars from a given category as possible. Categories include foods, first names of people, and animals.
Visual-Spatial Thinking (Gv)	
Spatial Relations	This measures visual-spatial thinking. The subject must identify, among a set of distracters, the pieces that make up an abstract stimulus figure. This subtest can be thought of as a motor-free visual-spatial task that would be useful to assess visual-spatial skills in those with motor impairments.
Picture Recognition	This is a visual memory task. The subject is shown a visual stimulus for 5 seconds (line drawings of objects); recall is tested by a recognition format (i.e., the subject must identify the remembered target among similar distracters). The use of similar objects as distracters eliminates the use of verbal mediation as a recall strategy (e.g., the subject must identify one particular window among several different windows).
Auditory Processing (Ga)	
Sound Blending	This is an auditory processing subtest that measures phonemic awareness. The subject is required to synthesize language sounds into meaningful wholes (i.e., separate syllables/phonemes must be blended to form a word).
Auditory Attention	This is a test of selective attention in the auditory modality. It measures the ability to overcome auditory distracters when processing auditory language, and as such, measures aspects of speech-sound discrimination. The subject listens to words while background noise increases, and must identify the target word on a page on which are also presented distracter items.
Fluid Reasoning (Gf)	
Concept Formation	This measures fluid reasoning, including categorical reasoning and inductive logic, as well as the executive function of set shifting. However, unlike tests such as the Category test, there is no learning of a specific rule over several trials based on examiner feedback. Each item demonstrates a particular rule that must be deduced from the stimuli. A new rule must be learned for each item.
Analysis-Synthesis	This is a test of general sequential (deductive) reasoning. The subject is given basic rules and instructions, and then must solve a series of formula-like problems consisting of colored boxes. The examinee uses examiner feedback to self-correct.
Processing Speed (Gs)	
Visual Matching	In this processing speed test presented in standard cancellation task format, the subject is presented with rows of numbers in which matching numbers must be crossed out, under timed conditions. The total score is the number correct.

(continued)

Table 6–168 Description of WJ III Cognitive Subtests, Grouped by CHC Factor (*continued*)

Subtests	Description
Decision Speed	This test of processing speed follows a cancellation task paradigm, but uses small line drawings of common objects instead of symbols or letters. The subject must locate two items that are similar conceptually, among distracters, line by line, under time constraints (e.g., shoe and boot). The total score is the number correct.
Short-Term Memory (Gsm)	
Numbers Reversed	This is a working memory test and a test of attentional capacity in the auditory modality. It employs the standard digits-backward paradigm.
Memory for Words	This is similar to a Digit Span task except that items are unrelated words instead of digits (e.g., "had-know-be-other"). Only the earliest items contain imaginable words, which makes the task highly dependent on auditory working memory. There is no backward condition.
Supplemental Subtests[a]	
Incomplete Words	This is a test of phonemic awareness and phonetic coding (i.e., auditory analysis and auditory closure). The subject hears words with one or more phonemes missing and must identify the word.
Auditory Working Memory	This is a working memory test and a test of divided attention in the auditory modality. The subject hears a series of digits and words (e.g., "cat, 2, dog, mouse, 7, 1") and must reorder the series into a two-part sequence starting with words and then digits.
Visual-Auditory-Learning Delayed	A long-term memory task, this is the delayed recall trial of the Visual-Auditory Learning task; recall of rebuses is tested 30 minutes to 8 days after presentation.
Rapid Picture Naming	This test measures processing speed and cognitive fluency in the verbal domain. The subject must name, as rapidly as possible, pictures of simple, common objects (e.g., carrot, shoe, duck). There is a two-minute time limit.
Planning	This is a test of executive functioning involving visual scanning. The subject must solve visual puzzles that involve tracing a complex pattern without removing the pencil from the paper or retracing lines. The functions required are somewhat like those required of maze-tracing tasks.
Pair Cancellation	This test is a test of sustained attention that is also purported to measure executive functioning and processing speed. This is a cancellation task that incorporates elements of CPT/go-no-go paradigms, and as such, requires sustained attention and response inhibition. The subject is presented with lines made up of multiple exemplars of three small drawings of a cup, a ball, and a dog, which are arranged in random order. The subject must circle the ball and the dog, but only if they are presented next to each other in a specific order, under time constraints. The total score is the number of correct pairs circled.

[a]Supplemental subtests, in conjunction with subtests from the Standard and Expanded batteries, are used to calculate standard scores for the five Clinical Clusters (see Table 6–166).

The test is best administered with the examiner sitting diagonally across from the subject, at one corner of the testing table. It is important to administer auditory subtests using a tape recorder and headphones (i.e., Sound Blending, Numbers Reversed, Incomplete Words, Auditory Working Memory, Auditory Attention, Memory for Words). Subtests are designed to be administered in the order provided, though flexibility is also permitted at the examiner's discretion.

Unlike some other intelligence tests, responses given in another language are credited on specific verbal subtests when examinees are English-dominant bilingual (Schrank et al., 2002). This includes Verbal Comprehension, General Information, Retrieval Fluency, and Rapid Picture Naming.

A Test Session Observation Checklist is provided on the front of the test form to check observations during the evaluation (e.g., level of cooperation, frustration tolerance). Although not intended as an actual rating scale, it was field tested in the normative sample for ease of use.

SCORING

Procedure

See manual. Additional scoring guidelines are provided in Schrank et al. (2002). Hand scoring is not possible with this version of the WJ. Raw scores must be entered into the computer program to obtain norm-based scores. However, examiners can quickly determine age and grade equivalents with the help of a table printed on the test form if immediate information on performance level is needed. The scoring program is easy to use and provides several options for reporting scores, including score tables, score profiles, and short verbal summary. Specific norms can also be chosen (e.g., age versus education).

Main Scores

The test yields several scores, including GIA, based on either the Standard or Extended battery, or on the three-subtest BIA battery (standard score format, with $M = 100$, $SD = 15$). The GIA/BIA score is not automatically computed in the scoring printout; it must be checked as an option in the "Score Report Options" box. As noted before, unlike other measures of intelligence that yield an IQ score that is the arithmetic mean of subtests, the GIA is conceptualized as a "distillate measure of psychometric *g*" (Schrank et al., 2002, p. 78). Each test making up the GIA is differentially weighted depending on age, based on factor-analytic research (see p. 79 in Schrank et al., 2002, for a table of weights by age). The *Gc* (Verbal Comprehension and General Information) and *Gf* tests (Concept Formation and Analysis-Synthesis) are the most heavily weighted as they are most predictive of *g* in factor-analytic research. This is an important point to remember when interpreting GIA scores. Specific *g* weights across age are presented in Appendix C of the Technical Manual.

Standard scores are also provided for each of the seven CHC factors, as well as for five Clinical Clusters (Phonemic Awareness, Working Memory, Broad Attention, Cognitive Fluency, Executive Processes). Two additional Clusters can be obtained by supplementing with specific WJ III ACH subtests (i.e., Delayed Recall Cluster, Knowledge Cluster).

Discrepancy Scores

Discrepancy scores can be calculated in several ways: (a) intraindividual (using both WJ III COG and WJ III ACH factors), (b) intracognitive (WJ III COG factors only), and (c) intra-achievement (WJ III ACH factors only). The scoring program presents all factor scores including their predicted scores based on multiple regression, along with information on whether the discrepancy was significant and/or rare in the normative sample. Specifically, the "Discrepancy *SD*" is a standardized z score indicating the magnitude of the discrepancy compared with the normative sample, while the "Discrepancy Percentile" indicates the percentage of the population with a similar discrepancy. In this way, information on statistical and clinical significance of discrepancies is readily available from the score printout. The magnitude of significance for discrepancies can be adjusted by the user.

Additional Scores

The scoring program also provides several additional scores. The Relative Proficiency Index (RPI) is a measure of the subject's level of proficiency on tasks similar to those that were tested. Schrank et al. (2002) note that this score is similar to visual acuity testing. In their example, 20/40 vision allows a person to see at 20 feet what a normally sighted person sees at 40 feet. Similarly, an RPI of 50/90 means that the subject can perform the task at a level of 50% proficiency when others in his or her age group are performing the task with 90% proficiency. The W score is a transformation of the Rasch ability scale that provides an equal-interval scale. Percentiles, standard scores, grade equivalents, age equivalents, z scores, T scores, stanine, normal curve equivalent, and CALP levels can also be derived using the scoring program (see Technical Manual for more information).

DEMOGRAPHIC EFFECTS

Age

WJ III scores show specific age-related changes that are fully described in the Technical Manual. Examples are shown graphically in Chapter 2 (Figure 2–1, as well as in Figure 6–28).

Gender and Ethnicity

Detailed analysis of the WJ III with regard to race, ethnicity, and gender is reviewed in the Technical Manual, indicating that there are no gender differences, and that it is overall a fair test (McGrew & Woodcock, 2001). To our knowledge, there are no independent studies on the use of the test in minorities or in countries other than the United States, although preliminary results indicate that Canadian and American children perform similarly on the test (L. Ford, personal communication, June 2005).

Education

As is the case for almost all IQ tests, persons who have more years of formal education tend to obtain higher scores; as a

Figure 6–28 Growth curves for the WJ III COG. *Source:* Reprinted with permission from McGrew & Woodcock, 2001.

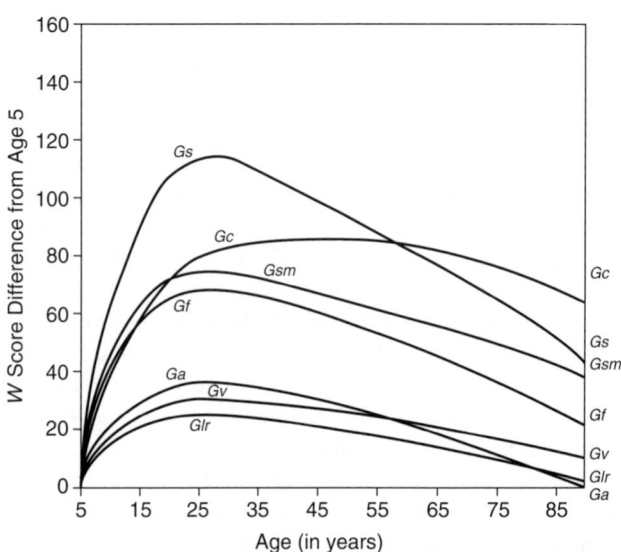

result, the WJ III provides norms spanning the range of education in adults. To our knowledge, there are no independent studies on educational effects apart from the general information presented in the manuals.

NORMATIVE DATA

Standardization Sample

Norms are extensive. Normative data are based on 8818 subjects in over 100 geographic regions in the United States. Individuals were randomly selected within a stratified sampling design that controlled for 10 specific community and individual variables and 13 socioeconomic status variables, and that approximated U.S. 2000 Census composition projections. The sample consisted of 1143 preschool subjects, 4784 kindergarten to twelfth-grade subjects, 1165 college and university subjects, and 1843 adult subjects. Individual subject data were then weighted to obtain a distribution of scores that mirrored the composition of the U.S. population. See Table 6–169 for information on the target percentages for norms composition during the WJ III standardization.

Age norms are provided for one-month intervals from age 24 months to 18 years, 11 months. One-year intervals are provided for ages 19 to 90+. Grade norms are also provided at one-month intervals from K.0 to 18.0. There are also separate norms for college and university students (two- and four-year college norms).

RELIABILITY

Internal Reliability

In most cases, as noted in the test description provided by the publisher, the reliability characteristics of the WJ III meet or exceed basic standards for both individual placement and programming decisions (McGrew & Woodcock, 2001). In the manual, split-half reliabilities were calculated for all the non-speeded subtests, and Rasch analysis procedures were used for calculating reliabilities of speeded subtests and subtests with multiple-point scoring (see Technical Manual for details). These range from .80 to .97. All of the Cluster (factor score) coefficients are high ($r = .81–.98$), and full-scale score reliabilities are very high (i.e., GIA reliabilities for Standard and Extended batteries are .97 and .98, respectively). Subtest score reliabilities are, for the most part, high; median reliabilities for two subtests are in the adequate range (i.e., $r = .76$ for Picture Recognition and $r = .74$ for Planning).

Standard Error of Measurement

SEMs for the Standard Battery GIA are less than three standard score points across all ages; for the BIA, it is less than 3.67. As expected, the SEM is smaller for the Extended Battery GIA, and SEMs for individual subtests are slightly larger. SEMs for clusters and subtests are provided in considerable detail in the

Table 6–169 Target Percentages for the WJ III Cognitive Normative Sample[a]

Sample type	National, stratified, random sample[b]
Number	8818
Age	2 to 90+ years
Community Size	
Central city and urban fringe	64%
Larger community and associated rural area	18%
Smaller community and associated rural area	18%
Geographic location	
Northeast	19%
Midwest	23%
South	36%
West	22%
Education[c]	
<9th grade	9%
< High school	14%
High school	33%
1–3 years of college	24%
Bachelor's degree	14%
Master's degree or higher	7%
Gender	
Males	48%
Females	52%
Race	
White	84%
Black	12%
American Indian	1%
Asian and Pacific Islander	4%
Hispanic origin	
Hispanic	10%
Non-Hispanic	90%
Occupational status	
Employed	64%
Unemployed	4%
Not in Labor Force	32%
Occupation	
Professional/managerial	29%
Technical/sales/administrative	30%
Service	14%
Farming/forestry/fishing	3%
Precision product/craft/repair	11%
Operative/fabricator/laborer	14%
Screening[d]	

Note: The grade-school sample was also stratified according to type of school (i.e., public, private, or home); the college/university sample was also stratified according to type of school (public or private) and college (two-year or four-year).
[a]These values represent the target percentages for each category, based on U.S. Census data; actual values differ because of lower numbers in some categories, along with deliberate oversampling in others. Final percentages in the standardization sample were therefore adjusted by case weighting. Details of the procedure are presented in McGrew and Woodcock, 2001, along with the actual percents attained and specific case weights. [b]Based on 2000 U.S. Census data, and collected between 1996 and 1999. [c]For the grade-school sample, data were stratified according to maternal and paternal education. [d]Subjects with less than one year experience in regular English-speaking classes were excluded from the school-age sample.

Source: Adapted from McGrew & Woodcock, 2001.

Table 6–170 Test-Retest Reliabilities for WJ III COG Speeded Subtests

Magnitude of Coefficient	Ages 7–11	Ages 14–17	Ages 26–79
Very high (.90+)	—	—	—
High (.80–.89)	Visual Matching Decision Speed Retrieval Fluency Pair Cancellation	Retrieval Fluency	Retrieval Fluency Rapid Picture Naming
Adequate (.70–.79)	Rapid Picture Naming	Visual Matching Decision Speed Rapid Picture Naming Pair Cancellation	Visual Matching Decision Speed
Marginal (.60–.69)	—	—	Pair Cancellation
Low (≤ .59)	—	—	—

Note: Test-retest interval is one day only.

Source: Adapted from McGrew & Woodcock, 2001.

Test-Retest Reliability

Technical Manual across each age band (one-year age bands for children, 10-year age bands for adults).

The temporal stability of the WJ III is for the most part good, but information is lacking for some important WJ III COG scores, including the GIA, BIA, factor scores, and several subtests. Tables 6–170 and 6–171 present reliabilities for WJ III COG subtests, as reported in the Technical Manual. When the less-than-one-year interval is considered, which is the standard interval presented in most test manuals, all subtests presented have at least adequate reliability. As expected, reliabilities are somewhat lower as the time interval increases, but many are still in the adequate range.

Note that the time intervals provided offer considerably more range than those typically provided in test manuals. In particular, the one-year and three- to 10-year intervals approx-imate more closely what might occur in a clinical context. Test-retest reliabilities for the speeded tests (Table 6–170) are based on a one-day testing interval of 59 subjects in three age groups. This short interval was chosen to minimize variability due to state or trait changes, according to the authors (McGrew & Woodcock, 2001).

Although these are not presented here, the Technical Manual also provides test-retest reliabilities by age for selected subtests. These are generally impressive, including those for preschoolers over significant time intervals (e.g., >1 year).

Practice Effects

Information on practice effects is not well detailed in the manual. Scores are provided in W-score format only, which complicates interpretation for those used to working exclusively with standard scores. See technical manual for details.

Table 6–171 Median Test-Retest Reliability for Selected WJ III COG Subtests for Three Time Intervals, Across Age

Magnitude of Coefficient	Less than 1 Year	1–2 Years	3–10 Years
Very high (.90+)	Synonyms/Antonyms[a]	Synonyms/Antonyms[a]	—
High (.80–.89)	Analysis-Synthesis Visual Matching	Visual Matching	Synonyms/Antonyms[a]
Adequate (.70–.79)	Concept Formation Memory for Words	Concept Formation Analysis-Synthesis	Incomplete Words Visual Matching
Marginal (.60–.69)	—	Incomplete Words Memory for Words	Concept Formation Analysis-Synthesis Memory for Words
Low (≤ .59)	—	—	—

[a]For this study, the Synonyms/Antonyms subtests included subtests B and C of the Verbal Comprehension test only.

Source: Adapted from McGrew & Woodcock, 2001.

Interrater Reliability

Interrater reliability information on the WJ III COG is not provided in the manual. This is because only a minority of subtests, all from the WJ ACH battery, require subjective judgment in scoring.

VALIDITY

Content Validity

WJ III items were developed with considerable technical sophistication. The Rasch single-parameter logistic test model, multiple regression, and factor analyses were used for item calibration, scaling, cluster composition, and validation (see McGrew & Woodcock, 2001, for a detailed discussion). Coverage of content is extensive, including tables detailing the CHC factor, stimuli, test requirements, and response requirements for each subtest (see Technical Manual).

Subtest and Factor Intercorrelations

Intercorrelations between WJ III factors range from about .20 to .60, suggesting that factor scores reflect related but distinct dimensions of cognition (McGrew & Woodcock, 2001).

Factor Structure

The Technical Manual presents extensive information on factor-analytic studies of the WJ III, including confirmatory factor analyses testing the fit of CHC models against simpler models of intelligence such as those underlying other IQ tests such as the WAIS-III, SB-IV, and CAS. The CHC model was the best model of fit. Other research supports the invariance of the factor structure across age (Taub & McGrew, 2004). Previous research on the WJ-R, including over 1000 clinical cases with psychiatric and neurological diagnoses (e.g., ADHD, depression, seizure disorder, traumatic brain injury), support its factor structure in non-normal populations (Dean & Woodcock, 1999).

WJ III Versus WJ-R

When the WJ III and WJ-R are administered concurrently, scores are about two points higher on the WJ III (Sanborn et al., 2003).

Correlation With Other Intelligence Batteries

The Technical Manual describes these in detail. In general, the WJ III correlates about .70 with other major intelligence tests. The standard full-scale score (GIA) correlates .71 with the WISC-III, .73 with the WPPSI-R, .76 with the SB-IV, .75 with the KAIT, and .72 with the DAS. Correlation with the WAIS-III is slightly lower (.67), possibly owing to restriction of range in the sample studied (McGrew & Woodcock, 2001).

Correlations involving the WJ III screener (BIA score), although slightly smaller (.60 to .68), support the construct validity of the BIA as an IQ screener (McGrew & Woodcock, 2001).

Measures of verbal ability from the WJ III are moderately to highly correlated with measures of verbal ability from other major intelligence batteries. Specifically, WJ III verbal scales (Verbal Ability-Extended, Verbal Ability-Standard, and the *Gc* measures of Comprehension-Knowledge and Knowledge) are correlated .71 to .79 with WISC-III VIQ and VCI, and .57 and .70 with the WPPSI-R VIQ. Correlations with WAIS-III, KAIT, SB-IV, and DAS verbal indices are between .60 and .71 (see manual for full details).

Interpretation of convergent and divergent validity data from the manual for the other WJ III factors is complicated by the fact that most other intelligence batteries do not measure all the CHC factors included in the WJ III, or else have index scores that combine different CHC factors (McGrew & Woodcock, 2001). However, of visual-spatial indices, the WJ III Visual Spatial Thinking cluster shows only a small correlation to the WISC-III POI ($r = .23$) in children, which the authors attributed to restriction of range. In contrast, correlations to WAIS-III POI, SB-IV Abstract/Visual Reasoning Composite, and WPPSI-R PIQ were moderately high (range .50–.60). The WJ III Thinking Ability indices (Standard and Extended) are best conceptualized as composite measures of multiple CHC abilities, and as such, correlate most highly with full-scale scores from other major intelligence batteries (see Technical Manual for details). Validity information for the Clinical Clusters is lacking.

Although this is not explicitly discussed in the Technical Manual, all the studies presented in the manual for validity purposes indicate that WJ III Standard GIA scores are usually lower than those of other intelligence tests. This is apparent across all ages, in samples ranging from approximately 100 to 150 individuals per age group. Specifically, scores for the WJ III Standard GIA were 2.2 points lower than the WPPSI-R, 3.9 to 4.1 points lower than the DAS, 3.9 lower than the SB-IV, 5.2 points lower than the WISC-III, 3.6 lower than the KAIT, and a full 8.5 lower than the WAIS-III. Differences between WJ III BIA and Full-Scale WAIS-III scores were larger than 10 points. Differences between the WJ III BIA and CAS Full-Scale scores were 5.1, again in the direction of lower WJ III scores.

Correlation With Tests of Achievement

When all other major IQ batteries are evaluated, the WJ III COG has some of the highest correlations with achievement ($r = .70$), along with the K-ABC and CAS ($r = .74$ and .70, respectively; Naglieri & Bornstein, 2003). However, the WJ III shares some common content with the WJ III Achievement Battery, which some argue may inflate ability-achievement correlations (Naglieri & Bornstein, 2003). Shared content includes picture vocabulary items as part of both the WJ III COG Verbal Comprehension and the WJ III ACH Picture

Figure 6–29 Relations between WJ III Clusters and Mathematics Achievement for each age group. *Note:* MC = Math Calculations cluster; MR = Math Reasoning cluster; White = no significant relations; Gray = moderately significant relations; Black = strong significant relations. *Source:* Reprinted with permission from Floyd et al., 2003.

WJ III Cluster and Mathematics Ability		Age Group													
		6	7	8	9	10	11	12	13	14	15	16	17	18	19
Comprehension-Knowledge (*Gc*)	MC					Gray	Gray	Gray	Gray	Gray	Gray	Gray	Gray	Gray	Gray
	MR	Gray	Gray	Gray	Gray	Black	Black	Black	Black	Black	Black	Black	Black	Black	Black
Long-term Retrieval (*Glr*)	MC		Gray	Gray											
	MR														
Visual-Spatial Thinking (*Gv*)	MC														
	MR														
Auditory Processing (*Ga*)	MC	Gray													
	MR														
Fluid Reasoning (*Gf*)	MC	Gray	Gray	Gray	Gray	Gray	Gray	Gray	Gray	Gray	Gray	Gray	Gray	Gray	Gray
	MR	Gray	Gray	Gray	Gray	Gray	Gray	Gray	Black	Black	Black	Black	Gray	Gray	Gray
Processing Speed (*Gs*)	MC	Gray	Black	Black	Black	Black	Black	Black	Black	Black	Black	Black	Gray	Gray	Gray
	MR	Gray	Gray	Gray	Gray					Gray	Gray	Gray	Gray	Gray	Gray
Short-term Memory (*Gsm*)	MC	Gray		Gray	Gray	Gray	Gray	Gray	Gray	Gray	Gray	Gray	Gray	Gray	Gray
	MR	Gray	Gray	Gray	Gray	Gray	Gray	Gray	Gray	Gray	Gray	Gray			
Working Memory	MC	Gray	Gray	Gray	Gray	Gray	Gray	Gray	Gray	Gray	Gray	Gray	Gray	Gray	Gray
	MR	Gray	Gray	Gray	Gray	Gray	Gray	Gray	Gray	Gray	Gray	Gray	Gray	Gray	Gray

Vocabulary subtests. Naglieri and Bornstein (2003) conclude that cognitive batteries that measure basic cognitive processes, using a lesser number of subtests, may be of equal utility in predicting achievement than a test such as the WJ III, which involves a large number of subtests measuring several factors.

Some WJ III COG clusters are good predictors of reading achievement, whereas others are best at predicting mathematics achievement. Figure 6–29 shows the associations between WJ III Clusters and mathematics achievement; see Evans et al. (2001), Floyd, Evans, & McGrew (2003), and Floyd, Shaver, & McGrew (2003) for full details.

Clinical Studies

The manual presents three datasets involving individuals with LD and ADHD. In one dataset, college students with LD (*N* = 84) obtained significantly lower scores on virtually every WJ III COG subtest compared with a non-LD group. In school-aged children with ADHD, performance on the Auditory Attention subtest was especially low. In a third sample composed of three groups (i.e., normal, LD, and ADHD children), use of WJ III COG subtests, in conjunction with the WJ III ACH, correctly identified 64% of the group, a substantial improvement over chance. Concept Formation, Visual Auditory Learning, Incomplete Words, and Rapid Picture Naming

helped to correctly classify subjects, along with WISC-III Digit Span. One study comparing gifted and nongifted students on the WJ III found that both groups had similar score profiles across CHC factor clusters despite consistently higher scores in the gifted group (Rizza et al., 2001).

Despite a fairly extensive body of research on the WJ-R, few independent studies on the validity of the WJ III have been published yet, due to its relatively recent publication date. Evidence on the WJ-R's ability to differentiate between patients with and without confirmed brain damage, and between closed head injury cases versus psychiatric diagnosis, is presented by Dean and Woodcock (1999). To our knowledge, there is no research on the use of the WJ III COG in clinical groups of interest to neuropsychologists (e.g., TBI, AD, epilepsy).

COMMENT

To date, the WJ III COG has had limited usage by neuropsychologists; this should change as more users become aware of its features and of its of impressive psychometric properties. The WJ III's theory-based roots are clearly evident in its score and test structure, and it has comprehensive, well-written manuals. The test provides a wealth of subtests to choose from (i.e., over 40 possible subtests in the combined WJ III

COG and WJ III ACH batteries), and is constructed in such a way as to allow tailored and flexible assessment. Norms are also extremely extensive (i.e., $N > 8000$). The age band is wide (2 to 90+), there are two kinds of college norms, and norms for certain age bands such as preschoolers rival those of tests developed exclusively for these groups (e.g., N of over 1000 for this age group alone). The test also allows derivation of scores based on age and education, which, while an obvious asset when testing children, is also useful in evaluating adults.

One major asset of the test is its use of complete normative data in ability-achievement comparisons. The WJ III does not rely on linkage groups (i.e., normative subsets administered both tests) or estimation methods (e.g., simple difference method), but on actual performance of all 8000+ subjects in the normative sample on the WJ III COG and the WJ III ACH. This is also appealing for comparing performance across subtests in situations where analyzing achievement-ability discrepancies is not the goal. For instance, the availability of 40 individual subtests conormed on the same large sample allows flexibility in building customized test batteries or else for accomplishing targeted comparisons of specific domains in individual patients.

Another major asset is that most subtests can be administered at all ages. The test can therefore safely be used as a single assessment tool for conducting longitudinal assessments across the age span, without confounding the comparison of performance at different ages with method variance arising from the use of different tests. In clinical settings, this means that a child's intellectual ability can be assessed with the same instrument from preschool to old age. The test also has impressive reliabilities, including data on extended testing intervals from 1 to 10 years, with large retest samples. (Note, however, that some important test-retest reliability coefficients are not provided in the manual, and that further information on practice effects is needed.)

Along with its advanced psychometric and technical features, the WJ III is a user-friendly instrument from a test administration standpoint; the two-easel format also makes the test portable and simple to use. Certain features also make it appropriate for special populations. Several subtests require only basic verbal or motor responding. For example, Verbal Comprehension subtests require only one-word answers. This makes the test useful for assessing individuals with motor impairments that interfere with lengthy verbal expression (e.g., cerebral palsy, facial injury). The WJ III also includes an almost motor-free measure of visual-spatial skills (Spatial Relations) and attention (Auditory Attention), both of which necessitate only pointing. Speed is only required on subtests specifically designed to measure processing speed; thus, patients with motor or cognitive impairments that interfere with response speed (e.g., MS) are not penalized on tests measuring other abilities. Conversely, this also means that in cases where these skills are crucial for answering the referral question, other tests that specifically assess verbal expression or the ability to use manipulatives under time constraints need to be supplemented.

The test appears especially useful for assessing high-functioning individuals because of the reduced likelihood of ceiling effects and the large range of item difficulty (Rizza et al., 2001). In particular, the executive/reasoning subtests (e.g., Analysis-Synthesis, Concept Formation) offer an alternative to tests such as the WCST and Category test, which may suffer from ceiling effects in high-functioning individuals.

Overall, WJ III subtests are quite short, an asset when time is limited or when testing individuals with limited tolerance for extended testing sessions (e.g., the very young, the very old, or the very impaired). The ease of administration, lack of separate examiner manual, and lack of manipulatives also facilitate training examiners—an asset when testing is to be accomplished by psychometrists or research assistants. This contrasts with most IQ batteries, which require extensive training in administration and scoring.

From a neuropsychological perspective, the WJ III also has certain strengths. Several subtests are based on common neuropsychological paradigms, including digit recall, cancellation tasks, and verbal fluency. The WJ III COG also includes several short subtests thought to measure aspects of executive functioning (e.g., Planning, Analysis-Synthesis). The ability to compare separate cluster scores (i.e., Executive Processes, Broad Attention, Working Memory) to overall ability is also of potential utility within a neuropsychological context.

Other aspects are not so useful for neuropsychological assessment. Data on WJ III scores in clinical groups of interest to neuropsychologists are lacking. Clinical Cluster scores do not yet have supporting convergent or divergent validity information. The test structure is not organized in an inherently familiar way for neuropsychologists (e.g., the verbal memory task is found in the WJ III ACH, but the visual memory task is found in the WJ III COG). In addition, some subtests are not designed from a neuropsychological framework. For instance, verbal memory subtests do not provide a recognition or multiple-choice trial to enable differentiation of retrieval versus encoding failure, and no information is provided on the impact of using delays ranging from 30 minutes to eight days for recall tests. The WJ III also uses omnibus scores for Attention/Processing Speed tests, which makes interpretation of performance problematic (i.e., poor performance may be due to slowness, inattention, or impulsivity). This criticism is not unique to WJ III, as many other measures not originally intended for neuropsychological usage are constructed similarly (e.g., CAS, Wechsler scales). Similarly, a naming task (Picture Vocabulary) is included in the four-part Verbal Comprehension subtest, but a separate naming score cannot be derived without administering the full Picture Vocabulary test from the WJ ACH.

Others have noted that the sheer number of scores available in the WJ III make it daunting to use (Schrank et al., 2002). Clearly, attaining familiarity with the test structure and all the subtests and scores requires a considerable amount of training time. A thorough understanding of the battery is significantly augmented by learning most aspects of the WJ III ACH as well. Learning the actual administration of individual subtests, however, is relatively simple. Some clinicians may therefore consider including two or four subtests as a supplement to their usual battery, since the norms for the WJ III are vastly superior to those of many commonly used neuropsychological tests assessing similar domains (e.g., WJ III COG Retrieval Fluency for verbal fluency, WJ ACH Picture Vocabulary as a naming task, WJ III ACH Understanding Directions as a Token Test alternative, etc.).

As noted previously, it is also important to note that the WJ III yields full-scale scores that are somewhat lower than those of some other IQ tests (e.g., two to eight points for the standard GIA, depending on age and comparison measure). Note that comparisons to the WISC-IV and WPPSI-III were not yet available as of this writing.

REFERENCES

Carroll, J. B. (1993). *Human cognitive abilities: A survey of factor-analytic studies.* New York: Cambridge University Press.

Carroll, J. B. (1997). The three-stratum theory of cognitive abilities. In D. P. Flanagan, J. L. Genshaft, & P. L. Harrison (Eds.), *Contemporary intellectual assessment: Theories, tests, and issues* (pp. 122–130). New York: The Guilford Press.

Cattell, R. B. (1941). Some theoretical issues in adult intelligence testing. *Psychological Bulletin, 38,* 592.

Cohen, J. (1959). The factorial structure of the WISC at ages 7-7, 10-6, and 13-6. *Journal of Consulting and Clinical Psychology, 23,* 285–299.

Dean, R. S., & Woodcock, R. W. (1999). *The WJ-R and Bateria-R in neuropsychological assessment (Woodcock-Johnson III research report No. 3).* Itasca, IL: Riverside Publishing.

Evans, J. J., Floyd, R. G., McGrew, K. S., & Leforgee, M. H. (2001). The relations between measures of Cattell-Horn-Carroll (CHC) cognitive abilities and reading achievement during childhood and adolescence. *School Psychology Review, 31*(2), 246–262.

Flanagan, D. P., McGrew, K. S., & Ortiz, S. O. (2000). *The Wechsler intelligence scales and Gf-Gc theory: A contemporary approach to interpretation.* Boston: Allyn & Bacon.

Floyd, R. G., Evans, J. J., & McGrew, K. S. (2003). Relations between measures of Cattell-Horn-Carroll (CHC) cognitive abilities and mathematics achievement across the school-age years. *Psychology in the Schools, 40*(2), 155–171.

Floyd, R. G., Shaver, R. B., & McGrew, K. S. (2003). Interpretation of the Woodcock–Johnson III Tests of Cognitive Abilities: Acting on evidence. In F. A. Schrank & D. P. Flanagan (Eds.), *WJ III clinical use and interpretation* (pp. 1–46, 403–408). New York: Academic Press.

Horn, J. L., & Noll, J. (1997). Human cognitive abilities: Gf-Gc theory. In D. P. Flanagan, J. L. Genshaft, & P. L. Harrison (Eds.), *Contemporary intellectual assessment: Theories, tests, and issues* (pp. 53–91). New York: The Guilford Press.

Ittenbach, R. F., Esters, I. G., & Wainer, H. (1997). The history of test development. In D. P. Flanagan, J. L. Genshaft, & P. L. Harrison (Eds.), *Contemporary intellectual assessment: Theories, tests, and issues* (pp. 17–31). New York: The Guilford Press.

Joseph, L. M., McCachran, M. E., & Naglieri, J. A. (2003). PASS cognitive processes, phonological processes, and basic reading performance for a sample of referred primary-grade children. *Journal of Research in Reading, 26*(3), 304–314.

Kamphaus, R. W., Petoskey, M. D., & Morgan, A. W. (1997). A history of intelligence test interpretation. In D. P. Flanagan, J. L. Genshaft, & P. L. Harrison (Eds.), *Contemporary intellectual assessment: Theories, tests, and issues* (pp. 32–47). New York: The Guilford Press.

Keith, T. Z., Kranzler, J. H., & Flanagan, D. P. (2001). What does the Cognitive Assessment System (CAS) measure? Joint confirmatory factor analysis of the CAS and the Woodcock-Johnson Tests of Cognitive Ability (3rd Edition). *School Psychology Review, 30*(1), 89–119.

Mather, N., & Woodcock, R. W. (2001). *Woodcock-Johnson III Tests of Cognitive Abilities examiner's manual.* Itasca, IL: Riverside Publishing.

McGrew, K. S. (1997). Analysis of the major intelligence batteries according to a proposed comprehensive Gf-Gc framework. In D. P. Flanagan, J. L. Genshaft, & P. L. Harrison (Eds.), *Contemporary intellectual assessment: Theories, tests, and issues* (pp. 151–179). New York: The Guilford Press.

McGrew, K. S., & Woodcock, R. W. (2001). *Woodcock-Johnson III technical manual.* Itasca, IL: Riverside Publishing.

Naglieri, J. A., & Bornstein, B. T. (2003). Intelligence and achievement: Just how correlated are they? *Journal of Psychoeducational Assessment, 21*(3), 244–260.

Rasch, G. (1960). *Probabilistic models for some intelligence and attainment tests.* Copenhagen, Denmark: Danish Institute for Educational Research.

Rizza, M. G., McIntosh, D. E., & McCunn, A. (2001). Profile analysis of the Woodcock-Johnson III Tests of Cognitive Abilities with gifted students. *Psychology in the Schools, 38*(5), 447–455.

Sanborn, K. J., Truscott, S. D., Phelps, L., & McDougal, J. L. (2003). Does the Flynn effect differ by IQ level in samples of students classified as learning disabled? *Journal of Psychoeducational Assessment, 21*(2), 145–159.

Schrank, F. A., Flanagan, D. P., Woodcock, R. W., & Mascolo, J. T. (2002). *Essentials of WJ III Cognitive Abilities assessment.* New York: John Wiley & Sons, Inc.

Schrank, F. A., & Woodcock, R. W. (2001). *WJ III Compuscore and Profiles program [computer software]. Woodcock-Johnson III.* Itasca, IL: Riverside Publishing.

Taub, G. E., & McGrew, K. S. (2004). A confirmatory factor analysis of the Cattell-Horn-Carroll theory and cross-age invariance of the Woodcock-Johnson Tests of Cognitive Abilities III. *School Psychology Quarterly, 19*(1), 72–87.

Woodcock, R. W., & Johnson, M. B. (1977). *Woodcock-Johnson Psycho-Educational Battery.* Itasca, IL: Riverside Publishing.

Woodcock, R. W., & Johnson, M. B. (1989a). *WJ-R Tests of Achievement.* Itasca, IL: Riverside Publishing.

Woodcock, R. W., & Johnson, M. B. (1989b). *WJ-R Tests of Cognitive Ability.* Itasca, IL: Riverside Publishing.

Woodcock, R. W., McGrew, K. S., & Mather, N. (2001a). *Woodcock-Johnson III Tests of Achievement.* Itasca, IL: Riverside Publishing.

Woodcock, R. W., McGrew, K. S., & Mather, N. (2001b). *Woodcock-Johnson III Tests of Cognitive Abilities.* Itasca, IL: Riverside Publishing.

7

Achievement Tests

Achievement tests are primarily used to assist in diagnosing learning disabilities. Traditionally, this has involved comparing IQ scores with achievement scores to derive an ability-achievement discrepancy. However, the ability-achievement discrepancy model is increasingly viewed as inadequate and obsolete due to several inherent limitations, including the technical and psychometric limitations of cutoff scores and discrepancies, the "wait to fail" model as the basis for diagnosis (versus prevention and intervention-responsiveness models), and the pervasive sociocultural factors that lead to overrepresentation of minorities in LD categories. (See recent reviews for more information on this important issue [e.g., Dombrowski et al., 2004; Fletcher et al., 2004; Francis et al., 2005; Lyon et al., 2005; Steubing et al., 2002].) Although the future of LD diagnosis appears to be poised for a major conceptual shift, some fundamentals remain, including the fact that achievement tests provide only one portion of the data required for making diagnostic decisions, and that learning disorders can only be identified with appropriate consideration of several important sources of information, including direct observation, intervention history, family history, and the instructional environment (e.g., impoverished versus enriched milieu).

Achievement tests are also useful adjuncts to the neuropsychological assessment in situations where diagnosing learning disorders is not the primary referral question. For example, most achievement batteries include language subtests that evaluate aspects of expressive and receptive language. These, in conjunction with existing neuropsychological tests, are of considerable utility for assessing patients with language disturbance (e.g., aphasic patients). In addition, most achievement batteries are well normed; many are superior, psychometrically, to neuropsychological tests developed for aphasia screening or language evaluation, and most boast reliabilities that rival those of IQ tests. Most also contain items that range from the most basic preacademic skills to high-level items suitable for high-education and high-IQ subjects. Because of linkages or conorming to IQ tests, achievement tests also allow users to compare cognitive domains covered in IQ tests with those covered in achievement batteries; this is useful for detecting individual strengths and deficits in patients with neurological disorders affecting reading, computation, or writing skills. Achievement batteries also allow neuropsychologists to estimate the functional skills of patients to determine the degree of assistance they will need in their daily lives. For example, when used in conjunction with other tests (e.g., executive functioning testing, adaptive behavior scales), achievement tests provide useful information that is relevant to many work situations (e.g., reading level, reading rate) and to independence in activities of daily living requiring functional academic skills, such as handling financial matters or reading directions. Estimating reading and math levels is also of utility for the assessment itself, to determine whether the patient has sufficient reading skills to complete self-report questionnaires (e.g., PAI, MMPI-2) or sufficient math skills to adequately perform non-achievement tests such as the PASAT (see reviews in this volume). Achievement tests such as the WRAT-3 Reading subtest have also been used to estimate premorbid intellectual abilities and to provide an estimate of literacy/quality of education. The latter is of considerable utility in assessing minorities (see the work of Manly, as reviewed in Chapter 2, and the *WRAT-3* review in this volume).

This chapter includes a small selection of achievement tests (see Table 7–1). We review two major achievement test batteries (WJ III ACH and WIAT-II), along with an academic screener (WRAT-3) and a reading test (GORT-4). Additional tests are well reviewed in other sources (e.g., Sattler, 2001). The WJ III ACH and WIAT-II are both comprehensive achievement batteries that assess reading (rate, decoding, and comprehension), mathematics (reasoning, computation), writing (spelling, prose writing), and language (receptive and expressive). The WJ III ACH, in particular, covers areas not traditionally thought of as "academic," but which are useful in the neuropsychological evaluation (e.g., receptive language, prose recall, naming), in addition to a wide coverage of academic skills. The WRAT-3, although it also assesses reading, spelling, and mathematics, is best viewed as a limited screening battery only. The GORT-4 provides a comprehensive assessment of reading skills.

Table 7–1 Overview of Achievement Tests

Test	Age Range	Tasks Included	Administration Time	Some Key Processes Thought to be Assessed	Internal Reliability	Test-Retest Reliability	Co-normed
WJ III ACH	2–90+	Letter-Word Identification, Word Attack, Reading Fluency, Passage Comprehension, Reading Vocabulary, Calculation, Math Fluency, Applied Problems, Quantitative Concepts, Spelling, Editing, Writing Fluency, Writing Samples, Story Recall, Picture Vocabulary, Understanding Directions, Oral Comprehension, Academic Knowledge, Story Recall—Delayed, Handwriting Legibility Scale, Writing Evaluation Scale, Spelling of Sounds, Sound Awareness, Punctuation/Capitalization	60–70 min (each subtest is 5 to 10 min); longer for Extended Battery	Basic Reading, Reading Fluency, Reading Comprehension, Math Calculation, Math Fluency, Math Reasoning, Basic Writing, Writing Fluency, Written Expression, Oral Expression, Listening Comprehension, Academic Knowledge	High to very high	High (not all reliabilities are reported in the manual)	Yes (WJ III COG)
WIAT-II[a]	4–85	Word Reading, Pseudoword Decoding, Reading Comprehension, Spelling, Written Expression, Numerical Operations, Mathematics Reasoning, Listening Comprehension, Oral Expression	45 min to 2 hours	Reading, Written Language, Mathematics, Oral Language	High to very high[b]	High to very high[b]	No (but has linking samples to the WPPSI-III, WISC-IV, and WAIS-III)
WRAT-3	5–74	Reading, Spelling, Arithmetic	15–30 min	Single-word decoding[c], Word spelling, Math computation	High to very high; lower for Arithmetic	Very high	No
GORT-4	6–18	Reading Rate, Reading Accuracy, Reading Fluency, Reading Comprehension	15–45 min	Reading speed, accuracy, and comprehension	Very high	High to very high[d]	No

[a] Also provides Supplemental scores for Target Words, Reading Speed, Alphabet Writing, Word Fluency (written), Word Count, and Word Fluency (oral). [b] In grades pre-K to 12; adult samples differ somewhat. [c] Has been used as an IQ estimate and to estimate literacy (see review in this volume). [d] Based on test-retest reliability of alternate forms.

When using achievement tests, it is important to note that scores may differ based on whether norms for age or for grade are used (i.e., grade-based norms may include children of several ages, particularly in the upper grades). Limitations of grade equivalents must also be kept in mind. These include the fact that grade equivalents are not comparable across subtests and do not represent equally spaced units; grade equivalents at the extremes of the distribution may be the result of interpolation rather than actual data. Additionally, obtaining a specific number of correct responses corresponding to a specific grade equivalent is not equivalent to mastering that grade's curriculum (Sattler, 2001).

REFERENCES

Dombrowski, S. C., Kamphaus, R. W., & Reynolds, C. R. (2004). After the demise of the discrepancy: Proposed learning disabilities diagnostic criteria. *Professional Psychology: Research and Practice, 35*(4), 364–372.

Fletcher, J. M., Coulter, W. A., Reschly, D. J., & Vaughn, S. (2004). Alternative approaches to the definition and identification of learning disabilities: Some questions and answers. *Annals of Dyslexia, 54*(2), 304–331.

Francis, D. J., Fletcher, J. M., Stuebing, K. K., Lyon, G. R., Shaywitz, B. A., & Shaywitz, S. E. (2005). Psychometric approaches to the identification of LD: IQ and achievement scores are not sufficient. *Journal of Learning Disabilities, 38*(2), 98–108.

Lyon, G. R. (2005). Why scientific research must guide educational policy and instructional practices in learning disabilities. *Learning Disabilities Quarterly, 28,* 140–143.

Sattler, J. M. (2001). *Assessment of children: Cognitive applications* (4th ed.). San Diego: Jerome M. Sattler, Publisher.

Stuebing, K. K., Fletcher, J. M., LeDoux, J. M., Lyon, G. R., Shaywitz, S. E., & Shaywitz, B. A. (2002). Validity of IQ-discrepancy classifications of reading disabilities: A meta-analysis. *American Educational Research Journal, 39,* 469–518.

The Gray Oral Reading Tests—Fourth Edition (GORT-4)

PURPOSE

The purpose of the GORT-4 is to measure reading skills (i.e., rate, accuracy, fluency, and comprehension).

SOURCE

The GORT-4 Examiner's Manual, Student Book (i.e., stimulus book with stories and comprehension questions), and Profile/Examiner's Record Booklets can be obtained from PRO-ED (www.proedinc.com). The cost for the Complete Kit is $198 US.

AGE RANGE

The age range is from 6 years to 18 years, 11 months.

DESCRIPTION

According to its authors, the original GORT (1963) was the most commonly used test of oral reading during the 1960s to 1980s (Wiederholt & Bryant, 2001). It was revised in 1986 (GORT-R), and then again in 1992 (GORT-3). The GORT-4 (Wiederholt & Bryant, 2001) is generally similar in format, content, and scoring to its predecessors, but includes new normative data, an extension of the floor with the addition of another story at the beginning of the test, and improved psychometric and validity information. Additionally, the Passage score has been renamed Fluency score to reflect current terminology, and the order of some of the stories has been altered.

There are two parallel forms (A and B) designed for retesting purposes, each containing 14 stories. The child is required to read each short story aloud. Following completion of the story, the story is removed from view and the child is shown a page with five questions, each with multiple-choice responses, which the examiner then reads to the subject. In this way, comprehension is also evaluated.

The GORT-4 is intended for four purposes: (1) to identify students who are significantly below their peers in oral reading proficiency, (2) to determine specific reading strengths and weaknesses, (3) to document progress as a result of reading interventions, and (4) for research purposes in school-age children (Wiederholt & Bryant, 2001). According to the test authors, the GORT-4 can be used as a stand-alone test or it can be used with a silent reading test (Gray Silent Reading Test, GSRT; Wiederhold & Blalock, 2000) or a battery designed to assess reading in detail (Gray Diagnostic Reading Tests—Second Edition, GDRT-2).

ADMINISTRATION

See manual. As the child reads, the examiner records the time taken to complete the story and the number of deviations from print during oral reading (i.e., substitutions, additions, omissions, or any other reading errors). Following this, the examiner records the number of correct answers to the multiple-choice comprehension questions. The examiner also provides difficult words for the subject if the subject takes more than five seconds without any audible attempt to read the word. If more than 20% of the words are provided in this way, the Comprehension score is 0. The maximum number of words allowed per story is provided in the response booklet. Skipping a line while reading is also recorded as a deviation and pointed out to the subject.

During administration, time in seconds and number of deviations from print are converted to Rate and Accuracy ratings (these range from 0 to 5; see p. 57 of the manual for details on how these ratings were derived from the normative score distribution) using a table at the bottom of each page in the Profile/Examiner's Booklet.

Ceilings and Basals

Rate and Accuracy scores are summed to provide Fluency scores, which are then used to establish the basal and ceiling. A separate basal and ceiling must also be obtained for the Comprehension score (i.e., the number of correct responses to multiple-choice comprehension questions). The Fluency basal is a Fluency score of 9 or 10 for any given story. The Fluency ceiling is a score of 2 or less for a story (note that Fluency scores are calculated by summing the Rate and Accuracy scores for each story, which are derived using a table for each story in the Examiner's Booklet). To establish the Comprehension basal and ceiling, the child is tested until three out of five comprehension items are missed for any one story. The examiner then goes back to the entry item and tests backwards to establish a basal (i.e., five out of five correct comprehension questions).

ADMINISTRATION TIME

The test takes 15 to 45 minutes.

SCORING

Main Scores

Five scores can be derived. There are four "subtest" scores (i.e., Rate, Accuracy, Fluency, and Comprehension; see Table 7–2), which are provided in scaled score format ($M = 10$, $SD = 3$), and a Composite score (Oral Reading Quotient, ORQ), which reflects overall oral reading ability and is computed in standard score format ($M = 100$, $SD = 15$). Age equivalents, grade equivalents, and percentiles can also be derived for each score, although the test authors do not recommend the use of age and grade equivalents for describing performance.

Table 7–2 List of GORT-4 Scores

GORT-4 Score	Definition
Rate	Total time taken to read each story orally
Accuracy	Number of pronunciation errors
Fluency	Total of rate and accuracy scores
Comprehension	Number of correct answers to multiple-choice comprehension questions
Oral Reading Quotient (ORQ)	Composite score obtained by summing Fluency and Comprehension scores; provides a measure of overall oral reading ability

Error Analysis

Additionally, an error analysis can be performed by calculating the frequency of specific error types during reading, using a worksheet included in the Record Form. Specific error classifications are Meaning Similarity, Function Similarity, Graphic/Phonemic Similarity, Multiple Sources, and Self-Correction. A tape recorder is recommended for recording and scoring specific errors. A minimum of 25 miscues is required for an accurate error analysis (see p. 21 of Examiner's Manual for more detail). Error analysis scores are reported as percentages. The authors note that some types of errors, including insertions, omissions, additions, and reversals, are characteristic of beginning readers and should not be used in planning reading interventions.

Repeat Testing

The procedure for comparing scores in retest situations is described on p. 37 of the manual. The authors recommend using only the ORQ score when assessing for differences over time as assessed by performance on the two alternate forms (but see *Comments*). A Difference score is computed (higher ORQ score – lower ORQ score) using a formula provided by Anastasi and Urbina (1997) that takes into account the measures' reliabilities. Statistically significant and clinically useful difference scores between GORT-4 and other language and intelligence tests are also presented in the manual, including the WISC-III, TONI-3, C-TONI, TACL-3, and TOLD-3.

DEMOGRAPHIC EFFECTS

Age

GORT-4 performance, as expected, is highly correlated to age ($r = .66–.74$; see manual).

Gender

To our knowledge, there are no gender effects on the test. The test manual reports mean scores of 101 and 100 for girls and boys in the standardization sample, respectively.

Ethnicity

The manual shows mean scores obtained by African American and Hispanic American children (i.e., ORQ = 95 and 96, respectively). No other information is provided on these groups. Although care was taken in the development of the test to avoid bias (see *Validity*), there are as yet no independent studies on the use of the test in minority groups. However, Craig et al. (2004) tested whether dialectal variations as a result of the use of African American English (AAE) in a group of African American children might be scored as reading errors on the GORT-3. They found that almost every child produced AAE features while reading passages from the GORT-3, and that older children produced fewer AAE features than did younger children. Scoring the test in the standard manner yielded an average score for African American students in the boundary between below average and average, whereas crediting AAE-related variations yielded performance in the average range. However, the actual mean score difference between scoring methods was only two points, and the score distributions for the two scoring methods were normally distributed, with about the same number of children falling below one *SD* from the mean for both scoring methods. As a result, the authors concluded that the test is an appropriate measure for assessing reading in African American children. However, individual clinicians might consider scoring the test in both ways to avoid overestimating reading errors in African American children or in other groups with specific English dialects.

NORMATIVE DATA

Standardization Sample

Norms are based on 1677 individuals tested between 1999 and 2000 in 28 U.S. states, stratified according to the 1997 U.S. Census according to geographic region, gender, race, ethnicity, parental income, and parental education. See Table 7–3 for specific sample characteristics. In each one-year age band from 6 to 18 years, 78 to 189 children were tested. Continuous norming was used to develop the standard scores (i.e., fitted values estimated for each six-month interval, using regression methods and smoothing).

RELIABILITY

Internal Consistency

Coefficient alphas were calculated at 13 age intervals using data from the entire normative sample; these were all very high (i.e., all approximated or exceeded .90; see manual). Reliabilities for Comprehension and ORQ were especially high (i.e., generally above .95 for all age groups). Alphas for selected subgroups from the normative sample presented in the manual are also very high (>.90); this includes racial/ethnic subgroups and children with learning disability or ADHD. Again, Comprehension and ORQ showed the highest reliabilities (i.e., almost all .98 or .99).

Standard Error of Measurement

GORT-4 *SEM*s are small, which is expected given the high reliabilities reviewed above. For the Rate, Accuracy, Fluency, and Comprehension scores, *SEM*s were 1 across age groups; *SEM*s for the ORQ were on average 3 (range 2 to 4; see manual).

Test-Retest Stability

Stability is reported in the manual for a group of 49 children tested over two weeks. Although this is not well explained in

Table 7–3 GORT-4 Normative Sample Characteristics

Number	1677
Age	6 to 18 years, 11 months[a]
Geographic location	
Northeast	21%
South	34%
Midwest	24%
West	22%
Sample type	National, stratified random sample[b]
Parental education	
Less than Bachelor's degree	72%
Bachelor's degree	21%
Master's, professional, doctoral degrees	7%
SES	Assessed by six different family income categories
Gender	
Males	47%
Females	53%
Race	
White	85%
Black	12%
Other	3%
Ethnicity	
Native American	1%
Hispanic	12%
Asian	2%
African American	12%
European American	72%
Other	1%
Residence	
Urban	83%
Rural	17%
Disability Status	
No disability	92%
Learning disability	2%
Speech-language disorder	<1%
Attention-deficit disorder	2%
Other handicap	2%
Screening	All students attending general classes were selected, including those with disabilities

[a]Based on 13 separate age bands. [b]Based on 1997 U.S. Census data, stratified by age, gender, race, ethnicity, geographic region, residence, income, parental education, and disability status.

Source: Adapted from Wiederholt & Bryant, 2001.

the manual, it appears that the children were administered Form A twice, followed by Form B twice, followed by Form A, then Form B. The authors called the last retesting (A then B) a "delayed alternate forms" administration. Reliability coefficient classifications are shown in Table 7–4. These indicate

Table 7–4 Magnitude of Test-Retest Reliability Coefficients for GORT-4 Scores

Magnitude of Coefficient	Form A to A	Form B to B	Form A to B
Very high (.90+)	Rate Accuracy Fluency	Rate Fluency ORQ	Rate Accuracy Fluency ORQ
High (.80–.89)	Comprehension ORQ	Accuracy Comprehension	—
Adequate (.70–.79)	—	—	Comprehension
Marginal (.60–.69)	—	—	—
Low (<.59)	—	—	—

Source: From Wiederholt & Bryant, 2001. Reprinted with permission.

high to very high test-retest reliability of most GORT-4 scores. Note that Comprehension reliability is lower when alternate forms are used ($r = .78$), but still within the acceptable range.

Practice Effects

Practice effects on the GORT-4 appear negligible (i.e., ≤1 on both the subtests and ORQ; see manual).

Alternate Form Reliability

According to the authors, alternate form reliability was maximized by using a linear equating procedure to equate scores on Forms A and B (see p. 52 of manual for details). Correlations between Forms A and B, averaged across age, were very high for Rate, Accuracy, and Fluency ($r \geq .94$) and high for Comprehension ($r = .85$). At some ages, correlations between forms for the Comprehension score were not as high (e.g., $r = .71$ at age 8), but still acceptable.

Interrater Reliability

Interscorer reliability, as reported in the test manual, is very high ($r = .94–.99$).

VALIDITY

Content Validity

GORT-4 item content was chosen on the basis of graded word lists to maximize content validity, and questions were chosen to cover the accepted types of comprehension (e.g., literal, inferential, critical, affective; see p. 74 of the manual for additional details). In addition, the passage dependency of the questions was tested to ensure that questions could not be correctly answered by guessing. Paragraphs were also assessed using readability formulas to ensure that they were properly organized in order of increasing difficulty. Conventional item analysis and differential item functioning analysis (to detect item bias with regard to gender, race, and ethnicity) were also used to select and order test items.

Subscore Intercorrelations

According to the manual, GORT-4 Accuracy and Rate are highly correlated ($r = .85$), whereas Comprehension correlates only moderately with Rate, Accuracy, and Fluency ($r = .39–.42$), which seems to show some support for the computation of separate Fluency and Comprehension scores.

Factor Structure

No factor analysis evidence is presented in the manual.

Correlation With Other Reading Tests

The manual lists 11 validity studies involving other reading tests as evidence of criterion-prediction validity. According to these studies, the GORT-4 composite reading score (ORQ) is highly correlated to the reading composite score from the GDRT-2 and GSRT ($r = .63$ and $.59$, respectively). Correlations between previous GORT versions and reading composites from other tests are also moderate to high ($r = .57–.74$; Test of Word Reading Efficiency, Iowa tests of Educational Development, California Achievement Tests—Fifth Edition, Diagnostic Achievement Battery—Second Edition). See *Comment* for further discussion of these validity studies.

The GORT-4 allows the assessment of three separate dimensions of reading—reading speed, decoding skills, and comprehension. Unfortunately, validity information on these separate subscores is limited. Correlations between GORT-3 and the TOWRE, a timed decoding test that does not allow separate comparisons for decoding skills and speed, are presented in the manual. These correlations were all moderate to high. In the case of Comprehension, the average correlation with other reading tests across studies was in the moderate range (i.e., $r = .45$; range, $r = .34–.75$). However, not all the tests presented in the manual assess comprehension per se, so it is unclear what the purpose of this section was other than to demonstrate that all the measures overlap to a moderate degree, as one would expect various reading tests to do. Only one study appears to test the validity of the Comprehension score separate from other reading skills; in it, the GORT-4 Comprehension score was only moderately correlated with the GDRT-2 Reading Comprehension Quotient ($r = .41$)

Correlation With Other Abilities

The authors note that previous research has found a robust correlation of about .50 between reading and spoken language, and of about .55 between reading and writing skills (see manual for details). No information on the GORT-4 is presented for either spoken or written language. However, in support of GORT-4 validity, the manual presents correlations between the GORT-R and the WISC-R Comprehension subtest for a small sample of children with severe learning disabilities ($r = .39–.45$; $N = 54$, grades K–2), along with similar correlations between an unstandardized measure of language and GORT-R scores. In three studies from 1992 using the GORT-3 (see manual), the median correlation between the ORQ and various tests of written language was high ($r = .59$). According to the authors, these studies provide "evidence of the GORT-4's construct-identification validity" (p. 88). Previous versions of the GORT also correlate moderately well with measures of rapid automatized naming, a skill that typically correlates between .40 and .60 with reading ability (see manual). However, more validation evidence would be of benefit.

Correlation With IQ

Some information is provided regarding the relationship of test scores to IQ. Correlations between the GORT-4 and the WISC-III in a group of 30 adolescents aged 13 to 16 indicate moderate correlations with all scores (VIQ = .54, PIQ = 46, FSIQ = .51; see manual). Averaged correlations for other versions of the GORT with the VIQ and FSIQ are somewhat higher (i.e., $r = .69$ and .65, respectively). Notably, some of these studies are based on small samples (e.g., $N = 18$) or restricted ages (e.g., grades 3–4).

Clinical Studies

Mean GORT-4 scores of various clinical groups (LD, emotionally disturbed, ADHD, and gifted) are presented in the manual. These indicate that the lowest ORQ was obtained in the LD group (ORQ = 82). All other groups had essentially normal performance, with above average performance in the gifted group (ORQ = 116). However, no other information is reported, apart from three studies reporting increases in GORT-R and GORT-3 performance after reading intervention, listed in the manual as evidence of the GORT-4's sensitivity to change. Information on sensitivity, specificity, and positive/negative predictive power is lacking, which would be crucial in determining the test's efficacy at detecting children with reading disabilities.

COMMENT

The GORT-4 uses paragraph reading as its testing paradigm. As noted in the manual, this format has face validity in that it mirrors the types of reading tasks that are used in school and in everyday life. Unlike many other reading tests that either are multifactorial, are one-dimensional, or confound decoding with response speed, the GORT-4 allows examiners to assess reading speed, decoding skills, and reading comprehension separately. This is an asset when testing neuropsychological populations where response speed is an issue. Additionally, the assessment of the three separate dimensions may be helpful in designing interventions to maximize reading performance in different individuals with reading problems. Norms are also considerable, and the test appears to have been well developed in terms of item content and test construction. Internal reliability is uniformly high and has been demonstrated in clinical groups. Test-retest stability is also excellent over short intervals. Some limitations need to be kept in mind when using the test. Although this should be obvious given the age limits of the norms (i.e., 18 years), the test is not appropriate for evaluating reading in adults (see Stevens & Price, 1999).

Administration

While administering the test, the examiner must keep track of failed items to establish two sets of basals and ceilings (i.e., one set for Fluency and one set for Comprehension, both with different basal/ceiling criteria). This can be difficult to do while simultaneously maintaining the interest of challenging patients (e.g., inattentive or off-task children). Testing length can also be prolonged with readers who have a slow reading rate but good comprehension.

Validity Data

As noted above, the reliability of the GORT-4 is sufficiently high to support its use as a diagnostic instrument. However, because reading tests are used to make diagnostic decisions that directly affect children, validity data are equally important. The validity information presented in the manual is not particularly comprehensive or extensive, and is somewhat limited by emphasizing studies based on prior versions. In addition, some of the validity studies reviewed include small Ns, limited age ranges, and in some cases, unstandardized tests. These provide some information on how the test correlates with composite measures of reading ability, but does not detail whether subscores correlate well to those of other tests measuring specific aspects of reading performance such as speed or accuracy. Validity information is provided for Form A only. It is also difficult for users to effectively review all the validity information because of the way studies are presented in the manual (i.e., identified by numbers in tables corresponding to information outlined in an appendix). Factor-analytic studies are not included to support the test score structure.

A related issue is whether Rate and Accuracy scores can be interpreted separately. For instance, a child might be an accurate but very slow reader who obtains a high Accuracy score but a low Rate score; this child would differ markedly from another child who obtains the reverse pattern of scores. Information on whether certain patterns of high and low scores are associated with specific types of reading disability, and guidelines regarding the interpretation of specific patterns of scores, would be helpful. Similarly, although touched upon in the manual, the clinical utility and predictive validity of miscues deserves additional study.

Repeat Testing and Correspondence Between Versions

More information is also needed on the stability of GORT-4 scores over time. The test-retest reliability data presented in the manual is for only a small sample of children of different ages, with no information on whether stability differs across age. Similarly, no information on whether children score lower on the GORT-4 than on the GORT-3, due to the re-norming of the measure, is provided in the manual. This information is crucial to clinicians for interpreting apparent score changes when reassessing children with the new test.

Use of Alternate Forms

At some ages, alternate form correlations were only in the .70 to .80 range. This means that at these ages, there is a portion of unique variance inherent in each form that could lead to children obtaining slightly different scores on the different forms. In a treatment situation, this could potentially complicate interpretation of posttreatment gains if different forms are administered pre- and posttreatment. In general, internal consistency correlations (>.90) as well as correlations for the same form administered twice (>.80) were higher than the intercorrelations of the two alternate forms at these ages. Notably, practice effects on the GORT-4 are practically nonexistent. For these reasons, clinicians might consider using the same form for testing posttreatment gains. Use of Form A would make the most sense, since there is virtually no validity information on Form B presented in the manual. Note that the manual recommends interpreting only ORQ in retest situations and using alternate forms.

Floor and Ceiling Effects

As is the case for many tests that assess skills that depend on schooling, the test likely has limited sensitivity and clinical utility in the youngest age band (6 years to 6 years, 5 months), given that not all children have been exposed to reading by their sixth birthday. In addition, the paragraph-reading format of the test does not allow more basic reading skills or prereading skills to be assessed, as is the case in other tests intended to cover a younger age group. This leads to floor effects. For instance, a Rate score of 0 yields a percentile of 16 in the youngest age band. There also appears to be a ceiling effect in the oldest age band (18 years to 18 years, 11 months) for some scores. For instance, the highest score possible for Rate and Comprehension for this group is 13 (84th percentile). While adequate for evaluating adolescents of average ability, this limits the use of the GORT-4 in the assessment of gifted older adolescents.

REFERENCES

Anastasi, A., & Urbina, S. (1997). *Psychological testing* (7th ed.). Upper Saddle River, NJ: Prentice-Hall.

Bryant, B. R., & Wiederholt, J. L. (1991). *Gray Oral Reading Tests—Diagnostic.* Austin, TX: PRO-ED.

Craig, H. K., Thompson, C. A., Washington, J. A., & Potter, S. L. (2004). Performance of elementary-grade African American students on the Grey Oral Reading Test. *Language, Speech, and Hearing Services in Schools, 35,* 141–154.

Stevens, K. B., & Price, J. R. (1999). Adult reading assessment: Are we doing the best with what we have? *Applied Neuropsychology, 6*(2), 68–78.

Wiederholt, J. L., & Blalock, G. (2000). *Gray Silent Reading Tests.* Austin, TX: PRO-ED.

Wiederholt, J. L., & Bryant, B. R. (2001). *Gray Oral Reading Tests—Fourth Edition: Examiner's manual.* Austin, TX: PRO-ED.

Wechsler Individual Achievement Test—Second Edition (WIAT-II)

PURPOSE

The Wechsler Individual Achievement Test—Second Edition (WIAT-II) is a comprehensive test battery intended to measure academic achievement.

SOURCE

The test can be obtained from The Psychological Corporation (www.wiatII.com). Materials include the Examiner's Manual, Scoring and Normative Supplement for Grades Pre-K to 12, Supplement for College Students and Adults, Stimulus Booklets 1 and 2, Word Card, Pseudoword Card, 25 Record Forms, and 25 Response Booklets. The scale costs about $340 US. Normative manuals and test editions for other countries, including Canada and the United Kingdom, can also be obtained from the publisher.

The Psychological Corporation provides various options for computer scoring, including a WIAT-II Scoring Assistant, and, to calculate ability-achievement discrepancies, various combined IQ/Achievement scoring programs (i.e., WISC-IV/WIAT-II, WAIS-III/WMS-III/WIAT-II). The cost is about $199 US. Training materials, including presentations and training CDs, are also available through the Web site.

AGE RANGE

The age range for administration differs somewhat, depending on the version used. For U.S. norms, the range includes ages 4 to 85 years and/or grades Pre-Kindergarten to 16. For Canadian norms, the age range extends from 5 to 19 years (i.e., adult norms are not yet available).

DESCRIPTION

Overview

The WIAT-II (The Psychological Corporation, 2002a) is a revision of the original WIAT (The Psychological Corporation, 1992). It is a comprehensive achievement battery intended to assist with diagnosis, eligibility/placement decisions, and intervention planning. It was specifically designed to cover each of the seven areas traditionally used to diagnose learning disabilities (i.e., word reading, reading comprehension, mathematics calculation, mathematics reasoning, listening comprehension, oral expression, and written expression) and to allow ability-achievement discrepancy analyses for purposes of diagnosing learning disabilities. The test yields five composite scores (Reading, Mathematics, Written Expression, Oral Language, and Total Composite) and Supplemental scores for some subtests (see Tables 7–5 and 7–6).

The WIAT-II is specifically designed to allow identification of significant achievement difficulties, and provides scores with a wide range to allow detection of low achievement levels (i.e., generally four standard deviations below the mean) as well as above-grade-level abilities (minimum of one standard deviation above the mean, with some subtests up to three standard deviations above the mean; but see *Comments*). Note that the WIAT-II is not intended to assess giftedness in older adolescents because of ceiling effects on some tests, as specified in the Examiner's Manual.

Changes to the WIAT

See Table 7–7 for a listing of specific changes from the WIAT. With regard to reading, the test was revised according to recommendations from the National Reading Panel (2000) and existing research on reading; these changes are outlined in the manual (e.g., separate reading rate and reading accuracy scores to assist in identifying different types of reading disability, addition of a measure of phonological decoding). Mathematics subtests were revised to be congruent with the Principles and Standards for School Mathematics (National Council of Teachers of Mathematics, 2000); other changes include the addition of multistep problem solving and items for preschoolers.

The revision of the written language subtests was undertaken to include words with varying morphological features (e.g., homonyms with context-dependent spelling). Written Expression includes timed alphabet writing, which is reportedly a strong predictor of skill acquisition in the primary grades (see Examiner's Manual for references), and covers a hierarchy of tasks selected to parallel the normal development of writing skills (i.e., alphabet writing, sentence combining, sentence generation, written word fluency).

According to the Examiner's Manual, Oral Language subtests were revised to mirror classroom demands, to help identify individuals in need of speech and language therapy, and to link language to reading. The inclusion of language tests in the battery is based on research suggesting that language skills are good predictors of reading skill in children.

The WIAT was criticized for inadequate floors and ceilings (Smith, 2001). Therefore, other aspects of the WIAT-II revision, in addition to updated norms, include an extended age range and the addition of items at each end of the difficulty spectrum to allow assessment of preacademic skills in preschoolers and of academic skills in adults.

A Qualitative Observations checklist was added to the Record Form to facilitate process analysis of performance during specific subtests. See Figure 7–1 for an example. A detachable Parent Report that describes subtest content and scores in lay language was also added to the Record Form. Scoring criteria were improved for subtests involving qualitative analysis (e.g., Reading Comprehension, Written Expression, Oral Expression).

Ability-Achievement Comparisons

The WIAT-II is linked (but not co-normed) with Wechsler intelligence scales to facilitate ability-achievement discrepancy analysis in the evaluation of learning disabilities. WIAT-II linking samples include the WAIS-III, WPPSI-III, and WISC-IV, as well as the older versions of these tests (i.e., WPPSI-R and WISC-III). Additionally, the WIAT-II is linked with the PAL-RW (Berninger, 2001) and the Academic Competence Evaluation Scales (DiPerna & Elliott, 2000). See *Normative Data* and *Comment* for a more detailed discussion.

ADMINISTRATION TIME

The test takes 45 minutes for young children and 1.5 to 2 hours for grades 3 to college/university level.

ADMINISTRATION

Materials

Administration requires blank paper for math and written tests, and eight pennies for Numerical Operations. Tape recording of responses is recommended for subtests requiring verbatim responses that must be qualitatively evaluated (Listening Comprehension, Oral Expression). Reading Comprehension may also require recording of verbatim responses for new test users. A tape is provided for examiners to learn the correct pronunciation of the Pseudoword Decoding test.

Table 7–5 WIAT-II Subtest Content and Grade Ranges

	Grade	Subtest Description
Reading Composite		
Word Reading	All	A single-word reading subtest that moves through several levels of difficulty: preschoolers and children in grades 1 and 2 are administered letter matching, letter naming, sound/phoneme discrimination, phoneme blending, and sound-letter correspondence tasks; grades 3 and up are administered a standard oral word reading task.
Pseudoword Decoding	1–16	Requires reading nonwords to measure phonological decoding and word attack skills.
Reading Comprehension	1–16	Early items consist of matching pictures to written words; later items involve answering questions about paragraphs; examinees can read the passages silently or aloud, and the passage remains visible to examinees as they answer comprehension questions; items are arranged in item sets based on grade level.*
Written Language Composite		
Spelling	1–16	Early items consist of name writing and letter/phoneme writing; later items proceed to a word dictation task.
Written Expression	All	This task includes items that reflect increasingly demanding aspects of written work: alphabet printing, sentence building, sentence generation with visual cues, and paragraph generation; items are arranged in item sets corresponding to grade level.*
Mathematics Composite		
Numerical Operations	K–16	Early items include number identification, matching, counting pennies, and number writing; later items consist of written computational math problems.
Mathematics Reasoning	All	The subject is asked to provide answers orally to questions involving math concepts (e.g., money, time, estimation, probability) based partially on information provided in visual form on the stimulus book.
Oral Language Composite		
Listening Comprehension	All	Composed of three sections: (1) *Receptive Vocabulary* (a four-picture receptive vocabulary test, similar to the PPVT-III), (2) *Sentence Comprehension* (a four-picture-choice auditory comprehension test), and (3) *Expressive Vocabulary* (requires the subject to provide words for an aurally presented definition matched to a picture cue).
Oral Expression	All	There are four tasks: (1) *Sentence Repetition* (administered only to young children in pre-K to grade 3), (2) *Word Fluency* (a verbal fluency task requiring the generation of as many words as possible in 60 seconds), (3) *Visual Passage Retell* (a story-generation task using visual cues; two items), and (4) *Giving Directions* (the child is asked to provide detailed directions to performing a specific task; with and without visual cueing; two items).*

*Supplemental scores available for these subtests are listed in Table 7-6.

Table 7–6 WIAT-II Standard Subtests That Yield Supplemental Scores

Standard Subtest	Supplemental Score
Reading Comprehension	Target Words
	Reading Speed
Written Expression	Alphabet Writing
	Word Fluency (written)
	Word Count
Oral Expression	Word Fluency (oral)

Administration

Users are highly encouraged to carefully read the three WIAT-II Manuals to familiarize themselves with these and other specifics of test administration. Selected administration points are highlighted below.

For some age/grade bands, different composites/subtests are available depending on whether age- or grade-based norms are used. Examiners should therefore plan their assessments with reference to the available norms for age and grade for the specific child they are testing. For instance, based on norms for age, three subtests are administered to 4-year-olds, four subtests to 5-year-olds, six subtests to 6-year-olds, and nine subtests to ages 7 and up. Grade-based norms call for a slightly different group of subtests, with four subtests for Pre-K, six subtests for K, and nine subtests for grades 1 and up. These differences should only matter when testing very young children or children whose age and grade do not match (e.g., a 6-year-old in Pre-K).

Subtest sequence should follow the order in the Record Form to conform to the standardization order. Subtest start points, stop points, and discontinue rules differ across subtests; these are indicated on the Record Form, on the Stimulus Booklets, and outlined on p. 24 of the Examiner's Manual. Discontinue criteria are generally six to seven failed responses.

Reading Comprehension is timed, and strict timing limits are used for Written Expression and Oral Expression. Timing is optional for Word Reading. Other subtests only employ timing guidelines, not actual time limits (i.e., the task must be completed within a given time limit, but the examinee is not timed).

Most subtests allow the examiner to record Qualitative Observations during testing, to provide process information. The examiner rates the subject on the frequency of certain specific error types or task approaches on a Likert scale.

Some specifics of administration should be noted. Unlike its predecessor, the WIAT-II uses item sets for Reading Comprehension and Written Expression instead of presenting items in order of increasing difficulty. Entry points are specified based on grade level, and all items are administered within the set. According to the authors, this ensures that each grade band covers various item types. However, the authors note that using the standard grade-based entry level may

result in unduly restricting the maximum score obtained by specific subjects whose academic knowledge may exceed their grade level (e.g., individuals who are self-taught). Therefore, in adults with limited education (less than nine years), modified administration instructions for Reading Comprehension and Written Expression should be used, as outlined in the Supplement (The Psychological Corporation, 2002c).

SCORING

Because of problems with the norms for Reading Comprehension, those who purchased the first printing of the norms manual (i.e., *Scoring and Normative Supplement for Grades Pre-K to 12* [2001]) must obtain a copy of the revised norms for Reading Comprehension (The Psychological Corporation, 2001).

Scoring instructions and U.S. normative data are contained in two manuals (*Scoring and Normative Supplement for Grades Pre-K to 12* and *Supplement for College Students and Adults*). Table numbers are identical in the two manuals to facilitate comparison across reference groups.

For subtests and composites, the test yields standard scores ($M = 100$, $SD = 15$) and percentile ranks for age and grade. There are four composite scores (see Table 7–5): Reading, Mathematics, Written Expression, and Oral Language. Note that the only composite available for 4-year-olds is Oral Language. However, if grade-based scores are used instead, both the Oral Language and Mathematics composites can be derived. These two composites can also be derived for 5-year-olds.

Standard scores are intended to range from 40 to 160; the actual range varies somewhat by age, grade, and subtest (see *Comment*). Age and grade equivalents, normal curve equivalents, stanines, quartile scores, and decile scores can also be derived.

Supplemental scores can also be derived for some subtests (see Table 7–6). Note that even though Listening Comprehension includes three subtasks (Receptive Vocabulary, Sentence Comprehension, and Expressive Vocabulary), separate Supplemental scores cannot be derived for each task. Similarly, only one of the three Oral Expression subtasks yields a Supplemental score (Word Fluency). Supplemental scores are described in quartile and/or decile form. Note that Reading Comprehension Supplemental scores can only be obtained by examinees who were administered their appropriate grade item set. According to the authors, Supplemental scores should not be used to make diagnostic decisions (see *Comment*).

For children and adolescents, age-based scores are provided for four-month intervals from ages 4 years to 13 years, 11 months, and in one-year intervals for ages 14 to 19 (see *Scoring and Normative Supplement for Grades Pre-K to 12*). For adults, scores are provided for five age bands: 17 to 19, 20 to 25, 26 to 35, 36 to 50, and 51 to 85 (see *Supplement for College Students and Adults*). Several tables are provided in these manuals to aid in score interpretation (e.g., significance of

Table 7–7 Processes Measured by the WIAT-II and WIAT

WIAT Subtest	Measures	WIAT-II Subtest	Measures
Basic Reading	• Accuracy of word recognition	Word Reading	• Letter identification • Phonological awareness • Alphabet principle (letter-sound awareness) • Accuracy of word recognition • Automaticity of word recognition
		Pseudoword Decoding	• Phonological decoding • Accuracy of word attack
Reading Comprehension	• Literal comprehension • Inferential comprehension	Reading Comprehension	• Literal comprehension • Inferential comprehension • Lexical comprehension • Reading rate • Oral reading accuracy • Oral reading fluency • Oral reading comprehension • Word recognition in context
Spelling	• Alphabet principle (sound-letter awareness) • Written spelling of regular and irregular words • Written spelling of homonyms integration of spelling and lexical comprehension)	Spelling	• Alphabet principle (sound-letter awareness) • Written spelling of regular and irregular words • Written spelling of homonyms (integration of spelling and lexical comprehension)
Written Expression	• Descriptive writing (evaluated on extension and elaboration, grammar and usage, ideas and development, organization, unity and coherence, and sentence structure and variety) • Narrative writing (evaluated on the same criteria as descriptive)	Written Expression	• Timed alphabet writing • Word fluency writing • Sentence combining • Sentence generation • Written responses to verbal and visual cues • Descriptive writing (evaluated on organization, vocabulary and mechanics) • Persuasive writing (evaluated on organization, vocabulary, theme development, and mechanics) • Writing fluency (based on word count)
Numerical Operations	• Numeral writing • Calculation (addition, subtraction, multiplication, division) • Fractions, decimals, algebra	Numerical Operations	• Counting • One-to-one correspondence • Numeral identification and writing • Calculation (addition, subtraction, multiplication, division) • Fractions, decimals, algebra
Mathematics Reasoning	• Quantitative concepts • Problem solving • Money, time, and measurement • Geometry • Reading and interpreting charts and graphs	Mathematics Reasoning	• Quantitative concepts • Multistep problem solving • Money, time, and measurement • Geometry • Reading and interpreting charts and graphs • Statistics and probability • Estimation • Identifying patterns

(*continued*)

Table 7–7 Processes Measured by the WIAT-II and WIAT (*continued*)

WIAT Subtest	Measures	WIAT-II Subtest	Measures
Listening Comprehension	• Receptive vocabulary • Listening literal comprehension • Listening-inferential	Listening Comprehension	• Receptive vocabulary • Expressive vocabulary • Listening-inferential comprehension
Oral Expression	• Expressive vocabulary • Giving directions • Explain steps in sequential tasks	Oral Expression	• Word fluency (oral) • Auditory short-term recall for contextual information • Story generation • Giving directions • Explaining steps in sequential tasks

Source: From The Psychological Corporation, 2002b.

differences and frequencies for subtest/average subtest discrepancies, significance of differences between subtests, and intersubtest scatter).

According to the *Supplement for College Students and Adults*, grade equivalents for adults (college age and adult) are only appropriate for adults who obtained standard scores of less than 85. Age equivalents are not provided for adults. As noted in *Administration*, special care must be employed in scoring results for adults with limited education (i.e., less than nine years; see *Comment* for further information on score interpretation).

Detailed information on scoring subtests that include subjective judgment (Reading Comprehension, Written Expression, and Oral Expression), including examples, can be found either in the *Scoring and Normative Supplement for Grades Pre-K to 12* (2002) or the *Supplement for College Students and Adults* (2002).

Note that for Reading Comprehension, specific item sets are administered according to grade level, which means that subtest scores for each set are weighted according to difficulty level before conversion to the Reading Comprehension standard score. Each of the Written Expression tasks must also be converted to quartiles before conversion to a standard score (i.e., Word Fluency, Paragraph Spelling Errors, Paragraph Punctuation Errors, Essay Spelling Errors, Essay Punctuation Errors). To derive the standard score for the Oral Expression subtest, Word Fluency must also first be weighted using tables in the Examiner's Manual. Given the multiple steps involved in scoring, use of the scoring software is highly recommended.

Qualitative Observations are not standardized and are intended for qualitative purposes only.

NORMATIVE DATA

There are several normative datasets for the WIAT-II, and the specifics regarding these datasets are somewhat scattered across the three main WIAT-II Manuals. Careful reading of all three manuals is therefore recommended. In some cases, the overlap

Figure 7–1 Example of WIAT-II Qualitative Observations Checklist. *Source:* From Record Form.

WORD READING QUALITATIVE OBSERVATIONS Note how frequently a behavior occurred by checking the appropriate box.	Never	Seldom	Often	Always	Not Observed
Substitutes a visually similar letter when identifying letters	☐	☐	☐	☐	☐
Provides nonword responses for rhyming words	☐	☐	☐	☐	☐
Pronounces words automatically	☐	☐	☐	☐	☐
Laboriously "sounds out" words	☐	☐	☐	☐	☐
Self-corrects errors	☐	☐	☐	☐	☐
Loses his/her place when reading words	☐	☐	☐	☐	☐
Makes accent errors	☐	☐	☐	☐	☐
Adds, omits, or transposes syllables when reading words	☐	☐	☐	☐	☐

Table 7–8 Ability-Achievement Linking Samples for the WIAT-II

Ability-Achievement Measures	Linking Sample Size	Age Range	IQ-WIAT-II Correlation
WPPSI-III and WIAT-II	208	4–7 years, 3 months	.78
WISC-IV and WIAT-II	550	6–16 years, 11 months	.87
WAIS-III and WIAT-II: K–12 Sample	95	16–19 years, 11 months	
WAIS-III and WIAT-II: College Sample	268	*	.71
WAIS-III and WIAT-II: Adult Sample	90**	***	.86

Note: IQ and achievement tests were not necessarily administered on the same day; Ability-Achievement correlations reflect the correlation between FSIQ and WIAT-II Total Achievement.

*Not indicated, but represents college students in grades 13–16. **Case weighting was applied to yield a final sample size of 100. ***Age unspecified.

Adapted from Wechsler, 2002a, Wechsler, 2003a, and The Psychological Corporation, 2002c.

between age-based and grade-based datasets is not clear, and norms for young adults seem to be available in three separate sources (e.g., K–12, college sample, and adult norms). As a result, gaining a full understanding of the different datasets and their uses demands considerable time and lends itself to confusion. This is even more of an issue for those using normative data for other countries (e.g., Canada or the United Kingdom) in addition to, or in place of, U.S. norms. This is because complete normative coverage is not always available, depending on the age of the examinee (e.g., as of this writing, there are no adult norms for the WIAT-II-Canadian).

Standardization—U.S. Normative Data

There are two main sets of U.S. norms: Pre-K to 12 and college and adult.

Pre-K to 12. U.S. norms include 4379 individuals; norms are stratified based on grade, age, gender, race/ethnicity, geographic region, and parental education according to 1998 Census data. This total includes individuals included in the grade-based norms (3600 individuals) and individuals included in the age-based norms (2950 individuals); 2171 participants were represented in both groups. The grade-based sample included 200 children in Pre-Kindergarten and aged 5 years; there were 300 participants in each of the other grades up to grade 8. Half of this sample was collected in the fall and half during the spring semester. Winter norms were extrapolated from this data for grades pre-K to 8. Grades 9 to 12 include 700 participants (200 each in grades 9 and 10, 150 each in grades 11 and 12). The age-based sample ranged from 4 years to 19 years, 11 months. Of the 2950 individuals in the age-based sample, 550 were aged 15 years to 19 years, 11 months; those attending college were excluded from this normative group.

College and Adult. These include a college sample composed of students in two-year colleges (*N* = 259) and students in four-year colleges/universities (*N* = 448).

The adult sample includes 500 participants from 17 to 85 years. Three age bands were case-weighted to produce a final standardization sample of 515. Five age bands of 100 individuals each were sampled (i.e., 17–20, 21–25, 26–35, 36–50, 51–85). These are detailed in the Supplement. Of these, 24% were in college, and 18% were in high school.

Linking Samples

Linking samples (Table 7–8) are provided for WIAT-II and the three main Wechsler tests (i.e., WPPSI-III, WISC-IV, and WAIS-III). The linking samples consist of individuals from the WIAT-II normative sample who were also administered a Wechsler IQ test for purposes of calculating ability-achievement discrepancies.

College and adult linking samples include 268 participants in college and 90 adults administered the WAIS-III and WIAT-II; the adult sample was case-weighted to better approximate the U.S. population (for a final total of 100 adults). Demographics of these samples are presented on p. 13 of the Supplement; the age for both groups is unspecified. Mean FSIQ of the college linking sample was 115, and that of the adult linking sample was 104. These are also presented in Table 7–8. Note that the adult sample is relatively small, given the age range it must cover.

Reading Comprehension Norms

According to the publisher, norms for the Reading Comprehension subtest were revised in November 2001 due to problems with the reverse rules when testing low-functioning subjects that resulted in overestimating scores. The revised Examiner's Manual with the newer norms for this subtest should have the word "Updated" in the upper right hand corner (publication date: 2002). How these norms were corrected is unclear.

RELIABILITY

Internal reliability

Grades Pre-K to 12. Internal reliability of the WIAT-II in this sample is for the most part excellent. Note that split-half reliability coefficients are presented for all subtests except Written Expression and Oral Expression, where stability coefficients were substituted (i.e., these tests cannot be split into two equivalent halves; see Examiner's Manual). Split-half coefficients for all remaining composite scores are very high for both grade- and age-based scores (i.e., $r = .94–.98$). In particular, the Total Composite score reliability is consistently very high across grade and age ($r = .98$). Of the four other composites, the Reading Composite is consistently high across all ages (i.e., $r = .97–.99$), which clearly exceeds the recommended standard of .95 for tests used for diagnostic purposes. The Mathematics and Written Language Composites have coefficients of .94 to .95 across age, with slightly higher or lower coefficients at different grades/ages; however, these too appear high enough for diagnostic decision making. While still high, reliabilities are slightly lower for the Oral Language Composite across grade and age categories ($r = .83–.91$).

At the subtest level, most reliabilities are in the high to very high range (>.80–.90). As expected given the very high Reading Composite reliability, the reading subtests have very strong reliability coefficients ($r = .97$; Word Reading and Pseudoword Decoding). Oral Expression subtest reliabilities are in the high range across age and grade ($r = .88–.89$). The reliability for Listening Comprehension is lower, particularly at age 4 and in the spring semester of pre-K ($r = .71$ and .72, respectively). However, it is important to note that reliabilities for ages 4 and 5 are estimates only, based on age 6/grade 1 data, due to insufficient sample size (see pp. 106–108, Examiner's Manual).

College and Adult. WIAT-II reliabilities in this sample are for the most part excellent, apart from slightly lower reliabilities for grade-based scores. Specifically, total Composite score reliability is very high for all five age bands ($r = .98$; see manual). Of the domain composites, Reading and Mathematics have very high average reliability across age ($r = .98$ and .96, respectively); composite reliabilities are also very respectable for Written Expression and Oral Language ($r = .92$ and .88, respectively).

At the subtest level, age-based reliability scores are very high for reading and mathematics subtests, high for Listening Comprehension, and acceptable for Written Expression and Oral Expression ($r = .77$ and .75, respectively, for the latter).

For grade-based scores (i.e., two or four years of college), reliability coefficients are somewhat lower. None of the composite score reliabilities, including that of the Total Composite, was higher than .95, and those for Mathematics and Oral Language were in the low .80s. At the subtest level, some subtests had reliabilities that were marginal (Reading Comprehension, Written Expression, Oral Expression; $r = .60–.69$). Subtest reliabilities are all very high for Word Reading, Numerical Operations, and Pseudoword Decoding ($r = >.90$), though none reach above .95.

Standard Error of Measurement

In the pre-K to grade 12 sample, consistent with the size of their respective reliability coefficients, *SEM*s across age and grade for the Total Composite score and Reading Composite are small (one to two standard score points). Mathematics and Written Language Composite *SEM*s are less than 4 (i.e., 3.4–3.8), while the *SEM* for Oral Language is slightly larger (i.e., four to five points), consistent with the slightly lower reliability for this subtest.

At the subtest level, the reading tasks (Word Reading and Pseudoword Decoding) have the smallest *SEM*s (i.e., two to three points) and Listening Comprehension has the largest *SEM*s (i.e., six to eight points), particularly in the youngest age/grade bands. *SEM*s for ages 4 to 5 and grades Pre-K to K are estimates only.

In the college and adult sample, *SEM*s for the age-based normative data are generally comparable to those for the pre-K to grade 12 norms. Grade-based (two- and four-year college) *SEM*s are slightly larger than those based on age, with Written Expression and Oral Expression having the largest *SEM*s (7 in the age-based sample, 8 to 9 in the grade-based sample). In the grade-based sample, Reading Comprehension *SEM*s are also considerable (i.e., 8) compared with other subtests involving reading (i.e., 4 to 5).

Test-Retest Reliability

Grades Pre-K to 12. Temporal stability is for the most part impressive in this sample. To test stability, 297 individuals in three age bands (6–9, 10–12, and 13–19) were tested twice with the WIAT-II over an average interval of 10 days (see manual). Composite stability was uniformly very high for all ages (>.91). Stability coefficients for the Reading Composite and Total score at all ages were particularly high (i.e., $r = .97–.98$). Overall, stability was high to very high for all subtests (see Table 7–9 for reliability classifications across age). Test-retest reliability information for younger children (ages 4 to 5/grades Pre-K to K) is not reported.

College and Adult. To test stability, 76 individuals were administered the WIAT-II twice over a mean interval of 11 days (age band, 17–20 years; see manual). Very high reliability was obtained for Total, Reading, and Mathematics composites (>.90), and only adequate stability for the Written Language composite. Subtest test-retest coefficients are shown in Table 7–9. At the subtest level, most reliabilities were high to very high; only Written Expression and Oral Expression had reliabilities that were only in the adequate range.

Practice Effects

In the Pre-K to grade 12 sample, on average, practice effects are relatively minimal (i.e., two to five standard score points; see manual). In the college and adult sample, practice effects

Table 7–9 Magnitude of Test-Retest Reliability Coefficients for WIAT-II Scores in Four Age Groups

Magnitude of Coefficient	Ages 6–9	Ages 10–12	Ages 13–19	Adults (17–20 yrs)
Very high (.90+)	Word Reading Numerical Operations Reading Comprehension Spelling Pseudoword Decoding Math Reasoning	Word Reading Numerical Operations Reading Comprehension Spelling Pseudoword Decoding Math Reasoning Listening Comprehension	Word Reading Numerical Operations Reading Comprehension Spelling Pseudoword Decoding Math Reasoning Listening Comprehension	Word Reading Numerical Operations Spelling Math Reasoning Listening Comprehension
High (.80–.89)	Written Expression Listening Comprehension Oral Expression	Written Expression Oral Expression	Written Expression Oral Expression	Reading Comprehension Pseudoword Decoding
Adequate (.70–.79)	—	—	—	Written Expression Oral Expression
Marginal (.60–.69)	—	—	—	
Low (<.59)	—	—	—	—

Note: Coefficients were corrected for variability.

on age-based standard scores are also minimal (one to four points) for subtests and composites (see manual).

Interscorer Reliability

Grades Pre-K to 12. Interrater reliability is higher for Reading Comprehension and Oral Expression than for Written Expression. Specifically, Reading Comprehension interrater reliability was very high ($r = .94$) in a large subsample of protocols scored twice (see Examiner's Manual), as were intraclass correlations for Oral Expression ($r = .96$). Intraclass correlations for Written Expression ranged from .71 to .94 ($M = .85$).

College and Adult. Interscorer reliability is very high for Reading Comprehension ($r = .94$); reliabilities for Written Expression were high in the adult age bands ($r = .80–.93$) but lower for college grades ($r = .72–.90$). Reliabilities for Oral Expression were high to very high across samples ($r = .88–.97$; see manual for more details).

VALIDITY

Content

According to the publishers, the WIAT-II content was based on comprehensive surveys of achievement test users, recommendations from experts, and review of the literature. The test was field-tested, and an empirically based item analysis was performed, including item response theory. Start points, stop points, and discontinue rules were all derived empirically based on standardization data. The rationale for inclusion of specific domains is well explained, as detailed in *Description.*

Composite and Subtest Intercorrelations

Grades Pre-K to 12. WIAT-II score intercorrelations are provided for each age group in the Examiner's Manual. Overall, composite scores are moderately to highly intercorrelated at all ages ($r = .51–.93$). The Total score is most highly correlated with the Reading composite (.86–.93). At the subtest level, Reading Composite subtests are highly intercorrelated at all age groups. Intercorrelations between subtests making up Mathematics and Written Expression Composites are also generally high. Only the Oral Language Composite has subtest intercorrelations that are generally below .50. Specifically, the correlations between Listening Comprehension and Oral Expression were below .50 for ages 10, 11, 12, and 14, and below .30 for ages 15 and 17 to 19. This raises some questions about the interpretation of the Oral Language composite as a unitary construct in these age ranges.

College and Adult. A similar pattern is obtained in this age group. Math and written language subtests are highly intercorrelated ($r = .73$ and .62, respectively; see manual). Reading subtests are also moderately to highly intercorrelated ($r = .47–.67$). As is the case with the Pre-K to 12 sample, the Oral Language subtests are only modestly intercorrelated ($r = .31$). In the adult sample, math subtests intercorrelations are very high ($r = .84$); those for Oral Language subtests are lower ($r = .54$).

Correlation With Intelligence Tests

Grades Pre-K to 12. As would be expected, the WIAT-II demonstrates strong correlations with FSIQ scores from Wechsler IQ tests (i.e., $r = .71–.87$; see also Table 7–8). Correlations between the WIAT-III and VIQ are in many cases higher than those involving FSIQ, likely due to the fact that the WIAT-II exhibits lesser correlations with PIQ. This is consistent with prior research indicating that the PIQ is a poor predictor of academic achievement in comparison to the VIQ (Kamphaus, 2001), including mathematics achievement. (Note, however, that subtests tapping fluid abilities may be good predictors of mathematics achievement; see *WJ III COG* review, in this volume, for an example.)

At the composite level, VIQ appears to be one of the stronger predictors of WIAT-II achievement. In preschoolers, FSIQ and VIQ are most highly correlated with the WIAT-II Oral Language composite, while PIQ shows higher correlations with the Mathematics composite. In school-age children, VIQ appears to be the strongest predictor of WIAT-II composites, including those purported to measure mathematics skills ($r = .59–.86$). Compared with VIQ and FSIQ, PIQ demonstrates only moderate to high correlations with all the WIAT-II composite scores, including both verbally based (Reading, Written Expression, Oral Language) and nonverbal achievement scores (Mathematics). In older adolescents assessed with the WAIS-III, overall intelligence and overall achievement are highly correlated ($r = .88$). The only noticeable difference between VIQ and PIQ is that VIQ is more highly associated with the Reading composite than is the PIQ. Both VIQ and PIQ are highly related to Mathematics, Written Language, and Oral Expression composites (see manual).

College and Adult. Correlations with WAIS-III FSIQ are high for all WIAT-II composites ($r = .62–.86$) except for a moderate correlation for Written Language in the college sample ($r = .46$) that the authors attribute to a restriction in range. WIAT-II/WAIS-III correlations are presented in Table 7–9. As is the case in the younger age sample, VIQ is a better predictor of achievement than is PIQ for WIAT-II composites in this age group.

Comparison of the WIAT-II with the WIAT

Correlations between the two versions are high for Reading and Mathematics composites ($r = .91$ and .87, respectively), but considerably lower for those subtests that were significantly revised (i.e., $r = .45$, Written Expression; $r = .29$, Oral Expression). These findings are based on data from 70 children administered both measures (age 7–15) described in the Examiner's Manual. WIAT scores were generally higher than WIAT-II scores, though this was not always the case (e.g., Written Expression). Mean differences between versions were minimal for most subtests (one to three points) except for Oral Language, which showed a 9.4 point difference between versions, and the mean WIAT Oral Expression subtest score was almost 10 points higher than its WIAT-II equivalent. These results suggest care in interpreting Written Language and Oral Language retest scores in children originally tested with the WIAT and retested with the WIAT-II.

Correlations With Other Achievement Measures

Grades Pre-K to 12. Correlations between the WIAT-II and various tests of achievement are reviewed in the Examiner's Manual, including the PAL-RW (Berninger, 2001). Correlations between the WRAT-3 subtests and corresponding WIAT-II composites (e.g., WRAT-3 Reading and WIAT-II Reading) are all high ($r = .70–.79$), and the mean scores were within one standard score point ($N = 36$). However, correlations to noncorresponding composites (e.g., WRAT-3 Reading with WIAT-II Math) are not reported, so it is difficult to assess whether these support the discriminant validity of the composite scores. In the case of the DAS, less agreement was found between WIAT-II Reading composite and DAS Word Reading ($r = .31$). In a group of young children ($N = 64$, age 4–7 years), PPVT-III scores were more strongly correlated with the WIAT-II Reading subtests and Reading Composite ($r = .60–.75$) than with Listening Comprehension, a subtest that employs a similar testing format in one of its subtasks ($r = .44$; $N = 64$).

WIAT-II composites also correlated highly with corresponding scores from group-administered achievement tests that use multiple-choice response formats ($r \geq .60$; Stanford Achievement Tests, Ninth Edition, Harcourt Educational Measurement, 1996; Metropolitan Achievement Tests, Eighth Edition, Harcourt Educational Measurement, 1999). Again, correlations for noncorresponding tests were not reported in the manual; this limits interpretation of discriminant validity.

Correlations With Intelligence Tests

College and Adult. Correlations with the WJ-R were high for composites ($r = .73–.79$) for 48 college students described in the manual. Subtests measuring similar domains were correlated to a moderate to high degree. Notably, correlations between reading comprehension subtests were only .49, which indicates that the presentation mode and format of reading comprehension subtests may be important in determining the final score in a diagnostic situation (the WJ-R differs in its presentation mode in that the subject must provide missing words from a written passage). Similar results were obtained for written expression subtests ($r = .47$). WJ-R scores were also higher on average (i.e., over 10 points for the reading composite), which may relate to the year in which it was standardized (1989). Lesser differences are expected with the newer revision (WJ III).

Correlations With School Grades

WIAT-II correlations with school grades are also reviewed in the Examiner's Manual for 313 school-age students. The test publisher notes that school grades reflect an element of subjectivity that is not present in standardized tests due to the variability in grade assignment across individual teachers. However, tests of achievement should correlate well with school grades because the ultimate purpose of achievement tests is to predict school achievement, to correctly identify those who will need specific interventions. The Examiner's Manual presents data for grades 1 to 6 (primarily reading, mathematics, and spelling) and 7 to 12 (primarily English and mathematics).

The Total Composite was a good predictor of grades in several content domains, including reading grades and spelling grades ($r = .60$ and $.57$, respectively). Interestingly, correlations between reading grades and Written Language and Oral Language composites were slightly higher ($r = .57$ and $.53$, respectively) than those involving Reading and Mathematics composites ($r = .46$, and $.45$, respectively).

At the subtest level, reading grades were not as highly correlated with reading subtests ($r = .40–.44$) as they were to subtests measuring other aspects of language-based instruction, including Spelling, Written Expression, and Listening Comprehension ($r = .52, .56,$ and $.51$). Spelling grade was also more related to the WIAT-II Total Composite than to the Spelling subtest itself ($r = .34$). In adolescents, English grade was most correlated to the Written Language Composite ($r = .43$); correlations between English grades with individual reading subtests were only modest ($r = .23–.27$), while math grades were most related to the Math Reasoning subtest and Total Composite score ($r = .51$ and $.48$, respectively). These data have implications for using WIAT-II scores to predict school achievement in individual patients in that specific subtests/composites were not always the best predictors of grades in corresponding content domains.

Clinical Groups

Grades Pre-K to 12. Studies with clinical groups reported in the Examiner's Manual support the validity of the WIAT-II; these include small groups of children with giftedness, mental retardation, learning disability, and ADHD.

Gifted children ($N = 123$) showed an average WIAT-II Total score of almost 125, with the highest scores attained on the Mathematics composite (124) and the lowest on the Oral Language composite (118) compared with matched controls. Although these numbers are not technically consistent with giftedness, these numbers are in the expected range, given that the WIAT-II is not intended to measure giftedness and has ceiling effects that would attenuate high scores in older adolescents. Composite and subtest means were all consistently below 70 in a group of children with mild mental retardation ($N = 36$); in this group, the highest score was on the Oral Language composite (i.e., 63).

Two groups of children with learning disabilities are also described. In a group of children with reading disabilities ($N = 162$), the Reading Composite was 24 points lower than that of a matched control group. Written Language differences were also large (almost 23 points) as were those for Mathematics (almost 20 points). In a group with learning disabilities not specific to reading ($N = 81$), the Mathematics Composite was lowest (i.e., by almost 24 points) compared

with a matched control group. However, the Reading and Written Language composites were also significantly lower (about 22 points each). In both these learning disability groups, the Oral Language composite was least different between groups (about 10 points), and the smallest group difference at the subtest level was for Oral Expression (six to seven points).

In a group with ADHD ($N = 178$), the Written Language and Mathematics Composites were both significantly lower than those of a matched control group by about eight points. The Reading Composite was about six points lower, and the Oral Language Composite again showed the least discrimination between groups (three points); this was also the case in a comorbid ADHD/learning disabilities group ($M = 51$). In a group of young children with expressive language impairments (with or without receptive difficulties; $N = 49$, ages 5–8), the Reading Composite was most depressed when compared with matched controls (approximately 19 points), and one of its subtests, Pseudoword Decoding, showed the largest discrimination between groups (16 points). Of note, the Oral Language composite only differed between groups by nine points, even though this composite is specifically intended to measure language skills.

Percentages of children in each of these clinical groups obtaining subtest and composite scores below a significant clinical cutoff of 70 are presented on pages 141 and 142 of the Examiner's Manual. The data indicate that 53% of a reading disability group obtained broadly normal scores (i.e., >70) on the WIAT-II composites, along with 48% of a nonreading learning disability group, 87% of an ADHD group, 71% of an ADHD/LD group, and 80% of a speech/language impairment group. None of the mental retardation group obtained scores above 70 on any composite. Notably, matched controls had a very low base rate of impaired scores on WIAT-II composites (i.e., maximum of 10% with impaired scores, depending on the sample, or 90% or more correctly identified by the test). In sum, although the WIAT-II provides preliminary evidence of strong specificity (i.e., few normal individuals are incorrectly classified), the sensitivity of its composites to disorders of reading (and particularly language) deserve further study.

The original WIAT's Written Expression appears less sensitive than the written expression subtest of the WJ-R in identifying children for special education services (Brown et al., 2000), but has better psychometric properties than the equivalent PIAT-R score (Muenz et al., 1999). With regard to math, the original WIAT yielded higher scores than its equivalent Key Math-Revised scale in African American students (Wickes et al., 1999). Further independent research is needed to confirm whether these or other findings also apply to the WIAT-II.

College and Adult. Two studies reported in the Supplement support the use of the WIAT-II in assessing learning disabilities in this age group. In 41 college students with reading disabilities compared with matched controls, the lowest composite score was Reading ($M = 74$), while the Mathematics composite was within normal limits. At the subtest level, the largest differences were for Word Reading and Pseudoword Decoding, which were both over 27 points lower in the learning disabled group; Reading Comprehension differences were not as large, suggesting that this subtest is less sensitive to reading disabilities in this age group. Although the authors note that language skills are related to reading disabilities, there were no significant differences in Oral Language composite scores between groups. In a group of 22 college students with learning disabilities other than reading, the pattern was reversed, with the lowest scores occurring in subtests and composites relating to mathematics. Although of interest, these data contribute little to our understanding of the WIAT-II's diagnostic utility in identifying reading disorders in adults, because of a lack of inclusion of classification accuracy statistics (i.e., sensitivity, specificity, positive predictive power, etc.).

COMMENT

The WIAT-II's psychometric properties are sound, it is well-grounded in research and theory, and because of its links to the Wechsler scales, it is likely to remain one of the main tools for assessing academic skills in children and adults. Its strengths include extensive norms, an easy-to-administer format with attractive and portable materials, and strong reliability and validity evidence for the majority of composites. However, the WIAT-II has some significant limitations that users should be aware of.

Usability

Although relatively simple to administer for experienced examiners, the test itself is quite complex in terms of its scoring and normative sets. Although users should familiarize themselves with all three WIAT-II Manuals to competently administer and interpret the test, this is a daunting task due to the volume and complexity of the information provided. Although the publisher has endeavored to make the manuals user-friendly and appealing, from a user's perspective, the sheer volume of information can be overwhelming, and some of this information (i.e., similarities and differences of adult linking samples) is somewhat scattered within and across the different manuals. Scoring Written Expression can be quite lengthy, and requires careful attention to guidelines in the manual.

Use of the software for scoring is highly recommended given the number of scores and steps involved, but this should not absolve users from fully familiarizing themselves with the test manuals and specific score ranges across age/grade bands for the different WIAT-II subtests.

Normative Data

Some of the criticisms leveled against the WIAT, the WIAT-II's predecessor, still stand. These include the use of case-weighting to adjust the standardization samples and linking samples, and

the limited demographic details on linking samples (Smith, 2001). One of the most salient limitations, in our view, is the somewhat fractionated linking samples, which arise because the WIAT-II appeared during the process of restandardization of all the major Wechsler IQ tests. As of this writing, the only currently used Wechsler scale that was actually normed at the same time as the WIAT-II is the WAIS-III. For other linking samples, ability-achievement discrepancies rest on data from standardization efforts that occurred after publication of the WIAT-II (i.e., WPPSI-III and WISC-IV). In addition, all of the WIAT-II linking samples represent relatively small subsamples compared to the size of the full standardization samples involved. For example, the adult linking sample for the WAIS-III consists of 90 cases, which is a relatively small sample given the age range over which it extends. Ideally, ability-achievement scores should be based on normative samples that were collected contemporaneously (Reynolds, 1990), so that preexisting differences between scale means caused by the Flynn effect do not confound score discrepancies. (Note that cohort effects are clearly an issue for WIAT-II ability-achievement discrepancies involving the WISC-III and WPPSI-R.)

Although this is clearly stated in the manuals, it is important to note that the WIAT-II is not "co-normed" with Wechsler IQ tests. A truly co-normed IQ-achievement normative dataset, such as that employed by the WJ III, collected contemporaneously on the entire standardization sample, would have been preferable. The Examiner's Manual notes that examiners should be fully cognizant of the known limitations of ability-achievement discrepancies in diagnosing learning disabilities (Reynolds, 1990; see also Kamphaus, 2001).

Floor and Ceiling Effects

The manual states that the WIAT-II allows detection of severe achievement difficulties because its floor is low enough to detect performances four standard deviations below the mean across subtests. Although this is true for most school-age ranges, floor effects are evident at both ends of the age spectrum. For example, floor effects are present for older adults on Pseudoword Decoding (i.e., the lowest possible score in adults over 51 years of age is 72). For floor and ceiling effects in other age groups, see later discussion.

Use of the WIAT-II With Preschoolers and Children at School Entry

One of the goals of the revision was to allow comprehensive assessment of preacademic skills to "facilitate early identification and intervention in young children at risk for academic failure" (Examiner's Manual, p. 2). To do this, the publishers extended the age range down to 4 years and added a number of simple items to extend the floor of the test. Although these additions have not made the test suitable for assessing preacademic delays in preschoolers, they have improved the test for use in school-entry-age children (e.g., age 6/grade 1). Specifically, the score ranges at the youngest ages are clearly insufficient for detecting preacademic delays, particularly in preschoolers with low average or lower intelligence, because of significant floor effects (e.g., in 4-year-olds, the lowest possible standard score for Word Reading is 84; for Math Reasoning, it is 70). In contrast, at age 6, the lowest scores for these subtests are 64 and 56, respectively, due to the inclusion of the very easy items designed for preschoolers. Therefore, although the inclusion of easy items to extend the age range resulted in a better floor for children at school entry (age 6/grade 1), floor effects are significant enough to question the use of the test in assessing 4- or 5-year-olds with suspected achievement delays.

Other issues limit its use in this age group. Although it is designed as a comprehensive assessment, the WIAT-II only allows evaluation of one composite score in 4-year-olds (Oral Language, based on two subtests) and two composites in 5-year-olds (Oral Language and Mathematics, based on four subtests). In addition, it is important to note that in this age group, internal reliability coefficients and *SEM*s for the Oral Language composite are partially based on an estimate from the data of older children, not on actual reliability data for this age group. Further, test-retest reliability is entirely lacking for this age group on all subtests. Obviously, assessing preacademic skills in preschoolers is not an easy task. However, in the younger age/grade bands, a better choice might be batteries specifically aimed at assessing preacademic skills and language in preschoolers, with demonstrated reliability and validity.

Users should also be cognizant that floor effects are also present on some subtests for school-age children. For instance, Pseudoword Decoding has, according to the test publisher's Web site, a "natural floor" for children below grade 3, due to the fact that reading skills are developing during this time. This results in an overestimation of scores for grades 1 to 2. The Web site recommends that when interpreting data for first-grade children, Word Reading be used instead of Pseudoword Decoding.

Use of the WIAT-II With Adolescents and Adults

Ceilings are a problem for assessing high-functioning older adolescents. For example, in grade 12, the maximum possible scores for Pseudoword Decoding and Word Reading are 124 and 118, respectively. Therefore, the test is not suitable for assessing giftedness in older adolescents or adults. Other achievement batteries are a better choice in this age range (e.g., WJ III). This limitation is clearly stated in the Examiner's Manual.

The choice of norms in young adults (e.g., around age 19) is extremely confusing. For instance, for individuals aged 17 to 19, five different norms tables can be used (Pre-K to 12: Age Based; Pre-K to 12: Grade Based; College: Two Year; College: Four Year; or Adult). Although not explicitly stated, it appears that the Pre-K to 12 norms should be used for all high school students up to age 19, even those whose age overlaps with the adult norms. With college students, college norms should also be chosen carefully, because two- and four-year college students in the standardization sample ob-

tained different raw scores on all subtests except Pseudoword Decoding (Supplement, p. 14). Strangely, the adult norms also include individuals who were enrolled in college and high school, though it appears that these norms might be more appropriate for young adults who are not currently in school. More guidance on the choice of norms for young adults would be helpful.

Diagnosing Learning Disability and Use of Ability-Achievement Discrepancies

In conducting this kind of analysis, age-based standard scores must be used to compute ability-achievement discrepancies. If the purpose is to compare the student's scores with those of peers in the same grade, grade-based scores should be used. According to the Supplement, differences between grade- and age-based standard scores are expected due to differences in the normative groups used to derive these scores. It is unclear what procedure should be followed when one encounters a discrepancy between age- and grade-based discrepancy analyses. However, this problem is not unique to the WIAT-II. In particular, the WIAT-II presents problems because of the additional complication of different linking samples for different age groups and slightly different age- and grade-based normative groups.

The manual recommends that the Total Achievement score be interpreted with caution and not be used in ability-achievement discrepancy analyses because of "the diverse nature of the scores that it represents" (p. 149). According to the Examiner's Manual, the Total Composite score appears to be a strong predictor of school success as measured by school grades, and is more correlated with reading grades than the Reading composite or reading subtests. This suggests that, despite the manual's recommendation, the prediction of a child's potential in reading (as measured by school grades) should take into account the Total Composite score (and possibly, scores for other language-based composites) in addition to the Reading composite. With regard to diagnosing reading disability, the publisher indicates that "a low score in *either* Word Reading or Pseudoword Decoding is indicative of a Basic Reading deficit" (FAQs, publisher's Web site). However, the actual diagnostic sensitivities of these subtests is unknown. Further, when used together to detect learning disability, the sensitivity of all the WIAT-II composite scores is clearly below par (see *Validity, Clinical Studies*), even though its specificity appears good. Users should also check subtest floors for specific age ranges when interpreting scores in children suspected of learning disabilities, as floor effects may attenuate ability-achievement discrepancies at some ages. Further research on the diagnostic utility of the test, particularly independent studies, is clearly needed.

Supplemental Scores

The publisher states that Supplemental scores are intended to delineate areas of strengths and weaknesses, but should not be used for diagnosis or eligibility decisions. Instead, these can be used by IEP teams to design accommodations for students (publisher's Web site). However, interpretation of Supplemental scores is not recommended due to the lack of reliability and validity evidence. This means that reading scores for accuracy (Total Words) and speed (Reading Rate) should not be used to diagnose specific types of reading disability, despite the fact that these scores were added to the WIAT-II to help differentiate between reading disability subtypes. The lack of psychometric validation for Supplemental scores is also unfortunate for neuropsychologists, as two of the Supplemental scores are of particular relevance (i.e., oral and written Word Fluency).

Language Assessment and the WIAT-II

Some specific limitations of the Oral Language composite and subtests should be mentioned. Although the manual states that these can help identify individuals in need of speech and language therapy, Oral Language scores should be used with caution in diagnosing speech and language delays and language-based learning disabilities. The Oral Language composite has weaker psychometric properties than the other WIAT-II composites, including modest intercorrelations of composite subtests at some ages and a reliability level that is inadequate for diagnostic decision making. Most important, this composite, along with other WIAT-II composites, identified only a small fraction of children with speech/language impairments in a clinical study described in the manual (see *Validity, Clinical Groups*). Similarly, the Oral Language composite did not discriminate well between learning disability groups and matched controls, or in younger children, between those with and without language impairment (see *Validity, Clinical Groups*).

Listening Comprehension and Oral Expression subtests contain "subtasks" that each assess somewhat distinct abilities and employ only a small number of items, presumably to keep each subtest short. This likely results in a subtest and composite score that is multifactorial in nature. There may be utility in using a multifactorial score to predict a multifactorial ability such as school achievement, but less utility when determining the specific linguistic strengths and weaknesses for diagnostic or intervention purposes. Use of more established tests, upon which some subtasks appear to be modeled (e.g., PPVT-III), may therefore be preferable when making diagnostic decisions. Also note that one of the Oral Expression tasks presents visual cues, some of which may facilitate word retrieval in some subjects. Until there is more research on the WIAT-II language subtests, users may therefore look to other tests designed specifically for assessing language in children where language deficits are presumed to underlie a learning disability.

Reading Comprehension Subtest

Again, users who purchased the first printing of the test should be aware of a problem with the early norms for Reading Comprehension (see *Normative Data*) and obtain updated normative information and scoring programs.

Unlike most other subtests, Reading Comprehension employs item sets to facilitate administration and keep testing time reasonably short. However, the item set format has inherent limitations when assessing low-functioning children whose abilities may not match their grade-based start point. The provision of visual cues for some items, and the use of a combined overall score reflecting comprehension, decoding, and speed, also limit usability. Given the weaker sensitivity of the Reading Comprehension subtest to reading disability (see *Validity*), reading disability diagnoses based on Reading Comprehension scores alone are not recommended.

Other Features

More evidence is needed regarding the utility of the Parent Report, which some users believe may raise the risk that parents are not provided with a full narrative report or feedback session. However, these forms may be useful for structuring feedback to parents, and serve as a reminder to translate the test results into relevant terms for parents. The Qualitative Observations may best be viewed as a useful way of keeping track of process elements of performance. However, as is the case for observational measures during testing, some elements are difficult to rate because they may represent covert behaviors (e.g., "uses context clues when decoding unknown words"). Additionally, although the WIAT-II is intended to allow a more process-based assessment, these ratings should be used with considerable caution in diagnostic decision making because their psychometric properties and predictive validity are unknown.

REFERENCES

Berninger, V. (2001). *Process assessment of the learner: Test battery for reading and writing.* San Antonio, TX: The Psychological Corporation.

Brown, M. B., Giandenoto, M. J., & Bolen, L. M. (2000). Diagnosing written language disabilities using the Woodcock-Johnson tests of educational achievement—revised and the Wechsler Individual Achievement Test. *Psychological Reports, 86*(1), 197–204.

DiPerna, J. C., & Elliott, S. N. (2000). *Academic Competence Evaluation Scales—manual K-12.* San Antonio, TX: The Psychological Corporation.

Individuals with Disabilities Education Act Amendment of 1997, 20 U.S.C. 1400 *et seq.* (Fed. Reg. 64, 1999).

Kamphaus, R. W. (2001). *Clinical assessment of child and adolescent intelligence* (2nd ed.). Boston: Allyn & Bacon.

Muenz, T. A., Ouchi, J. C., & Cole, J. C. (1999). Item analysis of written expression scoring systems from the PIAT-R and the WIAT. *Psychology in the Schools, 36*(1), 31–40.

National Council of Teachers of Mathematics. (2000). *Principles and standards for school mathematics.* Reston, VA: Author.

National Reading Panel. (2000). *Teaching children to read: An evidence-based assessment of the scientific research literature on reading and its implications for reading instruction (NIH Publication*

No. 00-4754). Washington, DC: National Institute of Child Health and Human Development.

The Psychological Corporation. (1992). *Wechsler Individual Achievement Test*. San Antonio, TX: Author.

The Psychological Corporation. (2001). *Administering and calculating conversion scores for Reading Comprehension*. San Antonio, TX: Author.

The Psychological Corporation. (2002a). *Wechsler Individual Achievement Test—Second Edition*. San Antonio, TX: Author.

The Psychological Corporation. (2002b). *Wechsler Individual Achievement Test—Second Edition: Examiner's manual*. San Antonio, TX: Author.

The Psychological Corporation. (2002c). *Wechsler Individual Achievement Test—Second Edition: Supplement for college students and adults*. San Antonio, TX: Author.

The Psychological Corporation. (2002d). *Wechsler Individual Achievement Test—Second Edition: Canadian scoring and normative supplement for grades K–16*. San Antonio, TX: Author.

Reynolds, C. R. (1990). Conceptual and technical problems in learning disability diagnosis. In C. R. Reynolds & R. W. Kamphaus (Eds.), *Handbook of psychological and education assessment of children: Intelligence and achievement* (pp. 571–592). New York: Guilford Press.

Smith, J. K. (2001). *Essentials of individual achievement assessment*. New York: John Wiley & Sons.

Wechsler, D. (1997). *Wechsler Adult Intelligence Scale—Third Edition*. San Antonio, TX: The Psychological Corporation.

Wechsler, D. (2002). *Wechsler Preschool and Primary Scale of Intelligence—Third Edition technical and interpretive manual*. San Antonio, TX: The Psychological Corporation.

Wechsler, D. (2003). *Wechsler Intelligence Scale for Children—Fourth Edition technical and interpretive manual*. San Antonio, TX: The Psychological Corporation.

Wickes, K., & Slate, J. R. (1999). Math and reading tests: Dissimilar scores provided by similar measures for African-American students. *Research in the Schools, 6*(1), 41–45.

Wide Range Achievement Test—3 (WRAT-3)

PURPOSE

The WRAT-3 is an individually administered screening test of academic achievement.

SOURCE

The test, including the two Alternate Forms, Manual, and Reading/Spelling Cards, can be ordered from Psychological Assessment Resources (PAR; www.parinc.com), at a cost of approximately $150 US. A computer scoring program is also available for about $129 US.

AGE RANGE

The age range is 5 years to 74 years, 11 months.

DESCRIPTION

The WRAT has a long history; it traces its roots to 1936, when it was developed to serve as an adjunct to the Wechsler-Bellevue (Smith, 2001). Revisions appeared in 1946, 1965, 1976, 1978 (WRAT, Jastak & Jastak, 1978), 1984 (WRAT-R, Jastak & Wilkinson, 1984), and most recently, in 1993. This latest revision, the WRAT-3 (Wilkinson, 1993), differs only slightly in item content from its predecessors. As Smith (2001) observed, despite its known limitations (see *Comment*), it remains one of the most frequently used measures of academic achievement (Harrison et al., 1994; Hutton et al., 1992; Sellers & Medler, 1992). Surveys place it among the top ten tests used by neuropsychologists (e.g., Camara et al., 2000). In one survey, the WRAT Reading subtest was ranked as the most used reading test for adult neuropsychological evaluations, used by almost 75% of respondents (Stevens & Price, 1999).

According to its author, the goal of the WRAT-3 is to "measure the codes which are needed to learn the basic skills of reading, spelling and arithmetic," and in conjunction with a test of general intelligence, to aid in the determination of learning disability (manual, p. 10).

The test consists of three subtests: Reading, Spelling, and Arithmetic. The Reading subtest measures letter and word recognition. The Spelling subtest measures name writing, letter writing, and single-word dictation. The Arithmetic subtest measures counting, basic arithmetic, and written computation. The same form is administered to all ages and is available in two alternate versions (Blue and Tan). Both versions can also be administered in a single session (Combined Form). According to the author, the Combined Form provides a finer breakdown of grade scores and can be used to provide "more opportunity for performance observation" for those interested in qualitative aspects of performance (manual, p. 9). However, most users administer only one of the forms.

ADMINISTRATION TIME

Each form takes about 15 to 30 minutes.

ADMINISTRATION

See *Source*. The test is very easy to administer. Each subtest has two sections (easy items for those aged 5 to 7 years and harder items for those 8 years and older). For Reading and Spelling, reverse and discontinue rules are known as the "5/10 Rules." The "5" means that if an individual 8 years or over obtains a score of less than 5, then the easy items must be administered. The "10" rule refers to the discontinue criterion of 10 consecutive failed responses. Examinees are given 15 minutes to complete the Arithmetic subtest. Despite the test's apparent simplicity, users should be aware that the most common error in using the test consists of improperly establishing basal and ceiling levels (Peterson et al., 1991; see also *Scoring*).

The Reading test must be administered individually, but the Spelling and Arithmetic tests may be administered in a small group setting. The three subtests can be given in any order (but see *Normative Data*).

SCORING

For each subtest, the total number correct is recorded. Raw scores for each task can be converted to standard scores ($M = 100, SD = 15$) and percentiles using tables in the manual for each of the Blue, Tan, and Combined forms. Absolute scores, grade scores, stanines, scaled scores, T scores, and normal curve equivalents are also provided. There is no general composite score for overall performance across the three domains.

Standard scores range from 45 to 155 for most ages (but see *Comment*). As noted previously, despite its ease of scoring, users of the WRAT-3 may be prone to scoring errors. Surprisingly, in a small sample of WRAT-R protocols, 95% of protocols had scoring errors, with an average of three errors per protocol (Peterson et al., 1991).

DEMOGRAPHIC EFFECTS

Age

WRAT-3 scores show an expected developmental curve; mean test scores show a steady increase until the 45- to 54-year-old age group. After this age, when cross-sectional data are considered, scores begin to decline (see manual).

Gender

There are no reported gender effects on the test.

Ethnicity

There is a lack of information on whether the WRAT-3 is appropriate for use in cross-cultural contexts. Item bias studies were performed on the WRAT-R only, which indicated that there was a "slight, but consistent" bias against non-whites for the Arithmetic subtest. The WRAT-3 Arithmetic was therefore lengthened to 15 minutes to reduce the effect of speed, which was felt to contribute to the effect. However, no information on whether this was successful in reducing bias is provided in the manual.

Education

Academic tests are invariably related to educational level. However, WRAT-3 norms are not broken down by education, nor are education effects described in the manual. One study reported that in adults with schizophrenia, WRAT-3 Reading scores were moderately related to education ($r = .38$; Wilk et al., 2004).

IQ

Correlations to IQ tests shown in the manual (i.e., WISC-III, WAIS-R) indicate moderate to high association with IQ for the Combined form (i.e., .49–.60; see also Lucas et al., 2003). See also *Validity*.

NORMATIVE DATA

Standardization Sample

The WRAT-3 was standardized on a large American sample ($N = 4433$) stratified according to age, regional residence, gender, and ethnicity based on 1990 U.S. Census data. Norms were collected in 1992 and 1993. There are approximately 100 individuals in each age band. See Table 7–10 for sample characteristics.

Individuals in the normative sample were administered the Blue and Tan versions in counterbalanced order. The manual notes that Spelling and Arithmetic tests could be administered in small groups, and in larger groups in the adult sample "if the examiner felt that the examination conditions did not affect test performance" (p. 28). Although the author states that the subtests can be administered in any order, no information is presented on whether subtests were administered in a specific order in the standardization sample (see *Comment* for further discussion).

RELIABILITY

Internal Consistency

This varies somewhat with age and test form. As would be expected given the higher number of items, the Combined form has the highest reliability at all ages. Median reliabilities across age for Combined Reading, Spelling, and Arithmetic are .95, .95, and .92, respectively. Across age, Combined form reliabilities are highest at the older age ranges (i.e., most are larger than .90). Only the Reading Combined and Spelling Combined forms have reliabilities that exceed .95 at certain ages (see manual for details). Reliability for Combined Arithmetic is marginally adequate in the youngest age band ($r = .72$ for age 5).

For the Blue form, median reliabilities for Reading, Spelling, and Arithmetic are high to very high (.86–.91). As with the Combined form, reliabilities also tend to increase with age. Reading reliability coefficients are above .90 for almost all ages, though none is above .95. Blue Spelling reliabilities across age are also high, particularly in the oldest age bands (.83–.95). Blue Mathematics reliabilities are slightly lower (.69–.92), with only a marginal reliability in the lowest age band ($r = .69$, age 5). Tan form reliabilities are quite similar to those of the Blue form across age.

Table 7–10 WRAT-3 Normative Sample Characteristics

Number	4433
Age	5 to 74 years, 11 months[a]
Geographic location	According to four main regions in the United States: North Central, South, East, and West
Sample type	National, stratified random standardization sample[b]
Education/parental education	Not specified
SES	Based on occupation (see below)
Gender	
Males	51%
Females	49%
Race	
White	72%
Black	14%
Hispanic	11%
Other	4%
Occupational group/parent occupational group	
Managerial and professional	25%
Technical, sales, and administrative support	31%
Precision production, craft, and repair	13%
Operators, fabricators, and laborers	15%
Service, farming, and fishing occupations	16%
Screening	Special education students were not excluded; subjects were only excluded if they were physically unable to respond to test items.

[a]Based on 23 separate age bands, with smaller age bands in younger subjects to adequately capture developmental progression of skills. [b]Based on 1990 U.S. Census data, stratified by age, gender, race, ethnicity, geographic region, and socioeconomic level.

Source: Adapted from Wilkinson, 1993.

Standard Error of Measurement

Average *SEM*s across age range from three to four points for Combined Reading, Spelling, and Arithmetic. *SEM*s for Blue and Tan Reading and Spelling are about 5 points, and about 6 points for Blue and Tan Arithmetic. *SEM*s are largest for the youngest age band, where Arithmetic *SEM*s are about 8 points. According to Smith (2001), the WRAT-3 *SEM*s are large compared to other achievement tests.

Test-Retest Reliability

Stability is reported as very high: 142 children (aged 6–16) from the standardization sample were administered the WRAT-3 after a one-month interval (see manual). Corrected test-retest correlations ranged from .91 to .98. There is no stability information on adults apart from a one-year test-retest study of the stability of WRAT-3 Reading in adults with TBI; reliability in this case was very high ($r = .88$; Orme et al., 2004), and considerably higher than that of other neuropsychological tests such as the Trail Making Test and Logical Memory ($r = .41$ and .57, respectively, in this study). The mean score increase for the TBI sample was 4.4 points (see also *Validity, Clinical Studies*).

Alternate Form Reliability

According to the author, Blue and Tan forms were in part constructed using items that were used in previous editions of the WRAT. There are also several new items on each test to increase the difficulty level and provide parallel content in both forms. Alternate form reliability is reported to be high, with a median correlation of .98. As shown in the manual, all correlations are above .80 across age. However, scores obtained with these forms are not identical. The Tan form reportedly yields slightly higher standard scores at certain ages (Smith, 2001), and the two forms do not measure exactly the same skills in the Arithmetic task (Mabry, 1995).

VALIDITY

Content

According to the author, content validity is supported by the use of Rasch item analyses (see manual for details). Unlike other achievement tests, WRAT-3 content does not appear to have been selected on the basis of current school curricula. Some reviewers have vehemently criticized the lack of rationale or theoretical background for item content and the fact that items dating back 60 years are still included, despite major changes in educational standards and concepts (e.g., Mabry, 1995).

The WRAT-3 also assesses fewer skills than other academic screeners. Kamphaus (2001) notes that the term "Wide Range" is a misnomer that might give users the false impression that the test is more comprehensive than it is, and it is unclear what the test actually measures due to the lack of construct definition.

The WRAT-3 does not require sentence or paragraph reading, nor does it assess comprehension. As noted by Mabry (1995), the test simply assesses the pronunciation of isolated words. Oddly, the lack of a reading comprehension requirement is noted as a strength by its author. Similarly, Mabry (1995) noted that the Arithmetic subtest provides an insufficient coverage of the arithmetic domain, and includes only one item per type; item types also differ by form (e.g., only the Tan form includes a compound interest and a logarithm item). Further, the speeded nature of the test may complicate interpretation (Mabry, 1995).

Another problem specific to non-U.S. users is a lack of correspondence with curricula in other English-speaking countries, and the lack of non-U.S. norms. The Arithmetic subtest in particular is of questionable use since students may not have been exposed to some of the skills. For instance, because of the metric system, there is a lesser emphasis on fractions and more stress on decimals in countries such as Canada (Sheehan, 1983).

Subtest Intercorrelations

The various skills measured by the WRAT-3 show moderate to high intercorrelations. Reading and Spelling are more highly correlated to each other than to Arithmetic at all ages (median correlation of .87, versus .66 and .70).

Comparison With Previous WRAT Versions

Care should be taken when comparing scores from current and previous editions. Although the WRAT-3 correlates highly with the WRAT-R (corrected r's = .79–.99), WRAT-3 raw scores are lower than those of the WRAT-R because there are fewer items on the WRAT-3. Standard scores for the WRAT-R are about 8 to 11 points lower than those of the older 1978 WRAT. Whether standard scores are equivalent between the WRAT-3 and WRAT-R is unknown, although WRAT-3 scores are expected to be slightly lower due to the Flynn effect.

Correlation With IQ

WRAT-3 scores correlate moderately with WISC-III Full-Scale IQ scores (r = .57–.66), with the highest correlations between VIQ and Reading/Spelling (r = .69–.70; see manual). Correlations with the WAIS-R, presented in the manual, are similar to those reported for the WISC-III. To our knowledge, there are no data involving newer versions of these Wechsler tests (i.e., WAIS-III or WISC-IV).

In clinical populations of children referred for academic problems, WRAT-3 and IQ are also moderately to highly correlated (Smith et al., 1995; Vance & Fuller, 1995). Very high agreement was found between IQ (K-BIT) and all three WRAT-3 subtests in a group of adults with developmental disabilities (Powell et al., 2002).

Correlation With Other Achievement Tests

Moderate to high correlations are found between the WRAT-3 and relevant subtests of the group-administered California Test of Basic Skills—4th Edition, California Achievement Test, and the Stanford Achievement Test (see manual). In adults, Flanagan at al. (1997) reported equivalent mean scores for reading and mathematics for the WRAT-3, Mini-Battery of Achievement (MBA; Woodcock et al., 1994), and K-FAST (Kaufman & Kaufman, 1994). However, WRAT-3 Reading showed slightly less convergent validity with regard to correlations with other reading tests (r = .31–.48), compared to WRAT-3 Arithmetic and other arithmetic tests (r = .52–.54). Evidence of concurrent validity has also been found in clinical populations. In children with reading disability, mean scores are similar between the WRAT-3 and corresponding subtests of the WIAT (Smith & Smith, 1998).

The WRAT-3 tasks should be considered equivalent to *subtests* of other achievement batteries, not to composite scores that measure a broader domain of academic knowledge. For example, Arithmetic is similar to Applied Problems from the WJ III and to Numerical Operations from the WIAT-II, but the WRAT-3 score for Arithmetic cannot be directly compared to the Mathematics composite scores from either battery. Further, because of mean score difference between the instruments, WRAT-3 scores cannot be directly compared to those from Wechsler tests (e.g., Ward, 1995). Given its limitations, other academic screeners are preferred for determining ability-achievement discrepancies (e.g., WJ III, WIAT-II).

Correlation With Other Domains

In adults with developmental disabilities, WRAT-3 scores were highly related to a measure of receptive vocabulary (PPVT-III), but only modestly to verbal memory (CVLT; Powell et al., 2002).

Clinical Studies

The WRAT-3 appears moderately sensitive to differences of academic skill. The manual reports on 111 children in special education programs for gifted, learning disabled, and educable mentally handicapped children, matched to individuals from the standardization sample. In discriminant analyses, the WRAT-3 provided correct group membership predictions for 72% to 85% of the children in special education. Notably, only 56% of the normal children were correctly classified. WRAT-3 group means were consistent with the children's designation in a particular program (e.g., a Blue Reading mean score of 121 for the gifted children versus 58 for the educable mentally handicapped children).

WRAT-3 Arithmetic may be a marker for dyscalculia in dementing disorders. WRAT-3 Arithmetic scores are related to MMSE scores in patients with AD ($r = .48$; Martin et al., 2003), and are more sensitive to AD severity than WAIS-III Arithmetic. Specifically, while controls obtain scores in the average range, patients with mild AD have mildly depressed scores ($M = 91$, $SD = 7$) and patients with moderate AD have low scores ($M = 73.4$, $SD = 11.5$).

Estimating Premorbid Intelligence With the WRAT-3

Reading tests are frequently used as estimates of premorbid intelligence to determine the existence and extent of cognitive decline following brain damage (see Chapter 6 for more discussion of this issue). In fact, this was the number one usage reported by neuropsychologists in a survey of reading tests (Stevens & Price, 1999). WRAT-R Reading scores have been used in this manner to predict premorbid WAIS-R scores (e.g., Johnstone & Wilhelm, 1996; Johnstone et al., 1996; Kareken et al., 1995). However, WRAT-R scores were found to underestimate at the higher IQ ranges and overestimate at the lower IQ ranges.

Like its predecessor, WRAT-3 Reading is also sometimes used as an IQ estimate (e.g., Ahles et al., 2003), as well as used to estimate premorbid IQ. There is a fair amount of evidence suggesting that the WRAT-3 Reading subtest, like other reading tests, is more immune to the effects of brain damage than other neuropsychological tests, and that as a result, it may be used as an estimate of premorbid ability (i.e., as a "hold" test; see below). For example, the WRAT-3 Reading test is highly related to other word-based premorbid IQ estimators such as Spot-the-Word Test ($r = .65$) and NART ($r = -.81$ with C-AUSNART, or Contextual Australian NART; Lucas et al., 2003; see also Griffin et al., 2002, for similar findings).

Although it is a moderate predictor—accounting for about 33% of the variance in IQ—the WRAT-3 is not as effective as the Spot-the-Word Test or NART at predicting IQ (Griffin et al., 2002; Lucas et al., 2003). It is also significantly less effective than combined prediction methods involving IQ subtests and demographics (e.g., OPIE, or the Australian version, the SPIE). Overall, Griffin et al. (2002) found that WRAT-3 Reading underestimated WAIS-R FSIQ compared with other established methods (i.e., NAART, OPIE), particularly in individuals with above-average intelligence. However, the WRAT-3 was better at predicting IQ in individuals with below-average intelligence, compared with the other estimation methods. This may be because the WRAT-3 has a low floor but significant ceiling effects in adults.

When used in combination with other estimation methods, the WRAT-3 only adds about 2% to 3% of the variance in predicting premorbid IQ, and, like other estimation methods,

carries a large SE_E when used for estimating IQ (Lucas et al., 2003). Caution is therefore suggested in making inferences about individual patients' premorbid abilities.

Is the WRAT-3 a "Hold" Test?

Orme et al. (2004) found that after one year, WRAT-3 Reading score increases were related to the severity of TBI, with mild, moderate, and severe groups increasing about three, four, and nine points, respectively. In other words, the most significantly impaired patients demonstrated the largest increases in WRAT-3 Reading. This raises some questions about the WRAT-3's validity as a "hold" test. However, WRAT-3 scores were much more stable than those of other neuropsychological tests, which provides partial evidence for its use in this capacity, at least in individuals with moderate to mild impairments. Because WRAT-3 scores of severely impaired patients taken in the acute period of a TBI may underestimate premorbid ability, other estimation methods may therefore be more appropriate in these patients (Orme et al., 2004; see also Chapter 6.

In individuals with schizophrenia, WRAT-3 Reading scores are significantly more intact than Total scores from the RBANS, a neuropsychological screening battery. Specifically, WRAT-3 Reading scores are almost a full SD above Total RBANS scores (i.e., mean difference of 18 points, or 87.9, $SD = 15.5$ versus 69.9, $SD = 13.4$), with 89% of cases showing higher WRAT-3 than RBANS scores. However, the significant correlation between WRAT-3 Reading scores and RBANS ($r = .52$) suggests that WRAT-3 scores are not completely immune to the effects of neurological/neuropsychiatric compromise (Wilk et al., 2004; see also Orme et al., 2004).

There is evidence that literacy (as measured by the WRAT-3) captures an aspect of educational experience (i.e., quality of education) that is not accounted for by years of education alone, and that it can add to the prediction of how minority groups should perform on cognitive tests (Manly et al., 1999, 2002). For example, Manly et al. (2002) found that African American elders obtained significantly lower scores than Whites on measures of memory, abstract reasoning, fluency, and visual-spatial skills even though the groups were matched on years of education. However, after adjusting for the WRAT-3 Reading score, the overall effect of race was greatly reduced and racial differences on all tests except category fluency and a drawing measure became nonsignificant.

There is also evidence that cognitive change over time is better predicted by literacy (as measured by WRAT-3 Reading) than by years of education. That is, literacy may be a powerful indicator of brain reserve, with higher levels increasing protection against cognitive decline. Manly et al. (2003) found that after accounting for age at baseline and years of education, older adults with low levels of literacy defined by WRAT-3 Reading scores had a steeper decline in verbal recall (Buschke SRT) over a four-year period as compared with elders with high literacy.

COMMENT

The main assets of the WRAT-3 are its ease of administration, scoring, and brevity (Smith, 2001). The test is also quite portable. At best, it is an acceptable screening measure of basic academic skills (Cohen & Spenciner, 1998; Sattler, 2001) but should not be used for diagnostic purposes, where a comprehensive assessment is required (e.g., WIAT-II, WJ III ACH; see *Validity, Content*). Consequently, describing an examinee's reading level based on WRAT-3 scores may be misleading (Stevens & Price, 1999; see *Validity*).

Some users employ the Reading subtest to determine whether an examinee has sufficient reading ability to complete standardized questionnaires such as the MMPI or PAI; however, there is no evidence that the test is useful for this purpose, and reading comprehension tests would be more appropriate in this regard (Stevens & Price, 1999). The Reading subtest may have a limited place in neuropsychological assessment in providing an estimate of premorbid ability or of literacy levels (see *Validity* for discussion). However, users should not prioritize "quickness at the expense of quality" (Stevens & Price, 1999, p. 69); there are a number of well-constructed, comprehensive reading tests available, many of which may be superior to the WRAT-3 for most clinical usages.

Psychometric Issues

Although it demonstrates good reliability, the WRAT-3 has weaker validity (Salvia & Ysseldyke, 2001). It is important to note that the WRAT-3 norms were collected over 15 years ago, which is a major limitation compared with tests with norms collected more recently (e.g., WJ III, WIAT-II). Overall, the normative sample is not well described, and the lack of information on education is a major omission. In addition, the manual states that in some instances, norms for Spelling and Arithmetic were gathered through group administration; however, no data are presented on whether this administration variant affected scores. Similarly, although the manual indicates that subtests can be administered in any order, no supporting data are presented, and the order used in the standardization is not indicated. The 10-item discontinue rule has also been deemed excessive (Smith, 2001).

Cross-Cultural Usage

There is a lack of information on whether the WRAT-3 is appropriate for use in cross-cultural contexts. Mabry (1995) noted that the potential for bias is a major shortcoming. However, there is some evidence that the WRAT-3 Reading may be useful in the assessment of minority groups as an adjustment factor for neuropsychological measures. Specifically, WRAT-3 Reading may have more relevance than years of education in populations where years of education is confounded by factors such as differing quality of education across cultural/racial groups (see Manley et al., 2002, 2003).

Floor and Ceiling Effects

There are significant floor effects for 5-year-olds for Reading and Spelling, but not Arithmetic (e.g., a 5-year-old with a Reading score of 0 would obtain a standard score of 76). Because of significant ceiling effects on the Reading task in older adolescents and adults (e.g., at age 17, the maximum score obtainable is 125), the WRAT-3 is not suitable for assessing the full range of giftedness in this age group. Note, too, that in some adult age bands, the maximum score is only in the high average range (e.g., 117 in 35- to 44-year-olds). In younger children, maximum score ranges are acceptable (e.g., 130 up to 155). On average, the Arithmetic task appears to have suitable floors and ceilings at all age levels.

REFERENCES

Ahles, T. A., Saykin, A. J., Noll, W. W., Furstenberg, C. T., Guerin, S., Cole, B., & Mott, L. A. (2003). The relationship of APOE genotype to neuropsychological performance in long-term cancer survivors treated with standard dose chemotherapy. *Psycho-Oncology, 12,* 612–619.

Camara, W. J., Nathan, J. S., & Puente, A. E. (2000). Psychological test usage: Implications in professional psychology. *Professional Psychology: Research and Practice, 31*(2), 141–154.

Cohen, L. G., & Spenciner, L. J. (1998). *Assessment of children and youth.* New York: Addison Wesley Longman.

Flanagan, D. P., McGrew, K. P., Abramowitz, E., Lehner, L., Untiedt, S., Berger, D., & Armstrong, H. (1997). Improvement in academic screening instruments? A concurrent validity investigation of the K-FAST, MBA and WRAT-3. *Journal of Psychoeducational Assessment, 13,* 99–112.

Griffin, S. L., Rivera Mindt, M., Rankin, E. J., Ritchie, A. J., & Scott, J. G. (2002). Estimating premorbid intelligence: Comparison of traditional and contemporary methods across the intelligence spectrum. *Archives of Clinical Neuropsychology, 17,* 497–507.

Harrison, P. L. (1994). Review of the Wide Range Achievement Test—Revised. In J. C. Impara & L. L. Murphy (Eds.), *Buros desk reference: Psychological assessment in the schools.* Lincoln, NE: Buros Institute of Mental Measurements.

Hutton, J. B., Dubes, R., & Muir, S. (1992). Assessment practices of school psychologists: Ten years later. *School Psychology Review, 21,* 271–284.

Jastak, J., & Jastak, S. (1978). *The Wide Range Achievement Test.* Wilmington, DE: Jastak Associates.

Jastak, S., & Wilkinson, G. S. (1984). *The Wide Range Achievement Test—Revised.* Wilmington, DE: Jastak Associates.

Johnstone, B., Callahan, C. D., Kapila, C. J., & Bouman, D. E. (1996). The comparability of the WRAT-R Reading test and NAART as estimates of premorbid intelligence in neurologically impaired patients. *Archives of Clinical Neuropsychology, 11,* 513–519.

Johnstone, B., & Wilhelm, K. L. (1996). The longitudinal stability of the WRAT-R Reading subtest: Is it an appropriate estimate of premorbid intelligence? *Journal of the International Neuropsychological Society, 2,* 282–285.

Kamphaus, R. W. (2001). *Clinical assessment of child and adolescent intelligence* (2nd ed.). Boston: Allyn and Bacon.

Karaken, D. A., Gur, R. C., & Saykin, A. J. (1995). Reading on the Wide Range Achievement Test—Revised and parental education as predictors of IQ: Comparison with the Barona formula. *Archives of Clinical Neuropsychology, 10,* 147–157.

Kaufman, A. S., & Kaufman, N. L. (1994). *Kaufman Functional Academic Skills Test.* Circle Pines, MN: American Guidance Service.

Klimczak, N. C., Bradford, K. A., Burright, R. G., & Donovick, P. J. (2000). K-FAST and WRAT-3: Are they really different? *The Clinical Neuropsychologist, 14*(1), 135–138.

Leverett, J. P., Lassiter, K. S., & Buchanan, G. M. (2002). Correlations for the Stroop Color and Word Test with measures of reading and language achievement. *Perceptual and Motor Skills, 94*(4), 459–466.

Lucas, S. K., Carstairs, J. R., & Shores, E. A. (2003). A comparison of methods to estimate premorbid intelligence in an Australian sample: Data from the Macquarie University Neuropsychological Normative Study (MUNNS). *Australian Psychologist, 38*(3), 227–237.

Mabry, L. (1995). Review of the Wide Range Achievement Test 3. In J. C. Conoley & J. C. Impara (Eds.), *The twelfth mental measurements yearbook* (pp. 1108–1110). Lincoln, NE: Buros Institute of Measurements.

Manly, J. J., Jacobs, D. M., Sano, M., Bell, K., Merchant, C. A., Small, S. A., & Stern, Y. (1999). Effect of literacy on neuropsychological test performance on nondemented education-matched elders. *Journal of the International Neuropsychological Society, 5,* 191–202.

Manly, J. J., Jacobs, D. M., Touradji, P., Small, S. A., & Stern, Y. (2002). Reading level attenuates differences in neuropsychological test performance between African American and White elders. *Journal of the International Neuropsychological Society, 8,* 341–348.

Manly, J. J., Touradji, P., Tang, M.-X., & Stern, Y. (2003). Literacy and memory decline among ethnically diverse elders. *Journal of Clinical and Experimental Neuropsychology, 25*(5), 680–690.

Martin, R. C., Annis, S. M., Darling, L. Z., Wadley, V., Harrell, L., & Marson, D. C. (2003). Loss of calculation abilities in patients with mild and moderate Alzheimer's disease. *Archives of Neurology, 60,* 1585–1589.

Orme, D. R., Johnstone, B., Hanks, R., & Novack, T. (2004). The WRAT-3 Reading subtest as a measure of premorbid intelligence among persons with brain injury. *Rehabilitation Psychology, 49*(3), 250–253.

Peterson, R. C., Smith, G. E., Waring, S. C., Ivnik, R. J., Tangelos, E. G., & Kokmen, E. (1999). Mild cognitive impairment: Clinical characterization and outcome. *Archives of Neurology, 56,* 303–308.

Peterson, D., Stege, H., Slate, J. R., & Jones, C. H. (1991). Examiner errors on the WRAT-R. *Psychology in the Schools, 28,* 205–208.

Powell, S., Plamondon, R., & Retzlaff, P. (2002). Screening cognitive abilities in adults with developmental disabilities: Correlations of the K-BIT, PPVT-3, WRAT-3 and CVLT. *Journal of Developmental and Physical Disabilities, 14*(3), 239–246.

Ross, J. L., Roeltgen, D., Feuillan, P., Kushner, H., & Cutler, G. B. (2000). Use of estrogen in young girls with Turner syndrome: Effects on memory. *Neurology, 54,* 164–170.

Salvia, J., & Ysseldyke, J. E. (2001). *Assessment* (8th ed.). Boston: Houghton Mifflin.

Sattler, J. M. (2001). *Assessment of children: Cognitive applications.* San Diego: J. M. Sattler, Publisher.

Sellers, A. H., & Medler, J. D. (1992). A survey of current neuropsychological assessment procedures used for different age groups. *Psychotherapy in Private Practice, 11,* 47–57.

Sheehan, T. D. (1983). Re-norming the WRAT: An urban Ontario sample. *Ontario Psychologist, 15,* 16–33.

Slate, J. R. (1996). Interrelations of frequently administered achievement measures in the determination of specific learning disabilities. *Learning Disabilities Research and Practice, 11,* 86–89.

Smith, J. K. (2001). *Essentials of individual achievement assessment.* New York: John Wiley & Sons.

Smith, T. D., & Smith, B. L. (1998). Relationship between the Wide Range Achievement Test 3 and the Wechsler Individual Achievement Test. *Psychological Reports, 83,* 963–967.

Smith, T. D., Smith, B. L., & Smithson, M. M. (1995). The relationship between the WISC-III and the WRAT3 in a sample of rural referred children. *Psychology in the Schools, 32,* 291–295.

Stevens, K. B., & Price, J. R. (1999). Adult reading assessment: Are we doing the best with what we have? *Applied Neuropsychology, 6*(2), 68–78.

Vance, B., & Fuller, G. B. (1995). Relations of scores on WISC-III and WRAT3 for a sample of referred children and youth. *Psychological Reports, 76,* 371–374.

Ward, A. W. (1995). Review of the Wide Range Achievement Test 3. In J. C. Conoley & J. C. Impara (Eds.), *The twelfth mental measurements yearbook* (pp. 1110–1111). Lincoln, NE: Buros Institute of Measurements.

Wilk, C. M., Gold, J. M., Humber, K., Dickerson, F., Fenton, W. S., & Bucanan, R. W. (2004). Brief cognitive assessment in schizophrenia: Normative data for the Repeatable Battery for the Assessment of Neuropsychological Status. *Schizophrenia Research, 70,* 175–186.

Wilkinson, G. S. (1993). *Wide Range Achievement Test 3.* Wilmington, DE: Wide Range, Inc.

Woodcock, R. W., McGrew, K., & Werder, J. (1994). *The Mini-Battery of Achievement.* Itasca, IL: Riverside.

Woodcock-Johnson III Tests of Achievement (WJ III ACH)

PURPOSE

The Woodcock-Johnson III Tests of Achievement (WJ III ACH) are a test battery designed to assess academic achievement in children and adults.

SOURCE

The WJ III ACH (Woodcock et al., 2001a) can be ordered from Riverside Publishing Company (www.riverpub.com). The test can be purchased in combination with the WJ III COG (see review in this volume) or separately ($485 US). Computer scoring (WJ III Compuscore and Profiles Program) is about $125 US. Additional report writing software is also available (WJ III Report Writer). Several training options for learning WJ III administration and scoring are available through the web site, including self-study materials (training manuals, CD-ROMs, and training videos), group training sessions, and workshops offered throughout the United States and Canada. An online Resource Center also provides regular updates on the WJ III in the form of newsletters and research

Table 7–11 General Content Domain and Organization of the WJ III ACH Subtests

General Domain	Clusters	WJ III ACH Subtests
Reading	Basic Reading Skills	Letter-Word Identification *Word Attack*
	Reading Comprehension	Passage Comprehension *Reading Vocabulary*
Mathematics	Math Calculations Skills	Calculation Math Fluency[a]
	Math Reasoning	Applied Problems *Quantitative Concepts*
Written Language	Basic Writing Skills	Spelling *Editing*
	Written Expression	Writing Fluency Writing Samples
Oral Language	Oral Expression	Story Recall[a] *Picture Vocabulary*
	Listening Comprehension	Understanding Directions[a] *Oral Comprehension*
Knowledge	Academic Knowledge	*Academic Knowledge* (General Information—WJ III COG)
Supplemental Subtests		Story Recall-Delayed[a] Handwriting Legibility Scale Writing Evaluation Scale *Spelling of Sounds*[a] *Sound Awareness*[a] *Punctuation/Capitalization*

Note: Tests in italics are from the Extended Battery.
Together, each of the three Standard subtests under the general domains of Reading, Mathematics, and Written Language form the three Broad domains (e.g., Broad Reading consists of Letter-Word Identification, Reading Fluency, and Passage Comprehension). WJ III ACH Clusters represent other ways of organizing the subtests; see Table 7–12.
[a]New subtests.

bulletins; these can be downloaded in Adobe format (www
.riverpub.com/products/clinical/wj3).

AGE RANGE

The age range is from 2 to 90+ years.

DESCRIPTION

Background

The WJ III is the third revision of the original Woodcock-Johnson Psycho-Educational Battery first published in 1977 (Woodcock & Johnson, 1977; see review of *WJ III COG*, in this volume). The original WJ was the first conormed IQ/achievement battery ever published (Mather et al., 2001). Unlike the original WJ, which was not theory-based (Schrank et al., 2002), the Cattell-Horn-Carroll (CHC) theory of intelligence provided the "blueprint" for the WJ III (McGrew & Woodcock, 2001; see Chapter 6 for description of CHC theory). The WJ-R (Woodcock & Johnson, 1989a, 1989b) was based on an earlier version of CHC theory (i.e., *Gf-Gc* theory). The WJ III ACH measures five broad CHC abilities: Reading-Writing (*Grw*), Mathematics (*Gq*), Comprehension-Knowledge (*Gc*), Auditory Processing (*Ga*), and Long-Term Retrieval (*Glr*; Mather et al., 2001).

Test Structure and Theoretical Underpinnings

The WJ II ACH allows interpretation at the broad and specific level and allows for combining subtests to measure different domains. For instance, the test yields a global achievement estimate (Total Achievement), as well as composite index scores reflecting five broad areas: reading, mathematics, written language, knowledge, and oral language. The first three broad areas (i.e., reading, mathematics, and written language) yield Broad index scores combining subtests that focus on three levels of skill: basic skills, fluency, and application. Subtests can also be rearranged into functional "clusters" that are useful for interpretive purposes (McGrew & Woodcock, 2001; see Tables 7–11 and 7–12).

There are 22 subtests in all. Depending on which subtests are selected, the test can either be administered as a Standard Battery (tests 1 to 12) or as an Extended Battery (Standard Battery, along with tests 13 to 22). The examiner chooses which areas to assess more fully. Scores can be derived at several levels of interpretation (i.e., overall performance, factor scores, clinical cluster scores, and subtest scores). The WJ III

Table 7–12 Additional WJ III ACH Clusters

Domain	
Broad Reading	Letter-Word Identification
	Reading Fluency
	Passage Comprehension
Broad Math	Calculation
	Math Fluency
	Applied Problems
Broad Written Language	Spelling
	Writing Fluency
	Writing Samples
Oral Language-Standard	Story Recall
	Understanding Directions
Oral Language-Extended	Story Recall
	Understanding Directions
	Picture Vocabulary
	Oral Comprehension
Phoneme/Grapheme Knowledge	*Word Attack*
	Spelling of Sounds
Academic Skills	Letter-Word Identification
	Spelling
	Math Calculation
Academic Fluency	Reading Fluency
	Math Fluency
	Writing Fluency
Academic Applications	Passage Comprehension
	Applied Problems
	Writing Samples

Note: Extended Battery subtests are shown in italics.

ACH is designed to be administered with its companion test, the WJ III Tests of Cognitive Abilities (WJ III COG; Woodcock et al., 2001b; see review in this volume), but can also be used in other contexts. See Table 7–13 for a description of subtests and content domains.

The WJ III differs from other achievement tests in that each of the subtests comprising each factor are described as "qualitatively different" from each other (McGrew & Woodcock, 2001, p. 11). That is, each subtest measures a unique Stratum I ability, but each subtest also reflects a broader Stratum II ability. The multifaceted nature of factors is intended to increase validity and generalizability of scores (Schrank et al., 2002) and to reduce the risk inherent to generalizing from a single narrow aspect of ability to a multifaceted ability (McGrew & Woodcock, 2001). See *Source* for more details.

Like other achievement tests, the WJ III is intended to be used to (a) diagnose learning disabilities, (b) determine discrepancies (intra-achievement, and ability-achievement), (c) plan educational programs, and (d) assess change over time. The test allows users to select the type of ability-achievement discrepancy desired. Predicted Achievement, General Intellectual Ability, or Oral Language Ability can all be selected as the basis of comparison (see Technical Manual for more details). The test also allows derivation of two types of discrepancy estimators that may be needed for state or provincial funding

eligibility criteria: (1) distance from the average level of ability for the normative sample and (2) percentage of the population identified as having a severe discrepancy.

The WJ III is designed to be administered following the principle of selective testing (i.e., matching the tests to the specific referral question). Thus, test selection may be based on the need for a full-scale score or on those specific clusters or factors that require evaluation (Schrank et al., 2002). The WJ III ACH has alternate forms (A and B). Except for a few exceptions in the youngest age bands (see Table 7–14), tasks can be given to all ages. Examples of items from the WJ III ACH are given in Figure 7–2.

WJ III Versus WJ-R

See *WJ III COG* in this volume. The WJ III has been revised to include seven new subtests (see Table 7–11). Oral language tests, originally in the cognitive battery of the WJ-R, are now part of the WJ III ACH. In addition, ability-achievement comparisons using the conormed WJ III COG have been expanded to include comparisons of oral language and academic performance, among other features. Test materials have also been redesigned (see *Administration*).

ADMINISTRATION TIME

The Standard Battery takes 60 to 70 minutes. Each subtest takes 5 to 10 minutes to administer.

ADMINISTRATION

See Mather and Woodcock (2001), Mather and Jaffe (2002), and Mather et al. (2001). For ease of testing and portability, the test itself consists of only two folding easels, with no associated manipulatives. Easel size has also been reduced from the previous edition to further facilitate portability. Test items are colorful and of interest to young test takers. Administration is straightforward, requiring simple entry-level guidelines based on age and/or grade, and, in general, a six-item basal and ceiling rule. All instructions are presented on the easel on the examiner's side, which eliminates the need for a separate Examiner's Manual. A cassette tape is provided for standardized administration of auditory subtests.

The test is best administered with the examiner sitting diagonally across from the subject, at one corner of the testing table. It is important to administer auditory subtests using a tape recorder and headphones (e.g., Story Recall, Understanding Directions). Subtests are designed to be administered in the order provided, though flexibility is also permitted at the examiner's discretion. In fact, the test easel is constructed like a binder so that subtests can be reordered if needed. Unlike other achievement tests, responses provided in another language are credited on specific verbal subtests when examinees are English-dominant bilingual (Schrank et al., 2002).

A Test Session Observation Checklist is provided on the front of the test form to check observations during the evaluation

Table 7–13 WJ III ACH Content and Task Demands

Area	Test Name	Description	Task Demands
Reading	Test 1: Letter-Word Identification	Measures an aspect of reading decoding	Requires identifying and pronouncing isolated letters and words
	Test 2: Reading Fluency	Measures reading speed	Requires reading and comprehending simple sentences and then deciding if the statement was true or false by marking yes or no (three-minute time limit)
	Test 9: Passage Comprehension	Measures reading comprehension of contextual information	Requires reading a short passage and supplying a key missing word
	Test 13: Word Attack	Measures aspects of phonological and orthographic coding	Requires applying phonic and structural analysis skills in pronouncing phonically regular nonsense words
	Test 17: Reading Vocabulary	Measures reading vocabulary and comprehension	Requires reading and providing synonyms or antonyms, or solving analogies
	Test 21: Sound Awareness	Measures four aspects of phonological awareness: rhyming, deletion, substitution, and reversal	Requires analyzing and manipulating phonemes
Math	Test 5: Calculation	Measures the ability to perform mathematical computations	Requires calculation of simple to complex mathematical facts and equations
	Test 6: Math Fluency	Measures aspects of number facility and math achievement	Requires rapid calculation of single-digit addition, subtraction, and multiplication facts (three-minute time limit)
	Test 10: Applied Problems	Measures the ability to analyze and solve practical math problems and mathematical reasoning	Requires comprehending the nature of the problem, identifying relevant information, performing calculations, and stating solutions
	Test 18: Quantitative Concepts	Measures aspects of quantitative reasoning and math knowledge	Requires pointing to or stating answers to questions on number identification, sequencing, shapes, symbols, terms, and formulas
Written Language	Test 7: Spelling	Measures the ability to spell dictated words	Requires writing the correct spelling of words presented orally
	Test 8: Writing Fluency	Measures aspects of automaticity with syntactic components of written expression	Requires formulating and writing simple sentences rapidly (seven-minute time limit)
	Test 11: Writing Samples	Measures quality of meaningful written expression and ability to convey ideas	Requires writing sentences in response to a series of demands that increase in difficulty
	Test 16: Editing	Measures the ability to identify and correct errors in spelling, usage, punctuation, and capitalization	Requires identifying errors in short written passages and correcting them orally
	Test 20: Spelling of Sounds	Measures aspects of phonological/orthographic coding	Requires spelling nonsense words that conform to conventional English spelling rules
	Test 22: Punctuation and Capitalization	Measures knowledge of punctuation and capitalization rules	Requires inserting punctuation and capitals into written words
	(WES) Writing Evaluation Scale	Measures writing skills by informal, analytic evaluation of longer, more complex passages	Requires writing an essay or composition
	(H) Handwriting	Measures writing legibility	Requires producing legible handwriting
Oral Language	Test 3: Story Recall	Measures aspects of language development, listening ability, and meaningful memory	Requires listening to passages and recalling story elements
	Test 4: Understanding Directions	Measures aspects of language development and listening ability	Requires pointing to objects in pictures after listening to instructions of increasing linguistic complexity

(continued)

Table 7–13 WJ III ACH Content and Task Demands (*continued*)

Area	Test Name	Description	Task Demands
	Test 14: Picture Vocabulary	Measures aspects of word knowledge	Requires naming familiar to less familiar pictured objects
	Test 15: Oral Comprehension	Measures aspects of listening ability and language development	Requires listening to a short passage and providing the missing final word
	Test 12: Story Recall-Delayed	Measures aspects of meaningful memory	Requires recalling elements of stories presented earlier in Test 3
Academic Knowledge	Test 19: Academic Knowledge	Measures acquired knowledge in content areas of science, social studies, and humanities	Requires providing an oral response to orally presented questions; many items provide visual stimuli

Source: From Mather et al., 2001. Reproduced by permission. Copyright © 2001 by John Wiley & Sons, Inc., New York. All rights reserved.

(e.g., level of cooperation, frustration tolerance). Although not intended as a standardized rating scale, it was field tested in the normative sample for ease of use.

SCORING

Procedure

The process for describing and reporting WJ III scores is shown in Figure 7–3. See manual, Mather & Jaffe (2002), and

Table 7–14 WJ III ACH Subtests for Preschoolers and Young Children

Test Name/Number	2	3	4	5	6	7
1: Letter-Word Identification	✓	✓	✓	✓	✓	✓
3: Story Recall		✓	✓	✓	✓	✓
4: Understanding Directions		✓	✓	✓	✓	✓
7: Spelling		✓	✓	✓	✓	✓
9: Passage Comprehension		✓	✓	✓	✓	✓
10: Applied Problems	✓	✓	✓	✓	✓	✓
12: Story Recall-Delayed			✓	✓	✓	✓
13: Word Attack				✓	✓	✓
14: Picture Vocabulary	✓	✓	✓	✓	✓	✓
15: Oral Comprehension	✓	✓	✓	✓	✓	✓
19: Academic Knowledge	✓	✓	✓	✓	✓	✓
21: Sound Awareness			✓	✓	✓	✓
2: Reading Fluency					✓	✓
5: Calculation				✓	✓	✓
6: Math Fluency						✓
8: Writing Fluency						✓
11: Writing Samples				✓	✓	✓
16: Editing					✓	✓
17: Reading Vocabulary				✓	✓	✓
18: Quantitative Concepts	✓	✓	✓	✓	✓	✓
20: Spelling of Sounds					✓	✓
22: Punctuation and Capitalization					✓	✓

Source: From Mather et al., 2001. Reproduced by permission. Copyright © 2001 by John Wiley & Sons, Inc., New York. All rights reserved.

Mather et al. (2001) for further details. Complete hand scoring is not possible with this version of the WJ; norm-based scores are only provided through computer scoring. If immediate information on performance level is needed during test administration, examiners can quickly determine age and grade equivalents with the help of a table printed on the test forms.

The scoring program is easy to use and provides several options for reporting scores, including score tables, score profiles, and short verbal summary. Specific norms can also be chosen (e.g., age versus education). Data can also be saved in ASCII format for transfer to other programs.

Main Scores

The test yields several scores, including a Total Achievement score based on either the Standard or Extended Battery, as well as Broad Ability scores for specific clusters (standard score format, with $M = 100$, $SD = 15$). See manual for complete description of all possible score types for composites and subtests (e.g., percentile, W scores, etc.), as well as the *WJ III COG* review in this volume.

Discrepancy Scores

Discrepancy scores can be calculated in several ways, including (1) intra-individual (using both WJ III COG and ACH factors) and (2) intra-achievement (WJ III ACH factors only) comparisons. The scoring program presents all factor scores along with their predicted scores based on multiple regression, along with information on whether the discrepancy was significant and/or rare in the normative sample. Specifically, the "Discrepancy *SD*" is a standardized *z* score indicating the magnitude of the discrepancy compared with the normative sample, while the "Discrepancy Percentile" indicates the percentage of the population with a similar discrepancy. In this way, information on statistical and clinical significance of discrepancies is readily available from the score printout. The magnitude of significance (e.g., .05, .01) for discrepancies can be adjusted by the user.

Figure 7–2 Examples of items from the WJ III ACH. *Source:* Reprinted with permission from Mather & Jaffe, 2002.

Test 1: Letter-Word Identification
The task requires identifying and pronouncing isolated letters and words.

g   r   cat   palm

Test 2: Reading Fluency (timed)
The task requires rapidly reading and comprehending simple sentences.

The sky is green.	YES (NO)
You can sit on a chair.	(YES) NO
A bird has four wings.	YES (NO)

Test 3: Story Recall (taped)
The task requires listening to passages of gradually increasing length and complexity and then recalling the story elements.

Martha went to the store to buy groceries. When she got there, she discovered that she had forgotten her shopping list. She bought milk, eggs, and flour. When she got home she discovered that she had remembered to buy everything except the butter.

Test 4: Understanding Directions
The task requires pointing to objects in a picture after listening to instructions that increase in linguistic complexity.

Point to the man on the bike. Go.

Before you point to the third car, point to the tree closest to a corner. Go.

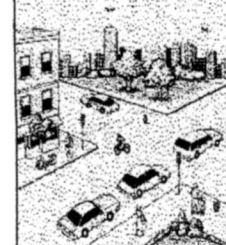

Test 5: Calculation
The task includes mathematical computations from simple addition facts to complex equations.

$$2 + 4 =   \qquad 3x + 3y = 15$$

Test 6: Math Fluency (timed)
The task requires rapid recall or calculation of simple, single-digit addition, subtraction, and multiplication facts.

$$\begin{array}{ccc} 8 & 7 & 6 \\ -3 & +7 & \cdot 9 \end{array}$$

Test 7: Spelling
The task requires the written spelling of words presented orally.

Spell the word "horn." She played the horn in the band. Horn.

Test 8: Writing Fluency (timed)
The task requires quickly formulating and writing simple sentences using three given words and a picture prompt.

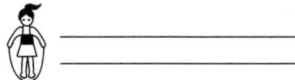

books   _____
likes   _____
read   _____

Test 9: Passage Comprehension
The task requires reading a short passage silently and then supplying a key missing word.

The boy _____ off his bike. (Correct: fell, jumped)

The book is one of a series of over eighty volumes. Each volume is designed to provide convenient _____ to a wide range of carefully selected articles.
(Correct: access)

Test 10: Applied Problems
The task involves analyzing and solving practical mathematical problems.

Bill had $7.00. He bought a ball for $3.95 and a comb for $1.20. How much money did he have left?

Test 11: Writing Samples
The task requires writing sentences in response to a variety of demands. The sentences are evaluated based on the quality of expression.

Write a sentence to describe the picture.

Test 12: Story Recall—Delayed
The task requires the student to recall, after a 30-minute to 8-day delay, the story elements presented in the Story Recall test.

Yesterday you heard some short stories. I am going to read a few words from the story and I want you to tell me what you remember about the rest of the story. "Martha went to the store . . ."

Additional Scores

The scoring program also provides several additional scores. The Relative Proficiency Index (RPI) is a measure of the subject's level of proficiency on tasks similar to those that were tested. Schrank et al. (2002) noted that this score is similar to visual acuity testing. In their example, 20/40 vision allows a person to see at 20 feet what a normally sighted person sees at 40 feet. Similarly, an RPI of 50/90 means that the subject can perform the task at a level of 50% proficiency when others in his or her age group are performing the task with 90% proficiency. The W score is a transformation of the Rasch ability scale that provides an equal-interval scale. Percentiles, standard scores, grade equivalents, age equivalents, z scores,

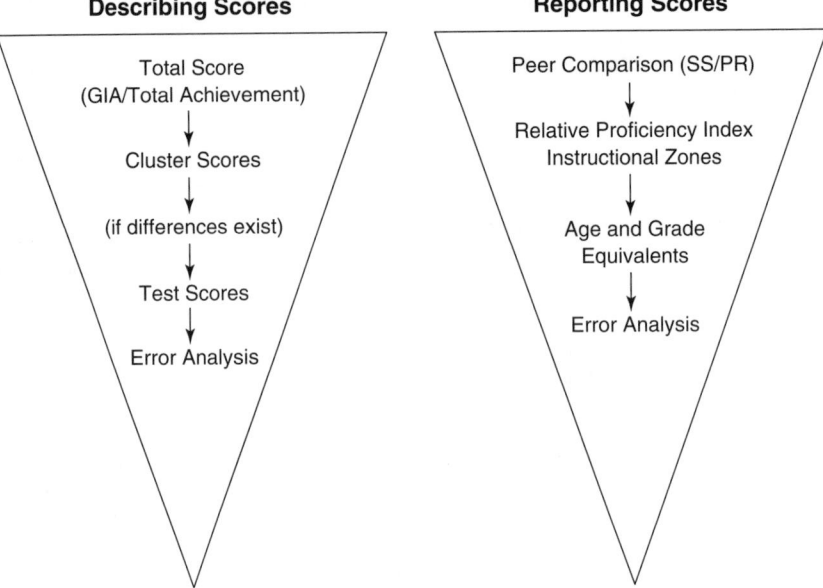

Describing Scores

Total Score
(GIA/Total Achievement)
↓
Cluster Scores
↓
(if differences exist)
↓
Test Scores
↓
Error Analysis

Reporting Scores

Peer Comparison (SS/PR)
↓
Relative Proficiency Index
Instructional Zones
↓
Age and Grade
Equivalents
↓
Error Analysis

Figure 7–3 Process for describing and reporting WJ III scores. *Source:* Reprinted with permission from Mather & Jaffe, 2002.

T scores, stanines, normal curve equivalent, and CALP levels can also be derived using the scoring program (see Technical Manual for more information). The various score options are also discussed in detail in Mather and Jaffe (2002) and Mather et al. (2001).

DEMOGRAPHIC EFFECTS

Age

WJ III scores show specific age-related changes that are fully described in the Technical Manual. An example is shown graphically in the *WJ III COG* review and in Chapter 1 (see also Figures 2–1 and 6–28).

Gender and Ethnicity

Detailed analysis of the WJ III with regard to race, ethnicity, and gender is reviewed in the Technical Manual, indicating that there are no gender differences, and that it is overall a fair test (Woodcock & McGrew, 2001a). To our knowledge, there are no independent studies on the use of the test in minority groups.

Education

As expected for a test measuring academic achievement, persons who have more years of formal education tend to obtain higher scores; as a result, the WJ III tests provide norms spanning the range of education in adults. To our knowledge, there are no independent studies on educational effects on the test apart from the general information presented in the manuals.

NORMATIVE DATA

Standardization Sample

Norms are extensive. Normative data are based on 8818 subjects in over 100 geographic regions in the United States. Individuals were randomly selected within the stratified sampling design that controlled for 10 specific community and individual variables and 13 socioeconomic status variables and approximates U.S. 2000 Census composition projections. The sample consisted of 1143 preschool subjects, 4784 kindergarten to twelfth-grade subjects, 1165 college and university subjects, and 1843 adult subjects. Individual subject data were then weighted to obtain a distribution of scores that mirrored the composition of the U.S. population. See Table 7–15 for information on the target percentages for norms composition during the WJ III standardization.

Age norms are provided for one-month intervals from age 24 months to 18 years, 11 months. One-year intervals are provided for ages 19 to 90+. Grade norms are also provided at one-month intervals from kindergarten to grade 18. There are also separate norms for college and university students (two- and four-year college norms).

RELIABILITY

Internal Reliability

In most cases, as noted in the test description provided by the publisher, the reliability characteristics of the WJ III meet or exceed basic standards for both individual placement and programming decisions (McGrew et al., 2001). Split-half reliabilities are reported for all the nonspeeded subtests, and Rasch analysis procedures were used for calculating reliabilities

Table 7–15 Target Percentages for the WJ III Cognitive Normative Sample[a]

Sample type	National, stratified, random sample[b]
Number	8818
Age	2 to 90+ years
Community size	
Central city and urban fringe	64%
Larger community and associated rural area	18%
Smaller community and associated rural area	18%
Geographic location	
Northeast	19%
Midwest	23%
South	36%
West	22%
Education[c]	
<9th Grade	9%
Less than high school	14%
High school	33%
1–3 years of college	24%
Bachelor's degree	14%
Master's degree or higher	7%
Sex	
Males	48%
Females	52%
Race	
White	84%
Black	12%
American Indian	1%
Asian and Pacific Islander	4%
Hispanic Origin	
Hispanic	10%
Non-Hispanic	90%
Occupational Status	
Employed	64%
Unemployed	4%
Not in labor force	32%
Occupation	
Professional/managerial	29%
Technical/sales/administrative	30%
Service	14%
Farming/forestry/fishing	3%
Precision product/craft/repair	11%
Operative/fabricator/laborer	14%
Screening	Only partially detailed in manual (see source)

[a]These values represent the target percentages for each category, based on U.S. Census data, during standardization of the test; actual values differ because of lower numbers in some categories, along with deliberate oversampling in others. Final percentages in the standardization sample are therefore adjusted by case weighting. Details of the procedure are presented in McGrew and Woodcock (2001), along with the actual percent of target attained and specific case weights. [b]Based on 2000 U.S. Census data, and collected between 1996 and 1999. [c]For the grade-school sample, data was stratified according to maternal and paternal education. The grade-school sample was also stratified according to type of school (i.e., public, private, or home); the college/university sample was also stratified according to type of school (public or private) and college (two-year or four-year).

Source: Adapted from McGrew & Woodcock, 2001.

of speeded subtests and subtests with multiple-point scoring (see Technical Manual for details).

Total Achievement reliability is very high (r = .98); all other cluster scores are over .80, with most over .90. Standard Battery subtest reliabilities range from .81 to .94; Extended Battery subtest reliabilities range from .76 to .91. Separate reliability data across age for each of the subtests are also shown in the Technical Manual. One-day test-retest reliability for the speeded subtests indicate that the Writing Fluency subtest demonstrates lower reliability in younger children (7–11 years, r = .76) than either the Reading Fluency or Math Fluency, which demonstrate high to very high one-day test-retest correlations across age (r's >.80). These are shown on p. 39 of the Technical Manual.

Standard Error of Measurement

*SEM*s for the Total Achievement standard score across age generally range between two and three standard score points, with the largest *SEM* at the youngest ages (e.g., *SEM* = 3.97 at age 5). Standard errors of measurement for clusters and subtests across age are provided in considerable detail in the Technical Manual. These are for the most part acceptable or better.

Test-Retest Reliability

The temporal stability of the WJ III is for the most part good, but only selected WJ III ACH subtests are presented in the manual (i.e., information is lacking for other major scores such as Total Achievement and cluster scores). Tables 7–16 and 7–17 present reliabilities from the Technical Manual for one-day and less than one-, one- to two-, and three- to 10-year intervals. When the less than one-year interval is considered, all subtests except Writing Fluency have high reliability. As expected, reliabilities are somewhat lower as the time interval increases, but are still high. See *Internal Reliability* for one-day test-retest reliability estimates for speeded tests based on 59 subjects in three age groups. This short interval for speeded tests was chosen to minimize variability due to state or trait changes, according to the authors (McGrew et al., 2001).

Note that the time intervals provided offer considerably more range than those typically provided in test manuals. In particular, the one-year and three- to 10-year intervals approximate more closely what might occur in a clinical context. They by necessity in some cases involve comparison of different test versions given the large time span involved. See the Technical Manual for test-retest reliabilities for selected subtests, by age.

Practice Effects

While the amount of information for stability coefficients provided in the Technical Manual is impressive, information on the magnitude of practice effects is provided in W-score

Table 7-16 One-Day Test-Retest Reliabilities for WJ III ACH Speeded Subtests

Magnitude of Coefficient	Ages 7–11	Ages 14–17	Ages 26–79
Very high (.90+)	Reading Fluency Math Fluency	—	Reading Fluency Math Fluency
High (.80–.89)	—	Reading Fluency Math Fluency Writing Fluency	Writing Fluency
Adequate (.70–.79)	Writing Fluency	—	—
Marginal (.60–.69)	—	—	—
Low (≤.59)	—	—	—

Adapted from McGrew & Woodcock, 2001.

format only, which complicates interpretation for those used to working exclusively with standard scores. A more detailed analysis of practice effects would improve the test's utility in retest situations.

Interrater Reliability

Only a minority of subtests from the WJ III ACH battery require subjective judgment in scoring. These involve writing (Writing Samples, Writing Fluency, and Handwriting). While the others show good reliability, Handwriting demonstrates only moderate reliability; the manual therefore recommends that this subtest be scored jointly by two raters (see McGrew & Woodcock, 2001, for further discussion).

Alternate Form Reliability

Correlations between Forms A and B are high across age ($r = .80–.96$). Development of the alternate forms (A and B) followed a detailed, empirically based process with regard to

item difficulty, standard error, and Rasch analysis. See Technical Manual for details.

VALIDITY

Content Validity

WJ III items were developed with considerable technical sophistication. Rasch single-parameter logistic test model, multiple regression, and factor analyses were used for item calibration, scaling, cluster composition and validation (see McGrew & Woodcock, 2001, for detailed discussion). As well, coverage of content is extensive, including tables detailing the CHC factor, stimuli, test requirements, and response requirements for each subtest (see Technical Manual).

Subtest and Factor Intercorrelations

Intercorrelations between WJ III factors range from about .20 to .60, suggesting that factor scores reflect related but distinct dimensions of cognition (McGrew & Woodcock, 2001).

Table 7-17 Test-Retest Reliability for Selected WJ III ACH Subtests for Three Time Intervals, Across Age

Magnitude of Coefficient	Less than 1 Year	1 to 2 Years	3 to 10 Years
Very high (.90+)	Academic Knowledge Letter-Word Identification	Academic Knowledge Letter-Word Identification	—
High (.80–.89)	Passage Comprehension Applied Problems Spelling/Punctuation and Capitalization[a]	Applied Problems Spelling/Punctuation and Capitalization[a]	Academic Knowledge Letter-Word Identification Passage Comprehension Applied Problems Spelling/Punctuation & Capitalization[a]
Adequate (.70–.79)	—	Passage Comprehension	—
Marginal (.60–.69)	—	—	—
Low (≤.59)	—	—	—

[a]Reflects a combination of the separate WJ III Spelling and Punctuation and Capitalization subtests.

Source: Adapted from McGrew & Woodcock, 2001.

Intercorrelations by age are presented in Appendix D of the Technical Manual.

Factor Structure

See *WJ III COG.*

WJ III Versus WJ-R

See *WJ III COG.*

Correlation With IQ

In general, the WJ III ACH correlates highly with major intelligence tests, especially the WJ III COG ($r = .70$). Note, however, that correlations between the WJ III COG and ACH may be slightly inflated because the two batteries share some common content (Naglieri & Bornstein, 2003; see *WJ III COG* in this volume for additional discussion; see also Evans et al., 2001; Floyd et al., 2003; and Joseph et al., 2003).

Correlation With Other Tests of Achievement

The test demonstrates high correlations with other achievement batteries in normal and clinical samples such as ADHD. For example, the Total Achievement score correlates .79 with the KTEA Battery Composite, and .65 with the WIAT Total Achievement Composite (see Technical Manual for more details).

Clinical Studies

Despite a fairly extensive body of research on the WJ-R, few independent studies on the validity of the WJ III ACH have been published yet, which is partially due to its relatively recent publication date. See *WJ III COG* for related studies, and the Technical Manual for some data involving clinical groups.

COMMENT

Like the WJ III COG, the WJ III ACH is a state-of-the-art achievement battery that is vastly superior to many tests in common usage. It is a solid, theory-driven instrument with impressive psychometric and research-based features and comprehensive, well-written manuals. Its theory-based roots are clearly evident in its score and test structure. Used with the WJ III COG, the ACH provides a wealth of subtests to chose from (i.e., over 40 possible subtests in the combined COG and ACH batteries), and is constructed in such as way as to allow tailored and flexible assessment. Norms are also extremely impressive (i.e., $N > 8000$). The age band is wide (2 to 90+), there are two kinds of college norms, and norms for certain age bands such as preschoolers rival those of tests developed exclusively for these groups (i.e., $N \geq 1000$). The test also allows derivation of scores based on age and education, which, while an obvious asset when testing children, is also useful in evaluating adults.

One major asset of the test is its use of complete normative data in ability-achievement comparisons. Specifically, unlike other major test batteries, the WJ III does not rely on linkage groups (i.e., normative subsets administered both tests) or estimation methods (e.g., simple difference method) to compare IQ and achievement. Instead, the test uses actual scores from all 8000+ subjects in the normative sample, since all were administered both the WJ III COG and the WJ III ACH.

Another major asset is that most subtests can be administered to most ages, including, in most cases, children as young as 2 years of age. The test can therefore safely be used as a single assessment tool for conducting longitudinal assessments across the age span, without confounding the comparison of performance at different ages with method variance arising from the use of different tests. The test also has impressive reliabilities, including data on extended testing intervals from one to 10 years, with large retest samples. (Note, however, that some important test-retest reliability coefficients are not provided in the manual.)

Along with its advanced psychometric and technical features, the WJ III is a user-friendly instrument from a test administration standpoint; the two-easel format also makes the test portable and simple to use. Certain features also make it appropriate for special populations. Several subtests require only basic verbal or motor responding. Speed is only required on subtests specifically designed to measure processing speed; thus, patients with motor or cognitive impairments that interfere with response speed are not penalized on tests measuring other abilities. Other features make it useful for assessing giftedness, including lack of penalties for time and reduced likelihood of ceiling effects because of the large range of item difficulty (Rizza et al., 2001). Subtests are also quite short, which is helpful for brief evaluations or for those who have difficulty staying on task. Clearly, attaining familiarity with the test structure and all the subtests and scores requires a considerable amount of training time. Although it can be used in conjunction with other IQ tests such as the WISC-IV and WAIS-III, a thorough understanding of the WJ III ACH is much enhanced by a working knowledge of the WJ III COG. In contrast, learning the actual administration of individual subtests is relatively simple.

From a neuropsychological perspective, the WJ III also has certain assets. Several subtests are based on common neuropsychological paradigms. For example, the WJ III ACH contains an alternative to the Token Test (i.e., Understanding Directions), and a verbal memory test that, with regression techniques, adjusts for the delay interval employed (i.e., Story Recall). The naming task (Picture Vocabulary) is also of considerable utility because it can be compared to other conormed domains. Similarly, the ability to compare separate cluster scores from both aspects of the battery (COG and ACH) is also of potential utility within a neuropsychological context. As noted in our review of the WJ III COG, some WJ III ACH subtests include domains not usually sampled in academic batteries (e.g., Verbal Memory).

Other aspects are not so useful for neuropsychological assessment. The Cluster scores do not yet have sufficient validity data, and data on clinical groups of interest to neuropsychologists for the test as a whole is lacking. In addition, some subtests are not designed from a neuropsychological framework. For instance, verbal memory subtests do not provide a recognition or multiple-choice trial to enable differentiation of retrieval versus encoding failure, and no information is provided on the impact of using delays ranging from 30 minutes to eight days for recall tests. In addition, some of the domains lack face validity for neuropsychologists. For example, the Oral Expression cluster is made up of Story Recall, a memory task, and Picture Vocabulary, a naming task. Others have noted that the sheer number of scores available in the WJ III make it daunting to use (Schrank et al., 2002). However, the test remains an impressive assessment tool suitable for most situations requiring diagnostic evaluation of academic skills.

REFERENCES

Carroll, J. B. (1993). *Human cognitive abilities: A survey of factor-analytic studies.* New York: Cambridge University Press.

Carroll, J. B. (1997). The three-stratum theory of cognitive abilities. In D. P. Flanagan, J. L. Genshaft, & P. L. Harrison (Eds.), *Contemporary intellectual assessment: Theories, tests, and issues* (pp. 122–130). New York: The Guilford Press.

Cattell, R. B. (1941). Some theoretical issues in adult intelligence testing. *Psychological Bulletin, 38,* 592.

Cohen, J. (1959). The factorial structure of the WISC at ages 7-7, 10-6, and 13-6. *Journal of Consulting and Clinical Psychology, 23,* 285–299.

Dean, R. S., & Woodcock, R. W. (1999). *The WJ-R and Bateria-R in neuropsychological assessment (Woodcock-Johnson III research report No. 3).* Itasca, IL: Riverside Publishing.

Evans, J. J., Floyd, R. G., McGrew, K. S., & Leforgee, M. H. (2001). The relations between measures of Cattell-Horn-Carroll (CHC) cognitive abilities and reading achievement during childhood and adolescence. *School Psychology Review, 31*(2), 246–262.

Flanagan, D. P., McGrew, K. S., & Ortiz, S. O. (2000). *The Wechsler intelligence scales and Gf-Gc theory: A contemporary approach to interpretation.* Boston: Allyn & Bacon.

Floyd, R. G., Evans, J. J., & McGrew, K. S. (2003). Relations between measures of Cattell-Horn-Carroll (CHC) cognitive abilities and mathematics achievement across the school-age years. *Psychology in the Schools, 40*(2), 155–171.

Horn, J. L., & Noll, J. (1997). Human cognitive abilities: Gf-Gc theory. In D. P. Flanagan, J. L. Genshaft, & P. L. Harrison (Eds.), *Contemporary intellectual assessment: Theories, tests, and issues* (pp. 53–91). New York: The Guilford Press.

Ittenbach, R. F., Esters, I. G., & Wainer, H. (1997). The history of test development. In D. P. Flanagan, J. L. Genshaft, & P. L. Harrison (Eds.), *Contemporary intellectual assessment: Theories, tests, and issues* (pp. 17–31). New York: The Guilford Press.

Joseph, L. M., McCachran, M. E., & Naglieri, J. A. (2003). PASS cognitive processes, phonological processes, and basic reading performance for a sample of referred primary-grade children. *Journal of Research in Reading, 26*(3), 304–314.

Kamphaus, R. W., Petoskey, M. D., & Morgan, A. W. (1997). A history of intelligence test interpretation. In D. P. Flanagan, J. L. Genshaft, & P. L. Harrison (Eds.), *Contemporary intellectual assessment: Theories, tests, and issues* (pp. 32–47). New York: The Guilford Press.

Keith, T. Z., Kranzler, J. H., & Flanagan, D. P. (2001). What does the Cognitive Assessment System (CAS) measure? Joint confirmatory factor analysis of the CAS and the Woodcock-Johnson Tests of Cognitive Ability (3rd Edition). *School Psychology Review, 30*(1), 89–119.

Mather, N., & Jaffe, L. E. (2002). *Woodcock-Johnson III: Reports, recommendations, and strategies.* New York: John Wiley & Sons.

Mather, N., Wendling, B. J., & Woodcock, R. W. (2001). *Essentials of WJ III Tests of Achievement assessment.* New York: John Wiley & Sons, Inc.

Mather, N., & Woodcock, R. W. (2001). *Woodcock-Johnson III Tests of Achievement examiner's manual.* Itasca, IL: Riverside Publishing.

McGrew, K. S. (1997). Analysis of the major intelligence batteries according to a proposed comprehensive Gf-Gc framework. In D. P. Flanagan, J. L. Genshaft, & P. L. Harrison (Eds.), *Contemporary intellectual assessment: Theories, tests, and issues* (pp. 151–179). New York: The Guilford Press.

McGrew, K. S., & Woodcock, R. W. (2001). *Woodcock-Johnson III technical manual.* Itasca, IL: Riverside Publishing.

Naglieri, J. A., & Bornstein, B. T. (2003). Intelligence and achievement: Just how correlated are they? *Journal of Psychoeducational Assessment, 21*(3), 244–260.

Rasch, G. (1960). *Probabilistic models for some intelligence and attainment tests.* Copenhagen, Denmark: Danish Institute for Educational Research.

Rizza, M. G., McIntosh, D. E., & McCunn, A. (2001). Profile analysis of the Woodcock-Johnson III Tests of Cognitive Abilities with gifted students. *Psychology in the Schools, 38*(5), 447–455.

Sanborn, K. J., Truscott, S. D., Phelps, L., & McDougal, J. L. (2003). Does the Flynn effect differ by IQ level in samples of students classified as learning disabled? *Journal of Psychoeducational Assessment, 21*(2), 145–159.

Schrank, F. A., Flanagan, D. P., Woodcock, R. W., & Mascolo, J. T. (2002). *Essentials of WJ III Cognitive Abilities assessment.* New York: John Wiley & Sons, Inc.

Schrank, F. A., & Woodcock, R. W. (2001). *WJ III Compuscore and Profiles Program [computer software]. Woodcock-Johnson III.* Itasca, IL: Riverside Publishing.

Taub, G. E., & McGrew, K. S. (2004). A confirmatory factor analysis of the Cattell-Horn-Carroll theory and cross-age invariance of the Woodcock-Johnson Tests of Cognitive Abilities III. *School Psychology Quarterly, 19*(1), 72–87.

Woodcock, R. W., & Johnson, M. B. (1977). *Woodcock-Johnson Psycho-Educational Battery.* Itasca, IL: Riverside Publishing.

Woodcock, R. W., & Johnson, M. B. (1989a). *WJ-R Tests of Achievement.* Itasca, IL: Riverside Publishing.

Woodcock, R. W., & Johnson, M. B. (1989b). *WJ-R Tests of Cognitive Ability.* Itasca, IL: Riverside Publishing.

Woodcock, R. W., McGrew, K. S., & Mather, N. (2001a). *Woodcock-Johnson III Tests of Achievement.* Itasca, IL: Riverside Publishing.

Woodcock, R. W., McGrew, K. S., & Mather, N. (2001b). *Woodcock-Johnson III Tests of Cognitive Abilities.* Itasca, IL: Riverside Publishing.

8

Executive Functions

ISSUES OF DEFINITION

Executive function is a shorthand description of a complex set of processes that have been broadly and variously defined. This breadth and complexity is illustrated in the following characterizations from recent volumes in neuropsychology:

> Executive functions are intrinsic to the ability to respond in an adaptive manner to novel situations . . . and can be conceptualized as having four components: (1) volition; (2) planning; (3) purposive action; and (4) effective performance (Lezak et al., 2004, p. 11).

> [Executive functions are] metacognitive capacities that allow an individual to perceive stimuli from his or her environment, respond adaptively, flexibly change direction, anticipate future goals, consider consequences, and respond in an integrated or common-sense way, utilizing all these capacities to serve a common purposive goal (Baron, 2004, p. 135).

> Executive functions are a collection of processes that are responsible for guiding, directing, and managing cognitive, emotional, and behavioural functions, particularly during active, novel problem solving (Gioia et al., 2000, p. 1).

Although variously defined, most investigators believe executive processes are part of a system that acts in a supervisory capacity in the overall hierarchy of brain processing (Burgess & Shallice, 1997) and encompasses skills necessary for purposeful, goal-directed behavior (e.g., Baron, 2004; Gioia et al., 2001; Lezak et al., 2004; Luria, 1966; Stuss & Benson, 1986, 1987). Shallice (1990) has fine-tuned the concept further, arguing that executive functions are not in maximal use for the execution of routine, well-learned behaviors, but rather they are especially called upon in novel, unfamiliar contexts where no previously established routines exist. That is, when confronted with novel or complex circumstances, the individual must develop new strategies and monitor their effectiveness.

Thus, executive dysfunctions may manifest in a constellation of problems in everyday life. They may include inappropriate social behavior; problems with decision making and showing good judgement; difficulties with devising, following, and shifting plans; problems with organization; distractibility; and difficulties in situations involving various aspects of memory (e.g., remembering to carry out intended actions at a future time (Burgess & Shallice, 1997; Gioia et al., 2000). Executive dysfunction may be reflected in test performances by poor initiation, poor planning and organization, poor inhibition, difficulty shifting, poor working memory, inflexibility, perseveration, difficulties generating and implementing strategies, difficulty correcting errors or using feedback, and carelessness (Anderson, 1998).

CORRESPONDENCE TO FRONTAL LOBE PROCESSES

Research on executive functions and many of the measures that are in common use have their roots in the study of patients with frontal lobe lesions. It has been known for a long time that patients with damage to the frontal lobes exhibit marked changes in the regulation of their behavior. The famous case of Phineas Gage, first reported by John Harlow in 1868, demonstrated that severe problems in behavioral control can occur with damage to the frontal lobes. Although some of these patients show remarkably intact performance on various neuropsychological tests, they tend to show, as a group, some impairments on a variety of measures such as the WCST, Category Test, Stroop, and Fluency tests. However, review of the literature suggests that these measures are not sufficiently sensitive or specific to frontal lobe lesions (see Table 8–1). Although the frontal lobes play an important role in behavioral regulation, such findings indicate that the anatomical term "frontal lobe" and the functional term "executive" are not synonymous. To avoid confusion, anatomical labels for tasks should be avoided.

Table 8–1 Characteristics of Tests of Executive Function

Test	Ages Assessed	Tasks Included in Batteries	Administration Time	Some Key Processes Thought to Be Assessed	Test-Retest Reliability	Evidence of Sensitivity to Frontal Damage	Evidence of Ecological Ability
BADS	16–87	• Rule Shift Cards • Action Program • Key Search • Temporal Judgment • Zoo Map • Modified Six Elements • Dysexecutive Questionnaire	30 min	Organization and planning	All but Key Search have less than acceptable stability coefficients (<.70)	No—but BADS impaired in a variety of conditions thought to affect executive functioning	Yes
CANTAB	4–90	• Motor Screening • Matching to Sample • Delayed Matching to Sample • Pattern Recognition Memory • Spatial Recognition Memory • Paired Associate Learning • Spatial Span • Spatial Working Memory • Big Little Circle • Intra-Extra Dimensional Shift • Rapid Visual Information Processing • Reaction Time • Stockings of Cambridge	5–10 min per task	Learning and memory Working memory Planning Set-shifting Speed Sustained attention Fluid intelligence	Most test-retest correlations marginal or low	Yes—depending on the task; but no information on sensitivity and specificity	NA
Category Test	5–80		Full version: 40 min Short version: 20 min	Abstraction ability Nonverbal reasoning	Marginal to high	No	NA

Test	Age range	Subtests	Function measured	Time	Reliability	Validity	
Cognitive Estimation Test/Biber Cognitive Estimation Test	17+		Generate estimates of time, quantity, weight, distance	5 min	<.60	Mixed	No
D-KEFS	8–89	• Trail Making Test • Verbal Fluency • Design Fluency • Color-Word Interference • Sorting Test • Twenty Questions • Word Context Test • Tower Test • Proverbs	Set-shifting/switching/inhibition Response generation Concept formation Categorization, effective use of feedback Deductive reasoning, integration of information Planning, rule learning	90 min for complete battery	Depending on task, correlations range from low (e.g., Trail Making, Design Fluency) to adequate/high (e.g., Letter and Category Fluency total correct)	Some evidence that patients with frontal lesions are impaired on some tasks compared with controls	NA
Design Fluency	5–72		Response (design) generation	15 min	Adequate (.70) for total number of drawings in fixed condition but poor for other conditions	Yes—but deficits can also occur with lesions to nonfrontal regions	NA
Five-Point Test	6+		Response (design) generation	5–7 min	Not reported	Yes—but no information regarding sensitivity and specificity	NA
Hayling & Brixton	Hayling: 8–80; Brixton: 18–80		Hayling; Response inhibition; fluid ability Brixton: Rule derivation, shifting; fluid ability	5 min for each	Adequate for overall scores	Hayling—promising Brixton—mixed	Hayling— Yes Yes Brixton—NA
Ruff Figural Fluency	7–70		Response (design) generation; memory for temporal order; speed, nonverbal reasoning	10 min	Adequate to high for total number of unique designs; poor for perseverative error and ratio scores	Affected more by anterior than posterior damage but impairment can occur with	No

(continued)

Table 8–1 Characteristics of Tests of Executive Function (*continued*)

Test	Ages Assessed	Tasks Included in Batteries	Administration Time	Some Key Processes Thought to Be Assessed	Test-Retest Reliability	Evidence of Sensitivity to Frontal Damage	Evidence of Ecological Ability
						nonfrontal lesions and some patients with frontal damage do not show impairment	
SOPT	7–65 but depends on the version		20 min	Speed Working memory	Poor to adequate	Yes—but no information regarding sensitivity and specificity	Yes
Stroop	5–90 but depends on the version		5 min	Inhibition Fluid ability Speed	Adequate for the interference trial	Yes—but poor specificity sensitivity	Yes
Verbal Fluency	2–95 but depends on the version		5 min	Response generation Working memory Speed Semantic memory	Adequate	Yes—but poor sensitivity and specificity	Yes
WCST	5–89		15–30 min	Shifting	Generally low	Yes—but poor sensitivity and specificity	Yes

In fact, Baddeley (1998; Baddeley & Wilson, 1988) proposed the concept of a "dysexecutive syndrome" explicitly to allow the discussion of function to be separated from the question of anatomical location of such function. They base their argument on the grounds that

- Executive processes need not be unitary;
- The frontal lobes represent a large and multifaceted area of the brain, which is unlikely to be unitary in function;
- Executive processes are likely to involve links between different parts of the brain and hence are unlikely to be exclusively associated with a frontal function;
- Consequently patients may conceivably have executive deficits without clear evidence of frontal damage; and
- Patients with frontal lesions will not always show executive deficits.

CONSTRUCT VALIDITY PROBLEM

Cognitive tasks particularly dependent on executive processes are presumed to impose substantial demands on self-directed planning and strategy formation and require goal-directed and nonhabitual responses (Henry & Crawford, 2004). However, there is no clear consensus on what tasks should be used to measure executive processes. Rabin et al. (2005) recently surveyed 747 neuropsychologists about their test usage patterns with regard to executive functioning. Table 8–2 presents the top 10 most frequently used instruments in this domain. The majority of respondents appear to be using the WCST, with modest consensus regarding other instruments. Thus, the top three instruments (i.e., WCST, ROCF, and Halstead Category Test) saw use by 75.5%, 41%, and 40% of respondents, respectively. However, such an approach is problematic for a number of important reasons.

The first issue relates to concerns of task impurity. Essentially the problem is that any executive task must involve nonexecutive cognitive processes simply because, by definition, executive functions operate on other cognitive processes (Miyake et al., 2000a). In some cases, the nonexecutive component may play a critical role, thereby skewing results. For example, successful performance on the WCST requires adequate visual processing, basic numerical ability, some rule induction abilities, the ability to process feedback, working memory, the ability to shift mental set, and an adequate motivation level. In other words, there are many ways for performance to be compromised, and it may be difficult to tease out whether failure is due to executive or other components. Thus, it is critical to bear in mind that task failure does not automatically signify executive impairment. Of note, the D-KEFS is a new measure that attempts to isolate component skills underlying failure on a variety of tasks.

Another serious problem is that construct validities of these "executive" tests are often not well established. Unfortunately, clinicians often choose tests based on their face validity rather than their psychometric properties. For example, Kafer and Hunter (1997) gave 130 normal adults four tests purported to measure planning/problem solving: the Tower of London, the Six Elements Test, the Twenty Questions Test, and the Rey Osterrieth Complex Figure. A structural equation modeling approach suggested that the four tasks are measuring different, unrelated constructs, begging the question as to what clinicians are assessing when they administer these tests to clinical populations. In fact, the extent to which subjects actually do careful planning in performing tasks such as the Tower of London or Hanoi may be quite limited (Miyake et al., 2000a, 2000b). Thus, if a patient shows impaired performance on an executive test (e.g., Tower Test), it is incorrect to assume that the patient has impaired "planning" ability.

Table 8–2 Top 10 Executive Functioning Instruments

Rank	Instrument	N	Percentage of Responses	Percentage of Respondents
1	WCST	494	15.1	75.5
2	ROCF	268	8.2	42.0
3	Halstead Category Test	262	8.0	40.1
4	Trail Making Test	260	7.9	39.8
5	COWAT	154	4.7	23.5
6	WAIS-R/WAIS-III/WASI Block Design	114	3.5	22.8
7	WAIS-R/WAIS-III	111	3.4	17.0
8	Stroop Test	110	3.4	16.8
9	WAIS-R/WAIS-III Picture Arrangement	78	2.4	11.9
10	Porteus Maze Test	76	2.3	11.6

Source: From Rabin et al., 2005. Reprinted with permission of Elsevier.

Additional difficulties arise when "alternate" or slightly different versions of the same test are used. For example, Shilling et al. (2002) gave four different versions of the Stroop test to the same groups of young-old and old-old normal adults. They found no evidence that the relative sizes of the Stroop effects that individuals showed on any of these tasks predicted the sizes of the effects that they showed on any of the others. That is, at the level of individual participants, there was no evidence of construct validity as defined by the Stroop paradigm.

Understanding the precise nature of the processes implicated in task performance is critical because there is growing evidence that executive functioning is not unitary (e.g., Baddeley, 1998; Burgess & Shallice, 1997). Recently, Miyake et al. (2000b) showed that executive functioning can be fractionated into three more basic executive processes: (1) shifting back and forth between multiple tasks or mental sets ("shifting"), (2) monitoring incoming information for relevance to the task at hand and then appropriately updating the informational content by replacing old, no longer relevant information with newer, more relevant information ("updating"), and (3) deliberately inhibiting dominant, automatic, or prepotent responses ("inhibition"; Miyake et al., 2000a, 2000b). While these three operations share some common element, Miyake et al. (2000b) found that they are somewhat separable, with different complex executive tests loading heavily on just one or two of these specific operations. Thus, the WCST tapped primarily the "shifting" ability while the "inhibition ability" proved the main contributor for the Tower of Hanoi task. Miyake et al. (2000b) acknowledged that it may be possible to decompose the target executive processes further and that the choice of their three component processes, while reasonable, is not exhaustive; other important basic functions need to be added (e.g., the coordination of multiple tasks).

The clinical significance of these findings is clear: When choosing tasks, it is important first to specify the target executive process and to evaluate carefully the assessment tools, considering the specific executive components they are thought to measure. Table 8–1 lists some commonly used measures, along with the primary aspects of functioning that they appear/purport to assess. Readers are referred to the validity sections of each test, described later in this volume, for a more detailed examination of the cognitive processes implicated in the performance of these tasks. We stress, however, that despite the proposals as to what constructs the various test measure, there is often a paucity of independent research indicating what these tasks truly measure.

Another important point is that one should not assume that a single task captures executive disturbance. Because the executive system is composed of a number of different processes that can be impaired singly or in combination in any one patient, assessment requires multiple measures (e.g., Burgess & Shallice, 1994). Simply relying on a commonly used complex task like the WCST as a general measure of executive functioning will not suffice.

LOW RELIABILITY OF EXECUTIVE MEASURES

Another complication arises from the fact that executive tasks tend to show test-retest reliabilities that are generally below levels considered acceptable in clinical practice (see Table 8–1) and lower than those found in other domains (Lowe & Rabbitt, 1998). Rabbitt et al. (2001) have argued that excellent frontal tests may depend for their sensitivity on their novelty and high attentional demands. Thus, in clinical practice they are one-shot tests that can only be used once with any particular patient. It also means that the more efficiently a test measures executive deficits, the less useful it is for longitudinal studies of cognitive change (Rabbitt et al., 2001).

A possible explanation for the low test-retest reliabilities (Lowe & Rabbitt, 1998) is that performance on these novel tasks can abruptly improve as soon as an individual discovers an optimal strategy, but will improve less, or not at all, if no strategy is found, and may even deteriorate if a suboptimal strategy is attempted. Therefore, practice effects will markedly differ between individuals and test-retest reliability will be low.

Regardless of the reasons for the low test-retest results, one needs to take their reliabilities into account when interpreting a patient's performance. First, low test-retest reliability limits the utility of particular tests for diagnostic purposes. Second, such findings limit the levels of associations between scores on different tests, rendering pattern analysis problematic. Finally, the dilemma arises of how to interpret change over time (e.g., the effects of clinical interventions, the progress of pathologies) as well as expected developmental changes.

Miyake et al. (2001a) suggest that difficulties of low reliability can be partly circumvented by the use of multiple tasks for each executive process of interest. The use of multiple measures may also help with the task impurity problem because the idiosyncratic, nonexecutive task requirements have less influence. Thus, the use of multiple measures may provide a more accurate, reliable picture of the specific skills that are affected.

RELATIONS TO MEASURES OF INTELLIGENCE

The relationship between executive function and intelligence has a long history. The work of Hebb and Penfield (1940) and Teuber (1972) suggested that functions like planning and monitoring of behavior could be severely disrupted despite preserved intelligence (determined by the Wechsler scales). On the other hand, Duncan et al. (1995) have shown that individuals with lesions of the frontal lobes perform well on the WAIS-R, yet present with lower g when g is measured by a test of fluid intelligence (the Culture Fair Test). Indeed, intelligence (particularly fluid ability) proves to be a major contributor to performance on many of the tasks listed in Table 8–1. Obonsawin et al. (2002) have recently shown that many executive measures (Tower of London, Cognitive Estimates, Uses for Common Objects, Stroop, Verbal Fluency, PASAT) load on the same factor in healthy individuals, and the score for this factor correlates highly (.66–.73) with FSIQ ($r = .73$), *VIQ* ($r = .66$), and PIQ ($r = .66$) of the WAIS-R. However, performance on the modified WCST was not related to Wechsler IQ scores, suggesting that it may be assessing more specific cognitive operations. It is also worth noting that while differences in IQ (as measured by the Wechsler test) clearly account for substantial proportions of the variance in tests of executive function (as well as other functions), they do not account for all of the variance on any single measure in healthy adults, suggesting that these neuropsychological tests assess cognitive processes beyond those captured by traditional IQ tests (Diaz-Asper et al., 2004).

In practical terms, because measures of executive function tend to overlap considerably with measures of intelligence (particularly fluid ability), proper interpretation of test results requires attention to an individual's performance on measures of fluid and crystallized ability. Conceivably, low scores on executive tasks may be a proxy for low intelligence, rather than reflecting a specific "executive" deficit. Further, as Henry and Crawford (2004) note, it is the pattern of deficits across measures (e.g., verbal fluency, crystallized ability, processing speed) that is important to determine whether deficits on executive measures qualify as differential deficits.

BEHAVIORAL RATINGS

A major difficulty in assessing executive dysfunction within formal examinations is that this format typically allows the patient little room for discretionary behavior. The challenge for the clinician, therefore, is how to transfer initiation, planning, and judgment from the examiner to the patient within the structured testing situation (Lezak et al., 2004). Some measures, presented in this volume (see also Table 8–1), may allow the patient to demonstrate some components of executive dysfunction. However, performance-based measures assess the potential or capacity of the individual but are devoid of the environmental supports (or distractions) that may facilitate (or hinder) an individual in functioning in daily life. Interviews with the patient, the family or other persons familiar with the patient may bring some of these issues to light. Specialized questionnaires completed by persons familiar with the patient (e.g., the DEX included as part of the BADS; the BRIEF; and the SIB-R, described in the section *Assessment of Mood, Personality, and Adaptive Functions*) have also been developed and appear to tap aspects that may not be measured by standard tests of executive functioning (e.g., the individual's capacity to function with or without support or distraction in their regular milieu). They also sample behavior over a longer time frame than is afforded by standard clinical measures. In short, standard tests and questionnaires may identify somewhat different manifestations of executive dysfunction, and both measures should be included in the assessment.

RECOMMENDATIONS FOR ASSESSMENT

On the basis of their review, Miyake et al. (2000a) offered five suggestions for the assessment of executive functions in clinical settings. We include a few others as well. These are shown in Table 8–3.

Table 8–3 Recommendations for Clinical Assessment of Executive Functions

Recommendations	Rationale
1. Do not confuse "frontal" with "executive" tests.	They do not mean the same thing.
2. Understand the specific cognitive functions tapped by each executive task.	Executive processes are somewhat separable. The target process should be specified first and then appropriate tasks selected.
3. Use multiple measures.	This helps to alleviate task impurity and low reliability problems.
4. Use simpler tasks.	Most standard tests are complex, making it difficult to isolate the processes underlying impaired performance.
5. Control strategies.	Complex tasks can be performed in multiple ways. Controlling the strategies people use increases confidence in the abilities assessed and may improve reliability.
6. Test IQ as well as other basic processes such as speed.	In this way, one can determine whether the impairment qualifies as a differential deficit.
7. Include questionnaires.	Performance-based measures and questionnaires may sample different aspects of a patient's functioning and over different time frames.

Source: The first five points are from Miyake et al., 2000a.

REFERENCES

Anderson, V. (1998). Assessing executive functions in children: Biological, psychological, and developmental considerations. *Neuropsychological Rehabilitation, 8,* 319–349.

Baddeley, A. D. (1998). The central executive: A concept and some misconceptions. *Journal of the International Neuropsychological Society, 4,* 523–526.

Baddeley, A. D., & Wilson, B. (1988). Frontal amnesia and the dysexecutive syndrome. *Brain and Cognition, 7,* 212–230.

Baron, I. S. (2004). *Neuropsychological evaluation of the child.* New York: Oxford University Press.

Burgess, P. W., & Shallice, T. (1994). Fractionnement du syndrome frontal. *Revue de Neuropsychologie, 4,* 345–370.

Burgess, P. W., & Shallice, T. (1997). *The Hayling and Brixton tests.* Thurston, Suffolk: Thames Valley Test Company.

Diaz-Asper, C. M., Schretlen, D. J., & Pearlson, G. D. (2004). How well does IQ predict neuropsychological test performance in normal adults? *Journal of the International Neuropsychological Society, 10,* 82–90.

Duncan, J., Burgess, P., & Emslie, H. (1995). Fluid intelligence after frontal lobe lesions. *Neuropsychologia, 33,* 261–268.

Gioia, G. A., Isquith, P. K., Guy, S. C., & Kenworthy, L. (2000). *BRIEF: Behavior Rating Inventory of Executive Function Professional Manual.* Lutz, FL: PAR.

Hebb, D. O., & Penfield, W. (1940). Human behaviour after extensive removal from the frontal lobes. *Archives of Neurology and Psychiatry, 44,* 421–438.

Henry, J. D., & Crawford, J. R. (2004). A meta-analytic review of verbal fluency performance following focal cortical lesions. *Neuropsychology, 18,* 284–295.

Kafer, K. L., & Hunter, M. (1997). On testing the face validity of planning/problem-solving tasks in a normal population. *Journal of the International Neuropsychological Society, 3,* 108–109.

Lezak, M. D., Howieson, D. B., & Loring D. W. (2004). *Neuropsychological assessment* (4th ed.). New York: Oxford University Press.

Lowe, C., & Rabbitt, P. (1998). Test/retest reliability of the CANTAB and ISPOCD *Neuropsychologia, 36,* 915–923.

Luria, A. R. (1966). *Higher cortical functions in man.* New York: Basic Books.

Miyake, A., Emerson, M. J., & Friedman, N. P. (2000a). Assessment of executive functions in clinical settings: Problems and recommendations. *Seminars in Speech and Language, 21,* 169–183.

Miyake, A., Frieman, N. P., Emerson, M. J., Witzki, A. H., & Howerter, A. (2000b). The unity and diversity of executive functions and their contributions to complex "frontal lobe" tasks: A latent variable analysis. *Cognitive Psychology, 41,* 49–100.

Obonsawin, M. C., Crawford, J. R., Page, J., Chalmers, P., Cochrane, R., & Low, G. (2002). Performance on tests of frontal lobe function reflect general intellectual ability. *Neuropsychologia, 40,* 970–977.

Rabbitt, P., Lowe, C., & Shilling, V. (2001). Frontal tests and models for cognitive aging. *European Journal of Cognitive Psychology, 13,* 5–28.

Rabin, L. A., Barr, W. B., & Burton, L. A. (2005). Assessment practices of clinical neuropsychologists in the United States and Canada: A survey of INS, NAN, and APA division 40 members. *Archives of Clinical Neuropsychology, 20,* 33–65.

Shallice, T. (1990). *From neuropsychology to mental structure.* New York: Cambridge University Press.

Shilling, V. M., Chetwynd, A., & Rabbitt, P. M. A. (2002). Individual inconsistency across measures of inhibition: An investigation of the construct validity of inhibition in older adults. *Neuropsychologia, 40,* 605–619.

Stuss, D. T., & Benson, D. F. (1986). *The frontal lobes.* New York: Raven Press.

Stuss, D. T., & Benson, D. F. (1987). The frontal lobes and control of cognition and memory. In E. Perecman (Ed.), *The frontal lobes revisited* (pp. 141–158). New York: IRBN Press.

Teuber, H. L. (1972). Unity and diversity of frontal lobe functions. *Acta Neurobiologica Experimentalis (Warsaw), 32,* 615–656.

Behavioral Assessment of the Dysexecutive Syndrome (BADS)

PURPOSE

The purpose of this battery is to predict everyday problems arising from executive disturbances.

SOURCE

The kit includes the manual, test materials, and 25 scoring and rating sheets and can be ordered from Harcourt Assessment, Inc., 19500 Bulverde Road, San Antonio, TX, 78259 (http://harcourtassessment.com), at a cost of about $399 US. A version for children, aged 8 to 16 years (BADS-C) has also been developed.

AGE RANGE

The BADS can be given to individuals aged 16 to 87 years.

DESCRIPTION

The authors (Wilson et al., 1996) note that most neuropsychological tests consist of an explicit task to solve, a short trial, examiner-prompted task initiation, and well-defined task success. Rarely are patients required to organize or plan their behavior over longer time periods or to set priorities in the face of two or more competing tasks despite the fact that these sorts of executive abilities are a large component of everyday activities. BADS presents a collection of six tests that are thought to be similar to real-life activities and that could cause difficulty for some patients with the dysexecutive syndrome (DES). In addition, a questionnaire (the Dysexecutive Questionnaire, DEX) given to both the patient and a rater are also included. The DEX is not technically part of the BADS in the sense that it is not formally used in the calculation of the profile score for the battery. The following six subtests make up the BADS (see Table 8–4):

Table 8–4 Description of BADS Tasks

Task	Description	Scoring
Rule Shift Cards Test	Uses 21 spiral-bound nonpicture playing cards. In the first part of the test, the subject is asked to say "Yes" to a red card and "No" to a black card. This rule, typed on a card, is left in full view throughout to reduce memory constraints. In the second part, the subject must "forget" the first rule and concentrate on applying a new rule. The subject is asked to respond "Yes" if the card that has just been turned over is the same color as the previously turned card and "No" if it is a different color. This new, typed rule is left in full view of the subject.	The measures are time taken and number of errors on the second trial.
Action Program Test	Requires five steps to its solution. The subject is presented with a rectangular stand; in one end is set a large transparent beaker with a removable lid that has a small central hole in it. The beaker is two-thirds full of water. Into the other end of the stand is set a thin transparent tube at the bottom of which is a small piece of cork. To the left of the stand is placed an L-shaped metal rod, which is not long enough to reach the cork, and a small screw-top container, with its lid unscrewed and lying beside it. Subjects are asked to get the cork out of the tube using any of the objects in front of them without lifting up the stand, the tube, or the beaker, and without touching the beaker lid with their fingers. There is no time limit.	A profile score is obtained according to the number of stages completed.
Key Search	Subjects are presented with a piece of paper with a square in the middle and a small black dot below. They are told to imagine that the square is a large field and that they have lost their keys. They are asked to draw a line, starting at the black dot, to show where they would walk to search the field to make absolutely certain that they would find their keys.	The time required and efficiency of the search plan are evaluated.
Temporal Judgment	The task comprises four short questions concerning commonplace events that take a few seconds (e.g., how long does it take to blow up a party balloon?) to several years (how long do most dogs live?).	Each of the four questions is scored 0 or 1.
Zoo Map Test	Subjects show how they would visit a series of designated locations on a map of a zoo, following certain rules. The first trial consists of a high-demand version of the task in which the planning abilities of the subject are rigorously tested. In the second, low demand trial, the subject is simply required to follow the instructions to produce an error-free performance.	The profile score reflects the sequence produced, the number of errors made, and the time to task completion.
Modified Six Elements Test	The subject is given instructions to do three tasks (dictating or describing an event, arithmetic, and picture naming), each of which is divided into two parts, called A and B. The subject is required to attempt at least something from each of the six subtasks within a 10-minute period. In addition, the subject is told that there is one rule that must not be broken: Subjects are not allowed to do the two parts of the same task consecutively.	The profile score is based on the number of tasks completed, the number of tasks where rule breaks were made, and the time spent on any one task.
Dysexecutive Questionnaire (DEX)	The DEX is a 20-item questionnaire that samples four broad areas of changes: emotional or personality changes, motivational changes, behavioral changes, and cognitive changes. Items include statements such as: "I act without thinking, doing the first thing that comes to mind" or "I have difficulty thinking ahead and planning for the future." Each item is scored on a five-point (0–4) Likert scale, ranging from "Never" to "Very Often." The questionnaire compares responses in two versions, one of which is designed to be completed by the subject (DEX-Self) and another by a relative or a caregiver who has close, preferably daily, contact with the subject (DEX-Other).	

1. The Rule Shift Cards Test uses non-picture playing cards and examines the subject's ability to respond correctly to a rule and to shift from one rule to another. The test, therefore, is a measure of the ability to shift from one rule to another and of working memory.
2. The Action Program Test was adapted from a task originally described by Klosowaska (1976) and requires the individual to solve a novel problem by developing a five-step plan of action.
3. In the Key Search Test, subjects are presented with a task of finding something that they have lost. The efficiency of the search strategy is evaluated.
4. The Temporal Judgment Test comprises four short questions concerning commonplace events. The task evaluates the individual's ability to make reasonable guesses or estimates.
5. The Zoo Map Test requires subjects to show how they would visit a series of designated locations on a map of a zoo, following certain rules. Planning ability is evaluated.
6. The Modified Six Elements Test is modeled after a task developed by Shallice and Burgess (1991) and requires individuals to organize their activities to carry out six tasks in a limited time period and without breaking certain rules.

The 20-item DEX purports to assess a number of characteristics including abstract thinking problems, impulsivity, confabulation, perseveration, planning problems, euphoria, lack of insight, apathy, disinhibition, distractibility, knowledge-response dissociation, lack of concern, and unconcern for social rules. Each item is scored on a five-point Likert scale ranging from *never* to *very often*.

ADMINISTRATION

Instructions for administration are given in the BADS Manual. Some items have timed components. The scoring sheet prompts the examiner about various aspects of the administration and scoring procedures.

ADMINISTRATION TIME

The entire test can be given in about one-half hour.

SCORING

Scoring guidelines are found in the BADS Manual. The method of scoring was devised so that a "profile" score, ranging from 0 to 4, is calculated for each test. An overall profile score for the whole battery is obtained by adding together the individual profile scores for each test. The DEX, however, is not formally part of the BADS in the sense that it is not used in the calculation of the profile score for the battery. Rather, it is used to supplement information obtained on the battery,

through the provision of additional qualitative information. Therefore, any subject who completes the whole battery will obtain a BADS profile score within the range of 0 to 24. Although it is recommended that all six tests of the BADS be administered to obtain the total BADS profile score, it is possible to prorate on the basis of five tests.

The profile or overall score can be converted (using Table 5 in the BADS Manual) into a standardized score with a mean of 100 and a standard deviation of 15. In this way, it is possible to classify BADS performance as either being impaired, borderline, low average, average, high average, or superior. The overall profile score is evaluated with reference to three age groups (40 or less, 41–65, 65–87).

DEMOGRAPHIC EFFECTS

Age

Age affects task performance, with poorer overall scores for subjects aged 65 years and above (Wilson et al., 1996).

Other

The authors do not report on the potential influences of gender, education, or intelligence. For the temporal judgment task, there is evidence that older participants score marginally worse than younger adults; gender and verbal intelligence (measured by the Spot-the-Word task of the SCOLP) appear unrelated to performance (Gillespie et al. 2002).

NORMATIVE DATA

Standardization Sample

Description of the sample is sparse (see Table 8–5). Wilson et al. (1996) normed the test on a group of 216 healthy individuals (age, $M = 46.6$, $SD = 19.8$) in each of three ability bands (below average, average, above average according to the NART; mean NART FSIQ = 102.7; $SD = 16.2$; range 69–129) and balanced to have approximately equal numbers of men and women in each of these bands from each of four age groups (16–31, 32–47, 48–63, and 64+; age, $M = 58.93$, $SD = 15.35$; education, $M = 13.83$ years, $SD = 2.70$). The actual composition (N, number of males and females) of each of these bands is not provided. Although the overall score is evaluated with reference to age, no age-based norms are provided for the individual subtests.

Examination of Table 8–6 suggests that performance was at ceiling for some of the tasks (especially Action Program, Six Elements, and Rule Shift). Gillespie et al. (2002) examined a group of 101 community-dwelling older adults who were negative by self-report of neurological disorder (age, $M = 71.2$ years; range 56–89 years) on the temporal judgment tasks. The median score was 2, a value similar to that reported by Wilson et al. (1996). Garden et al. (2001) examined younger ($M = 38.20$, $SD = 3.44$; range 31–46) and

Table 8–5 Characteristics of the BADS Normative Sample

Number	216
Age	16–87 years
Geographic location	England
Sample type	Volunteers selected to comprise approximately equal numbers in each of three NART IQ-based ability bands: below average (≤89), average, (90–109), and above average (110+), Mean NART FSIQ = 102.7 (SD = 16.2, range 69–129)
Education	Not reported
SES	Not reported
Gender	Balanced to have approximately equal numbers of men and women in each of the IQ bands from each of four age groups: 16–31, 32–47, 48–63, and 64+.
Race/ethnicity	Not reported
Screening	Reported to be neurologically healthy but screening method not provided

Source: Adapted from Wilson et al., 1996.

older ($M = 59.60$, $SD = 4.27$; range 53–64) normal adults on a variant of the Six Elements task. There were no midlife declines in task performance. Younger adults had better rule recall but were more likely to break the rule to prioritize the beginning of tasks.

The authors provide no normative data for the DEX. Evans et al. (1997) examined a small group of normal controls ($N = 26$; age, $M = 39.1$, $SD = 19.02$; mean estimated NART IQ = 110.3, $SD = 8.95$) and reported DEX-Self ratings ($M = 21.81$, $SD = 8.16$) and DEX-Other ratings ($M = 11.25$, $SD = 6.71$). The relationship of the "other" raters to the controls is not reported. More recently, Chan (2001) recruited a sample of 93 healthy Hong Kong Chinese participants (29 males, 64 females) between the ages of 18 and 50 years

Table 8–6 BADS Subtest Means and Standard Deviations for Normal Controls ($N = 216$)

	Mean (SD)
Profile Total	18.05 (3.05)
Action Program	3.77 (0.52)
Key Search	2.60 (1.32)
Modified Six Elements	3.52 (0.80)
Rule Shift Cards	3.56 (0.87)
Zoo Map	2.44 (1.13)
Temporal Judgment	2.15 (0.91)

Source: Adapted from Wilson et al., 1998.

($M = 34.7$, $SD = 10.39$) and their relatives. The reported dysexecutive behaviors by the participants (self and relatives) are summarized in Table 8–7. The values are reported to be similar to those obtained in the United Kingdom (Chan & Manly, 2002).

RELIABILITY

Internal Consistency

Bennett et al. (2005) reported a Cronbach alpha coefficient of .60 for the total profile score. Gillespie et al. (2002) noted that the number of items in the Temporal Judgment task is too small for its internal consistency to be examined. Even when this subtest is omitted, the reliability of the overall score is low (.63; Bennett et al., 2005).

Test-Retest Reliability

Wilson et al. (1996) report that 29 normals were retested on the battery (excluding the DEX) as well as three other executive tasks (Modified Card Sorting Test, Cognitive Estimation Task, and FAS) after an interval of six to 12 months. Test-retest correlations for the BADS tests ranged from −.08 (Rule Shift Cards) to .71 (Key Search), which is generally below acceptable levels. Test-retest reliability for the overall score was not reported. Ceiling effects in conjunction with small sample size likely adversely affected the correlation calculations.

Low to moderate correlations between testing occasions were also found for the other executive tasks. In general, there was a tendency for slight improvement on repeat testing.

The authors also reported an alternative method of determining test-retest reliability. They calculated the percentage agreement of the same score being achieved on both occasions. Percentage agreement also tended to be low. On only two tasks (Action Program and Rule Shift Cards) did more than 70% the sample achieve the same score on both testing occasions.

Similar results were obtained with shorter retest intervals in a patient sample. Jelicic et al. (2001) studied the temporal stability of the Dutch version of the BADS (excluding the DEX) in a sample of 22 adult psychiatric patients. All patients were given the BADS twice with an interval of 3 weeks. Test-retest correlations ranged from very low (e.g., .22, Action Program) to high (.85, overall score). All but one of the tasks (Key Search: $r = .84$) had less than acceptable (<.70) stability coefficients. On the repeat administration, patients obtained higher scores (about one point) on one test (Action Program) as well as on the total BADS (about two points).

Interrater Reliability

Wilson et al. (1996) report that 25 normal individuals were tested with a second tester present on the six BADS tasks (excluding the DEX). Interrater reliability was high (above .88).

Table 8–7 Reported Measures of the DEX and DEX-R (Relative-Rated) Versions in a Nonclinical Sample

Items	DEX			DEX-R		
	Mean	(SD)	Range	Mean	(SD)	Range
1. Abstract thinking problems	1.28	(0.85)	0–4	1.08	(0.81)	0–3
2. Impulsivity	1.04	(0.79)	0–3	0.94	(0.88)	0–4
3. Confabulation	0.61	(0.77)	0–3	0.75	(0.88)	0–3
4. Planning problems	1.52	(0.79)	0–4	1.34	(1.03)	0–4
5. Euphoria	1.27	(0.86)	0–4	1.25	(0.95)	0–4
6. Temporal sequencing problems	1.24	(0.72)	0–3	0.91	(0.78)	0–3
7. Lack of insight and social awareness	0.90	(0.81)	0–4	0.79	(0.77)	0–3
8. Apathy and lack of drive	1.37	(0.89)	0–4	1.30	(0.96)	0–3
9. Disinhibition	0.70	(0.62)	0–2	0.60	(0.67)	0–3
10. Variable motivation	0.78	(0.77)	0–4	0.83	(0.92)	0–3
11. Shallowing of affective responses	1.29	(0.82)	0–4	1.14	(1.06)	0–3
12. Aggression	0.94	(0.83)	0–4	1.18	(0.95)	0–3
13. Lack of concern	0.98	(0.76)	0–2	0.83	(0.81)	0–4
14. Perseveration	1.10	(0.85)	0–3	0.96	(0.88)	0–4
15. Restlessness-hyperkinesis	0.75	(0.90)	0–3	0.68	(0.76)	0–3
16. Inability to inhibit response	1.10	(0.73)	0–4	1.13	(0.88)	0–4
17. Knowing-doing dissociation	0.97	(0.78)	0–4	0.85	(0.86)	0–3
18. Distractibility	1.61	(0.94)	0–4	1.11	(0.91)	0–4
19. Poor decision-making ability	1.38	(0.82)	0–4	1.18	(0.94)	0–4
20. No concern for social rules	1.31	(1.00)	0–4	1.20	(1.04)	0–4
Total scores	22.13	(8.86)	4–49	20.61	(10.52)	0–48

Note: Range of score in each item is 0–4; range of total score is 0–80.

Source: From Chan, 2001. Reprinted with the permission of the British Psychological Society.

DEX

Internal consistency is reported to be high (>.90; Bennett et al., 2005). No information is provided regarding the inter-rater reliability for the DEX-Other rating or test-retest reliability for DEX-Self or Other forms.

VALIDITY

BADS Tasks

Correlations With Other Neuropsychological Tests. Norris and Tate (2000) examined healthy individuals and a mixed group of neurological patients (traumatic brain injury, multiple sclerosis) and found moderate correlations between BADS scores and other measures of executive function (e.g., WCST, TMT B, Porteus Mazes, Rey copy strategy, Cognitive Estimation, COWA). In particular, the overall score and the Action and Rule Shift subtests showed small to moderate correlations (.20–.54) with all these executive tasks. While the Zoo ($r = .41$) and Key ($r = .28$) tasks did show a statistically significant relation with another measure sampling the similar domain of planning (Porteus Mazes), the Temporal Judgment task had low and nonsignificant correlations with the executive tasks, including another measure of cognitive estimation

($r = .11$). There appears to be little relationship between performance on the BADS tests and memory test scores (as measured by the Rivermead; Evans et al., 1997).

Clinical Findings. Performance on the BADS is impaired in a variety of conditions thought to impact adversely executive functioning, including chronic alcoholism (Moriyama et al., 2002), schizophrenia (Evans et al., 1997; Ihara et al., 2000; Krabbendam et al., 1999; Wilson et al., 1998), and attention-deficit/hyperactivity disorder (Clark et al., 2000). Wilson et al. (1996, 1998) report that the overall BADS profile score differentiated the performance of healthy controls from a group of 76 patients with neurological disorders, most with closed head injury. In addition, the performance of neurological patients was poorer than that of controls on all six of the individual tests making up the BADS.

Shallice and Burgess (1991) described several atypical behaviors (e.g., spending a disproportionately long time on one subtask, misinterpreting task instructions) in patients with frontal lobe damage performing the Six Elements task. However, Garden et al. (2001) reported that unusual behaviors may be seen in healthy as well as patient populations.

The BADS appears comparable to standard executive tasks in discriminating between neurological (patients with TBI, MS) and nonneurological participants (Norris & Tate, 2000).

Significant group differences were observed on three subtests (Action, Zoo, and Six Elements), along with the total profile score and two other measures (Porteus Mazes, COWA). Correct classification with the BADS of non-brain-damaged individuals was good (84%), but classification success for the neurologically impaired individuals (patients with TBI or multiple sclerosis) was poorer (64%). The overall classification rate was 74%. Similar results were obtained for other executive tasks (e.g., Porteus Mazes, COWA).

Ecological Validity. Wilson et al. (1996) reported that there were moderate negative correlations between the DEX ratings of others and performance on the six individual tests; that is, poor awareness of deficit was correlated with poor executive functioning on each BADS test. There was also a moderate correlation between WAIS-R FSIQ and others' rating, although the magnitude of this correlation (−.42) was less than that of the BADS total profile score (−.62). None of the BADS tests, total profile score, or FSIQ correlated with the patients' ratings of their perception of the presence of everyday executive problems. In short, performance on the BADS appears to be associated with objective ratings of everyday executive problems among brain-injured individuals. While WAIS-R IQ is moderately correlated with these ratings, the BADS profile score appears more highly correlated with the objective ratings.

There is additional evidence of ecological validity of portions of the BADS. Bennett et al. (2005) examined patients who had sustained head injuries and found a moderate association between various BADS subtests (particularly Action Program, Modified Six Elements) and DEX ratings made by clinicians. Clark et al. (2000) reported that performance on the Six Elements Test by adolescents showed moderate correlations with parent ratings of hyperactivity/distractibility. Further, Norris and Tate (2000) found that performance on the Action, Zoo, and Six Elements tests predicted clinicians' ratings of everyday role functioning (measured by the Role Functioning Scale; McPheeters, 1984) in neurological patients. Standard measures (COWA, errors on the Progressive Matrices) failed to predict role functioning. However, contrary to the findings by Wilson et al. (1996), BADS subtests did not show the expected relationships with ratings of others on the DEX.

DEX

Factor-Analytic Findings. Factor analysis of others' ratings on the DEX has suggested that the questionnaire measures change in at least three (Wilson et al., 1996) or more possibly five (Burgess et al., 1998; Chan, 2001) areas. Wilson et al. (1996) reported that there were three factors underlying the symptoms reported by caregivers and these represented behavioral, cognitive, and emotional components. They indicated that the only significant predictor of each of the factors was the BADS profile score. Performance on the Cognitive Estimation Test, WCST (Nelson version), NART FSIQ, and WAIS-R FSIQ and age did not predict DEX factors. By contrast, Burgess et al. (1998) reported a five-factor solution among a heterogeneous group of neurological patients. The five factors represented inhibition, intentionality, executive memory, positive affect, and negative affect. The first three factors were well correlated with executive tasks, whereas the latter two factors were much less well correlated. Chan (2001) found a somewhat similar five-factor solution among healthy Hong Kong Chinese: inhibition, intentionality, knowing-doing dissociation, in-resistance, and social regulation. Modest-moderate correlations were obtained between the factors and other standard tests of executive function.

Clinical Findings. The DEX (self- and other reports) is sensitive to the presence of mild to moderate TBI (Chan & Manly, 2001). DEX ratings made by professionals are also linked to severity of injury (Bennett et al., 2005). Its ability to discriminate frontal from nonfrontal focal lesion groups remains to be determined.

The difference between the DEX-Self and DEX-Other may prove a useful measure of insight. Wilson et al. (1996) gave the DEX and BADS tasks to a mixed neurological sample, most with traumatic brain injury. Neurological patients, as a group, rated themselves on the DEX as having fewer problems than their significant others or clinicians reported—a pattern expected following brain injury where problems of reduced insight are evident (Wilson et al., 1996). Similar findings have been reported by others (Alderman et al., 2001; Burgess et al., 1998).

The ability of the DEX to predict scores on other putative executive functioning measures is conflicting. Evans et al. (1997) found that patients with schizophrenia as well as a mixed group of brain-injured individuals were rated by their caregiver, but not by themselves, as having significant behavioral problems. Surprisingly, for the patients with schizophrenia there was no clear relation between BADS test performance and DEX ratings. For the brain-injured group, however, there was a strong correlation between the overall BADS profile score and the DEX ratings.

Similarly, Burgess et al. (1998) found that in a general neurological population, the DEX-Other score correlated with impairment on many neuropsychological measures. By contrast, the DEX-Other/Self discrepancy score, a crude measure of insight, was related to executive test scores (e.g., WCST, Trails, Six Elements), but not with memory test scores or measures of intellectual status or naming ability. Chan and Manly (2001) reported that in patients with mild-moderate TBI, the DEX Other-Self discrepancy score was significantly correlated with Six Elements Test performance (poorer insight-poorer performance) and proved a stronger correlate than either the DEX-Self or DEX-Other alone. There was no significant relationship with the Tower of Hanoi test.

By contrast, Norris and Tate (2000) reported that the DEX-Other's association with a different rating of patient functioning (in work, independent living, and the social domain) was not significant. Bogod et al. (2003) evaluated patients with traumatic brain injury and found little relation between the DEX (other or self-ratings) and a structured interview measure of awareness of deficit (SADI; Fleming et al., 1996). They did find a moderate relation (.40) between a discrepancy score calculated from the DEX self- and other ratings and the SADI. Further, only the SADI, not the DEX discrepancy score, was able to identify severity of head injury better than chance or could be predicted by the executive function measures (Stroop errors, go-no-go, Self-Ordered Pointing Test). Thus, their findings failed to support previous results (Burgess et al., 1998; Wilson et al., 1996), suggesting that the DEX discrepancy and "other" scores are associated with executive functioning. They did find that the DEX discrepancy score shared a modest negative relation with IQ (−.33).

The conflicting findings may reflect, at least in part, the nature of the rater. Bennett et al. (2005) found that the DEX could identify executive dysfunction (on the BADS) in an acute rehabilitation setting provided it was completed by professionals (neuropsychologists, occupational therapists). Ratings by family members proved less sensitive to executive dysfunction, while patient ratings were not associated with any BADS test variables.

COMMENT

The evidence suggests that the BADS has ecological validity and may be a useful tool for picking up executive difficulties that manifest in everyday functioning. The battery, however, is in need of further study.

The normative data base is poorly described, and apart from age, there is little or no information on the impact of various demographic influences. Although the overall score is evaluated relative to age, no age-based norms are available for the individual subtests. Accordingly, there is at present no way to evaluate individual subtest performance.

Reliability of the individual tests tends to be poor. Wilson et al. (1996) suggested that the test-retest correlations may not be high on these tests because at retest, they are no longer assessing novelty, a critical aspect of the dysexecutive syndrome. They note that in patients with memory or attentional difficulties, performance may be less susceptible to reduced novelty effects as they may have little or no recall of attempting the tests before and as a consequence, reliability estimates should be better. This proposal, however, remains to be tested. In the meantime, given the generally low stability coefficients of most of the subtests of the BADS (except Key Search), they should not be used for characterizing strengths and weaknesses or for repeat testing.

Further, evidence supporting the interpretability of some of the tasks (in particular, Temporal Judgment) is weak. Rather, greater weight should be placed on the overall score, which appears to possess better psychometric properties, both in terms of reliability and validity.

BADS tests appear to have been selected because they captured some nonroutine problem-solving ability and were similar to real-life activities that might cause difficulty for some patients with executive disturbances (Wilson et al., 1996).

These tasks are complex, and poor performance on them can arise for many reasons. While not denying the clinical utility of the tasks, the precise nature of the processes implicated in performance on these tasks is not known. Future work should include additional studies of reliability (e.g., test-retest reliability in neurologically impaired populations) and validity (e.g., the relation of the different tasks to each other, their relation to nonexecutive function tasks, including measures of intellectual status and spatial ability). Whether all of the BADS tasks are equally useful in identifying executive dysfunction is also not clear. There is some evidence that one or two subtests (e.g., Six Elements, Action Program) may be just as sensitive to executive dysfunction as the entire battery (Bennett et al., 2005). Further, ceiling effects appear on some of the tasks, raising the concern that subtle deficits may go undetected (see also Norris & Tate, 2001).

The DEX provides one of the few rating scales available to quantify everyday executive behaviors, including awareness of deficit. It is cost-efficient, allows evaluation of self-other report discrepancies, and requires minimal supervision by the examiner (Malloy & Grace, 2005). It also appears useful in non-English-speaking contexts (e.g., Hong Kong; Chan & Manly, 2002). However, there is conflicting evidence of its validity, perhaps in part a reflection of who does the rating. There is some evidence that family members may not always provide the most accurate assessment of executive dysfunction and that in some cases (e.g., acute rehabilitation setting), a better estimate is obtained when professionals, rather than caregivers, are used as raters (Bennett et al., 2005). Family members are nonetheless more accurate raters than patients.

Further, there is little published information regarding the reliability of the DEX. In addition, normative data are limited—a distinct limitation since there is evidence that nonclinical samples can present with dysexecutive-like behaviors in everyday life (Chan, 2001). Finally, users should note that the instructions for completing the DEX do not specify a time frame, so it is possible that some raters adopt a long-term perspective, assessing the patient's premorbid rather than current behavior—a situation that can be easily avoided by providing more specific instructions with the DEX (Bennett et al., 2005).

REFERENCES

Alderman, N., Dawson, K., Rutterford, N. A., & Reynolds, P. J. (2001). A comparison of the validity of self-report measures amongst people with acquired brain injury: A preliminary study of the usefulness of EuroQol-5D. *Neuropsychological Rehabilitation, 11,* 529–537.

Bennett, P. C., Ong, B., & Ponsford, J. (2005). Measuring executive dysfunction in an acute rehabilitation setting: Using the dysexecutive questionnaire (DEX). *Journal of the International Neuropsychological Society, 11,* 376–385.

Bogod, N. M., Mateer, C. A., & MacDonald, S. W. S. (2003). Self-awareness after traumatic brain injury: A comparison of measures and their relationship to executive functions. *Journal of the International Neuropsychological Society, 9,* 450–458.

Burgess, P. W., Alderman, N., Evans, J., Emslie, H., & Wilson, B. A. (1998). The ecological validity of tests of executive function. *Journal of the International Neuropsychological Society, 4*, 547–558.

Chan, R. K. C. (2001). Dysexecutive symptoms among a non-clinical sample: A study with the use of the dysexecutive questionnaire. *British Journal of Psychology, 92*, 551–565.

Chan, R. C. K., & Manly, T. (2002). The application of "dysexecutive syndrome" measures across cultures: Performance and checklist assessment in neurologically healthy and traumatically brain-injured Hong Kong Chinese volunteers. *Journal of the International Neuropsychological Society, 8*, 771–780.

Clark, C., Prior, M., & Kinsella, G. J. (2000). Do executive function deficits differentiate between adolescents with ADHD and oppositional defiant/conduct disorder? A neuropsychological study using the Six Elements Test and Hayling Sentence Completion Test. *Journal of Abnormal Child Psychology, 28*, 403–414.

Evans, J. J., Chua, S. E., McKenna, P. J., & Wilson, B. A. (1997). Assessment of the dysexecutive syndrome in schizophrenia. *Psychological Medicine, 27*, 1–12.

Fleming, J. M., Strong, J., & Ashton, R. (1996). Self-awareness of deficits in adults with traumatic brain injury. How best to measure? *Brain Injury, 10*, 1–15.

Garden, S. E., Phillips, L. H., & MacPherson, S. E. (2001). Midlife aging, open-ended planning, and laboratory measures of executive function. *Neuropsychology, 15*, 472–482.

Gillespie, D. C., Evans, R. I., Gardener, E. A., & Bowen, A. (2002). Performance of older adults on tests of cognitive estimation. *Journal of Clinical and Experimental Neuropsychology, 24*, 286–293.

Ihara, H., Berrios, G. E., & McKenna, P. J. (2000). Dysexecutive syndrome in schizophrenia: A cross-cultural comparison between Japanese and British patients. *Behavioral Neurology, 12*, 209–220.

Jelicic, M., Henquet, C. E. C., Derix, M. M. A., & Jolles, J. (2001). Test-retest stability of the Behavioral Assessment of the Dysexecutive Syndrome in a sample of psychiatric patients. *International Journal of Neuroscience, 110*, 73–78.

Klosowaska, D. (1976). Relation between ability to program actions and location of brain damage. *Polish Psychological Bulletin, 7*, 245–255.

Krabbendam, L., de Vugt, M. E., & Derix, M. M. A. (1999). The Behavioral Assessment of the Dysexecutive Syndrome as a tool to assess executive functions in schizophrenia. *The Clinical Neuropsychologist, 13*, 370–375.

Malloy, P., & Grace, J. (2005). A review of rating scales for measuring behaviour change due to frontal systems damage. *Cognitive and Behavioral Neurology, 18*, 18–27.

McPheeters, H. L. (1984). Statewide mental health outcome evaluation: A perspective of two southern states. *Community mental Health Journal, 20*, 44–55.

Moriyama, Y., Mimura, M., Kato, M., Yoshino, A., Hara, T., Kashima, H., Kato, A., & Watanabe, A. (2002). Executive dysfunction and clinical outcome in chronic alcoholics. *Alcoholism: Clinical & Experimental Research, 26*, 1239–1244.

Norris, G., & Tate, R. L. (2000). The Behavioral Assessment of the Dysexecutive Syndrome (BADS): Ecological, concurrent and construct validity. *Neuropsychological Rehabilitation, 10*, 33–45.

Shallice, T., & Burgess, P. (1991). Deficits in strategy application following frontal lobe damage in man. *Brain, 114*, 727–741.

Wilson, B. A., Alderman, N., Burgess, P. W., Emslie, H., & Evans, J. J. (1996). *Behavioral Assessment of the Dysexecutive Syndrome.* Bury St. Edmunds, England: Thames Valley Test Company.

Wilson, B. A., Evans, J. J., Emslie, H., Alderman, N., & Burgess, P. (1998). The development of an ecologically valid test for assessing patients with a dysexecutive syndrome. *Neuropsychological Rehabilitation, 8*, 213–228.

CANTAB

PURPOSE

The purpose of Cambridge Neuropsychological Test Automated Batteries (CANTAB) is to provide an evaluation of cognitive abilities including visual memory, visual attention, working memory, and planning.

SOURCE

The software can be ordered from Cambridge Cognition Ltd, Turnbridge Court, Turnbridge Lane Bottisham, Cambridge, England CB5 9DU UK (www.cantab.com). It runs on standard Windows-based PC systems. The cost is £1500 for a 12-month unlimited use license (other prices are available for different test options; contact info@cantab.com). Although the individual may use the mouse for responding, a touch screen is required as the tests are designed and validated for use with it. A press pad is preferred for some of the tasks (MTS, RVP, RTI), although the spacebar on the keyboard can be used.

AGE RANGE

The age range is from 4 to about 90 years. Most of the studies are with adults, including the elderly. There are, however, increasing reports of use of the battery with children (e.g., Hughes et al., 1994; Kempton et al., 1999) as young as age 4 years (e.g., Luciana & Nelson, 1998, 2002). Luciana and Nelson (2002) note that 4-year-olds were very difficult to test on the CANTAB, perhaps due to the nature of the tasks or to lapses in motivation and fatigue. They note that ease of administration improves dramatically for 5-year-olds, although complete ease of administration occurred by about age 9 years.

DESCRIPTION

The software comprises one screening test and 12 principal tests from the CANTAB[1] system (Fray et al., 1996; Robbins et al., 1994, 1998; Sahakian & Owen, 1992), which takes as its starting point well-documented paradigms used in animal research of memory. The original theoretical impetus of CANTAB was to bridge the gap that exists between human and animal experimental research such that direct comparisons of cognitive deficits observed in brain-damaged patients with those observed in animals bearing selective lesions could be made. Thus, the authors adapted paradigms developed by investigators such as Gaffan (1974), Mishkin (1982), and

Petrides (1987) and their colleagues for testing models of memory in rodents and infrahuman primates (e.g., delayed matching to sample, conditional associative learning, radial maze). In addition, tests were added based on methodological advances in neuropsychological assessments of humans. The aim was to provide a componential analysis of particular cognitive functions in the assessment of elderly and dementing individuals.

The tasks, shown in Table 8–8 and Figure 8–1, cover a wide range of cognitive domains, including visual memory, attention, working memory, and planning. They are graded in nature, allowing for a wide range of ability while avoiding ceiling or floor effects. The use of a computer ensures that testing is given in a standardized manner with standardized feedback, and both accuracy and speed can be evaluated. The tests can be run individually. Alternatively, a schedule comprising a number of tests may be set up. When a test is run, there is a choice of "clinical" or "parallel" modes. Clinical mode is the standard form when comparisons with the normative data are to be made. The parallel modes (alternate forms) are intended for repeat testing. Measures for each task may be displayed in a window, printed out in summary reports and data sheets, or saved to a disk, including into a file format suitable for further analysis (e.g., Excel). In addition, detailed trial-by-trial results may also be saved to disk for further analysis.

ADMINISTRATION

Directions for administering the tests appear in the test administration guide. The examiner enters the subject details (e.g., name, age, gender, NART score) and selects a schedule comprising the required test(s). The examiner sits next to the examinee and provides necessary instructions. It is possible to pause or abort the test by pressing the "Esc" key.

ADMINISTRATION TIME

The approximate administration times for each test are provided in Table 8–8.

SCORING

The examiner can choose whether to output all the summary outcome measures or a limited subset. The examiner can also choose to include standard score data in the summary data sheet. In this case, following the raw score, the z score and percentile are provided along with information regarding the peer comparison group (age, NART, gender, N). The test results can be compared against all subjects in the normative database that have a score for the measure in question. Alternatively, CANTAB will attempt to narrow the basis of comparison to include only peers within matching age and NART ranges and of the same gender. The program will choose the best peer group it can with an N of over 30 for the particular measure in question. Age is prioritized over NART, and NART

over gender, when choosing the best peer group. The examiner can also customize some options (e.g., widening peer group to include all ages). There are no composite or factor scores.

DEMOGRAPHIC EFFECTS

Age

Performance tends to improve during childhood, reaching its peak between ages 20 and 29 and then declining with advancing age (De Luca et al., 2003; Luciana & Nelson, 2002; Robbins, 1994). However, developmental trajectories differ depending upon the task/function. For example, planning ability (as measured by the Stocking task) shows steady improvement through early adolescence, while attentional set-shifting ability shows a much swifter maturational path, with adult levels of competence appearing by age 8 to 10 years (De Luca et al., 2003; Luciana & Nelson, 2002). Robbins et al. (1998) reported that the Intradimension/Extradimensional Shift task and the Stockings of Cambridge are more sensitive to aging than any of the other CANTAB measures. However, Rabbitt and Lowe (2000) found that scores from neither test correlated with age between 60 and 80 years. Rather, the most age-sensitive tests in the CANTAB battery were the memory tasks. Correlations between memory task scores and age, however, were modest. The most age-sensitive memory performance indices were those from the Paired Associates task, which accounted for more than 10% of age-related variance between individuals. No other memory test accounted for more than 1% of age-related variance.

IQ

Scores tend to be poorer in those with lower IQ levels (De Luca et al., 2003; Luciana & Nelson, 2002; Robbins et al., 1994).

Gender

Robbins et al. (1994) reported men were slightly but significantly better than women on the Spatial Recognition task. Men also had a clear advantage over women on the Spatial Working Memory task (De Luca et al., 2003; Robbins et al., 1994) and the Stockings task (De Luca et al., 2003). By contrast, women were slightly but significantly faster than men at the simultaneous component of the Delayed Matching to Sample task (Robbins et al., 1994).

NORMATIVE DATA

Standardization Sample

The CANTAB normative database was created from over 2000 control subjects (aged 4–90) who participated in various research studies, with most being from English-speaking U.K. residents. No information is provided in the manual regarding gender or average NART estimated IQ.

Table 8–8 CANTAB Tasks

Test	Purpose	Task Demands	Approximate Time
Motor Screening (MOT)	Screens for visual, movement, and comprehension problems; introduces subject to computer	A series of crosses are shown in different locations on the screen and subject must touch the crosses in turn.	3 min
Matching to Sample Visual Search (MTS)	Tests the ability to match visual samples	Subject is shown an abstract pattern as well as similar patterns. Subject must touch the one pattern that matches the target.	9 min
Delayed Matching to Sample (DMS)	A test of perceptual matching, immediate and delayed visual memory, in a four-choice simultaneous and delayed recognition memory paradigm	Subject is shown a complex pattern (made up of four sub-elements), and then four patterns. Subject must touch the pattern that matches the sample. One of the choice patterns is identical to the sample, one is a novel distractor pattern, one has the shape of the sample and the colors of the distractor, and the fourth has the colors of the sample and the shape of the distractor. In some trials the sample and choice patterns are shown simultaneously, whereas in others, there is a delay (0, 4, or 12 seconds).	10 min
Pattern Recognition Memory (Immediate/Delayed) (PRM)	Two separate tests of visual pattern recognition in a two-choice forced discrimination paradigm	Subject is presented with a series of 12 visual patterns in the center of the screen. In the recognition phase, subject must choose between the old and a novel pattern. Each response is accompanied by an auditory tone, and visual feedback is provided in the form of a tick for a correct response and a cross for an incorrect response. This procedure is repeated with 12 new patterns.	5 min each
Spatial Recognition Memory (SRM)	A test of spatial recognition memory in a two-choice forced discrimination paradigm	A white square appears in sequence at five different locations. In the recognition phase, subject must identify, by touching one of two squares, which of these locations had been occupied by a square. Feedback is provided. The procedure is repeated three times using new target and distracter locations.	5 min
Paired Associate Learning (PAL)	Assesses conditional learning of pattern-location associations. The number of patterns placed correctly on the first presentation of each trial gives an index of list memory. The number of repeat, reminder presentations needed for the subject to learn all the associations provides a measure of list learning.	White boxes are shown on the screen, each opened in a randomized order. In one (or more) is a pattern. Subject must remember patterns associated with different locations, and during the test phase, as each pattern is presented, touch the appropriate location. After three correct sets with a single pattern, the number of patterns are increased to two for two sets, then to three for two sets, then to six, and finally eight for one set each.	10 min
Spatial Span (SSP)	Like Corsi memory span	A pattern of white squares is shown. Some squares change in color in a variable sequence. After each sequence, subject must touch each of the target boxes in the same order. The number of boxes in the sequence is increased from two at the start of the test to nine by the end.	5 min each

(continued)

417

Table 8–8 CANTAB Tasks (continued)

Test	Purpose	Task Demands	Approximate Time
Spatial Working Memory (SWM)	A self-ordered task requiring retention and manipulation of spatial information in working memory	By process of elimination, subject has to find one blue token in each of a number of boxes and use them to fill up the right column. Subject decides the order in which boxes are visited. The key instruction is that once a token has been taken from a box, the box will not be used again. Returning to an empty box already sampled on this search is an error.	8 min
Big Little Circle (BLC)	Trains subject to follow a simple rule and reverse a rule; usually given before IED	Subject is presented with pairs of circles, one large and one small. Subject is trained to touch the small circle and then after 20 trials to touch the larger circle.	3 min
Intra/Extradimensional Shift (IED)	Test of rule acquisition and reversal, requiring visual discrimination, attentional set formation, maintenance, and shifting	Subject is presented with two complex stimuli and must learn which of the stimuli is correct by touching it. Two artificial dimensions are used: color-filled shapes and white lines. Two stimuli (one correct, one incorrect) are displayed, initially each of only one dimension, then each of both dimensions (first adjacent, then overlapping). Feedback teaches the subject which stimulus is correct, and after six correct responses, the stimuli and/or rules are changed. These shifts are initially intradimensional (e.g., color-filled shapes remain the only relevant dimension), then later extradimensional (white lines become the only relevant dimension).	7 min
Rapid Visual Information Processing (RVP)	A test of sustained attention	A white box appears in the center of the screen, inside which digits from 2 to 9 appear in a pseudorandom order, at the rate of 100 digits per minute. Subject must detect target odd or even sequences of digits and register responses by pressing the space bar.	7 min
Reaction Time (RTI)	Measures simple and choice reaction time	In SRT, subject holds the press-pad down, then releases it and touches the screen when a yellow dot appears. In CRT, the yellow dot may appear in any one of five locations.	5 min
Stockings of Cambridge (SOC)	Spatial planning test based on the Tower of London	Subject must use balls in the lower display to copy the pattern in the upper display in the minimum number of moves possible. There are two parts to the test: a passive movement copying stage and an active planning and execution task. For both stages, the display is the same.	10 min

Other Normative Data

Recently, Luciana and Nelson (2002) have provided normative data from healthy children ages 4 to 12 years for six of the tasks (Motor Screening, Spatial Memory Span, Self-Ordered Search, Tower of London, Pattern Recognition and Intradimensional/Extradimensional Set-Shifting). De Luca et al. (2003) provided normative data for four of the CANTAB tasks (Spatial Span, Spatial Working Memory, Tower of London, Intradimensional/Extradimensional Set-Shifting). The data are based on

Figure 8–1 Sample items of standard CANTAB tasks. *Source:* Courtesy of Cambridge Cognition Ltd.

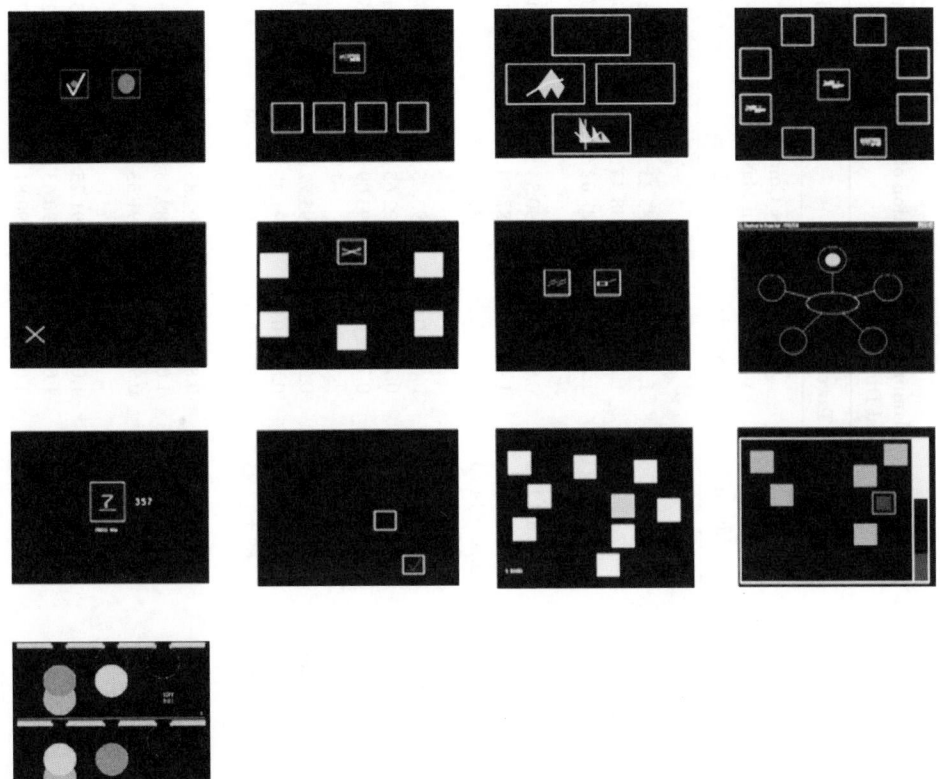

194 healthy Australian individuals, aged 8 to 64 years. The data are shown in Table 8–9.

RELIABILITY

Internal Consistency

In 4- to 12-year-old children, internal consistency is reported to be adequate to high, ranging from .73 for a measure of RT latency to .95 on the self-ordered search task (Luciana, 2003).

Test-Retest Reliability and Practice Effects

Estimates of test-retest reliability and practice effects were obtained for many of the CANTAB measures on a sample of 162 elderly volunteers, ranging in age from 60 to 80 years (Lowe & Rabbitt, 1998). Volunteers performed CANTAB tests in randomized order on two occasions separated by an interval of about four weeks. As shown in Table 8–10, many of the CANTAB measures have poor test-retest reliability. Correlations that fell within adequate or higher levels (.70+) were the accuracy measure for the two-choice Pattern Recognition task, the average number of trials to succeed on the Paired Associated Learning task, and the total errors to extradimensional shift on the Intra/Extradimensional Shift task. The rest of the tests had test-retest reliabilities that were marginal or low. Modest practice effects were evident on most of the tasks.

The relative unreliability of many of the tasks, particularly on tasks thought to tap working memory and planning, likely relates to the fact that marked improvements in performance can occur on tests of executive function once appropriate strategies are found, but improvement will be less or not at all if a suboptimal strategy is attempted. Rabbitt et al. (2001) stressed that the tasks may not be poorly defined or ill-chosen; rather, excellent tests of executive ability may depend for their sensitivity on their novelty, restricting their use to a single occasion. Nonetheless, the relative unreliability of the tasks limits the extent to which it is possible to use them for diagnostic purposes and to index changes over time, the progress of pathologies, or the effects of clinical interventions (Lowe & Rabbitt, 1998).

Alternate Form Reliability

This is not provided for the various tests reported in the manual.

VALIDITY

Factor-Analytic Findings

Robbins et al. (1998) examined the factor structure of some of the CANTAB subtests (Paired Associate Learning, Delayed Matching to Sample, Pattern Recognition, Matching to Sample,

Table 8-9 Means and Standard Deviations for the CANTAB Tasks Organized According to Age Group and Gender

	N	Short-Term Memory Capacity and Sequencing Ability	Working Memory			Strategic Planning and Organization of Goal-Directed Behavior			Attentional Set-Shifting
		Spatial Span	Spatial Working Memory			Tower of London			ID/ED
		Span	Within Search Errors	Between Search Errors	Strategy	% Perfect Solutions	Average Excess Moves Per Trial	% Completed in Maximum Moves	Level Completed
8–10									
Male	13	5.71 ± 0.91	2.46 ± 3.13	44.38 ± 13.05	16.85 ± 3.08	64.06 ± 10.36	1.30 ± 0.40	85.23 ± 8.04	8.50 ± 1.09
Female	16	5.56 ± 1.09	1.31 ± 1.62	43.88 ± 10.12	17.75 ± 2.32	59.17 ± 8.47	1.24 ± 0.39	88.33 ± 6.19	8.79 ± 0.87
Total	29	5.63 ± 0.10	1.83 ± 2.44	44.10 ± 11.31	17.34 ± 2.68	61.34 ± 9.50	1.26 ± 0.39	87.02 ± 7.05	8.60 ± 0.97
11–14									
Male	13	6.46 ± 1.51	1.31 ± 1.60	26.92 ± 16.98	15.92 ± 4.11	72.16 ± 12.92	0.97 ± 0.58	90.34 ± 10.22	8.46 ± 1.20
Female	16	6.00 ± 1.20	1.06 ± 1.00	38.94 ± 15.34	16.25 ± 4.19	60.27 ± 13.56	1.40 ± 0.47	87.50 ± 6.93	8.19 ± 0.98
Total	29	6.21 ± 1.29	1.17 ± 1.28	33.55 ± 16.93	16.10 ± 4.08	65.50 ± 14.33	1.21 ± 0.55	88.75 ± 8.46	8.31 ± 1.07
15–19									
Male	21	7.76 ± 1.34	0.81 ± 1.66	14.14 ± 11.53	14.19 ± 3.68	81.53 ± 12.57	0.69 ± 0.52	93.45 ± 6.98	8.73 ± 0.94
Female	18	6.63 ± 1.50	1.17 ± 1.42	26.61 ± 18.47	15.50 ± 4.83	78.47 ± 12.17	0.77 ± 0.37	92.65 ± 7.73	8.63 ± 0.76
Total	39	7.23 ± 1.51	0.97 ± 1.55	19.90 ± 16.19	14.79 ± 4.24	80.16 ± 12.33	0.72 ± 0.45	93.09 ± 7.23	8.68 ± 0.85
20–29									
Male	19	7.05 ± 1.19	0.74 ± 1.52	8.05 ± 7.63	10.63 ± 5.52	81.56 ± 15.37	0.57 ± 0.53	95.72 ± 5.91	8.42 ± 1.47
Female	20	7.05 ± 1.64	1.05 ± 1.54	19.60 ± 14.55	15.75 ± 3.27	75.66 ± 11.95	0.84 ± 0.46	91.45 ± 7.30	8.75 ± 0.79
Total	39	7.05 ± 1.41	0.90 ± 1.52	13.97 ± 12.94	13.26 ± 5.15	78.69 ± 13.95	0.70 ± 0.51	93.59 ± 6.89	8.59 ± 1.16
30–49									
Male	21	6.41 ± 1.40	1.38 ± 1.99	20.19 ± 18.93	14.10 ± 4.27	76.70 ± 14.71	0.80 ± 0.52	92.85 ± 8.90	8.86 ± 0.64
Female	18	5.63 ± 1.07	2.53 ± 2.43	28.29 ± 21.98	15.29 ± 5.41	69.74 ± 13.05	1.03 ± 0.53	89.58 ± 6.78	8.84 ± 0.50
Total	39	6.05 ± 1.30	1.89 ± 2.24	23.82 ± 20.48	14.63 ± 4.78	73.48 ± 14.24	0.91 ± 0.53	91.35 ± 8.06	8.85 ± 0.57
50–64									
Male	6	5.33 ± 0.52	2.83 ± 1.72	32.83 ± 9.62	16.50 ± 3.62	71.25 ± 20.06	1.03 ± 0.50	91.25 ± 7.13	8.33 ± 0.82
Female	13	4.92 ± 0.95	3.00 ± 3.98	37.31 ± 17.06	17.62 ± 3.62	69.27 ± 15.18	1.06 ± 0.60	90.63 ± 8.64	8.23 ± 1.30
Total	19	5.05 ± 0.85	2.95 ± 3.37	35.89 ± 14.97	17.25 ± 3.56	69.85 ± 16.12	1.05 ± 0.55	90.81 ± 8.00	8.26 ± 1.15

Source: From De Luca et al., 2003. Reprinted with the kind permission of Psychology Press.

Table 8–10 Test-Retest Coefficients for CANTAB Tasks

Magnitude of Coefficient	Test
Very high (.90+)	
High (.80–.89)	Pattern Recognition no. correct
	PAL—Average trials to success
Adequate (.70–.79)	ID/ED—Total errors to ED shift
Marginal (.60–.69)	PAL—First Memory Score
	SOC—No. of trials in optimum solution
	SWM—Total errors
	Spatial Span
Low (≤.59)	Spatial Recognition no. correct
	DMS Total
	DMS—No delay
	DMS—4-second delay
	DMS—12-second delay
	SOC—Av No. moves: four moves problem
	SOC—Av No. moves: five moves problem
	ID/ED—Total errors to ID shift

Source: From Lowe & Rabbit, 1998. Reprinted with permission from Elsevier.

Spatial Working Memory, Stockings of Cambridge [Tower of London], Spatial Span, Spatial Recognition, Intra/Extradimensional Shift) and a measure of fluid intelligence (the AH4) in a large group ($N = 787$) of elderly volunteers, aged 55 to 80 years. They found evidence for a six-factor model. Factor 1 represented general learning and memory ability and comprised scores from Paired Associate Learning, Pattern Recognition, Delayed Matching to Sample (accuracy), and the Matching to Sample visual search task (accuracy). Factor 2 represented executive processes including Spatial Working Memory, Spatial Span, and Stockings of Cambridge. Factor 3 loaded mainly on latency measures (Delayed Matching to Sample, Matching to Sample, and Stockings of Cambridge). Factor 4 captured other aspects of executive and planning functions represented by the Stockings of Cambridge. Factor 5 represented attentional set formation, maintenance, and shifting on the Intra-/Extradimensional shift task, while Factor 6 incorporated error scores of the Delayed Matching to Sample tasks. Of note, while there was some clustering among executive tasks and memory tests, there was also considerable independence among the different executive measures. Further, the attention set-shifting task, Intra/Extradimensional Shift, loaded on a separate factor from all other tests in the battery, suggesting that the various "frontal" tasks are measuring different aspects of executive function.

Rabbitt and Lowe (2000) also found that Intra/Extradimensional Shift scores did not correlate with scores on any other CANTAB task in a healthy elderly sample. In addition, principal components analysis suggested some evidence of separation of executive and memory factors. Two executive tests (Spatial Working Memory, Stockings of Cambridge) loaded on a factor separate from the memory tests, which were split across two factors. The separation of factors incorporating scores from executive and memory measures is consistent with the analyses reported by Robbins et al. (1998).

In adults, when the entire battery is factor analyzed, a measure of fluid intelligence (AH 42) shows considerable loading on factors tapping visual memory and learning (Factor 1) and executive functioning (Factor 2; Robbins et al., 1998). In children (Luciana & Nelson, 2003), some CANTAB measures (Spatial Memory Span, number of Tower of London perfect solutions, percent correct on Pattern Recognition) show modest associations ($r = .27–.39$) with measures of fluid (WISC-III Block Design) and crystallized (e.g., WISC-III Vocabulary) ability.

Clinical Studies

The CANTAB tests have been used with a variety of populations (e.g., Fray & Robbins, 1996; Joyce & Robbins, 1991; Owen et al., 1991, 1992, 1993, 1995, 1996; Sahakian et al., 1990), and there is evidence that CANTAB tasks are differentially sensitive to disturbances in various brain systems. For example, Owen et al. have reported that patients with lesions of the temporal lobe are unaffected on the tower (SOC) and set-shifting tasks (IED), while those with frontal lesions are impaired. Patients with early Alzheimer's disease (AD) are relatively unaffected on the Intra/Extradimensional Shift task, whereas those early in the course of Huntington's disease show severe impairment. In Parkinson's disease, the Intra/Extradimensional Shift test reveals impairment independent of motor ability, and this is ameliorated by conventional dopaminergic medication. Neurosurgical patients with localized excisions of the frontal lobes are also impaired on the Spatial Working Memory task (Owen et al., 1991, 1995, 1996). While spatial working memory impairments may also be observed following temporal lobectomy or unilateral amygdalo-hippocampectomy, the deficits are both qualitatively and quantitatively different (e.g., tend to be seen only with increasing task difficulty) from those observed after frontal lobe damage. As might be expected, tests of Pattern Recognition Memory, Delayed Matching to Sample, and Paired Associated Learning appear sensitive to temporal lobe damage (Owen et al., 1995). Further, patients with mild or moderate AD are impaired on tests of Pattern and Spatial Recognition, Delayed Matching to Sample, and Paired Associate Learning (Sahakian et al., 1990; Sahgal et al., 1991), and the tests appear capable of distinguishing between different stages of severity of the disease (Sahgal et al., 1991). The paired associate task appears to be particularly sensitive to changes early in the course of AD. Fowler et al. (2002) assessed elderly individuals at six-month intervals over a two-year period and found that the Paired Associate Learning task was an especially effective tool for the early, preclinical detection of AD. In almost all cases, this identification was possible well before significant deterioration was noted on standard neuropsychological tests (e.g., WMS-R, COWA, RAVLT). Similar findings have been reported by Blackwell et al. (2004).

Rabbitt and Lowe (2000) found that performance on memory tasks (the Paired Associate Learning and Spatial Recognition) was the most sensitive to normal aging even when general fluid ability (measured by the Cattell Culture Fair Intelligence Test, CCF) was taken into account. In contrast, performance on executive tasks (Stockings of Cambridge, Spatial Working Memory, Intra/Extradimensional Shift) was generally not related to age; rather, fluid intelligence scores predicted performance on these tests. These results provide additional evidence that the executive and memory tests in the CANTAB are sensitive to changes in different sets of functional processes.

The CANTAB also appears sensitive to a variety of toxic substances. Joyce and Robbins (1991) reported that chronic alcoholics, who had been abstinent for at least three years, showed mild deficits in tests of planning (SOC) and spatial working memory. Maruff et al. (1998) found deficits in Pattern and Spatial Recognition Memory and Paired Associate Learning in individuals who sniff gasoline but who do not have acute toxic encephalopathy. In addition, the memory deficits were reduced (but not necessarily eliminated) with abstinence.

A number of studies have also been published characterizing the neuropsychological profiles of various other conditions including autism (Ozonoff et al., 2004), schizophrenia (e.g., Pantelis et al., 1997), depression (Elliott et al., 1996; Sweeney et al., 2000; Weiland-Fiedler et al., 2004), ADHD (Kempton et al., 1999), obsessive-compulsive disorder (Nielen & Den Boer, 2003; Veale et al., 1996), and antisocial personality (Dolan & Park, 2002). For example, Pantelis et al. (1997) compared patients with chronic schizophrenia, normal controls, and patients with neurological disorders (frontal lobe lesions, temporal lobe lesions, Parkinson's disease) on the Spatial Span, Spatial Working Memory, and Stockings of Cambridge tasks. The patients with schizophrenia were impaired on all three tasks in comparison with matched control subjects. The pattern of results was qualitatively similar to the impairment found in the patients with focal frontal lesions and, to a lesser extent, similar to that found in patients with Parkinson's disease. The findings provided support for the notion of dysfunction of frontostriatal circuits in schizophrenia. Dolan and Park (2002) reported that individuals diagnosed with antisocial personality disorder showed deficits on tests of planning (Stockings of Cambridge), set-shifting (Intra/Extradimensional Shift), and Delayed Matching to Sample. The deficits were similar to those observed in unmedicated children with ADHD (Kempton et al., 1999), raising the question of the role of ADHD in explaining some of the executive deficits observed in antisocial personality disorder. The battery has also been used to chart the development of memory and executive functions in children (Luciana, 2003).

Proficiency in English does not impact performance, supporting its use with individuals who have compromised verbal skills. For example, comparison of children who spoke English as a primary or second language revealed no differences in CANTAB performance (Luciana & Nelson, 2002).

The stimuli are fairly large, and mild visual impairment does not appear to significantly impact performance (Luciana & Nelson, 2002).

COMMENT

The particular strength of the CANTAB battery is that it incorporates a wide variety of executive and memory tasks, which have not been selected on the basis of informed intuition or clinical tradition, but rather are adaptations for use with humans of paradigms developed on animals with damage to specific brain areas, principally frontal and temporal regions (Lowe & Rabbitt, 1998). The battery has also been used with a wide variety of populations (including neurological and psychiatric), varying in level of ability and age. The fact that the same tasks can be applied across the lifespan is a very positive feature. That said, very young children (e.g., 4-year-olds) do have difficulty with the computerized battery (Luciana & Nelson, 2002). The CANTAB does not require facility with English (e.g., Luciana & Nelson, 2002) and has been used with populations (e.g., aboriginals in Australia) with no or limited exposure to psychological or educational testing (Maruff et al., 1998). Thus, it can be used with illiterate individuals, individuals with weak verbal skills, or individuals from different cultures. It also controls for problems with movement by including measures of motor speed, and the graded nature of the tasks reduces the likelihood of floor and ceiling effects. It is portable and can be taken to the patient's bedside or house, in addition to being used in the laboratory or clinic (Fray & Robbins, 1996). Further, the use of a computer ensures that testing is given in a uniform manner with standardized feedback and detailed recording of accuracy and latency. It (particularly the Paired Associate Learning task) appears sensitive for detecting the early effects of progressive, neurodegenerative disorders such as Alzheimer's and Parkinson's disease.

The normative base is also large. However, its description is sparse. Reliability information on alternate forms is lacking. Further, the low test-retest reliability of many of the CANTAB measures limits their ability to characterize strengths and weaknesses and to monitor changes in functioning. Only Pattern Recognition and Paired Associate Learning appear to be sufficiently reliable for clinical use (see Table 8–10). Rabbitt et al. (Lowe & Rabbitt, 1998; Rabbitt et al., 2001) have made a compelling argument for why tests of executive functioning might be expected to show low test-retest reliabilities, namely, that tests of executive functions are maximally sensitive under conditions of novelty. Nonetheless, reliability studies need to address the dilemma of how to interpret changes over time relative to expected practice effects as well as expected developmental changes in cognitive skill (Luciana & Nelson, 2002). It is also important to bear in mind that information on test-retest reliability currently exists for adult but not pediatric populations.

Several other issues deserve mention. While there are many positive features associated with computerized assessment, it is also possible that such administration can mask deficits that would otherwise be apparent in some populations. For example, some individuals (e.g., those with autism) may perform better when faced with a computer than with a person, tapping cognitive functions at a level that is rarely demanded in real-life settings (Luciana, 2003). Further, the CANTAB software is programmed to ignore irrelevant responses. Accordingly, this design feature may limit its ability to index problems with behavioral regulation (Hughes & Graham, 2002). Finally, a major strength of the CANTAB is also a weakness: The battery is almost exclusively nonverbal in its response requirements and in the nature of stimulus presentation, limiting conclusions that can be drawn about a patient's verbal functioning (Luciana, 2003).

NOTE

1. CANTAB Eclipse includes two new tests: Affective Go/No-Go Test, which presents a series of word pairs from three affective categories (positive, negative, neutral) and the examinee must identify the category of a word according to two target affective category options, and Verbal Recognition Memory Test, which assesses immediate and delayed memory of a word list under free recall and forced choice recognition conditions.

REFERENCES

Blackwell, A. D., Sahakian, B. J., Vesey, R., Semple, J. M., Robbins, T. W., & Hodges, J. R. (2004). Detecting dementia: Novel neuropsychological markers of preclinical Alzheimer's disease. *Dementia Geriatric Cognitive Disorders, 17,* 42–48.

De Luca, C. R., Wood, S. J., Anderson, V., Buchanan, J-O, Proffitt, T. M., Mahony, K., & Pamelis, C. (2003). Normative data from the CANTAB I. Development of executive function over the lifespan. *Journal of Clinical and Experimental Neuropsychology, 25,* 242–254.

Dolan, M., & Park, I. (2002). The neuropsychology of antisocial personality disorder. *Psychological Medicine, 32,* 417–427.

Elliott, R., Sahakian, B. J., McKay, A. P., Herrod, J. J., Robbins, T. W., & Paykel, E. S. (1996). Neuropsychological impairments in unipolar depression: The influence of perceived failure on subsequent performance. *Psychological Medicine, 26,* 975–989.

Fowler, K. S., Saling, M. M., Conway, E. L., Semple, J. M., & Louis, W. J. (2002). Paired associate performance in the early detection of DAT. *Journal of the International Neuropsychological Society, 8,* 58–71.

Fray, P. J., & Robbins, T. W. (1996). CANTAB battery: Proposed utility in neurotoxicology. *Neurotoxicology and Teratology, 18,* 499–504.

Fray, P. J., Robbins, T. W., & Sahakian, B. J. (1996). Neuropsychiatric applications of CANTAB. *International Journal of Geriatric Psychiatry, 11,* 329–336.

Gaffan, D. (1974). Recognition impaired and association intact in the memory of monkeys after transection of the fornix. *Journal of Comparative Physiology and Psychology, 86,* 1100–1109.

Huges, C., & Graham, A. (2002). Measuring executive functions in childhood: Problems and solutions? *Child and Adolescent Mental Health, 7,* 131–142.

Hughes, C., Russell, J., & Robbins, T. W. (1994). Evidence for executive dysfunction in autism. *Neuropsychologia, 29,* 709–723.

Joyce, E., & Robbins, T. W. (1991). Frontal lobe function in Korsakoff and non-Korsakoff alcoholics: Planning and spatial working memory. *Neuropsychologia, 29,* 709–723.

Kempton, S., Vance, A., Maruff, P., Luk, E., Costin, J., & Pantelis, C. (1999). Executive function and attention deficit hyperactivity disorder: Stimulant medication and better executive function performance in children. *Psychological Medicine, 29,* 527–538.

Lowe, C., & Rabbitt, P. (1998). Test/re-test reliability of the CANTAB and ISPOCD neuropsychological batteries: Theoretical and practical issues. *Neuropsychologia, 36,* 915–923.

Luciana, M. (2003). Practitioner review: Computerized assessment of neuropsychological function in children: Clinical and research applications of the Cambridge Neuropsychological Testing Automated Battery (CANTAB). *Journal of Child Psychology and Psychiatry, 44,* 649–663.

Luciana, M., & Nelson, C. A. (1998). The functional emergence of prefrontally-guided working memory systems in four- to eight-year-old children. *Neuropsychologia, 36,* 273–293.

Luciana, M., & Nelson, C. A. (2002). Assessment of neuropsychological functioning through use of the Cambridge Neuropsychological Testing Automated Battery: Performance in 4- to 12-year-old children. *Developmental Neuropsychology, 22,* 595–624.

Maruff, P., Burns, C. B., Tyler, P., Currie, B. J., & Currie, J. (1998). Neurological and cognitive abnormalities with chronic petrol sniffing. *Brain, 121,* 1903–1917.

Mishkin, M. (1982). A memory system in the monkey. *Philosophical Transactions of the Royal Society of London. 298,* 85–95.

Nielen, M. M. A., & Den Boer, J. A. (2003). Neuropsychological performances of OCD patients before and after treatment with fluoxetine: Evidence for persistent cognitive complaints. *Psychological Medicine, 33,* 917–925.

Owen, A. M., Beksinska, M., James, M., Leigh, P. N., Summers, B. A., Marsden, C. D., Quinn, N. P., Sahakian, B. J., & Robbins, T. W. (1993). Visuospatial memory deficits at different stages of Parkinson's disease. *Neuropsychologia, 31,* 627–644.

Owen, A. M., James, M., Leigh, P. N., Summers, B. A., Marsden, C. D., Quinn, N. P., Lange, K. W., & Robbins, T. W. (1992). Fronto-striatal cognitive deficits at different stages of Parkinson's disease. *Brain, 115,* 1727–1751.

Owen, A. M., Morris, R. G., Sahakian, B. J., Polkey, C. E., & Robbins, T. W. (1996). Double dissociations of memory and executive functions in working memory task following frontal lobe excision, temporal lobe excision or amygdalo-hippocampectomy in man. *Brain, 119,* 1597–1615.

Owen, A. M., Roberts, A. C., Polkey, C. E., Sahakian, B. J., & Robbins, T. W. (1991). Extra-dimensional versus intra-dimensional set shifting performance following frontal lobe excisions of amygdalo-hippocampectomy in man. *Neuropsychologia, 29,* 993–1006.

Owen, A. M., Sahakian, B. J., Semple, J., Polkey, C. E., & Robbins, T. W. (1995) Visuospatial short term recognition memory and learning after temporal lobe excisions, frontal lobe excision or amygdalo-hippocampectomy in man. *Neuropsychologia, 33,* 1–24.

Ozonoff, S., Cook, I., Coon, H., Dawson, G., Joseph, R. M., Klin, A., McMahon, W. M., Minshew, N. J., Munson, J. A., Pennington, B. F., Rogers, S. J., Spence, M. A., Tager-Flusberg, H., Volkmar, F. R., & Wrathall, D. (2004). Performance on Cambridge Neuropsychological Test Automated Battery subtests sensitive to frontal lobe function in people with autistic disorder: Evidence from the collaborative programs of excellence in autism network. *Journal of Autism & Developmental Disorders, 34,* 139–150.

Pantelis, C., Barnes, T. R., Nelson, H. E., Tanner. S., Weatherley, L., Owen, A. M., & Robbins, T. W. (1997). Frontal-striatal cognitive deficits in patients with chronic schizophrenia. *Brain, 120,* 1823–1843.

Petrides, M. (1987). Conditional learning and the primate frontal cortex. In E. Perecman (Ed.), *The frontal lobes revisited* (pp. 91–108). New York: IRBN Press.

Rabbitt, P., & Lowe, C. (2000). Patterns of cognitive ageing. *Psychological Research, 63,* 308–316.

Rabbitt, P., Lowe, C., & Shilling, V. (2001). Frontal tests and models for cognitive ageing. *European Journal of Cognitive Psychology, 13,* 5–28.

Robbins, T. W., James, M., Owen, A. M., Sahakian, B. J., Lawrence, A. D., McIness, L., & Rabbitt, P. M. A. (1998). A study of performance on tests from the CANTAB battery sensitive to frontal lobe dysfunction in a large sample of normal volunteers: Implications for theories of executive functioning and cognitive aging. *Journal of the International Neuropsychological Society, 4,* 474–490.

Robbins, T. W., James, M., Owen, A. M., Sahakian, B. J., McInnes, L., & Rabbitt, P. (1994). Cambridge Neuropsychological Test Automated Battery (CANTAB): A factor analytic study of a large sample of normal elderly volunteers. *Dementia, 5,* 266–281.

Sahakian, B. J., Downes, J. J., Eagger, S., Evenden, J. L., Levy, R., Philpot, M. P., Roberts, A. C., & Robbins, T. W. (1990). Sparing of attentional relative to mnemonic function in a subgroup of patients with dementia of the Alzheimer type. *Neuropsychologia, 28,* 1197–1213.

Sahakian, B. J., & Owen, A. M. (1992). Computerized assessment in neuropsychiatry using CANTAB. *Journal of the Royal Society of Medicine, 85,* 399–402.

Sahgal, A., Sahakian, B. J., Robbins, T. W., Wray, C. J., Lloyd, S., Cook, J. H., McKeith, I. G., Disley, J. C. A., Eagger, S., Boddington, S., & Edwardson, J. A. (1991). Detection of visual memory and learning deficits in Alzheimer's disease using the Cambridge Neuropsychological Test Automated Battery. *Dementia, 2,* 150–158.

Sweeney, J. A., Kmiec, J. A., & Kupfer, D. J. (2000). Neuropsychological impairments in bipolar and unipolar mood disorders on the CANTAB neurocognitive battery. *Biological Psychiatry, 48,* 674–684.

Veale, D. M., Sahakian, B. J., Owen, A. M., & Marks, I. M. (1996). Specific cognitive deficits in tests sensitive to frontal lobe dysfunction in obsessive-compulsive disorder. *Psychological Medicine, 26,* 1261–1269.

Weiland-Fiedler, P., Erickson, K., Waldeck, T., Luckenbaugh, D. A., Pike, D., Bonne, O., Charney, D. S., & Neumeister, A. (2004). Evidence for continuing neuropsychological impairments in depression. *Journal of Affective Disorders, 82,* 253–258.

Category Test (CT)

PURPOSE

This test measures a patient's abstraction or concept formation ability, flexibility in the face of complex and novel problem solving, and capacity to learn from experience.

SOURCE

Manual Version

The Halstead-Reitan version of the test (Halstead-Reitan Category Test, HRCT) requires a projection box, examiner's control panel, and projector and can be obtained from Reitan Neuropsychology Lab, P.O. Box 66080, Tucson, AZ 85728-6080. The projection box, examiner's control panel, projector, and slides cost $1380 US. Recording forms are $25 US per package (100/package).

Booklet Version

The booklet version of the Adult form (Booklet Category Test, BCT, 2nd Edition; DeFilippis & McCampbell, 1997) can be ordered from Psychological Assessment Resources (PAR), PO Box 998, Odessa, FL 33556 (http://www.parinc.com), at a cost of $455 US. The kit includes a Professional Manual, two-volume set of Stimulus Plates, and 50 Response Booklets. A booklet form of the Children's Category Test (CCT), appropriate for ages 5 years through 16 years (Boll, 1993), can be ordered from Harcourt Assessment (www.harcourtassessment .com) for $399 US. Western Psychological Services also offers a short form of the adult version (Short Category Test, SCT; Wetzel & Boll, 1987) at a cost of $175 US.

Computer Version

A program (developed by Choca, Laatsch, Garside, & Arnemann) with a number of different versions (e.g., standard, Russell's Short Form, Intermediate, and the new Adaptive Category Test that automatically jumps to the next subtest when it has enough information to predict performance on that subtest) is available through MHS, 65 Overlea Blvd., Suite 210, Toronto, Ontario, M4H 1P1 (http://www.mhs.com), at a cost of $360 US. PAR also offers computer versions of the Category Test (DeFilippis & PAR staff). The computer program allows the examiner to give any of three versions of the test: the standard 208-item version and two short-form versions, one consisting of 120 items, the other of 108 items. The price from PAR is $475 US.

AGE RANGE

The adult version was developed for use with individuals aged 15 years, 6 months and older, although adequate normative data are only available for individuals aged 20 to 85 years. An intermediate version covers the age range from 9 years to 15 years, 6 months, while the children's version is available for ages 5 to 8 years.

DESCRIPTION

The Category Test was developed by Halstead (1947) to assess the ability to conceptualize qualities such as size, shape, number, position, and color. It is also part of the Reitan test battery (Halstead-Reitan Category Test, HRCT; Reitan & Davison, 1974). The original version included 336 items organized into nine subtests. In 1948 (D. Wolfson, January 27, 2005, Neuropsychology Listserv), Reitan reduced it to seven sets of items, with a total of 208 items presented via a slide projector. Each set is organized on the basis of a different principle, such as number of objects, spatial position of an odd stimulus, etc. For example, the first set shows Roman numerals from I to IV and the patient is asked to indicate the number (1 to 4) on the response key that the design suggests (see Figure 8–2). Subjects must use feedback they receive from their correct and incorrect guesses on the series of items in each subtest to infer the underlying principle behind the subtest. No clues are given as to what the principle might be. Therefore, the test requires the deduction of a classification principle by means of response-contingent feedback, the use of the principle while it remains effective, and the ability to abandon the principle when it is no longer effective. The adult version covers the age range 15 years, 6 months and older. An intermediate version (Reed et al., 1965) covers the age range 9 years to 15 years, 6 months and includes 168 items, divided into six subtests. A children's version (Reitan, 1964) consisting of 80 items, arranged into five subtests, is available for ages 5 to 8 years.

One problem with the slide version of the test is that it relies on expensive and unwieldy equipment that may break down and is difficult to use at bedside examinations. Booklet (DeFilippis & McCampbell, 1979, 1991, 1997) and computer forms of the test are available (see *Source*). There is some evidence that these forms yield results that are equivalent to the original slide version (Choca & Morris, 1992; DeFilippis & McCampbell, 1979, 1991, 1997; Holz et al., 1996; Mercer et al., 1997). The booklet form by DeFilippis and McCampbell is very popular, and much of the recent literature uses this version with adults. It is the version that we use.

Figure 8–2 Example of item from CT.

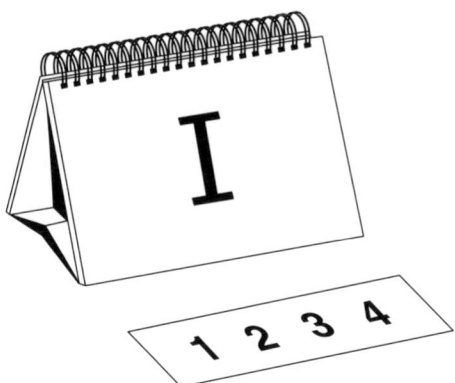

Short Forms

Another problem is that impaired subjects can take a long time (up to two hours) to complete the test. Short forms of the adult version of the Category Test have been developed (e.g., Boyle, 1986; Caslyn et al., 1980; Charter et al., 1997; Gregory et al., 1979; Labreche, 1983; Russell & Levy, 1987; Wetzel & Boll, 1987). The Short Category Test, Booklet Format (SCT) developed by Wetzel and Boll (1987) consists of 100 items. There is some evidence that the SCT functions in a similar fashion as the HRCT in terms of its psychometric properties, discriminative ability, and relation to standard neuropsychological tests (Gelowitz & Paniak, 1992). It also appears to produce scores (T scores but not raw scores) similar to the booklet version developed by DeFillipis and McCampbell (Gontkovsky & Souheaver, 2002; but see *Comment*). The short form developed by Charter et al. (1997) appears problematic, at least in patients with traumatic brain injuries. Hogg et al. (2001) found that prediction errors from the short to the long form were quite large (10 points or more) for a significant proportion (about 25%) of their sample.

An attempt has also been made to shorten the forms given to adolescents. The Children's Category Test (CCT; Boll, 1993) is available in booklet format and consists of two levels: Level 2 is given to children aged 9 to 16 years and consists of six subtests and 83 items as opposed to 168 items in the original version; Level 1 is given to children aged 5 to 8 years and consists of five subtests and 80 items, the same number as in the original version. The internal structure of the test was not changed by Boll, although the administration method is different because the stimuli are presented in booklet format. Also, the colors white and black have been substituted for the original red and green to avoid problems for children who are color blind. Boll (1993) contends that scores on the original and CCT versions are highly correlated (.88) and that the versions are therefore parallel forms. We use the CCT.

ADMINISTRATION

Manual Versions

The instructions for the Adult, Intermediate, and Children's versions are provided in Figure 8–3. The apparatus for presenting the test items to the subject consists of a slide projector, a console with a viewing screen for rearview projection, and the examiner's control board. The subject must find the underlying principle by choosing one out of four presented stimuli. The subject responds by pressing one of four levers, numbered 1, 2, 3, and 4 (colored knobs for children), corresponding to the four stimuli, arranged from left to right, and placed on the apparatus immediately below the screen.

The test items are projected from the slide projector. The slides begin with eight Roman numeral items varying from I to IV. Because the keys on the subject's board are numbered, this first subtest serves to associate the items on the screen with the subject's response keys, as well as to acquaint the

Figure 8–3 Instructions for Manual Standard HRCT Versions.

Adult Manual Version—Standard HRCT Version

Say to the patient: *On this screen you are going to see different geometrical figures and designs. Something about the pattern on the screen will remind you of a number between 1 and 4. On the keyboard in front of you (pointing) the keys are numbered 1, 2, 3, and 4. You are to press down on the key that is the same number that the pattern on the screen reminds you of. That is, if the picture on the screen reminds you of the number 1, pull key number 1. If the picture on the screen reminds you of the number 2, pull key number 2. And so on. For example, what number does this remind you of?*

Put on the first slide. If the subject says "one," ask the subject which key he or she should press. After the subject has pressed the number 1 key, say: *The bell you have just heard tells you that you got the right answer. Every time you have the right answer you will hear the bell ring.* Instruct the subject to try one of the other keys to find out what happens when an incorrect key is pressed. Then say: *The buzzer is what you hear when you have the wrong answer. In this way, you will know each time whether you have the right or wrong answer. However, for each picture on the screen you get only one choice. If you make a mistake we just go right on to the next picture.*

Proceed with Subtest I. Say: *Now which key would you pick for this picture?* After Subtest I, say: *That was the end of the first subtest. This test is divided into seven subtests. In each subtest there is one idea or principle that runs throughout the entire subtest. Once you have figured out what the idea or principle in the subtest is, by using this idea you will get the right answer each time. Now we are going to begin the second subtest. The idea in it may be the same as in the practice set, or it may be different. We want you to figure it out.*

Proceed with Subtest II. After Subtest II, say: *That was the end of the second subtest and, as you probably noticed, you don't necessarily have to see a number to have a number suggested to you. You saw squares, circles, and other figures. Also, as you may or may not have noticed, in each of these subtests, there is one idea or principle that runs throughout. Once you figure out the idea, you continue to apply it to get the right answer. Now we are going to start the third subtest. The idea may be the same as the last one or it may be different. I want to see if you can figure out what the idea is and then use it to get the right answer. Remember, the idea remains the same throughout the subtest. I will tell you when we complete one subtest and are ready to begin a new one.*

Proceed with Subtest III. In Subtest IV, after slide #6 (the first slide without numbers), say: *This is still the same group, but now the numbers are missing. The principle is still the same.* After Subtests III, IV, and V, say: *That was the end of that subtest. Now we are going to begin the next one. The idea in it may be the same as the last one or it may be different. We want you to figure it out.*

After Subtest VI, say: *In the last subtest there is no one idea or principle that runs throughout the group because it is made up of items you have already seen in preceding subtests. Try to remember what the right answer was the last time you saw the pattern and give that same answer again.*

Intermediate Manual Version—Standard HRCT Form

The instructions for the standard version are similar to those given previously. Note, however, that the task consists of six subtests. Following Subtest V, say: *That was the end of the fifth subtest and now we are going to begin the last one. In this last subtest, there is no one idea or principle that runs throughout the subtest because it is made up of pictures that you have seen before. Try to remember what the right answer was the first time that you saw the picture and then give that same answer again.*

Children's Version—Standard HRCT Form

For this version of the test, the numbered key discs are replaced by colored ones. The sequence 1, 2, 3, and 4, changes to Red, Blue, Yellow, and Green. Say: *On this screen you will see pictures of different figures and designs. Each picture will make you think of a color, either red, blue, yellow, or green. On this keyboard in front of you, you will notice that the keys are different colors. This one is red, this one is blue, this one is yellow, and this one is green (pointing). Press down on the key that has the same color as the color you think of when you look at the picture. For example, what color does this make you think of?*

Flash on the first picture—red circle. If the subject says "red," ask which key he or she would press. When the subject presses the key, say: *That is the bell, which means that you got the right answer. Try another key and see what happens when you get the wrong answer.*

After the subject does this, say: *That is the buzzer, which means you got the wrong answer. This way you will know each time whether you are right or wrong, but for each design you may press only one key. If you make a mistake we will go right on to the next one. Let's try some of these.*

After the first subtest, say: *That completes the first group of pictures. Now we are going to start the next group. You will have to try to figure out the right reason for picking one key or another. If you are able to figure out the reason why your answers are right or wrong it will help, because the reason stays the same all the way through the group.* Proceed with the second subtest.

Then say: *Now we are going to start the third group. This group may be different from the one you just finished or it may be the same. Let's see if you can figure out the right answers.*

Proceed with the fourth subtest using the same type of introductory comments as with the third subtest. Before beginning the fifth subtest, say: *Now we are going to start the last group. This group will test your memory since it is made up of pictures that you have already seen. Try to remember what the right answer was the first time you saw the picture and give the same answer again.* Do not hesitate to comment favorably at any time during the test when the subject answers correctly.

subject with the test procedure and to relieve test anxiety. A correct response produces a chime; an incorrect response produces a buzzer sound. Between each subtest or group there is one blank frame.

The master off-on switch is located on the left of the examiner's control board. When this switch is turned on, the screen and examiner's control board are ready for use. A hand control switch controlling item presentation is located at the right of the examiner's control board. When this switch is depressed once quickly, a new item will replace the previous item on the screen. Do *not* keep the switch depressed. A four-way control switch corresponding to the subject's four response keys is located in the center of the examiner's control board. To provide feedback to the subject (i.e., to engage the chime for correct responses and the buzzer for incorrect responses), the examiner must set the switch to the appropriate numbered slot for each item. The proper setting of this switch for each item is indicated on a record blank. The examiner must always set the answer key before changing the slide.

As a general rule, any part of the instructions may be repeated when the examiner believes it necessary. The purpose is to give the subject a clear understanding of the problem he or she is facing and the rules involved in its solution. The principles themselves are never given to a subject, but when working with subjects who are extremely impaired in their ability to form concepts, it may become necessary to urge them to study the picture carefully; to ask for their descriptions of the stimulus material, which are then followed by examiner questions such as, "Does that give you any idea of what might be the right answer?"; to urge them to try to notice and remember how the pictures change, since this often provides clues to the underlying principle; and to try to think of the reason when they answer correctly. However, examiners should not provide information relevant to the solution of the problems presented by the test. The only information of this kind comes from the bell or buzzer following each response.

Impaired subjects sometimes find the test trying and frustrating. The examiner should make every effort to encourage the subject to continue working at the task. If a subject shows no sign of making progress on the first 20 items of any one of Subtests III through VI and *also* gives evidence of extreme frustration with the task, it is better to discontinue the subtest at this point and prorate the error scores (linear extrapolation) than run the risk of not being able to complete the test.

Some additional points should be mentioned briefly:

1. Although speed is not a factor and subjects should not be hurried, neither should they be permitted to take an unduly long time to respond and thus affect the continuity of the test.
2. The examiner should always be alert to the slide on the screen, not only to monitor the subject's performance, but also to ensure correct slide order.
3. The testing room should be somewhat darkened, yet light enough for the examiner to record errors.

4. The subject should sit directly in front of the screen. The colors particularly may be difficult to see from an angle.

Booklet Versions (Booklet Category Test, Short Category Test, Children's Category Test)

See *Source*. Briefly, the examiner presents a series of stimulus pages in sequence. The patient responds by pointing to or verbally identifying one of four colors (for subjects aged 5–8 years) or one of four numerals (for subjects aged 9 years and older) printed on a separate response card. The examiner says "correct" or "incorrect" following each response.

ADMINISTRATION TIME

Full-length versions for adults, including the commonly used BCT, require about 40 minutes, although impaired individuals may take as long as two hours. Abbreviated versions, including the version for children (CCT), take about 20 minutes.

SCORING

The total number of errors are recorded. Raw error scores must be converted initially to scaled scores and then to demographically corrected T scores for use with the Heaton et al. (2004) norms (see *Normative Data*). For the SCT and CCT, error raw scores are converted to T scores and percentile ranks.

DEMOGRAPHIC EFFECTS

Age

Not surprisingly, error scores decline as children mature, particularly after about age 10 years (e.g., Boll, 1993; Nesbit-Greene & Donders, 2002), and increase with advancing years (e.g., Golden et al., 1998; Heaton et al., 2004; Leckliter & Matarazzo, 1989; Mitrushina et al., 2005; Sherrill-Pattison et al., 2000; Sweeney & Johnson, 2001).

IQ/Education

Scores are negatively affected by lower levels of educational achievement (e.g., Golden et al., 1998; Greiffenstein & Baker, 2003; Leckliter & Matarazzo, 1989; but see Mitrushina et al., 2005, who reported that education did not contribute to test scores beyond its association with age in their dataset) and IQ (e.g., Golden et al., 1998; Leckliter & Matarazzo, 1989; Mitrushina et al., 2005; Nesbit-Greene & Donders, 2002; Titus et al., 2002). Education impacts performance even after accounting for neurological variables (e.g., brain injury severity; Sherrill-Pattison et al., 2000).

Gender

Gender has little impact on test scores (Rosselli et al., 2001; Sherrill-Pattison et al., 2000).

Ethnicity/Acculturation

Performance is affected by level of acculturation, with less acculturated individuals obtaining lower scores (Arnold et al., 1994; Manly et al., 1998).

Overview

Heaton et al. (2004) report that in adults aged 20 to 85 years, age accounts for the largest amount of the variance (29% in Caucasians, 42% in African Americans) in test scores, followed by education (13% in Caucasians, 4% in African Americans) and then gender (1% in Caucasians, 2% in African Americans).

NORMATIVE DATA

Adult Versions

For the 208-item version of the CT, Reitan recommends a cutoff error score of 50 to 51 for adults. Ranges of scores for varying degrees of impairment have been defined for the standard form (Reitan & Wolfson, 1985; Table 8–11). These data are inadequate because no information was provided regarding the normative sample on which these guidelines were based.

Russell and Starkey (1993) developed the Halstead-Russell Neuropsychological Evaluation System (HRNES), which includes the HRCT. The HRNES computer scoring system evaluates an individual's performance relative to a sample that consists of 576 brain-damaged individuals and a comparison group of 200 individuals. The data are further partitioned into seven age groups and four levels of education/IQ. Caution is needed when using the scoring program since the "normal" group is based on individuals who had negative neurological examinations. However, Russell (2003) has pointed out that records of these subjects were reexamined about one year after initial testing to verify that no neurological condition, undetected at the time of the original testing, had become evident.

Mitrushina et al. (2005) provide age-based metanorms, based on 1579 participants, aged 16 to 79 years. The sample size is large, but the data are not broken down by variables (e.g., education/IQ) that have been shown to impact CT performance. It is also worth noting that the data derive from 11 studies dating largely from the 1970s to the 1980s, and the inclusion of old normative sets may introduce the potential for

Table 8–11 Severity Ranges for the Standard Form of the Adult CT (Errors)

	Perfectly Normal	Normal	Mildly Impaired	Severely Impaired
CT	0–25	26–45	46–65	65+

Source: From Reitan & Wolfson, 1985.

Table 8–12 Characteristics of the Category Test Normative Sample provided by Heaton et al. (2004)

Number	1212
Age	20–85 years[a]
Geographic location	Various states in United States and Manitoba, Canada
Sample type	Individuals recruited as part of multicenter studies
Education	0–20 years[b]
Gender	
Male	56.8%
Female	43.2%
Race/ethnicity	
Caucasian	634
African American	578
Screening	Subjects completed structured interview and reported no history of learning disability, neurological disorder, serious psychiatric disorder, or alcohol or drug abuse.

[a]Age: 20–34, 35–39, 40–44, 45–49, 50–54, 55–59, 60–64, 65–69, 70–74, 75–79, 80–89.
[b]Education: 7–8, 9–11, 12, 13–15, 16–17, 18–20.

considerable score inflation (i.e., Flynn effect, see Chapter 2, *Norms Selection*).

Heaton et al. (2004) also provide normative data based on 1212 healthy adults between 20 and 85 years of age. Their data may be preferred as they are provided separately for Caucasians and African Americans and are broken down by age, education, and gender (see Table 8–12). Note, however, that participants were tested over a period of about 25 years and it is not known to what extent they include dated norms.

Because intellectual level correlates with CT performance, IQ scores can be used to predict expected CT error scores and to determine if obtained scores are suspect. Titus et al. (2002) developed regression equations to predict CT error scores from WAIS-III VIQ, PIQ, and FSIQ scores. The equations for predicting HCT scores and predictor tables for VIQ, PIQ, and FSIQ are shown in Table 8–13. Cutoff scores were calculated by averaging the standard deviations of CT scores in their study with standard deviations observed in prior studies using normal individuals. Doubling and rounding the average standard deviation ($SD = 15$) created cutoff scores that were two standard deviations above the projected means for each IQ level. Note that the equations were developed using a sample of 51 Caucasian university students (mean age = 19.51, range 17–34 years). Accordingly, it is difficult to generalize these findings to minority group members and individuals of younger or older ages.

For the SCT (Wetzel & Boll, 1987), normative data are based on a relatively small number of healthy individuals ($N = 120$). The manual provides tables broken down by age (45 years and younger; 46 years and older). A raw score cutoff of 41 is recommended for subjects aged 45 and younger,

Table 8–13 Predicted CT Error Scores

Observed IQ	VIQ		PIQ		FSIQ	
	Predicted CT	Cutoff	Predicted CT	Cutoff	Predicted CT	Cutoff
150	10	40	9	39	6	36
145	12	42	11	41	9	39
140	14	44	14	44	11	41
135	16	46	16	46	14	44
130	18	48	19	49	17	47
125	20	50	21	51	19	49
120	22	52	23	53	22	52
115	24	54	26	56	25	55
110	27	57	28	58	27	57
105	29	59	31	61	30	60
100	31	61	33	63	33	63
95	33	63	36	66	35	65
90	35	65	38	68	38	68
85	37	67	40	70	41	71
80	39	69	43	73	43	73
75	42	72	45	75	46	76
70	44	74	48	78	49	79
65	46	76	50	80	51	81
60	48	78	53	83	54	84
55	50	80	55	85	57	87
50	52	82	57	87	59	89

Regression equations are as follows:

(1) $CT = -.427$ (WAIS-III VIQ) $+ 73.552$, $R^2 = .084$, $SE = 16.86$
(2) $CT = -.486$ (WAIS-III PIQ) $+ 81.77$, $R^2 = .112$, $SE = 16.60$
(3) $CT = -.534$ (WAIS-III FSIQ) $+ 86.00$, $R^2 = .129$, $SE = 16.51$

Source: Adapted from Titus et al., 2002.

while a cutoff score of 46 is suggested for subjects aged 46 and older. Gontkovsky and Souheaver (2002) suggest that these cutoffs may require downward adjustment to increase sensitivity.

The computer version by DeFillipis (PAR) uses the norms provided by Heaton et al. in their 1991 manual. Thus, the sample size is smaller and the data are not presented separately for Caucasians and African Americans. The program by Choca et al. (MHS) uses a simple cutoff of 51 errors or above as suspect, although the user is advised to adopt a more sophisticated approach and refer to demographically corrected norms (J. Choca, personal communication, May 23, 2003).

Intermediate and Children's Versions

Several investigators (e.g., Klonoff & Low, 1974; Knights, 1966; Spreen & Gaddes, 1969; Trites, 1977) have provided data for children on the standard slide HRCT version. Findeis and Weight (1994) presented metanorms for the CT based on a total *N* of 964, and these are shown in Table 8–14. However, the data have questionable clinical utility because they are 30 to 40 years old (based on articles published from 1965–1990) and were obtained from middle-upper-class children of above-average psychometric intelligence (average FSIQ of 112.87).

Table 8–14 Norms for the Category Test by Age

	Age										
	5	6	7	8	9	10	11	12	13	14	15
Mean	27.40	26.00	20.56	12.35	53.56	46.58	40.88	35.12	36.29	30.81	30.6
SD	9.1	12.7	8.9	6.7	17.4	18.6	16.3	16.0	16.4	12.0	12.3

Errors: Ages 5–8 (80 items), 9–15 (168 items).

Source: Data for ages 5–14 derived from Findeis and Weight, 1995, in Nussbaum & Bigler, 1997; for ages 15, data are derived from Spreen & Gaddes, 1969, and are based on a population of normal schoolchildren (*N* = 41).

Table 8–15 Characteristics of the Children's Category Test Normative Sample provided by Boll (1993)

Number	920
Age	5–16 years[a]
Geographic location	Representative of the four major U.S. geographic regions in proportions specified in 1988 U.S. Census data
Sample type	Stratified according to race/ethnicity, parent education, and geographical region representative of the proportions of the U.S. population of children according to 1988 Census data
Parent education	Stratified according to four categories: ≤ 11 years, HS, 1–3 years college, 4 or more years college
Gender	
Male	461
Female	459
Race/ethnicity	
Caucasian	69.7%
African American	14.7%
Hispanic	11.9%
Other	3.7%
Screening	Sample drawn from both public and private school settings. Students receiving mainstream special services in school settings were not excluded from testing. Only children who could understand and speak English were tested.

[a]Age: Norms are provided by yearly intervals. In age groups 5–12 there were 80 children per age group, and in age groups 13–16 years, there were 70 children per age group.

Boll (1993) provides more up-to-date norms for the booklet form of the CCT based on a very large sample representative of the school-aged population of the United States as reported in the 1988 Census data population of children ($N = 920$) in 12 age groups ranging from 5 through 16 years of age. Stratification variables included race/ethnicity, geographic region, and parent/guardian education. The characteristics of the sample are shown in Table 8–15. These norms establish a higher standard than those reported by Klonoff and Low (1974), in line with the trend for increased average performance of individuals over time (Flynn, 1984).

The CCT and the CVLT-C were standardized and normed on the same population of children and both provide age-corrected standard scores. Using the standardization sample, Donders (1998) has determined the base rates of specific discrepancies as well as the level of discrepancy required for statistical significance. These data are provided in Tables 8–16 and 8–17. On average, in children between the ages of 9 and 16 years, a discrepancy of about nine points is required for statistical significance at the .05 level and discrepancies of about 16 T-score points should be considered clinically significant. Donders noted that it was just as common for the CCT score

Table 8–16 Differences (in T scores) Between CCT Total and CVLT-C Total Indices Required for Statistical Significance

Age	Level of Significance	Difference Required
5–8	.10	6.72
	.05	8.66
9–16	.10	6.79
	.05	8.76

Source: Adapted from Donders, 1998. For more detailed breakdown by age, see Donders.

Table 8–17 Cumulative Percentages of the Standardization Sample Obtaining Various Discrepancies Between CCT Total and CVLT-C Total T scores

Difference	Ages 5–8 Years	Ages 9–16 Years
0	4	2
1	11	8
2	16	15
3	20	21
4	26	27
5	30	33
6	35	39
7	41	45
8	46	51
9	50	55
10	55	60
11	59	63
12	64	67
13	66	71
14	68	74
15	72	77
16	76	80
17	78	84
18	82	87
19	85	89
20	88	91
21	90	94
22	91	95
23	93	95
24	94	96
25	95	97
26	96	97
27	97	97
28	98	98
29	98	98
30	98	99
31	98	99
32	99	99
≥33	100	100
M	10.85	10.06
SD	7.99	7.33

Source: From Donders, 1998. Reprinted with the permission of Cambridge University Press.

to be higher than the CVLT-C score as vice versa. CVLT-C T scores that exceeded the CCT score by 17 or more points occurred in only 9.83% of the standardization sample, whereas 10.67% of the sample had a discrepancy of that magnitude in the opposite direction.

RELIABILITY

Internal Consistency

The odd-even split-half method and coefficient alpha have been used to calculate internal consistency values for the 208-item version of the CT. High reliability coefficients were obtained for the total score (>.95) for samples of normal and brain-damaged adults (Charter et al., 1987; Lopez et al., 2000; Moses, 1985; Shaw, 1966). Reliabilities for Subtest I ($r = .46$) and II ($r = .65$) were unacceptable for clinical purposes. Reliability coefficients were high for the other subtests (.77–.95; Lopez et al., 2000). For the booklet versions, SCT and CCT, split-half reliability coefficients for the total score are slightly lower (.81 on the SCT; .88 for Level 1 and .86 for Level 2 of the CCT), although still respectable (Boll, 1993; Wetzel & Boll, 1987).

Choca et al. (1997) argue that there is an especially abrupt jump from the difficulty levels of Subtest I and II to that of Subtest III of the CT. In fact, there is evidence that the items for Subtest I and II are too easy (evaluated according to the number of individuals passing an item) and show poor discrimination (low correlation between test item and total score; Lopez et al., 2000). Most of the other test items from the other subtests were within established criteria for item difficulty and the discrimination index.

Test-Retest Reliability

With intact individuals, test-retest reliability is marginal to high over short (three weeks) or longer intervals (up to one year; $r = .60$–.85; Bornstein et al., 1987; Dikmen et al., 1999; Matarazzo et al., 1974), with low values perhaps due to a restriction in the range of scores and a learning effect (Russell, 1992). When severely impaired neurological patients are considered, the Category Test has high retest reliability, above .90, even after intervals of two years (Goldstein & Watson, 1989; Matarazzo et al., 1974). In the case of children and persons with schizophrenia, correlation coefficients are somewhat lower and range from .63 to .75 (Boll, 1993; Goldstein & Watson, 1989). Long-term follow-up (about 15 years) of a group of children with learning disabilities revealed only modest correlations (about .4) and a decline in error scores, although it should be noted that a shift was made from the intermediate to the adult form for the second test administration (Sarazin & Spreen, 1986).

Practice Effects

It should be noted that the coefficients mean only that subjects were ranked in more or less the same order on both administrations, not that subjects achieved the same scores on both administrations. In fact, significant changes or practice effects emerge, even in moderately impaired neurological patients (Boll, 1993; DeFilippis & McCampbell, 1997; Dodrill & Troupin, 1975). Thus, the absence of improvement (practice effects) may be an indicator of abnormality.

In normal adults (age, $M = 32.3$ years, $SD = 10.3$; VIQ, $M = 105$, $SD = 10.8$; PIQ, $M = 105.0$, $SD = 10.5$), following short retest intervals (about three weeks), an average raw score change of 23.5 ($SD = 18.5$) points has been noted (Bornstein et al., 1987). The average percentage of change in relation to initial performance was about 46%. Dikmen et al. (1999) report an average decline in errors of about 10 points in a sample of 384 normal or neurologically stable individuals (aged 15–83 years, $M = 34.2$, $SD = 16.7$) who were retested about nine months after initial testing.

Table 8–18 provides information to determine if there has been substantial change taking practice into account. One first subtracts the mean T2 − T1 change (column 3) from the difference between the two testings for the individual and then compares it to 1.64 times the standard deviation of the difference (column 4). The 1.64 comes from the normal distribution and is exceeded in the positive or negative direction only 10% of the time if indeed there is no real change in clinical condition. Dikmen et al. (1999) also note that many factors influence practice effects. In general, younger, better-educated people, those with initial competency, or a short interval between testings have bigger improvements in test scores. In addition, regression to the mean also occurs, with a large positive change for people initially scoring poorly and a much smaller improvement or even deterioration for those initially scoring well.

Table 8–18 Test-retest Data Based on a Sample ($N = 384$) of Normal or Neurologically Stable Adults, Aged 15–83 ($M = 34.2$, $SD = 16.7$)

Category Test	Time 1 (1)		Time 2 (2)		T2 − T1 (3)	(4)	
N	M	SD	M	SD	M	SD	r
384	40.97	26.07	30.42	25.01	−10.54	14.13	.85

Interval is about 9 months.

Source: Adapted from Dikmen et al., 1999.

In children, a reduction in the total number of raw errors (about six points on Level 1, about eight points on Level 2) occurs following a retest interval of about one month, although this varies by IQ level (Boll, 1993). Children of low ability show little benefit from prior experience with the test; children of above-average IQ also show little improvement because they are at ceiling. By contrast, children of average ability are most likely to benefit from practice.

VALIDITY

Correlation With Other Measures

The total score of the CT (adult and child versions) shows moderate relations with the Full-Scale IQ and particularly the Performance subtests (Block Design, Object Assembly) of the Wechsler intelligence scales (Berger, 1998; Golden et al., 1998; Klonoff, 1971; Lansdell & Donnelly, 1977; Nesbitt-Greene & Donders, 2002; Titus et al., 2002). The new Matrix Reasoning and Letter-Number Sequencing subtests of the WAIS-III also show moderate/high relations (about .35–.58; Dugbarty et al., 1999; Titus et al., 2002). While some suggest that it may not distinguish an ability that is separate from nonverbal reasoning (Lansdell & Donnelly, 1977), others (Donders, 1996; Titus et al., 2002) have reported only a modest amount of shared variance, about 11% to 13%, between Wechsler PIQ and total CT score.

Further, there is a modest association between the CT and neuropsychological measures of learning and memory (Bertram et al., 1990; Boll, 1993; Fischer & Dean, 1990), providing some evidence of the test's value as a measure of learning ability. It does not, however, assess learning as a pure ability construct. Research with the CCT and the CVLT-C suggests that they measure fairly different aspects of children's cognition, sharing less than 15% of common variance at any age level, and that statistically significant differences between the standard scores of these two tests are not uncommon (Donders, 1998). The CT also shows little/modest relation (.14–.38) with academic performance (Boll, 1993; Rosselli et al., 2001).

Factor-Analytic Findings

Despite the fact that the CT is composed of several subtests, clinical interpretations and most studies tend to rely (perhaps incorrectly) on a single composite score. There is general agreement that the CT is a complex measure, loading on a number of different factors. Several studies, using a variety of different samples (e.g., people with schizophrenia, people with brain damage, patient controls), have suggested that the CT measures at least two factors, identified as spatial position reasoning (Subtests III, IV, and VII), and proportional reasoning (Subtests V and VI and sometimes VII; Allen et al., 1999; Donders, 2001; Johnstone et al., 1997). The subtests loading on the spatial positioning factor are affected by age, whereas performance on the subtests loading on the proportional

reasoning factor are affected more by education and appear sensitive to severity of head injury (Donders, 2001). Donders (2001) also noted that Subtest III was in the range of chance for more than one-third of the sample, without any relationship to injury variables (see also Nesbitt-Greene & Donders, 2002). He suggested dropping this task, given the lack of criterion validity.

The children's booklet version of the test (CCT) is also multifactorial in nature (Donders, 1999; Nesbitt-Greene & Donders, 2002). A two-factor solution was found in the standardization sample for both the younger (ages 5–8) and older (ages 9–16) age groups, although the nature of the constructs measured was different between the two versions of the test. Nesbitt-Greene and Donders (2002) also identified a two-factor solution for the CCT in 9- to 16-year-olds who had suffered traumatic head injury. Factor 1 was composed primarily of Subtest IV, V, and VI, whereas Factor 2 was defined primarily by Subtests III and VI. Factor 1, but not 2, demonstrated sensitivity to severity of head injury. Subtests I and II did not load strongly on either factor, a finding that also emerged in the study of the standardization sample (Donders, 1999). The summary score proved unrelated to neurological or demographic variables (Donders & Nesbitt-Greene, 2004). Nesbitt-Greene and Donders (2002; Donders & Nesbitt-Greene, 2004) caution that reliance on the summary total score may impede diagnostic accuracy. Unfortunately, norm-based subtest scores are not available.

There is additional evidence in pediatric populations that the summary T score may not always provide useful diagnostic information. In 5- to 8-year-old children with traumatic brain injury, only Subtests III and V (but not Subtest IV) of the CCT-1 varied in a consistent and meaningful manner with levels of injury severity and postinjury psychometric intelligence (Moore et al., 2004). Further, about 21% of the sample performed at chance level on Subtest IV, a task that did not demonstrate any criterion validity. The authors concluded that when a substantial proportion of the total errors (e.g., ≥50%) on the CCT-1 pertain to errors from Subtest IV and errors on Subtest V that require recall of items from Subtest IV, the composite T score of the CCT-1 should not be interpreted.

Clinical Studies

The CT is sensitive to a variety of brain disturbances (see Choca et al., 1997, for a review) and is almost as sensitive as the full Halstead-Reitan battery in determining the presence or absence of neurological damage (Adams & Trenton, 1981). However, other tests that depend more heavily on memory or speed of processing (e.g., CVLT-II/CVLT-C) may prove more sensitive to various disorders (e.g., head injury) and/or injury severity (Hoffman et al., 2000; Donders & Giroux, 2005; Donders & Nesbitt-Greene, 2004). As noted above, combining subtests into a single summary score may also limit its sensitivity (Donders & Nesbitt-Greene, 2004; Moore et al., 2004; Nesbitt-Greene & Donders, 2002).

Impairment on the CT shows no consistent relation to specific location or laterality of brain damage (Anderson et al., 1995; Bornstein, 1986; Demakis, 2004; Doehring & Reitan, 1962; Donders, 2001; Hom & Reitan, 1990; Klove, 1974; Lansdell & Donnelly, 1977; Pendleton & Heaton, 1982; Reitan & Wolfson, 1995a), although it was originally designed to detect frontal lobe damage (Halstead, 1947). Diminished performance also occurs in depressed individuals (Savard et al., 1980; but see Ruttan & Heinrichs, 2003) and those with schizophrenia (Goldstein et al., 2002; Steindl & Boyle, 1995).

In terms of predictive validity, Barreca et al. (1999) found that stroke survivors who made few errors on the CT subsequently showed the greatest improvement in arm and hand function.

Malingering

A patient's effort may be evaluated on the Category Test in a number of ways. Bolter (personal communication, 1995; J. Sweet, November 2, 2005) identified 18 items on the HCT that most normal and neurologically impaired individuals pass note: subsequently, four items (Subtest IV: 22, 32; Subtest VI: 26, 27) were eliminated on cross-validation. The eighteen items that form the Bolter Validity Index (VI) include one item from Subtest I (6), two items from Subtest II (9, 18), two items from Subtest IV (22, 32), three items in Subtest V (27, 30, 33), seven in Subtest VI (4, 18, 21, 24, 26, 27, 30), and three in Subtest VII (6, 10, 13). Approximately 97% of normal and neurologically impaired individuals failed two or fewer of the 18 items. Tenhula and Sweet (1996) reported that a cutoff of more than three infrequently missed items was reasonably effective (84% hit rate, 51% sensitivity, 98% specificity) in discriminating brain-injured individuals from normals instructed to malinger (see also DiCarlo et al., 2000). Trueblood and Schmidt (1993), however, did not find a significant difference between suspected malingerers and brain-injured controls in the number of "rare errors." It may be that this indicator occurs rarely, and therefore its presence would suggest invalidity while its absence would not substantiate a test protocol's validity (Trueblood & Schmidt, 1993).

Tenhula and Sweet (1996) also suggested that an excessive number of errors on Subtests I, II, and VII might also raise the suspicion of malingering. DiCarlo et al. (2000), using a simulation paradigm, confirmed that a decision rule of more than error on Subtests I and II was a fairly accurate indicator of malingering. This indicator correctly classified 76% of all simulators and all of the controls as well as individuals who had suffered a traumatic brain injury (mean GCS about 12). However, Williamson et al. (2003) reported that it may be difficult to distinguish malingerers from moderate-severely injured patients on the basis of these criteria. Forrest et al. (2004) recommend a more liberal cutoff of two or more errors on these subtests to reduce the likelihood of false positives. It is worth noting in this context that factor-analytic findings (see Donders, 2001; Johnstone et al., 1997) reveal Subtests I and II to be conceptually different from the other CT subtests and

unrelated to injury severity. In addition, very few normals or brain-injured individuals make errors on items in these subtests (see also Forrest et al., 2004), a fact that had been noted many years ago by Simmel and Counts (1957; see the excellent review by Sweet & King, 2002).

Performance inconsistency may also suggest suboptimal effort. Reitan and Wolfson (1996) gave the CT on two occasions to litigants and nonlitigants who complained of having suffered a traumatic brain injury. Nonlitigants improved their performance on the second test session, making on average 10 fewer errors. By contrast, litigants made about 14 more errors on the second administration.

The CT validity indicators appear appropriate for use with a variety of neurological populations, including those with TBI (Forrest et al., 2004). Note, however, that they have been evaluated in individuals typically with average to above educational achievement. Accordingly, the indicators should be used cautiously with individuals of limited education/IQ. In addition, Williamson et al. (2003) noted considerable discrepancies in those head-injured individuals identified as malingering by the CT and by the Word Memory Test (WMT). The classifications based upon the CT (but not the WMT) appeared to be confounded by true neurocognitive impairment, particularly in those who suffered severe brain injuries. In short, the CT indices may suggest but do not confirm motivational status and should not be used in isolation (Sweet & King, 2002).

COMMENT

The CT has a long history of use in neuropsychology and remains a very popular test. Lees-Haley et al. (1996) found that the CT was administered 32% of the time by neuropsychologists conducting forensic evaluations and ranked as the eighth most frequently administered test. Camara et al. (2000) found that the CT ranked ninth in frequency of use by neuropsychologists, and Rabin et al. (2005) recently reported that the CT was the third most commonly used measure of executive functioning (following the WCST and ROCF). The booklet version by DeFilippis appears to be in much wider use than the original slide version. The booklet form of the children's version, the CCT, is also recommended for clinical use given its relatively short administration time, good normative base, and good predictive accuracy (see also Donders, 1996). The booklet forms have the added advantage of being relatively inexpensive and highly portable.

A number of efforts have been made to shorten the Category Test. However, as Mitrushina et al. (2005) pointed out, the validity of the shortened versions are based on analyses derived from administration of the entire CT. Studies that actually administered a shortened version are needed, and it remains to be determined whether they do indeed show psychometric properties and discriminative ability similar to the long form.

The evidence suggests that the CT is robust to alterations in instrumentation (slide, booklet, computer). With regard to the computer versions, the advantages include error-free test administration as well as the collection of additional data, such as reaction time and number of perseverations. However, as computer-related anxiety increases, error scores and response latencies may also increase (Browndyke et al., 2002). Heaton et al.'s 1991 norms tend to be used for the computer versions; however, interpretation may be problematic in individuals who may present with computer-related anxiety.

Although Reitan and Wolfson (1995b) have asserted that adjusting raw scores according to demographic variables may not be a valid procedure when evaluating individuals with brain impairment, the available literature (e.g., Sherrill-Pattison et al., 2000) suggests that norms that consider demographic background are likely to reflect more accurately the neuropsychological status of the patients. The relative advantage appears to be primarily in the reduced likelihood of misclassifying an individual as impaired when none might exist (Sherrill-Pattison et al., 2000; Sweeney, 1999).

The CT is a multifactorial task and combining subtest scores into a composite measure may limit diagnostic information. A two-factor solution has been found for the adult and children's versions. Unfortunately, norm-based data are not available for these factor-based scores. Development of reliable norms at the subtest level has been recommended (Moore et al., 2004; Nesbitt-Greene & Donders, 2002).

Significant practice effects can be expected on the CT when individuals are retested. Failure to show improvement may signal abnormality and/or suboptimal effort. An excessive number of errors, particularly on Subtests I and II, are also suspicious.

Comparison Between the Category Test and the WCST

Both the Category Test and Wisconsin Card Sort Test (WCST) require, in part, the deduction of a classification principle by means of response-contingent feedback, the use of the principle while it remains effective, and the ability to abandon the principle when it is no longer effective. The two tests, however, are not identical (Adams et al., 1995; Bond & Buchtel, 1984; Donders & Kirsch, 1991; Gelowitz & Paniak, 1992; Golden et al., 1998; King & Snow, 1981; O'Donnell et al., 1994; Pendleton & Heaton, 1982; Perrine, 1993) and show only a modest amount of common variance (Golden et al., 1998; Perrine, 1993). Perrine (1993) suggested that the two tests relate to different facets of concept formation. The WCST is related to attribute identification, which entails discrimination of relevant features, while the CT is more related to rule learning, which assesses the deduction of classification rules. Similarly, based on factor analysis with the WAIS-R subtests, Golden et al. (1998) suggested that the CT appears to reflect spatial analytic skills (loading with the Performance subtests), while the WCST measures loaded on factors independent of the other tasks. Bond and Buchtel (1984) pointed out that the perceptual abstraction abilities that are required by the CT are more difficult than those required by the WCST.

On the other hand, the WCST requires the subject to realize that the correct matching principle shifts periodically without warning. The CT makes no such demand. The WCST also provides a measure of perseverative tendencies while the CT does not. Adams et al. (1995) reported that in alcoholic patients, Subtest VII of the HCT correlated with glucose metabolism in cingulate, dorsolateral, and orbitomedial regions of the frontal lobe. Number of categories achieved on the WCST correlated only with glucose metabolism in the cingulate region. On the other hand, Anderson et al. (1995) examined the MRI scans of 68 traumatically brain-injured patients and found that while both CT and WCST performance were associated with brain injury, neither appeared related to volume of focal frontal damage, presence or absence of frontal damage, or degree of nonspecific structural (atrophic) changes.

The use of one or both of these tests depends on the diagnostic question. For example, if the examiner wishes to examine for perseverative tendencies, then the WCST should be chosen. On the other hand, if the examiner wishes for a more difficult and sensitive measure of abstraction ability, then the CT is the preferred measure. Because of order of administration effects (Brandon & Chavez, 1985; Franzen et al., 1993), the clinician should consider which of the two instruments will provide the best information regarding the referral question and should use only that test for the patient.

REFERENCES

Adams, K. M., Gilman, S., Koeppe, R., Klain, K., Junck, L., Lohman, M., Johnson-Greene, D., Berent, S., Dede, D., & Kroll, P. (1995). Correlation of neuropsychological function with cerebral metabolic rate in subdivisions of the frontal lobes of older alcoholic patients measured with [^{18}F]Fluorodeoxyglucose and positron emission tomography. *Neuropsychology, 9*, 275–280.

Adams, R. L., & Trenton, S. L. (1981). Development of a paper-and-pen form of the Halstead Category Test. *Journal of Consulting and Clinical Psychology, 49*, 298–299.

Allen, D. N., Goldstein, G., & Mariano, E. (1999). Is the Halstead Category Test a multidimensional instrument? *Journal of Clinical and Experimental Neuropsychology, 21*, 237–244.

Anderson, C. V., Bigler, E. D., & Blatter, D. D. (1995). Frontal lobe lesions, diffuse damage, and neuropsychological functioning of traumatic brain-injured patients. *Journal of Clinical and Experimental Neuropsychology, 17*, 900–908.

Arnold, B. R., Montgomery, G. T., Castaneda, I., & Longoria, R. (1994). Acculturation and performance of Hispanics on selected Halstead-Reitan neuropsychological tests. *Assessment, 1*, 239–248.

Barreca, S. R., Finlayson, A. J., Gowland, C. A., & Basmajian, J. V. (1999). Use of the Halstead Category Test as a cognitive predictor of functional recovery in the hemiplegic upper limb: A cross-validation study. *The Clinical Neuropsychologist, 13*, 171–181.

Berger, S. (1998). The WAIS-R factors: Usefulness and construct validity in neuropsychological assessments. *Applied Neuropsychology, 5*, 37–42.

Bertram, K. W., Abeles, N., & Snyder, P. J. (1990). The role of learning in performance on Halstead's Category Test. *The Clinical Neuropsychologist, 4*, 244–252.

Boll, T. (1993). *Children's Category Test.* San Antonio, TX: The Psychological Corporation.

Bond, J. A., & Buchtel, H. A. (1984). Comparison of the Wisconsin Card Sorting Test and the Halstead Category Test. *Journal of Clinical Psychology, 40,* 1251–1254.

Bornstein, R. A. (1986). Contribution of various neuropsychological measures to detection of frontal lobe impairment. *International Journal of Clinical Neuropsychology, 8,* 18–22.

Bornstein, R. A., Baker, R. B., & Douglass, A. B. (1987). Short-term retest reliability of the Halstead-Reitan battery in a normal sample. *The Journal of Nervous and Mental Disease, 175,* 229–232.

Boyle, G. L. (1986). Clinical neuropsychological assessment: Abbreviating the Halstead Category Test of brain dysfunction. *Journal of Clinical Psychology, 42,* 615–625.

Brandon, A. D., & Chavez, E. L. (1985). Order and delay effects on neuropsychological test presentation: The Halstead Category and Wisconsin Card Sorting Tests. *International Journal of Clinical Neuropsychology, 7,* 152–153.

Browndyke, J. N., Albert, A. L., Malone, W., Schatz, P., Paul, R. H., Cohen, R. A., Tucker, K. A., & Gouvier, W. D. (2002). Computer-related anxiety: Examining the impact of technology-specific affect on the performance of a computerized neuropsychological assessment measure. *Applied Neuropsychology, 4,* 210–218.

Camara, W. J., Nathan, J. S., & Puente, A. E. (2000). Psychological test usage: Implications in professional psychology. *Professional Psychology: Research and Practice, 31,* 141–154.

Caslyn, D. A., O'Leary, M. R., & Chaney, E. F. (1980). Shortening the Category Test. *Journal of Consulting and Clinical Psychology, 48,* 788–789.

Charter, R. A., Adkins, T. G., Alekoumbides, A., & Seacat, G. F. (1987). Reliability of the WAIS, WMS, and Reitan Battery: Raw scores and standardization scores corrected for age and education. *The International Journal of Clinical Neuropsychology, 9,* 28–32.

Charter, R. A., Swift, K. M., & Blusewicz, M. J. (1997). Age- and education-corrected, standardized short form of the Category Test. *The Clinical Neuropsychologist, 11,* 142–145.

Choca, J. P., Laatsch, L., Wetzel, L., & Agresti, A. (1997). The Halstead Category Test: A fifty year perspective. *Neuropsychology Review, 7,* 61–75.

Choca, J., & Morris, J. (1992). Administering the Category Test by computer: Equivalence of results. *The Clinical Neuropsychologist, 6,* 9–15.

DeFilippis, N. A., & McCampbell, E. (1979, 1991, 1997). *Manual for the Booklet Category Test.* Odessa, FL: Psychological Assessment Resources.

Demakis, G. J. (2004). Frontal lobe damage and tests of executive processing: A meta-analysis of the Category Test, Stroop Test, and Trail-Making Test. *Journal of Clinical and Experimental Neuropsychology, 26,* 441–450.

DiCarlo, M. A., Gfeller, J. D., & Oliveri, M. V. (2000). Effects of coaching on detecting feigned cognitive impairment with the Category Test. *Archives of Clinical Neuropsychology, 15,* 399–413.

Dikmen, S. S., Heaton, R. K., Grant, I., & Temkin, N. R. (1999). Test-retest reliability and practice effects of expanded Halstead-Reitan neuropsychological test battery. *Journal of the International Neuropsychological Society, 5,* 346–356.

Dodrill, C. B., & Troupin, A. S. (1975). Effects of repeated administrations of a comprehensive neuropsychological battery among chronic epileptics. *Journal of Nervous and Mental Disease, 161,* 185–190.

Doehring, D. G., & Reitan, R. M. (1962). Concept attainment of human adults with lateralized cerebral lesions. *Perceptual and Motor Skills, 14,* 27–33.

Donders, J. (1996). Validity of short forms of Intermediate Halstead Category Test in children with traumatic brain injury. *Archives of Clinical Neuropsychology, 11,* 131–137.

Donders, J. (1998). Performance discrepancies between the Children's Category Test (CCT) and the California Verbal Learning Test-Children's Version. (CVLT-C) in the standardization sample. *Journal of the International Neuropsychological Society, 4,* 242–246.

Donders, J. (1999). Latent structure of the Children's Category Test at two age levels in the standardization sample. *Journal of Clinical and Experimental Neuropsychology, 21,* 279–282.

Donders, J. (2001). Clinical utility of the Category Test as a multidimensional instrument. *Psychological Assessment, 13,* 592–594.

Donders, J., & Giroux, A. (2005). Discrepancies between the California Verbal Hearing Test: Children's Version and the Children's Category Test after pediatric traumatic brain injury. *Journal of the International Neuropsychological Society, 11,* 386–390.

Donders, J., & Kirsch, N. (1991). Nature and implications on the Booklet Category Test and Wisconsin Card Sorting Test. *The Clinical Neuropsychologist, 5,* 78–82.

Donders, J., & Nesbitt-Greene, K. (2004). Predictors of neuropsychological test performance after pediatric traumatic brain injury. *Assessment, 11,* 275–284.

Dugbarty, A. T., Sanchez, P. N., Rosenbaum, J. G., Mahurin, R. K., Davis, M., & Townes, B. (1999). WAIS-III Matrix Reasoning test performance in a mixed clinical sample. *The Clinical Neuropsychologist, 13,* 396–404.

Findeis, M. K., & Weight, D. G. (1994). *Meta-norms for two forms of neuropsychological test batteries for children.* Unpublished paper, Brigham Young University.

Fischer, W. E., & Dean, R. S. (1990). Factor structure of the Halstead Category Test by age and gender. *International Journal of Clinical Neuropsychology, 12,* 180–183.

Forrest, T. J., Allen, D. N., & Goldstein, G. (2004). Malingering indexes for the Halstead Category Test. *The Clinical Neuropsychologist, 18,* 334–347.

Franzen, M. D., Smith, S. S., Paul, D. S., & MacInnes, W. D. (1993). Order effects in the administration of the Booklet Category Test and Wisconsin Card Sorting Test. *Archives of Clinical Neuropsychology, 8,* 105–110.

Flynn, J. R. (1984). The mean IQ of Americans: Massive gains 1932-1978. *Psychological Bulletin, 95,* 29–51.

Gelowitz, D. L., & Paniak, C. E. (1992). Cross-validation of the Short Category Test-Booklet Format. *Neuropsychology, 6,* 287–292.

Golden, C. J., Kushner, T., Lee, B., & McMorrow, M. A. (1998). Searching for the meaning of the Category Test: A comparative analysis. *International Journal of Neuroscience, 93,* 141–150.

Goldstein, G., Minshew, N. J., Allen, D. N., & Seaton, B. E. (2002). High-functioning autism and schizophrenia: A comparison of an early and late onset neurodevelopment disorder. *Archives of Clinical Neuropsychology, 17,* 461–475.

Goldstein, G., & Watson, J. R. (1989). Test-retest reliability of the Halstead-Reitan Battery and the WAIS in a neuropsychiatric population. *The Clinical Neuropsychologist, 3,* 265–273.

Gontkovsky, S. T., & Souheaver, G. T. (2002). T-score and raw-score comparisons in detecting brain dysfunction using the Booklet Category Test and the Short Category Test. *Perceptual and Motor Skills, 94,* 319–322.

Gregory, R. J., Paul, J. J., & Morrison, M. W. (1979). A short form of the Category Test for adults. *Journal of Clinical Psychology, 35,* 795–798.

Greiffenstein, M. F., & Baker, W. J. (2003). Premorbid clues? Preinjury scholastic performance and present neuropsychological functioning in late postconcussion syndrome. *The Clinical Neuropsychologist, 17,* 561–573.

Halstead, W. C. (1947). *Brain and intelligence.* Chicago: University of Chicago Press.

Heaton, R. K., Miller, S. W., Taylor, M. J., & Grant, I. (1991, 1992, 2004). *Revised comprehensive norms for an expanded Halstead-Reitan Battery: Demographically adjusted neuropsychological norms for African American and Caucasian adults.* Lutz, FL: PAR.

Hoffman, N., Donders, J., & Thompson, E. H. (2000). Novel learning abilities after traumatic head injury in children. *Archives of Clinical Neuropsychology, 15,* 47–58.

Hogg, J. R., Johnstone, B., Weishaar, S., & Petroski, G. F. (2001). Application of a short form of the Category Test for individuals with a traumatic brain injury: A cautionary note. *The Clinical Neuropsychologist, 15,* 129–133.

Holz, J. L., Gearhart, L. P., & Watson, C. G. (1996). Comparability of scores on projector- and booklet-administration of the Category Test in brain-impaired veterans and controls. *Neuropsychology, 10,* 194–196.

Hom, J., & Reitan, R. M. (1990). Generalized cognitive function after stroke. *Journal of Clinical and Experimental Neuropsychology, 12,* 644–654.

Johnstone, B., Holland, D., & Hewett, J. E. (1997). The construct validity of the Category Test: Is it a measure of reasoning or intelligence? *Psychological Assessment, 9,* 28–33.

King, M. C., & Snow, W. G. (1981). Problem-solving task performance in brain-damaged subjects. *Journal of Clinical Psychology, 38,* 400–404.

Klonoff, H. (1971). Factor analysis of a neuropsychological battery for children aged 9 to 15. *Perceptual and Motor Skills, 32,* 603–616.

Klonoff, H., & Low, M. (1974). Disordered brain function in young children and early adolescents: Neuropsychological and electroencephalographic correlates. In R. Reitan & L.A. Davidson (Eds.), *Clinical neuropsychology: Current status and applications.* New York: Wiley and Sons.

Klove, H. (1974). Validation studies in adult clinical neuropsychology. In R. Reitan & L. Davison (Eds.), *Clinical neuropsychology: Current status and application.* New York: Wiley and Sons.

Knights, R. M. (1966). *Normative data on tests for evaluating brain damage in children from 5 to 14 years of age.* Research Bulletin No. 20, Department of Psychology, University of Western Ontario, London, Canada.

Labreche, T. M. (1983). *The Victoria revision of the Halstead Category Test.* Unpublished doctoral dissertation, University of Victoria, Victoria, British Columbia, Canada.

Lansdell, H., & Donnelly, E. F. (1977). Factor analysis of the Wechsler Adult Intelligence Scale and the Halstead-Reitan Category and Tapping Tests. *Journal of Consulting and Clinical Psychology, 3,* 412–416.

Leckliter, I. N., & Matarazzo, J. D. (1989). The influence of age, education, IQ, gender, and alcohol abuse on Halstead-Reitan neuropsychological test battery performance. *Journal of Clinical Psychology, 45,* 484–512.

Lees-Haley, P. R., Smith, H. H., Williams, C. W., & Dunn, J. T. (1996). Forensic neuropsychological test usage: An empirical survey. *Archives of Clinical Neuropsychology, 11,* 45–51.

Lopez, M. N., Charter, R. A., & Newman, J. R. (2000). Psychometric properties of the Halstead Category Test. *The Clinical Neuropsychologist, 14,* 157–161.

Manly, J. J., Miller, S. W., Heaton, R. K., Byrd, D., Reilly, J., Velasquez, R. J., Saccuzzo, D. P., Grant, I., & the HIV Neurobehavioral Research Center (HNRC) group. The effect of African-American acculturation on neuropsychological test performance in normal and HIV-positive individuals. *Journal of the International Neuropsychological Society, 4,* 291–302.

Matarazzo, J. D., Wiens, A. N., Matarazzo, R. G., & Goldstein, S. G. (1974). Psychometric and test-retest reliability of the Halstead impairment index in a sample of healthy, young, normal men. *Journal of Nervous and Mental Disease, 158,* 37–49.

Mercer, W. N., Harrell, E. H., Miller, D. C., Childs, H. W., & Rockers, D. M. (1997). Performance of brain-injured versus healthy adults on three versions of the Category Test. *The Clinical Neuropsychologist, 11,* 174–179.

Mitrushina, M. N., Boone, K. B., Razani, J., & D'Elia, L. F. (2005). *Handbook of normative data for neuropsychological assessment* (2nd ed.). New York: Oxford University Press.

Moore, B. A., Donders, J., & Thompson, E. H. (2004). Validity of the Children's Category Test-Level 1 after pediatric traumatic brain injury. *Archives of Clinical Neuropsychology, 19,* 1–9.

Moses, J. A. (1985). Internal consistency of standard and short forms of three itemized Halstead-Reitan neuropsychological battery tests. *The International Journal of Clinical Neuropsychology, 3,* 164–166.

Nesbitt-Greene, K., & Donders, J. (2002). Latent structure of the Children's Category Test after pediatric traumatic head injury. *Journal of Clinical and Experimental Neuropsychology, 24,* 194–199.

O'Donnell, J. P., MacGregor, L. A., Dabrowski, J. J., Oestreicher, J. M., & Romero, J. J. (1994). Construct validity of neuropsychological tests of conceptual and attentional abilities. *Journal of Clinical Psychology, 50,* 596–600.

Pendleton, M. G., & Heaton, R. K. (1982). A comparison of the Wisconsin Card Sorting Test and the Category Test. *Journal of Clinical Psychology, 38,* 392–396.

Perrine, K. (1993). Differential aspects of conceptual processing in the Category Test and Wisconsin Card Sorting Test. *Journal of Clinical and Experimental Neuropsychology, 15,* 461–473.

Rabin, L. A., Barr, W. B., & Burton, L. A. (2005). Assessment practices of clinical neuropsychologists in the United States and Canada: A survey of INS, NAN, and APA division 40 members. *Archives of Clinical Neuropsychology, 20,* 33–66.

Reed, H. B. C., Reitan, R. M., & Klove, H. (1965). Influence of cerebral lesions on psychological test performances of older children. *Journal of Consulting Psychology, 29,* 247–251.

Reitan, R. M. (1964). *Manual for administration of neuropsychological batteries for children (aged 5 though 8).* Indianapolis: IN: Author.

Reitan, R. M., & Davison, L. A. (1974). *Clinical neuropsychology: Current status and applications.* Oxford: V. H. Winston & Sons.

Reitan, R. M., & Wolfson, D. (1985). *The Halstead-Reitan neuropsychological test battery: Theory and clinical interpretation.* Tucson, AZ: Neuropsychology Press.

Reitan, R. M., & Wolfson, D. (1995a). Category Test and Trail Making Test as measures of frontal lobe functions. *The Clinical Neuropsychologist, 9,* 50–56.

Reitan, R. M., & Wolfson, D. (1995b). Influence of age and education on neuropsychological test results. *The Clinical Neuropsychologist, 9,* 151–158.

Reitan, R. M., & Wolfson, D. (1996). The question of validity of neuropsychological test scores among head-injured litigants: Development of a dissimulation index. *Archives of Clinical Neuropsychology, 11,* 573–580.

Rosselli, M., Ardila, A., Bateman, J. R., & Guzman, M. (2001). Neuropsychological test scores, academic performance, and developmental disorders in Spanish-speaking children. *Developmental Neuropsychology, 20*, 355–373.

Russell, E. W. (1992). Reliability of the Halstead Impairment Index: A simulation and reanalysis of Matarazzo et al. (1974). *Neuropsychology, 6*, 251–259.

Russell, E. W. (2003). The critique of the HRNES in the handbook of normative data for neuropsychological assessment. *Archives of Clinical Neuropsychology, 18*, 177–180.

Russell, E. W., & Levy, M. (1987). Revision of the Halstead Category Test. *Journal of Consulting and Clinical Psychology, 55*, 898–901.

Russell, E. W., & Starkey, R. I. (1993). *Halstead Russell Neuropsychological Evaluation System (HRNES)*. Los Angeles: Western Psychological Services.

Ruttan, L. A., & Heinrichs, R. W. (2003). Depression and neurocognitive functioning mild traumatic brain injury patients referred for assessment. *Journal of Clinical and Experimental Neuropsychology, 25*, 407–419.

Sarazin, F. F-A., & Spreen, O. (1986). Fifteen-year stability of some neuropsychological tests in learning disabled subjects with and without neurological impairment. *Journal of Clinical and Experimental Neuropsychology, 8*, 190–200.

Savard, R. J., Rey, A. C., & Post, R. M. (1980). Halstead-Reitan Category Test in bipolar and unipolar affective disorders: Relationship to age and phase in illness. *Journal of Nervous and Mental Disease, 168*, 297–304.

Shaw, D. J. (1966). The reliability and validity of the Halstead Category Test. *Journal of Clinical Psychology, 37*, 847–848.

Sherrill-Pattison, S., Donders, J., & Thompson, E. (2000). Influence of demographic variables on neuropsychological test performance after traumatic brain injury. *The Clinical Neuropsychologist, 14*, 496–503.

Simmel, M. S., & Counts, S. (1957). Some stable determinants of perception, thinking, and learning: A study based on the analysis of a single test. *Genetic Psychology Monographs, 56*, 3–157.

Spreen, O., & Gaddes, W. H. (1969). Developmental norms for 15 neuropsychological tests age 6 to 15. *Cortex, 5*, 170–191.

Steindl, S. R., & Boyle, G. J. (1995). Use of the Booklet Category Test to assess abstract concept formation in schizophrenic disorders. *Archives of Clinical Neuropsychology, 10*, 205–210.

Sweeney, J. E. (1999). Raw, demographically altered, and composite Halstead-Reitan Battery data in the evaluation of adult victims of nonimpact acceleration forces in motor vehicle accidents. *Applied Neuropsychology, 6*, 79–87.

Sweeney, J. E., & Johnson, A. M. (2001). Age and neuropsychological status following exposure to violent nonimpact acceleration forces in MVAs. *Journal of Forensic Neuropsychology, 2*, 31–40.

Sweet, J. J., & King, J. H. (2002). Category Test validity indicators: Overview and practice recommendations. *Journal of Forensic Neuropsychology, 3*, 241–274.

Tenhula, W. N., & Sweet, J. J. (1996). Double cross-validation of the Booklet Category Test in detecting malingered traumatic brain injury. *The Clinical Neuropsychologist, 10*, 104–116.

Titus, J. B., Retzlaff, P. D., & Dean, R. S. (2002). Predicting scores of the Halstead Category Test with the WAIS-III. *International Journal of Neuroscience, 112*, 1099–1114.

Trites, R. L. (1977). *Neuropsychological test manual*. Ottawa, Ontario: Royal Ottawa Hospital.

Trueblood, W., & Schmidt, M. (1993). Malingering and other validity considerations in the neuropsychological evaluation of mild head injury. *Journal of Clinical and Experimental Neuropsychology, 15*, 578–590.

Wetzel, L., & Boll, T. J. (1987). *Short Category Test, Booklet Format*. Los Angeles: Western Psychological Services.

Williamson, D. J. G., Green, P., Allen, L., & Rohling, M. L. (2003). Evaluating effort with the Word Memory Test and Category Test—or not: Inconsistencies in a compensation-seeking sample. *Journal of Forensic Neuropsychology, 3*, 19–44.

Cognitive Estimation Test (CET)

PURPOSE

This test is used to assess the ability to generate effective problem-solving strategies.

SOURCE

There is no commercial source. Users may refer to the following text to design their own material.

AGE RANGE

The age range is 17+.

DESCRIPTION

Shallice and Evans (1978) focused attention on the ability of brain-damaged patients, particularly those with frontal lobe damage, to produce adequate cognitive estimates. They designed a test that requires subjects to respond to questions that do not have readily apparent answers. For example, answering questions such as "What is the average length of a man's spine?" requires selecting an appropriate plan and of checking the plausibility of the estimate but does not require performing any complex computation.

Shallice and Evans (1978) provided preliminary normative data based on a sample of 25 British neurologically intact individuals. Axelrod and Millis (1994) revised the task. They adapted the task for use with North American populations, eliminated items that required nonnumerative responses, and provided an empirically based, standardized scoring method. They presented response ranges for each item and assigned deviation scores of 0, 1, and 2, corresponding to percentile ranges (deviation score of 0 corresponding to answers between the 16th and 84th percentile, etc.). They also provided some preliminary normative data. The test consists of 10 items, shown in Figure 8–4. The deviation scoring system is shown in Figure 8–5.

Figure 8–4 CET. *Source:* From Axelrod & Millis, 1994. Reprinted with permission of Sage Publications.

Please answer the following questions in the space provided. Although you may not know the exact answer, make a best guess. Be sure to complete all items.

1. How tall is the Empire State Building? feet
2. How fast do race horses gallop? miles per hour
3. How long is the average necktie? feet, inches
4. What is the average length of a man's spine? feet, inches
5. How tall is the average woman? feet, inches
6. How heavy is a full-grown elephant? pounds
7. How much does one quart of milk weigh? pound(s)
8. How fast does a commercial jet fly? miles per hour
9. On average, how many TV programs are there on any one channel between the hours of 6 PM and 11 PM?
10. What is the average temperature in Anchorage, Alaska, on Christmas Day? degrees F.

Total Deviation score =

Figure 8–5 CET deviation scoring sheet. *Source:* From Axelrod & Millis, 1994. Reprinted with permission of Sage Publications.

Response	Deviation	Response	Deviation
Empire State Building (ft)		**Elephant Weight (lbs)**	
<78	2	<500	2
78–499	1	500–1000	1
500–3555	0	1001–4999	0
3556–66,900	1	5000–20,880	1
>66,900	2	>20,880	2
Race Horse (mph)		**Quart of Milk Weight (lbs)**	
<5	2	<0.3	2
5–20	1	0.3–0.99	1
21–49	0	1.0–2.2	0
50–100	1	2.3–5.0	1
>100	2	>5.0	2
Necktie Length (inches)		**Speed of Commercial Jet (mph)**	
<10.5	2	<83	2
10.5–18	1	83–250	1
19–47	0	251–787	0
48–70	1	788–6720	1
>70	2	>6720	2
Spine Length (inches)		**Number of TV Shows**	
<12	2	<1.3	2
12–24	1	1.3–5.0	1
25–42	0	5.1–9.9	0
43–64	1	10–88	1
>64	2	>88	2
Height of Woman (inches)		**Temperature in Anchorage (°F)**	
<60.5	2	<−37	2
60.5–64.0	1	−37 to −10	1
64.1–65.9	0	−9 to +32	0
66.0–68.0	1	+33 to +59	1
>68	2	>59	2

Figure 8–6 BCET items and instructions. *Source:* From Bullard et al., 2004. Reprinted with permission of Elsevier.

1. How many seeds are there in a watermelon?
2. How much does a telephone weigh?
3. How many sticks of spaghetti are there in a one-pound package?
4. What is the distance an adult can walk in an afternoon?
5. How high off a trampoline can a person jump?
6. How long does it take a builder to construct an average-sized house?
7. How much do a dozen medium-sized apples weigh?
8. How far could a horse pull a farm cart in one hour?
9. How many brushings can someone get from a large tube of toothpaste?
10. How many potato chips are there in a small, one-ounce bag?
11. How long would it take an adult to hand-write a one-page letter?
12. What is the age of the oldest living person in the United States?
13. How long is a tablespoon?
14. How much does a bridge (folding) chair weigh?
15. How long does it take to iron a shirt?
16. How long is a giraffe's neck?
17. How many slices are there in a one-pound loaf?
18. How much does a pair of men's shoes weigh?
19. How much does the fattest man in the United States weigh?
20. How long does it take for fresh milk to go sour in the refrigerator?

It is unlikely that anyone would know the exact answer to any of the above questions, so please give your best guess. Provide only a single guess to each, not a range. For example, do not write "between 10 and 20," or "about 50." In addition to the number, be sure to indicate how many "what." In other words, do not just write "30." Write "30 miles" or "30s" or 30 pounds," etc. Please answer every question no matter how unsure you are or how unusual the question seems.

The Biber Cognitive Estimation Test (BCET; Bullard et al., 2004) represents an attempt to establish quantitative rather than subjective judgments of normality for items in several content areas. Thus, it consists of 20 items, five in each category of time/duration, quantity, weight, and distance/length. The items are shown in Figure 8–6. To define the normally acceptable response range, items were given to normal volunteers, and the responses that fell within the 5th to 95th percentile were considered normal; those that fell outside those percentiles were considered abnormal.

ADMINISTRATION

CET

The examiner provides a response sheet with the test questions and requests that the patient complete the questions with "best guesses" in the spaces provided. There is no time limit.

BCET

The instructions for the BCET are provided in Figure 8–6. There is no time limit.

ADMINISTRATION TIME

Each test requires about 5 minutes.

SCORING

CET

Each response is compared with answers provided on the Deviation Scoring Sheet (Figure 8–5). The deviation scores for each CET item were developed from percentiles based on the mean performance of the standardization sample (e.g., deviation score of 0 for responses between the 16th and 84th percentiles; deviation score of 1 for responses between the 2nd and 16th as well as 84th to 98th percentiles; deviation score of

Table 8–19 BCET Item Statistics

Item	Category	Units	5th percentile	95th percentile
1	Quantity	Seeds	30	1000
2	Weight	Pounds	0.5	10
3	Quantity	Sticks	50	500
4	Distance/length	Miles	2.7	25
5	Distance/length	Feet	3	20
6	Time/age	Months	0.4	8
7	Weight	Pounds	1.5	9.3
8	Distance/length	Miles	1	15
9	Quantity	Brushings	34.2	250
10	Quantity	Chips	10	93
11	Time/age	Minutes	5	33
12	Time/age	Years	102	122.9
13	Distance/length	Inches	1.5	10
14	Weight	Pounds	0.90	15.9
15	Time/age	Minutes	2	20
16	Distance/length	Feet	2.5	15
17	Quantity	Slices	12	30.6
18	Weight	Pounds	0.7	5
19	Weight	Pounds	350	1200
20	Distance/length	Days	4	21

Source: From Bullard et al., 2004. Reprinted with the permission of Elsevier.

2 for responses less than the 2nd and greater than the 98th percentiles). The total deviation score is computed by summing item deviation scores for all 10 CET items. Thus, higher deviation scores imply more impaired (bizarre) performance.

O'Carroll et al. (1994) use a somewhat different scoring system, with each response being scored from 0 (good estimate) to 3 (bizarre).

BCET

Table 8–19 shows the item number, category, units of measurement, and percentile ranges. Responses that fall within the 5th to 95th percentile are considered normal; those that fall outside of those percentiles are considered abnormal. The number of items within the normal range is the total score.

DEMOGRAPHIC EFFECTS

Age

In adults, age has no effect on performance on the CET (Axelrod & Millis, 1994; Gillespie et al., 2002; O'Carroll et al., 1994) or the BCET (Bullard et al., 2004).

Education/IQ

On the CET, level of education impacts performance (Axelrod and Millis, 1994), with deviation scores being lower for individuals with more education. CET scores are moderately related to general intellectual ability (e.g., NART errors, $r = .30$), with lower IQ linked to poorer CET performance (Dias-Asper

et al., 2004; Gillespie et al., 2002; O'Carroll et al., 1994). No education or fund of information effects have been found for the BCET (Bullard et al., 2004).

Gender

On the CET, some (O'Carroll et al., 1994) have reported that females perform worse than males, whereas others (Gillespie et al., 2002) have noted no relationship between gender and estimation ability. On the BCET, gender effects are not found in healthy individuals; however, in patients with dementia, female patients with dementia performed slightly better in the time domain than their male counterparts (Bullard et al., 2004).

NORMATIVE DATA

CET

Axelrod and Millis (1994) reported that the average deviation score for a sample of 164 adults (age, $M = 39.0$, $SD = 16.1$; education, $M = 16.2$ years, $SD = 2.8$; 74% female, 26% male; 75% Caucasian, 23% black, 2% other) was 4.4 ($SD = 2.2$). Factually correct responses for each item on the CET result in a total deviation score of 3, which falls within one standard deviation of the sample mean.

In general, deviation scores were lower for individuals with more education (see Table 8–20).

O'Carroll et al. (1994) provide normative data for a 10-item British version of the CET. The data are based on a sample of 150 healthy individuals, aged 17 to 91 years (education,

Table 8–20 Mean Deviation Score for Cognitive Estimation
Performance Across Education groups

Education Level	N	Mean Deviation Score	SD
≤12	16	5.9	2.3
13–15	32	4.8	2.1
16	32	4.2	2.4
17–18	37	3.8	1.9
≥19	25	4.2	2.0

Source: From Axelrod & Millis, 1994. Reprinted with permission of Sage Publications.

$M = 11.6$ [2.9] years), living in the United Kingdom. Mean
CET score for the entire sample was 5.3 ($SD = 3.6$).

BCET

In the initial development of the BCET with 113 healthy normal individuals (age, $M = 37.3$, $SD = 16.1$, range 17–85; education, $M = 16.5$, $SD = 2.6$; 42% male, 95% Caucasian), the
authors reported a mean score of 18.9 ($SD = 1.1$) and a range
of 16 to 20. Cross-validation in a second sample of 49 healthy
individuals (age, $M = 40.3$, $SD = 14$, range 17–78; education,
$M = 13.7$, $SD = 3.1$; 39% male, 90% Caucasian) suggested that
a cutoff score of three standard deviations below the mean
(i.e., below 15.6) would be more appropriate.

Some data are available for school-age children, 5 to 16
years, on this version (Fein et al., 1998) and are reported in
Baron (2004).

RELIABILITY

Internal Consistency

The broad content represented in the CET appears to be multidimensional. Item-total correlations range from –.16 to .57
for the American (Axelrod & Millis, 1994) and the British version (Gillespie et al., 2002). O'Carroll et al. (1994) found that
the internal consistency of the British version of the CET was
.40 (Cronbach's alpha) and .35 (Guttman split-half reliability coefficient). Ross et al. (1996) examined reliability in an
American college sample ($r = 158$) and reported that internal
consistency was low (Cronbach's alpha = .37).

For the BCET, Bullard et al. (2004) reported that there was
insufficient variability within healthy controls to assess internal consistency. In patients with dementia, values are marginally acceptable, revealing a Crohnbach's alpha of .62 and a
Guttman split-half of .74.

Test-Retest Reliability

For the CET, Ross et al. (1996) retested 44 individuals following about 37.5 days ($SD = 17.5$). The coefficient of stability for
the CET was low ($r = .57$). On average, slightly better scores
were obtained at retest ($M = 4.7$, $SD = 2.1$) than at initial

examination ($M = 5.3$, $SD = 2.3$), suggesting a modest practice effect. Test-retest reliability information is not available
for the BCET.

Interrater Reliability

O'Carroll et al. (1994) reported that the interrater reliability
coefficient was high ($r = .91$) for a group of 50 healthy subjects given the British version of the CET in which responses
were scored from 0 (good estimate) to 3 (bizarre estimate).

VALIDITY

Factor-Analytic Findings

O'Carroll et al. (1994) examined the factor structure of their
British version of the CET. Principal component analysis followed by varimax rotation resulted in five factors being extracted from this 10-item scale.

Correlations With Other Measures

Correlations between the CET and other executive function
tests tend to be modest. For example, Ross et al. (1996) reported that in normal people, CET performance has low correlations to other putative measures of executive functioning
(COWAT, $r = -.22$; Design Fluency, $r = -.19$; Ruff Figural Fluency, $r = -.27$; Porteus Mazes, $r = .24$; Stroop, $r = .22$; Trails B,
$r = .27$; WCST, $r = .19$; Tower of Hanoi, $r = .03$). Similar results have been reported by others in a variety of populations
(e.g., patients with AD, MS, and Korsakoff's; older adults;
Brand, Fujiwara, et al., 2003; Canellopoulou & Richardson,
1998; Kopelman, 1991; Shoqueirat et al., 1990). The CET has
been found to be unrelated to one measure of estimation (the
Temporal Judgment Test of the BADS; Gillespie et al., 2002)
and moderately related ($r = .47$) to others (Luria Memory Test
in which individuals must estimate the number of words they
will recall following each trial of a word list: Freeman et al.,
1995; affective judgements where individuals must judge the
valence of words: Brand, Fujiwara, et al., 2003). The relations
of the BCET to measures of executive functioning have not
yet been reported.

Level of intelligence or general knowledge contributes significantly to CET performance (Brand, Fujiwara, et al., 2003;
Freeman et al., 1995; Gillespie et al., 2002; Kopelman, 1991;
Ross et al., 1996; Shoqueirat et al., 1990; Taylor & O'Carroll,
1995). For example, Shoqueirat et al. (1990) found in amnesic patients that CET performance was significantly worse
in those with lower IQs (FSIQ, $r = -.62$), and Kopelman
(1991) reported that in Alzheimer and Korsakoff patients,
CET performance was significantly correlated with measures
of premorbid (NART, $r = -.40$) and current intelligence
(Full-Scale IQ, $r = -.53$). Taylor and O'Carroll (1995) also
noted that CET scores were moderately related to education,
IQ (NART errors), and social class in both normal and neurological populations.

General cognitive status is also related to BCET performance. Bullard et al. (2004) reported that the BCET total score was moderate/highly correlated (.46–.53) with the total score of MMSE in normals and patients with dementia. Somewhat surprisingly, in their sample of healthy individuals, measures of abstract reasoning, fund of general information, and fund of numerical information showed no relationship to test performance. This issue requires examination in a more diverse sample.

Aspects of memory appear to be involved in cognitive estimation. Kopelman (1991) noted a relation between CET performance and measures of retrograde and anterograde memory (.32–.67). Others (Freeman et al., 1995; Mendez et al., 1998) have also described an association between CET performance and memory test scores in neurological patients. Numerical ability and the capacity to construct and/or make appropriate use of mental images may also be important (Canellopoulou & Richardson, 1998; Mendez et al., 1998; but see Goldstein et al., 1996, & Shallice & Evans, 1978, who failed to find a relation with arithmetic ability). Naming ability does not impact performance (Goldstein et al., 1996).

Clinical Findings

Shallice and Evans (1978) gave their version of the CET to 96 patients with localized cerebral lesions. Patients with anterior lesions performed significantly worse (gave significantly more bizarre answers) than the posterior group on this task. They suggested that the difficulty shown by the patients reflected a deficit in the selection and regulation of cognitive planning. In contrast, the only other study to directly compare patients with anterior and posterior lesions failed to support Shallice and Evans' claim. Taylor and O'Carroll (1995) compared a group of patients with discrete frontal lesions (confirmed via CT or MRI) with a group with localized nonfrontal lesions. No significant difference in CET performance was observed between the anterior and posterior lesioned groups, calling into question the sensitivity of the CET to anterior brain dysfunction. Mendez et al. (1998) gave the CET to patients with frontotemporal dementia (FTS) and Alzheimer's disease (AD). Both groups gave more extreme answers than controls and, contrary to expectation, AD patients gave more extreme estimates than the patients with FTD.

Impaired CET performance has been found in patients with Korsakoff's syndrome (Brand, Fujiwara, et al., 2003; Brand, Kalbe, et al., 2003; Kopelman, 1991; Shoqueirat et al., 1990; Taylor & O'Carroll, 1995; but see Leng & Parkin, 1988), prenatal exposure to alcohol (Kopera-Frye et al., 1996), Alzheimer's disease (Brand, Kalbe, et al., 2003; Goldstein et al., 1996; Kopelman, 1991; Mendez et al., 1998; Nathan et al., 2001), postencephalitic amnesia (Kopelman, 1991; Shoqueirat et al., 1990), and patients with anterior communicating artery aneurysm (AcoAA; Leng & Parkin, 1988).

Axelrod and Millis (1994) reported that patients with severe head injuries were impaired on the CET relative to a sample of medical outpatients. They suggested that a cutoff ≥7 produced the best differentiation of patients from controls and resulted in an overall correct classification rate of 78%. It is worth noting, however, that in this study, patients with TBI had significantly less education than controls, raising the concern that the test may be more sensitive to education than to brain injury. Measures of anxiety and depression appear unrelated to cognitive estimation (Freeman et al., 1995).

Impairments on the BCET have been reported in patients with probable dementia of the Alzheimer's type (Bullard et al., 2004), Parkinson's disease (Bullard et al., 2004), and schizophrenia (Jackson et al., 2001), and in children diagnosed with autism (Liss et al., 2000).

There is some evidence that various dimensions (e.g., estimation of time, quantity, size, weight) may be differentially affected in various disorders. For example, Brand, Kalbe, et al. (2003) constructed their own CET version and found that in AD patients, the dimensions of size and weight were the most affected, while patients with Korsakoff's syndrome had the most difficulties in estimating time questions.

Ecological Validity

Burgess et al. (1998) reported that in a mixed group of adult neurological patients, the CET (version by Shallice & Evans, 1978) was one of the few putative measures of executive function that failed to correlate significantly with rated everyday executive problems.

COMMENT

Many activities in daily life depend critically on providing adequate guesses or estimations. One might suspect, for example, that accurate time estimates would be necessary for planning a day's activities (Bullard et al., 2004). Whether the CET/BCET captures this important component of reasoning is uncertain. The relation of the CET to other measures of executive function appears modest, raising concerns about whether this measure taps executive processing. Rather, general intellectual status, one's fund of general knowledge, and ability to retrieve information from memory seem to be important contributors to performance, along with numerical reasoning and mental visualization.

There may be a gender bias in the CET items, with females performing worse than males. Note that the Axelrod and Millis norms (1994) were developed on a largely female sample, making them problematic for use with males.

The CET is brief and easily administered; however, it can hardly be described as a reliable and valid tool. The BCET appears to have somewhat better psychometric properties, although this remains to be examined in more diverse samples (e.g., aging samples). Further, studies with patient populations are needed to investigate its theoretical and clinical relevance.

REFERENCES

Axelrod, B. N., & Millis, S. R. (1994). Preliminary standardization of the Cognitive Estimation Test. *Assessment, 1,* 269–274.

Baron, I. S. (2004). *Neuropsychological evaluation of the child.* New York: Oxford University Press.

Brand, M., Fujiwara, E., Kalbe, E., Steingass, H-P., Kessler, J., & Markowitsch, H. (2003). Cognitive estimation and affective judgements in alcoholic Korsakoff patients. *Journal of Clinical and Experimental Neuropsychology, 25,* 324–334.

Brand, M., Kalbe, E., Fujiwara, E., Huber, M., & Markowitsch, H. J. (2003). Cognitive estimation in patients with probably Alzheimer's disease and alcoholic Korsakoff patients. *Neuropsychologia, 41,* 575–584.

Bullard, S. E., Fein, D., Gleeson, M. K., Tischer, N., Mapou, R. L., & Kaplan, E. (2004). The Biber Cognitive Estimation Test. *Archives of Clinical Neuropsychology, 19,* 835–846.

Burgess, P. W., Alderman, N., Evans, J., Emslie, H., & Wilson, B. A. (1998). The ecological validity of tests of executive function. *Journal of the International Neuropsychological Society, 4,* 547–558.

Canellopoulou, M., & Richardson, J. T. E. (1998). The role of executive function in imagery mnemonics: Evidence from multiple sclerosis. *Neuropsychologia, 36,* 1181–1188.

Diaz-Asper, C., Schretlen, D. J., & Pearlson, G. D. (2004). How well does IQ predict neuropsychological test performance in normal adults. *Journal of the International Neuropsychological Society, 10,* 82–90.

Fein, D., Gleeson, M. K., Bullard, S., Mapou, R., & Kaplan, E. (1998). *The Biber Cognitive Estimation test.* Paper presented to the 29th Annual Meeting of the International Neuropsychological Society, Honolulu, HI.

Freeman, M. R., Ryan, J. J., Lopez, S., & Mittenberg, W. (1995) Cognitive estimation in traumatic brain injury: Relationships with measures of intelligence, memory, and affect. *International Journal of Neuroscience, 83,* 269–273.

Gillespie, D. C., Evans, R. I., Gardener, E. A., & Bowen, A. (2002). Performance of older adults on tests of cognitive estimation. *Journal of Clinical and Experimental Neuropsychology, 24,* 286–293.

Goldstein, F. C., Green, J., & Presley, R. M. (1996). Cognitive estimation in patients with Alzheimer's disease. *Neuropsychiatry, Neuropsychology, & Behavioral Neurology, 9,* 35–42.

Jackson, C. T., Fein, D., Essock, S. M., & Mueser, K. T. (2001). The effects of cognitive impairment and substance abuse on psychiatric hospitalizations. *Community Mental Health Journal, 37,* 303–312.

Kopelman, M. (1991). Frontal dysfunction and memory deficits in the alcoholic Korsakoff syndrome and Alzheimer-type dementia. *Brain, 114,* 117–137.

Kopera-Frye, K., Dehaene, S., Streissguth, A. P. (1996). Impairments of number processing induced by prenatal alcohol exposure. *Neuropsychologia, 34,* 1187–1196.

Leng, N. R. C., & Parkin, A. J. (1988). Double dissociation of frontal dysfunction in organic amnesia. *British Journal of Clinical Psychology, 27,* 359–362.

Liss, M., Fein, D., Bullard, S., Robins, D., & Waterhouse, L. (2000). Cognitive estimation in individuals with pervasive developmental disorders. *Journal of Autism and Developmental Disabilities, 30,* 613–618.

Mendez, M. F., Doss, R. C., & Cherrier, M. M. (1998). Use of the Cognitive Estimations Test to discriminate frontotemporal dementia from Alzheimer's disease. *Journal of Geriatric Psychiatry & Neurology, 11,* 2–6.

Nathan, J., Wilkinson, D., Stammers, S., & Low, J. L. (2001). The role of tests of frontal executive functioning in the detection of mild dementia. *International Journal of Geriatric Psychiatry, 16,* 18–26.

O'Carroll, R., Egan, V., & Mackenzie, D. M. (1994). Assessing cognitive estimation. *British Journal of Clinical Psychology, 33,* 193–197.

Ross, T. P., Hanks, R. A., Kotasek, R. S., & Whitman, R. D. (1996). *The reliability and validity of a modified Cognitive Estimation Test.* Paper presented to the International Neuropsychological Society, Chicago.

Shallice, T., & Evans, M. E. (1978). The involvement of the frontal lobes in cognitive estimation. *Cortex, 14,* 292–303.

Shoqeirat, M. A., Mayes, A., MacDonald, C., Meudell, P., & Pickering, A. (1990). Performance on tests sensitive to frontal lobe lesions by patients with organic amnesia: Leng and Parkin revisited. *British Journal of Clinical Psychology, 29,* 401–408.

Taylor, R., & O'Carroll, R. (1995). Cognitive estimation in neurological disorders. *British Journal of Clinical Psychology, 34,* 223–228.

Delis-Kaplan Executive Function System (D-KEFS)

PURPOSE

The D-KEFS consists of a set of nine tasks designed to assess the component processes of executive functioning.

SOURCE

The kit includes the Examiner and Technical Manuals, Stimulus Booklet, Sorting Cards (three sets of six cards each), one tower stand with five color disks for the Tower Test, 25 Record Forms, 25 Design Fluency Response Booklets, and 25 Trail Making Response Booklet sets (each set contains 25 Response Booklets for the five Trail Making conditions). The kit can be ordered from the Psychological Corporation, 19500 Bulverde Road, San Antonio, TX, 78259 (http://harcourtassessment.com) and costs about $525 US. Scoring software is also available for $199 US.

AGE RANGE

With one exception, the D-KEFS tests can be used with individuals aged 8 to 89 years. The Proverbs Test was designed for adolescents and adults aged 16 to 89 years.

DESCRIPTION

The D-KEFS (Delis et al., 2001) was designed to detect even mild forms of executive dysfunction. It includes nine tests that derive from existing experimental and clinical measures. The

Table 8–21 D-KEFS Tests and Their Functions

D-KEFS Tests	Description	Key Functions Assessed
Trail Making Test	The examinee has to scan letters and numbers and mark the number 3 (Condition 1), connect the number in ascending order (Condition 2), connect just the letters in alphabetical order (Condition 3), switch between connecting numbers and letters (Condition 4), and draw a line over a dotted line as quickly as possible (Condition 5).	Assesses visual scanning, number sequencing, letter sequencing, number-letter switching, and motor speed
Verbal Fluency Test	The examinee is asked to say words that begin with a specified letter (Letter Fluency), say words that belong to a designated semantic category (Category Fluency) and alternate between saying words from two different semantic categories (Category Switching).	Fluent productivity in the verbal domain
Design Fluency Test	The examinee is presented rows of boxes containing an array of dots and must make as many designs as possible in one minute by connecting filled dots (Condition 1), by connecting unfilled dots only (Condition 2), and by alternating connections between filled and unfilled dots (Condition 3).	Fluent productivity in the nonverbal domain
Color-Word Interference Test	A variant of the Stroop procedure in which the examinee names color patches (Condition 1), reads words that denote colors printed in black ink (Condition 2), names the ink color in which color words are printed (Condition 3), and switches back and forth between naming the dissonant ink colors and reading the conflicting words (Condition 4).	Inhibition of an overlearned response and flexibility
Sorting Test	In Condition 1 (Free Sorting), the examinee is asked to sort six cards into two groups, according to as many rules as possible. In Condition 2 (Sort Recognition), the examinee has to identify and describe the correct rules the examiner used to generate the sort.	Problem-solving, verbal and nonverbal concept formation, and flexibility of thinking on a conceptual task
Twenty Questions Test	The examinee is presented with a stimulus page containing 30 common objects and has to ask the fewest number of yes/no questions to identify the target.	Categorical processing and ability to use feedback to guide problem solving
Word Context Test	Examinee has to discover the meaning of made-up words based on cues given in sentences.	Deductive reasoning, verbal abstract thinking, and hypothesis testing
Tower Test	The examinee's task is to move five disks across three pegs to build a target tower in the fewest number of moves possible.	Planning, rule learning, and inhibition
Proverb Test	The examinee has to interpret proverbs orally (Free Inquiry) and select the best interpretation from four alternatives (Multiple Choice).	Metaphorical thinking and generating versus comprehending abstract thought

tests are listed in Table 8–21 along with brief descriptions of each and the key functions purported to be assessed. The tests embrace a process-oriented approach so that each task provides multiple scores to delineate the source of any difficulties. For example, the D-KEFS Sorting Test yields five primary measures and more than 20 optional measures of different components of problem-solving skills. In this way, the examiner can isolate the fundamental components resulting in impaired performance and can assess the fundamental skill itself.

The authors introduced a number of features to increase the sensitivity of the tests to mild brain damage. Thus, they included a number of switching conditions in the tasks. For example, in addition to traditional Stroop procedures of naming color patches, reading color words in black ink, and naming the ink color in which a color word is written (an interference condition), a fourth condition is added in which the examinee is asked to switch between naming the dissonant ink color and reading the actual word. Because patients with frontal lobe damage may have difficulty disengaging their attention from salient aspects of their physical environment, the authors added capture stimuli to several of the test materials, inviting more automatic, effortless responding. For example, on the switching version Trail Making Test where the examinee must alternate connecting numbers and letters in sequence, two pairs of capture stimuli were placed strategically in each quadrant of the stimulus page. For instance, a 4 is printed immediately adjacent to the 3 along the same path as the B-to-3 connection. Further, to maximize detection of subtle executive deficits, processing demands of tasks were increased. For example, the D-KEFS Sorting Test requires the examinee to identify a maximum of 16 different conceptual rules for sorting the card sets.

The D-KEFS was designed to be used in a flexible manner. Thus, the tests can be used singly or in combination with other D-KEFS tests. In addition, the examiner might decide to omit a test condition.

An alternate form is provided for three of the tests that are most susceptible to practice effects: Sorting, Twenty Questions, and Verbal Fluency.

ADMINISTRATION

Instructions for administration are given in the stimulus booklet or record booklet. The D-KEFS Examiner's Manual is not needed during administration. The examiner prompts, discontinue rules, and time limits are clearly displayed to examiners in the Stimulus Booklet and/or Record Form.

ADMINISTRATION TIME

About 90 minutes are required for the entire battery (Schonfeld et al., 2001).

SCORING

Scoring guidelines for each test are found in the Examiner's Manual and the Record Form. For most of the measures, raw scores are converted to age-scaled scores, with a mean of 10 and a standard deviation of three. For some process measures (e.g., error or ratio measures), the raw scores have limited ranges in normal populations. Thus, the raw scores are converted to cumulative percentile ranks corrected for each of 16 age groups. A few measures (e.g., set-loss errors on the Verbal Fluency Test) have limited raw-score ranges and showed almost no age effects across the normative sample. In those cases, raw scores are converted to cumulative percentile ranks corrected for the entire normative sample.

The D-KEFS includes contrast measures that quantify relative performance on (a) a baseline task and a higher level task (e.g., Trail Making Contrast = Number-Letter Switching minus Motor Speed) or (b) two higher level tasks (e.g., Verbal Fluency Contrast = Letter Fluency minus Category Fluency). Scaled-score differences are treated like raw scores and are converted to a new scaled score, with a mean of 10 and a standard deviation of three. In addition, some measures are combined into new scaled scores so that tasks that are thought to measure similar cognitive functions can be evaluated (e.g., Design Fluency Composite = Condition 1 Filled Dots plus Condition 2 Empty Dots). Given that the two individual scaled scores that are subtracted or added to yield a contrast or composite scaled score are already age corrected, the derived contrast and composite scaled score are corrected for the entire sample.

The D-KEFS distinguishes between "primary" and "optional" measures. Primary measures are so designated because they either provide a global overall characterization of performance on that task or they provide process scores for key components of the task. If the examiner must score the protocol manually, then he or she may choose to compute mostly the primary measures. However, an analysis of both the primary and optional measures is recommended by the authors for a more comprehensive assessment of executive functions.

The D-KEFS Scoring Assistant software computes the standardized scores for both the primary and optional measures of the standard and alternate forms.

DEMOGRAPHIC EFFECTS

Age

Age affects performance on the D-KEFS (Technical Manual; Wecker et al., 2000), with individuals in the youngest (8–10 years) and oldest (70–89 years) age groups obtaining the lowest scores. Performance on measures that are highly dependent on speed of processing tend to peak in the adolescent and young-adult groups, whereas performance on tests of verbal conceptual reasoning tends to peak in the adult age groups.

Education/IQ

The impact of these variables is not reported.

Gender

The impact of this variable is not reported.

Ethnicity

The impact of this variable is not reported.

Table 8–22 Characteristics of the D-KEFS Normative Sample

Number	1750
Age	8–89 years[a]
Geographic location	From geographic regions in proportions consistent with the 2000 U.S. Census data
Sample type	Based on a representative sample of the U.S. population stratified on the basis of age, gender, race/ethnicity, educational level, and geographic region
Education	<8 to >16 years and consistent with U.S. Census proportions; for examinees aged 8–19 years, parent education was used
Gender	Roughly an equal number of males and females in each age group with the exception that the older age groups included more women than men, in proportions consistent with 2000 U.S. Census data
Race/ethnicity	The proportions of Whites, African Americans, Hispanics and other racial/ethnic groups were based on racial/ethnic proportions within each age band according to 2000 U.S. Census data
Screening	Screened via self-report for sensory, substance abuse, medical, psychiatric, or motor condition that could potentially affect performance

[a]The sample was divided into the following age groups: 8, 9, 10, 11, 12, 13, 14, 15, 16–19, 20–29, 30–39, 40–49, 50–59, 60–69, 70–79, 80–89 years. The N in each age band ranges from 70–175, depending on the age group.

NORMATIVE DATA

Standardization Sample

The D-KEFS was normed on a sample of 1750 individuals, aged 8 to 89 years, selected to match the U.S. population in terms of age, gender, race/ethnicity, education, and geographic region. For examinees aged 8 to 19 years, the mean parental education level was used. The characteristics of the standardization sample are shown in Table 8–22.

For the alternate forms, a normative equating study was conducted with a sample of 286 individuals (105 males, 181 females; ages 16–89 years, $M = 47.5$, $SD = 23.5$; 83.9% Caucasian; 88.5% with 12 or more years of education) who were given both the standard and alternate forms in counterbalanced order. Norms for each alternate form were derived from the linear transformations of the standard form normative values for each age group; however, use of the norms may be problematic given the low correlations between forms for many of the key variables (see *Reliability*). The norms for the younger age groups (below age 16 years) were estimated from relationships of scores on the two forms observed in the adolescent sample.

RELIABILITY

Internal Consistency

Internal consistency was evaluated for primary measures in the normative sample (Technical Manual). As is shown in Table 8–23, coefficients range from inadequate (e.g., Verbal Fluency Category Switching total correct) to adequate/high (e.g., Twenty Questions Initial Abstraction), depending upon the particular measure and the age group.

Test-Retest Reliability

The authors indicate that the test-retest studies of the standard form of the D-KEFS were based on a sample of 101 cases, distributed across all the age groups. The time between administrations ranged from nine to 74 days, with an average of about 25 days. Test-retest correlations ranged from low (e.g., Trail Making, Design Fluency) to adequate/high (e.g., Letter and Category Fluency total correct; see Table 8–23). Practice effects are evident for most of the tasks, with gains of about 1 to 2 scaled score points on each task.

Alternate Form Reliability

The D-KEFS provides alternate forms for the Sorting, Verbal Fluency, and Twenty Questions Tests. The two forms were given in counterbalanced order to 286 individuals, ranging in age from 16 to 89 years ($M = 47.5$, $SD = 23.5$). The Technical Manual provides means, standard deviations, and correlations for the key variables of the standard and alternate forms. As shown in Table 8–24, correlations between forms for key variables vary from low (e.g., Twenty Questions) to high (e.g., Letter Fluency total correct).

Interrater Reliability

In general, scoring criteria are clear. However, scoring of some of the tasks (e.g., Proverbs, Twenty Questions, Word Context) requires some judgment on the part of the examiner. This aspect remains to be evaluated.

VALIDITY

Task Intercorrelations

The authors report (Technical Manual) numerous within- and between-task correlational analyses broken down by specified age bands of the normative sample. The magnitude of the correlations of scores within tasks varies greatly by task, measure, and age group. In general, primary measures derived from the same test correlate more highly than scores across tests. Correlations between tasks tend to be low. For example, median correlations among summary scores for Sorting, Tower, Letter Fluency, and Figural Fluency tasks were .25 for

Table 8–23 Magnitude of Reliability Coefficients for D-KEFS Tests

	Internal Consistency	**Test-Retest**
Very high (.90+)		
High (.80–.89)	**Verbal Fluency:** Condition 1 Letter Fluency Total Correct **Twenty Questions:** Initial Abstraction **Proverb Test:** Total Achievement	**Verbal Fluency:** Condition 1 Letter Fluency Total Correct
Adequate (.70–.79)	**Trail Making:** Combined Number & Letter Sequencing Composite **Color Word:** Combined Color Naming + Word Reading Composite **Sorting:** Condition 1 Free Sorting Confirmed, Condition 2 Free Sorting Description Condition 3 Sorting Recognition Total	**Trail Making:** Condition 5 Motor Speed Seconds to Complete **Verbal Fluency:** Condition 2 Category Fluency Total Correct **Color-Word:** Condition 1 Color Naming Seconds to Complete, Condition 3 Inhibition Seconds to Complete **Word Context:** Total First Trial Consistency Correct **Proverb Test:** Total Achievement
Marginal (.60–.69)	**Verbal Fluency:** Condition 2 Category Fluency, Condition 3 Category Switching Total Switching **Word Context:** Total Consecutively Correct **Tower Test:** Total Achievement	**Color-Word:** Condition 2 Word Reading Seconds to Complete, Condition 4 Inhibition/Switching Seconds to Complete **Trail Making:** Combined Number + Letter Sequencing
Low (≤.59)	**Trail Making:** Conditions 1–4 **Verbal Fluency:** Category Switching Total Correct **Twenty Questions:** Total Weighted Achievement	**Design Fluency** **Sorting Test** **Twenty Questions** **Tower Test:** Total Achievement **Verbal Fluency:** Condition 3 Category Switching Total Correct and Total Switching Accuracy

20- to 49-year-olds and .33 for 50- 89-year-olds. These relatively low values suggest that the tasks are not interchangeable (Delis et al., 2001). They also raise the possibility that the executive functioning construct in this test battery has weak convergent validity (Salthouse et al., 2003).

The D-KEFS provides many process variables including several measures reflecting initiation of problem-solving behavior (e.g., the number of attempted sorts on the Sorting Test, and the number of total responses generated on the Verbal and Design Fluency Tests). The correlations among these measures are surprisingly low (.1–.3), given that they are purported to measure a similar underlying construct. Indicators of speed of processing also tend to be low across tasks (typically <.20). Various errors (e.g., repetition, set loss) are quantified and normed on several of the D-KEFS tests, and the correlations among tasks are also low. These low correlations raise concerns regarding the meaning of the various scores and the possibility that measures that have the same label (e.g., repetition, set-loss errors) may in fact measure different constructs. To date, factor-analytic studies have not been reported.

Table 8–24 Correlations Between Standard and Alternate Forms

Test Measure	r
Verbal Fluency	Ranges from .44 (Condition 3 Category Switching Total Switching Accuracy) to .83 (Condition 1 Letter Fluency Total Correct)
Sorting Test	Ranges from .39 (Condition 1 Free Sorting Description Total Score) to .72 (Condition 2 Sort Recognition Total Description Score)
Twenty Questions Test	Ranges from .25 (Total Questions Asked) to .61 (Total Abstraction Score)

Source: Adapted from Delis et al., 2001.

Correlations With Other Tests of Executive Functioning

The authors report only one study comparing the D-KEFS with another measure of executive function. A correlational study (Technical Manual) with the WCST involving a small number of participants ($N = 23$, age range 19–78) found moderate/high correlations (.31–.59) between WCST measures (number of categories completed) and various D-KEFS measures from the nine tests (including the D-KEFS Sorting Test). The number of perseverative responses on the WCST showed a more variable pattern of associations with the D-KEFS. The implication is that the D-KEFS and WCST are assessing similar, though not identical, processes.

Correlations With Other Neuropsychological Domains

The D-KEFS and a measure of episodic memory, the CVLT-II, were given to a sample of 292 individuals, aged 16 to 89 years (Technical Manual). The vast majority of the correlations were low and similar in magnitude to those among purported executive measures. For example, correlations with measures of recall across Trials 1 to 5 were .28 for Sorting, .23 for Tower, .32 for Letter Fluency, and .27 for Design Fluency. Because these values are within the same range as the correlations of the executive function variables with one another (see previous discussion), these data provide weak evidence for discriminant validity (Salthouse et al., 2003).

Clinical Studies

Several studies have documented that performance on the D-KEFS is adversely affected by frontal lobe lesions. Thus, Baldo et al. (2001) found that patients with frontal lobe lesions were impaired, compared with healthy controls, on both Verbal and Design Fluency tasks. Patients with left frontal lesions performed worse than patients with right frontal lesions on the Verbal Fluency task, but the two groups performed comparably on the Design Fluency task. Both patients and control participants were impacted similarly by the switching conditions. That is, patients were able to switch as effectively as controls, when they were explicitly instructed to do so. More recently, Baldo et al. (2004) reported that patients with focal frontal lesions were impaired on the Twenty Questions Test, asking significantly more questions than controls in their attempt to guess the target items. In addition, poor performance on this measure of problem solving was strongly associated with a fewer number of correct sorts on another concept-formation task, the Sorting Test. Keil et al. (2005) have recently reported that patients with frontal lobe (particularly left-sided) lesions were significantly impaired on the Word Context Test relative to a group of age- and education-matched controls. Unfortunately, in all of these studies, patients with lesions outside of the frontal lobes were not evaluated, leaving open the question of the specificity of their findings.

Recently, McDonald et al. (2005) evaluated the Trail Making Test in patients with frontal lobe epilepsy (FLE) and compared their performance with that of patients with temporal lobe epilepsy (TLE). They found that patients with FLE were impaired in both speed and accuracy on the switching condition relative to patients with TLE and controls. The two patient groups did not differ from controls on the four baseline conditions of the test, designed to assess visual scanning, motor speed, number sequencing, and letter sequencing.

Declines in executive functioning as assessed by D-KEFS tests have also been documented in other patient groups. Subcortical ischemic vascular disease is associated with mild impairment on an abbreviated version of the D-KEFS Sorting Test in nondemented elderly individuals (Kramer et al., 2002). Children diagnosed with FAS show poor performance on the D-KEFS Color-Word Interference, Trail Making, Tower, and Word Context Tests (Mattson et al., 1999). Prenatal exposure to alcohol (with and without FAS) also impairs Verbal and Design Fluency performance, even when IQ is controlled (Schonfeld et al., 2001). These latter findings are consistent with other literature suggesting that children with early heavy alcohol exposure display executive deficits.

Age differences have been documented on the Sorting Test, with older adults producing fewer correct sorts, whether required to generate them without cues (Free Sorting condition) or from groupings of stimuli created by the examiner (Sort Recognition condition; e.g., see *Source*). The reduction in concept identification in older adults appears to be due in part to diminished working memory for previous sorts. Thus, Hartman et al. (2004) have shown that age differences are reduced when cues are provided to test-takers such that they could view the verbal descriptions of their previous sorts, helping them monitor and organize information necessary for decision making.

Executive function tests call upon many component skills, and the claim of the test authors is that the D-KEFS will assist in the clear delineation of the affected processes in individuals and groups. In line with their claim, Wecker et al. (2000) showed that age accounted for a significant portion of the variance on the Stroop interference condition, even when simpler component processes (color naming, word reading) were accounted for. Similarly, Wecker et al. (2005) have recently reported that age affects cognitive switching—on Trail Making, Design Fluency, and Verbal Fluency—when component skills were controlled.

Whether the D-KEFS is sensitive to even mild forms of executive dysfunction, as intended by the authors, is not known. It is also not clear whether the D-KEFS can distinguish different executive dysfunction profiles. The authors report (Technical Manual) some preliminary findings suggesting that the D-KEFS can distinguish cortical (Alzheimer's) from subcortical (Huntington's) disorders. However, the sample sizes were very small (nine in each group) and the study lacks the appropriate controls (e.g., matching groups for dementia severity). In short, additional study of validity is needed.

COMMENT

The D-KEFS is a new measure that purports to assess important dimensions of executive functioning, with a wide array of tasks/measures. The tests have numerous interesting features including the emphasis on task switching (e.g., Trails, Verbal Fluency, Design Fluency) and the inclusion of tasks/measures that may isolate those component skills underlying test failure (e.g., inclusion of measures of motor speed and visual scanning as part of the Trail Test, asking the patient to describe his or her sorting strategy on the Sorting Test). The availability of a single, comprehensive set of age-based normative data is also an asset, although norms corrected for other potentially important variables (e.g., education) are not yet available. Because all of the tests were normed on the same reference group, the standardized scores of these tests can be directly compared (see also Homack et al., 2005). As a consequence, it may be possible to distinguish different profiles of executive disturbance. Unfortunately, data are not provided to determine whether discrepancies between tasks are significant or unusual.

Alternate forms are also available for three of the tasks. However, examiners should note that intercorrelations for many of the measures are low, raising concern regarding the use of some of the alternate form scores. With the exception of Verbal Fluency (Condition 1 Letter Fluency total correct, Condition 2 Category Fluency total correct), most show correlations that are inadequate as evidence of the concordance of the alternate forms. Users should also note that normative data for the alternate form in children younger than age 16 years are based on estimated data.

Other analyses provided in the Technical Manual raise concerns about the internal consistency and test-retest properties of many measures, which suffer perhaps due to limited ranges and skewed distributions in normal individuals. Further, reliability data are not provided for the various optional measures. In addition, no information is provided regarding interrater reliability. These issues require additional study, particularly in clinical populations. Table 8–23 provides a rough guide as to the measures that have adequate reliability, although the clinician should check the Technical Manual with respect to the particular age band needed. Internal consistency of a number of tests (e.g., Letter Fluency) appears to be sufficiently high for clinical decision making. Due to low test-retest reliabilities, the Design Fluency, Sorting, Tower, and Twenty Questions Tests are not recommended for longitudinal assessment.

According to the authors, a key asset of the D-KEFS is that it provides measures to assist the clinician in parsing and understanding patient behavior. However, only a few studies have appeared in the literature evaluating its utility in clinical populations. Whether the measures actually assess frontal/executive functioning (see, e.g., , Salthouse et al., 2003) and are clearly an improvement in comparison to more standard methods requires additional study. A recent study (Baldo et al., 2001) of patients with lesions in the frontal lobe found no firm evidence for incremental validity for switching conditions used in the fluency tests. By contrast, other studies suggest a more positive picture. Thus, an earlier version of the D-KEFS Sorting Test, called the California Card Sorting Test, proved better able than the WCST to characterize the different capacities of various patient populations (PD, MS, chronic alcoholism; e.g., Beatty & Monson, 1990, 1996; Beatty et al., 1993; see also Delis et al., 2004). Similarly, a recent study of a patient with ventromedial prefrontal damage by Cato et al. (2004) suggests that the patient's deficits may have gone undetected if error measures provided by the D-KEFS had not been evaluated. Recent work by Wecker et al. (2000, 2005) suggests that a unique relationship exists between aging and cognitive flexibility (switching) on tests such as Trail Making, Design Fluency, and Verbal Fluency that cannot be accounted for by age-related declines on more basic component skills and demographic factors (e.g., IQ, education, gender). Such evidence is encouraging and suggests that the test has clinical utility.

The authors intended the D-KEFS as a flexible instrument and indicated that only some tests and conditions need be given to a particular patient. This flexibility, however, may be problematic when interpretations of isolated tests are based on a battery that was apparently given in its entirety to the normative sample. This issue requires additional study.

Finally, the clinician should note that the D-KEFS does not represent a theoretically driven or comprehensive set of measures of executive function. Delis et al. (2004) admit that the D-KEFS was never intended to assess all aspects of executive/frontal lobe functioning. They state (D-KEFS Examiner's Manual, p. 14) that their choice was guided by tasks that "in either experimental studies or clinical practice, have demonstrated sensitivity in the detection of frontal-lobe dysfunction." There is, however, no rationale provided as to why these nine tests were chosen and other techniques were not (e.g., behavioral ratings, estimation, risk-taking procedures).

REFERENCES

Baldo, J. V., Delis, D. C., Wilkins, D. P., & Shimamura, A. P. (2004). Is it bigger than a breadbox? Performance of patients with prefrontal lesions on a new executive function test. *Archives of Clinical Neuropsychology, 19*, 407–419.

Baldo, J. V., Shimamura, A. P., Delis, D. C., Kramer, J., & Kaplan, E. (2001). Verbal and design fluency in patients with frontal lobe lesions. *Journal of the International Neuropsychological Society, 7*, 586–596.

Beatty, W. W., Katzung, V. M., Nixon, S. J., & Moreland, V. J. (1993). Problem-solving deficits in alcoholics: Evidence from the California Card Sorting Test. *Journal of Studies on Alcohol, 545*, 687–692.

Beatty, W. W., & Monson, N. (1990). Problem-solving in Parkinson's disease: Comparison of performance on the Wisconsin and California Card Sorting Test. *Journal of Geriatric Psychiatry and Neurology, 3*, 163–171.

Beatty, W. W., & Monson, N. (1996). Problem solving by patients with multiple sclerosis: Comparison of performance on the Wisconsin and California Card Sorting Test. *International Journal of Clinical Neuropsychology, 2*, 132–140.

Cato, M. A., Delis, D. C., Abildskov, T. J., & Bigler, E. (2004). Assessing the elusive cognitive deficits associated with ventromedial prefrontal damage: A case of a modern-day Phineas Gage. *Journal of the International Neuropsychological Society, 10,* 453–465.

Delis, D. C., Kaplan, E., & Kramer, J. H. (2001). *Delis-Kaplan Executive Function System.* San Antonio, TX: The Psychological Corporation.

Delis, D. C., Kramer, J. H., Kaplan, E., & Holdnack, J. (2004). Reliability and validity of the Delis-Kaplan Executive Function System: An update. *Journal of the International Neuropsychological Society, 10,* 301–303.

Hartman, M., Nielsen, C., & Stratton, B. (2004). The contributions of attention and working memory to age differences in concept identification. *Journal of Clinical and Experimental Neuropsychology, 26,* 227–245.

Homack, S., Lee, D., & Riccio, C. A. (2005). Test review: Delis-Kaplan Executive Function System. *Journal of Clinical and Experimental Neuropsychology, 27,* 500–609.

Keil, K., Baldo, J., Kaplan, E., Kramer, J., & Delis, D. C. (2005). Role of frontal cortex in inferential reasoning: Evidence from the Word Context Test. *Journal of the International Neuropsychological Society, 11,* 426–433.

Kramer, J. H., Reed, B. R., Mungas, D., Weiner, M. W., & Chui, H. C. (2002). Executive dysfunction in subcortical ischaemic vascular disease. *Journal of Neurology, Neurosurgery & Psychiatry, 72,* 217–220.

Mattson, S. N., Goodman, A. M., & Caine, C. (1999). Executive functioning in children with heavy prenatal alcohol exposure. *Alcoholism: Clinical & Experimental Research, 23,* 1808–1815.

McDonald, C. R., Delis, D. C., Norman, M. A., Tecoma, E. S., & Iragui-Madoz, V. J. (2005). Impairment in set-shifting specific to frontal-lobe dysfunction? Evidence from patients with frontal-lobe or temporal-lobe epilepsy. *Journal of the International Neuropsychological Society, 11,* 477–481.

Salthouse, T. A., Atkinson, T. M., & Berish, D. E. (2003). Executive functioning as a potential mediator of age-related cognitive decline in normal adults. *Journal of Experimental Psychology: General, 132,* 566–594.

Schmidt, M. (2003). Hit or miss? Insight into executive functions. *Journal of the International Neuropsychological Society, 9,* 962–964.

Schonfeld, A. M., Mattson, S. N., Lang, A., Delis, D. C., & Riley, E. P. (2001). Verbal and nonverbal fluency in children with heavy prenatal alcohol exposure. *Journal of Studies on Alcohol, 62,* 239–246.

Wecker, N. S., Kramer, J. H., Hallam, B. J., & Delis, D. C. (2005). Mental flexibility: Age effects on switching. *Neuropsychology, 19,* 345–352.

Wecker, N. S., Kramer, J. H., Wisniewski, A., Delis, D. C., & Kaplan, E. (2000). Age effects on executive ability. *Neuropsychology, 14,* 409–414.

Design Fluency Test

PURPOSE

This test uses the production of novel abstract designs to measure executive functioning.

SOURCE

No specific material is required.

AGE RANGE

The test can be given to individuals aged 5 to 72 years.

DESCRIPTION

Design Fluency (Jones-Gotman, 1991; Jones-Gotman & Milner, 1977) was developed as a nonverbal analog to word fluency tasks. The task requires the patient to generate as many different abstract designs as possible. The test is composed of a free-response condition, lasting five minutes, in which few restrictions are imposed on design generation, and a fixed-response condition, lasting four minutes, in which the patient must produce designs that contain exactly four lines or components. A modification of the fixed-condition task is also part of the Halstead Russell Neuropsychological Evaluation System (HRNES; Russell & Starkey, 1993, 2001).

ADMINISTRATION

The instructions provided in the original article are somewhat vague. More detailed instructions are provided in Figure 8–7 (from M. Jones-Gotman, personal communication, April 1995).

ADMINISTRATION TIME

The entire test takes about 15 minutes to administer. The time limits are five minutes for the free condition and four minutes for the fixed condition.

SCORING

There is one basic score for each condition: a *novel output score*, which is defined as the total output (total number of drawings) minus the sum of all perseverative responses, nameable drawings, and drawings with the wrong number of lines.

To score the Design Fluency Test, first determine the perseverative responses. These include rotations or mirror-image versions of previous drawings, variations on a theme, complicated drawings that differ from previous ones by small details, and scribbles. The perseverative responses must be scored harshly and then subtracted from the total number drawn; the remaining drawings should then be all quite different from one another. Occasionally, the patient might reproduce the drawing made by the examiner. This is not counted as a perseverative error.

For nameable drawings, the examiner will have asked "What is this?" for at least one drawing at the end of each condition. Most often patients will deny knowing what the drawing represents, but they sometimes answer with the name of a concrete object or a letter that has been elaborated, etc. The examiner must also use his or her own judgment when something looks obviously nameable.

For each of the two conditions, the final novel output score is the number of drawings remaining after perseverations and rule-breaking items (nameable, wrong number of lines) have

Use a stopwatch and have the patient comfortably seated before giving the instructions. If more than one page is used per condition, provide new blank paper and place the old one so that the patient can always see what he or she has already drawn. Always use a ballpoint pen to avoid erasures. Use a separate page for examples provided during the instructions, and hide that page after giving the directions. Draw the examples one under the other to illustrate what is expected from the patient.

A. Free Condition (five minutes)

I want you to do some drawing for me. This test is different from others that you have done, because in this test you must make up the drawings in your head. Do not make drawings that represent something. Do not draw anything you have ever seen before. Do not make drawings that anybody could name; if you draw something that can be named I won't count it. Instead, what you must do is to make up designs out of your head. For example, you could draw something like this:

It's nothing, I just made it up. Or you could draw something like this: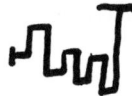

It's also nothing and I made it up. But if you were to draw, for example, something like this:

I would call it a star and I would not count it. The only other thing that is not accepted is scribbling. If you draw

And then

each might be slightly different from the other, but they do not require much effort from you and they are too much alike, so they are also not accepted and wouldn't count in your score. All of your drawings must be <u>very different</u> from each other.

Do you have any questions? When I say go, begin drawing. Make as <u>many different</u> drawings as you can in five minutes. You can start here, and draw them in columns like I have done. Go.

Remove the examiner's drawings from the patient's view. It is important to watch while the patient draws, so that warnings can be given at the appropriate moment. One warning only is given for each of the following: Scribbling (*That is a scribble. Remember scribbling is not allowed.*); Nameable Drawing (*I can name that. It's a _____. Do not make drawings that represent something.*); Too Similar to a Previous Drawing (*That is too much like . . .* indicate which one *. . . remember, all of your drawings must be very different from each other.*); Too Elaborate (*Remember, you must make as many different drawings as you can.*) At the end, always question at least one design to probe for nameable drawings (*What is this?*).

B. Four-Line Condition (four minutes)

Give the patient a separate sheet of paper and write "4 lines" at the top. Use your instruction page to draw examples. Count the lines aloud while drawing the examples in this condition.

There is a second part to this test. It is like the first one because again you have to make up designs that you invent yourself, but this time each design must be made with exactly four lines. I will show you what I mean by 'a line' for the purposes of this test.

(continued)

Figure 8–7 *(continued)*

Obviously, a straight line like this /

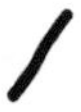

will count as one line. Whenever you draw a sharp angle, such as this ⌐¹₂

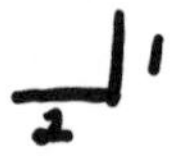

it will make two lines, whether you lift your pen or not. You can also draw a curved line, like this (

or like this)

or you can even draw a sort of double curve, like this ∫

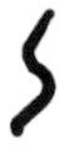

but avoid making lines that would be difficult to count, such as this ∮

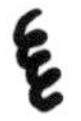

or this ⌇

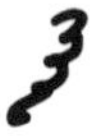

because I must be able to count the lines in your drawing easily. One other thing: A circle O

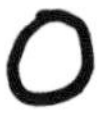

counts as one line, too. So, here is an example of what you could do. You could draw like this, for example ᡒ⌐|

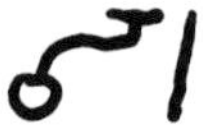

(count components while drawing); or for another example you could draw this:)X(

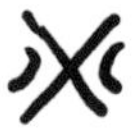

    Just like in the first part of the test, you must not make drawings that can be named or that represent anything. Just make up abstract designs, using exactly four lines in each one. Now, when I say go, make as many different designs as you can in four minutes. Go.

    As before, remove the examiner's drawings from the patient's view. Watch the patient so that warnings can be given at the appropriate moment. *One* warning only is given for *each* of the following: Too Similar to a Previous Drawing *(That is too much like . . . indicate which one . . .remember, all of your drawings must be very different from each other)*; Nameable Drawings (often a letter or a square in this condition); Wrong Number of Lines (count the lines aloud and remind patient to use exactly four lines). Question at least one drawing at the end to probe for nameable designs that you may not recognize as such *(What is this?)*.

been subtracted. This represents the patient's real output of novel designs. The two conditions are not added together. Although the first one may be the more sensitive of the two with regard to frontal lobe dysfunction, Jones-Gotman recommends retaining the two conditions. She found that the fixed condition was particularly sensitive in patients with subcortical dementia (Jones-Gotman, March 1995, personal communication).

Jones-Gotman (1990) noted that it is normal to produce some drawings that are too similar to others, although normal individuals produce relatively few perseverations (see *Normative Data*). Furthermore, the greater the total number is of drawings produced, the higher the likelihood is that some will be repeated. The drawings of an individual may also have a certain resemblance, reflecting the individual's style; however, Jones-Gotman suggests that this is quite different from the pathological repetitiveness or perseveration that is often seen in the productions made by patients with right frontal dysfunction.

Of note, Harter et al. (1999) have developed an expanded scoring system to allow more reliable scoring of the number of novel designs, complexity of designs, variations in designs, and concrete, perseverative, and scribbled responses.

Table 8–25 Mean Acceptable Novel Output by Adults on the Design Fluency Test—Free and Fixed Conditions

Age	N	Free Condition			Fixed Condition		
		M	*SD*	Range	*M*	*SD*	Range
14–55	45	15.5	6.1	9.5–21.7	18.9	5.6	13.3–24.5
58–72	10	11.8	4.4	7.4–16.2	12.6	4.3	8.3–16.9

Source: From Jones-Gotman, personal communication, June 1995.

DEMOGRAPHIC EFFECTS

Age

The literature suggests improvement in scores during the childhood years and then decreased performance with advancing age (Jones-Gotman, 1990; Levin et al., 1991; Mittenberg et al., 1989). Others, however (e.g., Turner, 1999; Varney et al. 1996), have found no significant correlation between number of novel designs and age. Daigneault et al. (1992) found only a higher incidence of perseverative errors in older adults (ages 45–65) without any reduction in the number of correct designs. They suggest that fluency and the ability to generate strategies remain intact with advancing age; rather, it is the regulation of behavior on the basis of preceding responses that is affected.

Education/IQ

Some have found no or little effect of education or IQ on the mean number of novel designs (Harter et al., 1999; Turner, 1999; Varney et al., 1996), whereas others (Diaz-Asper et al., 2004) have noted that productivity improves with increasing FSIQ.

Gender

Some report no gender differences (Demakis & Harrison, 1997; Harter et al., 1999; Varney et al., 1996), although Harter et al. (1999) found college men to produce more designs than their female counterparts.

NORMATIVE DATA

Adults

Jones-Gotman (personal communication, June 1995) has collected normative data for adults on both the free (five-minute) and fixed or four-line (four-minute) condition. The data are shown in Table 8–25. Carter et al. (1998) obtained similar data for a slightly larger sample of adults (*N* = 66; age, *M* = 25.06 years, *SD* = 7.83, range 19–56; education, *M* = 15.21, *SD* = 1.60; WAIS-R FSIQ = 100.85, *SD* = 11.07) using the revised scoring criteria described previously (free condition: mean novel output = 13.9, *SD* = 6.3; mean perse-

verative errors = 7.1, *SD* = 7.8; fixed condition: mean novel output = 16.7, *SD* = 6.1; mean perseverative errors = 6.4, *SD* = 5.5). Normals make one or no nameable errors (Carter et al., 1998; Varney et al., 1996) and produce very few designs (less than three) with an incorrect number of lines on the fixed condition (Carter et al., 1998).

Children

Jones-Gotman (1990) tested 324 school children between the ages of 5 and 14 years in the free condition. The mean numbers of acceptable drawings produced in five minutes for each age group are shown in Table 8–26.

Other researchers have provided data for both children and adults (Daigneault et al., 1992; Franzen & Petrick, 1995; Levin et al., 1991; Varney et al., 1996; Woodward et al., 1992). The values reported are generally higher than those reported here and likely reflect the strictness with which the scoring criteria are applied (Jones-Gotman, personal communication April 1995).

RELIABILITY

Test-Retest Reliability and Practice Effects

Ross et al. (1996) retested college students following a one-month interval and found stability coefficients for the free condition to be low, ranging from *r* = .10 (nameable drawings) to .56 (total number of drawings). Coefficients of stability for the fixed condition ranged from *r* = .12 (nameable drawings) to .70 (total number of drawings). Somewhat higher values were reported by Harter et al. (1999). In

Table 8–26 Mean Number of Acceptable Drawings by Children on the Design Fluency Test—Free Condition

Age	N	M	SD
5–6	52	3.2	2.0
7–8	68	6.2	3.2
9–10	68	8.0	3.2
11–14	68	9.4	3.9

Source: From Jones-Gotman, 1990, and personal communication, April 1995.

that study, college students were retested following a one-month interval and test-retest reliability ($r = .69$) for number of novel designs in the free condition approached the recommended range. Scoring parameters of concreteness ($r = .91$) and complexity of the protocol ($r = .77$) were relatively stable.

Previous exposure to the task resulted in both an increase in design production characterized by more total and novel designs (about seven designs in the free or fixed condition: Ross et al., 1996; two novel designs in the free condition: Harter et al., 1999), as well as an increase in test-taking efficiency, marked by a relative decrease in the proportion of perseverative responses.

Interrater Reliability

When the original scoring criteria described in Jones-Gotman and Milner (1977) are used, there is marginal to adequate interrater agreement (.64 for novel output in the free condition and .71 in the fixed condition) and rater consistency for the majority of scoring parameters in both conditions (Woodward et al., 1992). These scoring criteria do not, however, produce sufficient reliability for clinical use. Varney et al. (1996) gave the test to 86 patients who suffered closed head injuries and 87 normal controls. Two independent raters agreed 90% of the time with respect to the novel design score in the free condition. In a study with a college sample, Ross et al. (1996) found good to fair interrater reliability with regard to total ($r = .98$) and novel (about .69) responses. Perseverations and other rule violations showed poor interrater agreement (.21–.48).

The supplementary scoring criteria presented previously (see *Scoring*) enhance overall reliability. Jones-Gotman (1991) assessed scoring reliability in a study of 324 children and 50 adults. Three judges scored all tests independently. Correlation coefficients between judges were above .74. Carter et al. (1998) had three raters independently score Design Fluency protocols from 66 normal adults according to these revised criteria. They found that interrater reliability was good to excellent (intraclass correlation coefficients ranging from .73–.99) for novel output scores and perseverative errors. However, nameable errors and designs with the incorrect number of lines yielded lower reliability coefficients (.42–.50). Other expanded scoring instructions also result in high interrater reliabilities (Harter et al., 1999).

VALIDITY

Correlations Between Conditions

Moderately strong correlations (.55–.78) have been reported between the free and fixed conditions in samples of healthy individuals, suggesting that they are measuring similar but not identical functions (Demakis & Harrison, 1997; Franzen & Petrick, 1995). Scores on the Design Fluency and Ruff Figural Fluency Tests are modestly correlated (Demakis & Harrison, 1997), although the fixed condition is more robustly

related to the Ruff Figural Fluency Test than the free condition (.38 versus .25).

Correlations With Verbal Fluency

The degree of association with word fluency appears to depend on the nature of the sample. Positive, but weak, correlations ($r = <.20$) have been noted between design and verbal fluency (COWA) measures in healthy individuals, suggesting that the two measures are dissociable (Demakis & Harrison, 1997; Franzen & Petrick, 1995; see also Harter et al., 1999). Slightly higher agreement has been reported by Varney et al. (1996) in a sample of 86 patients with closed head injuries. Novel design performance in the free condition showed a modest relation with verbal fluency ($r = .34$). Whereas 47% of the patients performed defectively on Design Fluency, only 13% performed defectively on the COWA. Turner (1999), however, reported moderately strong relations (.65–.76) between Design Fluency and Word Fluency (COWA) as well as Ideational Fluency tasks in normals as well as individuals with autism.

Correlations With Other Measures

The cognitive operations underlying the task are not well understood. Creating novel designs is a complex task and likely involves several cognitive processes, including creativity, and constructional abilities (Bigler et al., 1988), as well as working memory for keeping track of items that have already been produced, shifting set from one design to the next, all while inhibiting repetition of a design (Foldi et al., 2003).

The fixed condition correlates moderately with measures of speed (Trails A, $r = -.39$) and inhibition (Stroop color-word interference trial, $r = .36$; Franzen & Petrick, 1995). The free condition shows strong relations with visual constructional and memory tasks such as the copy and recall of the Rey figure (.60; Mickanin et al., 1994). However, poor performance is not simply a matter of general mental impairment or problems with speed (Harter et al., 1999; Varney et al., 1996).

Clinical Studies

Jones-Gotman (1991) and Jones-Gotman and Milner (1977) showed that patients with right frontal or central damage are the most impaired on the task, although patients with lesions in other brain regions (e.g., right temporal, left frontal) also generate fewer novel designs than normals (see also Butler et al., 1993). The patients with right frontal or central damage have difficulty in two different ways: They simply create few new designs and/or tend to make numerous perseverative errors (see also Canavan et al., 1985).

The test appears to be sensitive to a variety of neurological conditions that can impact executive (or frontal lobe) functioning. Thus, the test has been useful in detecting dementias involving the frontal lobe (FTD; Canavan et al., 1985; Neary et al., 1990), particularly those with right-sided frontotemporal dementia (Boone et al., 1999), and is sensitive to even minor closed head injury. Varney et al. (1996) reported that patients with closed head injuries, even of a mild nature, tend to produce fewer novel designs in the free condition than normal controls. Impairment in Design Fluency has also been found in patients with AD (Bigler et al., 1988; Harter et al., 1999; Mickanin et al., 1994), MS (Tong et al., 2002), ALS (Abrahams et al., 2000; for number of rule violations only), and autism (Turner, 1999), and in pain sufferers following bilateral anterior cingulotomy (Cohen et al., 1999). Patients with idiopathic Parkinson's, however, appear relatively intact on the test (Auriacombe et al., 1993).

Elfgren and Risberg (1998) made regional cerebral blood flow (rCBF) measurements in frontal and frontotemporal regions in normal individuals during performance of the Design Fluency task. Regional cerebral blood flow augmentation was seen in both frontal lobes compared with baseline (Elfgren & Risberg, 1998). This was particularly evident when subjects used a visual-spatial strategy to generate designs. A mixed strategy (a visual-spatial strategy combined with thoughts about nameable objects) engaged the left frontal lobe.

Depression does not affect performance (Crews et al., 1999), at least among outpatient women not receiving antidepressants. Obsessionality, however, is associated with reduced design fluency (Mataix-Cols et al., 1999).

COMMENT

One of the common criticisms of the test (Ruff et al., 1987) has been that the scoring criteria are difficult to interpret and overly subjective. To address these difficulties, Jones-Gotman (see previous discussion) provided more detailed administration and scoring criteria. When such strict scoring criteria are used, the novel output scores and perseverative errors appear to be reliably scored. Other aspects (e.g., nameable errors, designs with the wrong number of lines) show poor interrater agreement. Further, temporal stability of the original DFT scoring parameters is low (and below that of other figural fluency tests such as the RFFT). With more detailed scoring criteria, test-retest reliability of the DFT improves (Harter et al., 1999). Note, too, that the norms for older adults are based on a very small sample of individuals and should be used with considerable caution.

The task does show some association with other measures of fluency, suggesting that they tap some common, though not identical, abilities. For example, in contrast to verbal fluency measures, designs are not taken from meaningful semantic or phonological stores, but must be generated as newly created responses (Foldi et al., 2003). Further, the Design Fluency task does not demand that the subject fully formulate the idea behind each response before beginning to produce that response; that is, they may generate "on the go" (Turner, 1999). Such an approach may result in a high rate of perseverative responding as the subject begins his or her response without stopping to plan the response fully, and therefore is more susceptible to be attracted to the salience of a previous response. By contrast, on Verbal Fluency tasks, the subject must first begin by generating some idea in a complete way.

Further, the other measures of nonverbal fluency (Five Point, Ruff Figural Fluency) cannot be considered alternate versions of Design Fluency. Designs that would be considered unique on the Ruff Figural Fluency task or the Five Point test would be viewed as repetitions on the Design Fluency test.

Scores for the free condition appear to be most sensitive to neurological impairment, likely due to its relatively unstructured format. The task appears sensitive to frontal lobe impairment, but there is less support that it is especially sensitive to right frontal lobe functioning. In addition, interpretation may be problematic in those patients with visual-constructional or motor deficits.

REFERENCES

Abrahams, S., Leigh, P. N., Harvey, A., Vythelingum, G. N., Grise, D., & Goldstein, L. H. (2000). Verbal fluency and executive dysfunction in amyotrophic lateral sclerosis (ALS). *Neuropsychologia, 38,* 734–747.

Auriacombe, S., Grossman, M., Carvell, S., Gollomp, S., Stern, M. B., & Hurtig, H. I. (1993). Verbal fluency deficits in Parkinson's disease. *Neuropsychology, 7,* 182–192.

Bigler, E. D., Schultz, R., Grant, M., Knight, G., Lucas, J., Roman, M., Hall, S., & Sullivan, M. (1988). Design fluency in dementia of the Alzheimer's type: Preliminary findings. *Neuropsychology, 2,* 127–133.

Boone, K. B., Miller, B. L., Lee, A., Berman, N., Sherman, D., & Stuss, D. T. (1999). Neuropsychological patterns in right versus left frontotemporal dementia. *Journal of the International Neuropsychological Society, 5,* 612–622.

Butler, R. W., Rorsman, I., Hill, J. M., & Tuma, R. (1993). The effects of frontal brain impairment on fluency: Simple and complex paradigms. *Neuropsychology, 7,* 519–529.

Canavan, S., Janota, I., & Schurr, P. H. (1985). Luria's frontal lobe syndrome: Psychological and anatomical considerations. *Journal of Neurology, Neurosurgery, and Psychiatry, 48,* 1049–1053.

Carter, S. L., Shore, D., Harnadek, M. S., & Kubu, C. S. (1998). Normative data and interrater reliability of the Design Fluency Test. *The Clinical Neuropsychologist, 12,* 531–534.

Cohen, R. A., Kaplan, R. F., Zuffante, P., Moser, D. J., Jenkines, M. A., Salloway, S., & Wilkinson, H. (1999). Alteration of intention and self-initiated action associated with bilateral anterior cingulotomy. *Journal of Neuropsychiatry and Clinical Neuroscience, 11,* 444–453.

Crews, W. D., Harrison, D. W., & Rhodes, R. D. (1999). Neuropsychological test performances of young depressed outpatient women: An examination of executive functions. *Archives of Clinical Neuropsychology, 14,* 517–529.

Daigneault, S., Braun, C. M. J., & Whitaker, H. A. (1992). Early effects of normal aging on perseverative and nonperseverative prefrontal measures. *Developmental Neuropsychology, 8,* 99–114.

Demakis, G. J., & Harrison, D. W. (1997). Relationships between verbal and nonverbal fluency measures: Implications for assessment of executive functioning. *Psychological Reports, 81,* 443–448.

Diaz-Asper, C., Schretlen, D. J., & Pearlson, G. D. (2004). How well does IQ predict neuropsychological test performance in normal adults. *Journal of the International Neuropsychological Society, 10,* 82–90.

Elfgren, C. I., & Risberg, J. (1998). Lateralized frontal blood flow increases during fluency tasks: Influence of cognitive strategy. *Neuropsychologia, 36*, 505–512.

Foldi, N. S., Helm-estabrookds, N., Redfield, J., & Nickel, D. G. (2003). Perseveration in normal aging: A comparison of perseveration rates on design fluency and verbal generative tasks. *Aging, Neuropsychology and Cognition, 10*, 268–280.

Franzen, M. D., & Petrick, J. D. (1995). *Preliminary norms for Design Fluency.* Paper presented to the 103rd meeting of the American Psychological Association, New York.

Harter, S. L., Hart, C. C., & Harter, G. W. (1999). Expanded scoring criteria for the Design Fluency Test: Reliability and validity in neuropsychological and college samples. *Archives of Clinical Psychology, 14*, 419–432.

Jones-Gotman, M. (1990). Presurgical psychological assessment in children: Special tests. *Journal of Epilepsy, 3*, 93–102.

Jones-Gotman, M. (1991). Localization of lesions by neuropsychological testing. *Epilepsia, 32*, S41–S52.

Jones-Gotman, M., & Milner, B. (1977). Design fluency: The invention of nonsense drawings after focal cortical lesions. *Neuropsychologia, 15*, 653–674.

Levin, H. S., Culhane, K. A., Hartmann, J., Harword, H., Ringholtz, G., Ewing-Cobbs, L., & Fletcher, J. M. (1991). Developmental changes in performance on tests of purported frontal lobe functioning. *Developmental Neuropsychology, 7*, 377–395.

Mataix-Cols, D., Barrios, M., Sanchez-Turet, M., & Vallejo, J. (1999). Reduced design fluency in subclinical obsessive-compulsive subjects. *Journal of Neuropsychiatry & Clinical Neurosciences, 11*, 395–397.

Mickanin, J., Grossman, M., Onishi, K., Auriacombe, S., & Clark, C. (1994). Verbal and nonverbal fluency in patients with probable Alzheimer's disease. *Neuropsychology, 8*, 385–394.

Mittenberg, W., Seidenberg, M., O'Leary, D. S., & DiGiulio, D. V. (1989). Changes in cerebral functioning associated with normal aging. *Journal of Clinical and Experimental Neuropsychology, 11*, 918–932.

Neary, D., Snowden, J. S., Mann, D. M. A., Northen, B., Goulding, P. J., & Macdermott, N. (1990). Frontal lobe dementia and motor neuron disease. *Journal of Neurology, Neurosurgery, and Psychiatry, 53*, 23–32.

Ross, T. P., Axelrod, B. N., Hanks, R. A., Kotasek, R. S., & Whitman, R. D. (1996). *The interrater and test-retest reliability of the Design Fluency and Ruff Figural Fluency Tests.* Paper presented to the 24th meeting of the International Neuropsychological Society, Chicago.

Ruff, R. M., Light, R. H., & Evans, R. (1987). The Ruff Figural Fluency Test: a normative study with adults. *Developmental Neuropsychology, 3*, 37–51.

Russell, E. W., & Starkey, R. I. (1993, 2001). *Halstead Russell Neuropsychological Evaluation System (HRNES-R).* Los Angeles: Western Psychological Services.

Tong, B. S., Yip, J. T. H., Lee, T. M. C., & Li, L. S. W. (2002). Frontal fluency and memory functioning among multiple sclerosis patients in Hong Kong. *Brain Injury, 16*, 987–995.

Turner, M. A. (1999). Generating novel ideas: Fluency performance in high-functioning and learning disabled individuals with autism. *Journal of Child Psychology and Psychiatry, 40*, 189–201.

Varney, N. R., Roberts, R. J., Struchen, M. A., Hanson, T. V., Franzen, K. M., & Connell, S. K. (1996). Design fluency among normals and patients with closed head injury. *Archives of Clinical Neuropsychology, 11*, 345–353.

Woodward, J. L., Axelrod, B. N., & Henry, R. R. (1992). Interrater reliability of scoring parameters for the Design Fluency Test. *Neuropsychology, 6*, 173–178.

Five-Point Test

PURPOSE

This test requires production of novel designs under time constraints.

SOURCE

Users may make up their own stimuli as described later. There are a number of adaptations of the Five-Point Test, including the Ruff Figural Fluency Test (Ruff, 1988; Ruff et al., 1987), the D-KEFS Design Fluency Test (Delis et al., 2001), and the NEPSY Design Fluency Test (Korkman et al., 1998) described elsewhere in this volume.

AGE RANGE

For the version using a five-minute time limit, norms are available for children 6 to 13 years. For the version using a three-minute time limit, data are available for individuals aged 11 years to adulthood.

DESCRIPTION

Figural fluency tests have been developed as nonverbal analogs to word fluency tasks. One of the first figural fluency

tasks, Jones-Gotman and Milner's Design Fluency Test (1977; see review earlier in this chapter), has several problems that restrict its widespread use (Lee et al., 1997). These include inadequate normative data and difficulty in interpreting the performance of patients with visual-constructive or motor deficits. In addition, cognitively impaired patients often have difficulty understanding the task demands. In an attempt to overcome some of these limitations, Regard et al. (1982) provided an alternative figural fluency task, the Five-Point Test. This task consists of a sheet of paper ($8\frac{1}{2} \times 11$") with 40 dot matrices arranged in eight rows and five columns. The matrices are identical to the five-dot arrangement on dice (see Figure 8–8). Patients are asked to produce as many different figures as possible by connecting the dots within each rectangle.

Regard et al. (1982) allowed the subjects five minutes to perform the task. Using the Regard et al. stimuli, Lee et al. (1994) adapted the task to use a three-minute limit to make it more comparable to the time limits used for the Controlled Oral Word Association (COWA) test.

ADMINISTRATION

The examiner places a protocol sheet in front of the patient and indicates that the object is to produce as many different

Figure 8–8 Five-Point Test.

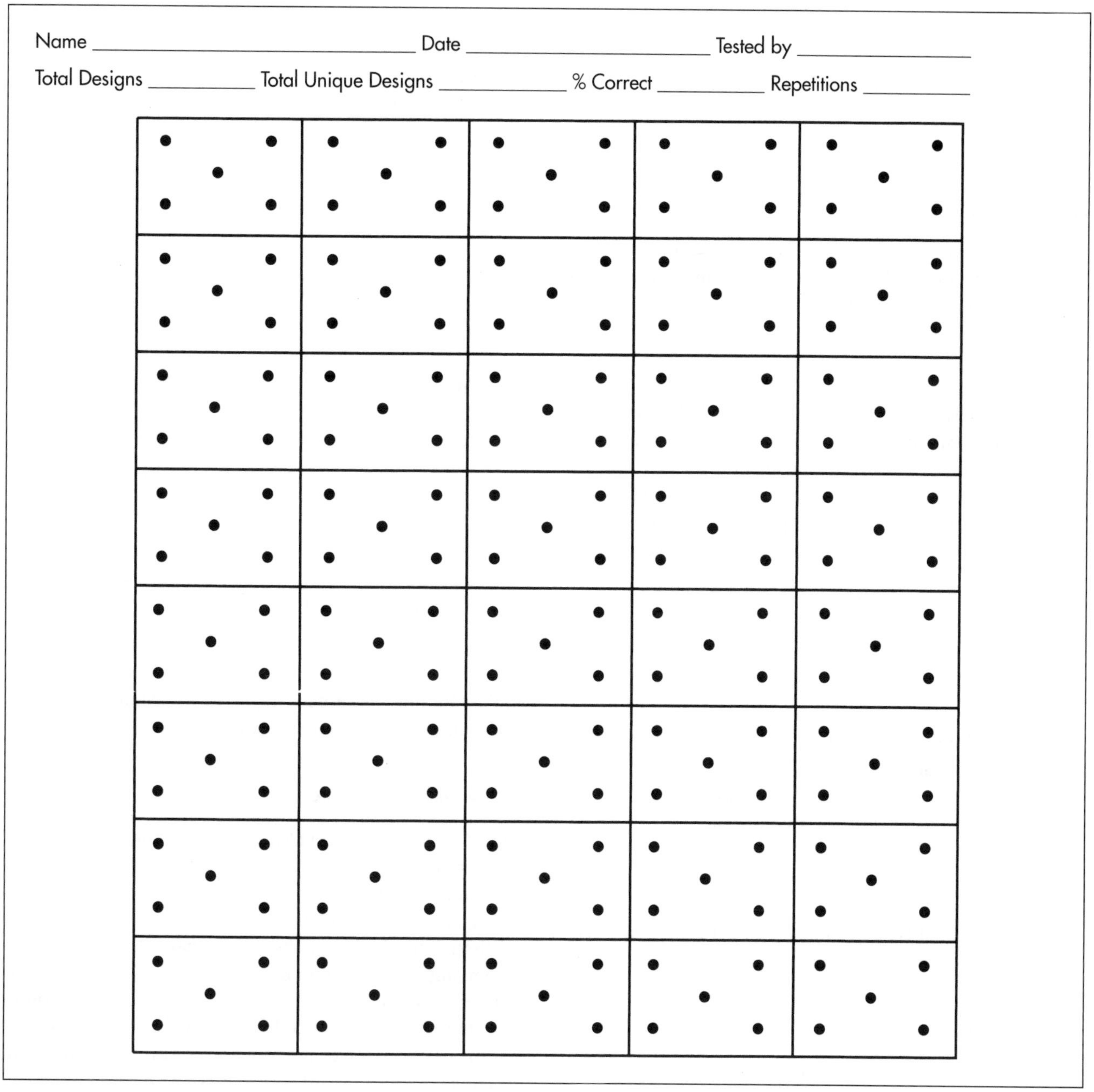

Name _____ Date _____ Tested by _____

Total Designs _____ Total Unique Designs _____ % Correct _____ Repetitions _____

figures or designs as possible in three minutes by connecting the dots in each rectangle. The patient is also informed that only straight lines are to be used, that all lines must connect dots, that no figures are to be repeated, and that only single lines are to be used. One warning is given on the first (and only the first) violation of each of these rules. The rules are not repeated on any further infraction.

At the start of the test, two sample solutions are drawn by the examiner. We typically draw the first sample design using all five dots and the second using just two dots to demonstrate to the patient that he or she can make either simple or complex designs using some or all of the dots. The patient is permitted to copy the sample designs drawn by the examiner. Most patients do not use more than two test sheets. When a patient exhausts a page, the examiner smoothly and quickly gives the patient a second page while repositioning the first page so that the subject can easily see it.

Patients often ask whether a seemingly trivial variation of a design constitutes a unique production. The examiner should reassure the patient that the second design counts. Another frequent question is whether all dots need to be used. The examiner should repeat that the patient need not use all dots.

Table 8–27 Five-Point Test (Three-Minute Time Limit): Mean Unique Designs and Perseverations in Adults

N	Unique Designs	Perseverations	% Perseverations
62	31.95 (8.4)	1.39 (1.8)	4.82 (6.6)

Source: Adapted from Lee et al., 1997.

ADMINISTRATION TIME

The entire test takes about five to seven minutes to administer. The time limit for the test itself is three or five minutes, depending on the age of the client.

SCORING

A number of scores can be calculated, including the total number of unique designs and the number of repeated designs (perseverations). Patients who are more productive have a greater opportunity to make more perseverative errors, so to adjust for this, the percentage of perseverative errors ([perseverative errors/total unique designs] × 100) can also be calculated.

DEMOGRAPHIC EFFECTS

Age

Age has little impact on test scores in adults (Glosser & Goodglass, 1997; Lee et al., 1997; Santa Maria et al., 2001) or adolescents (Risser & Andrikopoulos, 1996). However, in children, performance improves with age (Regard et al., 1982).

Gender

Gender does not affect performance (Lee et al., 1997; Regard et al., 1982; Risser & Andrikopoulos, 1996).

Education/IQ

Although the impact of education appears limited (Glosser & Goodglass, 1990; Lee et al., 1997; Santa Maria et al., 2001), IQ appears correlated with the number of unique designs produced ($r = .64$; Lee et al., 1997).

NORMATIVE DATA

Adults

Normative data based on a sample of 62 adults with psychiatric disorders (age, $M = 35.4$, $SD = 10.3$; education, $M = 13.4$ years, $SD = 3.4$; mean FSIQ = 109.1, $SD = 11.9$) are provided by Lee et al. (1997) and are shown in Table 8–27. The distribution of the percentage of perseverative errors (with percentile ranks) produced by these individuals is shown in Table 8–28.

Table 8–28 Five-Point Test (Three-Minute Time Limit): Percentile Ranks Associated With the Percentage of Perseverative Errors in Non-Neurologically Impaired Adults

Percent of Perseverations	Cumulative Percentile
0	100
1	56
2	56
3	48
4	39
5	32
6	31
7	27
8	27
9	21
10	21
11	16
12	15
13	11
14	6
15 (cutoff score)	6
16	5
17	0

Source: Adapted from Lee et al., 1997.

Similar findings have been reported by Santa Maria et al. (2001) in a sample of undergraduates.

Children and Adolescents

Regard et al. (1982) provided data (total number of figures, number of rotated figures, number of self-corrections) for the five-minute version. Their sample consisted of normal children aged 6 to 13 years. The data are shown in Table 8–29.

Risser and Andrikopoulos (1996) gave the original five-minute and the three-minute task to a sample of 30 healthy children, aged 11 years, 9 months to 14 years, 8 months ($M = 13$ years). Scores on both versions were highly correlated, and the performance of the adolescents was similar to that of the adults (see also Regard et al., 1982). The data for the three-

Table 8–29 Five-Point Test (Five-Minute Time Limit): Total Number of Figures (Means and Standard Deviations)

Group (Mean Age)	N	Total Figures
Grade 1 (6.3)	20	22.48 (12.56)
Grade 3 (8.4)	20	30.10 (9.92)
Grade 5 (10.6)	20	37.35 (8.99)
Grade 7 (12.4)	20	44.00 (8.71)

Source: From Regard et al., 1982. Reproduced with permission of the publisher. © Perceptual and Motor Skills.

minute and five-minute versions are shown in Table 8–30. No rule-breaking errors were noted on either version.

RELIABILITY

Data on reliability are not available.

VALIDITY

Correlations With Other Tests

The test is moderately correlated to measures of verbal fluency, suggesting that the verbal and nonverbal fluency measures tap similar though not identical functions (Regard et al., 1982; Risser & Andrikopoulos, 1996) as the amount of variance unexplained is rather large (more than 70%).

The Five-Point Test and its variant (an untimed version by Glosser & Goodglass, 1990) are also moderately to highly (.4–.7) correlated with visual-spatial and visual-constructive measures (e.g., Picture Completion, Block Design) and measures of executive control (e.g., Wisconsin Card Sorting Test), but not with linguistic function (Glosser & Goodglass, 1990).

Factor-analytic findings in patients with seizure disorders (Helmstaedter et al., 1996) suggested that the number correct loaded together with other tasks tapping attention and speed (e.g., mazes-time, letter cancellation, word fluency) while errors loaded on a response inhibition factor (mazes-errors, Stroop Interference).

Clinical Studies

There is some evidence that the Five-Point Test is sensitive to brain damage generally and to frontal lobe pathology specifically. Lee et al. (1997) gave the test to 196 patients with neurologic disease (mostly patients with intractable partial complex seizures) and 62 patients with psychiatric disorder. Psychiatric patients produced significantly more unique designs and a lower percentage of perseverative errors than patients with neurological disorder. Among neurological patients, individuals with frontal lobe disease and nonfrontal lobe lesions both produced fewer unique designs than psychiatric patients but did not differ from each other. Patients with frontal lobe disease were, however, distinguished from nonfrontal lobe disease neurologic patients and psychiatric patients by producing a significantly higher percentage of perseverative errors. There were no significant differences between patients with left and right frontal damage, although there was a trend for patients with right-sided involvement to perform more poorly than their left-sided counterparts (see also Glosser & Goodglass, 1990). Similarly, Helmstaedter et al. (1996) found that patients with frontal lobe epilepsy made more errors (perseveration, rule breaks) than patients with temporal lobe epilepsy. Others, however, have failed to find that the Five-Point Test is particularly sensitive to right frontal lobe damage (Tucha et al., 1999). Reduced performance has been documented in patients with obsessive-compulsive disorder, a disorder that is thought to reflect frontostriatal dysfunction (Schmidtke et al., 1998).

Regard et al. (1982) originally used a five-minute interval. The three-minute version, however, appears to accomplish the same discriminatory goals as the five-minute version and, because of its brevity and high correlation with the five-minute version, is more attractive (Lee et al., 1997; Risser & Andrikopoulos, 1996). However, if the time limits for the test are increased, then progressive decreases in the number of unique designs and increases in perseverative errors as a function of time can be expected (Santa Maria et al., 2001).

COMMENT

Use of this task is limited by the lack of data on reliability. There is some evidence of construct validity as the task does show moderate relations with other fluency tests (i.e., Verbal Fluency). Its relation to other measures of nonverbal fluency (e.g., Design Fluency, Figural Fluency) remains to be determined. A difference between the Five-Point test and the Design Fluency test developed by Jones-Gotman and Milner (1977) lies in the degree of structure provided for the patient. While designs generated in the Five-Point Test may be counted as valid and novel, the same productions would likely be viewed as repetitions in the Design Fluency task. That is, the Design Fluency measure may place greater demands on the ability to generate novel productions. On the other hand, it may be more difficult to score in a standardized manner.

The Ruff Figural Fluency Test stimuli were designed to vary in level of difficulty (e.g., through the use of interference). The research (Ruff, 1988) revealed, however, no significant differences among the five parts of the test, and only the total scores are provided in the manual. Thus, it appears that the use of multiple trials on the Ruff Figural Fluency Test may be redundant and unnecessary (Lee et al., 1997). On the other hand, the Ruff Figural Fluency task has the advantage of a larger psychometric base (e.g., a larger normative base, information on reliability is available) than the Five-Point Test. Further, an untimed version of the Five-Point Test (e.g., Glosser & Goodglass, 1990) may be more appropriate to use when time constraints could unduly penalize patients (e.g., with patients who have had a stroke or who have Parkinson's disease). Finally, it should be noted that variants of the Five-Point Test are included in both the NEPSY and the D-KEFS. However, in both cases, reliability coefficients are low.

Table 8–30 Five-Point Test (Three-Minute and Five-Minute Versions): Mean Scores for Adolescents, aged 11–14 years (Mean 13 years)

Version	Unique Designs	No. of Perseverations
Three-minute	29.5 (7.77)	1.27 (1.76)
Five-minute	42.6 (11.45)	2.57 (2.97)

Source: Adapted from Risser & Andrikopoulos, 1996.

REFERENCES

Delis, D. C., Kaplan, E., & Kramer, J. H. (2001). *Delis-Kaplan Executive Function System*. San Antonio, TX: The Psychological Corporation.

Glosser, G., & Goodglass, H. (1990). Disorders in executive control functions among aphasic and other brain-damaged patients. *Journal of Clinical and Experimental Neuropsychology, 12*, 485–501.

Helmstaedter, C., Kemper, B., & Elger, C. E. (1996) Neuropsychological aspects of frontal lobe epilepsy. *Neuropsychologia, 34*, 399–406.

Jones-Gotman, M., & Milner, B. (1977). Design fluency: The invention of nonsense drawings after focal cortical lesions. *Neuropsychologia, 15*, 653–674.

Korkman, M., Kirk, U., & Kemp, S. (1998). *NEPSY: A Developmental Neuropsychological Assessment Manual*. San Antonio, TX: The Psychological Corporation.

Lee, G. P., Loring, D. W., Newell, J., & McCloskey, L. (1994). Figural fluency on the Five-Point Test: Preliminary normative and validity data. *International Neuropsychological Society Program and Abstracts, 1*, 51.

Lee, G. P., Strauss, E., Loring, D. W., McCloskey, L., & Haworth, J. M. (1997). Sensitivity of figural fluency on the Five-Point Test to focal neurological disease. *The Clinical Neuropsychologist, 11*, 59–68.

Regard, M., Strauss, E., & Knapp, P. (1982). Children's production of verbal and nonverbal fluency tasks. *Perceptual and Motor Skills, 55*, 839–844.

Risser, A. H., & Andrikopoulos, J. (1996). *Regard's Five-Point Test: Adolescent cohort stability*. Paper presented to the International Neuropsychological Society, Chicago.

Ruff, R. (1988). *Ruff Figural Fluency Test*. San Diego, CA: Neuropsychological Resources.

Ruff, R. M., Light, R., & Evans, R. (1987). The Ruff Figural Fluency Test: A normative study with adults. *Developmental Neuropsychology, 3*, 37–51.

Santa Maria, M. P., Martin, J. A., Morrow, C. M., & Gouvier, W. D. (2001). On the duration of spatial fluency measures. *International Journal of Neuroscience, 7*, 586–596.

Schmidtke, K., Schorb, A., Winkelmann, G., & Hohagen, F. (1998). Cognitive frontal lobe dysfunction in obsessive-compulsive disorder. *Society of Biological Psychiatry, 43*, 666–673.

Tucha, O., Smely, C., & Lange, K. W. (1999). Verbal and figural fluency in patients with mass lesions of the left or right frontal lobes. *Journal of Clinical and Experimental Neuropsychology, 21*, 229–236.

The Hayling and Brixton Tests

PURPOSE

These two tests are thought to assess behavioral regulation. The Hayling Test evaluates initiation speed as well as response suppression, while the Brixton Spatial Anticipation Test is a rule attainment task.

SOURCE

The kit includes the manual, Brixton Test Stimulus Book, and 25 scoring sheets and can be ordered from Harcourt Assessment, www.harcourtassessment-uk.com, at a cost of about £131 or $246 US.

AGE RANGE

The Hayling Test can be used with children aged 8 to 15 years and adults aged 18 to 80 years. The Brixton can be used with adults aged 18 to 80 years.

DESCRIPTION

The authors (Burgess & Shallice, 1997) developed these tasks to be sensitive to symptoms of executive disturbance. Each test can be given singly or in combination. The Hayling Test consists of two sets of 15 sentences, each having the last word missing. In the first part, Section 1, the examiner reads each sentence aloud and the patient has to complete the sentence as quickly as possible. For example, "The old house will be torn . . . (patient says) down." This section yields a simple measure of response speed. In the second part, Section 2, the patient is faced with the more novel task of completing the sentence with a word that is unconnected to the sentence in every way. For example, "The captain wanted to stay with the sinking . . . (patient says) light bulb." Therefore, the patient has to inhibit a strongly activated (automatic) response before generating a new response. This section yields two scores, an error score and a measure of response speed. In addition, performance on all three measures (response latencies from Sections 1 and 2 and error score from Section 2) can be combined into an overall score.

The Brixton Spatial Anticipation Test is a rule attainment task based on the WCST. However, in contrast to the WCST, the rule that is currently in operation cannot be triggered by any perceptually salient aspect of the stimuli. It consists of a 56-page Stimulus Booklet, each page showing the same basic array of 10 circles set in two rows of five, with each circle numbered from one to 10. On each page, one of the circles is filled with a blue color. The position of this filled circle changes from one page to the next. The changes in position are governed by a series of simple rules, which vary without warning. The patient is shown one page at a time and is asked to decide where the next filled position will be, by trying to see a pattern or rule based on what he or she has seen on previous pages. The test does not require verbal responses; rather, the patient can point to a position. The total errors are recorded.

ADMINISTRATION

Instructions for administration are given in the manual. The scoring sheet prompts the examiner about scoring procedures.

ADMINISTRATION TIME

Each test takes about five minutes to give.

SCORING

Scoring guidelines for each test are found in the manual. For the Hayling Test, response latencies are recorded in whole second units and are not rounded up. Therefore, a time between 0 and .99 seconds is recorded as 0. The raw score for Section 1 is the sum of all the individual latencies and is converted to a scaled score (range: 1—Impaired to 7—High average) using Table A on the scoring sheet. Section 2 time measures are scored in the same way as Section 1 is. This score is then converted to a scaled score (range: 1—Impaired to 8—Good) using Table B on the scoring sheet.

Each response on Section 2 is classed as falling into one of three categories. The first is where the word produced is completely unconnected to the sentence and is given zero points. The second type of response is classed as a Category B error. This is where the response is somewhat connected to the meaning of the sentence, but is not a direct sentence completion. The third type of response is a Category A error. This is where the patient completes the sentence in an entirely plausible manner. The number of Category A errors is converted to an "A score" and the number of Category B errors is converted to a "B score" using tables on the score sheet. The A and B scores are summed and this "converted" score is transformed to a scaled score (range: 1—Impaired to 8—Good) by means of Table C on the score sheet. The sum of the three scaled scores (from Sections 1 and 2) can be converted to an overall scaled score (range: 1—Impaired to 10—Very superior; 6 is average) by means of Table E on the score sheet. Additional error scoring criteria for each sentence are provided in an appendix of the manual.

For the Brixton Test, the total number of errors is converted to a scaled score (range: 1—Impaired to 10—Very superior). However, the patient's answer to the first item is disregarded as this is a guess. Only accuracy, not response latency, is recorded for the Brixton.

DEMOGRAPHIC EFFECTS

Age

Age impacts performance on both the Hayling and Brixton tasks (Andres & Van der Linden, 2000; Bielak et al., in press; Burgess & Shallice, 1997), although in one study (Andres & Van der Linden, 2000) older adults (aged 60–70 years) were significantly slower than younger participants (aged 20–30 years) in Hayling Section A, but not B.

IQ/Education

Higher IQ is linked to fewer errors (Bielak et al., in press; Burgess & Shallice, 1997; Clark et al., 2000) and reduced time required on Section B relative to Section A (Clark et al., 2000). Education also affects Hayling and Brixton scores, although less so than age (Bielak et al., in press). Burgess and Shallice recommend that the tests be used with caution in individuals with relatively low educational achievement or who premorbidly would fall within the bottom 15% of the population on measures of general intelligence (i.e., IQ $\leq$ 85).

Gender

Gender does not significantly impact Hayling scores (Bielak et al., in press; Burgess & Shallice, 1997), although Bielak et al. (in press) found that being female was associated with more errors on the Brixton. In this study, age accounted for about 11% of the variance while education and gender contributed about 2% and 1%, respectively.

NORMATIVE DATA

Standardization Sample

Burgess and Shallice (1997) normed the Hayling on a group of 118 healthy individuals, aged 18 to 80 ($M = 45.3$, $SD = 18.1$) living in the United Kingdom. The NART estimated IQ for a subsample ($N = 71$) of these individuals was in the above-average range (110.9, $SD = 6.7$). Characteristics of the sample are shown in Table 8–31. Note that low NART performers were excluded from study. Therefore, a scaled score of 6, which is "average" for all three measures yielded by the Hayling Test, is the score that would be expected to be achieved by a person 45 years old and of "average" ability (Burgess & Shallice, 1997).

Table 8–31 Characteristics of the Hayling Normative Sample

Number	118
Age	18–80 years[a]
Geographic location	England
Sample type	A mix of patient relatives, volunteers for research studies, people from a job-employment program, and nonacademic staff at a university; mean NART FSIQ of 71 subjects = 110.9 ($SD = 6.7$)
Education	Not reported
SES	Not reported
Gender	
Females	61
Males	57
Race/ethnicity	Not reported
Screening	Reported to have no history of neurologic or psychiatric disorders or drug/alcohol abuse problems but method used to screen not reported; low-NART performers excluded

[a]Age distributions as follows: 18–45, $N = 48$; 46–65, $N = 51$; 66–80, $N = 19$.

Source: Adapted from Burgess & Shallice, 1997.

Table 8–32 Characteristics of the Brixton Normative Sample

Number	121
Age	18–80 years[a]
Geographic location	England
Sample type	A mix of patient relatives, volunteers for research studies, people from a job-employment program, and nonacademic staff at a university; mean NART FSIQ of a subsample of 73 subjects = 109.9 (SD = 7.1)
Education	Not reported
SES	Not reported
Gender	
Females	67
Males	54
Race/ethnicity	Not reported
Screening	Reported to have no history of neurologic or psychiatric disorders or drug/alcohol abuse problems but method used to screen not reported; low-NART performers excluded

[a]Age distributions as follows: 18–45, N = 58; 46–65, N = 45; 66–80, N = 18.

Source: Adapted from Burgess & Shallice, 1997.

The Brixton was normed on a sample of 121 healthy people, aged 18 to 80 (M = 45.6, SD = 17.8). The NART estimated IQ of a subsample was in the upper end of the average range (Brixton: 109.9, SD = 7.1, N = 73). Characteristics of the sample are shown in Table 8–32. As with the Hayling, low NART performers were excluded from study.

For each test, age, IQ, and age- and IQ-related 5% cutoff scores are provided in an appendix of the test manual.

Other Normative Data

Adults. Bielak et al. (in press) have recently provided normative data on a larger sample of 457 typically aging older community-dwelling adults (53–90 years). The sample was well educated (education, M = 15.23; SD = 2.86), predominantly female (69.8%), and Caucasian (98.2%), and considered English their native tongue (90.2%). Individuals with MMSE scores of 24 or less, moderate/severe visual or auditory impairment even with corrective aids, and a history of significant neurological or psychiatric disorders were excluded. The data for the Hayling Test are presented in Table 8–33 using overlapping midpoint age ranges to constitute the groups. The values for the Hayling time scores are somewhat lower than those reported by Burgess and Shallice (1997).

Table 8–34 provides the data for Brixton Test based on the same sample. The scores are generally consistent with those reported by others (Andres & Van der Linden, 2000; Burgess & Shallice, 1997).

Children. Baylis and Roodenrys (2000) gave both tests to a small group (N = 15) of healthy children, ranging in age from 8 to 12 years (M = 9.61, SD = .91) of average IQ (Raven's SPM percentile rank = 65.47, SD = 20.90). Clark et al. (2000) tested a group of 26 adolescents aged 12 to 15 years (M = 14.0, SD = .8). The data are shown in Table 8–35.

RELIABILITY

Hayling Test

Internal Consistency. Burgess and Shallice (1997) report that split-half reliability coefficients were variable (.35–.83)

Table 8–33 Hayling: Response Latencies and Error Scores by Age Midpoints

Variable	Midpoint Age 57	Midpoint Age 60	Midpoint Age 65	Midpoint Age 70	Midpoint Age 75	Midpoint Age 80	Midpoint Age 85
Age range	53–60	55–65	60–70	65–75	70–80	75–85	80–90
M	57.34	60.19	64.80	69.93	75.11	79.47	82.69
N	88	167	161	141	128	105	55
Time to Section 1							
M	4.49	5.24	5.25	4.57	6.56	8.62	9.13
(SD)	(5.21)	(6.65)	(6.30)	(4.34)	(7.77)	(8.64)	(6.41)
Time to Section 2							
M	19.93	20.83	24.80	34.38	40.41	43.65	51.38
(SD)	(16.43)	(19.24)	(21.43)	(33.23)	(40.45)	(41.48)	(41.89)
Category A errors							
M	0.83	0.82	0.76	0.87	1.03	1.05	1.11
(SD)	(1.04)	(0.98)	(0.91)	(1.01)	(1.18)	(1.28)	(1.41)
Category B errors							
M	2.43	2.23	2.52	3.33	3.36	3.30	3.64
(SD)	(2.25)	(2.15)	(2.27)	(2.63)	(2.53)	(2.34)	(2.67)

Note: Times are rounded down to nearest second and out of 15 trials.

Source: From Bielak et al., in press. Reprinted with permission of Elsevier.

Table 8–34 Brixton Test: Total Number of Errors by Age Midpoints

Variable	Midpoint Age 57	Midpoint Age 60	Midpoint Age 65	Midpoint Age 70	Midpoint Age 75	Midpoint Age 80	Midpoint Age 85
Age range	53–60	55–65	60–70	65–75	70–80	75–85	80–90
M	57.30	60.19	64.72	69.98	75.17	79.36	82.72
N	89	172	165	143	134	107	53
Errors score							
M	16.1	17.23	17.93	18.71	21.19	22.92	24.08
(SD)	(5.32)	(6.86)	(7.37)	(6.93)	(8.08)	(8.53)	(7.37)

Source: From Bielak et al., in press. Reprinted with permission of Elsevier.

for healthy adults but respectable for patients with anterior lesions (Hayling 1 time: .93, Hayling 2 time: .80, errors: .72). There is no information available for pediatric populations.

Test-Retest Reliability and Practice Effects. This was assessed in a group of 31 healthy adults retested between two days and four weeks after the first assessment (Burgess & Shallice, 1997). Reliabilities were adequate for the overall score (.76) and Hayling 2 time (.78) but weak for the other scores (Hayling 1 time: .62, errors: .52). Practice effects were not reported.

Interrater Reliability. Significant judgment is required in terms of assigning responses to particular categories. Unfortunately, no information is provided in the test manual regarding interrater reliability. One study (Andres & Van der Linden, 2000) noted that two raters agreed on only 76.5% of 1425 responses.

Brixton Test

Internal Consistency. Split-half reliability in healthy individuals is marginal (.62; Burgess & Shallice, 1997).

Test-Retest Reliability. This was assessed in a group of 31 healthy people retested either two days or four weeks after the first assessment (Burgess & Shallice, 1997). Reliability was adequate (.71). No information is provided regarding the nature of any practice effects.

VALIDITY

Correlations Between Hayling and Brixton Tests

Correlations between the tasks tend to be low in community-dwelling older adults (r = .12 or less; Bielak et al., in press; de Frias et al., in press). However, de Frias et al. (in press) noted that these tests (along with the Stroop and Color Trails tasks) share some common variance at the latent construct level, even though they appear quite disparate based on zero-order correlations. Burgess and Shallice (1997) reported that in healthy individuals, the strongest correlation between the Hayling and Brixton tests (between Hayling overall score and Brixton) was reduced from .35 to .14 when the effects attributable to age and IQ (as measured by the NART) were partialed from the analysis. Similar results have been reported by Andres and Van der Linden (2000). In their study of healthy individuals, a modest correlation between error scores on both tests (.33) was no longer significant after controlling for the effect of age.

The implication of these findings is that the two tests probably measure somewhat different cognitive processes, an interpretation supported by a previous study (Burgess & Shallice, 1994), which reported individual cases with frontal lobe lesions who showed double dissociations on the Hayling and Brixton Tests. Temple and Sanfilippo (2003) reported that children with Klinefelter's syndrome demonstrated impaired performance on a modified Hayling Test but were unimpaired on the Brixton task. By contrast, Marczewski et al. (2001) found that in patients with schizophrenia, performance on

Table 8–35 Hayling and Brixton Means and Standard Deviations for Healthy Children

Measure	Ages 8–12[a] Mean	Ages 8–12[a] SD	Ages 12–15[b] Mean	Ages 12–15[b] SD
Hayling Section 1 errors	.53	.74		
Hayling Section 2 errors	4.20	1.97	1.0	2.1
Section 2 minus Section 1 latencies			10.1	19.4
Brixton errors	17.47	7.12		

Source: From [a]Baylis & Roodenrys, 2000, based on a sample of 15 healthy children aged 8–12 years. [b]Clark et al., 2000, based on a sample of 26 healthy children aged 12–15 years.

the two tasks was correlated (about .70), even when age and medication were partialed out. In normal controls, the correlation between tasks was trivial (.17) when the effects of age were partialed out, consistent with the findings of Burgess and Shallice (1997) and Andres & Van der Linden (2000).

Hayling Test and Correlations With Other Measures

The Hayling Test shows moderate relations to other measures of executive function including the Six Elements Test (.40–.65; Clark et al., 2000) and the Tower of London (.40, Andres & Van der Linden, 2000; .64, Marczewski et al., 2001). Hayling scores show more of a relationship with measures of fluid (.27) than crystallized (.16) intelligence (Bielak et al., in press; de Frias et al., in press).

Hayling Test and Clinical Studies

Burgess and Shallice (1997) claim that the task is sensitive to frontal lobe dysfunction. Thus, they found that patients with lesions including, but not exclusive to, the frontal cortex were slower in the two sections and made more errors on the second section than controls and patients with posterior lesions. The posterior group did not differ from controls. In line with these findings, functional imaging evidence (PET) in normal individuals indicates that activation of the left prefrontal regions (frontal operculum, inferior frontal gyrus) and right anterior cingulate is associated with response suppression and selection on Section 2 of this task (Nathaniel-James et al., 1997). During response initiation (Section 1), activation is evident in left prefrontal, left middle temporal, and right anterior cingulate gyri. Noel et al. (2001) also reported a relationship between Hayling Test performance and regional cerebral blood flow (rCBF) measures in the bilateral inferior and medial frontal gyrus in alcoholic patients.

By contrast, there is other evidence indicating that other brain structures in addition to the frontal lobe contribute to task performance. Collette et al. (2002) found that in patients with Alzheimer's disease (AD), those with hypometabolism restricted to posterior cerebral areas and those with hypometabolism in both posterior and anterior regions obtained similar scores. Andres and Van der Linden (2001) compared patients with discrete lesions to the frontal lobe who were in the postacute phase (when mass effects are reduced) with controls. The number of errors committed in Section 2 was equivalent, despite a longer response latency in the frontal group. That is, patients with frontal lesions could inhibit a prepotent response, but it took them longer.

Performance is impaired in a variety of conditions thought to disrupt executive functioning, including Alzheimer's disease (Collette et al., 2000, 2002), alcoholism (Noel et al., 2001), schizophrenia (Marczewski et al., 2001), Parkinson's disease (Bouquet et al., 2003), Klinefelter's syndrome (Temple & Sanfilippo, 2003), and attention-deficit/hyperactivity disorder (ADHD; Baylis & Roodenrys, 2000; Clark et al., 2000). Of note, children with learning disorders or with oppositional defiant/conduct disorders perform like healthy controls on this task, suggesting its potential utility in diagnosing ADHD distinct from comorbid disorders (Baylis & Roodenrys, 2000; Clark et al., 2000).

Advancing age also is associated with poorer performance (Bielak et al., in press), especially on Section 2 (Andres & Van der Linden, 2000), with elderly individuals being more likely to complete a sentence with an entirely plausible response. Controlling for processing speed attenuated age-related differences. Correlations between Hayling errors in Section 2 and age decreased from .33 to .28 but were nonetheless significant (Andres & Van der Linden, 2000). Similarly, controlling for fluid intelligence reduced, but did not eliminate, the test's correlation with age (Bielak et al., in press). This suggests that age-related differences on this task are linked to more specific factors than processing speed and fluid ability (at least when these factors are considered individually).

Hayling and Ecological Validity

There is some evidence of ecological validity. Test performance in adolescents shows moderate correlations ($r =$ about .30) with parental ratings of hyperactivity/distractibility (Clark et al., 2000). In patients with schizophrenia, social impulsivity symptoms are moderately linked to performance on the Hayling Sentence Completion task (Chan et al. 2004).

Brixton Test and Correlations With Other Measures

The test is related to other measures of executive function. Thus, Marczewski et al. (2001) noted moderately strong correlations between the Brixton and Tower of London Tests (.58) in patients with schizophrenia, raising the possibility that the ability to anticipate or plan or inhibit is important. Other executive processes such as rapid alternation between mental sets may also play a role. In patients with eating disorders, the task loaded on the same factor as Trails B (Tchanturia et al., 2004).

Brixton errors show a moderate relation with fluid intelligence ($r = -.34$), while the correlation with crystallized ability is low ($r = -.08$; Bielak et al., in press; de Frias et al., in press).

Brixton Test and Clinical Studies

According to the test authors, patients with anterior lesions (including but not limited to the frontal lobe) made more errors than patients with posterior lesions and controls on this task. Moreover, the patients with anterior lesions showed an abnormally high incidence of bizarre-guessing responses. The patients with posterior lesions did not differ from controls. However, Andres and Van der Linden (2001) found that patients with lesions strictly confined to the frontal lobes did not differ from controls on this task. Also of note, they did not make more bizarre responses than controls.

Impaired performance has been reported in disorders thought to adversely impact executive processes including schizophrenia (Marczewski et al., 2001) and eating disorders (Tchanturia et al., 2004). However, children with ADHD or learning disabilities perform adequately on this task (Baylis & Roodenrys, 2000).

Aging adversely impacts performance, with older adults making more errors (but not specifically more bizarre responses) than younger adults (Andres & Van der Linden, 2000; Bielak et al., in press; de Frias et al., in press). Moreover, the age effect persists (albeit slightly diminished) even after statistical control of processing speed (Andres & Van der Linden, 2000) and fluid intelligence (Bielak et al., in press). Crystallized intelligence (measured by a vocabulary task) appears to contribute little to age-related differences on this task (Bielak et al., in press).

COMMENT

Both tasks are easy to give and are well tolerated by patients. Both seem to tap somewhat different executive abilities (e.g., Hayling: inhibition, Brixton: planning), although neither is a pure measure. For example, the Hayling likely also requires planning (searching for a novel response) and the Brixton likely necessitates inhibition (to stop responding according to the rule that is no longer relevant).

The Brixton does not require verbal ability, a feature that may enhance its utility with patients who have language-related deficits. However, psychometric data (reliability, validity, practice effects) are limited in adults and nonexistent in children. Note, too, that for both tasks, normative data are based on samples with IQ at the upper end of the spectrum, which limits their applicability.

More information is available for the Hayling Test. The task is sensitive to frontal lobe functioning and is related to other measures of executive function. However, the specific cognitive components contributing to performance are not clear. It has been proposed that the generation of nonsensical words is facilitated by heuristic strategies such as using objects in the room (Burgess & Shallice, 1997). Whether the use of such strategies actually improves performance is not known.

Recent normative reports (e.g., Baylis & Roodenrys, 2000; Bielak et al., in press; Clark et al., 2000) have extended the utility of the task; however, a larger normative sample is needed at both ends of the age continuum.

Internal consistency is marginal, while temporal stability is barely adequate. Further, no information is available regarding practice effects, limiting its use for repeat testing. Information regarding interrater reliability of the Hayling is also scant. Our impression is that responses can be very difficult to score and clearer guidelines are needed. The scoring of the responses can also be influenced by cultural differences. For example, responding "stripes" to the item "He bought them in the candy" would be considered a Category B error, as "candy stripes" is a common phrase in England, referring to striped pants. However, this same response would not form a common phrase in Canada, and therefore would not be scored as a Category B error.

It should also be noted that both the Brixton and Hayling tasks are relatively simple and fairly structured, suggesting that patients with executive disturbances may not show significant impairment on either of these tasks (Andres & Van der Linden, 2001). Finally, the scaled score systems are quite different from those used in most other tests. Both the Brixton and Hayling Tests use Sten scores as a metric to express performance (Crawford & Henry, in press). Although these have the advantage of simplicity, they are coarse-grained (the difference between Sten scores correspond to 0.5 of an SD), and thus, potentially meaningful differences between raw scores are obscured (Crawford & Henry, in press).

REFERENCES

Andres, P., & Van der Linden, M. (2000). Age-related differences in supervisory attentional system functions. *Journal of Gerontology: Psychological Sciences, 55B*, P373–P380.

Andres, P., & Van der Linden, M. (2001). Supervisory attentional system in patients with focal frontal lesions. *Journal of Clinical and Experimental Neuropsychology, 23*, 225–239.

Baylis, D. M., & Roodenrys, S. (2000). Executive processing and attention deficit disorder: An application of the supervisory attentional system. *Developmental Neuropsychology, 17*, 161–180.

Bielak, A. A. M., Mansueti, L., Strauss, E., & Dixon, R. A. (in press). Performance on the Hayling and Brixton Tests in older adults: Norms and correlates. *Archives of Clinical Neuropsychology.*

Bouquet, C. A., Bonnaud, V., & Gil, R. (2003). Investigation of supervisory attentional system functions in patients with Parkinson's disease using the Hayling task. *Journal of Clinical and Experimental Neuropsychology, 25*, 751–760.

Burgess, P. W., & Shallice, T. (1994). Fractionnement du syndrome frontal. *Revue de Neuropsychologie, 4*, 345–370.

Burgess, P. W., & Shallice, T. (1997). *The Hayling and Brixton tests.* Thurston, Suffolk: Thames Valley Test Company.

Chan, R. C. K., Chen, E. Y. H., Cheung, E. F. C., & Cheung, H. K. (2004). Executive dysfunctions in schizophrenia: Relationships to clinical manifestation. *Eur. Arch. Psychiatry Clin Neurosci, 254*, 256–262.

Clark, C., Prior, M., & Kinsella, G. J. (2000). Do executive function deficits differentiate between adolescents with ADHD and oppositional/defiant/conduct disorder? A neuropsychological study using the Six Elements Test and Hayling Sentence Completion Test. *Journal of Abnormal Child Psychology, 28*, 403–414.

Collette, F., Van der Linden, M., Delrue, G., & Salmon, E. (2002). Frontal hypometabolism does not explain inhibitory dysfunction in Alzheimer disease. *Alzheimer Disease & Related Disorders, 16*, 228–238.

Collette, F., Van der Linden, M., & Salmon, E. (2000). Relationships between cognitive performance and cerebral metabolism in Alzheimer's disease. *Current Psychology Letters, 1*, 55–69.

Crawford, J. R., & Henry, J. D. (in press). Assessment of executive dysfunction. In P. E. Halligan & N. Wad (Eds.), *Effectiveness of cognitive rehabilitation.* Oxford: Oxford University Press.

De Frias, C. M., Dixon, R. A., & Strauss, E. (in press). Structure of four executive functioning tests in healthy older adults. *Neuropsychology.*

Marczewski, P., Van der Linden, M., & Laroi, F. (2001). Further investigation of the supervisory attentional system in schizophrenia: Planning, inhibition, and rule abstraction. *Cognitive Neuropsychiatry, 6*, 175–192.

Nathaniel-James, D. A., Fletcher, P., & Frith, C. D. (1997). The functional anatomy of verbal initiation and suppression using the Hayling Test. *Neuropsychologia, 35*, 559–566.

Noel, X., Paternot, J., Van der Linden, M., Sferrazza, R., Verhas, M., Hanak, C., Kornreich, C., Martin, P., De Mol, J., Pelc, I., & Verbanck, P. (2001). Correlation between inhibition, working memory and delimited frontal area blood flow measured by –super (99m)-Tc-Bicisate Spect in alcohol-dependent patients. *Alcohol & Alcoholism, 36*, 556–563.

Tchanturia, K., Anderluh, M. B., Morris, R. G., Rabe-Hesketh, S., Collier, D. A., Sanchex, P., & Treaure, J. L. (2004). Cognitive flexibility in anorexia nervosa and bulimia nervosa. *Journal of the International Neuropsychological Society, 10*, 513–520.

Temple, C. M., & Sanfilippo, P. M. (2003). Executive skills in Klinefelter's syndrome. *Neuropsychologia, 41*, 1547–1559.

Ruff Figural Fluency Test (RFFT)

PURPOSE

This test measures the production of novel designs under time constraints.

SOURCE

The test (including manual and 25 test booklets) can be ordered from PAR (http://www.parinc.com), at a cost of $112 US. There are a number of similar tests, including the Five-Point Test (Regard et al., 1982), the Design Fluency tasks found in the D-KEFS (Delis et al., 2001), and the NEPSY (Korkman et al., 1998), described elsewhere in this volume.

AGE RANGE

The age range is from 7 to 70 years.

DESCRIPTION

Figural fluency tests (Jones-Gotman & Milner, 1977; Regard et al., 1982) have been developed as nonverbal analogs to word fluency tasks. Ruff (1996, 1998) developed a variant of the Five-Point Test (Regard et al., 1982; described elsewhere in this volume) that consists of five parts. The test is made up of five pages (parts), each consisting of 35 five-dot matrices, arranged in seven rows and five columns on an 8½ × 11" sheet of paper. Each part (1–5) consists of a different stimulus pattern of dots (see Figure 8–9). Parts 2 and 3 contain the dot pattern of Part 1 with various distractors (Part 2: triangles, Part 3: lines); Parts 4 and 5 contain variations of the original dot pattern (without distracting elements). Each stimulus sheet is preceded by a page containing three samples of the specific stimulus to allow the respondent an opportunity to practice. The task in each part is to draw as many unique designs as possible in a one-minute interval, by connecting the dots in the different patterns. If the same design is repeated, then this is scored as a perseverative error.

ADMINISTRATION TIME

The entire test takes about 10 minutes to administer. The time limit for each of the five parts is one minute.

SCORING

The number of unique designs and perseverations appear to be fairly consistent among the five parts of the test, suggesting no significant practice or learning effects. Accordingly, only total test scores are evaluated. Standard RFFT indices include:

- The total number of unique designs;
- The total number of perseverative errors across the five parts of the test; and
- An error ratio calculated by dividing the total number of perseverative errors by the total number of unique designs.

Ruff (1996, 1998) suggests that the error ratio represents an index of planning efficiency by assessing the degree to which an individual is able to minimize repetition while maximizing unique productions.

The total number of unique designs and error ratio are converted to T scores and descriptive ranges (Impaired to Very Superior) by means of age-based appendices provided in the RFFT Manual. Raw score educational corrections are available for each of the age groups, and these corrections are listed in the tables for both total unique designs and error ratios.

Qualitative scores to assess strategy have recently been suggested (Ross et al., 2003). These are defined as three or more consecutive designs for which the subject has employed a systematic process to generate designs. These "strategic clusters" are categorized as two types: a rotational strategy that involves simply rotating a drawing systematically clockwise or counterclockwise within the array of dots to make it appear differently in each square, or an enumerative strategy whereby subjects enumerate upon a design by systematically adding or removing one line. In addition to the production strategy scores, two other indices of production strategy were developed: mean cluster size (reflecting the extent to which an examinee applied a single strategy across consecutive designs) and percentage of designs used in strategies (the number of designs incorporated into production strategies divided by the number of designs overall including perseverations).

Figure 8–9 Examples of dot patterns in Parts 1 to 5 of the RFFT. *Source:* Reprinted with permission from Ruff, 1998.

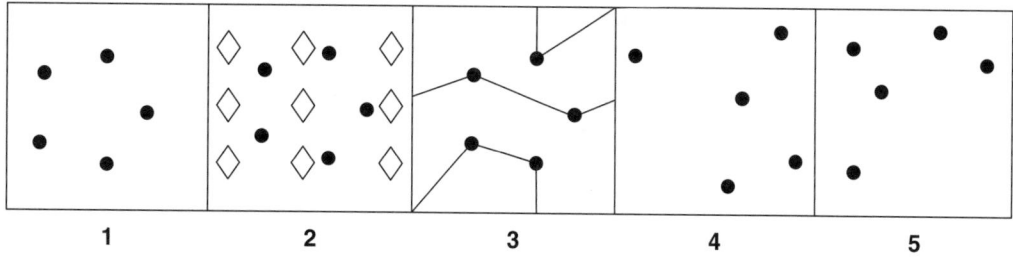

DEMOGRAPHIC EFFECTS

Age

The RFFT is sensitive to differences in age (Evans et al., 1985; Fama et al., 1998; Lee, 2003; Ruff et al., 1987; Salthouse et al., 2003; Vik & Ruff, 1988). Performance is better in young versus old adults. Studies with pediatric populations suggest an age-related increase in figural fluency (Evans et al., 1985; Vik & Ruff, 1988). Older children produce more designs than younger children and are also more likely to use strategies (Vik & Ruff, 1988).

Education/IQ

Education and IQ (Ruff et al., 1987) impact performance in adults with higher scores in those with higher education/reasoning ability. Bright children are also more likely to use a strategic approach (Vik & Ruff, 1988).

Gender

Gender differences have not been found in children or adults (Demakis & Harrison, 1997; Evans et al., 1985).

NORMATIVE DATA

Adults

Standardization Data. Normative data provided in the test manual are based on a sample of 358 healthy individuals (197 women, 161 men) ranging in age from 16 to 70 years. Test scores (Total Number of Unique Designs, Error Ratio) are evaluated according to four age (16–24, 25–39, 40–54, 55–70) and three educational groupings (≤12 years, 13–15 years, ≥16 years). Table 8–36 shows the characteristics of the sample.

Other Normative Data. Lee (2003) provides normative data for a sample of 178 healthy, Cantonese-speaking individuals living in Hong Kong (ages 20–70+).

Children's Norms

Evans et al. (1985) provide data for a sample of children and adults of above-average intellectual level (average WISC-R,

WAIS-R Vocabulary scores of 12 or greater). The data are presented in Table 8–37.

RELIABILITY

Test-Retest Reliability

In normal individuals, the test-retest reliability coefficient for the total number of unique designs is acceptable/high over intervals of three weeks to 12 months (.71–.88; Basso et al., 1999; Demakis, 1999; Evans et al., 1985; Ross et al., 2003; Ruff et al., 1987). The reliability coefficients for the number of perseverative errors and ratio score, however, are low (.36–.48; Basso et al., 1999; Evans et al., 1985; Ross et al., 2003; Ruff et al., 1987). Reliability coefficients for qualitative (production

Table 8–36 Characteristics of Ruff Figural Fluency Standardization Sample

Number	358
Age	
16–24	80
25–39	101
40–54	92
55–70	85
Geographic location	65% from California; 30% Michigan; 5% eastern U.S. seaboard
Sample type	Volunteers
Education	
≤12	116
13–15	128
≥16	114
Gender	
Male	161
Female	197
Race/ethnicity	Not reported
Screening	Subjects excluded with a positive history of psychiatric hospitalization, chronic polydrug abuse, or neurological disorder

Source: Adapted from Ruff, 1996.

Table 8–37 Ruff Figural Fluency Scores by Age

Mean Age	N	Total Unique Designs	Total Perseveration Errors	Error Ratio
7.7	22	46.0 (10.8)	5.6 (4.2)	.12
9.8	22	59.1 (15.1)	5.5 (5.2)	.09
11.8	18	71.7 (15.3)	4.4 (2.4)	.06
22.8	20	112.9 (19.5)	4.7 (3.9)	.04

Data are based on a sample of individuals of above average intelligence.

Source: Adapted from Evans et al., 1985.

strategy) scores are acceptable (.70 and above), with the exception of the mean cluster size (.51; Ross et al., 2003).

Practice Effects

Significant practice effects emerge on this test. With relatively short intervals (about three weeks), university students show a gain of about 17 designs (Demakis, 1999). Following retest intervals of one to six months, normal individuals tend to increase the number of unique designs by about eight designs (in children, one to three points depending on their age), although there tends to be no commensurate increase in perseverations (Ross et al., 1996, 2003; Ruff et al., 1987; Vik & Ruff, 1988). Similarly, over longer retest intervals (12 months), normal adults produce more unique designs (an increase of seven T-score points or 6.81 designs), with no change in the ratio of perseverative errors to unique designs (Basso et al., 1999). Intelligence level (average or above) does not mediate performance increments across time; however, the inclusion of low-average individuals is needed to more fully examine whether intelligence level mediates improvement (Basso et al., 1999).

Basso et al. (1999) used reliable change methodology to estimate the range of change in T scores that might be expected while accounting for measurement error and practice effects. Table 8–38 shows the mean estimated true scores at 12 months together with the standard error of prediction (SE$_p$) and resulting 90% confidence interval. Note the large range of retest scores that may fall within the 90% confidence interval. An individual could increase or decrease performance by as much as 10 T-score units without displaying meaningful changes in performance. In this sample of community-dwelling healthy men, no individual obtained a score that reflected significant improvement or decline. To use the confidence intervals, the 90% confidence band should be summed with an individual's estimated true score ($Y_{TRUE} = M + r[Y_{OBS} - M]$), where M is the sample mean of the test and Y_{OBS} is the actual score obtained by the individual. Significant changes reflect the frequency of obtained scores that fall above or below the confidence interval.

Interrater Reliability

In a university sample, Ross et al. (1996, 2003) found excellent interrater reliability for standard ($r = .80–.98$) scoring parameters of the Ruff Figural Fluency Test. Interrater agreement was also very good for qualitative scores (.79–.95). However, Berning et al. (1998) also examined a college sample and found that interrater reliability was excellent for unique designs (.93), adequate for the number of design perseverations (.74), and low for error ratios (.66). Reliabilities improved with practice.

VALIDITY

Correlation Within Test Scores

The perseveration and error ratio scores are highly correlated ($r = .89$); however, the number of unique designs shows only small correlations with the error ratio score ($r = -.24$) and the number of perseverative designs ($r = .06$; Ross et al., 2003). The qualitative indices are all positively associated with the number of unique designs, with the total number of strategic clusters exhibiting the highest correlation ($r = .50$). Rotational strategy use is correlated more highly ($r = .47$) with unique design output than enumerative strategy use ($r = .21$). Strategy

Table 8–38 Descriptive Statistics and Confidence Intervals for Ruff Figural Fluency Estimated True Scores at 12-Month Follow-Up

	M	r$_{y1y2}$	SE$_p$	90% CI	Significant Increases	Significant Decreases
Unique Designs	58.66	.71	6.22	±10	0	0
Ratio Score	49.20	.39	7.64	±13	0	0

Based on a sample of 50 community-dwelling healthy males, for the most part Caucasian, ranging in age from 20–59 ($M = 32.5$, $SD = 9.27$) and mean education of 14.98 years ($SD = 1.93$).

Source: From Basso et al., 1999. Reprinted with the kind permission of Psychology Press.

utilization, however, does not influence perseverative responding (Ross et al., 2003).

Correlation With Other Tests

The various figural fluency tasks are not interchangeable. Scores on the RFFT are modestly correlated with those of other figural fluency tasks (Demakis & Harrison, 1997; Hanks et al., 1996), including the Design Fluency Test. The fixed condition of the Design Fluency Test is more robustly related to the RFFT than the free condition (.38 versus .25; Demakis & Harrison, 1997).

Performance on the RFFT is less consistently related to phonemic fluency (COWA; Demakis & Harrison, 1997; Fama et al., 1998; Ruff et al., 1987) than semantic fluency (Fama et al., 1998), although even with the latter task, the coefficients tend to be modest/moderate in size (.28–.67; Fama et al., 1998). In short, the RFFT cannot simply be viewed as a nonverbal analog to verbal fluency tasks. The tasks are measuring similar as well as unique components.

RFFT scores are moderately correlated with measures of general cognitive status such as the Performance IQ of the WAIS-R (about .38; Ruff et al., 1987), the MMSE (.38–.55; Fama et al., 1998, 2000), and the NART (.45; Fama et al., 1998). There is evidence that reduced motor speed contributes to poorer scores on the RFFT; however, it does not fully account for impaired performance (Evans et al., 1985; Fama et al., 1998; Milders et al., 2003; Ruff et al. 1987). Memory for temporal order also appears to be moderately associated with design fluency performance (Parkin et al., 1995).

Factor-Analytic Findings

Studies (Ruff, 1996, 1998) in normal people suggest that the total unique designs measure loads on two factors: general intelligence (WAIS-R) and attention/speed (Ruff 2 & 7, Finger Tapping). The ratio of perseverative errors to unique designs (Error Ratio) loads on a planning factor (Rey Copy, Grooved Pegboard, WCST). In a mixed clinical sample (TBI, patients with schizophrenia), error scores load on two factors, labeled as complex intelligence (WAIS-R) and planning ability (Ruff Light Trail Learning Test, Ruff 2 & 7). However, the latter tasks seem to tap learning/memory/attention/speed more so than planning ability.

Salthouse et al. (2003) recently examined executive functioning constructs in healthy adults by combining standard neuropsychological tasks and cognitive process approaches. Structural equation analyses suggested that verbal fluency (FAS) was more closely related to speed and vocabulary abilities, whereas Ruff Figural Fluency was more closely related to fluid intelligence and speed abilities.

Clinical Studies

The RFFT is sensitive to severity of injury, with greater fluency deficits in those with severe, as compared to moderate, brain injuries (Ruff et al., 1986). Patients with moderate/severe trau-matic brain injuries tend to produce fewer designs than controls but do not seem more likely to break the rules (Milders et al., 2003). Fluency is also affected in individuals with Parkinson's disease (Fama et al., 1998), although improvement is seen following pallidotomy regardless of the side of the surgery (Lacritz et al., 1999). Further, design generation is reduced in those individuals with prenatal exposure to alcohol, beyond what might be expected on the basis of general intellectual status (Connor et al., 2000). Perseveration, however, appears to reflect level of IQ, at least in this population. Patients with AD are also impaired on the RFFT (Fama et al., 1998, 2000) as are patients with AIDS (Basso & Bornstein, 2003).

Fluency performance tends to be affected more by anterior than posterior cerebral compromise (Ruff et al., 1994; Suchy et al., 2003). For example, Suchy et al. (2003) examined patients with focal seizures and reported that the test demonstrated a better than chance classification of patients into frontal and temporal groups (using receiver operating curve [ROC] analyses). The most optimal cutoff was a T score of 39 for total unique designs, correctly identifying 50% of the patients with frontal seizure foci and 69.7% of the patients with temporal seizure foci, for an overall hit rate of 67%.

The influence of laterality is not certain. Based on an examination of a sample of 30 patients (27 with closed head injury), Ruff et al. (1994) claimed that the test was useful diagnostically, accurately classifying 60% of the right frontal cases and 96% of the nonright frontal cases. Bartolic et al. (1999) reported that negative mood induction (presumed to be associated with increased right hemisphere activity) resulted in better figural than verbal fluency, whereas the converse pattern resulted during a positive mood. Recently, Foster et al. (2005) reported that healthy university students who perform poorly on the RFFT exhibit heightened right frontal delta magnitude as compared with those who perform well. Unfortunately, left-sided activity was not measured in this study; nor was activity at other brain sites (e.g., posterior).

Others, however, have not noted an association between laterality and performance (Fama et al., 2000; Suchy et al., 2003). For example, in patients with AD, fluency was selectively associated with bilateral frontal gray matter volumes, suggesting that both regions contribute to the generation of nonverbal exemplars (Fama et al., 2003). Similarly, Suchy et al. (2003) reported that the RFFT was sensitive to both left and right frontal impairment in patients with epilepsy.

Ecological/Predictive Validity

No significant association was found between performance on the RFFT and behavioral ratings of patients who sustained moderate/severe head injuries (Milders et al., 2003).

Malingering

Individuals instructed to feign symptoms of head injury tend to depress their performance on the test (Demakis, 1999). Interestingly, these individuals improved their performance in a consistent manner when retested three weeks later, suggesting that they may not have had an effective strategy for such a task.

COMMENT

The various figural fluency tasks are not interchangeable. In comparison to the Design Fluency task, the RFFT is highly structured and places more of a reward on the number of responses generated than on their uniqueness (Hanks et al., 1996). Further, the RFFT does not have a graded scoring system that allows one to distinguish a truly unique design from a response that is a simple permutation (Hanks et al., 1996). Thus, mirror rotations are scored as correct. Indices regarding production strategy have recently been proposed (Ross et al., 2003); however, their clinical utility remains to be established. Whether the RFFT is more or less sensitive than Design Fluency to various neurobehavioral deficits that affect anterior brain regions is also not known.

Figural fluency tests have been developed as nonverbal analogs to word fluency tasks. However, the evidence indicates that the tasks are not simple analogs of one another. Some (Suchy et al., 2003) have proposed that the RFFT is a more sensitive measure of general frontal lobe functioning than verbal fluency as the RFFT appears compromised by both right and left frontal lobe lesions, whereas verbal fluency is affected more by left frontal lesions (but see Ruff et al., 1994). Suchy et al. (2003) suggest that the RFFT may be a more novel task than verbal fluency, and therefore may place greater demands on executive functioning in general.

The Ruff Figural Fluency Test stimuli were designed to vary in level of difficulty (e.g., through the use of interference). The research (Ruff et al., 1987) reveals, however, no significant differences among the five parts of the test, and only the total scores are provided in the manual. Thus, it appears that the use of multiple trials on the Ruff Figural Fluency Test may be redundant (Lee et al., 1997) but may ensure better reliability.

Normative data are available for both adults and children. However, the normative base is not extensive (e.g., cell sizes <50 when adults are classed in terms of both age and education, no norms for adults above age 70, limited data in children and adolescents). In addition, there is no information on the effects of ethnicity.

There is substantial interrater and test-retest reliability when the number of unique designs or various qualitative scores related to strategy production are considered. The reliability for perseverative errors, error ratios, and mean cluster size tend to be too low for clinical use. On retesting, normal individuals tend to produce a somewhat higher number of unique patterns. To measure change over time in a clinical setting, the reliable change data provided by Basso et al. (1999) may be of some help. Users should bear in mind, however, that their sample was predominantly Caucasian males who ranged in age from 20 to 59 years and were relatively well educated. Accordingly, these data may not be applicable to other groups, particularly elderly individuals.

REFERENCES

Bartolic, E. I., Basso, M. R., Schefft, B. K., Glauser, T., & Titanic-Schefft, M. (1999). Effects of experimentally-induced emotional states on frontal lobe cognitive task performance. *Neuropsychologia, 37,* 677–683.

Basso, M. R., & Bornstein, R. A. (2003). Effects of past noninjection drug abuse upon executive function and working memory in HIV infection. *Journal of Clinical and Experimental Neuropsychology, 25,* 893–903.

Basso, M. R., Bornstein, R. A., & Lang, J. M. (1999). Practice effects on commonly used measures of executive function across twelve months. *The Clinical Neuropsychologist, 13,* 283–292.

Berning, L. C., Weed, N. C., & Aloia, M. S. (1998). Interrater reliability of the Ruff Figural Fluency Test. *Assessment, 5,* 181–186.

Connor, P. D., Sampson, P. D., Bookstein, F. L., Barr, H. M., & Streissguth, A. P. (2000). Direct and indirect effects of prenatal alcohol damage on executive function. *Developmental Neuropsychology, 18,* 331–354.

Delis, D. C., Kaplan, E., & Kramer, J. H. (2001). *Delis-Kaplan Executive Function System.* San Antonio, TX: The Psychological Corporation.

Demakis, G. J. (1999). Serial malingering on verbal and nonverbal fluency and memory measures: An analog investigation. *Archives of Clinical Neuropsychology, 14,* 401–410.

Demakis, G. J., & Harrison, D. W. (1997). Relationships between verbal and nonverbal fluency measures: Implications for assessment of executive functioning. *Psychological Reports, 81,* 443–448.

Evans, R., Ruff, R. M., & Gualtieri, C. (1985) Verbal fluency and figural fluency in bright children. *Perceptual and Motor Skills, 61,* 699–709.

Fama, R., Sullivan, E. V., Shear, P. K., Cahn-Weiner, D. A., Marsh, L., Lim, K. O., Yesavage, J. A., & Tinklenberg, J. R. (2000). Structural brain correlates of verbal and nonverbal fluency measures in Alzheimer's disease. *Neuropsychology, 14,* 29–40.

Fama, R., Sullivan, E. V., Shear, P. K., Cahn-Weiner, D. A., Yesavage, J. A., Tinklenberg, J. R, & Pfefferbaum, A. (1998). Fluency performance patterns in Alzheimer's disease and Parkinson's disease. *The Clinical Neuropsychologist, 12,* 487–499.

Foster, P. S., Williamson, J. B., & Harrison, D. W. (2005). The Ruff Figural Fluency Test: Heightened right frontal lobe delta activity as a function of performance. *Archives of Clinical Neuropsychology, 20,* 427–434.

Hanks, R. A., Allen, J. B., Ricker, J. H., & Deshpande, S. A. (1996). Normative data on a measure of design fluency: The Make a Figure Test. *Assessment, 3,* 459–466.

Jones-Gotman, M., & Milner, B. (1977). Design fluency: The invention of nonsense drawings after focal cortical lesions. *Neuropsychologia, 15,* 653–674.

Korkman, M., Kirk, U., & Kemp, S. (1998). *NEPSY: A Developmental Neuropsychological Assessment Manual.* San Antonio, TX: The Psychological Corporation.

Lacritz, L. H., Cullum, C. M., Frol, A. B., Dewey Jr., R. B., & Giller, C. A. (2000). Neuropsychological outcome following unilateral stereotactic pallidotomy in intractable Parkinson's disease. *Brain and Cognition, 42,* 364–378.

Lee, G. P., Strauss, E., Loring, D. W., McCloskey, L., & Haworth, J. M. (1977). Sensitivity of figural fluency on the Five Point Test to focal neurological disease. *The Clinical Neuropsychologist, 11,* 59–68.

Lee, T. M. C. (2003). *Normative data: Neuropsychological measures for Hong Kong Chinese.* The University of Hong Kong Neuropsychology Laboratory.

Milders, M., Fuchs, S., & Crawford, J. R. (2003). Neuropsychological impairments and changes in emotional and social behavior following severe traumatic brain injury. *Journal of Clinical and Experimental Neuropsychology, 25,* 157–172.

Parkin, A. J., Walter, B. M., & Hunkin, N. M. (1995). Relationship between normal aging, frontal lobe function, and memory for temporal and spatial information. *Neuropsychology, 9,* 304–312.

Regard, M., Strauss, E., & Knapp, P. (1982). Children's production of verbal and nonverbal fluency tasks. *Perceptual and Motor Skills, 55,* 839–844.

Ross, T. P., Axelrod, B. N., Hanks, R. A., Kotasek, R. S., & Whitman, R. D. (1996). *The interrater and test-retest reliability of the Design Fluency and Ruff Figural Fluency tests.* Paper presented to the 24th meeting of the International Neuropsychological Society, Chicago.

Ross, T. P., Foard, E. L., Hiott, F. B., & Vincent, A. (2003). The reliability of production strategy scores for the Ruff Figural Fluency Test. *Archives of Clinical Neuropsychology, 18,* 879–891.

Ruff, R. (1996, 1998). *Ruff Figural Fluency Test.* Odessa, FL: PAR.

Ruff, R. M., Allen, C. C., Farrow, C. E., Niemann, H., & Wylie, T. (1994). Figural fluency: Differential impairment in patients with left versus right frontal lobe lesions. *Archives of Clinical Neuropsychology, 9,* 41–45.

Ruff, R. M., Evans, R., & Marshall, L. M. (1986). Impaired verbal and figural fluency after head injury. *Archives of Clinical Neuropsychology, 1,* 87–101.

Ruff, R. M., Light, R., & Evans, R. (1987). The Ruff Figural Fluency Test: A normative study with adults. *Developmental Neuropsychology, 3,* 37–51.

Salthouse, T. A., Atkinson, T. M., & Berish, D. E. (2003). Executive functioning as a potential mediator of age-related cognitive decline in normal adults. *Journal of Experimental Psychology: General, 132,* 566–594.

Suchy, Y., Sands, K., & Chelune, G. J. (2003). Verbal and nonverbal fluency performance before and after surgery. *Journal of Clinical and Experimental Neuropsychology, 25,* 190–200.

Vik, P., & Ruff, R. M. (1988). Children's figural fluency performance: Development of strategy use. *Developmental Neuropsychology, 4,* 63–74.

Self-Ordered Pointing Test (SOPT)

PURPOSE

This test is used to assess the capacity to regulate behavior by using plans and strategies.

SOURCE

There is no commercial source. Users may refer to the following text and figures to design their own material. Alternatively, they may contact Michael Petrides, Ph.D., Montreal Neurological Institute, Department of Psychology, 3801 University Street, Montreal, Quebec H3A 2B4, for the exact stimuli.

AGE RANGE

The representational version can be given to individuals aged 7 to 12 and 19 to 35 years. The version using abstract designs can be given to adults aged 20 to 35 and 45 to 65 years.

DESCRIPTION

In the self-ordered pointing test (SOPT; Petrides & Milner, 1982), the same set of stimulus items is arranged in different layouts on as many different pages as there are items, and subjects are required to point to a different item on each page without repeating an item already pointed to. The task requires that the individual initiate and execute a sequence of responses, maintain a record of responses, and monitor performance. Petrides and Milner (1982) found that SOPT performance was sensitive to frontal lobe lesions and concluded that the task makes significant demands on working memory since participants must constantly compare responses already made with those remaining to be made.

Petrides and Milner (1982) used four tasks differing in the type of stimulus material: abstract designs, representational drawings, high-imagery words, and low-imagery words. Usually, however, only one of the tasks is given. Subjects are presented with a binder containing sheets of paper (8½×11"), each one showing a single type of stimuli (e.g., representational drawings). The binder is divided into four consecutive sections, consisting of six, eight, 10, and 12 stimulus sheets, with a blank sheet between each section. Three consecutive trials of each section are administered. A different set of drawings is used for each of the four sections. Within each section, the same drawings are used, but they are arranged differently on each stimulus sheet. The positions of the drawings are randomly determined for each sheet of paper, but the layout remains constant (i.e., for six-item: 2 × 3, for eight-item: 2 × 4). For example, the first six-item section contains six pages displaying the same six drawings in a different random order on each sheet. The second eight-item section displays a new set of eight drawings on eight separate sheets, and so on.

The stimuli used in the longest list (12 items) of Petrides and Milner's abstract designs task are shown in Figure 8–10. Stimuli used in the shortest list (six items) of a representational drawings task are shown in Figure 8–11.

On each trial, subjects are instructed to point to one of the drawings with the restriction that they should point to a different one on each trial. The demand on working memory is increased by having the subjects perform each section three times before moving on to the next section.

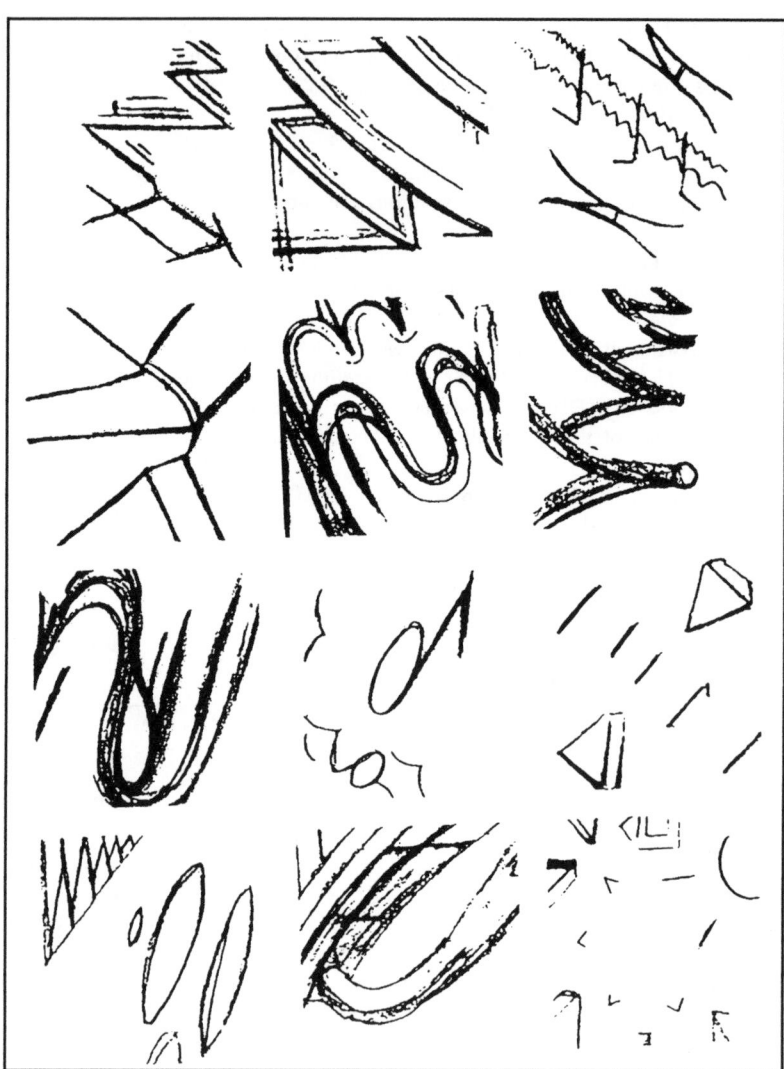

Figure 8–10 Stimuli used in the longest list (12 items) of the abstract designs task. *Source:* From Petrides & Milner, 1982.

ADMINISTRATION

Instruct the patient as follows:

> *Look, here are six pictures. I have pages with the same pictures but they are in different places each time. See, the orange is up here* (point to orange on first page), *but now it is down here* (point to orange on second page). *I want you to point to one picture on each page. I want you to point to a different picture each time. Once you point to a picture, you can't choose it again. Do you understand? Point to a picture on this page.* There is no practice trial.

The examiner turns the sheets to maintain a comfortable pace. Testing begins only after it is clear that the patient understands the task. When the patient encounters the first blank sheet (indicating completion of that trial), the patient is instructed to start all over again. The examiner says, "Now we are going to do it again beginning with a different one than last time." Again, the examiner emphasizes that the patient is not to touch any stimulus more than once, but can touch the stimuli in any order.

The patient is not allowed to respond consistently to the same location on any given trial, because by adopting such a strategy the patient merely has to recognize the recurrence of a given item in that location rather than plan a sequence of responses. The patient is also not allowed to verbalize items as he or she points. There is no time limit.

ADMINISTRATION TIME

About 20 minutes are required for the task.

SCORING

The examiner records the order in which the stimuli are touched on the record sheet (see Figure 8–12). An error is

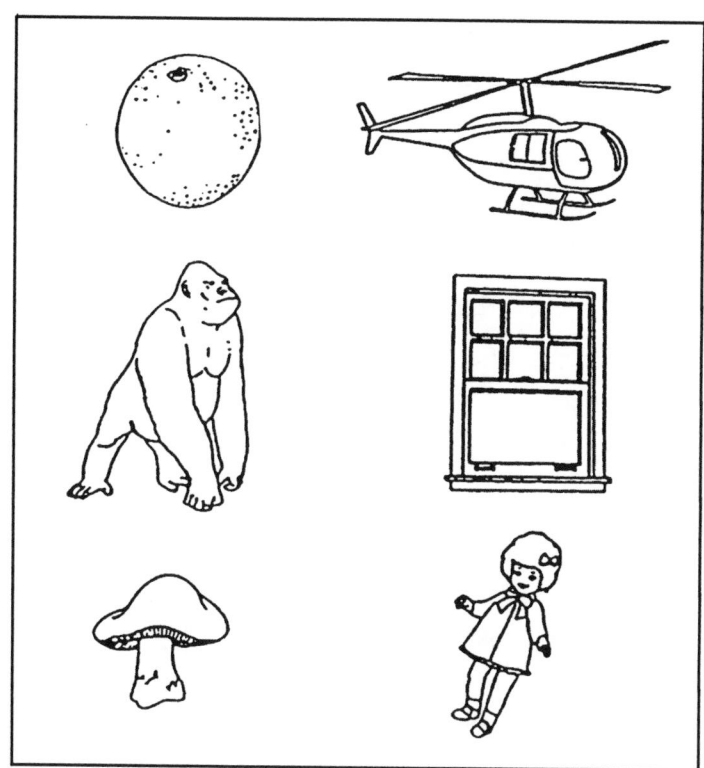

Figure 8–11 Stimuli used in the shortest list (six items) of representational drawings task. *Source:* From M. Kates, M. L. Smith, & E. Vriesen, April 1997.

recorded each time the subject selects a picture chosen previously in that trial. The number of errors is readily evident since there will be two or more numbers recorded for a particular item. The total number of errors summed across the four sections (6- to 12-item sets) is recorded.

DEMOGRAPHIC EFFECTS

Age

In adults, performance declines with advancing age (Bryan & Luszcz, 2002; Daigneault & Braun, 1993; Daigneault et al., 1992; Haut et al., 1999; Shimamura & Jurica, 1994; West et al., 1998), with declines evident by midlife (by about age 50; Garden et al., 2001). In children, errors decline with increasing age (Archibald & Kerns, 1999).

Gender

Gender has little effect on SOPT performance in adults (Daigneault and Braun, 1993) or children (Archibald & Kerns, 1999).

Education/IQ

IQ is only minimally related to scores in children (about .20; Archibald & Kerns, 1999).

NORMATIVE DATA

Adults

Twenty-two adults, aged 19 to 35 years ($M = 24.1$), of average IQ ($M = 102$) made 4.68 ($SD = 2.53$) errors on the representational drawings task (Smith et al., 1996; see Table 8–39).

Normative data for the abstract designs condition are provided by Daigneault et al. (1992). A group of 70 healthy young adults aged 20 to 35 (education, $M = 12.36$ years, $SD = 2.09$) made on average 15.2 errors ($SD = 6.22$). A group of 58 healthy older adults, aged 45 to 65 years, made about 21.67 ($SD = 5.58$) errors.

Children

On the representational designs task, Archibald and Kerns (1999) reported that 89 healthy children, aged 6.9 to 12 years, made about 14.09 ($SD = 5.29$) errors. Their data are shown in Table 8–39.

Somewhat better performance was found by Shue and Douglas (1992), although the sample was smaller. Shue and Douglas (1992) reported that 24 normal children (age, $M = 10.3$, $SD = 1.54$; Wechsler IQ, $M = 96.88$, $SD = 11.57$) made an average of 9.31 errors ($SD = 4.55$) on the representational task. They made an average of 24.15 errors ($SD = 25.15$) when abstract drawings were used as stimuli.

Figure 8–12 Sample score sheet for SOPT. *Source:* From Mary Lou Smith, April 1997.

Six-Item Set
doll
gorilla
helicopter
mushroom
orange
window   Errors ____

Eight-Item Set
ball
basket
belt
bowl
flag
kettle
tiger
wagon   Errors ____

10-Item Set
banana
couch
ear
envelope
giraffe
guitar
motorcycle
mountain
pot
sandwich   Errors ____

12-Item Set
bottle
bow
brush
candle
fence
finger
hanger
moon
purse
squirrel
strawberry
toaster   Errors ____

RELIABILITY

Test-Retest Reliability

Information on test reliability is sparse. When 18 children were retested on the representational designs task following a four-month interval, reliability was acceptable (.76; Archibald & Kerns, 1999). However, Bryan & Luszcz (2001) presented healthy adults with three trials of a modification of Shimamura and Jurica's (1994) 16-item version of the SOPT. They reported that the reliability across the three trials was only .38.

VALIDITY

Correlations With Other Tests

The task is assumed to assess executive functioning and may be distinguished from other tasks that require the patient to execute a particular response sequence, such as the Knox cubes in the WMS-R Visual Memory Span subtest, in that the SOPT requires patients to plan, sequence, initiate, and monitor their own pointing responses, rather than follow a sequence dictated by the examiner (Rich et al., 1996). Working

Table 8–39 SOPT Errors as a Function of Age on the Representational Task

	7	8	9	10	11	12	24 (19–35)
N	15	12	13	25	8	16	22
M	18.07	16.41	13.92	12.72	11.88	12.00	4.68
SD	6.64	6.65	3.57	4.44	4.16	3.20	2.53

Source: From Archibald & Kerns, 1999, Based on a sample of 89 children, mean age = 10.03 years (SD = 1.72; range 6.9–12.91) and mean K–BIT IQ = 109.76 (SD = 10.49, range 88–144); Smith et al., 1996, based on a sample of 22 adults, aged 19–35 years (M = 24.1) of average IQ (M = 102).

memory is thought to be a critical component of task success.

The literature suggests that in adults, SOPT performance is associated with scores on some other measures of executive function. Thus, Daigneault et al. (1992) reported that in normal individuals, the SOPT (abstract designs condition) correlated moderately with the WCST ($r = .33$), the Porteus Mazes ($r = .38$), and the Stroop Test ($r = .36$). Similarly, Bryan and Luszcz (2001) found SOPT performance to be related (.23–.52) to measures of executive function (e.g., Stroop, WCST, verbal fluency) and working memory (e.g., backward word span) in normal adults. However, the best predictor was speed of information processing (e.g., Digit Symbol), which accounted for 22% of the variance. After controlling for speed, executive function and working memory tasks no longer predicted SOPT performance. The implication is that SOPT performance may rely more on speed of information processing than on working memory. By contrast, Pukrop et al. (2003) found that the SOPT loaded on the same factor as other measures of working memory (e.g., Letter-Number Span) in normals as well as in patients with schizophrenia; measures of speed (e.g., Digit Symbol, Trails B) loaded on a different dimension.

In addition to working memory and speed of processing, other factors including memory capacity can impact SOPT performance. Schmitter-Edgecombe and Chaytor (2003) reported that in normal adults, errors on the SOPT (abstract designs) were associated with a measure of working memory (Reading Span Test); by contrast, in patients with severe closed head injury, visual memory impairment (i.e., WMS-R Visual Reproduction II subtest) was the primary factor associated with poor SOPT performance.

In children, SOPT scores correlate moderately well (.26–.46) with executive function measures that reflect inhibitory capacity and working memory (e.g., Go-No Go, Stroop, Delayed Alternation/Nonalternation; Archibald & Kerns, 1999). IQ shows only a small relation to SOPT performance (Archibald & Kerns, 1999).

Clinical Studies

Patients with frontal lobe lesions are impaired on the SOPT, whereas patients with temporal lobe lesions not extending beyond the pes of the hippocampus (i.e., involving only the anterior temporal neocortex, the amygdala, and/or the pes hippocampus) perform normally (Petrides & Milner, 1982). However, patients with radical hippocampectomies exhibit material-specific deficits on the SOPT that correspond to the side of the lesion. Thus, the ability to carry out the general task demands of the SOPT requires intact frontal lobe functioning, whereas success on material-specific SOPT tasks requires intact left or right hippocampal functioning for verbal or nonverbal material, respectively. Petrides et al. (1993a, 1993b) have also observed PET rCBF activation of middordso-lateral frontal cortex when normal individuals must monitor a series of responses within working memory. This is consistent with data from nonhuman primates showing that lesions limited to the mid-dorsolateral frontal cortex (areas 46 and 9) give rise to severe impairment on analogous tasks (Petrides, 1991, 1995).

In line with findings of age-related changes in the frontal lobes, a number of authors (e.g., Bryan & Luszcz, 2001; Chaytor & Schmitter-Edgecombe, 2004; Daigneault et al., 1992, 1993; Garden et al., 2001; McPherson et al., 2002; Shimamura and Jurica, 1994; West et al., 1998) have demonstrated an impairment, in the form of more errors and an increase in perseveration, on versions of the SOPT in adults aged 40 years and older. Daigneault and Braun (1993) suggest that, with advancing age, there is significantly less effective exploitation of top-down clustering strategy. That is, young adults seem to benefit significantly from the use of strategy, whereas older individuals do not. Bryan and Luszcz (2001), however, found no age difference in the frequency of use of a clustering strategy. West et al. (1998) also noted that older adults tended to make more errors of a perseverative nature, suggesting a deficit in monitoring information in working memory (i.e., keeping track of those items selected and those not). More recently, Chaytor and Schmitter-Edgecombe (2004) reported no age differences in strategy use between old and young adults. There was also no evidence to suggest that age differences in SOPT performance were due to differences in the ability to overcome proactive interference. Rather, only processing speed and monitoring explained age differences in SOPT performance.

Given the integral connections between prefrontal cortex and the striatum, one might expect compromised functioning in patients with primary pathology in the basal ganglia. Gabrielli et al. (1996) gave a version of the SOPT (10-, 12-, and 14-word tests) to untreated patients with Parkinson's disease (PD) and to normal controls. Parkinson's disease patients made more errors than controls on tests of self-ordered pointing, temporal ordering, and free recall but were not impaired on tests of recognition memory and semantic memory. West et al. (1998) also noted impaired performance in PD patients, using the representational objects version of the SOPT. There was no relation between SOPT and CVLT recognition memory scores. Rich et al. (1996) found that patients with Huntington's disease (HD) made more SOPT errors than controls. Further, performance on the task showed a moderate correlation with activities of daily living. Patients with greater impairment in everyday life made proportionately more errors.

Some investigators have proposed that frontal lobe/executive dysfunction may serve as a conceptual model for disorders such as attention-deficit/hyperactivity disorder (ADHD). In support of this hypothesis, Shue and Douglas (1992) reported that ADHD children differed significantly from normal controls on measures such as the WCST and the SOPT, but not on tests of temporal lobe function (e.g., Wechsler Memory Scale).

Impaired performance on variants of the SOPT has also been noted in other conditions thought to impair executive functioning, including PKU (Channon et al., 2004; Smith et al., 1996), closed head injury (Schmitter-Edgecombe & Chaytor, 2003), and schizophrenia (Chey et al., 2002; Pukrop et al., 2003), and among drug users seropositive for HIV, particularly those who were symptomatic (Farinpour et al., 2000).

Of note, among drug users, scores on measures of mood (Beck Depression Inventory, State Trait Anxiety Inventory) did not correlate significantly with SOPT performance (Farinpour et al., 2000). Sleep deprivation (35 hours) also does not appear to affect performance, at least in young adults (Harrison & Horne, 2000).

COMMENT

The evidence suggests that damage to parts of the frontal lobe (particularly dorsolateral regions) resulting from injury, a neurodegenerative disease, or as part of the aging process contributes to poor performance. Studies from both normal and clinical studies generally link poor performance on the SOPT with deficiencies in working memory, speed of processing, or visual memory. Thus, limited short-term capacity and slowed speed of processing could influence SOPT performance by resulting in fewer representations in working memory that are available for active monitoring; alternatively, limited ability to remember the designs selected earlier in the trial could be the salient problem (Schmitter-Edgecombe & Chaytor, 2003). Failure to monitor accurately the progression of items through the trial could also contribute to deficient performance (e.g., Chaytor & Schmitter-Edgecombe, 2004; West et al., 1998). Reduced ability to inhibit task-irrelevant thoughts could also interfere with task performance. That is, the inability to inhibit the information from previous trials (proactive interference) could overload working memory performance on the current trial (Chaytor & Schmitter-Edgecombe, 2004). The specific factor(s) leading to deficient SOPT performance in particular clinical populations requires additional study.

Normative data are sparse for both the representational and abstract designs tasks and more extensive normative studies with larger sample sizes are needed. In addition, the influence of demographic variables (e.g., education, IQ, ethnicity) requires study.

Poor reliability is a common problem of executive function tasks (see *Introduction*) since strategies will change once tasks are no longer novel (i.e., after the first time they are performed). Not surprisingly, temporal stability of the SOPT can be less than optimal (Bryan & Luszcz, 2001). However, the fact that some researchers (Archibald & Kerns, 1999) report acceptable values suggests that additional studies are required to determine the factors (e.g., procedural modifications, populations) attenuating test-retest reliability coefficients.

A number of variants appear in the literature and one version is included in the CANTAB (discussed elsewhere in this volume). However, research is needed to determine if the SOPT variants are measuring similar cognitive processes.

REFERENCES

Archibald, S. J., & Kerns, K. A. (1999). Identification and description of new tests of executive functioning in children. *Child Neuropsychology, 5*, 115–129.

Bryan, J., & Luszcz, M. A. (2001). Adult age differences in self-ordered pointing task performance: Contributions from working memory, executive function and speed of information processing. *Journal of Clinical and Experimental Neuropsychology, 23*, 608–619.

Channon, S., German, E., Cassina, C., & Lee, P. (2004). Executive functioning, memory, and learning in phenylketonuria. *Neuropsychology, 18*, 613–620.

Chaytor, N., & Schmitter-Edgecombe, M. (2004). Working memory and aging: A cross-sectional and longitudinal analysis using a self-ordered pointing task. *Journal of the International Neuropsychological Society, 10*, 489–503.

Chey, J., Lee, J., Kim, Y.-S., Kwon, S-M., & Shin, Y-M. (2002). Spatial working memory span, delayed response and executive function in schizophrenia. *Psychiatry Research, 110*, 259–279.

Daigneault, S., & Braun, C. M. (1993). Working memory and the Self-Ordered Pointing Task: Further evidence of early prefrontal decline in normal aging. *Journal of Clinical and Experimental Neuropsychology, 15*, 881–895.

Daigneault, S., Braun, C. M., & Whitaker, H. A. (1992). Early effects of normal aging on perseverative and non-perseverative prefrontal measures. *Developmental Neuropsychology, 8*, 99–114.

Farinpour, R., Martin, E. M., Seidenberg, M., Pitrak, D. L., Pursell, K. J., Mullane, K. M., Novak, R. M., & Harrow, M. (2000). Verbal working memory in HIV-seropositive drug users. *Journal of the International Neuropsychological Society, 6*, 548–555.

Gabrieli, J. D. E., Singh, J., Stebbins, G. T., & Goetz, C. G. (1996). Reduced working memory span in Parkinson's disease: Evidence for the role of a frontostriatal system in working and strategic memory. *Neuropsychology, 10*, 322–332.

Garden, S. E., Phillips, L. H., & MacPherson, S. E. (2001). Midlife aging, open-ended planning, and laboratory measures of executive function. *Neuropsychology, 15*, 472–482.

Harrison, Y., & Horne, J. A. (2000). Sleep loss and temporal memory. *The Quarterly Journal of Experimental Psychology, 53A*, 271–279.

Haut, M. W., Chen, S-H., & Edwards, S. (1999). Working memory, semantics, and normal aging. *Aging, Neuropsychology and Cognition, 6*, 179–186.

Macpherson, S. E., Phillips, L. H., & Della Sala, S. (2002). Age, executive function, and social decision making: A dorsolateral prefrontal theory of cognitive aging. *Psychology and Aging, 17*, 598–609.

Petrides, M. (1991). Monitoring of selections of visual stimuli and the primate frontal cortex. *Proceedings of the Royal Society of London (Biol), 246*, 293–298.

Petrides, M. (1995). Impairments on nonspatial self-ordered and externally ordered working memory tasks after lesions of the mid-dorsal part of the lateral frontal cortex in the monkey. *Journal of Neuroscience, 15,* 359–375.

Petrides, M., Alivisatos, B., Meyer, E., & Evans, A. (1993a). Functional activation of the human frontal cortex during the performance of verbal working memory tasks. *Neurobiology, 90,* 878–882.

Petrides, M., Alivisatos, B., Evans, A., & Meyer, E. (1993b). Dissociation of human mid-dorsolateral from posterior dorsolateral frontal cortex in memory processing. *Society for Neuroscience Abstracts, 90,* 873–877.

Petrides, M., & Milner, B. (1982). Deficits on subject-ordered tasks after frontal- and temporal-lobe lesions in man. *Neuropsychologia 20,* 249–262.

Pukrop, R., Matuschek, E., Ruhrmann, S., Brockhaus-Dumke, A., Tendolkar, I., Bertsch, A., & Klosterkotter, J. (2003). Dimensions of working memory dysfunction in schizophrenia. *Schizophrenia Research, 62,* 259–268.

Rich, J. B., Blysma, F. W., & Brandt, J. (1996). Self-ordered pointing performance in Huntington's disease patients. *Neuro-psychiatry, Neuropsychology and Behavioral Neurology, 9,* 99–106.

Schmitter-Edgecombe, M., & Chaytor, N. S. (2003). Self-ordered pointing performance following severe head injury. *Journal of Clinical and Experimental Neuropsychology, 25,* 918–932.

Shimamura, A. P., & Jurica, P. J. (1994). Memory interference effects and aging: Findings from a test of frontal lobe function. *Neuropsychology, 8,* 408–412.

Shue, K. L., & Douglas, V. I. (1992). Attention deficit hyperactivity disorders and the frontal lobe syndrome. *Brain and Cognition, 20,* 104–124.

Smith, M. L., Klim, P., Mallozzi, E., & Hanley, W. (1996). A test of the frontal specificity hypothesis in the cognitive performance of young adults with phenylketonuria. *Developmental Neuropsychology, 12,* 327–341.

West, R., Ergis, A-M., Winocur, G., & Sant-Cyr, J. (1998). The contribution of impaired working memory monitoring to performance of the Self Ordered Pointing Task in normal aging and Parkinson's disease. *Neuropsychology, 12,* 546–554.

Stroop Test

PURPOSE

This measure of cognitive control assesses the ease with which a person can maintain a goal in mind and suppress a habitual response in favor of a less familiar one.

SOURCE

There are a number of versions of the Stroop test that are commercially available. Psychological Assessment Resources, Inc. (www.parinc.com) offers versions developed by Golden (1978) for adults at a cost of $104 US (includes Examiner's Manual; Golden & Freshwater, 2002) and a version for children (Golden et al., 2003) at a cost of $104 US. PAR also offers another version developed by Trenerry et al. (1989) for use with individuals, aged 18 to 50+, at a cost of $124 US.

The Victoria version of the test can be ordered from the Psychology Clinic, University of Victoria, PO Box 1700, Victoria, B.C. (http://web.uvic.ca/psyc/testsale) for approximately $40 US (e-mail: psychtest@uvic.ca). Alternatively, users may make their own cards as described later.

The Stroop task is also included in the D-KEFS described elsewhere in this volume (Color-Word Interference Test) and can be used with individuals aged 8 to 89 years. The CAS also includes a subtest modeled after the Stroop paradigm (i.e., Expressive Attention), also described elsewhere in this book, suitable for ages 8 to 17, and a pictorial version for younger children, ages 5 to 7.

Other Language Versions

The Golden version is available for Spanish-speaking individuals, aged 18 to 65, in Artiola I Fortuny et al. (1999). The Victoria version has been translated into Cantonese for use with adults ages 20 to 70+ (Lee, 2003).

AGE RANGE

We describe here the Victoria version for ages 18 to 94 and the Golden version for ages 5 to 90.

DESCRIPTION

This measure of selective attention and cognitive flexibility was originally developed by Stroop (1935), although the paradigm dates back to the work of Cattell in the late 1800s (Mitrushina et al., 2005). Stroop's version consisted of three white cards, each containing 10 rows of five items. There are four parts to the test. In Part 1, the subject reads randomized color names (blue, green, red, brown, purple) printed in black type. In Part 2, the subject reads the color names (blue, green, red, brown, purple) printed in colored ink (blue, green, red, yellow), ignoring the color of the print (the print color never corresponds to the color name). In Part 3, the subject has to name the color of squares (blue, green, red, brown, purple). In Part 4, the subject is given the card used in Part 2, but this time, the subject must name the color in which the color names are printed and disregard their verbal content. Of major interest is the subject's behavior when presented with colored words printed in nonmatching colored inks. Stroop reported that normal people can read color words printed in colored ink as fast as when the words are presented in black ink (Part 2 versus Part 1). However, the time to complete the task increases significantly when the subject is asked to name the color of the ink rather than read the word (Part 4 versus Part 3). This decrease in color-naming speed is called the "color-word interference effect."

A number of versions of the Stroop Test have been developed (e.g., Comalli et al., 1962; Comalli-Kaplan version described in Strickland et al., 1997, and Mistrushina et al., 2005; Dodrill, 1978; Golden, 1976, 1978; Graf et al., 1995; Trenerry et al., 1989; also see D-KEFS, Delis et al., 2001, and CAS, Naglieri & Das, 1997). Thus, tests differ in the number of cards used. For example, sometimes the card containing color words printed in black ink is omitted (e.g., Trenerry et al., 1989), and sometimes a congruent color card is included in which the color words are printed in their congruent ink colors (e.g., Graf et al., 1995). Tests also differ in the use of colored patches/dots (e.g., Comalli version, Victoria version, D-KEFS) or colored X's (Golden, 1976; Graf et al., 1995), the number of items on each test card (e.g., 24 per card on the Victoria version, 50 items on the D-KEFS version, 100 items on the Golden and Comalli versions), and the number of colors used (e.g., three in the versions by Comalli, Delis et al., and Graf et al.; four in the Victoria and Golden versions; and five in the original form used by Stroop). The D-KEFS also includes a fourth condition that requires the patient to switch back and forth between naming the dissonant ink colors and reading the conflicting words. Limitations of these various versions include the lack of normative data for error scores (Golden, 1978; Naglieri & Das, 1997; Trenerry et al., 1989), failure to correct for generalized slowing on the interference trial (Trenerry et al., 1989), the lack of detailed age-corrected normative data (Trenerry et al., 1989), and the lack of data for children (Victoria version, Trenerry et al., 1989).

Victoria Stroop Test (VST)

The Victoria version (Regard, 1981) is similar to that devised by Perret (1974) and has several advantages (Troyer et al., in press). First, it is brief. In contrast to other versions, which have a large number of items (i.e., 60–112) on each component task, the Victoria Stroop Test (VST) has only 24 items on each of three tasks (naming the color of dots, of neutral words, and of color words printed in contrasting colors). There is evidence that shorter test durations may be preferable for identifying individuals who have difficulty with this task. Klein et al. (1997) found that on a 100-item version of the Stroop task, older adults showed greater interference than younger adults and that this effect was more pronounced on the first 40 items than on the last 60 items. Thus, not only does the VST require less administration time, but it may be ideal for detecting difficulties with response inhibition because the examinee does not get extended practice with the task. Second, scores that are relatively independent of cognitive speed can be evaluated, including an error score and an interference (ratio) score that corrects for generalized slowing. Third, a reasonable normative data base is available (see later discussion). Finally, the VST is in the public domain, and users may make their own stimuli.

The VST consists of three 21.5 × 14 cm cards, each containing six rows of four items (Helvetica, 28 point). The rows are spaced 1 cm apart. In Part D (Dots), the subject must name as quickly as possible the color of 24 dots printed in blue, green, red, or yellow. Each color is used six times, and the four colors are arranged in a pseudorandom order within the array, each

color appearing once in each row. Unlike the original Stroop Test, Part W (Words) is similar to Part D, except that the dots are replaced by common words (when, hard, and over), printed in lowercase letters. The subject is required to name the colors in which the stimuli are printed, and to disregard their verbal content. Part C (Colors) is similar to Parts D and W, but here the colored stimuli are the color names "blue, green, red, and yellow" printed in lowercase so that the print color never corresponds to the color name (e.g., "red" is written in blue ink). This latter task thus requires the individual to inhibit an automatic reading response and to produce a more effortful color-naming response. The interference effect is determined by calculating the extra time required to name colors in the interference task in comparison to the time required to name colors in the control task.

Stroop Color and Word Test

The Golden version (Golden, 1978; Golden & Freshwater, 2002) is used frequently and is also considered here. It consists of a Word Page with 100 color words (red, green, blue) printed in black ink, a Color Page with 100 Xs printed in either red, green, or blue ink, and a Color-Word Page with 100 words from the first page (red, green, blue) printed in colors from the second page (the color and the word do not match). The patient looks at each sheet and moves down the columns, reading words or naming the ink color as quickly as possible within a time limit (45 seconds). The test yields three scores based on the number of items completed on each of the three stimulus sheets. In addition, an interference score can also be calculated.

The Comalli Version

This version (Comalli et al., 1962) consists of three 24 × 24 cm white cards, each containing 100 items (10 × 10). The first card contains the words red, blue, and green printed in black ink, randomly selected and arranged in 10 rows of 10 items each. The second card contains patches of the colors red, blue, and green randomly selected and presented in a 10 × 10 array. The third card contains color names printed in a discrepant ink color. Time to completion on each of the three conditions is used as the independent variable. The Comalli-Kaplan modification requires that the color-naming card be presented first and that errors be recorded. The rationale underlying this modification is that (a) individuals who are color blind can be quickly identified and (b) the procedure maximizes the interference effect by presenting the word reading condition just prior to the interference task. Normative data are provided in Mitrushina et al. (2005). A Spanish translation of the Comalli-Kaplan version has been developed for use with children, ages 6 to 12 years (Armengol, 2002). The D-KEFS version incorporates the Comalli-Kaplan modification and is described elsewhere in this book, as is the CAS.

ADMINISTRATION

Victoria Version

In this version, the three cards are always presented in the same sequence: Dots (Part D), Words (Part W), and Colors (Part C). The subject is instructed to read or call out the color name as quickly as possible. The examiner starts the timer immediately after providing instructions, and instructs as follows:

Part D. "*Name the colors of the dots as quickly as you can. Begin here and go across the rows from left to right.*" Direct the patient's eyes across the rows from left to right.

Part W. "*This time, name the colors of the words as quickly as you can. Begin here and go across the rows from left to right.*" Clarify, if necessary: "*Name the colors in which the words are printed.*"

Part C. "*Again, name the colors in which the words are printed as quickly as you can.*" Clarify if necessary: "*Don't read the word, tell me the color in which the word is printed.*"

The errors in color naming on each part are corrected by the examiner immediately, if not spontaneously corrected by the patient. The subject is then instructed to go on as rapidly as possible. The examiner notes the number of errors and time taken for each section.

Golden Version

See *Source*. For the Word-Reading trial (p. 1), examinees are asked to read down the columns starting with the top word in the left-most column. In the Color-Naming trial (p. 2), examinees are instructed to name the color of the item with all other instructions being identical to those of the previous trial. During the Color-Word Interference trial (p. 3), examinees are asked to read down the columns, naming the color of the words, ignoring the printed word. For all trials, examinees are asked to complete the trials as quickly as possible. Errors are indicated by the examiner, cueing the participant to correct the error and continue. After 45 seconds, the item last named on each stimulus sheet (trial) is noted. Errors are not counted.

ADMINISTRATION TIME

The approximate time required is five minutes for each version.

SCORING

Victoria Version

For each part, the examiner records both the time to complete and the number of errors. Spontaneous corrections are scored as correct. Figure 8–13 shows a sample scoring sheet.

Researchers have typically relied on a difference score, defined as the difference in the amount of time required for the interference card (e.g., Part C) versus the color card (e.g., Part D; MacLeod, 1991). Graf et al. (1995) contend that a difference score is not independent of age-related slowing and recommend the use of a ratio index of interference (e.g., Card C/ Part D; see also Verhaeghen & De Meersman, 1998).

Golden Version

This version produces three scores: The word-reading (W) score consists of the number of items completed in 45 seconds on p. 1; the color-naming (C) score is made up of the number of items completed in 45 seconds on p. 2; and the color-word (CW) score is made up of the number of items completed on p. 3. An interference score is also calculated.

The scoring system for adults incorporates adjusted scores derived from the prediction of normal performance based on an individual's age and years of education. Thus, predicted word (W), color (C), and color-word (CW) are determined from tables (I–III) provided the test manual. The age/education adjusted scores are then subtracted from the raw scores to yield a residual score for each measure. These residual scores are translated into T scores ($M = 50$, $SD = 10$) using another table (IV) in the manual. A derived score, the color-word minus predicted color-word score, is used as the measure of interference (interference T score) for individuals aged 15 and older (using Tables V and VI in the manual). For ages 5 to 14 years, an interference score is derived from the difference between the color-word T score and the color T score. For the three basic scores, higher T scores reflect better performance. For the interference score, lower scores (a T score of 40 or less) are generally indicative of problems.

Franzen (2000) cautions that there is insufficient information about the appropriateness or the size of the samples used in the derivation of these standardized scores (see also *Normative Data*). In addition, Chafetz and Matthews (2004) have questioned the theoretical model underlying Golden's interference score used for adults. They note that the interference score is based on the assumption that the brain *adds* word-reading to color-naming processes to produce the results on the CW card (i.e., the time to read a CW item is an additive function of the time to read a word plus the time to name a color). However, discussion of the Stroop effects in neuropsychology has not been about addition, but about inhibition or suppression. Consistent with this notion, they propose a different interference score based on the notion that the time to read a CW item reflects the time to *suppress* the reading of a word plus the time to name a color.

DEMOGRAPHIC EFFECTS

Age

Age has a significant impact on the interference score on the Victoria version ($r = .41$; Troyer et al., in press). A recent

Figure 8–13 Sample Score Sheet for the Victoria Stroop Test.

Name _____ Date _____

Age _____

Dots:

G	B	Y	R
Y	R	G	B
B	G	Y	R
B	Y	R	G
R	G	B	Y
Y	G	B	R

Colors:

G	B	Y	R
Y	R	G	B
B	G	Y	R
B	Y	R	G
R	G	B	Y
Y	G	B	R

Words:

G	B	Y	R
Y	R	G	B
B	G	Y	R
B	Y	R	G
R	G	B	Y
Y	G	B	R

	Time	*Errors*
Dots		
Colors		
Words		

compilation of six datasets, comprising 490 adults, revealed that age accounted for a significant amount of variability in the interference scores on the Golden version ($r^2 = .79$; Mitrushina et al., 2005). In children, the correlation between age and the interference score on the Golden version is .29 (Golden & Golden, 2002). In adults, aging appears to be linked with a slowing in color naming and an increase in the Stroop interference effect, expressed as difference (e.g., C-D), ratio (e.g., C/D), or error scores (but see *Validity*). In children, interference is minimal when children are just beginning to learn to read and increases (in the first few grades) as children gain in reading fluency. Thereafter it declines gradually as they gain control over the automatic response of reading (on the Comalli and D-KEFS; Armengol, 2002; Comalli et al., 1962; but see Golden & Golden, 2003, for a different pattern), showing adult levels by about age 13 years (Delis et al., 2001).

Gender

Although women tend to have superior color-naming skills (Strickland et al., 1997; Stroop, 1935), gender differences on the color-word interference card are not always present (Anstey et al., 2000; Armegnol, 2002; Connor et al., 1988; Golden, 1978, Golden & Freshwater, 2002; Golden & Golden, 2003; Ivnik et al., 1996; Strickland et al., 1997; Troyer et al., in press; but see Moering et al., 2004) or are minimal (Lucas et al., 2005).

Education/IQ

Education shows a modest relation (<.30) to the Stroop interference score in adults (Anstey et al., 2000; Ivnik et al., 1996; Steinberg et al., 2005; Troyer et al., in press; but see Mitrushina et al., 2005). In African Americans, Moering et al. (2004) found that education had the strongest effect on Stroop scores, accounting for 8% to 26% of the variance, followed by gender (0–5.7%) and age (.06 = –1.56%). However, Lucas et al. (2005) examined African Americans and reported that both age and education each accounted for about 8% to 9% of the variance in performance on the interference trial. IQ shows a stronger relationship to test scores than education (Steinberg et al., 2005). Although correlations with years of education decrease as task complexity increases (reading color names versus naming incongruent ink colors), correlations with intelligence increase across these conditions (Steinberg et al., 2005). In general, the higher an individual's intelligence (particularly fluid intelligence) scores are, the less interference they are likely to experience (Shilling et al., 2002).

Ethnicity/Language

Ethnicity also impacts test scores, with African Americans performing at a lower level than Caucasians even when edu-

cation is taken into account (Moering et al., 2004). Performance tends to be slower in bilinguals (Spanish-English) than in monolinguals, particularly in the color-naming condition (Rosselli et al., 2002).

NORMATIVE DATA

Victoria Version

Normative data, using overlapping age groups, are based on 272 healthy, community-dwelling adults, ages 18 to 94, living in Victoria, British Columbia, or Toronto, Ontario (64% females; mean education about 13 years; Troyer et al, in press). They were recruited from a university-based older-adult subject pool, senior centers, and advertisements posted in the community and at the university. Participants were interviewed to screen for neurological disorders (e.g., loss of consciousness exceeding one hour, stroke, epilepsy, multiple sclerosis) and psychiatric disorders (e.g., depression or anxiety requiring hospitalization) that could affect cognitive functioning. All were fluent in English. Scaled scores (2–18) and percentiles were determined for time and error scores and these are shown in Tables 8–40 to 8–44.

Golden Version—Adults

Standardization Sample. Normative data are based on a sample of individuals ranging from 15 to 90 years. However, the characteristics of the sample (e.g., sample size, gender distribution, and age groupings) are not clearly provided in the manual (see Table 8–45). The 2002 manual (page 6) merely notes that "the work reported in the initial manual (Golden, 1978) has been updated and expanded using an additional 300 normals ranging from age 15–90 (mean = 38.23, sd = 15.42) with education levels ranging from 2–20 years (mean = 12.04, sd = 3.84) collected over the past twenty years." Mitrushina et al. (2005) also note that the norms presented in the 1978 manual derived from data from Golden's own studies as well as from normative data provided by Stroop (1935), Jensen (1965), and Comalli et al. (1962). However, the procedures and formats used by others differed from Golden's (e.g., subjects completed the entire stimulus card rather than stopping at 45 seconds, used colored rectangles rather than colored Xs, used a wall chart presentation rather than a standard page presented up close to the subject).

Other Normative Data. Ivnik et al. (1996) provide normative data for the three conditions based on a sample of 356 Caucasian individuals of average IQ (Mayo FSIQ= 106.2, *SD* = 14.0), aged 56 to 94 years. Participants were independently functioning, community-dwelling persons who had been recently examined by their personal physician and who had no active neurological or psychiatric disorder with potential to

Table 8–40 Scaled Score Equivalents for VST Dot Time Scores (in Seconds), by Age Group

Age	18–39 (29)	30–49 (40)	40–59 (50)	50–64 (57)	60–69 (65)	65–74 (70)	70–79 (75)	75–84 (80)	80–94 (87)
Mean	11.0	11.1	12.3	12.0	12.1	13.3	14.2	15.1	15.9
SD	2.5	1.9	2.4	2.3	2.3	3.6	3.9	3.8	4.2
SS									
17	<7				<8	<9	<9	<9	<9
16	7	<8	<8	<8	8	9	9	9	9
15	8	8	8	8	9	10	10	10	10
14			9	9	10			11	11
13	9	9	10	10		11	11	12	12
12		10			11		12	13	13
11	10		11	11		12	13	14	14
10		11	12	12	12	13	14	15	15–16
9	11	12	13	13	13	14	15	16	17
8	12	13	14	14	14	15	16–17	17	18–19
7	13	14	15	15	15	16–17	18–19	18–20	20–21
6	14–15	15–16	16	16	16–17	18–20	20–21	21–22	22–23
5	16–17	17	17	17	18–19	21–27	22–27	23–27	24–29
4	18	18	18	18	20	28–29	28–29	28–29	>29
3	19	19	19	19	21	30	>29	>29	
2	>19	>19	>19	>19	>21	>30			

Note: Midpoint ages are shown in parentheses. Overlapping age groups were used. Total $N = 272$. Education information was not recorded for the youngest age groups. Mean education was as follows: Ages 40–59: 13.2 ($SD = 3.0$); 50–64: 13.2 (2.4); 60–69: 13.6 (2.5); 65–74: 13.6 (2.9); 70–79: 12.9 (2.8); 75–84: 12.1 (2.7); 80–94: 11.5 (3.1).

Source: From Troyer et al., in press. Reprinted with the kind permission of Psychology Press.

Table 8–41 Scaled Score Equivalents for VST Neutral Word Time Scores (in Seconds), by Age Group

Age	18–39 (29)	30–49 (40)	40–59 (50)	50–64 (57)	60–69 (65)	65–74 (70)	70–79 (75)	75–84 (80)	80–94 (87)
Mean	13.0	13.9	15.2	15.4	15.9	16.9	18.6	20.7	22.1
SD	2.9	2.6	2.9	3.2	5.1	5.1	5.4	6.7	6.0
SS									
17			<10	<10	<10	<11	<11		
16	<9	<10	10	10	10	11	11–12	<14	<14
15	9	10	11	11	11	12	13	14	14
14	10	11		12	12	13	14	15	15
13	11		12	13	13		15	16	16
12		12	13			14	16	17	17–18
11	12	13	14	14	14	15	17	18	19–20
10	13	14	15	15	15	16	18	19	21–22
9	14	15	16	16	16	17	19	20–22	23–24
8	15	16	17	17	17	18–19	20–21	23–25	25–26
7	16–17	17	18	18	18	20–21	22–23	26–29	27–29
6	18–19	18–19	19	19–20	19–24	22–24	24–29	30–33	30–33
5	20	20	20	21–26	25–41	25–41	30–41	34–45	34–45
4	21	21	21–24	27–28	42–45	42–45	42–46	>45	>45
3	22	>21	>24	>28	>45	>45	>46		
2	>22								

Note: Midpoint ages are shown in parentheses.

Source: From Troyer et al., in press. Reprinted with the kind permission of Psychology Press.

Table 8–42 Scaled Score Equivalents for VST Color Word Time Scores (in Seconds), by Age Group

Age	18–39 (29)	30–49 (40)	40–59 (50)	50–64 (57)	60–69 (65)	65–74 (70)	70–79 (75)	75–84 (80)	80–94 (87)
Mean	22.1	25.7	27.8	28.5	29.4	32.6	37.1	43.3	50.4
SD	7.2	9.0	8.2	9.5	9.0	9.6	11.9	17.7	23.9
SS									
17	<11	<15	<15	<15	<15	<19	<19	<22	<22
16	11	15	15–17	15–17	15–17	19–20	19–21	22	22–25
15	12–13	16	18	18	18–19	21	22–23	23–24	26–28
14	14–15	17	19	19	20	22	24	25–26	29–30
13	16	18	20–21	20–21	21–22	23–25	25–28	27–29	31–32
12	17–18	19–20	22–23	22–23	23–24	26–28	29–31	30–32	33–36
11	19	21–22	24–25	24–25	25–26	29–31	32–34	33–36	37–44
10	20–22	23–24	26–27	26–28	27–29	32–33	35–39	37–44	45–53
9	23–24	25–28	28–30	29–30	30–33	34–36	40–42	45–52	54–59
8	25–28	29–33	31–34	31–37	34–37	37–41	43–47	53–63	60–68
7	29–30	34–38	35–39	38–42	38–42	42–44	48–55	64–66	69–83
6	31–35	39–48	40–48	43–51	43–56	45–57	56–65	67–74	84–112
5	36–48	49–50	49–51	52–57	57–58	58–68	66–69	75–109	113–137
4	>48	>50	>51	58–59	>58	69–70	70–71	110–112	>137
3				>59		>70	>71	>112	
2									

Note: Midpoint ages are shown in parentheses.

Source: From Troyer et al., in press. Reprinted with the kind permission of Psychology Press.

Table 8–43 Scaled Score Equivalents for VST Interference Scores, by Age Group

Age	18–39 (29)	30–49 (40)	40–59 (50)	50–64 (57)	60–69 (65)	65–74 (70)	70–79 (75)	75–84 (80)	80–94 (87)
Mean	2.0	2.3	2.3	2.4	2.5	2.6	2.7	2.9	3.2
SD	0.6	0.8	0.7	0.8	0.8	0.9	1.0	1.0	1.6
SS									
18							<1.2	<1.2	<1.5
17		<1.1	<1.2	<1.2	<1.3	<1.4	1.2–1.3	1.2–1.3	1.5
16	<1.1	1.1–1.2	1.2	1.2	1.3–1.4	1.4	1.4–1.5	1.4–1.5	1.6–1.7
15	1.1–1.2	1.3	1.3–1.4	1.3–1.4	1.5–1.6	1.5–1.6	1.6	1.6–1.8	1.8
14	1.3	1.4–1.5	1.5	1.5–1.6	1.7–1.8	1.7–1.8	1.7–1.9	1.9–2.0	1.9–2.0
13	1.4–1.5	1.6–1.7	1.6–1.7	1.7–1.8	1.9	1.9	2.0	2.1	2.1–2.2
12	1.6–1.7	1.8–1.9	1.8–1.9	1.9–2.0	2.0	2.0–2.1	2.1	2.2	2.3
11	1.8–1.9	2.0–2.1	2.0–2.1	2.1	2.1	2.2	2.2–2.4	2.3–2.4	2.4–2.7
10	2.0–2.1	2.2–2.3	2.2–2.4	2.2–2.4	2.2–2.4	2.3–2.5	2.5–2.6	2.5–2.8	2.8–3.4
9	2.2–2.3	2.4–2.5	2.5–2.6	2.5–2.7	2.5–2.7	2.6–2.8	2.7–3.0	2.9–3.3	3.5–3.6
8	2.4–2.5	2.6–2.8	2.7–2.8	2.8–3.2	2.8–3.2	2.9–3.2	3.1–3.5	3.4–3.9	3.7–3.9
7	2.6–2.8	2.9–3.7	2.9–3.7	3.3–3.7	3.3–3.7	3.3–4.0	3.6–4.1	4.0–5.0	4.0–5.1
6	2.9–3.5	3.8–3.9	3.8–3.9	3.8–4.0	3.8–4.1	4.1–5.0	4.2–5.0	5.1–5.5	5.2–5.5
5	3.6–4.0	4.0–4.5	4.0–4.5	4.1–4.7	4.2–4.7	5.1–6.0	5.1–6.0	5.6–6.1	5.6–10.0
4	4.1–4.2	4.6	4.6	4.8–4.9	4.8–4.9	6.1–6.3	6.1–6.4	6.2–6.5	>10.0
3	>4.2	>4.6	>4.6	>4.9	>4.9	>6.3	>6.4	>6.5	
2									

Note: Midpoint ages are shown in parentheses. Interference scores were calculated as the number of seconds required to complete the Color Word task divided by the number of seconds required to complete the Dot task.

Source: From Troyer et al., in press. Reprinted with the kind permission of Psychology Press.

Table 8–44 Means and Cumulative Percentages Associated With Raw Error Scores on VST Color Word Task, by Age Group

Age	18–39 (29)	30–49 (40)	40–59 (50)	50–64 (57)	60–69 (65)	65–74 (70)	70–79 (75)	75–84 (80)	80–94 (87)
Mean	0.8	0.8	0.7	0.6	0.5	0.6	1.1	1.7	2.1
SD	1.0	1.0	1.0	1.0	0.9	1.2	1.6	1.8	2.0
Errors									
0	100	100	100	100	100	100	100	100	100
1	47	50	43	35	27	33	47	64	79
2	19	24	22	19	14	17	29	45	50
3	9	9	4	5	4	5	18	28	32
4	3		2	3	2	2	6	11	16
5						2	5	8	10
6						2	3	6	8
7						2	2	4	8
8									3

Note: Midpoint ages are shown in parentheses.

Source: From Troyer et al., in press. Reprinted with kind permission of Psychology Press.

affect cognition. Data are stratified by age using the midpoint interval technique. The data are shown in Tables 8–46 to 8–56. Education contributes minimally to test performance (correlations <.30 between age and the three test trials). Nonetheless, a computational formula is also provided (Table 8–57) to derive age- and education-corrected scaled scores.

IQ is more strongly related to performance than education. Steinberg et al. (2005) have reanalyzed data from the Mayo Clinic's Older Americans Normative Studies (MOANS) and provided age (55+) and IQ-adjusted percentile equivalents of MOANS age-adjusted Stroop scores. Readers should note that all FSIQs are MAYO age-adjusted scores which are based on the WAIS-R, not the WAIS-III. Given the upward shift in scores (Flynn effect) with the passage of time, use of the WAIS-R FSIQ rather than the WAIS-III might result in a given Stroop score appearing less favorable. The interested reader is referred to their article for the relevant tables.

Table 8–45 Characteristics of the Stroop Adult Normative Sample Provided by Golden and Freshwater, 2002

Number	300+
Age	15–90 years
Geographic location	Not reported
Sample type	Not reported
Education	2–20 years
Gender	Not reported
Race/ethnicity	Not reported
Screening	Not reported

Mitrushina et al. (2005) recently compiled six datasets comprising 490 adults, aged 25 to 74 years. Data for the word-reading and color-naming conditions were sparse and therefore were not analyzed. Metanorms are provided for the interference condition only.

Normative data for older African Americans have recently been provided by Moering et al. (2004) and Lucas et al. (2005). The data by Lucas et al. (2005) are shown here given the somewhat larger normative sample (303 versus 236), a somewhat wider age range (56–94 versus 60–84), and the availability of conormed tests (see *RAVLT, BNT, Verbal Fluency, MAE Token, TMT,* and *JLO,* elsewhere in this volume). Their data for Stroop raw scores are shown in Tables 8–58a and b and are based on a sample of 303 African-American community-dwelling participants from the MOAANS (Mayo African American Normative Studies) project in Jacksonville, Florida. Participants were predominantly female (75%), ranged in age from 56 to 94 years ($M = 69.6$, $SD = 6.87$), and varied in education from 0 to 20 years of formal education ($M = 12.2$, $SD = 3.48$). They were screened to exclude those with active neurological, psychiatric, or other conditions that might affect cognition. Table 8–58a presents the age scaled scores and Table 8–58b provides the computational formula used to calculate age- and education-adjusted MOAANS scaled scores. The authors urge that their data be used with caution since the number of very old adults is somewhat small and they used a sample of convenience, which may not represent the full range of cultural and educational experiences of the African American community.

Golden Version—Children

Standardization Sample. Golden and Golden (2003) provide norms derived from a sample of 182 children, ranging in

Table 8–46 Golden Version: MOANS Scaled Scores for Persons Whose Ages Range From 56 to 62

Scaled Scores	Raw Scores Earned Stroop Word	Stroop Color	Stroop C/W	Percentile Ranges
2	<60	<41	<17	<1
3	60–63	41–42	17–18	1
4	64–65	43–44	19–20	2
5	66–72	45–50	21–23	3–5
6	73–77	51–54	24–25	6–10
7	78–82	55–59	26–28	11–18
8	83–88	60–64	29–30	19–28
9	89–93	65–66	31–34	29–40
10	94–101	67–71	35–38	41–59
11	102–107	72–75	39–40	60–71
12	108–111	76–81	41–43	72–81
13	112–116	82–85	44–47	82–89
14	117–122	86–88	48–49	90–94
15	123–125	89–91	50–55	95–97
16	126–129	92–93	56–57	98
17	130–139	94–104	58–62	99
18	>139	>104	>62	>99
Type of score for each test	Correct Count	Correct Count	Correct Count	
Age range (years) used for each test's norms	56–66	56–66	56–66	
Normative sample size (N) for each test	160	160	160	

Source: From Ivnik et al., 1996. Reprinted with the kind permission of Psychology Press.

Table 8–47 Golden Version: MOANS Scaled Scores for Persons Whose Ages Range From 63 to 65

Scaled Scores	Raw Scores Earned Stroop Word	Stroop Color	Stroop C/W	Percentile Ranges
2	<58	<39	<16	<1
3	58	39–40	16	1
4	59	41–43	17	2
5	60–68	44–48	18–21	3–5
6	69–76	49–53	22–23	6–10
7	77–81	54–58	24–26	11–18
8	82–86	59–61	27–29	19–28
9	87–91	62–64	30–32	29–40
10	92–98	65–70	33–36	41–59
11	99–103	71–73	37–39	60–71
12	104–109	74–80	40–42	72–81
13	110–115	81–82	43–45	82–89
14	116–122	83–86	46–48	90–94
15	123–125	87–89	49–51	95–97
16	126–127	90–92	52–54	98
17	128–132	93–104	55–62	99
18	>132	>104	>62	>99
Type of score for each test	Correct Count	Correct Count	Correct Count	
Age range (years) used for each test's norms	59–69	59–69	59–69	
Normative sample size (N) for each test	206	206	206	

Source: From Ivnik et al., 1996. Reprinted with the kind permission of Psychology Press.

Table 8–48 Golden Version: MOANS Scaled Scores for Persons Whose Ages Range From 66 to 68

| | Raw Scores Earned | | | |
| | | Stroop | | Percentile |
Scaled Scores	Word	Color	C/W	Ranges
2	<58	<32	<16	<1
3	58	32–40	16	1
4	59	41–42	17	2
5	60–68	43–47	18–21	3–5
6	69–74	48–51	22	6–10
7	75–80	52–57	23–26	11–18
8	81–85	58–59	27–29	19–28
9	86–91	60–63	30–31	29–40
10	92–97	64–69	32–35	41–59
11	98–103	70–72	36–38	60–71
12	104–109	73–78	39–42	72–81
13	110–115	79–81	43–44	82–89
14	116–122	82–85	45–47	90–94
15	123–125	86–87	48–50	95–97
16	126–127	88–90	51–52	98
17	128–131	91–104	53–60	99
18	>131	>104	>60	>99
Type of score for each test	Correct Count	Correct Count	Correct Count	
Age range (years) used for each test's norms	62–72	62–72	62–72	
Normative sample size (N) for each test	152	152	152	

Source: From Ivnik et al., 1996. Reprinted with the kind permission of Psychology Press.

Table 8–49 Golden Version: MOANS Scaled Scores for Persons Whose Ages Range From 69 to 71

| | Raw Scores Earned | | | |
| | | Stroop | | Percentile |
Scaled Scores	Word	Color	C/W	Ranges
2	<44	<24	<16	<1
3	44–46	24–30	16	1
4	47–50	31–41	17	2
5	51–59	42–45	18–19	3–5
6	60–71	46–48	20–21	6–10
7	72–79	49–52	22–24	11–18
8	80–83	53–57	25–27	19–28
9	84–87	58–60	28–29	29–40
10	88–94	61–65	30–32	41–59
11	95–98	66–71	33–35	60–71
12	99–103	72–76	36–39	72–81
13	104–111	77–81	40–44	82–89
14	112–120	82–85	45	90–94
15	121–125	86–87	46–50	95–97
16	126–127	88–90	51–52	98
17	128–131	91–104	53–60	99
18	>131	>104	>60	>99
Type of score for each test	Correct Count	Correct Count	Correct Count	
Age range (years) used for each test's norms	65–75	65–75	65–75	
Normative sample size (N) for each test	134	134	134	

Source: From Ivnik et al., 1996. Reprinted with the kind permission of Psychology Press.

Table 8–50 Golden Version: MOANS Scaled Scores for Persons Whose Ages Range From 72 to 74

| | Raw Scores Earned | | | |
| | Stroop | | | Percentile |
Scaled Scores	Word	Color	C/W	Ranges
2	<42	<24	<4	<1
3	42–45	24–30	4–6	1
4	46–48	31–39	7–15	2
5	49–56	40–41	16–17	3–5
6	57–63	42–44	18–20	6–10
7	64–76	45–49	21–22	11–18
8	77–81	50–53	23–26	19–28
9	82–85	54–58	27–28	29–40
10	86–93	59–63	29–31	41–59
11	94–96	64–67	32–33	60–71
12	97–100	68–71	34–36	72–81
13	101–105	72–74	37–40	82–89
14	106–111	75–80	41–44	90–94
15	112–115	81	45	95–97
16	116–122	82–84	46–49	98
17	123–130	85–90	50–52	99
18	>130	>90	>52	>99
Type of score for each test	Correct Count	Correct Count	Correct Count	
Age range (years) used for each test's norms	68–78	68–78	68–78	
Normative sample size (N) for each test	124	124	124	

Source: Ivnik et al., 1996. Reprinted with the kind permission of Psychology Press.

Table 8–51 Golden Version: MOANS Scaled Scores for Persons Whose Ages Range From 75 to 77

| | Raw Scores Earned | | | |
| | Stroop | | | Percentile |
Scaled Scores	Word	Color	C/W	Ranges
2	<42	<23	<4	<1
3	42–45	23	4–6	1
4	46–48	24–26	7–13	2
5	49–54	27–39	14–15	3–5
6	55–63	40–43	16–17	6–10
7	64–72	44–48	18–21	11–18
8	73–80	49–51	22–25	19–28
9	81–84	52–55	26–27	29–40
10	85–91	56–60	28–30	41–59
11	92–96	61–65	31–32	60–71
12	97–98	66–70	33–34	72–81
13	99–105	71–73	35–38	82–89
14	106–110	74–80	39–42	90–94
15	111–115	81	43–45	95–97
16	116–122	82–84	—	98
17	123–130	85–90	46	99
18	>130	>90	>46	>99
Type of score for each test	Correct Count	Correct Count	Correct Count	
Age range (years) used for each test's norms	71–81	71–81	71–81	
Normative sample size (N) for each test	111	111	111	

Source: Ivnik et al., 1996. Reprinted with the kind permission of Psychology Press.

Table 8–52 Golden Version: MOANS Scaled Scores for Persons Whose Ages Range From 78 to 80

| Scaled Scores | Raw Scores Earned | | | Percentile Ranges |
| | Stroop | | | |
	Word	Color	C/W	
2	<41	<23	<4	<1
3	41–44	23	4–6	1
4	45–48	24–26	7–13	2
5	49–52	27–39	14	3–5
6	53–63	40–41	15	6–10
7	64–70	42–45	16–20	11–18
8	71–76	46–48	21–22	19–28
9	77–82	49–51	23–25	29–40
10	83–88	52–57	26–28	41–59
11	89–93	58–60	29	60–71
12	94–96	61–65	30–32	72–81
13	97–98	66–71	33–36	82–89
14	99–104	72–75	37–39	90–94
15	105	76–80	40–43	95–97
16	106–109	81	44	98
17	110–114	82	45	99
18	>114	>82	>45	>99
Type of score for each test	Correct Count	Correct Count	Correct Count	
Age range (years) used for each test's norms	74–84	74–84	74–84	
Normative sample size (N) for each test	88	88	88	

Source: Ivnik et al., 1996. Reprinted with the kind permission of Psychology Press.

Table 8–53 Golden Version: MOANS Scaled Scores for Persons Whose Ages Range From 81 to 83

| Scaled Scores | Raw Scores Earned | | | Percentile Ranges |
| | Stroop | | | |
	Word	Color	C/W	
2	<41	<23	<4	<1
3	41–44	23	4	1
4	45–47	24–25	5–6	2
5	48–52	26–30	7–10	3–5
6	53–63	31–39	11–15	6–10
7	64–69	40–42	16	11–18
8	70–74	43–45	17–19	19–28
9	75–80	46–49	20–22	29–40
10	81–86	50–53	23–25	41–59
11	87–91	54–56	26–28	60–71
12	92–96	57–59	29–30	72–81
13	97–98	60–64	31–32	82–89
14	99–104	65–71	33–38	90–94
15	105	72–78	39–40	95–97
16	106–109	79–80	41–43	98
17	110–114	81	44	99
18	>114	>81	>44	>99
Type of score for each test	Correct Count	Correct Count	Correct Count	
Age range (years) used for each test's norms	>76	>76	>76	
Normative sample size (N) for each test	79	79	79	

Source: Ivnik et al., 1996. Reprinted with the kind permission of Psychology Press.

Table 8–54 MOANS Scaled Scores for Persons Whose Ages Range From 84 to 86

| | Raw Scores Earned | | | |
| | Stroop | | | Percentile |
Scaled Scores	Word	Color	C/W	Ranges
2	<41	<23	<4	<1
3	41–44	23	4	1
4	45–47	24–25	5–6	2
5	48–52	26–30	7–10	3–5
6	53–63	31–39	11–15	6–10
7	64–69	40–42	16	11–18
8	70–74	43–45	17–19	19–28
9	75–80	46–49	20–22	29–40
10	81–86	50–53	23–25	41–59
11	87–91	54–56	26–28	60–71
12	92–96	57–59	29–30	72–81
13	97–98	60–64	31–32	82–89
14	99–104	65–71	33–38	90–94
15	105	72–78	39–40	95–97
16	106–109	79–80	41–43	98
17	110–114	81	44	99
18	>114	>81	>44	>99
Type of score for each test	Correct Count	Correct Count	Correct Count	
Age range (years) used for each test's norms	>76	>76	>76	
Normative sample size (N) for each test	79	79	79	

Source: Ivnik et al., 1996. Reprinted with the kind permission of Psychology Press.

Table 8–55 MOANS Scaled Scores for Persons Whose Ages Range From 87 to 89

| | Raw Scores Earned | | | |
| | Stroop | | | Percentile |
Scaled Scores	Word	Color	C/W	Ranges
2	<41	<23	<4	<1
3	41–44	23	4	1
4	45–47	24–25	5–6	2
5	48–52	26–30	7–10	3–5
6	53–63	31–39	11–15	6–10
7	64–69	40–42	16	11–18
8	70–74	43–45	17–19	19–28
9	75–80	46–49	20–22	29–40
10	81–86	50–53	23–25	41–59
11	87–91	54–56	26–28	60–71
12	92–96	57–59	29–30	72–81
13	97–98	60–64	31–32	82–89
14	99–104	65–71	33–38	90–94
15	105	72–78	39–40	95–97
16	106–109	79–80	41–43	98
17	110–114	81	44	99
18	>114	>81	>44	>99
Type of score for each test	Correct Count	Correct Count	Correct Count	
Age range (years) used for each test's norms	>76	>76	>76	
Normative sample size (N) for each test	79	79	79	

Source: Ivnik et al., 1996. Reprinted with the kind permission of Psychology Press.

Table 8–56 MOANS Scaled Scores for Persons Whose Ages Range From 90 to 97

| Scaled Scores | Raw Scores Earned | | | Percentile Ranges |
| | Stroop | | | |
	Word	Color	C/W	
2	<41	<23	<4	<1
3	41–44	23	4	1
4	45–47	24–25	5–6	2
5	48–52	26–30	7–10	3–5
6	53–63	31–39	11–15	6–10
7	64–69	40–42	16	11–18
8	70–74	43–45	17–19	19–28
9	75–80	46–49	20–22	29–40
10	81–86	50–53	23–25	41–59
11	87–91	54–56	26–28	60–71
12	92–96	57–59	29–30	72–81
13	97–98	60–64	31–32	82–89
14	99–104	65–71	33–38	90–94
15	105	72–78	39–40	95–97
16	106–109	79–80	41–43	98
17	110–114	81	44	99
18	>114	>81	>44	>99
Type of score for each test	Correct Count	Correct Count	Correct Count	
Age range (years) used for each test's norms	>76	>76	>76	
Normative sample size (*N*) for each test	79	79	79	

Source: Ivnik et al., 1996. Reprinted with the kind permission of Psychology Press.

age from 5 to 14 years, predominantly female. The sample sizes in each age group are modest (15–39), and apart from information regarding age, the sample is not well described (see Table 8–59).

RELIABILITY

Test-Retest Reliability and Practice Effects

Bullock et al. (unpublished data) tested university students twice on the Victoria version, with a one-month interval between test sessions. Reliability coefficients were high: Coefficients of .90, .83, and .91 were found for the three parts of the test. However, experience with the test does affect performance. Students showed significant practice effects. On the second administration, performance improved by about two seconds on Parts D and W and by about five seconds on Part C.

Similar results have been reported for other versions of the test (e.g., Delis et al., 2001; Dikmen et al., 1999; Feinstein et al., 1994; Graf et al., 1995; Naglieri & Das, 1997; Neyens & Aldenkamp, 1996; Sachs et al., 1991; Stroop, 1935; Trenerry

et al., 1989), including the Golden version (Connor et al., 1988; Franzen et al., 1987; Golden, 1975), although reliabilities for the interference trial tend to be in the marginal/adequate range. Thus, Golden (1975) reported reliabilities of .89 (Word), .84 (Color), and .73 (Color-Word; $N = 450$) for a group-administered version of the test, and reliabilities of .86, .82, and .73, respectively ($N = 30$), for the individual version.

Table 8–57 Computational Formula for Age- and Education-Corrected MOANS Scaled Score

Age- and education-corrected MOANS scaled score
= k (constant) + (W_1 × Age-MOANS Scaled Score)
− (W_2 × number of years of formal schooling).
The specific values are:

Stroop	K	W_1	W_2
Word	3.47	1.10	0.34
Color	1.88	1.10	0.23
C/W	1.38	1.09	0.19

Source: From Ivnik et al., 1996. Reprinted with the kind permission of Psychology Press.

Table 8–58a MOAANS Age-based Stroop Norms in African American Adults

Ages	56–62			63–65			66–68			
Scaled Score	Word	Color	C-W	Word	Color	C-W	Word	Color	C-W	Percentile Ranges
2	0–45	0–32	0–3	0–45	0–32	0–3	0–37	0–23	0–3	<1
3	46–48	—	4–5	46–48	—	4	38–44	24–32	4	1
4	49–51	33	6–8	49–51	33	—	45–46	33	—	2
5	52–62	34–38	9–12	52–62	34–38	5–8	47–50	34–36	5–8	3–5
6	63–67	39–44	13–14	63–66	39–44	9–12	52–64	37–41	9–10	6–10
7	68–73	45–49	15–16	67–71	45–48	13–15	65–69	42–47	11–14	11–18
8	74–79	50–52	17–20	72–76	49–52	16–18	70–74	48–50	15–16	19–28
9	80–83	53–57	21–23	77–82	53–57	19–21	75–79	51–55	17–20	29–40
10	84–90	58–62	24–28	83–88	58–62	22–26	80–87	56–61	21–25	41–59
11	91–96	63–69	29–31	89–95	63–67	27–29	88–92	62–64	26–28	60–71
12	97–101	70–73	32–36	96–99	68–72	30–34	93–97	65–71	29–32	72–81
13	102–107	74–76	37–38	100–106	73–76	35–37	98–105	72–76	33–37	82–89
14	108–112	77–80	39–40	107–109	77–79	38–40	106–107	77–79	38–39	90–94
15	113–123	81–82	41–42	110–121	80–82	41–42	108–110	80–82	40–42	95–97
16	124–125	83–85	43–44	122–125	83–84	43–44	111–112	83	43–44	98
17	126–130	86–89	—	126–130	85–88	—	113–121	84–87	—	99
18	131+	90+	45+	131+	89+	45+	122+	88+	45+	>99
N	106	106	106	128	128	128	165	165	165	

Ages	69–71			72–74			75–77			
Scaled Score	Word	Color	C-W	Word	Color	C-W	Word	Color	C-W	Percentile Ranges
2	0–34	0–20	0–3	0–34	0–20	0–3	0–34	0–20	0–3	<1
3	35–44	21–30	4	35–37	21–25	4	35–37	21–25	4	1
4	45–46	31	—	38–46	26–29	—	38–42	26–27	—	2
5	47–49	32–34	5–8	47–48	30–33	5–8	43–47	28–32	5–8	3–5
6	50–63	35–40	9–10	49–60	34–37	9–10	48–58	33–36	9–10	6–10
7	64–67	41–44	11–13	61–66	38–43	11–13	59–64	37–41	11–13	11–18
8	68–73	45–49	14–16	67–70	44–47	14–16	65–70	42–46	14–16	19–28
9	74–78	50–54	17–19	71–76	48–51	17–19	71–76	47–50	17–18	29–40
10	79–87	55–60	20–24	77–87	52–59	20–24	77–87	51–59	19–23	41–59
11	88–92	61–62	25–27	88–92	60–62	25–26	88–92	60–61	24–26	60–71
12	93–97	63–68	28–31	93–97	63–67	27–29	93–96	62–64	27–29	72–81
13	98–101	69–73	32–36	98–101	68–73	30–32	97–101	65–73	30–32	82–89
14	102–106	74–78	37–38	102–106	74–78	33–37	102–105	74–78	33–36	90–94
15	107–109	79–82	39–42	107–109	79–82	38–39	106–109	79–82	37–38	95–97
16	110	83	43	110	83	40–42	110	83	—	98
17	111–112	84–87	44	111–112	84–87	43	111–112	84–87	39–43	99
18	113+	88+	45+	113+	88+	44+	113+	88+	44+	>99
N	182	182	182	156	156	156	119	119	119	

Ages	78+			
Scaled Score	Word	Color	C-W	Percentile Ranges
2	0–30	0–20	0–3	<1
3	31–37	21–23	4	1
4	38–42	—	—	2
5	43–47	24–26	5–8	3–5
6	48–57	27–33	9–10	6–10
7	58–61	33–39	11–12	11–18
8	62–69	40–42	13–15	19–28
9	70–74	43–48	16–17	29–40
10	75–83	49–55	18–20	41–59
11	84–90	56–59	21–24	60–71
12	91–95	60–64	25–27	72–81
13	96–99	65–70	28–29	82–89
14	100–103	71–76	30–31	90–94
15	104–107	77–79	32–34	95–97
16	108–109	80–81	35–36	98
17	—	82–83	37–38	99
18	110+	84+	39+	>99
N	78	78	78	

Table 8–58b Computational Formula for Age- and Education-Corrected MOAANS Scaled Scores

	K	W_1	W_2
Word Reading	2.49	1.10	0.29
Color Color Naming	2.82	1.09	0.31
Stroop Interference	2.77	1.08	0.28

Age- and education-corrected MOAANS Scaled Scores ($MSS_{A\&E}$) can be calculated for Stroop scores by using aged-corrected MOAANS scaled scores (MSS_A) and education (expressed in years completed) in the following formula: $MSS_{A\&E} = K + (W_1 \times MSS_A) - (W_2 \times EDUC)$

Source: From Lucas et al., 2005. Reprinted with the kind permission of the Mayo Foundation for Medical Education and Research.

However, the intertest interval and the characteristics of the subjects were not described. Franzen et al. (1987) gave the Golden version to 62 healthy individuals on two occasions, spaced one or two weeks apart. The coefficients were .83 for the Word score, .74 for the Color score, and .67 for the Color-Word score. Like the Victoria version, there were significant increases in scores, with gains in number of correct responses of about five points on the Word and Color trials and four points on the Color-Word trial. These increases may not affect interpretation of the results if interpretation is based on pattern and not level because all scores increase consistently (Connor et al., 1988; but see Feinstein et al., 1994, who found marked practice effects on the Color-Naming and Interference trials but not on the Color-Reading trial). The reason for the improvement in performance is not certain but may reflect an active learning process that suppresses distraction and/or a habituation of competing responses (Reisberg et al., 1980).

Alternate Form Reliability

Although Stroop (1935) made an equivalent form of the test by printing the cards in reverse order, most examiners have generally retested subjects with the same set of cards. Sachs

Table 8–59 Characteristics of the Stroop Children's Normative Sample Provided by Golden and Freshwater, 2002

Number	182
Age	5–14 years[a]
Geographic location	Not reported
Sample type	Not reported
Parental education	Not reported
Gender	Not specified but biased toward females
Race/ethnicity	Not reported
Screening	Not reported

[a]*N* in each age group: 5: 17, 6: 21, 7: 21, 8: 39, 9: 15, 10: 21, 11–12: 25; 13–14: 23

et al. (1991) developed five equivalent forms of the Dodrill version. The reliability coefficient for parallel forms was .82. Due to the presence of significant practice effects, examiners interested in documenting change by repeat measurement on the same or alternate forms should ensure that patients have sufficient practice with the test, at least more than one practice trial (Franzen et al., 1987; Sachs et al., 1991). Connor et al. (1988) reported that the increases tend to become asymptotic after three administrations.

VALIDITY

Correlations Within the Test

Correlations among test trials tend to be moderate in normal individuals for the Victoria version (Pineda & Merchan, 2003) and moderate/high for the Golden version (Chafetz & Matthew, 2004), suggesting that they are tapping similar, although not totally identical, abilities.

Correlation With Other Tests

The interference score correlates moderately well with other measures of attention including omission errors on continuous performance tasks ($R^2 = .31$; Weinstein et al., 1999) and the PASAT (MacLeod & Prior, 1996). The interference score is moderately related to other measures of prepotent response inhibition such as the stopping probability ($r = .33$) and time (.56) of the stop-signal task (May & Hasher, 1998; also see Friedman & Miyake, in press) and the difference score between Trails A and B (.55; May & Hasher, 1998).

The inhibition-related function tapped by the Stroop appears similar to another inhibitory function, the ability to resist or resolve interference from irrelevant information in the external environment. However, it seems to tap a different inhibitory process than that involved in resistance to proactive interference (i.e., the ability to resist memory intrusions from previously relevant information; Friedman & Miyake, in press).

Working memory contributes to Stroop interference. Recently, Kane and Engle (2003) reported that individual differences in working memory capacity predict performance on the Stroop task, indicating the importance of goal maintenance in the face of competition from habit. These authors propose a dual-mechanism view of the Stroop effect. That is, Stroop interference may reflect a failure to maintain the task goal of ignoring the word dimension. Interference may also reflect the time-consuming process of resolving response competition in service of a successfully activated goal.

Other factors such as conceptual ability and speed of processing are also important (Anstey et al., 2002; Graf et al., 1995; MacLeod & Prior, 1996; Sherman et al., 1995; Shum et al., 1990). For example, Anstey et al. (2002) found that in healthy older adults, Stroop interference loads on the same factor as a measure of fluid intelligence, the Raven's Progressive Matrices. Similarly, Graf et al. (1995) reported that in healthy older adults, Stroop interference loads on the same factor as several WAIS subtests that measure speed of processing and conceptual abilities (Digit Symbol, Block Design, Similarities).

There is additional evidence that Stroop interference needs to be interpreted within the context of mental speed. For instance, in normal elderly individuals, 85% of age-related variance in the Stroop incongruent condition is due to overall processing speed (Salthouse & Meinz, 1995). Further, in clinical samples, Stroop interference loads on factors that appear to represent speed of processing (e.g., Digit Symbol, Trails A, FAS) rather than executive functions as measured by tests such as WCST and Trails B (Bondi et al. 2002; Boone et al. 1998).

The interference trial also invokes the semantic system and perhaps aspects of planning. Bondi et al. (2002) noted that in normal individuals, the interference trial loaded on a factor representing semantic knowledge (FAS, BNT, vocabulary) and attention (Digit Span). Similarly, Hanes et al. (1996) found that in patients with schizophrenia, Parkinson's disease, and Huntington's disease, Stroop interference showed strong relations with performance on a semantic (Category) fluency task ($r = .58$) and the number of trials to completion on the Tower of London ($r = .65$), but only modest or little relations with other tasks, such as delayed recall of the Rey figure ($r = .31$) and peg placement on the Purdue Pegboard ($r = .12$).

Clinical Studies

Increased interference has been found in a variety of patient groups thought to have executive disturbance, including schizophrenia (Hanes et al., 1996; Moritz et al., 2002), Parkinson's disease (Hanes et al., 1996), Huntington's disease (Hanes et al., 1996; Snowden et al., 2001), Friedreich's ataxia (White et al., 2000), age-associated memory impairment (Hanninen et al., 1997), prenatal exposure to alcohol (Connor et al., 2000), chronic alcoholism (Dao-Castellana et al., 1998), HIV infection (Castellon et al., 2000), benign focal childhood epilepsy (Chevalier et al., 2000), and ADHD (Homack & Riccio, 2004; Reeve & Schandler, 2001; but see Perugini et al., 2000). Head-injured patients are typically slower to respond on all subtasks, although they do not consistently demonstrate disproportionate difficulty on the interference condition (e.g., Batchelor et al., 1995; Felmingham et al., 2004; McLean et al., 1983; Ponsford & Kinsella, 1992; Rios et al., 2004).

The interference effect can be elicited more readily in mildly head-injured patients with a more challenging version of the Stroop test (Batchelor et al., 1995; Bohnen et al., 1992). The modification (Bohnen et al., 1992; see also *D-KEFS*) consists of drawing rectangular lines around a random selection of one-fifth of the items comprising the Color-Word subtest. On the boxed items, subjects are required to read the word rather than name the color of the print. Thus, task complexity is increased by requiring flexibility in directing attention to the naming and reading of the different items. Aloia et al. (1997) suggest, however, that a more drastic modification may be necessary to elicit interference.

Increased Stroop interference is also associated with dementia (e.g., Bondi et al., 2002; Nathan et al., 2001; Spieler et al., 1996). The breakdown in inhibitory processes appears to occur early in the course of AD, and the magnitude of the interference effect increases with increasing severity of dementia (Bondi et al., 2002; Koss et al., 1984). However, the correlations between Stroop performance and dementia severity tend to be modest in size (about .30), suggesting that the task may be less useful in tracking disease progression than for the early detection of AD. Increased interference has also been reported in nondemented patients with subcortical lacunar infarcts, with the extent of white matter signal hyperintensity correlated to Stroop performance (Kramer et al., 2002).

The prefrontal cortex appears to be highly sensitive to the effects of increasing age (West & Bell, 1997). Because this region is considered critical for adequate Stroop performance (see *Neuroanatomical Correlates*), one might expect increased interference with advancing age. However, studies of aging and Stroop interference have been somewhat contradictory (Troyer et al., in press). Graf et al. (1995) found no effect of age on the ratio index of interference in adults aged 65 or older, but they only examined older adults. Using a broader sample, aged 12 to 83 years, Uttl and Graf (1997) found a small influence of age in the incongruent condition. They interpreted the age effects in Stroop interference as due to age-related decline in processing speed (indexed also by color naming and by word reading), and not as evidence of a selective age-related decline in specific cognitive functions, such as cognitive flexibility and control (see also Salthouse & Meinz, 1995). Others, however, have found an age-related increase in interference even when generalized slowing is taken into account (e.g., Troyer et al., in press; Wecker et al., 2000). Increased errors with age have also been reported (Delis et al., 2001; Troyer et al., in press), suggesting that age-related decrements on the Stroop task are related to cognitive processes (e.g., response inhibition) other than or perhaps in addition to generalized slowing. Shilling et al. (2002) has suggested that age-related declines in fluid intelligence may be sufficient to explain age-related changes in Stroop.

There are, however, other challenges to the identification of aging effects on the Stroop task with deficits in executive functioning. Antsey et al. (2002) recently reported that age differences in Stroop performance were explained entirely by color vision performance (see later discussion), suggesting the operation of a more general biological aging process.

Diminished performance on the Stroop test has also been documented in depressed patients (Kalska et al., 1999; Moritz et al., 2002; Nathan et al., 2001; Raskin et al., 1982; but see Crews et al., 1999), particularly those with bipolar as opposed to unipolar depression (Borkowska & Rybakowski, 2001) and in anxious patients (Batchelor et al., 1995; but see Vingerhoets et al., 1995, who found no relation between psychological distress and cognitive performance in patients before or after open-heart surgery). The implication is that the clinician should not necessarily conclude that poor performance on the task is syndrome specific.

It should also be noted that the manual for the Golden version of the Stroop (2002) suggests various interpretive hypotheses for patterns obtained on the three scores. However, little support is given in the manual (but see Golden & Golden, 2002, for some preliminary data with regard to children with learning disabilities, attention deficit, and psychiatric problems).

With regard to predictive validity, baseline interference scores on the Golden version are predictive of functional status at one-year follow-up in patients with vascular dementia (Boyle et al., 2004).

Diagnostic Validity

The test's utility in cases of mild head injury is questionable. Sensitivity, specificity, efficiency (i.e., number of subjects correctly classified, defined as true positives + true negatives/N), positive predictive power, negative predictive power, and odds ratios for the Golden version of the Stroop Test were examined by Cicerone and Azulay (2002) in a group of patients with postconcussion syndrome (PCS) and matched controls, screened for symptom exaggeration. These are reproduced in Table 8–60. Values for various impairment levels were calculated, with impairment defined as 1.5 SDs below the mean. The Stroop speed and in particular interference variables showed limited sensitivity, which indicates that they would have limited utility in *ruling out* the presence of PCS. However, their high specificity suggests considerable utility in *ruling in* PCS (i.e., persons without PCS are unlikely to have impaired scores). The positive predictive power of the speed score was strong, indicating the diagnostic utility of impaired scores on the test. According to criteria set by the authors (i.e., odds ratio equal to or greater than three, lower limit of the confidence interval greater than one), the speed scores (particularly Stroop Color subtest) showed reliable, positive associations with PCS. Values for the interference score were not strongly supportive of its diagnostic utility in this group.

Neuroanatomical Correlates

Neuroimaging and electrophysiological studies have shown that the frontal lobe is the most consistent region of activation (Brown et al., 1999; Dao-Castellana et al., 1998; Mead et al., 2002; West & Bell, 1997). In line with these findings, patients with focal frontal lesions tend to show greater than normal levels of interference on Stroop tests (Mellier & Fessard, 1998; Stuss et al., 2001; Vendrell et al., 1995; but see Wildgruber et al., 2000, who found sensitivity to be poor), including the Victoria version (Perret, 1981; Regard, 1981). A recent meta-analysis (Demakis, 2004) compared patients with frontal lobe damage with those with damage to posterior brain regions. Significant differences between groups were found for all trials of the Stroop (weighted effect sizes of −.33 for Word, −.36 for Color, −.45 for Color-Word). However, use of Stroop performance alone was not sufficient to discriminate between frontal and nonfrontal groups. In fact, the amount of overlap between the distributions of these two groups at these effect sizes was about 70% to 79%, indicating little separation of groups and thus relatively poor sensitivity (true positives) and specificity (true negatives). Because it is incorrect to discuss

Table 8–60 Diagnostic Utility of the Stroop Test (Golden Version) in Postconcussion Syndrome: Sensitivity, Specificity, Efficiency, Positive Predictive Power, Negative Predictive Power, and Diagnostic Accuracy (Odds Ratio and 90% Confidence Interval) for Scores Greater than −1.5 SDs Below the Mean

	Stroop C	Stroop CW	Stroop Interference
Sensitivity	25.0	22.5	3.2
Specificity	96.6	93.3	100.0
Efficiency[a]	60.7	57.4	50.8
Positive predictive power	88.9	77.8	100.0
Negative predictive power	55.8	53.8	53.8
Odds ratio	7.1	3.5	3.0
90% confidence interval	1.5–32.8	1.3–9.5	0.3–45.3

Note: The base rate of postconcussion syndrome in this sample was 50%; the sample included 32 postconcussive patients screened for exaggeration and 32 matched controls.
[a]Refers to the number of subjects correctly classified (true positives + true negatives / N).

Source: Adapted from Cicerone & Azulay, 2002.

frontal lobe functioning as global concept (Stuss et al., 2001), researchers have sought to identify the contributions of different subregions.

A variety of frontal sites have been proposed as critical for recruiting cognitive control in the Stroop task, including the lateral prefrontal cortex and the anterior cingulate cortex (ACC; e.g., Brown et al., 1999; Kerns et al., 2004; Ravnkilde et al., 2002; Stuss et al., 2001). Based on fMRI studies of normal individuals, Kerns et al. (2004) have suggested that the prefrontal cortex is involved in implementing control processes to overcome conflict, whereas the ACC detects conflicts between plans of action and implements a conflict-monitoring function.

Although frontal systems appear critical, the task is mediated by a more broadly based system. Stroop performance is associated with AD pathology in the hippocampus and a number of neocortical regions including posterior cerebral areas (Bondi et al., 2002; Collette et al., 2002). Further, fMRI activations obtained in healthy adults during performance of the Stroop task include not only the frontal region but also inferior temporal and parietal cortices as well as the caudate nuclei (Peterson et al., 2002).

Vision, Reading, and Stroop Performance

Visual competence is important. In older adults, results may be confounded by age-related declines in visual acuity or color vision (Anstey et al., 2000, 2002; van Boxtel et al., 2001). Van Boxtel et al. (2001) examined adults aged 52 to 84 and noted that after adjustment for age, gender, and educational level, low contrast sensitivity was associated with more time needed on word naming, red/green color weakness was linked to slower color naming, and reduced distant acuity was associated with slower performance on the interference card. Half of the variance in Stroop performance explained by age alone could also be explained by visual function variables. Obviously, color blindness precludes use of this test; however, these findings suggest that even subtle defects in visual function of the type observed in normal aging can impact Stroop performance.

The amount of interference also depends on the subject's familiarity with the stimuli and the semantic relatedness of the material (e.g., pictures versus words; Graf et al., 1995). The degree of automaticity of the reading response is also a critical factor. Cox et al. (1997) recommend that interpretation of the interference score as a measure of response inhibition be restricted to those whose single word readings are at least equal to their Full-Scale IQs.

Time-of-Day Effects

Time of testing (i.e., level of circadian arousal) may also impact the magnitude of the Stroop effect, at least in older adults. May and Hasher (1998) reported that Stroop interference is equivalent in young adults (ages 17–21) tested in the morning or the evening. However, when older adults (ages

63–76) are tested at their nonoptimal times (i.e., evening), inhibitory efficiency is compromised.

Malingering

Van Gorp et al. (1999) reported that probable malingerers take significantly more time to complete the color naming and interference trials than nonmalingerers, although the task does not reliably identify those who are malingering. Lu et al. (2004) noted that the Stroop test may be particularly useful in patients complaining of complete illiteracy. They describe six patients who claimed that they were unable to perform the Word-Reading trial, but on the Color-Word Interference trial, they all committed errors by reading the written words. Five of the six patients also performed substantially slower on the Interference trial relative to the Color-Naming trial, indicating that they were in fact inhibiting a reading response. These authors indicate that a complaint of total reading disability is rare; however, when such a complaint arises, failure to suppress the Stroop effect may be a valuable diagnostic tool to test the veracity of this symptom presentation.

COMMENT

The Stroop paradigm is one of the oldest and most widely used techniques to examine attention and response inhibition (MacLeod, 1991). Multiple versions of the Stroop test exist (see *Description*), and this diversity poses significant challenges for the clinician since they may not be tapping the same underlying processes (Salthouse & Meinz, 1995; Shilling et al., 2002). For example, Salthouse and Meinz (1995) found that correlations between difference scores on three different Stroop tasks were low to moderate in size. Similarly, Shilling et al. (2002) reported that sensitivity to interference on one of four different Stroop tasks did not predict sensitivity to interference on the others. The level of individual consistency in performance will depend on the similarity of the tasks used. Whether the various Stroop versions popular in clinical contexts yield scores that are highly correlated with one another is not known.

Several issues need to be considered in identifying an appropriate Stroop version for a particular client. In addition to the stimulus properties and number of trials included in a task, a variety of other factors may influence the incidence and extent of Stroop interference and the likelihood of engaging particular neural systems. Stroop (1935) employed neutral and incongruent conditions to measure interference. If no baseline (neutral) condition is employed, interpretation of Stroop results as measuring interference is not warranted (Henik, 1996). The incongruent condition measures general performance (e.g., general slowness) and also interference; if only one condition is given, it is impossible to tease them apart. Sometimes, patients are given the card used for the incongruent condition and are asked once to read the word and ignore the color, and as a second condition, they are asked to name the color and ignore the word (e.g., Dodrill, 1978; Trenerry et al., 1989). This comparison is also problematic since it confounds differences between tasks and interference (Henik, 1996). For example, the difference between color naming and word reading could reflect interference of color on word or word on color.

Some (e.g., Spieler et al., 1996) have expressed concern that blocked trials (i.e., separate trials where all items are either congruent or incongruent) such as occur on the Victoria and Golden Stroop Tests might allow participants to develop strategies to focus on the relevant dimensions of the stimuli. However, such a design format (as opposed to mixing of congruent and incongruent trials as in the D-KEFS) may strengthen the test's sensitivity to various clinical conditions (e.g., dementia) because such strategies are less likely to be used by such patients (Bondi et al., 2002). On the other hand, such blocked presentations of incongruent trials may minimize working memory involvement because the task demands remain consistent across trials, making it easier for the individuals to keep the goal in mind. Every incongruent stimulus therefore reinforces the goal, to ignore the word, and so the task environment acts in place of the central executive (Kane & Engle, 2003).

The choice of Stroop version needs to be guided, in part, by the adequacy of the normative base. There is insufficient information regarding the adult normative sample provided by Golden (1978; Golden & Freshwater, 2002); rather, the normative sets published by Ivnik et al. (1996), Steinberg et al. (2005), and Moering et al. (2004) appear preferable. Note, however, that the norms typically apply to older adults. Norms for young and middle-aged adults are sparse. For the Victoria version, the normative set provided by Troyer et al. (in press) is recommended and can be used with adults across a wide age range. However, the Victoria version lacks data for children and adolescents and the standardization sample in Golden's Children's version is small and not well described. The CAS includes Stroop tasks for individuals aged 5 to 17 years. A key asset of the D-KEFS is that norms are available for individuals aged 8 to 89 years.

There are a number of techniques to analyze test time. Difference scores between conditions are often used but may not be sufficiently independent of general slowing. To overcome baseline differences in response speed, a proportion score, which takes into account the individual's baseline speed, is recommended.

The model underlying the interference score in the Golden version has recently been questioned. Golden (1978) assumes an additive model where the time to read a CW item is an additive function of the time to read a word plus the time to name a color. By contrast, Chafetz and Matthews (2004) propose that the time to read a CW item reflects the time to suppress the reading of a word plus the time to name a color. This model appears to provide a better fit with clinical and lifespan (maturational) data.

Error analysis of the Stroop is less common than examination of time scores but is available for some versions (e.g., Victoria, D-KEFS). Brain disorders may impair word or color processing or cause distractibility, slowing, perseveration, or indifference. These various qualities may influence the susceptibility to error and therefore, analysis of errors may be particularly important in neurologically impaired populations (Stuss et al., 2001).

The psychological mechanisms underlying the task include working memory, speed of processing information, semantic activation, and the ability to strengthen one response characteristic. The test taps somewhat different abilities than other executive measures (e.g., WCST). Therefore, adequate assessment requires the use of more than one test of executive function (e.g., Boone et al., 1998; Pineda & Merchan, 2003). The neural basis for performance of the different conditions, especially the incongruent condition, are not certain, although there is evidence from disparate sources of the importance of the frontal lobes, in particular the anterior cingulate cortex and the lateral prefrontal cortex. Bear in mind, however, that while frontal systems appear critical, task performance depends on a more broadly based system.

Intact visual function is critical since results may be confounded by impairments in color vision and visual acuity. Stroop test results should be interpreted with caution in older people (Anstey et al., 2002; Van Boxtel et al., 2001), and in some age groups (e.g., over age 90 years), the task is likely not suitable (Anstey et al., 2000).

The finding that older adults show reliable differences over the course of the day (May & Hasher, 1998) is also important. Time of testing must be considered in the administration of the Stroop to allow appropriate assessment of behavior in both single-test and test-retest situations. It is also possible that normative data needs to be reevaluated with testing time controlled (May & Hasher, 1998).

Finally, the interference trial (at least in the Golden version) has only marginal/acceptable reliability. Accordingly, this score should not be used as the basis of diagnostic decisions without supplementation by other data.

REFERENCES

Aloia, M. S., Weed, N. C., & Marx, B. (1997). Some construct network effects of modifying the Stroop Color and Word Test. *The Clinical Neuropsychologist, 11*, 54–58.

Antsey, K. J., Dain, S., Andrews, S., & Drobny, J. (2002). Visual abilities in older adults explain age-differences in Stroop and fluid intelligence but not face recognition: Implications for the vision-cognition connection. *Aging, Neuropsychology, & Cognition, 9*, 253–265.

Anstey, K. J., Matters, B., Brown, A. K., & Lord, S. R. (2000). Normative data on neuropsychological tests for very old adults living in retirement villages and hostels. *The Clinical Neuropsychologist, 14*, 309–317.

Armegnol, C. G. (2002). Stroop test in Spanish: Children's norms. *The Clinical Neuropsychologist, 16*, 67–80.

Artiola I Fortuny, L., Romo, D. H., Heaton, R. K., & Pardee III, R. E. (1999). *Manual de normas y procedimemientos para la bateria neuropsicologia en espanol.* The Netherlands: Swets & Zeitlinger.

Batchelor, J., Harvery, A. G., & Bryant, R. A. (1995). Stroop Color Word Test as a measure of attentional deficit following mild head injury. *The Clinical Neuropsychologist, 9*, 180–186.

Bohnen, N., Jolles, J., & Twijnstra, A. (1992). Modification of the Stroop Color Word Test improves differentiation between patients with mild head injury and matched controls. *The Clinical Neuropsychologist, 6*, 178–188.

Bondi, M. W., Serody, A. B., Chan, A. S., Eberson-Schumate, S. C., Delis, D. C., Hansen, L. A., & Salmon, D. P. (2002). Cognitive and neuropathologic correlates of Stroop Color-Word Test performance in Alzheimer's disease. *Neuropsychology, 16*, 335–343.

Boone, K. B., Ponton, M. O., Gorsuch, R. L., Gonzalez, J. J., & Miller, B. L. (1998). Factor analysis of four measures of prefrontal lobe functioning. *Archives of Clinical Neuropsychology, 13*, 585–595.

Borkowska, A., & Rybakowski, J. (2001). Neuropsychological frontal lobe tests indicate that bipolar depressed patients are more impaired than unipolar. *Bipolar Disorders, 3*, 89–94.

Boyle, P. A., Paul, R. H., Moser, D. J., & Cohen, R. A. (2004). Executive impairments predict functional declines in vascular dementia. *The Clinical Neuropsychologist, 18*, 75–82.

Brown, G. G., Kindermann, S. S., Siegle, G. J., Granholm, E., Wang, E. C., & Bukton, R. B. (1999). Brain activation and pupil response during covert performance of the Stroop Color Word task. *Journal of the International Neuropsychological Society, 5*, 308–319.

Castellon, S. A., Hinkin, C. H., & Myers, H. F. (2000). Neuropsychiatric disturbance is associated with executive dysfunction in HIV-1 infection. *Journal of the International Neuropsychological Society, 6*, 336–347.

Chafetz, M. D., & Matthews, L. H. (2004). A new interference score for the Stroop test. *Archives of Clinical Neuropsychology, 19*, 555–567.

Chevalier, H., Metz-Lutz, M-N., & Segalowitz, S. J. (2000). Impulsivity and control of inhibition in benign focal childhood epilepsy. *Brain and Cognition, 43*, 86–90.

Cicerone, K. D., & Azulay, J. (2002). Diagnostic utility of attention measures in postconcussion syndrome. *The Clinical Neuropsychologist, 16*, 280–289.

Collette, F., Van der Linden, M., Delrue, G., & Salmon, E. (2002). Frontal hypometabolism does not explain inhibitory dysfunction in Alzheimer disease. *Alzheimer Disease & Associated Disorders, 16*, 228–238.

Comalli Jr., P. E., Wapner, S., & Werner, H. (1962). Interference effects of Stroop Color-Word Test in childhood, adulthood and aging. *Journal of Genetic Psychology, 100*, 47–53.

Connor, A., Franzen, M., & Sharp, B. (1988). Effects of practice and differential instructions on Stroop performance. *International Journal of Clinical Neuropsychology, 10*, 1–4.

Connor, P. D., Sampson, P. D., Bookstein, F. L., Barr, H. M., & Streissguth, A. P. (2000). Direct and indirect effects of prenatal alcohol damage on executive function. *Developmental Neuropsychology, 18*, 331–354.

Cox, C. S., Chee, E., Chase, G. A., Baumgardner, T. L., Schuerholz, L. J., Reader, M. J., Mohr, J., & Denkla, M. B. (1997). Reading proficiency affects the construct validity of the Stroop Test Interference Score. *The Clinical Neuropsychologist, 11*, 105–110.

Crews, W. D., Harrison, D. W., & Rhodes, R. D. (1999). Neuropsychological test performances of young depressed outpatient women: An examination of executive functions. *Archives of Clinical Neuropsychology, 14*, 517–529.

Dao-Castellana, M. H., Samson, Y., Legaugt, F., Martinot, J. L., Aubin, H. J., Crouzel, C., Feldman, L., Barrucand, D., Rancurel, G., Feline, A., & Syrota, A. (1998). Frontal dysfunction in neurologically normal chronic alcoholic subjects: Metabolic and neuropsychological findings. *Psychological Medicine, 28*, 1039–1048.

Delis, D. C., Kaplan, E., & Kramer, J. H. (2001). *Delis-Kaplan Executive Function System.* San Antonio, TX: The Psychological Corporation.

Demakis, G. J. (2004). Frontal lobe damage and tests of executive processing: A meta-analysis of the Category Test, Stroop Test, and Trail-Making Test. *Journal of Clinical and Experimental Neuropsychology, 26*, 441–450.

Dikmen, S. S., Heaton, R. K., Grant, I., & Temkin, N. R. (1999). Test-retest reliability and practice effects of expanded Halstead-Reitan Neuropsychological Test Battery. *Journal of the International Neuropsychological Society, 5*, 346–356.

Dodrill, C. B. (1978). A neuropsychological battery for epilepsy. *Epilepsia, 19*, 611–623.

Feinstein, A., Brown, R., & Ron, M. (1994). Effects of practice on serial tests of attention in healthy subjects. *Journal of Clinical and Experimental Neuropsychology, 16*, 436–447.

Felmingham, K. L., Baguley, I. J., & Green, A. M. (2004). Effects of diffuse axonal injury on speed of information processing following severe traumatic brain injury. *Neuropsychology, 18*, 564–571.

Franzen, M. D. (2000). *Reliability and validity in neuropsychological assessment* (2nd ed.). New York: Kluwer Academic/Plenum Publishers.

Franzen, M. D., Tishelman, A. C., Sharp, B. H., & Friedman, A. G. (1987). An investigation of the test-retest reliability of the Stroop Color-Word Test across two intervals. *Archives of Clinical Neuropsychology, 2*, 265–272.

Friedman, N. P., & Miyake, A. (in press). The relations among inhibition and interference control functions: A latent variable analysis. *JEP: General.*

Golden, C. J. (1975). A group version of the Stroop Color and Word Test. *Journal of Personality Assessment, 39*, 502–506.

Golden, C. J. (1976). Identification of brain disorders by the Stroop Color and Word Test. *Journal of Clinical Psychology, 32*, 654–658.

Golden, C. J. (1978). *Stroop Color and Word Test: A manual for clinical and experimental uses.* Chicago, IL: Stoelting Co.

Golden, C. J., & Freshwater, S. M. (2002). *Stroop Color and Word Test: Revised examiner's manual.* Wood Dale, IL: Stoelting Co.

Golden, C. J., Freshwater, S. M., & Golden, Z. (2003). *Stroop Color and Word Test Children's Version for ages 5–14.* Wood Date, IL: Stoelting Co.

Golden, Z. L., & Golden, C. J. (2002). Patterns of performance on the Stroop Color and Word Test in children with learning, attentional, and psychiatric disabilities. *Psychology in the Schools, 39*, 489–495.

Graf, P., Uttl, B., & Tuokko, H. (1995). Color- and picture-word Stroop tests: Performance changes in old age. *Journal of Clinical and Experimental Neuropsychology, 17*, 390–415.

Hanes, K. R., Andrewes, D. G., Smith, D. J., & Pantelis, C. (1996). A brief assessment of executive control dysfunction: Discriminant validity and homogeneity of planning, set shift, and fluency measures. *Archives of Clinical Neuropsychology, 11*, 185–191.

Hanninen, T., Hallikainen, M., Koivisto, K., Partanen, K., Laakso, M. P., Riekkinen, P. J., & Soininen, H. (1997). Decline of frontal lobe functions in subjects with age-associated memory impairment. *Neurology, 48*, 148–153.

Henik, A. (1996). Paying attention to the Stroop effect. *Journal of the International Neuropsychological Society, 2,* 467–470.

Homack, S., & Riccio, C. A. (2004). A meta-analysis of the sensitivity and specificity of the Stroop Color and Word Test with children. *Archives of Clinical Neuropsychology, 19,* 725–743.

Ivnik, R. J., Malec, J. F., Smith, G. E., & Tangalos, E. G. (1996). Neuropsychological test norms above age 55: COWAT, BNT, MAE token, WRAT-R reading, AMNART, Stroop, TMT, and JLO. *The Clinical Neuropsychologist, 10,* 262–278.

Jensen, A. (1965). Scoring the Stroop test. *Acta Psychologica, 24,* 398–408.

Kalska, H., Punamaki, R-L., Makinen-Pelli, T., & Saarinen, M. (1999). Memory and metamemory functioning among depressed patients. *Applied Neuropsychology, 6,* 96–107.

Kane, M. J., & Engle, R. W. (2003). Working-memory capacity and the control of attention: The contributions of goal neglect, response competition, and task set to Stroop interference. *Journal of Experimental Psychology: General, 132,* 47–70.

Kerns, J. G., Cohen, J. D., MacDonald, A. W., Cho, R. Y., Stenger, V. A., & Carter, C. S. (2004). Anterior cingulate conflict monitoring and adjustments in control. *Science, 303,* 102–123.

Klein, M., Ponds, R. W. H. M., Houx, P. J., & Jolles, J. (1997). Effect of test duration on age-related differences in Stroop interference. *Journal of Clinical and Experimental Neuropsychology, 19,* 77–82.

Koss, E., Ober, B. A., Delis, D. C., & Friedland, R. P. (1984). The Stroop Color-Word Test: Indicator of dementia severity. *International Journal of Neuroscience, 24,* 53–61.

Kramer, J. H., Reed, B. R., Mungas, D., Weiner, M. W., & Chui, H. C. (2002). Executive dysfunction in subcortical ischaemic vascular disease. *Journal of Neurology, Neurosurgery and Psychiatry, 72,* 217–220.

Lee, T. M. (2003). *Normative data: Neuropsychological measures for Hong Kong Chinese.* The University of Hong Kong Neuropsychology Laboratory.

Lu, P. H., Boone, K. B., Jiminez, N., & Razami, J. (2004). Failure to inhibit the reading response on the Stroop test: A pathognomic indicator of suspect effort. *Journal of Clinical and Experimental Neuropsychology, 26,* 180–189.

Lucas, J. A., Ivnik, R. J., Smith, G. E., Ferman, T. J., Willis, F. B., Petersen, R. C., & Graff-Radford, N. R. (2005). Mayo's Older African Americans Normative Studies: Norms for Boston naming test, Controlled Oral Word Association, Category Fluency, Animal Naming, Token Test, WRAT-3 Reading, Trail Making Test, Stroop Test, and Judgement of Line Orientation. *The Clinical Neuropsychologist, 19,* 243–269.

MacLeod, C. M. (1991). Half a century of research on the Stroop effect: An integrative review. *Psychological Bulletin, 109,* 163–203.

MacLeod, D., & Prior, M. (1996). Attention deficits in adolescents with ADHD and other clinical groups. *Child Neuropsychiatry, 2,* 1–10.

May, C. P., & Hasher, L. (1998). Synchrony effects in inhibitory control over thought and action. *Journal of Experimental Psychology: Human Perception and Performance, 24,* 363–379.

McLean, A., Temkin, N. R., Dikmen, S., & Wyler, A. R. (1983). The behavioral sequelae of head injury. *Journal of Clinical Neuropsychology, 5,* 361–376.

Mead, L. A., Mayer, A. R., Bobholz, J. A., Woodley, S. J., Cunningham, J. M., Hammeke, T. A., & Rao, S. M. (2002). Neural basis of the Stroop interference task: Response competition or selective attention. *Journal of the International Neuropsychological Society, 8,* 735–742.

Mellier, D. & Fessard, C. (1998). Preterm birth and cognitive inhibition. *European Review of Applied Psychology, 48,* 13–17.

Mitrushina, M. M., Boone, K. B., Razani, J., & D'Elia, L. F. (2005). *Handbook of normative data for neuropsychological assessment* (2nd ed.). New York: Oxford University Press.

Moering, R. G., Schinka, J. A., Mortimer, J. A., & Graves, A. B. (2004). Normative data for elderly African Americans for the Stroop Color and Word Test. *Archives of Clinical Neuropsychology, 19,* 61–71.

Moritz, S., Birkner, C., & Kloss, M. (2002). Executive functioning in obsessive-compulsive disorder, unipolar depression, and schizophrenia. *Archives of Clinical Neuropsychology, 17,* 477–483.

Naglieri, J. A., & Das, J. P. (1997). *Cognitive assessment systems interpretive handbook.* Itaska, IL: Riverside.

Nathan, J., Wilkinson, D., Stammers, S., & Low, J. L. (2001). The role of tests of frontal executive functioning in the detection of mild dementia. *International Journal of Geriatric Psychiatry, 16,* 18–26.

Neyens, L. G. J., & Aldenkamp, A. P. (1996). Stability of cognitive measures in children of average ability. *Clinical Neuropsychology, 2,* 161–170.

Perret, E. (1974). The left frontal lobe of man and the suppression of habitual responses in verbal categorical behavior. *Neuropsychologia, 12,* 323–330.

Perugini, E. M., Harvey, E. A., Lovejoy, D. W., Sandstrom, K., & Webb, A. H. (2000). The predictive power of combined neuropsychological measures for attention-deficit/hyperactivity disorder in children. *Child Neuropsychology, 6,* 101–114.

Peterson, B. S., Kane, M. J., Alexander, G. M., Lacadie, C., Skudlarski, P., Leung, H-C., May, J., & Gore, J. C. (2002). An event-related fMRI study interference effects in the Simon and Stroop tasks. *Cognitive Brain Research, 13,* 427–440.

Pineda, D. A., & Merchan, V. (2003). Executive function in young Colombian adults. *International Journal of Neuroscience, 113,* 397–410.

Ponsford, J., & Kinsella, G. (1992). Attentional deficits following closed head injury. *Journal of Clinical and Experimental Neuropsychology, 14,* 822–828.

Raskin, A., Friedman, A. S., & DiMascio, A. (1982). Cognitive and performance deficits in depression. *Psychopharmacology Bulletin, 18,* 196–202.

Ravnkilde, B., Videbech, P., Rosenberg, R., Gjedde, A., & Gade, A. (2002). Putative tests of frontal lobe function: A PET-study of brain activation during Stroop's test and verbal fluency. *Journal of Clinical and Experimental Neuropsychology, 24,* 534–547.

Reeve, W. V, & Schandler, S. L. (2001). Frontal lobe functioning in adolescents with attention deficit disorder. *Adolescence, 36,* 749–765.

Regard, M. (1981). *Cognitive rigidity and flexibility: A neuropsychological study.* Unpublished Ph.D. dissertation, University of Victoria.

Reisberg, D., Baron, J., & Kemler, D. G. (1980). Overcoming Stroop interference: Effects of practice on distractor potency. *Journal of Experimental Psychology: Human Perception and Performance, 6,* 14–150.

Rios, M., Perianez, J. A., & Munoz-Cespedes, J. M. (2004). Attentional control and slowness of information processing after severe traumatic brain injury. *Brain Injury, 18,* 257–272.

Rosselli, M., Ardila, A., Santisi, M. N., Arecco, A. D. R., Salvatierra, J., Conde, A., & Lenis, B. (2002). Stroop effect in Spanish-English bilinguals. *Journal of the International Neuropsychological Society, 8*, 819–827.

Sachs, T. L., Clark, C. R., Pols, R. G., & Geffen, L. B. (1991). Comparability and stability of performance of six alternate forms of the Dodrill-Stroop Color-Word Test. *The Clinical Neuropsychologist, 5*, 220–225.

Salthouse, T. A., & Meinz, E. J. (1995). Aging, inhibition, working memory, and speed. *Journal of Gerontology, 50*, 297–306.

Sherman, E. M. S., Strauss, E., Spellacy, F., & Hunter, M. (1995). Construct validity of WAIS-R factors: Neuropsychological test correlates in adults referred for possible head injury. *Psychological Assessment, 7*, 440–444.

Shilling, V. M., Chetwynd, A., & Rabbitt, P. M. A. (2002). Individual inconsistency across measures of inhibition: An investigation of the construct validity of inhibition in older adults. *Neuropsychologia, 40*, 605–619.

Shum, D. H. K., McFarland, K. A., & Bain, J. D. (1990). Construct validity of eight tests of attention: Comparison of normal and closed head injured samples. *The Clinical Neuropsychologist, 4*, 151–162.

Snowden, J., Craufurd, D., Griffiths, H., Thompson, J., & Neary, D. (2001). Longitudinal evaluation of cognitive disorder in Huntington's disease. *Journal of the International Neuropsychological Society, 7*, 33–44.

Spieler, D. H., Balota, D. A., & Faust, M. E. (1996). Stroop performance in healthy younger and older adults and in individuals with dementia of the Alzheimer's type. *Journal of Experimental Psychology: Human Perception and Performance, 22*, 461–479.

Steinberg, B. A., Bieliauskas, L. A., Smith, G. E., & Ivnik, R. J. (2005). Mayo's Older Americans Normative Studies: Age- and IQ-adjusted norms for the Trail-Making Test, the Stroop Test, and MAE Controlled Oral Word Association Test. *The Clinical Neuropsychologist, 19*, 329–377.

Strickland, T. L., d'Elia, L. F., James, R., & Stein, R. (1997). Stroop Color-Word performance of African Americans. *The Clinical Neuropsychologist, 11*, 87–90.

Stroop, J. R. (1935). Studies of interference in serial verbal reaction. *Journal of Experimental Psychology, 18*, 643–662.

Stuss, D. T., Floden, D., Alexander, M. P., Levine, B., & Katz, D. (2001). Stroop performance in focal lesion patients: Dissociation of processes and frontal lobe lesion location. *Neuropsychologia, 39*, 771–786.

Trenerry, M. R., Crosson, B., DeBoe, J., & Leber, W. R. (1989). *Stroop Neurological Screening Test*. Odessa, FL: Psychological Assessment Resources.

Troyer, A. K., Leach, L., & Strauss, E. (in press). Aging and response inhibition: Normative data for the Victoria Stroop Test. *Aging, Neuropsychology and Cognition*.

Uttl, B., & Graf, P. (1997). Color Word Stroop Test performance across the adult life span. *Journal of Clinical and Experimental Neuropsychology, 19*, 405–420.

Van Boxtel, M. P. J., ten Tusscher, M. P. M., Metsemakers, J. F. M., Willems, B., & Jolles, J. (2001). Visual determinants of reduced performance on the Stroop Color-Word Test in normal aging adults. *Journal of Clinical and Experimental Neuropsychology, 23*, 620–627.

Van Gorp, W. G., Humphrey, L. A., Kalechstein, A., Brumm, V. L., McMullen, W. J., Stoddard, M., & Pachana, N. A. (1999). How well do standard clinical neuropsychological tests identify malingering? A preliminary analysis. *Journal of Clinical and Experimental Neuropsychology, 21*, 245–250.

Vendrell, P., Junqué, C., Pujol, J., Jurado, M. A., Molet, J., & Grafman, J. (1995). The role of prefrontal regions in the Stroop task. *Neuropsychologia, 33*, 341–352.

Verhaeghen, P., & De Meersman, L. (1998). Aging and the Stroop effect: A meta-analysis. *Psychology & Aging, 13*, 120–126.

Vingerhoets, G., De Soete, G., & Jannes, C. (1995). Relationship between emotional variables and cognitive test performance before and after open-heart surgery. *The Clinical Neuropsychologist, 9*, 198–202.

Wecker, N. S., Kramer, J. H., Wisniewski, A., Delis, D. C., & Kaplan, E. (2000). Age effects on executive ability. *Neuropsychology, 14*, 409–414.

Weinstein, M., Silverstein, M. L., Nader, T., & Turnbull, A. (1999). Sustained attention and related perceptuomotor functions. *Perceptual and Motor Skills, 89*, 387–388.

West, R., & Bell, M. A. (1997). Color-word interference and electroencephalogram activation: Evidence for age-related decline of the anterior attention system. *Neuropsychology, 11*, 421–427.

White, M., Lalonde, R., & Botez-Marquard, T. (2000). Neuropsychologic and neuropsychiatric characteristics of patients with Friedreich's ataxia. *Acta Neurologica Scandinavica 102*, 222–226.

Wildgruber, D., Kischka, U., Fassbender, K., & Ettlin, T. M. (2000). The frontal lobe score: Part II: Evaluation of its clinical validity. *Clinical Rehabilitation, 14*, 272–278.

Verbal Fluency

OTHER TEST NAMES

Other test names include Controlled Oral Word Association (COWA), Word Fluency, Letter Fluency, FAS-Test, Category Fluency, Phonemic Fluency, Semantic Fluency, Controlled Verbal Fluency, and Thurstone Word Fluency Test.

PURPOSE

This test evaluates the spontaneous production of words under restricted search conditions (verbal association fluency).

SOURCE

No specific material is required. Users may design their own materials and use the norms presented here, or purchase the test as part of larger standardized batteries, such as the following:

Phonemic Fluency Tasks

Phonemic fluency tasks are part of the Multilingual Aphasia Examination (CFL and PRW; Benton et al., 1994), the Neurosensory Center Comprehensive Examination for Aphasia

(NCCEA-FAS; Spreen & Benton, 1977), the DKEFS, KBNA, and the NEPSY. The MAE, D-KEFS, KBNA, and NEPSY are described elsewhere in this volume. Norms for FAS and Animal Fluency are also sold by PAR (www.parinc.com) (Gladsjo, Schuman, Miller, et al., 1999, manual costs $27 US; Heaton et al., 2004, manual costs $174 US).

Semantic Fluency Tasks

Semantic fluency tasks are also part of the RBANS (fruits and vegetables), WJ III COG (food, first names, animals), CELF-4 (animals, foods, jobs), DKEFS (animals and boys names, alternative version: clothing and girls names; switching condition: fruits and furniture, alternate version: vegetables and musical instruments), and NEPSY (animals and foods). Animal Fluency is also a subtest of the BDAE, the CERAD (Consortium for the Establishment of a Registry for Alzheimer's Disease) dementia battery (Morris et al., 1989), and the 7 Minute Screen (Solomon et al., 1998). The KBNA includes animals and first names. PAR (www.parinc.com) also sells norms for FAS and animal fluency (Gladsjo, Schuman, Miller, et al., 1999; Heaton et al., 2004).

Alternate Language Versions

Phonemic fluency (PMR) is included in the battery of tests for Spanish-speaking individuals developed by Artiola I Fortuny et al. (1999), and as part of NEUROPSI, a neuropsychological battery normed on a sample of Spanish speakers residing in Mexico (Ostrosky-Solis et al., 1999). Several other groups have developed norms for other languages. For example, norms for Hebrew semantic (animals, fruits and vegetables, and vehicles) and phonemic (bet, gimel, and shin) fluency have recently been provided by Kave (2005). Normative data for Cantonese-speaking adults are available for semantic fluency (fruits/vegetable) in Lee (2003). Kosmidis et al. (2004) assessed healthy adults in Greece on measures of semantic (animals, fruits, and objects) and phonemic fluency. Gonzalez et al. (2005) provide normative data for a semantic fluency task (naming of animals with four legs) for a sample of older (60+) Latinos of predominantly Mexican ancestry. Some norms for Spanish speakers on phonemic and semantic fluency tasks are also provided later (see *Normative Data*).

Other Fluency Tests

There are a number of alternatives to conventional fluency tests. For example, Warrington (2000) developed the Homophone Meaning Generation Test (HMGT), which involves providing multiple definitions for a series of homophones (e.g., bear/bare). Crawford et al. (1995) developed an Excluded Letter Fluency task (ELF) that requires generation of words that do not contain a specified vowel (e.g., examinees have to generate words that do not contain the letter *e*). The Uses for Common Objects task (UCO; Getzels & Jackson,

1961) or "alternate uses" task requires the generation of unusual uses for everyday objects (e.g., a brick).

AGE RANGE

Table 8–61 shows the tasks for which we provide normative data. The table also provides a listing of the tasks and age ranges included in some batteries and manuals.

DESCRIPTION

Phonemic and semantic fluency tasks have a long history of use in psychology, dating from the work of Thurstone (1938).

Phonemic Fluency

For this version, the examinee must produce orally as many words as possible beginning with a specified letter during a fixed period of time, usually one minute. As Marshall (1986) pointed out, the label "Word Fluency" is misleading since verbal productivity in conversation or in continuous sentences is not measured. Instead, the test measures timed production of individual words under restricted search conditions (e.g., a given letter of the alphabet). Thus, to avoid confusion with the fluency/nonfluency dimension of speech, Benton et al. (1994) prefer the term "Controlled Oral Word Association" (COWA). However, the test is often known under the general term of "verbal fluency."

F, A, and S are the most commonly used letters for this popular test, although other letter combinations are also used. These include C, F, and L and P, R, and W (e.g., Benton et al., 1994), and B, H, and R (Delis et al., 2001). The choice of letter set affects the results to some extent because of differences in letter difficulty and word frequency for each letter (Borkowski et al., 1967; see *Alternate Form Reliability* for a detailed discussion of letter equivalence across versions). For younger children, words beginning with "sh" have also been used to avoid the reliance on spelling skills (Halperin et al., 1989). Other variants of administration may be found in the literature. For example, Tucha et al. (1999) report using just the letter "S" from the FAS test and proceeding with that letter for a trial duration of three minutes, while Jurado et al. (2000) used all three letters, but expanded the trial length to 90 seconds for each letter.

Semantic Fluency

The most common category is "animals" and the examinee is asked to produce as many animal names as possible within a one-minute interval. Food names (fruits and vegetables) and "things in the kitchen," "things in a supermarket," "things to wear," "things that get you from one place to another," "first names," etc., have also been used. Other versions of the test require a combination of phonetic and semantic fluency ("animal names that begin with 'a'"; Heller & Dobbs, 1993) and

Table 8–61 Word Generation Tasks and Ranges of Ages Included in Normative Sets Provided Here and in Select Instruments/Manuals

Task	Provided Here	Ages	Other Sources	Ages
Phonemic Fluency	FAS	7–95	Heaton et al. (2004)/ Gladsjo et al., (1999a, b)	20–85
			Mitrushina et al. (2005)	18–74
	CFL	6–97		
	PRW	6–12		
	"sh"	6–12		
	FAS, BHR		D-KEFS	8–89
	S F		NEPSY	7–12
	C		KBNA	20–89
Semantic Fluency	Animals	7–95	Heaton et al. (2004)/ Gladsjo et al., (1999)	20–85
			Mitrushina et al. (2005)	25–87
	Vegetables	50–79		
	Fruits	50–79		
	Food	6–12; 60–80+		
	Clothing	60–80+		
	Animals, fruits, and vegetables (combined)	56–95+		
	Animals and foods and jobs-occupations (combined)		CELF-4	5–21
	Animals and boys names (combined)/ clothing and girls names (combined)		D-KEFS	8–89
	Switching: Fruits and furniture/ vegetables and musical instruments			
	Animals, foods to eat or drink		NEPSY	3–12
	Fruits and vegetables (combined)		RBANS	20–89
	Foods to eat or drink and first names and animals (combined)		WJ III	2–80+
	Animals and first names (combined)		KBNA	20–89
Written Fluency	S and C	6–18	Heaton et al. (2004)	20–85

"action fluency" (verb naming: things that people do; Piatt, Fields, Paolo, & Troester, 1999; Piatt, Fields, Paolo, Koller, et al., 1999; Woods et al., 2005) or a "switching format," which requires the individual to alternate between categories, such as fruits and furniture (e.g., Baldo et al., 2001; Delis et al., 2001) or colors and birds (Newcomb, 1969) in an attempt to increase demands on executive functions.

Written Word Fluency

This variant was first used by Thurstone as part of his exploration of primary mental abilities (1938), allowing five minutes for each letter. The patient is first required to write as many words beginning with a specific letter (i.e., the letter "S") in a period of five minutes. Next, the person is required to write as many four-letter words as possible that begin with the letter "C" during a four-minute trial. Since the test is somewhat lengthy and dependent on basic spelling skills and intact motor ability, it is not suitable for younger children (although norms are available for as low as age 6) and patients with motor impairment. Because of the frequent presence of a dominant-side hemiparesis in poststroke aphasic patients,

this written test has been used only infrequently in aphasia examinations.

ADMINISTRATION

Phonemic Fluency

See Figure 8–14 for specific instructions.

Semantic Fluency

See Figure 8–15 for specific instructions.

Written Fluency

See Figure 8–16 for specific instructions.

ADMINISTRATION TIME

The administration of phonemic and semantic fluency takes about five minutes. Written fluency takes longer, about 10 minutes.

Figure 8–14 Instructions for Phonemic Fluency.

Use a stopwatch and have the patient comfortably seated before giving the following instructions: *I will say a letter of the alphabet. Then I want you to give me as many words that begin with that letter as quickly as you can. For example, if I say "b" you might give me "bad, battle, bed. . . ." I do not want you to use words that are proper names such as "Boston, Bob, or Buick." Also, do not use the same word with different ending such as "eat" and "eating." Any questions? (pause). Begin when I say the letter. The first letter is F. Go ahead.*

Begin timing immediately.

Allow one minute for each letter (F, A, and S). Say *"Fine"* or *"Good"* after each one-minute performance. If the examinee stops before the end of the minute, encourage him or her to try to think of more words. If there is a silence of 15 seconds, repeat the basic instructions, and the letter.

For scoring purposes, write down the actual words in the order in which they are produced. If repetitions occur that may be acceptable if an alternate meaning was intended by the examinee ('Four" and "for," "sun" and "son"), ask what was meant by this word at the end of the one-minute period.

Administer all three letters: F, A, and S.

SCORING

Phonemic Fluency

The total correct is the sum of all admissible words for the three letters. Slang terms and foreign words that are part of standard English ("faux pas" or "lasagna") are acceptable. Inadmissible words under these instructions (e.g., proper names, wrong words, variations, repetitions) are not counted as correct.

Semantic Fluency

The total correct is the sum of all admissible words for the semantic category. For animal category fluency, names of extinct, imaginary, or magic animals are admissible, but given names for animals like "Fido" and "Morris" are not. Inadmissible words under these instructions (e.g., proper names, wrong words, variations, repetitions) are not counted as correct.

Written Fluency

The individual obtains a score of one point for each word; duplicate words do not earn points. The score is the sum of scores for Part A (S words) and Part B (C words). Misspelled words are counted as correct (Bryan Kolb, personal communication, January 31, 2005, gives a score of 1 if the error does not affect the correctness of the word). The examiner should ask the client about any words not written clearly. If an individual has written a word that does not resemble the one he or she says it is, it may be counted anyway provided that the word the patient meant to write meets the criteria specified in the instructions (Heaton et al., 2004).

Evaluating Performance Based on Errors

Errors should be reviewed carefully because they may provide clues to certain types of disorders, for example, repetitions of previous responses (recurrent or ideational perseverations), reverting back to a previous category (stuck in set), repeating the same item over and over (continuous perseveration), intrusions (of other letters or from another category), paraphasias, or spelling errors.

Evaluating Strategy

The order of words produced also provides clues to processes underlying reduced test performance (see *Validity*). Based on studies of patients with AD, Chertkow and Bub (1990) concluded that effective verbal fluency performance requires (a) an intact semantic store for supplying a knowledge base of related words and (b) an effective search process to access and retrieve this information. Thus, poor performance on verbal fluency tasks can result from deterioration of a stored

Figure 8–15 Instructions for Semantic Fluency.

Say: *I am going to tell you the names of some things you can find in the kitchen: spoons, knives, forks, plates, faucet. Can you think of other things in the kitchen?*

Allow the examinee to name other things, and correct if he or she produces incorrect responses, explaining the task once again. Then say: *Now, tell me the names of as many animals as you can. Name them as quickly as possible.*

Allow one minute. If the examinee discontinues before the end of the period, encourage him or her to produce more names. If there is a pause of 15 or more seconds, repeat the instructions and give the starting word *"dog."* Start timing immediately after instructions have been given, but allow extra time in the period if instructions are repeated. Write down the actual words in the order in which they are produced.

Figure 8–16 Instructions for Written Fluency.

Part A

Say: *You have five minutes to write down as many words as you can that begin with the letter "S." I do not want you to use words that are proper names. Also, do not use the same word with different ending such as "eat" and "eating. It does not matter if your words are spelled correctly. I am only interested in how many words you can get down on paper.*

Allow 5 minutes.

Part B

Say: *Now, this part is harder. You are to write words that begin with the letter "C" and have only four letters in them. You have four minutes to write as many words as possible. Again, do not use proper names; however, on this part you are allowed to use different forms of the same word, as long as they all have four letters.*

knowledge base or from an inefficient search (e.g., not generating search strategies, or not shifting to new searches when previous ones are exhausted). These store and search processes were operationalized by Troyer et al. (1997) as clustering and switching, respectively. According to Troyer et al., optimal fluency performance involves clustering or generating words within a subcategory and, when a subcategory is exhausted, switching to a new subcategory. Clustering involves phonemic analysis on phonemic fluency and semantic categorization on semantic fluency, and is thought to be a relatively automatic process. Switching involves cognitive flexibility in shifting from one subcategory to another and is thought to involve a relatively effortful process. Decreased clustering has been related to temporal lobe disturbance, while switching implicates frontal functioning, although some inconsistencies in this pattern have been noted (see section on *Validity*).

The rules for scoring cluster size and switches are provided in Troyer (2000; Troyer et al., 1997). Briefly, on phonemic fluency, clusters are defined as successively generated words that begin with the same first two letters, differing only by a vowel sound, or are homonyms. On animal fluency, clusters are successively generated words belonging to the same semantic subcategories, such as African animals, Australian animals, North American wild animals, pets, and individual zoological categories, such as birds, canines, insects, etc. On phonemic fluency, only phonemic clusters are counted, and on semantic fluency, only semantic clusters are counted. The size of the cluster is counted beginning with the second word in each cluster. The mean cluster size is calculated by summing the size of each cluster and dividing by the number of clusters. Switches are calculated as the number of transitions between clusters, including single words. Repetitions and intrusions are included in the calculations of cluster size and switches. More detailed approaches to verbal fluency scoring have been presented by others (e.g., Abwender et al., 2001; Giovannetti et al. 2001; Giovannetti-Carew et al. 1997).

While most healthy people produce the majority of their responses at the beginning of the time allotted per trial and trail off over time (Delis et al., 2001; Fernaeus & Almquist, 1998), others may have difficulty with task initiation or maintenance; yet others who are prone to some performance anxiety may show a little flustering at the start, but then produce the bulk of their responses later in the trial. This can be explored by noting (with a line) and counting the number of words in each 15-second block and referring to Delis et al. (2001), who provide normative data for each of the four 15-second blocks.

DEMOGRAPHIC EFFECTS

Age

Performance on phonemic fluency improves during childhood, with a dramatic increase between the ages of 5 and 7 years. The increase peaks at about age 30 to 39 and shows a mild decline in old age (Backman et al., 2004; Delis et al., 2001; Elias et al. 1997; Gladsjo, Schuman, Evans, et al., 1999; Heaton et al., 2004; Kave, 2005; Kosmidis et al., 2004; La Rue et al., 1999; Loonstra et al., 2001; Lucas et al., 2005; Mack et al., 2005; Matute et al., 2004; Mitrushina et al., 2005; Riva et al., 2000; Tombaugh et al., 1999; Troyer, 2000; Yeudall et al., 1986). Age also has an impact on category fluency (Acevado et al., 2000; Backman et al., 2004; Delis et al., 2001; Fillenbaum et al., 2001; Gladsjo, Schuman, Evans, et al., 1999; Harrison et al., 2000; Kempler et al., 1998; Kosmidis et al., 2004; Lucas et al., 1998; Marcopulos et al., 1997; Matute et al., 2004; Ratcliff et al., 2003; Riva et al., 1999; Tombaugh et al., 1999; Troyer, 2000), although in comparison to letter fluency, the developmental rise in childhood is not as steep (Delis et al., 2001), tending to stabilize by about age 11 to 12 (Sauzeon et al., 2004) and showing a steady decline from about age 20 on (Mitrushina et al., 2005). Some have reported that in adults, aging is more strongly related to the number of words generated on semantic fluency than phonemic fluency tasks, with poorer performance associated with increasing age (Brickman et al., 2005; Crossley et al., 1997; Kozora & Cullum, 1995; Mathuranath et al., 2003; Ravdin et al., 2003; Troyer, 2000).

Education

Educational level exerts a significant influence on both phonemic and semantic fluency tasks with higher levels of education associated with better performance (e.g., Acevado et al., 2000; Anstey et al., 2000; Backman et al., 2004; Brickman et al., 2005; Crossley et al., 1997; Dursun et al., 2002; Fillenbaum et al., 2001; Gladsjo, Schuman, Miller, et al., 1999; Harrison et al., 2000; Ivnik et al., 1996; Kave, 2005; Kempler et al., 1998; Kosmidis et al., 2004; La Rue et al., 1999; Lannoo & Vingerhoets, 1997; Loonstra et al., 2001; Lucas et al., 1998, 2005; Mack et al., 2005; Marcopulos et al., 1997; Mathuranath et al., 2003; Mitrushina et al., 2005; Ruff et al., 1996; Sliwinski & Buschke, 1999; Steinberg et al., 2005; Stricks et al., 1998; Troyer, 2000; Yeudall et al., 1986). In one large-scale study, for example, healthy older individuals at the highest educational level (i.e., 13 or more years of education) produced more than twice as many words as those in the lowest educational level (i.e., 0–6 years; Crossley et al., 1997).

Tombaugh et al. (1999) reported that for phonemic fluency (e.g., FAS), education (21.7%) accounted for more variance than age (11.85%), while for semantic (e.g., animal) naming, the opposite relationship existed (education = 13.6%; age = 23.4%). Similar findings have been reported by Heaton et al. (2004). Among Hebrew speakers, age proved the best predictor of performance on both phonemic and semantic fluency tasks but it accounted for a greater share of the variance in semantic than in phonemic fluency (Kave, 2005). Kosmidis et al. (2004), however, failed to find such a differential effect in a Greek sample. In that sample, education was the most influential demographic factor on both semantic and phonemic tasks.

On the Thurstone Written Fluency task, education accounts for more variance (about 14%) than age (about 9%) among Caucasians (Heaton et al., 2004). Similar results emerge in African Americans (Heaton et al., 2004).

Reading Level

Reading level shows a small correlation with category (animal) fluency ($r = .26$), but a moderate relationship with phonemic (FAS) fluency ($r =$ about .47; Johnson-Selfridge et al., 1998). The level of literacy may differentially impact performance depending upon the particular semantic task chosen. Gonzales da Silva et al. (2004) noted that literacy had little impact on a supermarket fluency task, but a significant impact on animal fluency, perhaps reflecting differences in cultural background.

Gender

Many authors find little evidence of gender differences on the number of words generated on phonemic and semantic fluency (Anstey et al., 2000; Backman et al., 2004; Brickman et al., 2005; Fillenbaum et al., 2001; Glasjo et al., 1999; Harrison et al., 2000; Heaton et al., 2004; Ivnik et al., 1996; Kave, 2005; Kozora & Cullum, 1995; Lucas et al., 1998, 2005; Mack et al., 2005; Mathuranath et al., 2003; Mitrushina et al., 2005; Riva et al., 2000; Schum et al., 1989; Tombaugh et al., 1999; Troyer, 2000; Yeudall et al., 1986). However, some have reported that females (especially well-educated ones) perform better than men on letter fluency (Anderson et al., 2001; Barr, 2003; Crossley et al., 1997; Elias et al., 1997; La Rue et al., 1999; Ruff et al., 1996). Recent meta-analytic findings, based on an aggregate sample of 17,625 healthy individuals, confirm a small advantage on letter fluency for women ($M = 35.14$, $SD = 12.59$) in comparison with men ($M = 33.28$, $SD = 12.96$; Loonstra et al., 2001). While animal fluency may not be affected by gender (but see Sliwinski & Buschke, 1999, who found men to show superior performance), other categories (e.g., fruits and vegetables) may show gender differences (Acevado et al., 2000; Kosmidis et al., 2004).

A Spanish study examining written word fluency of 234 11- to 14-year-old high school children (Codorniu-Raga & Vigil-Colet, 2003) reported a minor gender effect in favor of boys.

Ethnicity/Language/Geographical Region

On average, studies find significant effects of ethnicity (Caucasian, African American) on both letter and animal fluency tasks, with Caucasian ethnicity associated with better performance even when income, education, and WRAT-R Reading scores are taken into account (e.g., Gladsjo, Schuman, Evans, et al., 1999; Johnson-Selfridge et al., 1998; but see Fillenbaum et al., 2001). Other studies have reported differences between Hispanic and non-Hispanic older adults on both letter fluency (Loewenstein et al., 1995; Taussig et al., 1992) and category fluency (Jacobs et al., 1997; La Rue et al. 1999), with higher scores in non-Hispanics. There are also some cross-linguistic differences in the type of words produced (e.g., English monolinguals generate more wild animals while Spanish monolinguals generate more birds and insects; on letter fluency, grammatical words are more frequently produced in English than in Spanish; Rosselli et al., 2002).

Kempler et al. (1998) explored the effects of ethnicity on animal fluency performances in a sample of 317 healthy individuals between 54 and 99 years of age. They found a striking difference between Hispanic and Vietnamese immigrants, with the Vietnamese producing the most animal names and the Spanish speakers producing the fewest. They attributed the difference to the predominance of one-syllable animal names in Vietnamese and multisyllable animal names in Spanish.

Figure 8–17 Predicted FAS score from NART.

Predicted WF = 57.5 − 0.76 × NART errors, SE_E = 9.09; also see www.psyc.abdn.ac.uk

The impact of bilingualism (Spanish-English) has been studied by Rosselli et al. (2002). They found that bilinguals generated fewer words than the monolingual English in the animal naming condition, but not the FAS condition. Rosselli et al. (2002) hypothesized that the bilingual participants experienced interference between the two languages. Semantic fluency only includes the recall of concrete nouns, while phonemic fluency does not. Concrete nouns may share more elements of their representations across languages than nonconcrete words. Semantic fluency tasks may therefore promote more language interference.

Geographical region may also impact performance. Fillenbaum et al. (2001) reported that older African Americans living in North Carolina produced fewer animals than their peers in Indianapolis, perhaps a reflection of differences in quality of education and/or acculturation.

IQ

Intellectual level is related to both phonemic and semantic fluency (Diaz-Asper et al., 2004). Tombaugh et al. (1999) reported a modest correlation of .25 between FAS and the WAIS-R Vocabulary subtest in a large sample of healthy individuals. Vocabulary scores were not highly correlated with total number of animals named ($r = .17$). Harrison et al. (2000) reported a modest relationship between WAIS-R IQ and phonemic fluency (FAS; .33) and semantic fluency (animals; .29) in a sample of healthy people. In clinical samples, correlations between phonemic fluency and WAIS-R Full-Scale, Verbal and Performance scores are higher, ranging between .49 and .59 (Lacy et al., 1996).

IQ shows a stronger relationship to phonemic fluency than does education (Steinberg et al., 2005). Further, the association becomes stronger as IQ increases (Steinberg et al., 2005).

Moderately high correlations (.41 – .46) have been reported between NAART/NART and COWA-CFL/FAS scores in undergraduates (Ross, 2003) and in older adults (Harvey & Seigert, 1999). In a British normative sample, Crawford et al. (1992) found a correlation of .67 between FAS and the National Adult Reading Test (NART), but not with age (see also Bird et al., 2004). They suggested that expected scores in letter fluency could be predicted on the basis of NART scores (see Figure 8–17).

The comparison of their normal group with a neurological sample showed a significantly better discrimination when expected word fluency scores were used. A table to convert NART errors to predicted FAS scores is presented in Table 8–62. Users should keep in mind that this table is based on a study with the British NART and healthy British subjects; however, a similar relationship is likely to apply to North American individuals and the NAART.

Senior et al. (2001) reported moderate relations between the SCOLP Spot-the-Word (STW) and FAS ($r = .38$) scores in a normal sample of individuals living in Australia. Accordingly, using multiple regression techniques, they suggested that STW raw scores could be used to predict expected raw scores on verbal fluency tasks. The equation to predict FAS is shown in Figure 8–18.

The reader should consult the section on the SCOLP described elsewhere in this book to determine whether the FAS-STW discrepancy between obtained and expected is unusual.

Table 8–62 Conversion of NART (N) errors to predicted FAS-COWA scores

N-WF	N-WF	N-WF	N-WF	N-WF	N-WF
0–57	9–51	18–44	27–37	36–30	45–23
1–57	10–50	19–43	28–36	37–29	46–23
2–56	11–49	20–42	29–35	38–29	47–22
3–55	12–48	21–42	30–35	39–28	48–21
4–54	13–48	22–41	31–34	40–27	49–20
5–54	14–47	23–40	32–33	41–26	50–19
6–53	15–46	24–39	33–32	42–26	
7–52	16–45	25–38	34–32	43–25	
8–51	17–45	26–38	35–31	44–24	

Note: Error scores refer to NART, not the NAART. The NAART has 61 rather than 50 items.

Source: From Crawford et al., 1992. Reprinted with the permission of the British Journal of Clinical Psychology, © British Psychological Society.

Figure 8–18 FAS prediction from STW scores.

$$\text{FAS predicted} = .757 \,(\text{STW raw}) + .77 \,(\text{years of education}) - 4.747, \, SE_E = 10.8$$

NORMATIVE DATA

Normative Data for Adults

Phonemic Fluency—FAS. Loonstra et al. (2001) provide metanorms for FAS derived from 32 studies comprising a total of 17,625 English speakers. The studies were either normative studies or studies in which a control group of normal participants were used. The authors note that in several of these studies, the criteria of normality were quite vague or based only on self-report and that demographic data were incomplete in a number of cases. The data are stratified by age, level of education, and gender and are shown in Table 8–63. Although the increased sample size results in more stable score norms, the data do not allow for simultaneous consideration of various influences such as age and education. The values are somewhat lower than those reported by Mitrushina et al. (2005) in their compilation of 18 studies, based on a total of 3469 participants, aged 18 to 74 years. Differences in values perhaps reflect differences in study inclusion criteria. Mitrushina et al. (2005) employed more stringent criteria for inclusion of studies in their meta-analysis (e.g., those without demographic descriptions were excluded from analysis). Use of the tables provided by Mitrushina et al. (2005) allows evaluation of scores with respect to both age and education.

The normative data provided by Gladsjo and Heaton (Gladsjo, Schuman, Evans, et al. 1999; Gladsjo, Schuman, Miller, et al., 1999; Heaton et al. 2004) are based on a large sample (N = 768 in Gladsjo, Schuman, Evans, et al., 1999; Gladsjo, Schuman, Miller, et al., 1999; N = 1148 in Heaton et al., 2004) of healthy Caucasians and African Americans, aged 20 to 101 years, with a mean educational level of about 13.6 years (SD = 3.1; range 0–20 years). Use of their data allows simultaneous consideration of age, education, and ethnicity.

Tombaugh et al. (1999) provide normative data based on a sample of 1298 community-dwelling (Canada) healthy individuals, ranging in age from 16 to 95 years, with no evidence of cognitive impairment. English was the first language for all participants. The normative data allow simultaneous consideration of both age and level of education and are shown in Table 8–64. The values are broadly consistent with data provided in other normative reports (e.g., Bolla et al., 1990; Gladsjo, Schuman, Evans, et al., 1999; Gladsjo, Schuman, Miller, et al., 1999; Heaton et al., 2004; Harrison et al., 2000; Kozora & Cullum, 1995, Loonstra et al., 2001; Mitrushina et al., 2005; Yeudall et al., 1986).

Phonemic Fluency—CFL. The original norms (Benton et al., 1994) were collected in the 1960s in Iowa. Updated norms published by Ruff et al. (1996) were collected for CFL-COWA in the mid-1980s (Iverson et al., 1999). They are based on 360 individuals, ranging in age between 16 and 70 years and in education from 7 to 22 years, with equal cell size for gender and education groups (Table 8–65). It is important to use the updated norms since they establish a higher standard than the original norms, reflecting a general increase in performance with the passage of time (the Flynn effect). Thus, use of the updated norms will result in a higher proportion of patients being classed as impaired. They also found that three or more perseverative or repetition errors were unusual, occurring in less than 5% of their sample.

Others have extended normative reports to include different age ranges and/or specific subgroups. For example, Ivnik et al. (1996) provide age- and education-corrected scores for CFL for use with older adults, aged 56 to 95+. Note that these norms are derived from a large sample (N = 743) of Caucasian individuals living in an economically advantaged region of the United States. The WAIS FSIQ was 106.2 (SD = 14, range 76–138) and the mean WMS-R General Memory Index was 106.2 (SD = 14.2, range 65–143), suggesting that a broad range of general cognitive ability was represented within this sample. Their data are shown in Table 8–66 along with an equation to adjust scores for education level. Midpoint intervals were used to maximize the available information. Note that MOANS scores have a mean of 10 and an SD of three.

Table 8–63 Metanorms for FAS Totals

Category	N	M	SD
Gender			
Males	7310	33.28	12.96
Females	9172	35.14	12.59
Age			
<40	634	43.51	9.44
40–59	9202	34.24	12.48
60–79	5294	32.31	12.70
80–95	433	29.37	13.05
Education			
0–12	1357	30.07	13.09
>12	588	41.14	12.37
Overall	17,625	34.78	12.82

Note: Norms derived from 32 studies comprising 17,625 English speakers.

Source: From Loonstra et al., 2001. Reprinted with the permission of Lawrence Erlbaum Associates.

Table 8–64 Norms for FAS Stratified for Age (16–59, 60–79, and 80–95 Years) and Years of Education (0–8, 9–12, and 13–21)

Percentile Score	Age 16–59 Years			Age 60–79 Years			Age 80–95 Years		
	Education (Years)			Education (Years)			Education (Years)		
	0–8 (N = 12)	9–12 (N = 268)	13–21 (N = 242)	0–8 (N = 76)	9–12 (N = 292)	13–21 (N = 185)	0–8 (N = 75)	9–12 (N = 102)	13–21 (N = 46)
90	48	56	61	39	54	59	33	42	56
80	45	50	55	36	47	53	29	38	47
70	42	47	51	31	43	49	26	34	43
60	39	43	49	27	39	45	24	31	39
50	36	40	45	25	35	41	22	29	36
40	35	38	42	22	32	38	21	27	33
30	34	35	38	20	28	36	19	24	30
20	30	32	35	17	24	34	17	22	28
10	27	28	30	13	21	27	13	18	23
M	38.5	40.5	44.7	25.3	35.6	42.0	22.4	29.8	37.0
(SD)	(12.0)	(10.7)	(11.2)	(11.1)	(12.5)	(12.1)	(8.2)	(11.4)	(11.2)

Source: From Tombaugh et al., 1999, with permission of Elsevier.

Table 8–65 Letter (CFL) Fluency in Adults, age 16–70 Years by Education Level

Education	Men (N = 180)		Women (N = 180)		Both Genders (N = 360)	
	M	SD	M	SD	M	SD
13 years or less	36.9	9.8	35.9	9.6	36.5	9.9
13–15 years	40.5	9.4	39.4	10.1	40.0	9.7
16 years and more	41.0	9.3	46.5	11.2	43.8	10.6
All education levels	39.5	9.8	40.6	11.2	40.1	10.5

Source: From Ruff et al., 1996, with permission of Elsevier.

Table 8–66 CFL MOANS Norms for Persons Aged 56–97

Percentile Ranges	56–62	63–65	66–68	69–71	72–74	75–77	78–80	81–83	84–86	87–89	90–97	Scaled Score
<1	<13	<13	<13	<13	<12	<11	<6	<6	<6	<5	<5	2
1	13–16	13–16	13–16	13–14	12	11	6–8	6–8	6	5	5	3
2	17–18	17–18	17	15	13–15	12–13	9–10	9–10	7–10	6–10	6–10	4
3–5	19–20	19–20	18–20	16–19	16–19	14–19	11–15	11–15	11–15	11–15	11–15	5
6–10	21–25	21–24	21–23	20–22	20–22	20–22	16–21	16–19	16–18	16–18	16–18	6
11–18	26–28	25–26	24–25	23–25	23–24	23–24	22–23	20–23	19–22	19–22	19–22	7
19–28	29–31	27–29	26–29	26–28	25–28	25–28	24–26	24–25	23–25	23–24	23	8
29–40	32–33	30–32	30–32	29–31	29–31	29–31	27–30	26–30	26–29	25–28	24–26	9
41–50	34–39	33–37	33–37	32–36	32–36	32–36	31–35	31–35	30–35	29–35	27–34	10
60–71	40–42	38–40	38–40	37–39	37–39	37–39	36–39	36–39	36–39	36–39	35–37	11
72–81	43–45	41–44	41–44	40–43	40–43	40–43	40–43	40–43	40–42	40–42	38–41	12
82–89	46–51	45–49	45–49	44–49	44–49	44–49	44–48	44–48	43–48	43–48	42–48	13
90–94	52–56	50–56	50–56	50–56	50–56	50–56	49–52	49–52	49–52	49–52	49–51	14
95–97	57–62	57–62	57–62	57–61	57–61	57–61	53–61	53–60	53–59	53–58	52–56	15
98	63–67	63–67	63–67	62–67	62–66	62–64	62–64	61–62	60–62	59–61	57	16
99	68–71	68–71	68–71	68–71	67–70	65–70	65–70	63–70	63–67	62–63	58	17
>99	>71	>71	>71	>71	>70	>70	>70	>70	>67	>63	>58	18
N	174	257	201	215	250	282	309	293	242	165	100	

Age- and education-corrected MOANS scaled score ($MSS_{A\&E}$) is calculated from a person's age-corrected MOANS scaled score (MSS_A) and that person's education expressed in years of formal schooling completed as follows: $MSS_{A\&E} = 3.50 + (1.16 \times MSS_A) - (0.40 \times Education)$. Mean FSIQ about 106, range 76–138.

Source: From Ivnik et al., 1996, based on Mayo's Older Normative Studies (MOANS). Reprinted with the kind permission of Psychology Press.

Steinberg et al. (2005) have recently reanalyzed data from the Mayo Clinic's Older Americans Normative Studies (MOANS) and provided age (55+) and IQ-adjusted percentile equivalents of MOANS age-adjusted CFL scores. Readers should note that all FSIQs are Mayo age-adjusted scores which are based on the WAIS-R, not the WAIS-III. Given the upward shift in scores (Flynn effect) with the passage of time, use of the WAIS-R FSIQ rather than the WAIS-III might result in a given fluency score appearing less favorable. The interested reader is referred to their article for the relevant tables.

Ravdin et al. (2003) provide data for a sample of 149 community–dwelling, well-educated older adults (aged 60–91, $M = 76.67$, $SD = 6.27$; education, $M = 15.57$, $SD = 2.67$) of superior intellectual ability (AMNART score, $M = 120.44$, $SD = 5.74$). The majority (117/149) were women and all were healthy and screened for evidence of cognitive decline. Their normative data are most applicable to highly educated women and are generally consistent with the age- and education-corrected values reported by Ivnik et al. (1996).

Stricks et al. (1998) provide data for CFL based on a more ethnically diverse sample. They assessed 566 older English-speaking adults living in the New York City area, screened as nondemented by a physician. Individuals with neurological conditions that might affect cognition were also excluded. Approximately 4% were Hispanic, and 60% were African American. About 68% were female. In addition, a group of 378 nondemented, disease-free Spanish speakers (largely of Caribbean origin) were tested in Spanish using the letters ABS. The ABS mean scores are also provided in Table 8–67.

Lucas et al. (2005) have recently provided age- and education-adjusted normative data based on 308 African American community-dwelling participants from the MOAANS (Mayo African American Normative Studies) project in Jacksonville, Florida. Participants were predominantly female (75%), ranged in age from 56 to 94 years ($M = 69.6$, $SD = 6.87$) and varied in education from 0 to 20 years of formal education ($M = 12.2$, $SD = 3.48$). They were screened to exclude those with active neurological, psychiatric or other conditions that might affect cognition. Their data are shown in Table 8–68a. The computational formula for age- and education-corrected MOAANS scaled is shown in Table 8–68b. The authors suggest caution in the use of their norms since there was limited representation of the oldest participants and they used a regional convenience sample of volunteers that may not represent the full range of cultural and educational experiences of the African-American community.

Semantic Fluency—Animals, Vegetables, and Fruits/Animals, Foods, and Clothing. Gladsjo and Heaton (Gladsjo, Schuman, Evans, et al., 1999; Gladsjo, Schuman, Miller, et al., 1999; Heaton et al., 2004) provide norms for animal fluency derived from a large sample ($N = 768$ in Gladsjo, Schuman, Evans, et al., 1999; Gladsjo, Schuman, Miller, et al., 1999; $N = 1148$ in Heaton et al., 2004) of healthy Caucasians and African Americans, aged 20 to 101 years, with a mean educational level of about 13.6 years ($SD = 3.1$; range 0–20 years). Use of their data allows simultaneous consideration of age, education, and ethnicity.

Mitrushina et al. (2005) compiled 11 studies for animal naming, consisting of 2843 participants, aged 25 to 87 years. Data are corrected for age only as education did not account for a significant amount of variance.

Tombaugh et al. (1999) collected norms for animal fluency, based on a subset ($N = 735$) of the Canadian sample

Table 8–67 Letter and Category (Animals, Foods, and Clothing) Fluency in English-speaking (CFL) and Spanish-speaking (ABS) Older Adults

Age	60–69						70–79						80+						Total		
Education	<9			9+			<9			9+			<9			9+					
	M	SD	N	M	SD	N	M	SD	N	M	SD	N	M	SD	N	M	SD	N	M	SD	N
English CFL mean	7.8	4.5	21	10.6	4.3	93	6.1	2.8	91	10.1	4.4	200	5.6	2.9	58	9.1	4.6	102	8.8	4.4	566
Spanish ABS mean	6.7	3.3	67	8.0	3.5	21	6.3	2.7	162	9.1	2.9	47	6.2	2.9	57	9.1	5.4	25	7.0	3.3	378
English Category Mean	14.3	3.1	21	16.5	4.7	93	12.1	3.8	92	14.6	4.2	200	9.8	3.4	60	12.5	4.1	101	13.6	4.5	567
Spanish Category Mean	11.6	3.2	74	12.8	2.5	21	11.2	3.2	180	13.2	3.5	47	10.4	3.2	67	11.8	4.3	25	11.5	3.3	413

Tested in English: <9 years of education: Mean age = 77.5 (6.8), mean years of education = 6.1 (2.1), 75% Black, 3.5% Hispanic; 9+ years of education: Mean age = 75.1 (6.6), mean years of education = 12.7 (2.6), 52.8% Black, 4.7% Hispanic. Tested in Spanish: <9 years of education: Mean age = 74.5 (6.0), mean years of education = 4.5 (2.7), 8% Black, 99.3% Hispanic; 9+ years of education: Mean age = 75.4 (7.0), mean years of education = 12.0 (3.0), 5.9% Black, 66.9% Hispanic.

Source: Adapted from Stricks et al., 1998.

Table 8–68a MOAANS Age-Based Norms for C, F, and L in African American Adults

Scaled Score	56–62	63–65	66–68	69–71	72–74	75–77	78+	Percentile Ranges
2	0–7	0–7	0–6	0–6	0–5	0–5	0–5	<1
3	8–10	8–10	7–10	7–10	6–10	6–10	6–7	1
4	11–12	11–12	11	—	—	—	8–10	2
5	13–14	13–14	12–14	11–13	11–12	11–12	11–12	3–5
6	15–16	15–16	15–16	14–16	13–15	13–15	13–15	6–10
7	17–21	17–20	17–20	17–20	16–19	16–19	16–17	11–18
8	22–23	21–22	21–22	21–22	20–22	20–22	18–21	19–28
9	24–27	23–26	23–26	23–26	23–25	23–25	22–23	29–40
10	28–33	27–31	27–31	27–31	26–31	26–30	24–28	41–59
11	34–36	32–36	32–36	32–36	32–36	31–36	29–32	60–71
12	37–41	37–41	37–40	37–40	37–40	37–40	33–37	72–81
13	42–47	42–45	41–44	41–44	41–44	41–44	38–41	82–89
14	48–53	46–52	45–50	45–50	45–50	45–50	42–49	90–94
15	54–56	53–56	51–55	51–55	51–55	51–53	50–51	95–97
16	57–61	57–60	56–60	56–60	56–60	54–55	52	98
17	62+	61–62	61–62	61–62	61	56–58	53	99
18	—	63+	63+	63+	62+	59+	54+	>99
N	108	130	167	183	159	120	80	

Source: Adapted from Lucas et al., 2005. Reprinted with the permission of the Mayo Foundation for Medical Education and Research.

(aged 16–95) described above (FAS). The data are stratified on the basis of age and years of education and are shown in Table 8–69. The data are similar to those provided in other normative reports (e.g., Gladsjo, Schuman, Evans, et al., 1999; Gladsjo, Schuman, Miller, et al., 1999; Heaton et al., 2004; Mitrushina et al., 2005).

Many clinicians supplement the animal naming trial with additional categories, such as fruits and vegetables, to sample a greater range of behavior and parallel the three trials often given in phonemic fluency tasks. Lucas et al. (1998) provide age- and education-corrected normative data for 412 community-dwelling, Caucasian individuals, aged 56 to 95+, for this version. Each person was examined by his or her personal physician and found to have no active medical, neurological, or psychiatric disorder with potential to affect cognition. The data (sum of the three trials) are shown in Table 8–70. Midpoint intervals were used to maximize the

Table 8–68b Computational Formula for Age- and Education-Corrected MOAANS Scaled Scores

	K	W_1	W_2
CFL	2.97	1.19	0.41

Age- and education-corrected MOAANS scaled scores ($MSS_{A\&E}$) can be calculated for CFL scores by using aged-corrected MOAANS scaled scores (MSS_A) and education (expressed in years completed) in the following formula: $MSS_{A\&E} = K + (W_1 \times MSS_A) - (W_2 \times EDUC)$

Source: Adapted from Lucas et al., 2005. Reprinted with the permission of the Mayo Foundation for Medical Education and Research.

available information. Note that MOAANS scaled scores have a mean of 10.0 and a standard deviation of three. Although education accounted for a relatively small proportion of raw score variance, some may wish to adjust for its effects. To this end, a regression-based formula is also presented in the table.

The lack of ethnic and cultural diversity of the participants (mainly Caucasians living in economically advantaged parts of North America) in the studies by Tombaugh et al. (1999) and Lucas et al. (1998) limits the use of these norms in individuals who do not share similar backgrounds. Lucas et al. (2005) have provided age- and education-adjusted category fluency normative data based on 304 African American community-dwelling participants from the MOAANS (Mayo African American Normative Studies) project in Jacksonville, Florida. As noted above (see *Phonemic Fluency—CFL*), participants were predominantly female (75%), ranged in age from 56 to 94 years ($M = 69.6$, $SD = 6.87$), and varied in education from 0 to 20 years of formal education ($M = 12.2$, $SD = 3.48$). They were screened to exclude those with active neurological, psychiatric, or other conditions that might affect cognition. Two sets of age-corrected normative data are shown in Table 8–71a: One set is presented for the combined total number of words produced across all three categories (animals, fruits, and vegetables) and the second set provides norms for animal naming alone. Table 8–71b shows the computational formula used to calculate age- and education-corrected scaled scores.

Acevedo et al. (2000) provide norms for English speakers ($N = 316$; age, $M = 69.1$, $SD = 6.9$; education, $M = 14.4$, $SD = 2.5$) as well as Spanish speakers ($N = 237$; age, $M = 64.9$, $SD = 7.7$; education, $M = 13.4$, $SD = 3.2$, range 8–17+), aged 50 to 79 years, for three categories in the order of administration:

Table 8–69 Norms for Animals Stratified for Age (16–59, 60–79, and 80–95 Years) and Years of Education (0–8, 9–12, and 13–21)

	Age 16–59 Years			Age 60–79 Years			Age 80–95 Years		
	Education (Years)			Education (Years)			Education (Years)		
	0–8 (N = 4)	9–12 (N = 109)	13–21 (N = 78)	0–8 (N = 61)	9–12 (N = 165)	13–21 (N = 94)	0–8 (N = 75)	9–12 (N = 103)	13–21 (N = 46)
Percentile Score									
90		26	30	20	22	25	18	19	24
75		23	25	17	19	22	16	17	20
50		20	23	14	17	19	13	14	16
25		17	18	12	14	16	11	12	14
10		15	16	11	12	13	9	11	12
M		19.8	21.9	14.4	16.4	18.2	13.1	13.9	16.3
(SD)		(4.2)	(5.4)	(3.4)	(4.3)	(4.2)	(3.8)	(3.4)	(4.3)

Source: From Tombaugh et al., 1999. Reprinted with the permission of Elsevier.

animals, vegetable, and fruits. The values for English speakers are similar to those reported by Lucas et al. (1998). Data for Spanish speakers are provided in Table 8–72. The sample comprised community-dwelling individuals living in Florida who were screened (e.g., with the MMSE, the Hamilton Depression Rating Scale) to include only cognitively intact individuals.

Stricks et al. (1998) also provide normative data for healthy English speakers and Spanish speakers (aged 65–80+) asked to generate animals, foods, and clothing. The values are somewhat lower than those reported by Acevedo et al. (2000), perhaps reflecting differences in categories requested and a wider

range of educational attainment in the Stricks et al. (1998) study. Their normative data for category fluency are shown in Table 8–67 separately for English-speaking and Spanish-speaking individuals.

Written Fluency. Heaton et al. (2004) provide norms separately for two ethnicity groups (Caucasians, African Americans) organized by age, gender, and education. The samples are large (295 Caucasians, 409 African Americans), cover a wide range in terms of age (20–85 years) and education (0–20 years), and exclusion criteria are specified. T scores less than 40 are classed as impaired.

Table 8–70 Combined Animals, Fruits, and Vegetables: MOANS Norms for Persons Aged 56–95+

Percentile Ranges	<69	69–71	72–74	75–77	78–80	81–83	84–86	87–89	90+	Scaled Score
<1	<24	<22	<18	<13	<13	<13	<13	<6	<4	2
1	24	22–23	18–21	13–19	13–17	13–15	13	6–13	4–9	3
2	25	24	22–23	20–22	18–20	16–20	14–19	14–19	10–13	4
3–5	26–27	25	24–25	23	21–23	21–22	20–22	20–21	14–17	5
6–10	28–31	26–29	26–29	24–26	24–26	23–25	23–25	22–25	18–20	6
11–18	32–37	30–33	30–31	27–30	27–29	26–29	26–28	26–28	21–24	7
19–28	38–39	34–38	32–35	31–33	30–31	30–31	29–30	29–30	25–27	8
29–40	40–42	39–41	36–38	34–36	32–34	32–33	31–32	31–32	28–29	9
41–50	43–48	42–46	39–42	37–40	35–38	34–37	33–36	33–36	30–33	10
60–71	49–50	47–49	43–45	41–44	39–41	38–39	37–39	37–38	34–37	11
72–81	51–55	50–51	46–49	45–48	42–45	40–44	40–43	39–41	38–40	12
82–89	56–58	52–57	50	49	46–49	45–48	44–47	42–46	41–44	13
90–94	59–62	58–61	51–57	50–55	50–53	49–52	48–52	47–50	45–48	14
95–97	63–65	62–64	58–63	56–61	54–58	53–55	53–55	51–54	49–52	15
98	66	65	64–65	62–64	59–63	56–57	56–57	55	53–55	16
99	67–74	66–72	66–72	65–71	64–71	58–71	58–71	56–61	56–58	17
>99	>74	>72	>72	>71	>71	>71	>71	>61	>58	18
N	77	102	129	156	196	215	201	167	99	

Age- and education-corrected MOANS scaled score (MSS$_{A\&E}$) is calculated from a person's age-corrected MOANS scaled score (MSS$_A$) and that person's education expressed in years of formal schooling completed as follows: MSS$_{A\&E}$ = 1.83 + (1.09 × MSS$_A$) − (0.21 × Education). Mean Mayo Verbal Comprehension Factor Score about 107.7, *SD* = 12.7.

Source: Adapted from Lucas et al., 1998, based on Mayo's Older Normative Studies (MOANS).

Table 8–71a MOAANS Age-Based Category (Animals, Fruits and Vegetables) and Animal Fluency Norms in African American Adults

Scaled Score	56–62		63–65		66–68		69–71		72–74		75–77		78+		Percentile Ranges
	C	A	C	A	C	A	C	A	C	A	C	A	C	A	
2	0–19	0–6	0–19	0–1	0–19	0–1	0–19	0–1	0–17	0–1	0–17	0–1	0–16	0–1	<1
3	20–22	—	20–22	2–6	20–21	2–6	20–21	2–6	18–19	2–6	18–19	2–6	17–19	2–4	1
4	23	7	23	—	22–23	—	22	—	20–21	—	20	—	20	5–6	2
5	24	—	24	7	24	7	23–24	7	22–24	7	21–24	7	21–23	7	3–5
6	25–29	8–9	25–28	8	25–28	8	25–27	8	25–27	8	25–26	8	24	8	6–10
7	30	10	29–30	9–10	29–30	9–10	28–29	9–10	28–29	9–10	27–29	9	25–27	9	11–18
8	31–33	11	31–33	11	31–33	11	30–32	11	30–32	11	30–32	10–11	28–29	—	19–28
9	34–37	12–14	34–36	12	34–36	12	33–35	12	33–34	12	33–34	12	30–33	10	29–40
10	38–42	15–16	37–40	13–15	37–39	13–14	36–39	13–14	35–38	13	35–38	13	34–35	11–12	41–59
11	43–45	17	41–43	16	40–42	15	40–41	15	39–41	14–15	39–41	14–15	36–39	13–14	60–71
12	46–48	18–19	44–46	17–18	43–44	16–17	42–44	16–17	42–43	16	42–43	16	40	15	72–81
13	49–53	20–21	47–49	19–20	45–47	18–19	45–47	18	44–46	17–18	44–46	17–18	41–42	16	82–89
14	54–57	22–23	50–53	21	48–51	20	48–51	19–20	47–49	19	47	19	43–46	17–18	90–94
15	58–60	24	54–58	22–24	52–54	21–22	52–54	21–22	50–54	20–21	48–54	20–21	47–51	19	95–97
16	—	25	59–60	25	55–57	23–24	55–57	23–24	55–57	22–24	55–56	22–24	52–54	20–23	98
17	61–64	26–28	61–64	26–28	58–63	25–27	58–63	25–27	58–59	—	57	—	55–57	24	99
18	65+	29+	65+	29+	64+	28+	64+	28+	60+	25+	58+	25+	58+	25+	>99
N	107	107	129	129	165	165	181	181	155	155	118	118	79	79	

Source: Adapted from Lucas et al., 2005. Reprinted with permission of the Mayo Foundation for Medical Education and Research.

Table 8–71b Computational Formula for Age- and
Education-Corrected MOAANS Scaled Scores

	K	W_1	W_2
Category fluency	2.00	1.11	0.23
Animal fluency	1.84	1.11	0.24

Age- and education-corrected MOAANS scaled scores
($MSS_{A\&E}$) can be calculated for fluency scores by using
aged-corrected MOAANS scaled scores (MSS_A)
and education (expressed in years completed)
in the following formula:

$$MSS_{A\&E} = K + (W_1 \times MSS_A) - (W_2 \times EDUC)$$

Source: Adapted from Lucas et al., 2005. Reprinted with permission
of the Mayo Foundation for Medical Education and Research.

Discrepancies Between Phonemic (FAS) and Semantic (Animal) Fluency. Discrepancies in phonemic (FAS) and category (animal) fluency may be of diagnostic value (see *Validity*). Accordingly, Gladsjo, Schuman, Evans, et al. (1999) and Gladsjo, Schuman, Miller, et al. (1999) provide the frequency of letter (FAS)-category (animal) fluency T-score discrepancies of different magnitudes. Relatively large differences between phonemic (L or Letter) and semantic (C or Category) fluency were not uncommon: 10% of the total sample had a L > C T-score difference of 18 or more, or had a L < C T-score difference of 19 or greater. Letter-category fluency discrepancy score was not significantly related to participant's age, education, gender, or ethnicity. The D-KEFS also allows the examiner to contrast phonemic (e.g., FAS) and category (e.g., animals, boys names) fluency conditions.

Clustering and Switching. According to Troyer (2000), increasing age is associated with slightly larger cluster sizes and with reduced switches and words generated (see also Kosmidis et al., 2004). Education showed small effect sizes with regard to switching and clustering, while effects regarding gender were minimal.

Normative data for clustering and switching are provided by Troyer (2000) for tests of phonemic fluency (FAS or CFL) and semantic fluency (animals and supermarket) based on a sample of 411 healthy adults between the ages of 18 and 91 years. Percentiles for individual raw scores can be obtained by adding relevant corrections and looking up the corresponding corrected score in Table 8–73. For example, consider a 50-year-old woman with 13 years of education. If she produced a cluster size of 0.35 on the FAS, her corrected score would be calculated as $0.35 + 50(-.001) + 13(-0.015) + 0.094 = 0.20$. This places her at about the 50th percentile.

Normative Data in Children and Adolescents

Phonemic Fluency—FAS. Normative data for healthy school children have been provided by Gaddes and Crockett (1975) and Anderson et al. (1997). These norms appear to be higher than those reported by Delis et al. (2001).

The sample, aged 7 to 13, studied by Anderson et al. (1997) is well described and contemporary, and their data are provided in Table 8–74. The sample includes approximately 50 participants (approximately half male, half female) in each age group. The sample attended primary and secondary schools in Melbourne, Australia, with school selection based on the need to include a broad range of socioeconomic groups. All children spoke English as their first language and had no previous history of neurological, sensory, or developmental disorders. Children

Table 8–72 Fluency Scores in Spanish Speakers by Gender and Age

	Men: Age (Years)			Women: Age (Years)		
	50–59 (N = 15)	60–69 (N = 32)	70–79 (N = 26)	50–59 (N = 49)	60–69 (N = 65)	70–79 (N = 50)
Task	M (SD)	M (SD)	M (SD)	M (SD)	M (SD)	M (SD)
Animals	15.5 (3.4)	18.0 (7.2)	15.4 (4.2)	16.6 (4.10)	16.7 (4.0)	16.7 (4.5)
Fruits	11.1 (3.0)	12.7 (3.9)	12.4 (3.2)	13.8 (3.1)	13.7 (3.2)	13.0 (3.8)
Vegetables	11.5 (3.4)	11.0 (3.70)	11.6 (4.2)	13.5 (3.6)	14.1 (3.7)	12.7 (3.3)
Total fluency	38.3 (7.8)	41.7 (12.3)	39.3 (9.9)	43.9 (8.2)	44.6 (8.6)	42.4 (9.5)

	Men: Education (Years)			Women: Education (Years)		
	8–12 (N = 39)	13–16 (N = 21)	17+ (N = 13)	8–12 (N = 66)	13–17 (N = 73)	17+ (N = 25)
Task	M (SD)	M (SD)	M (SD)	M (SD)	M (SD)	M (SD)
Animals	16.3 (5.4)	16.8 (5.2)	17.1 (7.7)	15.6 (4.2)	17.2 (3.8)	18.0 (4.5)
Fruits	12.2 (3.7)	12.8 (3.2)	11.5 (3.2)	12.6 (3.1)	14.1 (3.6)	14.5 (2.7)
Vegetables	11.8 (4.0)	10.6 (3.7)	10.9 (3.4)	13.1 (3.6)	13.8 (3.7)	13.8 (3.0)
Total fluency	40.3 (10.9)	40.2 (10.6)	39.5 (10.9)	41.2 (8.6)	45.1 (9.1)	46.4 (6.5)

Source: From Acevedo et al., 2000. Reprinted with the permission of Cambridge University Press.

Table 8–73 Corrections, Demographically Corrected Descriptive Data, and Percentiles for Fluency Scores

	Phonemic (FAS or CFL)			Animals		
	Cluster	Switches	Total	Cluster	Switches	Total
Age (years)	−0.001	+0.05	+0.04	−0.002	+0.05	+0.09
Ed (years)	−0.015	−0.38	−1.06	−0.023	−0.17	−0.51
Form (FAS)	+0.094	−2.67	−2.18	NA	NA	NA
Mean	0.24	23.9	28.6	0.75	9.8	18.1
SD	0.23	8.2	11.1	0.57	2.7	4.6
1st percentile	−0.16	6.6	4.3	−0.24	3.9	8.3
5th percentile	−0.06	10.2	11.4	0.01	5.8	10.9
16th percentile	0.01	15.6	17.0	0.23	7.3	13.5
25th percentile	0.08	18.7	20.6	0.40	7.9	14.9
50th percentile	0.19	23.3	28.7	0.64	9.6	17.9
75th percentile	0.35	29.7	36.6	1.12	11.6	21.2
84th percentile	0.44	32.3	39.3	1.39	12.4	22.8
95th percentile	0.73	37.6	47.6	1.89	14.7	26.7
99th percentile	0.97	43.2	57.4	2.43	16.7	29.3

Based on a sample 411 healthy community-dwelling adults, aged 18–91 years ($M = 59.8$, $SD = 20.7$), and level of education ranging from 5–21 years ($M = 13.9$, $SD = 2.9$).

Source: From Troyer, 2000. Reprinted with the kind permission of Psychology Press.

requiring special educational placement were also excluded from the sample. Data for a smaller sample of adolescents, 14 and 15 years (Anderson et al., 2001), are also provided in Table 8–74. Selection criteria were the same as in Anderson et al. (1997). Similar findings have been reported among Spanish-speaking children in Mexico (Matute et al., 2004).

Phonemic Fluency—CFL, PRW, and "sh." Schum et al. (1989) gave versions CFL and PRW to 229 children (98 males, 131 females), aged 6 to 12 years, with alternate versions (CFL or PRW) given to each successive child. Only children with PPVT-R standard scores between 80 and 120 were included ($M = 102.6$, $SD = 8.9$). Differences between the forms were nonsignificant and the scores were combined. The data are shown in Table 8–75.

Barr (2003) tested a sample of 100 high school athletes, aged 13 to 17 years ($M = 15.9$ years, $SD = 0.98$) on the CFL version. Females outperformed males. The data are shown in Table 8–76 and suggest that adult levels are obtained during this period.

The reader is referred to Table 8–77 for data on words beginning with "sh" (Halperin et al., 1989). Norms for phonemic fluency (S and F) can also be found in the NEPSY for ages 7 to 12.

Category Fluency. Halperin et al.'s (1989) norms for the production of animal names and food names are shown in Table 8–77. Riva et al. (2000) obtained similar animal naming norms for Italian children aged 5 to 11 years (approximately one point higher).

As noted in Table 8–61, the WJ III COG provides semantic fluency norms (combined for foods, first names of people, and animals) for ages ranging from 2 to 80+. Norms for semantic fluency (animals and foods) are also found in the

Table 8–74 Means and Standard Deviations for FAS Among School-Age Children

	Age								
	7	8	9	10	11	12	13	14	15
N	55	56	61	62	51	54	51	18	14
F	5.49 (2.6)	5.86 (2.7)	7.34 (3.0)	8.10 (2.7)	8.66 (3.3)	9.61 (2.9)	9.9 (3.3)		
A	4.55 (2.2)	5.07 (2.0)	6.20 (3.3)	6.68 (2.6)	7.49 (3.2)	8.98 (2.9)	7.8 (3.3)		
S	7.04 (2.8)	7.04 (2.8)	8.93 (3.7)	9.29 (3.26)	10.77 (3.5)	11.93 (3.7)	11.28 (3.5)		
Total	17.07 (6.0)	17.96 (6.2)	22.53 (8.6)	24.18 (6.5)	26.9 (7.8)	30.13 (8.2)	28.98 (8.2)	28.1 (1.7)	30.6 (1.0)
No. rule breaks	0.9	0.9	0.8	0.6	0.4	0.8	0.6		
No. repetitions	0.4	0.1	0.3	0.4	0.3	0.6	0.5		

Source: Adapted from Anderson et al., 1997: Ages 7–13; Anderson et al., 2001: Ages 14–15.

Table 8–75 CFL/PRW Means and Standard Deviations by Grade and Mean Age

Grade	Mean Age	N	Mean Fluency	SD
K	6.3	35	9.1	5.2
1	7.3	34	14.4	4.6
2	8.2	32	17.6	6.2
3	9.3	43	22.7	6.5
4	10.2	33	26.7	7.4
5	11.3	31	24.2	6.9
6	12.3	21	25.8	5.0

Source: Adapted from Schum et al., 1989.

NEPSY; these include preschoolers as well as school-age children (age range 3–12). Norms are provided for the categories individually and for both categories combined. The D-KEFS provides normative data for category fluency (animals and boys names combined, alternative version: clothing and girls names combined; switching condition: fruits and furniture, alternate version: vegetables and musical instruments) for ages 8 and older. Criterion-based norms for children aged 5 to 21 years for naming fluency in three categories (animals, transportation, types of work) can be found in the CELF-4.

Written Fluency. Table 8–78 presents norms for written word fluency in children, aged 6 to 18 years (Kolb & Wishaw, 1985).

Clustering and Switching. Sauzeon et al. (2004) evaluated children aged 7 to 16 years on semantic and phonemic fluency tasks. In letter fluency production, age modified both the number of switches and clusters formed, whereas in semantic fluency, only cluster size changed with age. These authors concluded that increasing letter fluency reflects the development of a strategic switching component (about age 11–12), whereas semantic fluency is associated with the enrichment of semantic knowledge between the ages of 6 and 16 and more efficient access to this knowledge after the age of 13 to 14 years.

RELIABILITY

Internal Reliability

Tombaugh et al. (1999) assessed the degree of internal consistency that existed among F, A, and S. Coefficient alpha was computed using the total number of words generated for each letter as individual items and was found to be high ($r = .83$). The same result ($r = .83$) was reported for C, F, and L (Ruff et al., 1996).

Test-Retest Reliability and Practice Effects

In healthy adults, test-retest correlations tend to be high, typically above .70, for both letter and semantic fluency, with short (e.g., one week) as well as long (e.g., five years) intervals (Basso et al., 1999; Dikmen et al., 1999; Harrison et al., 2000; Levine et al., 2004; Ross, 2003). For example, Tombaugh et al. (1999) found a test-retest reliability coefficient of .74 for FAS after an interval of more than five years in elderly individuals.

Table 8–76 Test Scores for CFL in Adolescents, aged 13–17 Years

	Total Sample ($N = 100$) Mean (*SD*)	Males ($N = 60$) Mean (*SD*)	Females ($N = 40$) Mean (*SD*)
Total words	35.3 (9.8)	33.1 (8.8)	38.7 (10.3)

Source: Adapted from Barr, 2003.

Table 8–77 Performance of Normal School Children on Naming Animals, Foods, and Words Beginning With "Sh"

	Animals			Foods		"Sh words"	
Age (Years)	N	M	SD	M	SD	M	SD
6	34	10.74	2.4	9.74	3.3	4.24	1.6
7	40	12.43	2.9	11.88	2.7	5.53	1.6
8	32	12.31	2.7	11.11	3.4	5.21	2.1
9	38	13.76	3.7	14.05	3.9	5.95	2.4
10	22	14.27	3.7	13.97	2.2	6.00	2.0
11	28	15.50	3.8	14.80	4.6	6.28	2.4
12	10	18.90	6.2	17.70	4.0	6.10	1.8

Source: From Halperin et al., 1989. Reprinted with the kind permission of Psychology Press.

Table 8–78 Children's Written Word Fluency—Thurstone Version

	Total			Female			Male		
Age	N	M	SD	N	M	SD	N	M	SD
6	80	9.28	4.47	40	9.85	4.58	40	8.70	4.33
7	133	15.87	8.22	72	17.22	8.20	61	14.26	8.00
8	197	21.52	9.29	85	23.72	10.34	112	19.85	8.05
9	208	25.93	10.18	90	28.41	9.93	118	24.03	10.01
10	189	29.98	11.92	86	33.16	11.83	103	27.32	11.39
11	146	37.08	11.98	75	39.03	10.57	71	35.01	13.07
12	140	40.58	13.00	84	44.52	12.98	56	34.61	10.61
13	167	45.07	14.10	76	51.37	13.65	91	39.81	12.26
14	175	48.46	14.72	85	52.64	14.30	90	44.52	14.08
15	120	47.35	15.22	51	51.57	13.38	69	44.23	15.88
16	69	48.28	13.69	28	53.43	10.54	41	44.76	14.56
17	79	49.65	17.51	37	53.65	17.63	42	46.12	16.83
18	30	61.47	15.29	18	64.22	14.98	12	57.33	15.42

Note: This test requires the person to write as many words as possible beginning with the letter "s" in five minutes, and as many four-letter words as possible beginning with the letter "c" in four minutes. Means are totals for both sets of responses.

Source: From Kolb & Whishaw, 1985. Reproduced with the permission of W. H. Freeman and Company & Worth Publishers.

Table 8–79a FAS Change Scores, Standard Deviations, and Reliability Coefficients

Measure	T1 Mean	SD	T2 Mean	SD	T2–T1	SD	r	p	Cohen's d
FAS	45.0	11.89	48.1	11.43	3.08	7.94	.77	.001	.26

Based on a sample of 145 well-educated men (education, $M = 16.4$, $SD = 2.3$), mostly Caucasians (age, $M = 38.8$, $SD = 7.9$).

Source: Adapted from Levine et al., 2004.

As might be expected, gains are seen following short retest intervals. Wilson et al. (2000) reported that fluency for the same letter or category shows a small but consistent increase across 20 successive administrations over a four-week period in normals as well as those with severe head injury.

Basso et al. (1999) noted no gains among 50 healthy males retested following a 12-month interval on FAS. However, Levine et al. (2004) reported gains of about three words for 145 healthy men (age, $M = 38.8$, $SD = 7.9$; education, $M = 16.4$, $SD = 2.3$, mostly Caucasians) reassessed with FAS across a wide time interval, four to 24 months (mean interval = 191 days, $SD = 38$). Table 8–79a shows the change score, standard deviation of the change score, and test-retest reliability coefficient for use in reliable change index (RCI) formulas. Table 8–79b shows a regression formula that can be used to estimate Time 2 scores. Neither the length of retest interval nor age

Table 8–79b Regression Equations for Estimating Retest Scores

Measure	Regression Equation	Residual SD
FAS	$14.84 + (.739 \times \text{Time 1 score})$	7.31

Source: Adapted from Levine et al., 2004.

contributed significantly to the regression equation. The impact of educational level, while significant, only contributed an additional 2% to the multiple regression equation. The residual standard deviation for the regression formula shown in Table 8–79b can be used to establish the normal range for retest scores. For example, a 90% confidence interval can be created around the scores by multiplying the residual standard deviation by 1.645, which allows for 5% of people to fall outside of both the upper and lower extremes. Individuals whose scores exceed the extremes are considered to have significant changes. Although test-retest reliabilities are reasonable for phonemic fluency, these findings suggest that relatively large changes in performance are required to conclude that real decline or improvement has occurred as opposed to being due to the effects of practice and random measurement error (see also Basso et al., 1999).

A similar picture emerges for category fluency. Bird et al. (2004) evaluated semantic (animals) fluency in 99 healthy adults (drawn from a larger sample of 188 healthy volunteers, aged 39–75 years; age, $M = 57.0$, $SD = 8.3$; education, $M = 13.1$, $SD = 3.7$) who were retested following a one-month interval. As Table 8–80 shows, small but reliable practice effects were seen. Reliable change indices were calculated as the standard deviations of the difference scores, multiplied by 1.645,

Table 8–80 Animal Fluency Test-Retest Reliability, Practice Effects, and Reliable Change Indices Corrected for Practice

Test	N	r	Mean T1 (SD)	Mean T2 (SD)	Lower RCI	Upper RCI
Animals	99	.56	23.4 (5.1)	24.7 (6.3)	–7.6	+10.5

Based on a sample of 99 normal adults, aged 39–75 years (M = 57.0 years, SD = 8.3) and 13.1 years of education (SD = 3.7). Retest interval was one month. RC indices are based on 90% confidence interval.

Source: Adapted from Bird et al., 2004.

Table 8–81 Verbal Fluency Test-Retest Effects in 81 Normal Individuals Assessed Following Intervals of About 11 Months

	Time 1 (1)		Time 2 (2)		T2–T1 (3)	(4)	(5)	(6)	T1, T2 (7)
Measure	M	(SD)	M	(SD)	M	(SD)	p	|T2–T1|/SD(T1)	r
Letter Fluency	43.25	10.75	44.47	10.36	1.22	7.85	.165	.11	.72

FAS and BDT given in counterbalanced manner. Mean age of sample about 29 years, mean education about 12 years.

Source: Adapted from Dikmen et al., 1999.

and by adding the mean change in score from Time 1 to Time 2. Therefore, 10% of the sample had a change in score that fell outside of the RCI corrected for practice. Note that the RCI is large, due to the considerable variability in performance that can be expected between assessments. Neither NART IQ nor age was related to the practice effect. As an example, suppose an individual obtains a baseline raw score of 20 on animal fluency. Repeat testing one month later following cognitive therapy reveals a score of 26. Examination of Table 8–80 indicates that a gain of six points does not exceed the upper limits (+10.5) of the 90% CI.

Ross (2003) examined the stability of COWA scores in a sample of 55 healthy college students who were retested over an average interval of six to seven weeks. He found that test-retest reliability for clustering and switching was poor (r_{icc} = .47 and .58, respectively), suggesting that any search process (strategic or otherwise) can vary considerably with each test administration.

For written word fluency (Thurstone version), Cohen and Stanczak (2000) reported a six-week retest reliability of .79 for 70 adult students (age, M = 20.62, SD = 4.36). There was a notable practice effect of an average eight-word gain on the second administration.

Alternate Form Reliability and Practice Effects

Ruff et al. (1996) gave alternate versions of phonemic fluency (CFL given in first test session, PRW given in second test session) to 120 subjects with an interval of six months. A significant correlation of .74 was reported, with an average gain of three words on the second administration. Because forms were not counterbalanced across participants, the authors

could not rule out differences between letter sets as an explanation for the three-word gain. Schum et al. (1989) gave these versions to children, aged 6 to 12 years, half receiving one form and half the other. They found few differences between the forms.

Wilson et al. (2000) suggested that practice effects can be reduced by changing the letter or category on each test occasion. The findings of Dikmen et al. (1999) are consistent with this proposal. They gave alternate forms (FAS, BDT) in a counterbalanced manner to 81 normal controls (mean age about 29 years, mean education about 12 years) with a retest interval of about 11 months. Reliability was adequate (.72), with only small practice effects noted. Table 8–81 provides information to assess change, taking practice into account. Using values in Table 8–81, one first subtracts the mean T2-T1 change (column 3) from the difference between the two testings for the individual and then compares it to 1.64 times the standard deviation of the difference (column 4). The 1.64 comes from the normal distribution and is exceeded in the positive or negative direction only 10% of the time if indeed there is no real change in clinical condition.

Barr (2003) gave 48 adolescents (aged 13–17 years) alternate versions (CFL on the first session and PRW on the second session) with an interval of about two months. Reliability was marginal (r = .68), with gains of about three words noted on the second administration (see table 8–80). Reliable change indices are shown in Table 8–82. The RCI is followed by the percentage of adolescents with a change score exceeding the lower limit. This value represents the level of raw score decline that is required to exceed what might be expected on the basis of normal error variance and the effects of practice. Upper limits are also listed to aid in interpretation of possible improvements.

Table 8–82 Test scores (COWA Total Words) in Adolescents at Baseline and Then About 60 Days Later and RCIs Followed by Percent of Sample With Scores Falling Below the Lower Limit

T1 Mean (*SD*)	T2 Mean (*SD*)	T2–T1 Mean (*SD*)	r	SEM	S difference	90% CI	80% CI	70% CI
36.3 (9.0)	39.7 (9.4)	3.42 (7.4)	.68	5.09	7.20	−8, +15 (6.3)	−6, +13 (10.4)	−4, +11 (16.7)

CFL given in first session, PRW in the second session.

Source: Adapted from Barr, 2003.

For example, an athlete obtains a baseline score of 36 on the COWA. Repeat testing within 48 hours of a concussion reveals a score of 29. Examination of Table 8–82 shows that that the observed decline of six points does not exceed the lower limit (−8) of the 90% CI; it does, however, exceed the 80% CI.

Interrater Reliability

Interrater reliability for scoring 125 CFL protocols of healthy subjects is high (.99; Ross, 2003). For the written Thurstone version, an interrater reliability of .98 was observed in university students (Cohen & Stanczak, 2000). For clustering and switching scores, Ross (2003) found near-perfect agreement among seven independent raters for 125 protocols of healthy subjects (.96 for total number of clusters; .99 for total number of switches; see also Abwender et al., 2001).

VALIDITY

Correlations Between Fluency Tasks

Correlations among phonemic fluency tasks (e.g., FAS, CFL) are high. Thus, studies of the equivalence of the letters FAS and CFL (Cohen & Stanczak, 2000; Lacy et al., 1996; Troyer, 2000) show that the two sets of letters are roughly comparable across different settings and groups (healthy, psychiatric, suspected CNS dysfunction), with correlations between forms ranging from .85 to .94. In general, differences between the letter sets appear to be small, as suggested in Table 8–71 (Troyer, 2000). For letters FAS and BHR, the correlation is .83 (Delis et al., 2001), and differences between versions appear to be negligible. The correlation between CFL and PRW is also high (.82; Benton et al., 1994) as are the correlations between written word fluency and phonemic fluency (FAS and CFL/PRW; *r* = .72 and .81, respectively; Cohen & Stanczak, 2000).

Correlations between forms using different semantic categories (e.g., animals and clothing, animals and foods) are moderately high (.66–.71; Delis et al., 2001; Riva et al., 1999); however, the values are not sufficiently high to establish equivalency among forms. Note, too, that demographic influences may differentially impact various categories (e.g., fruits and vegetables; Acevado et al., 2000).

Correlations within phonemic and semantic fluency tasks show higher indices of association than those between these two types of tests. In adults as well as children, phonemic fluency (e.g., FAS) scores correlate moderately (.34–.64) with category (e.g., animals, foods) fluency (Kave, 2005; Kosmidis et al., 2004; Matute et al., 2004; Riva et al., 1999; Johnson-Selfridge et al., 1998; Tombaugh et al., 1999). However, factor-analytic findings in children (Riva et al., 1999) reveal that both phonemic and category fluency tasks load on one factor.

Correlation With Other Cognitive Measures

Verbal fluency measures have a substantial verbal component. In fact, phonemic fluency was initially developed as a measure of Verbal IQ (Thurstone, 1938). Not surprisingly, correlations between .44 and .87 have been reported between phonemic fluency and VIQ (see Henry & Crawford, 2004a, for a review). Phonemic fluency shows a stronger relation to Verbal IQ (*r* = .42–.48) than does Performance IQ (*r* = .29–.36; Anderson et al., 2001; Steinberg et al., 2005). In children as well as adults, a closer relationship exists between naming (Boston Naming Test) and semantic fluency (.57–.68) than between naming and phonemic fluency (.43–.50; Henry et al., 2004; Riva et al., 2000). Thus, while performance on both phonemic and semantic fluency is dependent on the integrity of semantic memory, the relative contribution of this aspect of cognition to performance on the latter is substantially greater (Henry et al., 2004).

Some have reported that episodic verbal memory contributes to performance on tests of verbal fluency (e.g., Ruff et al., 1997; Somerville et al., 2000). However, there are reports of patients with dense amnesia who can perform at average or above-average levels on tests of verbal fluency (Dall'Ora et al., 1989), indicating that such tests can be performed adequately despite the presence of severe episodic memory deficits.

A number of factor-analytic findings in adults (Elias et al., 1997) and children (Anderson et al., 2001; Brocki & Bohli, 2004) have suggested that attentional control/working memory play an important role. Consistent with these findings, individuals who score high on a measure of working memory capacity generate more animal names than individuals who score low on the same measure (Rosen & Engle, 1997). Based on studies of healthy individuals performing verbal fluency tasks under various secondary load conditions, Rosen and Engle (1997) proposed that semantic fluency involves four retrieval components: (1) activation automatically spreading from the cue, (2) self-monitoring of output to prevent repetition and error, (3) suppression of previously retrieved responses, and (4) generation of cues to access new names. Although automatic activation is assumed to require little attention, the suppression of previous responses and monitoring for repetitions are particularly taxing on attention resources. Azuma (2004) noted that because words sharing first letters are unlikely to be organized in a network, phonemic fluency must involve somewhat different processes: self-monitoring to prevent errors, suppressing previous responses, and generating cues to access new items. Passive spreading activation would not be a viable retrieval process for letter fluency; rather, individuals must actively retrieve items, an attention-demanding process. According to this view, when resources are limited, other attention-demanding components (e.g., monitoring and suppression) may suffer, resulting in increases in perseverative errors.

The extent of the demands on attention may vary with the temporal duration of the task. Fernaeus and Almquist (1998) suggested that a two-factor model is needed to model word generation in the FAS test, which may generalize to other tests as well. They noted that FAS word production varies markedly across the one-minute span, with the number of words produced following a negatively accelerating curve approaching an asymptotic level after about 30 seconds. Initial responses appear to rely on a rapid access of words from semantic memory with little mental effort. These words load on the same factor as Digit Span and memory free recall. During the later phase of the test, word production seems to draw on an effortful and extensive search of semantic memory. These later responses were related to Wechsler Information, Similarities, and Vocabulary subtests.

Verbal fluency scores also need to be interpreted within the context of mental speed (see also Salthouse et al., 2003). For example, a factor analysis (Boone et al., 1998) of FAS and other tests (Wisconsin Card Sorting Test, Stroop Test, Auditory Consonant Test, WAIS-R, the Rey Complex Figure Test, and Wechsler Memory Scale subtests) in psychiatric patients and controls (Boone et al., 1998) revealed that FAS loaded on a "speeded processing" factor alongside performance on the Stroop Test and the Wechsler Digit Symbol subtest. The authors concluded that word fluency failure can have as much to do with an impairment in speed of information processing as with an impairment in the generation of lexical items.

Thus, individual differences in speed of processing are related to fluency performance, with relatively lower scores on fluency tasks associated with slowed processing speed. However, aging-related effects in fluency performance appear not to be mediated by declines in speed. Longitudinal studies (Ratcliff et al., 2003; Sliwinski & Buschke, 1999) show declines in fluency associated with advancing age. Although declines in processing speed are related to within-person declines in fluency (both phonemic and semantic), the magnitude of cognitive declines was not substantially attenuated by controlling for changes in processing speed.

Neuroanatomical Correlates

A number of studies have demonstrated that left frontal lesions impair performance on letter fluency tasks (e.g., Baldo et al., 2001; Levin et al., 2001; Milner, 1964; Perret, 1974; Ramier & Hecaen, 1970). A detailed exploration of brain-behavior relationships in fluency performances has been offered by Stuss et al. (1998). They found that as a group, left frontal lesions impair letter-based fluency, but not all patients with left frontal pathology are impaired. They noted that this is a large region, and there are likely to be important functional differences within this region. With the objective of defining more explicitly the brain-behavior relations of verbal fluency, they examined both phonemic (FAS) and category (animals) fluency performances in a sample of 74 adults with restricted brain lesions (all based upon CT and MRI findings). Those with lesions of the dorsolateral and/or striatal areas of the left frontal lobe were the most impaired. Superior medial frontal lobe regions of either hemisphere had a moderate impact on performance. Nonfrontal left hemisphere regions also have a role in letter fluency as left parietal lobe lesions were also associated with performance deficits. The same lesion sites produced impairments in category-based fluency, but so did lesions of right dorsolateral and inferior medial regions. In short, Stuss et al.'s work suggests that a number of regions are implicated in fluency performance with relevant processes including initiation and activation (supplementary motor area) and working memory (dorsolateral). Further, there are subtle differences in the neural networks underlying letter and semantic fluency.

Recent meta-analytic findings suggest that both phonemic and semantic fluency measures make comparable demands on frontal structures, but semantic fluency is also relatively more dependent on temporal structures (Henry & Crawford, 2004a; Henry et al., 2004). These authors (Henry & Crawford, 2004a) also noted that for frontal, but not nonfrontal patients, phonemic fluency deficits qualified as differential deficits when compared with IQ and psychomotor speed. Therefore, only for frontal patients can phonemic fluency deficits be regarded as executive dysfunction. Where there are nonfrontal injuries, the integrity of the semantic system and generalized impairment (e.g., slowing) must also be considered.

The lesion data are supported by activation studies in healthy individuals. For example, Gourovitch et al. (2000) examined PET-based regional cerebral blood flow patterns in a sample of 18 normal adult subjects under three conditions: phonemic fluency, semantic fluency, and a control (nonfluency) language task (i.e., generating days of the week and months of the year). Relative to control, participants activated similar brain regions during both fluency tasks, including the anterior cingulate, left prefrontal regions, thalamus, and cerebellum. However, subtle differences in activation patterns for phonemic versus semantic fluency were also described: relatively greater activation of left frontal cortex for phonemic fluency and relatively greater activation of left temporal cortex for semantic fluency.

Clinical Studies

Aphasia. Individuals with aphasia may produce fewer words in general or they may generate a number of words, including many errors (Spreen & Benton, 1977).

Head Injury. There is considerable evidence that neuropathologically, the frontal lobes are particularly vulnerable in TBI (e.g., Levin & Kraus, 1994). Because executive processes rely significantly on intact frontal structures, TBI should impact this aspect of cognition. Consistent with this notion, a recent meta-analysis of patients with TBI (Henry & Crawford, 2004b) found that as with patients with focal frontal (but not temporal) lobe injuries, TBI patients were comparably impaired on tests of phonemic and semantic fluency. The phonemic fluency deficit could not be accounted for by patients' level of premorbid or current level of Verbal IQ and was also substantially (although not significantly) in excess of the deficit on a measure of psychomotor speed (Trail Making Test A). Phonemic fluency was also significantly more sensitive to the presence of TBI than was the WCST. These authors also noted that while episodic memory deficits are widely regarded as the most prominent deficit associated with TBI, executive deficits, as manifested by impairments in fluency, are of at least comparable magnitude.

The test is also sensitive to severity of traumatic brain injury. For example, Iverson et al. (1999) examined CFL performances in a sample of 669 individuals (tested usually within the first week postinjury), categorized according to severity of head trauma: mild, moderate, or severe. The task was sensitive to reduced verbal fluency in all groups, and performance showed a clear relation to severity. In a longitudinal study of 122 5- to 15-year-old children with closed head injury, Levin et al. (2001) found that phonemic (COWA) fluency performance was poorer in younger children with severe injury than in older children. The word fluency studies with children are reviewed by Levin et al. (2000).

Dementia. There is evidence that semantic fluency is more useful than other tests (e.g., Trail Making Test) in the detection of dementia, although composite measures (e.g., MMSE) are better (Heun et al., 1998). The inclusion of verbal fluency measures has been recommended to increase the sensitivity of tests such as the MMSE (see *MMSE* elsewhere in this volume).

A number of studies have reported that discrepancies between letter and category fluency may be useful for the early detection of dementia and for distinguishing between cortical and subcortical dementias (Butters et al., 1987; Monsch et al., 1992, 1994). In patients with dementia of the Alzheimer type (AD), semantic fluency tends to be more affected than phonemic fluency (Butters et al., 1987; Epker et al., 1999; Henry & Crawford, 2004c; Henry et al., 2004; Monsch et al., 1992, 1994), reflecting disorganization or degradation in semantic knowledge. Meta-analytic findings suggest that patients with

Parkinson's disease (PD) also appear more impaired on semantic relative to phonemic fluency, although in patients with Alzheimer's disease (AD), the relative deficit in semantic fluency appears more pronounced (Henry & Crawford, 2004c; Henry et al., 2004). Patients with Huntington's disease (HD) appear to experience comparable deficits in these two types of fluency (Henry et al., 2005). Thus, although patients with PD or HD appear to experience particular difficulties with tasks reliant upon semantic memory, for patients with AD, the relative prominence of deficits in semantic versus phonemic fluency can be regarded as substantially greater.

It is important to bear in mind that discrepancies between semantic and phonemic fluency have limited diagnostic utility. Thus, Sherman and Massman (1999) found that a majority (66.8%) of their subjects with AD showed the expected advantage of letter (FAS) versus category (animal) fluency, but they also reported the presence of a sizeable minority of individuals where the opposite pattern was noted. The smaller group exhibiting the unexpected fluency pattern had higher MMSE scores; however, these two groupings did not show any difference in their performance on other neuropsychological measures using MMSE as a covariate. Further, Crossley et al. (1997) found that category fluency (animal naming) was more impaired than letter fluency at both mild and moderate states of dementia, but neither task differentiated AD from vascular dementia. Similarly, both groups display a similar pattern of impairment in fluency in the preclinical phase (Laukka et al., 2004).

The reason for the conflicting findings is not certain but may reflect differences in the anatomical site of the lesion, diagnostic accuracy, severity of impairment, small sample sizes, and the adequacy of the normative base. The presence of other disorders (e.g., depression) may present additional complications (Ravdin et al., 2003). Overall, the available literature suggests that use of dissociations in phonemic and semantic fluency patterns to support a specific diagnosis (e.g., of AD) may be problematic.

Mood and Thought Disorders. Depression has an impact on fluency, with lower levels of distress associated with higher fluency scores (Acevado et al., 2000; La Rue et al., 1999; but see Ravdin et al., 2003). A recent meta-analysis of 42 studies comprising 2206 participants (Henry & Crawford, 2005a) concluded that both phonemic and semantic fluency are broadly equivalent in the sensitivity to depression and that neither qualified as a differential deficit relative to psychomotor speed. Thus, for patients with depression, low scores on these fluency tasks may not reflect executive dysfunction or a degraded semantic store, but a more generalized impairment, such as cognitive slowing.

A recent meta-analysis (Henry & Crawford, 2005b) of studies comparing the performance of people with schizophrenia and healthy controls on tests of fluency suggested that neither phonemic nor semantic fluency deficits qualified as differential deficits relative to general intelligence or psychomotor speed.

Patient with schizophrenia were significantly more impaired on semantic relative to phonemic fluency. Henry and Crawford (2005b) concluded that deficits on tests of verbal fluency reflect a more generalized intellectual impairment and not particular deficits in executive control processes. Further, they suggested that the larger deficit for semantic relative to phonemic fluency suggests that, in addition to general retrieval difficulties, schizophrenia is associated with compromises to the semantic store.

Diagnostic Utility of Clustering/Switching Scores

Traditionally, the number of acceptable responses within the allotted time was used as the main variable in assessing performance on verbal fluency tests. However, fluency measures yield considerable qualitative information as well (e.g., coding of clustering and switching processes), and examination of the qualitative aspects of the output may help to clarify the nature of the deficient performance (e.g., Abwender et al., 2001; Troyer et al., 1997). Troyer et al. (1997) have proposed that clustering (i.e., contiguous words from the same subcategory) is related to temporal lobe processes such as retrieval from verbal memory, whereas switching (the ability to shift between clusters) implicates frontal processes involving mental flexibility and mental search processes.

In support of this proposal, impaired clustering performance has been found in patients with temporal lobectomy, whereas switching is impaired among patients with left dorsolateral and superior medial frontal lobe lesions (Troyer, Moscovitch, Winocur, Alexander, et al., 1998) and is decreased under conditions of divided attention (Troyer et al., 1997). Decreased switching is evident with advancing age (Kosmidis et al., 2004; Troyer et al., 1997) and is also seen in patient groups with presumed frontal dysfunction, including Parkinson's disease (perhaps restricted to those with dementia; Troester et al., 1998; Troyer, Moscovitch, Winocur, Leach, et al., 1998), Huntington's disease (Ho et al., 2002; Rich et al., 1999), multiple sclerosis (Troester et al., 1998), AIDS (Millikin et al., 2004), and schizophrenia (Robert et al., 1998; Zakzanis et al., 2000). Pallidotomy patients generate significantly fewer words on phonemic fluency (FAS, CFL) for up to a year following surgery (Troester et al., 2002; York et al., 2003). The impairment appears due to a decline in the total number of switches made on the test, rather than a decline in the number of clusters generated, and likely reflects disruption of frontostriatal neural circuits (Troester et al., 2002; York et al., 2003). There also appears to be an association between performance on switching indices (but not clustering indices) and on key neuropsychological tests thought to be sensitive to frontostriatal impairment (e.g., CANTAB IDED task, Stroop, TMT), at least in patients with HD (Ho et al., 2002).

Overall, the research has provided encouraging results with regard to the diagnostic utility of such a qualitative scoring technique. However, inconsistencies have been obtained. For example, Troyer, Moscovitch, Winocur, Leach, et al. (1998) reported that patients with Alzheimer's disease were impaired not only in clustering on phonemic fluency but also in both clustering and switching on semantic fluency. In addition, reservations about the utility of the clustering and switching measures have been raised by Epker et al. (1999). They examined individuals with Alzheimer's disease, Parkinson's disease, and older adults on both letter (FAS) and semantic (animals) fluency tasks. In addition to total words produced, the groups were compared on their use of clustering and switching strategies as defined by Troyer et al. (1997). The variable of total words was equal to or surpassed the other variables in distinguishing groups, suggesting that these qualitative verbal fluency measures may not provide significant additional information in terms of diagnostic utility, at least in individuals with dementing disorders of moderate severity. Qualitative fluency variables may be of greater utility in individuals with relatively mild cognitive dysfunction and possibly in patients with focal lesions. Finally, the precise interpretation of clustering and switching scores remains unresolved. For example, Demakis et al. (2003) has suggested that switching may not be a specific measure of executive processing but may just be tapping general cognitive functioning. Mayr (2002) has argued that the procedure introduced by Troyer et al (1997) does not allow an unambiguous dissociation between a general reduction in processing speed and a selective switching deficit. There is also some evidence based on correlational analyses with other tests presumed to test strategy use (CVLT, Ruff Figural Fluency) that clustering and switching can be further decomposed into subtypes that reflect different cognitive processes on phonemic versus semantic fluency tasks (Abwender et al., 2001). A more refined scoring system (e.g., Abwender et al., 2001) may improve our understanding of the cognitive processes underlying verbal fluency performance.

Error Scores

Among perseverative errors, recurrent perseverations are the most commonly observed, with greater frequency among individuals with a variety of neurological conditions including aphasia (Shindler et al., 1984), frontal lobe damage (Baldo & Shimamura, 1998), AD (Shindler et al., 1984; Suhr & Jones, 1998), and HD (Ho et al., 2002; Suhr & Jones, 1998). They are relatively rare in healthy adults (Ramage et al., 1999; see Azuma, 2004, for a review).

Ecological Validity

FAS-COWA has been successfully used in treatment studies. For example, a study by Sarno et al. (2005) compared FAS performance at 3, 6, 9, and 12 months in 18 poststroke moderately severe aphasics (BDAE severity rating of approximately 3.0) during the course of one year of intensive speech therapy. Scores at different times were highly correlated, though a steady and significant increase from 14.94 to 23.0 across the four tests was noted. Retesting at an average of 10 months after the end of treatment resulted in a mean of 19.17. The authors stress that word fluency was not a targeted part of speech therapy.

A study by Doesborgh et al. (2002) found evidence of ecological validity for semantic word fluency in that results were good predictors of actual communication skills as measured with the Nijmwegen Everyday Language Test (ANELT-A). Burgess et al. (1998) reported that in a mixed neurological sample, poor performance on fluency (FAS, animals) tasks was modestly reflected (.29–.35) in caregiver ratings of patients' problems in everyday life, and with the patients' lack of insight into their problems.

Written Word Fluency

Early studies of written word fluency were designed for individuals with frontal lobe disease (e.g., Milner's [1964] examination of patients with left and right frontal and temporal lobectomies in which she reported the test's sensitivity to left frontal lobe involvement).

Pendleton et al. (1982) examined written word fluency in a sample of 203 brain-damaged and 134 normal individuals. The authors reported that test performance was sensitive to cerebral involvement in general and that individuals with focal frontal lobe involvement performed more poorly than those with focal nonfrontal lesions. However, these authors also found that the task was unable to discriminate focal frontal from diffuse lesions. An analysis of written word fluency by Cohen and Stanczak (2000) compared data from 188 normal control subjects aged 18 to 60 years with archival data of 296 brain-damaged patients (etiologies predominantly TBI, CVA, seizure disorders, and neurodegenerative disorders). The brain-damaged and the neurologically intact subjects could be discriminated from each other with a sensitivity of 96.6% and a specificity of 37.5%, but performance did not clearly delineate left versus right, anterior versus posterior, and focal versus diffuse lesions.

COMMENT

Tests of verbal fluency have a venerable past. Thurstone (1938) included verbal fluency as part of the Primary Mental Abilities (PMA) Test. They are quick and simple and do not require any test material except a timer. Unlike most other tests, verbal fluency tasks do not have low ceilings when used in neurologically intact populations, making them popular for use in a variety of testing situations. The use of these tasks in aphasic and geriatric assessment is well established. The extension of these tests into the examination of executive functions in recent years has been found to have utility.

Clinicians have a choice of several types of fluency measures. The FAS and the MAE COWA both have had contemporary normative updating in large groups of individuals. Given the importance of factors such as age, education/intelligence, and ethnicity, the use of demographically adjusted norms is critical. Further, current norms are preferred since they establish a higher standard that will result in a higher sensitivity to impairment.

Alternate form reliability is high for phonemic versions (e.g., FAS, CFL), offering equivalent versions of this task (with some caveats). Test-retest reliability for total scores is also high, suggesting that verbal fluency tasks are appropriate for use when tracking change. However, poor stability (<.60) of cluster and switch scores (in healthy individuals) is problematic, suggesting that search processes can vary considerably with each test administration (Ross, 2003). This issue requires examination in neurologically impaired individuals.

Different semantic fluency measures are not equivalent and are differentially affected by various variables related to the individual. More normative studies have been published on animal fluency than on other category fluency tasks. Although affected by age and education, it is worth noting that animal fluency is not impacted by gender or depressed mood and is only minimally affected by the language of the examinee, suggesting that it may have wider use than other semantic categories (Acevedo et al., 2000). In general, age accounts for more variance on semantic than phonemic fluency tasks. The reason for the greater effect of age on semantic fluency may reflect the fact that fluency performance is a function of the size of the set being searched. Larger sets may be more vulnerable to a slowdown in search processes (Kave, 2005).

One procedural and interpretative problem with the use of category fluency, especially in comparison with letter fluency, is that performance is typically based upon a single trial, while letter fluency tasks proceed through several trials. This problem can be avoided if several trials for different categories are used. The greater number of responses will also yield more reliable results.

In healthy adults and children, category fluency tends to be somewhat easier than letter fluency (Kave, 2005; Kostidis et al., 2004; Mathuranath et al., 2003: Riva et al., 2000), although in very old individuals (80+), this pattern may no longer be valid (Ravdin et al., 2003). The reason for the discrepancy between tasks is not certain, although some (e.g., Riva et al., 2000) have suggested that phonemic fluency tasks may require greater organization and nonhabitual strategic capabilities (Riva et al., 2000; but see Henry & Crawford, 2004a). Azuma (2004) has argued that semantic categories follow hierarchical memory organization (they have natural subcategories that letter categories lack), thereby allowing organized searches. For example, when generating animals, the individual may sample from subdomains (e.g., farm animals, pets, jungle animals, etc.). By contrast, letter categories require nonheuristic searches, and therefore phonemic fluency places greater demands on effortful processes such as strategic organization and response inhibition.

Bear in mind that deficits on tests of verbal fluency do not by themselves provide evidence of executive dysfunction; rather, it is the pattern of deficits across fluency and other measures (e.g., Verbal IQ, Processing Speed) that is important. Rigorous assessment of this issue is critical to determine whether deficits on executive measures qualify as differential deficits (e.g., Henry & Crawford, 2004a, 2004b, 2004c; Henry et al., 2004). Comparison of the relative magnitude of deficits on phonemic and semantic fluency tasks may also provide clues regarding the prominence of executive and semantic memory dysfunction.

The verbal fluency test taps somewhat different abilities than other executive measures (e.g., WCST) and may be a more sensitive marker of executive dysfunction than the WCST (e.g., Henry & Crawford, 2004b). The psychological mechanisms underlying verbal fluency remain to be worked out. Word knowledge, episodic memory, working memory, speed of processing information, and effortful self-initiation appear to be integral components.

A single score is typically obtained for word generation tasks. However, studies of the temporal characteristics of such tasks (e.g., FAS) suggest that at least two separate scores are needed to give more detailed information about the functioning of memory retrieval. Thus, one score appears needed for the initial (semiautomatic retrieval) phase, while a second score is required for later (effortful retrieval) phases of the task (Fernaeus & Almquist, 1998). The version provided by Delis et al. (2001) allows examination of different parts of the retrieval process (each of the four 12-second intervals summed across phonemic and semantic fluency trials).

The neural bases for performance of the phonemic and semantic conditions are not certain, although there is evidence from disparate sources of the importance of the frontal lobes for both phonemic and semantic fluency. There also appear to be subtle differences with regard to neuroanatomic correlates underlying the letter and category fluency, with the latter also requiring intact temporal structures. Phonemic fluency is more sensitive to frontal dysfunction than the WCST (categories completed, perseverative errors) and has better specificity (Henry & Crawford, 2004a).

Finally, investigators/clinicians tend to rely on a quantitative measure of fluency performance. Whether evaluation of patterns of performance across letter/category tasks and qualitative assessment (e.g., clustering/switching) provides additional diagnostic information remains to be determined, particularly in cases with mild or focal disturbance. Further, despite some theoretically consistent findings in the literature, the precise meaning of these qualitative aspects of verbal fluency is not entirely clear. At present, such distinctions should not be used as the basis of diagnostic decisions without supplementation by other data.

REFERENCES

Abwender, D. A., Swan, J. G., Bowerman, J. T., & Connolly, S. W. (2001). Qualitative analysis of verbal fluency output: Review and comparison of several scoring methods. *Assessment, 8,* 323–336.

Acevedo, A., Loewenstein, D. A., Barker, W. B., Harwood, D. G., Luis, C., Bravo, M., Hurwitz, D. A., Aguero, H., Greenfield, L., & Duara, R. (2000). Category fluency test: Normative data for English- and Spanish-speaking elderly. *Journal of the International Neuropsychological Society, 6,* 760–769.

Anderson, V. A., Anderson, P., Northam, E., Jacobs, R., & Catroppa, C. (2001). Development of executive functions through late childhood and adolescence in an Australian sample. *Developmental Neuropsychology, 20,* 385–406.

Anderson, V., Lajoie, G., & Bell, R. (1997). *Neuropsychology assessment of the school-aged child.* Department of Psychology, University of Melbourne.

Anstey, K. J., Matters, B., Brown, A. K., & Lord, S. R. (2000). Normative data on neuropsychological tests for very old adults living in retirement villages and hostels. *The Clinical Neuropsychologist, 14,* 309–317.

Artiola I Fortuny, L., Romo, D. H., Heaton, R. K., & Pardee III, R. E. (1999). *Manual de normas y procedimeientos para la bateria neuropsicologia en espanol.* The Netherlands: Swets & Zeitlinger.

Azuma, T. (2004). Working memory and perseveration in verbal fluency. *Neuropsychology, 18,* 69–77.

Backman, L., Wahlin, A., Small, B. J., Herlitz, A., Winblad, B., & Fratiglioni, L. (2004). Cognitive functioning in aging and dementia: The Kugsholmen project. *Aging Neuropsychology & Cognition, 11,* 212–244.

Baldo, J. V., & Shimamura, A. P. (1998). Letter and category fluency in patients with frontal lobe lesions. *Neuropsychology, 12,* 259–267.

Baldo, J. V., Shimamura, A., Delis, D. C., Kramer, J., & Kaplan, E. (2001), Verbal and design fluency in patients with frontal lobe lesions. *Journal of the International Neuropsychological Society, 7,* 586–596.

Barr, W. B. (2003). Neuropsychological testing of high school athletes: Preliminary norms and test-retest indices. *Archives of Clinical Neuropsychology, 18,* 91–101.

Basso, M. R., Bornstein, R. A., & Lang, J. M. (1999). Practice effects on commonly used measures of executive function across twelve months. *The Clinical Neuropsychologist, 13,* 283–292.

Benton, A. L., Hamsher, K. deS., & Sivan, A. B. (1994). *Multilingual Aphasia Examination* (3rd ed.). San Antonio, TX: Psychological Corporation.

Bird, C. M., Papadopoulou, K., Ricciardelli, P., Rossor, M. N., & Cipolotti, L. (2004). Monitoring cognitive changes: Psychometric properties of six cognitive tests. *British Journal of Clinical Psychology, 43,* 197–210.

Bolla, K. I., Lindgren, K. N., Bonaccordy, C., & Bleecker, M. I. (1990). Predictors of verbal fluency (FAS) in the healthy elderly. *Journal of Clinical Psychology, 46,* 623–628.

Boone, K. B., Ponton, M. O., Gorsuch, R. L., Gonzales, J. J., & Miller, B. L. (1998). Factor analysis of four measures of prefrontal lobe functioning. *Archives of Clinical Neuropsychology, 13,* 585–595.

Borkowski, J., Benton, A., & Spreen, O. (1967). Word fluency and brain damage. *Neuropsychologia, 5,* 135–140.

Brickman, A. M., Paul, R. H., Cohen, R. A., Williams, L. M., MacGregor, K. L., Jefferson, A. L., Tate, D. F., Gunstad, J., & Gordon, E. (2005). Category and letter verbal fluency across the adult lifespan: Relationship to EEG theta power. *Archives of Clinical Neuropsychology, 20,* 561–573.

Brocki, K. C., & Bohlin, G. (2004). Executive functions in children aged 6 to 13: A dimensional and developmental study. *Developmental Neuropsychology, 26,* 571–593.

Burgess, P. W., Alderman, N., Evans, J., Emslie, H., & Wilson, B. A. (1998). The ecological validity of tests of executive function. *Journal of the International Neuropsychological Society, 4,* 547–558.

Butters, N., Granholm, E., Salmon, D. P., Grant, I., & Wolfe, J. (1987). Episodic and semantic memory: A comparison of amnesic and demented patients. *Journal of Clinical and Experimental Neuropsychology, 9,* 479–497.

Chertkow, H., & Bub, D. (1990). Semantic memory loss in dementia of the Alzheimer's type. *Brain, 113,* 397–417.

Codorniu-Raga, M. J. & Vigil-Colet, A. (2003). Sex differences in psychometric and chronometric measures of intelligence among young adolescents. *Personality and Individual Differences, 35,* 681–689.

Cohen, M. J. & Stanczak, D. E. (2000). On the reliability, validity, and cognitive structure of the Thurstone Word Fluency Test. *Archives of Clinical Neuropsychology, 15,* 267–279.

Crawford, J. R., Moore, J. W., & Cameron, I. M. (1992). Verbal fluency: A NART-based equation for estimation of premorbid performance. *British Journal of Clinical Psychology, 31,* 327–329.

Crawford, J. R., Wright, R., & Bate, A. (1995). Verbal, figural and ideational fluency in CHI. *Journal of the International Neuropsychological Society, 1,* 321.

Crossley, M., D'Arcy, C., & Rawson, N. S. B. (1997). Letter and category fluency in community-dwelling Canadian seniors: A comparison of normal participants to those with dementia of the Alzheimer or vascular type. *Journal of Clinical and Experimental Neuropsychology, 19,* 52–62.

Dall'Ora, P., Della Sala, S., & Spinnler, H. (1989). Autobiographical memory. Its impairments in amnesic syndromes. *Cortex, 25,* 197–217.

Delis, D. C., Kaplan, E., & Kramer, J. H. (2001). *Delis-Kaplan Executive Function System.* San Antonio, TX: Psychological Corporation.

Demakis, G. J., Mercury, M. G., Sweet, J. J., Rezak, M., Eller, T., & Vergenz, S. (2003). Qualitative analysis of verbal fluency before and after unilateral pallidotomy. *The Clinical Neuropsychologist, 17,* 322–330.

Diaz-Asper, C., Schretlen, D. J., & Pearlson, G. D. (2004). How well does IQ predict neuropsychological test performance in normal adults. *Journal of the International Neuropsychological Society, 10,* 82–90.

Dikmen, S. S., Heaton, R. K., Grant, I., & Temkin, N. R. (1999). Test-retest reliability and practice effects of expanded Halstead-Reitan neuropsychological test battery. *Journal of the International Neuropsychological Society, 5,* 346–356.

Doesborgh, S. J. C., Dippel, D. W. J., van Harskamp, F., Koudstaal, P. J., & Visch-Brink, E. G. (2002). The impact of linguistic deficit on verbal communication. *Aphasiology, 16,* 413–423.

Dursun, S. M., Robertson, H. A., Bird, D., Kutcher, D., & Kutcher, S. P. (2002). Effects of ageing on prefrontal temporal cortical network function in healthy volunteers as assessed by COWA: An exploratory survey. *Progress in Neuro-Psychopharmacology and Biological Psychiatry, 26,* 1007–1010.

Elias, M. F., Elias, P. K., D'Agostino, R. B., Silbershatz, H., & Wolf, P. A. (1997). Role of age, education and gender on cognitive performance in the Framingham Heart Study: Community-based norms. *Experimental Aging Research, 23,* 201–235.

Epker, M. O., Lacritz, L. H., & Cullum, M. C. (1999). Comparative analysis of qualitative verbal fluency performance in normal elderly and demented populations. *Journal of Clinical and Experimental Neuropsychology, 21,* 425–434.

Fernaeus, S-E., & Almquist, O. (1998). Word production: Dissociation of two retrieval modes of semantic memory across time. *Journal of Clinical and Experimental Neuropsychology, 20,* 137–143.

Fillenbaum, G. G., Heyman, A., Huber, M. S., Ganguli, M., & Unverzagt, F. W. (2001). Performance of elderly African American and white community residents on the CERAD neuropsychological battery. *Journal of the International Neuropsychological Society, 7,* 502–509.

Gaddes, W. H. & Crockett, D. J. (1975). The Spreen-Benton aphasia test: Normative data as a measure of normal language development. *Brain and Language, 2,* 257–280.

Getzels, J. W., & Jackson, P. W. (1962). *Creativity and intelligence.* New York: Wiley.

Giovanetti, T., Lamar, M., Cloud, B. S., Swenson, R., Fein, D., Kaplan, E., & Libon, D. J. (2001). Different underlying mechanisms for deficits in concept formation in dementia. *Archives of Clinical Neuropsychology, 16,* 547–560.

Giovanetti-Carew, T. G., Lamar, M., Cloud, B. S., Grossman, M., & Libon, D. J. (1997). Impairment in category fluency in ischaemic vascular dementia. *Neuropsychology, 11,* 400–412.

Gladsjo, J. A., Schuman, C. C. Evans, J. D., Peavy, G. M., Miller, S. W., & Heaton, R. K. (1999). Norms for letter and category fluency: Demographic corrections for age, education, and ethnicity. *Assessment, 6,* 147–178.

Gladsjo, J. A., Schuman, C. C. Miller, S. W., & Heaton, R. K. (1999). *Norms for letter and category fluency: Demographic corrections for age, education, and ethnicity.* Odessa, FL.: PAR.

Gonzalez, H. M., Mungas, D., & Haan, M. N. (2005). A semantic verbal fluency test for English- and Spanish-speaking older Mexican-Americans. *Archives of Clinical Neuropsychology, 20,* 199–208.

Gonzalez da Silva, C., Petersson, K. M., Faisca, L., Ingvar, M., & Reis, A. (2004). The effects of literacy and education on the quantitative and qualitative aspects of semantic verbal fluency. *Journal of Clinical and Experimental Neuropsychology, 26,* 266–277.

Gourovitch, M. L., Krikby, B. S., Goldberg, T. E., & Weinberger, D. R. (2000). A comparison of rCBF patterns during letter and semantic fluency. *Neuropsychology, 14,* 353–360.

Halperin, J. M., Healy, J. M., Zeitchik, E., Ludman, W. L., & Weinstein, L. (1989). Developmental aspects of linguistic and mnestic abilities in normal children. *Journal of Clinical and Experimental Neuropsychology, 11,* 518–528.

Harrison, J. E., Buxton, P., Husain, M., & Wise, R. (2000). Short test of semantic and phonological fluency: Normal performance, validity and test-retest reliability. *British Journal of Clinical Psychology, 39,* 181–191.

Harvey, J. A., & Siegert, R. J. (1999). Normative data for New Zealand elders on the Controlled Oral Word Association Test, Graded Naming Test, and the Recognition Memory Test. *New Zealand Journal of Psychology, 28,* 124–132.

Heaton, R. K., Miller, S. W., Taylor, M. J., & Grant, I. (2004). *Revised comprehensive norms for an expanded Halstead-Reitan battery: Demographically adjusted neuropsychological norms for African American and Caucasian adults.* Lutz, FL: PAR.

Heller, R. B., & Dobbs, A. R. (1993) Age differences in word finding in discourse and nondiscourse situations. *Psychology and Aging, 8,* 443–450.

Henry, J. D., & Crawford, J. R. (2004a). A meta-analytic review of verbal fluency performance following focal cortical lesions. *Neuropsychology, 18,* 284–295.

Henry, J. D., & Crawford, J. R. (2004b). A meta-analytic review of verbal fluency performance in patients with traumatic brain injury. *Neuropsychology, 18,* 621–628.

Henry, J. D., & Crawford, J. R. (2004c). Verbal fluency deficits in Parkinson's disease: A meta-analysis. *Journal of the International Neuropsychological Society, 10,* 608–622.

Henry, J. D., & Crawford, J. R. (2005a). A meta-analytic review of verbal fluency deficits in depression. *Journal of Clinical and Experimental Neuropsychology, 27,* 78–101.

Henry, J. D., & Crawford, J. R. (2005b). A meta-analytic review of verbal fluency deficits in schizophrenia relative to other neurocognitive deficits. *Cognitive Neuropsychiatry, 10,* 1–33.

Henry, J. D., Crawford, J. R., & Phillips, L. H. (2004). Verbal fluency performance in dementia of the Alzheimer's type: A meta-analysis. *Neuropsychologia, 42,* 1212–1222.

Henry, J. D., Crawford, J. R., & Phillips, L. H. (2005). A meta-analytic review of verbal fluency deficits in Huntington's disease. *Neuropsychology, 19,* 243–252.

Heun, R., Papassotiropoulos, A., & Jennssen, F. (1998). The validity of psychometric instruments for detection of dementia in the elderly general population. *International Journal of Geriatric Psychiatry, 13,* 368–380.

Ho, A. K., Sahakian, B. J., Robbins, T. W., Barker, R. A., Rosser, A. E., & Hodges, J. R. (2002). Verbal fluency in Huntington's disease: A longitudinal analysis of phonemic and semantic clustering and switching. *Neuropsychologia, 40,* 1277–1284.

Iverson, G. L., Franzen, M. D., & Lovell, M. R. (1999). Normative comparisons for the Controlled Oral Word Association Test following acute traumatic brain injury. *The Clinical Neuropsychologist, 13,* 437–441.

Ivnik, R., Malec, J. F., Smith, G. F., Tangelos, E. G. & Petersen, R. C. (1996). Neuropsychological tests' norms above age 55: COWAT, BNT, MAE token, WRAT-R reading, AMNART, Stroop, TMT, and JLO. *The Clinical Neuropsychologist, 10,* 262–278.

Jacobs, D. M., Sano, M., Albert, S., Schofield, P., Dooneief, G., & Stern, Y. (1997). Cross-cultural neuropsychological assessment: A comparison of randomly selected, demographically matched cohorts of English- and Spanish-speaking older adults. *Journal of Clinical and Experimental Neuropsychology, 19,* 331–339.

Johnson-Selfridge, M. T., Zalewski, C., & Aboudarham, J-F. (1998). The relationship between ethnicity and word fluency. *Archives of Clinical Neuropsychology, 13,* 319–325.

Jurado, M. A., Mataro, M., Verger, K., Bartumeus, E., & Junque, C. (2000). Phonemic and semantic fluencies in traumatic brain injury patients with focal frontal lesions. *Brain Injury, 14,* 789–795.

Kave, G. (2005). Phonemic fluency, semantic fluency, and difference scores: Normative data for adult Hebrew speakers. *Journal of Clinical and Experimental Neuropsychology, 27,* 690–699.

Kempler, D., Teng, E. L., Dick, M., Taussig, I. M., & Davis, D. S. (1998). The effects of age, education, and ethnicity on verbal fluency. *Journal of the International Neuropsychological Society, 4,* 531–538.

Kolb, B., & Whishaw, I. Q. (1985). *Fundamentals of human neuropsychology* (2nd ed.). New York: W.H. Freeman.

Kosmidis, M. H., Vlahou, C. H., Panagiotaki, P., & Kiosseoglou, G. (2004). The verbal fluency task in the Greek population: Normative data, and clustering and switching strategies. *Journal of the International Neuropsychological Society, 10,* 164–172.

Kozora, E., & Cullum, C. M. (1995). Generative naming in normal aging: Total output and qualitative changes using phonetic and semantic constraints. *The Clinical Neuropsychologist, 9,* 313–325.

La Rue, A., Romero, L. J., Ortiz, I. E., Liang, H. C., & Kindeman, R. D. (1999). Neuropsychological performance of Hispanic and non-Hispanic older adults: An epidemiologic survey. *The Clinical Neuropsychologist, 13,* 474–486.

Lacy, M. A., Gore, P. A., Pliskin, N. H. & Henry, G. K. (1996) Verbal fluency task equivalence. *The Clinical Neuropsychologist, 10,* 305–308.

Lannoo, E., & Vingerhoets, G. (1997). Flemish normative data on common neuropsychological tests: Influence of age, education, and gender. *Psychological Belgica, 37,* 141–155.

Laukka, E. J., Jones, S., Small, B. J., Fratiglioni, L., & Backman, L. (2004). Similar patterns of cognitive deficits in the preclinical phases of vascular dementia and Alzheimer's disease. *Journal of the International Neuropsychological Society, 10,* 382–391.

Lee, T. M. (2003). *Normative data: Neuropsychological measures for Hong Kong Chinese.* The University of Hong Kong: Neuropsychology Laboratory.

Levin, H., & Krauss, M. F. (1994). The frontal lobes and traumatic brain injury. *Journal of Neuropsychiatry and Clinical Neurosciences, 6,* 443–454.

Levin, H. S., Song, J., Chapman, S. B., & Harward, H. (2000). Neuroplasticity following traumatic diffuse versus focal brain injury in children. In H. S. Levin & J. Grafman (Eds.), *Cerebral reorganization of function after brain damage* (pp. 218–231). London: Oxford University Press.

Levin, H. S., Song, J., Ewing-Cobbs, L., Chapman, S. B., & Mendelsohn, D. (2001). Word fluency in relation to severity of closed head injury, associated frontal brain lesions, and age at injury in children. *Neuropsychologia, 39,* 122–131.

Levine, A. J., Miller, E. N., Becker, J. T., Selnes, O. A., & Cohen, B. A. (2004). Normative data for determining significance of test-retest differences on eight common neuropsychological instruments. *The Clinical Neuropsychologist, 18,* 373–384.

Loewenstein, D. A., Duara, R., Arguelles, T., & Arguelles, S. (1995). Use of the Fuld Object Memory Evaluation in the detection of mild dementia among Spanish-speaking and English-speaking groups. *American Journal of Geriatric Psychiatry, 3,* 448–454.

Loonstra, A. S., Tarlow, A. R., & Sellers, A. H. (2001). COWAT metanorms across age, education, and gender. *Applied Neuropsychology, 8,* 161–166.

Lucas, J. A., Ivnik, R. J., Smith, G. E., Bohac, D. L., Tangalos, E. G., Graff-Radford, N. R., & Peterson, R. C. (1998). Mayo's Older Americans Normative Study—category fluency norms. *Journal of Clinical and Experimental Neuropsychology, 20,* 194–200.

Lucas, J. A., Ivnik, R. J., Smith, G. E., Ferman, T. J., Willis, F. B., Petersen, R. C., & Graff-Radford, N. R. (2005). Mayo's Older African Americans Normative Studies: norms for Boston Naming Test, Controlled Oral Word Association, Category Fluency, Animal Naming, Token Test, WRAT-3 Reading, Trail Making Test, Stroop Test, and Judgement of Line Orientation. *The Clinical Neuropsychologist, 19,* 243–269.

Mack, W. J., Teng, E., Zheng, L., Paz, S., Chui, H., & Varma, R. (2005). Category fluency in a Latino sample: Associations with age, education, gender, and language. *Journal of Clinical and Experimental Neuropsychology, 27,* 591–598.

Marcopulos, B. A., McLain, C. A., & Giuliano, A. J. (1997). Cognitive impairment or inadequate norms? A study of healthy, rural, older adults with limited education. *The Clinical Neuropsychologist, 11,* 111–131.

Marshall, J. C. (1986). The description and interpretation of aphasic language disorder. *Neuropsychologia, 24,* 5–24.

Mathuranath, P. S., George, A., Cherian, P. J., Alexander, A., Sarma, S. G., & Sarma, P. S. (2003). Effects of age, education and gender on verbal fluency. *Journal of Clinical and Experimental Neuropsychology, 25,* 1057–1064.

Matute, E., Rosselli, M., Ardila, A., & Morales, G. (2004). Verbal and nonverbal fluency in Spanish-speaking children. *Developmental Neuropsychology, 26,* 647–660.

Mayr, U. (2002). On the dissociation between clustering and switching in verbal fluency: comment on Troyer, Moscovitch, Winocur, Alexander and Stuss. *Neuropsychologia, 40,* 562–566.

Millikin, C. P., Trepanier, L. L., & Rourke, S. B. (2004). Verbal fluency component analysis in adults with HIV/ AIDS. *Journal of Clinical and Experimental Neuropsychology, 26,* 933–942.

Milner, B. (1964). The effects of frontal lobectomy in man. In J. M. Warren & K. Akert (Eds.), *The frontal granular cortex and behavior.* New York: McGraw Hill.

Mitrushina, M. M., Boone, K. B., Razani, J., & D'Elia, L. F. (2005). *Handbook of normative data for neuropsychological assessment* (2nd ed.). New York: Oxford University Press.

Monsch, A. U., Bondi, M. W., Butters, N., Paulsen, J. S., Salmon, D. P., Brugger, P., & Swenson, M. R. (1994). A comparison of category and letter fluency in Alzheimer's disease and Huntington's disease. *Neuropsychology, 8,* 25–30.

Monsch, A. U., Bondi, M. W., Butters, N., & Salmon, D. P. (1992). A comparison of verbal fluency tasks in the detection of dementia of the Alzheimer type. *Archives of Neurology, 49,* 1253–1258.

Morris, J. C., Heyman, A., Mohs, R. C., Hughes, J. P., van Belle, G., Fullenbaum, G., et al. (1989). The Consortium to Establish a Registry for Alzheimer's Disease, part 1: Clinical and neuropsychological assessment of Alzheimer's disease. *Neurology, 39,* 1159–1165.

Newcomb, F. (1965). *Missile wounds of the brain.* London: Oxford University Press.

Ostrosky-Solis, F., Ardila, A., & Roselli, M. (1999). NEUROPSI: A brief neuropsychological test battery in Spanish with norms by age and educational level. *Journal of the International Neuropsychological Society, 5,* 413–433.

Pendleton, M. G., Heaton, R. K., Lehman, R. A. W., & Hulihan, D. (1982). Diagnostic utility of the Thurstone Word Fluency Test in neuropsychological evaluations. *Journal of Clinical Neuropsychology, 4,* 307–317.

Perret, E. (1974). The left frontal lobe of man and the suppression of habitual responses in verbal categorical behavior. *Neuropsychologia, 12,* 323–330.

Piatt, A. L., Fields, J. A., Paolo, A. M., Koller, W. C., Troester, A. I. (1999) Lexical, semantic, and action fluency in Parkinson's disease with and without dementia. *Journal of Clinical and Experimental Neuropsychology, 21,* 435–443.

Piatt, A. L., Fields, J. A., Paolo, A. M., & Troester, A. I. (1999). Action (verb naming) fluency as a unique executive function measure: Convergent and divergent evidence of validity. *Neuropsychologia, 37,* 1499–1503.

Ramage, A., Bayles, K. A., Helms-Estabrooks, N., & Cruz, R. (1999). Frequency in perseveration in normal subjects. *Brain and Language, 66,* 329–340.

Ramier, A. M., & Hecaen, H. (1970). Role respectif des attaintes frontales et la lateralisation lesionelle dans les deficits de la 'fluence verbale.' *Revue Neureologique Paris, 123,* 17–22.

Ratcliff, G., Dodge, H., Birzescu, M., & Ganguli, M. (2003). Tracking cognitive functioning over time: Ten-year longitudinal data from a community-based study. *Applied Neuropsychology, 10,* 76–88.

Ravdin, L. D., Katzen, H. L., Agrawal, P., & Relkin, N. R. (2003). Letter and semantic fluency in older adults: Effects of mild depressive symptoms and age-stratified normative data. *The Clinical Neuropsychologist, 17,* 195–202.

Rich, J. B., Troyer, A. K., Blysma, F. W., & Brandt, J. (1999). Longitudinal analysis of phonemic clustering and switching during word list generation in Huntington's disease. *Neuropsychology, 13,* 525–531.

Riva, D., Nichelli, F., & Devoti, M. (2000). Developmental aspects of verbal fluency and confrontation naming in children. *Brain and Language, 71,* 267–284.

Robert, P. H., Lafont, V., Medecin, I., Berthet, L., Thauby, S., Baudu, C., & Darcourt, G. (1998). Clustering and switching strategies in verbal fluency tasks: Comparison between schizophrenic and healthy subjects. *Journal of the International Neuropsychological Society, 4,* 539–546.

Rosen, V. M., & Engle, R. W. (1997). The role of working memory capacity in retrieval. *Journal of Experimental Psychology: General, 126,* 211–227.

Ross, T. P. (2003). The reliability of cluster and switch scores for the Controlled Oral Word Association Test. *Archives of Clinical Neuropsychology, 18,* 153–164.

Rosselli, M., Ardila, A., Salvatierra, J., Marquez, M., Matos, L., & Weekes, V. A. (2002). A cross-linguistic comparison of verbal fluency tests. *International Journal of Neuroscience, 112,* 759–776.

Ruff, R. M., Light, R. H., Parker, S. B., & Levin, H. S. (1996). Benton Controlled Oral Word Association Test: Reliability and updated norms. *Archives of Clinical Neuropsychology, 11,* 329–338.

Ruff, R. M., Light, R. H., Parker, S. B., & Levin, H. S. (1997). The psychological construct of word fluency. *Brain & Language, 57,* 394–405.

Salthouse, T. A., Atkinson, T. M., & Berish, D. E. (2003). Executive functioning as a potential mediator of age-related cognitive decline in normal adults. *Journal of Experimental Psychology: General, 132,* 566–594.

Sarno, M. T., Postman, W. A., Cho, Y. S., & Norman, R. (2005). Evolution of phonemic word fluency performance in post-stroke aphasia. *Journal of Communication Disorders, 38,* 83–107.

Sauzeon, H., Lestage, P., Raboutet, C., N'Kaoua, B., & Claverie, B. (2004). Verbal fluency output in children aged 7–16 as a function of the production criterion: Qualitative analysis of clustering, switching processes, and semantic network exploitation. *Brain and Language, 89,* 192–202.

Schum, R. L., Sivan, A. B., & Benton, A. (1989). Multilingual Aphasia Examination: Norms for children. *The Clinical Neuropsychologist, 3,* 375–383.

Senior, G., Douglas, L., & Dawes, S. (2001). *Discrepancy analysis: A new/old approach to psychological test data interpretation.* Presented at the 21st annual conference of the National Academy of Neuropsychology, San Francisco, CA.

Sherman, A. M., & Massman, P. J. (1999). Prevalence and correlates of category versus letter fluency discrepancies in Alzheimer's disease. *Archives of Clinical Neuropsychology, 14,* 411–418.

Shindler, A., Caplan, L., & Hier, D. (1984). Intrusions and perseverations. *Brain and Language, 23,* 148–158.

Sliwinski, M., & Buschke, H. (1999). Cross-sectional and longitudinal relationships among age, cognition, and processing speed. *Psychology and Aging, 14,* 18–33.

Solomon, P. R., Hirschoff, A., Kelly, B., Relin, M., Brush, M., DeVeaux, R. D., & Pendlebury, W. W. (1998). A 7 minute neurocognitive screening battery highly sensitive to Alzheimer disease. *Archives of Neurology, 55,* 349–355.

Somerville, J., Tremont, J., & Stern, R. A. (2000). The Boston Qualitative Scoring System as a measure of executive functioning in Rey-Osterrieth Complex Figure performance. *Journal of Clinical and Experimental Neuropsychology, 22,* 613–621.

Spreen, O., & Benton, A. L. (1977). *Neurosensory Center Comprehensive Examination for Aphasia.* Victoria, BC: Neuropsychology Laboratory, University of Victoria.

Steinberg, B. A., Bieliauskas, L. A., Smith, G. E., & Ivnik, R. J. (2005). Mayo's Older Americans Normative Studies: Age- and IQ-adjusted norms for the Trail-Making Test, the Stroop Test, and MAE Controlled Oral Word Association Test. *The Clinical Neuropsychologist, 19*, 329–377.

Stricks, L., Pittman, J., Jacobs, D. M., Sano, M., & Stern, Y. (1998). Normative data for a brief neuropsychological battery administered to English- and Spanish-speaking community-dwelling elders. *Journal of the International Neuropsychological Society, 4*, 311–318.

Stuss, D. T., Alexander, M. P., Hamer, L., Paumbo, C., Dempster, R., Binns, M., Levine, B., & Izukawa, D. (1998). The effects of focal anterior brain lesions on verbal fluency. *Journal of the International Neuropsychological Society, 4*, 265–278.

Suhr, J. A., & Jones, R. D. (1998). Letter and semantic fluency in Alzheimer's, Huntington's, and Parkinson's dementias. *Archives of Clinical Neuropsychology, 13*, 447–454.

Taussig, I. M., Henderson, V. W., & Mack, W. (1992). *Spanish translation and evaluation of a neuropsychological battery: Performance of Spanish and English-speaking Alzheimer's disease patients and normal comparison subjects.* Paper presented at the Gerontological Society of America.

Thurstone, L. L. (1938). *Primary Mental Abilities.* Chicago: University of Chicago Press.

Tombaugh, T. N., Kozak, J., & Rees, L. (1999). Normative data stratified by age and education for two measures of verbal fluency: FAS and animal naming. *Archives of Clinical Neuropsychology, 14*, 167–177.

Troester, A. I., Fields, J. A., Testa, J. A., Paul, R. H., Blanco, C. R., Hames, K. A., Salmon, D. P., & Beatty, W. W. (1998). Cortical and subcortical influences on clustering and switching in the performance of verbal fluency tasks. *Neuropsychologia, 36*, 295–304.

Troyer, A. K. (2000). Normative data for clustering and switching on verbal fluency tasks. *Journal of Clinical and Experimental Neuropsychology, 22*, 370–378.

Troester, A. I., Woods, S. P., Fields, J. A., Hanisch, C., & Beatty, W. W. (2002). Declines in switching underlie verbal fluency changes after unilateral pallidal surgery in Parkinson's disease. *Brain and Cognition, 50*, 207–217.

Troyer, A. K., Moscovitch, M., & Winocur, G. (1997). Clustering and switching as two components of verbal fluency: Evidence from younger and healthy adults. *Neuropsychology, 11*, 138–146.

Troyer, A. K., Moscovitch, M., Winocur, G., Alexander, M. P., & Stuss, D. (1998). Clustering and switching on verbal fluency: The effects of focal frontal- and temporal-lobe lesions. *Neuropsychologia, 36*, 449–504.

Troyer, A. K., Moscovitch, M., Winocur, G., Leach, L., & Freedman, M. (1998). Clustering and switching on verbal fluency tests in Alzheimer's disease and Parkinson's disease. *Journal of the International Neuropsychological Society, 4*, 137–143.

Tucha, O., Smely, C., & Lange, K. W. (1999). Verbal and figural fluency in patients with mass lesions of the left or right frontal lobes. *Journal of Clinical and Experimental Neuropsychology, 21*, 229–236.

Warrington, E. D. (2000). Homophone meaning generation: A new test of verbal switching for the detection of frontal lobe dysfunction. *Journal of the International Neuropsychological Society, 6*, 643–648.

Wilson, B. A., Watson, P. C., Baddeley, A. D., Emslie, H., & Evans, J. J. (2000). Improvement or simply practice? The effects of twenty repeated assessments on people with and without brain injury. *Journal of the International Neuropsychological Society, 6*, 469–479.

Woods, S. P., Scott, J. C., Sires, D. A., Grant, I., Heaton, R. K., Troster, A. I., & the HIV Neurobehavioral Research Center (HNRC) Group. (2005). Action (verb) fluency: Test-retest reliability, normative standards, and construct validity. *Journal of the International Neuropsychological Society, 11*, 408–415.

Yeudall, L. T., Fromm, D., Reddon, J. R., & Stefanyk, W. O. (1986). Normative data, stratified by age and sex for 12 neuropsychological tests. *Journal of Clinical Psychology, 42*, 918–946.

York, M. K., Levin, H. S., Grossman, R. G., Lai, E. C., & Krauss, J. K. (2003). Clustering and switching in phonemic fluency following pallidotomy for the treatment of Parkinson's disease. *Journal of Clinical and Experimental Neuropsychology, 25*, 110–121.

Zakzanis, K. K., Troyer, A. K., Rich, J. B., & Heinrichs, W. (2000). Component analysis of verbal fluency in patients with schizophrenia. *Neuropsychiatry, Neuropsychology, & Behavioral Neurology, 13*, 239–245.

Wisconsin Card Sorting Test (WCST)

PURPOSE

The purpose of this test is to assess the ability to form abstract concepts, to shift and maintain set, and to utilize feedback.

SOURCE

The test, including the WCST Manual-Revised and Expanded by Heaton et al. (1993), can be obtained from Psychological Assessment Resources, Inc. (www.parinc.com), for about $312 US. Unlimited-use scoring ($415 US) and administration on-screen and scoring software ($629 US) are also available from PAR. They also provide a shortened version, the WCST-64 Card version, developed by Kongs et al. (2000), for a cost of $236 US. The unlimited-use administration and scoring program (WCST-64: CV2) costs $529 US, whereas the scoring program alone costs $299 US. The WCST is also available for Spanish-speaking individuals in Artiola I Fortuny et al. (1999).

AGE RANGE

The test can be used with individuals aged 5 to 89 years.

DESCRIPTION

This test was developed by Berg and Grant (Berg, 1948; Grant & Berg, 1948) to assess abstraction ability and the ability to shift cognitive strategies in response to changing environmental contingencies. The test is considered a measure of executive function (Heaton et al., 1993) in that it requires strategic planning, organized searching, the ability to use environmental feedback to shift cognitive set, goal-oriented behavior, and the ability to modulate impulsive responding. Heaton et al. (1981, 1993) point out that there has been considerable interest in the test, in part because it provides information on several aspects of problem-solving behavior beyond such basic indices as task success or failure. Examples of such indices include the number of perseverative errors, the failure to maintain set, and the number of categories achieved. Heaton (1981) standardized the test instructions and scoring procedures and formally published it as a clinical instrument. In the updated manual (Heaton et al., 1993), scoring rules were refined, the recording form was revised, and normative data were provided for individuals aged 6 years, 5 months to 89 years.

The test consists of four stimulus cards, placed in front of the subject, the first with a red triangle, the second with two green stars, the third with three yellow crosses, and the fourth with four blue circles on them (see Figure 8–19). The subject is then given two packs each containing 64 response cards, which have designs similar to those on the stimulus cards, varying in color, geometric form, and number. The subject is told to match each of the cards in the decks to one of the four key cards and is given feedback each time whether he or she is right or wrong. No warning is provided that the sorting rule changes. There is no time limit to this test.

Short Form

The abbreviated form of the standard WCST, the WCST-64, (Axelrod, Woodard, et al., 1992; Kongs et al., 2000) involves giving only the first deck of 64 cards.

Modified Versions

Although most use Heaton's procedure, there are other versions of the test (e.g., Modified Card Sorting Test, Nelson, 1976; Milwaukee Card Sorting Test, Osmon & Suchy, 1996). Because the standard version includes some ambiguous stimuli that can be classed according to more than one category, the nature of the deficits leading to poor performance cannot always be clarified. Nelson (1976) removed the response cards that shared more than one attribute with the stimulus card, thus eliminating ambiguity. The task includes two sets of 24 cards and further reduces sorting requirements by asking individuals to produce only six consecutive successful sorts to complete a category. In addition, subjects are told when the target category is changed. A number of authors (Caffarra et al., 2004; Lineweaver et al. 1999; Obonsawin et al., 1999) have provided normative data for this version for use with adults (aged 20–90). Note, however, that Nelson's version changes the quality of the test and the literature indicates that the Modified Card Sorting Test and WCST are not entirely comparable and should be regarded as separate tests (de Zubicaray & Ashton, 1996; van Gorp et al., 1997). Although there is some evidence of validity in terms of its correlations to age and other test scores (e.g., Lineweaver et al., 1999; Rhodes,

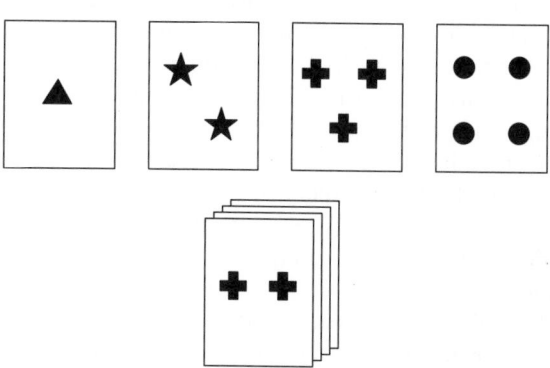

Figure 8–19 Example of WCST. *Note*: 1 Red Triangle; 2 Green Stars; 3 Yellow Crosses; 4 Blue Circles.

2004), test-retest reliability coefficients are low for this version (e.g., Bird et al., 2004; de Zubicaray et al., 1998; Lineweaver et al., 1999), suggesting that it is an unreliable tool for monitoring change in executive functioning over time.

The Milwaukee Card Sorting Test (Osmon & Suchy, 1996) requires that patients verbalize prior to sorting and provides additional scores that may be useful in characterizing a patient's difficulty in forming, maintaining, and switching mental set. Further research is needed, however, to evaluate the reliability and validity of this version. Normative data are also required. There are other rule derivation tests as well (e.g., *Brixton* and *D-KEFS* described elsewhere in this book; Weigl Test described in Lezak et al., 2004). A tactile version of the WCST for use with visually impaired individuals has also been developed (Beauvais et al., 2004).

Computer-Administered Versions

Computer implementation of the WCST is available (see *Source*). Artiola I Fortuny and Heaton (1996) report that the computerized (PAR) and standard versions yield fairly similar results in normal individuals. Similarly, Hellman et al. (1992) found no significant differences between computerized (Loong, 1990) and standard versions in a small and heterogeneous group of psychiatric patients. In contrast, others have not found equivalence on distributional properties (central tendency, variability, shape) of the scores between standard and computerized versions in normals (Feldstein et al., 1999). Further, Ozonoff (1995) reported that autistic children make fewer errors on the computer version (Loong, 1990). Given the various discrepancies in the literature, norms collected under standard administration conditions may not apply to computerized administrations.

ADMINISTRATION

See *Source*. Examinees should have normal or corrected vision and hearing sufficient to adequately comprehend the test instructions and to discriminate visually the stimulus parameters of color, form, and number. The two packs of cards are placed in front of the subject. The examiner instructs the subject to place each response card in piles below one of the four stimulus (key) cards, wherever he or she thinks it should go, and is told that the experimenter will then inform him or her whether the choice is "right" or "wrong." The subject is directed to make use of this information and to try to get as many cards "right" as possible. While it is permissible to clarify the meaning of the stimulus (key) cards and the manner in which the client is to respond, the examiner must never violate the integrity of the WCST by giving any indication of the sorting principles or the nature of the shift from one category to the next.

The subject is required to sort first to *color*, all other responses being called "wrong"; then, once 10 consecutive correct responses to color have been achieved, the required sorting principle shifts, without warning, to *form*; color responses are now "wrong." After 10 consecutive correct responses to form, the principle shifts to *number*, and then back to color once more. This procedure continues until the subject has successfully completed six sorting categories (color, form, number, color, form, number), or until all 128 cards have been placed.

Recording a performance, particularly if the patient works rapidly, can be difficult. Briefly, the recording form has 128 response items, each one "CFNO" (C = color, F = form, N = number, O = other). The examiner records the patient's response by making a slash through those dimensions that are the same on the response and stimulus cards. To assist in later scoring, the examiner consecutively numbers continuous correct responses, up to 10, in the space provided in the record booklet to the left of each item. Any time a patient interrupts

a sequence of correct responses by making an error, the examiner begins renumbering the next series with the number 1. In addition, a line is drawn under the last item when the criterion of 10 consecutive correct responses has been reached, and to indicate the new correct sorting category below that line.

ADMINISTRATION TIME

The time required is about 15 to 30 minutes.

SCORING

The WCST Record Booklet consists of four pages designed for recording information about the patient, recording the patient's responses to the WCST items, and calculating and recording WCST scores.

Scoring rules of the WCST, originally delineated by Heaton (1981), caused some confusion (Flashman et al., 1991). The revised manual (Heaton et al., 1993) provides detailed scoring criteria and clarifies common sources of difficulty. Scoring errors are common, even among experienced clinicians (Greve, 1993; Paolo et al., 1994). Errors are likely to occur when response cards match a stimulus card on two attributes (Paolo et al., 1994). Clinicians might consider purchasing computer scoring software to eliminate recording and scoring errors.

Performance is scored in a number of different ways. Table 8–83 provides an overview of various scores. For example, *Categories Completed* refers to the number of categories (i.e., each sequence of 10 consecutive correct matches to the criterion sorting category) completed during the test. Scores can

Table 8–83 Overview of Various WCST Scores

Score	Description
No. of Categories Completed	The number of sequences of 10 consecutive correct matches (maximum = 6)
Trials to Complete First Category	Total number of trials to complete first category
Perseverative Responses, Perseverative Errors	The number of items in which the patient persists in responding to a stimulus characteristic that is incorrect
Percent Perseverative Errors	The concentration of perseverative errors in relation to overall test performance (the number of trials given) multiplied by 100
Failure to Maintain Set	When a patient makes five or more consecutive correct matches but then makes an error before successfully completing the category
Percent Conceptual Level Responses	Consecutive correct responses occurring in runs of three
Learning to Learn	The subject's average change in conceptual efficiency across the successive stages (categories); based on percent error difference scores for each consecutive pair of adjacent categories

range from 0 for the subject who never gets the idea at all to 6, at which point the test is discontinued. When a person persists in responding to a stimulus characteristic that is incorrect, the response is said to match the "perseverated-to" principle and is scored as perseverative ("p"). Heaton et al. (1993) describe the situations that define the perseverated-to principle, and the reader should refer to their updated manual. Berry (1996) summarizes the relevant rules for scoring perseveration in a diagrammatic format that can also be used as an aid to scoring. The perseverative response may reveal an inability to relinquish the old category for the new one, or the inability to see a new possibility. The score for *Failure to Maintain Set* is the number of times the subject makes five or more correct responses in a row and then makes an error before successfully achieving a category. It indicates the inability to continue using a strategy that has been successful. *Percent Conceptual Level Responses* is defined as consecutive correct responses occurring in runs of three or more. It is thought to reflect some insight into correct sorting principles. The number of trials administered, total number correct, and total number of errors are also recorded. *Percent Errors, Percent Perseverative Responses, and Percent Nonperseverative Errors* can also be calculated to assist in research investigations. Use of these latter scores is not recommended for clinical interpretation, in part because reliabilities of these "percent" scores are lower than those of their respective basic scores.

There are a number of redundancies in the various WCST scores. For example, correlations are high between number of categories achieved and total number of errors (−.76 to −.89; e.g., Bowden et al., 1998; Iverson et al., 2000; Pineda & Merchan, 2003) and between perseverative errors and perseverative responses (.69–.95; Bowden et al., 1998; Iverson et al., 2000), and some of the scores (e.g., total errors) are linear combinations of other scores (perseverative errors and nonperseverative errors). The most common measures used to assess executive control on the WCST are the number of categories achieved and the number of perseverative errors. The measure of perseverative errors is marginally more sensitive to aging-related decline in comparison with categories achieved and may be a better metric of executive function if a single score from the WCST is to be used (Rhodes, 2004).

DEMOGRAPHIC EFFECTS

Age

Age has the strongest relationship to WCST performance compared with other demographic variables and accounts for about 20% of the variance in test scores (Heaton et al., 1993; Rhodes, 2004). Performance increases from 5 years through 19 years of age and remains fairly stable between the 20- to 50-year age decades. Declines in some aspects of performance (e.g., number of categories, number of perseverative errors) become apparent after age 60 (Axelrod & Henry, 1992; Axelrod et al., 1993; Beatty, 1993; Boone et al.,

1993; Chelune & Baer, 1986; Daigneault et al., 1992; Haaland et al., 1987; Heaton, 1981; Heinrichs, 1990; Laiacona et al., 2000; Levin et al., 1991; Levine et al., 1995; Parkin et al., 1995; Rosselli & Ardila, 1993; Shu et al., 2000; Snow, 1998; Welsh et al., 1988, 1991; see Rhodes [2004] for a recent meta-analysis).

Gender

The influence of gender is controversial. Most authors (e.g., Arffa et al., 1998; Heaton et al., 1993; Laiacona et al., 2000; Paniak et al., 1996; Rosselli & Ardilla, 1993; Shu et al., 2000, Snow, 1998) report that gender is not significantly related to WCST performance. By contrast, Boone et al. (1993) found that in an older sample, women tend to outperform men on the WCST.

Education

Educational level shows modest correlations with WCST scores (Boone et al., 1993; Boone, 1999; Heaton et al., 1993; Heinrichs, 1990) and appears to contribute a small but significant proportion of variance (about 4–7%) in addition to that explained by age (Heaton et al., 1993; Rhodes, 2004). For adults, there is a gradual increase in proficiency in WCST performance from lower to higher levels of education. In children, the father's education has a small effect (r about .20) on test scores (Shu et al., 2000).

IQ

A number of authors (e.g., Arffa et al., 1998; Boone, 1999; Chelune & Baer, 1986; Diaz-Asper et al., 2004; Heaton, 1981; Heinrichs, 1990; Paniak et al. 1996; Parkin et al. 1995) have documented a modest relation between IQ and WCST scores.

Ethnicity

Test results for Hispanic groups appear equivalent to those obtained with English-speaking individuals (Rey et al., 1999).

Other

Performance is also affected by vascular health status (Boone, 1999) and general socioeconomic/health-related conditions (Artiola I Fortuny et al., 1998).

NORMATIVE DATA

Standardization Data

Heaton et al. (1993) provide norms for individuals aged 6 years, 5 months to 89 years. The data were derived from a total group of 899 normal subjects aggregated from six samples. The characteristics of the sample are shown in Table 8–84. The educational level of the adult sample was somewhat

Table 8–84 Description of WCST Standardization Sample

Number	899
Age	6 years, 6 months–89 years, 11 months
Geographic location	United States
Sample type	Aggregate of six different samples:
	Sample 1—453 schoolchildren from southeast United States
	Sample 2—49 students age 18 years in southwest United States
	Sample 3—150 subjects aged 15–77 from Texas and Colorado
	Sample 4—50 subjects aged 58–84 from Colorado
	Sample 5—124 pilots aged 24–65 from Colorado
	Sample 6—73 adults aged 51–89 from Detroit
	384 adults age 20+ matched with 1995 projections of U.S. population with regard to age[a]
Education	6–20 years[b]
Gender	
Female	42%
Male	58%
Race/ethnicity	Not reported
Screening	Children were screened for a history of neurological dysfunction, learning disability, emotional disorder, and attention disorder; screening not reported for adults

[a]For the adult normative sample, subjects in the younger age ranges slightly are underrepresented while subjects in the older age ranges are slightly overrepresented in this sample. [b]Mean education of this sample is about three years higher ($M = 14.95$, $SD = 2.97$) than the U.S. population in 1987.

Source: Adapted from Heaton et al., 1993.

higher than that of the U.S. population in 1987. Note that information is not provided for a number of key variables (e.g., ethnicity, the method of screening adults).

Tables are provided (see source) based on the person's age or combination of age and years of education (for adults 20 years and older). Raw scores are converted to percentile scores. For some scores, corresponding standard scores ($M = 100$, $SD = 15$) and T scores ($M = 50$, $SD = 10$) are also recorded. Because both age and education influence performance, demographically corrected normative data are recommended (see Appendix D in source), particularly for diagnostic purposes. When making inferences about the adequacy of a person's capacity for everyday functioning (e.g., job placement), U.S. Census-based data for the general adult population (aged 20+) may be preferred (see Appendix C in source). Standard scores of 84 or below or T scores of 39 or below are considered to be in the impaired range. To assist in interpretation of the WCST performance, "base rate" information is also provided separately for adults, adolescents, and children (see Appendix E in source).

Some concerns have been raised about the adequacy of the norms for the WCST. Fastenau (1998) has argued that the norms create distortions, particularly for older adults, overcorrecting for age, making their performances look better than they really are. However, Heaton et al. (1999) have provided some evidence to suggest that their published norms do quite well in the older age range (but see later discussion).

Other Normative Data

Adult. A recent meta-analysis (Rhodes, 2004) of 34 studies published between 1990 and 2003 comprising about 3000 participants examined age-related differences in young (ages 20–35, $M =$ about 24 years, $SD = 3$; education, $M =$ about 14 years; $N =$ about 1350; 55% female,) and older (ages 55+, $M =$ about 71 years, $SD = 7$; education, $M = 13$ years; $N =$ about 1650; 58% female) healthy adults on the standard and the Nelson versions (Rhodes, 2004). The study documented robust age-related changes in performance on both versions for the number of categories achieved and the number of perseverative errors. The data are shown in Table 8–85 and appear to establish a higher standard than those reported by Heaton et al. (1993) for young as well as older adults. That is, the Heaton norms suggest that 11 perseverative errors is about average for young well-educated adults (20–29 years, 13–15 years of education) and 21 perseverative errors is average for older well-educated adults (70–74 years, 13–15 years of education).

For Spanish-speaking adults, the data provided by Artiola I Fortuny et al. (1999) are preferred. Normative data for Italians are also available (Laiacona et al., 2000).

Children. The WCST Manual includes norms for 459 normal children, ages 6 to 17 years. Paniak et al. (1996) have also provided data on 685 healthy Canadian children, ages 9 to 14 years, of normal verbal intelligence (mean WISC-III

Table 8–85 Meta-Norms for WCST

Variable	Older Participants (55+)	Younger Participants (20–35)
N	~1650	~1350
Mean categories achieved	3.99	5.58
SD	1.83	1.10
Mean perseverative errors	15.85	6.92
SD	11.44	5.04

Norms based on 34 studies comprising about 3000 healthy adults. The standard deviation refers to the mean of the standard deviations reported across all studies examined.

Source: From Rhodes, 2004.

Vocabulary scaled score = 10.3, SD = 2.69). The children showed general improvement with increasing age, but did not reach adult levels of performance, suggesting that the WCST is sensitive to age-related changes in executive ability, including those that occur in adolescence. For the age range from 9 to 14 years, the data reported by Paniak et al. (1996) are preferred over those by Heaton et al. (1993), Chelune and Baer (1986; N = 105), and Roselli and Ardilla (1993; N = 233) because their sample is larger and appears representative of the North American population with regard to verbal intelligence. The data are shown in Tables 8–86 and 8–87.

For children aged 5 to 8 years, the data collected in Bogota, Colombia, by Rosselli and Ardila (1993) on Spanish-speaking children are given in Table 8–88. No differences between socioeconomic groups were observed. The normative scores are somewhat higher than those reported by Chelune and Baer (1986) for a small American sample and by Shu et al. (2000) for a sample of children living in Taiwan.

WCST-64. Use of the standard WCST Manual's norms for 128 cards to estimate normative data from the WCST-64 is not recommended (Axelrod et al., 1997). Normative data have recently been published for the WCST-64 version (Kongs et al., 2000). The authors used the same data that had originally been included in the 1993 WCST Manual (Heaton et al., 1993). Demographically adjusted standard scores were generated via the continuous norming method.

Normative data from a sample (N = 303) of patients with acute, uncomplicated, mild head injuries have been provided by Iverson et al. (2000). They note that their data may be of value in interpreting test performance of individuals in the postacute period. The interested reader is referred to their article for the norms.

RELIABILITY

Test-Retest Reliability, Practice Effects, and Detection of Change

A group of 46 healthy children and adolescents were given the WCST on two occasions, spaced about one month apart

Table 8–86 Test Scores for Children on the WCST

	Age, in Years					
	9 (N = 80)	10 (N = 140)	11 (N = 131)	12 (N = 123)	13 (N = 96)	14 (N = 115)
ERR						
M	43.79	41.44	38.25	30.12	27.95	24.13
Mdn	42	42	34	24	23	18
SD	18.04	19.25	19.53	17.50	15.96	15.41
PERRES						
M	26.76	24.66	20.64	17.61	15.70	12.89
Mdn	23	22	17	13	11	9
SD	16.25	14.64	12.39	12.69	10.66	8.96
NONPER						
M	20.34	19.31	19.15	14.30	13.66	12.33
Mdn	17	18	15	11	11	9
SD	10.92	10.55	12.41	9.37	8.45	9.40
PERERR						
M	23.45	21.94	18.78	15.81	14.29	11.80
Mdn	21	20	16	12	10	9
SD	13.08	11.90	10.49	10.52	9.15	7.41

Note: ERR = errors; PERRES = perseverative responses; NONPER = nonperseverative errors; PERERR = perseverative errors.

Source: From Paniak et al., 1996. Reprinted with permission.

Table 8–87 Test Scores for Skewed Variables

| | Percentiles | WCST Variables | | |
		CATS	TTF	FMS
Age 9	>16	4–6	10–17	0–2
	11–16	2–3	18–22	3
	6–10	2	23–25	3–4
	2–5	1–2	26–78	4–5
	<1	0–1	79–128	6–21
Age 10	>16	4–6	10–17	0–2
	11–16	2–3	18–21	2–3
	6–10	2	22–37	3
	2–5	2	38–51	4
	<1	0–1	52–128	5–21
Age 11	>16	4–6	10–14	0–1
	11–16	3	15–19	2–3
	6–10	2–3	20–25	3
	2–5	1–2	32–63	3–4
	<1	0–1	64–128	5–21
Age 12	>16	5–6	10–12	0–1
	11–16	4	13–16	2
	6–10	2–4	17–19	2–3
	2–5	2	20–38	3
	<1	0–1	39–128	4–21
Age 13	>16	5–6	10–12	0–1
	11–16	4	13–15	2–3
	6–10	4	16–22	3
	2–5	3–4	23–31	3–5
	<1	0–2	32–128	6–21
Age 14	>16	6	10–15	0–1
	11–16	4–5	16–18	1–2
	6–10	4	19–21	2
	2–5	3–4	22–39	3–4
	<1	0–3	40–128	4–21

Note: CATS = categories achieved; TTF = trials to complete first category; FMS = Failure to maintain set.

Source: From Paniak et al., 1996. Reprinted with permission.

(Heaton et al., 1993). The investigators report generalizability coefficients that range from .37 (percent perseverative errors) to .72 (nonperseverative errors). It is also worth noting that the standard errors of measurement for WCST standard scores in normal children are quite large (e.g., 10.28 for perseverative responses; see *Source*). Thus, retesting in normal children may well yield different results and WCST scores should be interpreted with considerable caution.

In line with this notion are the findings of Paolo, Axelrod, & Troester (1996). They retested 87 normal elderly following an interval of about one year. To ensure that each participant displayed normal cognitive functions at both assessment probes, each participant had to have an initial DRS score greater than 130 and display no evidence of significant decline (i.e., a drop of 10 points or more). Stability coefficients were generally low, ranging from .12 on the Learning to Learn scale to .66 for the Total Number of Errors scale. The majority of individuals improved on retest, with five WCST scores demonstrating significant average retest gains of five to seven standard score points.

Paolo, Axelrod, and Troester (1996) also calculated standard error of prediction, standard error of difference, and abnormal test-retest discrepancy scores to assist in detecting possible meaningful changes in WCST scores on retest in older adults. Table 8–89 presents the 90% cutoff scores for WCST standard scores, with 5% of the cases falling in the positive direction (gain) and 5% falling in the negative direction (loss). To use the cutoff scores, the user must first convert the raw scores to normalized age- and education-corrected standard scores according to the WCST Manual (Heaton et al., 1993). Next, subtract the initial score from the score obtained on retest. If the difference score is negative, it reflects a loss on retest; if it is positive, it represents a retest gain. Next, compare the difference score to the cutoff values provided in Table 8–89. If the difference score equals or exceeds the tabled values, then the test-retest change is considered unusual, because it occurred in 5% or less of the normal sample. Note that the magnitude of the difference required for an unusual change on retest is quite large, typically more than one standard deviation.

Basso et al. (1999) retested a group of 50 healthy men (age, $M = 32.5$ years, $SD = 9.27$) following a 12-month interval and found that retesting resulted in significant improvement on nearly all indices, especially the number of trials needed to complete the test. On average, 101.12 cards were required at baseline, whereas only 84.74 trials were necessary 12 months later and the number of perseverative errors and responses decreased by nearly half on retesting (but see Tate et al., 1998, and Ferland et al., 1998, who found somewhat smaller practice effects in normal individuals when test intervals were about five months). The presence and magnitude of practice effects were similar among individuals of average and above-average IQ. The authors also calculated reliable change indices using the standard error of prediction to estimate the range of change in scores that might be expected while accounting for measurement error and practice effects. Table 8–90 shows the mean estimated true scores at 12 months together with the standard error of prediction (SE_P) and resulting 90% confidence interval. Note the wide range of retest scores that may fall within the 90% confidence interval and still reflect measurement error rather than meaningful change. For example, an individual could increase or decrease performance by as much as two categories, 17 errors, or nine perseverative errors without displaying meaningful change in performance (see also Tate et al., 1998, for similar findings). To use the confidence intervals, the 90% confidence band should be summed with an individual's estimated true score ($Y_{TRUE} = M + r[Y_{OBS} - M]$), where M is the sample mean of the test, Y_{OBS} is the actual score obtained by the individual, and r is the reliability coefficient. Significant changes reflect the frequency of obtained scores that fall above or below the confidence interval.

It has been argued that once a person with reasonably intact memory has figured out the category sorts and shift principle, the WCST no longer measures problem-solving ability

Table 8–88 WCST Scores for Children Aged 5–8 Years Grouped by Age and Socioeconomic Level

	Age 5–6 years ($N = 49$)				Age 7–8 years ($N = 63$)			
	High Socioeconomic Level		Low Socioeconomic Level		High Socioeconomic Level		Low Socioeconomic Level	
Variable	Score	SD	Score	SD	Score	SD	Score	SD
Categories achieved	4.2	1.8	4.2	2.2	4.9	1.7	4.4	1.9
Correct responses	66.9	15.1	67.0	17.8	67.8	11.6	70.5	14.4
Errors	46.1	23.0	51.6	24.7	48.4	20.9	48.4	23.0
Perseverative responses	21.7	11.3	29.5	21.7	19.1	8.7	24.4	18.2
Perseverative errors	21.3	15.7	25.3	10.6	17.9	8.1	20.9	10.5
Nonperseverative errors	24.6	17.6	25.9	12.0	30.5	16.3	27.2	17.1
Failure to maintain set	0.8	0.6	0.0	0.0	0.8	0.7	0.4	0.6

Source: Adapted from Rosselli & Ardila, 1993.

(Lezak et al., 2004). This suggests that the low stability of the WCST for normal people may reflect that, on retesting, it is no longer measuring problem-solving abilities in the same manner (Paolo, Axelrod, & Troester, 1996). It is unlikely that the specific progression of rule changes is remembered; rather, it is likely that procedural knowledge of test demands and effective test-taking strategies are retained, thereby shaping and enhancing subsequent performance (Basso et al., 1999). In clinical samples, however, reliability estimates may be considerably higher, suggesting that the test may be more sensitive to change in clinical than in nonclinical populations (but see Tate et al., 1998, who reported generally strong stability coefficients in the context of no significant change in performance over time in normal individuals).

In line with this notion, Ozonoff (1995) retested autistic and learning-disabled children over a two-and-a-half-year interval and reported test-retest generalizability coefficients greater than .90. Ingram et al. (1999) retested patients untreated for obstructive sleep apnea, a median of 12 days apart (range 1–71 days), and reported correlations ranging from .34 to .83, with a mean of .64. Perseverative errors and nonperseverative errors had high correlation coefficients (.83 and .80, respectively), while coefficients for trials to complete the first category ($r = .44$), failure to maintain set ($r = .50$), total correct ($r = .34$), and learning to learn ($r = .61$) were unacceptably low. Greve, Love, Sherwin, Mathias, Houston, et al.

(2002) examined temporal stability in survivors of severe TBI, whose conditions were stable (at least one year postinjury). The median retest interval was 53.7 weeks. On average, scores improved by about five T-score points. Stability coefficients were generally marginal/good ($>.60$) except for nonperseverative errors, categories completed, trials to first category, failure to maintain set, and learning to learn, which were all unacceptably low. They also provide 90% confidence intervals to determine whether the test-retest difference scores (Time 2 minus Time1) are unusual in TBI patients. The cutoff values for improvement and decline are shown in Table 8–91. A negative difference score indicates that the WCST score at Time 2 was lower than at Time 1. Depending on the variable, this can indicate improvement (e.g., total errors, perseverative responses, perseverative errors, and trials to complete the first category [TTF]) or decline (e.g., percentage conceptual level responses, number of categories, and learning to learn). The authors also noted that stability of the WCST-64 was poorer than for the standard WCST, and for most of the variables (except total errors and percentage conceptual level responses), below acceptable levels. As the authors note, in this study, the 64-card version was extracted from the standard version and these individuals had as much as twice the experience

Table 8–89 Cutoff Scores at the 90% Level of Abnormality for the Detection of Change on Retest in Older Adults

Scale	Loss	Gain
Total number of errors	18	35
Perseverative responses	12	30
Perseverative errors	15	35
Nonperseverative errors	29	40
Percent conceptual level response	24	35

Mean age of individuals was 68.79 years ($SD = 6.21$). The retest interval was on average 13.55 months ($SD = 2.19$). To calculate losses and gains, see *Reliability* section.

Source: From Paolo et al., 1996a. Reprinted with the permission of Sage Publications.

Table 8–90 Descriptive Statistics and Confidence Intervals for Estimated True Scores at 12-Month Follow-Up

	M	R_{y1y2}	SE_P	90% CI
Categories	5.42	.54	1.30	±2
Number of trials	84.73	.30	17.71	±29
Errors	16.68	.50	10.29	±17
Perseverative errors	8.43	.52	5.25	±9
% Conceptual responses	76.11	.54	15.74	±26
Perseverative responses	9.34	.50	6.65	±11
Learning to learn	.73	.36	3.63	±6
Failure to maintain set	.80	−.02	1.15	±2

Based on a sample of 50 community-dwelling healthy males, for the most part Caucasian, ranging in age from 20–59 ($M = 32.5$, $SD = 9.27$) and mean education of 14.98 years ($SD = 1.93$). For information on how to use these formulas, see *Reliability* section.

Source: From Basso et al., 1999. Reprinted with the permission of Psychology Press.

Table 8–91 Discrepancy Cutoff Scores for WCST-128 and WCST-64 variables

	WCST-128 Lower Bound	WCST-128 Upper Bound	WCST-64 Lower Bound	WCST-64 Higher Bound
T scores				
TE	−16	2	−16	8
PR	−27	7	−22	10
PE	−24	5	−20	10
NPE	−13	18	−15	12
%CLR	−16	2	−15	5
Raw Scores				
TE	−6	36	−8	17
PR	−20	58	−19	32
PE	−15	33	−15	20
NPE	−21	13	−9	9
%CLR	−39	12	−23	7
CAT	−5	1	−3	1
TTF	−15	100		
FMS	−3	3	−2	2
LL	−13	4	−38	8

Based on Time 2 minus Time 1 scores in a chronic traumatic brain injury sample. An individual difference score must be outside the 90% confidence interval—indicated by the Lower and Upper Bound—to indicate a significant change.

Source: Adapted from Greve et al., 2002a.

with the WCST-64 after Time 1 than would be the case if only the first 64 cards were given.

It is important to bear in mind that use of significant change indices provides the clinician with confidence that change has occurred. However, the inherent degree of unreliability in the WCST means that one cannot be certain that a change below the threshold of an index means that no change has occurred.

Alternate Form Reliability

Bowden et al. (1998) created an alternate form, with the order of correct sorting of cards changed. That is, participants were required to sort first to form, then color, then number. University students were given both versions in the same test session, with presentation order counterbalanced. Reliability coefficients were low (.63 and below). Therefore, use of alternate forms does not appear to improve reliability over retesting with the standard form administered twice.

Interrater Reliability

Interscorer and intrascorer reliability were excellent in some studies (interclass correlations above .83; Axelrod, Goldman, et al., 1992; Greve, 1993), whereas another study (Flashman et al., 1991) indicated that interscorer reliability on indices of perseveration was quite low (correlations not reported). The detailed criteria provided in the revised manual (Heaton et al., 1993) and/or the use of computer software may increase reliability, although this remains to be evaluated.

VALIDITY

Correlations Within Test

Numerous factor-analytic studies have been published (e.g., Bell et al., 1997; Goldman et al. 1996; Greve et al., 1993, 1998, 1999; Greve, Love, Sherwin, Mathias, Ramzinski, et al., 2002; Koren et al., 1998; Paolo et al., 1995; Salthouse et al., 1996, 2003; Sullivan et al., 1993; Wiegner & Donders, 1999), using a variety of populations (e.g., mixed psychiatric or neurologic patients, patients with schizophrenia, TBI, or CVA, normal elderly). Most have used exploratory factor analysis and have found evidence in favor of two or more factors, but more often, three factors are identified. These processes include the ability to shift set, problem solving/hypothesis testing, and response maintenance (Greve et al., 2005).

A recent large-scale confirmatory factor analysis from a mixed sample of neurological ($N = 620$) and psychiatric (228) patients and nonclinical controls (373) found support for the three-factor solutions reported in the exploratory factor analysis literature (Greve et al., 2005). However, only the first factor (comprising Perseverative Responses, Percentage Concept Level Responses, Categories Completed, and Total Correct), which reflects general executive functioning, appears statistically sound. The secondary factors (a: Percentage Concept Level Responses, Categories Completed, Total Correct, and Nonperseverative Errors [NPE]; b: Total Correct and Failure to Maintain Set [FMS]), while likely reflecting meaningful cognitive abilities, are less stable except when all subjects complete all 128 cards. That is, the WCST is sensitive to processes other than general executive functioning, but it does not appear to measure them well. The absence of abnormal NPE or FMS may have little clinical meaning, while their presence may indicate specific deficits worthy of follow-up. Greve et al. (2005) also suggest that having two termination criteria (i.e., completion of six categories or all 128 cards, whichever is first) has likely contributed to varied factor-analytic solutions reported in the literature. They recommend use of all 128 cards, since early discontinuation may result in some loss of useful information.

Correlations With Other Neuropsychological Tests

Although the interpretation of the factors appears reasonable, the specific cognitive processes underlying WCST performance remain to be established. General reasoning appears to play a role, albeit a modest one. For example, in adults as well as children, WCST performance shows modest relations with Full-Scale IQ (Ardila et al., 2000; Greve et al., 1999; Kizilbash & Donders, 1999; Koren et al., 1998; Sherman et al., 1995), although relations with specific IQ scores may vary. Thus, in normal children, perseveration on the WCST shows correlations of .30 to .37 with WISC-R Verbal and Full-Scale IQ (but not Performance IQ; Ardila et al., 2000). By contrast, in a heterogeneous pediatric sample, FSIQ and PIQ, but not VIQ, correlates modestly (.32–.44) with WCST performance (perseverative errors, perseverative responses, categories achieved; Kizilbash & Donders, 1999). In healthy adults, the total errors variable appears to be closely related to fluid intelligence (Salthouse et al., 2003).

Thus, the WCST measures some general reasoning ability that is somewhat related to psychometric intelligence. Its relation with measures of memory and attention/working memory is more controversial. For instance, some investigators (e.g., Koren et al., 1998; O'Donnell et al., 1994; Somerville et al., 2000; Vanderploeg et al., 1994) have reported that indices of perseveration on the WCST show modest correlations (.19–.42) with measures of attention/working memory (e.g., Part B of the Trail Making Test, Continuous Performance Test, Digit Span) and episodic memory (various indices of the CVLT). Further, factor-analytic findings in both healthy adults (e.g., Pukrop et al., 2003) as well as patients (e.g., Greve et al., 1998, 1999) have found that WCST scores loaded on the same factor as tasks that require speeded processing and aspects of working memory/attention involved in the comparison of information (e.g., Digit Symbol, Trails B, CPT).

On the other hand, Paolo et al. (1995) factor analyzed the WCST scores along with measures of attention and memory (Digit Span, CVLT, Logical Memory, Continuous Visual Memory Test). In neither normal elderly nor patients with Parkinson's disease did WCST scores load with the memory and attention/working memory measures. Similar findings have been reported by Boone et al. (1998) in a mixed clinical sample, with primarily psychiatric diagnoses.

Recently, Miyake, Friedman, et al. (2000) used a latent variable approach that suggested some separability of three more basic executive functions (e.g., mental set shifting, updating of information, inhibition) in healthy young adults. Structural equation modeling indicated that performance on the WCST was significantly predicted by the "shifting" ability. Once the "shifting" ability was taken into account, neither the "inhibition" nor "updating" abilities contributed to explanation of WCST performance. Fisk and Sharp (2004) reported findings consistent with those of Miyake, Friedman, et al. (2000) in a more age-heterogeneous sample. These findings show that one frequently mentioned executive function, namely shifting ability, contributes significantly to performance on this test, providing support for the commonly held view that the WCST is an executive task (Miyake, Emerson, et al., 2000).

Correlations With Other Measures of Executive Function

When the WCST is analyzed along with other measures of executive function, the WCST tends to load on a separate factor. For example, in individuals with autism (Minshew et al., 2002), the WCST (categories, perseverative errors) loaded on one factor, while other tasks (e.g., 20 Questions, Stanford-Binet Verbal and Pictorial Absurdities subtests, Category Test, Trail Making Test B) loaded on separate factors. Similar findings have been reported by others in healthy children (e.g., Welsh et al., 1991) and adults (e.g., Fisk & Sharp, 2004; Pineda & Merchan, 2003), as well as a heterogeneous group of patients seen for neuropsychological evaluation (Boone et al., 1998). The implication is that each task measures somewhat different aspects of the executive system.

The WCST appears to measure a dimension of conceptual processing similar, but not identical, to that of other tests of rule derivation such as the Weigl Test (Laiacona et al., 2000) and the Category Test (e.g., Golden et al., 1997; O'Donnell et al., 1994; Pendleton & Heaton, 1982; Perrine, 1993). Based on a factor analysis with the WAIS-R subtests in a mixed clinical sample, Golden et al. (1997) suggested that the Category Test reflects spatial analytic skills (loading with the Performance subtests), while the WCST measures loaded on factors independent of the other tasks. Perrine (1993) noted that the WCST was associated with attribute identification, which entails discrimination of relevant features (i.e., the correct answer is based on the stimulus attribute of color, form, or number). In the Category Test, the correct answer is based on identifying the correct principle or rule, regardless of the attributes of the stimuli. Perrine noted about 30% shared variance between the two procedures, suggesting considerable overlap but that these are separable abilities within conceptual reasoning. Minshew et al. (2002) have observed that the WCST is not entirely a concept identification task. Because the relevant principle changes unbeknownst to the test taker, a requirement is created for spontaneous evaluation and hypothesis formation, perhaps best assessed by the perseverative error score.

Additional evidence of separability derives from recent findings by MacPherson et al. (2002). They reported that aging impacts the WCST and other tasks dependent on dorso-lateral prefrontal regions (e.g., Self-Ordered Pointing, Delayed Response), but has little effect on tasks dependent on ventro-medial regions (gambling task, faux pas, emotional identifica-tion).

Clinical Studies

Adult Populations. In her classic study with the WCST, Milner (1963) found clear differences between patients with dorsolateral frontal excisions and those with orbitofrontal and posterior lesions. Patients with dorsolateral lesions showed an inability "to shift from one sorting principle to another, ap-parently due to perseverative interference from previous modes of response" (p. 99). Some subsequent studies, using patients and functional (PET or SPECT) and MRI imaging, have supported the notion that the WCST is sensitive to frontal lobe function (e.g., Arnett et al., 1994; Heaton et al., 1993; Rezai et al., 1993; Stuss et al., 2000; Weinberger et al., 1988), although others have not (Anderson et al., 1991; Ander-son et al., 1995; Axelrod et al., 1996; Cantor-Graae et al., 1993; Grafman et al., 1990; Hermann et al., 1988; Huber et al., 1992; Robinson et al., 1980; Strauss et al., 1993; Stuss et al., 1983). A recent meta-analysis (Demakis, 2003) comparing individuals with frontal lobe damage with those with posterior brain damage indicated significantly poorer performance for partic-ipants with frontal damage, particularly those with dorsolat-eral damage or with acute injuries (within one year). However, Demakis noted that even though effect sizes were reasonably large (e.g., $D = -1.3$ for patients with dorsolateral damage), the overlap in scores was fairly large (about 35%). That is, there was not enough separation between the distri-butions to classify frontal versus nonfrontal groups accurately. Others have also noted normal performance in some individ-uals with considerable frontal pathology (e.g., Anderson et al., 1991; Brazzelli et al., 1994; Eslinger & Damasio, 1985). In ad-dition, meta-analytic findings in patients with focal cortical excisions show that phonemic fluency is more strongly and specifically related to the presence of frontal lesions than the WCST scores (Henry & Crawford, 2004a).

There also appears to be little consistency in the literature with regard to laterality of dysfunction. Both Milner (1963) and Taylor (1979) suggested that the test is sensitive to func-tion in the dorsolateral areas of both frontal lobes, but more to the left than to the right side. However, some have reported ex-cessive impairment (typically in the form of more perservera-tion) in patients with right- as compared to left-sided damage (Bornstein, 1986; Drewe, 1974; Hermann et al., 1988; Lom-bardi et al., 1999; Robinson et al., 1980). Others (e.g., Horner et al. 1996; Martin et al., 2000; Stuss et al., 2000) found that the test is not differentially sensitive to laterality of temporal lobe epilepsy, but that about 40% of such patients displayed at least mild levels of impairment. Recent meta-analytic findings sug-gest no significant differences when those with right and left frontal damage are compared (Demakis, 2003).

Impaired performance has been documented in a number of conditions purported to involve disturbances in executive control, including autism (Minshew et al., 2002; Ozonoff, 1995; but see Goldstein et al., 2002), multiple sclerosis (Arnett et al., 1994; Beatty & Monson, 1996; in particular males with MS, Beatty & Aupperle, 2002), Parkinson's disease (Green et al., 2002; Henry & Crawford, 2004c; Monchi et al., 2004; Paolo et al., 1995; van Spaendonck et al., 1995), obsessive-compulsive disorder (Lacerda et al., 2003), Korsakoff's Syndrome (Brokate et al., 2003; Leng & Parkin, 1988), attention-deficit/hyperactivity disorder/impulsive type (Gansler et al., 1998), heavy alcohol use (Adams et al., 1995; Brokate et al., 2003), prenatal exposure to alcohol (Connor et al., 2000), and chronic cocaine and polydrug use (Rosselli & Ardila, 1996).

Aging-related declines are prominent on the WCST (see *Demographic Effects*). Some have proposed that the age differ-ences are linked to more fundamental age-related declines in working memory. For example, Hartman et al. (2001) found that age differences on the WCST were largely eliminated by reducing working memory demands. Specifically, older adults were provided explicit visual feedback about the immediately preceding sort (i.e., a cardboard arrow labelled YES or NO was placed above the most recent sort). However, others (Fris-toe et al., 1997; Salthouse et al., 1996) have suggested that age differences in performance on the WCST are the result of a more basic deficit in processing speed. Thus, Fristoe et al. (1997) gave the WCST as well as measures of working mem-ory and processing speed to both young and older adults. Their study suggested that age-related differences in WCST performance (on a factor defined by number of categories and percentage conceptual level responses) are related to both working memory and effective processing of feedback infor-mation, and both of these components are mediated by a speed of processing measure. They propose that age-related declines in speed of processing can lead to impaired WCST performance because of both limited time and simultaneity mechanisms. That is, lower processing speed results in fewer operations being successively executed (the limited time mech-anism results in incomplete encoding of WCST stimuli), and the results from earlier processing may not be available when later processing is complete (limited simultaneity mechanism may make feedback results of earlier WCST card sorts unavailable by the time encoding of current WCST items is complete).

Patients with TBI often perform poorly on the WCST, with severity of injury correlating moderately (.28–.49) with tradi-tional WCST variables (Anderson et al., 1995; King et al., 2002). However, a recent meta-analysis of 30 studies compris-ing 1269 TBI patients suggests that phonemic fluency is more sensitive to TBI than the WCST (categories completed, perse-verative errors; Henry & Crawford, 2004b) and may be a bet-ter measure of executive dysfunction in this population.

Individuals with schizophrenia demonstrate impaired lev-els of performance on the WCST (e.g., Beatty et al., 1994; Johnson-Selfridge & Zalewski, 2001; Koren et al., 1998; Moritz et al., 2002; Van der Does & Van den Bosch, 1992), although when Verbal IQ is taken into account, differences between patients and controls may disappear (Pukrop et al., 2003; also see Laws, 1999). The implication is that deficits on the WCST in this population may reflect a more generalized intellectual deficit and not particular difficulties with executive control (Henry & Crawford, 2005).

In addition, the literature suggests that depression (e.g., Borkowska & Rybakowski, 2001; Heinrichs, 1990; Martin et al., 1991; Moritz et al., 2002) or anxiety (Toren et al., 2000) may affect performance on the WCST, particularly as reflected in increased perseveration, failure to maintain set, and decreased percent conceptual level response. Depression is related to diminished problem-solving ability, and performance worsens as symptom severity increases. An obvious implication is that neuropsychological test batteries should include an assessment for mood disorder. If depressive or anxiety symptoms emerge, the clinician should not conclude that abnormal WCST test findings are indicative of specific neurological dysfunction since poor performance may occur in the context of mood disorders in the absence of any obvious specific neurological condition.

Of note, mental fatigue may result in lapses in executive control. Young healthy adults who work on cognitively demanding tasks for a considerable time (e.g., two hours) discover fewer categories and are more perseverative on the WCST, in comparison to nonfatigued individuals (van der Linden et al., 2003).

Finally, Ozonoff (1995) has pointed out that adequate performance on the WCST also requires a certain level of social awareness and motivation to attend to verbal feedback. This is an important aspect to consider when evaluating patients with social awareness or motivational deficits (e.g., autism).

Pediatric Populations. A factor-analytic study in children (aged 9–16 years) with traumatic head injuries suggested a three-factor solution, similar to that found in adults (Kizilbash & Donders, 1999). The presence of a reliable factor structure across adult and pediatric samples lends support to the contention of Chelune et al. (Chelune & Baer, 1986; Chelune & Thompson, 1987) that by age 9 to 10 years, the WCST measures similar constructs in adults and children.

There is some evidence (e.g., Brewer et al., 2001; Chelune & Thompson, 1987; Heaton et al., 1993; Kizilbash & Donders, 1999; Klorman et al., 1999; Lawrence et al., 2004; Levin et al., 1991, 1997; Romine et al., 2004; Snow, 1998) that the test may also be useful in identifying differences in developmental skill acquisition in various groups of children and adolescents (e.g., traumatic brain injury, seizure disorders, attention-deficit disorder, hydrocephalus, learning disorders). For example, WCST scores (e.g., number of categories, percent perseverative errors, response accuracy factor) are sensitive to both age and severity of traumatic brain injury (Kizilbash and Donders, 1999; Levin et al., 1997). Recent meta-analytic findings (Romine et al., 2004) confirm that children with ADHD show poorer performance as compared with controls on percent correct, total errors, and perseverative errors. Interestingly, failure to maintain set proved minimally sensitive to the presence of ADHD. In addition, the data showed that impairment on the WCST, while present in ADHD, was not unique to the disorder but occurred in other clinical groups as well (e.g., learning disorders, autism spectrum disorders). Finally, Bull et al. (1999) observed that children of high and low mathematical ability differed significantly on WCST measures after controlling for differences in reading ability and IQ.

Heaton et al. (1993) provide some clinical data suggesting that the test is sensitive (but not necessarily specific) to frontal lobe dysfunction in children and adolescents who have structural cerebral lesions. Similarly, Levin et al. (1997) reported that focal frontal lesion volume predicted WCST performance in children who suffered traumatic brain injuries. By contrast, Chase-Carmichael et al. (1999) did not find that the WCST was helpful in localizing the cerebral area of dysfunction in children with diverse neurological conditions.

Ecological/Predictive Validity

The test appears useful in predicting competency in meeting the demands of everyday life in adults as well as children. Thus, Burgess et al. (1998) reported that in a mixed group of adult neurological patients, the WCST (Nelson version) was predictive of behavioral and cognitive deficits reported by patients' caregivers. There is also some evidence that the WCST may have some value as a predictor of the capacity to manage independently outside of a hospital setting (Heinrichs, 1990), of occupational status of adults following severe head injury (Kibby et al., 1998), of vocational outcome (Nybo & Koskiniem, 1999), and of functional status at discharge from hospital following stroke (Greve et al., 1999). Similarly, in children, impairment on the WCST is associated with difficulties in real-world activities, including adaptive functioning following TBI (Levin et al., 1997) and problems in goal-directed behavior in children with ADHD (Lawrence et al., 2004)

Woods and Troster (2003) suggest that subtle executive dysfunction is evident during the immediate prodromal phase of dementia in Parkinson's disease (PD). They followed patients over a one-year interval and found that perseverations on the WCST demonstrated some diagnostic classification accuracy in identifying PD patients who later developed dementia from those who did not (overall predictive power of 68%). Similarly, long-term follow-up of individuals at risk for major mood disorder suggests an association between impairment on the WCST and subsequent development of bipolar disorder (Meyer et al., 2004).

Short Form

Although the use of a short form reduces reliability, the WCST-64 measures correlate highly (*r* values above .7) to corresponding scores on the long form (Axelrod, 2002; Donders & Wildeboer, 2004; Merrick et al., 2003; Sherer et al., 2003;

Smith-Seemiller et al., 2001; Vayalakkara et al., 2000). However, the WCST-64 may not produce results that are consistent with the full WCST on a case-by-case basis in adults. For example, in a mixed clinical sample, Axelrod (2002) observed that WCST-64 demographically adjusted scores capture about 59% of the full WCST scores when given a five-point margin of error. Based on these findings, Axelrod (2002) was guarded in his endorsement of the WCST-64 for regular clinical use. Sherer et al. (2003) were more optimistic. They noted that in patients who sustained TBI, scores were within 10 T scores of each other for only 72% of subjects. However, agreement in classification of performance as impaired (<40 T score) or not was good (86% received the same classification). Merrick et al. (2003) found that about one-quarter of a sample of adult patients who sustained TBI obtain WCST-64 perseverative response T scores that are more than 10 points below the corresponding WCST variable. The findings appeared to covary with age, with results from tests of older people showing stronger consistency between WCST/WCST-64 scores than those of younger adults (Donders & Wildeboer, 2004).

Conflicting reports have also been reported in children. For example, Smith-Seemiller et al. (2001) recommended caution in the use of the short form because they found that a high proportion of their heterogeneous pediatric sample was misclassified in terms of level of performance. By contrast, Donders and Wildeboer (2004) found that the WCST-64 could be used interchangeably with the original WCST in children (ages 10–16 years) with traumatic brain injury. This raises the possibility that the WCST-64 and the full WCST may covary differently across diagnostic groups.

There is some evidence that this short form is sensitive to deficits in AD and PD (Paolo, Axelrod, Troester, Blackwell, et al., 1996). In the acute recovery period following TBI (median time postinjury of 34 days), both the standard and short form are equally sensitive (or insensitive) to severity of injury, defined as length of coma (Merrick et al., 2003). The WCST appears to be more sensitive to impairment in the postacute phase following TBI (median time postinjury of three months) than the WCST-64, as a higher percentage of individuals produced impaired scores on the standard WCST (58% versus 32%; Sherer et al., 2003). The implication is that the long form may be the more appropriate test for patients whose disorders are more subtle. However, the WCST-64 performs comparably to the WCST in predicting level of disability in patients with TBI at discharge from inpatient rehabilitation (Sherer et al., 2003). Investigation of the WCST-64 scores to other measures of executive function such as verbal fluency, TMT-B, and the Category Test are needed (Sherer et al., 2003). A direct comparison of the factor structures for the two WCST versions in the same subjects would also be useful (Greve, 2001).

Malingering

Performance on the WCST may also be useful in detecting malingering. Patients suspected of incomplete effort tend to perform more poorly on WCST variables than those classified as having good effort (e.g., Greve, Bianchini, et al., 2002; King et al., 2002; Larrabee, 2003; but see Binder et al., 2003). For example, FMS scores greater than 1 are considered suspect (Suhr & Boyer, 1999), and Larrabee (2003) noted that no patient with moderate/severe head injury had scores greater than 3 FMS.

A number of formulas have been proposed (Bernard et al., 1996; King et al., 2002; Suhr & Boyer, 1999) that rely on the notion that individuals who malinger may suppress performance on obvious measures (e.g., number of categories) in comparison with subtle ones (e.g., perseverative errors) or may avoid too many consecutive correct responses (e.g., failure to maintain set). Although specificity tends to be good with these formulas, sensitivity is limited (Greve, Bianchini, et al., 2002; King et al., 2002). The Bernard formula shares a substantial amount of variance with the Suhr formula, suggesting that use of these formulas in combination does not enhance diagnostic accuracy (Greve, Bianchini, et al., 2002). Further, each approach may yield somewhat different results depending upon the chronicity and severity of the brain injury (King et al., 2002). The equations provided by Suhr and Boyer (1999) and King et al. (2002) appear to provide reasonably good classification rates in a variety of traumatically brain-injured samples and are shown in Table 8–92. However, in older adults (aged 55+), these formulas may result in a high rate of false positives and therefore may be inappropriate for use in this population (Ashendorf et al., 2003). Note, too, that Larrabee (2003) found that FMS alone worked more effectively than the Suhr and Boyer discriminant score in discriminating litigants identified as malingering from patients with moderate-severe TBI.

Table 8–92 WCST Logistic Regression Equation to Determine Incomplete Effort

King et al. (2002)		Suhr & Boyer (1999)
Logistic Regression Score	Probability of Incomplete Effort	Logistic Regression Score
4.29	0.99	4.69
2.90	0.95	3.68
2.13	0.90	3.16
1.74	0.85	2.41
1.32	0.80	1.69
1.09	0.75	1.43
0.87	0.70	1.17
0.57	0.65	.91
0.34	0.60	.42
0.20	0.55	.16
0.00	0.50	0.00

Logistic regression equation: $(-.752 \times$ categories completed$) + (.345 \times$ failure to maintain set errors$) - (.007\% \times$ conceptual level responses$) + 1.537$; Suhr & Boyer, 1999: $(-.75 \times$ # categories completed$) + (1.01 \times$ failure to maintain set$) + 3.16$.

Source: Adapted from King et al., 2002, and Suhr & Boyer, 1999.

COMMENT

The WCST is the most commonly used measure to assess executive function complaints (Rabin et al., 2005). It is important to bear in mind that executive functions are somewhat separable and that different executive functions contribute differently to various complex executive tasks (Miyake, Emerson, et al., 2000; Miyake, Friedman, et al., 2000; but see Salthouse et al., 2003, who raises questions about the meaning and distinctiveness of the component processes). Accordingly, relying simply on a task such as the WCST as a general measure of executive functioning does not suffice.

The nature of the cognitive processes underlying WCST success is complex. The task requires numerous skills including basic visual processing, numerical ability, rule induction ability, the ability to identify the most relevant stimulus attributes, speeded processing, the ability to maintain the current sorting category in working memory, the ability to shift mental set, and the appropriate motivational set. That shifting contributes significantly to WCST performance makes the widely accepted view that the WCST is an executive task somewhat defensible (Miyake, Emerson, et al., 2000). Nonetheless, any significant deficit in this or one or more of the other processes may lead to impairments on the WCST. That is, there are many different ways in which a patient can demonstrate impaired performance on this complex task.

In a related vein, performance can be impaired on this test for a variety of reasons, not all of which are related to the functions associated with the frontal lobes (Stuss et al., 2000). Thus, the WCST appears sensitive to frontal lobe damage; however, the WCST cannot be used by itself to predict a focal frontal lesion (e.g., Anderson et al., 1995; Demakis, 2003; Heaton et al., 1993; Henry & Crawford, 2004a; Mountain & Snow, 1993). Rather, it may be more plausible to conceive of the WCST as a multifactorial test that requires a distributed neural network (Stuss et al., 2000). In addition, there is evidence (Henry & Crawford, 2004a, 2004b) that other measures (e.g., phonemic fluency) may provide a better index of executive dysfunction because they are more sensitive and specific to frontal damage.

Users should bear in mind that the reliability of the WCST variables tends to be disappointingly low in normal individuals. Reliability estimates appear to be somewhat higher in clinical samples (e.g., perseverative errors), although not for all WCST measures (e.g., nonperseverative errors, categories completed, trials to first category, failure to maintain set, and learning to learn). Thus, clinicians may be misled by erroneous information and should be very cautious when interpreting individual scores or apparent patterns in test results.

Many of the WCST measures are highly redundant (e.g., perseverative responses, perseverative errors), suggesting that clinicians simply utilize variables considered representative of specific WCST dimensions (e.g., perseverative responses, failure to maintain set). Both categories achieved and perseverative errors are used with about equal consistency as predictors in studies of age-related changes in cognition or as measures of executive function. Rhodes (2004) suggests that the measure of perseverative errors committed is marginally more sensitive to age differences in comparison with categories achieved and may be the better metric of executive function if a single score from the WCST is to be used.

It can take a long time for some patients to complete the task. As a consequence, there has been increasing interest in the use of short forms, particularly the WCST-64. However, caution is advised in using the short form given the lack of correspondence between test scores in some studies. One reason for the limitations of short forms is that they are unable to account for the patterns of performance that emerge over the course of the test (e.g., improvement, decompensation; Smith-Seemiller et al., 2001). Possibly, the WCST-64 may be a reasonable substitute for the full-length version only at the ends of the age distribution (i.e., with children ≤16 or adults ≥60 years), whereas young adults can "catch on" to the task during the second deck of cards (Donders & Wildeboer, 2004). There is also evidence that the long form may be the more appropriate test for patients whose disorders are more subtle (Sherer et al., 2003). In a related vein, when administered in standard fashion, there are two termination criteria: completion of six categories or all 128 cards, whichever is first. Greve et al. (2005) have recommended routine use of all 128 cards, since early discontinuation may result in some loss of useful information.

Computerized versions are also available. However, clinicians and experimenters must use caution when basing conclusions on scores derived from computer versions (e.g., Feldstein et al., 1999; Rhodes, 2004). In addition, concerns regarding comparability of versions may be exacerbated when testing older adults, who have less facility and comfort with computer skills (Rhodes, 2004).

REFERENCES

Adams, K. M., Gilman, S., Koeppe, R., Klain, K., Junck, L., Lohman, M., Johnson-Greene, D., Berent, S., Dede, D., & Kroll, P. (1995). Correlation of neuropsychological function with cerebral metabolic rate in subdivisions of the frontal lobes of older alcoholic patients measured with [¹⁸F] fluorodeoxyglucose and positron emission tomography. *Neuropsychology, 9,* 275–280.

Anderson, C. V., Bigler, E. D., & Blatter, D. D. (1995). Frontal lobe lesions, diffuse damage, and neuropsychological functioning in traumatic brain-injured patients. *Journal of Clinical and Experimental Neuropsychology, 17,* 900–908.

Anderson, S. W., Damasio, H., Jones, R. D., & Tranel, D. (1991). Wisconsin Card Sorting Test performance as a measure of frontal lobe damage. *Journal of Clinical and Experimental Neuropsychology, 13,* 909–922.

Ardila, A., Pineda, D., & Rosseli, M. (2000). Correlation between intelligence test scores and executive function measures. *Archives of Clinical Neuropsychology, 15*, 31–36.

Arffa, S., Lovell, M., Podell, K., & Goldberg, E. (1998). Wisconsin Card Sorting Test performance in above average and superior school children: Relationship to intelligence and age. *Archives of Clinical Neuropsychology, 13*, 713–720.

Arnett, P. A., Rao, S. M., Bernardin, L., Grafman, J., Yetkin, F. Z., & Lobeck, L. (1994). Relationship between frontal lobe lesions and Wisconsin Card Sorting Test performance in patients with multiple sclerosis. *Neurology, 44*, 420–425.

Artiola I Fortuny, L. A., & Heaton, R. K. (1996). Standard versus computerized administration of the Wisconsin Card Sorting Test. *The Clinical Neuropsychologist, 10*, 419–424.

Artiola I Fortuny, L., Heaton, R. K., & Hermosillo, D. (1998). Neuropsychological comparisons of Spanish-speaking participants from the U.S.-Mexico border region versus Spain. *Journal of the International Neuropsychological Society, 4*, 363–379.

Artiola I Fortuny, L., Romo, D. H., Heaton, R. K., & Pardee III, R. E. (1999). *Manual de normas y procedimientos para la bateria neuropsicologia en espanol.* The Netherlands: Swets & Zeitlinger.

Ashendorf, L., O'Bryant, S. E., & McCaffrey, R. J. (2003). Specificity of malingering detection strategies in older adults using the CVLT and WCST. *The Clinical Neuropsychologist, 17*, 255–262.

Axelrod, B. N. (2002). Are normative data from the 64-card version of the WCST comparable to the full WCST? *The Clinical Neuropsychologist, 16*, 7–11.

Axelrod, B. N., Goldman, R. S., Heaton, R. K., Lawless, G., Thompson, L. L., Chelune, G. J., & Kay, G. G. (1996). Discriminability of the Wisconsin Card Sorting Test using the standardization sample. *Journal of Clinical and Experimental Neuropsychology, 18*, 338–342.

Axelrod, B. N., Goldman, R. S., & Woodard, J. L. (1992). Interrater reliability in scoring the Wisconsin Card Sorting Test. *The Clinical Neuropsychologist, 6*, 143–155.

Axelrod, B. N., & Henry, R. R. (1992). Age-related performance on the Wisconsin card sorting, similarities, and controlled oral word association tests. *The Clinical Neuropsychologist, 6*, 16–26.

Axelrod, B. N., Jiron, C. C., & Henry, R. R. (1993). Performance of adults ages 20 to 90 on the abbreviated Wisconsin Card Sorting Test. *The Clinical Neuropsychologist, 7*, 205–209.

Axelrod, B. N., Paolo, A. M., & Abraham, E. (1997). Do normative data from the full WCST extend to the abbreviated WCST? *Assessment, 4*, 41–46.

Axelrod, B. N., Woodard, J. L., & Henry, R. R. (1992). Analysis of an abbreviated form of the Wisconsin Card Sorting Test. *The Clinical Neuropsychologist, 6*, 27–31.

Basso, M. R., Bornstein, R. A., & Lang, J. M. (1999). Practice effects on commonly used measures of executive function across twelve months. *The Clinical Neuropsychologist, 13*, 283–292.

Beatty, W. W. (1993). Age differences on the California Card Sorting Test: Implications for the assessment of problem solving by the elderly. *Bulletin of the Psychonomic Society, 31*, 511–514.

Beatty, W. W., & Aupperle, R. L. (2002). Sex differences in cognitive impairment in multiple sclerosis. *The Clinical Neuropsychologist, 16*, 472–480.

Beatty, W. B., Jocic, Z., Monson, N., & Katzung, V. M. (1994). Problem solving by schizophrenic and schizoaffective patients on the Wisconsin and California Card Sorting Tests. *Neuropsychology, 8*, 49–54.

Beatty, W. W., & Monson, N. (1996). Problem solving by patients with multiple sclerosis: Comparison of performance on the Wisconsin and California Card Sorting Tests. *Journal of the International Neuropsychological Society, 2*, 134–140.

Beauvais, J. E., Woods, S. P., Delaney, R. C. & Fein, D. (2004). Development of a tactile Wisconsin Card Sorting Test. *Rehabilitation Psychology, 49*, 282–287.

Bell, M. D., Greig, T. C., Kaplan, E., & Bryson, G. (1997). Wisconsin Card Sorting Test dimensions in schizophrenia: Factorial, predictive, and divergent validity. *Journal of Clinical and Experimental Neuropsychology, 19*, 933–941.

Berg, E. A. (1948). A simple objective technique for measuring flexibility in thinking. *Journal of General Psychology, 39*, 15–22.

Bernard, L. C., McGrath, M. J., & Houston, W. (1996). The differential effects of simulating malingering, closed head injury, and other CNS pathology on the Wisconsin Card Sorting Test: Support for the "pattern of performance" hypothesis. *Archives of Clinical Neuropsychology, 11*, 231–245.

Berry, S. (1996). Diagrammatic procedure for scoring the Wisconsin Card Sorting Test. *The Clinical Neuropsychologist, 10*, 117–121.

Binder, L. M., Kelly, M. P., Villanueva, M. R., & Winslow, M. W. (2002). Motivation and neuropsychological test performance following mild head injury. *Journal of Clinical and Experimental Neuropsychology, 25*, 420–430.

Bird, C. M., Papadopoulou, K., Ricciardelli, P., Rossor, M. N., & Cipolotti, L. (2004). Monitoring cognitive changes: Psychometric properties of sex cognitive tests. *British Journal of Clinical Psychology, 43*, 197–210.

Boone, K. B. (1999). Neuropsychological assessment of executive functions: Impact of age, education, gender, intellectual level, and vascular status on executive test scores. In B. Miller & J. L. Cummings (Eds.), *The human frontal lobes: Functions and disorders* (pp. 247–260). New York: Guilford Press.

Boone, K. B., Gharffarian, S., Lesser, I. M., Hill-Gutierrez, E., & Berman, N. G. (1993). Wisconsin Card Sorting Test performance in healthy, older adults: Relationship to age, sex, education, and IQ. *Journal of Clinical Psychology, 49*, 54–60.

Boone, K. B., Ponton, M. O., Gorsuch, R. L., Gonzalez, J. J., & Miller, B. L. (1998). Factor analysis of four measures of prefrontal lobe functioning. *Archives of Clinical Neuropsychology, 13*, 585–595.

Borkowska, A., & Rybakowski, J. (2001). Neuropsychological frontal lobe tests indicate that bipolar depressed patients are more impaired than unipolar. *Bipolar Disorders, 3*, 88–94.

Bornstein, R. A. (1986). Contribution of various neuropsychological measures to detection of frontal lobe impairment. *International Journal of Clinical Neuropsychology, 8*, 18–22.

Bowden, S. C., Fowler, K. S., Bell, R. C., Whelan, G., Clifford, C., Ritter, A. J., & Long, C. M. (1998). The reliability and internal validity of the Wisconsin Card Sorting Test. *Neuropsychological Rehabilitation, 8*, 243–254.

Brazzelli, M., Columbi, N., Della Sala, S., & Spinnler, H. (1994). Spared and impaired cognitive abilities after bilateral frontal damage. *Cortex, 30*, 27–51.

Brewer, V. R., Fletcher, J. M., Hiscock, M., & Davidson, K. C. (2001). Attention processes in children with shunted hydrocephalus versus attention deficit-hyperactivity disorder. *Neuropsychology, 15*, 185–198.

Brokate, B., Hildebrandt, H., Eling, P., Fichtner, H., Rnge, K., & Timm, C. (2003). Frontal lobe dysfunction in Korsakoff's syndrome and chronic alcoholism: Continuity or discontinuity? *Neuropsychology, 17,* 420–428.

Bull, R., Johnston, R. S., & Roy, J. A. (1999). Exploring the roles of the visual-spatial sketch pad and central executive in children's arithmetical skills: Views from cognition and developmental neuropsychology. *Developmental Neuropsychology, 15,* 421–442.

Burgess, P. W., Alderman, N., Evans, J., Emslie, H., & Wilson, B. A. (1998). The ecological validity of tests of executive function. *Journal of the International Neuropsychological Society, 4,* 547–558.

Caffara, P., Vezzadini, G., Dieci, F., Zonato, F., & Venneri, A. (2004). Modified Card Sorting Test: Normative data. *Journal of Clinical and Experimental Neuropsychology, 26,* 246–250.

Cantor-Graae, E., Warkentin, S., Franzen, G., & Risberg, J. (1993). Frontal lobe challenge: A comparison of activation procedures during rCBF measurements in normal subjects. *Neuropsychiatry, Neuropsychology, and Behavioral Neurology, 6,* 83–92.

Chase-Carmichael, C. A., Ris, M. D., Weber, A. M., & Schefft, B. K. (1999). Neurologic validity of the Wisconsin Card Sorting Test with a pediatric population. *The Clinical Neuropsychologist, 13,* 405–413.

Chelune, G. J., & Baer, R. A. (1986). Developmental norms for the Wisconsin Card Sorting Test. *Journal of Clinical and Experimental Neuropsychology, 8,* 219–228.

Chelune, G. J., & Thompson, L. T. (1987). Evaluation of the general sensitivity of the Wisconsin Card Sorting Test among younger and older children. *Developmental Neuropsychology, 3,* 81–89.

Connor, P. D., Sampson, P. D., Bookstein, F. L., Barr, H. M., & Streissguth, A. P., (2000). Direct and indirect effects of prenatal alcohol damage on executive function. *Developmental Neuropsychology, 18,* 331–354.

Daigneault, S., Braun, C. M. J., & Whitaker, H. A. (1992). Early effects of normal aging on perseverative and non-perseverative prefrontal measures. *Developmental Neuropsychology, 8,* 99–114.

De Zubicaray, G., & Ashton, R. (1996). Nelson's Modified Card Sorting Test: A review. *The Clinical Neuropsychologist, 10,* 245–254.

De Zubicaray, G. I., Smith, G. A., Chalk, J. B., & Semple, J. (1998). The Modified Card Sorting Test: Test-retest stability and relationships with demographic variables in a healthy older adult sample. *British Journal of Clinical Psychology, 37,* 457–466.

Demakis, G. J. (2003). A meta-analytic review of the sensitivity of the Wisconsin Card Sorting Test to frontal and lateralized frontal brain damage. *Neuropsychology, 17,* 255–264.

Diaz-Asper, C., Schretlen, D. J., & Pearlson, G. D. (2004). How well does IQ predict neuropsychological test performance in normal adults. *Journal of the International Neuropsychological Society, 10,* 82–90.

Donders, J., & Wildeboer, M. A. (2004). Validity of the WCST-64 after traumatic brain injury in children. *The Clinical Neuropsychologist, 18,* 521–527

Drewe, E. A. (1974). The effect of type and area of brain lesion on Wisconsin Card Sorting Test performance. *Cortex, 10,* 159–170.

Eslinger, P. J., & Damasio, A. R. (1985). Severe disturbance of higher cortical function after frontal lobe ablation. *Neurology, 35,* 421–429.

Fastenau, P. S. (1998). Validity of regression-based norms: An empirical test of the comprehensive norms with older adults. *Journal of Clinical and Experimental Neuropsychology, 20,* 906–916.

Feldstein, S. N., Keller, F. R., Portman, R. E., Durham, R. L., Klebe, K. J., & Davis, H. P. (1999). A comparison of computerized and standard versions of the Wisconsin Card Sorting Test. *The Clinical Neuropsychologist, 13,* 303–313.

Ferland, M. B., Ramsay, J., Engeland, C., & O'Hara, P. (1998). Comparison of the performance of normal individuals and survivors of traumatic brain injury on repeat administrations of the Wisconsin Card Sorting Test. *Journal of Clinical and Experimental Neuropsychology, 20,* 473–482.

Fisk, J. E., & Sharp, C. A. (2004). Age-related impairment in executive functioning: Updating, inhibition, shifting, and access. *Journal of Clinical and Experimental Neuropsychology, 26,* 874–890.

Flashman, L. A., Horner, M. D., & Freides, D. (1991). Note on scoring perseveration on the Wisconsin Card Sorting Test. *The Clinical Neuropsychologist, 5,* 190–194.

Fristoe, N. M., Salthouse, T. A., & Woodard, J. L. (1997). Examination of age-related deficits on the Wisconsin Card Sorting Test. *Neuropsychology, 11,* 428–436.

Gansler, D. A., Fucetola, R., Krengel, M., Stetson, S., Zimering, R., & Makary, C. (1998). Are there cognitive subtypes in adult attention deficit/hyperactivity disorder? *The Journal of Nervous and Mental Disease, 186,* 776–781.

Golden, C. J., Kushner, T., Lee, B., & McMorrow, M. A. (1997). Searching for the meaning of the Category Test and the Wisconsin Card Sort Test: A comparative. *International Journal of Neuroscience, 93,* 141–150.

Goldman, R. S., Axelrod, B. N., Heaton, R. K., Chelune, G. J., Curtiss, G., Kay, G. G., & Thompson, L. L. (1996). Latent structure of the WCST with the standardization samples. *Assessment, 3,* 73–78.

Goldstein, G., Minshew, N. J., Allen, D. N., & Seaton, B. E. (2002). High functioning autism and schizophrenia. A comparison of an early and late onset neurodevelopmental disorder. *Archives of Clinical Neuropsychology, 17,* 461–475.

Grafman, J., Jones, B., & Salazar, A. (1990). Wisconsin Card Sorting Test performance based on location and size of neuroanatomical lesion in Vietnam veterans with penetrating head injury. *Perceptual and Motor Skills, 71,* 1120–1122.

Grant, D. A., & Berg, E. A. (1948). A behavioral analysis of degree of impairment and ease of shifting to new responses in a Weigl-type card sorting problem. *Journal of Experimental Psychology, 39,* 404–411.

Green, J., McDonald, W. M., Vitek, J. L., Evatt, M., Freeman, A., Haber, M., Bakay, R. A., Triche, S., Sirockman, B., & DeLong, M. R. (2002). Cognitive impairments in advanced PD without dementia. *Neurology, 59,* 1320–1324.

Greve, K. W. (2001). The WCST-64: A standardized short-form of the Wisconsin Card Sorting Test. *The Clinical Neuropsychologist, 15,* 228–234.

Greve, K. W. (1993). Can perseverative responses on the Wisconsin Card Sorting Test be scored accurately? *Archives of Clinical Neuropsychology, 8,* 511–517.

Greve, K. W., Bianchini, K. J., Hartley, S. M., & Adams, D. (1999). The Wisconsin Card Sorting Test in stroke rehabilitation: Factor structure and relationship to outcome. *Archives of Clinical Neuropsychology, 14,* 497–509.

Greve, K. W., Ingram, F., & Bianchini, K. J. (1998). Latent structure of the Wisconsin Card Sorting Test in a clinical sample. *Archives of Clinical Neuropsychology, 13,* 597–609.

Greve, K. W., Bianchini, K. J., Mathias, C. W., Houston, R. J., & Crouch, J. A. (2002). Detecting malingered performance with the Wisconsin Card Sorting Test: A preliminary investigation in traumatic brain injury. *The Clinical Neuropsychologist, 16*(2), 179–191.

Greve, K. W., Brooks, J., Crouch, J., Rice, W. J., Cicerone, K., & Rowland, L. (1993). Factorial structure of the Wisconsin Card Sorting Test. *The Clinical Neuropsychologist, 7*, 350–351.

Greve, K. W., Love, J. M., Sherwin, E., Mathias, C. W., Houston, R. J., & Brennan, A. (2002a). Temporal stability of the Wisconsin Card Sorting Test in a chronic traumatic brain injury sample. *Assessment, 9*, 271–277.

Greve, K. W., Love, J. M., Sherwin, E., Mathias, C. W., Ramzinski, P., & Levy, J. (2002). Wisconsin Card Sorting Test in chronic severe traumatic brain injury: Factor structure and performance subgroups. *Brain Injury, 16*, 29–40.

Greve, K. W., Stickle, T. R., Love, J. M., Bianchini, K. J., & Stanford, M. S. (2005). Latent structure of the Wisconsin Card Sorting Test: A confirmatory factor analytic study. *Archives of Clinical Neuropsychology, 20*, 355–364.

Haaland, K., Vranes, L. F., Goodwin, J. S., & Garry, J. P. (1987). Wisconsin Cart Sorting Test performance in a healthy elderly population. *Journal of Gerontology, 42*, 345–346.

Hartman, M., Bolton, E., & Fehnel, S. E. (2001). Accounting for age differences on the Wisconsin Card Sorting Test: Decreased working memory, not inflexibility. *Psychology & Aging, 16*, 385–399.

Heaton, R. K. (1981). *Wisconsin Card Sorting Test manual.* Odessa, FL: Psychological Assessment Resources, Inc.

Heaton, R. K., Avitable, N., Grant, I., & Mathews, C. (1999). Further cross-validation of regression-based neuropsychological norms with an update for the Boston Naming Test. *Journal of Clinical and Experimental Neuropsychology, 21*, 572–582.

Heaton, R. K., Chelune, G. J., Talley, J. L., Kay, G. G., & Curtis, G. (1993). *Wisconsin Card Sorting Test (WCST) manual, revised and expanded.* Odessa, FL: Psychological Assessment Resources.

Heinrichs, R. W. (1990). Variables associated with Wisconsin Card Sorting Test performance in neuropsychiatric patients referred for assessment. *Neuropsychiatry, Neuropsychology and Behavioral Neurology, 3*, 107–112.

Hellman, S. G., Green, M. F., Kern, R. S., & Christenson, C. D. (1992). Comparison of card and computer versions of the Wisconsin Card Sorting Test for psychotic patients. *International Journal of Methods in Psychiatric Research, 2*, 151–155.

Henry, J. D., & Crawford, J. R. (2004a). A meta-analytic review of verbal fluency performance following focal cortical lesions. *Neuropsychology, 18*, 284–295.

Henry, J. D., & Crawford, J. R. (2004b). A meta-analytic review of verbal fluency performance in patients with traumatic brain injury. *Neuropsychology, 18*, 621–628.

Henry, J. D., & Crawford, J. R. (2004c). Verbal fluency deficits in Parkinson's disease: A meta-analysis. *Journal of the International Neuropsychological Society, 10*, 608–622.

Henry, J. D., & Crawford, J. R. (2005). A meta-analytic review of verbal fluency deficits in schizophrenia relative to other neurocognitive deficits. *Cognitive Neuropsychiatry, 10*, 1–33.

Hermann, B. P., Wyler, A. R., & Richey, E. T. (1988). Wisconsin Card Sorting Test performance in patients with complex partial seizure of temporal lobe origin. *Journal of Clinical and Experimental Psychology, 10*, 467–476.

Horner, M. D., Flashman, L. A., Freides, D., Epstein, C. M., & Bakay, R. A. E. (1996). Temporal lobe epilepsy and performance on the Wisconsin Card Sorting Test. *Journal of Clinical and Experimental Neuropsychology, 18*, 310–313.

Huber, S. J., Bornstein, R. A., Rammohan, K. W., Christy, J. A., et al. (1992). Magnetic resonance imaging correlates of executive function impairments in multiple sclerosis. *Neuropsychiatry, Neuropsychology, and Behavioral Neurology, 5*, 33–36.

Ingram, F., Greve, K. W., Fishel Ingram, P. T., & Soukup, V. M. (1999). Temporal stability of the Wisconsin Card Sorting Test in an untreated patient sample. *British Journal of Clinical Psychology, 38*, 209–211.

Iverson, G. L., Slick, D. J., & Franzen, M. D. (2000). Clinical normative data for the WCST-64 following uncomplicated mild head injury. *Applied Neuropsychology, 7*, 247–251.

Johnson-Selfridge, M., & Zalewski, C. (2001). Moderator variables of executive functioning in schizophrenia: Meta-analytic findings. *Schizophrenia Bulletin, 27*, 305–313.

Kibby, M. Y., Schmitter-Edgecombe, M., & Long, C. J. (1998). Ecological validity of neuropsychological tests: focus on the California Verbal Learning Test and the Wisconsin Card Sorting Test. *Archives of Clinical Neuropsychology, 13*, 523–534.

King, J. H., Sweet, J. J., Sherer, M., Curtiss, G., & Vanderploeg, R. D. (2002). Validity indices within the Wisconsin Card Sorting Test: Application of new and previously researched multivariate procedures in multiple traumatic brain injury samples. *The Clinical Neuropsychologist, 16*, 506–523.

Kizilbash, A., & Donders, J. (1999). Latent structure of the Wisconsin Card Sorting Test after pediatric head injury. *Child Neuropsychology, 5*, 224–229.

Klorman, R., Hazel-Fernandez, L. A., Shaywitz, S. E., Fletcher, J. M., Marchione, K. E., Holahan, J. M., Stuebing, K. M., & Shaywitz, B. A. (1999). Executive functioning deficits in attention-deficit/hyperactivity disorder are independent of oppositional defiant or reading disorder. *Journal of the American Academy of Child & Adolescent Psychiatry, 38*, 1148–1155.

Kongs, S. K., Thompson, L. L., Iverson, G. L., & Heaton, R. K. (2000). *Wisconsin Card Sorting Test-64 Card Version.* Lutz, FL: Psychological Assessment Resources.

Koren, D., Seidman, L. J., Harrison, R. H., Lyons, M. J., Kremen, W. S., Caplan, B., Goldstein, J. M., Faraone, S. V., & Tsuang, M. T. (1998). Factor structure of the Wisconsin Card Sorting Test: Dimensions of deficit in schizophrenia. *Neuropsychology, 12*, 289–302.

Lacerda, A. L. T., Dalgalarrondo, P., Caetano, D., Haas, G. L., Camargo, E. E., Keshavan, M. S. (2003). Neuropsychological performance and regional cerebral blood flow in obsessive-compulsive disorder. *Progress in Neuro-Psychopharmacology & Biological Psychiatry, 27*, 657–665.

Laiacona, M., Inzaghi, M. G., De Tanti, A., & Capitani, E. (2000). Wisconsin card sorting test: A new global score, with Italian norms and its relationship with the Weigl sorting test. *Neurological Science, 21*, 279–291.

Larrabee, G. J. (2003). Detection of malingering using atypical performance patterns on standard neuropsychological tests. *The Clinical Neuropsychologist, 17*, 410–425.

Lawrence, V., Houghton, S., Douglas, G., Durkin, K., Whiting, K., & Tannock, R. (2004). Executive function and ADHD: A comparison of children's performance during neuropsychological testing and real world activities. *Journal of Attention Disorders, 7*, 137–149.

Laws, K. R. (1999). A meta-analytic review of Wisconsin Card Sort studies in schizophrenia: General intellectual deficits in disguise? *Cognitive Neuropsychiatry, 4*, 1–30.

Leng, N. R., & Parkin, A. J. (1988). Double dissociation of frontal dysfunction in organic amnesia. *British Journal of Clinical Psychology, 27*, 359–362.

Levin, H. S., Culhane, K. A., Hartmann, J., Evankovitch, K., Mattson, A. J., Harward, H., Ringholz, G., Ewing-Cobbs, L., & Fletcher, J. M. (1991). Developmental changes in performance on tests of purported frontal lobe functioning. *Developmental Neuropsychology, 7*, 377–395.

Levin, H. S., Song, J., Scheibel, R. S., Fletcher, J. M., Harvard, H., Lilly, M., & Goldstein, F. (1997). Concept formation and problem-solving following closed head injury in children. *Journal of the International Neuropsychological Society, 3*, 598–607.

Levine, B., Stuss, D. T., & Milberg, W. P. (1995). Concept generation: Validation of a test of executive functioning in a normal aging population. *Journal of Clinical and Experimental Neuropsychology, 17*, 740–758.

Lezak, M. D., Howieson, D. B., Loring, D. W., Hannay, H. J., & Fischer, J. S. (2004). *Neuropsychological assessment* (4th ed.). New York: Oxford University Press.

Lineweaver, T. T., Bondi, M. W., Thomas, R. G., & Salmon, D. P. (1999). A normative study of Nelson's (1976) modified version of the Wisconsin Card Sorting Test in healthy older adults. *The Clinical Neuropsychologist, 13*, 328–347.

Lombardi, W. J., Andreason, P. J., Sirocco, K. Y., Rio, D. E., Gross, R. E., Umhau, J. C., & Hommer, D. W. (1999). Wisconsin Card Sorting Test performance following head injury: Dorsolateral fronto-striatal circuit activity predicts perseveration. *Journal of Clinical and Experimental Neuropsychology, 21*, 2–16.

Loong, J. W. K. (1990). *The Wisconsin Card Sorting Test (IBM version).* San Luis Obispo, CA: Wang Neuropsychological Laboratory.

MacPherson, S. E., Phillips, L. H., & Della Sala, S. (2002). Age, executive function, and social decision making: A dorsolateral prefrontal theory of cognitive aging. *Psychology and Aging, 17*, 598–609.

Martin, D. J., Oren, Z., & Boone, K. (1991). Major depressives' and dysthymics' performance on the Wisconsin Card Sorting Test. *Journal of Clinical Psychology, 47*, 685–690.

Martin, R. C., Sawrie, S. M., Edwards, R., Roth, D. L., Faught, E., Kuzniecky, R. I., Morawetz, R. B., & Gilliam, F. G. (2000). Investigation of executive function change following anterior temporal lobectomy: Selective normalization of verbal fluency. *Neuropsychology, 14*, 501–508.

Merrick, E. E., Donders, J., & Wiersum, M. (2003). Validity of the WCST-64 after traumatic brain injury. *The Clinical Neuropsychologist, 17*, 153–158.

Meyer, S. E., Carlson, G. A., Wiggs, E. A., Martinez, P. E., Ronsaville, D. S., Kilmes-Dougan, B., Gold, P. W., & Radke-Yarrow, M. (2004). A prospective study of the association among impaired executive functioning, childhood attentional problems, and the development of bipolar disorder. *Development & Psychopathology, 16*, 461–476.

Milner, B. (1963). Effects of different brain lesions on card sorting. *Archives of Neurology, 9*, 90–100.

Minshew, N. J., Meyer, J., & Goldstein, G. (2002). Abstract reasoning in autism: A dissociation between concept formation and concept identification. *Neuropsychology, 16*, 327–334.

Miyake, A., Emerson, M. J., & Frieman, N. P. (2000). Assessment of executive functions in clinical settings: Problems and recommendation. *Seminars in Speech and Language, 21*, 169–183.

Miyake, A., Friedman, N. P., Emerson, M. J., Witzki, A. H., & Howerter, A. (2000). The unity and diversity of executive functions and their contributions to complex "frontal lobe" tasks: A latent variable analysis. *Cognitive Psychology, 41*, 49–109.

Monchi, O., Petrides, M., Doyon, J., Postuma, R. B., Worsley, K., & Dagher, A. (2004). Neural bases of set-shifting deficits in Parkinson's disease. *Journal of Neuroscience, 24*, 702–710.

Moritz, S., Birkner, C., Kloss, M., Jahn, H., Hand, I., Haasen, C., & Krausz, M. (2002). Executive functioning in obsessive-compulsive disorder, unipolar depression, and schizophrenia. *Archives of Clinical Neuropsychology, 17*, 477–483.

Mountain, M. A., & Snow, G. (1993). Wisconsin Card Sorting Test as a measure of frontal pathology: A review. *The Clinical Neuropsychologist, 7*, 108–118.

Nelson, H. E. (1976). A modified card sorting test sensitive to frontal lobe defects. *Cortex, 12*, 313–324.

Nybo, T., & Koskiniem, M. (1999). Cognitive indicators of vocational outcome after severe traumatic brain injury (TBI) in childhood. *Brain Injury, 13*, 759–766.

Obonsawin, M. C., Crawford, J. R., Page, J., Chalmers, P., Low, G., & Marsh, P. (1999). Performance on the Modified Card Sorting Test by normal, healthy individuals: Relationship to general intellectual ability and demographic variables. *British Journal of Clinical Psychology, 38*, 27–41.

O'Donnell, J. P., MacGregor, L. A., Dabrowski, J. J., Oestreicher, J. M., & Romero, J. J. (1994). Construct validity of neuropsychological tests of conceptual and attentional abilities. *Journal of Clinical Psychology, 50*, 596–600.

Osmon, D. C., & Suchy, Y. (1996). Fractionating frontal lobe functions: Factors of the Milwaukee Card Sorting Test. *Archives of Clinical Neuropsychology, 11*, 451–552.

Ozonoff, S. (1995). Reliability and validity of the Wisconsin Card Sorting Test in studies of autism. *Neuropsychology, 9*, 491–500.

Paniak, C., Miller, H. B., Murphy, D., Patterson, L., & Keizer, J. (1996). Canadian developmental norms for 9- to14-year-olds on the Wisconsin Card Sorting Test. *Canadian Journal of Rehabilitation, 9*, 233–237.

Paolo, A. M., Axelrod, B. N., Ryan, J. J., & Goldman, R. S. (1994). Administration accuracy of the Wisconsin Card Sorting Test. *The Clinical Neuropsychologist, 8*, 112–116.

Paolo, A. M., Axelrod, B. N., & Troster, A. I. (1996a). Test-retest stability of the Wisconsin Card Sorting Test. *Assessment, 3*, 137–143.

Paolo, A. M., Axelrod, B. N., Troster, A. I., Blackwell, K. T., & Koller, W. C. (1996b). Utility of a Wisconsin Card Sorting Test short form in persons with Alzheimer's and Parkinson's disease. *Journal of Clinical and Experimental Neuropsychology, 18*, 892–897.

Paolo, A. M., Troster, A. I., Axelrod, B. N., & Koller, W. C. (1995). Construct validity of the WCST in normal elderly and persons with Parkinson's disease. *Archives of Clinical Neuropsychology, 10*, 463–473.

Parkin, A. J., Walter, B. M., & Hunkin, N. M. (1995). Relationships between normal aging, frontal lobe function, and memory for temporal and spatial information. *Neuropsychology, 9*, 304–312.

Pendleton, M. G., & Heaton, R. K. (1982). A comparison of the Wisconsin Card Sorting Test and the Category Test. *Journal of Clinical Psychology, 38*, 392–396.

Perrine, K. (1993). Differential aspects of conceptual processing in the category test and Wisconsin Card Sorting Test. *Journal of Clinical and Experimental Neuropsychology, 15*, 461–473.

Pineda, D. A., & Merchan, V. (2003). Executive function in young Colombian adults. *International Journal of Neuroscience, 113*, 397–410.

Pukrop, R., Matuschek, E., Ruhrmann, S., Brockhaus-Dumke, A., Tendolkar, I., Bertsch, A., & Klosterkotter, J. (2003). Dimensions of working memory dysfunction in schizophrenia. *Schizophrenia Research, 62*, 259–268.

Rabin, L. A., Barr, W. B., & Burton, L. A. (2005). Assessment practices of clinical neuropsychologists in the United States and Canada: A survey of INS, NAN, and APA division 40 members. *Archives of Clinical Neuropsychology, 20*, 33–65.

Rey, G. J., Feldman, E., Rivas-Vazquez, R., Levin, B. E., & Benton, A. (1999). Neuropsychological test development and normative data on Hispanics. *Archives of Clinical Neuropsychology, 14*, 593–602.

Rezai, K., Andreasen, N. C., Alliger, R., Cohen, G., Swayze II, V., & O'Leary, D. S. (1993). The neuropsychology of the prefrontal cortex. *Archives of Neurology, 59*, 636–642.

Rhodes, M. G. (2004). Age-related differences in performance on the Wisconsin Card Sorting Test: A meta-analytic review. *Psychology and Aging, 19*, 482–494.

Robinson, A. L., Heaton, R. K., Lehman, R. A. W., & Stilson, D. W. (1980). The utility of the Wisconsin Card Sorting Test in detecting and localizing frontal lobe lesions. *Journal of Consulting and Clinical Psychology, 48*, 605–614.

Romine, C. B., Lee, D., Wolfe, M. E., Homack, S., George, C., & Riccio, C. A. (2004). Wisconsin Card Sorting Test with children: A meta-analytic study of sensitivity and specificity. *Archives of Clinical Neuropsychology, 19*, 1027–1041.

Rosselli, M., & Ardila, A. (1993). Developmental norms for the Wisconsin Card Sorting Test in 5- to 12-year-old children. *The Clinical Neuropsychologist, 7*, 145–154.

Rosselli, M., & Ardila, A. (1996). Cognitive effects of cocaine and polydrug abuse. *Journal of Clinical and Experimental Neuropsychology, 18*, 122–135.

Salthouse, T. A., Atkinson, T. M., & Berish, D. E. (2003). Executive functioning as a potential mediator of age-related cognitive decline in normal adults. *Journal of Experimental Psychology: General, 132*, 566–594.

Salthouse, T. A., Fristoe, N., & Rhee, S. H. (1996). How localized are age-related effects on neuropsychological measures? *Neuropsychology, 10*, 272–285.

Sherer, M., Nick, T. G., Millis, S. R., & Novack, T. A. (2003). Use of the WCST and the WCST-64 in the assessment of traumatic brain injury. *Journal of Clinical and Experimental Neuropsychology, 25*, 512–520.

Sherman, E. M., Strauss, E., Spellacy, F., & Hunter, M. (1995). Construct validity of WAIS-R factors: Neuropsychological correlates in adults referred for possible head injury. *Psychological Assessment, 7*, 440–444.

Shu, B-C., Tien, A. Y., Lung, F-W., & Chang, Y-Y. (2000). Norms for the Wisconsin Card Sorting Test in 6- to 11-year old children in Taiwan. *The Clinical Neuropsychologist, 14*, 275–286.

Smith-Seemiller, L., Arffa, S., & Franzen, M. D. (2001). Use of Wisconsin Card Sorting Test short forms with school-age children. *Archives of Clinical Neuropsychology, 16*, 489–499.

Snow, J. H. (1998). Developmental patterns and use of the Wisconsin Card Sorting Test for children and adolescents with learning disabilities. *Child Neuropsychology, 4*, 89–97.

Somerville, J., Tremont, J., & Stern, R. A. (2000). The Boston Qualitative Scoring System as a measure of executive functioning in Rey-Osterrieth Complex Figure performance. *Journal of Clinical and Experimental Neuropsychology, 22*, 613–621.

Strauss, E., Hunter, M., & Wada, J. (1993). Wisconsin Card Sort performance: Effects of age of onset and laterality of dysfunction.

Journal of Clinical and Experimental Neuropsychology, 15, 896–902.

Stuss, D. T., Benson, D. F., Kaplan, E.F., Weir, W. S., Naeser, M. A., Lieberman, I., & Ferrill, D. (1983). The involvement of orbitofrontal cerebrum in cognitive tasks. *Neuropsychologia, 21*, 235–248.

Stuss, D. T., Levine, B., Alexander, M. P., Hong, J., Palumbo, C., Hamer, L., Murphy, K. J., & Izukawa, D. (2000). Wisconsin Card Sorting Test performance in patients with focal frontal and posterior brain damage: Effects of lesion location and test structure on separable cognitive processes. *Neuropsychologia, 38*, 388–402.

Suhr, J. A., & Boyer, D. (1999). Use of the Wisconsin Card Sorting Test in the detection of malingering in student simulator and patient sample. *Journal of Clinical and Experimental Neuropsychology, 21*, 701–708.

Sullivan, E. V., Mathalon, D. H., Zipursky, R. B., Kersteen-Tucker, Z., Knight, R. T., & Pfefferbaum, A. (1993). Factors of the Wisconsin Card Sorting Test as measures of frontal-lobe function in schizophrenia and in chronic alcoholism. *Psychiatry Research, 46*, 175–199.

Tate, R. L., Perdices, M., & Maggiotto, S. (1998). Stability of the Wisconsin Card Sorting Test and the determination of reliability of change in scores. *The Clinical Neuropsychologist, 12*, 348–357.

Taylor, L. B. (1979). Psychological assessment of neurological patients. In T. Rasmussen & R. Marino (Eds.), *Functional neurosurgery*. New York: Raven Press.

Toren, P., Sadeh, M., Wolmer, L., Eldar, S., Koren, S., Weizman, R., & Laor, N. (2000). Neurocognitive correlates of anxiety disorders in children: A preliminary report. *Journal of Anxiety Disorders, 14*, 239–247.

Van der Does, A. J. W., & Van den Bosch, R. J. (1992). What determines Wisconsin Card Sorting performance in schizophrenia? *Clinical Psychology Review, 12*, 567–583.

Van der Linden, D., Frese, M., & Meijman, T. F. (2003). Mental fatigue and the control of cognitive processes: effects on perseveration and planning. *Acta Psychologia, 113*, 45–65.

Van Gorp, W. G., Kalechstein, A. D., Moore, L. H., Hinkin, C. H., Mahler, M. E., Foti, D., & Mendez, M. (1997). A clinical comparison of two forms of the card sorting test. *The Clinical Neuropsychologist, 11*, 155–160.

Van Spaendonck, K. P. M., Berger, H. J. C., Horstink, M. W. I. M., Borm, G. F., & Cools, A. R. (1995). Card sorting performance in Parkinson's disease: A comparison between acquisition and shifting performance. *Journal of Clinical and Experimental Neuropsychology, 17*, 918–925.

Vanderploeg, R. D., Schinka, J. A., & Retzlaff, P. (1994). Relationships between measures of auditory verbal learning and executive functioning. *Journal of Clinical and Experimental Neuropsychology, 16*, 243–252.

Vayalakkara, J., Devaraju-Backhaus, S., Bradley, J. D. D., Simco, E. R., & Golden, C. J. (2000). Abbreviated form of the Wisconsin Card Sort Test. *International Journal of Neuroscience, 103*, 131–137.

Weinberger, D. R., Berman, K. F., & Zec, R. F. (1988). Physiological dysfunction of dorsolateral prefrontal cortex in schizophrenia; I: Regional cerebral blood flow (rCBF) evidence. *Archives of General Psychiatry, 45*, 609–615.

Welsh, M. C., Groisser, D., & Pennington, B. F. (1988). *A normative-developmental study of performance on measures hypothesized to tap prefrontal functions.* Paper presented to the International Neuropsychological Society, New Orleans.

Welsh, M. C., Pennington, B. F., & Grossier, D. B. (1991). A normative-developmental study of executive function: A window on prefrontal function in children. *Developmental Neuropsychology, 7,* 131–149.

Wiegner, S., & Donders, J. (1999). Performance on the Wisconsin Card Sorting Test after traumatic brain injury. *Assessment, 6,* 179–188.

Woods, S. T., & Troster, A. I. (2003). Prodromal frontal/executive dysfunction predicts incident dementia in Parkinson's disease. *Journal of the International Neuropsychological Society, 9,* 17–24.

9

Attention

The brain has inherent limitations in the amount of information it can process at any one time. To function effectively, there must be a means to select specific information for further processing (Banich, 2004). In its simplest form, the term "attention" can be conceptualized as the gateway for information flow to the brain (Cohen, 1993). In most models, attention is a complex system of interacting components that allows the individual to filter relevant and irrelevant information in the context of internal drives and intentions, hold and manipulate mental representations, and monitor/modulate responses to stimuli. Attention therefore typically refers to a multifactorial set of processes that reach beyond the simple capacity to encode information.

Attention can be conceptualized as comprising several basic processes. These include sensory selection (filtering, focusing, automatic shifting), response selection (response intention, initiation and inhibition, active switching, and executive supervisory control), attentional capacity (structural and energetic capacity, arousal, effort), and sustained performance (fatigability, vigilance; Cohen, 1993). Attentional deficits may therefore result from a variety of deficits in one or more of these component processes (for more information on neuropsychological models of attention, see Banich, 2004; Baron, 2004; Cohen, 1993; Lezak et al., 2004; Lyon & Krasnegor, 1996).

Models of attention commonly divide attention into component processes such as alertness/arousal, focused attention, selective attention, divided attention, and sustained attention or vigilance. However, consensus on the exact meaning of these terms has not been reached, and some terms refer to overlapping or synonymous processes (e.g., "focused attention" and "selective attention"). Further, tests of attention typically measure more than one attentional process. Also complicating matters is the fact that attentional processes cannot be assessed in isolation. To maintain attention, the individual must attend to something. That "something" may vary across tests with regard to dimensions such as modality, complexity, and contextual relevance. The

target information may be language-based (e.g., letters or numbers), visual (e.g., squares), spatial (locations), or auditory (e.g., tones). Targets may be presented in one modality (visual or auditory), and responses may be required in the same or in a different modality (e.g., motor, verbal), which may add to task complexity and add additional interference effects. Many attention tests are themselves multifactorial, requiring aspects such as motor speed, information processing speed, verbal responding, or other capacity. Careful evaluation of the constituent requirements of each task, and the interaction of these parameters with patient characteristics, is therefore crucial for accurate interpretation of test performance. In particular, it is important to assess sustained attention (vigilance), as many attentional disorders only become evident over longer testing periods. The issue of practice effects and the need for dual baseline for some paradigms also needs to be considered. Like most cognitive processes, attentional processes change as the individual matures. An understanding of the developmental aspects of attentional functioning (including its interactions with executive function development) is also necessary for those working with children, but also for those working with older adults, to adequately take into consideration the developmental trajectory of attentional abilities in the later years.

From a conceptual and construct validity perspective, attention tasks may also overlap with other "distinct" neuropsychological domains such as executive function or memory. For example, to properly perform a "divided attention" task, the individual must demonstrate inhibition and switching capacity, component processes that easily fall under the executive function rubric. Similarly, "attention" overlaps with the executive function of "working memory." Thus, it can be argued that many existing neuropsychological tests of attention are a combination of attentional/executive functioning measures with lesser or greater need for switching, inhibition, and working memory, and that distinctions between current "attention tests" and "executive tests" are somewhat artificial. Similarly, early processing stages in memory paradigms ("encoding," "short-term memory," or "working memory") overlap conceptually with attention processes. In this way, first-exposure encoding trials in learning paradigms may inform more about working memory and attention than about overall learning capacity per se.

Attention is a central aspect of neuropsychological assessment, and attentional disorders affect a majority of patients with neurological disorders involving the brain. Indeed, some of the most sensitive measures used in the diagnosis of neurological disorders are tests of attention (e.g., Digit Symbol, Symbol Digit Modalities, PASAT). Thankfully, the field of standardized neuropsychological assessment has evolved from a lesser emphasis on attention to the availability of entire attentional batteries (e.g., TEA, TEACh). In this chapter, we present some of the main attentional measures. Table 9–1 on pages 548 and 549 lists these along with their strengths and weaknesses. Other tests such as the Stroop and Dichotic Listening, reviewed elsewhere in this volume, also measure aspects of attentional functioning.

In addition to these attention tests, most "stand-alone" neuropsychological batteries such as the Halstead-Reitan, NAB, and NEPSY also contain subtests specifically covering attentional functioning. Most IQ tests also cover at least some aspects of focused or selective attention (i.e., working memory) through subtests such as digit span tasks, cancellation tasks, or symbol substitution tasks (e.g., Wechsler tests, WJ III COG, SB5). Of note, the Cognitive Assessment System (CAS) provides a more thorough assessment of attention than most IQ tests. Many memory batteries also provide estimates of aspects of attentional functioning along with memory and learning (e.g., WRAML2, WMS III, CMS). However, it is important to note that only batteries designed specifically to measure attention (e.g., TEA and TEACh) sample most aspects of attention, including sustained attention and nonverbal attention, component processes that are overlooked in some batteries. Thus, in most cases, administering an IQ test and memory battery may allow one to rule out focused attention deficits, but not other kinds of attentional impairments.

Adequate assessment of attentional deficits also requires determining whether these deficits appear in daily life and whether they cause functional impairments. In children, administering parent and teacher questionnaires that assess for the presence of attention deficits in different settings (e.g., rating scales for ADHD and/or other rating scales such as the BRIEF; see *Assessment of Mood, Personality and Adaptive Functions* elsewhere in this volume) helps to determine whether attentional impairments are situation-specific or whether they cause functional interference in all settings. Although this is crucial in the differential diagnosis of ADHD, this is often helpful in most other situations as well. In adults, this can be accomplished using proxy ratings from other informants such as spouses, in addition to self-ratings.

REFERENCES

Banich, M. T. (2004). *Cognitive neuroscience and neuropsychology.* Boston: Houghton Mifflin.

Baron, I. S. (2004). *Neuropsychological evaluation of the child.* New York: Oxford University Press.

Cohen, R. A. (1993). *The neuropsychology of attention.* New York: Plenum Press.

Lezak, M. D., Howieson, D. B., & Loring, D. W. (2004). *Neuropsychological assessment* (4th ed.). New York: Oxford University Press.

Lyon, C. R., & Krasnegor, N. A. (1996). *Attention, memory and executive function.* Baltimore: Paul H. Brookes Publishing.

Brief Test of Attention (BTA)

PURPOSE

The Brief Test of Attention (BTA) is a test of auditory divided attention.

SOURCE

The test can be ordered from Psychological Assessment Resources, Inc., 16204 N. Florida Ave., Lutz, FL, 33549 (www.parinc.com; 1-800-331-TEST [8378]). The BTA Introductory Kit (Professional Manual, Stimulus Audio Tape, and 50 Scoring Forms) retails for $69 US.

AGE RANGE

The test manual includes norms for individuals aged 17 to 82; additional norms are available for children 6 to 14.

DESCRIPTION

The BTA (Schretlen, 1997) was initially developed in 1989 as a brief and easily administered test of attention. It was designed specifically to reduce the influence of confounding factors from task requirements that complicate the interpretation of attention tests (e.g., motor speed, visual scanning, memory; Schretlen, Bobholz, & Brandt 1996). In addition, the test is theory-based; it was developed following the model proposed by Cooley and Morris (1990), a framework for conceptualizing the task demands of attention tests. Thus, the BTA is conceived as a task that requires divided attention, using basic perceptual (distinguishing letters from numbers) and conceptual (counting from 1 to 12) task requirements. According to the author, the test is intended to detect attentional impairments, not as a tool for differentiating between levels of intact attention (Schretlen, 1997).

Table 9–1 Characteristics of Selected Tests of Attention

Test	Age Range	Tasks Included	Administration Time	Some Key Processes Thought to be Assessed	Internal Reliability	Test-Retest Reliability	Evidence of Sensitivity to Attentional Impairments	Evidence of Ecological Validity
Brief Test of Attention (BTA)	17–82[a]	—	10 min	Divided attention	Good	Low to adequate	Moderate	Good
Conners' Continuous Performance Test (CPT-II)	6–55+	Omissions Commissions Reaction Time Variability Index scores (see review for additional scores)	14 min	Sustained Attention Inhibitory Control/Impulsivity Response Speed	Acceptable to high	Limited	Moderate	Limited information
IVA+ Plus	6–99	Response Control scores Attention scores Attribute scores Symptomatic scores	13 min	Sustained Attention Inhibitory Control/Impulsivity Response Speed	N/A	Varies (see review)	Moderate	Limited information
PASAT	16–74	—	15–20 min	Divided Attention Sustained Attention Working Memory Information Processing Speed	Very high	Adequate to high	Good	Good
CHIPASAT	8–14	—	15–20 min	Divided Attention Sustained Attention Working Memory Information Processing Speed	Very high	Very High	Moderate	Limited information
CTMT	11–74 years, 11 months[b]	Trials 1 to 5 (each assessing different component of performance)	5–10 min	Attention Visual Scanning Executive Functioning	Composite: high; Trials: acceptable	Composite: high; Trials: acceptable	Limited information	Limited information
Ruff 2 & 7	16–70	Sustained Attention Selective Attention Discrepancy Analysis	5 min	Sustained Attention Selective Attention	High	Adequate to high	Good	Limited information
SDMT	8–91	—	5 min	Divided Attention Visual Attention Processing Speed	N/A	Varies (see review)	Good	Good

(continued)

Test	Age Range	Administration Time	Subtests/Scores	Attention Components	Norms	Reliability[c]	Validity	Clinical Utility
TEA	18–80	45–60 min	Map Search; Elevator Counting; Elevator Counting with Distraction; Visual Elevator; Elevator Counting with Reversal; Telephone Search; Telephone Switch while Counting; Lottery	Selective Attention; Sustained Attention; Attentional Control/Switching; Divided Attention	N/A	Most adequate to high[c]	Good	Good
TEA-Ch	6–16	60 min	Sky Search score; Creature Counting; Sky Search DT; Map Mission; Score DT; Walk, Don't Walk; Opposite Worlds; Code Transmission	Selective Attention; Sustained Attention; Attentional Control/Switching; Divided Attention	N/A	Most adequate to high[c]	Moderate	Limited information
T.O.V.A.	4–80	22 min	Omissions; Commissions; Response Time; Response Time Variability; D'; ADHD score; Postcommission Response Time; Anticipatory Responses; Multiple Responses	Sustained Attention; Inhibitory Control/Impulsivity; Response Speed	Varies (see review)	Varies (see review)	Good	Limited information
Trail Making Test	9–89	5–10 min	Part A: connect numbers; Part B: alternate numbers and letters	Visual search; Scanning; Sequencing; Switching; Speed	N/A	For the most part adequate	Good	Good

[a]Provisional norms for ages 6–14. [b]Norms for ages 8–10 are in press. [c]Reflects influences of both alternate form and test-retest reliability.

Source: Comprehensive Trail-Making Test. Reprinted with permission of PRO-ED, Inc., Austin, TX.

The test consists of two lists of alpha-numeric strings (e.g., "M-6-3-R-2"), presented on audiotape, that increase in length from four to 18 characters. In the first list (Form N), the subject's task is to disregard the letters and count how many numbers are presented aloud on the audiotape. In the second list (Form L), the same items are presented, but this time the examinee is instructed to disregard the numbers and count the number of letters. Unlike digit span tests, this test does not require the subject to recall which numbers (or letters) are presented. The test also does not require visual scanning or motor responding; for this reason, the BTA is suitable for assessing attention in populations with visual or motor impairments.

ADMINISTRATION

Materials

The test requires the BTA audiotape, an audio cassette player, and the Scoring Form; instructions are provided in the Professional Manual.

Instructions

See source for specific instructions (Schretlen, 1997). Both forms (N and L) are administered to all subjects. Test instructions should be read to the subject. One stimulus is presented per second; each trial is followed by five minutes of silence. Testing begins with two example items read by the examiner.

Discontinuing Testing

There are no discontinuation rules for the BTA. The author notes that this is because many examinees fail shorter lists but pass longer ones; list length and difficulty are thus not highly correlated. The test may be discontinued when a respondent fails all three trials of both samples. However, this discontinue criterion should only be applied to individuals under 75 years of age (see p. 9 of manual). Similarly, the manual states that the test can also be discontinued in individuals who do very well (i.e., greater than seven of 10 correct on the first form), because these individuals will almost always produce scores in the normal range when the entire test is administered (see *Normative Data* for more details). Because reliability is maximized by administering both forms, the manual indicates that some other task may be administered between forms if a subject finds the first form particularly frustrating.

ADMINISTRATION TIME

Each of the two lists takes about four or five minutes to administer and score; about 10 minutes are required for the entire test.

SCORING

Correct responses receive a score of 1. Thus, for each form, scores range from 0 to 10; the total score for the whole test

Table 9–2 Brief Test of Attention Percentile Classifications

Percentile	Classification
>74th	Above average
25th–74th	Average
10th–24th	Low average
2nd–9th	Borderline impaired
<2nd	Impaired

Source: Adapted from Schretlen, 1997.

ranges from 0 to 20. The total score is converted to a percentile using Appendix A in the manual. Normative scores are derived by age group. Because age ranges for the BTA overlap, users are instructed to select the age range with the midpoint corresponding to the examinee's age.

Impairment classifications based on BTA percentiles are presented in the manual, and in Table 9–2. Users should note that the highest possible percentile on the test is ">74."

DEMOGRAPHIC EFFECTS

Age

In normal adults, age is correlated with BTA performance. Performance tends to decline with advancing age, starting at about age 60.

Gender

Gender effects are also present; women score marginally higher than men (a difference of 0.8 points). Likewise, girls tend to slightly outperform boys (Schretlen, 1997).

Education

There are significant education effects on the test, which account for a small amount of variance (see later discussion).

Ethnicity

There are also subtle differences with regard to race/ethnicity on the BTA, with African American adults scoring on average about two points lower than Caucasian adults. However, African American adults mildly outperform Caucasians in the highest age group (0.4 points), but score slightly lower in the lower education groups (1.7–2.4 points).

Overview of Demographic Effects

When all factors are considered together, demographic variables account for approximately 17.5% of variance in BTA performance (i.e., 9% for age, 5% for ethnicity, 4% for education, and 1% for gender; Schretlen, 1997). Standardized scores are derived based only on age because of the minimal association with other demographic variables.

NORMATIVE DATA

Standardization Sample

Demographic characteristics of the normative sample are shown in Tables 9–3 and 9–4. Normative data are divided into 13 age groups from age 17 to 84. A clinical sample is also described in detail in the manual. Although percentile scores for children and clinical cases are not presented in the manual, these samples provide the basis for some reliability estimates. Children's norms based on the child sample are presented in Table 9–4, based on data presented in Schretlen et al. (1996).

Score Transformations

The manual indicates that after percentiles for each raw score were computed, slight inconsistencies in the progression of the percentile distribution across age were corrected.

Derivation of Discontinuation Cutoffs

Discontinuation cutoffs (see *Administration*) for use in determining whether administration of the abbreviated BTA (i.e., administration of the first form only) is sufficient were derived based on normative data as follows. The manual indicates that less than 1% of normal adults in the normative sample and 16.5% of the clinical sample scored less than 3 out of 10 correct on the first form of the BTA, which is the cutoff for abnormality. Of these, only one individual from the clinical sample obtained a nonabnormal score on the total BTA. This patient obtained a full BTA score in the borderline

Table 9–3 Characteristics of the Adult Normative
Sample for the BTA

Sample type	Combines data from three sources: a standardization sample ($N = 462$), research controls ($N = 187$), and individuals from a hypertension study ($N = 92$)
Number	667
Age	17 to 82 years
Geographic location	Baltimore, MD, and Buffalo, NY
SES	Not provided
Education	$M = 13.8$ ($SD = 2.6$)
Gender	
Men	37%
Women	63%
Race/ethnicity[a]	
White	82%
African American	18%
Other	0.3%
Screening	Dementia, severe psychiatric disorder, substance dependence[b]

[a]Data not recorded for 40 individuals in the sample. [b]Forty-five of the normal adults were not screened.

Table 9–4 Characteristics of the Child Normative
Sample for the BTA

Sample type	Children from a local elementary school
Number	74
Age	6 to 14 years
Geographic location	Location not specified, but presumably from Baltimore, MD, or Buffalo, NY
Parental education	Not specified
Education	
Second Grade	24
Fifth Grade	25
Eighth Grade	25
Gender	
Boys	51%
Girls	49%
Race/ethnicity	
White	95%
African American	5%
Other	0%
Screening	Not specified

Source: Adapted from Schretlen, 1997, and Schretlen et al., 1996a.

range (age 82); the remainder had abnormal scores on the full test, consistent with their abnormal score on the first form. Similarly, 27% of the clinical sample earned scores of greater than 7 out of 10 correct on the first BTA form; none of these had abnormal scores on the full test, although "several earned scores in the borderline range" (Schretlen, 1997, p. 10).

RELIABILITY

Internal Consistency

Based on the normative data (adults and children combined), the coefficient alpha for the whole test is high ($r = .80$), with lower coefficients for the separate forms ($r = .69$ and .65, respectively, for Forms L and N). When both the normative and clinical samples are combined ($N = 1231$), reliability estimates for the total test and separate forms are strong ($r = .90$ for the Total BTA, and .82 and .81, respectively, for Forms L and N; Schretlen, 1997). Separate internal reliability estimates for adults and children are not available.

Test-Retest Reliability

Test-retest stability is reported as .70 in a group of 60 older normal adults with mild hypertension, retested after a nine-month interval (Schretlen, 1997). Three-month stability data are also reported for a group of adolescent girls who received iron supplementation, described in the manual ($N = 78$). The test-retest correlation in this study was low ($r = .45$). The authors speculate that restriction of range may have lowered the coefficient in this case (only 14% of the group had scores below 15 of 20 on the BTA).

Practice Effects

Practice effects are minimal, with less than 5% of individuals showing retest changes exceeding ±4 or 5 points (Schretlen, 1997). However, it is unclear whether ceiling effects restrict the extent of practice effects.

Alternate Form Reliability

Although the two forms are designed to be used together, the correlation between Forms L and N is .65 for the normal sample ($N = 741$) and .79 for the combined normal-clinical sample ($N = 1328$). Forms L and N differ by less than 0.20 points in normals (Schretlen, 1997). The manual indicates that almost 95% of participants in the normal and clinical samples obtained L and N scores that were within three points of each other, which indicates that the two forms are equivalent in terms of difficulty. There are no order or practice effects between these forms in normals (Schretlen, 1997) or in patients with HD (Schretlen, Brandt, & Bobholz, 1996).

VALIDITY

Correlation With Other Attention Tests

Correlations and factor analyses involving other attention tests support the construct validity of the BTA. For instance, the BTA correlates slightly more with Digits Backward than with Digits Forward ($r = .53$ versus .43), and with Trails B than Trails A ($r = -.55$ versus .48). This is the case for both normal and patient groups (Schretlen, 1997; see also Wong, 1999). In normals, the BTA is highly correlated with all parts of the Stroop, not just the interference trial ($r = .66–.68$), suggesting that speed may be an important component of task success. In patients, the BTA correlates most highly with the Stroop interference trial (Schretlen, 1997).

In a principal components analysis with varimax rotation involving data for psychiatric patients ($N = 107$), the BTA emerged on an attention factor along with Digit Span, Digit Symbol, and all three Stroop components when examined with a number of other neuropsychological tests (Schretlen, 1997).

Correlation With Other Neuropsychological Tests

Correlation analyses and principal components analyses (Schretlen, Bobholz, & Brandt 1996) show that the BTA correlates more strongly with measures of attention than with other cognitive tasks such as the Rey-Osterrieth, Boston Naming Test, WMS-R Logical Memory, General Memory, and Delayed Memory Indices. In addition, Tagami and Strauss (1996) found, in a sample of 33 university students aged 18 to 44 years ($M = 22.12$, $SD = 6.33$), that scores on the BTA correlated significantly with scores on the first trial of the PASAT ($r = .55$). Whereas the PASAT showed a moderate relation with performance on the Wonderlic ($r = .33$), the BTA was unrelated to this brief measure of intellectual functioning ($r = .05$).

Clinical Studies

Schretlen, Brandt, and Bobholtz (1996) reported that nondemented patients with Huntington's disease performed poorly on the BTA compared with normal adults. Amnesic patients, however, were not impaired compared with controls, suggesting that the BTA does not require intact memory for successful performance. This study is also discussed in detail in the manual (Schretlen, 1997). Schretlen, Pearlson, and Anthony (1997) reported that BTA scores were also related to individual differences in cerebral volume as measured by MRI. Further, the effects of age on BTA performance may have been mediated by age-related differences in cerebral volume. In a study involving head injury patients, the BTA was found to be more sensitive to impairments in mild head injury patients than both Trails A and B (Wong, 1999).

Ecological Validity

In patients with severe mental disorders, the BTA appears to correlate highly with and account for more variance in functional competence (i.e., activities of daily living) than other tests of cognitive ability (e.g., VIQ, PIQ, FAS, HVLT; Schretlen, Jayaram, et al., 1997). In a group of adults with TBI, BTA scores were significantly related to psychosocial outcome (Schretlen, 1992); BTA scores, along with scores from the Cognitive Estimation Test, accounted for nearly 40% of the variance in psychosocial outcome. The BTA also appears to have potential as a screening instrument for driving capacity (Keyl et al., 1996).

COMMENT

The BTA is a theoretically based test of divided attention with features that make it appealing to busy clinicians. Its portability and brevity (less than 10 minutes) is useful for bedside examinations, and the lack of visual or motor components make it suitable for patients with severe visual or motor deficits. The test can be further abbreviated for those who do very poorly (i.e., the test can be discontinued after three failed trials, as long as age is less than 75 years), or for those who do very well (i.e., greater than 7 of 10 correct). However, it is recommended that the entire test be given to ensure adequate reliability, particularly since some patients in the clinical sample from the test manual who did well on the first form obtained borderline scores on the full test.

The test author emphasizes that the BTA measures only auditory selective and divided attention, not visual attention or other aspects of attentional functioning in the auditory

Table 9–5 Percent Cumulative Frequency of BTA Scores for Children

BTA Score	Age Range		
	6–8 years $N = 24$	9–11 years $N = 25$	12–14 years $N = 25$
20			100
19			96
18		100	84
17		96	84
16		88	72
15		76	68
14	100	72	36
13	96	52	24
12	88	44	20
11	75	36	12
10	63	28	8
9	58	12	8
8	50	8	4
7	33	8	
6	21		
5	13		
4	8		
3	4		
2	4		
1	4		
0	4		

Source: From Schretlen, Bobholz, & Brandt, 1996. Reprinted with the kind permission of Psychology Press.

information provided on whether Ns and gender distribution in each age band are equivalent, and overall gender distribution is uneven (i.e., 63% female). Norms taking into account education and gender may have also been helpful, although the author states that these variables accounted for minimal variance in test performance. More research is needed on the test's stability over time and on its use in ethnically diverse populations, particularly those that may not emphasize speed.

Lastly, a child sample is described in detail in the normative section, but no actual percentiles are provided for children. Children's norms are provided here from Schretlen, Bobholz, and Brandt (1996; see Table 9–5). The sample is geographically restricted and information on SES and parental education is lacking. Further, no information on reliability in children is provided and no validity information exists in children. The test should be used cautiously in this population until more research is conducted. Other measures would be preferable in diagnostic evaluations.

modality. Thus, the addition of other tests is required for a comprehensive evaluation of attention. The author also stresses that the BTA is primarily for screening for deficits in attention, not for measuring normal attentional functioning. This should be kept in mind when assessing gifted individuals, as ceiling effects may obscure superior ability.

Although most of the existing research on the BTA has been conducted by its author and colleagues, these studies cover an impressively diverse range of topics and appear to provide substantial support for the validity of the BTA in several clinical populations.

The adult normative sample is large and the manual is on the whole well written and comprehensive. However, there are some slight anomalies. For instance, the normative group extends up to age 82, not 84 as is printed in the manual (PAR, personal communication, December 2003). In addition, the normative sample is somewhat piecemeal. It is not a national, random stratified sample, is geographically restricted, and contains individuals with missing race/ethnicity data, as well as individuals who were not screened. Education levels are also not described, nor are screening procedures. There is no

REFERENCES

Cooley, E. L., & Morris, R. D. (1990). Attention in children: A neuropsychologically based model for assessment. *Developmental Neuropsychology, 6,* 239–274.

Keyl, P. M., Rebok, G. W., & Gallo, J. J. (1996). *Screening elderly drivers in general medical settings: Toward the development of a valid and feasible assessment procedure (final report).* Andrus Foundation of the NRTA/AARP.

Schretlen, D. (1992). Accounting for variance in long-term recovery from traumatic brain injury with executive abilities and injury severity [Abstract]. *Journal of Clinical and Experimental Neuropsychology, 14,* 77.

Schretlen, D. (1997). *Brief Test of Attention professional manual.* Odessa, FL: Psychological Assessment Resources.

Schretlen, D., Bobholz, J. H., & Brandt, J. (1996). Development and psychometric properties of the Brief Test of Attention. *The Clinical Neuropsychologist, 10,* 80–89.

Schretlen, D., Brandt, J., & Bobholz, J. H. (1996). Validation of the Brief Test of Attention in patients with Huntington's disease and amnesia. *The Clinical Neuropsychologist, 10,* 90–95.

Schretlen, D., Jayaram, G., Maki, P., Robinson, H., & devilliers, C. (1997). Functional correlates of neurocognitive deficits in adults with severe mental disorders [Abstract]. *Journal of the International Neuropsychological Society, 3,* 25.

Schretlen, D., Pearlson, G., & Anthony, J. (1997). *Individual differences in cerebral volume and BTA performance.* Unpublished data.

Tagami, Y., & Strauss, E. (1996). *The Brief Test of Attention: Relationship to the PASAT and to IQ.* B.A. Honours Thesis, University of Victoria.

Wong, T. M. (1999). Validity and sensitivity of the Brief Test of Attention with acute brain injury and mild head injury patients. [Abstract]. *Archives of Clinical Neuropsychology, 14*(8), 617–818.

Color Trails Test (CTT) and Children's Color Trails Test (CCTT)

PURPOSE

The Color Trails tests measure speed of attention, sequencing, mental flexibility, visual search, and motor function.

SOURCE

The Color Trails Test (CTT) is available from Psychological Assessment Resources, P.O. Box 998, Odessa, FL, for $99 US (www.parinc.com). The version for children, the CCTT, is available for $129 US.

Other Language Versions

The tests include a Spanish administration section. Norms are available for Cantonese-speaking adults (Lee, 2003) and Hispanics (Ponton et al., 2000).

AGE RANGE

The adult version is for individuals aged 18 to 89 years. The children's version (CCTT) is for ages 8 to 16 years. Limited normative data are also presented for children aged 5 years, 11 months to 7 years in the manual.

DESCRIPTION

The Color Trails Test (CTT; D'Elia et al., 1996; Llorente et al., 2003) is designed to minimize the influence of language so that it can be used in cross-cultural settings. It covers the child-to-adult age range, although data for age 17 are not provided. Part 1 is similar to the TMT Part A (reviewed in this volume), except that all odd-numbered circles are pink, and all even-numbered circles are yellow. Part 2 is similar to the TMT Part B; it shows all numbers from 1 to 25 (15 for children) twice (one sequence in yellow, the other in pink). The examinee is required to connect the numbers from 1 to 25 (15 for children), alternating between pink and yellow circles and disregarding the numbers in circles of the alternate color. For adults, three alternate forms for both parts are provided. However, Form A is the standard form for which normative data were collected. Therefore, Form A is the only form that should be used for clinical evaluation (Mitrushina et al., 2005). The alternate forms are considered experimental at present. For children, four alternate forms are available. Normative data are currently only available for Form K; it is therefore the standard one for administration (Llorente et al., 2003).

ADMINISTRATION

The administration, as described briefly in *Description*, is further detailed in the source. Prompts and corrections are given as in the TMT. Instructions can be presented nonverbally with visual cues. The authors caution that children must be able to recognize Arabic numerals 1 though 15, and they must be able to distinguish between the colors pink and yellow. They should also possess sufficient eye-hand coordination to use a pencil to connect the stimuli.

ADMINISTRATION TIME

About five to 10 minutes are needed.

SCORING

For the adult version, the time for the completion of Parts 1 and 2 is recorded in seconds. In addition, this test includes a qualitative scoring of number errors, near-misses, and prompts; further, an "interference index" (ratio of Part 2 minus 1 over Part 1 time scores) is calculated. Both Parts 1 and 2 require perceptual tracking of a sequence and speeded performance. However, Part 2 also requires divided attention. The interference index is an indicator of the need to elucidate the added task requirements of Part 2 and is thought to be a purer measure of the interference, attributable to the more complex divided attention and the alternating sequencing tasks required in Part 2.

Scores for the children's version are similar, although not totally identical (near-misses are not scored). Thus, the time for completion of Parts 1 and 2 are recorded, along with the number of prompts, errors, and an interference index. For both the adult and children's versions, scores are transformed to standard scores ($M = 100$, $SD = 15$), T scores, and percentiles. For the children's version, interpretive ranges and their rates of occurrence (baserate data) in the normative sample and children with learning disorders and/or ADHD are also provided.

NORMATIVE DATA

Influence of Demographic Variables

See *Source*. Increasing age adversely affects performance on both Part 1 and Part 2. Increasing education enhances performance on Part 2, but less so for Part 1 (Mitrushina et al., 2005). Gender does not impact performance (D'Elia et al., 1996). The means presented for African and Spanish Americans (D'Elia et al., 1996) suggest that these populations perform the CTT somewhat more slowly than Caucasian Americans. Lee (2003) has provided normative data based on a sample of 281 healthy Cantonese-speaking adults (20–70+) living in Hong Kong. Performance is somewhat faster (in 20- to 30-year-olds with high school education, 31 and 67 seconds for Part 1 and Part 2, respectively) than that of North American populations. See *Comment* for more discussion of ethnicity.

In children (age 5 years, 11 months to 16 years), a steady age progression is noted. There is evidence that female children complete Part 2 more quickly than males (Williams et al., 1995). However, Llorente et al. (2003) found only a small effect of gender ($r = .10$) on Part 1, with males performing better than females.

Normative Data

Adults. Normative data for the CTT (D'Elia et al., 1996) are based on the performance of 1528 healthy volunteers, including subsamples of 182 African Americans and 292 Hispanic Americans between the age of 18 years and 89 years, 11 months (see Table 9–6). These norms are presented separately for six education levels. Time in seconds for the CTT tends to be somewhat longer than for the TMT (e.g., in 20- to 30-year-olds, 37 and 82 seconds for Part 1 and Part 2, respectively, compared with about 23 and 50 seconds for the TMT A and TMT B, respectively).

Errors, near-misses, prompts, and an interference index of greater than 2.0 tend to occur only in the below 16th percentile range; that is, they are relatively rare in the standardization sample.

Children. Normative data are provided for ages 8 to 16 years based on a sample of 678 children (55% female) in Los Angeles (see Table 9–7). Children comprising the standardization cohort obtained an average PPVRT-R of 101.50 ($SD = 16.6$). Some data are also available in the manual for children aged 6 to 7 years, although the N is very small ($N = 17$) and the sample included children with mild neurological disorders, learning disability, or comorbid ADHD/learning disorder.

Table 9–6 Characteristics of the CTT Normative Sample Provided by D'Elia et al. (1996)

Number	1528
Age	18 to 89 years[a]
Geographic location	Various regions in the United States
Sample type	Most served as volunteers in other studies
Education	≤8–21 years[b]
Gender	
Male	88%
Female	12%
Race/ethnicity	
Caucasian	1054
African American	182
Hispanic	292
Screening	No reported history of medical, neurological, or psychiatric disorder or psychosocial condition that could interfere with neuropsychological test performance

[a]Age: 18–29, 30–44, 45–59, 60–74, 75–89 years. [b]Education: ≤8, 9–11, 12, 13–15, 16, 17–21 years.

Table 9–7 Characteristics of the CCTT Normative Sample Provided by Llorente et al. (2003)

Number	678
Age	8 to 16 years
Geographic location	Los Angeles
Sample type	Most (89%) right-handed from two high schools, one junior high, and one elementary school in Los Angeles representative of socioeconomic and cultural make-up of greater Los Angeles
Education	Elementary to high school
Gender	
Male	45%
Female	55%
Race/ethnicity	
Caucasian	309
African American	11
Hispanic	201
Other	105
Screening	No known history of medical, neurological, or psychiatric disorder or psychosocial condition that could interfere with neuropsychological test performance; children excluded if in special school placement due to attention or learning problems or if suffered from severe visual or physical handicaps

RELIABILITY

Test-Retest Reliability

For the CTT, two-week reliability is reported as marginal (.64) for Part 1, and acceptable to high (.79) for Part 2 (D'Elia et al., 1996). Several of the scores (e.g., errors, prompts, near-misses, interference index) have restrictions in range, reducing the magnitude of the reliability coefficients; these are not reported. Paired *t*-tests indicate that the interference index is significantly greater on the second test session (by less than one raw score point). No other CTT variables are significantly different across the two test sessions. Percentage agreement in clinical interpretation of the different variables between the first and second test sessions is good (varying from 77% for near-misses to 100% for the Part 1 and 2 time variables), suggesting relative stability across this short interval.

For the CCTT, test-retest reliability was assessed in a sample of children with ADHD following intervals of eight and 16 weeks and was found to be marginal to low ($r = .45–.68$; Llorente et al., 2003). However, the test authors report that diagnostic reliability (percentage agreement in clinical interpretation) was good for Part 1 and 2 time scores, at least in children with ADHD. Information regarding other scores (errors, prompts) is not provided. Information on practice effects is not reported.

Alternate Form Reliability

Llorente et al. (2003) reported high correlations between various forms (>.80) of the CCTT. However, mean score differences between the forms are not reported.

VALIDITY

Correlation With the TMT

Studies on the concordance between the Color Trails and standard TMT are somewhat conflicting. Maj et al. (1993) reported moderate correlations between CCT Parts 1 and 2 with TMT A and B of .41 and .50, respectively. Factor analysis of the CTT together with the TMT, the Color Figure Mazes, and the Stroop Test suggested that the CTT loaded on the same factor as Trails A and B in geriatric and nongeriatric samples (Uchiyama et al., 1994).

Somewhat more cautionary results have been reported by others working in non-American contexts. A study by Lee and Chan (2000) of 108 17- to 54-year-old Hong Kong Chinese individuals found strong correlations (.72) only in older individuals with higher education levels between Part B of the TMT and Part 2 of the CTT. The authors emphasize that the TMT and the CTT are tests of equivalent constructs only within specific age and education parameters. Lee et al. (2000) reported strong correlations between both parts of the CTT and TMT tasks (.72–.75) among English speakers but weak correlations (.25) between TMT A and Part 1 of the CCT among Chinese speakers, suggesting that language background may exert some mediating effect on performance. A study of 64 Turkish university students (mean age 22.67) reported that TMT A and CTT Part 1 are essentially equivalent tasks in this group; both measures rely almost exclusively on overlearned numerical sequencing abilities (Dugbarty et al., 2000). However, considerable differences between TMT B and CTT Part 2 in terms of time to completion and interference led the authors to conclude that the two tests are qualitatively different. They speculate that the fact that the CTT Part 2 has almost twice as many stimuli as the TMT B may introduce a higher emphasis on rapid visual scanning than on higher order cognitive flexibility.

In children, moderately high correlations (.69) have been found between the CCTT Part 1 and CCTT Part 2 (Williams et al., 1995). With regard to concurrent validity, moderately strong correlations (.67–.74) have been reported between the CCTT and the TMT in children aged 5 to 16 years, suggesting that they measure similar functional domains (Williams et al., 1975). However, they may not yield diagnostically similar results (Llorente et al., 2003).

There appear to be no effects on performance time when the CCTT and TMT are given sequentially in either order (Llorente et al., 2003).

Correlation to Other Neuropsychological Tests

The CCTT shows modest relations with a computerized measure of attention, the T.O.V.A. (.27–.55). Of note, the CCTT (and CCTT Part 2 in particular) shows a modest relationship with general intellectual skills, particularly the WISC-III Perceptual Organization Index (.41; Llorente et al., 2003).

Factor Structure

The internal structure of the CTT has been evaluated in the normative sample and in a sample of traumatic brain injury patients (D'Elia et al., 1996). The factor structures were somewhat divergent in the two samples, although both had four-factor solutions and factors that reflected speed of perceptual tracking and sequencing. Further, in both samples, the error, near-miss, and prompt variables appeared to tap constructs that are dissociable from those captured by the time variables. The authors suggested that these qualitative variables may capture different approaches to the speed-accuracy trade-off of CTT performance.

The internal structure of the CCTT in the normative sample suggests a three-factor solution (Llorente et al., 2003). The first factor, labeled speed of perceptual tracking and susceptibility to interference, is defined by high loadings of the two CCTT time variables and the interference index. Factor 2 is defined by high loadings of CCTT Part 2 prompts and sequence errors and is thought to reflect inattention and impulsivity. The third factor is defined by prompts and errors on CCTT Part 1 and is thought to reflect simple inattention. Similar factor structures emerge in children with mild head injury as well as in children who sustain physical trauma without injury to the head (Llorente et al., 2003).

Clinical Studies

Significant slowing on Parts 1 and 2 has been reported in patients with traumatic brain injuries (D'Elia et al., 1996) and HIV (Maj et al., 1993, 1994).

Llorente et al. (2003) provide some data suggesting that the CCTT can distinguish normal children from those with neurocognitive disorders (e.g., mild neurological disorders, unmedicated ADHD, learning disabled). Llorente et al. (2003) also report modest correlations (.39–.47) between CCTT time scores and select urine monoamines (dopamine, norepinephrine) in children diagnosed with ADHD.

COMMENT

The Color Trails is an interesting attempt to create a "culture-fair" version of the TMT by avoiding reliance on any alphabet and by aiming to be as free as possible from the influence of language. Task instructions can be given verbally as well as nonverbally. However, clients must be fairly fluent with Arabic numerals. While the test has been used in a variety of countries (e.g, Zaire, the United States, Germany, Kenya, Brazil,

Hong Kong), there are only a small number of studies on its culture fairness. Early work by Maj et al. (1993) demonstrated its sensitivity in discriminating between HIV seropositive and seronegative individuals of different cultures. Of note, while scores on TMT B were sensitive to different test sites, the CTT scores were not. The implication is that the CTT is more culturally fair than the TMT and may be preferred in cross-cultural assessment. Similar conclusions were reached by Lee et al. (2000). They found that Chinese-English bilingual and English monolingual individuals performed similarly on the CTT; however, Chinese participants performed more poorly on the TMT A than the English participants.

The normative samples are reasonably large. However, it is important to bear in mind that the adult normative sample is composed of samples of convenience (e.g., primarily males from various studies) and the child normative sample was drawn from a large urban center. These samples do not reflect the demographic characteristic of the general U.S. population.

Users should also note that the manual does not report whether ethnicity affects test scores, and there is some information that performance varies by ethnicity/geographical location (e.g., Caucasian, Hispanic, Cantonese). Thus, the use of norms imported from one foreign context to another is discouraged (Lee & Chan, 2000). To date, the CCTT appears not to have been used with children in nonwestern locations.

Test-reliability coefficients for time variables appear acceptable for the CTT but are less than optimal for the CCTT. Similar findings have been found for the TMT in children (see review in this volume). Given the lack of information regarding the CCTT error scores, caution is advised in their interpretation.

The CCT/CCTT is backed by some initial clinical studies but cannot be considered equivalent to the TMT, particularly with regard to the concordance of Part 2 to Part B of the TMT. Dugbarty et al. (2000) point out that the CTT Part 2 has almost twice as many stimuli as TMT B (49 versus 25 circles), which effectively makes it as much a measure of simple visual-perceptual scanning and susceptibility to visual distractors as a measure of higher order cognitive ability.

Perhaps equally important is the question of whether the CCT/CCTT is more sensitive to CNS disturbance than the TMT. It is also not known whether the test is better able than the TMT to discriminate among disorders.

REFERENCES

D'Elia, L. F., Satz, P., Uchiyama, C. L., & White, T. (1996). *Color Trails Test.* Odessa, FL: PAR.

Dugbarty, A. T., Townes, B. D. & Mahurin, R. K. (2000) Equivalence of the Color Trail Making Test in nonnative English-speakers. *Archives of Clinical Neuropsychology, 15,* 425–431.

Lee, T. M. (2003). *Normative data: Neuropsychological measures for Hong Kong Chinese.* Neuropsychology Laboratory, The University of Hong Kong, Hong Kong.

Lee, T. M., & Chan, C. C. H. (2000). Are Trail Making and Color Trails tests of equivalent constructs? *Journal of Clinical and Experimental Neuropsychology, 22,* 529–534.

Lee, T. M., Cheung, C. C. Y., Chan, J. K. P., & Chan, C. C. H. (2000). Trail Making across languages. *Journal of Clinical and Experimental Neuropsychology, 22,* 772–778.

Llorente, A. M., Williams, J., Satz, P., & D'Elia, L. F. (2003). *Children's Color Trails Test (CCTT).* Odessa, FL: PAR.

Maj, M., D'Elia, L. F., Satz, P., Janssen, R., Zaudig, M., Uchiyama, C., Galderisi, F., & Chervinsky, A. (1993). Evaluation of two new neuropsychological tests designed to minimize cultural bias in the assessment of HIV-1 seropositive persons: A WHO study. *Archives of Clinical Neuropsychology, 8,* 123–135.

Maj, M., Satz, P., Janssen, R., Zaudig, M., Starace, F., D'Elia, L., Sughondhabirom, B., Mussa, M., Naber, D., Ndetei, D., Schulte, G., & Sartorius, N. (1994). WHO neuropsychiatric AIDS study, cross-sectional phase II: Neuropsychological and neurological findings. *Archives of General Psychiatry, 51,* 51–61.

Mitrushina, M. N., Boone, K. B., Razani, J., & D'Elia, E. F. (2005). *Handbook of normative data for neuropsychological assessment* (2nd ed.). New York: Oxford University Press.

Ponton, M. O., Gonzales, J. J., Hernandez, I., Herrera, L., & Higareda, I. (2000). Factor analysis of the neuropsychological screening battery for Hispanics (NeSBHIS). *Applied Neuropsychology, 7,* 32–39.

Uchiyama, C. L., Mitrushina, M. N., D'Elia, L. F., Satz, P., & Mathews, A. (1994). Frontal lobe functioning in geriatric and nongeriatric samples: An argument for multimodal analyses. *Archives of Clinical Neuropsychology, 9,* 215–227.

Williams, J., Rickert, V., Hogan, J., Zolten, A. J., Satz, P., D'Elia, L. F., Asarnow, R. F., Zaucha, K., & Light, R. (1995). Children's Color Trails. *Archives of Clinical Neuropsychology, 10,* 211–223.

Comprehensive Trail Making Test (CTMT)

PURPOSE

The Comprehensive Trail Making Test (CTMT) is purported to measure attention, visual scanning, and executive functioning.

SOURCE

The CTMT (Examiner's Manual, test forms) can be obtained from PRO-ED (www.proedinc.com) at a cost of $90 US.

AGE RANGE

Norms for the CTMT range from ages 11 to 74 years, 11 months. Norms for ages 8 to 10 years are in press (C.R. Reynolds, personal communication, February 2005).

DESCRIPTION

The CTMT (Reynolds, 2002) was developed to address some of the shortcomings of the original Trail Making Test (see review in this volume). These include the need for improved norms and reliability, and increased sensitivity to detection of separate cognitive components underlying performance (Reynolds, 2002) while preserving the test's unique features such as ease of use, short administration time, and high sensitivity to brain dysfunction. In particular, the CTMT was intended to enhance sensitivity to executive dysfunction compared with the standard TMT paradigm with the inclusion of additional trials necessitating set shifting and inhibition and the addition of distractor stimuli within items. According to Reynolds (2002), the original TMT's norms are limited, and none reflects stratified random sampling based on U.S. Census information; many normative datasets also use different administration procedures (Mitrushina et al., 2005; Soukup et al., 1998; see also *TMT* review, in this volume). Further, the updated Heaton norms (i.e., Heaton et al., 2004), until now the largest norms available on the TMT, are based on samples of convenience collected as part of several studies and consist of older data collected over a period of over 25 years.

The CMT consists of five trials. The basic task is similar to the TMT. The examinee must connect a series of stimuli in order, as quickly as possible, using a pencil. The test includes additional distractor stimuli on some trials (empty circles, or circles with irrelevant line drawings) to increase the demands on inhibitory control, as well as set-shifting between stimulus format (numbers in Arabic numerals or spelled out) and between stimulus type (numbers and letters). Trial 1 is similar to the standard TMT A and Trial 5 is similar to TMT B, except that distractors (empty circles) are also included. See Table 9–8 for a detailed description of the five CTMT trials. Figure 9–1 shows sample items.

Table 9–8 Description of CTMT Trials

	Description
Trial 1	The examinee must draw a line connecting circles, within which are the numbers 1–25; similar to TMT A.
Trial 2	Same task as Trial 1, but with the addition of distractors (i.e., 29 empty circles).
Trial 3	Same task as Trial 1, but with the addition of two types of distractors (i.e., 13 empty circles and 19 circles with irrelevant drawings inside).
Trial 4	The examinee must draw a line connecting circles within which are the numbers 1–20; however, the examinee must randomly switch between numbers presented as Arabic numerals (i.e., 1, 7) and numbers that are spelled out (i.e., "nine").
Trial 5	The examinee must connect two sets of stimuli in alternating sequence: the numbers 1–13 and the letters A–L. The task is similar to TMT B; however, 50 distractors (i.e., empty circles) are also included on the page.

Note: TMT = Trail Making Test (reviewed elsewhere in this volume).

Source: Comprehensive Trail-Making Test. Reprinted with permission of PRO-ED, Inc., Austin, TX.

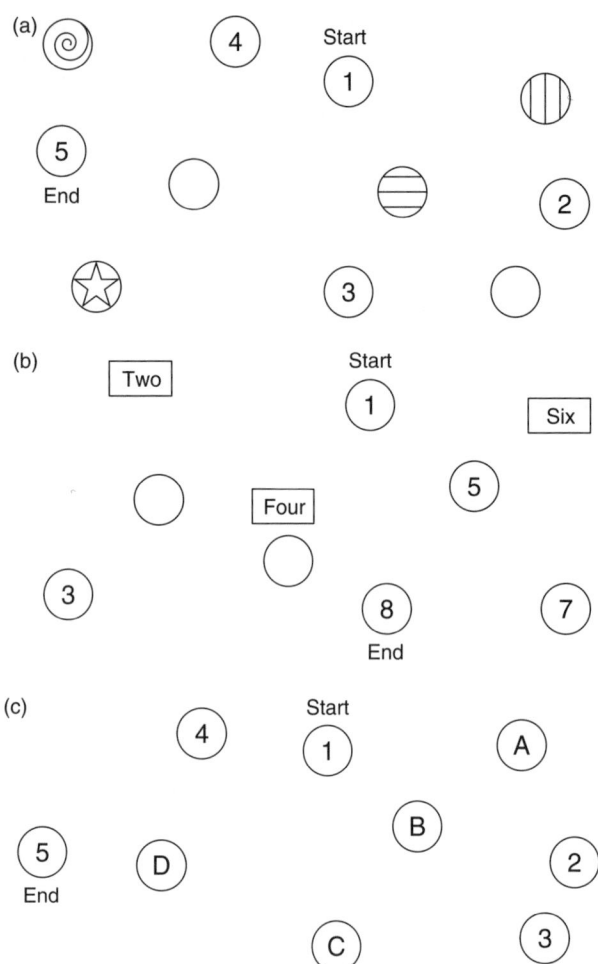

Figure 9–1 Sample CTMT Trials. (a) Trial 3, (b) Trial 4, (c) Trial 5.

In addition to format changes, the CTMT's array is more spatially complex than that of the TMT. Unlike the TMT, the CTMT stimulus pathway does not move progressively outward from the starting point but rather shifts direction as the examinee proceeds from stimulus to stimulus. Shifting between stimulus types also occurs on a random basis, unlike the TMT Part B, which requires alternate sequencing between stimulus sets. The test is therefore more demanding in terms of spatial scanning, sequencing, cognitive flexibility, and speed than the TMT (Moses, 2004).

ADMINISTRATION

See manual. Administration is simple and instructions are provided in the manual. A stopwatch, pencil, and Record Form are required. Each trial is preceded by a practice trial. Errors are corrected during administration, as is the case for the original TMT. Sample A precedes Trials 1 to 3, Sample B precedes Trial 4, and Sample C precedes Trial 5.

ADMINISTRATION TIME

The test takes 5 to 10 minutes to administer and score.

SCORING

Performance on the CTMT is based on the time taken to perform each trial. Raw scores are converted to normalized T scores ($M = 50$, $SD = 10$) and percentile ranks for each of the five trials. A CTMT Composite Index is then derived based on overall performance across trials. Scores can be prorated if less than five trials have been administered. Scores can be plotted on a profile on the Record Booklet.

Performance on a single CTMT trial can be evaluated against the average across-trial performance using tables in the manual. These indicate the magnitude of the difference required for statistical significance, which may yield important information regarding the component processes assessed by the test. Additionally, scores on the first three trials, which measure Simple Sequencing (see *Validity*) can be compared with scores on the last two trials, which measure Complex Sequencing. A methodology for evaluating the statistical significance of differences between these two domains is presented on p. 15 of the manual.

Although they can be recorded, errors do not yield standardized scores. This is due to the psychometric difficulties inherent in deriving standardized scores for behaviors that occur rarely in normals. However, the manual indicates that although further research is needed, the presence of two or more errors on any one trial may be strongly suggestive of abnormal performance and may indicate a frontal lobe deficit. However, this is not based on actual data involving the CTMT, and therefore should not be used as a basis for making clinical inferences.

Additional scores such as "quotients" (i.e., standard scores), z scores, stanines, and age equivalents can also be computed, though use of the latter is discouraged (see p. 23 of the manual for further discussion).

DEMOGRAPHIC EFFECTS

Age

CTMT scores are related to age, with faster performance from ages 11 to 29, a decrease in speed after age 30, and a more marked decrease after age 60, based on cross-sectional data from the standardization sample (Reynolds, 2002).

Gender

Gender does not affect scores on the CTMT; males and females score within two T-score points on the Composite Index, and within one point on the separate trials (Reynolds, 2002).

Ethnicity

The Composite score is also equivalent across ethnic groups (i.e., European, African, and Hispanic American). However, Hispanic Americans score five points lower on Trails 5 than European Americans (Reynolds, 2002).

Education

The effect of education on CTMT scores is not reported in the manual. However, correlations with education are reportedly minimal (C.R. Reynolds, personal communication, August 2004).

IQ

Correlations to standard IQ measures such as the Wechsler scales are unknown; however, correlations to the Draw-a-Person Intelligence Scoring (Reynolds & Hickman, 2002), a human figure drawing task, are small ($r = .16$, nonverbal IQ score; Reynolds, 2002).

NORMATIVE DATA

Standardization Sample

The CTMT standardization sample consists of 1664 individuals from 19 U.S. states, stratified by age (748 children and adolescents and 916 adults). Information on geographic region, age, gender, race, ethnicity, family income, parental education, and disability status closely parallel the composition of the U.S. population, based on U.S. Census information from 1998. Data were collected in 1999 and 2000. Cell sizes are considerable (range 79–106 for children; 104–205 for adults). As shown in Tables 9–9 and 9–10, the norms appear comprehensive and the sample characteristics are well described with regard to demographic factors such as ethnicity and education. Standard scores are derived based on age only.

RELIABILITY

Internal Consistency

Because it is a speeded test, conventional internal consistency measures such as alpha or split-half coefficients cannot be applied to the CTMT. Instead, the correlation between each trial and a composite of the other four trials were used as a reliability index reflecting sampling error, as described in detail in the manual (Reynolds, 2002). The Composite score, evaluated via a method outlined by Guildford (1954, as cited by Reynolds, 2002), attained very high reliability ($r = .92$). Reliabilities for the individual trials were also acceptable ($r = .70–.77$). Reliabilities for selected subgroups based on age, ethnicity, and clinical status (i.e., gifted, LD, and CVA) did not vary significantly from those obtained for the entire standardization sample.

Table 9-9 Characteristics of the CTMT Normative Sample: School-Age Sample

Sample type	National, stratified random sample
Number	748
Age	11 to 19 years, 11 months[a]
Geographic location	
Northeast	17%
Midwest	29%
South	35%
West	19%
Parental education	
Less than Bachelor's degree	81%
Bachelor's degree	12%
Master's, professional, or doctoral degree	7%
Gender	
Girls	374
Boys	374
Race	
White	79%
Black	15%
Other	6%
Ethnicity	
African American	15%
Hispanic American	10%
Asian American	2%
Native American	1%
Other	72%
Disability status	
No disability	92%
Learning disability	5%
Speech-language disorder	1%
Other disability	2%
Screening	None[b]

Note: Family income data are also provided on p. 18 of the manual (Reynolds, 2002). [a]Based on nine age groupings representing one-year intervals from age 11–19. [b]The percentage of individuals with disability is comparable to 1998 U.S. Census data presented in the manual.

Table 9-10 Characteristics of the CTMT Normative Sample: Adult Sample

Sample Type	National, stratified random sample
Number	916
Age	20 to 74 years, 11 months[a]
Geographic location	
Northeast	18%
Midwest	24%
South	35%
West	23%
Education	
Less than Bachelor's degree	76%
Bachelor's degree	16%
Master's, professional, or doctoral degree	8%
Gender	
Women	508
Men	408
Race	
White	85%
Black	11%
Other	4%
Ethnicity	
African American	12%
Hispanic American	8%
Asian American	2%
Native American	1%
Other	77%
Disability Status	
No disability	90%
Learning disability	6%
Speech-language disorder	2%
Other disability	2%
Screening	None[b]

Note: Family income data are also provided on p. 18 of the manual (Reynolds, 2002). [a]Based on eight age groupings: 20–29, 30–39, 40–49, 50–54, 55–59, 60–64, 65–69, and 70–74. [b]The proportion of individuals with disabilities is comparable to 1998 U.S. Census data presented in the manual.

Standard Error of Measurement (*SEM*)

*SEM*s are also acceptable for the Composite score (*SEM* = 3). *SEM*s for separate trials are larger (*SEM*s = 5–6, in T-score units), and expectedly yield a fairly large confidence interval (i.e., at the 95% confidence level, a T score of 50 with an *SEM* of 6 would yield a range between 38 and 62, or a percentile range of between the 12th and 88th percentile).

Test-Retest Reliability

Thirty adults were retested within a one-week period to provide test-retest stability estimates (age 20–57), as described in the manual. The Composite Index attained a high test-retest stability ($r = .84$), while results for the separate trials were in the acceptable range (i.e., $r = .70–.78$).

Practice Effects

Mean scores for the test-retest sample increased about three T-score points on the Composite Index, and between two and five points on the separate trials (i.e., a 0.3 *SD* improvement across scores; see manual).

Interrater Reliability

Interrater reliability is very high for the Composite score ($r = .99$) and for the separate trials ($r = .96–.98$; see manual for further details).

VALIDITY

Content Validity

The basic trail making paradigm upon which the CTMT is based is well validated (see *TMT*, in this volume). However, the additional features of the CTMT (i.e., addition of distractor stimuli and requirements for set-shifting) are new. Content review of the test by a panel of 10 expert neuropsychologists led to consensus that the test measures attention, executive control, visual search, sequencing, and inhibition (Reynolds, 2002).

Factor Structure

The manual indicates that the test comprises two main factors consisting of Simple Sequencing (Trials 1–3) and Complex Sequencing (Trials 4 and 5). The same two factors were found in additional analyses conducted across subgroups defined by gender and ethnicity (Reynolds, 2002).

Correlations With Other Neuropsychological Tests

Correlations between the CTMT and other attention tests, including the standard TMT, are not provided in the manual.

The CTMT appears to measure aspects of integration of visual-perceptual skill and speed, as shown by correlations with measures of visual perceptual and visual scanning/search from the Developmental Test of Visual Perception—Adolescents and Adults (Reynolds et al., 2002). Correlations with the RCFT copy trial are minimal ($r = <.10$), whereas moderate correlations are found between the CTMT and the RCFT recall trials ($N = 50$; Reynolds, 2002).

Clinical Studies

There are as yet no independent studies on the CTMT. However, the manual presents data on several clinical groups, including children characterized as gifted or learning disabled, and adults with CVA. These show the expected pattern of performance, with gifted children obtaining the highest scores and learning disabled and CVA patients the lowest (i.e., T-score $M = 55$, 42, and 33, respectively). At present, there are no data involving patients with primary difficulties with executive dysfunction or documented frontal lobe abnormalities. Sensitivity, specificity, and other diagnostic accuracy statistics for the test in different clinical populations are unknown.

COMMENT

The CTMT appears to be a test with good potential. Indeed, given that most normative datasets for the TMT do not meet contemporary professional standards (Reynolds, 2002), the CTMT is a worthwhile alternative due to its stratified normative sample and strong psychometric properties. In particular, the CTMT includes a well-written, comprehensive test manual that includes information not usually detailed for tests in common usage. This includes information on reliabilities by subgroup such as ethnicity and age (i.e., showing slightly increased reliability in some minority groups and in some clinical groups such as CVA), and factor structure by subgroups defined by variables such as gender and ethnicity. Discussions about reliability and validity are detailed, clear, and accessible to most readers. The normative sample is also of considerable size, is very well defined, and conforms to U.S. Census data. The test's ability to provide norm-based data on subcomponent processes should also allow a more precise delineation of performance compared with the standard TMT. The test does not seem to parcel motor speed from performance (e.g., as does the D-KEFS), but does allow interpretation of scores at several levels, including global performance, intersubtest differences, simple versus complex sequencing, and error analysis (Moses, 2004). Not all these levels of interpretation have been thoroughly validated. Further, given the relatively large *SEMs* for the separate trials, the more conservative approach to interpretation in a diagnostic clinical context would be to rely on the Composite Index.

Of concern, test-retest data are lacking for children, as is important information on the test's correlation to other attention tests and trail making tests (including the standard TMT) and to other executive measures (e.g., WCST). The latter is particularly important since one of the test's features versus other trail making tests is its proposed ability to better assess set-shifting and inhibition. In addition, the test yields two factors, but little is known about their relationship to other variables. Factor analyses including other tests and correlations with rating scales of attention and executive functioning (e.g., BRIEF; Conners' scales) are still needed, as are basic studies on the relationship between the CTMT and commonly used IQ tests such as the Wechsler scales. Research on the test's predictive validity is also needed.

REFERENCES

Heaton, R. K., Miller, S. W., Taylor, M. J., & Grant, I. (2004). *Revised comprehensive norms for an Expanded Halstead-Reitan Battery: Demographically adjusted neuropsychological norms for African American and Caucasian adults.* Lutz, FL: PAR.

Mitrushina, M. N., Boone, K. B., Razani, J., & D'Elia, E. F. (2005). *Handbook of normative data for neuropsychological assessment* (2nd ed.). New York: Oxford University Press.

Moses, J. A. (2004). Comprehensive Trail Making Test (CTMT). *Archives of Clinical Neuropsychology, 19,* 703–708.

Reynolds, C. R. (2002). *Comprehensive Trail-making Test.* Austin, TX: PRO-ED, Inc.

Reynolds, C. R., & Hickman, J. A. (2002). *Draw-A-Person intelligence scoring: The DAP:IQ.* Austin, TX: PRO-ED.

Reynolds, C. R., Pearson, N. A., & Voress, J. K. (2002). *Developmental Test of Visual Perception—Adolescent and Adult.* Austin, TX: PRO-ED.

Soukup, V. M., Ingram, F., Grady, J., & Schliess, M. (1998). Trail Making Test: Issues in normative data selection. *Applied Neuropsychology, 5,* 65–73.

Conners' Continuous Performance Test II (CPT-II)

PURPOSE

The Conners' Continuous Performance Test II (CPT-II) is a computerized test of sustained attention and response inhibition.

SOURCE

The CPT-II can be obtained from Harcourt Assessment—The Psychological Corporation. The program (which administers and scores the test) and manual cost about $495 US.

AGE RANGE

The CPT-II can be administered to individuals aged 6 to 55+ years.

DESCRIPTION

Overview

The term "continuous performance test" (CPT) is a general term that most often describes computerized paradigms that assess vigilance; actual testing parameters differ across CPTs. The CPT-II (Conners & MHS Staff, 2000) is the latest revision of the Conners' Continuous Performance Test, one of the most popular commercially available CPTs on the market (McGee et al., 2000). The CPT-II is one of the top 10 attention tests used by neuropsychologists and is the most frequently used CPT (Rabin et al., 2005).

The first CPT was developed by Rosvold et al. (1956). During sequential presentation of a series of letters, the examinee had to press a key when the letter "X" was presented, and inhibit responding to all other letters; a more difficult version required the subject to press a key only if the "X" was preceded by an "A." The test was a vigilance task because the subject had to maintain attention over long time intervals to detect infrequently occurring targets. Since publication of this early study, most CPTs have used the "X" or "A-then-X" task, or else have combined both paradigms within a single task. Traditional versions of the CPT use a fixed stimuli presentation rate, a fixed interval between targets, and a low target-to-distractor ratio (i.e., usually only 10% of stimuli are targets). Research on this paradigm has been relatively voluminous, in both the experimental and the clinical literature (for a review, see Riccio et al., 2001; 2002).

The CPT-II employs a different paradigm. First, the interval rate between stimulus presentations and the interstimulus event rate vary across trials. Second, the standard CPT paradigm was reversed so that the large majority of trials consist of targets instead of nontargets (i.e., it is a "not X" CPT). Thus, instead of responding relatively infrequently, as is the case in the classic CPT task, the examinee must press the space bar in response to all stimuli *except* the "X." The task therefore is fundamentally different than the standard CPT task because it requires the subject to maintain a continuous response set and then inhibit responding when a target is presented. According to the authors, increasing the target-to-nontarget ratio increases the number of possible correct responses, which then increases reliability. Further, the test becomes less susceptible to ceiling and floor effects. In the standard CPT paradigm, normal individuals with good sustained attention skills may attain almost perfect performance because there are so few targets to detect, and therefore few opportunities for omissions.

CPT-II Versus Previous Versions

The new CPT-II is similar to the old versions of the test (CPT Versions 3.0 and 3.1) in its basic paradigm. However, it has several improved features. The normative sample is larger and includes more adult cases; there is expansion of the clinical sample to include a Neurologically Impaired group; the signal detection measures have been revised; and the test is now designed to run on a Windows platform instead of DOS. A detailed explanation of specific changes to some of the variable calculations can be found in Appendix D of the test manual and are outlined in Table 9–11.

Diagnostic Utility

According to the authors, the CPT-II was designed primarily as a clinical instrument that can be used for screening, monitoring treatment effectiveness, and research. The authors clearly indicate that when used for clinical assessment, the

Table 9–11 Changes to the Conners' CPT-II Compared with Previous Versions of the Conners' CPT

New Features of the CPT-II

1. d' and *beta* are computed using a maximum likelihood approach that treats Reaction Time as an indicator of response confidence.
2. T scores for Hit Reaction Time and *beta* are no longer "inverted" (i.e., high T scores for Hit Reaction Time are associated with slow reaction times, and high T scores for *beta* are associated with a conservative response strategy that emphasizes avoidance of commission errors).
3. The ADHD Index and Neurological Index are used to assess the overall profile and to recommend a clinical or nonclinical classification.
4. Perseverations are included as a separate measure.
5. Perseverations are not included in the computation of Hit Reaction Time.
6. The very first trial is not included in CPT-II computations.

Note: A detailed explanation of the specific changes can be found in Appendix D of the test manual.

Source: Adapted from Conners & MHS Staff, 2000.

CPT-II should not be used as the only basis for diagnosis, but instead be used as part of a multimodal assessment that employs information from several sources.

ADMINISTRATION

See manual. The examinee is first administered a practice test (70 seconds), after which the test begins. Instructions are presented on the screen. According to the manual, the examiner "can quickly reiterate the instructions while the respondent reads them off the screen" (Conners & MHS Staff, 2000, p. 15). The examiner is expected to stay in the room during test administration, but to remain unobtrusive. Any questions from the examinee during testing should be answered with "I can answer that after you are finished. Please continue." An additional prompt is given if the subject appears distracted or leaves his or her seat. No further prompts are given.

The test is divided into six blocks to allow evaluation of changes over time. Each block is made up of three subblocks of 20 trials each. Letters are presented at varying speeds (1-, 2-, or 4-second intervals).

The manual states that when the CPT-II will be used to determine drug effectiveness, two baseline CPT-IIs should be administered prior to commencing treatment. A dual baseline procedure is usually employed when there is some degree of practice effect from baseline to retest, which is presumably less so on subsequent administrations (but see Lemay et al., 2004). However, no supporting evidence is given on the rationale underlying this recommendation.

ADMINISTRATION TIME

The test takes 14 minutes.

SCORING

Scores

CPT-II scores and descriptions are provided in Table 9–12. Additional information on the scores can be found in the manual.

Signal detection measures of d prime (d') and beta (β) are calculated using a newer method than in older studies, based on assumptions of non-normality and ROC curves (calculation via original signal detection equations as in prior versions is also an option; see pp. 19–20 of the manual for additional details).

T scores and percentiles can be obtained relative to three normative groups: (1) nonclinical cases, (2) an ADHD sample, and (3) a Neurologically Impaired clinical sample (excluding children and adolescents; see *Normative Data* for sample descriptions). A number of graphs and scoring options are available through the scoring program in addition to a narrative summary. Step-by-step interpretation guidelines are provided in the manual.

Confidence Indices and Performance Classification

The CPT-II provides two confidence index scores for classification purposes, depending on age, in addition to the Overall Index, a score from previous editions (see manual for details, and Table 9–12). On the score printout, these appear as "Confidence Index Associated With ADHD Assessment" and "Confidence Index Associated With Neurological Assessment." The definition of these indices is complex and not easily interpretable from information presented in the manual (some details can be found on pp. 67–70 and in Appendix A of the manual). These indices reflect results from discriminant function analyses that compare the examinee's score with nonclinical cases and with clinical cases (ADHD and/or Neurologically Impaired). As such, these scores provide an index of how deviant an individual's score pattern is from a nonclinical sample, and whether the obtained results match a clinical (ADHD or Neurologically Impaired) or nonclinical sample.

Figure 9–2 shows the variables that contribute to each Index score. In children aged 6 to 17, SE HRT is the main contributing variable in the "ADHD versus Nonclinical" discriminant function, based on the absolute value of the standard canonical coefficient, followed by Percent Commissions and Variability (other variables contribute to a lesser degree; see p. 138 of the manual for details). In adults, two functions are calculated: ADHD versus Nonclinical (where Percent Omissions, gender, and age are the largest contributors), and Neurologically Impaired versus Nonclinical (where SE HRT, d', and gender are the largest contributors).

Constructing Confidence Intervals for CPT-II Scores

In the manual, *SEM*s are presented in raw-score format, which makes it difficult to construct confidence intervals for T scores. We present *SEM*s in T-score format in Table 9–13, for use in constructing confidence intervals around CPT-II scores. Note that many of these are substantial, resulting in large confidence intervals around scores.

Score Interpretations

All of the CPT-II scores, with the exception of the Confidence Index and Overall Index, are presented in *converted* T-score and percentile form. This means that in most cases, higher T scores and percentiles indicate *worse* performance (i.e., the 90th percentile indicates the presence of significant attention problems). Note that possible exceptions are Hit Reaction Time and Beta, where a low score may also indicate problems, depending on performance on other scores.

A table is provided in the manual for interpreting T scores and percentiles, which range from "very good performance" to "markedly atypical." These guidelines are reproduced in Table 9–14. Note that norms for ages spanning 9 to 18 years

Table 9–12 Summary of CPT-II Scores

CPT-II Scores	Type of Deficit[a]	Description
Omissions	Inattention	Omissions are nontargets that the subject failed to respond to (i.e., failure to respond to all other letters except "X"). Although these may indicate severe difficulties, questions about the validity of the administration should be raised when T scores are above 100 (e.g., partially completed test, random responding, misunderstanding directions).
Commissions	Inattention or impulsivity	Commissions are targets ("X") that the subject erroneously responded to.
Hit RT	Inattention (slow); impulsivity (fast)	Reaction time to all non-"X" letters over all six time blocks, recorded to nearest millisecond and log transformed; high T scores indicate long response times.
Hit RT SE	Inattention	Log transformed; consistency of response times as measured by the standard error for responses to targets.
Variability	Inattention	Log transformed; measure of response time consistency calculated as the standard deviation of the standard error values for each sub-block.
Detectability (d')	Inattention	Provides information on how well the examinee discriminates between targets and nontargets (i.e., signal and noise).
Response Style (β)	Impulsivity	This score provides a measure of the examinee's response style (e.g., cautious versus risk-taking) expressed as a function of speed/accuracy trade-off (e.g., a tendency to respond very cautiously may ensure no commission errors are made, but at the cost of missing some targets). Higher Beta values indicate a more cautious response style.
Perseverations	Inattention	A response in which reaction time was less than 100 ms; these responses are assumed to be anticipatory, perseverative, random, or slow/inattentive (i.e., carried over from the previous response) because it is physiologically impossible to respond accurately in so short a time.
Hit RT Block Change	Inattention; vigilance	Slope generated by regression analyses using block as the independent variable and HRT and SE as the dependent variables (log transformed). Positive values indicate improved reaction time as the test progresses; high T scores indicate decreased vigilance over time.
Hit RT SE Block Change	Inattention; vigilance	Log transformed; positive values (i.e., a high T score) indicate less consistent reaction time as the test progresses; negative values indicate increasingly consistent reaction times as the test progresses.
Hit RT ISI Change	Inattention	Slope generated by regression analyses using ISI as the independent variable and HRT as the dependent variable (log transformed); assesses the ability to adapt to changing interstimulus intervals; positive values (high T scores) indicate that reaction times increased as the ISI increased; negative values indicate that reaction time decreased as the ISI increased.
Hit RT SE ISI Change	Inattention	Slope generated by regression analyses using ISI as the independent variable and HRT SE as the dependent variable (log transformed); positive values (i.e., a high T score) indicate less consistent reaction times during longer ISIs; negative values indicate increasingly consistent reaction times during longer ISIs.
Confidence Index	—	Provides an index of closeness of match to a clinical or nonclinical profile; provides the percentage of cases that would be correctly classified as clinical with a similar score (e.g., a confidence index of 90 indicates that 90 of 100 individuals with the profile would be clinical cases); the score is based on a discriminant function analysis; values between 40 and 60 are considered inconclusive.
Overall Index	—	An older method of calculating clinical significance based on logistic regression and weighting of CPT measures; details on this score can be obtained in Conners (1994).

Note: RT = reaction time; SE = standard error; ISI = interstimulus interval.
[a]Type of deficit suggested by each variable, according to the authors (Conners & MHS Staff, 2000).

Figure 9–2 Variable composition for discriminant functions for the CPT-II ADHD Index and Neurological Impairment Index. *Source:* Reprinted with permission from Conners & MHS Staff, 2000.

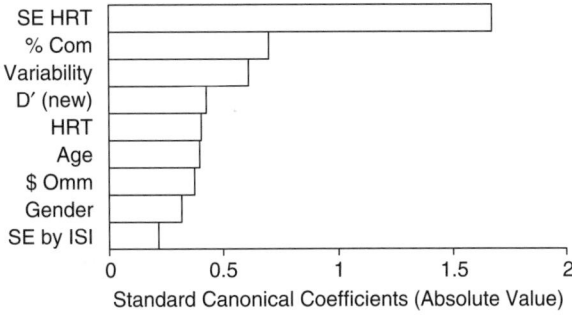

ADHD vs. Nonclinical, Ages 6–17: Contributions of Measures to Discriminant Function

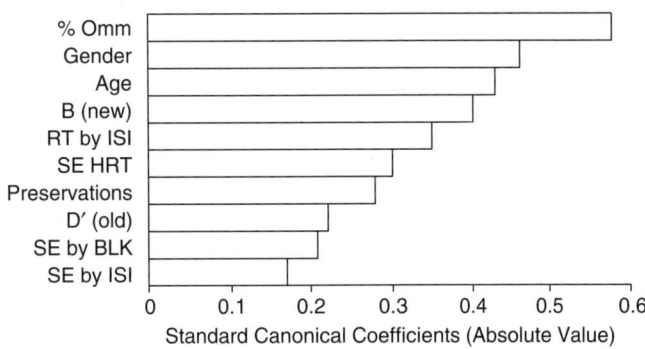

ADHD vs. Nonclinical, Ages 18+: Contributions of Measures to Discriminant Function

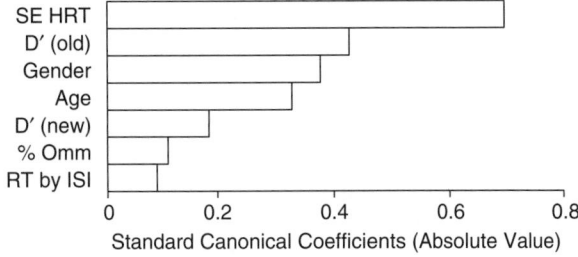

Neurological Impairment vs. Nonclinical: Contribution of Measures to Discriminant Function

are slightly elevated due to an oversampling of clinical cases. To compensate for this problem, lower cutoff criteria are suggested in the manual. Specifically, a T score of 60 or above should be interpreted as evidence of poor performance rather than the standard clinical cutoff of 70 (see manual, and *Comment*).

Scoring Features

The program can be set to different sensitivity cutoffs that will either minimize false positives or minimize false negatives in the scoring printout. Users can therefore customize these aspects of scoring, depending on the purpose of the evaluation. The default parameter is to "optimize overall hit rates," which assumes a 50% base rate of clinical cases.

According to the authors, this provides the best balance of false positives and negatives (for more information on this feature, see pp. 9 and 21 of the manual; also see discussion of sensitivity/specificity in *Validity* and *Comment*). Note that this baserate may not be the best match for all clinical settings. Unlike some scoring programs, the CPT-II has data-exporting features.

Repeat Assessment

The manual states that statistical information is provided on the significance of observed changes in the score printout (the Multiple Administrations report) in cases where the CPT-II has been administered twice (p. 17 of manual). This consists of a statement on whether the observed change meets the

Table 9–13 Standard Errors of Measurement for the CPT-II, in T-Score Units, for Purposes of Deriving Confidence Intervals for T Scores

Measure	SEM	90% CI (±)	95% CI (±)
Omissions	4.0	7	8
Comissions	5.9	10	12
Hit RT	6.7	11	13
Hit RT SE	5.9	10	12
Variability	6.3	10	12
d'	4.9	8	10
β	6.2	10	12
Perseverations	7.5	12	15
Hit RT Block Change	8.5	14	17
Hit SE Block Change	9.6	16	19
Hit RT ISI Change	7.0	12	14
Hit SE ISI Change	9.7	16	19

Note: Confidence index scores are not expressed as T scores, so they are not included in this listing.

Source: L. Spencer, personal communication, October 2001, Multi-Health Systems, Inc. (MHS, Inc.), North Tonawanda, NY. Reprinted wth permission.

Table 9–14 Guidelines for Interpreting CPT-II T Scores and Percentiles

T Score	Percentile	Guideline
65+	90+	Markedly atypical
60–64	85–89	Moderately atypical
55–59	70–84	Mildly atypical
45–54	31–69	Within the average range
40–44	15–30	Good performance
Under 40	Under 15	Very good performance

Note: Low T scores for Hit Reaction Time and *beta* can be associated with attention deficits. See manual for more details.

Source: Reprinted with permission from Conners & MHS Staff, 2000.

Jacobson-Truax criteria (see Chapter 1) for statistically significant change. Limited information is provided on how this is accomplished.

DEMOGRAPHIC EFFECTS

Age

Growth curves for the various CPT-II measures across the age range in the standardization sample show the expected developmental changes across age. Reaction time decreases from 6 to 17 years, stabilizes in adulthood, and then becomes progressively slower with advancing age (see Figure 9–3; note the truncation at age 55; it is likely that one would see a "U" shaped curve if there was an older age group included). A similar progression is observed for consistency of response times. Overall, errors of commission and omission are most frequent in children; omissions are minimal in adulthood. See also Conners et al. (2003) for a discussion of age effects.

Figure 9–3 Changes in CPT-II Performance across age. *Source:* Reprinted with permission from Conners & MHS Staff, 2000.

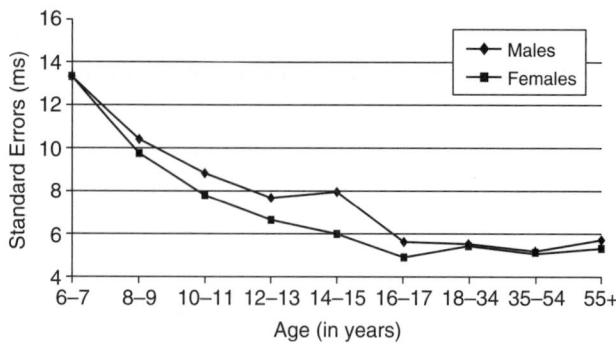

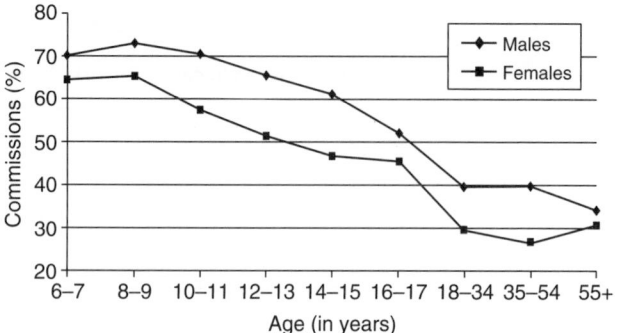

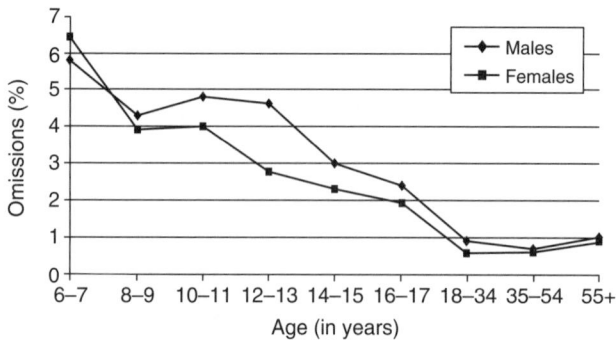

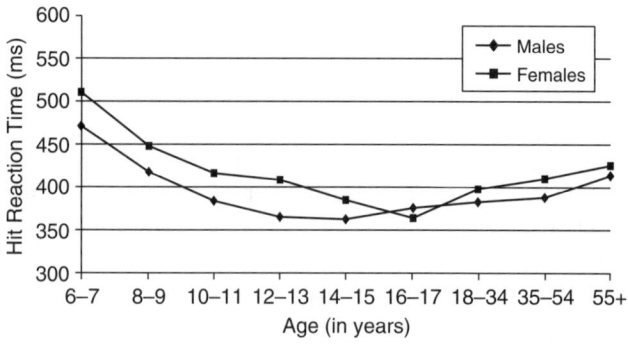

Gender

Males on average make more errors of commission than females at all ages (see *Comment* for discussion). There are also reaction time differences, with quicker reaction times in males (Conners et al., 2003). Gender effects have also been reported in clinical groups using the 1995 version (Robertson et al., 2003).

Ethnicity

CPT-II scores for African American and Asian American individuals taken from the multisite study comprising part of the standardization sample indicate few significant differences between minority groups, with most scores close to the standardization mean (i.e., T scores approaching 50). Actual means (but not standard deviations) are shown in the manual. Similarly, ethnicity was not a significant predictor of performance in the epidemiological study that forms one component of the standardization sample (Conners et al., 2003).

Education

To our knowledge, there is no information on the relationship between education and performance on the test in adults. However, educational effects are reportedly minimal on most CPTs, based on the limited research in this domain reviewed by Riccio et al. (2001).

IQ

Information on the relationship between IQ and CPT-II performance is not clear. The manual reports only one study from the standardization sample on an unspecified subgroup of 17 subjects. Correlations with IQ ranged from −.45 to .05, with a mean correlation of −.16. The manual does not indicate which correlations were associated with each CPT-II variable, and the sample size is insufficient to detect anything but large correlational effect sizes. An additional 19 subjects were administered a computerized IQ test (Computer Administered Aptitude Battery; Pepin & Loranger, 1996); similar results were obtained. Again, specific CPT-II variables were not identified, and the sample size was limited. General research on CPTs suggests that reaction time and reaction time variability are the variables most often inversely related to IQ (Riccio et al., 2001).

NORMATIVE DATA

Standardization Sample

Determining the exact composition of the CPT-II norms using information presented in the manual is not a straightforward task. The standardization sample is not a national, random, stratified sample. Rather, it consists of 1920 individuals (see Table 9–15 for overall sample characteristics), reflecting the combined data from two separate data collection efforts. The first component of the CPT-II norms was collected through a "multisite research study" involving both children and adults (see Table 9–16), and the second component was collected through an "epidemiological study," which included only children and adolescents (see Table 9–17). Information on education and SES are lacking.

Table 9–15 Characteristics of the CPT-II Normative Sample: Entire Combined Sample

Sample type	1108 cases through a multisite research study and 812 cases through an epidemiological study
Number	1920
Age	6 to 55+ years[a]
Geographic location	See below
Parental education	Unspecified
SES	Unspecified
Gender[b]	
Men	47%
Women	53%
Race/ethnicity	
White	47%
Black	27%
Asian	5%
Other	21%
Screening	Methods varied; see below

[a]Consisting of nine age groups (6–7, 8–9, 10–11, 12–13, 14–15, 16–17, 18–34, 35–54, 55+). [b]The gender distribution for ages 18+ is 71% female.

Source: Adapted from Conners & MHS Staff, 2000.

The two subsamples differ in major ways. First, CPT-II administration was conducted in the children's homes in the epidemiological study, whereas it was conducted in various sites outside the home in the multisite research study. Second, the

Table 9–16 Characteristics of the CPT-II Normative Sample, Part 1: Multisite Research Study Sample

Sample type	Multisite research study consisting of data collected in elementary, middle, and high schools, and from "organizations, science centers, and in controlled research settings"
Number	1108
Age	Unspecified
Geographic location	30 sites in the United States and Canada
Parental education	Unspecified
SES	Unspecified
Gender	Unspecified
Race/ethnicity	Unspecified
Screening	Not screened, except for nonsystematic exclusion of some cases; the manual reports that "some of the site coordinators, on relatively rare occasions, reported excluding some youths who had obvious attentional deficits or who had been diagnosed as such" (Conners & MHS Staff, 2000, p. 49).

Source: Adapted from Conners & MHS Staff, 2000.

Table 9–17 Characteristics of the CPT-II Normative Sample, Part 2: Epidemiological Study Sample[a]

Sample type	Epidemiological study
Number	816[b]
Age	9 to 17 years[c]
Geographic location	Rural area of North Carolina
Parental education	Unspecified
SES	Unspecified
Gender	
Boys	52%
Girls	48%
Race/ethnicity	
African American	58%
Caucasian	37%
Mixed/Other	5%
Screening	None; included oversampling of cases with psychopathology based on CBCL Externalizing, in a procedure described in Conners et al. (2003)

[a]Data collected in the child's home on laptop computer, as part of a larger study on psychopathology. [b]Excluding subjects with incomplete or missing CPT data (Conners et al., 2003). [c]As per Conners et al. (2003); the manual indicates an upper range of 18 years.

Source: Adapted from Conners et al., 2003, and Conners & MHS Staff, 2000.

epidemiological study involved a relatively specific, geographically limited sample of rural, largely African American children. Third, the epidemiological sample included an oversampling of cases with psychopathology. Thus, according to the manual, in the 9-to-18-year group ($N = 812$), 20% of the sample was selected because of high CBCL Externalizing scores because this was part of the recruitment criteria for the epidemiological study (see Conners et al., 2003, for specific procedures). According to the authors, this resulted in slightly

worse CPT-II performance in this subgroup compared with the remainder of the normative sample obtained through the multisite data collection initiative. As mentioned previously, the norms are therefore slightly elevated, and to compensate for this problem, lower cutoff criteria are suggested. Specifically, a T score of 60 or above should therefore be interpreted as evidence of poor performance rather than the standard clinical cutoff of 70.

Based on the combined sample (i.e., including both the multisite research study and the epidemiological study), normative data for children and adolescents is presented in two-year intervals (6–7, 8–9, 10–11, 12–13, 14–15, 16–17), and in three age bands for adults (18–34, 35–54, and 55+). Normative data are not equally distributed across ages. Although most age bands are well represented (i.e., approximately 150 to over 300 cases per age band), Ns are relatively smaller in the extreme age groups ($N = 88$ in the youngest age band, and $N = 54$ in the oldest age band). Although gender appears equally represented in the younger group (<18 years), there is an overrepresentation of women in the over-18 group (71%). Although the ethnic composition of the sample is described, there is no indication of its representativeness compared with the U.S. population. A cursory evaluation suggests an overrepresentation of minorities compared with recent U.S. Census data proportions. There is no information on whether the ethnic distribution is even across age bands in the combined sample.

Demographically Corrected Norms

Although Conners et al. (2003) did not find an effect of ethnicity on CPT-II performance, gender is a significant predictor of CPT-II performance, along with age. However, gender-based norms for the entire CPT-II standardization sample are not available. Gender-based norms for the epidemiological

Table 9–18 CPT-II Performance Based on Gender and Age for a Largely African American, Rural Sample of Children and Adolescents ($N = 816$)

Age Group		CPT-II Performance Measures											
		RT		RT(SE)		Errors of Comission (%)		Errors of Commission (%)		d'		β	
		Mean	SD	Mean	SD	Mean	SD	Mean	SD	Mean	SD	Mean	SD
9–11	Females	450.72	79.58	29.97	7.72	6.7	6.4	58.2	17.8	1.49	0.89	0.34	0.27
	Males	424.64	65.96	28.83	6.65	6.5	5.1	68.3	17.3	1.12	0.77	0.42	0.31
12–13	Females	416.64	66.26	26.49	5.12	3.5	3.1	52.3	20.6	1.91	0.87	0.23	0.22
	Males	384.21	55.86	24.85	5.79	5.4	4.7	66.3	16.9	1.27	0.76	0.34	0.25
14–15	Females	390.95	63.05	23.64	5.12	2.3	3.8	45.1	22.4	2.35	1.01	0.17	0.35
	Males	363.87	71.76	22.45	6.15	3.0	5.0	59.9	22.1	1.84	1.09	0.22	0.27
16–18	Females	378.44	56.08	22.54	4.14	2.1	3.4	40.5	22.2	2.54	0.95	0.12	0.13
	Males	365.59	57.28	22.50	4.29	2.9	3.0	53.6	18.9	2.00	0.85	0.18	0.17

Note: Sample includes an overrepresentation of cases with psychopathology.

Source: Reprinted with permission from Conners et al., 2003.

Table 9–19 Magnitude of Internal Test-Retest Reliability Coefficients for the CPT-II

Magnitude of Coefficient	Internal Reliability	Test-Retest Stability
Very high (.90+)	Hit RT Omissions	Confidence Index (Neuro)
High (.80–.89)	Commissions HT SE[a] *d* Prime	Omissions Confidence Index (ADHD)
Adequate (.70–.79)	Beta	*d* Prime
Marginal (.60–.69)	Variability	Commissions Hit RT SE Variability Beta
Low (< .59)		Hit RT Perseverations Hit RT Block Change (.28) Hit SE Block Change (.08) Hit RT ISI Change (.51) Hit SE ISI Change (.05)

Note: RT = reaction time; Neuro = neurologically impaired sample; SE = standard error; ISI = interstimulus interval.
[a]Not specified in manual, but presumably refers to Hit RT SE. Selected coefficients shown in parentheses.

Source: Adapted from Conners & MHS Staff, 2000.

sample are presented in Table 9–18. Note that the majority of the sample was African American.

Clinical Samples Used to Derive ADHD Index and Neurological Impairment Index

The clinical sample consists of two groups: an ADHD group ($N = 378$) and a Neurologically Impaired group (223 adults with various neurological impairments). According to the manual, no single set of diagnostic procedures was used to diagnose ADHD; these varied across the 30 sites involved in providing cases, although all reportedly followed DSM-IV criteria. The most common diagnosis in the Neurologically Impaired group was postconcussion disorder (29%); 21% had "organic brain syndrome," and the remainder had various neurological and medical diagnoses. The manual does not indicate whether cases were screened for motivational defects such as malingering. Half the sample was collected at a single site (Mid-Michigan Neuropsychology Services).

The ADHD sample appears fairly evenly distributed across age bands (18–72 cases per age band), and has a larger representation of males less than 18 years, as would be expected for this disorder. Gender composition is relatively well balanced in the adults with ADHD (>18 years). This is also the case for all ages of the adult Neurologically Impaired sample.

Score Transformations

Generally, raw scores from CPTs form negatively skewed distributions because of the high-level performance in most normals. CPT-II scores were corrected for skew prior to T-score transformation (see manual for more details).

RELIABILITY

Internal Consistency

Split-half reliability information is presented for seven variables based on 520 cases from the original 1994 standardization sample of the test (Version 3.0; Conners, 1994; see Table 9–19). Reliabilities are very high for Hit Reaction Time and Omissions ($r = .95$ and $.94$, respectively), high for Commissions, Standard Error, and *d* prime ($r = .83, 87$, and $.83$, respectively), and in the acceptable range for beta ($r = .73$). Internal reliability for the Variability measure is marginal ($r = .66$).

Standard Error of Measurement (*SEM*)

*SEM*s are reported for raw scores, based on the test-retest reliability estimate (see manual). These are divided by age bands that extend from 6 to 7 years to 55+ (note that the test-retest reliability sample had a mean age of 28 years). These *SEM* values are of limited clinical utility because they are presented in raw-score units; most clinicians will use T scores in determining confidence intervals for T scores. As noted previously (*Scoring*), *SEM*s in T-score units are presented in Table 9–13.

Test-Retest Reliability

Data from a small group of cases consisting of 10 non-clinical cases and 13 cases with various clinical diagnoses, with a mean age of 28 years, were used to assess test-retest stability over an average of three months (see manual). Two cases were excluded because they produced highly inconsistent data between administrations, which yielded a sample size of 21. Based on these data, only four CPT-II variables have stability coefficients that are adequate or better, with four variables demonstrating reliabilities sufficiently high to warrant clinical use in a diagnostic context. These include Omissions, *d* Prime, and Confidence Indexes for the Neurological Impaired and ADHD samples. The remainder of the many CPT-II scores had marginal or extremely low stability coefficients. Notably, some variables yielded reliability coefficients that were practically at chance (e.g., Hit SE Block Change, Hit SE ISI Change). Test-retest coefficients are shown in Table 9–19.

Practice Effects

Practice effects are not detailed in the manual. This is unfortunate, given the test's potential for use in situations where knowledge of practice effects is needed (i.e., pre-/post-treatment trials).

VALIDITY

Correlations With Attention Tests and Other Cognitive Abilities

The manual does not present correlations between the CPT-II and tests of attention (correlations to IQ are outlined in *Demographic Effects*). However, a small number of studies generally support the convergent validity of the CPT-II. Epstein et al. (2001) gave the 1992 version of the test (Conners, 1992) to adults with ADHD, adults with anxiety, and controls, along with two other measures of response inhibition (i.e., the Posner Visual Orienting Task and a variant of the Stop-Signal Task, a paradigm that measures the minimum amount of time required between the onset of the inhibitory response and the stopping of a response). CPT commissions were moderately to highly correlated with the other two measures of response inhibition ($r = .62$ and $.43$, respectively). In another study involving ADHD and reading disorders, a moderate correlation was obtained between the CPT Overall Index and total errors on an auditory CPT ($r = .39$; Keith, 1994). Concurrence rate between the two measures was 65%. Using a previous version of the test, Kerns et al. (2001) found that Beta was a strong predictor of the ability to estimate time in a mixed sample of children with ADHD and controls.

Barkley et al. (2001) conducted a factor analysis of the Conners' CPT and tests of executive functioning in a study involving 101 adolescents with ADHD/ODD and normal controls. CPT variables emerged on two separate factors: CPT Inattention (Omissions, Hit Rate SE, Variability of Hit Rate SE) and CPT Inhibition (Commissions, Hit Rate); a third factor was comprised of backward digit span and a variety of verbal/nonverbal fluency tasks.

Motor demands of the Conners' CPT exceed those of standard CPTs (McGee et al., 2000) because of the requirement for a continuous response set. However, Conners' CPT

performance appears unrelated to measures of visual processing speed or motor dexterity (McGee et al., 2000).

Because the Conners' CPT uses letter stimuli, McGee et al. (2000) investigated whether performance was related to phonological awareness, a core difficulty of children with reading disorders. They found a significant association between performance and phonological awareness, which they interpreted as a fundamental weakness in the test.

Correlations With ADHD Rating Scales

Research with the classic CPT paradigm indicates only moderate correlations with rating scales measuring similar constructs (e.g., Riccio et al., 2001). This is also the case with the CPT-II. Research reviewed in the manual based on the 1994 version indicates moderate correlations in some cases (e.g., Conners, 1997) and only limited correlations in others (e.g., Epstein et al., 1998). For example, in a study involving children with ADHD, children with reading disorders and clinical controls, omissions were related to hyperactivity ratings and externalizing behaviors, but the size of the correlations was modest ($r = .21–.26$), and the CPT Overall Index was unrelated to internalizing/externalizing behavior problems (McGee et al., 2000). In adults with ADHD and normal controls, no significant correlations were found between the Conners' CPT and self-reported ADHD symptoms on a DSM-IV diagnostic interview, although a small correlation between d' and inattention approached significance ($r = .23$; Epstein et al., 1998).

Diagnostic Utility of the CPT-II

Clinical utility of the CPT-II involves two issues: (1) whether the test discriminates between individuals with ADHD (or other clinical group) and normal controls, and (2) whether the test differentiates *between* clinical groups. Further, does the test provide strong evidence of clinical utility as shown by sensitivity/specificity data, or is clinical utility based on group studies alone? First, as is the case for other CPTs, group differences between individuals with ADHD and controls on the CPT-II are generally robust, but group differences between individuals with ADHD and other clinical disorders are not as reliable. Second, evidence regarding the CPT-II's sensitivity, specificity, and other indices of classification accuracy is less compelling.

Group Differences—ADHD

ADHD Versus Controls. Research supports the fact that individuals with ADHD, as a group, tend to perform worse on Conners' CPT measures than normal controls. In the CPT-II standardization sample, children and adolescents with ADHD performed worse on all the CPT-II variables except for commissions, when compared with the nonclinical group (Conners & MHS Staff, 2000). Barkley et al. (2001) found that adolescents with ADHD had higher scores on a Conners' CPT inattention factor than normal controls but did not differ on inhibition measures. With regard to the latter, the authors noted that the lack of differences between groups may have been due to a progressive normalization of inhibitory deficits in ADHD with age, or to a lack of sensitivity of the Conners' CPT to inhibitory problems in this age group. Prior research with other CPT paradigms have reported increased commission errors in adolescents with ADHD (e.g., Barkley et al., 1991), which raises the possibility that the Conners' CPT paradigm may be less sensitive than other versions to inhibitory deficits in adolescents with ADHD.

In the CPT-II standardization sample, adults with ADHD performed worse than the nonclinical group on all the CPT-II variables. Similar results have been obtained by other researchers studying adult ADHD (e.g., Epstein et al., 1998). Interestingly, expected performance decrements, based on prior research with the standard CPT paradigm, were not obtained in a group of adults with ADHD, which the authors interpreted as evidence that adults with ADHD do not have a sustained attention deficit (Epstein et al., 1998). In addition, adults with ADHD made the most errors during the short ISI, not the longest. It is not clear whether these reflect ADHD characteristics or task differences compared with traditional CPTs.

ADHD Versus Other Clinical Groups. With regard to differentiating between individuals with ADHD and other clinical groups, evidence is conflicting. The manual discusses a small number of studies on the clinical utility of the CPT-II, including a study involving the original standardization sample (Conners, 1994), which, according to the authors, showed significant differences between cases with ADHD and those with other clinical diagnoses on most of the CPT variables. In another study (McGee et al., 2000), the Conners' CPT did not discriminate ADHD children from those with reading disability (RD) or mixed clinical controls, with RD children performing worse on the Overall Index than those with ADHD. Specifically, children with ADHD and comorbid reading disorder had higher (i.e., more impaired) scores on the CPT, followed by children with reading disorder alone, ADHD alone, and lastly, clinical controls (McGee et al., 2000).

In adults from the CPT-II standardization data, the two clinical groups performed differently: compared with the ADHD group, the heterogeneous Neurologically Impaired group performed worse on omissions, reaction time, reaction time variability, and ISI variability (Conners & MHS Staff, 2000). Using an early edition of the test (i.e., Conners, 1992), Epstein et al. (2001) found a higher rate of commission errors in adults with ADHD compared with adults with anxiety disorders, which they interpreted as evidence for the deficit-specificity of the Conners' CPT. Other studies have not found differences between ADHD groups and other clinical groups such as patients with mild psychiatric disorder (e.g., Walker et al., 2000).

Sensitivity and Specificity in ADHD

Although the validity of the Conners' CPT appears to be supported by studies comparing group means of individuals with ADHD with those of controls, clinicians need information on the utility of the various scores in screening for ADHD, including data on sensitivity and specificity. Studies examining this question have found limited support for the utility of the CPT as a strong diagnostic screening device for ADHD. In one study, only slightly more than half of the ADHD children "failed" the CPT (according to the Overall Index cutoff); children who failed the CPT tended to have higher hyperactivity ratings (McGee et al., 2000). However, Perugini et al. (2000) reported adequate sensitivity, specificity, positive predictive power, and negative predictive power for the CPT (i.e., .75, .73, .67, and .80, respectively), with an overall predictive power of .80 in terms of the Overall Index's (1995 version) ability to differentiate children with ADHD from controls.

A small number of studies have examined the sensitivity and specificity of the Conners' CPT in detecting adult ADHD. The predictive power of the test was found to be poor in discriminating between ADHD and adults with mild psychiatric disorder (Walker et al., 2000). However, predictive power was increased when the Conners' CPT was combined with other neuropsychological tests (i.e., Stroop, Digit Symbol), and was even higher when these were combined with standardized questionnaires such as ADHD rating scales (i.e., sensitivity of 81% for ADHD, specificity of 85%). In contrast, the predictive power of the Conners' CPT when used alone (using two or more omission errors as a cutoff) was relatively inadequate in differentiating ADHD from psychiatric disorder (positive predictive power = 61%, negative predictive power = 67%). In another study, Epstein et al. (1998) concluded that the Conners' CPT had moderate clinical utility in differentiating ADHD adults from normal controls. Using discriminant function analysis, 33 of 60 adults were correctly classified as having ADHD; 55 of 72 normals were also correctly classified (sensitivity = 55%; specificity = 76%; positive predictive power = 66%; negative predictive power = 67%; kappa = .32).

Epstein et al.'s (1998) study with adults indicates that almost half of ADHD adults perform in the normal range, along with most normals (76%). They interpret these data as evidence of moderate clinical utility for the CPT. This translates into a positive predictive power of 66% for ADHD and a negative predictive power of 67%, which means that false negatives and false positives would both be approximately 30% (i.e., one in three erroneously classified). In most clinical contexts, this would be considered unacceptably high. The authors suggest caution in using the test for diagnosis in adult ADHD.

Group Differences

Clinical Groups Versus Controls. Research also supports group differences between various clinical groups and normal controls on the Conners' CPT. In one study, children with dyscalculia had higher Index scores, omission errors, and more inconsistent response times compared with controls (Lindsay et al., 2001). In a small group of adults with temporal lobe epilepsy evaluated for epilepsy surgery, Fleck et al.

(2002) found that patients had disproportionate increases in RT toward the end of the test compared with controls, despite normal accuracy scores on the Conners' CPT. In the adult CPT-II standardization data, the Neurologically Impaired group performed worse than the nonclinical group on all the CPT-II variables.

Sensitivity to Medications Effects

CPTs have traditionally shown sensitivity to drug effects in the treatment of ADHD (Riccio et al., 2001). Apart from limited data outlined in the manual involving previous versions of the test, there are as yet no studies on the CPT-II regarding sensitivity to medication effects in children with ADHD, although there is evidence that the 1995 version is sensitive to Ritalin-related improvement in attention in childhood cancer survivors (Thompson et al., 2001). The Conners' CPT also appears to be sensitive to improved performance associated with nicotine in neurologically impaired adults (White & Levin, 1999), normal adults (Levin et al., 1998), and adults with schizophrenia (Levin et al., 1996).

Other Clinical Groups

Using the Revised Children's Manifest Anxiety Scale, Epstein et al. (1997) found that physiological anxiety was associated with increased response inhibition (Beta) on the Conners' CPT, with the reverse effect for cognitive anxiety. Using the 1995 version, Robertson et al. (2003) found no deficits in CPT performance in adolescents with bipolar disorder or unipolar depression. Children with idiopathic epilepsy have also been studied using the 1995 version, where deficits were relatively common and tended to increase in frequency over time (Borgatti et al., 2004). There is also evidence that children with epilepsy may perform more poorly on an auditory CPT than on a visual CPT consisting of a modified version of the 1995 test (Taylor-Cooke et al., 2004), suggesting that neurologically compromised children may have more difficulty attending to information when presented in the auditory modality. The 1995 version has also been used to track attentional skills over time in children exposed in utero to cocaine (Bandstra et al., 2001) and to track the acute effects of radiotherapy in childhood cancer, where the test shows relative stability during treatment but decreased reaction time for younger children and slight increase in the Overall Index during treatment (Merchant et al., 2002).

COMMENT

In general, CPTs offer a quick, standardized method of assessing attention/executive functioning and are useful for treatment monitoring. As one of the few commercially available CPTs, the CPT-II has several strengths. It has relatively large norms, including expanded adult normative data and two new clinical samples (ADHD and Neurologically Impaired), though concerns remain concerning their exact composition.

The CPT-II may also be a better measure of impulsivity than other standard CPTs due to its different task requirements (Epstein et al., 1998). Some of its features, such as the inclusion of both long and short ISIs, may help elicit performance deficits in some diagnostic groups. Socioeconomic status effects appear minimal (McGee et al., 2000), though more research in this area is needed. From the standpoint of validity and clinical utility, it appears to differentiate between clinical and nonclinical cases at a group level and may show group differences between ADHD and neurological conditions in adults. The program itself is easy to use and has data-exporting features, which is an asset for researchers. However, users should be aware of certain limitations.

CPT-II Paradigm: Attention or Executive Functioning?

CPTs are one of the most popular and well-researched paradigms for measuring attention (Riccio et al., 2002). Consequently, there is a large amount of research and clinical data supporting the use of the traditional CPT in assessing attentional disturbances (e.g., Riccio et al., 2001; 2002). However, the CPT-II differs considerably from the classic CPT paradigm on which the majority of this research is based. Ballard (2001) discusses this problem in detail. Contrary to the original Rosvold et al. (1956) vigilance paradigm where targets were designed to be low-frequency events compared with nontargets, the CPT-II employs a high target-to-nontarget ratio (i.e., 90% of stimuli must be responded to). While the stimuli and task duration are similar, the CPT-II requires that the examinee *withhold* an ongoing response when a target is presented. Omissions may therefore occur when the examinee fails to maintain an ongoing response; it is not clear that this type of error is equally reflective of a deficit of vigilance, as is generally accepted for omissions on the traditional CPT paradigm. Further, commission errors on the CPT-II occur when the examinee continues to press the key (a habitual response, given the high target ratio) when a signal to stop appears ("X"). This type of error may reflect the inability to inhibit a habitual response (i.e., a perseverative deficit) rather than a primary problem with impulsivity, as commission errors on traditional CPTs are defined. Likewise, Conners et al. (2003) note that commission errors might reflect two separate and somewhat opposite problems: impulsivity or delayed responding from the previous trial (i.e., "sluggish responding"). Target rate may therefore affect the type of commission errors that are recorded (i.e., impulsive versus sluggish). Differentiating these two commission errors is not possible with the CPT-II.

From this evidence, it appears that the CPT-II may be a better measure of executive functioning (i.e., inhibitory control) than vigilance or attention per se and may therefore be associated with different brain systems than traditional CPTs (Ballard, 2001). Fortuitously, because inhibitory dyscontrol has replaced inattention as the core deficit in theories on ADHD (e.g., Barkley, 1997), this may make it especially useful in the assessment of ADHD—and possibly more useful than the traditional CPT paradigms intended to measure primarily vigilance, though research on the sensitivity and specificity of the CPT-II in ADHD is somewhat conflicting. Users should be aware of the specific task requirements in the CPT-II when evaluating populations where attention (i.e., vigilance), and not inhibitory control, may be selectively impaired.

Ballard's (2001) conceptualization of CPT-II commission errors as reflecting an inability to inhibit a habitual response suggests that the score may have potential as a measure of perseverative tendencies. Although this may be an interesting research question, the low reliability of the commissions variable limits its utility in the clinical context. Users should also note that the CPT-II "perseverations" variable has extremely low reliability/stability and may reflect a variety of error types as noted in the manual (e.g., anticipatory, perseverative, inattentive, random, etc.). Clinical use of this variable is not recommended.

Other aspects make the CPT-II fundamentally different from traditional CPT tasks. According to Ballard (2001), inherent characteristics of the CPT-II (i.e., slow event rate, high response rate, high probability of targets, and predictability of ISI changes within blocks) are associated, in CPT research, with fewer errors, faster reaction times, and less decrement in performance over time. Further, compared with traditional CPTs, the CPT-II does not show the expected changes in performance that are known to be associated with traditional CPTs as a result of environmental noise and anxiety. In addition, its decrement function (i.e., performance changes across blocks) differs significantly from that of traditional CPTs (Ballard, 2001; Epstein et al., 1998). Clinicians using the test should therefore be aware that results from the CPT-II may not be equivalent to those from traditional CPTs (Ballard, 2001), nor should scores from variants of the traditional paradigm be considered "alternate forms" of the same test (Borgaro et al., 2003).

Clinical Utility in Diagnosis

Research on traditional versions of the CPT has consistently indicated that CPT performance is symptom-specific but not disorder-specific (e.g., Corkum & Seigel, 1993; Riccio et al., 2001, 2002). Thus, despite high sensitivity to attentional dysfunction when clinical populations are contrasted to normals, CPTs yield impaired performances in many neurological, medical, and psychiatric disorders (e.g., Riccio & Reynolds, 2001; Riccio et al., 2001). Indeed, the American Academy of Pediatrics discourages the use of CPTs for ADHD diagnosis because of low sensitivity and specificity in this disorder (American Academy of Pediatrics, 2000). Other researchers agree: For example, McGee et al. (2000) state that reading-disordered children could be identified as ADHD "false positives" on the Conners' CPT, and conclude that the utility of the test in differential diagnosis of ADHD is questionable. This is also echoed by Epstein et al. (1998) in adults with ADHD. Riccio and Reynolds (2001) conclude that CPTs may

be useful tools in ruling out ADHD, though they should not be used as conclusive evidence.

Both CPT-II Confidence Indices (ADHD and Neurological) show good reliability, likely because several CPT-II scores contribute to these scores. In this way, they are somewhat akin to the composite scores found in other measures, since composite reliabilities almost invariably surpass those of individual subtests. However, CPT-II results should not be used as the primary evidence for diagnosing ADHD, and in this regard, the Confidence Index (ADHD) may be prone to misinterpretation. Lastly, CPT-II scores have relatively large *SEM*s, which should be taken into account when making diagnostic formulations involving CPT-II scores.

Normative Data

Compared with other large, published, standardized tests, the CPT-II norms are below standard (though not, as noted by Riccio et al., 2001, necessarily below that of other commercially available CPTs). These norms have several major shortcomings. Norms were not stratified according to Census data, and no SES or educational level data on the sample is presented in the manual. Only limited information is presented on geographic region (e.g., no information on rural/urban status), and not all the information is presented in the manual (note that Conners et al., 2003, include additional sample specifications). Further, a portion of the normative data was collected as part of an unrelated study in which a group of nonclinical child and adolescent participants were recruited on the basis of high CBCL scores, which resulted in poorer CPT scores for the group as a whole. More important, part of the CPT-II norms were collected in children's homes, while the remainder was collected in a variety of settings ranging from research studies to "science centers." These settings, particularly the home setting, differ substantially from the settings where the test is primarily intended for use (i.e., clinical settings), and likely introduces considerable variability in the scores obtained. We would add that the data collected in the home involved a sample that is not representative of the general population (i.e., consisting primarily of rural African American children). The dates of norming are not provided, and exclusionary criteria appear ad hoc. Other aspects of the norms are discussed above, including an overrepresentation of women. This, in particular, is problematic, given the evidence for significant gender effects on CPTs (see Conners, 2000; McGee et al., 2000; Riccio et al., 2001). Riccio et al. (2001) have recommended that CPT norms have equal numbers of males and females per age group, or else separate norms for each gender.

More information on recruitment procedures, including diagnostic procedures, are necessary for the ADHD clinical group. The Neurologically Impaired group is not well described, and its utility is not well elaborated. Almost one-third of individuals are reported to have postconcussion disorder; no further relevant information is provided for this group (e.g., severity, litigating/nonlitigating, time since injury). Given the likelihood of a high base rate of exaggeration in postconcussion patients, procedures to exclude malingering would have been preferable.

In their extensive review of CPTs, Riccio et al. (2001) pointed out that most, if not all, CPT data yield skewed distributions that should be scaled using standard scores with linear transformation and percentile ranks. This has been addressed in the CPT-II. They also recommended that due to developmental changes in attention and executive functions, norms be provided for four to six months from ages 5 to 15 years, one-year intervals from 15 to 20 years, and no more than five-year intervals for ages 20 and above. Previous Conners' versions had an overrepresentation of younger adults in the adult sample (18–30 years), despite known declines in attentional performance with advancing age (Riccio et al., 2001). The current version is somewhat improved in this regard, but still provides only three age bands in adults, with an overrepresentation of cases in the younger age bands. The appropriateness of the older age band for assessing elderly adults is unknown, as no upper age limit is provided in the manual. Our view is that given the limitations in the normative sample, the test should not be given to those aged 55 and above.

In reviewing the normative sample of the previous edition, Riccio et al. (2001) concluded that, like the normative samples of other commercially available CPT tests, the Conners' norms appeared to be based on a sample of convenience. This also appears to be the case for the CPT-II.

Psychometric Properties

Psychometric properties of the test could be improved. For example, split-half reliabilities are only reported for some variables, and are based on the 1994 standardization sample. The CPT-II test-retest sample is very small, contains both clinical and nonclinical cases, and is not well described. Based on these data, with the exception of omissions and the two indices, test-retest reliabilities of CPT-II variables are too low for clinical use involving diagnostic decision making (see Table 9–19). More information on practice effects and stability within different age groups are needed. Note that low reliability estimates are not necessarily found in all CPTs; internal reliability and test-retest stability coefficients of other CPTs have ranged from the acceptable to high range (e.g., Borgaro et al., 2003), including small-scale standardized versions of the CPT intended for clinical use (e.g., Seidel & Joschko, 1991).

REFERENCES

American Academy of Pediatrics. (2000). Clinical practice guideline: Diagnosis and evaluation of the child with attention-deficit/hyperactivity disorder (AC2002). *Pediatrics, 105*, 1158–1170.

Ballard, J. C. (2001). Assessing attention: Comparison of response-inhibition and traditional continuous performance tests. *Journal of Clinical and Experimental Neuropsychology, 23*(3), 331–350.

Bandstra, E. S., Morrow, C. E., Anthony, J. C., Accornero, V. H., & Fried, P. A. (2001). Longitudinal investigation of task persistence and sustained attention in children with prenatal cocaine exposure. *Neurotoxicology and Teratology, 23*, 545–559.

Barkley, R. A. (1997). *ADHD and the nature of self-control.* New York: Guilford Press.

Barkley, R. A., Anastopoulos, A. D., Guevremont, D. G., & Fletcher, K. F. (1991). Adolescents with attention deficit hyperactivity disorder: Patterns of behavioural adjustment, academic functioning, and treatment utilization. *Journal of the American Academy of Child and Adolescent Psychiatry, 30*, 752–761.

Barkley, R. A., Edwards, G., Laneri, M., Fletcher, K., & Metevia, L. (2001). Executive functioning, temporal discounting, and sense of time in adolescents with attention deficit hyperactivity disorder (ADHD) and oppositional defiant disorder (ODD). *Journal of Abnormal Child Psychology, 29*(6), 541–556.

Borgaro, S., Pogge, D. L., DeLuca, V. A., Bilginer, L., Stokes, J., & Harvey, P. D. (2003). Convergence of different versions of the continuous performance test: Clinical and scientific implications. *Journal of Clinical and Experimental Neuropsychology, 25*(2), 283–292.

Borgatti, R., Piccinelli, P., Montirosso, R., Donati, G., Rampani, A., Molteni, L., Tofani, A., Nicoli, F., Zucca, C., Bresolin, N., & Balottin, U. (2004). Study of attentional processes in children with idiopathic epilepsy by Conners' continuous performance test. *Journal of Child Neurology, 19*, 509–515.

Collings, R. D. (2003). Differences between ADHD inattentive and combined types on the CPT. *Journal of Psychopathology and Behavioral Assessment, 25*(3), 177–189.

Conners, C. K. (1992). *Continuous performance test computer program, version 2.0.* North Tonawanda, NY: Multi-Health Systems Inc.

Conners, C. K. (1994). *Conners' continuous performance test computer program 3.0 user's manual.* Toronto, ON: Multi-Health Systems, Inc.

Conners, C. K. (1997). *Conners' Rating Scales—Revised technical manual.* Toronto, ON: Multi-Health Systems Inc.

Conners, C. K., & MHS Staff. (2000). *Conners' continuous performance test (CPT II) computer programs for Windows™ technical guide and software manual.* North Tonawanda, NY: Multi-Health Systems Inc.

Conners, C. K., Epstein, J. N., Angold, A., & Klaric, J. (2003). Continuous performance test performance in a normative epidemiological sample. *Journal of Abnormal Child Psychology, 31*(5), 555–562.

Corkum, P., & Siegel, L. (1993). Is the continuous performance test a valuable research tool for use with children with attention deficit hyperactivity disorder? *Journal of Child Psychology and Psychiatry, 34*(7), 1217–1239.

Epstein, J. N., Goldberg, N. A., Conners, C. K., & March, J. (1997). The effects of anxiety on continuous performance test functioning in an ADHD clinical sample. *Journal of Attention Disorders, 2*, 45–52.

Epstein, J. N., Conners, C. K., Sitarenios, G., & Erhardt, D. (1998). Continuous performance test results in adults with attention deficit hyperactivity disorder (ADHD). *The Clinical Psychologist, 12*, 155–168.

Epstein, J. N., Erkanli, A., Conners, C. K., Klaric, J., Costello, J. E., & Angold, A. (2003). Relations between continuous performance test performance measures and ADHD behaviors. *Journal of Abnormal Child Psychology, 31*(5), 543–554.

Epstein, J. N., Johnson, D. E., Varia, I. M., & Conners, C. K. (2001). Neuropsychological assessment of response inhibition in adults with ADHD. *Journal of Clinical and Experimental Neuropsychology, 23*(3), 362–371.

Fleck, D. E., Shear, P. K., & Strakowski, S. M. (2002). A reevaluation of sustained attention performance in temporal lobe epilepsy. *Archives of Clinical Neuropsychology, 17,* 399–405.

Kerns, K. A., McInerney, R. J., & Wilde, N. J. (2001). Time reproduction, working memory, and behavioral inhibition in children with ADHD. *Child Neuropsychology, 7*(1), 21–31.

Lemay, S., Bedard, M.-A., Rouleau, I., & Tremblay, P.-L. G. (2004). Practice effect and test-retest reliability of attentional and executive tests in middle-aged to elderly subjects. *The Clinical Neuropsychologist, 18*(2), 284–302.

Levin, E. D., Conners, C. K., Silva, D., Hinton, S. C., Meck, W. H., March, J., & Rose, J. E. (1998). Transdermal nicotine effects on attention. *Psychopharmacology, 140,* 135–141.

Levin, E. D., Wilson, W., Rose, J. E., & McEvoy, J. (1996). Nicotine-haloperidol interactions and cognitive performance in schizophrenics. *Neuropsychopharmacology, 15,* 429–436.

Lindsay, R. L., Tomazic, T., Levine, M. D., & Accardo, P. J. (2001). Attentional function as measured by continuous performance task in children with dyscalculia. *Developmental and Behavioral Pediatrics, 22*(5), 287–292.

Loisier, B. J., McGrath, P. J., & Klein, R. M. (1996). Error patterns on the continuous performance test in non-medicated and medicated samples of children with and without ADHD: A meta-analytic review. *Journal of Child Psychology and Psychiatry, 37,* 971–987.

McGee, R. A., Clark, S. E., & Symons, D. K. (2000). Does the Conners' continuous performance test aid in ADHD diagnosis? *Journal of Abnormal Child Psychology, 28*(5), 415–424.

Merchant, T. E., Keihna, E. N., Miles, M. A., Zhu, J., Xiong, X., & Mulhern, R. K. (2002). Acute effects of irradiation on cognition: Changes in attention on a computerized continuous performance test during radiotherapy in pediatric patients with localized primary brain tumors. *International Journal of Radiation Oncology and Biological Physiology, 53*(5), 1271–1278.

Pepin, M., & Loranger, M. (1996). *Computer administered aptitude battery software program.* Toronto, ON: Multi-Health Systems Inc.

Perugini, E. M., Harvey, E. A., Lovejoy, D. W., Sandstrom, K., & Webb, A. H. (2000). The predictive power of combined neuropsychological measures for attention-deficit/hyperactivity disorder in children. *Child Neuropsychology, 6*(2), 101–114.

Rabin, L. A., Barr, W. B., & Burton, L. A. (2005). Assessment practices of clinical neuropsychologists in the United States and Canada: A survey of INS, NAN, and APA division 40 members. *Archives of Clinical Neuropsychology, 20,* 33–65.

Riccio, C. A., & Reynolds, C. R. (2001). Continuous performance tests are sensitive to ADHD in adults but lack specificity: A review and critique for differential diagnosis. In: authors *Adult attention deficit disorder: Brain mechanisms and life outcomes.* New York, NY: New York Academy of Sciences.

Riccio, C. A., Reynolds, C. R., & Lowe, P. A. (2001). *Clinical applications of continuous performance tests: Measuring attention and impulsive responding in children and adults.* New York: John Wiley & Sons.

Riccio, C. A., Reynolds, C. R., Lowe, P., & Moore, J. J. (2002). The continuous performance test: A window on the neural substrate of attention? *Archives of Clinical Neuropsychology, 17,* 235–272.

Robertson, H. A., Kutcher, S. P., & Lagace, D. C. (2003). No evidence of attentional deficits in stabilized bipolar youths relative to unipolar and control comparators. *Bipolar Disorders, 5,* 330–339.

Rosvold, H. E., Mirsky, A. F., Sarason, I., Bransome, E. D., & Beck, L. H. (1956). A continuous performance test of brain damage. *Journal of Consulting Psychology, 20,* 343–350.

Seidel, W. T., & Joschko, M. (1991). Assessment of attention in children. *The Clinical Neuropsychologist, 5*(1), 53–66.

Taylor-Cooke, P. A., & Fastenau, P. S. (2004). Effects of test order and modality on sustained attention in children with epilepsy. *Child Neuropsychology, 10*(3), 212–221.

Thompson, S. J., Leigh, L., Christensen, R., Xiong, X., Kun, L. E., Heideman, R. K., Reddick, W. E., Gajjar, A., Merchant, R., Pui, C.-H., Hudson, M. M., & Mulhern, R. K. (2001). Immediate neurocognitive effects of methylphenidate on learning-impaired survivors of childhood cancer. *Journal of Clinical Oncology, 19*(6), 1802–1808.

Walker, A. J., Shores, E. A., Trollor, J. N., Lee, T., & Sachdev, P. S. (2000). Neuropsychological functioning of adults with attention deficit hyperactivity disorder. *Journal of Clinical and Experimental Neuropsychology, 22*(1), 115–124.

White, H. K., & Levin, E. D. (1999). Four-week nicotine skin patch treatment effects on cognitive performance in Alzheimer's disease. *Psychopharmacology, 143,* 158–165.

Integrated Visual and Auditory Continuous Performance Test (IVA + Plus)

PURPOSE

The Integrated Visual and Auditory Continuous Performance Test (IVA + Plus) is a computerized test of sustained attention and response inhibition.

SOURCE

The IVA + Plus can be obtained from BrainTrain, Inc. 727 Twin Ridge Lane, Richmond, VA 23235 (Phone: 804-320-0105; 800-822-0538; Fax: 804-320-0242 e-mail: info@braintrain.com; www.braintrain.com). The unlimited-use program (which administers and scores the test) and Administration and Interpretation Manuals cost $1695 US.

Additional optional analyses and report writers can be added to the basic package for an extra cost. The IVA + Plus Investigator provides additional features including comparison of changes in quotient scores for up to six administrations, and is thus useful for assessing medication or treatment effects. An Interpretive Report Writer Package can also be obtained for an additional $299 US; this includes an ADHD Report, Standard Report, and Special Analyses Report. Foreign language presentation (French, German, Hebrew, Italian, Japanese, Mandarin, Russian, Spanish, and Taiwanese) for the auditory modality can be purchased for an additional $269 US. Note that a Microsoft USB mouse is required to ensure proper timing of reaction time data (an adapter cannot be used with a serial mouse port).

AGE RANGE

The IVA + Plus can be administered from ages 6 to adult; current norms extend up to age 99.

DESCRIPTION

Overview

The IVA + Plus is an auditory and visual CPT designed to measure two major domains: attention and response control (IVA + Plus; Sandford & Turner, 2004a, 2004b). The IVA + Plus is the updated version of the original IVA (Sandford & Turner, 1995). Although the test itself is the same, the newer version has additional features such as changes to the data printout and inclusion of a test interpretation flowchart in the Interpretation Manual from which the Standard and ADHD Interpretive Reports are derived. The new Interpretive Report Writers add additional scales to the basic test scales, including a scale reflecting overall mental concentration and data on the possibility that the test taker may be malingering (V. Sandford, personal communication, September 2004). According to the authors, the IVA + Plus is designed primarily to provide assistance in diagnosing ADHD, including differentiating among ADHD subtypes, but can also be used in the evaluation of other disorders involving attention and self-control difficulties. A secondary purpose is to allow tracking of treatment effects, including changes attributable to medication.

Parameters

The test itself is straightforward, and, like any good CPT, is "simple and boring" (Baerwald et al., 2001, p. 537). Two stimuli (i.e., the numbers "1" and "2") are presented pseudorandomly over 500 trials, alternating between visual and auditory modalities. There are 250 trials in each modality, presented either on the computer screen or via headphones. Each trial lasts 1.5 seconds. Stimulus display time is 167 ms for visual trials and 500 ms for auditory trials. The examinee is required to respond only to targets ("1") and to inhibit responding to nontargets ("2"), regardless of the modality in which the item appears.

Target frequency varies across the test. When targets are common, the demands on impulse control and inhibition are increased, thereby increasing the risk of commission errors. At other times, targets occur rarely, which increases attentional demands and confers a higher risk of omission errors.

The 500 trials are divided into five 100-trial blocks. During the first 50 trials of each block, 84% of the trials consist of targets ("1"), with only eight trials consisting of nontargets ("2"). During the second 50 trials, only 16% of the trials consist of targets, and the remaining 42 trials are nontargets. Visual and auditory presentations are equally represented within each block, but the intermixing of visual and auditory stimuli creates, according to the authors, a variable interstimulus interval when visual and auditory stimuli are considered separately (Sandford & Turner, 2004a).

Scores

The basic IVA + Plus provides a number of scores: six global composites (Full-Scale Response Control Quotient, Auditory Response Control Quotient, Visual Response Control Quotient, Full-Scale Attention Quotient, Auditory Attention Quotient, and Visual Attention Quotient) and 22 other scales measuring four broad categories (Response Control, Attention, Attribute, and Symptomatic). Primary scales make up the Quotient scales. In the case of Response Control, these include Prudence, Consistency, and Stamina. Primary scales for the Attention quotients include Vigilance, Focus, and Speed. Attribute and Symptomatic scores are designed to provide information on test-taking characteristics. The Attribute scales measure the test taker's optimum performance (i.e., visual versus auditory, high versus low target load), whereas the Symptomatic scales assess adherence to task requirements (i.e., as shown by random responding, motor speed impairments, and motivation/effort). The test also includes a scale measuring fine motor hyperactivity (Fine Motor Regulation). Additional scores are also provided through the software addons (e.g., Special Analyses, Investigator). Overall, the test yields an extremely large number of possible scores. See Table 9–20 for a description of the scores available through the basic package. IVA + Plus score labels are based on a positive interpretation of performance (e.g., "Vigilance" instead of "Inattention") to avoid negative connotations when providing feedback (Sandford & Turner, 2004b).

Features

Additional optional analyses and report writers can be added to the basic package. The IVA + Plus Investigator assists with comparing changes in quotient scores for up to six repeat administrations, and is thus useful for assessing medication or treatment effects. It provides statistical analysis of change scores in tabular format, indicating mild, moderate, or marked changes over time. The Report Writers provide a Standard Report, which is a narrative report designed for use with non-ADHD populations (e.g., head injury), and as such does not include statements about ADHD diagnosis. The ADHD Report classifies the profile as supporting or not supporting an ADHD diagnosis. The Special Analyses Report provides further detailing of individual performance according to additional scores such as Mental Concentration Analysis (four new scales: Reliability, Accuracy, Quickness, Stability), High and Low Demand Analysis, and Malingering Analysis.

ADMINISTRATION

See the Administration Manual (Sandford & Turner, 2004a). The test includes four phases: "warm-up" (two one-minute

Table 9–20 Summary of IVA Scores

IVA Quotient	IVA Scale	Description
Response Control[a]	Prudence	Assesses impulsivity/response inhibition; combines three types of commission errors
	Consistency	Assesses ability to stay on task; involves reliability and variability of response times
	Stamina	Assesses sustained attention; compares the mean reaction time of correct responses during the first 200 responses to that during the last 200 responses
Attention[a]	Vigilance	Measures attention; combines two different types of omission errors
	Focus	Assesses variability of response speed
	Speed	Provides information on the average reaction time for all correct responses
Attribute	Balance	Indicates the user's most efficient modality (i.e., auditory, visual, or both)
	Readiness	Indicates whether the user processes information more quickly under rapid conditions or under slower conditions
Symptomatic	Comprehension	Identifies random responding; is reportedly the most sensitive scale to ADHD
	Persistence	Assesses motivation or motor or mental fatigue
	Sensory/Motor	Identifies slow reaction that may impair performance
	Fine Motor Regulation	Measures fine motor hyperactivity via off-task mouse clicks; quantifies restlessness and fidgetiness

Note: Composite scores are shown in italics. [a]Full Scale, Auditory, and Visual Quotients; Full-Scale Response Control Quotient is based on both the Auditory Response Control Quotient and Visual Response Control Quotient; Full-Scale Attention Quotient is based on the Auditory Attention Quotient and the Visual Attention Quotient.

sessions consisting of simple visual and auditory reaction time tests to establish baseline reaction time), a 1.5-minute practice session, the test itself consisting of five sections of 100 visual and 100 auditory trials, and a "cool-down" phase (same as practice phase). Comparison of the latter to the "warm-up" phase allows a determination of the subject's motivation and fatigue.

The examinee should be seated in a stable, nonswivel chair. All instructions are spoken by the computer using digitized voice technology to maintain consistency across administrations. If the foreign-language option is used, instructions are posted on the computer screen only, and are presented verbally by the examiner. In the standard version, the only instruction the examiner can provide once the test has begun is "Keep working, do your best"; the examiner should not correct off-task behavior except for incorrect mouse use.

The examinee uses the mouse to respond, and the computer keyboard is moved out of the way so that it can be used by the examiner to set up the administration. A Microsoft USB mouse is required to ensure proper timing of reaction time data. Note that random mouse clicking by the subject during administration of test directions should not be stopped by the examiner, as these data contribute to the fine motor hyperactivity scale of the IVA + Plus. Auditory stimuli are presented via headphones. Use of speakers is not recommended by the authors.

The program allows the user to e-mail single record-protected test session data or an entire database to BrainTrain for consultation.

ADMINISTRATION TIME

The test itself takes 13 minutes. The entire test administration, including instructions and practice, requires a minimum of 20 minutes (Sandford & Turner, 2004a).

SCORING

Raw scores are converted to standard scores ($M = 100$, $SD = 15$) based on age and gender. According to the authors, the primary diagnostic scores are (a) the Full-Scale Response Control Quotient score and (b) the Full Attention Quotient score. Because these scores combine responses from the visual and auditory trials, modality-specific scores are also provided (i.e., Visual Response Control Quotient, Visual Attention Quotient, Auditory Response Control Quotient, and Auditory Attention Quotient). See Table 9–20 for a simplified description of scores (note that additional scores for the Special Analyses are not listed here). Score composition can be complex; see the Interpretive Manual for a full description of the calculations involved in each score. Table 9–21 shows the formulas for computing the various IVA + Plus scores. This is done automatically by the scoring program.

The IVA + Plus Investigator module allows the user to determine whether IVA quotients from test to retest are significantly different. The criterion for significant change is set at one SD (i.e., 15 points). Guidelines for describing change are provided (15–22 points: Mild Change; 30–37 points: Moderate Change; 45+ points: Marked Change; Sandford & Turner, 2004b, p. 95).

DEMOGRAPHIC EFFECTS

Age

Reaction time (Speed scale) across age generally follows a U-shaped curve, with rapid improvement between ages 5 and 7, a more gradual decrease in reaction time between ages 8 to 12, optimal performance in young adults, stability through adulthood, and then a slight slowing starting at age

Table 9–21 List of Formulae for Deriving IVA + Plus scores

AAQ	Auditory Attention Quotient (based on: VIA% + FOCA + MNA)
ARCQ	Auditory Response Control Quotient (based on: PRA% + CONA + STMA)
CONA	CONsistency Aud. SCALE ((Quartile 1 RT/ Quartile 3 RT) × 100)
CONV	CONsistency Vis. SCALE ((Quartile 1 RT/ Quartile 3 RT) × 100)
CMPA	CoMPrehension Auditory (Co + Om) SCALE (100 − ((IDIOERR#)/ (50 + 80) × 100))
CMPV	CoMPrehension Visual (Co + Om) SCALE (100 − ((IDIOERR#)/(60 + 80) × 100))
FAQ	Full-Scale Attention Quotient (based on: AAQ + VAQ)
FOCA	FOCus Auditory SCALE ((1 − (SD/MN)) × 100)
FOCV	FOCus Visual SCALE ((1 − (SD/MN)) × 100)
FRCQ	Full-Scale Response Control Quotient (based on: ARCQ + VRCQ)
HYP	HYPeractivity SCALE (XCL + LRT + ZRT + SCL) off-task behaviors
MNA	MeaN Auditory reaction time for all trials (Speed SCALE)
MNV	MeaN Visual RT for all trials (Speed SCALE, Max $N = 125$)
PRA%	PRudence Auditory SCALE Percent (100 − ((PRA# / 75) × 100))
PRV%	PRudence Visual SCALE Percent (100 − ((PRV# / 65) × 100))
RVAC	Ratio Visual/Auditory Combined RT × 100 (Balance SCALE)
RWCA	Ratio Warm-up/Cool-down Auditory RT × 100 (Persistence SCALE)
RWCV	Ratio Warm-up/Cool-down Visual RT × 100 (Persistence SCALE)
RFRA	Ratio Frequent/Rare Auditory RT × 100 (Readiness SCALE)
RFRV	Ratio Frequent/Rare Visual RT × 100 (Readiness SCALE)
SAAQ	Sustained Auditory Attention Quotient (Based on DEPA, SWFA, POA, IAA, ECAR, & EOAF)[a]
SMA	Sensory/Motor Auditory SCALE (better of Warm-up/Cool-down RT)
SMV	Sensory/Motor Visual SCALE (better of Warm-up/Cool-down RT)
STMA	STaMina Auditory SCALE RT((Sets 1 + 2)/(Sets 4 + 5) × 100)
STMV	STaMina Visual SCALE RT((Sets 1 + 2)/(Sets 4 + 5) × 100)
SVAQ	Sustained Visual Attention Quotient (Based on DEPV, SWFV, POV, IAV, ECVR, & EOVF)[a]
VAQ	Visual Attention Quotient (based on: VIV% + FOCV + MNV)
VIA%	Vigilance Auditory SCALE Percent (100 − ((VIA# /45) × 100))
VIV%	VIgilance Visual SCALE Percent (100 − ((VIV# / 45) × 100))
VRCQ	Visual Response Control Quotient (based on: PRV% + CONV + STMV)

Note: # = Number of errors; % = Percent of errors; A = Auditory mode; V = Visual mode; F = Frequent block–42 targets/block of 50 trials; R = Rare block–8 targets/block of 50 trials; Sets = Two blocks of 50 trials each; MN = Mean of reaction times; SD = Standard deviation of reaction times (N-1 correction factor); N = Number of cases to compute MN and SD; R = Ratio (used for warm up/cool down, visual/auditory, frequent/rare); RT = Reaction time in milliseconds.
[a]These scales refer to scales used in the Special Analyses and can be found in the Special Analyses Norms.

Source: From Sandford & Turner, 2004b. Reprinted with the permission of BrainTrain, Inc., Richmond. VA.

45 (Sandford & Turner, 2004b). Developmental trends for other IVA scores are not detailed in the manuals. In adults with ADHD, performance is also related to age ($r = .38$; Tinius, 2003).

Gender

The manual describes faster reaction times and higher commission error rates in men than in women (Sandford & Turner, 2004b), which supports the need for gender-based normative data.

Education

The test manuals do not provide information on the test's relationship to education in the normative sample. Tinius

(2003) found conflicting results: IVA performance was not correlated with education in controls or in adults with MTBI, but performance was related to education in ADHD ($r = .38$; Tinius, 2003).

IQ

IVA performance is not correlated with IQ in controls or in adults with MTBI (Tinius, 2003). However, in adults with ADHD, performance is highly related to IQ ($r = .64$; Tinius, 2003). See also *Comment*.

Ethnicity

Information on the effects of race/ethnicity is not available.

Table 9–22 Characteristics of the IVA + Plus Normative Sample

Number	1700
Age	6 to 99 years[a]
Geographic location	U.S. sample, unspecified location
Sample type	Unspecified
Education	Unspecified
Gender	Gender composition varies by age band
Race/ethnicity	Unspecified
Screening	Exclusion criteria included participation in therapy, history of learning disability, hyperactivity or attention problems, current medication usage, history of neurological problems (dementia, stroke or TBI), or inability to complete the test.

[a]Based on several age groupings: 6, 7, 8, 9, 10, 11, 12, 13, 14, 15, 16, 17–18, 19–21, 22–24, 25–29, 30–34, 35–39, 40–44, 45–54, 55–65, and 66–99.

NORMATIVE DATA

Standardization Sample

The standardization sample consists of 1700 individuals. The Interpretive Manual does not provide sufficient details concerning sample composition, including education, regional distribution, and ethnicity. See Table 9–22 for sample characteristics. Cell sizes based on age and gender are not entirely uniform, but range from 18 to 89, with most in the 30 to 40 range.

RELIABILITY

Internal Consistency

This is not reported in the manual.

Standard Error of Measurement (SEM)

Information on SEMs is not presented in the manual.

Test-Retest Reliability

The Interpretation Manual presents data on 70 normal volunteers tested twice over an interval of one to four weeks (age, $M = 22$ years, range 5–70; Sandford & Turner, 2004b). As shown in Table 9–23, composite quotient score reliability was marginal to adequate for the Attention quotients (i.e., $r = .66–.75$) but poor for all the Response Control scores (i.e., $r = .37–.41$). Certain primary score reliability coefficients were high (i.e., Mean Visual RT, Mean Auditory RT, Hyperactivity, Comprehension Visual Scale). However, reliabilities varied significantly in magnitude across scores, with several falling well below clinical standards (e.g., $r < .40$ for the Ratio Warm-Up/Cool-Down and Stamina scores; see Table 9–23). The manual indicates that variability in this sample was small (i.e.,

Table 9–23 Magnitude of Test-Retest Reliability Coefficients for the IVA + Plus

Magnitude of Coefficient	Test-Retest Reliability
Very high (.90+)	—
High (.80–.89)	Hyperactivity Comprehension Visual Scale Mean Auditory RT Mean Visual RT
Adequate (.70–.79)	*Full-Scale Attention Quotient* *Visual Attention Quotient* Comprehension Auditory Scale Sensory/Motor Visual Scale Vigilance Visual Scale Percent
Marginal (.60–.69)	*Auditory Attention Quotient* Prudence Visual Scale Percent Prudence Auditory Scale Percent Focus Visual Scale Focus Auditory Scale Consistency Auditory Scale Ratio Visual/Auditory Combined RT
Low (<.59)	*Full-Scale Response Control Quotient* *Auditory Response Control Quotient* *Visual Response Control Quotient* Ratio Warm-up/Cool-down Auditory RT Stamina Visual Scale RT Stamina Auditory Scale RT Vigilance Auditory Scale Percent Ratio Warm-up/Cool-down Visual RT Ratio Frequent/Rare Auditory RT Ratio Frequent/Rare Visual RT Consistency Visual Scale Sensory/Motor Auditory Scale

Note: Composite Quotient Scores are presented in italics.

error rates of 1–6%), which may have attenuated some of these correlations due to ceiling effects. Alternate means of assessing score stability are not provided (e.g., percent classification agreement from test to re-test).

Practice Effects

Practice effects, though present, are for the most part very small. For Composite Quotient scores, mean score changes are 3% or less (i.e., three or fewer standard score points; see manual).

VALIDITY

Correlations Among IVA + Plus Scores

The Interpretive Manual provides limited information on the intercorrelations among IVA + Plus scores. However, it states that of the primary scales measuring Response Control, only Prudence and Consistency are modestly correlated

($r = .33–.44$), and of the Attention scales, only Vigilance and Speed are correlated ($r = .25–.36$). The manual concludes that the primary scales are generally independent, which "helps to increase the power and sensitivity of the conglomerate global quotients" (Sandford & Turner, 2004b, p. 29). The lack of association between primary scales could also be interpreted as indicating that their respective quotients do not measure a unitary or homogenous domain. The Interpretive Manual also describes data on a subset of the normative sample, where the correlations for the six primary scales (i.e., Prudence, Consistency, Stamina, Vigilance, Focus, and Speed) were high ($r = .53–.86$; Sandford & Turner, 2004b, p. 105); why this differs from the correlations noted previously is not explained, but may have to do with score format (i.e., raw scores not adjusted for age would likely show higher correlations).

Factor Structure

The factor structure of the IVA + Plus is not reported in the manual; this would help confirm whether scores can be grouped into the six global composites and within the four broad domains specified by the test.

Correlations With Attention Tests

Information on the correlation between the IVA + Plus and other attention tests, including other CPTs, is lacking, apart from a small study (ADHD, $N = 26$; controls, $N = 31$) described in the Interpretive Manual (Sandford & Turner, 2004b). In this study, the percent of agreement between children identified as having ADHD by the IVA compared with the percent identified by other CPTs and rating scales was high (i.e., 90% concordance for T.O.V.A., 100% for the Gordon Diagnostic System [GDS; Gordon, 1983]), and between 92% and 100% for rating scales, including the Conners' Parent Rating Scale-39.

Correlations With Rating Scales

The IVA is not related to self-ratings of neuropsychological symptoms in adults with ADHD or MTBI (Tinius, 2003) using the NIS (Neuropsychological Impairment Scale; O'Donnell et al., 1994). Additional research on the concordance of IVA scores and standardized scales for assessing ADHD symptoms is needed.

Clinical Studies

Most CPTs can easily differentiate between individuals with ADHD and controls on a group level. What is more difficult to attain is diagnostic accuracy (i.e., positive predictive power, negative predictive power) and the ability to successfully differentiate individuals with ADHD from those with other clinical conditions. Surprisingly, there are few published studies on diagnostic utility of the IVA in children. The test authors indicate that the test has better diagnostic accuracy than other CPTs in differentiating children with ADHD from controls,

based on a lower false-positive rate, compared with the T.O.V.A. and GDS in a small, unpublished study involving children. Specifically, in a group of 26 children with ADHD and 31 controls, IVA + Plus sensitivity was 92%, specificity was 90%, positive predictive power was 89%, and negative predictive power was 93%. Corresponding values for other CPTs are not included for comparison. However, the false-negative rate of the IVA + Plus was 7.7%, in comparison to 12.5% for the T.O.V.A. and 36% for the GDS (Sandford & Turner, 2004b). To date, there exist no studies on the IVA's ability to differentiate between ADHD subtypes.

Adults with ADHD perform more poorly than controls on the IVA + Plus (Quinn et al., 2003; Tinius, 2003), although differences on Response Control scores are not always found (Quinn, 2003). This is of considerable significance, given that the Response Control scores form the basis for supporting specific ADHD subtype diagnoses in the Interpretive Manual (e.g., Combined subtype). As is the case with most CPTs, differentiation between clinical groups is less supported: adults with ADHD and adults with MTBI perform similarly on the test (Tinius, 2003).

Although individuals with MTBI perform more poorly than controls on the IVA, IVA performance is not related to markers of head injury severity in MTBI, such as time since injury (Tinius, 2003; note that this study makes no mention of exclusion of possible exaggerators). Adults with schizophrenia show asymmetrical attention deficits on the IVA (auditory more than visual) compared with patients with bipolar disorder; but both groups have impaired processing speed. Different patterns of cross-modal switching deficits are also shown for these patients on the IVA (Baerwald et al., 2001).

IVA scores reportedly improve following computerized attention training in ADHD (Slate et al., 1998). However, to our knowledge, there are no published studies on sensitivity to stimulant medication effects with the IVA, apart from a recent study comparing Ritalin to food supplements. In this case, both were effective at increasing IVA performance (Harding et al., 2003).

Malingering

Simulated malingerers perform more poorly on the IVA than adults with ADHD, with 81% of IVA subscales showing significant group differences, especially Vigilance and Comprehension scales (Quinn, 2003). Scores in the auditory modality are particularly sensitive, demonstrating excellent positive and negative predictive power (see Table 9–24). Unusually low IVA scores, such as T scores of 50 or below, may therefore suggest exaggeration. Note that subjects in this study were able to successfully simulate symptoms on ADHD rating scales (Quinn, 2003). This study requires replication in clinically defined groups.

COMMENT

The IVA + Plus is an interesting measure that combines several features of different CPTs. First, it provides variable

Table 9–24 Detection of Malingering on the IVA: Diagnostic Utility of Impairment Indexes

Impairment Index	Sensitivity	Specificity	PPP	NPP
Full-Scale Response Control >75 and				
Full-Scale Attention Quotient >37	81	91	88	87
Auditory Response Control >74 and				
Auditory Attention Quotient >44	94	91	88	95
Visual Response Control >76 and				
Visual Attention Quotient >40	81	74	68	85

Note: PPP = positive predictive power; NPP = negative predictive power.

Source: From Quinn, 2003.

interstimulus intervals designed to capture both impulse control and vigilance deficits, requiring the respondent at times to respond almost continuously (i.e., as do "response"-type CPTs or "not-X" CPTs such as the CPT-II or GDS) or, alternatively, to respond infrequently, like the more standard "X" CPT (e.g., T.O.V.A.; Sandford & Turner, 2004b). Second, stimuli are provided in both the auditory and visual modalities, which may increase sensitivity, given that auditory and visual CPTs may uncover attention deficits in different populations. It may also have utility in assessing populations where cross-modal switching difficulties are expected, such as patients with schizophrenia (see Baerwald et al., 2001). Other features are its ability to provide screening for simple reaction time deficits, including pre- and posttest reaction time to assess for fatigue, and its provision of a number of validity indicators. Additionally, its discrimination task is simpler than other CPTs such as the CPT-II or GDS (but not T.O.V.A.) because only a single nontarget ("2") is ever presented (Riccio et al., 2001). The Interpretive Manual is comprehensive and includes several discussions on the theoretical underpinnings of the IVA. It may also be of specific utility in detecting malingering of attention symptoms (Quinn, 2003).

Use of the IVA to diagnose ADHD is more problematic. The test itself is marketed as a tool for assisting in ADHD diagnosis. The Interpretive Manual specifies that the IVA should be used in conjunction with behavioral rating scales as corroborative evidence to support or refute an ADHD diagnosis. However, the emphasis on ADHD assessment (including flowcharts to aid in diagnosis) may lead some clinicians to erroneously assume that the IVA is more sensitive to ADHD than other instruments, or that it is able to differentiate between ADHD subtypes, a claim that is simply unsubstantiated. Users should keep in mind that CPTs may be useful tools in ruling out ADHD (Riccio et al., 2001), but should not be used as conclusive evidence of ADHD. Test-retest reliability of the test is also a concern. Despite the authors' interpretation of coefficients as showing that the test has demonstrated stability over time, limited reliability of some IVA scores preclude their use for clinical diagnosis. This includes the Response Control scores, which form the basis for some of the main ADHD interpretations. Our own opinion is that use of lengthy

interpretive reports, which the promotional materials claim are a strength of the IVA, are not necessarily an asset in clinical settings due to the risk of clinicians overinterpreting report conclusions, accepting results without critical analysis, and relying too much on the generated report over their own clinical judgment, which should integrate all other aspects of the evaluation.

The test can be difficult for younger children, and so may not be as useful for attentional screening in this age group (Sandford & Turner, 2004b); other CPTs may be more appropriate in this regard (e.g., T.O.V.A.). The manual also states that the test is designed to detect attentional and impulse control impairments, but not functioning above the very superior range. Although comprehensive, the manuals do not include enough information on some of its analyses, including the Malingering Analysis; however, this analysis is based on the occurrence of random responding and extreme scores, which can probably also be assessed using the validity scales and data from Quinn (2003).

The previous IVA version (Sandford & Turner, 1995) was criticized on several fronts: its norms were not stratified and appeared to represent a sample of convenience; the date of norming was not specified; sample ethnicity was not reported; geographic areas for norming were unclear; important demographic variables such as SES and education were not reported; internal consistency was unknown; no confidence levels were provided; and age intervals in the norming group were too wide (Riccio et al., 2001). As a result of these limitations, the previous version was deemed not to meet established standards for educational and psychological testing, and was viewed as presenting significant potential for misuse and misinterpretation of test results regarding ADHD diagnosis (Kane et al., 2001). Because the IVA + Plus uses the same normative sample as previous versions, many of these criticisms remain valid. However, when its limitations are understood and appropriately taken into account, the IVA does have significant potential in some contexts.

Users should also keep in mind other significant limitations. The test yields an incredibly large number of possible scores, based on a number of computations (see Table 9–21) whose rationale is not directly explained in the manual. This can make interpretation challenging. In addition, although there is a lengthy bibliography listed on its Web site, the majority of papers listed are not published in established journals, and some are not directly related to the IVA. The test itself could use more independent research, particularly in children and in different clinical groups. Gaining full familiarity with the test, its scores, and its interpretation requires a major time investment, as we have found for other CPTs reviewed in this manual.

Adjustment of scores for IQ is mentioned in the Interpretative Manual (Sandford & Turner, 2004b, p. 92), but no effects of IQ are reported for the normative sample (see *Demographic Effects*). The IQ adjustment technique involves using the individual's mental age to derive IVA scores rather than chronological age. However, the manual recommends that the technique be used with caution, as it depends on clinical judgment only and not on controlled research. The rationale is that ADHD may be underdiagnosed in gifted individuals and overdiagnosed in individuals with low IQ. Although this is an interesting premise, it requires further investigation.

The IVA + Plus Investigator module allows the user to determine whether IVA quotients from test to retest are significantly different. The criterion for significant change is set at one *SD* (i.e., 15 points). Although the use of the *SD* as a benchmark for change can provide a gross estimate, use of more sophisticated techniques such as reliable change methodology would be a useful option as it would take into account the reliability of the scores. There are also few published studies on the IVA + Plus's sensitivity to medication effects, an important feature for a test designed for use in ADHD.

REFERENCES

Baerwald, J. P., Tryon, W., & Sandford, J. (2001). Modal attention asymmetry in patients with schizophrenia and bipolar disorder. *Neuropsychology, 15*(4), 535–543.

Corkum, P., & Siegel, L. (1993). Is the continuous performance test a valuable research tool for use with children with attention deficit hyperactivity disorder? *Journal of Child Psychology and Psychiatry, 34*(7), 1217–1239.

Gordon, M. (1983). *The Gordon Diagnostic System.* DeWitt, NY: Gordon Systems.

Hagelthorn, K. M., Hiemenz, J. R., Pillion, J. P., & Mahone, F. M. (2003). Age and task parameters in continuous performance tests for preschoolers. *Perceptual and Motor Skills, 96*, 975–989.

Harding, K. L., Judah, R. D., & Gant, C. E. (2003). Outcome-based comparison of Ritalin® versus food-supplement treated children with ADHD. *Alternative Medicine Review, 8*(3), 319–330.

Kane, H., Whiston, S. C., & Wiese, M. J. (2001). *Review of the IVA.* Island Park, NJ: Buros Fourteenth Mental Measurements Yearbook.

O'Donnell, W. E., DeSoto, C. B., Desota, J. L., & Reynolds, D. M. (1994). *Neuropsychological impairment scales (NIS) manual.* Los Angeles, CA: Western Psychological Services.

Quinn, C. A. (2003). Detection of malingering in assessment of adult ADHD. *Archives of Clinical Neuropsychology, 18*, 379–395.

Riccio, C. A., Reynolds, C. R., & Lowe, P. A. (2001). *Clinical applications of continuous performance tests: Measuring attention and impulsive responding in children and adults.* New York: John Wiley & Sons, Inc.

Riccio, C. A., Reynolds, C. R., Lowe, P., & Moore, J. J. (2002). The continuous performance test: A window on the neural substrate of attention? *Archives of Clinical Neuropsychology, 17*, 235–272.

Sandford, J. A., & Turner, A. (1995). *Manual for the Integrated Visual and Auditory Continuous Performance Test.* Richmond, VA: Brain Train.

Sandford, J. A., & Turner, A. (2004a). *IVA+Plus™: Integrated Visual and Auditory Continuous Performance Test administration manual.* Richmond, VA: Brain Train, Inc.

Sandford, J. A., & Turner, A. (2004b). *IVA+Plus™: Integrated Visual and Auditory Continuous Performance Test interpretation manual.* Richmond, VA: Brain Train, Inc.

Sandford, J. A., Fine, A. H., & Goldman, L. (1995). *Validity study of the IVA: A visual and auditory CPT.* Paper presented at the 1995 annual convention of the American Psychological Association, New York.

Slate, S. E., Meyer, T. L., Burns, W. J., & Montgomery, D. D. (1998). Computerized cognitive training for severely emotionally disturbed children with ADHD. *Behavior Modification, 22*, 415–437.

Tinius, T. P. (2003). The Intermediate [sic] Visual and Auditory Continuous Performance Test as a neuropsychological measure. *Archives of Clinical Neuropsychology, 18*, 199–214.

Paced Auditory Serial Addition Test (PASAT) and Children's Paced Auditory Serial Addition Test (CHIPASAT)

PURPOSE

This test is a serial-addition task used to assess working memory, divided attention, and information processing speed.

SOURCE

There are several versions of the test. Ordering information for selected audiotape and computer versions is outlined in Table 9–25. Other versions of the PASAT are also in circulation.

AGE RANGE

The test can be administered to a broad age range. The 61-item-per-trial (Gronwall) version includes norms for ages 16 to 74 (Crawford et al., 1998; Stuss et al., 1987). The 50-item-per-trial (Levin) versions have norms for ages 20 to 68 (Diehr et al., 1998, 2003; Wiens et al., 1997). Norms for computerized versions depend on the version used.

The children's version (CHIPASAT) has norms extending from ages 8 to 14.5 years. The computerized CHIPASAT uses the same norms. Preliminary child norms are available for

Table 9–25 Ordering Information for Selected Versions of the PASAT and CHIPASAT

	Source	Comment	Age Range	Normative Data
Original Gronwall PASAT (61 items per trial)	Test Materials Sales Office Department of Psychology University of Victoria P.O. Box 1700 Victoria, BC, V8W 2Y2, Canada http://web.uvic.ca/psyc/testsale	This Gronwall audiotape version (including instructions and sample scoring sheet) can be ordered at cost of $50 US This version uses a New Zealand accent	16–74	Stuss et al., 1988 Crawford et al., 1998
Original Levin Version (50 items per trial)	This version is reportedly no longer available from Dr. Levin (T. Tombaugh, personal communication, October 2004).	Other versions of the same task exist, and older tapes are still in circulation	20–88	Wiens et al., 1997 Brittain et al., 1991 Roman et al., 1991
PASAT-50 PASAT-100 PASAT-200	Neurobehavioral Core Manager HIV Neurobehavioral Research Center University of California San Diego 9500 Gilman Drive Mail Code 0603-H La Jolla, CA 92093-0603H Telephone: 619-543-5000 Fax: 619-543-1235	A website to access a downloadable audio file and electronic copies of test forms is in development	20–68	Diehr et al., 1998, 2003
Children's version (CHIPASAT)	D. Johnson, Department of Child Life & Health University of Edinburgh 20 Sylvan Place Edinburgh EH9 1UW djohnso1@staffmail.ed.ac.uk	$50 US	8–14.5	Johnson et al., 1988
Adjusting-Paced Serial Addition Test (Adjusting-PSAT)	Not commercially available	An adjusting computerized version (Tombaugh, 1999)	—	N/A
Victoria Computerized Adaptation of the PASAT (Gronwall version)	Developed by Robert McInerney; can be downloaded from http://web.uvic.ca/psyc/, under "Test Sales"	Available for $100 Canadian; this version uses an American Midwestern accent; a French-Canadian version is also available from the author at www.RobertMcInerney.ca/software.html	*	None; norms from the Gronwall audiotape version are used instead
The Paced Visual Serial Addition Test (PVSAT)	Dr. Bruce J. Diamond P.O. Box 43592 Upper Montclair, NJ 07043 diamondb@wpunj.edu	A computerized visual version; other versions are available from the author, including adaptive visual and auditory versions	**	Diamond et al., 1997 Fos et al., 2000 Johnson et al., 1996.
Computerized CHIPASAT	Developed by Robert McInerney and D. Johnson; see www.RobertMcInerney.ca/software.html	A computerized CHIPASAT, using the standard CHIPASAT stimuli	*	None; norms from the CHIPASAT audiotape version are used instead

Note: There are other versions of the PASAT in circulation. This normative dataset list is not exhaustive, but rather presents the best normative datasets for each version. A computerized auditory version originally distributed by ForThought, Ltd. has also been described (Wingenfeld et al., 1999). However, this version may no longer be commercially available (S. Wigenfeld, personal communication, January 2004). There is also a nonnumerical version (PASOT; see Gow & Deary, 2004, available by contacting the authors). Users of audiotape versions should note that tape quality degrades with time and repeated copying.

*See audiotape version.
**Preliminary child norms range from age 3.5–8.

other computerized versions such as PVSAT, which uses an adaptive testing paradigm (ages 3.5–8.0; B. Diamond, personal communication, January 2004).

DESCRIPTION

The Paced Auditory Serial Addition Test (PASAT) was devised by Gronwall et al. (Gronwall, 1977; Gronwall & Sampson, 1974; Gronwall & Wrightson, 1974) to provide an estimate of speed of information processing. The paradigm is based on a procedure originally developed by Sampson (1956). Although Sampson's original procedure also included visual item presentation, Gronwall's pioneering use of the auditory version in assessing the effects of head injury has ensured that the auditory PASAT is used more often in neuropsychology (Royan et al., 2004).

In all versions, random series of numbers from 1 to 9 are presented, and the subject is instructed to consecutively add pairs of numbers such that each number is added to the one that immediately preceded it (i.e., the second number is added to the first, the third number to the second, the fourth number to the third, etc.). For example, if the stimulus "1" followed by "9" is presented, the examinee must respond "10"; if the next stimulus is "4," the examinee must respond "13" (i.e., by adding the "4" to the previous digit "9," not to the examinee's own response of "10"), and so on. This response requirement is sustained over numerous items until the end of the trial. The interstimulus interval (ISI) is then decreased, and the same process is repeated. The PASAT thus incrementally increases processing demands over trials by increasing the speed of stimulus input and decreasing the available response time.

The PASAT requires the examinee to sustain attention to the single digits, engage working memory by performing mental calculations involving single digits, and perform at an increasingly demanding, externally determined pace. The PASAT is considered a strong test of divided attention, sustained attention, and working memory because of the requirement to switch between two ongoing tasks (adding two digits and encoding the next presented digit) over several trials. The task's rapid, paced responding also requires information processing speed (Shucard et al., 2004). The paradigm evidently also requires basic arithmetic skills and numeracy. Thus, unlike previous conceptualizations of the test as measuring primarily information processing speed, recent thinking indicates that the PASAT is a demanding, multifactorial task.

Versions

There are now several different PASAT versions. These differ in two main ways: (1) modality (auditory or visual) and (2) administration format (audiotape versus computer administered). The number of items and actual ISIs also differ across certain PASAT versions, as may other task parameters. Most versions are, however, modeled on either the Gronwall (61 items per trial; Gronwall & Sampson, 1974) or Levin (50

items per trial; Levin et al., 1987) version. In this review, we will use the term "Gronwall" for 61-item versions and "Levin" for 50-item versions.

Short forms of the audio-taped PASAT have also been developed based on one-trial (PASAT-50) and two-trial (PASAT-100) administrations (Diehr et al., 2003). The children's version (CHIPASAT; Dyche & Johnson, 1991a, 1991b; Johnson et al., 1988) includes sums that never exceed 10. Computer versions offer either auditory or visual stimuli; the recording format for responses differs depending on the version (e.g., manually recorded versus computer recorded). See Table 9–26 for a summary of the response modalities, parameters, and corresponding norms for selected PASAT versions in common use.

Additional considerations for auditory versions are regional variations in spoken English. For example, Gronwall's original tape was created in New Zealand, whereas most Levin/50-item-per-trial versions were created in the United States (e.g., Diehr et al., 2003; Wiens et al., 1997). Others were created in Canada (e.g., Stuss et al., 1987) or Britain (e.g., CHIPASAT). A French-Canadian version also exists (see Table 9–25).

Other versions have been used in fMRI paradigms (e.g., Audoin et al., 2003; Lazeron et al., 2003) or have become core evaluation tools for MS studies (Cohen et al., 2002; Diamond et al., 1997; Fischer et al., 1999; Rao et al., 1991; Rudick et al., 1997). Recent innovations are the adaptive testing PASATs, which adjust ISIs based on examinee performance level (e.g., Adjusting-PSAT; Tombaugh, 1999).

ADMINISTRATION

Gronwall (61-Item-per-Trial) Version

Instructions are on the tape. Loudness should be well above threshold and adjusted to a comfortable listening level for each subject. For some very impaired subjects, the instructions may need to be reiterated and expanded by the examiner. See Figure 9–4 for specific instructions. The examiner records responses on the test protocol (Figure 9–5).

The test begins by a practice trial, followed by the first (2.4-second) trial. The examinee is warned before each trial that it will be faster than the previous one. The examiner allows at least 60 seconds between trials. Many patients find even the slower presentation trials (2.4 seconds, 2.0 seconds) difficult. Consequently, the two faster rates (1.6 seconds, 1.2 seconds) are given only if subjects perform adequately at the slower rates (i.e., above 20 items correct on the 2.0-second trial, or more than 40 correct on the 2.4-second trial).

Levin (50-Item-per-Trial) Versions

These include the original version developed by Levin (see Table 9–26 and Figure 9–6), and the modified version developed by Diehr et al. (i.e., PASAT-50, PASAT-100, and PASAT-200; 1998; 2003) using slightly different ISIs. Instructions for the latter are presented in Figure 9–7, along with the test form

Table 9–26 Summary of Characteristics of Selected PASAT Versions

	Author and/or Norms	Stimulus Modality	Response Modality	ISI	Items per Trial	Maximum Score per Trial	Items on Each Trial
Audiotape Versions							
Gronwall PASAT	Gronwall, 1977 Stuss et al., 1988 Crawford et al., 1998	Auditory	Verbal	2.4, 2.0, 1.6, 1.2 s	61	60	Repeated
Levin PASAT	Roman et al., 1991 Brittain et al., 1991 Wiens et al., 1997	Auditory	Verbal	2.4, 2.0, 1.6, 1.2 s	50	49	Unique
PASAT-200	Diehr et al., 1998	Auditory	Verbal	3.0, 2.4, 2.0, 1.6 s	50	49	Unique
PASAT-100	Diehr et al., 2003	Auditory	Verbal	3.0, 2.4, 2.0, 1.6 s	50	49	Unique
PASAT-50	Diehr et al., 2003	Auditory	Verbal	3.0, 2.4, 2.0, 1.6 s	50	49	Unique
CHIPASAT	Johnson et al., 1988	Auditory	Verbal	2.8[a], 2.4, 2.0, 1.6, 1.2 s	61	60	Repeated
Computer Versions							
Computerized PASAT	Wingenfeld et al., 1999[b]	Auditory	Verbal	2.4, 2.0, 1.6, 1.2 s			
PVSAT	Diamond et al., 1997 Fos et al., 2000	Visual	Verbal	2.4, 2.0, 1.6, 1.2 s[c]			
Adjusting-PSAT	Royan et al., 2004	Either	Verbal	Adjusts to individual's performance level			

Note: Duration of each spoken digit is about 0.4 seconds in the Gronwall version. For computer versions, see individual sources for items per trial, maximum score per trial, and items on each trial. [a]Used as practice trial only. [b]May no longer be commercially available. [c]Fos et al. (2000) report slightly different ISIs for the PVSAT (i.e., 2.5, 2.0, 1.5, 1.0 s).

Figure 9–4 Instructions for the PASAT (Gronwall Version).

(Instructions for the PASAT (Gronwall Version)

Oral and Written Demonstration

I am going to ask you to add together pairs of single-digit numbers. You will hear a tape-recorded list of numbers read one after the other. I will ask you to add the numbers in pairs and give your answers out loud. Although this is really a concentration task, and not a test to see how well you can add, it might help to do a little adding before I explain the task in more detail. Please add the following pairs of numbers together as fast as you can and give your answers out loud: 3,8 (11); 4,9 (13); 7,8 (15); 8,6 (14); 8,9 (17); 5,7 (12); 6,5 (11); 6,9 (15); 4,7 (11); 7,6 (13). Good. The task that I want you to do involves adding together pairs of numbers, just like you have done, except that the numbers will be read as a list, one after the other. Let me give you an example with a short, easy list. Suppose I gave you the following: 1, 2, 3, 4. Here is what you would do. After hearing the first two numbers on the list, which were 1 and 2, you would add these together and give your answer, 1+2 = 3. The next number on the list is 3, so when you heard it, you would add this number to the number right before it on the list, which was 2, and give your answer, 2+3 = 5. Are you following so far? The last number you heard is 4 (remember the list is 1,2,3,4), so you would add 4 to the number right before it, which was 3, and give your answer, 3+4 = 7. The important thing to remember is that you must add each number on the list to the number right before it on the list, and not to the answer you have just given. You can forget your answers as soon as you have said them. All you have to remember is the last digit that you have heard and add it to the next digit that you hear. OK? Let's try that short list again, only this time you say the answers. Ready? 1,2, (3), 3, (5), 4, (7). Now let's try another, longer practice list of numbers. This time the numbers on the list won't be in any particular order. Ready? 4,6, (10), 1, (7), 8, (9), 8, (16), 4, (12), 3, (7), 8, (11), 2, (10), 7, (9). Good.

If the subject has difficulty understanding the oral instruction, then provide a written demonstration. Say: That sounds complicated. Let me show you what I mean.

Write down a list of five numbers: 5, 3, 7, 4, 2. You see, you add the 5 and the 3 together, and say 8, then you have to forget the 8 and remember the 3. When the 7 comes along you add it to the 3, and say 10, and you have to remember the 7. All right, what do you say after 4?

Continue until the subject understands what he or she is to do. Say: It's very easy when all the numbers are written down for you. Try it with me saying some numbers to you.

See above list. Discontinue if the subject is unable to get at least the first three answers from the unpaced practice list correct, after two trials.

Paced Practice

Remember that I said the numbers would be tape-recorded? The task is not easy and no one is expected to get all of the answers right. The hard part is keeping up with the speed of the recording. However, if you can't answer in time, don't worry; just wait until you hear two more numbers, add them together and go on from there. OK? Any questions? I'll play a practice list of numbers and get you to give the answers.

Play to the end of the first practice list.

Test Trials

You see what I meant about the task measuring how well you can concentrate. It doesn't have anything to do with how smart you are. Now we'll try the first real trial. This trial is just the same as the practice trial you've just done, except that it is six times as long, so it goes on for almost two and a half minutes. Don't worry if you make adding mistakes or miss some answers. This is a difficult task. I want to see not only how long you can keep going without stopping, but also how quickly you can pick up again if you do stop. No one is expected to get all the answers. After this trial, we will take a break and then do another trial at a faster speed.

(Figure 9–8). Instructions for the Diehr et al. version are simpler and shorter than those for the Gronwall version. Also note that test administration is stopped and the instructions reiterated if the subject is found to engage in "chunking" responses. Chunking involves responding only to alternate items to reduce the working memory requirements of the task; see *Scoring* and *Comment* for further discussion of the effect of this strategy on performance.

CHIPASAT

Instructions are on the tape. The test begins with a demonstration involving four items, followed by a practice session involving 11 items, which the examiner also demonstrates on paper. Although the test has five trials, the first trial (i.e., 2.8 seconds) is not scored but is rather considered as another practice trial. The CHIPASAT test form is presented in Figure 9–9.

Figure 9–5 Gronwall PASAT form.

PASAT—Gronwall Version

Name _____   Date _____   Tested by _____

	2.4″	2.0″	1.6″	1.2″		2.4″	2.0″	1.6″	1.2″		2.4″	2.0″	1.6″	1.2″
7 (9)					8 (12)					5 (13)				
5 (12)					7 (15)					4 (9)				
1 (6)					1 (8)					8 (12)				
4 (5)					6 (7)					2 (10)				
9 (13)					3 (9)					1 (3)				
6 (15)					5 (8)					7 (8)				
5 (11)					9 (14)					5 (12)				
3 (8)					2 (11)					9 (14)				
8 (11)					7 (9)					1 (10)				
4 (12)					5 (12)					3 (4)				
3 (7)					3 (6)					6 (9)				
2 (5)					4 (7)					2 (8)				
6 (8)					7 (11)					9 (11)				
9 (15)					1 (8)					7 (16)				
3 (12)					5 (6)					8 (15)				
4 (7)					8 (13)					2 (10)				
5 (9)					3 (11)					4 (6)				
8 (13)					4 (7)					7 (11)				
6 (14)					6 (10)					6 (13)				
4 (10)					8 (14)					3 (9)				

	Total Correct	z	%ile
2.4″ Pacing	_____	_____	_____
2.0″ Pacing	_____	_____	_____
1.6″ Pacing	_____	_____	_____
1.2″ Pacing	_____	_____	_____

Other Versions

See respective sources. Specific parameters of administration differ among computerized versions. For example, for the Computerized PASAT (Wingenfeld et al., 1999) responses are recorded via a voice-activated computer recording, replayed, and then hand-scored for correctness of responding. For the Adjusting-PSAT (Tombaugh, 1999), the examinee responds orally, and the response is then typed into the computer by the examiner for automatic scoring of responses.

ADMINISTRATION TIME

Administration time depends on the version used. For the Gronwall version, about 15 to 20 minutes are required if all four trials are given. Levin versions are somewhat briefer, with

Figure 9–6 Form for the Levin version of the PASAT. *Source:* Courtesy of Dr. Julia Hannay.

PASAT—Levin Version

Name _____   Date _____
Education _____   Age _____ Sex _____

Series 1			Series 2			Series 3			Series 4		
9	—		2	—		4	—		3	—	
1	10		4	6		8	12		2	5	
4	5		5	9		6	14		6	8	
2	6		4	9		2	8		5	11	
8	10		3	7		2	4		4	9	
6	14		1	4		9	11		3	7	
5	11		8	9		3	12		1	4	
3	8		6	14		4	7		6	7	
4	7		9	15		5	9		5	11	
9	13		2	11		8	13		9	14	
1	10		9	11		1	9		8	17	
3	4		8	17		6	7		4	12	
6	9		6	14		3	9		2	6	
8	14		1	7		8	11		1	3	
2	10		3	4		6	14		2	3	
5	7		4	7		2	8		4	6	
1	6		5	9		4	6		9	13	
8	9		2	7		1	5		3	12	
6	14		1	3		9	10		6	9	
9	15		9	10		5	14		8	14	
2	11		4	13		1	6		5	13	
4	6		5	9		9	10		4	9	
3	7		6	11		8	17		3	7	
5	8		2	8		2	10		8	11	
6	11		3	5		5	7		2	10	
5	11		8	11		4	9		5	7	
8	13		4	12		6	10		1	6	
9	17		2	6		3	9		6	7	
4	13		1	3		6	9		9	15	
3	7		9	10		3	9		4	13	
1	4		8	17		2	5		8	12	
2	3		3	11		9	11		5	13	

(*continued*)

Figure 9–6 (*continued*)

	Series 1			Series 2			Series 3			Series 4	
6	8		5	8		1	10		9	14	
3	9		6	11		8	9		2	11	
4	7		9	15		5	13		6	8	
8	12		8	17		4	9		1	7	
9	17		4	12		9	13		3	4	
5	14		3	7		6	15		4	7	
1	6		2	5		2	8		2	6	
2	3		5	7		4	6		3	5	
8	10		1	6		3	7		9	12	
1	9		6	7		5	8		5	14	
2	3		1	7		8	13		6	11	
5	7		8	9		1	9		8	14	
3	8		5	13		5	6		1	9	
9	12		6	11		6	11		6	7	
6	15		3	9		9	15		4	10	
4	10		2	5		8	17		9	13	
3	7		9	11		3	11		2	11	
6	9		4	13		1	4		3	5	
No. Correct											

Figure 9–7 Instructions for the PASAT-200, PASAT-100 and PASAT-50. *Source:* Adapted from Diehr et al., 2003.

On the tape recording, you will hear a man's voice say numbers from 1 to 9. Add the first number that you hear to the second number that you hear and tell me the sum out loud. Then add the second number that you hear to the third number that you hear and tell me the sum out loud. Let's do some examples.

The examinee is given four sample sequences of four digits each orally. The instructions are repeated as needed, and participants who have trouble with the practice items are given additional practice items written on a piece of paper to clarify which digits are to be added together. Then the examinee is told: *The tape moves quickly so be sure to get your answer in before you hear the next number. If you get lost, be sure to pick up the addition as quickly as you can.*

The examinee is given encouragement to perform at his or her best and is given brief rests between the four sample sets of numbers if he or she appears frustrated. In addition, if an examinee initially uses a strategy of adding every other pair of numbers, the tape is stopped, the instructions repeated, and the tape restarted.

Figure 9–8 PASAT-50, PASAT-100, and PASAT-200 Forms. *Note:* This version consists of the Diehr et al. (2003) adaptation of the Levin version of the PASAT. *Source:* Courtesy of Dr. Mariana Cherner, April 2005.

ID _____   Visit No _____   Age _____   Education _____
Date ____/____/____   Staff ID _____   Gender _____   Ethnicity _____

PACED AUDITORY SERIAL ADDITION TASK

Channel 1 Correct/Response	Channel 2 Correct/Response	Channel 3 Correct/Response	Channel 4 Correct/Response
1. 9..........	2..........	4..........	3..........
2. 1..........10____	4..........6____	8..........12____	2..........5____
3. 4..........5____	5..........9____	6..........14____	6..........8____
4. 2..........6____	4..........9____	2..........8____	5..........11____
5. 8..........10____	3..........7____	2..........4____	4..........9____
6. 6..........14____	1..........4____	9..........11____	3..........7____
7. 5..........11____	8..........9____	3..........12____	1..........4____
8. 3..........8____	6..........14____	4..........7____	6..........7____
9. 4..........7____	9..........15____	5..........9____	5..........11____
10. 9..........13____	2..........11____	8..........13____	9..........14____
11. 1..........10____	9..........11____	1..........9____	8..........17____
12. 3..........4____	8..........17____	6..........7____	4..........12____
13. 6..........9____	6..........14____	3..........9____	2..........6____
14. 8..........14____	1..........7____	8..........11____	1..........3____
15. 2..........10____	3..........4____	6..........14____	2..........3____
16. 5..........7____	4..........7____	2..........8____	4..........6____
17. 1..........6____	5..........9____	4..........6____	9..........13____
18. 8..........9____	2..........7____	1..........5____	3..........12____
19. 6..........14____	1..........3____	9..........10____	6..........9____
20. 9..........15____	9..........10____	5..........14____	8..........14____
21. 2..........11____	4..........13____	1..........6____	5..........13____
22. 4..........6____	5..........9____	9..........10____	4..........9____
23. 3..........7____	6..........11____	8..........17____	3..........7____
24. 5..........8____	2..........8____	2..........10____	8..........11____
25. 6..........11____	3..........5____	5..........7____	2..........10____
26. 5..........11____	8..........11____	4..........9____	5..........7____
27. 8..........13____	4..........12____	6..........10____	1..........6____
28. 9..........17____	2..........6____	3..........9____	6..........7____
29. 4..........13____	1..........3____	6..........9____	9..........15____
30. 3..........7____	9..........10____	3..........9____	4..........13____
31. 1..........4____	8..........17____	2..........5____	8..........12____
32. 2..........3____	3..........11____	9..........11____	5..........13____
33. 6..........8____	5..........8____	1..........10____	9..........14____
34. 3..........9____	6..........11____	8..........9____	2..........11____
35. 4..........7____	9..........15____	5..........13____	6..........8____
36. 8..........12____	8..........17____	4..........9____	1..........7____
37. 9..........17____	4..........12____	9..........13____	3..........4____
38. 5..........14____	3..........7____	6..........15____	4..........7____
39. 1..........6____	2..........5____	2..........8____	2..........6____
40. 2..........3____	5..........7____	4..........6____	3..........5____
41. 8..........10____	1..........6____	3..........7____	9..........12____
42. 1..........9____	6..........7____	5..........8____	5..........14____
43. 2..........3____	1..........7____	8..........13____	6..........11____
44. 5..........7____	8..........9____	1..........9____	8..........14____
45. 3..........8____	5..........13____	5..........6____	1..........9____
46. 9..........12____	6..........11____	6..........11____	6..........7____
47. 6..........15____	3..........9____	9..........15____	4..........10____
48. 4..........10____	2..........5____	8..........17____	9..........13____
49. 3..........7____	9..........11____	3..........11____	2..........11____
50. 6..........9____	4..........13____	1..........4____	3..........5____
#Attempted: ☐☐	#Attempted: ☐☐	#Attempted: ☐☐	#Attempted: ☐☐
#Correct: ☐☐	#Correct: ☐☐	#Correct: ☐☐	#Correct: ☐☐
50-Item Score ☐☐ (Channel 1 correct)	100-Item score ☐☐ (Channel 1 + Channel 2 correct)		200-Item score ☐☐☐ (Total correct)

590

NAME: DATE OF BIRTH:

AGE: DATE OF TEST:

RESULTS SUMMARY:

                   TRIAL: 2.8 2.4 2.0 1.6 1.2

NUMBER CORRECT:

DEVIATION FROM NORM:

ERRORS:

OMISSIONS:

SEQUENCE:

DEMONSTRATION: 2 3 1 4
                  5 4 5

PRACTICE	REPEAT
1 3 4 2 5 3 2 4 1 1 3	1 3 4 2 5 3 2 4 1 1 3
4 7 6 7 8 5 6 5 2 4	4 7 6 7 8 5 6 5 2 4

CHIPASAT: 2.8	CHIPASAT: 2.4
1 2 5 1 4 5 1 5 3 5 2	1 2 4 1 3 5 5 2 3 4 1
3 7 6 5 9 6 6 8 8 7	3 6 5 4 8 10 7 5 7 5
2 4 5 2 3 2 3 2 4 1	2 5 1 4 5 1 5 3 5 2
4 6 9 7 5 5 5 5 6 5	3 7 6 5 9 6 6 8 8 7
1 3 5 3 3 1 5 4 4 5	2 4 5 2 3 2 3 2 4 1
2 4 8 8 6 4 6 9 8 9	4 6 9 7 5 5 5 5 6 5
2 4 1 2 1 4 2 2 3 5	1 3 5 3 3 1 5 4 4 5
7 6 5 3 3 5 6 4 5 8	2 4 8 8 6 4 6 9 8 9
5 2 1 4 3 4 5 1 4 5	2 4 1 2 1 4 2 2 3 5
10 7 3 5 7 7 9 6 5 9	7 6 5 3 3 5 6 4 5 8
2 3 2 3 5 4 4 1 3 3	5 2 1 4 3 4 5 1 4 5
7 5 5 5 8 9 8 5 4 6	10 7 3 5 7 7 9 6 5 9

NUMBER CORRECT: NUMBER CORRECT:

DEVIATION FROM NORM: DEVIATION FROM NORM:

ERRORS: ERRORS:

OMISSIONS: OMISSIONS:

SEQUENCE: SEQUENCE:

(*continued*)

Figure 9.9 *(continued)*

CHIPASAT: 2.0

2 1 4 2 2 3 5 5 2 1 4
   3 5 6 4 5 8 10 7 3 5

3 4 5 1 4 5 2 3 2 3
7 7 9 6 5 9 7 5 5 5

5 4 4 1 3 3 2 4 1 1
8 9 8 5 4 6 5 6 5 2

  3 2 4 3 1 5 1 2 4 1
  4 5 6 7 4 6 6 3 6 5

  3 5 5 2 3 4 1 2 5 1
  4 8 10 7 5 7 5 3 7 6

   4 5 1 5 3 5 2 2 4 5
   5 9 6 6 8 8 7 4 6 9

NUMBER CORRECT:

DEVIATION FROM NORM:

ERRORS:

OMISSIONS:

SEQUENCE:

CHIPASAT: 1.6

1 4 5 2 3 2 3 5 4 4 1
  5 9 7 5 5 5 8 9 8 5

3 3 2 4 1 1 3 2 4 3
4 6 5 6 5 2 4 5 6 7

1 5 1 2 4 1 3 5 5 2
4 6 6 3 6 5 4 8 10 7

3 4 1 2 5 1 4 5 1 5
5 7 5 3 7 6 5 9 6 6

3 5 2 2 4 5 2 3 2 3
8 8 7 4 6 9 7 5 5 5

2 4 1 1 3 5 3 3 1 5
4 6 5 2 4 8 8 6 4 6

NUMBER CORRECT:

DEVIATION FROM NORM:

ERRORS:

OMISSIONS:

SEQUENCE:

CHIPASAT: 1.2

1 4 5 1 5 3 5 2 2 4 5
  5 9 6 6 8 8 7 4 6 9

2 3 2 3 2 4 1 1 3 5
7 5 5 5 5 6 5 2 4 8

3 3 1 5 4 4 5 2 4 1
8 6 4 6 9 8 9 7 6 5

2 1 4 2 2 3 5 5 2 1
3 3 5 6 4 5 8 10 7 3

4 3 4 5 1 4 5 2 3 2
5 7 7 9 6 5 9 7 5 5

3 5 4 4 1 3 3 2 4 1
5 8 9 8 5 4 6 5 6 5

NUMBER CORRECT:

DEVIATION FROM NORM:

ERRORS:

OMISSIONS:

SEQUENCE:

an average time of about 11 minutes for full-length forms, and about six to eight minutes for short forms (PASAT-200, PASAT-100, and PASAT-50, respectively; Diehr et al., 2003).

SCORING

Scores

Several scores can be derived. These are considered in turn.

Total Number of Correct Responses. This is the most commonly used metric for PASAT performance. Scores are typically tallied by trial, in addition to a total score across trials. Note that using the total number of errors (not including omissions) rather than the number correct may be misleading, as the number of errors may decrease over trials. This occurs because examinees tend to respond to fewer items as trial difficulty increases (Wingenfeld et al., 1999).

To score the Gronwall version, the examiner records the number of correct responses per trial (i.e., at the four pacing rates). To be scored as correct, a response must be made before presentation of the next stimulus. The maximum score per trial is 60 (maximum total score = 240). The examiner should also compute the proportion of responses that were errors (summed across all trials). Note that omissions are also treated as errors. The proportion of errors should be less than 10%. If the proportion exceeds 20%, the PASAT is probably invalid. Incorrect answers may actually be relatively rare compared with omissions. For example, only one participant in the study by Wingenfeld et al. (1999) met the exclusion criterion of over 20% errors.

Most Levin or 50-items-per-trial versions use the total number correct per trial as the main outcome measure. To use the extensive norms developed by Diehr et al. (2003), the total number correct across trials must be computed (maximum score = 196). The total is then used to compute demographically corrected scores following the procedures outlined in Table 9–35.

To score the CHIPASAT, the total number of correct responses should be computed (Johnson et al., 1988). The percent correct per trial can also be computed; some have argued that this may provide a more precise measure of information processing ability (see Dyche & Johnson., 1991b).

Time per Correct Response. The practice of converting the total number of correct responses into "time per correct response" as a measure of processing speed, recommended in the previous edition of this text (see Spreen & Strauss, 1998), may yield inaccuracies. The approach involves dividing the duration of each trial by the number of correct responses for that trial. The problem is that the resulting score does not actually provide information on the speed at which responses occur (Tombaugh et al., 2004). Procedures that actually measure speed of response are preferred if information on processing speed is sought. To date, only computerized versions allow precise timing of response speed.

Dyad/Chunking Scoring. Additional scores have also been derived that are presumed to have higher sensitivity to impairment. One of these is the *dyad* score. A dyad is scored when two consecutive correct answers are given by the subject. The dyad score helps determine whether the examinee elected not to attempt every item presented by adopting a "chunking" strategy to improve performance (i.e., responding to every alternate item instead of to every consecutive item; Fisk & Archibald, 2001; Snyder et al., 1993). Because responding only to alternate items significantly reduces the working memory requirements of the task and allows a longer response time per correct item, an inaccurate estimate of information processing speed is therefore obtained if only the number of correct responses is considered. A percent dyad score (Fisk & Archibald, 2001; Snyder et al., 1993) can be computed, which consists of the percentage of total correct responses accounted for by dyads. See Figure 9–10 for an example and scoring instructions.

Chunking scores correspond to the number of correct responses that followed a skipped response (see Figure 9–10). Both control and clinical populations tend to use chunking strategies as task difficulty increases, as do younger children (Johnson et al., 1988). Note that the examiner must write down incorrect, correct, and omitted responses to derive dyad/chunking scores.

In this way, dyads reflect adherence to task demands, whereas chunking reflects the use of a compensatory strategy to compensate for difficulties keeping up with the pace of the task (Shucard et al., 2004). Thus, the percent dyad score does not reflect performance accuracy, but is instead a reflection of the individual's ability to follow task instructions (Shucard et al., 2004). For example, an individual with a high percent dyad score followed task instructions well (i.e., did not revert to responding to alternate items only), even if performance level was poor (as evidenced by few correct responses overall). This individual may actually have a better information processing capacity than another individual who attained a high overall performance (i.e., a high number correct) by circumventing the test's imposed pace with chunking.

Snyder and Cappelleri (2001) use a simpler technique that takes into account both performance level and strategy; they compute the mean number of dyads obtained across the four trials of the PASAT. This score appears to be more clinically sensitive than other more traditional PASAT scores (Snyder & Cappelleri, 2001).

Diehr et al. (2003) use a much simpler approach. Their instructions for the PASAT-200 simply require examiners to halt the testing session and repeat instructions if examinees begin engaging in chunking (Figure 9–7).

Computer-Derived Scores. Computer versions typically provide more scoring options, including tabulation of omitted responses, number of errors, number of suppression failures (i.e., adding to the sum of the last addition rather than to the last digit presented), number of strings of three consecutive correct responses, and longest sequence of correct responses

Figure 9–10 Dyad and chunking scoring for the PASAT. *Source:* Reprinted with permission from Shucard et al., 2004.

Dyad Score

- A correct response that is preceded by a correct response. The response to the first pair of numbers at each presentation rate, if correct, is scored as a dyad.
- Dyad scores are tallied to yield a total dyad score for each presentation rate. (Fisk and Archibald, 2001).

Chunking Score

- A correct response that is preceded by a skipped response.
- Chunking scores are tallied to yield a total chunking score for each presentation rate.

Other Score

- A correct response that is preceded by an incorrect response.
- Other scores are tallied to yield a total other score for each presentation rate.

Total dyad score + total chunking score + total other score = total correct.
Percent dyad = (total dyad score/total correct score) × 100
Percent Chunking = (total chunking score/total correct score) × 100

PASAT Dyad/Chunking Scoring Example:

Stimulus Sequence	Correct Response	Response given by participant	Scoring
2			
7	9	9 (correct)	Dyad
3	10	No response	No score
4	7	7 (correct)	Chunking
8	12	No response	No score
1	9	9 (correct)	Chunking
5	6	6 (correct)	Dyad
9	14	17 (incorrect)	No score
1	10	10 (correct)	Other*
3	4	4 (correct)	Dyad
2	5	5 (correct)	Dyad

*Not a dyad or chunking; this response is considered a correct score according to the standard PASAT scoring and is included in the total correct score.

(Wingenfeld et al., 1999). Note, however, that less is known about the psychometric properties and research correlates of these kinds of scores. Computer versions can also provide reaction time data, although these may not always be precise due to various computer limitations in some versions, such as lack of discrimination between actual responses and other sounds made by subjects (i.e., throat clearing), and lack of precision of reaction time data because of software/hardware constraints.

One recent innovation is the Adjusting-PSAT, which uses the temporal threshold (the shortest ISI yielding a correct response) in addition to the number of correct responses (Tombaugh, 1999). Among possible PASAT scores, it may be the variable that most closely captures the construct of information processing *speed* (see *Comment*).

DEMOGRAPHIC EFFECTS

Age

Age is related to PASAT performance in most samples (Brittain et al., 1991; Roman et al., 1991; Stuss et al., 1988; Wiens et al., 1997). The exceptions to this trend are studies involving young adults, which may suffer from restriction of range (e.g., Wingenfeld et al., 1999). In some studies, age effects may only become prominent after age 50 (e.g., Roman et al., 1991). Examination of normative data in this review indicates that the faster the rate of presentation, the worse the performance; this applies to all ages. (See also the discussion on numeric ability in *Validity*, which indicates cohort effects favoring older individuals.)

Age, and to a lesser extent arithmetic ability, also affects information-processing capacity in children. Older children achieve a greater number of correct responses in a given time than younger ones. Similarly, information-processing rate, as reflected in the average speed of response, improves exponentially with age, the greatest changes occurring in children aged 8 to 10 years (Johnson et al., 1988).

Education/IQ

Performance is correlated with education; the higher the educational level, the better the performance (Stuss et al., 1987, 1989). Similarly, performance is significantly related to IQ (Brittain et al., 1991; Crawford et al., 1998; Deary et al., 1991; Sherman et al., 1997; Wiens et al., 1997; see *Validity* for details). However, education effects have not been found in all studies. In contrast to the findings of Stuss et al. (1987), Brittain et al. (1991), using the Levin version, reported that education had little effect on performance on the Levin version. IQ effects, but not education effects, were reported in a recent, large normative study of the Levin version (Wiens et al., 1997). For a more thorough discussion of IQ effects, see *Validity*.

Gender

Males perform slightly better than females in some studies, but the effect is not considered clinically meaningful (Brittain et al., 1991; Wiens et al., 1997). In one large study, gender accounted for less than 1% of the variance in PASAT scores (Diehr et al., 2003). A lack of significant gender effect has also been reported for computerized versions (Wingenfeld et al., 1999). There is no gender effect in children (Johnson et al., 1988).

Ethnicity

Few studies have examined the effect of race/culture on PASAT performance. Brittain et al. (1991) found no significant race effects; however, race was not equally represented in all age ranges in this study (particularly older subjects), which complicates interpretation. In a large normative study using the Levin version, Wiens et al. (1997) found that ethnic differences on PASAT performance were actually due to the effects of IQ, age, and education rather than to race per se. Diehr et al. (2003) reported that age, education, and ethnicity were all significant predictors of short-form PASAT scores; demographically adjusted scores are therefore provided for this PASAT version (see later discussion).

NORMATIVE DATA

Gronwall Version

The original Gronwall norms are based on a sample of 80 individuals from New Zealand (Gronwall & Wrightson, 1974). Because this sample was predominantly male and not well described demographically, alternate norms are preferred.

Table 9–27 shows the demographic characteristics for the Gronwall version collected by Stuss et al. (1988); normative data are shown in Table 9–28. The normative data are based on samples of healthy North American adults. The data shown for young adults are similar to those reported by others (e.g., Gronwall, 1977; Weber, 1986) but somewhat lower than those provided by Crawford et al. (1998) on a U.K. sample.

Table 9–27 Characteristics of the Stuss et al. (1988) Normative Sample for the Gronwall Version of the PASAT

Sample type	Community volunteers
Number	90
Age	16 to 69 years
Geographic location	Ottawa, Canada
Education	Approximately 14 years
Gender	
Men	44
Women	46
Race/ethnicity	Not specified
Screening	No history of neurological and/or psychiatric disorder

Table 9–28 Stuss et al. (1988) Norms for the Gronwall Version of the PASAT

	Age in Years					
	16–29 (N = 30)		30–49 (N = 30)		50–69 (N = 30)	
Presentation	M	SD	M	SD	M	SD
2.4	47.4	10.1	43.4	10.2	43.5	13.6
2.0	42.0	12.5	41.9	10.2	35.6	14.6
1.6	36.0	13.0	33.1	12.2	30.8	15.9
1.2	27.4	9.9	24.6	10.6	21.2	14.4

Data derived from a sample of healthy, relatively well-educated adults.

Source: From Stuss et al., 1988.

Table 9–29 Characteristics of the Crawford et al. (1998) Normative Sample for the Gronwall Version of the PASAT

Sample type	Community volunteers
Number	152
Age	16 to 74 years ($M = 40.2$, $SD = 13.9$)
Geographic location	United Kingdom
SES	Social class based on occupation did not differ from census-derived social class of adult U.K. population.
Education	$M = 13.0$ ($SD = 2.9$)
Gender	
Men	77
Women	75
Race/ethnicity	Not specified
Screening	Via interview, for neurological, psychiatric, or major systemic disorder

The Crawford et al. (1998) sample characteristics and normative data are presented in Tables 9–29 and 9–30. Crawford et al. also provide regression equations to determine whether PASAT performance is discrepant with premorbid IQ (NART; Nelson, 1982) or current IQ (WAIS-R IQ; Table 9–31). The regression-based scoring program can be downloaded at Dr. Crawford's web site (http://www.abdn.ac.uk/~psy086/dept/psychom.htm). The regression method may be particularly useful in evaluating PASAT performance in individuals with

Table 9–30 Normative Data from Crawford et al. (1998) for the Gronwall Version of the PASAT for adults (U.K. Sample; Education = 13.0 years [SD = 2.9])

	Age		
	16–29 Years	30–49 Years	50–74 Years
N	38	78	36
Total PASAT	169.2	149.8	136.9
PASAT SD	30.12	40.29	43.79
PASAT SEM	9.38	12.54	13.63

Source: From Crawford et al., 1998.

modest premorbid intelligence, as low PASAT scores may not be indicative of acquired deficit in this population given the substantial association between IQ and PASAT scores. A case example of the use of this method is also described on p. 269 of Crawford et al. (1998).

Levin/50-Item Version

The two largest normative samples for the Levin version are provided by Wiens et al. (1997), and Diehr et al. (1998, 2003). The Diehr version is considered apart from the other normative datasets as it employed slightly different ISIs (3.0, 2.4, 2.0, and 1.6 seconds).

Demographic information and normative data for a large sample of healthy adults, stratified by IQ, are presented in Tables 9–32 and 9–33 as provided by Wiens et al. (1997). These norms are described as being based on the performance of "highly motivated" individuals; participants were generally well-educated applicants for civil service jobs. This primarily Caucasian sample does not extend past age 50 and is therefore inappropriate for older individuals.

Older norms for the 50-item Levin PASAT are provided by Brittain et al. (1991) and Roman et al. (1991). Brittain et al. (1991) provide data (total correct responses per trial as well as seconds per correct response) according to age and IQ, compiled from 526 normal healthy North American adults, ages 17 to 88 years. These norms cover a larger age range and are therefore still useful for evaluating older individuals. They are presented in Table 9–34. Norms provided by Roman et al. (1991), though not reproduced here, are based on a smaller group ($N = 143$) of North Americans of generally average to above-average IQ, aged 18 to 75 years. The norms are higher than those of Brittain et al.'s (1991) sample, perhaps reflecting IQ or education differences between the samples (i.e., the average education for the Roman et al. norms was 13 years).

Diehr et al.'s (1998) demographically corrected norms for the slightly modified Levin version (i.e., PASAT-200; see later discussion for PASAT-100 and PASAT-50 short forms) allow correction for age, education, and ethnicity, based on a large ($N = 560$), ethnically diverse sample. Interstimulus intervals for this version are 3.0, 2.4, 2.0, and 1.6 seconds.

Table 9–31 Predicted PASAT Scores Based on Premorbid IQ Estimate (NART*) and Current IQ (WAIS-R) at Different Ages

Predictors	Equations	Multiple R^2	SE_{est}	Discrepancy Required for One-Tailed Significance		
				.15	.10	.05
NART errors and age	$215.74 - (1.85 \times \text{NART}) - (.77 \times \text{Age})$	.52	34.87	35.9	44.6	57.2
WAIS-R FSIQ and age	$12.87 + (1.65 \times \text{FSIQ}) - (.87 \times \text{Age})$	.66	30.66	31.6	39.3	50.3

Note: These are one-tailed because only discrepancies suggesting that an examinee's PASAT performance is *below* their IQ are typically required in clinical practice.
*Nelson, 1982.

Source: From Crawford et al., 1998.

Table 9–32 Characteristics of the Wiens et al. (1997) Normative Sample for the Levin Version of the PASAT

Sample type	Civil service job applicants[a]
Number	821
Age	20 to 49 years ($M = 29.2$, $SD = 6.0$)
Geographic location	United States (Pacific Northwest)
Education	14.6 years[b]
Gender	
Men	672 (82%)
Women	149 (18%)
Race/ethnicity	
Caucasian	85.1%
African American	5.6%
Asian	3.9%
Hispanic	3.8%
Native American	1.6%
Screening	Basic academic skills and physical agility, medical screening for physical illness/limitation and substance abuse

[a]Norms collected over approximately 9 years. [b]Average IQ approximately 106 (WAIS-R).

The composition of the normative sample and procedure for score derivation are presented in Table 9–35; the test form is shown in Figure 9–8. Diehr et al. (1998) argue that in most contexts, demographically adjusted scores are preferred to IQ-corrected scores because, like PASAT performance, IQ may also be adversely affected by brain disease and injury.

Short Forms

Diehr et al. (2003) also provide demographically corrected PASAT scores for two short forms, based on either administering only the first trial (PASAT-50) or two first trials (PASAT-100) of the full-length version (PASAT-200). These short forms are based on normative data collected for the full-length administration. Procedures for calculating demographically corrected scores are presented in Table 9–35. The two-trial version (i.e., 100-item form) appears to be particularly promising (see *Comment*).

Dyad and Chunking Scoring

Although these scores are promising, extensive norms on these scoring variations are not available. At present, preliminary data exist on at least two control groups of healthy adults (Shucard et al., 2004; Snyder & Cappelleri, 2001).

CHIPASAT

Data for children aged 8 to 14.5 years on the CHIPASAT are provided by Johnson et al. (1988). Demographic information

and norms are provided in Tables 9–36 and 9–37. Data on correct responses per second, presumed to be a more precise measure of information processing speed by some authors, are available in Dyche & Johnson (1991b).

RELIABILITY

Internal Reliability

Cronbach's alpha for the four PASAT trials is very high in adults (i.e., $r = .90$; Crawford et al., 1998). In children, the CHIPASAT's split-half reliability is approximately .90 at different ages, implying high internal consistency (Johnson et al., 1988). It is also very high in adolescents ($r = .96$; Egan, 1988). Scores across the different pacings are highly correlated (r's between .76 and .95; MacLeod & Prior, 1996).

Test-Retest Reliability

Test-retest correlations following short retest intervals (7–10 days) are excellent ($r > .90$; McCaffrey et al., 1995). Others have reported slightly lower reliabilities over longer intervals such as four weeks, but test-retest reliability is at least adequate in these cases (i.e., $r = .73$ or larger; Schächinger et al., 2003). Long-term stability of over three months for the PASAT is excellent ($r = .83–.96$; Sjogren et al., 2000). In children, the CHIPASAT shows very high test-retest reliability for the overall mean score after a four-week interval, and good reliability across individual trials (range .78–.83; Dyche & Johnson, 1991a).

Practice Effects

There are significant practice effects on the PASAT (Gronwall, 1977; Schächinger et al., 2003). Normal subjects who are given the PASAT on two occasions, spaced one week apart, perform about 18% (or six points) higher on the second visit (Stuss et al., 1987). Similar practice effects have been reported in adults with traumatic brain injury (Stuss et al., 1989) and HIV infection (McCaffrey et al., 1995). In children (Dyche & Johnson, 1991a), performance improves about 20% at retest (mean difference of 3.8–7.3, depending on the trial).

Using the computerized Adjusting-PSAT, Baird et al. (submitted) found that practice effects were equally prominent whether the first retest occurred 20 minutes, one week, or three months after initial administration. Gains were maintained up to six months and were independent of stimulus modality (i.e., visual versus auditory) and type of number list (i.e., "easy" versus "hard" sums). Baird et al. suggest that the confounding effects of practice in retest situations may be lessened by performing a dual baseline (i.e., by administering the test twice during the initial session). Note that significant practice effects are reported for normals and specific patient groups when the PASAT is readministered several times *within* the same testing session (Johnson et al., 1997).

Gronwall (1977) reported that after the second presentation, practice effects tend to be minimal. However, this conclusion is

Table 9–33 Normative Data for the 50-Item per Trial Version of the PASAT, According to IQ

		Age		
		20–29 Years	**30–39 Years**	**40–49 Years**
FSIQ	80–89	$N = 27$	$N = 10$	$N = 0$
	Trial 1	42.1 (5.6)	40.9 (4.8)	—
	Trial 2	35.7 (6.1)	35.1 (6.8)	—
	Trial 3	28.2 (9.1)	31.1 (8.5)	—
	Trial 4	24.3 (7.4)	24.9 (7.0)	—
	Total	130.3 (22.4)	132.0 (24.0)	
FSIQ	90–99	$N = 116$	$N = 72$	$N = 7$
	Trial 1	42.0 (5.5)	40.8 (6.0)	33.7 (16.3)
	Trial 2	37.6 (6.9)	36.1 (8.2)	32.7 (11.8)
	Trial 3	32.5 (7.5)	31.6 (9.4)	27.1 (10.5)
	Trial 4	26.1 (7.0)	24.6 (7.9)	19.0 (6.5)
	Total	138.2 (22.9)	133.1 (27.9)	112.6 (39.9)
FSIQ	100–109	$N = 192$	$N = 94$	$N = 11$
	Trial 1	44.2 (4.4)	41.8 (6.5)	38.4 (8.8)
	Trial 2	40.4 (6.3)	37.8 (7.1)	36.4 (10.6)
	Trial 3	35.6 (7.1)	34.1 (8.0)	33.7 (10.8)
	Trial 4	29.9 (6.8)	28.5 (7.8)	26.4 (10.9)
	Total	150.1 (20.5)	142.2 (25.0)	135.1 (38.7)
FSIQ	110–119	$N = 95$	$N = 72$	$N = 11$
	Trial 1	44.7 (4.4)	43.9 (4.8)	41.9 (7.2)
	Trial 2	40.8 (6.8)	39.4 (7.5)	39.6 (7.0)
	Trial 3	37.6 (7.2)	36.4 (7.0)	35.0 (7.5)
	Trial 4	31.3 (7.3)	30.0 (7.4)	27.9 (8.2)
	Total	154.5 (22.8)	149.7 (23.5)	144.4 (27.2)
FSIQ	120–129	$N = 33$	$N = 44$	$N = 12$
	Trial 1	46.7 (2.5)	44.8 (5.4)	47.2 (2.3)
	Trial 2	43.7 (4.4)	40.7 (6.7)	43.7 (3.6)
	Trial 3	40.3 (6.4)	38.5 (7.0)	39.7 (7.6)
	Trial 4	35.1 (7.2)	31.7 (7.4)	32.1 (7.6)
	Total	166.0 (18.4)	155.6 (22.4)	162.7 (17.0)
FSIQ	130+	$N = 12$	$N = 7$	$N = 4$
	Trial 1	48.0 (1.4)	46.0 (3.9)	45.0 (3.7)
	Trial 2	46.5 (2.2)	39.7 (6.8)	43.8 (6.6)
	Trial 3	42.2 (6.3)	38.1 (6.8)	35.0 (5.2)
	Trial 4	35.2 (5.3)	30.7 (6.8)	28.8 (4.1)
	Total	171.8 (13.4)	154.6 (22.8)	152.5 (16.1)

Note: FSIQ based on WAIS-R.

Source: From Wiens et al., 1997. Reprinted with the kind permission of Psychology Press.

based on a study involving repeated administration of two different stimulus tapes. Feinstein et al. (1994) reported that younger subjects (aged 25–30 years) improved over a longer period compared with their older counterparts (41–57 years), who plateaued after six sessions spaced two to four weeks apart. However, significant methodological limitations, including the small number of subjects (10 normals), the administration of two versions at each testing session (auditory and visual, effectively doubling exposure to the paradigm), the use of visual examination versus statistical analysis, and the use of number of errors as dependent variables, limit conclusions that can be drawn from this study (Tombaugh, personal communication, June 2005).

Anecdotally, versions that employ unique number series on each trial (i.e., different number sets with increasing pace, as is the case in most 50-item versions) are thought to lead to lesser practice effects than those employing the same series of items for each trial. The latter includes most versions based on the Gronwall, 61-item paradigm. However, to date, there has been no convincing empirical evidence to support this assumption.

One explanation for the PASAT's significant practice effects is that examinees experience a reduction in subjective anxiety at retest due to familiarity with the testing paradigm, which accounts for suppressed performance at baseline and higher scores at retest (Dyche & Johnson, 1991a). There is no

Table 9–34 Normative Data from Brittain et al. (1991) in Mean Seconds per Correct Response

		IQ								
		<90			90–109			>109		
Age (years)		*N*	Time(s)	Errors	*N*	Time(s)	Errors	*N*	Time(s)	Errors
Trial 1										
<25	*M*	7	3.85	15.43	89	3.37	10.79	49	2.90	16.63
	SD		1.50	9.45		1.50	9.13		1.12	7.24
25–39	*M*	15	5.67	18.80	95	3.19	9.78	54	2.81	6.37
	SD		6.67	11.43		1.19	8.16		0.58	6.08
40–54	*M*	17	6.37	26.35	47	3.42	10.79	31	2.73	5.65
	SD		3.29	9.89		1.57	9.35		4.53	4.53
>54	*M*	18	6.56	28.83	54	4.97	21.78	50	3.80	14.24
	SD		2.65	6.84		2.05	10.45		1.66	10.36
Trial 2										
<25	*M*	7	3.52	18.71	89	3.20	14.84	49	2.90	11.06
	SD		1.13	9.16		1.74	8.66		1.75	8.81
25–39	*M*	15	4.21	20.47	95	3.15	14.98	54	2.65	10.74
	SD		2.88	10.24		1.43	8.28		0.55	6.81
40–54	*M*	17	5.72	28.06	47	3.14	15.15	31	2.57	9.97
	SD		3.10	8.57		1.12	8.48		0.52	7.18
>54	*M*	18	5.28	28.39	54	4.26	23.61	50	3.47	16.54
	SD		1.93	6.70		1.44	7.86		1.94	9.32
Trial 3										
<25	*M*	7	3.01	20.71	89	2.88	19.10	49	2.28	12.59
	SD		0.91	8.75		0.98	8.43		0.60	8.28
25–39	*M*	15	3.85	24.87	95	3.16	19.26	54	2.34	13.31
	SD		2.23	8.23		2.74	8.47		0.74	7.66
40–54	*M*	17	4.83	29.82	47	3.11	18.36	31	2.40	14.84
	SD		2.55	6.64		2.64	9.21		0.53	7.48
>54	*M*	18	4.15	28.50	54	3.49	25.04	50	3.27	20.90
	SD		1.51	4.87		0.97	6.08		1.99	8.50
Trial 4										
<25	*M*	7	3.38	29.00	89	2.67	24.22	49	2.07	18.59
	SD		1.56	7.21		1.03	7.77		0.59	7.52
25–39	*M*	15	3.07	28.67	95	3.35	25.64	54	2.20	20.61
	SD		0.75	5.47		5.86	7.14		0.56	7.18
40–54	*M*	17	4.60	32.76	47	2.70	25.34	31	2.28	21.61
	SD		2.71	6.90		0.85	6.68		0.54	7.13
>54	*M*	18	3.95	32.44	54	3.39	29.26	50	2.74	25.12
	SD		1.59	4.76		1.30	6.42		1.01	7.22
Total Trials										
<25	*M*	7	3.44	83.86	89	3.03	68.88	49	2.54	49.08
	SD		1.01	29.36		1.07	29.68		0.86	28.23
25–39	*M*	15	4.20	92.93	95	3.22	69.65	54	2.50	51.26
	SD		2.99	31.97		2.17	28.45		0.53	24.13
40–54	*M*	17	5.38	117.00	47	3.09	69.43	31	2.49	51.90
	SD		2.53	28.39		1.26	30.08		0.41	23.26
>54	*M*	18	4.98	118.06	54	4.02	99.76	50	3.32	76.82
	SD		1.44	20.37		1.13	27.01		1.41	31.59

Source: From Brittain et al., 1991. Reprinted with the kind permission of Psychology Press.

Table 9–35 Characteristics of the Diehr et al. (1998, 2003) Normative Sample and Procedure for Deriving Demographically Corrected PASAT-200, PASAT-100, and PASAT-50 Scores

Number	566
Age	20 to 68 years ($M = 39.7$, $SD = 12.1$)
Geographic location	Not specified, but presumably Southwestern United States/California
Sample type	Mixed (one group from a normative study, remainder consisting of controls from three different research studies)
Education	9 to 20 years ($M = 14.2$, $SD = 2.6$)[a]
Gender	
Men	61%
Women	39%
Race/ethnicity	
Caucasian	45%
African American	55%
Screening	History of neuropsychiatric condition (e.g., psychosis, developmental disability, substance abuse, TBI)

[a]Educational composition: 12% = <12 years; 21% = 12 years; 33% = 13–15 years; 34% = 16–20 years.

To obtain demographically corrected T scores, use the following values in the regression equations that follow. (Note that these values correspond to a PASAT version that employs ISIs of 3.0, 2.4, 2.0, and 1.6 seconds per digit. See Figures 9–7 and 9–8 for test administration instructions and test form)

Obtain the scaled score from the following conversion table, using the appropriate version. Then enter the appropriate values for education, age, and ethnicity (with the help of the values shown below) in the regression equation.

Scaled scores corresponding to total number of correct responses summed across trials for full-length and abbreviated PASAT versions (i.e., PASAT-200, PASAT-100, and PASAT-50), for use with demographic correction equations.

\multicolumn{3}{PASAT-200 Total}			\multicolumn{3}{PASAT-100 Total}			\multicolumn{3}{PASAT-50 Total}		
Min	Max	Scaled Score	Min	Max	Scaled Score	Min	Max	Scaled Score
24	33	2	0	19	2	0	10	2
34	44	3	20	21	3	11	12	3
45	55	4	22	29	4	13	16	4
56	66	5	30	39	5	17	19	5
67	77	6	40	46	6	20	24	6
78	88	7	47	52	7	25	29	7
89	99	8	53	59	8	30	33	8
100	110	9	60	68	9	34	37	9
111	121	10	69	73	10	38	41	10
122	132	11	74	79	11	42	44	11
133	142	12	80	84	12	45	46	12
143	153	13	85	89	13	47	47	13
154	164	14	90	92	14	48	48	14
165	175	15	93	94	15	49	49	15
176	186	16	95	96	16			
187	192	17	97	98	17			

Note: Min and Max values refer to total raw score across all trials.

Education (i.e., grade level of formal education completed; technical/vocational training are not counted as years of education)
Maximum values as follows:
High school = 12
GED = last high school grade completed
Two-year college = 14
Four-year college = 16
Master's/JD = 18
PhD/MD = 20

Ethnicity
Caucasian = 0
African American = 1

Regression Equations for Demographically Corrected T Scores

PASAT-200 T Score = $50.0 + (3.33 \times Scaled\ Score{-}10) + (0.1894 \times Age) - (0.8217 \times Education) + (7.314 \times Ethnicity)$

PASAT-100 T Score = $12.52 + (3.81 \times Scaled\ Score) + (0.24 \times Age) - (0.97 \times Education) + (6.72 \times Ethnicity)$

PASAT-50 T Score = $12.93 + (4.0 \times Scaled\ Score) + (0.23 \times Age) - (1.06 \times Education) + (5.87 \times Ethnicity)$

*PASAT-200 = four-trial, 50-item/trial version; PASAT-100 = two-trial, 15-item/trial version; PASAT-50 = one-trial, 50-item/trial version. All trials with ISIs = 3.0, 2.4, 2.0, and 1.6 seconds per digit. Each trial of 50 digits unique. Max raw score per trial = 49.

Note: The authors stress that care should be taken in using these formulas with subjects who have less than nine years of education, are of different ethnicity, or are younger than 20 or older than 68.

Source: From Diehr et al., 1998, 2003. Reprinted with the kind permission of Psychology Press.

Table 9–36 Characteristics of the Johnson et al. (1988) Normative Sample for the CHIPASAT

Sample type	Random selection from local schools
Number	315
Age	8 to 14 years, 6 months
Geographic location	London, United Kingdom
SES	Not reported
Parental education	Not reported
Gender	
Boys	148
Girls	167
Race/ethnicity	Not reported
Screening	Not reported

question that the PASAT does induce anxiety in some individuals (see *Validity*).

VALIDITY

Correlations Among Versions

Although more research is needed, among auditory versions, computerized and audiotape versions appear comparable (Wingenfeld et al., 1999). Additionally, short and long forms are highly correlated in healthy individuals (e.g., *r* = .86 for the PASAT-50 and *r* = .95 for the PASAT-100) and in HIV patients (Diehr et al., 2003).

Visual and auditory versions are also highly related. However, there are fundamental differences between the two paradigms that may yield different results in different clinical groups. The auditory (Gronwall) PASAT and visual PVSAT are highly correlated (i.e., *r* = .63–.73; Fos et al., 2000). PASAT and PVSAT also appear to have similar factor structures when evaluated with other attention tests (see later discussion). Note that Fos et al. (2000) found no order effects when both the auditory PASAT and PVSAT were administered to normals and individuals with TBI. However, modality-specific performance differences are found in some groups. For instance, deficits are found on both modalities of the test in patients with MS (Diamond et al., 1997), but not in chronic fatigue syndrome (Johnson et al., 1996).

Visual versions are thought to present less of an interference effect between modalities compared with auditory versions (Royan et al., 2004). Some have proposed that use of a similar input/output modality (verbal-auditory, in the standard version) leads to stimulus-response competition, especially as ISIs decrease over trials (Fos et al., 2000). This interference effect, when combined with demands on processing speed, is thought to underlie the PASAT's sensitivity in conditions such as head injury, and may explain why visual versions are generally easier than auditory versions (Royan et al., 2004). Versions that employ visual stimuli may not yield an interference effect due to use of alternate modalities for

stimulus and response (visual-verbal). When versions are compared, type of modality appears to be a larger moderator variable for PASAT performance than math skills (Tombaugh et al., 2004), even though the latter is a major factor in performance (see later discussion). Conversely, the visual version may be a purer measure of processing speed due to the lack of an interference effect and consequent demands on working memory (Tombaugh et al., 2004).

Ceiling effects may occur on trials with longer ISIs in some versions. This makes single-trial short forms based on longer ISIs (e.g., Diehr et al., 2003) less appropriate for higher functioning individuals. In the visual modality, Fos et al. (2000) found ceiling effects for the first two trials of the PVSAT, but no floor effects in a mixed sample of normal and head-injured college students, with the greatest increase in difficulty occurring from Trials 3 to 4 for both tests.

Correlations With Other Attention Tests

The PASAT is thought to measure a central information-processing capacity similar to that seen on divided-attention tasks (Gronwall & Sampson, 1974; Ponsford & Kinsella, 1992). Others note that the test consists of at least three components: working memory, information processing capacity, and information processing speed (Shucard et al., 2004).

There are a number of sources of corroborative evidence for construct validity of the PASAT. The test is moderately correlated to other measures of attention, such as Digit Span, Auditory Consonant Trigrams, d2 Test, Trail Making Test (particularly Trails B), Visual Search and Attention Test (VSAT), and Stroop test (Dyche & Johnson, 1991a; Gronwall & Wrightson, 1981; MacLeod & Prior, 1996; O'Donnell et al. 1994; Sherman et al. 1997), as well as to choice reaction time tasks (Deary et al., 1991; Schächinger et al., 2003). This has also been found in head-injured individuals with regard to the Freedom from Distractibility factor of the WAIS-R (Sherman et al., 1995). In normal individuals, the test appears to load on an attention-concentration factor, along with measures such as the Digit Span and WAIS-R Arithmetic (Crawford et al., 1998). However, math ability may account for more variance overall (Royan et al., 2004; Sherman et al., 1997; see later discussion).

In most factor-analytic studies involving clinical groups, the test also loads with other attention/processing speed tests. For instance, Larrabee and Curtiss (1995) found that the PASAT loaded on an attention, immediate memory, and information processing factor in a heterogeneous group of neuropsychology outpatients, along with Digit Span, Serial Digits, and WMS Mental Control. Likewise, the PASAT loaded on a sustained attention factor in a mixed sample of severe TBI patients and controls (Bate et al., 2001), along with TEA Lottery (sustained attention), Visual Elevator (attentional switching), and Digit Span Backward. In severely head-injured patients, the PASAT appears to load on the same factor as the Symbol Digit Modalities Test (Haslam et al., 1995). In patients with diabetes (Deary et al., 1991), the PASAT loads

Table 9–37 Normative Data for the Children's Version of the PASAT (i.e., CHIPASAT)

Age (Years)	CHIPASAT 2.4				CHIPASAT 2.0				CHIPASAT 1.6				CHIPASAT 1.2				CHIPASAT OVERALL				
	Correct Responses			Average Speed of Response in sec.	Correct Responses			Average Speed of Response in sec.	Correct Responses			Average Speed of Response in sec.	Correct Responses			Average Speed of Response in sec.	Correct Responses			Average speed of response in sec.	
	M	SD	%		M	SD	%		M	SD	%		M	SD	%		M	SD	%	M	SD
8–9 N=51	22.5	5.5	37.5	6.8	19.4	6.5	32.4	7.0	16.4	6.4	27.4	7.0	9.9	5.2	16.5	11.6	17.1	5.5	28.5	8.1	5.0
9–10 N=58	27.1	7.1	45.2	5.7	23.0	6.6	38.3	5.9	19.8	6.5	33.0	5.7	13.1	5.9	21.8	7.9	20.7	5.8	34.6	6.3	3.1
10–11 N=60	30.5	8.3	50.9	5.1	26.2	7.1	43.7	5.0	20.8	6.3	34.6	5.3	14.9	5.9	24.8	5.9	23.1	6.2	38.5	5.3	1.9
11–12 N=51	33.8	8.5	56.3	4.6	28.3	7.2	47.2	4.5	23.1	6.2	38.4	4.5	16.6	5.4	27.7	5.0	25.5	6.2	42.4	4.6	1.4
12–13 N=36	32.3	9.1	53.8	5.1	29.6	7.9	49.4	4.9	24.4	7.4	40.6	5.3	16.1	6.8	26.8	4.7	25.6	7.0	42.7	4.4	1.2
13–14 N=51	37.4	9.4	62.4	4.2	33.4	10.1	55.7	4.1	27.7	9.1	46.1	3.9	19.3	7.4	32.2	4.7	29.4	8.4	49.1	4.2	1.8
14–15 N=8	41.1	9.9	68.5	3.7	38.3	8.0	63.8	3.3	31.5	6.8	52.5	3.2	20.6	5.7	34.4	3.8	32.9	6.9	54.8	3.5	0.9

Source: From Johnson et al., 1988. Reprinted with permission from Blackwell Publishing/CANCOPY.

highest on the WAIS-R Freedom from Distractibility (FFD) factor. In schizophrenia spectrum disorders, the PASAT is highly related to performance on the WAIS-III Processing Speed Index and to sustained attention (d') on a continuous performance test (Townsend et al., 2001). The test also has been reported to load together with Trails B on a "focus-execute" factor (O'Donnell et al., 1994).

The test also appears to measure unique aspects of attentional functioning not measured by other paradigms. For instance, in one study, both PASAT and PVSAT loaded on a factor separate from other attentional measures such as Digit Span, Trails, and Stroop (Fos et al., 2000). Note that the factor structure may have been affected by method variance due to inclusion of multiple PASAT scores.

There is also some evidence that different PASAT speeds may index different processing stages. Deary et al. (1991) found that slower rates of presentation correlated moderately with scores from the RAVLT, whereas a faster rate showed little correlation with memory measures. In other studies, PASAT scores show only modest correlations with memory measures, and these are not consistently related to ISI (e.g., Sherman et al., 1997).

Correlations With IQ

Gronwall claimed that, although it is a cognitive task, the PASAT was only weakly correlated with intelligence (Gronwall & Sampson, 1974; Gronwall & Wrightson, 1981). Recent evidence indicates that correlations with IQ appear to be at least in the moderate range. For example, Crawford et al. (1998) gave the PASAT and WAIS-R to a sample of 152 healthy individuals. Principal components analysis revealed that the PASAT's loading on general intelligence was substantial and exceeded that of many WAIS-R subtests. Several studies have also found support for the test's significant association with IQ (Brittain et al., 1991; Deary et al., 1991; Sherman et al., 1997; Wiens et al., 1997).

Correlation With Mathematical Ability

Gronwall claimed that the PASAT was only weakly correlated with arithmetic ability (Gronwall & Sampson, 1974; Gronwall & Wrightson, 1981). Increasing evidence seems to indicate otherwise. Several studies indicate that the PASAT is moderately to highly correlated with numerical ability in both normal and clinical samples (e.g., .41–.68, Crawford et al., 1998; Sherman et al., 1997). For example, in head-injured patients, math-related tests (WAIS-R Arithmetic, WRAT-3 Mathematics) are the strongest unique predictors of PASAT performance (Sherman et al., 1997). Performance is also strongly related to math scores in the Adjusting-PSAT test, particularly when the auditory modality is used ($r = -.74$), with math accounting for 26% of the variance in threshold scores (i.e., the shortest ISI with a correct response; Royan et al, 2004). Other research also indicates that PASAT performance is related to reaction time on simple addition problems and to

recent attainment in school mathematics examinations and self-ratings of mental arithmetic skills (Chronicle & MacGregor, 1998).

The mechanism whereby higher arithmetic ability confers an advantage on the PASAT may be related to reaction time. Specifically, because shorter reaction time on math addition problems is associated with better PASAT performance (Chronicle & MacGregor, 1998), individuals who respond quickly to the addition problem have a longer time interval between items during which they can retain, recall, or rehearse the previous item. Conversely, individuals who take longer to compute the addition problem have minimal time in which to reactivate the previous digit, and hence are at a disadvantage (Chronicle & MacGregor, 1998). Interference and competition for cognitive resources between retention of the previously presented digit and computation with the current digit would also be more likely in subjects who take longer to respond, a situation that mirrors the increased difficulty level of shorter ISIs in all subjects as the test progresses.

Even though the addition skills involved in the PASAT appear basic, the degree of difficulty of the addition problem affects performance. Royan et al. (2004) and Tombaugh et al. (2004) found that item pairs yielding simple sums (i.e., sum = 2 to 10) yielded a higher proportion of correct responses compared with those requiring complex sums (sum = 11 to 18). Use of restricted number lists (e.g., sums = 2 to 10) may therefore reduce (but not eliminate) the impact of mathematical ability on PASAT performance (Royan et al., 2004: Tombaugh et al., 2004).

There may also be cohort effects on PASAT performance related to mathematical ability. Ward (1997) reported that the task was *less* easily accomplished by younger adults than by older adults. In their sample, younger adults performed worse on the PASAT compared with NART-matched older adults, despite better performance on other attention tasks. Ward concluded that cross-generational effects on numeracy favoring automaticity of memorized sums in older individuals may differentially affect PASAT performance depending on age cohort. Ward also noted that previous research indicates that simple addition is not necessarily accomplished in the same way by all individuals, by direct retrieval from memory. Rather, there is a range of strategies associated with different reaction times. This again raises questions about the role of numerical ability in PASAT performance. Crawford et al. (1998) noted that if cross-generational effects on numerical ability are present, these may attenuate the effect of age on PASAT performance, but likely not eliminate age effects altogether.

In children, CHIPASAT performance is moderately related to WISC-R Arithmetic, a subtest dependent on both math and attentional abilities (Dyche et al., 1991; Johnson et al., 1988). Because younger children may be less fluent in arithmetic, caution is needed in interpreting CHIPASAT performance of young children. Several children in the youngest age band were observed to count on their fingers in the normative sample (Johnson et al., 1988), which indicates that the test should only be reserved for children known to have adequate math ability and be used with caution in the youngest age group (8 to 9.5 years).

Clinical Studies

Head Injury. The PASAT is sensitive to mild concussion (Gronwall & Sampson, 1974; Gronwall & Wrightson, 1974) and appears to be a more sensitive indicator of information-processing capacity in head-injured patients than other standard measures of attention. These include the Attention/Concentration Index of the WMS-R (Crossen & Wiens, 1988), the Trail Making Test, and individual Wechsler subtests such as Digit Span (Cicerone, 1997). The test reportedly has high sensitivity in the context of severe head injury (Ponsford & Kinsella, 1992) and is related to time since head injury (Bate et al., 2001).

At the same time, a number of investigators (e.g., Levin et al., 1982; O'Shaughnessy et al., 1984; Sherman et al., 1997; Stuss et al., 1989) have reported no relation between the PASAT and measures of head-injury severity, such as PTA or loss of consciousness (LOC). For example, Stuss et al. (1989) found that in comparison with the PASAT and Trail Making Test, only the Auditory Consonant Trigrams explained more than 30% of the shared variance in PTA and coma duration (43% and 30%, respectively) in a group with severe head injuries. In a mild-concussion group, indices of head-injury severity were not correlated with the PASAT, and only the Auditory Consonant Trigrams distinguished patients from controls. Similarly, compared with other attention tests, the sensitivity of the PASAT to mild TBI is less than that of a continuous performance task, but clearly superior to that of other measures such as the TMT and Digit Span tasks, which do not employ an externally paced paradigm (Cicerone, 1997). Limited sensitivity to head injury has also been reported in samples with primarily high-functioning individuals, such as the college-educated head-injury sample evaluated by Fos et al. (2000).

Nevertheless, the PASAT appears to be more useful in identifying persistent postconcussion syndrome (PCS) compared with other attention tests (including Trails, Stroop, and Digit Span), possibly due to its combined requirements for working memory and processing speed. Classification accuracy estimates for PCS are provided in Table 9–38, based on data from Cicerone and Azulay (2002). A sensitivity of 56% has also been reported by Schmidt et al. (1994). In another study, 45% of patients with severe TBI obtained scores at or below the 10th percentile on the PASAT (Bradshaw et al., 1999). On the whole, the test appears to have better specificity than sensitivity, which suggests better utility in ruling out than ruling in PCS and TBI.

Less-than-ideal sensitivity of the PASAT in some studies may also relate to parameter differences across studies. For example, with regard to ISIs, while the easier trials (i.e., 2.4 seconds and 2.0 seconds) do not always yield group differences between individuals with severe TBI and controls, severe TBI

Table 9–38 Diagnostic Utility of the PASAT in Postconcussion Syndrome: Sensitivity, Specificity, Efficiency, Positive Predictive Power, Negative Predictive Power, and Diagnostic Accuracy (Odds Ratio and 90% Confidence Interval) for Scores Greater than −1.5 SDs Below the Mean

	PASAT[a]
Sensitivity	37.5
Specificity	84.4
Efficiency[b]	60.9
Positive predictive power	70.6
Negative predictive power	57.4
Odds ratio	3.1
90% Confidence interval	1.2–8.0

Note: The base rate of postconcussion syndrome in this sample was 50%; the sample included 32 postconcussive patients screened for exaggeration and 32 matched controls.
[a]Levin version; score = total number of correct responses on all four trials transformed to age-related z scores based on Roman et al. (1991) norms. [b]refers to the number of subjects correctly classified (True Positives + True Negatives / N).

Source: From Cicerone & Azulay, 2002. Reprinted with the kind permission of Psychology Press.

patients usually obtain lower scores on the more difficult trials (e.g., 1.6 seconds and 1.2 seconds; Bate et al., 2001). The PASAT's sensitivity to head injury may also relate, at least in part, to the type of injury sustained. Roman et al. (1991) suggest that the PASAT's ability to detect head injury is best in samples where injury is secondary to marked acceleration/deceleration forces and concomitant subcortical involvement, such as that following motor vehicle accidents. Head injuries secondary to assault, therefore, where acceleration/deceleration forces are less marked, and where associated subcortical or white matter damage is less extensive, are less likely to be associated with measurable impairments on the PASAT. Such an explanation, however, is unlikely to account for the findings of Sherman et al. (1997), who found that PASAT scores were unrelated to PTA or LOC in a sample consisting primarily of individuals who had been involved in motor vehicle accidents, and who had been screened for exaggeration.

Lastly, there may also be a self-selection bias in retrospective TBI/PCS studies, which complicates interpretation of findings. By definition, PASAT research studies include results of TBI patients who were able to finish the task. This is potentially problematic in that samples may overrepresent higher functioning individuals, given the PASAT's relatively high refusal/discontinuation rates in some patient groups (see later discussion).

Multiple Sclerosis. There is a large body of literature on PASAT performance in persons with MS (e.g., DeLuca et al., 1993; D'Esposito et al., 1996; Diamond et al., 1997; Fisk & Archibald, 2001). The test is commonly used in this population because rate of information processing is dependent on subcortical brain systems and white matter tracks, areas that are preferentially affected in this demyelinating disease (Fisk & Archibald, 2001). Deficits in performance in MS patients are hypothesized to occur because of slowed processing speed rather than working memory problems; as a result, the PASAT is more sensitive to impairment in MS than tasks that assess only working memory, such as Letter-Number Sequencing from the WAIS-III (Kalmar et al., 2004).

Because of its sensitivity to MS-related cognitive impairment, the PASAT has been recommended as a core measure in clinical trials involving MS patients. A 3.0-second-per-item, 60-item version constitutes part of the Multiple Sclerosis Functional Composite Score, which has been used in several multicenter MS outcome studies (Cohen et al., 2002; Fischer et al., 1999; Rudick et al., 1997). It is also a component of the Neuropsychological Screening Battery for Multiple Sclerosis (Rao et al., 1991).

There are issues regarding the sensitivity of different scores in this population. Some studies have not found differences between controls and MS patients (e.g., Fisk & Archibald, 2001; Staffen et al., 2002). However, this negative finding disappears when dyad scores are used to measure performance instead of number correct. For example, Fisk and Archibald (2001) found that, using the total correct score, differences between MS patients and controls actually decreased as speed demands increased, while differences in response strategy (i.e., answering only alternate items, a strategy measured using dyads/chunking scoring; see *Scoring*) increased as speed demands increased. In other words, they found that inability to adhere to the task requirements at later trials in MS patients artificially reduced the overall difficulty of the test. Both normals and MS patients tend to perform in this manner when task demands become excessive (Fisk & Archibald, 2001).

The PASAT is reportedly sensitive to treatment effects in MS (Cohen et al., 2002) and strongly correlated to total lesion volume (e.g., Hohol et al., 1997), especially when the mean number of dyads across the four trials is used as an outcome measure (Snyder & Cappelleri, 2001). The test is also sensitive to MS subtypes (see Aupperle et al., 2002, and Snyder et al., 2001, for further discussion).

Other Clinical Populations. The PASAT is sensitive to moderate hypoglycemia (Schächinger et al., 2003), a disorder that seems to increase reaction times and decrease accuracy by increasing omissions. Impaired PASAT performance has also been reported in chronic fatigue syndrome (Johnson et al., 1997). The PASAT is also particularly sensitive to the cognitive manifestations of schizophrenia spectrum disorders as seen in first-episode psychosis (Townsend et al., 2001) and schizotypal personality disorder (Mitropolou et al., 2002). The PASAT has also been used to examine cognitive function in chronic pain patients (Sjogren et al., 2000) and the cognitive effects of heading the ball in soccer players (Webbe et al., 2003). Patients with systemic lupus erythematosus, even without neurological impairment, perform below expectations when chunking scoring is used (Shucard et al., 2004).

Children. More research is needed on the utility of the CHIPASAT in children. However, improvements in CHIPASAT

performance are reported after renal transplantation in children (Mendley & Zelko, 1999).

Neuroanatomic Correlates

Mapping studies suggest that the PASAT activates several sites, consistent with its multifactorial task demands and sensitivity to several cognitive disorders (Lockwood et al., 2004). In particular, fMRI studies suggest that the PASAT activates a broad range of brain networks, including those important for attention and working memory (i.e., frontal and parietal areas; Lazeron et al., 2003).

Functional magnetic resonance imaging results suggest that different brain systems are activated in MS patients compared with controls (Staffen et al., 2002), even when PASAT performance is equivalent between groups. In controls, a visual version (PVSAT) activated the right cingulus gyrus (Brodmann area 32), whereas in MS patients, the right frontal cortex was activated along with areas in the left frontal lobe (Brodmann areas 6, 8, 9, 39). Increased effort on the part of MS patients to maintain normal performance levels and/or compensatory mechanisms recruiting other brain systems are thought to account for activation differences. Compensatory activation has been attributed to higher recruitment of executive systems (Audoin et al., 2003).

One important consideration in interpreting fMRI studies using the PASAT is the modality type (visual versus auditory) and the response type (e.g., use of paradigms that do not require an overt response to minimize movement artifact versus the standard approach). If the PASAT's sensitivity to neuropsychological deficits rests in its ability to elicit interference via the use of a single (verbal-auditory) stimulus-response channel rather than a dual (verbal-visual) channel (e.g., Royan et al., 2004; Tombaugh, et al., 2004; see *Comment*), fMRI studies that do not require an actual response from the subject to avoid motor artifacts may measure different abilities than the traditional auditory PASAT with verbal response. This possibility has not yet been systematically evaluated.

Impact of Anxiety, Task Difficulty, Mood, and Fatigue Effects

The PASAT has acquired the reputation of being an aversive task, even in normal individuals. It has also been used experimentally to induce stress (Lejuez et al., 2003) and to increase fatigue (Johnson et al., 1997). Diehr et al. (2003) even reported that several participants in their HIV longitudinal research preferred the lumbar puncture to the PASAT. In this study, over half of the sample reported significant discomfort associated with the full-length PASAT compared with 30% taking an abbreviated version. In a study involving MS patients, the PASAT was associated with the highest refusal/discontinue rate compared with other measures, with 17% of patients refusing to attempt the test and 6% of patients quitting in mid-administration (Aupperle et al., 2002). In another study, the PASAT was found to increase negative mood in normal individuals who were in a neutral or positive mood prior to the task. Further, those who were in a sad mood had poorer performance at the most rapid ISI (1.2 second) compared with those in a neutral mood, suggesting a negative effect of mood on performance (Holdwick & Wingenfeld, 1999). Anecdotal evidence also indicates that the CHIPASAT can be anxiety provoking for children (Dyche & Johnson, 1991b).

There is no doubt that the PASAT can be demanding and frustrating, and the clinical impression is that it may therefore not be appropriate for anxious individuals (Roman et al., 1991; Weber, 1986). The research reviewed previously, however, indicates that there may also be problems in administering the task to non-anxious individuals (see also Mathias et al., 2004). Modifications of the traditional PASAT such as short forms or use of the Adjusting-PSAT may be helpful in reducing discomfort by shortening the task. There is also a version that employs words instead of numbers ("day/night") to avoid the confound of mathematical skill level (PASOT). Although the test is less aversive to examinees, it is a less challenging task than the standard version (Gow & Deary, 2004), and therefore may not be as sensitive in some populations.

Although clinical impression suggests that fatigue adversely impacts performance, Johnson et al. (1997) found no evidence for fatigue effects when the PASAT was readministered four times within the same testing session. This applied both to normal controls and to patient groups whose conditions were associated with higher levels of fatigue, such as chronic fatigue syndrome, MS, and depression. Although self-ratings of fatigue worsened over administrations, these were not related to PASAT performance, which continued to improve over administrations due to a presumed practice effect (see *Reliability* for more information). Depression ratings were also not significantly related to PASAT performance in the patient groups. However, other studies indicate that depression is related to PASAT performance (e.g., Shawaryn et al., 2002). Indeed, in the context of MS, Demaree et al. (2003) conclude that depression increases the severity of processing speed deficits as measured by the PASAT.

Ecological Validity

The PASAT is reportedly related to the patient's subjective experience of symptoms (Gronwall, 1976), changes in the patient's personality (O'Shaughnessy et al., 1984), and readiness to return to work (Gronwall, 1977). It is also a strong predictor of employment status several years after head injury (Brooks et al., 1987). In MS patients, PASAT performance is also related to quality of life, particularly mental and emotional aspects of quality of life (Shawaryn et al., 2002) and to accident rate in driving simulations (Kotterba et al., 2003).

Malingering

The PASAT appears sensitive to dissimulation. Persons attempting to feign the effects of brain injury perform more poorly than nonmalingerers on the PASAT, at least at the longer interval of 2.0 seconds (Strauss et al., 1994). Studies using the PASAT in populations at risk for exaggeration (i.e., TBI, postconcussion disorder) should therefore employ techniques to identify individuals feigning cognitive dysfunction such as symptom validity testing.

COMMENT

The PASAT has now been used for many years as a measure of processing speed, divided attention, and working memory, and the evidence indicates that it is sensitive to the neurocognitive effects of several clinical conditions. It may also be particularly well suited to higher functioning individuals who may encounter ceiling effects on other attention tests. Specifically, because of its requirements for mathematical ability and its relationship to IQ and education, the test may best be conceptualized as a measure appropriate for average to above-average individuals (Wiens et al., 1997), including high-functioning children. Several recent, large normative datasets also increase the test's potential utility. We are particularly impressed by the PASAT-200, PASAT-100, and PASAT-50, by Diehr et al. (1998, 2003) because of the ability to adjust for demographic variables.

As is the case for all tests, users should be aware of the PASAT's unique limitations, which may make it less appropriate in certain circumstances or with certain patients. Screening for math ability is recommended when the PASAT is to be administered clinically. It should not be interpreted as measuring speed/attention in the context of difficulties with mathematics. Short forms of the PASAT (PASAT-50 and PASAT-100) appear promising, although one-trial versions may suffer from significant ceiling effects. The two-trial PASAT-100 is therefore preferred when short forms are needed.

Several versions of the test are available. While the most obvious differences across versions relate to different modality type, numbers of items per trial, and ISIs, actual item lists may also differ. Depending on the proportion of complex versus simple additions required in different number lists, this may also affect performance level. Careful selection of PASAT version, including selection of corresponding test forms, test parameters, and norms, is highly advised.

An additional consideration is test modality. As noted previously, several researchers have proposed that use of the same input/output modality (verbal-auditory, in the standard audiotape version) leads to stimulus-response competition, especially as ISIs decrease over trials (Fos et al., 2000). This interference effect, when combined with demands on processing speed, is thought to underlie the test's sensitivity to head injury and may explain why visual versions are usually easier than auditory versions (Royan et al., 2004: Tombaugh, et al., 2004). Versions that employ visual stimuli may not yield an interference effect due to use of alternate modalities for stimulus and response (i.e., visual-verbal). Visual versions may therefore be more appropriate for lower functioning individuals who would encounter floor effects on the standard auditory version. However, visual versions are not necessarily equivalent to each other. For instance, the visual mode of the Adjusting-PSAT employs a visual mask to prevent formation of afterimages, a manipulation that may not be used in other visual versions. Visual versions may also yield purer estimates of information processing speed, precisely because of the reduced demands on working memory.

With regard to audiotape versions, it is best to administer the audiotape that best matches the variation of spoken English used by the examinee (i.e., American tape to a U.S. patient). However, variations in standard English do not appear to affect performance; our own unpublished data suggest that similar scores are obtained in Canadian individuals regardless of whether an American or New Zealand accent is presented on the PASAT audiotape.

The type of score derived is also important. When people perform poorly on the PASAT, errors consist primarily of omissions, not incorrect responses (Schächinger et al., 2003; Wingenfeld et al., 1999). Mounting evidence suggests that the traditional scoring method (i.e., total number correct or time per correct response) may be inadequate in tapping working memory and processing speed. As mentioned previously, because examinees tend to use chunking strategies, selectively responding to alternate items at high presentation speeds as task demands increase, use of the total correct response score may lead to overestimation of ability in some examinees (Fisk & Archibald, 2001; Shucard et al., 2004; Snyder et al., 1993) by effectively allowing these examinees to circumvent the working memory and processing speed requirements of the test. Percent dyad or percent chunking scores are therefore recommended by some authors (e.g., Shucard et al., 2004); when the former is low and the latter high, the examinee is not following the imposed pace of the test. However, at present, these scores are restricted to research usage because comprehensive norms are not yet available. The PASAT-50, -100, and -200 (Diehr et al., 1998, 2003) avoid this problem altogether by requiring the examiner to halt and restart the administration if the examinee begins engaging in an alternate-item response strategy. The entire problem is completely eliminated with the use of paradigms such as the Adjusting-PSAT (see Royan et al., 2004).

Another point germane to scoring is the confusion surrounding the best way to estimate processing speed. Investigators and clinicians interested in a more precise estimate of processing speed should consider versions such as the Adjusting-PSAT (Royan et al., 2004; Tombaugh et al., 1999), which clearly measure the construct of speed somewhat separate from working memory (i.e., the shortest ISI with a correct response). Note that this version also eliminates the problem inherent in the differing sensitivity of various ISIs, since the ISI is continually adjusted to suit the patient's ability level. Unfortunately, this version is currently not commercially available.

With regard to other "speed" variables, reaction time on standard computer versions may also be promising and less affected by ceiling effects (Schächinger et al., 2003). However, because reaction time data depend on computer administration, users should be aware of any software/hardware limitations that may affect the reliability of reaction time data obtained

on specific computerized versions. Wingenfeld et al. (1999) also recommend caution in the use of computerized reaction time data that encode responses using voice-activated technology, as reaction times may be based on the examinee's first utterance (throat-clearing, sighing, etc.), rather than the first actual response.

Timing accuracy problems are by no means eliminated by use of audiotape versions, as repeated copying of audiotapes can decrease sound quality and alter ISIs. Users are therefore urged to check the accuracy of their PASAT audiotape ISIs, particularly if these tapes have been in use for some time. Tape quality decreases with repeated use, and copies of copies may lose precision with regard to timing. Consequently, users who employ the PASAT frequently should consider replacing tapes regularly. One recommendation is to replace the tapes twice per year if the test is used daily (R. McInerney, personal communication, March 2005).

Other issues include cross-generational differences in "number bond familiarity" (i.e., automaticity of simple addition skills), which may lead to better performance in older adults and overestimate information processing deficits in younger adults (Ward, 1997). This problem can be circumvented to some extent by using contemporary (and preferentially, local) norms so that the math instruction of the patient most closely matches that of the normative age band.

Lastly, the test requires fast speech responses, a feature that prevents its use with dysarthric or other speech-impaired patients (Weber, 1986). Further, it is not appropriate for excessively anxious individuals and may elicit negative reactions in nonanxious individuals. There is therefore the risk that it may be an inappropriate test for those already in a negative mood state, and that the test's effect on mood may affect performance independently of attentional deficits at the highest ISIs (Holdwick & Wingenfeld, 1999). The test may simply be refused or discontinued by some patients (Aupperle et al., 2002). Suggestions such as debriefing patients after the test or administering the PASAT late in the testing sequence so as not to adversely influence performance on other tests may be beneficial in reducing the adverse effects of the test on mood (Holdwick & Wingenfeld, 1999).

REFERENCES

Audoin, B., Ibarrola, D., Ranjeva, J.-P., Confort-Gouny, S., Malikova, I., Ali-Chérif, A., Pelletier, J., & Cozzone, P. (2003). Compensatory cortical activation observed by fMRI during a cognitive task at the earliest stage of MS. *Human Brain Mapping, 20,* 51–58.

Aupperle, R. L., Beatty, W. W., deNAP Shelton, F., & Gontkovsky, S. T. (2002). Three screening batteries to detect cognitive impairment in multiple sclerosis. *Multiple Sclerosis, 8,* 382–389.

Baird, B. J., Tombaugh, T. N., & Francis, M. (submitted). The effects of practice on speed of information processing using the Adjusting-PSAT (A-PSAT) and the Computerized Test of Information Processing (CTIP).

Bate, A. J., Mathias, J. L., & Crawford, J. R. (2001). Performance on the Test of Everyday Attention and standard tests of attention following severe traumatic brain injury. *The Clinical Neuropsychologist, 15*(3), 405–422.

Bradshaw, M., Stallings, G., Newbill, W., DaSilva, N., & Levin, H. (1999). Use of three tasks to classify working memory performance in patients with a history of severe traumatic brain injury. *Journal of the International Neuropsychological Society, 6*, 186–187.

Brittain, J. L., La Marche, J. A., Reeder, K. P., Roth, D. L., & Boll, T. J. (1991). Effects of age and IQ on Paced Auditory Serial Addition Task (PASAT) performance. *The Clinical Neuropsychologist, 5*, 163–175.

Brooks, D. N., McKinlay, W., Symington, C., Beattie, A., & Campsie, L. (1987). Return to work within the first seven years of severe head injury. *Brain Injury, 1*, 5–15.

Cicerone, K. D. (1997). Clinical sensitivity of four measures of attention to mild traumatic brain injury. *The Clinical Neuropsychologist, 11*(3), 266–272.

Cicerone, K. D., & Azulay, J. (2002). Diagnostic utility of attention measures in postconcussion syndrome. *The Clinical Neuropsychologist, 16*(3), 280–289.

Chronicle, E. P., & MacGregor, N. A. (1998). Are PASAT scores related to mathematical ability? *Neuropsychological Rehabilitation, 8*(3), 273–282.

Cohen, J. A., Cutter, G. R., Fischer, J. S., Goodman, A. D., Heidenreich, F. R., Kooijmans, M. F., Sandrock, A. W., Rudick, R. A., Simon, J. H., Simonian, N. A., Tsao, E. C., Whitaker, J. N., for the IMPACT Investigators. (2002). Benefit of interferon β-1a on MSFC progression in secondary progressive MS. *Neurology, 59*, 679–687.

Crawford, J. R., Obansawin, M. C., & Allan, K. M. (1998). PASAT and components of WAIS-R performance: Convergent and discriminant validity. *Neuropsychological Rehabilitation, 8*(3), 273–272.

Crossen, J. R., & Wiens, A. N. (1988). Residual neuropsychological deficits following head-injury on the Wechsler Memory Scale-Revised. *The Clinical Neuropsychologist, 2*, 393–399.

D'Esposito, M., Onishi, K., Thompson, H., Robinson, K., Armstrong, C., & Grossman, M. (1996). Working memory impairments in multiple sclerosis: Evidence from a dual-task paradigm. *Neuropsychology, 10*, 51–56.

Deary, I. J., Langan, S. J., Hepburn, D. A., & Frier, B. M. (1991). Which abilities does the PASAT test? *Personality and Individual Differences, 12*, 983–987.

DeLuca, J., Johnson, S. K., & Natelson, B. H. (1993). Information processing efficiency in chronic fatigue syndrome and multiple sclerosis. *Archives of Neurology, 50*, 301–304.

Demaree, J. A., Gaudino, E., & DeLuca, J. (2003). The relationship between depressive symptoms and cognitive dysfunction in multiple sclerosis. *Cognitive Neuropsychiatry, 8*(3), 161–171.

Diamond, B. J., DeLuca, J., Kim, H., & Kelley, S. M. (1997). The question of disproportionate impairments in visual and auditory information processing in multiple sclerosis. *Journal of Clinical and Experimental Neuropsychology, 19*, 34–42.

Diehr, M. C., Cherner, M., Wolfson, T. J., Miller, S. W., Grant, I., Heaton, R. K., and the HIV Neurobehavioral Research Center (HNRC) Group. (2003). The 50 and 100-item short forms of the Paced Auditory Serial Addition Task (PASAT): Demographically corrected norms and comparisons with the full PASAT in normal and clinical samples. *Journal of Clinical and Experimental Neuropsychology, 25*(4), 571–585.

Diehr, M. C., Heaton, R. K., Miller, W., & Grant, W. (1998). The Paced Auditory Serial Addition Task (PASAT): Norms for age, education and ethnicity. *Assessment, 5*(4), 375–387.

Dyche, G. E., & Johnson, D. A. (1991a). Development and evaluation of CHIPASAT, an attention test for children: II. Test-retest relia-bility and practice effect for a normal sample. *Perceptual and Motor Skills, 72*, 563–572.

Dyche, G. M., & Johnson, D. A. (1991b). Information-processing rates derived from CHIPASAT. *Perceptual and Motor Skills, 73*, 720–722.

Egan, V. (1988). PASAT: Observed correlations with IQ. *Personality and Individual Differences, 9*, 179–180.

Feinstein, A., Brown, R., & Ron, M. (1994). Effects of practice of serial tests of attention in healthy adults. *Journal of Clinical and Experimental Neuropsychology, 16*, 436–447.

Fischer, J. S., Rudick, R. A., Cutter, G. R., & Reingold, S. C. (1999). The Multiple Sclerosis Functional Composite measure (MSFC): An integrated approach to MS clinical outcome assessment. *Multiple Sclerosis, 5*, 244–250.

Fisk, J. D., & Archibald, C. (2001). Limitations of the Paced Auditory Serial Addition Test as a measure of working memory in patients with multiple sclerosis. *Journal of the International Neuropsychological Society, 7*, 363–372.

Fos, L. A., Greve, K. W., South, M. B., Mathias, C., & Benefield, H. (2000). Paced Visual Serial Addition Test: An alternative measure of information processing speed. *Applied Neuropsychology, 7*(3), 140–146.

Gow, A. J., & Deary, I. J. (2004). Is the PASAT past it? Testing attention and concentration without numbers. *Journal of Clinical and Experimental Neuropsychology, 26*(6), 723–736.

Gronwall, D. (1976). Performance changes during recovery from closed head injury. *Proceedings of the Australian Association of Neurologists, 5*, 72–78.

Gronwall, D. M. A. (1977). Paced Auditory Serial Addition Task: A measure of recovery from concussion. *Perceptual and Motor Skills, 44*, 367–373.

Gronwall, D. (1981). Information processing capacity and memory after closed head injury. *International Journal of Neuroscience, 12*, 171.

Gronwall, D. M. A., & Sampson, H. (1974). *The psychological effects of concussion.* New Zealand: Auckland University Press.

Gronwall, D., & Wrightson, P. (1974). Delayed recovery of intellectual function after minor head injury. *The Lancet, 2*, 605–609.

Gronwall, D., & Wrightson, P. (1981). Memory and information processing capacity after closed head injury. *Journal of Neurology, Neurosurgery, and Psychiatry, 44*, 889–895.

Haslam, C., Batchelor, J., Fearnside, M. R., Haslam, A. S., & Hawkins, S. (1995). Further examination of post-traumatic amnesia and post-coma disturbance as non-linear predictors of outcome after head injury. *Neuropsychology, 9*, 599–605.

Hohol, M. J., Guttman, C. R., Orav, J., Mackin, G. A., Kikinis, R., Khoury, S. J., Jolesz, F. A., & Weiner, H. L. (1997). Serial neuropsychological assessment and magnetic resonance imaging analysis in multiple sclerosis. *Archives of Neurology, 54*, 1018–1025.

Holdwick, D. J., & Wigenfeld, S. A. (1999). The subjective experience of PASAT testing: Does the PASAT induce negative mood? *Archives of Clinical Neuropsychology, 14*(3), 273–284.

Johnson, S. K., DeLuca, J., Diamond, B. J., & Natelson, B. H. (1996). Selective impairment of auditory processing in chronic fatigue syndrome: A comparison with multiple sclerosis and healthy controls. *Perceptual and Motor Skills, 83*, 51–62.

Johnson, S. K., Lange, G., DeLuca, J., Korn, L. R., & Natelson, B. (1997). The effects of fatigue on neuropsychological performance in patients with chronic fatigue syndrome, multiple sclerosis, and depression. *Applied Neuropsychology, 4*(3), 145–153.

Johnson, D. A., Roethig-Johnson, K., & Middleton, J. (1988). Development and evaluation of an attentional test for head-injured children: 1. Information processing capacity in a normal sample. *Journal of Child Psychology and Psychiatry, 2,* 199–208.

Kalmar, J. H., Bryant, D., Tulsky, D., & DeLuca, J. (2004). Information processing deficits in multiple sclerosis: Does choice of screening instrument make a difference? *Rehabilitation Psychology, 49*(3), 213–218.

Kinsella, G. J. (1998). Assessment of attention following traumatic brain injury: A review. *Neuropsychological Rehabilitation, 8,* 351–375.

Kotterba, S., Orth, M., Eren, E., Fangerau, T., & Sindern, E. (2003). Assessment of driving performance in patients with relapsing-remitting multiple sclerosis by a driving simulator. *European Neurology, 50*(3), 160–4.

Larrabee, G. J., & Curtiss, G. (1995). Construct validity of various verbal and visual memory tests. *Journal of Clinical and Experimental Neuropsychology, 17,* 536–547.

Lazeron, R. H. C., Rombouts, S. A. R. B., de Sonneville, L., Barkhof, F., & Scheltens, P. (2003). A paced visual serial addition for fMRI. *Journal of the Neurological Sciences, 213,* 29–34.

Lejuez, C. W., Kahler, C. W., & Brown, R. A. (2003). A modified computer version of the Paced Auditory Serial Addition Task (PASAT) as a laboratory-based stressor. *Behavior Therapist, 26*(4), 290–293.

Levin, H. S., Benton, A. L., & Grossman, R. G. (1982). *Neurobehavioral consequences of closed head injury.* New York: Oxford University Press.

Levin, H. S., Mattis, S., Ruff, R. M., Eisenberg, H. M., et al. (1987). Neurobehavioral outcome following minor head injury: A three-center study. *Journal of Neurosurgery, 66,* 234–243.

Lockwood, A. H., Linn, R. T., Szymanski, H., Coad, M. L., & Wack, D. S. (2004). Mapping the neural systems that mediate the Paced Auditory Serial Addition Task (PASAT). *Journal of the International Neuropsychological Society, 10,* 26–34.

MacLeod, D., & Prior, M. (1996). Attention deficits in adolescents with ADHD and other clinical groups. *Child Neuropsychology, 2,* 1–10.

Mathias, C. W., Stanford, M. S., & Houston, R. J. (2004). The physiological experience of the Paced Auditory Serial Addition Task (PASAT): Does the PASAT induce autonomic arousal? *Archives of Clinical Neuropsychology, 19,* 543–554.

McCaffrey, R. J., Cousins, J. P., Westervelt, H. J., Martnowicz, M., Remick, S. C., Szebenyi, S., Wagle, W. A., Bottomley, P. A., Hardy, C. J., & Haase, R. F. (1995). Practice effect with the NIMH AIDS Abbreviated Neuropsychological Battery. *Archives of Clinical Neuropsychology, 10,* 241–250.

Mendley, S. R., & Zelko, F. A. (1999). Improvements in specific aspects of neurocognitive performance in children after renal transplantation. *Kidney International, 56,* 318–323.

Mitropoulou, V., Harvey, P. D., Maldari, L. A., Moriarty, P. J., New, A. S., Silverman, J. M., & Siever, L. J. (2002). Neuropsychological performance in schizotypal personality disorder: Evidence regarding diagnostic specificity. *Biological Psychiatry, 52*(12), 1175–1182.

Nelson, H. E. (1982). *National Adult Reading Test (NART): Test manual.* Windsor: NFER Nelson.

O'Donnell, J. P., MacGregor, L. A., Dabrowski, J. J., Oestreicher, J. M., & Romero, J. J. (1994). Construct validity of neuropsychological tests of conceptual and attentional abilities. *Journal of Clinical Psychology, 50,* 596–600.

O'Shaughnessy, E. J., Fowler, R. S., & Reid, V. (1984). Sequelae of mild closed head injuries. *The Journal of Family Practice, 18,* 391–394.

Ponsford, J., & Kinsella, G. (1992). Attentional deficits following closed-head injury. *Journal of Clinical and Experimental Neuropsychology, 14,* 822–838.

Rao, S. M., Leo, G. J., Bernardin, L., Unverzagt, F. (1991). Cognitive dysfunction in multiple sclerosis: Frequency, patterns and prediction. *Neurology, 41,* 685–691.

Roman, D. D., Edwall, G. E., Buchanan, R. J., & Patton, J. H. (1991). Extended norms for the Paced Auditory Serial Addition Task. *The Clinical Neuropsychologist, 5,* 33–40.

Royan, J., Tombaugh, T. N., Rees, L., & Francis, M. (2004). The Adjusting-Paced Serial Addition Test (Adjusting-PSAT): Thresholds for speed of information processing as a function of stimulus modality and problem complexity. *Archives of Clinical Neuropsychology, 19,* 131–143.

Rudick, R., Antel, J., Confavreux, C., Cutter, G., Ellison, G., Fischer, J., Lubin, F., Miller, A., Petkau, J., Rao, S., Reingold, S., Snydulko, K., Thompson, A., Wallenberg, J., Weinshenker, B., & Willoughby, E. (1997). Recommendations from the National Multiple Sclerosis Society Clinical Outcomes Assessment Task Force. *Annals of Neurology, 42,* 379–382.

Sampson, H. (1956). Pacing and performance on a serial addition task. *Canadian Journal of Psychology, 10,* 219–225.

Schächinger, H., Cox, D., Linder, L., Brody, S., & Keller, U. (2003). Cognitive and psychomotor function in hypoglycemia: Response error patterns and retest reliability. *Pharmacology, Biochemistry and Behavior, 75,* 915–920.

Schmidt, M., Trueblood, W., Merwin, M., & Durham, R. L. (1994). How much do attention tests tell us? *Arch Clin Neuropsychol. 9*(5), 383–394.

Shawaryn, M. A., Schiaffino, K. M., LaRocca, N. G., & Johnston, M. V. (2002). Determinants of health-related quality of life in multiple sclerosis: The role of illness intrusiveness. *Multiple Sclerosis, 8,* 310–318.

Sherman, E. M. S., Strauss, E., & Spellacy, F. (1997). Testing the validity of the Paced Auditory Serial Addition Test (PASAT) in adults with head injury. *The Clinical Neuropsychologist, 11,* 34–45.

Sherman, E. M. S., Strauss, E., Spellacy, F., & Hunter, M. (1995). Construct validity of WAIS-R factors: Neuropsychological correlates in adults referred for possible head injury. *Psychological Assessment, 7,* 440–444.

Shucard, J. L., Parrish, J., Shucard, D. W., McCabe, D. C., Benedict, R. H. B., & Ambrus, J. (2004). Working memory and processing speed deficits in systemic lupus erythematosus as measured by the Paced Auditory Serial Addition Test. *Journal of the International Neuropsychological Society, 10,* 35–45.

Sjogren, P., Thomsen, A., & Olsen, A. (2000). Impaired neuropsychological performance in chronic nonmalignant pain patients receiving long-term oral opioid therapy. *Journal of Pain and Symptom Management, 19*(2), 100–108.

Snyder, P. J., Aniskiewicz, A. S., & Snyder, A. M. (1993). Quantitative MRI correlates and diagnostic utility of multi-modal measures of executive control in multiple sclerosis. *Journal of Clinical and Experimental Neuropsychology, 15,* 18.

Snyder, P. J., & Cappelleri, J. C. (2001). Information processing speed deficits may be better correlated with the extent of white matter sclerotic lesions in multiple sclerosis than previously suspected. *Brain and Cognition, 46,* 279–284.

Snyder, P. J., Cappelleri, J. C., Archibald, C. J., & Fisk, J. D. (2001). Improved detection of differential information-processing speed deficits between two disease-course types of multiple sclerosis. *Neuropsychology, 15*(4), 617–625.

Spreen, O., & Strauss, E. (1998). *A compendium of neuropsychological tests* (2nd ed.). New York: Oxford University Press.

Staffen, W., Mair, A., Zauner, H., Unterrainer, J., Niederhofer, H., Kutzelnigg, A., Ritter, S., Golaszewski, S., Iglseder, B., & Ladurner,

G. (2002). Cognitive function and fMRI in patients with multiple sclerosis: Evidence for compensatory cortical activation during an attention task. *Brain, 125,* 1275–1282.

Strauss, E., Spellacy, F., Hunter, M., & Berry, T. (1994). Assessing believable deficits on measures of attention and information processing capacity. *Archives of Clinical Neuropsychology, 9,* 483–490.

Stuss, D. T., Stethem, L. L., Hugenholtz, H., & Richard, M. T. (1989). Traumatic brain injury: A comparison of three clinical tests and analysis of recovery. *The Clinical Neuropsychologist, 3,* 145–156.

Stuss, D. T., Stethem, L. L., & Pelchat, G. (1988). Three tests of attention and rapid information processing: An extension. *The Clinical Neuropsychologist, 2,* 246–250.

Stuss, D. T., Stethem, L. L., & Poirier, C. A. (1987). Comparison of three tests of attention and rapid information processing across six age groups. *The Clinical Neuropsychologist, 1,* 139–152.

Tombaugh, T. N. (1999). *Administrative manual for the Adjusting-Paced Serial Addition Test (Adjusting-PSAT).* Carleton University, Ottawa, Ontario.

Tombaugh, T. N., Rees, L., Baird, B., & Kost, J. (2004). The effects of list difficulty and modality of presentation on a computerized version of the Paced Serial Addition Test (PSAT). *Journal of Clinical and Experimental Neuropsychology, 26*(2), 257–265.

Townsend, L. A., Malla, A. K., & Norman, R. G. (2001). Cognitive functioning in stabilized first-episode psychosis patients. *Psychiatry Research, 104,* 119–131.

Van Zomeren, A. H., & Brouwer, W. H. (1992). Assessment of attention. In J. R. Crawford, D. M. Parker, & W. McKinlay (Eds.), *Handbook of neuropsychological assessment* (pp. 241–266). Hove, UK: Lawrence Erlbaum Associates Ltd.

Ward, T. (1997). A note of caution for clinicians using the Paced Auditory Serial Addition Task. *British Journal of Clinical Psychology, 36,* 303–307.

Webbe, F., & Ochs, S. R. (2003). Recency and frequency of soccer heading interact to decrease neurocognitive performance. *Applied Neuropsychology, 10*(1), 31–41.

Weber, M. A. (1986). *Measuring attentional capacity.* Unpublished Ph.D. Thesis. University of Victoria.

Wiens, A. N., Fuller, K. H., & Crossen, J. R. (1997). Paced Auditory Serial Addition Test: Adult norms and moderator variables. *Journal of Clinical and Experimental Neuropsychology, 19*(4), 473–483.

Wingenfeld, S. A., Holdwick, D. J., Davis, J. L., & Hunter, B. B. (1999). Normative data on computerized Paced Auditory Serial Addition Task performance. *The Clinical Neuropsychologist, 13*(3), 268–273.

Ruff 2 & 7 Selective Attention Test (2 & 7 Test)

PURPOSE

The Ruff 2 & 7 Selective Attention Test (2 & 7 Test) is a test of sustained and selective attention.

SOURCE

The test can be ordered from Psychological Assessment Resources, Inc. (www.parinc.com). The Ruff 2 & 7 Introductory Kit (Professional Manual and 50 Test Booklets) retails for $139 US.

AGE RANGE

Test norms range from 16 to 70 years of age.

DESCRIPTION

The Ruff 2 & 7 Test (2 & 7 Test) is based on the premise that selective attention (i.e., the ability to select relevant stimuli while ignoring irrelevant information) can be assessed by comparing automatic and controlled processing with minimal demands on other cognitive processes such as memory (Cicerone & Azulay, 2002). The test is based on the theories of Logan et al. (Logan, 1988; Logan & Klapp, 1991; Logan & Stadler, 1991), which posit two processes through which attention is allocated: automatic processing and effortful processing.

The test itself is a paper-and-pencil cancellation task that consists of a set of 20 trials administered consecutively in 15-second intervals. For each trial, the examinee is required to make a line through specific targets (always the numbers 2 and 7) while ignoring other letters or numbers (see Figure 9–11).

Two types of trials are presented: *Automatic Detection* trials, where the target numbers are presented among distractor letters, and *Controlled Search* trials, where the target numbers are presented among other numbers. According to the authors, target selection is automatic in the first condition because targets (numbers) differ categorically from distractors (letters). This categorical difference between letters and numbers is overlearned, and hence subject to automatic processing even in semiliterate individuals (Ruff & Allen, 1996). In the second condition, because both targets and numbers belong to the same stimulus category (numbers), working memory and effortful processing of stimulus characteristics are required to effectively select targets from distractors.

According to the authors, specific cerebral regions are assumed to be associated with different components of the 2 & 7 Test. Deficits in specific domains are hypothesized to be associated with right hemisphere dysfunction (e.g., Test Speed and Accuracy), while others (e.g., Automatic Detection) are thought to measure functioning in posterior (temporoparietal) and anterior (prefrontal) systems (e.g., Controlled Search; Ruff & Allen, 1996).

ADMINISTRATION

Materials

The test requires only the Test Booklet, a brightly colored pencil or pen, and a stopwatch.

Figure 9–11 Sample item from the Ruff 2 & 7 Test. *Source:* Reprinted with permission from Ruff et al., 1992.

```
2GOXC7MJ7HZRNGAS2YWQ2LHBZGJNV7ET2PRVMJ
H STQ2C7KLWC7XMT7KTR2AVPIWOC2GJ7LS2BNVW
7TQXR2PH7FDABM2WHKAST2OPHWED2TRNEQX2PK

3107894470537638 152365697 0 891578436286
3286154280912 91 8 9281376453 7 80467962912
8391837894659 14 7 0 8671303910 2338941 2655
```

Instructions

See *Source.* There are 10 Automatic Detection trials and 10 Controlled Search trials, presented semirandomly in the test booklet. Instructions are provided verbatim. Test items are presented on the back of the Test Booklet. Each of the 20 trials consists of a line of alpha-numeric characters; the examinee is given 15 seconds to cross out as many targets as possible within the time limit, working from left to right. After 15 seconds, the examiner indicates the end of the trial by saying "Next," and the examinee must begin canceling targets on the next line of the Test Booklet.

ADMINISTRATION TIME

The entire test takes about five minutes to administer.

SCORING

Several scores can be derived from the test. These are generally based on errors of omission (hits) and commission (incorrect responses), but are more complex than these basic categories. A summary and description of test scores is shown in Table 9–39, which supplements score descriptions found in the manual. Sustained attention is measured primarily by the Total Speed

Table 9–39 Summary and Description of Ruff 2 & 7 Scores

Construct	2 & 7 Test Variable	Computation of Variables
Sustained Attention	Total Speed	Sum of Automatic Detection Speed T score and Controlled Search Speed T score
	Total Accuracy	Sum of Automatic Detection Accuracy T score and Controlled Search Accuracy T score
Selective Attention	Automatic Detection Speed	Total number of targets correctly identified on the 10 Letter trials
	Automatic Detection Accuracy	Total number of targets correctly identified on the 10 Letter trials, divided by the number of targets plus errors on the Letter trials, multiplied by 100
	Controlled Search Speed	Total number of targets correctly identified on the 10 Digit trials
	Controlled Search Accuracy	Total number of targets correctly identified on the 10 Digit trials, divided by the number of targets plus errors on the Digit trials, multiplied by 100
Discrepancy Analysis	Speed Difference	Automatic Detection Speed T score minus Controlled Search Speed T score
	Accuracy Difference	Automatic Detection Accuracy T score minus Controlled Search Accuracy T score
	Total Difference	Total Speed T score minus Total Accuracy T score

Source: From Ruff & Allen, 1996. Reproduced by special permission of the Publisher, Psychological Assessment Resources, Inc., 16204 North Florida Avenue, Lutz, FL 33549, from the *Ruff 2 & 7 Selective Attention Test* by Ronald M. Ruff, Ph.D., and C. Christopher Allen, Ph.D. Copyright 1986, 1996 by PAR, Inc. Further reproduction is prohibited without permission from PAR, Inc.

and Total Accuracy scores, while selective attention is measured by the Automatic Detection and Controlled Search scores.

Scoring is accomplished by first determining the number of hits (i.e., the number of targets correctly identified among the 10 possible targets for each row); this is called the Speed score. The Accuracy score is based on hits as well as the Error score. The latter includes errors of omissions (i.e., missed targets, which are only counted for those characters prior to the respondent's last correct response) and errors of commissions (incorrectly identified targets or false alarms).

DEMOGRAPHIC EFFECTS

Age

Age is moderately correlated with Automatic Detection Speed and Controlled Search Speed ($r = -.41$ and $-.38$, respectively; see manual; note that "speed" in this context refers to number of targets rather than response time per se). There are no significant age effects on any Accuracy measures.

Gender

According to the manual, there are no gender effects on the test.

Education

There are education effects on performance; these are relatively small for Automatic Detection Speed and Controlled Search Speed, as reported in the manual ($r = .19–.24$). However, these are sufficient enough to warrant education-based norms. There are no significant education effects on any Accuracy measures. Education may contribute to higher test-retest gains (Lemay et al., 2004; see *Practice Effects*).

Ethnicity

Information on the effects of race and ethnicity on performance is unavailable.

IQ

Correlations with FSIQ are negligible (Ruff & Allen, 1996). However, when demographically corrected scores are considered, modest correlations with PIQ are found in normals ($r = .22–.25$).

NORMATIVE DATA

Standardization Sample

The standardization sample is described in Table 9–40. Because gender does not affect test scores, norms are presented by age and education in the test manual. Limited information is presented in the manual regarding ethnicity composition and data collection procedures.

Table 9–40 Characteristics of the Ruff 2 & 7 Test Normative Sample

Sample type	Recruited as part of larger standardization study[a]
Number	360
Age	16 to 70 years[b]
Geographic location	
California	65%
Michigan	30%
Eastern Seaboard	5%
Education	7–22 years[c]
SES	Not reported
Gender	
Men	180
Women	180
Race/ethnicity	Details not provided[d]
Screening	Exclusion based on reported history of psychiatric disorder, substance abuse, or neurological disorder

[a]San Diego Neuropsychological Test Battery (Baser & Ruff, 1987; Ruff & Crouch, 1991). [b]Four age groups (16–24, 25–39, 40–54, and 55–70 years). [c]Three educational bands (≤12 years, 13–15 years, ≥16 years); proportions within each age band are not reported. [d]The manual indicates that the sample "roughly approximated the 1980 U.S. census proportions with regards to race" (Manual, p. 13).

Score Transformations

Norms were developed by using demographically corrected T scores in a method similar to that used by Heaton et al. (1991) for the Halstead-Reitan Battery. This is described in detail in the manual. No demographic corrections were needed for the Accuracy scores due to the lack of significant age or education effects on this variable.

Other Normative Datasets

Additional normative data are presented in Table 9–41, based on data collected by Lemay et al. (2004). These are based on the performance of 37 French-Canadian, older individuals (age range 52–80, age, $M = 67.4$, $SD = 7.8$). Average education was 13 years ($SD = 4.4$, range 6–22 years). In this case, the test was administered in French. Data are presented for three consecutive testing sessions, with a testing interval of 14 days between each session. Total Speed, Total Accuracy, and Processing are shown as age- and education-corrected scores. Raw Speed and Accuracy scores are also presented separately for automatic detection and controlled search blocks.

RELIABILITY

Internal Consistency

Alpha coefficients and split-half coefficients for the standardization sample ($N = 360$) are high, indicating strong internal

Table 9–41 Test-Retest Means, and Reliability Coefficients for Ruff 2 & 7 Test Scores in a Group of Older Adults

	Session 1		Session 2		Session 3		T_{1-2}	T_{1-3}	T_{2-3}	ICC
	Mean	(SD)	Mean	(SD)	Mean	(SD)				
Total Speed	274.32	(41.49)	294.43	(43.42)	300.38	(49.46)	.94	.86	.92	.82
Total Accuracy	94.15	(5.72)	95.25	(4.42)	96.47	(2.93)	.73	.55	.86	.68
Processing	1.241	(.162)	1.229	(.159)	1.186	(.153)	.66	.60	.71	.64
CS Speed	112.19	(19.08)	120.95	(19.13)	125.46	(22.60)	.94	.88	.92	.81
AD Speed	130.32	(25.61)	141.68	(27.87)	143.16	(30.87)	.92	.85	.91	.84
CS Accuracy	92.59	(5.58)	93.74	(5.44)	94.80	(4.30)	.53	.50	.78	.59
AD Accuracy	96.63	(3.50)	96.98	(2.52)	97.54	(2.07)	.54	.34	.64	.50

Note: The sample consisted of 37 French Canadian adults (52–80 years) tested in French.

Source: From Lemay et al., 2004.

reliability (all coefficients ≥.80; see manual). Coefficients for Controlled Search Speed and Automatic Detection Speed are especially strong (i.e., >.95).

Standard Error of Measurement (SEM)

SEMs based on alpha coefficients for Controlled Search and Automatic Detection Accuracy are relatively small (approximately four points; see manual). SEMs for each age group for the Speed scores range from one to two T-score points. When generalizability coefficients are used as the basis of calculation, SEM estimates are lower (i.e., one to three points).

Test-Retest Reliability

Most Ruff 2 & 7 Test variables have adequate to high reliability (see Table 9–42). Overall, test-retest reliability is higher for Speed scores than for Accuracy scores (Ruff & Allen, 1996). Stability estimates are based on 120 individuals from the normative sample with a retest interval of six months (i.e., five subjects from each of the 24 subgroups defined by age, education, and gender).

Over repeated sessions, reliability is excellent for some scores but not others, at least in older adults. Lemay et al. (2004) administered the test three times to older adults, with intersession intervals of 14 days, and reported correlation coefficients of over .85 for speed scores (see Table 9–41). However, reliability was modest for Processing scores and low for all Accuracy scores. The authors therefore suggested that use of Accuracy scores for repeat assessments should be avoided.

Practice Effects

Practice effects are about 10 raw-score points according to preliminary data presented by Ruff et al. (1986). Lemay et al. (2004) report that all Ruff 2 & 7 Speed scores are especially sensitive to practice effects; however, test-retest gains drop considerably after the second test session (see Table 9–41). Age and education do not appear to be related to the size of practice effects on the test, except in the case of Speed scores, where education is positively correlated with greater test-retest gains across testing sessions ($r = .37$; Lemay et al., 2004). However, the sample was restricted in terms of age (52–80 years). A wider age range (including young adults)

Table 9–42 Magnitude of Test-Retest Reliability Coefficients for the Ruff 2 & 7 (N = 120)

Magnitude of Coefficient	Stability Coefficients	Generalizability Coefficients
Very high (.90+)	Automatic Detection Speed Controlled Search Speed	Automatic Detection Speed Controlled Search Speed Controlled Search Accuracy Total Speed Total Accuracy
High (.80–.89)	Controlled Search Accuracy	Automatic Detection Accuracy
Adequate (.70–.79)	Automatic Detection Accuracy	
Marginal (.60–.69)		
Low (≤.59)		

Note: Stability coefficients consist of test-retest correlation coefficients corrected for restriction of range and variability (PAR, personal communication, December 2003).

may well reveal that age impacts the size of the practice effect.

VALIDITY

Content Validity

Test content appears to rest on a substantial theoretical foundation (see *Description*). Bias analyses (i.e., determination of extent of differential performance across groups defined by factors such as ethnicity) are lacking.

Factor Structure

Three main factors are found in healthy adults: Speed of Processing (Controlled Search Speed, Automatic Detection Speed), Controlled Processing (Speed Difference, Accuracy Difference, Controlled Search Accuracy), and Automatic Processing (Automatic Detection Accuracy, Accuracy Difference; Ruff & Allen, 1996).

Correlations With Other Tests of Attention

Processing speed is an important contributor to performance. When demographically corrected scores are considered, the Ruff 2 & 7 Test is most highly correlated with Digit Symbol in normals ($r = .35–.40$). Smaller correlations are found with block span tests ($r = .18–.24$) and with trail learning tests included in the San Diego Neuropsychological Battery (see manual for details; Baser & Ruff, 1987). The test does not appear to correlate with other tests of attention in normals (e.g., Digit Span, Stroop, Seashore Rhythm; Ruff & Allen, 1996).

In samples including clinical cases such as TBI, the Ruff 2 & 7 appears to correlate highly with other selective attention tests from the Test of Everyday Attention (TEA; $r = .62$ and $-.69$, for Map Search and Telephone Search, respectively; Bate et al., 2001). Significant correlations with TEA subtests measuring different attentional components such as attentional switching, divided attention, and sustained attention, although not as large, are also substantial ($r = .30$ to $-.57$).

Principal components analysis of the 2 & 7 Test and other tests of attention indicates that the test loads on a visual selective attention factor, along with measures such as the Stroop, Symbol Digit Modalities Test, and two selective attention tests from the TEA (i.e., Map Search and Telephone Search; Bate et al., 2001).

Correlations With Other Neuropsychological Tests

Minor correlations with word fluency are reported ($r = .17–.22$), but not with other executive functioning tests such as the WCST. Correlations with motor speed and conventional memory tests, both visual and auditory, are negligible

(Ruff & Allen, 1996). However, when present, motor or psychomotor slowing may contribute to lower total Speed scores (Ruff, 1994; Ruff & Allen, 1996). See *Demographic Effects* for information on the test's correlation to IQ.

In a mixed group of patients with schizophrenia and TBI, Controlled Search Speed loaded on an attention factor while the Speed Difference score loaded on a planning and flexibility factor, suggesting a greater role for planning and flexibility in some clinical groups (Baser & Ruff, 1987).

Clinical Studies

Accuracy is reportedly lower in the controlled versus automatic detection conditions in individuals with lesions in the frontal lobes versus those with posterior lesions ($N = 30$; Ruff & Allen, 1996; Ruff et al., 1992). The test also appears sensitive to injury severity in adults with TBI (Allen & Ruff, 1990; Bate et al., 2001) as well as in children with TBI (Nolin & Mathieu, 2001), who show selective deficits in controlled versus automatic processing. The 2 & 7 Test has also been used to discriminate between AIDS and AIDS-related complex patients, and between AZT- and placebo-treated groups at follow-up (Schmitt et al., 1988). The test has also been employed in studies of toxic exposure (Tröster et al., 1991) and shows promise for use in medical trials where a rapid assessment protocol that maximizes the likelihood of compliance is needed. This has been demonstrated in the case of an outcome trial for patients with brain metastases, where the test shows an excellent pretreatment compliance rate ($\geq 90\%$), and adequate posttreatment compliance rate ($\geq 70\%$) after whole-brain radiation (Regine et al., 2004).

The Ruff 2 & 7 Test has also been studied in psychiatric conditions (Baser & Ruff, 1987; Judd & Ruff, 1993; Ruff, 1994; Weiss, 1996). Severely depressed inpatients appear to have selective deficits on the test, typically showing poor total Speed but average total Accuracy scores (Allen et al., 1996, as cited by Ruff & Allen, 1996). Expected percentiles for inpatients and outpatients with major depression are shown on p. 35 of the manual. This table may be useful in the evaluation of depressed individuals suspected of having an additional neurological condition affecting attention (e.g., head injury, dementia), as severely impaired performance in total Accuracy and total Speed would not be expected to result from depression alone.

Ecological Validity

The 2 & 7 Test was found to be a good predictor of return to school or employment after TBI (Ruff et al., 1993).

Diagnostic Utility

Diagnostic accuracy has been examined by Cicerone and Azulay (2002) in a group of patients with postconcussion syndrome (PCS) and matched controls, screened for symptom

Table 9–43 Diagnostic Utility of the Ruff 2 & 7 Selective Attention Test in Postconcussion Syndrome: Sensitivity, Specificity, Efficiency, Positive Predictive Power, Negative Predictive Power, and Diagnostic Accuracy (Odds Ratio and 90% Confidence Interval) for Scores Greater than −1.5 SDs Below the Mean

	Ruff 2 & 7 Speed	Ruff 2 & 7 Accuracy
Sensitivity	9.9	12.5
Specificity	100	82.8
Efficiency[a]	52.5	45.9
Positive predictive power	100	44.4
Negative predictive power	50.0	46.2
Odds ratio	7.0	0.7
90% Confidence interval	1.8–87.4	0.2–2.2

Note: The base rate of postconcussion syndrome in this sample was 50%; the sample included 32 postconcussive patients screened for exaggeration and 32 matched controls.

[a]Refers to the number of subjects correctly classified (True Positives + True Negatives/N)

Source: From Cicerone & Azulay, 2002. Reprinted with the kind permission of Psychology Press.

exaggeration. Sensitivity, specificity, efficiency (i.e., number of subjects correctly classified, defined as true positives + true negatives/N), positive predictive power, negative predictive power, and odds ratios for the Ruff 2 & 7 Test are reproduced in Table 9–43. Values for various impairment levels were calculated in this study, with impairment defined as 1.5 SDs below the mean. The 2 & 7 Test speed and efficiency variables showed limited sensitivity, which indicates that they would have limited utility in *ruling in* the presence of PCS. However, their high specificity suggests considerable utility in *ruling out* PCS (i.e., persons without PCS are unlikely to have impaired scores). The positive predictive power of the Speed score was strong, indicating the diagnostic utility of impaired scores on the test. According to criteria set by the authors (i.e., odds ratio equal or greater than three, lower limit of the confidence interval greater than one), the speed score showed a reliable, positive association with PCS. Using the most conservative estimate (i.e., the lower limit of the confidence interval of the odds ratio), PCS patients were almost twice as likely to have an impaired Speed score than controls. Conversely, values for the Accuracy score were not supportive of its diagnostic utility in this group.

COMMENT

Like other paper-and-pencil cancellation tasks, the Ruff 2 & 7 is brief and quite portable, which makes it ideal for quick bedside examinations. Unlike some other cancellation tasks, it has well-defined theoretical underpinnings and is based on a relatively extensive research literature. Further, it may be more sensitive to deficits in sustained attention than commonly used brief attention tests (e.g., Digit Symbol, Symbol Digit Modalities) because of its slightly longer administration time. However, this proposal requires investigation. Performance is also relatively uninfluenced by other cognitive domains such as IQ, memory/learning, language ability, and motor speed (Ruff & Allen, 1996). This is not always the case for other attention tests. Overall, the test shows good convergent and

divergent validity, and its diagnostic utility is supported by data presented by Cicerone and Azulay (2002) and reproduced here. Again, many other tests in clinical practice lack this crucial information.

Overall, the psychometric properties of the test appear sound. The authors employed careful selection of subjects for test-retest reliability studies (representative in terms of age, education, and gender), and, unlike many tests that report stability data for only short retest intervals, the 2 & 7 provides stability data on a longer test interval that is likely more useful clinically (i.e., six-month stability). The manual includes step-by-step interpretation guidelines, beginning with ruling out interpretive confounds, normative comparisons, ipsative comparisons, and neuropsychological interpretation. Users are encouraged to read these sections carefully.

There is also a fairly extensive research literature on the use of the test in several diverse clinical populations. Although the samples are relatively small, the manual also provides tables for use in clinical evaluation, including base rates of impairment in patients with focal cerebral lesions (p. 36 of the manual) and base rates of impairment in individuals with preexisting depression (p. 35 in the manual). The latter would be of clinical utility in the diagnosis of neurological conditions affecting attention in individuals with coexisting depression. Additionally, although normative data for children are lacking, it has been found to be sensitive to attentional deficits in children with TBI (Nolin & Mathieu, 2001). Normative data for children may therefore be an asset for future revisions of the test.

Despite these strengths, the Ruff 2 & 7 also has some limitations. The main issue is that the normative sample does not represent a national, stratified random sample, which suggests caution in interpreting scores of individuals who differ substantially from the characteristics outlined in Table 9–40. Additionally, the effects of race/ethnicity on performance are unknown. There are also significant ceiling effects for Accuracy (e.g., 11% of individuals in the normative sample had scores at ceiling on the Automatic Detection and Controlled

Search conditions; see also Lemay et al., 2004), but floors appear quite adequate. Notably, test-retest reliability for Controlled Search Accuracy and Automatic Detection Accuracy is marginal to low (see Table 9–41). On the other hand, as noted by the authors, because of ceiling effects these coefficients may represent underestimates (Ruff & Allen, 1996). Nevertheless, caution is recommended in the interpretation of these scores in retesting situations. Practice effects also need to be considered, even in those variables with good reliability over time.

The variable names can engender confusion in novel users. For instance, the "speed" variables (i.e., Automatic Detection Speed, Controlled Search Speed, Total Speed) actually reflect the number of correct hits, not speed of responding per se. As well, there is no way of evaluating subtypes of incorrect responses (e.g., errors of commission versus errors of omission), which many researchers consider, for better or for worse, as conceptually separate entities. Additional research is needed to replicate the results of studies employing lesion groups to provide support for neuroanatomical correlates of the test suggested by the authors.

REFERENCES

Allen, C. C., & Ruff, R. M. (1990). Self-rating versus neuropsychological performance in moderate versus severe head injury patients. *Brain Injury, 4*, 7–17.

Baser, C. A., & Ruff, R. R. (1987). Construct validity of the San Diego Neuropsychological Test Battery. *Archives of Clinical Neuropsychology, 2*, 13–32.

Bate, A. J., Mathias, J. L., & Crawford, J. R. (2001). Performance on the Test of Everyday Attention and standard tests of attention following severe traumatic brain injury. *The Clinical Neuropsychologist, 15*(3), 405–422.

Cicerone, K. D. (1996). Attention deficit and dual task demands after mild traumatic brain injury. *Brain Injury, 10*, 79–90.

Cicerone, K. D., & Azulay, J. (2002). Diagnostic utility of attention measures in postconcussion syndrome. *The Clinical Neuropsychologist, 16*(3), 280–289.

Heaton, R. K., Grant, I., & Matthews, C. G. (1991). *Comprehensive Norms for an Expanded Halstead-Reitan Battery: Demographic corrections, research findings, and clinical applications.* Odessa, FL: Psychological Assessment Resources.

Judd, P. H., & Ruff, R. M. (1993). Neuropsychological dysfunction in patients with borderline personality disorder. *Journal of Personality Disorders, 7*, 275–284.

Lemay, S., Bedard, M.-A., Rouleau, I., & Tremblay, P.-L. G. (2004). Practice effect and test-retest reliability of attentional and executive tests in middle-aged to elderly subjects. *The Clinical Neuropsychologist, 18*(2), 284–302.

Logan, G. D. (1988). Toward an instance theory of automatization. *Psychological Review, 95*, 492–527.

Logan, G. D., & Klapp, S. T. (1991). Automatizing alphabet arithmetic: Is extended practice necessary to produce automaticity? *Journal of Experimental Psychology: Learning, Memory and Cognition, 17*, 179–195.

Logan, G. D., & Stadler, M. A. (1991). Mechanism of performance improvement and consistent mapping memory search: Automaticity or strategy search? *Journal of Experimental Psychology: Learning, Memory, and Cognition, 17*, 478–496.

Nolin, P., & Mathieu, F. (2001). L'importance de la sensibilité des mesures neuropsychologiques dans l'identification des déficits chez des enfants ayant subi un traumatisme craniocérébral léger. *Revue de neuropsychologie, 11*(1), 23–38.

Regine, W. F., Schmitt, F. A., Scott, C. B., Dearth, C., Patchell, R. A., Nichols, R. C., Gore, E. M., Franklin, R. L., Suh, J. H., & Mehta, M. P. (2004). Feasibility of neurocognitive outcome evaluations in patients with brain metastases in a multi-institutional cooperative group setting: Results of radiation therapy oncology group trial BR-0018. *International Journal of Radiation Oncology and Biology and Physiology 58*(5), 1346–1352.

Ruff, R. M. (1994). What role does depression play on the performance of the Ruff 2 & 7 Selective Attention Test? *Perceptual and Motor Skills, 78*(1), 63–66.

Ruff, R. M., & Allen, C. C. (1996). *Ruff 2 & 7 Selective Attention Test professional manual.* Odessa, FL: Psychological Assessment Resources, Inc.

Ruff, R. M., & Crouch, J. A. (1991). Neuropsychological test instruments in clinical trials. In E. Mohr & P. Brouwers (Eds.), *Handbook of clinical trials: The neurobehavioral approach* (pp. 89–119). Lisse, The Netherlands: Swets & Zeitlinger.

Ruff, R. M., Evans, R. W., & Light, R. H. (1986). Automatic detection versus controlled search: A paper and pencil approach. *Perceptual and Motor Skills, 62*, 407–416.

Ruff, R. M., Marshall, L. F., Crouch, J. A., Klauber, M. R., Levin, H. S., Barth, J. T., Kreutzer, J., Blunt, B. A., Foulkes, M. A., Eisenberg, H. M., Jane, J. A., & Marmarou, A. (1993). Predictors of outcome following severe head injury: Follow-up data from the TCDB. *Brain Injury, 7*, 101–111.

Ruff, R. M., Neimann, H., Allen, C. C., Farrow, C. E., & Wylie, T. (1992). The Ruff 2 & 7 Selective Attention Test: A neuropsychological application. *Perceptual and Motor Skills, 75*(3, Pt 2), 1311–1319.

Schmitt, F. A., Bigley, J. W., McKinnis, R., Logue, P. E., Evans, R. W., Drucker, J. L., & the AZT Collaborative Working Group. (1988). Neuropsychological outcome of Zidovudine (AZT) treatment of patients with AIDS and AIDS-related complex. *New England Journal of Medicine, 319*, 1573–1578.

Tröster, A. I., Ruff, R. M., & Watson, D. P. (1991). Dementia as a neuropsychological consequence of chronic occupational exposure to polychlorinated biphenyls (PCBs). *Archives of Clinical Neuropsychology, 6*, 301–318.

Weiss, K. M. (1996). A simple clinical assessment of attention in schizophrenia. *Psychiatry Research, 60*, 147–154.

Symbol Digit Modalities Test (SDMT)

PURPOSE

The test is used to assess divided attention, visual scanning, tracking, and motor speed.

SOURCE

The kit (including manual and 25 test forms) can be ordered from Western Psychological Services at a cost of $94 US. A Spanish version, the Test de Simbolos y Digitos (Arribas, 2002), is also available.

AGE RANGE

The test can be administered from ages 8 to 91.

DESCRIPTION

The Symbol Digit Modalities Test (SDMT; Smith, 1991), originally published in 1973, revised in 1982, and now in its eighth printing (1973–2000), was developed by Aaron Smith as a screening measure for cerebral dysfunction in children and adults. The original task can be found in the Army beta test and originated even earlier, in 1915 (Tulsky et al., 2003). A coding key is presented consisting of nine abstract symbols, each paired with a number, and the respondent is required to scan the key and write down the number corresponding to each symbol, as rapidly as possible. Wechsler reversed the task requirements (i.e., the respondent must write down the symbol rather than the digit) to create the Digit Symbol subtest. The test can be administered either in written or oral form. Group administration of the written form is also possible.

The SDMT has been used as a test of divided attention (Ponsford & Kinsella, 1992) but requires complex visual scanning and tracking (Shum et al., 1990), perceptual speed, motor speed, and memory (Laux & Lane, 1985; Lezak, 1995). Because SDMT responses consist of overlearned numbers, the written response is simpler than that required by Digit Symbol, which requires the subject to write unfamiliar symbols. However, from an attentional perspective, Digit Symbol may be somewhat easier than the SDMT (Glosser et al., 1977). On Digit Symbol, cues to spatial location are contained in the key since stimulus items (numbers) are arranged in arithmetic progression across the page. In the case of the SDMT, the sequence of symbols is random, with no cues to spatial location contained within the key (Glosser et al., 1977).

Alternate forms have been developed (e.g., Royer, 1971; Royer et al., 1981; Uchiyama et al., 1994), as well as a version enabling measurement of incidental learning (Uchiyama et al., 1994). The test has also been adapted for computer use (e.g., Feinstein et al., 1994), including versions adapted as part of computerized assessment packages for sports-related concussion such as the Immediate Post-Concussion Assessment and Cognitive Testing (ImPACT; Maroon et al., 2000) and Concussion Resolution Index (CRI; Erlanger et al., 2003).

ADMINISTRATION

Standard Procedure

See manual. The test form is placed before the patient, and the examiner reads the instructions that are provided in the SDMT Manual. As in the older versions of the Wechsler Digit Symbol subtest, 90 seconds are allowed to complete the trial. In the written version, the patient fills in the numbers that correspond with symbols (i.e., "marks") according to the key provided at the top of the page. In the oral version, the examiner records the numbers spoken by the patient. When administering both forms of the test, the recommended procedure is to give the written version first.

Incidental Learning

In the Uchiyama et al. (1994) incidental recall version, following standard administration, the examinee is given a new sheet composed of a line of 15 symbols in which all nine original symbols are included at least once. The line consists of the last line of the standard SDMT form (Eric Miller, personal communication, March 2005). The examinee is then asked to fill in the number associated with the symbols, from memory. In those cases where a symbol is presented more than once and the examinee is inconsistent with regard to providing the correct response, credit is given as long as the item was correctly identified on one of the trials.

Barncord and Wanlass (1999) note that administering the test using a washable marker and a plastic sheet protector on the standard single-use form is also an option. This variant on administration does not significantly affect test scores but is preferable from an ecological standpoint.

ADMINISTRATION TIME

About five minutes are required for the entire test.

SCORING

Scores

The number of correct substitutions within the 90-second interval is recorded. The maximum score is 110 on each form (i.e., written and oral).

Interpretation

SDMT scores that fall 1 to 1.5 *SD* below the mean should be considered suggestive of cerebral dysfunction (Smith, 1991).

DEMOGRAPHIC EFFECTS

Age

SDMT scores decline with advancing age on both written and oral forms (see *Source*; Bowler et al., 1992; Emmerson et al., 1990; Feinstein et al., 1994; Gilmore et al., 1983; Richardson & Marottoli, 1996; Selnes et al., 1991; Stones & Kozma, 1989; Uchiyama et al., 1994; Yeudall et al., 1986), perhaps reflecting changes in speed of motor response and speed of information processing, including symbol encoding, visual search (Gilmore et al., 1983), and memory (Joy et al., 2004).

Gender

Smith (1991) reported that gender affects performance, with girls outperforming boys. This has also been demonstrated in non-Western children (Jinabhai et al., 2004). In general, both boys and girls show consistently higher oral than written scores for ages 8 to 13 years. However, the gender-based difference between written and oral scores diminishes as age increases, particularly from ages 14 to 17 years.

In adults, gender differences have not always been found (Gilmore et al., 1983; Waldmann et al., 1992), though some report that females outperform males (see *Source*; Laux & Lane, 1985; Polubinski & Melamed, 1986; Yeudall et al., 1986). Although this has led to the conclusion that the influence of gender is not of sufficient magnitude to justify separate male and female norms (i.e., less than one-third of a standard deviation difference between genders), other evidence indicates otherwise. For example, in a large community-based study (N >7000), women outperformed men on the SDMT; when mediating variables such as education and health status were accounted for, the gender difference was even more pronounced (Jorm et al., 2004). That is, better health and education cannot account for better female performance.

IQ and Education

Performance improves with increasing IQ (Nielsen et al., 1989; Uchiyama et al., 1994; Waldmann et al., 1992; Yeudall et al., 1986). This underscores the need to consider intellectual level, particularly when dealing with low- or high-ability individuals. Better-educated subjects (13 years of school or more) have higher scores than less-educated individuals (12 years of school or less; see *Source*; Richardson & Marottoli, 1996; Selnes et al., 1991; Uchiyama et al., 1994; Yeudall et al., 1986). Education effects have also been found in clinical groups such as schizophrenia (Chan et al., 2004). Accordingly, the SDMT Manual presents the means and standard deviations by age and educational level (≤12 years versus 13+ years of education).

Ethnicity

Level of acculturation for African American individuals is related to SDMT performance, but seemingly less so for the oral version (Kennepohl et al., 2004). Uchiyama et al. (1994) also report an effect of ethnicity on SDMT scores, but caution that their results are based on a mostly Caucasian sample.

Children from rural South Africa obtain comparatively lower scores on the SDMT (Jinabhai et al., 2004). The authors note that factors such as educational deprivation and poverty may serve as moderators for presumed ethnic differences on the test.

NORMATIVE DATA

Standardization Sample: Adults

Smith (see *Source*) provides data based on a sample of 1307 normal adults, aged 18 to 78 years, presented by age and education (12 years or less and 13 years or more). See Table 9–44 for sample characteristics. Note that the data for the oral form are based on administration shortly after the written form. More important, users should note that the norms shown in the manual are, as of this writing, over 30 years old and appear to consist of a sample of convenience collected in a nonsystematic, nonstandardized manner, including data collected for a 1975 dissertation, and data collected by psychologists participating in a neuropsychology workshop. Other normative sources are therefore preferable.

Table 9–44 Characteristics of the Symbol Digit Modalities Test Normative Sample: Adults

Sample type	From two sources: adult volunteers for a 1975 doctoral dissertation ($N = 420$), and normal volunteers obtained by psychologists in private practice who participated in a workshop on clinical neuropsychology in Ann Arbor, Michigan; each psychologist contributed 20 participants ($N = 887$)
N	1307
Age	18–78 years[a]
Geographic location	New Jersey and Michigan, United States
Education	
12 years or less	477
13 years or more	830
Gender	Details unspecified, but gender reportedly evenly distributed
Race/ethnicity	Unspecified
Screening	Individuals with apparent handicaps or reported neurological involvement were excluded, or based on a double simultaneous stimulation screening test performance

[a]Based on six age groupings: 18–24, 25–34, 35–44, 45–54, 55–64, and 65+.

Source: Adapted from Smith, 1982.

Table 9–45 Normative Data for the Oral SDMT for a Large, Community-Based Sample by Gender ($N = 7,485$)

Age	Women			Men		
	N	Education	Score	N	Education	Score
20–24	1241	14.7	64.90 (9.89)	1163	14.5	62.82 (10.19)
40–44	1338	14.5	60.71 (9.42)	1192	14.8	58.98 (9.09)
60–64	1232	13.3	49.95 (10.0)	1319	14.2	49.39 (9.52)

Source: From Jorm et al., 2004. Reprinted with permission from Elsevier.

Other Normative Datasets for Adults

Given gender effects favoring women on the SDMT, gender-specific norms are recommended. Jorm et al. (2004) provide data for the oral version on a large, community-based sample of over 7000 individuals from Australia selected from the electoral roll of the region, with relatively high education (about 14 years). Data for women and men are presented separately in Table 9–45; three age cohorts are provided (20–24, 40–44, and 60–64). Note that these data were collected between 1999 and 2001, which is considerably more recent than the original SDMT standardization sample.

Table 9–46 shows normative data for older individuals (>75 years) according to education level, provided by Richardson and Marottoli (1996). The data derive from a sample of urban drivers (age, $M = 81.47$, $SD = 3.3$; education, $M = 11.02$, $SD = 3.68$).

Because it includes finer distinctions based on IQ and education, the large dataset ($N > 3000$) provided by Uchiyama et al. (1994) may also be of considerable utility. Norms are provided based on age, education (including highly educated individuals with >16 years of education), and estimated IQ (<90, 91–110, and ≥111). Norms for the standard form (Form 1) and for an alternate form (Form 2; Figure 9–12), based on a large sample of 3509 homosexual and bisexual HIV-seronegative men, are presented in Table 9–47. The sample was 85% Caucasian, 9% African American, 5% Hispanic Caucasian, and 1% other. Norms for the Incidental Learning trial are also presented in Table 9–47. Note that these data are based only on men, and that Form 2 may be slightly more difficult than the standard form (see *Reliability*). See also Levine et al. (2004) for test-retest norms and reliable change information.

Table 9–46 Symbol Digit Modalities Test Norms for Older Adults

	Age 76–80		Age 81–91	
Education	<12	>12	<12	>12
N	26	24	18	33
Mean	20.08	32.75	21.25	28.84
SD	9.08	10.16	9.48	8.93

Source: From Richardson & Marottoli, 1996. Reprinted with the kind permission of Psychology Press.

Hinton-Bayre et al. (1997, 1999) and Hinton-Bayre and Geffen (in press) also provide norms for alternate SDMT versions for male contact sport athletes, including reliable change information. The forms are reproduced in Figures 9–13 and 9–14a, b, and c.

For adults of above-average IQ, norms provided by Yeudall et al. (1986) may be appropriate, based on a Canadian sample of healthy, well-educated volunteers of above-average IQ, aged 15 to 40 years ($N = 255$). The data are stratified by age and gender, and are presented in Table 9–48. The data for the written form are similar to those reported by Smith (see *Source*) and Uchiyama et al. (1994), but the oral scores are somewhat

Figure 9–12 Symbol Digit Modalities Alternate Form (Uchiyama et al., 1994 norms.) *Source:* Courtesy of Eric Miller, Ph.D. (February 2005).

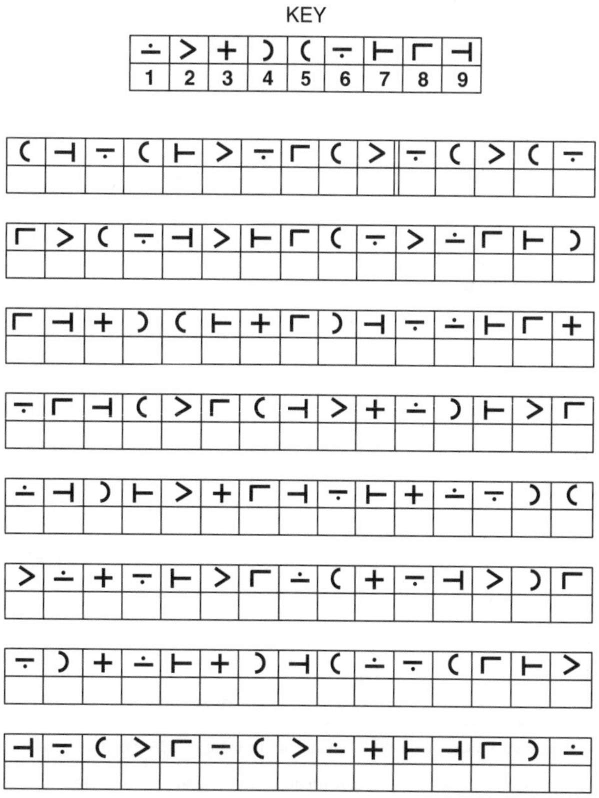

higher than those reported by Smith, perhaps reflecting differences in intellectual status between the samples.

Nielsen et al. (1989) give data on the written version based on a sample of 99 Danish individuals who underwent minor surgery (mean WAIS-R IQ = 98.61, SD = 12.21) and were tested as outpatients. The scores are somewhat lower than those reported by Smith, possibly the result of differences in cultural and general intellectual factors (see Table 9–49). The possible influence of psychological distress should also be kept in mind, but these norms could have some utility when assessing individuals in medical settings. Users should note, however, that the data were collected about 20 years ago.

Standardization Sample: Children

Smith provides data, by gender and age, based on a sample of 3680 normal children aged 8 to 17 years (see Table 9–50 for sample characteristics). The children were in the Omaha, Nebraska, school system. While the sample might be considered representative of urban Omaha, the scores may not be applicable to more ethnically diverse or rural populations. Note, too, that all written scores were derived from group administration of the test. The mean scores for the oral SDMT were also obtained when this version was the only test given.

Other Normative Datasets for Children

Norms for 1249 Spanish-speaking children are provided for the Spanish version of the test, the Test de Simbolos y Digitos (Arribas, 2002), and are reproduced in Table 9–51. Norms for

South African Zulu children are shown in Table 9–52. These means are considerably lower than those provided in the SDMT Manual.

RELIABILITY

Internal Reliability

Internal reliability information is not reported, likely because it is a timed task.

Test-Retest Reliability

Test-retest reliability for the SDMT is respectable. Smith (1991) reports that 80 normal adults were given two administrations of the written and oral forms with an average retest interval of 29 days. The test-retest correlations were .80 for the written SDMT and .76 for the oral version. Similar values are found in studies on sports concussion (i.e., r = .70; Echemendia et al., 1999, as cited in Erlander et al., 2003), although the values reported by Hinton-Bayre et al. (1999) are considerably higher (r = .91). Retest stability over longer intervals is also good. In a large study involving men (N >1000), Uchiyama et al. found strong test-retest coefficients at six months (r = .79). Retest coefficients for longer test intervals, based on smaller numbers of participants, were also acceptable (r = .72 at one year and two years; N = 39).

Test-retest reliability of the incidental learning trial developed by Uchiyama et al. is not uniformly strong (r = .46, .52, and .71, for six-month, one-year, and two-year retest reliability, respectively; 1994). Hinton-Bayre et al. (1997) found that

Table 9–47 Symbol Digit Modalities Test Norms for Men (N = 3509) According to IQ and Education (Includes High Education and Low/High IQ Individuals)

	Standard Form		Form 2	Incidental Recall	
	N	M (SD)	M (SD)	N	M (SD)
Age-Based Norms					
20–29	481	57.31 (10.11)	56.12 (11.56)	212	6.36 (2.38)
30–39	1596	56.11 (9.26)	53.55 (10.32)	795	6.18 (2.39)
40–49	952	52.96 (9.26)	52.21 (9.87)	600	5.53 (2.47)
>50	252	50.14 (8.18)	46.79 (8.08)	191	4.86 (2.42)
Education-Based Norms					
<16 years	1144	53.26 (9.97)	51.05 (10.54)	653	5.67 (2.51)
16 years	875	55.90 (8.78)	53.96 (10.32)	441	6.15 (2.39)
>16 years	1249	55.80 (9.43)	53.51 (10.02)	691	5.83 (2.44)
Estimated IQ-Based Norms					
<90	71	47.31 (7.51)	41.67 (8.69)	31	4.19 (2.18)
91–110	729	53.83 (8.73)	50.86 (9.16)	251	5.84 (2.32)
≥111	877	58.70 (8.95)	55.30 (10.49)	248	6.63 (2.16)

Note: Estimated IQ based on WAIS-R estimates from the Shipley-Hartford Test. Form 2 is shown in Figure 9–12; the Incidental Recall trial is the last line of the standard form.

Source: From Uchiyama et al., 1994. Reprinted with the kind permission of Psychology Press.

Figure 9–13 Instructions and Description of the Hinton-Bayre et al. Alternate Forms used in Sports Concussion Research. *Source:* Courtesy of Hinton Bayre and Geffen, March 2005.

New Alternate Forms of the
SYMBOL DIGIT MODALITIES TEST (SDMT)
Original designed by Aaron Smith (1973)

These forms have been developed maintaining the scale and layout of the original SDMT form. The visual array of the test form has been maintained. Thus, the same scoring key as used for the original may be used on the forms provided. In the original form there are three pairs of mirror-image symbols. The numbers these symbols are associated with are 1 and 8, 2 and 9, and 3 and 5. The array for each form presented also reflects this, but symbol pairs are varied across form and differ from each other and the original. Standard instructions from the revised manual (Smith, 1982) were used in the development of these alternate forms. Unlike the original, which was printed on U.S. letter paper, these forms are to be printed on A4 (210 mm × 297 mm) paper.

Preliminary data concerning alternate form equivalence are available in:

Hinton-Bayre, A. D., Geffen, G., & McFarland, K. (1997). Mild head injury and speed of information processing: A prospective study of professional rugby league players. *Journal of Clinical and Experimental Neuropsychology, 19(2),* 275–289.

Hinton-Bayre, A. D., & Geffen, G. (in press). Comparability, reliability, and practice effects on alternate forms of the Digit Symbol Substitution and Symbol Digit Modalities Tests. *Psychological Assessment.*

Contents

1. SDMT—Form B
2. SDMT—Form C
3. SDMT—Form D

When printing, ensure that bottom margin is set such that the form and copyright information does not print.

If you have any further queries, please contact:

Anton Hinton-Bayre, PhD
Cognitive Psychophysiology Laboratory
Edith Cavell Building
University of Queensland Medical School
Herston Rd, Herston
Queensland Australia 4006
Ph. +61 7 3511 6564
Fax. +61 7 3365 5564
s309339@student.uq.edu.au

Gina Geffen, PhD
Cognitive Psychophysiology Laboratory
Edith Cavell Building
University of Queensland Medical School
Herston Rd, Herston
Queensland Australia 4006
Ph. +61 7 3365 5562
Fax. +61 7 3365 5564
geffen@psy.uq.edu.au

Figure 9–14a SDMT Form B. © Cognitive Psychophysiology Laboratory. Courtesy of A. Hinton Bayre and G. Geffen.

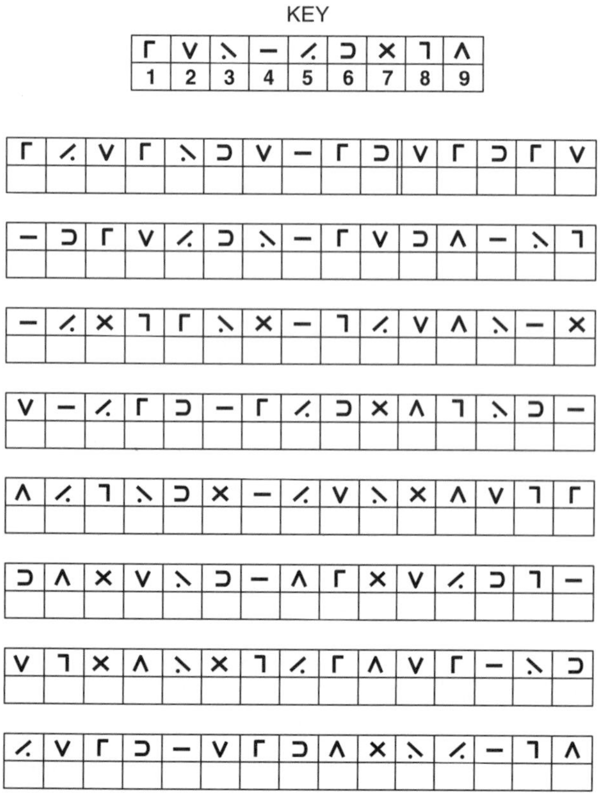

Figure 9–14c SDMT Form D. © Cognitive Psychophysiology Laboratory. Courtesy of A. Hinton Bayre and G. Geffen.

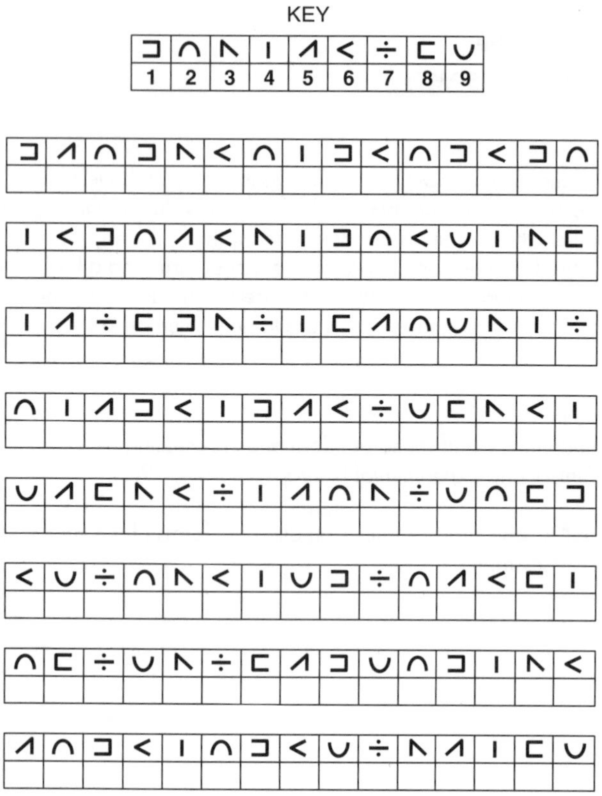

Figure 9–14b SDMT Form C. © Cognitive Psychophysiology Laboratory. Courtesy of A. Hinton Bayre and G. Geffen.

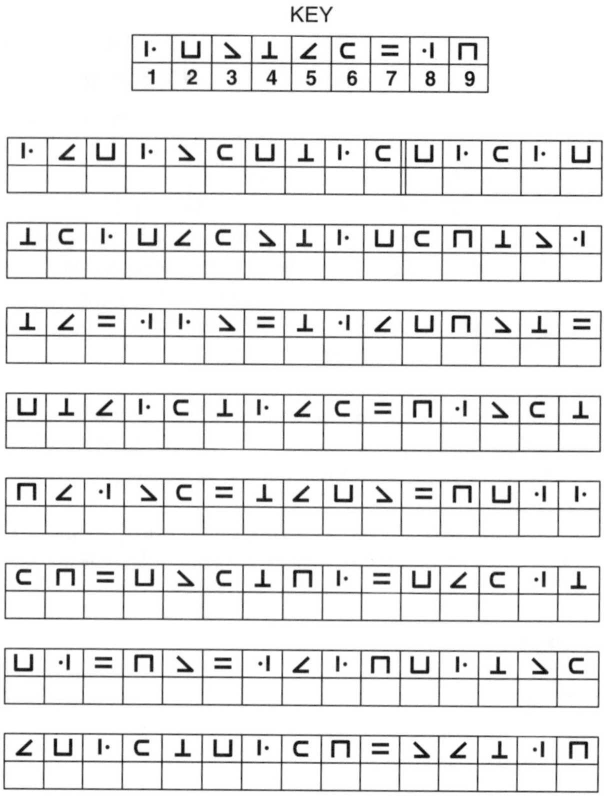

use of a derived index score for accuracy (i.e., percentage correct) yielded lower reliabilities than the number correct score (Hinton-Bayre et al., 1997).

Test-retest reliability information for children is not available. However, scores tend to be higher on the oral form when it is administered after the written form in this age group, especially in the younger children (Smith, 1991).

Practice Effects

The test manual reports gains of about four points at retest (Smith, 1991). Hinton-Bayre et al. (1997), using alternate forms, found a 2% increase in number correct over repeat assessment. Uchiyama et al. (1994), however, noted no significant practice effects when the written version was given at yearly intervals over a two-year period, suggesting relative stability over longer time intervals. Hinton-Bayre et al. (1999) found that the size of the practice effect was dependent on the retesting interval, with alternate forms not fully eliminating practice effects. They consequently recommend two baseline assessments prior to using the SDMT to assess concussion in athletes.

Assessing Reliable Change

Norms for assessing change can be found in Levine et al. (2004), based on a sample similar to the normative sample

Table 9–48 Symbol Digit Modalities Norms for Adults, by Age and Gender, for a Well-Educated, High IQ Sample

		Age			
		15–20	21–25	26–30	31–40
N		62	73	48	42
Education		12.2	14.8	15.5	16.5
FSIQ		118	116	120	122
SDMT	Men				
	Oral	69.97 (10.58)	73.08 (9.88)	68.38 (13.69)	61.96 (7.13)
	Written	57.31 (9.40)	61.00 (9.96)	59.08 (7.92)	52.22 (6.96)
SDMT	Women				
	Oral	71.70 (11.84)	76.59 (10.91)	70.58 (5.73)	69.17 (9.67)
	Written	61.78 (13.66)	63.93 (6.78)	60.58 (4.68)	58.67 (7.24)

Note: FSIQ based on WAIS.

Source: From Yeudall et al., 1986. Reproduced by permission. Copyright © 1986 John Wiley & Sons, Inc., New York. All rights reserved.

used by Uchiyama et al. (1994). The sports concussion literature also provides RCI cutoffs for the SDMT, using forms specific to the particular study (see Erlinger et al., 2003; Hinton-Bayre & Geffen, in press; and Hinton-Bayre et al., 1997, 1999 for additional details).

Alternate Form Reliability

Hinton-Bayre et al. (1997) developed three new written forms, including the three mirrored pairs of symbols appearing in the original, that appear to be equivalent to the standard form (see also Hinton-Bayre & Geffen, in press). These are reproduced in Figures 9–14a, b, and c.

Comparison of the standard form and the alternate form (Form 2; Figure 9–12) developed by Uchiyama et al. (1994) indicates that these forms are not equivalent in level of difficulty. Although the two forms are related ($r = .74$), Form 2 is more difficult than the original SDMT. However, use of form-specific normative data, which the authors provide, alleviates this problem to some extent (see Table 9–47). Form 2 may also be less reliable in longer term follow-ups (i.e., two years). Royer et al.'s alternate forms (1977, 1981) vary in difficulty from the standard form; these cannot therefore be used in serial evaluations.

Table 9–49 Symbol Digit Modalities Norms From a Danish Outpatient Sample ($N = 99$)

	Age Range		
	20–29	30–39	40–54
N	35	27	37
Mean	52.43	53.26	44.41
SD	8.43	8.83	10.61
Range	36–77	35–72	23–67

Source: Reprinted with permission from Nielsen et al., 1989.

VALIDITY

Written Versus Oral Administration

Written and oral forms, although highly correlated, are not necessarily interchangeable. In normal adults, the correlation between written and oral forms is above .78 (Smith, 1991). Likewise, Ponsford and Kinsella (1992) report a correlation of .88 in head-injured patients. However, despite relatively high intercorrelation, mean scores on the two forms may differ. In children, a general tendency to produce higher oral scores is found for all age groups, with the largest score gains evident in the earlier years (Smith, 1991; note that the written version

Table 9–50 Characteristics of the Symbol Digit Modalities Test Normative Sample: Children

Sample type	Children recruited from public schools selected to reflect demographic composition of urban Omaha, Nebraska; proportional representation of low, middle, and upper-middle class schools
N	3680
Age	8 to 17 years[a]
Geographic location	Omaha, Nebraska
Education	Grades 3–12
Gender	
Boys	Written: 1874; Oral: 784
Girls	Written: 1806; Oral: 795
Race/ethnicity	Unspecified
Screening	Exclusion criteria were mental retardation, brain damage, emotional disturbance, or severe visual impairment.

[a]Based on one-year age bands; data also presented in two-year age bands.

Table 9–51 Children's Norms for the Spanish Version of the Symbol Digit Modalities Test

Age	Score Level[a]				Mean	SD	N
	Very Low	Low	Normal	High			
Written SDMT							
8	0–18	19–21	22–36	37–110	29.04	7.07	106
9	0–21	22–25	26–40	41–110	33.07	7.66	161
10	0–24	25–29	30–47	48–110	38.61	9.29	167
11	0–30	31–34	35–52	53–110	43.37	8.62	137
12	0–25	26–32	33–60	61–110	46.36	13.86	120
13	0–34	35–39	40–60	61–110	50.19	10.31	124
14	0–35	36–40	41–60	61–110	50.36	9.76	87
15	0–36	37–41	42–63	64–110	52.69	10.89	100
16	0–39	40–45	46–66	67–110	55.90	10.71	149
17	0–41	42–46	47–68	69–110	57.40	10.66	97
Oral SDMT							
8	0–22	22–26	22–44	45–110	35.50	8.75	106
9	0–27	28–32	33–49	50–110	40.97	8.69	152
10	0–33	34–38	39–59	60–110	49.23	10.40	145
11	0–37	38–42	43–63	64–110	53.02	10.12	126
12	0–38	39–44	45–67	68–110	55.87	11.69	101
13	0–45	46–50	51–70	71–110	60.32	10.12	114
14	0–45	46–50	51–70	71–110	60.21	9.79	81
15	0–46	47–52	53–76	77–110	64.57	11.85	68
16	0–52	53–58	59–80	81–110	69.15	11.07	107
17	0–51	52–57	58–83	84–110	70.75	12.85	79

[a]Score level intervals: Very Low: [0, Mean − 1.5 (SD)]; Low: [Very Low, Mean − 1 (SD)]; Normal: [Low, High]; High: [Mean + 1.5 (SD), Max].

Source: From Arribas, 2002. Reproduced with permission and authorization of TEA Ediciones, S.A. Madrid, Spain. 2002.

was group-administered in this study). Yeudall et al. (1986) also found higher scores for the oral version (about 11 points) in 225 volunteers aged 15 to 40 years.

Correlation With Other Attention Tests

The SDMT is very similar in format to the Wechsler Digit Symbol/Coding subtest. Accordingly, correlations between the two tests for different populations have ranged from about .62 to .78 (e.g., Bowler et al., 1992; Hinton-Bayre et al., 1997; Lewandowski; 1984), to as high as .91 (Morgan & Wheelock, 1992). In the latter case, the tests were administered to 45 individuals referred for neuropsychological examination.

Table 9–52 Means and Standard Deviations for the Written SDMT for Rural, Low SES, South African Zulu Children (*N* = 806)

	Age		
	8 years	9 years	10 years
Boys	14.1 (6.2)	14.2 (6.1)	14.8 (6.9)
Girls	15.2 (6.4)	15.3 (6.6)	16.7 (7.9)

Source: Adapted from Jinabhai et al., 2004.

Despite their very high intercorrelation, SDMT raw scores are usually lower than those for Digit Symbol, likely the result of the increased difficulty of the SDMT (see Glosser et al., 1977), since in contrast to the Symbol Digit task, the key does not have any internal structure (i.e., no numerical progression to aid scanning).

The SDMT primarily assesses the scanning and tracking aspect of attention, tapping aspects of performance similar to those of Letter Cancellation, Trail Making, Digit Symbol, and choice reaction-time tests (McCaffrey et al., 1988; Ponsford & Kinsella, 1992; Royan et al., 2004; Shum et al., 1990). The test is also moderately to highly correlated with scores on the Adjusting PSAT (Royan et al., 2004).

The test has also been found to measure aspects of selective attention, as shown by relationships to the TEA (Bate et al., 2001; Chan et al., 2003). For example, it loads highly on a factor described as Visual Selective Attention along with measures such as Stroop, TEA Map Search, TEA Telephone Search, and Ruff 2 & 7 (Bate et al., 2001; Chan, 2000).

In athletes, it appears to load with other processing speed tasks (Erlanger et al., 2003). In a study on concussed athletes, the test loaded on a Speed/Reaction Time factor with other measures of processing speed and reaction time, separate from a second factor measuring memory (Iverson et al., in press). However, the test appears more highly related to processing speed than simple reaction time in this population (Erlanger et al., 2003). In adolescents at risk for alcoholism, the test correlates moderately with some (e.g. verbal fluency, WCST, and Stroop; $r = .26–.35$) but not other (e.g., Tower of Hanoi) executive functioning tasks (Nigg et al., 2004).

Clinical Studies

The SDMT is extremely sensitive to brain insult in adults as well as children. In particular, due to its sensitivity and its frequent use in research paradigms, it has become one of the most commonly used tests in the standardized evaluation of individuals with TBI, MS, HD, and concussion (see later discussion). Impaired performance has also been associated with a number of other conditions, including epilepsy (Campbell et al., 1981); stroke (see *Source*); organic solvent exposure (Bowler et al., 1992); Parkinson's disease (Starkstein et al., 1989); aging, exercise, dietary fat intake, general fitness, and the P3 component of event-related brain potentials (Emmerson et al., 1990; Morris et al., 2004; Stones & Kozma, 1989); substance abuse (McCaffrey et al., 1988; O'Malley et al., 1992); schizophrenia (Chan et al., 2004); HIV (Sacktor et al., 1999, 2003); sleep apnea (Verstraeten et al., 2004); and cognitive impairments in children of alcoholics (Nigg et al., 2004). It is also sensitive to the identification of individuals with progressive disease among adults treated for brain tumors (Torres et al., 2003), and has been used in neurotoxicity research to determine the cognitive effects of exposure to jet engine oil emissions by aircraft crew (Coxon, 2002) and in epilepsy research to determine cognitive effects of antiepileptic drugs (Meador et al., 2003).

Traumatic Brain Injury (TBI).   Ponsford and Kinsella (1992) found that the oral version of the SDMT was the single best indicator of information processing impairments in TBI, compared with other tasks such as reaction time, Stroop, and PASAT. Significant group differences are found on the SDMT between individuals with TBI and controls, and the task differentiates between individuals who are early versus late in the recovery process (Bate et al., 2001). The test is sensitive to the cognitive effects of diffuse axonal injury (DAI) in patients with severe TBI (Felmingham et al., 2004), and is related to ventricular enlargement (a marker of DAI) in individuals with TBI (Johnson et al., 1994). The test is sensitive to recovery in severe TBI patients with DAI (Felmingham et al., 2004), and predicts change in level of daily functioning five years after TBI (Hammond et al., 2004). The test also has utility in assessing persisting postconcussion symptoms (Chan, 2001; Chan et al., 2003).

The SDMT is sensitive to the effects of concussion in athletes (e.g., Erlanger et al., 2003; Hinton-Bayre et al., 1997, 1999; Zillmer, 2003), including change over time (Hinton-Bayre et al., 1999) and rate of recovery for injuries differing in severity (e.g.,

Mrazik et al., 2000). It is part of standard batteries for use in sports in determining return-to-play (Lovell & Collins, 1998). As noted previously, this includes versions adapted as part of computerized assessment packages for sports-related concussion (e.g., ImPACT, Maroon et al., 2000; CRI, Erlanger et al., 2003).

Multiple Sclerosis (MS).   The test is frequently used in MS research. It is part of standardized batteries for MS such as the Screening Examination for Cognitive Impairment (Beatty et al., 1995; Solari et al., 2002) and the Brief Repeatable Battery of Neuropsychological Tests (BRB-N; Rao & the Cognitive Function Study Group of the National Multiple Sclerosis Society, 1990), along with the PASAT, Selective Reminding Test, COWA, and other well-known neuropsychological tests. Among these, it has been demonstrated to be the most strongly associated with neuroimaging indices of disease, including central atrophy (accounting for approximately half the shared variance in patients with mild to moderate cognitive impairment; Christodoulou et al., 2003). Among the BRB-N tests, it is the most sensitive to visual memory problems in MS (Dent & Lincoln, 2000).

The SDMT has also been used to differentiate between MS subtypes (e.g., Huijbregts et al., 2004). In one study, it was the most sensitive measure for screening neuropsychological impairments in MS patients as part of an at-home, comprehensive evaluation package (Einarsson et al., 2003). The test also correlates with hypothalamic-pituitary-adrenal axis dysregulation in MS (Heesen et al., 2002) and to the presence of lesions in the internal capsule (Tsolaki et al., 1994).

Huntington's Disease (HD).   The SDMT has also been used in HD research and is part of standard assessment methods for the disease, including the Unified Huntington's Disease Rating Scale (UH-DRS; Huntington's Study Group, 1996). Like Digit Symbol, the SDMT is one of the few tests sensitive to cognitive impairments in asymptomatic carriers of the HD gene (Lemiere et al., 2002). It is therefore an important tool for assessing the earliest symptoms of HD, and correlates with radiological evidence of caudate atrophy in HD patients (Starkstein et al., 1988). The SDMT has also been used to track disease progression and identify markers of disease severity: for example, the rate of progression of HD is estimated at 2.1 SDMT points per year (Mahant et al., 2003). In patients with HD, disability is predicted by cognitive impairment as measured by the SDMT and by negative motor features, not positive motor features such as chorea and dystonia (Mahant et al., 2003). SDMT performance is also related to the presence of obsessive-compulsive symptoms in patients with HD (Anderson et al., 2001).

Validity Studies in Children

Despite the large standardization sample for this age group, there are few published reports on the use of the test in children. The manual presents some limited data on various clinical groups, including children with stuttering, whose performance does not differ from controls.

Malingering

The medical-legal context may affect performance on the SDMT. Lees-Hayley (1990) gave the test to 20 personal injury litigants with no history of brain injury and no claim for brain injury. One-half of the subjects scored in the potentially impaired range (that is, at or below −1.5 SD from the mean). Accordingly, administration of symptom validity tests or other tools to assess effort and motivation is recommended to clarify interpretation when assessing medico-legal or forensic patients.

COMMENT

The SDMT is easy to administer, quick, and reliable. Its oral administration is an asset in evaluating individuals with manual impairments, and its written form is useful for individuals with speech disorders. When used in group administrations, it is quick and economical, and can be used to screen for neurocognitive difficulties in children and adults, or for specific purposes such as obtaining pre-season baseline performance estimates in athletes (e.g., Hinton-Bayre et al., 1997). Most important, it is one of the most sensitive tests in neuropsychology, with a large number of research studies documenting its ability to detect cognitive impairment, changes in functioning, disease progression, and disability in a variety of clinical populations. Its sensitivity to cognitive impairment has also made it a mainstay of several standardized batteries for assessing specific clinical populations such as MS, HD, and sports-related concussion. Despite the publication of many tests of attention and processing speed since it was first published, the SDMT remains a crucial tool for neuropsychologists.

One important point concerning norms should be mentioned, and this is that the original adult norms are outdated and based on what appears to be a sample of convenience (see Table 9–44). Alternate norm sources, notably the gender-specific data from Jorm et al. (2004) and other IQ- and education-stratified norms, may be more appropriate.

The oral version may be less susceptible to cultural effects; however, it may provide higher scores than the written version in some cases. Surprisingly, despite its large normative sample in children ($N > 3000$), published studies on its validity and utility in children are few, and reliability data are lacking.

As was noted by Smith (1991), written and oral substitution tasks require the integration of several complex cognitive abilities involved in visual, motor, speech, and mental functions. However, Bate et al. (2001) note that due to its multifactorial nature, it is difficult to differentiate between specific attentional deficits and deficits in speed of information processing when performance is impaired on the SDMT. Note that this may be an asset of the test compared with tests

measuring narrower aspects of ability in that it confers sensitivity across several different populations.

REFERENCES

Anderson, K. E., Louis, E. D., Stern, Y., & Marder, K. S. (2001). Cognitive correlates of obsessive and compulsive symptoms in Huntington's disease. *American Journal of Psychiatry, 158,* 799–801.

Arribas, D. (2002). *SDMT, digit and symbol test (Test de Símbolos y Dígitos).* Madrid: TEA Ediciones.

Barncord, S. W., & Wanlass, R. L. (1999). Paper or plastic: Another ecological consideration in neuropsychological assessment. *Applied Neuropsychology, 6*(2), 121–122.

Bate, A. J., Mathias, J. L., & Crawford, J. R. (2001). Performance on the Test of Everyday Attention and standard tests of attention following severe traumatic brain injury. *The Clinical Neuropsychologist, 15*(3), 405–422.

Beatty, W. W., Paul, R. H., Wilbanks, S. L., Hames, K. A., Blanco, C. R., & Goodkin, D. E. (1995). Identifying multiple sclerosis patients with mild or global cognitive impairment using the screening examination for cognitive impairment (SEFCI). *Neurology, 45,* 718–723.

Bowler, R., Sudia, S., Mergler, D., Harrison, R., & Cone, J. (1992). Comparison of Digit Symbol and Symbol Digit Modalities Tests for assessing neurotoxic exposure. *The Clinical Neuropsychologist, 6,* 103–104.

Campbell Jr., A. L., Bogen, J. E., & Smith, A. (1981). Disorganization and reorganization of cognitive and sensorimotor functions in cerebral commissurotomy. *Brain, 104,* 493–511.

Chan, R. C. K. (2000). Attentional deficits in patients with closed head injury: A further study of the discriminative validity of the Test of Everyday Attention. *Brain Injury, 14,* 227–236.

Chan, R. C. K. (2001). Base rate of post-concussion symptoms among normal people and its neuropsychological correlates. *Clinical Rehabilitation, 15*(3), 266–273.

Chan, R. C. K., Hoosain, R., & Lee, T. M. C. (2003). Are there subtypes of attentional deficits in patients with persisting postconcussive symptoms? A cluster analytical study. *Brain Injury, 17*(2), 131–148.

Chan, M. W. C., Yip, J. T. H., & Lee, T. M. C. (2004). Differential impairment on measures of attention in patients with paranoid and nonparanoid schizophrenia. *Journal of Psychiatric Research, 38*(2), 145–152.

Christodoulou, C., Krupp, L. E., & Liang, Z. (2003). Cognitive performance and MR markers of cerebral injury in cognitively impaired MS patients. *Neurology, 60*(11), 1793–1798.

Coxon, L. (2002). Neuropsychological assessment of a group of BAe 146 aircraft crew members exposed to jet engine oil emissions. *Journal of Occupational Health Safety (Austria and New Zealand), 18*(4), 313–319.

Dent, A., & Lincoln, N. (2000). Screening for memory problems in multiple sclerosis. *British Journal of Clinical Psychology, 39*(3), 311–315.

Einarsson, U., Gottberg, K., & Fredrikson, S. (2003). Multiple sclerosis in Stockholm county: A pilot study exploring the feasibility of assessment of impairment disability and handicap by home visits. *Clinical Rehabilitation, 17*(3), 294–303.

Emmerson, R. Y., Dustman, R. E., Shearer, D. E., & Turner, C. W. (1990). P3 latency and symbol digit performance correlations in aging. *Experimental Aging Research, 15,* 151–159.

Erlanger, D., Feldman, D., Kutner, K., Kaushik, T., Kroger, H., Festa, J., Barth, J., Freeman, J., & Broshek, D. (2003). Development and validation of a web-based neuropsychological test protocol for sports-related return-to-play decision-making. *Archives of Clinical Neuropsychology, 18,* 293–316.

Feinstein, A., Brown, R., & Ron, M. (1994). Effects of practice on serial tests of attention in healthy subjects. *Journal of Clinical and Experimental Neuropsychology, 16,* 436–447.

Felmingham, K. L., Baguley, I. J., & Green, A. M. (2004). Effects of diffuse axonal injury on speed of information processing following a severe traumatic brain injury. *Neuropsychology, 18*(3), 564–571.

Gilmore, G. C., Royer, F. L., & Gruhn, J. J. (1983). Age differences in symbol-digit substitution task performance. *Journal of Clinical Psychology, 39,* 114–124.

Glosser, G., Butters, N., & Kaplan, E. (1977). Visuoperceptual processes in brain-damaged patients on the digit symbol substitution task. *International Journal of Neuroscience, 7,* 59–66.

Gottschalk, L. A., Bechtel, R. J., & Maguire, G. A. (2000). Computerized measurement of cognitive impairments and associated neuropsychiatric dimensions. *Comprehensive Psychiatry, 41*(5), 326–333.

Hammond, F. M., Grattan, K. D., & Sasser, H. (2004). Five years after traumatic brain injury: A study of individual outcomes and predictors of change in function. *NeuroRehabilitation, 19*(1), 25–35.

Heesen, C., Gold, S. M., & Raji, A. (2002). Cognitive impairment correlates with hypothalamo-pituitary-adrenal axis dysregulation in multiple sclerosis. *Psychoneuroendocrinology, 27*(4), 505–517.

Hinton-Bayre, A. D., & Geffen, G. (in press). Comparability, reliability, and practice effects on alternate forms of the Digit Symbol and Symbol Digit Modalities Tests. *Psychological Assessment.*

Hinton-Bayre, A. D., Geffen, G., & McFarland, K. (1997). Mild head injury and speed of information processing: A prospective study of professional rugby league players. *Journal of Clinical and Experimental Neuropsychology, 19,* 275–289.

Hinton-Bayre, A. D., Geffen, G., Geffen, L. B., McFarland, K. A., & Friis, P. (1999). Concussion in contact sports: Reliable change indices of impairment and recovery. *Journal of Clinical and Experimental Neuropsychology, 21*(1), 70–86.

Huijbregts, S. C. J., Kalkers, N. F., de Sonneville, L. M. J., de Groot, V., Reuling, I. E. W., & Polman, C. H. (2004). Differences in cognitive impairment of relapsing, remitting, secondary, and primary progressive MS. *Neurology, 63,* 335–339.

Huntington Study Group. (1996). Unified Huntington's Disease Rating Scale: Reliability and consistency. *Movement Disorders, 11,* 136–142.

Iverson, G. L., Lovell, M. R., & Collins, M. W. (in press). Validity of ImPact for measuring processing speed following sports-related concussion. *Journal of Clinical and Experimental Neuropsychology.*

Jinabhai, C. C., Taylor, M., Rangongo, M. F., Mkhize, N. J., Anderson, S., Pillay, B. J., & Sullivan, K. R. (2004). Investigating the mental abilities of rural Zulu primary school children in South Africa. *Ethnicity & Health, 9*(1), 17–36.

Johnson, S. C., Bigler, E. D., Burr, R. B., & Blatter, D. D. (1994). White matter atrophy, ventricular dilation, and intellectual functioning following traumatic brain injury. *Neuropsychology, 8,* 301–315.

Jorm, A. F., Anstey, K. J., Christensen, H., & Rodgers, B. (2004). Gender differences in cognitive abilities: The mediating role of health state and health habits. *Intelligence, 32,* 7–23.

Joy, S., Kaplan, E., & Fein, D. (2004). Speed and memory in the WAIS-III Digit Symbol-Coding subtest across the adult lifespan. *Archives of Clinical Neuropsychology, 19,* 759–767.

Kennepohl, S., Shore, D., & Nabors, N. (2004). African American acculturation and neuropsychological test performance following traumatic brain injury. *Journal of the International Neuropsychological Society, 10*(4), 566–577.

Laux, L. F., & Lane, D. M. (1985). Information processing components of substitution test performance. *Intelligence, 9*(2), 111–136.

Lees-Haley, P. R. (1990). Contamination of neuropsychological testing by litigation. *Forensic Reports, 3,* 421–426.

Lemiere, J., Decruyenaere, M., & Evers-Kiebooms, G. (2002). Longitudinal study evaluating neuropsychological changes in so-called asymptomatic carriers of the Huntington's disease mutation after 1 year. *Acta Neurologica Scandinavica, 106*(3), 131–141.

Levine, A. J., Miller, E. N., Becker, J. T., Selnes, O. A., & Cohen, B. A. (2004). Normative data for determining significance of test-retest differences on eight common neuropsychological instruments. *The Clinical Neuropsychologist, 18,* 373–384.

Lewandowski, L. J. (1984). The Symbol Digit Modalities Test: A screening instrument for brain-damaged children. *Perceptual and Motor Skills, 59,* 615–618.

Lezak, M. D. (1995). *Neuropsychological assessment* (3rd ed.). New York: Oxford University Press.

Lovell, M. R., & Collins, M. W. (1998). Neuropsychological assessment of the college football player. *Journal of Head Trauma Rehabilitation, 13,* 9–26.

Mahant, N., McCusker, E. A., Byth, K., and the Huntington Study Group. (2003). Huntington's disease: Clinical correlates of disability and progression. *Neurology, 61*(8), 1085-1092.

Maroon, J. C., Lovell, M. R., Norwig, J., Podell, K., Powell, J. W., & Hartl, R. (2000). Cerebral concussion in athletes: Evaluation and neuropsychological testing. *Neurosurgery, 47,* 659–672.

Martin, E. M., Pitrak, D. L., Pursell, K. J., Mullane, K. M., & Novak, R. M. (1995). Delayed recognition memory span in HIV-1 infection. *Journal of the International Neuropsychological Society, 1*(6), 575–580.

McCaffrey, R. J., Krahula, M. M., Heimberg, R. G., Keller, K. E., & Purcell, M. J. (1988). A comparison of the Trail Making Test, Symbol Digit Modalities Test, and the Hooper Visual Organization Test in an inpatient substance abuse population. *Archives of Clinical Neuropsychology, 3,* 181–187.

Meador, K. J., Loring, D. W., Hulihan, J. F., Kamin, M., Karim, R., & CAPSS-027 Study Group. (2003). Differential cognitive and behavioural effects of topiramate and valproate. *Neurology, 60*(9), 1483–1488.

Morgan, S. F., & Wheelock, J. (1992). Digit Symbol and Symbol Digit Modalities Tests: Are they directly interchangeable? *Neuropsychology 4*(6), 327–330.

Moriyama, Y., Mimura, M., & Kato, M. (2002). Executive dysfunction and clinical outcome in chronic alcoholism. *Alcoholism: Clinical & Experimental Research, 26*(8), 1239–1244.

Morris, M. C., Evans, D. A., & Bienias, J. L. (2004). Dietary fat intake and 6-year cognitive change in an older biracial community population. *Neurology, 62*(9), 1573–1579.

Mrazik, M., Ferrara, M. S., & Peterson, C. L. (2000). Injury severity and neuropsychological and balance outcomes of four college athletes. *Brain Injury, 14*(10), 921–931.

Nielsen, H., Knidsen, L., & Daugbjerg, O. (1989). Normative data for eight neuropsychological tests based on a Danish sample. *Scandinavian Journal of Psychology, 30,* 37–45.

Nigg, J. T., Glass, J. M., & Wong, M. M. (2001). Neuropsychological executive functioning in children at elevated risk for alcoholism: Findings in early adolescence. *Journal of Abnormal Psychology, 113*(2), 302–314.

O'Bryant, S. E., Hilsabeck, R. C., & McCaffrey, R. J. (2003). The recognition memory test: Examination of ethnic differences and norm validity. *Archives of Clinical Neuropsychology, 18*(2), 135–143.

O'Malley, S., Adams, M., Heaton, R. K., & Gawin, F. (1992). Neuropsychological impairment in chronic cocaine abusers. *American Journal of Drug and Alcohol Abuse, 18*, 131–144.

Polubinski, J. P., & Melamed, L. E. (1986). Examination of the sex difference on a symbol digit substitution task. *Perceptual and Motor Skills, 62*, 975–982.

Ponsford, J., & Kinsella, G. (1992). Attentional deficits following closed head injury. *Journal of Clinical and Experimental Neuropsychology, 14*, 822–838.

Rao, S. M., in collaboration with the Cognitive Function Study Group of the National Multiple Sclerosis Society. (1990). *A manual for the Brief, Repeatable Battery of Neuropsychological Tests in Multiple Sclerosis.* Milwaukee, WI: Medical College of Wisconsin.

Richardson, E. D., & Marottoli, R. A. (1996). Education-specific normative data on common neuropsychological indices for individuals older than 75 years. *The Clinical Neuropsychologist, 10*, 375–381.

Royan, J., Tombaugh, T. N., & Rees, L. (2004). The Adjusting-Paced Serial Addition Test (Adjusting-PSAT): Thresholds for speed of information processing as a function of stimulus modality and problem complexity. *Archives of Clinical Neuropsychology, 19*(1), 131–143.

Royer, F. L. (1971). Spatial orientational and figural information in free recall of visual figures. *Journal of Experimental Psychology, 91*, 326–332.

Royer, F. L., Gilmore, G. C., & Gruhn, J. J. (1981). Normative data for the symbol substitution task. *Journal of Clinical Psychology, 37*, 608–614.

Sacktor, N. C., Lyles, R. H., Skolarsky, R. L., Anderson, D. E., McArthur, J. C., McFarlane, G., Selnes, O. A., Becker, J. T., Cohen, B., Wesch, J., & Miller, E. N. (1999). Combination antiretroviral therapy improves psychomotor speed performance in HIV-seropositive homosexual men. *Neurology, 52*(8), 1640–1647.

Saktor, N., Skolavsky, R. L., Tarwater, P. M., McArthur, J. C., Selnes, O. A., Becker, J., et al. (2003). Response to systemic HIV viral load suppression correlates with psychomotor speed performance. *Neurology, 61*(4), 567–569.

Selnes, O. A., Jacobson, L., Machado, A. M., Becker, J. T., Wesch, J., Miller, E. N., Visscher, B., & McArthur, J. C. (1991). Normative data for a brief neuropsychological screening battery. *Perceptual and Motor Skills, 73*, 539–550.

Shum, D. H. K., McFarland, K. A., & Bain, J. D. (1990). Construct validity of eight tests of attention: Comparison of normal and closed head injured samples. *The Clinical Neuropsychologist, 4*, 151–162.

Smith, A. (1991). *Symbol Digit Modalities Test.* Los Angeles, CA: Western Psychological Services.

Solari, A., Mancuso, L., Motta, A., Mendozzi, L., & Serrati, C. (2002). Comparison of two brief neuropsychological batteries in people with multiple sclerosis. *Multiple Sclerosis, 8*, 169–176.

Starkstein, S. E., Brandt, J., Folstein, S., Strauss, M., Berthier, M. L., Pearlson, G. D., et al. (1988). Neuropsychological and neuroradiological correlates in Huntington's disease. *Journal of Neurology, Neurosurgery and Psychiatry, 51*, 1259–1263.

Torres, I. J., Mundt, A. J., & Sweeney, P. J. (2003). A longitudinal neuropsychological study of partial brain radiation in adults with brain tumors. *Neurology, 60*(7), 1113–1118.

Tsolaki, M., Drevelegas, A., Karachristianou, S., Kapinas, K., Divanoglou, D., & Routsonis, K. (1994). Correlation of dementia, neurological and MRI findings in multiple sclerosis. *Dementia, 5*(1), 48–52.

Tulsky, D. S., Saklofske, D. H., & Zhu, J. (2003). Revising a standard: An evaluation of the origin and development of the WAIS-III. In D. S. Tulsky, D. H. Saklofske, R. K. Heaton, R. Bornstein, & M. F. Ledbetter (Eds.), *Clinical interpretation of the WAIS-III and WMS-III* (pp. 43–92). New York: Academic Press.

Uchiyama, C. L., D'Elia, L. F., Delinger, A. M., Selnes, O. A., Becker, J. T., Wesch, J. E., Chen, B. B., Satz, P., Van Gorp, W., & Miller, E. N. (1994). Longitudinal comparison of alternate versions of the Symbol Digit Modalities Test: Issues of form comparability and moderating demographic variables. *The Clinical Neuropsychologist, 8*, 209–218.

Verstnaeten, E., Cluydts, R., Pevernagie, D., & Hoffman, G. (2004). Executive function in sleep apnea: Controlling for attentional capacity in assessing executive attention. *Sleep, 27*(4), 685–93.

Yeudall, L. T., Fromm, D., Reddon, J. R., & Stefanyk, W. O. (1986). Normative data stratified by age and sex for 12 neuropsychological tests. *Journal of Clinical Psychology, 42*, 918–946.

Zillmer, E. A. (2003). The neuropsychology of repeated 1- and 3-meter springboard diving among college athletes. *Applied Neuropsychology, 10*(1), 23–30.

Test of Everyday Attention (TEA)

PURPOSE

The Test of Everyday Attention (TEA) is a battery of eight tasks intended to measure attentional processes in adults.

SOURCE

The test can be ordered from Harcourt Assessment (http://www.harcourt-uk.com) at a cost of £271 or $514 US. A Cantonese version normed in Hong Kong has also been described (Chan et al., 2002). There is also an Italian standardization (Cantagallo & Zoccolotti, 1998).

AGE RANGE

The test can be administered to young and older adults; normative subjects range in age from 18 to 80 years. A version for children, the Test of Everyday Attention for Children (TEA-Ch; Manly et al., 1999) is also available (see review in this volume).

DESCRIPTION

The TEA (Robertson et al., 1994) is an eight-subtest test battery designed to assess various attentional components (selective attention, sustained attention, attentional switching, and

Table 9–53 Summary of TEA Subtests

Score	Attention Factor	Description
Map Search	Selective	This is similar in format to a cancellation task; examinees are required to search a visually cluttered display (a realistic map) to identify targets (symbol for restaurant or gas station) among distractors (other symbols and map characters). Testing time is 2 min; the total score is the number of correctly identified target symbols.
Elevator Counting	Sustained	This is an auditory sustained attention task. Examinees are instructed to count a series of tape-presented tones; the premise is that examinees are on an elevator that has a defective floor-indicator, and they must determine what floor they are on by keeping track of the number of tones that sound every time a new floor had been reached.
Elevator Counting with Distraction	Selective/Working Memory	Examinees must follow the instructions for Elevator Counting but count only the low tones while ignoring the high tones.
Visual Elevator	Attentional Switching	This is a visual attentional switching task that requires examinees to switch from an ongoing response (counting forward), when a specific signal is presented (down or up arrow), to a new response style (counting backward). Stimuli are "elevator floors" presented in a stimulus book along with arrows to signal the response switch. Time and accuracy are recorded.
Elevator Counting with Reversal	Attentional Switching/ Working Memory	This subtest uses the same paradigm as the Visual Elevator subtest but presents stimuli aurally instead of visually. "Floors" consist of low tones, up and down arrows are replaced by high and low tones, respectively.
Telephone Search	Selective	This is a visual attention task that requires examinees to search for targets among distractors in a simulated telephone directory.
Telephone Switch while Counting	Sustained/Divided	This is a dual task paradigm in which subject must engage in Telephone Search while simultaneously counting strings of tones presented on an audiotape.
Lottery	Sustained	This is similar in format to an auditory continuous performance test; subjects are instructed to listen to a tape with a series of consecutive letters and numbers, and then to provide the letters that precede a target (two 5s in a row). Targets occur infrequently. The premise is that examinees are listening to a news broadcast listing winning lottery numbers. The test is 10 min long.

Source: Reprinted with permission from Robertson et al., 1994.

divided attention; see Table 9–53). According to the authors, one of the aims of the TEA is to provide a measure with clinical utility that can assist in predicting recovery of function and daily life function after brain damage.

The TEA has several advantages over other tests of attention. It is based mainly on the attentional model by Posner and Peterson (1990), which proposes three attentional systems: orientation, vigilance, and selection. The TEA is designed to measure the last two systems (Bate et al., 2001). To do so, it employs familiar materials in tasks that approximate everyday activities. The TEA is also highly portable and, unlike some attention tests, does not require a computer for administration. The test itself is presented as a mock trip to Philadelphia (in the American version), during which the examinee must perform a series of tasks that would be appropriate in that context (e.g., using a map, finding information in a telephone directory). Three alternate forms are provided for repeat assessment.

ADMINISTRATION TIME

The entire TEA battery takes 45 to 60 minutes.

ADMINISTRATION

See test manual.

Materials

In addition to the test kit, a stopwatch, a black nonpermanent marker (provided in the test kit), and an audiocassette player are required. Extra paper for the Lottery subtest is also needed. The maps and telephone directory are encased in clear plastic so that examinees can mark directly on the stimulus materials. Responses are then wiped off with a damp sponge.

Instructions

Instructions are provided verbatim, after which the examiner may paraphrase if the examinee does not appear to understand task demands. Subtests are administered in a fixed order.

Special Populations

According to the authors, none of the TEA subtests are affected by hearing impairments, with the exception of the

Table 9–54 Summary of Score Ratings for TEA
Elevator Counting

Score Range	Rating
7	Normal
6	Doubtful
5 or less	Definitely abnormal

Source: Reprinted with permission from Robertson et al., 1994, p. 15.

Elevator Counting with Distraction subtest, which showed slightly lower scores in a group of examinees with mild hearing impairment (see test manual). The authors note that, if there are doubts about an examinee's visual acuity, Map Search should not be administered.

Repeat Assessment

Three versions are provided for use in repeat assessments (Versions A, B, and C). Version A is always to be administered first. For a discussion of repeat assessment with the TEA, see *Reliability* and *Comment*.

SCORING

Scores

Score calculations are detailed in the test manual. Scaled scores ($M = 10$, $SD = 3$) and percentiles are derived for each subtest based on normative data presented in the manual. Although the range of scores is from 1 to 19, some subtests have a slightly more restricted range in some age groups due to floor and ceiling effects (see *Comment*). Because of the significant ceiling effect for Elevator Counting (i.e., no normal examinees in the standardization sample made more than one error), there are no scaled score or percentile conversions for

this subtest. Instead, raw scores are assigned an abnormality rating (see Table 9–54). There are no composite scores.

Score Interpretation and Discrepancy Analyses

The manual describes in detail how each subtest should be interpreted and how performance deficits on each task might translate into everyday activities. Crawford et al. (1997) have developed additional tables to assist in clinical interpretation of subtests scores (see Tables 9–55 and 9–56). Table 9–55 shows the size of the difference between each subtest and an individual's mean subtest score on the TEA required for statistical significance. Table 9–56 shows the size of the difference between subtest and mean subtest score that is expected to occur in less than a given percentage of the normal population. These tables can be used in profile analysis to determine significant strengths and weaknesses on the TEA. A computer program can also be downloaded from Dr. Crawford's website and used to calculate these differences for any combination of TEA subtests (http://www.abdn.ac.uk).

DEMOGRAPHIC EFFECTS

Age

Age effects, although present, are not well detailed in the manual.

Gender

There are reportedly no gender differences on any of the subtests (see test manual).

Ethnicity

There is scant information on the test's use in ethnically diverse populations apart from the work of Chan et al. (2002)

Table 9–55 Difference Between TEA Subtest Score and Mean Score on All Subtests Required for Statistical Significance

TEA Subtest	SE$_{diff}$	Critical Value for a Given p			
		.15	.10	.05	.01
Map Search	1.11	2.56	2.73	2.99	3.55
EC with Distraction	1.48	3.41	3.64	3.99	4.73
Visual Elevator	1.48	3.41	3.64	3.99	4.73
EC with Reversal	1.59	3.65	3.89	4.27	5.07
Telephone Search (TS)	1.11	2.56	2.73	2.99	3.55
TS—Dual Task	1.72	3.97	4.22	4.64	5.50
Lottery	1.35	3.10	3.30	3.63	4.30

Note: Size of difference (regardless of sign) between each subtest and an individual's mean subtest score on the TEA required for statistical significance at the .15, .10, .05 and .01 levels. Mean subtest performance must include the individual subtest being compared in addition to all the other subtests. For determination of significant differences using shorter TEA forms, a computer program may be used (see text). EC = Elevator Counting; SE$_{diff}$ = standard error of the difference.

Source: From Crawford et al., 1997. Reproduced with permission from the *British Journal of Clinical Psychology,* © The British Psychological Society.

Table 9–56 Expected Difference Between TEA Subtest Score and Mean Score on All Subtests in a Normal Population

TEA Subtest	SD_{Da}	Percentage of Healthy Population			
		15	10	5	1
Map Search	2.61	3.76	4.29	5.12	6.74
EC with Distraction	2.37	3.42	3.89	4.65	6.12
Visual Elevator	2.40	3.46	3.94	4.71	6.20
EC with Reversal	2.21	3.18	3.62	4.33	5.70
Telephone Search (TS)	2.18	3.14	3.57	4.27	5.62
TS–Dual Task	2.56	3.68	4.20	5.02	6.60
Lottery	2.46	3.54	4.03	4.81	6.34

Note: Size of difference (regardless of sign) between each subtest and an individual's mean subtest score on the TEA such that it would be expected to occur in less than 15, 10, 5 and 1 percent of the healthy population; the standard deviation of the difference is also presented. Mean subtest performance must include the individual subtest being compared in addition to all the other subtests. For determination of significant differences using shorter TEA forms, a computer program may be used (see text). EC = Elevator Counting; SD_{Da} = Standard deviation of the difference.

Source: From Crawford, et al., 1997. Reproduced with permission from the *British Journal of Clinical Psychology*, © The British Psychological Society.

in Hong Kong, where the TEA was generally considered culturally appropriate for Hong Kong Chinese, with some reservations regarding its use in other regions (see *Normative Data*).

Education/IQ

To our knowledge, the influence of education on the test has not been studied. The manual presents correlations between the TEA and the NART as an estimate of verbal intelligence. For number correct, correlations are small (i.e., $r < .30$) for all TEA subtests except Visual Elevator, which is moderately related to NART scores ($r = .39$).

NORMATIVE DATA

Standardization Sample

Overall, the normative sample is not well described (see Table 9–57). The standardization sample (Version A) consists of 154 adults ranging in age from 18 to 80 (69 men, 85 women). The norms are stratified into four age bands (18–34, 35–49, 50–64, and 65–80 years) and two educational levels. The latter are based on scores obtained on the NART (i.e., above or below a score of 100; Nelson, 1982); however, NART scores are estimates of IQ, which may differ from actual education levels. Further, NART score distributions are uneven in the sample (i.e., 65% of the sample had an estimated IQ > 100), leading to an overrepresentation of high-IQ individuals in the TEA norms. Nevertheless, the authors note that this is not likely to cause a problem in score interpretation because of the low correlation between TEA scores and estimated verbal intelligence (see *Validity*). However, TEA score equivalence between high- and low-NART scorers is needed to support this conclusion. Overall, cell sizes are modest ($N = 33$ to 39) in each of

the four age bands. In some age/education groupings, cell sizes are quite small (e.g., $N = 11$ adults at age 50 to 64 years with IQ < 100). Information on norms collection procedure, screening, socioeconomic status, race/ethnicity, and geographic location is not provided. Note that the number of individuals in the norming samples for Version C ($N = 39$) is considerably smaller than for Version A or B (see Table 9–57).

Table 9–57 Characteristics of the Test of Everyday Attention (TEA) Normative Sample

Sample type	Recruitment process not reported; sample is described only as consisting of "normal volunteers"
Number[a]	
Version A	154
Version B	118
Version C	39
Age	18 to 80 years
Geographic location	Presumably England; region not specified
Education	Based on NART score (see Estimated IQ)
Estimated IQ[b]	
Below 100	35%
Above 100	65%
Socioeconomic status	Not reported
Gender	
Men	45%
Women	55%
Race/Ethnicity	Not reported
Screening	Not reported

[a]Divided into four age-bands and two educational bands (NART-based).
[b]Based on NART scores.

Source: Adapted from Robertson et al., 1994.

Table 9–58 Norms and Alternate Form Reliability for the Cantonese version of the TEA

Subtest	Version A (N = 49)		Version B (N = 35)		Pearson Correlation Coefficient (N = 35)
	Mean	(SD)	Mean	(SD)	
Map Search in 1 min	51.69	(10.89)	51.57	(9.81)	0.753**
Map Search in 2 min	73.69	(6.96)	74.31	(3.97)	0.690**
Elevator Counting	6.93	(0.47)	7.00	(0.00)	—a
Elevator Counting with Distraction	8.90	(1.42)	9.14	(1.26)	0.857**
Visual Elevator (number correct)	8.69	(1.29)	8.82	(0.95)	0.462**
Visual Elevator (time per switch)	3.07	(1.04)	2.99	(1.01)	0.939**
Elevator With Reversal	8.18	(1.81)	8.63	(1.54)	0.805**
Telephone Search (time per target)	2.69	(1.40)	2.41	(0.48)	0.841**
Dual task decrement	0.84	(1.34)	0.83	(0.77)	0.591**
Lottery task	9.31	(1.62)	9.63	(0.64)	0.194**

aUnable to calculate due to no variance in the sample.

**$p < 0.01$

Source: From Chan, 2000, p. 903. Reproduced with the permission of Edward Arnold Publishers Ltd.

Score Derivations

Norms construction is detailed in the test manual. Power transform techniques were employed (see manual). Based on the techniques used, it appears that raw score distributions for some subtests were non-normal.

Other Normative Datasets

A Cantonese version normed on 49 Chinese individuals living in Hong Kong has also been described (Chan et al., 2002). Norms are presented in Table 9–58. According to a subsample of individuals surveyed in the normative study, the TEA was generally considered culturally appropriate for Hong Kong Chinese. However, the authors note reservations about the applicability of this version of the test to individuals from mainland China and the suitability of some subtests for individuals who have never traveled abroad, given the travel theme of some of the tasks.

RELIABILITY

Internal Reliability

No information on internal reliability of TEA subtests is provided in the manual, probably because of the speeded nature of the tasks.

Standard Error of Measurement (SEM)

SEMs are not reported in the manual.

Test-Retest Reliability

Users should note that test-retest reliability information for repeat administrations of Version A are not provided. Instead, stability information for the TEA is based on Versions A and B administered sequentially. Consequently, these coefficients reflect both alternate form reliability and test-retest reliability. Coefficients are provided in the manual for a subgroup of 118 individuals from the normative sample who were retested after a 1-week interval. Of these, 39 individuals were then administered Version C in a third session one week after Version B. One-week test-retest reliability data for 74 patients with unilateral stroke is also described. Table 9–59 presents this information in terms of the magnitude of the coefficients obtained.

Overall, test-retest coefficients are substantial (acceptable to high), but some subtests have marginal to poor stability (e.g., Telephone Search While Counting; see Table 9–59). Although stability correlations are not presented for the Elevator or Lottery subtests due to large ceiling effects in the standardization sample, the authors report in the test manual that percentage agreement at retest for these two subtests was substantial (i.e., 96% and 82%, respectively), "allowing for a difference of 1 between first and second scores." It is unclear what is meant by "1," but presumably this refers to one standard deviation (1 SD), as is the case for the children's version (see TEA-Ch).

Despite the low reliability of the Telephone Search While Counting task, the authors note that this measure may nonetheless be "invaluable" clinically because of its sensitivity and because of the fact that some patient groups have extreme difficulty with it. However, no data are presented in the manual to support the clinical sensitivity of this subtest (but see Validity).

In a reliability study involving the Cantonese version of the test (Chan et al., 2002), test-retest reliability was adequate to high for most TEA subtests. However, Visual Elevator (number correct), Telephone Search While Counting, and Lottery all showed poor reliability in this sample (r < .60). Reliability for Elevator Counting could not be computed because of the lack of variance in sample scores.

Table 9–59 Magnitude of Test-Retest Reliability Coefficients and Percentage Agreement for the TEA

Magnitude of Coefficient	Test-Retest Coefficients (Normal Controls, Version A then B)	Test-Retest Coefficients (Normal Controls, Version B then C)	Test-Retest Coefficients (Stroke Patients)
Very high ≥. 90)	—	Telephone Search (raw score)	Visual Elevator (raw accuracy score)
High (.80 to .89)	Map Search Telephone Search (raw score)	Map Search	Map Search Elevator Counting Elevator Counting with Distraction
Adequate (.70 to .79)	Elevator Counting with Distraction Visual Elevator	Visual Elevator	Telephone Search (raw score) Lottery
Marginal (.60 to .69)	Elevator Counting with Reversal	Elevator Counting with Distraction Elevator Counting with Reversal Telephone Search while Counting (dual task decrement)	—
Low (≤. 59)	Telephone Search while Counting (dual task decrement)	—	Telephone Search while Counting (dual task decrement)

Note: Stability coefficients are not provided for normal controls on Elevator Counting and Lottery because of significant ceiling effects. Data are unavailable for stability of Visual Elevator timing scores and Elevator Counting With Reversal in stroke patients.

Practice Effects

No practice effect information (i.e., means and SDs) appears to be presented in the manual, in terms of quantifying the increase in scores that occurs when Version A is followed by Version B, in scaled score format. Note that Version A followed by B is the testing paradigm used to assess test-retest effects; Version A–Version A effects are unknown. According to the manual, practice effects are automatically taken into account when scaled scores are derived for Version B. However, no information on the clinical significance of Version A–Version B scaled score differences (e.g., frequencies of various difference scores in the standardization sample) is presented in the manual.

The manual shows the expected practice effects when Version C is administered after Version B. These vary across subtests, with the largest practice effect obtained for Map Search 1-min score ($M = 4.5$ points, $SD = 8.4$) and the smallest for Visual Elevator accuracy ($M = 0$, $SD = 1.58$). Because of the limited number of subjects administered Version C ($N = 39$), interpretation of repeat assessments involving Version C is made with reference to the average practice effect across subjects, rather than by age group.

VALIDITY

Content Validity

The TEA is one of the few tests based on an established theory of attention (Bate et al., 2001). Rationales for content are detailed in the test manual. No information on bias studies across subgroups (e.g., gender, ethnicity) is presented in the manual.

Factor Structure

To our knowledge, there are no studies on the factor structure of the test except for combined studies that include other measures (see following discussion).

Relationship to Other Measures of Attention

In a related paper (Robertson et al., 1996), the authors provide correlations between selected TEA subtests and conventional attention tests (Stroop, Trails B, PASAT, WCST, WMS Digit Span Backward). Tests that measure sustained attention (Lottery, Elevator Counting) or divided attention (Telephone Search While Counting) were not included because the authors believed that no plausible validated tests of these attentional abilities exist. All of the selected correlations presented are in the moderate to high range ($r = .42$ to $.63$). However, because not all correlations were provided, it is difficult to determine whether these correlational analyses also support the discriminant validity of the attentional components as measured by the TEA.

In a paper by Chan et al. (2002) using the Hong Kong version of the test, TEA subtests showed significant correlations with a number of attention and executive functioning tests (Trails, Color Trails, Symbol Digit Modalities Test, Modified Six Elements Test, Digits Backward, Stroop, Design Fluency, Word Fluency). In another study involving a combined group of normal controls and individuals with severe head injury, Bate et al. (2001) found that two TEA subtests (Elevator Counting, Elevator Counting With Distraction) did not correlate with any established measures of attention. However, the majority of TEA subtests correlated with established measures of attention such as, Stroop, PASAT, and Ruff Selective Attention Test.

The manual describes a principal components analysis with varimax rotation of TEA subtests along with other tests of attention (d2 Visual Search Task, Stroop, Trail Making Test, PASAT, WCST—Nelson Version, Digit Span Backward). This yielded a four-factor solution in the standardization sample. The factors were (a) visual selective attention/speed (Map Search, Telephone Search, d2 Visual Search Task, Stroop, Trails B), (b) attentional switching (Visual Elevator, WCST), (c) sustained attention (Lottery, Elevator Counting, Telephone Search While Counting), and (d) auditory-verbal working memory (Elevator Counting With Reversal, Elevator Counting With Distraction, Digits Backward, PASAT). The first two factors are hypothesized to reflect Posner and Peterson's (1990) selection system, and the sustained attention factor to reflect the vigilance system (Bate et al., 2001).

Using the Hong Kong version, Chan et al. (2002) found somewhat similar factors in normal controls using the TEA in combination with other tests. Both the selective and the sustained attention factors were replicated, and the attentional switching factor was partially replicated with Visual Elevator subtest loading on this factor in both solutions. However, the auditory-verbal working memory factor (Robertson et al., 1994) was not replicated. In a mixed group of normal examinees and patients with severe head injury, Bate et al. (2001) also replicated the visual selective attention factor, attentional switching factor, and sustained attention factor using the TEA and established measures of attention. As in the Chan et al. (2002) study, these authors did not find support for the auditory-verbal working memory factor; rather, the dual task paradigm (Telephone Search While Counting) loaded on a separate factor deemed to reflect divided attention.

In one study, the dual performance task (Telephone Search While Counting) was moderately correlated with another dual performance task involving simultaneous digit span recall and crossing out, and both tasks emerged together in a factor analysis of executive tasks and autobiographical memory tests (Greene et al., 1995).

Correlations With IQ

The manual presents correlations between the TEA and NART (as an estimate of verbal intelligence). Correlations are small (i.e., <.30) for all TEA subtests except Visual Elevator (number correct). This subtest was moderately related to NART scores ($r = .39$).

Clinical Studies

The TEA is increasingly used in clinical research on attention, including patients with dementia, stroke, traumatic brain injury (TBI), and psychiatric disorders. Overall, the TEA appears to be useful in discriminating patients with cognitive deficits from controls, but as with many tests of attention, it is less useful in differentiating between clinical conditions (see also Clayton, 1999). For example, the sensitivity and specificity of

Map Search from the TEA is good in terms of differentiating individuals with mild cognitive impairment or dementia from healthy matched controls, but the test does not differentiate well between the two conditions (De Jager et al., 2003). This is not entirely unexpected, because individuals with mild cognitive impairment and those with dementia of the Alzheimer type (AD) represent a continuum of impairment rather than two distinct populations. In addition, the common effect of disordered executive functioning in the two disorders may also obscure group differences (Royall, 2004). In a small group of patients with early AD, Greene et al. (1995) found that the dual performance task from the TEA (Telephone Search While Counting) was sensitive to disease stage in early AD; this subtest was significantly lower in AD patients with mild signs of dementia than in those with minimal signs. In a study involving patients with progressive supranuclear palsy (PSP) described in the manual (Esmonde et al., in press, as cited by Robertson et al., 1996), two TEA subtests (Lottery and Elevator Counting With Distraction) best discriminated between PSP patients and age-matched controls, compared with other neuropsychological tests.

The TEA is sensitive to the effects of stroke. Older patients with unilateral stroke perform more poorly on all TEA subtests than age-matched controls. In younger stroke patients (ages 50–64 years), this is also true for most of the TEA subtests; exceptions are Elevator Counting, Telephone Search (time per target), and Lottery (see manual for details). Impaired performance on the TEA has also been reported in patients with sustained small white matter infarcts (Van Zandvoort et al., 2003).

Impaired performance has been reported in patients with closed head injury (CHI). The test has also been employed in cluster analyses involving CHI patients (Chan et al., 2003). The manual describes 15 patients with moderate or severe CHI who were administered the TEA (mean of 17 days PTA, seen 14 months after injury). Compared with age- and NART-matched controls, CHI patients had poorer scores on TEA subtests measuring selective and sustained attention (Map Search, Telephone Search, Telephone Search While Counting, and Lottery). Chan (2000) also found that individuals with CHI obtained lower scores on all TEA subtests except Elevator Counting compared with matched controls on a Cantonese version of the test.

In contrast, Bate et al. (2001) found that only three TEA subtests measuring primarily selective attention (Map Search, Visual Elevator, and Telephone Search) discriminated between a group of individuals with severe TBI and a matched control group. Compared with other TEA subtests and other attention tests, only the Map Search test, along with the Stroop, clearly differentiated between individuals with severe head injury and normal controls when shared variance was taken into account (Bate et al., 2001). Results are shown in Table 9–60. Selection of two tests or subtests from each of the attention domains would provide a comprehensive, nonoverlapping assessment of attention in TBI.

Table 9–60 TEA and Other Attention Tests That Can Be Used in a Comprehensive Assessment of Attentional Factors in Patients With Traumatic Brain Injury (TBI)

Factor	Roberston et al. 1996	Chan et al. 2000	Bate et al., 2001
Visual selective attention	Map Search Telephone Search Stroop Cancellation Task (d2 Total)	Map Search Telephone Search Stroop SDMT (oral) Elevator Counting with Reversal	Map Search Telephone Search Stroop SDMT (oral) Ruff (2s and 7s) Selective Attention Test
Attentional switching	Visual Elevator (number correct) Wisconsin	Visual Elevator (time) Elevator Counting with Distraction	Elevator Counting with Reversal Elevator Counting with Distraction
Sustained attention	Lottery Elevator Counting Telephone Search while Counting (dual task decrement)	Lottery Elevator Counting Digit Span Backward	Lottery Visual Elevator (correct) Digit Span Backward PASAT (2s)
Auditory-Verbal	Elevator Counting with Reversal		
Working memory	Elevator Counting with Distraction Digit Span Backward PASAT (2s)		
Divided attention		Telephone Search while Counting (dual task decrement)	Telephone Search while Counting (dual task decrement) Elevator Counting

Note: At least two subtests from each of the domains are recommended for a comprehensive, nonoverlapping assessment of attention in TBI.

Source: From Bate, et al., 2001. Reprinted with the kind permission of Psychology Press.

The test has also been used in individuals with psychiatric disorders. Clayton et al. (1999) found that individuals with obsessive-compulsive disorder (OCD) displayed a selective attention deficit on the TEA (i.e., poor performance on three of four selective attention subtests), compared with patients with panic disorder and nonclinical controls. Pleva and Wade (2002) found that university students with high obsessionality scored lower on some TEA subtests than did those with low obsessionality, with the largest differences obtained on the Visual Elevator subtest.

One study showed significant differences on only one TEA subtest (Map Search 2) in Ecstasy users with a polydrug history. This effect size was large, and dosage was related to attentional impairment on other TEA subtests (Zakzanis et al., 2002). Recently, the test was also used to show the substantial heterogeneity of attention profiles across individuals with learning disability (Sterr, 2004).

Ecological Validity

Moderate correlations between an attention questionnaire completed by close relatives (the Rating Scale of Attentional Behaviour; Ponsford and Kinsella, 1992) and two TEA subtests (Map Search and Elevator Counting) were obtained in the group of 80 stroke patients described in the manual ($r = -.30$

and $-.45$, respectively). The correlations for other TEA subtests are not presented. However, the authors note that other conventional measures of attention (Stroop, PASAT, Digit Span Backward) did not correlate consistently with the attentional rating scale. Using the Hong Kong version, the TEA was generally not significantly correlated with either the Dysexecutive Questionnaire (DEX, from the BADS test) or the Cognitive Failures Questionnaire (CFQ; Broadbent et al., 1982). Only the Visual Elevator and Lottery subtests were related to ratings on the CFQ.

Robertson et al. (1994) examined relationships between TEA subtests and measures of functional status in the stroke group presented in the manual ($N = 80$). The Map Search and Elevator Counting subtests were moderately correlated with two measures of activities of daily living (Barthel Index, Wade & Collin, 1988; Extended Activities of Daily Living Scale, Nourri & Lincoln, 1987), with rs ranging from .34 to .48. Correlations with other TEA subtests are not presented. However, the authors note that, unlike the TEA, other conventional measures of attention (Stroop, PASAT, Digit Span Backward) did not correlate consistently with these functional measures. The TEA has also been used as an outcome measure in evaluating the efficacy of a visual retraining program designed to improve driving skills after stroke (Mazer et al., 2003).

COMMENT

The TEA authors should be commended for attempting to address some of the major weaknesses of established tests of attention; namely, their multifactorial nature, their poor ecological validity, and their lack of theoretical basis (Bate et al., 2001). The TEA is one of the few tests based on an established theory of attention (Bate et al., 2001) that also strives for ecological validity. The TEA embeds its subtests in the novel and imaginative format of a mock holiday using materials that simulate real-life tasks. This is an asset because, as the authors note, a major factor predicting satisfaction with neuropsychological assessment is the perceived relevance of the tests (Bennett-Levy et al., 1994). The TEA test manual is generally well written; additional information on the test can be found in a published study by the authors (Robertson et al., 1996). Many of the subtests have proved useful in studies involving several clinical groups.

The dual task subtest is considered an important addition to the assessment of attention (Bate et al., 2001) and the conormed subtests enable accurate cross-domain comparisons. Profile analysis is also possible using the tables developed by Crawford et al. (1997) and the related computer program (see Tables 9–55 and 9–56). There are, however, some limitations.

Psychometric Limitations

The normative sample is not well described. Important information on the test's relationship to IQ, education, gender, and ethnicity is limited or lacking. Not enough information is provided on the test's reliability. In addition, the selective influence of practice effects on TEA subtests cannot be assessed based on the information presented in the manual. Although norms for Version B appear to already take into account the practice effect, there remain questions about the equivalence of test forms.

The procedures required for determining the significance of changes at retest are not well described, and one must read several separate portions of the manual to understand them. Further, there are no guidelines for determining the clinical significance of Version A versus Version B scaled score differences when individuals are retested. As noted by the authors, caution must be employed in interpreting Version C scores due to the small number of individuals administered this version in the standardization sample. Given the small size of this sample, we would recommend against using Version C in clinical practice.

Although the test appears to have considerable potential in the clinical evaluation of attention problems based on group studies of various neuropsychological populations, information on the sensitivity, specificity, and positive/negative predictive power for various disorders involving attention are lacking. In addition, some subtests have poor test-retest reliability (e.g., Telephone Search While Counting); therefore, despite their potential utility in a clinical context, these tasks must be employed with caution in the diagnostic assessment of attentional problems. Further information on the construct validity of Elevator Counting and Elevator Counting With Distraction would also be helpful.

Floor and Ceiling Effects

Ceiling effects are clearly apparent on the Elevator Counting subtest, on which normal individuals achieve virtually perfect performance. However, ceiling effects are also apparent on other tasks; for example, the highest score that can be obtained by the youngest age group on the Elevator Counting With Reversal subtest is a scaled score of 13. Ceiling effects were noted on several subtests in a study involving university students (Preva & Wade, 2002), suggesting that caution should be used in interpreting scores in high-achieving patients.

In older individuals, floor effects are evident on a number of subtests. For example, in the oldest age range of the normative sample, the lowest score possible (i.e., a score of 0) is equivalent to a scaled score of 7 on the Elevator Counting With Reversal subtest. Floors also appear to differ depending on whether Version A or Version B is employed. Users should note that on some subtests, Version B has a slightly higher floor, which means that examinees obtaining very poor scores on Version A might obtain slightly higher scaled scores on Version B due to the restriction in range in some Version B subtests. For example, in the oldest age group, the minimum scaled score for Version A Map Search 2 is a scaled score of 1, but the minimum scaled score for Version B is 5. However, these differences do not appear to be consistent across subtests (for Map Search B, the reverse is true: in the oldest age group, the minimum score for Version A is a scaled score of 6, whereas the minimum score for Version B is 3). Although these differences may be minimal when normal to high-level individuals are assessed, they can potentially cause interpretation problems for low-functioning individuals and when trying to evaluate change.

Clinical Use and Interpretation

Additional information on the neuroanatomical correlates of some subtests is needed, particularly because the test is based on a theory of attention that posits separate neuroanatomical systems for separate attentional systems. In addition, the TEA contains subtests that are multifactorial in nature (Bate et al., 2001), which complicates the interpretation of poor performance on some subtests. Adjustments for motor speed and processing speed, a feature of the children's version, would be a welcome addition to any revision of the test.

Bate et al. (2001) recommended caution in the interpretation of the TEA factor structure because of the lack of correspondence between some subtests and the attentional factor they are presumed to measure (see *Validity*). However, the selective attention, the sustained attention, and possibly the attention switching factors seem fairly well replicated in the three studies that examined this question (Robertson et al., 1996; Chan et al., 2002; Bate et al., 2001).

Bate et al. (2001) listed the factor analytical solutions obtained to date, including relevant TEA subtests by domain along with other established measures of attention (see Table 9–60). This table might be of clinical utility in choosing combinations of TEA subtests and established attentional tests to ensure that the evaluation covers the attentional factors identified in previous studies. These authors recommended that two subtests or tests from each factor in the table be chosen to provide an adequate assessment of attention. Additional reference to the reliability information provided in Table 9–58 would also be useful in selecting subtests that are reliable in addition to having sensitivity to specific attentional dimensions.

REFERENCES

Bate, A. J., Mathias, J. L., & Crawford, J. R. (2001). Performance on the Test of Everyday Attention and standard tests of attention following severe traumatic brain injury. *The Clinical Neuropsychologist, 15*(3), 405–422.

Bennett-Levy, J., Klein-Boonschate, M. A., Batchelor, J., McCarter, R., & Walton, N. (1994). Encounters with Anna Thompson: The consumer's experience of neuropsychological assessment. *The Clinical Neuropsychologist, 8*, 219–238.

Broadbent, D. E., Cooper, P. F., FitzGerald, P., & Parkes, K. R. (1982). The Cognitive Failures Questionnaire (CFQ) and its correlates. *British Journal of Clinical Psychology, 21*, 1–16.

Cantagallo, A., & Zoccolotti, P. (1998). *Il Test dell'Attenzione nella vita Quotidiana (T.A.Q.): Il contributo alla standardizzazione italiana.* [A contribution on the Italian standardization of the Test of Everyday Attention.] *Rassegna di Psicologia, 15*(3), 137–147.

Chan, R. C. (2000). Attentional deficits in patients with closed head injury: A further study of the discriminative validity of the Test of Everyday Attention. *Brain Injury, 14*(3), 227–236.

Chan, R. C. (2002). Reliability and validity of the Cantonese version of the Test of Everyday Attention among normal Hong Kong Chinese: A preliminary report. *Clinical Rehabilitation, 16*, 900–909.

Chan, R. C. K., Hoosain, R., Lee, T. M. C., Fan, Y. M., & Fong, D. (2003). Are there sub-types of attentional deficits in patients with persisting post-concussive symptoms? A cluster analytical study. *Brain Injury, 17*(2), 131–148.

Clayton, I. C., Richards, J. C., & Edwards, C. J. (1999). Selective attention in obsessive-compulsive disorder. *Journal of Abnormal Psychology, 108*, 171–175.

Crawford, J. R.., Sommerville, J., & Robertson, I. H. (1997). Assessing the reliability and abnormality of subtest differences on the Test of Everyday Attention. *British Journal of Clinical Psychology, 36*, 609–617.

De Jager, C. A., Hogervorst, E., Combrinck, M., & Budge, M. M. (2003). Sensitivity and specificity of neuropsychological tests for mild cognitive impairment, vascular cognitive impairment and Alzheimer's disease. *Psychological Medicine, 33*, 1039–1050.

Esmonde, T., Giles, E., Gibson, M., & Hodges, J. R. (in press). Neuropsychological performance, disease severity and psychiatric symptoms in progressive supranuclear palsy. *Journal of Neurology, Neurosurgery and Psychiatry.*

Greene, J. D. W., Hodges, J. R., & Baddeley, A. D. (1995). Autobiographical memory and executive function in early dementia of the Alzheimer's type. *Neuropsychologia, 33*, 1647–1670.

Manly, T., Robertson, I. H., Anderson, V., & Nimmo-Smith, I. (1999). *TEA-Ch: The Test of Everyday Attention for Children.* Bury St. Edmunds, UK: Thames Valley Test Company.

Mazer, B. L., Sofer, S., Korner-Bitensky, N., Gelinas, I., Hanley, J., & Wood-Dauphinee, S. (2003). Effectiveness of a visual attention retraining program on the driving performance of clients with stroke. *Archives of Physical Medicine and Rehabilitation, 84*, 541–550.

Nelson, H. (1982). *The National Adult Reading Test (NART).* Windsor, UK: NFER.

Nourri, F. M., & Lincoln, N. B. (1987). The extended activities of daily living scale for stroke patients. *Clinical Rehabilitation, 1*, 301–305.

Pleva, J., & Wade, T. D. (2002). An investigation of the relationship between responsibility and attention deficits characteristic of obsessive-compulsive phenomena. *Behavioural and Cognitive Psychotherapy, 30*, 399–414.

Ponsford, J., & Kinsella, G. (1992). The use of a rating scale of attentional behaviour. *Neuropsychological Rehabilitation, 1*, 241–257.

Posner, M. I., & Peterson, S. E. (1990). The attention system of the human brain. *Annual Review of Neuroscience, 13*, 25–42.

Robertson, I. H., Ward, T., Ridgeway, V., & Nimmo-Smith, I. (1994). *The Test of Everyday Attention.* Bury St. Edmunds, England: Thames Valley Test Company.

Robertson, I. H., Ward, T., Ridgeway, V., & Nimmo-Smith, I. (1996). The structure of human attention: The Test of Everyday Attention. *Journal of the International Neuropsychological Society, 2*, 525–534.

Royall, D. R. (2004). Letter to the editor. *Psychological Medicine, 34*, 761–762.

Sterr, A. M. (2004). Attention performance in young adults with learning disabilities. *Learning and Individual Differences, 14*, 125–133.

Van Zandvoort, M., De Haan, E., Van Gijn, J., & Kappelle, L. J. (2003). Cognitive functioning in patients with a small infarct in the brainstem. *Journal of the International Neuropsychological Society, 9*, 490–494.

Wade, D. T., & Collin, C. (1988). The Barthel ADL index: A standard measure of physical disability? *International Disability Studies, 10*, 64–67.

Zakzanis, K. K., Young, D. A., & Radkhoshnoud, N. F. (2002). Attentional processes in abstinent methylenedioxymethamphetamine (Ecstasy) users. *Applied Neuropsychology, 9*(2), 84–91.

Test of Everyday Attention for Children (TEA-Ch)

PURPOSE

The Test of Everyday Attention for Children (TEA-Ch) is a battery of nine tasks intended to measure attentional processes in children and adolescents.

SOURCE

The tests can be ordered from Harcourt Assessment (http://www.harcourt-uk.com) at a cost of $703 US.

AGE RANGE

The TEA-Ch can be administered to children between the ages of 6 and 16 years.

DESCRIPTION

The TEA-Ch (Manly et al., 1999) is a modification of the Test of Everyday Attention (TEA; Robertson et al., 1994–1999), adapted for use with children. The test's theoretical foundation is that attention consists of a system of separate attentional processes that may be differentially affected in different disorders. Unlike many commercially available attention tests, it consists of an entire test battery designed to assess various attentional components. According to the authors, the TEA-Ch has several other advantages over other tests of attention. It is theoretically driven, includes multiple subtests to assess each attentional dimension, presents stimuli in both auditory and visual modalities, minimizes the involvement of other cognitive processes in the assessment process (e.g., motor speed, verbal comprehension, reading), and uses game-like materials designed to maximize ecological validity and test engagement (see Figures 9–15 through 9–17 for examples). It is also highly portable and, unlike

Figure 9–15 Stimuli for Sky Search and Sky Search DT subsets of the TEA-Ch. Children are asked to search for pairs in which the two spacecrafts are the same. *Source:* Reprinted with permission from Manly et al., 2001, p. 1069.

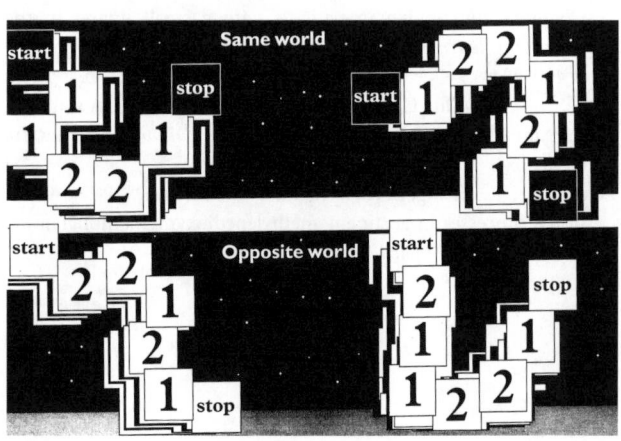

Figure 9–16 TEA-Ch Sky Search Motor Control stimulus sheet. *Source:* Reprinted with permission from Manly et al., 2001, p. 1070.

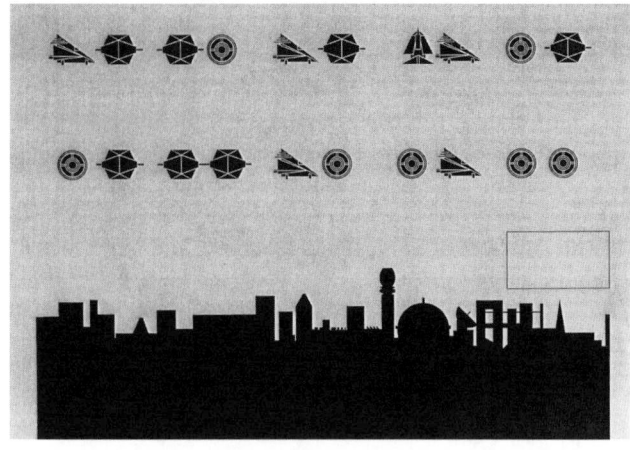

some attention tests, does not require a computer for administration.

The nine subtests assess three attention factors: focused (selective) attention, sustained attention, and attentional control/switching (see Table 9–61). The first four subtests can also be administered as a brief screener that covers each of the attentional factors and provides a measure of dual task performance.

ADMINISTRATION TIME

The entire TEA-Ch battery takes approximately 1 hour. The manual does not provide estimated testing time for the four-subtest screener.

Figure 9–17 Item from the TEA-Ch Creature Counting subset. *Source:* Reprinted with permission from Manly et al., 2001, p. 1070.

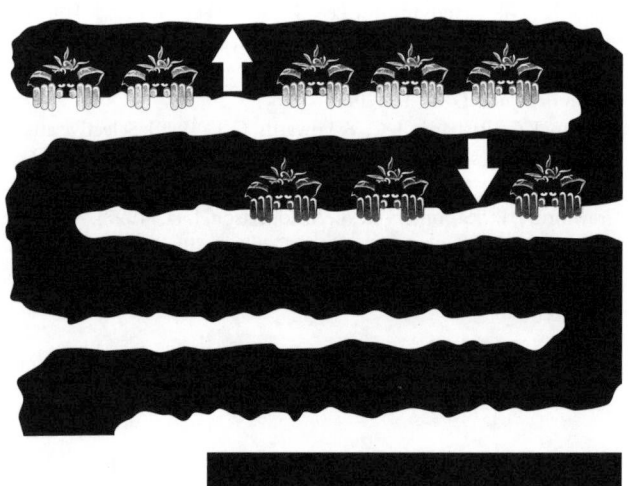

Table 9–61 Summary of TEA-Ch Subtests

Score	Attention Factor	Description
Sky Search	Selective/Focused	This is similar to a paper-and-pencil cancellation task. In the first part of the test, examinees are instructed to circle targets (identical spaceship pairs) on a large plastic sheet that also includes distractors (dissimilar spaceship pairs) under time constraints. The second part of the task is designed to control for motor speed only: on a second sheet, children are simply instructed to circle targets (no distractors are presented). The final score is adjusted for motor speed based on performance on the second part of the test.
Score!	Sustained	This is similar to an auditory continuous performance task. Children are instructed to count the number of "scoring" sounds heard on a tape, as if they were keeping score on a computer game. Targets are interspersed with long gaps, which maximizes the need for sustained attention.
Creature Counting	Control/Switching	This is an attentional switching task that requires children to suppress an ongoing response (counting forward) when a specific signal is presented (down or up arrow) and switch to a new response style (counting backward). Stimuli are colorful "aliens" presented along a path (i.e., "burrow") in a stimulus book. Time and accuracy are recorded.
Sky Search DT	Sustained-Divided	In this task, children are required to do two previous subtests simultaneously (Sky Search and Score!) to determine whether a significant decrement in performance occurs when divided attention is required.
Map Mission	Selective/Focused	Also similar to a cancellation test; children are required to search a visually cluttered display (a realistic map) to identify targets (symbol for restaurant or gas station) among distractors (other symbols and map characters). Testing time is 1 min.
Score DT	Sustained	This subtest combines the Score! Subtest with a second auditory sustained attention task that is similar to a continuous performance task (i.e., a long news broadcast during which animal names are mentioned). The children are told to focus on the counting required for the Score! Subtest while simultaneously attending to the animal names. This subtest therefore requires children to selectively allocate attentional resources.
Walk, Don't Walk	Sustained/Response Inhibition	This is similar to a go/no-go paradigm in that children must listen to an auditory signal to determine whether to "step forward" on a visual array, using a pen to mark their progress. Both a "go" signal and a "no-go" signal are presented, and the child must inhibit his or her motor response only to the "no-go" signal.
Opposite Worlds	Control/Switching	This task employs congruent and noncongruent conditions to measure the ability to suppress a habitual response in a way that approximates a Stroop paradigm. Children are shown two sets of numbers (alternating 1s and 2s), which must be "read" in two different ways, depending on whether the numbers are presented in the "Same World" (conventional meaning of the numbers) or "Opposite World" (opposite meaning of the numbers; i.e., 2s must be read as 1s and vice versa). The time taken to make the cognitive reversal on the "Opposite World" task is the main measure; speed of processing is controlled by subtracting performance on the "Same World" task.
Code Transmission	Sustained	This is an auditory continuous performance task. Children must listen to a tape with a series of consecutive numbers and are instructed to provide the number that preceded a target (two 5s in a row). Targets occur infrequently. The subtest takes 12 min and is designed to be monotonous.

Note: DT = Dual Task.

ADMINISTRATION

See test manual.

Materials

In addition to the test kit, a stopwatch, a black nonpermanent marker (provided in the test kit), and an audiocassette player are required.

Instructions

Instructions are provided verbatim, after which the examiner asks the child to explain the test instructions to ensure comprehension. If the child does not understand task demands, the examiner can then paraphrase the directions. Because the test was normed in Australia, Baron (2001) recommended minor modifications of standard instructions for North American children (e.g., "mark" instead of "tic," "at the end of each part" instead of "at the end of each go").

Special Populations

According to the authors, caution should be employed in interpreting results from children with difficulties in speech production on the Creature Counting and Opposite Worlds subtests because of the requirement for rapid verbal response. Similar caution should be used in interpreting results of Map Mission, Sky Search DT, and Walk Don't Walk in children with slowed motor functioning because of the requirement for rapid motor response on these subtests. Although the test has a relatively low correlation with IQ, the authors also note that data are lacking on the TEA-Ch performance of children with below-average IQ, so caution should also be used in interpreting scores of these children. In addition, the manual discusses how strategy use can yield spuriously high or low time-per-target scores on Sky Search, a situation that should be clarified by careful observation. Hearing difficulties should be assessed before the Score DT subtest is administered, given its high demand for auditory discrimination. Similarly, children whose first language is not English or who have receptive language impairments should not be administered this subtest.

Repeat Assessment

The manual recommends using the alternate form (Version B) if a retest is required, and 95% confidence bands accounting for the expected practice effect are provided in the manual for interpretation of obtained scores. For some tests, changes would have to be quite large to be considered clinically significant; for example, for Sky Search DT, a difference in scaled scores of 10 points is necessary (see *Reliability* and *Comment* for further discussion of this approach).

SCORING

Scores

Scaled scores ($M = 10$, $SD = 3$) and percentiles are derived for each subtest based on normative data presented in the manual. There are no composite scores. Detailed scoring instructions on how to derive scaled scores adjusted for motor or processing speed for specific subtests are provided in the manual.

DEMOGRAPHIC EFFECTS

Age

There are moderate to high age effects on the TEA-Ch, depending on the subtest. For the most part, there appears to be a plateauing of skills during adolescence that is a result of developmental factors, ceiling effects, or both (Manly et al., 2001).

Gender

Gender effects are minimal. Boys perform moderately better on Creature Counting timing score, and girls outperform boys on Sky Search in some age bands (Manly et al., 2001).

Ethnicity and Socioeconomic Status

To our knowledge, there are no studies involving the use of the test in ethnically diverse populations, nor have bias analyses been carried out. However, the test is not significantly correlated with socioeconomic status (SES), at least in the standardization sample (Manly et al., 2001).

IQ

The test's correlation with FSIQ is not known. The manual reports generally minimal correlations between TEA-Ch subtests and an abbreviated IQ estimate comprising Vocabulary, Similarities, Block Design, and Object Assembly from the WISC-III. However, this estimate did not include Freedom from Distractibility or Processing Speed Wechsler subtests, which may yield higher TEA-Ch/IQ correlations (see also *Validity*). No information is available yet on the TEA-Ch's correlation with the WISC-IV.

NORMATIVE DATA

Standardization Sample

See Table 9–62. The standardization sample consisted of 293 Australian children between the ages of 6 and 16 years, arranged into six age bands (6–7, 7–9, 9–11, 11–13, 13–15, and 15–16 years). Although the overall number of examinees is substantial, breakdown by age and gender causes some cells to be modest in size ($N = 13$ to 30 per age band), with some age bands somewhat underrepresented (e.g., $N = 13$ for girls and $N = 16$ for boys in the oldest age band). Although the manual does not indicate why this was needed, separate norms are provided for boys and girls for each subtest. As noted earlier, Manly et al. (2001) found gender effects on only a few TEA-Ch subtests. Short-form WISC-III IQ tests administered to a subset of the sample ($N = 160$) indicated that the sample had slightly above-average IQ in all age bands except the two older age bands (13+ years), in which IQs were average. Information on parental education and ethnic composition of the normative sample is not provided in the manual. However, Manly et al. (2001) indicated that the mean SES of the sample was 4.04 of a possible 7 (where 1 is the highest SES and 7 is the lowest score) according to an Australian SES system (Daniel, 1983). SES was not related to TEA-Ch scores.

Table 9–62 Characteristics of the TEA-Ch Normative Sample

Sample type	Children recruited from state schools
Number	293
Age	6 years to 15 years 11 months[a]
Geographic location	Melbourne, Australia
Parental education	Not reported
Prorated IQ (median)	
Age 6	110
Age 7 to 8	112
Age 9 to 10	114
Age 11 to 12	105
Age 13 to 14	103
Age 15 to 16	98
Socioeconomic status	4.04 (*SD* = 1.2, range = 1.7 to 6.6)[b]
Gender (%)	
Boys	50%
Girls	50%
Race/Ethnicity	Not reported
Screening	Exclusion: Head injury or neurological illness, developmental delay or sensory loss, referral for attention or learning problems, or assessed as having special education needs

[a]Divided into six age bands.
[b]Based on parental occupation, as coded in Daniel's Scale of Occupational Prestige (Daniel, 1983); a high occupational status is coded as 1, and a low status is coded as 7 on this scale.

Source: Adapted from Manly, T., et al., 1999.

Score Conversion

Norms construction is detailed in the manual. Power transform techniques were employed (see p. 32 of the test manual for further details). Scores for some subtests were non-normally distributed. Skew and kurtosis values for the subtests are described in a separate paper by the authors (Manly et al., 2001).

RELIABILITY

Internal Consistency

No information on internal reliability of TEA-Ch subtests is provided in the manual, most likely because of the speeded nature of the tasks.

Test-Retest Reliability

Test-retest reliability information for 55 children is provided for alternate forms administered in sequence (Version A then B), but not for the same form administered twice. These coefficients therefore reflect both test-retest and alternate form reliability. The test interval was less than 20 days. According to the authors, raw scores from Version B were scaled using the transforms established from the larger sample of Version A scores. Reliability correlations are based on raw scores after adjustment for age. These are presented in Table 9–63. With some exceptions, most reliabilities are adequate to high. For three subtests, correlations are not presented because of ceiling effects. Instead, the percentage agreement within one standard deviation (3 scaled score points) for the first and second testing was used instead (see Table 9–63). These values indicate that approximately one fourth of children received scores at retest that were one standard deviation larger or smaller than their baseline score.

Practice Effects

The manual provides 95% confidence bands based on the expected practice effect for retest values involving baseline testing with Version A and retesting with Version B (Manly et al., 1999). Scores outside the range are presumed to reflect clinically significant change. Actual means, standard deviations, and scaled score differences for the retest sample are not presented. Depending on the subtest, a difference of 2 to 7 scaled score points is needed to indicate a significant drop in performance, and a difference of 5 to 10 scaled score points is

Table 9–63 Magnitude of Test-Retest Reliability Coefficients and Percentage Agreement for the TEA-Ch

Magnitude of Coefficient	Test-Retest Coefficients	Percentage Agreement
Very High (≥.90)	—	—
High (.80 to .89)	Sky Search—Time per target Sky Search—Decrement Same World—Time Opposite World—Time	—
Adequate (.70 to .79)	Sky Search—Attention score Creature Counting—Accuracy Code Transmission	Score! (76%) Score DT (71%) Walk Don't Walk (71%)
Marginal (.60 to .69)	Map Mission	—
Low (≤.59)	Creature Counting—Timing	—

Note: Percentage agreement within 1 *SD* is provided for subtests with ceiling effects.

needed to indicate a significant increase in performance. The manual indicates that particular caution should be applied when using longer testing intervals or if more than one retest is required.

Alternate Forms Reliability

No specific information on the reliability of Version B is provided in the manual. As noted earlier, test-retest reliability also combines alternate form reliability because test-retest reliability is based on first administration with Version A, followed by retest with Version B (see test manual).

VALIDITY

Subtest Intercorrelations

No information on subtest intercorrelations is provided in the manual.

Factor Structure

As described in the manual, a three-factor model of sustained and selective attention and executive control was entered as the a priori model and was found to be supported by the data. A one-factor model reflecting a single latent variable was not supported in a structural equation modeling study by the authors involving the normative sample (see Figure 9–18; Manly et al., 2001). No other factor models or structure in other populations have been investigated.

Correlations With IQ

For the most part, correlations with IQ are minimal, but moderate correlations are reported between Creature Counting and IQ ($r = .31$), as well as small correlations between Map Mission, Walk Don't Walk, Code Transmission, and IQ ($r = .17$ to $.25$) using a four-subtest WISC-III IQ test administered to 160 children from the normative sample. Users should note that this abbreviated IQ estimate (Vocabulary, Similarities, Block Design, and Object Assembly) did not include any subtests from the WISC-III Freedom from Distractibility or Processing Speed indices. Inclusion of these subtests might have yielded higher TEA-Ch/IQ correlations.

Correlations With Other Attention Tests

The test manual describes the performance of 96 children from the normative sample who were also administered measures of selective attention (Stroop), selective attention and attentional switching (Trail Making Test), and impulsivity (Matching Familiar Figures Test [MFFT]; Arizmendi, Paulsen & Domino, 1981). The same data were also presented in detail in a separate paper by the authors (Manly et al., 2001).

Although several subtests were significantly correlated with these measures, examination of the correlations between tests reveals that many TEA-Ch subtests were related to attention tests that are not ostensibly measuring similar attentional dimensions. For example, although some TEA-Ch attentional control/switching subtests (i.e., Creature Counting, Opposite Worlds) were moderately related to the MFFT ($r = .08$ to $.35$), so were most of the TEA-Ch sustained attention subtests ($r = .10$ to $.40$). Similarly, although none of the attentional control/switching subtests had very large correlations with Trails B, a test purported to measure attentional switching, other subtests such as Sky Search and Code Transmission, assumed to measure primarily selective and sustained attention, respectively, had substantial correlations with this test ($r = .45$ and $r = .40$, respectively). Overall, these apparent discrepancies are not unexpected and may simply reveal the multidimensional aspects of the criterion measures employed. In addition, neither the Stroop, Trails, nor MFFT is a suitable measure of sustained attention. Therefore, validity information on the relationship between the TEA-Ch and other validated measures of sustained attention such as continuous

Figure 9–18 Structural Equation Model of TEA-Ch performance. *Source:* Reprinted with permission from Manly et al., 2001, p. 1075.

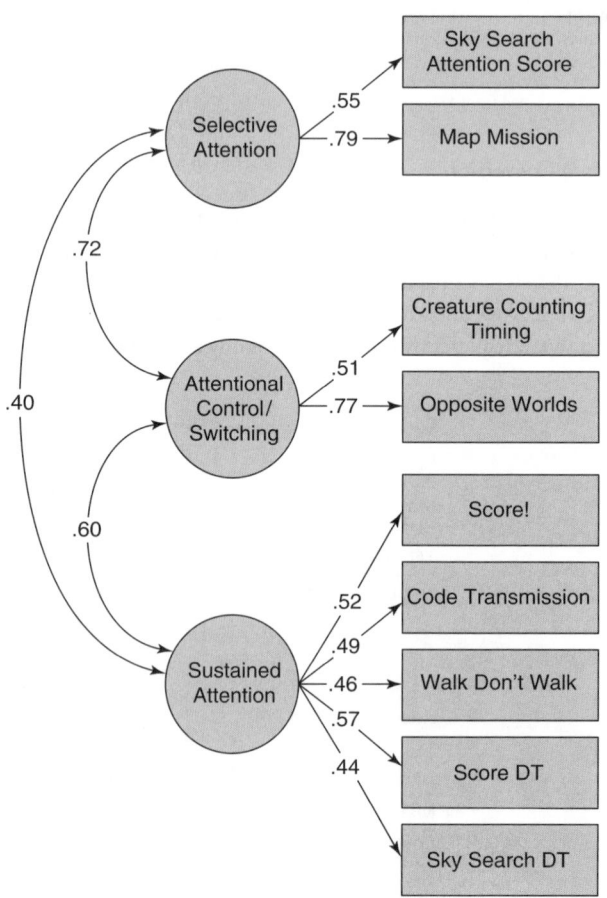

performance tests (CPTs) is needed, given that a number of TEA-Ch subtests are designed to measure this attentional dimension (i.e., Score!, Score DT, Walk Don't Walk, Code Transmission, and Sky Search DT).

Correlations With Achievement

Usually, correlations between attention tests and achievement tests are fairly minimal (although there are exceptions). This is also the case with the TEA-Ch. Correlations with the WRAT-R were generally modest (i.e., $r = .06$ to $.28$), as described in the manual, for 160 children from the normative sample. Correlations between WRAT-R Arithmetic and Sky Search DT and Creature Counting accuracy were slightly higher, attaining a medium correlational effect size ($r = .33$ and $r = .40$, respectively).

Correlations With Rating Scales

The manual does not provide correlations with standardized rating scales of attention.

Clinical Studies

Overall, studies with relevant clinical groups are encouraging, but important information on the test's diagnostic accuracy using classification accuracy statistics (i.e., sensitivity, specificity) are lacking. The manual describes the performance of 24 boys with attention-deficit/hyperactivity disorder (ADHD). They performed Sky Search as well as matched controls did, which the authors interpreted as demonstrating the lack of selective attention deficits in ADHD. All other subtests were performed more poorly by ADHD patients than by matched controls. Other studies have found poor performance on TEA-Ch sustained attention and attention control subtests for children with ADHD compared with clinical controls (Heaton et al., 2001) or with normal controls (Manly et al., 2001). No differences between groups on selective attention subtests (Sky Search, Map Mission) were reported in these studies either.

ADHD subtypes reportedly do not perform differently on TEA-Ch subtests (Heaton et al., 2001). Although no studies comparing children's scores before and after stimulant medication have yet been conducted, ADHD children receiving stimulant medication did not perform differently than those not receiving medication on TEA-Ch subtests in one study (Heaton et al., 2001). However, inherent differences between medicated and nonmedicated children may have accounted for the lack of differences, because this study did not employ randomization to groups.

Another study using a pilot version of the TEA-Ch found no differences between children with learning disorders and those with ADHD or normal controls, apart from visual selective attention problems (Villella et al., 2001) and auditory sustained attention problems on a subtest that was not included in the final version of the test. However, this study comprised very small group sizes (10 children per group).

The test manual describes the performance of 18 children with traumatic brain injury (TBI), whose mean Glasgow Coma Scale score was approximately 5 (of a possible 15) and whose mean coma duration was almost 7 days (i.e., moderate to severe TBI). These children had difficulty with Sky Search and Map Mission compared with controls, even after performance was adjusted for motor speed. This group was also described in a published study involving the test's authors (Anderson et al., 1998). Compared with normal controls, TBI children had significant deficits in selective attention, sustained attention, and attentional control on the TEA-Ch; these persisted even 6 years after injury.

COMMENT

Among currently available attention tests for children, the TEA-Ch is unique in allowing a multidimensional assessment of attention that is grounded in theory and research on attentional processes. The manual includes a thorough discussion of attention and of the specific ways in which attentional problems can manifest on each subtest. It also includes detailed explanations of subtest task requirements to facilitate interpretation. However, even though the battery is relatively easy to use, because of the theory-laden underpinnings of some of the tasks, users should read the manual in detail and be familiar with a paper by the authors that includes information on test development and standardization not included in the manual (Manly et al., 2001). Baron (2001) noted that novice users may also encounter difficulty interpreting discrepant results such as variable performance across factors purported to measure a single attentional dimension.

The TEA-Ch has several practical features: it employs imaginative, game-like stimuli that are likely to be interesting to children, does not require a computer, and is highly portable, which makes it useful for bedside and school evaluations. It also allows statistical correction for motor and processing speed, a feature that many commonly used attention tests typically omit. However, the test has some limitations.

Norms

North American users should be aware that norms are not based on North American samples but consist of an Australian sample that is predominantly of above-average IQ (although this differs by age band; see Table 9–62). Additionally, no information on ethnic distribution, SES, or parental education is provided in the manual itself, although a separate study by the authors did describe the SES level of the sample (Manly et al., 2001). Caution is therefore advised when using the norms in populations that differ markedly from the standardization sample. Additional caution is also recommended in interpreting scores of older adolescents, given significant ceiling effects in this age group and restricted cell sizes.

Reliability

Although a number of TEA-Ch subtests show adequate to strong test-retest reliability, some subtests have marginal to poor reliability (see Table 9–63), which makes their use questionable in the diagnostic assessment of children. Further, not enough information is provided in the manual on the psychometric properties of Version B, which the authors recommend should be used for retesting purposes. Given the inherent difficulties in interpreting retests involving alternate forms (see Lineweaver & Chelune, 2003), test-retest reliabilities involving readministrations of Version A would be useful to users, particularly those who see children for multiple assessments (e.g., stimulant medication efficacy trials). Guidelines regarding the procedure to be used when testing involves more than two assessments and test-retest reliabilities over intervals longer than 20 days are also needed.

Validity

More validity information on the test would be useful. The manual does not report subtest intercorrelations or correlations with standardized attention scales (i.e., Conners, ADHD-RS), nor does it present correlations to criterion measures of sustained attention such as CPTs or cancellation tasks. This information would be useful to clinicians, because these measures are typically also used as additional components of an attentional workup. Further, the test requires replication of its factor structure, both in normal controls and in clinical groups such as ADHD patients, particularly because, as Heaton et al. (2001) noted, divided attention may constitute a separate factor in ADHD populations. As was noted by Baron (2001), information on the positive predictive power, negative predictive power, sensitivity, specificity, and neuroanatomical correlation of the TEA-Ch is also currently lacking.

Although the authors describe the test as measuring three distinct attentional factors, no composite scores can be derived for these factors. Information on sensitivity and validity of the four-subtest screener is also lacking. Further, the authors' suggestion that the TEA-Ch may have better ecological validity than other attention tests has not yet been empirically tested. Additional studies, including independent studies conducted by researchers other than the test authors, are also needed, as are studies in diverse neuropsychological conditions of childhood.

Ceiling and Floor Effects

Floor and ceiling effects are not discussed in the manual except for a short section on reliability, in which Score!, Score DT, and Walk Don't Walk are mentioned as subtests with ceiling effects. However, the authors described ceiling and floor effects in considerable detail in a published paper (Manly et al., 2001). They indicated that, in the youngest age band, no floor effects were observed for Score!, Score DT, Code Transmission, or Walk Don't Walk subtests (i.e., no scores of 0). However, 7 (18%) of 38 children in the normative sample in this age band obtained a score of 0 on the Creature Counting subtest. With regard to ceilings, 72% of children scored at ceiling on the Score! subtest in the oldest age band. Rates of children obtaining ceiling-level scores on the remaining subtests are lower but in some cases are still not negligible: 24%, 37%, 10%, and 34% on Score DT, Code Transmission, Walk Don't Walk, and Creature Counting, respectively. Only the Map Mission subtest had no children scoring at ceiling among adolescents older than 15 years of age (Manly et al., 2001). Although most subtests provide an appropriate range of scores, users should review the maximum and minimum scores that can be obtained in specific age bands to avoid interpretation errors (e.g., the lowest score possible for a 6-year-old girl on the Creature Counting test is a scaled score of 7).

REFERENCES

Anderson, V., Fenwick, T., Manly, T., & Robertson, I. (1998). Attentional skills following traumatic brain injury in childhood: A componential analysis. *Brain Injury, 12*(11), 937–949.

Arizmendi, T., Paulsen, K., & Domino, G. (1981). The Matching Familiar Figures Test: A primary, secondary and tertiary evaluation. *Journal of Clinical Psychology, 37*, 812–818.

Baron, I. S. (2001). Test of Everyday Attention for Children. *Child Neuropsychology, 7*(3), 190–195.

Daniel, A. (1983). *Power, privilege and prestige: Occupations in Australia.* Melbourne, Australia: Longman-Chesire.

Heaton, S. C., Reader, S. K., Preston, A. S., Fennell, E. B., Puyana, O. E., Gill, N., & Johnson, J. H. (2001). The Test of Everyday Attention for Children (TEA-Ch): Patterns of performance in children with ADHD and clinical controls. *Child Neuropsychology, 7*(4), 251–264.

Lineweaver, T. T., & Chelune, G. J. (2003). Use of the WAIS-III and WMS-III in the context of serial assessments: Interpreting reliable and meaningful change. In D. S. Tulsky, D. H. Saklofske, G. J. Chelune, R. K. Heaton, R. Ivnik, R. Bornstein, A. Prifitera, & M. F. Ledbetter (Eds.), *Clinical interpretation of the WAIS-III and WMS-III* (pp. 303–337). New York: Academic Press.

Manly, T., Anderson, V., Nimmo-Smith, I., Turner, A., Watson, P., & Robertson, I. H. (2001). The differential assessment of children's attention: The Test of Everyday Attention for Children (TEA-Ch), normative sample and ADHD performance. *Journal of Child Psychology, Psychiatry and Allied Disciplines, 42*(8), 1065–1081.

Manly, T., Robertson, I. H., Anderson, V., & Nimmo-Smith, I. (1999). *TEA-Ch: The Test of Everyday Attention for Children.* Bury St. Edmunds, England: Thames Valley Test Company.

Robertson, I. H., Ward, T., Ridgeway, V., & Nimmo-Smith, I. (1994–1999). *The Test of Everyday Attention.* Bury St. Edmunds, England: Thames Valley Test Company.

Villella, S., Anderson, J., Anderson, V., Robertson, I. H., & Manly, T. (2001). Sustained and selective attention in children with attention deficit/hyperactivity disorder and specific learning disabilities. *Clinical Neuropsychological Assessment, 21*, 1–23.

Test of Variables of Attention (T.O.V.A.)

PURPOSE

The Test of Variables of Attention (T.O.V.A.) is a computerized test of sustained attention and impulsivity.

SOURCE

The T.O.V.A. can be obtained from Universal Attention Disorders, Inc. (http://www.tovatest.com) or through other distributors such as Psychological Assessment Resources (http://www.parinc.com) and Western Psychological Services (http://www.wpspublish.com). The cost is $375 US for the Visual T.O.V.A. and $395 US for the Visual and Auditory T.O.V.A. (T.O.V.A.-A); the kit includes test manuals, IBM software, Microswitch Scorebox, and five Interpretation Reports. Additional "scoring credits" (i.e., pay-per-use costs) are $10 to $15 US and are accessed through an automated ordering system.

AGE RANGE

The T.O.V.A. can be administered to persons aged 4 through 80 years (note that 4- and 5-year-olds are given a briefer test). The T.O.V.A.-A can be administered to children and adolescents ages 6 to 19 years.

DESCRIPTION

Overview

The T.O.V.A. is a computerized continuous performance test (CPT) formerly known as the Minnesota Computer Assessment. It has several versions: a visual CPT (T.O.V.A.), an auditory CPT (T.O.V.A.-A), and a screening or preschool version offered as part of the standard T.O.V.A. (Greenberg, 1988–2000). The T.O.V.A. is a CPT with minimal stimulus processing requirements; stimuli consist of only two simple geometric forms (see Figure 9–19). The test uses brief stimulus presentations and short interstimulus intervals and lasts longer than most CPTs, conditions some believe are most likely to differentiate children with attention-deficit/hyperactivity disorder (ADHD) from control children (Corkum & Siegel, 1993, as cited in Forbes, 1998). According to the authors, the T.O.V.A. can be used in several ways: as an attention measure in the context of neuropsychological evaluation, to screen for attentional disorders, as a key component in the diagnosis of attentional disorders, to measure response to medication, to titrate dosage, and to monitor treatment over time (Greenberg et al., 2000).

Testing Paradigm

The T.O.V.A. paradigm consists of a monochromatic square within which is a small square; targets occur when the small square is at the top of the large square, and nontargets occur

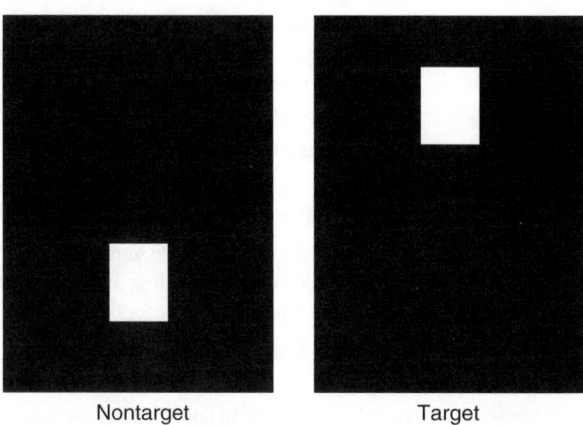

Figure 9–19 T.O.V.A. test stimuli. *Source:* Reprinted with permission from Leark et al., 1988–1999, p. 3.

Nontarget   Target

when it is at the bottom (see Figure 9–19). For the T.O.V.A.-A, two distinct tones are used to differentiate the target from the nontarget. The test requires use of a switchbox with a single button, connected to a computer via a parallel port. The examinee presses the button every time a target is presented. The switchbox device ensures accuracy in timing (i.e., ±1 ms variance), unlike response devices used in other CPTs (mouse, spacebar, or keyboard), which may introduce additional variability (Leark et al., 1999). This device also minimizes the motor component of the task and, because the keyboard can be moved out of reach of the examinee, prevents impulsive examinees from inadvertently pressing other computer keys and disrupting the test session, as can be the case with CPTs that use the space bar or the mouse.

The test consists of four intervals; during the first two intervals, the target appears on 22.5% of the trials (stimulus-infrequent condition). During the second two intervals, the target appears on 77.5% of the trials (stimulus-frequent condition). The interstimulus interval is reduced, which means that the examinee must respond more quickly in addition to responding more frequently. Thus, the first half of the test is designed to maximize demands on sustained attention (and elicit errors of omission), whereas the second half demands inhibitory control (and elicits errors of commission). Preschoolers (ages 4 and 5 years) are given only quarters 1 and 3 of the T.O.V.A.; the T.O.V.A.-A is too difficult for this age range.

T.O.V.A. Rating Scales

The T.O.V.A. also includes several rating scales to be completed by the examiner, as well as forms for conducting an interview, tracking treatment effects, and, for adults, a self-report form. There is also a diagnostic checklist. These forms are found in the T.O.V.A. manuals (*Professional Guide* and *Clinical Guide*).

Table 9–64 Summary of T.O.V.A. Scores

T.O.V.A. Score	Description
Omissions	Measures inattention; reflects missed targets; calculated as the ratio of correctly identified targets to the actual number of targets, minus anticipatory responses toward targets, presented as a percentage
Commissions	Measures impulsivity and disinhibition; reflects responses to nontargets; calculated as the ratio of incorrect responses (to nontargets) to the actual number of nontargets, minus anticipatory responses to nontargets, presented as a percentage
Response time	Provides the mean time taken to respond correctly to targets, in milliseconds, reported for each quarter, half, and total
Response time variability	Measures consistency of response time; consists of the *SD* of the mean correct response times, for each quarter, half, and total
d′	Measures response sensitivity, with regard to the ratio of the hit rate to false-alarm rate; measures performance decrement according to signal detection theory, accuracy of signal-to-noise discrimination (see p. 5 of the *Professional Guide* for details)
ADHD score	Compares the subject's performance to that of an ADHD sample, according to a formula presented in the *Professional Guide* (p. 6).
Postcommission response time	Mean time taken to respond to targets immediately after a commission error, in milliseconds
Anticipatory responses	Responses occurring when the subject responds within 200 ms after stimulus presentation; these are not included in omissions, commissions, response times, or response variability; calculated as a percentage of the total stimuli
Multiple responses	Occurs when the microswitch is pressed more than once per stimulus presentation; calculated as the sum of multiple responses, regardless of whether the response was to a target or nontarget

Note: See *Professional Guide* (Lleark et al., 1999) for further details.

ADMINISTRATION TIME

The test takes about 22 minutes.

ADMINISTRATION

See test manual. The examiner reads the test instructions. The test begins with a 3-min practice session. The examiner should remain present for the entire administration (Leark et al., 1999). Prompting is not permitted during the test itself. Although this is not explicitly stated in the *Professional Guide* (Leark et al., 1999), additional instructions provided in the *Clinical Guide* (Greenberg et al., 2000) state that the T.O.V.A. should be administered in the morning and that the test should be the first test administered, consistent with standardization procedures. Details on computer requirements and software can be found in the user's manual (Dupuy & Cenedela, 2000).

SCORING

Scores

The T.O.V.A. yields a number of different scores (see Table 9–64). The ADHD score is based on a combination of scores found to have superior predictive ability in detecting ADHD based on receiver operating characteristic (ROC) analyses

(Leark et al., 1999). Note that the omission error score is not simply the number of missed targets but instead is a ratio score, as is the commission score.

Variables are presented as raw scores, standard deviations, and z-scores for quarters, halves, and total test. Raw scores are converted to standard scores ($M = 100$, $SD = 15$) based on age and gender.

Validity and Interpretation

Test performance is evaluated for validity and is deemed invalid if it meets one of the criteria shown in Table 9–65. Detailed interpretive information can be found in the *Professional Guide* (Leark et al., 1999) and *Clinical Guide* (Greenberg et al., 2000). The authors recommend that scores be adjusted for IQ, according to a procedure outlined in the manuals (but see *Comment*).

Table 9–65 Criteria for Determining Invalidity of a T.O.V.A. Administration

1. Response time or variability of zero for any half, quarter, or total
2. Test interrupted by the user
3. Excessive anticipatory responses
4. Omission/commission errors of 100% for any half, quarter, or total

DEMOGRAPHIC EFFECTS

Age

T.O.V.A. performance follows a curvilinear progression across age. The age-related decrease in commission errors is particularly evident on the second half of the test. Response time and response time variability also decrease in a curvilinear manner with age, particularly in the second half of the test (Leark et al., 1999). Note that response times and variability should increase with age in older adults; however, there may have been too few adults in this age group in the normative sample to demonstrate an effect. In clinical groups such as children with ADHD, there is a significant correlation between age and number of multiple responses, indicating that younger children make more multiple responses (Forbes, 1998). Age effects are also found on the T.O.V.A.-A (Leark et al., 1999).

Gender

There are gender effects for percentage omissions, percentage commissions, and mean response time. Males tend to have faster reaction times and to make more errors of omission and commission than females (Greenberg & Waldman, 1993). Gender-based differences in errors of commission are particularly salient on the second half of the test (Leark et al., 1999).

Table 9–66 Characteristics of the Original T.O.V.A. (Visual) Normative Sample—Children and Adolescents

Sample type	Children from several suburban public grade and high schools, from one early education screening project, and from one rural high school
Number	1340
Age (years)	4 to 19[a]
Geographic location	Minneapolis, Minnesota
Socioeconomic status (SES)	Unspecified[b]
Gender (no.)	
Males	631
Females	709
Race/Ethnicity (%)	
Caucasian	99%
Other	1%
Screening	Exclusion based on a score >2SDs from the mean on the Conners Parent-Teacher Questionnaire Abbreviated form, use of psychotropic medication, or participation in a special education program

[a]Based on 2-year age groupings: 4–5, 6–7, 8–9, 10–11, 12–13, 14–15, 16–17, and 18–19 years.
[b]Children were living in areas that were predominantly middle to upper-middle SES (Riccio et al., 2001).

On the T.O.V.A.-A, males make more commission errors and have shorter reaction times than females (Leark et al., 1999).

Ethnicity

Although the impact of ethnicity on test scores has not been directly studied, the test has been used in cultures other than that of the normative sample, including Senegalese children (Boivin, 2002) and children from Laos (Boivin et al., 1996).

Education

Education effects in adults have not been adequately studied.

IQ

Research on the relationship between IQ and T.O.V.A. performance is conflicting. For example, T.O.V.A. performance is not related to IQ in young adults with or without ADHD (Weyandt et al., 2002) or in children with ADHD (Chae, 1999). However, it is related to K-ABC performance in Lao children (Boivin et al., 1996), and, when samples include gifted children, IQ accounts for up to 26% of omission error variance and 25% of response sensitivity (Chae et al., 2003). See *Validity* and *Comment* for further discussion.

NORMATIVE DATA

Standardization Sample

The norms for the T.O.V.A. (Visual) are based on data from 1596 individuals aged 4 to 80+ years, from two sources: an original sample (N = 775; Greenberg & Waldman, 1993) and a second sample that was later added to the original pool (N = 821; Greenberg & Crosby, 1992, as cited in Leark et al., 1999). Sample characteristics for these combined norms are presented in Tables 9–66 and 9–67 for children and adults, respectively. Note that the sample is primarily Caucasian and exclusively from Minnesota. Education level is not specified for the adults. The year in which data were collected is not provided.

Users should also note that some cell sizes are extremely restricted for adult males; for example, there are only four men in the 30- to 39-year age band, and only eight in the 50- to 59-year and 80+ years age bands. Riccio et al. (2001) note that the 6- to 18-year groups are overrepresented and males and females are not equally represented across the age bands, with the number of males in each age group dropping significantly after age 19. Nonequivalence of gender composition across age bands is not optimal because there are gender effects for some variables. Users should note that the examinees in the 18- to 19-year age band were recruited from high schools, so this may not be a suitable comparison group for college students of the same age.

Norms for the T.O.V.A.-A are based on the performance of 2551 children and adolescents, ages 6 to 19 years.

Table 9–67 Characteristics of the T.O.V.A. (Visual) Normative Sample—Adults

Sample type	Volunteer undergraduates from three liberal arts colleges and adults living in six adult community settings
Number	250
Age (years)	20 to 80+[a]
Geographic location	Minnesota
Socioeconomic status (SES)	Unspecified[b]
Education	Unspecified
Gender	
Males	31%
Females	69%
Race/Ethnicity	
Caucasian	99%
Other	1%
Screening	Exclusion based on use of psychotropic medication, history of central nervous system (CNS) disorder or CNS injury

[a]Based on 10-year age groupings: 20–29, 30–39, 40–49, 50–59, 60–69, 70–79, and 80+.
[b]Participants were living in areas that were predominantly middle to upper-middle SES (Riccio et al., 2001).

See Table 9–68 for sample composition. Norms are not provided for 4- and 5-year-olds because the task is too difficult for them (Leark et al., 1999). According to Riccio et al. (2001), the sample distribution across age and sex is fairly uniform for ages 6 to 18 years, with approximately 160 individuals per age band. However, there is overrepresentation of males in the 19-year-old age band (69%), and the number

Table 9–68 Characteristics of the T.O.V.A.-A Normative Sample

Sample type	Three suburban public schools
Number	2,551
Age (years)	6 to 19[a]
Geographic location	Minneapolis, Minnesota
Socioeconomic status (SES)	Not reported[b]
Gender	Not clearly specified
Race/Ethnicity	
Caucasian	99%
Other	1%
Screening	Exclusion based on a score >2SDs from the mean on the Conners, Parent-Teacher Questionnaire Abbreviated form, use of psychotropic medication, or participation in a special education program

[a]Based on one-year age groupings.
[b]Children were living in areas that were predominantly White and middle to upper-middle SES (Riccio et al., 2001).

of examinees is considerably smaller ($n = 32$) than in other age bands. There are no adults norms for the T.O.V.A.-A beyond 19 years of age.

Norms are not provided for any of the rating scales described in the test manuals.

RELIABILITY

Internal Consistency

Internal consistency, assessed by correlational analyses showing the degree of association between the first and second halves of the test in the standardization sample, is highest for reaction time and reaction time variability ($r = .88$ and $r = .83$, respectively), moderate for omissions ($r = .75$), and less optimal for commissions and d' ($r = .57$ and $r = .60$, respectively; Leark et al., 1999). Similar values are obtained for the T.O.V.A.-A (see Table 9–69 for details). Comparisons of the first and second halves of the test to the total score yield larger coefficients, as would be expected. Internal consistency coefficients for correct responses, assessed in children with ADHD, calculated in the same manner, are considerably higher ($r = .93$ to .96; Llorente et al., 2001).

Standard Error of Measurement (*SEM*)

*SEM*s are provided in the manual on pages 25 and 30 for the T.O.V.A. and T.O.V.A.-A, respectively (Leark et al., 1999). These appear to be provided in raw score format, which makes it difficult to compare *SEM*s across variables or to construct confidence intervals around standard scores. Instead, we recommend using the values provided by Leark et al. (2004). These are reproduced in Table 9–70 and are based on test-retest data (see later discussion). As shown, *SEM*s are quite considerable for commissions and response time and would result in fairly large confidence intervals. Note that most test manuals use *SEM*s derived from internal reliability estimates, which typically result in smaller values.

Test-Retest Reliability

The authors provide test-retest coefficients for a 90-minute retest interval on 24 children from the standardization group (Greenberg et al., 2000). Reaction time stability was very high ($r = .93$), and stability for the remainder of the T.O.V.A. variables was moderate to high ($r = .77$ to .80). The authors report that practice effects are negligible. Data for longer intervals are not presented in the manual. Recently, the authors published test-retest coefficients in healthy children for the four main T.O.V.A. variables at two time intervals (90 min and 1 week) in healthy children. These are shown in Table 9–71. Test-retest stability was adequate to high for all four variables.

Test-retest correlations based on a group of children with ADHD receiving effective stimulant medication dosages indicate adequate reliability for only a subset of T.O.V.A. variables after 2 months; 4-month stability is lower still, with only

Table 9–69 Internal Reliability Coefficients for the T.O.V.A. and T.O.V.A.-A in Normal Subjects

Test Segment	Omission	Commission	Response Time	Response Time Variability	D'
T.O.V.A.					
Half 1 vs. Half 2	.75	.57	.88	.83	.60
Half 1 vs. Total	.85	.73	.93	.89	.72
Half 2 vs. Total	.98	.97	.99	.99	.93
Half 1 vs. Total	.88	.71	.89	.92	.72
Half 2 vs. Total	.88	.93	.99	.99	.99
T.O.V.A.-A					
Half 1 vs. Half 2	.74	.42	.81	.82	.65
Half 1 vs. Total	.80	.90	.88	.87	.75
Half 2 vs. Total	.99	.77	.99	.99	.97
Half 1 vs. Total	.99	.90	.88	.87	.75
Half 2 vs. Total	.99	.77	.99	.99	.97

Source: Adapted from Leark et al., 1988–1999.

response time showing adequate reliability (Llorente et al., 2001). See Table 9–72 for actual reliabilities in this sample.

Practice Effects

In Llorente's study on ADHD (2001), response time and response time variability showed good reproducibility of individual scores across visits; however, there was a bias for all standard scores to increase toward the average range with repeated administrations over time. This suggests a practice effect. This conflicts with information provided in the manual, which suggests that practice effects on the T.O.V.A. are negligible to nonexistent. Indeed, a recent study (Leark et al., 2004) suggested substantial practice effects on commissions, with fewer commissions at retest for both short and longer time

intervals (see Table 9–70). The means for healthy children in Table 9–71 can be used to construct reliable change intervals adjusted for practice effects when using the test in a test-retest paradigm (see Chapter 1). In addition, users may want to consider a dual-baseline approach when using the test in treatment trials. However, one would have to show that giving this test twice actually eliminates practice effects.

VALIDITY

Factor Structure

Factor analyses for the T.O.V.A. and T.O.V.A.-A are described in the test manual based on the standardization sample (Leark et al., 1999). Using principal components involving data for the

Table 9–70 Means, Reliabilities, and *SEMs* for Two Testing Intervals for the T.O.V.A. in Healthy Children

T.O.V.A. Score	First Time		Second Time			
	M	*SD*	*M*	*SD*	*r*	*SEM*
Scores for the 90-min interval (N = 31)						
Omission	95.95	15.40	96.95	14.68	.70	8.22
Commission	95.29	14.32	107.12	11.54*	.78	7.03
Response time	96.66	15.43	92.36	20.07*	.84	6.00
Response time variability	99.94	16.43	101.48	20.12	.87	5.41
Scores for the 1-week interval (N = 33)						
Omission	90.39	21.85	91.42	21.86	.86	5.61
Commission	92.39	19.95	105.88**	15.37	.74	7.65
Response time	94.63	15.55	90.85	21.05	.79	6.87
Response time variability	97.70	18.32	98.64	20.94	.87	5.41

*p < .05.
**p < .01.

Source: From Leark, R.A., et al., 2004. Reprinted with the permission of Sage Publications Inc.

Table 9–71 Test-Retest Reliability for the T.O.V.A. for Two Time Intervals in Healthy Children

	Time Interval	
Magnitude of Coefficient	90 min (N = 31)	1 Week (N = 33)
Very high (≥. 90)	—	—
High (.80 to .89)	Response time	Omissions
	Response time variability	Response time variability
Adequate (.70 to .79)	Omissions	Commissions
	Commissions	Response time
Marginal (.60 to .69)	—	—
Low (≤ .59)	—	—

Note: Reliabilities based on a sample of healthy school children from Southern California.

Source: Adapted from Leark et al., 2004.

quarters, halves, and full test, the authors found three factors for the T.O.V.A.: response time (consisting of response time, variability, and d'), commission errors, and omission errors.

A factor analysis of the T.O.V.A.-A yielded a five-factor solution with a similar response time factor (response time and variability) but with further breakdown of omissions and commissions based on stimulus-frequent and stimulus-infrequent conditions. The different factor solutions suggest that test modality affects the underlying constructs being measured (Riccio et al., 2001). Comparison of the visual and auditory T.O.V.A. in the standardization sample indicates that about twice as many omissions are made on the auditory version but that more commissions are made on the visual test. Response times are also faster on the visual test, but variability is greater on the auditory version (Leark et al., 1999).

In Lao children, principal components analysis of TPT, K-ABC, and T.O.V.A. showed that the T.O.V.A. loads on a factor composed of T.O.V.A. omissions, T.O.V.A. commissions, and TPT Memory Location (Boivin et al., 1996).

Correlations With Other Attention Tests

In children and adults with ADHD, correlations between the T.O.V.A. and Wechsler index scores and subtests purported to measure attention or response speed, including FFD, PSI, and subtests such as Coding, Symbol Search, and Digit Span (Chae, 1999; Weyandt et al., 2002) are negligible. This is perhaps not surprising, because they probably measure different aspects of attention (e.g., vigilance versus selective attention). There are as yet no published correlational data on the relationship between the T.O.V.A. and other CPTs. However, in an unpublished study described in the IVA manual, the T.O.V.A. identified 90% of children with ADHD who were identified by the IVA (Sandford & Turner, 2004).

Correlations With Attention Rating Scales

Correlations between the T.O.V.A. and rating scales measuring ADHD symptoms are not always high, as is true for most CPTs. In addition, as with most CPTs, correlations to rating scales do not support the hypothesis that errors of omission and errors of commission measure distinct domains (Forbes, 1998). Forbes (1998) concludes that the T.O.V.A. and teacher ratings are measuring important but somewhat different dimensions of ADHD, and that both contribute unique information. Nevertheless, concordance between T.O.V.A.-based ADHD and criteria of the *Diagnostic and Statistical Manual of Mental Disorders* (4th ed.; DSM-IV) for ADHD is reportedly

Table 9–72 Long-Term Test-Retest Reliability for the T.O.V.A. in Children with ADHD

	Time Interval	
Magnitude of Coefficient	2 Months	4 Months
Very high (≥.90)	—	—
High (.80 to .89)	—	—
Adequate (.70 to .79)	Commissions	Response time
	Response time	
	Response time variability	
Marginal (.60 to .69)	—	Omissions
		Response time variability
Low (≤ .59)	Omissions	Commissions

Note: N = 63.

Adapted from Llorente et al., 2001.

high ($r = .84$; Llorente et al., 2001). In one study, concordance between physician-based and T.O.V.A.-based ADHD diagnoses was 72%, considerably higher than that obtained for another CPT, the Conners' 1994 CPT (Monastra et al., 2001; see additional discussion of ADHD later).

Correlations With IQ

As noted previously, data on the relationship between the T.O.V.A. and measures of general intellectual ability are conflicting. There is minimal correlation between T.O.V.A. and FSIQ, VIQ, or any of the other WISC-III index scores in children with ADHD (Chae, 1999) or in young adults with or without ADHD (Weyandt et al., 2002). However, with regard to subscales, Chae (1999) found that T.O.V.A. Inattention was related to PIQ and FSIQ ($r = -.44$ to $-.45$) and was significantly related to performance on WISC-III visual-spatial subtests (i.e., Picture Arrangement, Object Assembly) in children with ADHD. It was also found to relate to cognitive ability as measured by the K-ABC in Senegalese children (Boivin et al., 1996). Further, T.O.V.A. performance was related to IQ when samples included gifted children, with IQ accounting for up to 26% of omission error variance and 25% of response sensitivity (Chae et al., 2003).

Correlations With Language

Unlike other commercially available CPTs, the T.O.V.A. does not include letters. This is assumed to reduce the influence of language/letter familiarity on test performance. To this effect, the T.O.V.A. is not related to language as measured by the PPVT-R (Forbes, 1998) and is generally not related to achievement as measured by the WRAT-3, although T.O.V.A. variability has been reported to be related to Reading ($r = .37$; Chae, 1999).

Clinical Studies

Group studies indicate impairments on specific T.O.V.A. variables in young adults with ADHD compared with controls (i.e., omission errors, Weyandt et al., 2002; see also Weyandt et al., 1998). Similarly, impairments are found in terms of omissions, commissions, reaction time, variability, decrement in performance over time, and ADHD score in adolescents with ADHD (Chae et al., 2001), and in variability and reaction time in children with ADHD (Schatz et al., 2001). However, the ADHD score does not appear to differentiate between gifted ADHD and gifted non-ADHD children (Chae et al., 2003), although group differences are found in response time and variability. Forbes (1998) reported differences between a group of individuals with ADHD and a mixed group including patients with various clinical diagnoses.

The T.O.V.A. *Professional Guide* describes in detail unpublished data supporting the test's sensitivity and specificity (Leark et al., 1999). A small number of published studies have also examined this question. In one study, the T.O.V.A. and the Conners' rating scale were equally sensitive for identifying ADHD, but the T.O.V.A. had a significantly higher false-positive rate (Schatz et al., 2001). Specifically, despite 86% accuracy in identifying children with ADHD, about 30% of normal controls scored in the abnormal range (Schatz et al., 2001). None of the controls scored in the abnormal range on the Conners' rating scale. In this study, variability was the only useful diagnostic predictor capable of distinguishing ADHD children from normal subjects using the recommended T-score cutoff value of 65 (sensitivity, 86%; specificity, 70%; false-positive rate, 30%; miss rate, 14%). This variable detected about 65% of the ADHD children in the sample (35% were missed with this variable alone). Changing the cutoff value did not alleviate the T.O.V.A.'s discriminability problem (Schatz et al., 2001), because increasing the cutoff in an attempt to decrease the false-positive rate adversely affected the test's hit rate. A false-positive rate of 25% has also been reported in other studies (Schatz et al., 2002). Despite this, the T.O.V.A. appears to improve classification accuracy when those incorrectly classified by rating scales are reclassified based on T.O.V.A. results (Forbes, 1998). Likewise, among gifted children, the T.O.V.A. identifies fewer children as having ADHD than do ADHD rating scales; this suggests some utility in reducing the risk of overdiagnosis in this group (Chae et al., 2003).

If diagnostic accuracy is compared with regard to differentiating ADHD from other clinical disorders, the T.O.V.A., like other CPTs, does not fare well. In one study, the T.O.V.A. showed good discriminability between a group with ADHD and another group with various clinical diagnoses, but demonstrated limited specificity on an individual level. Although it correctly identified 80% of an ADHD sample as having ADHD, it also incorrectly identified 72% to 86% of a clinical sample without ADHD (Forbes, 1998). Rating scales may be better able to accurately differentiate between ADHD subgroups (Forbes, 1998).

The T.O.V.A. is sensitive to the effects of Ritalin in ADHD (Monastra et al., 2002; Li & Wang, 2000) and to the effects of EEG biofeedback in children with ADHD (Monastra et al., 2002). The test has also been used in Chinese children with ADHD, in whom it demonstrated sensitivity to medication effects (Li & Wang, 2000).

Research on genetic susceptibility to ADHD has shown that T.O.V.A. performance is related to the specific allele of a gene implicated in the metabolism of amine neurotransmitters, including dopamine (long MAO-A allele; see Manor et al., 2002a). Interestingly, differences between affected individuals and controls disappear when affected individuals are tested while taking Ritalin (Manor et al., 2002b). The T.O.V.A. has also been used in studies of ADHD in neurofibromatosis, where it demonstrated sensitivity to medication effects (Mautner et al., 2002), including in children with IQs lower than 80. Notably, in a triple-blind, placebo-controlled, crossover study on sensitivity to differences in Ritalin dosage (twice versus three times a day), T.O.V.A. improvements appeared marginal compared with teacher and parent rating scales (Stein et al., 1996).

Although the emphasis in T.O.V.A. research is often on ADHD, the test shows considerable utility in other disorders. For instance, children with autism demonstrate deficits in response time variability on the T.O.V.A. (Schatz et al., 2002). Gifted children perform better with regard to omissions, commissions, variability, sensitivity, and ADHD scores but show response times similar to those of control children (Chae et al., 2003). Lastly, young delinquents perform more poorly than controls on all T.O.V.A. variables except response time (Chae et al., 2001).

The T.O.V.A. is sensitive to the effects of cerebral malaria in children (Boivin, 2002); in affected children, coma duration, age at episode, and time since episode account for 31% of the variance in T.O.V.A. percentage omission errors. The test is also sensitive to the effects of sickle cell disease (DeBaun et al., 1998; Schatz et al., 1999). T.O.V.A. performance is decreased both in children with anterior lesions and in those with diffuse lesions (Schatz et al., 1999). In this population, T.O.V.A. scores have 86% sensitivity and 81% specificity in identifying individuals with silent cerebral infarcts and 95% sensitivity in identifying overt stroke; this is considerably higher than the values reported for other neuropsychological tests (DeBaun et al., 1998).

In one study, although children exposed prenatally to alcohol perform more poorly than controls on the T.O.V.A., the T.O.V.A. did not add any additional unique variance to predicting group membership when other attention measures (CBCL and WISC-III) were included (Lee et al., 2004).

The T.O.V.A. has also been used to assess postconcussion symptoms in children with mild head injury (Yeates et al., 1999) and to assess for dopaminergic medication effects in children with restless leg/periodic limb movements in sleep (Walters et al., 2000). The T.O.V.A. is also sensitive to the effect of glucose on attentional performance in normal adults (Flint & Turek, 2003).

Malingering

Subjects instructed to fake ADHD on the T.O.V.A. typically produce excessive omission and commission errors, longer response time, more variability and poorer d' scores than controls (Leark et al., 2002). Exaggeration should therefore be ruled out with the use of other techniques (e.g., symptom validity tests) when performance on the T.O.V.A. is grossly impaired.

COMMENT

The T.O.V.A. has several assets. These include its nonverbal format and its requirement for few complex cognitive processes except for sustained attention, response inhibition, up/down visual discrimination, and motor response because it employs a very simple discrimination task. In addition, because it uses geometric stimuli instead of letters or numbers, the T.O.V.A. may minimize cultural differences (Boivin et al.,

1996) and is appropriate for young children and adults with letter or number identification difficulties. Its length (as one of the longest commercially available CPTs) and short interstimulus presentation rate may confer some advantage in detecting attentional impairments. Further, an impressive number of studies have documented its use in various clinical populations, including efficacy in medication trials and other clinical paradigms.

Users should note that most of the studies on the T.O.V.A. have investigated the visual version, not the T.O.V.A.-A, and that modality does affect construct validity, as was suggested by the differing factor structures in visual and auditory versions (Leark et al., 1999). Therefore, study results on the T.O.V.A. may not necessarily apply to the T.O.V.A.-A.

On the other hand, the test does not actually include an additional stimulus manipulation designed specifically to elicit inhibition errors (as do A-X-CPTs that require responding to targets but only if preceded by a specific cue, or non-X-CPTs requiring continuous responding, such as the Conners' CPT-II), except for a more rapid presentation rate in the second half of the test. It is therefore not clear whether it measures constructs similar to those measured by CPTs employing inhibition tasks (e.g., CPT-II, GDS) or whether it is as useful in populations in which inhibition deficits are central (see Riccio et al., 2001, and Ballard, 2001, for a discussion of this issue). However, the reduced complexity of the T.O.V.A. make it easier to use in cognitively impaired populations and in the very young. In fact, it is one of the few commercially available CPTs with norms extending down to the preschool level.

Studies on the sensitivity and specificity of the T.O.V.A. suggest that, although the test might be good at detecting inattention (hit rate), it is not as good at detecting the resulting impairments of functioning in daily life, which rating scales such as the Conners' scales are best at (Schatz et al., 2001). Therefore, the T.O.V.A. can be seen as one component of a comprehensive ADHD evaluation that would also include confirmation of impairment in daily functioning via questionnaires. The authors in fact recommend that the test be used, in concert with other sources of information within a comprehensive ADHD workup.

From a psychometric perspective, the T.O.V.A. norms' skewed sex distribution may lead to error (Riccio et al., 2001). Depending on the age band, norms are inadequate for adults, and sometimes grossly so (i.e., $N = 4$ for 30- to 39-year-olds). Further, some standard scores for males in the older age groups are artificially inflated because of small sample size and lack of subject errors. In addition, Riccio et al. (2001) found that the 10-year age bands for adults may be too broad to properly detect age-related changes in CPT performance. No education information on the adult normative sample is provided. Therefore, use of the test is best restricted to children and adolescents, for whom the norms are more extensive and education effects less relevant. However, in both of these age groups, because of the demographic characteristics of the sample (e.g., primarily Caucasian), generalizations across socioeconomic status and ethnicity should be made with caution (Riccio et al., 2001). Use of the rating forms is not recommended because of the lack of reliability and validity data, although these could be used qualitatively to supplement observations.

Retest reliability data are available for several time intervals (90-minute, 1-week, 2 months, and 4 months in ADHD children), although the level of reliability is not uniformly acceptable across all scores. Nevertheless, Llorente et al. (2001) concluded that test-retest reliabilities are generally satisfactory in ADHD children while acknowledging that coefficients fall below standards for clinical decision making. They concluded that T.O.V.A. scores from single test sessions should be interpreted with caution, given the substantial variability in scores from testing to testing (note that this may be a feature of ADHD or of children in general). Conducting two baseline evaluations and selecting the higher score may be useful in this regard when assessing medication efficacy in individual children (see Mautner et al., 2002).

Most CPTs can easily differentiate between individuals with ADHD and controls on a group level. What is more difficult to attain is diagnostic accuracy (i.e., positive predictive power, negative predictive power) and the ability to successfully differentiate individuals with ADHD from those with other clinical conditions. In the case of the T.O.V.A., studies indicate good sensitivity to attentional disturbance but limited utility in terms of differentiating between individuals with ADHD and those with other conditions, or among ADHD subtypes. Because of its high sensitivity, the T.O.V.A. may overdiagnose ADHD in some children (see Schatz et al., 2001). Further, the false-positive rate may be unacceptably high, underlining the authors' contention that the test should be used as only one component of a comprehensive assessment for ADHD.

The adjustment for IQ recommended in the manuals is not entirely supported by research findings. IQ was not related to T.O.V.A. performance in several studies, albeit perhaps in part because of restricted ranges in some cases. Alternatively, the lack of association with IQ may occur because, unlike other CPTs, the T.O.V.A. employs simple stimuli and a simple response paradigm and therefore has low cognitive demands (Weyandt et al., 2002). However, there is still some evidence that higher cutoff values may be necessary to identify ADHD in gifted children because of the better overall performance of these children on the T.O.V.A. (Chae et al., 2003).

The authors clearly indicate that the test is to be used as one component of a comprehensive diagnostic workup for ADHD, which should include a history, physical/neurological screening examination, evaluation of classroom/work environment, structured interview, and behavioral ratings, and that the test measures attentional characteristics that can be affected by a number of factors (Greenberg et al., 2000).

Nevertheless, as of this writing, the interpretation report states that, on reports of individuals with high ADHD scores, performance "is suggestive of ADHD." Although the *Clinical Guide* indicates that this does not necessarily mean that the person has ADHD, the statement may increase the risk of misuse of T.O.V.A. results in individuals unfamiliar with complex diagnostic issues.

Notably, the T.O.V.A. manuals could be better organized. In addition, the *Clinical Guide* contains recommendations that are not necessarily supported by published data. This includes the claims that use of the T.O.V.A. to titrate medication dosage dramatically increases efficacy (Greenberg et al., 2000) and that dosage adjustments should be based on T.O.V.A. results rather than on rating scales because rating scales are insensitive to dosage levels involved in improving inattention. However, because improvements in real life are sought, use of rating scales to titrate dosage may better accomplish these goals (Michael Kirkwood, personal communication, October 2004), and this is the accepted standard in stimulant medication efficacy research. Other information in the manuals is of interest but needs to be substantiated by actual research. This includes the claim that athletes may have extremely short reaction times (i.e., <100 ms), and that the auditory version may be useful for subjects with extensive video game experience or for highly trained athletes (Greenberg et al., 2000).

REFERENCES

Ballard, J. C. (2001). Assessing attention: Comparison of response-inhibition and traditional Continuous Performance Tests. *Journal of Clinical and Experimental Neuropsychology, 23*(3), 331–350.

Boivin, M. J. (2002). Effects of early cerebral malaria on cognitive ability in Senegalese children. *Developmental and Behavioral Pediatrics, 23*(5), 353–364.

Boivin, M. J., Chounramany, C., Giordani, B., Xaisida, S., Choulamountry, L., Pholsena, P., Crist, C., & Olness, K. (1996). Validating a cognitive ability testing protocol with Lao children for community development applications. *Neuropsychology, 10*(4), 588–599.

Chae, P. K. (1999). Correlation study between WISC-III scores and T.O.V.A. performance. *Psychology in the Schools, 36*(3), 179–185.

Chae, P. K., Jung, H. O., & Noh, K. S. (2001). Attention deficit hyperactivity disorder in Korean juvenile delinquents. *Adolescence, 36*(144), 707–725.

Chae, P. K., Kim, J. H., & Noh, K. S. (2003). Diagnosis of ADHD among gifted children in relation to KEDI-WISC and T.O.V.A. performance. *Gifted Child Quarterly, 47*(3), 192–201.

Corkum, P. V., & Siegel, L. S. (1995). Is the Continuous Performance Task a valuable research tool for use with children with Attention-Deficit-Hyperactivity Disorder? *Journal of Child Psychology and Psychiatry, 34*(7), 1217–39.

DeBaun, M. R., Schatz, M. J., & Koby, M. (1998). Cognitive screening examination for silent cerebral infarcts in sickle cell disease. *Neurology, 50*(6), 1678–1682.

Dupuy, T., & Cenedela, M. (2000). *Test of Variables of Attention: User's Guide*. Los Alamitos, Calif.: Universal Attention Disorders.

Flint, R. W., & Turek, C. (2003). Glucose effects on a continuous performance test of attention in adults. *Behavioural Brain Research, 142*, 217–228.

Forbes, G. B. (1998). Clinical utility of the Test of Variables of Attention (T.O.V.A.) in the diagnosis of attention-deficit/hyperactivity disorder. *Journal of Clinical Psychology, 54*(4), 461–467.

Greenberg, L. M. (1988–2000). *T.O.V.A.® Continuous Performance Test*. Los Alamitos, CA: Universal Attention Disorders.

Greenberg, L. M., & Crosby, R. D. (1992). *A summary of developmental normative data on the T.O.V.A. ages 4 to 80+*. Unpublished manuscript.

Greenberg, L. M., & Waldman, I. D. (1993). Developmental normative data on the Test of Variables of Attention (T.O.V.A.). *Journal of Child and Adolescent Psychiatry, 34*(6), 1019–1030.

Greenberg, L. M., Kindschi, C. L., & Corman, C. M. (2000). *Test of Variables of Attention: Clinical Guide*. Los Alamitos, CA: Universal Attention Disorders.

Lee, K. T., Mattson, S. N., & Riley, E. P. (2004). Classifying children with heavy prenatal alcohol exposure using measures of attention. *Journal of the International Neuropsychological Society, 10*, 271–277.

Leark, R. A., Dixon, D., Hoffman, T., & Huynh, D. (2002). Fake bad test response bias effects on the Test of Variables of Attention. *Archives of Clinical Neuropsychology, 17*, 335–342.

Leark, R. A., Dupuy, T. R., Greenberg, L. M., Corman, C. L., & Kindschi, C. L. (1988–1999). *Test of Variables of Attention: Professional Guide*. Los Alamitos, Calif.: Universal Attention Disorders.

Leark, R. A., Wallace, D. R., & Fitzgerald, R. (2004). Test-retest reliability and standard error of measurement for the Test of Variables of Attention (T.O.V.A.) with healthy school-age children. *Assessment, 11*(4), 285–289.

Li, X., & Wang, Y. (2000). A preliminary application of the Test of Variables of Attention (T.O.V.A.) in China. *Chinese Mental Health Journal, 14*(3), 149–152.

Llorente, A. M., Amado, A. J., Voigt, R. G., Berretta, M. C., Fraley, J. K., Jensen, C. L., & Heird, W. C. (2001). Internal consistency, temporal stability, and reproducibility of individual index scores of the Test of Variables of Attention in children with attention-deficit/hyperactivity disorder. *Archives of Clinical Neuropsychology, 16*, 535–546.

Manor, I., Tyano, S., Mel, S., Eisenberg, J., Bachner-Melman, R., Kotler, M., & Ebstein, R. P. (2002a). The short DRD4 repeats confer risk to attention deficit hyperactivity disorder in a family-based design and impair performance on a continuous performance test (T.O.V.A.). *Molecular Psychiatry, 7*, 626–632.

Manor, I., Tyano, S., Mel, S., Eisenberg, J., Bachner-Melman, R., Kotler, M., & Ebstein, R. P. (2002b). Family-based and association studies of monoamine oxidase A and attention deficit hyperactivity disorder (ADHD): Preferential transmission of the long promoter-region repeat and its association with impaired performance on a continuous performance test (T.O.V.A.). *Molecular Psychiatry, 7*, 626–632.

Mautner, V. F., Kluwe, L., Thakker, S. D., Leark, R. A. (2002). Treatment of ADHD in neurofibromatosis type 1. *Developmental Medicine and Child Neurology, 44*, 164–170.

Monastra, V. J., Lubar, J. F., & Linden, M. (2001). The development of quantitative electroencephalographic scanning process for attention deficit-hyperactivity disorder: Reliability and validity studies. *Neuropsychology, 15*(1), 136–144.

Monastra, V. J., Monastra, D. M., & George, S. (2002). The effects of stimulant therapy, EEG biofeedback, and parenting style on primary symptoms of attention-deficit/hyperactivity disorder. *Applied Psychophysiology and Biofeedback, 27*(4), 231–249.

Riccio, C. A., Reynolds, C. R., & Lowe, P. A. (2001). *Clinical applications of continuous performance tests: Measuring attention and impulsive responding in children and adults*. New York: John Wiley & Sons.

Sandford, J. A., & Turner, A. (1994–2004). *IVA+Plus™: Integrated Visual and Auditory Continuous Performance Test Interpretation Manual*. Richmond, Va.: BrainTrain.

Schatz, A. M., Ballantyne, A. O., Trauner, D. A. (2001). Sensitivity and specificity of a computerized test of attention in the diagnosis of attention-deficit/hyperactivity disorder. *Assessment, 8*(4), 357–365.

Schatz, A. M., Weimer, A. K., & Trauner, D. A. (2002). Attention differences in Asperger syndrome. *Journal of Autism and Developmental Disorders, 32*(4), 333–336.

Schatz, J., Craft, S., Koby, M., Siegel, M., Resar, L., Lee, R. R., Chu, J. Y., Launius, G., Dadash-Zadehm, M., & DeBaun, M. (1999). Neuropsychologic deficits in children with sickle cell disease and cerebral infarction: Role of lesion site and volume. *Child Neuropsychology, 5*(2), 92–103.

Stein, M. A., Blondis, T. A., Schnitzler, E. R., O'Brien, T., Fishkin, J., Blackwell, B., Szumowski, E., & Roizen, N. J. (1996). Methylphenidate dosing: Twice daily versus three times daily. *Pediatrics, 98*, 748–756.

Walters, A. S., Mandelbaum, D. E., Lewin, D. S., Kugler, S., England, S. J., Miller, M., and the Dopaminergic Therapy Study Group. (2000). Dopaminergic therapy in children with restless legs/periodic limb movement in sleep and ADHD. *Pediatric Neurology, 22*, 182–186.

Weyandt, L. L., Mitzlaff, L., & Thomas, L. (2002). The relationship between intelligence and performance on the Test of Variables of Attention (T.O.V.A.). *Journal of Learning Disabilities, 35*(2), 114–120.

Weyandt, L. L., Rice, J. A., Linterman, H. I., Mitzlaff, L., & Emert, E. (1998). Neuropsychological performance of a sample of adults with ADHD, developmental reading disorder, and controls. *Developmental Neuropsychology, 14*, 643–656.

Yeates, K. O., Luria, J., Bartkowski, H., Rusin, J., Martin, L., & Bigler, E. D. (1999). Postconcussive symptoms in children with mild closed head injuries. *Journal of Head Trauma Rehabilitation, 14*(4), 337–350.

Trail Making Test (TMT)

OTHER TEST NAMES

Alternative names for this test are Trail Making Test (TMT), Partington Pathways, and Oral Trail Making Test.

PURPOSE

The TMT is a measure of attention, speed, and mental flexibility.

SOURCE

The TMT can be purchased from Reitan Neuropsychology Laboratory, P.O. Box 66080, Tucson AZ 85728 (http://www.reitanlabs.com). The administration manual and 100 copies of parts A and B for adults cost $50 US; for older children, $50 US. As Lezak et al. (2004) noted, the TMT is in the public domain and can be reproduced without permission. The Oral TMT, described later, does not require specific material.

Other Versions

Arabic (Stanczak et al., 2001), Chinese (Lu & Bigler, 2000), and Hebrew (Axelrod et al., 2000) versions of the TMT are also available. A Symbol Trail Making Test (Barncord & Wanlass, 2001) was developed for populations who have no familiarity with the Arabic numerical system.

The Delis-Kaplan Executive Function Scale (D-KEFS) and CAS also include subtests modeled after the TMT (e.g., Planned Connections; see descriptions elsewhere in this volume). Others (Davis et al., 1989; D'Elia et al., 1996; Espy & Cwik, 2004; Llorente et al., 2003; Reynolds, 2002; Stanczak & Triplett, 2003; Stanczak et al., 1998) have developed variants of the TMT for adults and children. Both the Color Trails (D'Elia et al., 1996) and the Comprehensive Trail Making Test (Reynolds, 2002) are considered elsewhere in this volume.

AGE RANGE

The age range for the Intermediate Version of the TMT is 9 to 14 years, and that of the Adult Version is 15 to 89 years. For the Oral TMT, the age range is 15 to 89 years.

DESCRIPTION

TMT

The test, originally constructed in 1938 as "Partington's Pathways" or the "Divided Attention Test" (Partington & Leiter, 1949) was part of the Army Individual Test Battery (1944). It was adapted by Reitan (1955) and added to the Halstead Battery. It requires the subject to connect, by making pencil lines, 25 encircled numbers randomly arranged on a page in proper order (Part A) and 25 encircled numbers and letters in alternating order (Part B). The test has two forms: the Child (Intermediate) Form for ages 9 to 14 years and the Adult Form for ages 15 years and older.

Others (Franzen et al., 1996; Lewis & Rennick, 1979) have constructed alternate forms of the TMT for repeat testing—for example, by simply reversing the order of the sequences.

Oral TMT

Ricker and Axelrod (Abraham et al., 1996; Ricker & Axelrod, 1994; Ricker et al., 1996) recommend an oral version of the TMT as an alternative for special populations for whom the drawing form may be inappropriate, such as individuals with motor deficits (e.g., arthritis) or with visual impairment. The patient is merely asked to count from 1 to 25 in Part A and to alternate between numbers and letters progressively up to 13 in Part B. The authors gave both the oral and written versions in counterbalanced order to individuals in three age groups; the mean ages and standard deviations (SDs) were 18.9 ± 1.1 years for group 1; 31.9 ± 8.9 years for group 2, and 83.5 ± 6.6 years for group 3. They converted raw scores to T scores demographically corrected for age, education, and gender and found a consistent relationship between oral and written versions across age groups. In addition, correlations between versions (oral, written) for each form were moderately strong ($r = -.68$ for part A; $r = -.72$ for part B).

ADMINISTRATION

Administration guidelines for the TMT (standard and oral versions) are provided in Figures 9–20 and 9–21. A number of authors (e.g., Heaton et al., 2004; Lucas et al., 2005) include a time limit of 5 min (300 s) on Part B to reduce testing time and participant frustration. Participants who cannot complete Part B within 5 min are assigned a time of 300 or 301 s.

The standard procedure includes practice exercises for Parts A and B. Thompson et al. (1999) analyzed practice times and provided tables to assist the clinician in deciding whether to administer the remainder of that particular part of the TMT or to discontinue in the case of severely impaired patients. A 20-s Part A practice time cutoff resulted in optimal prediction of successful completion (<180 s) for TMT Part A; a Part B practice time cutoff of 30 s proved optimal in predicting successful completion (<300 s) of TMT Part B.

ADMINISTRATION TIME

About 5 to 10 minutes are needed for test administration.

Figure 9–20 Instructions for TMT.

Part A

Sample A. When ready to begin the test, place the Part A test sheet in front of the subject, give the subject a pencil, and say: *On this page* (point) *are some numbers. Begin at number 1* (point to "1") *and draw a line from 1 to 2,* (point to "2"), *2 to 3* (point to "3"), *3 to 4* (point to "4"), *and so on, in order, until you reach the end* (pointing to the circle marked "END"). *Draw the lines as fast as you can. Do not lift the pencil from the paper. Ready! Begin!*

If the subject makes a mistake on Sample A, point it out and explain it. The following explanations of mistakes are acceptable:

1. *You started with the wrong circle. This is where you start* (point to "1").
2. *You skipped this circle* (point to the one omitted). *You should go from number 1* (point) *to 2* (point), *2 to 3* (point), *and so on, until you reach the circle marked "END"* (point).
3. *Please keep the pencil on the paper, and continue right on to the next circle.*

After the mistake has been explained, the examiner marks out the wrong part and says: *Go on from here* (point to the last circle completed correctly in the sequence).

If the subject still cannot complete Sample A, take the subject's hand and guide the pencil (eraser end down) through the trail. Then say: *Now you try it. Put your pencil, point down. Remember, begin at number 1* (point), *and draw a line from 1 to 2* (point to "2"), *2 to 3* (point to "3"), *3 to 4* (point to "4"), *and so on, in order until you reach the circle marked "END"* (point). *Do not skip around but go from one number to the next in the proper order. If you make a mistake, mark it out. Remember, work as fast as you can. Ready! Begin!*

If the subject succeeds this time, go on to Part A of the test. If not, repeat the procedure until the subject does succeed or it becomes evident that he or she cannot do it.

If the subject completes the sample item correctly, and in a manner which shows that he or she knows what to do, say: *Good! Let's try the next one.* Turn the page and give Part A of the test.

Say, *On this page are numbers from 1 to 25. Do this the same way. Begin at number 1* (point) *and draw a line from 1 to 2* (point to "2"), *2 to 3* (point to "3"), *3 to 4* (point to "4"), *and so on, in order until you reach the end* (point). *Remember, work as fast as you can. Ready! Begin!*

Start timing. If the subject makes an error, call it to his or her attention immediately, and have the subject proceed from the point where the mistake occurred. Do not stop timing.

If the examinee completes Part A without error, remove the test sheet. Record the time in seconds. Errors count only in the increased time of performance. Then say: *"That's fine. Now we'll try another one."* Proceed immediately to Part B, sample.

Part B

Sample B. Place the test sheet for Part B, sample side up, flat on the table in front of the examinee, in the same position as the sheet for Part A was placed. Point with the right hand to the sample and say: *On this page are some numbers and letters. Begin at number 1* (point) *and draw a line from 1 to A* (point to "A"), *A to 2* (point to "2"), *2 to B* (point to "B"), *B to 3* (point to "3"), *3 to C* (point to "C"), *and so on, in order until you reach the end* (point to circle marked "END"). *Remember, first you have a number* (point to "1"), *then a letter* (point to "A"), *then a number* (point to "2"), *then a letter* (point to "B"), *and so on. Draw the lines as fast as you can. Ready! Begin!*

If the subject makes a mistake on Sample B, point it out and explain it. The following explanations of mistakes are acceptable:

1. *You started with the wrong circle. This is where you start* (point to "1").
2. *You skipped this circle* (point to the one omitted). *You should go from 1* (point) *to A* (point), *A to 2* (point), *2 to B* (point), *B to 3* (point), *and so on until you reach the circle marked "END"* (point). If it is clear that the subject intended to touch the circle but missed it, do not count it as an omission, but caution him or her to touch the circle.
3. *You only went as far as this circle* (point). *You should have gone to the circle marked "END"* (point).
4. *"Please keep the pencil on the paper and go right on to the next circle."*

After the mistake has been explained, the examiner marks out the wrong part and says: *Go on from here* (point to the last circle completed correctly in the sequence).

If the subject still cannot complete Sample B, take the subject's hand and guide the pencil (eraser end down) through the circles. Then say: *Now you try it. Remember, you begin at number 1* (point) *and draw a line from 1 to A* (point to "A"), *A to 2* (point to "2"), *2 to B* (point to "B"), *B to 3* (point to "3"), *and so on until you reach the circle marked "END"* (point). *Ready! Begin!*

If the subject succeeds this time, go on to Part B of the test. If not, repeat the procedure until the subject does succeed or it becomes evident that he or she cannot do it.

If the subject completes the sample item correctly, say: *Good. Let's try the next one.* Turn the page over and proceed immediately to Part B, and say: *On this page are both numbers and letters. Do this the same way. Begin at number 1* (point) *and draw a line from 1 to A* (point to "A"), *A to 2* (point to "2"), *2 to B* (point to "B"), *B to 3* (point to "3"), *3 to C* (point to "C"), *and so on, in order, until you reach the end* (point to circle marked "END"). *Remember, first you have a number* (point to "1"), *then a letter* (point to "B"), *and so on. Do not skip around, but go from one circle to the next in the proper order. Draw the lines as fast as you can. Ready! Begin!*

Start timing. If the subject makes an error, immediately call it to his or her attention and have the subject proceed from the point at which the mistake occurred. Do not stop timing.

If the subject completes Part B without error, remove the test sheet. Record the time in seconds. Errors count only in the increased time of performance.

Figure 9–21 Instructions for the Oral TMT. *Source:* Adapted from Abraham et al., 1996.

Trails A
I would like you to count from 1 to 25 as quickly as you can. 1, 2, 3, 4, and so on. Ready? Begin.

Trails B
Now, I would like you to count again, but this time you are to switch between numbers and letters when you count. 1, A, 2, B, 3, C, and so on until you reach number 13. Ready? Begin.

If the patient makes an error on either task, direct him or her back to the last correct item and to start from there. Time to completion is the score for both the forms A and B.

SCORING

TMT

Scoring is expressed in terms of the time in seconds required for completion of each of the two parts of the test. Because of the difference in cognitive test demands between Part A and Part B, some examiners also calculate derived scores: the Trails B/Trails A ratio and a Trails B – Trails A difference score (Lamberty et al., 1994). Both parts require perceptual tracking of a sequence and speeded performance, but Part B also requires divided attention. The ratio and difference scores are attempts to elucidate the added task requirements of Part B and are thought to be purer measures of the more complex divided attention and alternating sequencing tasks required in Part B.

Oral Version

TMT-B scores are transformed to written equivalents by multiplying them by 2.44 (written equivalent = oral TMT-B × 2.44; Ricker et al., 1996).

DEMOGRAPHIC EFFECTS

TMT

Age. Performance on Trails A and B is affected by age, with performance declining with advancing age (Backman et al., 2004; Drane et al., 2002; Hester et al., 2005; Lannoo & Vingerhoets, 1997; Lucas et al., 2005; Miatton et al., 2004; Mitrushina et al., 2005; Tombaugh, 2004). Longitudinal examination also reveals decline with advancing age, with greater variability between individuals with increasing age (Ratcliff et al., 2003). Interestingly, the age-related differences are localized to the speed with which the tasks can be completed; age is unrelated to accuracy (Backman et al., 2004). Further, the magnitude of the age-related effect appears to be similar for TMT-A and TMT-B (Backman et al., 2004).

Education/IQ. Lower levels of educational achievement (Clark et al., 2004; Greiffenstein & Baker, 2003; Hester et al., 2005; Lannoo & Vingerhoets, 1997; Lucas et al., 2005; Miatton et al., 2004; Mitrushina et al., 2005; Tombaugh, 2004; but see Backman et al., 2004) and lower IQ (Diaz-Asper et al., 2004) are associated with poorer test scores. IQ shows a moderate relationship with test performance, with associations becoming stronger, as IQ increases (Steinberg et al., 2005). The effect of IQ appears slightly more pronounced on Part B (Dodrill, 1987; Steinberg et al., 2005; Warner et al., 1987). For example, Steinberg et al. (2005) reported correlations with FSIQ of .37 for Part A and .50 for Part B.

Gender. Gender has little impact on performance in adults (Hester et al., 2005; Lanno & Vingerhoets, 1997; Lucas et al., 2005; Mitrushina et al., 2005; Tombaugh, 2004). Sex-related differences also appear to be minimal in children (Anderson et al., 1997), although Barr (2003) found a female advantage among adolescents.

Ethnicity/Culture. Cultural/linguistic variables may affect test scores. Lee et al. (2000) found that English monolinguals performed TMT-A faster than Chinese-English bilinguals did, suggesting that language background may exert some effect on task performance. Manly et al. (1998) reported that use of Black English among African Americans was associated with poor performance on Trails B. They suggested that unacculturated African Americans may take more time to complete Trails B because of the lack of saliency of this type of timed sequencing task within traditional African American culture. Others have also reported that ethnicity affects test scores (Lucas et al., 2005; Horton & Roberts, 2003; Roberts & Horton, 2001); however, Arnold et al. (1994) found no acculturation differences between Anglo American, Mexican American, and Mexican subjects). Examiner ethnicity may also have an effect on test scores. Kennepohl et al. (2004) found that African Americans who had high mistrust of Caucasians performed worse on Trails A when tested by a Caucasian examiner.

Relative Contributions. A recent study of normal individuals by Tombaugh (2004) found that age accounted for 31% and 35% of the variance for Trails A and B, respectively, whereas education accounted for only 3% and 7%. Gender accounted for less than 1%. Heaton et al. (2004) reported similar results: age accounted for 25% of the variance for both Trails A and B among Caucasians (26% and 29%, respectively, in African Americans); education accounted for 10% and 16% of the variance in Caucasians (6% and 8% in African Americans), whereas gender accounted for less than 1%. Similarly, Mitrushina et al. (2005) found that age is a stronger predictor than education of both TMT-A and TMT-B scores, although both variables make significant contributions. The influence of gender was negligible. Lucas et al. (2005) reported that both age and education made moderate, and roughly comparable, contributions to performance in African Americans; however, they evaluated a restricted age range (56+ years). As with the other studies, the amount of variance explained by gender was minimal.

The influence of demographic variables tends to be less in clinical populations. For example, Horton and Roberts (2003) found that, in a substance abuse population, demographic variables accounted for only a small percentage of variance for TMT-A (9%) and TMT B (12%). Similarly, Sherrill-Pattison et al. (2000) reported that, in patients with traumatic brain injury (TBI), duration of coma had a greater impact on TMT-B than did demographic variables. Nonetheless, education and, to a lesser extent, age accounted for a significant proportion of the variance in raw scores in subjects with TBI, and correction of test scores for demographic variables (age, education) led to greater accuracy when classifying individuals with mild-moderate TBI. Sherrill-Pattison et al. (2000) argued that use of values corrected for age and education should more accurately reflect the neuropsychological status of the patient than interpretations that are based exclusively on raw data.

Oral TMT

Increasing age is mildly associated with poorer performance on TMT-B ($r = .21$; Ruchinskas, 2003). The most notable associations, however, occur with education (TMT-A, $r = -.27$; TMT-B, $r = -.55$) and with general cognitive status as indexed by the MMSE (TMT-A, $r = -.21$; TMT-B, $r = -.66$; Ruchinskas, 2003).

NORMATIVE DATA

TMT — Adults/Adolescents

This popular test is backed by a large number of normative studies. Mitrushina et al. (2005) list no less than 46 normative studies. The use of cutoff scores designating "organic impairment," as suggested by Reitan and Wolfson (1985, 1988; e.g., >85/86 s for Part B) and by Matarazzo et al. (1974; >40 s for Part A, >91 s for Part B), has been abandoned by most authors in favor of actual normative data.

Table 9–73 Characteristics of the Trails Normative Sample

Number	1212
Age (years)	20 to 85[a]
Geographic location	Various states in United States and Manitoba, Canada
Sample type	Individuals recruited as part of multicenter studies
Education (years)	0 to 20[b]
Gender	
Male	56.8%
Female	43.2%
Race/Ethnicity (no.)	
Caucasian	634
African American	578
Screening	No reported history of learning disability, neurological disorder, serious psychiatric disorder, or alcohol or drug abuse

[a]Age bands: 20–34, 35–39, 40–44, 45–49, 50–54, 55–59, 60–64, 65–69, 70–74, 75–79, and 80–89 years.
[b]Education groups: 7–8, 9–11, 12, 13–15, 16–17, and 18–20 years.

Source: From Heaton et al., 2004.

Heaton et al. (2004) provide norms separately for Caucasians and African Americans organized by age, gender, and education. The samples are large and cover a wide range in terms of age and education, and exclusion criteria are specified (see Table 9–73). Users should note, however, that these data derive from several separate studies, some of which were conducted many years ago. Note also that individuals "generally" were given a maximum of 300 s to complete Part B. If the TMT-B was discontinued before completion, the time score (in seconds) was prorated by dividing 300 s by the number of circles completed and then multiplying the resulting "time per circle" figure by 25. T scores less than 40 were classed as impaired.

Other age- and education-based norms are also available. Mitrushina et al. (2005) collected data from 28 studies for Trails A and 29 for Trails B, reflecting data points for each part based on a total of 6317 participants aged 16 to 89 years for Part A, and 6360 for Part B.

Tombaugh (2004) recently provided normative data based on a large sample ($N = 858$) of healthy, community-dwelling individuals aged 20 to 89 years living in Canada. The education level varied from 5 to 25 years ($M = 12.6$, $SD = 2.7$). All persons scored higher than 23 ($M = 28.6$, $SD = 1.5$) on the MMSE and lower than 14 ($M = 4.1$, $SD = 3.4$) on the Geriatric Depression Scale. The data, stratified by age and education, are shown in Table 9–74. A series of regression analyses revealed that education accounts for virtually none of the variance in the 25-to-54 age range. However for Trails B, education becomes progressively more important with increasing age. These observations, as well as the fact that most of the participants in the 25-to-54 age range were relatively

Table 9–74 Percentiles of Trails A and B Scores for Each Normative Group

Percentile	Education 0–12 Years		Education 12+ Years		Total	
	Trail A	Trail B	Trail A	Trail B	Trail A	Trail B
Age group 18–24 (university students; n)					*155*	
90					16	35
80					17	38
70					19	41
60					20	44
50					22	47
40					23	49
30					25	54
20					27	61
10					31	66
Age group 25–34 (n)					*33*	
90					14	33
80					17	38
70					19	45
60					21	48
50					23	50
40					25	53
30					27	58
20					33	63
10					40	67
Age group 35–44 (n)					*39*	
90					16	40
80					20	45
70					23	50
60					24	53
50					26	58
40					28	60
30					32	62
20					36	70
10					46	87
Age group 45–54 (n)					*41*	
90					19	42
80					23	50
70					27	59
60					29	62
50					31	64
40					33	68
30					34	72
20					38	75
10					50	84
Age group 55–59 (n)	*58*		*37*		*95*	
90	25	56	22	42	23	56
80	27	64	24	56	25	58
70	29	66	25	57	27	64
60	31	71	26	61	30	66
50	32	74	30	65	32	73
40	34	81	32	71	33	74
30	38	87	33	74	35	83
20	40	98	37	81	40	90
10	50	105	53	102	53	104

(continued)

Table 9–74 Percentiles of Trails A and B Scores for Each Normative Group (*continued*)

	Education 0–12 Years		Education 12+ Years		Total	
Percentile	Trail A	Trail B	Trail A	Trail B	Trail A	Trail B
Age Group 60–64 (n)	55		31		86	
90	21	56	22	45	22	48
80	24	58	25	48	24	56
70	26	62	26	53	26	59
60	30	67	27	59	29	62
50	33	72	31	60	32	68
40	37	75	33	66	34	72
30	40	79	35	71	37	77
20	43	92	37	77	42	84
10	45	96	43	87	45	96
Age Group 65–69 (n)	65		32		95	
90	24	60	26	52	25	56
80	30	71	28	57	29	62
70	32	74	30	63	31	70
60	36	81	31	67	32	73
50	39	86	32	68	37	76
40	40	93	34	71	39	83
30	44	103	39	73	42	91
20	47	110	40	75	45	104
10	56	137	45	77	53	121
Age Group 70–74 (n)	76		30		106	
90	25	70	26	59	26	64
80	30	79	29	63	30	76
70	35	74	31	68	34	81
60	37	83	33	80	36	85
50	38	95	36	84	38	97
40	42	101	41	85	41	105
30	46	112	42	103	45	112
20	52	146	46	109	49	138
10	57	172	71	112	61	159
Age Group 75–79 (n)	74		34		108	
90	30	78	22	57	27	65
80	37	92	27	59	34	79
70	39	96	34	66	38	88
60	45	107	37	73	40	98
50	50	120	40	87	46	115
40	53	140	43	105	50	128
30	56	156	46	126	54	148
20	61	167	58	141	58	163
10	72	189	66	178	70	185
Age Group 80–84 (n)	84		34		118	
90	31	72	37	89	31	84
80	39	101	38	100	39	101
70	43	112	41	111	42	111
60	49	119	46	113	47	116
50	53	140	48	128	52	133
40	59	154	56	131	58	144
30	66	176	58	139	63	159
20	78	204	64	151	75	193
10	90	259	101	227	93	241

(continued)

Table 9–74 Percentiles of Trails A and B Scores for Each Normative Group (*continued*)

Percentile	Education 0–12 Years		Education 12+ Years		Total	
	Trail A	Trail B	Trail A	Trail B	Trail A	Trail B
Age Group 85–89 (n)	*16*		*13*		*29*	
90	37	89	35	70	36	81
80	39	95	42	81	39	87
70	43	112	49	87	47	95
60	47	132	52	90	51	121
50	55	143	53	121	54	138
40	56	188	60	143	56	150
30	63	194	67	156	65	194
20	72	214	78	212	68	199
10	94	317	125	290	120	296

Source: From Tombaugh, 2004. Reprinted with the permission of Elsevier.

well educated, led to the decision to divide only the older age groups into two education levels (0–12 and 12+ years). Some caution should be exercised in interpreting scores from the oldest age group (age 85–89) because of the restricted sample size. It should also be noted that all members of the youngest group (age 18–24) were university students. The normative values reported by Tombaugh (2004) suggest a higher standard than those provided by Mitrushina et al. (2005) but appear broadly similar to those provided by Heaton et al. (2004).

Lucas et al. (2005) recently provided age- and education-adjusted normative data based on 303 African-American community-dwelling participants from the Mayo African American Normative Studies (MOAANS) project in Jacksonville, Florida. Participants were predominantly female (75%), ranged in age from 56 to 94 years ($M = 69.6$, $SD = 6.87$), and varied in education from 0 to 20 years of formal education ($M = 12.2$, $SD = 3.48$). They were screened to exclude those with active neurological, psychiatric, or other conditions that might affect cognition. A time limit of 300 s was used on Part B; participants who required additional time were assigned a time of 301 s. Table 9–75a presents their data, and Table 9–75b provides the computational formula used to calculate age- and education-adjusted MOAANS scaled scores. Lucas et al. (2005) reported that about 15% of their sample performed above the discontinuation cutoff of 300 s on Part B, suggesting that examination of speed alone may not be fully informative for understanding the performance of older African Americans. Consequently, they also provide frequency distributions of error scores on Parts A and B. About 36% of their sample made two or more errors on TMT-B, whereas it was much less common for that number of errors to be made on Part A (3% of the normative sample). Less than 10% of their sample made four or more errors on Part B.

Examination of MOAANS normative estimates for TMT-B reveal a substantial floor effect, probably because of the truncation of higher scores (i.e., longer completion times) resulting

from the use of an a priori time limit (300 s). Overall, the relatively large number of study participants who discontinued TMT-B suggests that poor performance on this measure may not be a reliable indicator of cognitive dysfunction in older African Americans (Lucas et al., 2005). The reasons for this poor performance are uncertain but may reflect culturally related factors such as information processing style, perceived task relevance, importance of speed versus accuracy, quality of educational experiences, and presence of general medical factors (Lucas et al., 2005). The authors urged that their data be used with caution, because the number of very old adults is somewhat small and their sample of convenience may not represent the full range of cultural and educational experiences of the African American community.

Most normative reports for adults adjust for age and education. Given that IQ is more strongly related to performance than education, Steinberg et al. (2005) have reanalyzed data from the Mayo Clinic's Older Americans Normative Studies (MOANS) and provided age- (55+) and IQ-adjusted percentile equivalents of MOANS age-adjusted TMT scores. Readers should note that all FSIQs are MAYO age-adjusted scores, which are based on the WAIS-R, not the WAIS-III. Given the upward shift in scores (Flynn effect) with the passage of time, use of the WAIS-R FSIQ rather than the WAIS-III may result in a given TMT score appearing less favorable. The interested reader is referred to their article for the relevant tables.

Barr (2003) provided data on a sample of 100 young athletes (60 males, 40 females), with a mean age of 15.9 years ($SD = 0.98$). The sample was largely Caucasian (88%). All spoke English as their native language and were in good academic standing. Females tended to outperform males on Part B. The data are similar to those given by Yeaudall et al. (1987) and are shown in Table 9–76.

Difference and Ratio Scores. Some authors (Axelrod et al., 2000; Golden et al., 1981; Hester et al., 2005; Lamberty et al., 1994) have proposed that analyzing the difference score (B – A)

Table 9-75a MOAANS TMT Norms in African American Adults, By Age Group

Scaled Score Test Part	56–62 years A	56–62 years B	63–65 years A	63–65 years B	66–68 years A	66–68 years B	69–71 years A	69–71 years B	72–74 years A	72–74 years B	75–77 years A	75–77 years B	78+ years A	78+ years B	Percentile Ranges
2	120+	—	121+	—	121+	—	121+	—	125+	—	202+	—	227+	—	<1
3	112–119	—	117–120	—	117–120	—	117–120	—	118–124	—	184–201	—	202–226	—	1
4	93–111	—	101–116	—	107–116	—	113–116	—	—	301+	—	301+	183–201	—	2
5	88–92	301+	90–100	301+	95–106	301+	102–112	301+	112–117	285–299	122–183	295–300	154–182	—	3–5
6	76–87	247–300	80–89	260–300	86–94	270–300	89–101	285–300	97–111	267–284	113–121	257–294	121–153	301+	6–10
7	67–75	239–246	74–79	246–259	76–85	255–271	79–88	268–284	81–96	239–266	87–112	221–256	114–120	—	11–18
8	58–66	189–238	62–73	196–245	67–75	218–254	72–78	239–267	73–80	202–238	75–86	156–220	82–113	288–300	19–28
9	48–57	150–188	53–61	169–195	57–66	183–217	60–71	191–238	62–72	155–201	65–74	126–155	71–81	259–287	29–40
10	41–47	109–149	44–52	121–168	48–56	135–182	49–59	147–190	51–61	121–154	51–64	112–125	53–70	194–258	41–59
11	38–40	97–108	39–43	103–120	43–47	111–134	43–48	115–146	45–50	111–120	45–50	102–111	46–52	155–193	60–71
12	34–37	82–96	36–38	86–102	38–42	100–110	39–42	104–114	41–44	101–110	41–44	88–101	41–45	123–154	72–81
13	31–33	70–81	31–35	72–85	33–37	79–99	33–38	95–103	34–40	88–100	34–40	73–87	34–40	111–122	82–89
14	28–30	56–69	28–30	60–71	30–32	71–78	30–32	73–94	30–33	73–87	30–33	69–72	30–33	98–110	90–94
15	25–27	52–58	26–27	52–59	27–29	54–70	27–29	69–72	28–29	69–72	28–29	59–68	28–29	91–97	95–97
16	—	50–51	25	50–51	25–26	52–53	25–26	54–68	25–27	59–68	25–27		24–27	88–90	98
17	22–24	46–49	23–24	46–49	23–24	50–51	23–24	50–53	23–24		23–24		23	78–71	99
18	<22	<46	<23	<46	<23	<50	<23	<50	<23	<59	<23	<59	<23	<71	>99
n	107	107	129	129	165	165	181	181	155	155	118	118	77	77	

Source: Adapted from Lucas et al., 2005. Reprinted with permission of the Mayo Foundation for Medical Education and Research.

Table 9–75b Computational Formula for Age- and Education-Corrected MOAANS Scaled Scores

	K	W$_1$	W$_2$
Trails A	2.93	1.12	0.35
Trails B	3.10	1.19	0.40

Note: Age- and education-corrected MOAANS Scaled Scores (MSS$_{A\&E}$) can be calculated for TMT scores by using age-corrected MOAANS Scaled Scores (MSS$_A$) and education (expressed in years completed) in the following formula: MSS$_{A\&E}$ = K + (W$_1$ × MSS$_A$) – (W$_2$ × EDUC).

Source: Adapted from Lucas et al., 2005. Reprinted permission of the Mayo Foundation for Medical Education and Research.

or the ratio between Part A and Part B (B:A) might also be useful in interpreting TMT protocols. Lamberty et al. (1994) reported that ratio scores greater than 3.0 were found more frequently in impaired people, whereas ratios of less than 2.5 were considered to be within normal limits. However, demographic variables can affect derived TMT indices (Drane et al., 2002), although the impact of age and education may be reduced if ratio scores are considered (Hester et al., 2005). Therefore, scores that take into account demographic variables are likely to result in less erroneous interpretation than simple fixed cutoffs. Tom Tombaugh (personal communication, July 20, 2003) has provided ratio (percentage; B/A × 100) and difference score (B – A) data based on his large sample (*N* = 858) of healthy, community-dwelling individuals aged 20 to 89 years (described earlier). The data are shown in Tables 9–77 and 9–78. As is evident in the tables, derived scores tend to increase, particularly after age 70 years. In addition, derived scores tend to be smaller for subjects with more years of education (but see Drane et al., 2002, and Roberts & Horton, 2002, who reported no impact of education on derived scores).

TMT—Children

A number of investigators (e.g., Findeis & Weight, 1994; Klonoff & Low, 1974; Knights, 1970; Knights & Norwood, 1980; Reitan, 1971; Trites, 1977) have provided data for children. However, the data, including the metanorms provided by Findeis and Weight (1994), are based on articles published between 1960 and 1990; given their age, these norms must be used with caution. See earlier discussion for normative data sets involving adolescents.

Table 9–76 Scores of Adolescents (Mean Age = 15.9 Years, *SD* = 0.98) on the Adult Form of the TMT

		Trails A		Trails B	
	N	Mean	SD	Mean	SD
Males	60	23.2	7.6	56.5	18.9
Females	40	21.4	4.9	47.2	12.4

Source: Adapted from Barr, 2003.

Table 9–77 Total Scores (Mean and *SD*) for Two Derived Measures on the TMT Parts A and B

Age Group (Years)	Ratio % (B/A%)	Difference Score (B – A)
18–24	224.79 (71.40)	26.03 (12.08)
25–54	218.22 (65.48)	29.60 (12.95)
55–59	234.06 (73.05)	41.20 (1942)
60–64	223.93 (54.50)	38.41 (16.45)
65–69	230.47 (68.51)	42.07 (20.82)
70–74	261.68 (90.80)	61.43 (30.72)
75–79	263.33 (96.56)	73.23 (39.64)
80–84	263.20 (72.17)	89.44 (45.42)
85–89	261.93 (90.47)	95.31 (62.17)

Source: Tom Tombaugh, personal communication, July 20, 2003.

Anderson et al. (1997) provided more current normative data based on a sample of 392 children, aged 7 to 13.11 years, with approximately equal numbers of males and females in each age group. Children with a history of neurological, developmental, or psychiatric disorders and those requiring special educational assistance were excluded. The data are shown in Table 9–79.

Oral TMT

The oral version is performed considerably faster than the written version (Ricker & Axelrod, 1994). One way to evaluate the TMT-B score is to transform it to a written equivalent (see *Scoring*) and then evaluate it using the demographically based norms described earlier (e.g., Heaton et al., 2004; Tombaugh, 2004). Alternatively, some normative data were provided by Ricker and Axelrod (1994) based on small samples of healthy individuals (mean education not reported; see Table 9–80). Somewhat faster times were recently reported by Ruchinksas (2003) for a sample of 27 healthy older adults aged 60 years and older (*M* = 70.3, *SD* = 6.4) with mean education of 12.5 years (*SD* = 2.9): TMT-A, *M* = 7.0 s, *SD* = 1.7; TMT-B, *M* = 35.1 s, *SD* = 14.4.

RELIABILITY

TMT

Test-Retest Reliability. This varies with the age range and population studied but is for the most part adequate, at least for Part B. In young adults retested after an interval of 3 weeks, reliability was low for Part A (.55) but adequate for Part B (.75) (Bornstein et al., 1987). Matarazzo et al. (1974) gave the test twice, 12 weeks apart, and reported reliability coefficients of .46 and .44 (Parts A and B, respectively) for young, healthy, normal males. Dikmen et al. (1999) examined 384 normal or neurologically stable adults (age 15–83 years, *M* = 34.2, *SD* = 16.7) who were retested about 11 months after the initial test session. Coefficients were adequate for Part A

Table 9–78 Derived Scores for Each Normative Group on the TMT Parts A and B

	Education 0–12 Years		Education 12+ Years		Total	
Percentile	B/A%	B − A	B/A%	B − A	B/A%	B − A
Age group 18–24 (University Students)						
90					150	13
80					172	15
70					182	18
60					196	21
50					206	23
40					222	26
30					245	30
20					271	35
10					313	43
Age Group 25–54						
90					135	13
80					164	18
70					188	22
60					203	26
50					210	29
40					222	32
30					238	37
20					256	41
10					309	46
Age Group 55–59						
90	153	23	152	12	153	22
80	167	27	167	25	168	26
70	200	31	178	26	187	30
60	214	34	194	30	212	32
50	225	39	221	33	223	36
40	235	43	232	37	233	41
30	261	50	243	46	258	48
20	303	59	292	51	292	54
10	335	75	336	61	333	68
Age Group 60–64						
90	168	24	154	16	160	21
80	175	28	163	20	173	25
70	191	34	167	25	180	28
60	213	35	189	28	208	33
50	230	36	213	31	214	35
40	246	40	222	33	240	39
30	261	49	232	36	255	45
20	280	51	244	44	264	50
10	312	60	259	51	285	56
Age Group 65–69						
90	147	23	151	21	151	23
80	177	34	157	24	177	26
70	185	38	179	26	185	34
60	221	41	190	27	197	38
50	231	46	196	31	221	41
40	249	53	197	36	235	46
30	275	60	217	38	266	51
20	297	65	262	46	284	60
10	351	94	274	48	344	81

(continued)

Table 9–78 Derived Scores for Each Normative Group on the TMT Parts A and B (*continued*)

Percentile	Education 0–12 Years		Education 12+ Years		Total	
	B/A%	B − A	B/A%	B − A	B/A%	B − A
Age Group 70–74						
90	172	34	151	28	165	32
80	198	41	182	29	193	38
70	206	45	191	34	205	41
60	224	49	201	38	211	45
50	244	55	210	41	230	50
40	287	72	216	44	260	57
30	320	81	231	49	295	76
20	382	104	275	68	334	83
10	429	121	343	77	406	117
Age Group 75–79						
90	176	36	165	26	173	31
80	190	43	176	27	184	37
70	211	50	189	35	201	43
60	222	64	224	38	223	52
50	238	71	249	43	247	66
40	251	82	260	63	259	76
30	296	91	268	77	287	83
20	346	119	293	83	329	105
10	405	131	349	112	376	128
Age Group 80–84						
90	196	43	172	45	190	44
80	214	54	194	47	213	52
70	226	65	215	55	222	56
60	242	69	223	55	232	67
50	262	83	228	70	249	73
40	269	103	244	73	265	91
30	281	111	275	91	281	106
20	305	126	297	104	302	124
10	364	168	382	130	365	164
Age Group 85–89						
90	197	47	128	15	152	28
80	208	51	152	28	187	48
70	219	71	180	43	213	52
60	249	77	200	52	223	71
50	274	96	223	54	248	83
40	294	108	244	85	267	100
30	337	125	248	109	285	124
20	350	136	286	135	338	134
10	470	253	337	164	359	181

Note: B/A% = ratio of scores on Trails A and Trails B expressed as a percentage. B − A = difference score. Readers can convert B − A scores into a percent difference change score (B − A/A × 100) by subtracting 100 from the B/A% score.

Source: Tom Tombaugh, personal communication, July 22, 2003.

(.79) and high for Part B (.89). Similar findings were reported by Levine et al. (2004) in a well-educated, mostly Caucasian sample of male subjects (.70 for A and B). In older adults, 1-year test-retest reliabilities were low for part A (.53–.64) and somewhat higher for part B (.67–.72) (Mitrushina & Satz, 1991; Snow et al. 1988).

Reliabilities in clinical groups are sometimes not as strong. Goldstein and Watson (1989) found similar reliability coefficients (.69 to .94 for Part A, .66 to .86 for Part B) for various neurological groups but inadequate reliability in persons with schizophrenia (.36 for Part A, .63 for Part B). Matarazzo et al. (1974) found that, after 12 weeks, reliability coefficients were

Table 9–79 Normative Data for Children on the TMT (Intermediate Version): Time Score in Seconds (Mean and *SD*)

	Age and No. of Subjects						
	7 Years (56)	8 Years (56)	9 Years (62)	10 Years (62)	11 Years (51)	12 Years (54)	13 Years (51)
Trails A							
Time	30.9 (15.9)	26.6 (11.5)	22.8 (11.8)	18.1 (5.0)	15.8 (4.9)	20.1 (17.0)	15.7 (9.1)
Mean Errors	.20	.30	.20	.10	.10	.10	.10
Trails B							
Time	97.9 (113.4)	69.0 (32.2)	58.1 (29.5)	44.5 (19.9)	43.6 (29.1)	33.6 (19.3)	30.6 (11.6)
Mean Errors	.9	.9	.4	.7	.4	.4	.4

Source: From Anderson et al., 1997. Reprinted with the permission of the authors.

marginal to adequate for older adults with diffuse cerebrovascular disease (*r* = .78 for Part A and *r* = .67 for Part B in 60-year-old patients). In contrast, Bardi et al. (1995) reported inadequate reliability over repeated administrations. They gave the test four times over an 18-month period to cognitively stable HIV-positive adults and found retest reliability to range from .49 to .50 for Trails A and from .54 to .62 for Trails B. Dodrill and Troupin (1975) reported 6- to 12-month reliability coefficients for individuals with epilepsy ranging between .67 and .89 for Part A, and between .30 and .87 for Part B; the highest values were obtained at the fourth repeat administration. Overall, these studies indicate that, although reliability of the test can be high, it is not a uniformly reliable measure across populations and time intervals.

TMT reliability has also been studied in children with varying results. A meta-analysis by Leckliter et al. (1992) concluded that TMT Part A is reliable but that Part B may be less reliable across the 9- to 14-year age range. Others have found Part B to be more reliable. In adolescents retested after an interval of 60 days, test-retest correlations were reported to be low to marginal (Trails A, *r* = .41; Trails B, *r* = .65; Barr, 2003). Neyens & Aldenkamp (1996) evaluated Dutch children (ranging in age from 4 to 12 years) three times, with a test-retest interval of 6 months. Stability coefficients were good for Part B but poor for part A.

Practice Effects. Over short retest intervals, practice effects emerge; however, these seem to disappear after several administrations. For example, Bornstein et al. (1987) retested a sample of healthy adults after a 3-week interval and noted

Table 9–80 Raw Scores (Mean and *SD*) on the Oral TMT in Three Age Groups

	Young Adults	Middle-Aged Adults	Older Adults
Age (years)	18.9 (1.1)	31.9 (8.9)	83.5 (6.6)
n	20	18	20
Trails A	6.4 (0.9)	6.4 (1.0)	10.6 (0.8)
Trails B	24.1 (10.6)	22.8 (10.6)	40.2 (5.6)

Source: Adapted from Ricker & Axelrod, 1994.

significant improvement (about 3 s) for Part A only. However, Dye (1979) and Stuss et al. (1987, 1988) reported significant practice effects after a 1-week interval for both parts (see Table 9–81), and Durvasula et al. (1996) found continuing improvement for both parts during repeat testing at 6-month intervals which flattened off after five administrations. McCaffrey et al. (1993) found steady improvement across three assessments followed by a sudden decrement on the fourth session.

Barr (2003) retested a sample of 48 adolescent athletes (age 13–17 years; *M* = 15.96, *SD* = .94) and found that they improved their scores (by about 2 s on Part A and 6 s on Part B) after a retest interval of 60 days (see Table 9–82). Reliable change indices (RCIs) are shown in Table 9–83. All RCIs are followed by the percentage of adolescents with change scores exceeding the lower limit. This value represents the level of raw score decline that is required to exceed what might be expected on the basis of normal error variance and the effects of practice. Upper limits are also listed to aid in interpretation of possible improvements.

After longer intervals, TMT scores show little or only modest change, at least in healthy adults. For example, Basso et al. (1999) retested a group of 50 healthy men after a 12-month interval and found that retesting had no effect on performance. The presence and magnitude of practice effects were similar among individuals of average and above-average IQ. The authors also calculated RCIs using the standard error of prediction to estimate the range of change in scores that might be expected while accounting for measurement error and practice effects. They noted that a wide range of retest scores could fall within the 90% confidence interval and still reflect measurement error rather than meaningful change. An individual could increase or decrease performance by as much as 24 s on Part B without displaying meaningful change in performance.

Similar findings were reported by Levine et al. (2004). Drawing from a database of 605 well-educated, mostly Caucasian men (education *M* = 16.4 years, *SD* = 2.3; age *M* = 39.5 years, *SD* = 8.7), they used the regression approach to derive estimates of change. The retest interval ranged from 4 to 24 months. Table 9–84 shows the regression formulas used to

Table 9–81 Completion Time in Seconds (Mean and *SD*) for TMT Parts A and B by Age, Based on Two Test Sessions Spaced 1 Week Apart

n	Age	Education (years)	Trails A		Trails B	
			Test 1	Test 2	Test 1	Test 2
30	16–29	14.1	21.48 (6.44)	19.68 (7.32)	48.77 (18.66)	42.18 (15.54)
30	30–49	14.9	27.58 (9.43)	22.95 (6.23)	61.30 (17.88)	61.52 (22.79)
30	50–69	13.2	36.73 (13.68)	29.30 (14.73)	76.97 (30.52)	67.10 (28.37)

Source: Adapted from Stuss et al., 1988.

Table 9–82 Completion Time in Seconds (Mean and *SD*) for TMT Parts A and B by Adolescents aged 13 to 17 Years, Based on Two Test Sessions Spaced About 60 Days Apart

	T1	T2	T2 – T1	*r*	*SEM*	S_{diff}
Part A sec.	21.4 (5.4)	19.3 (5.4)	−2.14 (5.9)	.41	4.16	5.88
Part B sec.	50.1 (17.3)	44.9 (15.6)	−5.83 (13.8)	.65	10.22	14.45

Source: Adapted from Barr, 2003.

estimate Time 2 scores. The residual *SD*s for the regression formulas are also shown and can be used to establish the normal range for retest scores. For example, a 90% confidence interval can be created around the scores by multiplying the residual *SD* by 1.645, which allows for 5% of people to fall outside of both the upper and lower extremes. Individuals whose scores exceed the extremes are considered to have significant changes. The length of the retest interval did not contribute significantly to the regression equation.

Dikmen et al. (1999) retested a sample of 384 normal or neurologically stable adults (age *M* = 34.1, *SD* = 16.7; education *M* = 12.1, *SD* = 2.6; 66% male) after retest intervals of about 9 months (range, about 2–16 months) and also noted that mean difference scores were small. However, some individuals did show large differences, as reflected in the large *SD* of the difference score (see Table 9–85). This table also provides information needed to determine whether there has been substantial change (RCI) taking practice effects into account. One first subtracts the mean score change for all subjects (T2 − T1) from the difference between the two testings for the individual and then compares the resulting value to 1.64 times the standard deviation of the difference. The 1.64 comes from the normal distribution and is exceeded in the

positive or negative direction only 10% of the time if indeed there is no real change in clinical condition.

Alternate Form Reliability. Charter et al. (1987) created an alternate form by changing numbers and letters but leaving the circles in place and reported reliability coefficients of .89 and .92 for Parts A and B, respectively. Alternate forms called TMT-C and TMT-D have also been proposed (des Rosiers and Kavanaugh, 1987; Franzen,1996; Franzen et al., 1996), with reported reliabilities of .80, and .78. McCracken and Franzen (1992) showed that the original and the alternate forms (TMT-C and TMT-D) contributed similar variance in factor analyses with other tests. However, TMT-D is slightly more difficult than TMT-B (LoSasso et al., 1998).

Interrater Reliability. For the TMT, interrater reliability has been reported as .94 for Part A and .90 for Part B (Fals-Stewart, 1991).

Oral TMT

Test-retest reliability and practice effects for the oral version need to be established.

Table 9–83 Adjusted RCIs (in Seconds) calculated for 90%, 80%, and 70% Confidence Intervals and Percentage of a Sample of Adolescents aged 13 to 17 Years With Change Scores Falling Below the Lower Limit

	90% CI	80% CI	70% CI
Part A	−12 to +8 (4.2%)	−10 to +5 (12.5%)	−8 to +4 (12.5%)
Part B	−30 to +18 (0%)	−24 to +13 (4.2%)	−21 to +9 (14.2%)

Source: Adapted from Barr, 2003.

Table 9–84 Regression Equations for Estimating Retest (Time 2) Scores

Measure	Regression Equation	Residual *SD*
Trails A	9.55 + (.545 × Time 1 score)	5.35
Trails B	21 + (.553 × Time 1 score)	11.61

Note: Based on a sample of 605 well-educated men (education *M* = 16.4, *SD* = 2.3), mostly Caucasians (age *M* = 39.5, *SD* = 8.7).

Source: Adapted from Levine et al., 2004.

Table 9–85 TMT Test-Retest Data (Mean and *SD*) Based on a Sample (*N* = 384) of Normal or Neurologically Stable Adults, aged 15 to 83 years (*M* = 34.2, *SD* = 16.7)

Trail Making Test	Time 1	Time 2	T2 − T1	SD_{diff}	r
Part A	26.52 (11.66)	25.56 (11.66)	−.96	7.54	.79
Part B	72.05 (45.22)	68.19 (46.13)	−3.86	21.64	.89

Note: In order to reduce testing time and patient fatigue, time limits were imposed on Part A (100 s) and Part B (300 s). The mean test-retest interval was about 9 months. One first subtracts the mean change (T1 score − T2 score) from the difference between the two testings for the individual and then compares this value to 1.64 times the standard deviation of the difference. The 1.64 comes from the normal distribution and is exceeded in the positive or negative direction only 10% of the time if indeed there is no real change in clinical condition.

Source: Adapted from Dikmen et al., 1999.

VALIDITY

TMT

Part A Versus Part B.   Parts A and B correlate moderately well with each other ($r = .31 − .60$), suggesting that they measure similar although somewhat different functions (Heilbronner et al., 1991; Pineda & Merchan, 2003; Royan et al., 2004). In addition to switching between numbers and letters in Part B, the actual distances between circles are longer in Part B than in Part A (Part B requires 56.9 cm more line length). Part B also includes more visual interference: there are 11 items within a 3-cm distance from the lines to be drawn in Part A, and 28 such items in Part B. Hence, Part B makes greater demands on visual search and motor speed than Part A does (Gaudino et al., 1995; Woodruff et al., 1995). Therefore, a low score on Trails B relative to Trails A does not necessarily imply reduced cognitive efficiency but may reflect the increased demands on motor speed and visual-perceptual processes.

Not only do the spatial arrangements and item sets differ between Parts A and B, but Part A is always given first. This feature also may complicate evaluation of the cognitive aspects involved in the test. Taylor (1998) gave the test to a heterogeneous sample of 100 patients. Half received the test in standard order and half in reversed order. The only significant difference was a higher B/A ratio in the reverse order group, reflecting slightly slower performance on TMT-B and slightly quicker performance on TMT-A in that group. Miner and Ferraro (1998) found similar order effects in undergraduates. However, the difference between standard and reverse-order groups in these studies tended to be small and fairly insignificant in clinical terms, suggesting that performance on the complex component of TMT-B is not crucially dependent on the accumulation of proactive interference from the preceding simpler component. The implication is that Trails B can be used in isolation. Whether diagnostic accuracy is unchanged when Trails B is used in isolation requires further study (Franzen, 2000).

Relations With Other Measures.   Evidence from several sources points to the TMT as a test of attentional abilities, including visual search and visual-spatial sequencing or scanning abilities, as well as speed. For example, Royan et al. (2004) reported that TMT-B correlated moderately well with scores on other measures of speeded processing (i.e., Symbol Digit Modality Test and a variant of the PASAT). O'Donnell et al. (1994) examined neuropsychiatric patients and performed a factor analysis of Trails B, Category Test, Wisconsin Card Sorting Test (WCST), Visual Search and Attention Test (VSAT), and the Paced Serial Addition Test (PASAT). They found that TMT-B loaded on a "focused mental processing speed" factor together with the VSAT and PASAT. Shum et al. (1990) reported high loadings on a visuomotor scanning factor, the first of three factors of tests of attention; other tests loading on this factor were the Digit Symbol Test, Letter Cancellation, and the Symbol-Digit Modality Test. Construct validity for visual search was also established by correlations (.36 to .93) with an object-finding test and a hidden pattern test obtained in 92 aphasic and nonaphasic patients (Ehrenstein et al., 1982). In this study, the test did not correlate with verbal tests (Token Test, Peabody Picture Vocabulary Test, and Picture Naming).

Executive control also plays a role. Kortte et al. (2002) used regression analysis of the TMT and the WCST with Veterans Administration patients to clarify what best predicts Trails B performance. They concluded that Part B is more sensitive to cognitive flexibility (percentage of perseverative errors on the WCST) than to ability to maintain set (failure to maintain set score on the WCST). Arbuthnott and Frank (2000) found that TMT performance (particularly the B:A index) correlated strongly with another set-switching task. They concluded that the "cost" for alternating switches was especially large for participants with a B/A ratio greater than 3. The authors interpreted their results as evidence that the ratio represents an index of executive function. However, inhibitory functioning (measured by a negative priming task) proved unrelated to task performance on Part A or B in undergraduates (Miner & Ferraro, 1998).

The TMT measures more than psychometric intelligence. Ardila et al. (2000) administered the TMT together with the Spanish version of the WISC-R, the Verbal Fluency Test, and the WCST to 50 Spanish-speaking children in Columbia who were of average intelligence and 13 to 16 years old. They found a significant negative correlations only between TMT-B errors and the WISC vocabulary subtest and between TMT-A time and Performance IQ; however, the correlations were low (about .30).

The test appears to be less affected by visual acuity than by motor speed and dexterity. A study of patients with mixed neuropsychiatric diagnoses (Schear & Sato, 1989) investigated the question of how TMT-B performance is affected by near visual acuity, motor speed, and dexterity. Visual acuity was measured with a vision tester, motor speed with the finger-tapping test, and dexterity with the Grooved Pegboard Test. Although visual acuity showed a modest correlation (−.27) with TMT-B (see also Skeel et al., 2003), motor speed and dexterity showed significant correlations with the test (−.42 and .46, respectively). In addition, only the motor tests were significant predictors of TMT performance in a regression analysis.

LoSasso et al. (1998) found that, in normal adults, execution of the TMT with the nonpreferred hand did not result in a clinically meaningful decline in performance. One implication is that patients with dominant hand paralysis may be tested using the nondominant hand. The authors noted, however, that generalizeability of these findings to elderly individuals or to patients with unilateral brain damage, who may lack some interhemispheric neural pathways important to modulating performance in the dominant hand, should be made with caution. Further, although the active hand may obscure items during task administration, left-handed examinees were not disproportionately affected in this study.

Circadian arousal is related to TMT performance, at least in older adults (May & Hasher, 1998). The difference in response time for Part B versus Part A was equivalent in young adults (aged 17–21) tested in the morning or the evening. However, when older adults (aged 63–76) were tested at their nonoptimal time (i.e., evening), processing was compromised.

Sensitivity to Neurocognitive Deficits.   Reitan and Wolfson (2004) recommended the TMT, particularly TMT-B, as a useful indicator of neurological integrity in both adults and children. In fact, they suggested that the task may serve as a useful screen to identify those in need of more comprehensive assessment. In support of their proposal, the test has been found to be sensitive to a variety of disorders, including heterogeneous neurological damage (Reitan & Wolfson, 1995, 2004), alcoholism (Grant et al., 1984, 1987), polysubstance abuse (McCaffrey et al., 1988), lead exposure (Stewart et al., 1999), HIV infection (Di Sclafani et al., 1997), fragile X syndrome (Moore et al., 2004), and academic difficulties (Reitan & Wolfson, 2004).

The test is also sensitive to closed-head injury (des Rosiers & Kavanagh, 1987). TMT completion times increase with increasing severity of head injury (Dikmen et al., 1995; Iverson et al., 2002; Martin et al., 2003). Felmingham et al. (2004) noted that diffuse axonal injury is associated with slowed performance in patients with severe TBI. They also recommended the use of a ratio score, because slower performance on TMT-A appeared to underlie deficits in TMT-B. That is, slowing of information processing speed appeared to be responsible for difficulties on more complex cognitive tasks. Errors and types of errors did not discriminate between head-injured patients and normal controls (Klusman et al., 1989). Although Iverson et al. (2002) reported that TMT ratio scores (but not errors) increased with injury severity, Martin et al.(2003) reported that the B/A ratio did not demonstrate sensitivity to injury severity.

Longitudinal studies reveal that there is marked heterogeneity of TMT outcome after moderate to severe head injury. Five years after injury, a substantial proportion of individuals with moderate to severe TBI show normal TMT performance, although a significant number continue to show deficits on the test. Millis et al. (2001) found that about 43% of such individuals showed marked impairment on TMT-A, and about 33% demonstrated such deficits on TMT-B. Contrary to conventional wisdom that recovery tends to occur within the first year, Millis et al. (2001) noted that substantial recovery occurred in some individuals several years after injury, although in some cases late decline was also apparent. Older age at the time of injury appeared to be an important risk factor for neuropsychological outcome.

The test's utility in cases of mild head injury is questionable. Sensitivity, specificity, efficiency (i.e., number of subjects correctly classified, defined as the number of true-positive results plus the number of true-negative results divided by the total number of subjects), positive predictive power, negative predictive power, and odds ratios for the TMT were examined by Cicerone and Azulay (2002) in a group of patients with postconcussion syndrome (PCS) and matched controls, screened for symptom exaggeration. These are reproduced in Table 9–86. Values for various impairment levels were calculated, with impairment defined as 1.5 *SD* below the mean. The TMT-A and TMT-B speed variables showed poor sensitivity, which indicates that they would have limited utility in ruling out the presence of PCS. However, their high specificity suggests considerable utility in ruling in PCS (i.e., persons without PCS are unlikely to have impaired scores). The positive predictive power of the speed score was strong, indicating the diagnostic utility of impaired scores on the test. According to criteria set by the authors (i.e., odds ratio ≥3, lower limit of the confidence interval >1), the Trails A score showed a reliable, positive association with PCS. Using the lower limit of the confidence interval of the odds ratio, a patient at least 3 months after injury with impaired performance on the TMT-A (i.e., at 1.5 *SD*s below the mean) is about three times more likely to exhibit PCS than a person with intact performance on this measure. Values for the Trails B score were less strongly supportive of its diagnostic utility in this group.

Table 9–86 Diagnostic Utility of the TMT in Postconcussion Syndrome: Sensitivity, Specificity, Efficiency, Positive Predictive Power, Negative Predictive Power and Diagnostic Accuracy (Odds Ratio and 90% Confidence Interval) for Scores Greater than 1.5 SDs below the Mean

	Trails A	Trails B
Sensitivity	31.3	14.3
Specificity	100	100
Efficiency[a]	64.1	57.8
Positive Predictive Power	90.9	100
Negative Predictive Power	59.3	54.2
Odds Ratio	30.3	13.0
90% Confidence Interval	2.7–339.7	1.1–152.6

Note: The base rate of postconcussion syndrome in this sample was 50%; the sample included 32 postconcussive patients screened for exaggeration and 32 matched controls.
[a]Refers to the number of subjects correctly classified ([True Positives + True Negatives]/N).

Source: Adapted from Cicerone & Azulay, 2002.

Poor discrimination was also reported by Iverson et al. (2005). They noted that patients with acute, uncomplicated mild TBI could not reliably be differentiated by the TMT from patients with substance abuse problems. The implication is that poor performance in mild TBI after injury may well reflect the contribution of premorbid difficulties.

Both cross-sectional and longitudinal studies have revealed that performance declines with advancing age (see *Demographic Effects*). Salthouse & Fristoe (1995) and Salthouse et al. (2000) investigated the relations of variants of the TMT with age and other cognitive variables (including vocabulary, spatial relations, Raven's PM, memory, and perceptual speed) in a sample of normal adults. They concluded that aspects related to perceptual speed are responsible for much of the individual differences of the test, and particularly for the age-related individual differences (see also Backman et al., 2004). There is also some evidence from positron emission tomography that change in dopaminergic neurotransmission (decline in D_2 receptor binding) is a more important factor than chronological age in accounting for variation in cognitive performance (on Trails A) across the adult lifespan (Backman et al., 2000).

As might be expected, the test is sensitive to dementing disorders such as Alzheimer's disease (Cahn et al., 1995; Chen et al., 2000; Lafleche and Albert, 1995). However, the task does not distinguish adequately among dementing disorders. For example, Barr et al. (1992) reported that time scores were high in patients with Alzheimer's disease and in patients with cerebrovascular dementia, but the difference between the two groups was not significant.

Neuroanatomical Correlates. Studies have explored the relationship between the TMT and localized brain dysfunction, particularly frontal lobe abnormalities. Early on, larger than normal differences between Parts A and B were interpreted as indicative of left lateralized lesions (Lewinsohn, 1973; Wheeler & Reitan, 1963), but other studies have not confirmed this (Heilbronner et al., 1991; Hom & Reitan, 1990; Schreiber et al., 1976; Wedding, 1979). Another interpretation has been that such differences indicate difficulties in the ability to execute and modify a plan of action (Annlies et al., 1980; Eson et al., 1978) or to maintain two trains of thought at the same time, which may possibly be related to frontal lobe damage (Lezak, 1983; Reitan, 1971). Some authors (e.g., Libon et al., 1994; Ricker et al., 1996) have found that Part B (in both the written and oral versions) is closely related to other tests of executive function (e.g., WCST) and to frontal lobe dysfunction (Ricker et al., 1996; but see Reitan & Wolfson, 1994, 1995). A recent meta-analysis (Demakis, 2004) compared patients with frontal damage to those with damage to posterior brain regions. Significant differences between groups were found for Trails A but not for Trails B (weighted effect size = −.23 and −.16, respectively). However, use of Trails A alone was not sufficient to discriminate between those with frontal versus nonfrontal brain injury. In fact, the amount of overlap between the distributions of these two groups at this effect size was about 85%, indicating little separation of groups and thus relatively poor sensitivity and specificity.

It may be that the Trails B is indeed sensitive to damage to specific frontal subregions, but, because these are aggregated with other frontal regions, this is not evident in meta-analytic research. Stuss et al. (2001) found notable slowing of TMT in patients with frontal lobe injury but concluded that error analysis provided a more useful method of categorizing performance: all patients who made more than one error on Trails B had frontal lesions. Patients with damage in dorsolateral frontal cortex were most impaired. The area of the frontal lobe that appeared to be least involved in TMT-A or TMT-B was the inferior (ventromedial/orbitofrontal) region.

Studies in Non-Neurological Populations. Patients with schizophrenia tend to show deficits on the TMT (Moritz et al., 2002; Woelwer, 2002; Zalla et al., 2004), as do patients with obsessive-compulsive disorder (Moritz et al., 2002). Major depression also affects performance negatively, particularly on Part B (Elderkin-Thompson et al., 2003; Naismith et al., 2003; Schopp et al., 2001; Veil, 1997). Elderly patients with depression did poorly on Trails B even after the depression had lifted after 6 months of treatment (King et al., 1991, 1995). Steffens et al. (2001) noted that depressed geriatric patients tended to make errors even after feedback after the first error. TMT performance as part of an attention/mental tracking factor was also found to be related to depression measured with the BDI in survivors of severe deprivation in prisoners-of-war camps, but not to weight loss sustained during imprisonment (Sutker et al., 1995). However, Zalla et al. (2004) observed no differences between euthymic bipolar patients and normal controls.

Table 9–87 Cutoff Values for Abnormality Data for Time to Completion Scores for the TMT

	TMT-A Time (Percentile)			TMT-B Time (Percentile)			TMT B/A Ratio (Percentile)		
	10th	5th	1st	10th	5th	1st	10th	5th	1st
Total Clinical Sample (*N* = 571)	52	63	86	155	200	288	1.66	1.49	1.25

Note: Age *M* = 34.7, *SD* = 15; Education *M* = 11.8, *SD* = 1.8.

Source: Adapted from Iverson et al., 2002.

Predictive/Ecological Validity. TMT performance is associated with vocational outcome in adulthood after childhood TBI. Those working full-time tend to perform faster on TMT-B (Nybo et al., 2004). Similar findings were reported for injury incurred in adulthood (Atchison et al., 2004). In addition, psychosocial outcome of head injury can be predicted by TMT-A and TMT-B (Acker & Davis, 1989; Colantonio et al., 2000; Millis et al., 1994; Ross et al., 1997). The TMT (Parts A and B) also appears useful for predicting instrumental activities of daily living in community-dwelling older adults (Cahn-Weiner et al., 2002; Bell-McGinty et al., 2002) and in cognitively impaired older adults (Baum et al., 1996; Boyle et al., 2004; Tierney et al., 2001). For example, Tierney et al. (2001) confirmed the ecological validity of TMT-B in a study of cognitively impaired people who live alone: the test was significantly related to self-care deficits, use of emergency services, experiencing harm, and loss of property as judged by independent raters and primary care physicians.

In combination with a test of visual acuity, the MMSE, and clock drawing, the TMT-A showed 85% specificity and 80% sensitivity when used to predict real-world road test performance in the elderly (De Raedt, 2001).

Malingering. A number of authors have found differences in TMT performance between individuals with genuine injuries and both experimental and suspected malingerers, with TMT performance suppressed in malingerers (Binder et al., 2003; Goebel, 1983; Ruffolo et al., 2000; Youngjohn et al., 1995). Recently, Iverson et al. (2002) examined a group of 571 patients with acute TBI and developed cutoff scores (scores falling at or below the 5th percentile) that could be considered suspicious for possible exaggeration (see Table 9–87). The performances of 228 patients involved in head injury litigation were compared to these cutoff values; 160 of these patients were considered to have provided adequate effort on cognitive tests, and the remaining 69 were suspected of inadequate effort based on symptom validity tests. Using cutoff scores at the 5th percentile, Iverson et al. (2002) noted that suspected malingerers consistently performed more poorly than controls on both Part A and Part B of the TMT. Although the TMT-A and TMT-B time-to-completion scores appeared to be reasonable indicators of

poor effort at the group level, this held true only when those with very mild head injury were considered. At the level of individual classification, the scores were unlikely to detect malingerers (sensitivity = 7.1%–18.5%), and there was a low degree of confidence in the classification of nonmalingerers (negative predictive value range, 66.4% to 78.2%). There was also little benefit in the use of the ratio scores to identify poor effort (see also Martin et al., 2003). The authors concluded that scores that fall in the range of possible biased responding can be considered "red flags" for the clinician because they do not make biological or psychometric sense. However, the sensitivity of the TMT to deliberate exaggeration is very low, so that clinicians who rely on this test to identify poor performance will fail to identify the vast majority of cases. Similar findings have been reported by others (e.g., Van Gorp et al., 1999; O'Bryant et al., 2003). Specialized tasks (symptom validity tests) appeared better able to detect malingering, at least in a simulation study (Merten et al., 2004).

Errors tend to be few even in patients with severe head injuries (Iverson et al., 2002; Ruffolo et al., 2000). Iverson et al. (2002) found it unusual for individuals with moderate to severe TBI to demonstrate two or more errors on Part A, and four or more errors on Part B; less than about 5% of the clinical sample obtained a similar score. Therefore, a large number of errors may alert the examiner to malingering.

Oral TMT

Ricker et al. (1996) found this version to be sensitive to anterior lesions in stroke patients, but they found no difference for right versus left lateralized lesions. Oral TMT also correlated with another measure of executive control (WCST percent perseverative errors, *r* = .35) but not with phonemic fluency (COWA, *r* = .17). The authors interpreted these findings to argue against a significant impact of expressive language on oral TMT-B performance.

Ricker, Axelrod, and colleagues (Abraham et al., 1996; Ricker and Axelrod, 1994; Ricker et al., 1996) suggested that, despite removal of the written component, the version still obtains clinically useful information. They recommended that the oral version of the TMT should be given if the times for the standard TMT exceed normal limits. They argued that, if

Oral TMT is also slow, it is likely that cognitive set shifting is impaired. If the Oral TMT is within normal limits, the deficit is more likely to be found in the visual-perceptual and motor components of the test.

COMMENT

The TMT is one of the five measures most commonly used by neuropsychologists (Camara et al., 2000; Rabin et al., 2005). As a measure of attention, it ranks as the top instrument, and in the domain of executive functioning, it ranks fourth in terms of frequency of use (Rabin et al., 2005). Reitan and Wolfson (2004) claimed that Trails B is second only to the Category Test in the Halstead-Reitan Battery as a general and consistent indicator of neurological integrity. Its sensitivity to neurological impairment is probably related to the complex set of skills required for successful performance (Franzen, 2000). The weakness, however, is that one cannot be certain of the basis for poor performance.

Lezak et al. (2004) noted that the imprecision of the scoring system (e.g., the time taken by the examiner to note and point out errors, the speed taken by the patient in making the correction) probably contributes to the reduced reliability of the test. Over short retest intervals, significant practice effects are evident. Over longer retest intervals (e.g., 1 year), practice effects appear negligible, and relatively large variations in performance may reflect the confounding effects of measurement error. Because of practice effects and measurement error, clinicians are encouraged to use reliable change methodology in the evaluation of repeat assessments.

It is worth bearing in mind that older adults show reliable differences over the course of the day (May & Hasher, 1998). Therefore, time of testing must be considered in the administration of the task to allow appropriate assessment of behavior in both single-test and test-retest situations. It is also possible that normative data need to be reevaluated with testing time controlled (May & Hasher, 1998).

Some have proposed that analysis of the difference score (B – A) or the ratio between Part A and Part B (B:A) might also be useful in interpreting TMT protocols, because such a manipulation controls for general speed of processing when interpreting TMT-B. However, information on their reliability is not available, and their utility requires additional investigation. Information on the reliability of error scores is also lacking. Of note, errors tend to be relatively infrequent in individuals with moderate to severe head injury. Accordingly, their presence in litigants claiming head injury may raise the concern of suboptimal performance.

The Oral TMT is a variation that omits the visual-motor component of the TMT and is suitable for patients with visual or severe motor handicaps. There is some evidence from stroke patients that this version is unrelated to expressive language functioning (Ricker et al., 1996). However, retest data are lacking. Further, many older adults find this task difficult, particularly those with low education and those whose MMSE scores are even mildly impaired (Ruchinskas, 2003).

REFERENCES

Abraham, E., Axelrod, B. N., & Ricker, J. H. (1996). Application of the oral Trail Making Test to a mixed clinical sample. *Archives of Clinical Neuropsychology, 11,* 697–701.

Acker, M. B., & Davis, J. R. (1989). Psychology test scores associated with late outcome in head injury. *Neuropsychology, 3,* 1–10.

Anderson, V., Lajoie, G., & Bell, R. (1997). *Neuropsychology assessment of the school-aged child.* Department of Psychology, Royal Children's Hospital, Melbourne, Australia.

Annelies, A., Pontius, A. A., & Yudowitz, L. B. (1980). Frontal lobe system dysfunction in some criminal actions as shown with the Narratives Test. *Journal of Nervous and Mental Disease, 168,* 111–117.

Arbuthnott, K., & Frank, J. (2000). Trail Making Test, Part B as a measure of executive control: Validation using a set-switching paradigm. *Journal of Clinical and Experimental Neuropsychology, 22,* 518–528.

Ardila, A., Pineda, D., & Rosselli, M. (2000). Correlation between intelligence test scores and executive function measures. *Archives of Clinical Neuropsychology, 15,* 31–36.

Army Individual Test Battery: Manual of directions and scoring. (1944). Washington, D. C.: War Department, Adjutant General's Office.

Arnold, B. R., Montgomery, G. T., Castaneda, I., & Longoria, R. (1994). Acculturation and performance of Hispanics on selected Halstead-Reitan neuropsychological tests. *Assessment, 1,* 239–248.

Atchison, T. B., Sander, A. M., Struchen, M. A., High, W. M., Roebuck, T. M., Contant, C. F., Wefel, J. S., Novack, T. A., & Sherer, M. (2004). Relationship between neuropsychological test performance and productivity at 1-year following traumatic brain injury. *The Clinical Neuropsychologist, 18,* 249–265.

Axelrod, B. N., Aharon-Peretz, J., Tomer, R., & Fisher, T. (2000) Creating interpretation guidelines for the Hebrew Trail Making Test. *Applied Neuropsychology, 7,* 186–188.

Backman, L., Ginovart, N., Dixon, R. A., Wahlin, T. B., Wahlin, A., Halldin, C., & Farde, L. (2000). Age-related cognitive deficits mediated by changes in the striatal dopamine system. *American Journal of Psychiatry, 157,* 635–637.

Backman, L., Wahlin, A., Small, B. J., Herlitz, A., Winblad, B., & Fratiglioni, L. (2004). Cognitive functioning in aging and dementia: The Kungsholmen Project. *Aging, Neuropsychology and Cognition, 11,* 212–244.

Bardi, C. A., Hamby, S. L., & Wilkins, J. W. (1995). Stability of several brief neuropsychological tests in an HIV+ longitudinal sample [Abstract]. *Archives of Clinical Neuropsychology, 10,* 295.

Barncord, S. W., & Wanlass, R. L. (2001). The Symbol Trail Making Test: Test development and utility as a measure of cognitive impairment. *Applied Neuropsychology, 8,* 99–103.

Barr, A., Benedict, R., Tune, L., & Brandt, J. (1992). Neuropsychological differentiation of Alzheimer's disease from vascular dementia. *International Journal of Geriatric Medicine, 7,* 621–627.

Barr, W. B. (2003). Neuropsychological testing of high school athletes: Preliminary norms and test-retest indices. *Archives of Clinical Neuropsychology, 18,* 91–101.

Basso, M. R., Bornstein, R. A., & Lang, J. M. (1999). Practice effects on commonly used measures of executive function across twelve months. *The Clinical Neuropsychologist, 13,* 283–292.

Baum, C., Edwards, D., Yonan, C., & Storandt, M. (1996). The relation of neuropsychological test performance to performance on functional tasks in dementia of the Alzheimer type. *Archives of Clinical Neuropsychology, 11,* 69–75.

Bell-McGinty, S., Podell, K., Baird, A., & Williams, M. J. (2002). Standard measures of executive function in predicting instrumental activities of daily living in older adults. *International Journal of Geriatric Psychiatry, 17*, 828–834.

Binder, L. M., Kelly, M. P., Villanueva, M. R., & Winslow, M. W. (2003). Motivation and neuropsychological test performance following mild head injury. *Journal of Clinical and Experimental Neuropsychology, 25*, 420–430.

Bornstein, R. A., Baker, G. B., & Douglas, A. B. (1987). Short-term retest reliability of the Halstead-Reitan Battery in a normal sample. *Journal of Nervous and Mental Disease, 175*, 229–232.

Boyle, P. A., Paul, R. H., Moser, D. J., & Cohen, R. A. (2004). Executive impairments predict functional declines in vascular dementia. *The Clinical Neuropsychologist, 18*, 75–82.

Cahn, D. A., Salmon, D. P., Butters, N., Wiederholt, W. C., Corey-Bloom, J., Edelstein, S. L., & Barrett-Connor, E. (1995). Detection of dementia of the Alzheimer type in a population-based sample: Neuropsychological test performance. *Journal of the International Neuropsychological Society, 1*, 252–260.

Cahn-Weiner, D. A., Boyle, P. A., & Malloy, P. F. (2002). Tests of executive function predict instrumental activities of daily living in community-dwelling older individuals. *Applied Neuropsychology, 9*, 187–191.

Camara, W. J., Nathan, J. S., & Puente, A. E. Psychological test usage: Implications in professional psychology. *Professional Psychology: Research and Practice, 31*, 141–154.

Charter, R. A., Adkins, T. G., Alekoumbides, A., & Seacat, G. F. (1987). Reliability of the WAIS, WMS, and Reitan Battery: Raw scores and standardized scores corrected for age and education. *International Journal of Clinical Neuropsychology, 9*, 28–32.

Chen, P., Ratcliff, G., Belle, S. H., Cauley, J. A. De Kosky, S. T., Ganguli, M., & Phil, D. (2000). Cognitive tests that best discriminate between presymptomatic AD and those who remain nondemented. *Neurology, 55*, 1847–1853.

Cicerone, K. D., & Azulay, J. (2002). Diagnostic utility of attention measures in postconcussion syndrome. *The Clinical Neuropsychologist, 16*, 280–289.

Clark, M. S., Dennerstein, L., Elkadi, S., Guthrie, J. R., Bowden, S. C., & Henderson, V. W. (2004). Normative data for tasks of executive function and working memory for Australian-born women aged 56-67. *Australian Psychologist, 39*, 244–250.

Colantonio, A., Ratcliff, G., Chase, S., & Escobar, M. (2000). Is cognitive performance related to level of community integration many years after traumatic brain injury? *Brain and Cognition, 44*, 19–20.

Davis, R. D., Adams, R. E., Gates, D. O., & Cheramie, G. M. (1989). Screening for learning disabilities: A neuropsychological approach. *Journal of Clinical Psychology, 43*, 402–409.

D'Elia, L. F., Satz, P., Uchiyama, C. L., & White, T. (1996). Color Trails Test. Odessa, Fla.: PAR.

Demakis, G. J. (2004). Frontal lobe damage and tests of executive processing: A meta-analysis of the Category Test, Stroop Test, and Trail-Making Test. *Journal of Clinical and Experimental Neuropsychology, 26*, 441–450.

De Raedt, R. (2001). Short, cognitive neuropsychological test battery for first-tier fitness-to-drive assessment of older adults. *Clinical Neuropsychologist, 15*, 329–336.

Des Rosiers, G., & Kavanagh, D. (1987). Cognitive assessment in closed head injury: Stability, validity and parallel forms for two neuropsychological measures of recovery. *International Journal of Clinical Neuropsychology, 9*, 162–173.

Diaz-Asper, C., Schretlen, D. J., & Pearlson, G. D. (2004). How well does IQ predict neuropsychological test performance in normal adults. *Journal of the International Neuropsychological Society, 10*, 82–90.

Dikmen, S. S., Heaton, R. K., Grant, I., & Temkin, N. R. (1999). Test-retest reliability and practice effects of expanded Halstead-Reitan Neuropsychological Test Battery. *Journal of the International Neuropsychological Society, 5*, 346–356.

Dikmen, S. S., Machamer, J. E., Winn, H. R., & Temkin, N. R. (1995). Neuropsychological outcome at 1-year post head injury. *Neuropsychology, 9*, 80–90.

Di Sclafani, V., Mackay, R. D. S., Meyerhoff, D. J., Norman, D., Weiner, M. W., & Fein, G. (1997). Brain atrophy in HIV infection is more strongly associated with CDC clinical stages than with cognitive impairment. *Journal of the International Neuropsychological Society, 3*, 276–287.

Dodrill, C. B. (1987). *What's normal?* Presidential address, Pacific Northwest Neuropsychological Association. Seattle, WA.

Dodrill, C. B., & Troupin, A. S. (1975). Effects of repeated administration of a comprehensive neuropsychological battery among chronic epileptics. *Journal of Nervous and Mental Disease, 161*, 185–190.

Drane, D. L., Yuspeh, R. L., Huthwaite, J. S., & Klingler, L. K. (2002). Demographic characteristics and normative observations for derived Trail Making indices. *Neuropsychiatry, Neuropsychology, and Behavioral Neurology, 15*, 39–43.

Durvasula, R. S., Satz, P., Hinkin, C. H., et al. (1996). Does practice make perfect? Results of a six-year longitudinal study with semi-annual testing [Abstract]. *Archives of Clinical Neuropsychology, 11*, 386.

Dye, O. A. (1979). Effects of practice on Trail Making Test performance. *Perceptual and Motor Skills, 48*, 296.

Ehrenstein, W. H., Heister, G., & Cohen, R. (1982). Trail Making Test and visual search. *Archiv fuer Psychiatrie und Nervenkrankheiten, 231*, 333–338.

Elderkin-Thompson, V., Kumar, A., Bilker, W. B., Dunkin, J. J., Mintz, J., Moberg, P. J., Mesholam, R. I., & Gur, R. E. (2003). Neuropsychological deficits among patients with late-onset minor and major depression. *Archives of Clinical Neuropsychology, 18*, 529–549.

Eson, M. E., Yen, J. K., & Bourke, R. S. (1978). Assessment of recovery from serious head injury. *Journal of Neurology, Neurosurgery and Psychiatry, 41*, 1036–1042.

Espy, K. A., & Cwik, M. F. (2004). The development of a Trail Making test in young children: The TRAILS-P. *The Clinical Neuropsychologist, 18*, 411–422.

Fals-Stewart, W. (1991). An interrater reliability study of the Trail Making Test (Part A and B). Unpublished manuscript.

Felmingham, K. L., Baguley, I. J., & Green, A. M. (2004). Effects of diffuse axonal injury on speed of information processing following severe traumatic brain injury. *Neuropsychology, 18*, 564–571.

Findeis, M. K., & Weight, D. K. (1994). Meta-norms for two forms of neuropsychological test batteries for children. Unpublished manuscript, Brigham Young University, Provo, Utah.

Franzen, M. D. (1996). Cross-validation of the alternate forms reliability of the Trail Making Test [Abstract]. *Archives of Clinical Neuropsychology, 11*, 390.

Franzen, M. D. (2000). *Reliability and validity in neuropsychological assessment.* New York: Kluwer Academic/Plenum Publishers.

Franzen, M. D., Paul, D., & Iverson, G. L. (1996). Reliability of alternate forms of the Trail Making Test. *The Clinical Neuropsychologist, 10*, 125–129.

Gaudino, E. A., Geisler, M. W., & Squires, N. K. (1995). Construct validity in the Trail Making Test: What makes Trail B harder? *Journal of Clinical and Experimental Neuropsychology, 17,* 529–535.

Goebel, R. A. (1983). Detection of faking on the Halstead-Reitan neuropsychological test battery. *Journal of Clinical Psychology, 39,* 731–742.

Golden, C. J., Osmon, D. C., Moses, J. A., & Berg, R. A. (1981). *Interpretation of the Halstead-Reitan Neuropsychological Test Battery.* New York: Grune & Stratton.

Goldstein, G., & Watson, J. R. (1989). Test-retest reliability of the Halstead-Reitan battery and the WAIS in a neuropsychiatric population. *The Clinical Neuropsychologist, 3,* 265–273.

Grant, I., Adams, K. M., & Reed, R. (1984). Aging, abstinence, and medical risk in the prediction of neuropsychological deficit among long-term alcoholics. *Archives of General Psychiatry, 41,* 710–716.

Grant, I., Reed, R., & Adams, K. M. (1987). Diagnosis of intermediate-duration and subacute organic mental disorders in abstinent alcoholics. *Journal of Clinical Psychiatry, 48,* 319–323.

Greiffenstein, M. F., & Baker, W. J. (2003). Premorbid clues? Preinjury scholastic performance and present neuropsychological functioning in late postconcussion syndrome. *The Clinical Neuropsychologist, 17,* 561–573.

Heaton, R. K., Miller, S. W., Taylor, M. J., & Grant, I. (2004). *Revised comprehensive norms for an expanded Halstead-Reitan battery: Demographically adjusted neuropsychological norms for African American and Caucasian adults.* Lutz, Fla: PAR.

Heilbronner, R. L., Henry, G. K., Buck, P., Adams, R. L., & Fogle, T. (1991). Lateralized brain damage and performance on Trail Making A and B, Digit Span Forward and Backward, and TPT memory and location. *Archives of Clinical Neuropsychology, 6,* 251–258.

Hester, R. L., Kinsella, G. J., Ong, B., & McGregor, J. (2005). Demographic influences on baseline and derived scores from the Trail Making Test in healthy older Australian adults. *The Clinical Neuropsychologist, 19,* 45–54.

Hom, J., & Reitan, R. M. (1990). Generalized cognitive function after stroke. *Journal of Clinical and Experimental Neuropsychology, 12,* 644–654.

Horton, A. M., & Roberts, C. (2003). Demographic effects on the Trail Making Test in a drug abuse treatment sample. *Archives of Clinical Neuropsychology, 18,* 49–56.

Iverson, G. T., Lange, R. T., & Franzen, M. D. (2005). Effects of mild traumatic brain injury cannot be differentiated from substance abuse. *Brain Injury, 19,* 11–18.

Iverson, G. L., Lange, R. T., Green, P., & Franzen, M. (2002). Detecting exaggeration and malingering with the Trail Making Test. *The Clinical Neuropsychologist, 16,* 398–406.

Kennepohl, S., Shore, D., Nabors, N., & Hanks, R. (2004). African American acculturation and neuropsychological test performance following traumatic brain injury. *Journal of the International Neuropsychological Society, 10,* 566–577.

King, D. A., Caine, E. D., Conwell, Y., & Cox, C. (1991). Predicting severity of depression in the elderly at six-months follow-up: A neuropsychological study. *Journal of Neuropsychiatry and Clinical Neurosciences, 3,* 64–66.

King, D. A., Cox, C., Lyness, J. M., & Caine, E. D. (1995). Neuropsychological effects of depression and age in an elderly sample: A confirmatory study. *Neuropsychology, 9,* 300–408.

Klonoff, H., & Low, M. (1974). Disordered brain function in young children and early adolescents: Neuropsychological and electroencephalographic correlates. In R. M. Reitan & L. A. Davison (Eds.), *Clinical neuropsychology: Current status and applications.* New York: Wiley.

Klusman, L. E., Cripe, L. I., & Dodrill, C. B. (1989). Analysis of errors on the trail making test. *Perceptual and Motor Skills, 68,* 1199–1204.

Knights, R. M. (1970). Smoothed normative data on tests for evaluating brain damage in children. Unpublished manuscript, Department of Psychology, Carleton University, Ottawa, Ont.

Knights, R. M., & Norwood, J. A. (1980). Revised smoothed normative data on the neuropsychological test battery for children. Unpublished manuscript. Department of Psychology, Carleton University, Ottawa, Ont.

Kortte, C. B., Horner, M. D., & Windham, W. K. (2002) The Trail Making Test, Part B: Cognitive flexibility or ability to maintain set? *Applied Neuropsychology, 9,* 106–109.

Lafleche, G., & Albert, M. S. (1995). Executive function deficits in mild Alzheimer's disease. *Neuropsychology, 9,* 313–320.

Lamberty, G. J., Putnam, S. H., Chatel, D. M., Beliauskas, L. A., & Adams, K. S. (1994). Derived Trail Making Test indices: A preliminary report. *Neuropsychiatry, Neuropsychology, and Behavioral Neurology, 7,* 230–234.

Lannoo, E., & Vingerhoets, G. (1997). Flemish normative data on common neuropsychological tests: Influence of age, education, and gender. *Psychological Belgica, 37,* 141–155.

Leckliter, I. N., Forster, A. A., Klonoff, H., & Knights, R. M. (1992). A review of reference group data from normal children for the Halstead-Reitan Battery for older children. *The Clinical Neuropsychologist, 6,* 201–229.

Lee, T. M. C., Cheung, C. C. Y., Chan, J., & Chan, C. C. H. (2000). Trail making across languages. *Journal of Clinical and Experimental Neuropsychology, 22,* 772–778.

Levine, A. J., Miller, E. N., Becker, J. T., Selnes, O. A., & Cohen, B. A. (2004). Normative data for determining significance of test-retest differences on eight common neuropsychological instruments. *The Clinical Neuropsychologist, 18,* 373–384.

Lewinsohn, P. M. (1973). Psychological assessment of patients with brain injury. Unpublished manuscript, University of Oregon, Eugene, Ore.

Lewis, R. F., & Rennick, P. M. (1979). *Manual for the Repeatable Cognitive-Perceptual-Motor Battery.* Grosse Pointe Park, Mich.: Axon.

Lezak, M. D. (1983). *Neuropsychological assessment* (2nd ed.). New York: Oxford University Press.

Lezak, M. D., Howieson, D. B., & Loring, D. W. (2004). *Neuropsychological assessment* (4th ed.). New York: Oxford University Press.

Libon, D. J., Glosser, G., Malamut, B. L., Kaplan, E., Goldberg, E., Swenson, R., & Sands, L. P. (1994). Age, executive functions, and visuospatial functioning in healthy older adults. *Neuropsychology, 8,* 38–43.

Llorente, A. M., Williams, J., Satz, P., & d'Elia, L. F. (2003). *Children's Color Trails Test (CCTT).* Odessa, Fla: PAR.

LoSasso, G. L., Rapport, L. J., Axelrod, B. N., & Reeder, K. P. (1998). Intermanual and alternate-form equivalence on the Trail Making Tests. *Journal of Clinical and Experimental Neuropsychology, 20,* 107–110.

Lu, L., & Bigler, E. D. (2000). Performance on original and a Chinese version of Trail Making Part B: A normative bilingual sample. *Applied Neuropsychology, 7,* 243–246.

Lucas, J. A., Ivnik, R. J., Smith, G. E., Ferman, T. J., Willis, F. B., Petersen, R. C., & Graff-Radford, N. R. (2005). Mayo's Older African

Americans Normative Studies: Norms for Boston Naming Test, Controlled Oral Word Association, Category Fluency, Animal Naming, Token Test, WRAT-3 Reading, Trail Making Test, Stroop Test, and Judgment of Line Orientation. *The Clinical Neuropsychologist, 19*, 243–269.

Manly, J. L., Miller, S. W., Heaton, R. K., Byrd, D., Reilly, J., Velasquez, R. J., Saccuzzo, D. P., Grant, I., and the HIV Neurobehavioral Research Center (HNRC) Group. (1998). The effect of African American acculturation on neuropsychological test performance in normal and HIV-positive individuals. *Journal of the International Neuropsychological Society, 4*, 291–302.

Martin, T. A., Hoffman, N. M., & Donders, J. (2003). Clinical utility of the Trail Making Test ratio score. *Applied Neuropsychology, 10*, 163–169.

Matarazzo, J. D., Wiens, A. N., Matarazzo, R. G., & Goldstein, S. G. (1974). Psychometric and clinical test-retest reliability of the Halstead Impairment Index in a sample of healthy, young, normal men. *Journal of Nervous and Mental Disease, 158*, 37–49.

May, C. P., & Hasher, L. (1998). Synchrony effects in inhibitory control over thought and action. *Journal of Experimental Psychology: Human Perception and Performance, 24*, 363–379.

McCaffrey, R. J., Ortega, A., & Haase, R. F. (1993). Effects of repeated neuropsychological assessments. *Archives of Clinical Neuropsychology, 8*, 519–524.

McCaffrey, R. J., Krahula, M. M., Heimberg, R. G., Keller, K. E., et al. (1988). A comparison of the Trail Making Test, Symbol Digit Modalities Test, and the Hooper Visual Organization Test in an inpatient substance abuse population. *Archives of Clinical Neuropsychology, 3*, 181–187.

McCracken, L. M., & Franzen, M. D. (1992). Principal-components analysis of the equivalence of alternate forms of the Trail Making Test. *Psychological Assessment, 4*, 235–238.

Merten, T., Henry, M., & Hilsabeck, R. (2004). Symptomvalidierungsstests in der neuropsycholgischen diagnostic: Eine analogstudie. *Zeitschrift fur Neuropsychologie, 15*, 81–90.

Miatton, M., Wolters, M., Lannoo, E., & Vingerhoets, G. (2004). Updated and extended normative data of commonly used neuropsychological tests. *Psychologica Belgica, 44*, 189–216.

Millis, S. R., Rosenthal, M., & Lourie, I. F. (1994). Predicting community integration after traumatic brain injury with neuropsychological measures. *International Journal of Neuroscience, 79*, 165–167.

Millis, S. R., Rosenthal, M., Novack, T. A., Sherer, M., Nick, T. G., Kreutzer, J. S., High, W. M. Jr., & Ricker, J. H. (2001). Long-term neuropsychological outcome after traumatic brain injury. *Journal of Head Trauma Rehabilitation, 16*, 343–355.

Miner, T., & Ferraro, F. R. (1998). The role of speed of processing, inhibitory mechanisms, and presentation order in Trail-Making Test performance. *Brain and Cognition, 38*, 246–253.

Mitrushina, M., & Satz, P. (1991). Effect of repeated administration of a neuropsychological battery in the elderly. *Journal of Clinical Psychology, 47*, 790–801.

Mitrushina, M. N., Boone, K. B., Razani, J., & D'Elia, L. F. (2005). *Handbook of normative data for neuropsychological assessment* (2nd ed.). New York: Oxford University Press.

Moore, C. J., Daly, E. M., Schmitz, N., Tassone, F., Tysoe, C., Hagerman, R. J., Hagerman, P. J., Morris, R. G., Murphy, K. C., & Murphy, D. G. (2004). A neuropsychological investigation of male permutation carriers of fragile X syndrome. *Neuropsychologia, 42*, 1934–1947.

Moritz, S., Birkner, C., Kloss, M., Holger, J., Hand, I., Haasen, C., & Krausz, M. (2002). Executive functioning in obsessive-compulsive disorder, unipolar depression, and schizophrenia. *Archives of Clinical Neuropsychology, 17*, 477–483.

Naismith, S. L., Hickie, I. B., Turner, K., Little, C. L., Winter, V., Ward, P. B., Wilhelm. K., Mitchell, P., & Parker, G. (2003). Neuropsychological performance in patients with depression is associated with clinical, etiological and genetic risk factors. *Journal of Clinical and Experimental Neuropsychology, 25*, 866–877.

Neyens, L. G. J., & Aldenkamp, A. P. (1996). Stability of cognitive measures in children of average ability. *Clinical Neuropsychology, 2*, 161–170.

Nybo, T., Saino, M., & Muller, K. (2004). Stability of vocational outcome in adulthood after moderate to severe preschool brain injury. *Journal of the International Neuropsychological Society, 10*, 719–723.

Partington, J. E., & Leiter, R. G. (1949). Partington's Pathway Test. *The Psychological Service Center Bulletin, 1*, 9–20.

Pineda, D. A., & Merchan, V. (2003). Executive function in young Colombian adults. *International Journal of Neuroscience, 113*, 397–410.

O'Bryant, S. E., Hilsabeck, R. C., Fisher, J. M., & McCaffrey, R. J. (2003). Utility of the Trail Making Test in the assessment of malingering in a sample of mild traumatic brain injury litigants. *The Clinical Neuropsychologist, 17*, 69–74.

O'Donnell, J. P., McGregor, L. A., Dabrowski, J. J., Oestreicher, J. M., & Romero, J. J. (1994). Construct validity of neuropsychological tests of conceptual and attentional abilities. *Journal of Clinical Psychology, 50*, 596–600.

Rabin, L. A., Barr, W. B., & Burton, L. A. (2005). Assessment practices of clinical neuropsychologists in the United States and Canada: A survey of INS, NAN, and APA Division 40 members. *Archives of Clinical Neuropsychology, 20*, 33–65.

Ratcliff, G., Dodge, H., Birzescu, M., & Ganguli, M. (2003). Tracking cognitive functioning over time: Ten-year longitudinal data from a community-based study. *Applied Neuropsychology, 10*, 76–88.

Reitan, R. M. (1955). The relation of the Trail Making Test to organic brain damage. *Journal of Consulting Psychology, 19*, 393–394.

Reitan, R. M. (1971). Trail Making Test results for normal and brain-damaged children. *Perceptual and Motor Skills, 33*, 575–581.

Reitan, R. M., & Wolfson, D. (1985). The Halstead-Reitan Neuropsychological Test Battery. Tucson, Ariz.: Neuropsychology Press.

Reitan, R. M., & Wolfson, D. (1988). Traumatic Brain Injury. Vol. II: Recovery and Rehabilitation. Tucson, Ariz.: Neuropsychology Press.

Reitan, R. M., & Wolfson, D. (1994). A selective and critical review of neuropsychological deficits and the frontal lobes. *Neuropsychology Review, 4*, 161–198.

Reitan, R. M., & Wolfson, D. (1995). Category Test and Trail Making Test as measures of frontal lobe functions. *Clinical Neuropsychologist, 9*, 50–56.

Reitan, R. M., & Wolfson, D. (2004). Trail Making Test as an initial screening procedure for neuropsychological impairment in older children. *Archives of Clinical Neuropsychology, 19*, 281–288.

Reynolds, C. (2002). Comprehensive Trail Making Test. Austin, Tex.: Pro-Ed.

Ricker, J. H., & Axelrod, B. N. (1994). Analysis of an oral paradigm for the Trail Making Test. *Assessment, 1*, 47–51.

Ricker, J. H., Axelrod, B. N., & Houtler, B. D. (1996). Clinical validation of the oral Trail Making Test. *Neuropsychiatry, Neuropsychology, and Behavioral Neurology, 9*, 50–53.

Roberts, C., & Horton, A. M. (2001). Demographic effects on the Trail Making Test in hallucinogen abusers. *International Journal of Neuroscience, 110*, 91–97.

Roberts, C., & Horton, A. M. (2002). Derived Trail Making Test indices in a sample of amphetamine abusers. *International Journal of Neuroscience, 112*, 575–584.

Ross, S. R., Millis, S. R., & Rosenthal, M. (1997). Neuropsychological prediction of psychosocial outcome after traumatic brain injury. *Applied Neuropsychology, 4*, 165–170.

Royan, J., Tombaugh, T. N., Rees, L., & Francis, M. (2004). The Adjusting-Paced Serial Addition Test (Adjusting-PSAT): Thresholds for speed of information processing as a function of stimulus modality and problem complexity. *Archives of Clinical Neuropsychology, 19*, 131–143.

Ruchinskas, R. A. (2003). Limitations of the oral Trail Making Test in a mixed sample of older adults. *The Clinical Neuropsychologist, 17*, 137–142.

Ruffulo, L. F., Guilmette, T. J., & Willis, W. G. (2000). Comparison of time and error analysis on the Trail Making Test among patients with head injuries, experimental malingerers, patients with suspect effort on testing, and normal controls. *Clinical Neuropsychologist, 14*, 223–230.

Salthouse, T. A., & Fristoe, N. M. (1995). Process analysis of adult age effects on a computer-administered Trail Making Test. *Neuropsychology, 9*, 518–528.

Salthouse, T., Toth, J., Daniels, K., Parks, C., Pak, R., Wolbrette, M., & Hocking, K.J. (2000). Effects of aging on efficiency of task switching in a variant of the Trail Making Test. *Neuropsychology, 14*, 102–111.

Schear, J. M., & Sato, S. D. (1989). Effects of visual acuity and visual motor speed and dexterity on cognitive test performance. *Archives of Clinical Neuropsychology, 4*, 25–33.

Schopp, L. H., Shigaki, C. L., Johnstone, B., & Kirkpatrick, H. A. (2001). Gender differences in cognitive and emotional adjustment to traumatic brain injury. *Journal of Clinical Psychology in Medical Settings, 8*, 181–188.

Schreiber, D. J., Goldman, H., Kleinman, K. M., Goldfader, P. R., & Snow, M. Y. (1976). The relationship between independent neuropsychological and neurological detection of cerebral impairment. *Journal of Nervous and Mental Disease, 162*, 360–365.

Sherrill-Pattison, S., Donders, J., & Thompson, E. (2000). Influence of demographic variables on neuropsychological test performance after traumatic brain injury. *Clinical Neuropsychologist, 14*, 496–503.

Shum, D. H. K., McFarland, K. A., & Bain, J. D. (1990). Construct validity of eight tests of attention: Comparison of normal and closed head injury samples. *Clinical Neuropsychologist, 4*, 151–162.

Skeel, R. L., Nagra, A., Van Voorst, W., & Olson, E. (2003). The relationship between performance-based visual acuity screening, self-reported visual acuity, and neuropsychological performance. *The Clinical Neuropsychologist, 17*, 129–136.

Snow, W. G., Tierney, M. C., Zorzitto, M. L., Fisher, R. H., & Reid, D. W. (1988). One-year test-retest reliability of selected neuropsychological tests in older adults [Abstract]. *Journal of Clinical and Experimental Neuropsychology, 10*, 60.

Stanczak, D. E., & Triplett, G. (2003). Psychometric properties of the mid-range expanded Trail Making Test: An examination of learning-disabled and non-learning-disabled children. *Archives of Clinical Neuropsychology, 18*, 107–120.

Stanczak, D. E., Lynch, M. D., NcNeil, C. K., & Brown, B. (1998). The Expanded Trail Making Test: Rationale, development, and psychometric properties. *Archives of Clinical Neuropsychology, 13*, 473–487.

Stanczak, D. E., Stanczak, E. M., & Amadella, A. W. (2001). Development and initial validation of an Arabic version of the expanded Trail Making Test: Implications for cross-cultural assessment. *Archives of Clinical Neuropsychology, 16*, 141–149.

Steffens, D. C., Wagner, H. R., Levy, R. M., Horn, K. A., & Krishnan, K. (2001). Performance feedback deficit in geriatric depression. *Biological Psychiatry, 50*, 358–363.

Steinberg, B. A., Bieliauskas, L. A., Smith, G. E., & Ivnik, R. J. (2005). Mayo Older Americans Normative Studies: Age- and IQ-adjusted norms for the Trail-Making Test, the Stroop Test, and MAE Controlled Oral Word Association Test. *The Clinical Neuropsychologist, 19*, 329–377.

Stewart, W. F., Schwartz, B. S., Simon, D., Bola, K. I., Todd, A. C., & Links, J. (1999). Neurobehavioral function and tibial and chelatable lead levels in 543 former organolead workers. *Neurology, 52*, 1610–1617.

Stuss, D. T., Bisschop, S. M., Alexander, M. P., Levine, B., Katz, D., & Izukawa, D. (2001). The Trail Making Test: A study in focal lesion patients. *Psychological Assessment, 13*, 230–239.

Stuss, D. T., Stethem, L. L., & Pelchat, G. (1988). Three tests of attention and rapid information processing: An extension. *The Clinical Neuropsychologist, 2*, 246–250.

Stuss, D. T., Stethem, L. L., & Poirier, C. A. (1987). Comparison of three tests of attention and rapid information processing across six age groups. *The Clinical Neuropsychologist, 1*, 139–152.

Sutker, P. B., Vasterling, J. J., Brailey, K., & Allain, A. N. (1995). Memory, attention, and executive deficits in POW survivors: Contributing biological and psychological factors. *Neuropsychology, 9*, 118–125.

Taylor, R. (1998). Order effects within the Trail Making and Stroop tests in patients with neurological disorders. *Journal of Clinical and Experimental Neuropsychology, 20*, 750–754.

Thompson, M. D., Scott, J. G., Dickson, S. W., Schoenfeld, J. D., Ruwe, W. D., & Adams, R. L. (1999). Clinical utility of the Trail Making Test practice time. *Clinical Neuropsychologist, 13*, 450–455.

Tierney, M. C., Charles, J., Jaglai, S., Snow, W. G., Szalai, J. P., Spizziri, F., & Fisher, R. H. (2001). Identification of those at greatest risk of harm among cognitively impaired people who live alone. *Aging, Neuropsychology, and Cognition, 8*, 182–191.

Tombaugh, T. N. (2004). Trail Making Test A and B: Normative data stratified by age and education. *Archives of Clinical Neuropsychology, 19*, 203–214.

Trites, R. L. (1977). *Neuropsychological test manual.* Ottawa, Ont.: Royal Ottawa Hospital.

Van Gorp, W. G., Humphrey, L. A., Kalechstein, A., Brumm, V. L., McMullen, W. J., Soddard, M., & Pachana, N. A. (1999). How well do standard clinical neuropsychological tests identify malingering? A preliminary analysis. *Journal of Clinical and Experimental Neuropsychology, 21*, 245–250.

Veil, H. O. F. (1997). A preliminary profile of neuropsychological deficits associated with major depression. *Journal of Clinical and Experimental Neuropsychology, 19*, 587–603.

Warner, M. H., Ernst, J., Townes, B. D., Peel, J., & Preston, M. (1987). Relationship between IQ and neuropsychological measures in neuropsychiatric populations: Within-laboratory and cross-cultural replications using WAIS and WAIS-R. *Journal of Clinical and Experimental Neuropsychology, 9*, 545–562.

Wedding, D. (1979). A comparison of statistical, actuarial, and clinical models used in predicting presence, lateralization, and type of brain damage in humans. Unpublished Ph.D. dissertation, University of Hawaii.

Wheeler, L., & Reitan, R. M. (1963). Discriminant functions applied to the problem of predicting cerebral damage from behavioral tests: A cross-validation study. *Perceptual and Motor Skills, 16,* 681–701.

Woelwer, W. (2002). Impaired Trail-Making Test-B performance in patients with acute schizophrenia is related to inefficient sequencing of planning and acting. *Journal of Psychiatric Research, 36,* 407–416.

Woodruff, G. R., Mendoza, J. E., Dickson, A. L., Blanchard, E., & Christenberry, L. B. (1995). The effects of configural differences on the Trail Making Test [Archives]. *Archives of Clinical Neuropsychology, 10,* 408.

Yeudall, L. T., Reddon, J. R., Gill, D. M., & Stefanyk, W. O. (1987). Normative data for the Halstead-Reitan neuropsychological tests stratified by age and sex. *Journal of Clinical Psychology, 43,* 346–367.

Youngjohn, J. R., Burrows, L., & Erdal, K. (1995). Brain damage or compensation neurosis? The controversial post-concussion syndrome. *Clinical Neuropsychologist, 9,* 112–123.

Zalla, T., Joyce, C., Szoke, A., Schurhoff, F., Pillon, B., Komano, O., Perez-Diaz, F., Bellivier, F., Alter, C., Dubois, B., Rouillon, F., Houde, O., & Leboyer, M. (2004). Executive dysfunctions as potential markers of familial vulnerability to bipolar disorder and schizophrenia. *Psychiatry Research, 121,* 207–217.

10

Memory

CONCEPTUAL MODEL

Memory refers to the complex processes by which the individual encodes, stores, and retrieves information. *Encoding* refers to the processing of information to be stored, whereas *consolidation* refers to the strengthening of the representations while they are stored. For a memory to be useful, however, one must be able to *retrieve* it (Banich, 2004). Studies of normal people and patients with amnesia have revealed that memory is not unitary but rather consists of a variety of different forms, each mediated by different component processes which in turn are subserved by different neural mechanisms (Moscovitch, 2004). Although many models have been proposed to explain these processes, there is some consistency with respect to the major components in current models, and these are shown in Figure 10–1.

WORKING MEMORY

Whereas *long-term memory* refers to the permanent or more stable storage of memories, *working memory* (replacing the older terms, short-term or immediate memory) is conceived of as a limited-capacity store for retaining information over the short term (seconds to 1–2 minutes) and for performing mental operations on the contents of this store. The contents of working memory may originate from sensory inputs but also may be retrieved from long-term memory. In either case, working memory contains information that can be acted on and processed, not merely maintained by rehearsal, although this is one aspect of working memory (Gazzaniga et al., 2002). Working memory allows information to guide behavior in the absence of external cues (Goldman-Rakic, 1993) and ensures that information will be available until it can be effectively encoded into long-term memory.

That working memory and long-term memory can be dissociated is shown by the fact that amnesic people (e.g., patients with Korsakoff's syndrome or with lesions to the medial temporal lobes) have a normal digit span (7 ± 2 digits) as well as a normal backward span (in which the digits must be recalled in reverse order; Wilde et al., 2004). They are impaired, however, at retaining and recalling even a subspan list of words after a short interval that is filled with distracting activity— that is, they are impaired in terms of their long-term memory (Moscovitch, 2004). In addition, there are individuals with relatively pure working memory deficits (e.g., reduced auditory span) who appear to have normal long-term memory (e.g., Shallice & Warrington, 1970).

One of the most prominent and clearly articulated models of working memory dates to the work of Baddeley and Hitch (1974) (see Figure 10–2). In this model, working memory is fractionated into a supervisory controlling system (the central executive) aided by two peripheral "slave" systems: the phonological (or articulatory) loop, which is involved in the temporary storage and processing of speech-based material, and its visual equivalent, the visual-spatial sketchpad (Baddeley, 1986, 2000). Baddeley (2003) recently added a third component, the episodic buffer—a limited-capacity store that binds together information to form integrated episodes. The central executive controls the slave systems and forms strategies for using the information that they contain. Therefore, it is conceptualized as a limited-capacity attention control system that is responsible for strategy selection and control and coordination of cognitive processes to facilitate complex cognitive activities such as learning, comprehending, and reasoning (see also the "supervisory attentional system," e.g., Shallice, 1982). Within this schema, tasks such as digit span are thought to be managed primarily by the phonological loop, whereas tasks such as spatial span require the visual-spatial sketchpad. Involvement of the central executive is expected to occur, for example, when the individual must perform mental arithmetic, prepare an ambitious meal (breaking away from well-learned stereotypes and switching to new retrieval plans), or devise cues to search for items in memory.

The phonological loop is assumed to be defective in the type of patient studied by Shallice and Warrington (1970);

Figure 10–1 Hypothesized structure of memory.

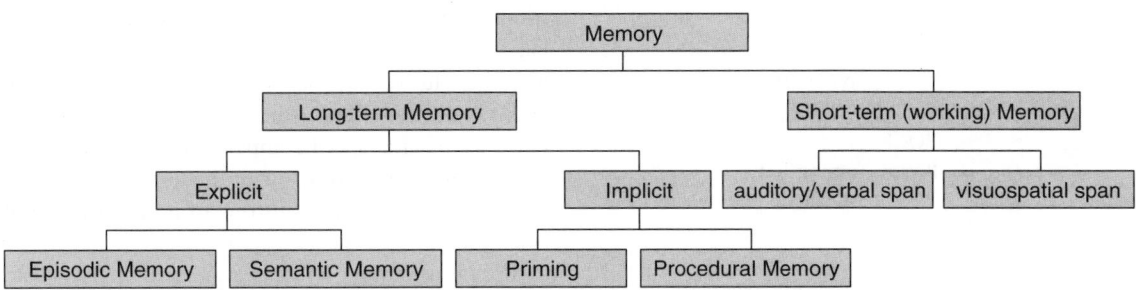

that is, individuals with reduced auditory span but intact long-term memory. General cognitive disruption does not occur, presumably because the central executive is intact in such patients.

Researchers stress that working memory capacity is an important moderating variable of learning (Kyllonen, 1987; Kyllonen & Christal, 1990). It is important to note, however, that factors outside working memory, including processing speed and the knowledge base, can also affect an individual's ability to learn new information (Donders & Minnema, 2004; Kyllonen, 1987; Salthouse et al., 1996).

LONG-TERM MEMORY

Long-term memory is typically split into two major divisions: *explicit* (conscious or declarative) memory and *implicit* (unconscious or nondeclarative or procedural) memory (Tulving & Schacter, 1990; Schacter & Tulving, 1994). Explicit memory refers to intentional or conscious recollection of previous experiences. In a typical explicit memory task, patients are shown a series of words, pictures, or some other set of material to be remembered and are later given a recall or recognition task that requires them to think back to the study episode in order to produce or select a correct response.

Implicit memory, by contrast, refers to a heterogeneous collection of abilities (e.g., priming, skill learning or procedural memory, habit formation) that are manifested across a wide range of situations. Priming acts within the perceptual system with words and objects. An example of priming is when the individual is better able to generate words from fragments if the words were seen previously rather than not seen previously. Learning to ride a bike and acquiring reading skills are examples of procedural memory. Implicit memory involves a facilitation or change in test performance that is attributable to information or skills acquired during a prior study episode, even if the individual is not required to, and may even be unable to, recollect the study phase. For example, having studied a set of words or pictures, amnesic patients perform poorly when their memory is tested explicitly with recall or recognition tasks. However, their memory for studied items may be normal if they are tested implicitly, by determining how performance is altered by the study experience without making any explicit reference to the study episode. Although they cannot recall or recognize the items studied, amnesics do perceive them more quickly and accurately than items that they did not study, or they complete them better when they are degraded (e.g., filling in the missing letters in a word or completing the lines in a picture). Performance on these implicit tasks indicates that the information about the studied items is held in memory even if the patient does not have conscious access to it (Moscovitch, 2004).

Unfortunately, results from practice surveys indicate that neuropsychologists typically use explicit rather than implicit measures as part of their routine assessment battery. Table 10–1 shows the results of a recent survey of test usage among neuropsychologists. None of the top 10 measures taps implicit memory. Rather, they are mostly measures of explicit memory, although some include tests of working memory (e.g., Digit Span). In short, current theoretical knowledge is not well integrated in clinical assessment, and, as a consequence, important information regarding patient functioning is likely missed (Spaan et al., 2004).

Figure 10–2 The Working Memory model proposed by Baddeley & Hitch (1974).

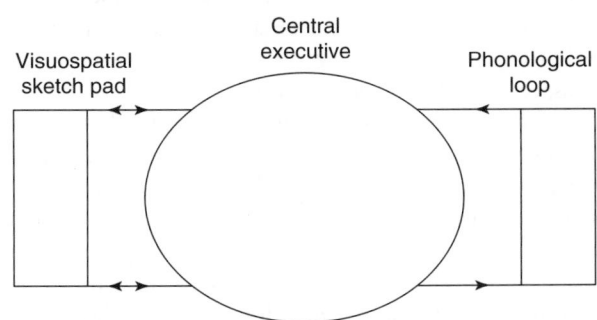

EPISODIC MEMORY

Explicit memory can be broken down further into two subsystems: episodic and semantic memory (Tulving, 1972). Episodic memory refers to the system that enables conscious *recollection* of specific personal events (episodes) as well as the

Table 10–1 Top 10 Memory Instruments in a Recent Survey of Neuropsychologists

Rank	Instrument
1	WMS-R/WMS-III
2	CVLT/CVLT-II
3	ROCF
4	Boston Naming Test
5	WAIS-R, WAIS-III
6	COWA
7	RAVLT
8	WMS-R/WMS-III Logical Memory
9	WMS-R/WMS-III Digit Span
10	Warrington Recognition Memory Test

Source: Adapted from Rabin et al., 2005.

contexts (time and place) in which they occurred. Examples of episodic memory include events in one's personal history, such as the birth of a child or a dissertation defense. Clinical measures of learning and memory are most commonly measures of episodic memory and typically involve free recall, cued recall, and recognition of lists of items (e.g., words, pictures, faces). Almost all of the tests shown in Table 10–2 are measures of episodic memory, relying heavily on the capacity of recollection.[1] That is, they require the person to consciously recollect the content of past experiences as well as their spatial-temporal context.

It is important to distinguish recollection, which is closer to what is meant by episodic memory, from another type of explicit memory, namely *familiarity* with a past event. Familiarity refers to recognition that an event occurred in the past without the information needed to place it in a specific context. For example, familiarity is the kind of memory that occurs when one encounters a person whom one recognizes as familiar but cannot place the individual or the encounter in a particular time or place (Moscovitch et al., 2005). This type of memory shares attributes with episodic memory in that it is memory for a particular bit of information linked to an episode, but it lacks a defining spatial-temporal context (Moscovitch et al., 2005). This distinction, which has gained in importance in the past decade, is also supported by neuropsychological and neurophysiological studies which suggest that these two processes (episodic recollection and feelings of familiarity) may depend on different neuroanatomic regions (see *Neuroanatomical Correlates*). For example, the relatively preserved recognition as opposed to recall performance of some amnesics on forced-choice tasks such as the Warrington Recognition Memory Test may reflect the fact that such a procedure relies less on recollection (*remembering* the content and context of an event) and more on assessment of a relatively automatic feeling of familiarity (simply *knowing* that it happened) (Baddeley et al., 2001).

Historically, hemispheric differences in episodic memory processing have been suggested, with verbal memory processed by left temporal lobe structures and nonverbal memory han-

dled by right hemisphere structures (Milner, 1975). As a consequence, the collection of episodic memory tests may be further subdivided according to the type of task (i.e., verbal or nonverbal). However, evidence for such laterality effects has proved to be rather elusive (e.g., Barr et al., 1997, 2004; Lee et al., 1989), and it is unclear whether difficulties in documenting the existence of material specific impairments in nonverbal memory are the result of problems with the test procedures or of lack of validity of the entire construct of nonverbal memory (Barr et al., 2004).

Episodic memory tests can also be differentiated according to the degree of inherent organization of the material to be memorized and the mode of reproduction (Spaan et al., 2003). Tasks that require recall of semantically unrelated material (e.g., an unrelated list of words such as the RAVLT or Buschke SRT) are thought to be more difficult because they require more effortful strategies for encoding and retrieval than do story recall tasks (e.g., WMS-III Logical Memory) or semantically related word lists (e.g., CVLT-II, HVLT-R). In the latter types, the material to be reproduced already possesses a meaningful structure, aiding recollection processes. Tasks that require recognition of previously presented items (e.g., Warrington Recognition Memory Test, WMS-III Faces, Word Lists, Verbal Paired Associates) are easiest in that they require the least amount of retrieval effort. However, recognition can be complicated by the introduction of semantically, phonologically, or visually similar distractors (e.g., BVMT-R, CVLT-II, CVLT-C, HVLT-R, RAVLT); this approach may allow the examiner to evaluate specific recognition memory components (e.g., false alarm rate, response bias in which the examinee says "yes" or "no" to every item) that may affect overall accuracy.

Many of the tests include both delayed recall and recognition trials (e.g., BVMT-R, Buschke SRT, CVLT, CMS, HVLT-R, RAVLT, ROCF, WMS-III, WRAML) to explore whether a deficit relates more to the storage rather than the retrieval of information. Some list-learning tasks also include an interference list (e.g., CVLT, CMS, RAVLT, WMS-III) to assess whether forgetting is adversely affected by increased susceptibility to proactive or retroactive interference.

The most sophisticated verbal episodic memory measure is the CVLT-II/CVLT-C. Not only does it assess overall level of achievement (e.g., Trials 1–5 correct, short and long delayed recall, recognition), but it also measures qualitative aspects of performance, such as error types, learning strategies, and mechanisms of memory failure. However, reliability coefficients tend to be low for process-oriented variables, suggesting that users need to be cautious in drawing inferences regarding the qualitative aspects of a client's performance.

As noted earlier, recognition memory itself reflects at least two underlying processes, one recollective and based on the capacity to associate the recognized item with some aspect of its original presentation ("remembered" items), and the other more automatic ("known" items) and possibly based on a general feeling of familiarity (Baddeley et al., 2001). There are some methods that distinguish between recollection and

Table 10–2 Characteristics of Measures of Memory

Test	Ages Assessed (Years)	Administration Time (Excluding Delays, min)	Key Processes	Some Measures Obtained	Test-Retest Reliability	Practice Effects	Alternate Versions Available
Autobiographical Memory Interview	18–80	20–30	Explicit memory of remote personal facts and events	Recall of facts and events from childhood, early adult life, and recent life	NA	Unknown	No
BVRT	6–97 (Administration A)	5–10	Explicit recall of designs; copying and recognition test formats are also available	Total number correct; number of errors	High	Conflicting findings	Yes
BVMT-R	18–79	15	Explicit recall of designs and their locations presented over repeated trials; recognition of designs also tested	Learning, delayed recall; recognition (including false alarms)	Marginal to high depending on the measure	Yes, but small	Yes
Brown-Peterson Task	9–84 depending on the version	10	Working memory	Number correct	NA	Yes, but small	Yes
Buschke SRT	5–15, 18–91	Adults: 30 Children: 10	Explicit recall and recognition of words presented over multiple trials	Working memory, long-term memory, retrieval	NA	Yes, in healthy people but not in the neurologically impaired	Yes
CVLT-II	16–89	20	Explicit recall and recognition of semantically related words presented over multiple trials	Immediate and delayed recall, retrieval efficacy, acquisition rate, learning strategy, proactive and retroactive interference, motivation	High for scores of level of performance; low for scores of process/ strategy	Yes	Yes
CVLT-C	4–16 years 11 months	15–20	Explicit recall and recognition of semantically related words presented over multiple trials	Immediate and delayed recall, retrieval efficacy, acquisition rate, learning strategy, proactive and retroactive interference	Variable— depends on the measure; marginal to adequate for List A Total	Yes	No

(continued)

Table 10–2 Characteristics of Measures of Memory (*continued*)

Test	Ages Assessed (Years)	Administration Time Excluding Delays, min	Key Processes	Some Measures Obtained	Test-Retest Reliability	Practice Effects	Alternate Versions Available
CMS	5–16	30–45 for main subtests; 10–15 for supplemental subtests	Working memory, explicit recall and recognition of verbal and visual material	Working memory, immediate and delayed recall and recognition, learning	Variable—depends on the measure; high for general memory, attention/concentration, and verbal immediate memory	Yes	No
Doors and People	16–80+	35–40	Explicit recall and recognition of verbal and visual material	Long-term memory of visual and verbal material, forgetting	NA	NA	No
HVLT-R	13–80+	15	Explicit recall and recognition of semantically related words presented over multiple trials	Long-term memory, recognition (including false alarms), forgetting	Adequate for total recall in adults only	Yes	Yes
RMT	Words: 18–70 Faces: 18–93	15	Explicit recognition of verbal and visual material	Long-term memory, motivation	Marginal for words; adequate for faces	Yes	No
RAVLT	6–97	10–15	Explicit recall and recognition of unrelated words presented over multiple trials	Working and long-term memory, learning, recognition (including false alarms), forgetting, proactive and retroactive interference, temporal order, motivation	Marginal to adequate for total recall, Trial 5, and delayed recall trials	Yes	Yes

Test	Age range	Time (min)	Description	What is measured	Reliability	Validity	Normed
Rey-O	6–93	10–15	Explicit recall and recognition of a complex figure, constructional ability	Long-term memory, learning, recognition (including false alarms), forgetting, strategy, motivation	Adequate to high for intervals of 6 months or less	Yes	Yes
RULIT	16–70	20	Learning and recall of visual-spatial information (route)	Learning, recall	NA	NA	Yes
RBMT-II/C	5–94	25	Recall and recognition of objects and events, prospective memory, orientation	Recall, recognition, prospective memory, orientation Number correct	High for patients especially if profile scores used	Yes	Yes
Sentence Repetition	3–86	10–15	Working memory	Working memory	Adequate to high	NA	Yes
WMS-III	16–89	30–35 for primary subtests; 15–20 for optional subtests	Working memory, explicit recall and recognition of auditory and visual information	Working memory, immediate and delayed recall and recognition of auditory and visual material, personal semantic information, orientation, learning, forgetting, proactive and retroactive interference	Marginal to high, depending on the measure	Yes	No
WRAML2	5–90	60 for core battery; 20 for screening battery	Working memory, explicit recall and recognition of verbal and visual information	Working memory, recall and recognition of verbal and visual material	Low to high depending on the measure	Yes	No

Note: NA = not available.

familiarity, although currently these have not been incorporated into standard clinical measures. One method of accessing the recollective component is through asking the subject to decide whether the item they have recognized is "remembered" or whether it is simply "known" to have been presented (Gardiner & Java, 1993). A second approach is based on requiring the subject to make a judgment based on list membership; the instructions and interfering lists are so arranged that, under certain circumstances a knowledge of list membership will help, but in others it will hinder performance—the so-called *process dissociation method* developed by Jacoby (1994).

SEMANTIC MEMORY

Semantic memory refers to a person's general knowledge about the world, including facts, concepts, and vocabulary. For example, semantic memory reflects knowing what chairs are (even though they may look very different), that animals and vegetables are fundamentally different, who is the president of the United States, and other similar facts and concepts. As opposed to episodic memory, semantic memory is not context dependent. That is, the knowledge is remembered in the absence of any recollection of the specific circumstances surrounding the learning. Examples of semantic memory measures include category fluency tasks, word identification (e.g., Vocabulary), and object naming tasks (e.g., Boston Naming Test) (Spaan et al., 2003).

Semantic memory can also refer to knowledge one has about oneself (personal semantics), such as where one went to school, whom one married, where one lived, and who one's friends were. For example, the Autobiographical Memory Inventory includes a component (personal semantic schedule) that assesses patients' recall of facts from their own past life.

NEURAL CORRELATES

Only a brief overview is provided here. For a more extensive overview of the neural substrates of memory, the reader is referred to other sources such as Banich (2004), Kolb & Whishaw (2003), Markowitsch (2000), Moscovitch et al. (2005), and Schacter et al. (2000).

A variety of neural correlates have been proposed for the various components of memory. *Memory acquisition* refers to the sensory uptake of information, its initial encoding, and further consolidation (the creation of a stronger representation over time). Sensory uptake engages the appropriate sensory receptors (e.g., hair cells in the cochlea, rods and cones in the retina), reaching the cortical level (via various subcortical routes and waystations, such as the thalamus), where the information undergoes additional sensory analysis and is maintained over the short term in cortical association areas, particularly prefrontal and posterior neocortex, such as the

parietal and inferior temporal cortex. This statement is qualified by reserving it to those forms of information that are acquired explicitly, that is, as episodic memories (Markowitsch, 2000). One significant question regarding working memory concerns whether there is a single, content-independent central executive that subserves the coordination, manipulation, and updating of the contents of the slave systems (Moscovitch & Umilta, 1990; Schacter et al., 2000). Petrides and his colleagues (Owen et al., 1996) have argued for a two-stage model of working memory, with ventrolateral regions subserving the maintenance and evaluation of representations held in working memory and dorsolateral regions handling the monitoring and manipulation of these representations. The implication is that the dorsolateral prefrontal cortex performs functions that resemble the putative operations of a shared central executive (Schacter et al., 2000).

The limbic system is viewed as engaged in the transfer of episodes and facts for long-term storage in cortical networks. With regard to semantic memory, there is evidence for neuroanatomic segregation of semantic domains (e.g., knowledge of animate and inanimate objects may require different cortical regions; Warrington & Shallice, 1984; Martin et al., 1996) with the semantic attributes of a stimulus likely stored near the cortical regions that underlie perception of those attributes (Banich, 2004; Schacter et al., 2000). Retrieval is seen as engaging a combination of frontal-temporal-polar regions, with the left hemisphere dominating retrieval of factual information and the right hemisphere (particularly prefrontal, medial temporal, and parietal areas) dominating retrieval of episodic information (Markowitsch, 2000; Schacter et al., 2000).

The traditional view of memory consolidation is that the medial temporal lobes, particularly the hippocampus and possibly the diencephalon, are temporary memory structures, needed only for memory retention and retrieval until memories are consolidated in neocortex and other structures, where they are permanently stored and from which they can be retrieved directly (Moscovitch et al., 2005; Nadel & Moscovitch, 1997; Nadel et al., 2000). In this view, memory storage initially requires hippocampal linking of dispersed neocortical storage sites, but, over time, this need dissipates and the hippocampal component is rendered unnecessary (Nadel et al., 2000). This change in function over time is held to account for the retrograde amnesia gradients (deficits in memory stretching back to some point before the onset of the amnesia) that are often seen in patients with hippocampal damage. Contrary to the traditional consolidation model, Nadel and Moscovitch (1997) argued that the function of the medial temporal system is not temporally limited; rather, it is needed to represent even old memories in rich, multifaceted detail, be it autobiographical or spatial, for as long as the memory exists (i.e., for episodic memory). Semantic (gist) information can be established in the neocortex and will survive damage to the hippocampal system if enough time has elapsed. The medial temporal lobe system may aid in the initial formation of these neocortical

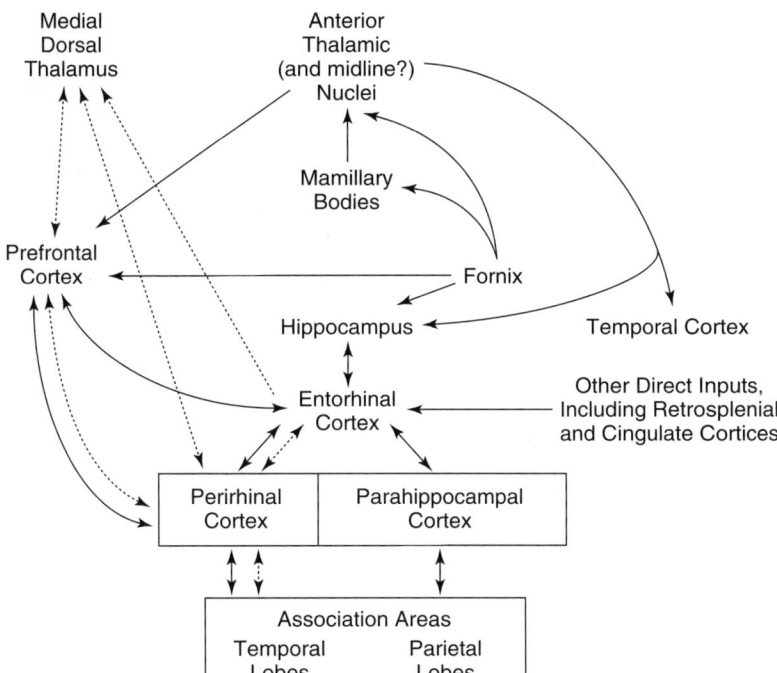

Figure 10–3 Hippocampal complex and linkages.
Source: Reprinted with permission from
Moscovitch et al., 2005.

representations, but, once formed, they can exist on their own (Moscovitch, 2004; Moscovitch et al., 2005). In support of their theory, Nadel et al. (2000) reported a neuroimaging study showing that retrieval of very remote (25-year-old) memories elicits as much activation in the hippocampus as does retrieval of quite recent memories. In addition, they showed that, in patients with temporal lobe damage, deficits in episodic details can be observed even for very remote memories. They also note that their theory provides a better account than does traditional consolidation theory of very long retrograde memory impairments observed in some amnesics.

Moscovitch (2004) has argued that both encoding and retrieval of consciously apprehended information via the hippocampus and related structures is obligatory and automatic, yet we know from experience that we have some control over what we encode and retrieve from memory. He suggested that "other structures, particularly those in the frontal lobes, control the information delivered to the medial temporal and diencephalic system at encoding, initiate and guide retrieval, monitor, and help interpret and organize the information that is retrieved. By operating on the medial temporal and diencephalic system, the frontal lobes act as *working-with-memory* structures that control the more reflexive medial temporal and diencephalic system and confer a measure of intelligence and direction to it" (p. 8).

Regions within the medial temporal lobe are clearly implicated in the formation of new memories for events. Investigators have also focused on differences among the structures in

the medial temporal lobe, proposing that subregions might contribute to different aspects of explicit memory. As noted earlier (see *Episodic Memory*), recognition memory is thought to reflect at least two underlying processes, one recollective and the other more automatic and possibly based on a feeling of familiarity. Aggleton and Brown (1999) proposed that these two memory processes depend on different regions within the medial temporal lobe. Specifically, they suggested that the hippocampus supports recollection, whereas the perirhinal system supports familiarity-based recognition (see Figure 10–3). Thus, recognition based on familiarity can survive hippocampal damage but not damage to the perirhinal cortex.

Finally, with regard to implicit memory, the evidence indicates that the structures implicated in explicit memory, the medial temporal lobes and diencephalon, are not needed. Instead performance is mediated by a variety of structures, depending on the type of implicit memory called upon. On tests of perceptual implicit memory, the test stimulus resembles the studied target perceptually (e.g., a perceptually degraded version of the target, or even an identical repetition), and performance is mediated by the same unimodal posterior cortical regions that are involved in perceiving the stimuli (Moscovitch, 2004). On tests of conceptual implicit memory, the test stimulus resembles the target semantically (e.g., having studied the word "horse," the participant may be asked to make a semantic decision to the word at test, or to produce it in response to the word "animal"). Here, performance is mediated by conceptual systems in the lateral temporal lobe and inferior frontal cortex (Moscovitch, 2004). The structures identified as crucial for procedural memory (e.g., learning rules, motor sequences, conditioned responses) include the basal ganglia and cerebellum (Markowitsch, 2000; Moscovitch, 2004).

RELIABILITY AND PRACTICE EFFECTS

Interpretation of memory measures can be difficult because test-retest reliability coefficients are often less than optimal (see Table 10–2), in part perhaps because of ceiling effects, fluctuations in motivation, or changes in strategy—factors that can attenuate correlations. Regardless of the reasons, low test-retest reliability restricts the utility of particular measures for diagnostic purposes, renders pattern analysis problematic, and limits the ability to evaluate change over time. Therefore, users should focus on those measures for which high reliability has been demonstrated. Scores of overall level of performance (e.g., total recall, index as opposed to subtest scores) tend to be the most reliable. The difficulties of low reliability can be partly circumvented by the use of multiple tasks for abilities of interest. In this way, a more accurate, reliable picture can be obtained of the specific processes that are affected.

As Table 10–2 shows, memory tests are influenced by practice effects. Gains tend to be less on measures of working memory than on tests of explicit memory. For example, on the WMS-III, mean subtest gains on the episodic memory subtests were about 1 to 3 scaled score points among 16- to 54-year-olds retested after an interval of about 5 weeks. Subtests making up the working memory index (Spatial Span, Letter Number Sequencing) showed gains of less than one-half point (The Psychological Corporation, 2002).

One approach to counter the effects of practice is to allow participants to repeat the test until they are familiar with the requirements and their performance has stabilized. There is evidence that practice effects tend to be maximal between the first and second assessments, with performance tending to stabilize after the second assessment (e.g., Beglinger et al., 2005; Hinton-Bayre et al., 1997; Rapport et al., 1997). Accordingly, one option is to use a dual baseline approach, whereby the individual is tested twice and performance in any subsequent assessments is compared with scores from the second test session. However, this approach may not be suitable for all tests or all participants. In addition, the problem of imperfect test-retest reliability must still be considered.

The use of alternate forms tends to reduce but not always eliminate practice effects (e.g., BVMT-R, Buschke SRT; see also Beglinger et al., 2005; Wilson et al., 2000). Lineweaver and Chelune (2003) noted that, although alternate forms may control for one source of the effects of practice, namely content, they do not control for procedural learning and other factors that contribute to the overall practice effect. They further warned that rote use of alternate forms may lull the practitioner into ignoring other issues that could affect test-retest change, such as reliability and error. The use of two separate forms may increase error and make interpretation of test-retest change scores more difficult.

Yet another approach is to use statistical methods (e.g., reliable change indices, standardized regression-based change scores) to evaluate test scores from repeated administrations (Lineweaver & Chelune, 2003). These methods take into account the reliability and stability of test measures. True change is inferred if the observed change is rare—that is, if it falls outside a set confidence interval (e.g., 90%). These methods are gaining in popularity in the neuropsychology literature, including memory assessment.

NOTE

1. Some are measures of working memory (e.g., Brown-Peterson, Sentence Repetition). The RULIT (a trail learning task) may involve a combination of episodic and procedural memory.

REFERENCES

Aggleton, J. P., & Brown, M. W. (1999). Episodic memory, amnesia, and the hippocampal-anterior thalamic axis. *Behavioral and Brain Sciences, 2,* 425–190.

Baddeley, A. D. (1986). *Working memory.* Oxford: Clarendon Press/ Oxford University Press.

Baddeley, A. (2000). Short-term and working memory. In E. Tulving & F. I. M. Craik (Eds.), *The Oxford handbook of memory* (pp. 77–92). New York: Oxford University Press.

Baddeley, A. D. (2003). Working memory: Looking back and looking forward. *Nature Reviews: Neuroscience, 4,* 829–839.

Baddelely, A. D., & Hitch, G. (1974). Working memory. In G. H. Bower (Ed.), *The psychology of learning and motivation* (Vol. 8, pp. 47–90). San Diego: Academic Press.

Baddeley, A., Vargha-Khadem, F., & Mishkin, M. (2001). Preserved recognition in a case of developmental amnesia: Implications for the acquisition of semantic memory? *Journal of Cognitive Neuroscience, 13,* 357–369.

Banich, M. T. (2004). *Cognitive neuroscience and neuropsychology* (2nd ed.). Boston: Houghton Mifflin.

Barr, W. B., Chelune, G. J., Hermann, B. P., et al. (1997). The use of figural reproduction tests as measures of nonverbal memory in epilepsy surgery candidates. *Journal of the International Neuropsychological Society, 3,* 435–443.

Barr, W., Morrison, C., Zaroff, C., & Devinsky, O. (2004). Use of the Brief Visuospatial Memory Test-Revised (BVMT-R) in neuropsychological evaluation of epilepsy surgery candidates. *Epilepsy & Behavior, 5,* 175–179.

Beglinger, L. J., Gaydos, B., Tangphao-Daniels, O., Duff, K., Kareken, D. A., Crawford, J., Fastenau, P. S., & Siemers, E. R. (2005). Practice effects and the use of alternate forms in serial neuropsychological testing. *Archives of Clinical Neuropsychology, 20,* 517–529.

Donders, J., & Minnema, M. T. (2004). Performance discrepancies on the California Verbal Learning Test—Children's Version (CVLT-C) in children with traumatic brain injury. *Journal of the International Neuropsychological Society, 10,* 482–488.

Gardiner, J. M., & Java, R. I. (1993). Recognizing and remembering. In A. F. Collingers, S. E. Gathercole, M. A. Conway, & P. E. Morris (Eds.), *Theories of memory* (pp.163–188). Hove, U. K.: Erlbaum.

Gazzaniga, M. S., Ivry, R. B., & Mangun, G. R. (2002). *Cognitive neuroscience: The biology of the mind* (2nd ed.). New York: W. W. Norton.

Goldman-Rakic, P. S. (1993). *Working memory and the mind: Readings from Scientific American Magazine* (pp. 67–77). New York: W. H. Freeman.

Hinton-Bayre, A. D., Geffen, G. M., & McFarland, K. A. (1997). Mild head injury and speed of information processing: A prospective study of professional rugby league players. *Journal of Clinical and Experimental Neuropsychology, 19,* 275–289.

Jacoby, L. I. (1994). Measuring recollection: Strategic versus automatic influences of associative context. In C. Umilta & M. Moscovitch (Eds.), *Attention and performance: XV. Conscious and non-conscious information processing* (pp. 661–680). Cambridge: MIT Press.

Kolb, B., & Whishaw, I. Q. (2003). *Fundamentals of human neuropsychology* (5th ed.). New York: Worth Publishers.

Kyllonen, P. C. (1987). Theory-based cognitive assessment. In J. Zeidner (Ed.), *Human productivity enhancement: Organizations, personnel, and decision making* (Vol.2, pp. 338–381). New York: Praeger.

Kyllonen, P. C., & Christal, R. E. (1990). Reasoning ability is (little more than) working memory capacity? *Intelligence, 14,* 389–433.

Lee, G. P., Loring, D. W., & Thompson, J. L. (1989). Construct validity of material-specific memory measures following unilateral temporal lobe ablations. *Psychological Assessment, 1,* 192–197.

Lineweaver, T. T., & Chelune, G. J. (2003). Use of the WASI-III and WMS-III in the context of serial assessments: Interpreting reliable and meaningful change. In D. Tulsky, R. K. Saklofske, G. Heaton, G. Chelune, R. A. Ivnik, R. A. Bornstein, A. Prifitera, & M. Ledbetter (Eds.). *Clinical interpretation of the WAIS-III and WMS-III* (pp. 303–337). San Diego, Calif.: Academic Press.

Markowitsch, H. J. (2000). Neuroanatomy of memory. In E. Tulving & F. I. M. Craik (Eds.), *The Oxford handbook of memory* (pp 465–484). New York: Oxford University Press.

Martin, A., Wiggs, C. L., Ungerleider, L. G., & Haxby, J. U. (1996). Neural correlates of category-specific knowledge. *Nature, 379,* 649–652.

Milner, B. (1975). Psychological aspects of focal epilepsy and its neurosurgical management, *Advances in Neurology, 8,* 299–321.

Moscovitch, M. (2004). Amnesia. In N. B. Smesler & O. B. Baltes (Eds.), *The international encyclopedia of social and behavioral sciences* (Vols. 1–26). Oxford: Pergamon/Elsevier Science.

Moscovitch, M., & Umilta, C. (1990). Modularity and neuropsychology: Modules and central processes in attention and memory. In M. F. Schwartz (Ed.), *Modular deficits in Alzheimer's disease* (pp. 1-59). Cambridge, Mass.: MIT Press/ Bradford.

Moscovitch, M., Westmacott, R., Gilboa, A., Addis, D. P., Rosenbaum, S., Viskontas, I., et al. (2005). Hippocampal complex contribution to retention and retrieval of recent and remote episodic and semantic memories: Evidence from behavioral and neuroimaging studies of healthy and brain-damaged people. In N. Ohta, C. M. MacLeod, & B. Uttl (Eds.), *Dynamic cognitive processes* (pp. 333–380). Tokyo: Springer-Verlag.

Nadel, L., & Moscovitch, M. (1997). Memory consolidation, retrograde amnesia and the hippocampal complex. *Current Opinion in Neurobiology, 7,* 217–227.

Nadel, L., Samsonovich, A., Ryan, L., & Moscovitch, M. (2000). Multiple trace theory of human memory: Computational, neuroimaging, and neuropsychological results. *Hippocampus, 10,* 352–368.

Owen, A. M., Evans, A. C., & Petrides, M. (1996). Evidence for a two-stage model of spatial working memory processing within the lateral frontal cortex: A positron emission tomography study. *Cerebral Cortex, 6,* 31–38.

Rabin, L. A., Barr, W. B., & Burton, L. A. (2005). Assessment practices of clinical neuropsychologists in the United States and Canada: A survey of INS, NAN, and APA Division 40 members. *Archives of Clinical Neuropsychology, 20,* 33–65.

Rapport, L. J., Brines, D. B., Axelrod, B. N., & Theisen, M. E. (1997). Full Scale IQ as a mediator of practice effects: The rich get richer. *The Clinical Neuropsychologist, 11,* 375–389.

Salthouse, T. A., Fristoe, N., & Rhee, S. H. (1996). How localized are age-related effects on neuropsychological measures? *Neuropsychology, 10,* 272–285.

Schacter, D. L., & Tulving, E. (1994). *Memory systems.* Cambridge, Mass.: MIT Press.

Schacter, D. L., Wagner, A. D., & Buckner, R. L. (2000). Memory systems of 1999. In E. Tulving and F. I. M. Craik (Eds.), *The Oxford handbook of memory* (pp. 627–643). New York: Oxford University Press.

Shallice, T. (1982). Specific impairments of planning. *Philosophical Transactions of the Royal Society London B, 298,* 199–209.

Shallice, T., & Warrington, E. K. (1970). Independent functioning of verbal memory stores: A neuropsychological study. *Quarterly Journal of Experimental Psychology, 22,* 261–273.

Spaan, P. E. J., Raaijmakers, J. G. W., & Jonker, C. (2003). Alzheimer's disease versus normal ageing: A review of the efficiency of clinical and experimental memory measures. *Journal of Clinical and Experimental Neuropsychology, 25,* 216–233.

The Psychological Corporation. (2002). *WAIS-III/ WMS-III technical manual.* San Antonio, Texas: Harcourt Assessment.

Tulving, E. (1972). Episodic and semantic memory. In E. Tulving & W. Donaldson (Eds.), *Organization and memory.* New York: Academic Press.

Tulving, E., & Schacter, D. L. (1990). Priming and human memory systems. *Science, 247,* 301–306.

Warrington, E. K., & Shallice, T. (1984). Category specific semantic impairments. *Brain, 107,* 829–854.

Wilde, N. J., Strauss, E., & Tulsky, D. S. (2004). Memory span on the Wechsler Scales. *Journal of Clinical and Experimental Neuropsychology, 26,* 539–549.

Wilson, B. A., Watson, P. C., Baddeley, A. D., Emslie, H., & Evans, J. J. (2000). Improvement or simply practice? The effects of twenty repeated assessments on people with and without brain injury. *Journal of the International Neuropsychological Society, 6,* 469–479.

Autobiographical Memory Interview (AMI)

PURPOSE

The Autobiographical Memory Interview (AMI) is used to assess retrograde amnesia, the inability to remember events and facts preceding injury or illness.

SOURCE

The test (including a test manual and 25 scoring sheets) can be ordered from Harcourt Assessment (http://www.harcourt.uk.com) at a cost of £81 or $152 US.

AGE RANGE

According to the authors, the test is appropriate across the adult age range from 18 years to old age.

DESCRIPTION

This test was devised by Kopelman et al. (1990) to assess the intactness of a client's remote memory, including the pattern of any deficit and its temporal gradient (e.g., relative sparing of early compared with more recent memories). The AMI consists of a semistructured interview schedule encompassing two components. The first, called the personal semantic schedule (PSS), assesses patients' recall of non-event-based *facts* from their own past life, relating to childhood (e.g., names of schools or teachers), early adult life (e.g., name of first employer, date and place of wedding), and more recent facts (e.g., holidays, journeys, previous hospitalizations). This is used as a measure of semantic memory. The second component, called the autobiographical incidents schedule (AIS), assesses patients' recall of specific *events or incidents*, including detailed contextual information such as time and place, three each from the same three time periods (e.g., an incident while at primary school, an incident from college or the first job, and an event that took place while on holiday in the last 5 years). This is used as a measure of episodic memory.

The test constrains patients to produce memories from these three specific time periods. In addition, the early time period can be subdivided into three time periods (0–5, 5–11, and 11–18 years), although norms are not available to support this level of discrimination. Thus, the test allows a measurement of the pattern of autobiographical memory deficit and the detection of any temporal gradient in retrograde amnesia.

ADMINISTRATION

See source. The examiner asks questions and records responses on the scoring sheet as close to verbatim as possible. Instructions for administering the AMI appear in the test manual. If a patient fails to produce any memory, some specific prompts may be used, and these are provided on the answer sheet (see AMI scoring sheet). It may be preferable to tape-record the interview, but this is not obligatory.

ADMINISTRATION TIME

About 20 to 30 minutes is required for the test.

SCORING

Items in the PSS are assigned a score from 1 to 3 points. Each PSS subsection (i.e., childhood, early adult life, and recent life) is scored with a possible 21 points, for a maximum total of 63 points. Partial credit can be given for many of the items.

On the AIS, 3 points are given for an episodic memory, specific in time and place; 2 points for a specific memory in which time and place are not recalled, or for a less specific event in which time and place are recalled; 1 point for a vague personal memory; and no points for no response or a response based purely on general knowledge (semantic memory). Examples are provided in the appendix of the AMI manual. Scores for each AIS subsection range from 0 to 9, and the maximum total score is 27.

DEMOGRAPHIC EFFECTS

Age

According to the test authors, age does not affect performance (Kopelman et al., 1990).

Gender

Effects of gender are not reported.

Education/IQ

The authors state that IQ (estimated by the NART) does not affect performance (in all cases, correlations were less than .25). However, in patients with multiple sclerosis (MS), general cognitive ability, as indexed by Raven's Colored Progressive Matrices, shows a moderately strong correlation with scores on both components of the AMI ($r = .65$ to .69; Kenealy et al., 2002).

Ethnicity

Effects of ethnicity are not reported.

NORMATIVE DATA

Standardization Sample

Kopelman et al. (1990) provide cutoff points based on a small sample ($N = 34$) of healthy adults. The sample is not well described (see Table 10–3) but apparently consisted of healthy participants in two studies (Kopelman, 1989; Kopelman et al., 1989; M. Kopelman, personal communication, February 16, 2005). They included healthy relatives of some of the amnesic patients, inhabitants of a sheltered accommodation unit for the elderly in South London, nonacademic staff of the Institute of Psychiatry, and two control subjects living in Oxford. The age range was 20 to 78 years.

The authors report that, based on the performance of healthy controls, scores of 12 or less on the AIS and 47 or less on the PSS indicate abnormal memory, because none of the control subjects scored below these values.

RELIABILITY

Internal Reliability

No information on internal reliability is provided.

Table 10–3 Characteristics of the AMI Normative Sample

Number	34
Age (years)	20–78
Geographic location	England
Sample type	Healthy relatives of amnesic patients, inhabitants of a sheltered accommodation unit for the elderly in South London, nonacademic staff of the Institute of Psychiatry, and two control subjects living in Oxford
Education	Not reported
Socioeconomic status (SES)	Not reported
Gender	Not reported
Race/Ethnicity	Not reported
Screening	Reported to be healthy, but screening method not reported

Source: Adapted from Kopelman, 1989; Kopelman et al., 1989; Kopelman et al., 1990.

Test-Retest Reliability

No information on test-retest reliability is currently available.

Interrater Reliability

Kopelman et al. (1990) state that interrater reliability is high. Three raters independently scored written descriptions of memories recalled. The correlations between pairs of testers varied between .83 and .86. Viskontas et al. (2000) reported an intraclass correlation of .75 for responses scored by two individuals.

Kopelman et al. (1990) suggest that, for clinical use, scoring appears to be sufficiently reliable for it to be based on a single rater. For research purposes, however, a very precise measure is needed, and the authors suggest that it may be preferable to use two raters. If they disagree by 1 point or less, the mean score should be taken. If they disagree by more than 1 point, they should discuss the response together before coming to an agreed score.

VALIDITY

Relations Within the Test

In a group of amnesic patients ($N = 62$), the correlation between the PSS and the AIS was about .60 (Kopelman et al., 1990). When normal and memory-impaired groups were merged, increasing the variability in performance, the two components of the AMI correlated highly (.77), casting some doubt on the usefulness of interpreting episodic and semantic components of the test as two distinct dimensions. However, dissociations between semantic and episodic memory have been reported on the AMI in various patient groups, including

those with MS (Paul et al., 1997; Kenealy et al., 2002—albeit the dissociations were different in the two studies) and those with temporal lobe epilepsy (Viskontas et al., 2000).

Correlations With Other Measures

The AMI tends to correlate moderately well with other remote memory tests (e.g., Prices Test, News Recall, Famous Personality), suggesting that the AMI and other retrograde memory tests are measuring similar but not necessarily identical components of memory (Kopelman et al., 1990; see also Brandt & Benedict, 1993). Moderate to high correlations between the AMI and the WMS MQ, as an index of anterograde impairment, have also been reported and ranged from .32 to .35 in patients with Korsakoff's disease and from .52 to .65 in those with Alzheimer's disease (Kopelman, 1989).

Clinical Studies

The AMI discriminates amnesics from healthy controls. Kopelman et al. (1989, 1999) tested patients with memory deficits (including those associated with Korsakoff's disease, herpes encephalitis, or frontal lobe lesions) who were matched in estimated premorbid intelligence (NART) and age with control subjects. Patients showed reduced capacity for new learning (on WMS Logical Memory, the Recognition Memory Test, and the Rivermead Behavioral Memory Test) and showed impaired remote memory when assessed on the AMI as well as other measures of remote memory, such as the Prices test (in which subjects must estimate the prices of common objects) and the Crovitz Test of Autobiographical Memory.

Impaired performance has also been found in other populations. For example, people with schizophrenia showed significant impairment on this measure (Corcoran & Frith, 2003). In addition, patients with MS, particularly those with advanced disease, showed deficits in autobiographical memory (Paul et al., 1997). Kenealy et al. (2002) found that about two thirds of severely affected individuals (Expanded Disability Status Scale, $M = 8.5$, $SD = 0.4$) showed impairment on the AMI. Further, memory for episodic incidents was more disturbed than that for personal semantic information. There is also evidence that temporal lobe damage or dysfunction, caused by recurrent seizures or surgical excision, results in impaired personal episodic memory but intact personal semantic memory (Viskontas et al., 2000).

Autobiographical memory is thought to contribute to self-knowledge (e.g., knowledge about one's traits) and self-narratives (stories about oneself), enabling a sense of continuity of identity. Not surprisingly, both personal semantic and personal incident memory are significantly impaired in Alzheimer's disease (Addis & Tippett, 2004; Kopelman, 1989); however, Addis and Tippett (2004) also found that loss of some components of autobiographical memory, particularly memory for childhood and early adulthood, may help drive some changes in identity in these patients.

Autobiographical memory may also contribute to how people think about the beliefs and intentions of others. In patients with schizophrenia, robust relationships were found between scores achieved on the AMI and performance on tests of theory of mind tasks (Corcoran & Frith, 2003).

Temporal Gradients

A number of authors have reported that patients with Alzheimer's disease show a temporal gradient on the AMI, with preserved older memories and impaired recent memories; however, the conclusion as to whether this affects personal semantic memory (Addis & Tippett, 2004; Kopelman, 1989) or personal incidents memory (Graham & Hodges, 1997) has varied, perhaps reflecting differences in dementia severity (and extent of damage to the hippocampal complex). According to Graham and Hodges (1997), patients with semantic dementia (i.e., with primary progressive aphasia) whose lesions involve the left temporal neocortex with sparing of the hippocampal region showed the reverse temporal pattern for both personal semantic and autobiographical events: The patients were able to produce more detailed information from the recent past than from their childhood or early adulthood. This double dissociation in performance on autobiographical components of the AMI is compatible with the notion that hippocampal structures and the neocortex play temporally distinct roles in long-term storage.

Patients with advanced MS also show a disruption in the temporal gradient, with lower scores for recent than for childhood recall on both components of the test (Kenealy et al., 2002). The gradient, however, is not as steep as that reported for either Alzheimer's or Korsakoff's patients.

Cases have also been reported that manifest more extensive and flat gradients. Kopelman et al. (1999) found a relatively low, flat temporal gradient for the recall of both personal semantic facts and autobiographical incidents in patients with frontal lobe pathology (unilateral or bilateral), perhaps due to an impairment in the strategic recall of remote memories (see also Eslinger, 1998). They suggested that the retrieval deficits associated with frontal lobe pathology may make a contribution to the extensive remote memory impairment seen in patients with Korsakoff's disease.

Kopelman et al (1999) also reported a relatively flat gradient in patients with herpes encephalitis who had extensive bilateral damage to the temporal lobes. In line with these findings, Viskontas et al. (2000) argued that damage to the medial temporal lobes results in significant impairment to autobiographical episodic memory. They found that patients with temporal lobe epilepsy have impaired personal episodic memory but intact personal semantic memory. There was no evidence of a temporal gradient: the loss encompassed all time periods equally, extending to even early childhood. Findings were believed to be better explained by the multiple trace theory of hippocampal function in memory (Nadel & Moscovitch, 1997) than by traditional consolidation theory. According to the multiple trace theory, the hippocampal complex rapidly binds novel information and experience into a coherent memory trace composed of hippocampal elements active at the time of encoding and the neocortical (or other) neurons that represent the events' features or components. Personal semantic memories are more resistant than episodic memories because of multiple traces established through many retrieval attempts in the past and/or the evolution of independent semantic traces via the same mechanism. In contrast, autobiographical episodes are more vulnerable because fewer complete traces are laid down.

Authenticity of the Memories

Kopelman et al. (1989, 1990, 1999) checked patients' recall against a number of corroborative sources. They reported that, although some inaccuracy and confabulation occurs, the amount is small. They suggested that detailed checking of responses with relatives is probably not necessary for routine assessments, except for patients who are clearly confabulating. Paul et al. (1997) also found that MS patients and healthy controls rarely confabulate on the AMI.

COMMENT

The AMI has several advantages. First, it assesses information that any person is likely to possess and is not dependent on an individual's interest in current affairs or inclination to read the newspaper or watch television. Second, the test content does not quickly become out of date and require restandardization, because the content itself is provided by the examinee. Third, the AMI measures personal semantic and episodic memories, permitting examination of the possible differential effects of brain damage on these two types of autobiographical memory (Viskontas et al., 2000).

On the other hand, the AMI does not assess remote memory on a year-by-year basis, and as a result some deficits may go undetected. In addition, information regarding reliability is sparse, and the normative base is small and poorly described. Whereas age and education appear not to affect performance, IQ may have an effect (Kenealy et al., 2002). The influence of sex and ethnicity or cultural factors remains to be determined. Because the task necessitates verbal report, the effects of language deficits require study. Of note, retrieval deficits appear to influence performance.

REFERENCES

Addis, D. R., & Tippett, L. (2004). Memory of myself: Autobiographical memory and identity in Alzheimer's disease. *Memory, 12*, 56–74.

Brandt, J., & Benedict, R. H. B. (1993). Assessment of retrograde amnesia: Findings with a new public events procedure. *Neuropsychology, 7*, 217–227.

Corcoran, R., & Frith, C. D. (2003). Autobiographical memory and theory of mind: Evidence of a relationship in schizophrenia. *Psychological Medicine, 33*, 897–905.

Eslinger, P. J. (1998). Autobiographical memory after temporal lobe lesions. *Neurocase, 4,* 481–495.

Graham, K. S., & Hodges, J. R. (1997). Differentiating the roles of the hippocampal complex and the neocortex in long-term memory storage: Evidence from the study of semantic dementia and Alzheimer's disease. *Neuropsychology, 11,* 77–89.

Kenealy, P. M., Beaumont, J. G., Lintern, T. C., & Murrell, R. C. (2002). Autobiographical memory in advanced multiple sclerosis: Assessments of episodic and personal semantic memory across three time spans. *Journal of the International Neuropsychological Society, 8,* 855–860.

Kopelman, M. D. (1989). Remote and autobiographical memory, temporal context memory, and frontal atrophy in Korsakoff and Alzheimer patients. *Neuropsychologia, 27,* 437–460.

Kopelman, M. D., Stanhope, N., & Kingsley, D. (1999). Retrograde amnesia in patients with diencephalic, temporal lobe or frontal lesions. *Neuropsychologia, 37,* 939–958.

Kopelman, M. D., Wilson, B. A., & Baddeley, A. D. (1989). The Autobiographical Memory Interview: A new assessment of autobiographical and personal semantic memory in amnesic patients. *Journal of Clinical and Experimental Neuropsychology, 11,* 724–744.

Kopelman, M., Wilson, B., & Baddely, A. (1990). *The Autobiographical Memory Interview.* Bury St. Edmunds, England: Thames Valley Test Company.

Nadel, L., & Moscovitch, M. (1997). Memory consolidation, retrograde amnesia and the hippocampal complex. *Current Opinion in Neurobiology, 7,* 217–227.

Paul, R. H., Blanco, C. R., Hames, K. A., & Beatty, W. W. (1997). Autobiographical memory in multiple sclerosis. *Journal of the International Neuropsychological Society, 3,* 246–251.

Viskontas, I. V., McAndrews, M. P., & Moscovitch, M. (2000). Remote episodic memory deficits in patients with unilateral temporal lobe epilepsy and excisions. *Journal of Neuroscience, 20,* 5853–5857.

Benton Visual Retention Test (BVRT-5)

OTHER TEST NAMES

Other test names for the Benton Visual Retention Test (BVRT-5) are the Visual Retention Test—Revised (VRT-5) and the Benton-Test.

PURPOSE

The purpose of this test is to assess visual memory, visual perception, and visual-constructive abilities.

SOURCE

The manual (5th edition; Sivan, 1992) for the drawing administrations, design cards (forms C, D, and E bound together, with easel support), and 25 record forms can be obtained from Harcourt Assessment, Inc., 19500 Bulverde Road, San Antonio, TX 78259 (http://www.harcourtassessment.com) at a cost of $199 US. The German version (Der Benton-Test; Sivan & Spreen, 1996) includes the multiple-choice version; stimulus booklets and answer sheets can be obtained from Testzentrale, im Hogrefe Verlag GmbH & Co. KG, Robert-Bosch-Breite 25, 37079 Goettingen, Germany (http://www.testzentrale.de) at a cost of about $128 US.

AGE RANGE

Table 10–4 shows the tasks for which normative data are provided. The table also provides a listing of the age ranges of the norms included in the test manual.

DESCRIPTION

There are two main administration modes for the BVRT, requiring either drawing or multiple-choice responses from the examinee (see Table 10–4). The drawing administrations of the BVRT have three alternate forms (C, D, and E) that are roughly of equivalent difficulty (see *Reliability* for details). Each form is composed of 10 designs; the first two designs in each form consist of one major geometric figure, and the other eight designs consist of two major figures and a smaller peripheral figure. An example of the latter type is shown in Figure 10–4.

There are four main types of administration. Under Administration A, the standard (and most commonly used) procedure, each design is displayed for 10 s and then withdrawn. Immediately after this, the subject is required to reproduce the design from memory at his or her own pace on a blank piece of paper. Administration B is similar to A except that each design is exposed for only 5 s. Administration C (copying) requires the subject to copy each of the designs without removing the stimulus card from sight. In Administration D, each design is exposed for 10 s and the subject must reproduce the design after a 15-s delay.

Two additional multiple-choice forms (F and G) are available only in the German edition of the test; they are used to measure the subject's recognition, rather than reproduction, ability (Administration M). Because of its minimal reliance on language, Administration M is also appropriate for non-English-speaking individuals. The multiple-choice administration can be used for people with or without motor handicaps, to determine whether an individual's disability lies in the area of memory, perception, or drawing ability.

ADMINISTRATION

Drawing Administrations

See test manual. Briefly, for Administrations A through D, the subject is given 10 blank, white pieces of paper measuring 21.5 × 14 cm. The subject either reproduces each design from memory (Administrations A, B, and D) or copies each design

Table 10–4 Administration Forms of the BVRT

Mode	Alternate Forms	Administration	Exposure Duration(s)	Task	Age Range (Years) for Norms Provided Here	Sivan (1992)
Drawing	C, D, E	A	10	After each exposure, subject draws the design from memory	6–11; 17–97	8–80+ years
Drawing	C, D, E	B	5	After each exposure, subject draws the design from memory	—	16–60 years
Drawing	C, D, E	C	—	Subject copies each design	6–11	Adults: ages not reported; Children: 5 years 6 months to 13 years
Drawing	C, D, E	D	10	Subject reproduces design after 15-s delay	—	—
Multiple-choice	F, G	M	10	Subject chooses the design from a four-choice display	20–86	—

(Administration C). Drawings should be numbered in the right-hand corner by the examiner after completion, to identify the spatial orientation of the drawing and the specific design that was drawn (Wellman, 1985).

Multiple-Choice Administrations

See test manual (Sivan & Spreen, 1996). For Administration M, each of the 15 stimulus cards, consisting of one to three geometric figures, is exposed for 10 s. Immediately after each exposure, the stimulus card is withdrawn and the subject is shown a multiple-choice card with four similar stimuli labeled A, B, C, and D; the examinee must choose (point to or name by letter) the one that is identical to the stimulus card.

There are also other administrations. In Administration O, the stimulus card is removed, and after 15 s the examinee is

Form C, Design 8

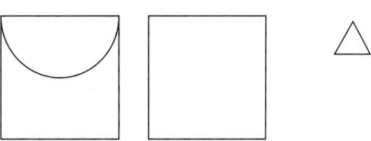

asked to make the choice. Administration P (form discrimination) is used primarily with children; the stimulus card is shown at the same time as the M-Choice card. In Administration PR, the examinee draws all 10 stimulus figures according to Administration C and then is shown the M-Choice cards and asked to indicate which of the figures he or she has drawn.

ADMINISTRATION TIME

The time required for each administration is about 5 to 10 minutes.

SCORING

Scoring is accomplished according to explicit criteria that are detailed in the manual (Sivan, 1992; Sivan & Spreen, 1996). Briefly, two scoring systems (the number of correct reproductions and the error score) are available for the evaluation of a subject's performance on the drawing forms (Administrations A through D). The number correct score has a range of 0 to 10, because each of the 10 designs is scored on an all-or-none basis and given a credit of 1 or 0. Principles underlying the scoring of the designs, together with specific scoring samples illustrating correct and incorrect reproductions, are presented in the test manual. The scoring of errors allows for both quantitative and qualitative analysis of a subject's performance. Six major types of errors are noted: (a) omissions, (b) distortions, (c) perseverations, (d) rotations, (e) misplacements, and (f) size errors. Each major category contains a variety of specific error subtypes. Provision is also made for noting right- and left-sided errors. Scoring is recorded and summarized on the record form. This form allows the examiner to indicate the correct designs and to summarize the types of errors made on each design.

For the multiple-choice administration, the number of correct choices (of a possible 15) is recorded.

DEMOGRAPHIC EFFECTS

Administration A

Age. Age is the strongest predictor of performance on Administration A, accounting for 9% to 18% of the variance in test scores (Coman et al., 1999; Youngjohn et al., 1993). Scores show a progressive rise from age 6 years (Rosselli et al., 2001; but see Snow, 1998, who found little difference between ages 9 and 13 years) until a plateau is reached at the age of 14 or 15 years (Sivan, 1992). This plateau is maintained into the third decade of life, after which a progressive decline in performance occurs, beginning at age 40 to 50 years (Arenberg, 1978; Giambra et al., 1995; Resnick et al., 1995; Robertson-Tchabo & Arenberg, 1989; Youngjohn et al., 1993; also see Coman et al., 2002, for a recent review). The threshold for marked decline in level of performance appears to be about age 75 years (Coman et al., 2002). Variability in BVRT performance increases with aging, although the increases are not significant (Coman et al., 2002).

Gender. Most studies have found that gender has little effect on performance (Coman et al., 1999, 2002; Giambra et al., 1995; Resnick et al., 1995; Rosselli et al., 2001; Shichita et al., 1986; Youngjohn et al., 1992).

Education/IQ. Performance on the BVRT shows a moderate to high correlation with intelligence ($r = .3$ to $.7$; Benton, 1974; Dougherty et al., 2003; Randall et al., 1988) and with education (Coman et al., 2002; Robertson-Tchabo & Arenberg, 1989; Youngjohn et al., 1993). The effects of education interact with those of age. For example, among older adults, the performance of highly educated individuals tends to decline less with age than that of examinees with limited education. In older adults with moderate to severe cognitive deficits, however, the more generalized effects of neurological insult override any protective effect of education, so that BVRT performance is adversely affected regardless of age or educational level (Coman et al., 1999, 2002).

Occupation. Occupational status is another important consideration. Dartigues et al. (1992) found in 2720 healthy elderly community residents that BVRT results corresponded strongly with lifetime occupation regardless of education level; in particular, farmers, domestic service employees, and blue-collar workers showed poor memory two to three times more often than people with professional or managerial occupations.

Administration M

Age. Adult levels are obtained by about age 12 years (Sivan & Spreen, 1996). In general, adults tend to make two or fewer errors. Performance declines with advancing age (Miatton et al., 2004; Tuokko & Woodward, 1996).

Gender. Gender effects tend to be minimal (Miatton et al., 2004; Tuokko & Woodward, 1996; Wagner, 1992).

Education/IQ. Performance is affected by education (Le Carret et al., 2003; Miatton et al., 2004). Le Carret et al. (2003) suggested that the better performance of those with higher educational level is partly mediated by their ability to use a more strategic search of the targets in memory. In children, a moderate relationship with IQ has been reported ($r = .48$; Wagner, 1992).

Ethnicity. Differences between older Caucasian and African American individuals (Manly et al., 1998) and between older Spanish-speaking and English-speaking adults (Jacobs et al., 1997) have been reported, with Caucasians and English speakers scoring higher even after education and various medical conditions were taken into account. However, if quality of education was taken into consideration, differences between Caucasians and African Americans were eliminated (Manly et al., 2002).

NORMATIVE DATA

Administration A

Adults. Data for adults (aged 15–69 years) are presented in the manual (Sivan, 1992). The norms are given by age and IQ level. Note that the data are based on the performance of 600 examinees evaluated more than 40 years ago by Benton (1963), and no information is provided regarding their education, gender, or method of recruitment. The majority were inpatients and outpatients of hospitals in Iowa City, Iowa, with no evidence or history of psychosis, no evidence of cerebral injury or disease except for mental retardation, and no serious physical depletion as a consequence of somatic disease. The manual includes additional normative information based on two studies (Arenberg, 1978; Benton et al., 1981) that extended the norms to old age. The Arenberg data were based solely on male subjects, stratified by age group but not by education, and normative information was provided for mean number of errors only. The data from Benton et al. (1981) were presented in terms of means, standard deviations, and range of scores for number of errors and number correct.

Coman et al. (1999) refined the norms collected by Benton in 1981 for the age range 55 to 97 years ($N = 156$; age $M = 71$

Table 10–5 Normative Expected Scores: BVRT (Administration A), Number Correct (N = 156 Normal Subjects)

Age (Years)	Years of Education (SD = 1.6 for Each Cell)										
	8	9	10	11	12	13	14	15	16	18	20
55	6.54	6.72	6.90	7.09	7.27	7.46	7.64	7.82	8.01	8.38	8.74
60	6.09	6.28	6.46	6.64	6.82	7.01	7.19	7.37	7.56	7.92	8.29
65	5.65	5.83	6.01	6.20	6.38	6.56	6.74	6.92	7.10	7.47	7.83
70	5.21	5.39	5.57	5.75	5.93	6.11	6.29	6.47	6.65	7.01	7.37
75	4.77	4.95	5.12	5.30	5.48	5.66	5.84	6.02	6.20	6.56	6.91
80	4.32	4.50	4.68	4.86	5.03	5.21	5.39	5.57	5.75	6.10	6.46
85	3.88	4.06	4.23	4.41	4.59	4.76	4.94	5.12	5.29	5.65	6.00
90	3.44	3.61	3.79	3.96	4.14	4.31	4.49	4.67	4.84	5.19	5.54
95	3.00	3.17	3.34	3.52	3.69	3.87	4.04	4.21	4.39	4.74	5.08

Source: From Coman et al., 1999. Reprinted with the kind permission of Psychology Press.

years, SD = 8.40; education M = 14, SD = 3.31) by providing adjustments for age and education (see Table 10–5). Participants were reported to be healthy, to be primarily Caucasian, and to have an average of 12.67 years of education (SD = 3.46, range = 4–20 years). There were 31 males and 125 females. Note that the sample was largely female, and cell sizes were very small at the extremes of the age distributions (e.g., N = 6 for ages 55–64 years, N = 29 for ages 85+). The authors cautioned that the window of greatest accuracy encompasses ages 63 to 79 years and 11 to 17 years of education.

Similar results, shown in Table 10–6, were obtained in a study of 1128 subjects, ages 17 to 84 years, by Youngjohn et al. (1993). The sample consisted of 464 males and 664 females who were well-educated (M = 16.01 years, SD = 2.29, range = 12–25 years). All completed a health history questionnaire, and those with evidence or history of physical, psychiatric, or neurological conditions that would affect memory

were excluded. The average score of examinees on a measure of mood was within the nondepressed range.

The choice of which normative dataset to use for estimating the performance level of a given patient depends on the patient's particular demographic characteristics. Where datasets overlap (ages 55–70 years), the set provided by Youngjohn et al. (1993) is preferred, given its larger sample size. In addition, their norms are preferred for relatively young, highly educated adults. The tables provided by Coman et al. (1999) may be more applicable to older adults with limited education. Of note, Coman et al. (1999) also provided expected scores for normal older adults with memory concerns, as well as for a group with mixed neurological disorders.

Children. Norms for Administration A are provided in the test manual (Sivan, 1992) for children and adolescents aged 8 to 14 years and are based on expectations given IQ

Table 10–6 Mean Number of Correct Responses and Errors by Age and Education Level for BVRT Administration A

Age	Education 12–14 Years			Education 15–17 Years			Education 18+ Years		
	n	M	SD	n	M	SD	n	M	SD
Number Correct									
18–39	29	7.59	1.52	27	8.04	1.19	18	8.11	1.28
40–49	18	7.11	1.53	23	7.78	1.54	19	7.42	1.22
50–59	130	6.66	1.47	146	7.08	1.70	133	7.55	1.53
60–69	129	6.18	1.67	159	6.70	1.47	134	6.80	1.55
70+	53	5.62	1.73	54	6.06	1.84	49	6.22	1.57
Number of Errors									
18–39	29	3.38	2.37	27	2.52	1.70	18	2.67	1.78
40–49	18	4.22	2.62	23	3.48	2.78	19	3.74	2.47
50–59	130	4.90	2.42	146	4.21	2.85	133	3.64	2.76
60–69	129	5.55	2.74	159	4.99	2.78	134	4.93	2.87
70+	53	7.28	3.55	54	7.74	4.34	49	6.33	3.63

Source: Adapted from Youngjohn et al., 1993. Data are derived from 1128 well-educated volunteers aged 17–84 years.

Table 10–7 Children's Performance (Mean and *SD*) on the BVRT Administration A, Form D, and Administration C, Form C (*N* = 290 Spanish-speaking Normal Children)

	Age (Years)					
	6–7 (*n* = 83)		8–9 (*n* = 121)		10–11 (*n* = 86)	
Test	M	SD	M	SD	M	SD
Administration C						
Copy correct	7.85	2.18	8.73	1.52	8.97	0.98
Copy errors	2.40	2.52	1.31	1.63	1.02	1.00
Administration A						
Memory correct	4.27	1.52	5.16	1.54	6.06	1.67
Memory errors	9.02	2.01	7.33	2.93	5.66	3.29

Source: Adapted from Rosselli et al., 2001.

level. The sample is poorly described; for example, no information is provided regarding sample size, gender distribution, or method for determining IQ.

More recently, Rosselli et al. (2001) provided normative data based on a sample of 290 children (140 boys, 149 girls), aged 6 to 11 years, who were attending a middle-class school in Bogota, Columbia. None of the participants was intellectually deficient. Performance was somewhat better than that reported by Sivan (1992), perhaps reflecting cultural differences or the rise in test scores with the passage of time (i.e., the Flynn effect). The data provided by Rosselli et al. (2001) are shown in Table 10–7 and are preferred given their recency.

Administration B

According to the manual (Sivan, 1992), the norms were generated from the performance of 103 medical patients with no evidence of neurological damage. The data probably date back to the 1960s. Based on these data, the test manual suggests that 1 point should be subtracted from the expected number correct score for Administration A.

Administration C

Adults. Normative data, dating from the 1960s and derived from the performance of 200 medical patients with no history or evidence of cerebral disease, are provided in the test manual (Sivan, 1992). For adults, only rounded error scores without standard deviations are provided. In general, adults of average intellectual ability are reported to make two or fewer errors on this form of the test. Robinson-Whelen (1992) reported means of 9.38 (number correct) and 0.65 (number of errors) for a group of 122 older adults with an average of 12.8 years of education (mean age, 72 years). This suggests that less than one error is made, even in elderly subjects.

Children. For children aged 7 to 13 years, the exact number correct and error scores with standard deviations are given in the manual. These data probably date to the 1960s. Additional data gathered by Brasfield (1971) and by Beames and

Russell (1970) for young children, aged 5 to 6 years, are also summarized in the manual (Sivan, 1992). However, given the 40-year time span since these norms were collected, recent normative data are preferred. Scores for Spanish-speaking children, aged 6 to 11 years, in Bogota, Columbia (Rosselli et al., 2001) were somewhat higher than those reported by Sivan (1992), and the data are shown in Table 10–7. There is a rapid rise in performance between the ages of 5 and 9 years, and a much slower rise between ages 10 and 13. The performance of 13-year-old children is reported to be very close to the adult level.

Administration D

Adults. The test manual (Sivan, 1992) indicates that normal adults obtain number correct scores about 0.4 points less with Administration D (10-s exposure, 15-s delay) than with Administration A. No norms are available for children for Administration D.

Administration M

Adults. Form G is easier than Form F, and the two forms are differentially affected by age and education (see *Reliability*). On Form F, younger people and those with higher education performed better. Form G was affected only by age, with elderly examinees performing worse (Lannoo & Vingerhoets, 1997; Miatton et al., 2004). Miatton et al. (2004) presented data for each form separately, using a sample of Flemish people (aged 20–86 years) who, based on a standardized interview, had no history of cardiovascular, neurological, or psychiatric disease and were taking no psychoactive medications. The data are shown in Tables 10–8 (Form F) and 10–9 (Form G).

RELIABILITY

Internal Consistency

Cronbach's alpha coefficients were reported to be .76 for Form C, .79 for Form D, and .79 for Form E number correct (Steck et al., 1990) for Administration A. For number of errors,

Table 10–8 Normative Data for BVRT Form F According to Age and Education

	Education ≤ 12 Years			Education > 12 Years		
	20–30 (n = 22)	30 ≤ 50 (n = 21)	>50 (n = 22)	20–30 (n = 42)	30 ≤ 50 (n = 30)	>50 (n = 14)
Mean (SD)	13.2 (1.3)	13.1 (1.5)	11.2 (2.3)	13.9 (1.2)	13.1 (1.3)	12.4 (2.1)
Percentile Rank						
10th	11.3	11	7	12.3	12	9
20th	12	12	9	13	12	11
30th	12	12	9.9	14	12	11
40th	13	12	11	14	13	12
50th	13.5	13	12	14	13	12.5
60th	14	14	12	14	13	13
70th	14	14	13	15	14	14
80th	14	15	13	15	14	15
90th	15	15	14	15	15	15

Source: Adapted from Miatton et al., 2004.

the corresponding values were .71, .82, and .80. Steck et al. (1990) also noted that internal consistency rose to .91 when all 30 items (Form C + D + E) were administered. Steck (2005) recently developed two 20-item parallel forms (items taken from all three forms) that also showed high reliability. Split-half reliability of the multiple-choice forms (Administration M) was .76 according to Sivan & Spreen (1996). However, internal consistency of this format was reported to be low in children, mean age about 10 years; only five of the items allowed differentiation between those who achieved a good versus a bad performance on the complete test (Wagner, 1992).

Test-Retest Reliability and Practice Effects

Initial examination of test-retest reliability for Administration A was reported to be high in adults (.85; Benton, 1974), although details regarding the sample and duration of retest interval were not provided. More recent work suggests that reliability may be less than optimal. Youngjohn et al. (1992) retested healthy volunteers, aged 17 to 82 years, after an interval of about 21 days and reported that test-retest reliability was low (r = .57 for number correct; r = .53 for number of errors).

Practice effects of retesting are in dispute. Botwinick et al. (1986) found virtually no change in scores for 64- to 81-year-olds tested four times at 18-month intervals. Similarly, Lezak (cited in Lezak et al., 2004) gave three administrations to healthy control subjects 6 and 12 months apart and found no significant differences between either number correct or error score means. Coefficients of concordance between scores obtained for each administration were .74 for number correct and .77 for errors. By contrast, Larrabee et al. (1986) found an improvement of more than 1 point on retesting of 60- to 90-year-olds after 10 to 13 months. Similar findings were reported by Youngjohn et al. (1992) in their sample of adults (aged 17–82 years) retested after an interval of about 3 weeks.

Snow et al. (1988) reported low test-retest reliability coefficients in a sample of 100 older adults, mean age = 67.1, retested after 1 year for both copy and multiple-choice versions (r = .52 and .53, respectively).

Alternate Form Reliability

Sivan (1992) reported correlation coefficients ranging from .79 to .84 among the three forms (C, D, and E) of the test. There is some evidence (Breidt, 1970) that Form D is slightly more difficult than Form C for the memory but not the copying task, with Form E occupying an intermediate position, although other studies found virtually no difference among these forms (Brown & Rice, 1967; Weiss, 1974).

For the multiple-choice administration (M), alternate-form reliability (Forms F and G) is reported to be good (.80, Sivan & Spreen, 1996). However, higher scores were reported for Form G in Flemish adults, and the two forms are differentially

Table 10–9 Normative Data for BVRT Form G According to Age

	20–30 (n = 35)	30 ≤ 50 (n = 38)	>50 (n = 60)
Mean (SD)	14.3 (0.7)	14.1 (0.9)	13.0 (1.9)
Percentile Rank			
10th	13	13	10
20th	14	13	11
30th	14	14	12
40th	14	14	13
50th	14	14	13
60th	14.6	15	14
70th	15	15	14
80th	15	15	15
90th	15	15	15

Source: Adapted from Miatton et al., 2004.

influenced by demographic factors (Lannoo & Vingerhoets, 1997; Miatton et al., 2004).

Interrater Reliability

For the drawing administrations of the BVRT, interscorer agreement for number correct and the total error score is reportedly high (>.95; Dougherty et al., 2003; Swan et al., 1990; Wahler, 1956). Interrater agreement for some qualitative aspects of the scoring system was also good (omissions, .96; perseverations, .88; rotations, .88), but it was less acceptable for scoring of misplacement and size errors (Swan et al., 1990). The introduction of augmented scoring rules and examples in the current edition of the test manual may improve this situation. However, estimates based on the revised scoring guidelines are not yet available.

VALIDITY

Relations Among Formats

As might be expected, number correct and error scores are highly correlated (Benton, 1974; Vakil et al., 1989). The various formats appear to be measuring similar, but not totally identical, skills. There is a moderate relation ($r = .41$ to $.52$) between performance levels on the copying task (Administration C) and the memory task (Administration B; Benton, 1974). Positive correlations, ranging from .40 to .83, have also been reported between immediate reproduction (Administration A) and delayed reproduction (Administration D) versions (Benton, 1974). The correlation between the multiple-choice and reproduction forms is .55 (Sivan & Spreen, 1996).

Relations With Other Measures

Factor analyses have revealed that the BVRT (Administration A) loads primarily on a visual-perceptual-motor factor, and only secondarily on a memory-concentration-attention factor (Crook and Larrabee, 1988; Larrabee et al., 1985). A second factor analytic study (Larrabee & Crook, 1989) found that the test loaded on two factors, "vigilance" and "psychomotor speed," when analyzed in the context of other memory tests and measures of everyday memory performance. In children and adolescents with learning disorders, low coefficients (<.25) were found between the BVRT (Administration A) and verbal memory measures (Selective Reminding Test; Snow, 1998), and BVRT test scores loaded on the same factor as the Bender-Gestalt, a measure of visual-motor ability.

Moses (1986), however, showed that Administration A and the multiple-choice administration both loaded on a first factor representing primarily memory skills and on a second factor described as attention span and perceptual-analytic ability. The copying form (Form C) loaded primarily on the second factor. A replication study with 162 neuropsychiatric patients (Moses, 1989) confirmed that the BVRT copy and

memory scores form separable factorial components. Executive control processes appear to play a role in BVRT performance. There is evidence that impulsivity (e.g., commission errors on continuous performance tasks) impairs performance on the BVRT (Administration A), at least in adolescents with disruptive behavior disorder (Dougherty et al., 2003).

Of note, some of the items on the multiple-choice version of the BVRT can be correctly completed without viewing the target stimuli, merely by solving the task as an oddity problem (Blanton & Gouvier, 1985). Therefore, the validity of the test may be compromised in subjects who respond strategically rather than by relying on visual memory. Franzen (1989) recommended that the examiner interview the subject after the test to determine the type of strategy that was used.

Clinical Studies

Numerous studies have examined BVRT performance in various diagnostic groups (e.g., Heaton et al., 1978; Marsh & Hirsch, 1982; Schwerd & Salgueiro-Feik, 1980; Tamkin & Kunce, 1985; Zonderman et al., 1995). Overall, these studies showed that the standard version of the test (Administration A) is sensitive to the presence of neurobehavioral disturbance, although its diagnostic ability is not high. Steck et al. (1990) reported that even a 30-item version did not show significant score or type-of-error differences among small groups of adults with depression, schizophrenia, alcoholism, or brain damage, although all groups showed error scores well above those of 145 healthy control subjects.

Impairment on the standard administration (A) of the BVRT has been reported in subjects with a variety of conditions thought to affect memory, including those with head injury (Levin et al., 1990), subjects with the relapsing-remitting form of multiple sclerosis (Rugglieri et al., 2003), gene carriers of Huntington's disease not clinically diagnosed with the disorder (Witjes-Ane et al., 2003), polydrug abusers (Amir & Bahri, 1999), postmenopausal women not treated with estrogen replacement therapy (Resnick et al., 1997), and older men with both the apolipoprotein E allele and magnetic resonance imaging signs of brain atrophy (Carmelli et al., 2000).

Patients with subcortical dementia (associated with Parkinson's disease) and cortical dementia (Alzheimer's disease, or AD) are impaired on the standard form (Administration A) of the BVRT (Kuzis et al., 1999). Of note, the test is sensitive to even mild forms of dementia. Robinson-Whelen (1992) reported significant differences between normal controls and patients with very mild or moderate dementia for both Administration A and Administration C. Omission errors were significantly higher on both administrations in demented patients, although other error types also showed significant differences. Storandt et al. (1986) also reported that patients with mild AD showed significantly more errors on Administration C ($M = 3.3$, $SD = 5.1$) than did age-matched controls. Further, 2½ years later, the error score had climbed rapidly ($M = 13.5$, $SD = 11.7$), whereas the scores of controls showed virtually no change.

There is evidence that performance on the BVRT (Administration A) can predict the development of AD more than a decade before diagnosis (Kawas et al., 2003; Zonderman et al., 1995). Kawas et al. (2003) reported that subjects who scored six or more errors on the BVRT had about twice the risk of developing AD than did subjects with zero to five errors, up to 15 years before the diagnosis of AD. No single error type was consistently associated with the risk of AD in the intervals before diagnosis. However, others tasks (e.g., Letter Cancellation) appeared to be better predictors of short-term (within 2 years) conversion to dementia (Amieva et al., 2004). Swan et al. (1996) found the BVRT to be a significant predictor of mortality in a follow-up study of older adults, even in the context of a regression analysis including health factors such as cancer, cardiovascular disease, systolic blood pressure, and cholesterol level.

The clinical impression is that patients with right posterior lesions tend to be most impaired on the reproduction administrations of the BVRT, but the evidence is inconsistent (Sivan, 1992). For example, both DeRenzi et al. (1977) and Vakil et al. (1989) found that patients with right- and left-hemisphere lesions did not differ on Administration A, although their performance was significantly worse than that of a control group. With a 15-s delay (Administration D), however, right-hemisphere patients showed more impairment than left-hemisphere patients on number correct but not on error score. Vakil et al. (1989) argued that this finding justifies the use of both scores. By contrast, Mann et al. (1989) found a relationship between magnetic resonance imaging lesion volume in patients with multiple sclerosis and impairment of BVRT performance. Patients with lesions in both hemispheres showed impairment, but there was a trend for more impairment to be related to left parietal lobe lesions. The copying version (Administration C) and the multiple-choice version (Administration M) of the BVRT do not distinguish among examinees in terms of hemispheric side of lesion (Arena & Gainotti, 1978).

Studies with children showed that the standard administration of the test discriminates well between reading-delayed and normal fifth-graders (Arnkelsson, 1993). It may also be of value in distinguishing among children with subtypes of learning disabilities (Snow, 1998).

Ecological Validity

Baum et al. (1996) conducted a canonical analysis of a variety of measures of activities of daily living and a set of neuropsychological tests. The BVRT had a loading of .85 (memory) and .69 (copying) on the first canonical variate, indicating good ecological validity in this AD population. Poor performance on the BVRT may also signify problems in decision making (assessed via Bechara's Card Test) in patients with AD (Torralva et al., 2000) and problems in vocational outcome after severe traumatic brain injury in childhood (Nybo & Koskiniem, 1999). However, in normal schoolchildren, BVRT copy and memory scores were not related to school grades (Rosselli et al., 2001).

The test has also been used in case study designs to estimate the effect of memory training in patients with brain trauma (Kaschel, 1994) and in alcoholics (Unterholzner et al., 1992) and of cognitive/communicative training in schizophrenics (Roder et al., 1987). In a group design ($N = 168$), John et al. (1991) found that significant improvement compared with controls during an alcohol detoxification program occurred mainly during the first week, whereas subsequent weeks did not show further improvement.

Malingering

Simulators and litigants suspected of malingering produce fewer correct responses and more errors than brain-damaged subjects. In particular, they produce more distortion errors than do brain-damaged patients (Benton & Spreen, 1961; Suhr et al., 1997), depressed patients, or patients with somatoform disorders (Suhr et al., 1997).

COMMENT

This popular test has been in use since 1946 (Benton, 1946) and has stimulated numerous psychometric and clinical studies. The BVRT has a number of advantages (Wellman, 1985). These include short administration time, precise scoring criteria, excellent interrater reliability, acceptable internal reliability (at least for forms used with Administration A), and the availability of alternate forms. Further, because of its multiple-choice, drawing from memory, and copying administrations, the examiner may be able to discriminate among perceptual, motor, and memory deficits.

Clinical studies have demonstrated the sensitivity of the BVRT (particularly Administration A) to age-related cognitive decline, dementia, head injury, and learning disabilities, although the test's sensitivity to right hemisphere lesions is less compelling. Examination of the pattern of errors may be useful in detecting neglect.

Users should be aware of specific limitations regarding the norms. Some of the normative data provided in the 1992 manual were compiled more than 40 years ago. More recent studies have updated most of these norms and are preferred. The test has been used not only with English-speaking populations but also in countries such as China, Egypt, India, and Venezuela. The reader is referred to Mitrushina et al. (2005) for normative reports for these and other countries. However, the breadth of normative data varies by administration type (more extensive for Administration A); users should therefore select specific administration formats with regard to the norms available for the specific age and education range they require. It is also important to bear in mind that reliance on a simple measure of educational achievement (highest grade attained) does not capture the extent of discrepancies in educational experience between (and within) various ethnic groups. One way to avoid faulty interpretations may be to adjust for reading recognition (Manly et al., 2002).

Note that a ceiling effect appears evident on Administrations A and M in young and middle-aged adults of above-average education, and, therefore, results should be interpreted with caution in this group. Test-retest reliability information is conflicting and is limited to adults. In addition, cultural effects have been examined systematically only for a multiple-choice format.

In addition, the specific construct measured by the BVRT remains to be determined. Although performance is intended to measure nonverbal memory, some of the geometric figures can be verbalized (Arenberg, 1978), and some items on the multiple-choice version can be solved strategically (Blanton & Gouvier, 1985). Further, the reproduction administrations may be more closely associated with visual-perceptual- motor ability than with visual memory.

REFERENCES

Amieva, H., Letenneur, L., Dartigues, J. F., Rouch-Leroyer, I., Sourgen, C., D'Alchee-Biree, F., Dib, M., Barberger-Gateau, P., Orgogozo, J. M., & Fabrigoule, C. (2004). Annual rate and predictors of conversion to dementia in subjects presenting mild cognitive impairment criteria defined according to a population-based study. *Dementia and Geriatric Cognitive Disorders, 18,* 87–93.

Amir, T., & Bahri, T. (1999). Effect of polydrug abuse on sustained attention, visuographic function, and reaction time. *Social Behavior and Personality, 27,* 289–296.

Arena, R., & Gainotti, G. (1978). Constructional apraxia and visuoperceptive disabilities in relation to laterality of lesions. *Cortex, 14,* 463–473.

Arenberg, D. (1978). Differences and changes with age in the Benton Visual Retention Test. *Journal of Gerontology, 33,* 534–540.

Arnkelsson, G. B. (1993). Reading-retarded Icelandic children: The discriminant validity of psychological tests. *Scandinavian Journal of Educational Research, 37,* 163–174.

Baum, C., Edwards, D., Yonan, C., & Storandt, M. (1996). The relation of neuropsychological test performance to performance on functional tasks in dementia of the Alzheimer type. *Archives of Clinical Neuropsychology, 11,* 69–75.

Beames, T. B., & Russell, R. L. (1970). *Normative data by age and sex for five preschool tests.* Neuropsychology Laboratory, University of Victoria.

Benton, A. L. (1946). *A Visual Retention Test for clinical use.* New York: Psychological Corporation.

Benton, A. L. (1963). *Revised Visual Retention Test: Clinical and experimental applications* (3rd ed.). New York: Psychological Corporation.

Benton, A. L. (1974). *Revised Visual Retention Test* (4th ed.). New York: Psychological Corporation.

Benton, A. L., & Spreen, O. (1961). Visual Memory Test: The simulation of mental incompetence. *Archives of General Psychiatry, 4,* 79–83.

Benton, A. L., Eslinger, P. J., & Damasio, A. R. (1981). Normative observations on neuropsychological test performances in old age. *Journal of Clinical Psychology, 3,* 33–42.

Blanton, P. D., & Gouvier, W. D. (1985). A systematic solution to the Benton Visual Retention Test: A caveat to examiners. *International Journal of Clinical Neuropsychology, 7,* 95–96.

Botwinick, J., Storandt, M., & Berg, L. (1986). A longitudinal, behavioral study of senile dementia of the Alzheimer type. *Archives of Neurology, 43,* 1124–1127.

Brasfield, D. M. (1971). *An investigation of the use of the Benton Visual Retention Test with preschool children.* M. A. Thesis, University of Victoria.

Breidt, R. (1970). Möglichkeiten des Benton-Tests in der Untersuchung psychoorganischer Störungen nach Hirnverletzungen. *Archiv für Psychologie, 122,* 314–326.

Brown, L. F., & Rice, J. A. (1967). Form equivalence analysis of the Benton Visual Retention Test in children with low IQ. *Perceptual and Motor Skills, 24,* 737–738.

Carmelli, D., DeCarli, C., Swan, G. E. (2000). The joint effect of apolipoprotein E epsilon4 and MRI findings on lower-extremity function and decline in cognitive function. *Journals of Gerontology—Series A: Biological Sciences & Medical Sciences, 55A,* M103–M109.

Coman, E., Moses, J. A., & Kraemer, H. C. (1999). Geriatric performance on the Benton Test: Demographic and diagnostic considerations. *The Clinical Neuropsychologist, 13,* 66–77.

Coman, E., Moses, J. A., Kraemer, H. C., Friedman, L., Benton, A. L., & Yesavage, J. (2002). Interactive influences on BVRT performance level: Geriatric considerations. *Archives of Clinical Neuropsychology, 17,* 595–610.

Crook, T. H., & Larrabee, G. J. (1988). Interrelationship among everyday memory tests: Stability of factor structure with age. *Neuropsychology, 2,* 1–12.

Dartigues, J. F., Gagnon, M., Mazaux, J. M., & Barberger-Gateau, P. (1992). Occupation during life and memory performance in nondemented French elderly community residents. *Neurology, 42,* 1697–1701.

DeRenzi, E., Faglioni, P., & Previdi, P. (1977). Spatial memory and hemispheric locus of lesion. *Cortex, 13,* 424–433.

Dougherty, D. M., Mathias, C. M., March, D. M., Greve, K. W., Bjork, J. M., & Moeller, F. G. (2003). Commission error rates on a continuous performance test are related to deficits measured by the Benton Visual Retention Test. *Assessment, 10,* 3–12.

Franzen, M. D. (1989). *Reliability and validity in neuropsychological assessment.* New York: Plenum Press.

Giambra, L. M., Arenberg, D., Zonerman, A. B., Kawas, C., & Costa, P. T. (1995). Adult life span changes in immediate visual memory and verbal intelligence. *Psychology and Aging, 10,* 123–139.

Heaton, R., Baade, L. E., & Johnson, K. L. (1978). Neuropsychological test results associated with psychiatric disorders in adults. *Psychological Bulletin, 85,* 141–162.

Jacobs, D. M., Sano, M., & Albert, S. (1997). Cross-cultural neuropsychological assessment: A comparison of randomly selected, demographically matched cohorts of English- and Spanish-speaking older adults. *Journal of Clinical and Experimental Neuropsychology, 19,* 331–339.

John, U., Veltrup, C., Schnofl, A., Wetterling, T., Kanitz, W. D., & Dilling, H. (1991). Gedächtnisdefizite Alkoholabhängiger in der ersten Woche der Abstinenz. *Zeitschrift für klinische Psychologie, Psychopathologie und Psychotherapie, 39,* 348–356.

Kaschel, R. (1994). *Neuropsychologische Rehabilitation von Gedächtnisleistungen.* Weinheim, Germany: Beltz Psychologie Verlags Union.

Kawas, C. H., Corrada, M. M., Brookmeyer, R., Morrison, A., Resnick, S. M., Zonderman, A. B., & Arenberg, D. (2003). Visual memory predicts Alzheimer's disease more than a decade before diagnosis. *Neurology, 60,* 1089–1093.

Kuzis, G., Sabem L., Tiberti, C., Merello, M., Leiguarda, R., & Starkstein, S. E. (1999). Explicit and implicit learning in patients with Alzheimer's disease and Parkinson disease with dementia. *Neuropsychiatry, Neuropsychology, and Behavioral Neurology, 12,* 265–269.

Lannoo, E., & Vingerhoets, G. (1997). Flemish normative data on common neuropsychological tests: Influence of age, education, and gender. *Psychological Belgica, 37,* 141–155.

Larrabee, G. J., & Crook, T. H. (1989). Dimensions of everyday memory in age-associated memory impairment. *Psychological Assessment, 1,* 92–97.

Larrabee, G. J., Kane, R. L., Schuck, J. R., & Francis, D. J. (1985). Construct validity of various memory testing procedures. *Journal of Clinical and Experimental Neuropsychology, 7,* 239–250.

Larrabee, G. J., Levin, H. S., & High, W. M. (1986). Senescent forgetfulness: A quantitative study. *Developmental Neuropsychology, 2,* 373–385.

Le Carret, N., Rainville, C., Lechevaliier, N., Lafont, S., Letenneur, L., & Fabrigoule, C. (2003). Influence of education on the Benton Visual Retention Test performance as mediated by a strategic search component. *Brain and Cognition, 53,* 408–411.

Levin, H. S., Gary, H. E., & Eisenberg, H. M. (1990). Neurobehavioral outcome 1 year after severe head injury: Experience of the Traumatic Coma Data Bank. *Journal of Neurosurgery, 73,* 699–709.

Lezak, M. D., Howieson, D. B., & Loring, D. W. (2004). *Neuropsychological assessment* (4th ed.). New York: Oxford University Press.

Manly, J. J., Jacobs, D. M., Sano, M., Bell, K., Merchant, C. A., Small, S., & Stern, Y. (1998). Cognitive test performance among nondemented elderly African Americans and Whites. *Neurology, 50,* 1238–1245.

Manly, J. J., Jacobs, D. M., Touradji, P., Small, S. A., & Stern, Y. (2002). Reading level attenuates differences in neuropsychological test performance between African American and white elders. *Journal of the International Neuropsychological Society, 8,* 341–348.

Mann, U., Staedt, D., Kappos, L., Wense, A. V. D., & Haubitz, I. (1989). Correlation of MRI findings and neuropsychological results in patients with multiple sclerosis. *Psychiatry Research, 29,* 293–294.

Marsh, G. G., & Hirsch, S. H. (1982). Effectiveness of two tests of visual retention. *Journal of Clinical Psychology, 38,* 115–118.

Miatton, M., Wolters, M., Lannoo, E., & Vingerhoets, G. (2004). Updated and extended normative data of commonly used neuropsychological tests. *Psychologica Belgica, 44,* 189–216.

Mitrushina, M. M., Boone, K. B., Razani, J., & D'Elia, L. F. (2005). *Handbook of Normative Data for Neuropsychological Assessment* (2nd ed.). New York: Oxford University Press.

Moses, J. A. (1986). Factor structure of Benton's tests of visual retention, visual construction, and visual form discrimination. *Archives of Clinical Neuropsychology, 1,* 147–156.

Moses, J. A. (1989). Replicated factor structure of Benton's tests of visual retention, visual construction, and visual form discrimination. *International Journal of Clinical Neuropsychology, 11,* 30–37.

Nybo, T., & Koskiniem, M. (1999). Cognitive indicators of vocational outcome after severe traumatic brain injury (TBI) in childhood. *Brain Injury, 13,* 759–766.

Randall, C. M., Dickson, A. L., & Plasay, M. T. (1988). The relationship between intellectual function and adult performance on the Benton Visual Retention Test. *Cortex, 24,* 277–289.

Resnick, S. M., Metterm J. E., & Zonderman, A. B. (1997). Estrogen replacement therapy and longitudinal decline in visual memory: A possible protective effect. *Neurology, 49*(6), 1491–1497.

Resnick, S. M., Trotman, K. M., Kawas, C., & Zonderman, A. B. (1995). Age-associated changes in specific errors on the Benton Visual Retention Test. *Journals of Gerontology: Psychological Sciences, 50B,* P171–P178.

Robertson-Tchabo, E. A., & Arenberg, D. (1989). Assessment of memory in older adults. In T. Huntert & C. Lindley (Eds.), *Testing older adults.* Austin, Tex.: Pro-Ed.

Robinson-Whelen, S. (1992). Benton Visual Retention Test performance among normal and demented older adults. *Neuropsychology, 6,* 261–269.

Roder, V., Studer, K., & Brenner, H. (1987). Erfahrungen mit einem integrierten psychologischen Therapieprogramm zum Training kommunikativer und kognitiver Fähigkeiten in der Rehabilitation schwer chronisch schizophrener Patienten. *Schweizer Archiv für Neurologie und Psychiatrie, 138,* 31–44.

Rosselli, M., Ardila, A., Bateman, J. R. (2001). Neuropsychological test scores, academic performance, and developmental disorders in Spanish-speaking children. *Developmental Neuropsychology, 20,* 355–373.

Rugglieri, R. M., Palermo, R., Vitello, G., Gennuso, M., Settipani, N., & Piccoli, F. (2003). Cognitive impairment in patients suffering from relapsing-remitting multiple sclerosis with EDSS < 3.5. *Acta Neurological Scandinavica, 108,* 323–326.

Shichita, K., Hatano, S., Ohashi, Y., & Shibata, H. (1986). Memory changes in the Benton Visual Retention Test between ages 70 and 75. *Journal of Gerontology, 41,* 385–386.

Schwerd, A., & Salgueiro-Feik, M. (1980). Untersuchung zur Diagnostischen Validität des Benton-Test bei Kindern und Jugendlichen. *Zeitschrift für Kinder und Jugendpsychiatrie, 8,* 300–313.

Sivan, A. B. (1992). *Benton Visual Retention Test* (5th ed.). San Antonio, Tex.: The Psychological Corporation.

Sivan, A. B., & Spreen, O. (1996). *Der Benton-Test* (7th ed.). Berne, Switzerland: Verlag Hans Huber.

Snow, J. (1998). Clinical use of the Benton Visual Retention Test for children and adolescents with learning disabilities. *Archives of Clinical Neuropsychology, 13,* 629–636.

Snow, W. G., Tierney, M. C., Zorzito, M. L., Fisher, R. H., & Reid, D. W. (1988). *One-year test-retest reliability of selected neuropsychological tests in older adults.* Paper presented to the International Neurological Society, New Orleans.

Steck, P. H. (2005). A revision of A. L. Benton's Visual Retention test (BVRT) in two parallel forms. *Archives of Clinical Neuropsychology, 20,* 409–416.

Steck, P., Beer, U., Frey, A., Frühschütz, H. G., & Körner, A. (1990). Testkritische Überprüfung einer 30-Item Version des Visual Retention Tests nach A. L. Benton. *Diagnostica, 36,* 38–49.

Storandt, M., Botwinick, J., & Danzinger, W. L. (1986). Longitudinal changes: Patients with mild SDAT and matched healthy controls. In L. W. Poon (Ed.), *Handbook for clinical memory assessment of older adults.* Washington, D. C.: American Psychological Association.

Suhr, J., Tranel, D., Wefel, J., & Barrash, J. (1997). Memory performance after head injury: Contributions of malingering, litigation status, psychological factors, and medication use. *Journal of Clinical and Experimental Neuropsychology, 19,* 500–514.

Swan, G. E., Carmelli, D., & Larue, A. (1996). *Psychomotor speed and visual memory as predictors of 7-year all-cause mortality in older adults.* Paper presented at the meeting of the International Neuropsychological Society, Chicago.

Swan, G. E., Morrison, E., & Eslinger, P. J. (1990). Interrater agreement on the Benton Visual Retention Test. *The Clinical Neuropsychologist, 4,* 37–44.

Tamkin, A. S., & Kunce, J. T. (1985). A comparison of three neuropsychological tests: The Weigl, Hooper, and Benton. *Journal of Clinical Psychology, 41,* 660–664.

Torralva, T., Dorrego, F., Sabe, L., Chemerinski, E., & Starkstein, S. E. (2000). Impairments of social cognition and decision making in Alzheimer disease. *International Psychogeriatrics, 12,* 359–368.

Tuokko, H., & Woodward, T. S. (1996). Development and validation of the demographic correction system for neuropsychological measures used in the Canadian Study of Health and Aging. *Journal of Clinical and Experimental Neuropsychology, 18,* 479–616.

Unterholzner, G., Sagstetter, E., & Bauer, M. G. (1992). Mehrstufiges Trainingsprogramm (MKT) zur Verbesserung kognitiver Funktionen bei chronischen Alkoholikern. *Zeitschrift für klinische Psychologie, Psychopathologie und Psychotherapie, 40,* 378–395.

Vakil, E., Blachstein, H., Sheleff, P., & Grossman, S. (1989). BVRT-Scoring system and time delay in the differentiation of lateralized hemispheric damage. *International Journal of Clinical Neuropsychology, 11,* 125–128.

Wagner, H. (1992). The Benton test in school counselling diagnostics. *Acta Paedopsychiatrica, 55,* 179–181.

Wahler, H. J. (1956). A comparison of reproduction errors made by brain-damaged and control patients on a memory-for-designs test. *Journal of Abnormal and Social Psychology, 52,* 251–255.

Weiss, A. A. (1974). Equivalence of three alternate forms of Benton's Visual Retention Test. *Perceptual and Motor Skills, 38,* 623–635.

Wellman, M. M. (1985). Benton Revised Visual Retention Test. In D. J. Keyser & R. C. Sweetland (Eds.), *Test critiques.* Kansas City, Mo.: Test Corporation of America.

Witjes-Ane, M. N. W., Vegter-Vander Vlis, M., van Vugt, J. P. P., Lanser, J. B. K., Hermans, J., Zwinderman, A. H., van Ommen, G. J. B., & Roos, R. A. C. (2003). Cognitive and motor functioning in gene carriers for Huntington's disease: A baseline study. *Journal of Neuropsychiatry and Clinical Neuroscience, 15,* 7–16.

Youngjohn, J. R., Larrabee, G. J., & Crook, T. H. (1992). Test-retest reliability of computerized, everyday memory measures and traditional memory tests. *The Clinical Neuropscyhologist, 6,* 276–286.

Youngjohn, J. R., Larrabee, G. J., & Crook, T. H. (1993). New adult- and education-correction norms for the Benton Visual Retention Test. *The Clinical Neuropsychologist, 7,* 155–160.

Zonderman, A. B., Giamba, L. M., Arenberg, D., Resnick, S. M., & Costa, P. T. (1995). Changes in immediate visual memory predict cognitive impairment. *Archives of Clinical Neuropsychology, 10,* 111–123.

Brief Visuospatial Memory Test—Revised (BVMT-R)

PURPOSE

The Brief Visuospatial Memory Test—Revised (BVMT-R) measures visual learning and memory using a multiple-trial list-learning paradigm.

SOURCE

The test (including test manual, stimuli, and 25 scoring sheets) can be ordered from Psychological Assessment Resources, Lutz, Florida (http://www.parinc.com), at a cost of $247 US.

AGE RANGE

The test can be given to individuals aged 18 to 79 years.

DESCRIPTION

Tests that require subjects to learn and retain a series of verbal items presented over repeated trials are common in neuropsychology. However, figural learning tests are less typical. The BVMT-R is a multiple-trial figural learning test devised by Benedict and colleagues (Benedict, 1997; Benedict & Groninger, 1995; Benedict et al., 1996) and modeled after the Visual Reproduction subtest of the Wechsler Memory Scale (Russell Revision), but with alternate forms.

The test consists of six alternate forms that yield measures of immediate recall, rate of acquisition, delayed recall, and recognition. The patient is shown an 8×11-inch plate containing six simple geometric visual designs in a 2×3 matrix. The matrix is presented for 10 s, after which time the patient is asked to reproduce (on a blank sheet of paper) as many of the designs as possible, in the same location as they appeared on the display. There is no time limit for recall. The patient is then asked to complete two additional learning trials using the same plate and is encouraged to improve his or her performance. After 25 min of distracting tasks, the patient is asked to reproduce the designs again. This delayed recall trial is followed by a recognition trial in which the individual is shown 12 designs (each printed on a 3×5-inch card), one at a time. The patient is asked to respond "yes" to those designs that were included in the original matrix and "no" to foils. This yes/no delayed recognition task includes six targets and six nontargets.

ADMINISTRATION

The instructions for administering the BVMT-R are provided in the test manual. Briefly, the examiner presents the displays and reads the instructions. Recall performance is recorded on a scoring sheet for each of the immediate recall trials (Trials 1 to 3) and for the delayed recall and recognition trials.

ADMINISTRATION TIME

About 15 min is required for the test, excluding the delay interval.

SCORING

Each response is evaluated in terms of two dimensions: accuracy and location. Two points are awarded for each reproduction that

Table 10–10 Overview of BVMT-R Scores

BVMT-R Variable	Description
Trials 1–3	Raw scores range from 0 to 12 for each trial and reflect accuracy and correct placement
Total learning	Sum of scores across the three trials
Learning	The best of Trial 2 or 3 minus the Trial 1 score
Delayed recall	Raw scores range from 0 to 12 and reflect recall of designs after 25-min delay
Percent retained	Scores range from 1 to 100 and reflect the amount originally learned that was retained across the delay
Recognition hits	Number of target figures correctly recognized; scores range from 0 to 6
Recognition false alarms	Number of distractors incorrectly recognized as targets; scores range from 0 to 6
Recognition discrimination index	Recognition hits minus recognition false alarms; scores range from −6 to 6
Recognition response bias	Scores range from 0.00 to 1.00 and reflect the tendency (or lack of) to answer "yes" to a recognition item

is correct with regard to accuracy and location. One point is given if the reproduction is correct with regard to accuracy but incorrectly placed or is incorrect but recognizable as the target and correctly placed. If the drawing is incorrect (not present or present but not recognizable), 0 points are given. Scoring examples for each design are provided in the manual. The maximum total for each recall trial is 12.

As shown in Table 10–10, a number of different scores are derived. The recall scores are combined to form three additional measures of learning and memory. The total immediate recall score is the sum of Trials 1 to 3. The learning score is the best of Trials 2 and 3 minus the Trial 1 score. The percent retained after delay is calculated as Trial 4 recall divided by the best of Trials 2 and 3. Finally, measures of target discriminability and response bias are calculated from the total number of true- and false-positive responses obtained from the delayed recognition trial. The discrimination index is the number of true-positives minus the number of false-positives. The response bias measure ranges from 0 to 1, with higher scores reflecting a liberal as opposed to a conservative response bias.

Raw scores on Trials 1 to 3, total recall, learning, and delayed recall are converted to T scores and percentile equivalents. Scores on percent retained, recognition hits, false alarms, discrimination index, and response bias all had highly skewed distributions in the normative sample, and only percentile rank ranges were calculated for these scores (e.g., 6th–10th percentile).

DEMOGRAPHIC EFFECTS

Age

Benedict et al. (1996) reported that age was moderately correlated with single-trial recall scores ($r = −.44$ to $−.50$). Correlations between age and recognition performance were not significant. On average, age accounted for about 11% of the variance in BVMT-R scores (Benedict, 1997).

Gender

Gender did not influence most aspects of recall and recognition performance (Benedict, 1997).

Education/IQ

Correlations with education were weak (<.20; Benedict et al., 1996). The proportion of variance in age-adjusted scores accounted for by years of education was about 1% (Benedict, 1997). IQ showed a moderate relation with BVMT-R recall but not with recognition discrimination measures (Diaz-Asper et al., 2004).

NORMATIVE DATA

Standardization Sample

Table 10–11 shows the characteristics of the standardization sample. Based on the significant relationships between age and BVMT-R scores and the insignificant relationships with other demographic variables (i.e., gender and years of education), normative values are provided in the manual subdivided according to age (Benedict, 1997). Normative tables were constructed using the method of overlapping-midpoint age cells. Separate normative data are also given for a subset of the normative sample ($n = 377$) selected to reflect the age distributions of the U.S. population for the year 2000. Base-rate data are also provided that show the proportion of normal

Table 10–11 Characteristics of the BVMT-R Normative Sample

Number	588
Age (years)[a]	18–84; $M = 38.6$, $SD = 18$
Geographic location	United States
Sample type	Two distinct samples: (a) 171 college students and (b) 417 community participants who responded to advertisements
Education	$M = 13.4$, $SD = 1.8$
Gender (%)	
Male	35.7
Female	64.3
Race/Ethnicity (%)	
Caucasian	82.0
African	14.5
Other	3.6
Screening	University students were not screened, but all were in acceptable academic standing; community participants were screened with structured interview, and those with neurological or psychiatric disorders or substance dependence were excluded; also, participants aged 60 years and older were required to score at least 25/30 on the MMSE

[a]Age ranges: 18–22, 20–24, 22–26, 24–28, 26–30, 28–32, 30–34, 32–36, 34–38, 36–40, 38–42, 40–44, 42–46, 44–48, 46–50, 48–52, 50–54, 52–56, 54–58, 56–60, 58–62, 60–64, 62–66, 64–68, 66–70, 68–72, 70–74, and 72–79 years.

subjects and patients with neurological disorders who fall within the various score ranges.

RELIABILITY

Test-Retest Reliability

Benedict (1997) retested 71 participants with the same form after an interval of about 56 days ($SD = 10.0$ days). Ceiling effects were found for the recognition task and for the percent retained score for both test sessions. Accordingly, test-retest data are presented in the test manual for trial (Trials 1, 2, and 3) and recall (total, delayed) data. Reliability coefficients vary by measure and test form. When the sample is combined across the six test forms, reliability coefficients are marginal to high, ranging from .60 for Trial 1 to .84 for Trial 3. The reliability coefficient for the total recall score is .80.

Alternate-Form Reliability

Benedict et al. (1996) randomly assigned the six different test forms to a large sample of healthy individuals ($N = 457$). In

addition, a sample of 18 college students completed all six forms at weekly intervals. Both between-groups and within-subjects analyses revealed equivalence of the alternate forms.

Practice Effects

Depending on the form, gains of 2 to 4 raw score points were evident in total recall scores when healthy participants (age $M = 43.5$ years, $SD = 9.6$; education $M = 13.6$ years, $SD = 1.7$) were retested after an interval of about 56 days ($SD = 10$) (Benedict, 1997).

Benedict and Zgaljardic (1998) found that healthy older adults (aged 57–82 years, $M = 63.3$, $SD = 6.8$) who were administered the same form every 2 weeks improved significantly over four sessions, showing gains of about 9 points in total recall.

There are also subtle practice effects with the use of alternate forms. Healthy college students, administered alternate forms at intervals of 6 weeks, improved their BVMT-R total recall scores from 28.9 ($SD = 3.1$) in session 1 to 30.8 ($SD = 1.8$) by session 6, a difference of about five T scores (Benedict et al., 1996). Older adults improved their total recall from 18.8 ($SD = 5.0$) on session one to 22.1 ($SD = 5.6$) by session four (Benedict & Zgaljardic, 1998), a difference of about seven T scores.

Interrater reliability

This is reported to be high, greater than .90 (Benedict, 1997).

VALIDITY

Relationship With Other Measures

Benedict et al. (1996) found, in patients with either nonlateralized cerebral pathology or psychiatric disease, that indices of learning and delayed recall correlated most strongly with other tests of explicit memory, such as the Hopkins Verbal Learning Test, the Visual Reproduction subtest of the WMS-R, and Rey Figure recall ($r = .65$ to $.80$); less strongly with a measure of visuospatial construction, the copy portion of the Rey figure ($r = .65$ to $.66$); and moderately with measures of expressive language, FAS word fluency, and the Boston Naming Test ($r = .24$ to 54). The findings suggest that the BVMT-R, like other visual memory tests, involves both verbal and nonverbal processes. On the other hand, in a factor analysis that also included the Trail Making Test, Controlled Oral Word Association Test, VMI, and Hopkins Verbal Learning Test, the BVMT-R loaded on a separate factor, suggesting that it does measure visuospatial learning and memory in a mixed clinical sample with a reasonable degree of specificity (Benedict et al., 1996). However, support for this proposal is weakened because of the distortion introduced by the use of multiple scores from the same test (method variance problem; Larrabee, 2003).

Clinical Studies

Impaired performance has been noted in a variety of conditions thought to affect memory, including HIV infection, dementia of the Alzheimer type (AD), and vascular dementia (VaD) (Benedict et al., 1996, 1999). None of the BVMT-R measures, however, discriminated between AD and VaD patients. Poor test performance was also noted in patients with multiple sclerosis (Benedict et al., 2001) and in patients with epilepsy (Barr et al., 2004). However, the test was not able to discriminate lateralized disturbances. That is, presurgical candidates with left or right temporal lobe seizures did not differ in their patterns of performance on the learning, delayed recall, or recognition trials (Barr et al., 2004).

COMMENT

In summary, this task has a number of advantages, including its brevity, the availability of six equivalent forms, and the inclusion of learning, delayed recall, and recognition components. Reliability is good, and the test has demonstrated validity in a number of clinical groups. In addition, normative data are based on a wide age range, 18 to 85 years.

On the other hand, motor (drawing) responses are required, limiting its use to those who do not have motor deficits. It may also be difficult to disentangle visual-constructional deficits from memory problems. An optional copy trial can be given after the recognition trial, but normative data are not provided.

Users should be aware of some limitations of the scoring system and normative data. First, responses are evaluated with regard to both accuracy and spatial location. Surprisingly, these aspects are combined in the scoring (and in the normative data). Research is needed to determine whether separate consideration of these two dimensions would improve diagnostic accuracy. Second, the distribution of scores on some of the measures is skewed, rendering interpretation of some scores (e.g., the discrimination index) problematic. Third, the literature suggests that IQ is moderately related to most of the BVMT measures. Accordingly, poor performance must be interpreted with considerable caution in those with below-average IQ (Diaz-Asper et al., 2004).

The available evidence suggests that the BVMT-R is useful in detecting memory impairment in a variety of clinical groups. However, the ability of the test to characterize the unique learning and memory deficits associated with various disorders requires additional study.

REFERENCES

Barr, W., Morrison, C., Zaroff, C., & Devinsky, O. (2004). Use of the Brief Visuospatial Memory Test-Revised (BVMT-R) in neuropsychological evaluation of epilepsy surgery candidates. *Epilepsy and Behavior, 5,* 175–179.

Benedict, R. H. B. (1997). *Brief Visuospatial Memory Test—Revised.* Odessa, Fla.: Psychological Assessment Resources.

Benedict, R. H. B., Dobraski, M., & Goldstein, M. Z. (1999). A preliminary study of the association between changes in mood and cognition in a mixed geriatric psychiatry sample. *Journal of Gerontology: Psychological Sciences, 54B,* P94–P99.

Benedict, R. H. B., & Groninger, L. (1995). Preliminary standardization of a new visuospatial memory test with six alternate forms. *The Clinical Neuropsychologist, 9,* 11–16.

Benedict, R. H. B., & Zgaljardic, D. J. (1998). Practice effects during repeated administrations of memory tests with and without alternate forms. *Journal of Clinical and Experimental Neuropsychology, 20,* 339–352.

Benedict, R. H. B., Priore, R. L., Miller, C., Munschauer, F., & Jacobs, L. (2001). Personality disorder in multiple sclerosis correlates with cognitive impairment. *Journal of Neuropsychiatry and Clinical Neuroscience, 13,* 70–76.

Benedict, R. H. B., Schretlen, D., Groninger, L., Dobraski, M., & Shpritz, B. (1996). Revision of the Brief Visuospatial Memory Test: Studies of normal performance, reliability, and validity. *Psychological Assessment, 8,* 145–153.

Diaz-Asper, C., Schretlen, D. J., & Pearlson, G. D. (2004). How well does IQ predict neuropsychological test performance in normal adults. *Journal of the International Neuropsychological Society, 10,* 82–90.

Larrabee, G. J. (2003). Lessons on measuring construct validity: A commentary on Delis, Jacobson, Bondi, Hamilton, and Salmon. *Journal of the International Neuropsychological Society, 9,* 947–954.

Brown-Peterson Task

OTHER TEST NAME

The typical task uses three-letter trigrams (consonants) read aloud by the examiner. The task is sometimes called Auditory Consonant Trigrams and is abbreviated as CCC in written form. Tasks using words have also been used.

PURPOSE

The purpose of the Brown-Peterson test is to assess short-term or working memory.

SOURCE

There is no commercial source for this test. Users can refer to the following information to make their own material.

AGE RANGE

The test can be used with individuals aged 9 to 84 years, depending on the version. Table 10–12 shows a listing of various versions and the age ranges for which normative data are available.

Table 10–12 Brown-Peterson Tasks and Age Ranges Included in Normative Datasets

	Age Range (Years)
Provided Here	
CCC Version by Paniak (1997)	5–15
CCC Version by Stuss (1987, 1988)	16–69
Four Word Version by Morrow & Ryan (2002)	18–65
Other Sources	
CCC Version by Boone (in Mitrushina et al., [2005])	45–83

DESCRIPTION

The Brown-Peterson task (Brown, 1958; Peterson & Peterson, 1959) is considered to be a measure of working memory in that it requires on-line maintenance of information no longer available from sensory input in the face of simultaneous activation of cognitive processes that compete for attentional resources (Fleming et al., 1995). The typical task requires participants to recall a series of items after variable delays during which they complete an interference task (e.g., mental addition or subtraction). Often three-letter trigrams or four-letter words with retention intervals ranging from 5 to 30 s are used. Because the delayed recall of material requires maintenance rehearsal, the interference task usually decreases recall performance as the delay increases, producing what is termed a forgetting function. The amount of processing resources required by the interpolated task also affects the forgetting function: The number of items correctly recalled decreases with increasing demands from the interference task.

In the version described by Stuss et al. (1987, 1988, 1989; see Figure 10–5), a consonant trigram (e.g., GRX) is presented to the subject verbally at a rate of one letter per second, followed immediately by a two- or three-digit random number (e.g., 167). The subject is asked to count backward, out loud, by threes starting from this number, for interval delays of 9, 18, or 36 s used at random. At the end of the interval, the subject is asked to recall the trigram. Five trials are given for each delay period, with intertrial delays of 2 to 5 s. The delays of 9, 18, and 36 s are intended to minimize any ceiling effect, although others use different intervals (e.g., Boone uses the same stimuli but with intervals of 3, 9, and 18 s). Dependent measures are the total number of letters correctly recalled at each of the three delay intervals.

Paniak et al. (1997) developed a version of the task that is appropriate for children aged 9 to 15 years (see Figure 10–6). Delays of 3, 9, and 18 s are used. Having the children count backward by threes proved too difficult for them. Accordingly, the children count backward by ones instead, and the random numbers always comprise only two digits. The task has also been adapted to the Turkish language for use with adults (Anil et al., 2003).

A version called the Four Word Short-Term Memory Test (FWSTM) that uses four unrelated words and delays of 5, 15, and 30 s has also been normed for adults aged 18 to 65 (Morrow & Ryan, 2002) and is shown in Figure 10–7.

ADMINISTRATION

CCC — Adult Version

The instructions provided here are adapted from Stuss (personal communication, May 1994). Three consonants are presented, as shown in Figure 10–5. The individual must remember these consonants after intervals of 0, 9, 18, and 36 s. During the intervals of 9, 18, and 36 s, the examinee is required to count backward aloud by threes from different numbers (e.g., 100-97-94). If this is too difficult, variations may be used, such as counting backward by ones; however, this may affect the use of norms.

The consonants are read by the examiner at the speed of one consonant per second. The individual is not allowed to repeat the consonants aloud at any time. After the presentation of the third consonant, the examiner immediately initiates the counting backward by counting aloud himself or herself, urging the individual to do likewise. The examiner then stops counting. If the subject stops counting before the prescribed delay interval, the examiner again counts out loud with the subject. It is important that interference be sustained throughout the delay interval by the client himself or herself.

All intervals are timed, the timing beginning after presentation of the last consonant. The examiner signals when the consonants are to be recalled by some prescribed movement or sign (e.g., a knock on the table).

The instructions are shown in Figure 10–8.

CCC — Children's Version

Three consonants are presented, as shown in Figure 10–6. The instructions are shown in Figure 10–9.

FWSTM

The instructions to the examinee are shown in Figure 10–10. The words are read aloud to the individual at the rate one word per second.

ADMINISTRATION TIME

The time required is about 10 min.

SCORING

Record the responses verbatim. The number of letters correctly remembered is tallied for each category of delay interval. The

Figure 10–5 Auditory Consonant Trigrams sample score sheet—Adults. *Source*: Adapted from D. Stuss, personal communication, May, 1994.

Stimulus	Starting Number	Delay (Seconds)	Response	Number Correct
QLX	—	0		
SZB	—	0		
HJT	—	0		
GPW	—	0		
DLH	—	0		
XCP	75	18		
NDJ	28	9		
FXB	194	36		
JCN	20	9		
BGQ	167	18		
KMC	180	36		
RXT	82	18		
KFN	47	9		
MBW	188	36		
TDH	51	9		
LRP	117	36		
ZWS	141	18		
PHQ	89	9		
XGD	91	18		
CZQ	158	36		
Total Number Correct				
0-s delay				
9-s delay				
18-s delay				
36-s delay				

Figure 10–6 Auditory Consonant Trigrams sample score sheet—Children. Note that children are instructed to count backward by ones instead of by threes (see text). *Source:* Adapted from Paniak et al., 1997.

Stimulus	Starting Number	Delay (Seconds)	Response	Number Correct
XTN	—	0		
TQJ	—	0		
LNP	—	0		
SJH	—	0		
KPW	—	0		
NKR	94	18		
FBM	69	9		
KXQ	53	3		
GQS	46	9		
DLX	47	18		
BFM	48	3		
ZDK	55	18		
WGP	62	9		
ZDL	38	3		
RLB	22	9		
QDH	35	3		
GWB	47	18		
CSJ	39	9		
FMH	77	18		
HFZ	49	3		
Total Number Correct				
0-s delay				
3-s delay				
9-s delay				
18-s delay				
Total				

Figure 10–7 Four Word Short-Term Memory Test. *Source:* From Morrow & Ryan, 2002. Reprinted with the kind permission of Psychology Press.

Item		Time (Seconds)	Count	Number Correct and Time		
				5 s	15 s	30 s
1	LEMON JAR STEER ZONE	5	100			
2	STAIN LAWN COTTAGE ANGEL	15	100			
3	MALE LANE PIGEON CRACK	30	100			
4	MOUSE PINT LEAF PRIEST	5	262			
5	POT CREW CHEST SNAKE	15	315			
6	ACID SHED KITTEN GRADE	15	554			
7	DAISY TUNE RAG LOAN	30	487			
8	COLLAR LUNCH AGENT SPEAR	5	548			
9	STOVE PAINTER CROW GRAPE	30	731			
10	BAR MINERAL NEEDLE LAMB	5	443			
11	FAN HAMMER STUMP PARLOR	15	174			
12	TRUNK ANT CHEESE HEN	30	336			
13	LACE HUNTER KETTLE BRICK	30	709			
14	NAVY PILLOW PRINCESS DEER	15	214			
15	TRUCK TUBE GLOVE PEARL	5	716			

Number correct for 5 s   _____

Number correct for 15 s   _____

Number correct for 30 s   _____

ADMINISTER ALL ITEMS. CIRCLE CORRECT WORDS: WRITE INCORRECT WORDS TO THE LEFT.

order in which the consonants are recalled does not matter for scoring purposes. The maximum score at each delay interval for the CCC task is 15. To calculate the total score, add the number of consonants recalled correctly on each trial, including those from the 0-second delay trials. The maximum score obtainable is 60.

For the FWSTM task, there is a total possible score of 20 for each of the three retention intervals.

DEMOGRAPHIC EFFECTS

Age

In normal individuals, age shows little relation with test scores on the CCC version (Bherer et al., 2001; Stuss et al. 1987; but see *Validity*). An age difference has been observed by some in overall recall but not in the slope of the forgetting function on

Figure 10–8 Instructions for Auditory Consonant Trigrams—
Version for Adults.

Instruct as follows: *I'm going to say three letters of the alphabet, which I want you to remember. When I signal
you, like this (give sign), you tell me what the letters
were. Sometimes, after I say the letters, you must count
backward from a number by threes, like this: 100-97-
94. Count out loud, and continue until I give you the signal to tell me the letters. I'll tell you each time what the
number is from which you should count backward.*

Let's try one for practice. F-D-B. 98-95-. . . . (The examiner immediately starts counting and urges that the
subject to do so as well. After the defined delay interval,
the examiner signals the subject to say the letters). *That's
right. You start counting with me, and keep on counting
out loud until I give the signal. Then try to remember the
three letters.* The examinee is not instructed to repeat the
letters in the exact order.

Figure 10–10 Instructions for the Four Word Short-Term
Memory Test. *Source:* From Morrow & Ryan, 2002. Reprinted with
the kind permission of Psychology Press.

*I'm going to read you four words, which I would like you
to try to remember. In order to make this task more difficult, however, after I read the fourth word, I'm going to
read a three-digit number, like 100. As soon as I read
that number, I want you to begin counting backwards by
threes as rapidly and as accurately as you can. I want
you to continue doing that until I tell you to stop. At that
point you'll tell me what the four words were.*

*How good are you at counting backwards by threes?
Let's try it. Start from 100.* (Provide practice).

*Before we begin, I want to quickly review what you'll
be doing. First, you'll hear four words—and I want you
to try to remember those. Then you'll hear a number,
and I want you to count backward by threes. After a
while, I'll tell you to stop, and you'll tell me the words.*

Here are the first words I want you to remember.

the Stuss version (Floden et al., 2000). On the Boone version, age accounted for only a modest amount (6%) of unique test score variance in a sample of healthy older adults (Boone et al., 1998). Similar findings were reported for the word version (Morrow & Ryan, 2002). On the children's version, scores improved with age (Paniak et al., 1997).

Gender

Gender does not contribute to test performance in adults (Anil et al., 2003; Boone, 1999; Morrow & Ryan, 2002) or in children (Paniak et al., 1997).

Education/IQ

There are conflicting reports regarding the impact of education in healthy adults. Some authors (Boone, 1999; Stuss et al., 1987) have found that education shows little relation with scores on

Figure 10–9 Instructions for Auditory Consonant Trigrams—
Version for Children.

Say to the child: *I am going to say three letters, and
when I am through, I am going to knock like this (give
sign). When I do, I want you to say the letters back.* Present the first five (0-delay) trials. Then say: *This time, I
am going to say three letters followed immediately by a
number. As soon as you get the number, I want you to
start counting backward by ones out loud, like this: 29-
28-27. Continue counting out loud until I knock as before.* Demonstrate knocking on the desk. *When I knock, I
want you to recall the three letters. Do you have any
questions?*

the test. Others (Anil et al., 2003; Bherer et al., 2001; Morrow & Ryan, 2002) found an effect of education in healthy adults, with scores improving as education level increased. In head-injured patients, education correlated significantly with the results from the 9- and 18-s delay trials, explaining 38% and 45% of the shared variance, respectively (Stuss et al., 1989).

IQ does affect test scores. Boone (1999) reported that FSIQ accounted for 17% of test score variance in a sample of healthy older adults.

NORMATIVE DATA

Norms for Adults—CCC Version

Age-based normative data for healthy, well-educated ($M = 14.4$, $SD = 2.63$) adults aged 16 to 69 years were provided by Stuss et al. (1987, 1988) and are shown in Table 10–13. With this technique, normal subjects have essentially perfect recall with no distraction delay. In general, the greater the delay, the worse the performance.

Mitrushina et al. (2005) provide normative data on a variant in which items are the same as in the Stuss version but delay intervals are 3, 9, and 18 s. The data (total correct) are based on a sample of 155 older adults, aged 45 to 84 years, and are stratified by IQ and age. Note, however, that about one third of the sample (51/155) had some evidence of vascular illness, which has an impact on test performance.

Norms for Children—CCC Version

Paniak et al. (1997) provided normative data based on 715 Canadian students (326 males, 389 females), aged 9 to 15 years, from Edmonton, Alberta. Estimated verbal intelligence (based on the WISC-R Vocabulary subtest) was within the

Table 10–13 Performance of Healthy Adults (Mean and *SD*) on the Auditory Consonant Trigrams Test on Two Separate Occasions (1 Week Apart) by Age

Visit	16–29 Years (*n* = 30)		30–49 Years (*n* = 30)		50–69 Years (*n* = 30)	
	1st	2nd	1st	2nd	1st	2nd
9-s delay	12.03 (2.24)	12.57 (2.03)	12.00 (2.52)	12.10 (2.85)	11.47 (2.33)	11.70 (2.28)
18-s delay	11.37 (2.82)	12.27 (2.41)	10.50 (3.11)	12.00 (2.59)	10.23 (2.46)	10.67 (2.92)
36-s delay	9.43 (2.71)	10.93 (2.88)	9.90 (3.04)	11.10 (2.37)	8.67 (2.85)	8.57 (3.54)

Note: Second visit data are based on an alternative form of the test (see text).

Source: Adapted from Stuss et al., 1988.

average range, near the mean of the WISC-III normative sample. The data are shown in Table 10–14. Note that even though the test was simpler than the adult version, scores appear not to have reached adult levels by age 15 years.

Norms for Adults—FWSTM

Morrow and Ryan (2002) provided norms based on a large group (*N* = 35) of healthy men and women (95% Caucasian) who were native English speakers 18 to 65 years of age. Individuals were excluded if they had a neurological or medical disorder that might affect cognition. Those with a history of drug or alcohol abuse or dependence were also excluded. The norms were stratified by age and education and were established using an overlapping-midpoint interval strategy. Table 10–15 presents the data. Note, however that the sample of older adults was quite small and the data should be used with considerable caution.

Table 10–14 Auditory Consonant Trigrams Test Scores (Mean and *SD*) for Children, by Age

Delay (in Sec)	9 Years (*n* = 82)	10 Years (*n* = 140)	11 Years (*n* = 32)	12 Years (*n* = 122)	13 Years (*n* = 96)	14 Years (*n* = 115)	15 Years (*n* = 28)
0	15.0 (0.2)	14.9 (0.3)	14.9 (0.4)	14.9 (0.4)	14.9 (0.4)	15.0 (0.1)	14.9 (0.3)
3	9.9 (2.7)	10.5 (2.6)	10.9 (2.3)	11.5 (2.5)	12.2 (2.0)	12.1 (2.0)	12.1 (1.9)
9	6.6 (2.6)	6.9 (2.7)	7.8 (2.4)	8.6 (2.6)	9.9 (2.8)	10.1 (2.6)	10.9 (2.2)
18	5.7 (2.5)	6.0 (2.1)	6.7 (2.4)	7.8 (2.6)	8.7 (2.9)	9.3 (2.6)	9.5 (2.8)
Total	37.1 (6.2)	38.2 (6.0)	40.3 (6.0)	42.8 (6.2)	45.8 (6.5)	46.4 (5.6)	47.4 (5.5)

Source: From Paniak et al., 1997; reprinted with the kind permission of Psychology Press.

Table 10–15 FWSTM Mean, *SD*, and Ranges of Raw Scores (in Seconds) by Education Levels and Overlapping Age Groups at Delays of 5, 15, and 30 s.

Age in Years (Midpoint and Range)	Education (Years)	*n*	5 s		15 s		30 s	
			Mean (*SD*)	Range	Mean (*SD*)	Range	Mean (*SD*)	Range
25 (18–30)	≤12	32	13.0 (3.5)	5–20	10.4 (4.0)	3–19	8.4 (4.1)	1–19
	>12	77	15.4 (3.0)	7–20	12.2 (4.1)	3–20	10.7 (4.1)	3–20
35 (28–38)	≤12	51	13.1 (3.5)	5–20	10.3 (3.8)	3–19	8.5 (4.8)	0–19
	>12	75	15.8 (2.8)	8–20	12.7 (4.2)	4–20	11.0 (4.1)	3–19
39 (35–47)	≤12	60	13.9 (3.6)	3–20	10.7 (3.6)	4–19	9.1 (4.1)	1–19
	>12	92	15.0 (3.1)	6–20	11.9 (4.0)	4–20	10.1 (4.0)	1–19
48 (45–57)	≤12	24	12.6 (3.6)	3–17	9.1 (2.9)	3–16	8.3 (3.3)	2–15
	>12	26	14.6 (3.3)	7–19	11.0 (3.5)	5–18	9.2 (4.2)	1–16
59 (54–65)	≤12	13	13.9 (1.9)	11–18	9.5 (2.2)	7–15	8.4 (3.4)	4–13
	>12	7	14.9 (2.4)	11–19	11.0 (4.3)	3–17	9.7 (2.9)	6–13

Source: From Morrow & Ryan, 2002. Reprinted with the kind permission of Psychology Press.

RELIABILITY

Internal Consistency

Cronbach's alpha was calculated for the Turkish version of the CCC version and found to be high (.85).

Test-Retest Reliability and Practice Effects

Stuss et al. (1987, 1989) gave the CCC test and an alternate form to both normal subjects ($n = 90$) and head-injured individuals ($n = 26$) on two separate occasions with an intersession duration of 1 week. There is no mention of whether the two forms were given in counter-balanced order, and correlation coefficients between versions are not reported. However, given the nonmeaningful nature of the stimuli (unrelated letters), no differences in forms are expected. Both healthy and neurologically impaired subjects scored significantly higher on their second visit than they did on their first, although the effects appeared to be small (see Table 10–13). No information regarding the word version is provided.

VALIDITY

Relation With Other Measures

Impairments in a number of domains, including memory, attention, and possibly aspects of executive function can lead to lower performance. Floden et al. (2000) reported that in older adults (age $M = 71$ years, $SD = 5.2$) test scores correlated only with memory (e.g., WMS-R Paired Associate, CVLT Total) but not with executive measures (e.g., FAS, Stroop). Boone et al. (1998) gave the task along with a variety of other neuropsychological tasks to a mixed clinical sample, largely individuals with psychiatric diagnoses. The CCC task loaded largely with verbal IQ and tests of attention (Digit Span). Correlations with other measures of executive function (e.g., WCST, Stroop, FAS) were modest. Anil et al. (2003) reported that, in normal individuals, Digit Span Backward raw scores were significantly and positively correlated ($r = .54$ to $.57$) with CCC scores at each delay interval. Finally, Kopelman and Stanhope (1997) reported that, in patients with diencephalic, frontal, or temporal damage, scores on a word version of the task correlated moderately well with modified WCST percent perseverations ($r = -.38$), but correlations with other executive function measures (card-sorting categories, FAS, Cognitive Estimation) were nonsignificant. Information regarding construct validity in pediatric populations is not yet available.

Clinical Studies

Impaired performance on the Brown-Peterson task is observed in a variety of conditions that are thought to adversely impact memory as well executive functioning, including Alzheimer's disease (Corkin, 1982; Dannenbaum et al., 1988; Morris, 1986;

Sebastian et al., 2001), Parkinson's disease (Graceffa et al., 1999), herpes encephalitis, Korsakoff's syndrome (Cermak & Butters, 1972: Leng & Parkin, 1989), anterior communicating artery aneurysms (Kopelman & Stanhope, 1997; Parkin et al., 1988), frontal leucotomy (Stuss et al., 1982), schizophrenia (Anil et al., 2003), multiple sclerosis and chronic fatigue syndrome (Johnson et al., 1998), adult ADHD inattentive type (Gansler et al., 1998), prenatal exposure to alcohol (Connor et al., 2000), and sleep deprivation (Forest & Godbout, 2000).

The effect of aging on task performance is complex, with numerous studies failing to find age-related effects. However, negative results may be a function of the specific procedure employed, in particular the lack of control of the distractor task. The typical clinical version (described here) allows for differences in rehearsal opportunity, task difficulty, and amount of information to be processed, because the distraction trial is self-paced. Floden et al. (2000) pointed out that, if participants are able to rehearse the items in memory despite the distracting task, recall may reflect primary memory without working memory input. Further, if the distractor task is unpaced, then individuals who perform at a slow rate will be exposed to fewer interposed stimuli and less retroactive interference. The interaction between level of difficulty of the distractor task and patient characteristics is another potential confound. If the interpolated activity is heavily dependent on working memory, then those individuals with compromise to working memory systems may find the distractor task particularly demanding.

If these factors are controlled, age differences in overall recall and in the slope of the forgetting function are observed—which is not true with the clinical, self-paced version. The age difference occurs only at the point at which recall becomes more dependent on long-term memory (i.e., after the 3-s delay but by the 18-s delay) and does not worsen as the delay increases (i.e., between 19 and 60 s). There is no evidence of an age-related increase in the rate of forgetting from short-term memory (Floden et al., 2000). This pattern is consistent with current conceptions of age-related changes in memory function (i.e., large age differences in long-term memory relative to working memory; Floden et al., 2000).

A number of researchers (Parkin et al., 1988; Stuss et al., 1982) have suggested that the test is particularly sensitive to frontal lobe or frontal/brainstem system deficits. Correlation with regard to frontal-lobe disturbance, however, has not been perfect. First, Winocur et al. (1984) examined a patient with a lesion restricted to the thalamus who showed impairment on the Brown-Peterson task. Second, Parkin (1984) noted that postencephalitic amnesics often have frontal involvement but, in general, show normal performance on the task. Third, performance on the task was found to be impaired in some patients with anterior communicating artery aneurysms and not in others (for a review, see DeLuca & Diamond, 1995). In addition, Corsi (cited in Frisk & Milner, 1990) found that temporal lobectomy patients showed an increased slope of the forgetting function at delays after 3 s, suggesting that the task may be sensitive to temporal lobe disturbance.

Stuss et al. (1989) found that the test does distinguish normal individuals from patients with traumatic brain injury. The longer the duration of posttraumatic amnesia or coma, the worse the performance on the Auditory Consonant Trigrams test. In comparison with the PASAT and the Trail Making Test, only the CCC was sufficiently sensitive to differentiate patients with mild concussion from their control group.

COMMENT

The Brown-Peterson task captures an everyday experience; namely, momentary distraction and the subsequent loss of very recent information (Crowder, 1982). Forgetting is thought to be influenced by both proactive and retroactive interference, as well as the success with which the distractor task blocks rehearsal (Morris, 1986). It has been proposed that retention of the material to be remembered on the task involves mainly maintenance rehearsal, making significant demands on central-processing resources (see also Valler & Baddeley, 1984). Therefore, one reason the distractor task causes forgetting is that it uses up central-processing resources that would otherwise be devoted to rehearsing the to-be-remembered items (Morris, 1986).

However, there are problems with the clinical version that reflect poor control of the distractor task (Floden et al., 2000). That is, the clinical version allows for differences in rehearsal opportunity, task difficulty, and amount of information to be processed, because the distraction trial is self-paced. Unless these factors are controlled (e.g., by using a paced distractor task), it is difficult to know what the results mean. Confounding variables such as the degree of retroactive interference and task difficulty may permit individuals to compensate for working memory impairments and thereby inflate their recall performance. Only in studies where the interpolated task is paced and is successful in suppressing rehearsal can performance be interpreted in terms of component processes (Floden et al., 2000).

Despite these problems, the task has been helpful in identifying dysfunction after frontal and medial temporal damage. In addition to quantitative analyses of performance, qualitative assessments (e.g., omissions, intrusions, confusions, perseverations) are possible although rarely reported. Such errors may aid in determining which cognitive mechanisms are deficient. For example, intrusions have been found to predominate in patients with Korsakoff's syndrome (Kopelman, 1985). An increase in perseverations has been reported in patients with AD, suggesting problems in the central executive in updating the contents of working memory (Sebastian et al., 2001).

Various letter versions are available. For children aged 9 to 15 years the version by Paniak is appropriate, whereas for individuals aged 16 to 44 years normative data are available for the Stuss version. Both Boone and Stuss provided norms for individuals aged 45 to 69 years, although the version by Boone may be preferred because the data are stratified by both age and IQ. Beyond age 69 years, normative data are available only for the Boone version.

Only limited information on reliability is available in adults. Accordingly, test data may best be used to support findings from other measures. In addition, because of the lack of reliability and validity information in children, the task should be interpreted with caution in this age group.

REFERENCES

Anil, A. E., Kivircik, B. B., Batur, S., Kabakci, E., Kitis, A., Guven, E., Basar, K., Turgut, T. I., & Arkar, H. (2003). The Turkish version of the Auditory Consonant Trigram test as a measure of working memory: A normative study. *The Clinical Neuropsychologist, 17,* 159–169.

Bherer, L., Belleville, S., & Peretz, I. (2001). Education, age, and the Brown-Peterson technique. *Developmental Neuropsychology, 19,* 237–251.

Boone, K. B. (1999). Neuropsychological assessment of executive functions: Impact of age, education, gender, intellectual level, and vascular status on executive test scores. In B. L. Miller & J. L. Cummings (Eds.), *The human frontal lobes: Functions and disorders.* New York: Guilford Press.

Boone, K. B., Ponton, M. O., Gorsuch, R. L., Gonzales, J. J., & Miller, B. L. (1998). Factor analysis of four measures of prefrontal lobe functioning. *Archives of Clinical Neuropsychology, 13,* 585–595.

Brown, J. (1958). Some tests of the decay of immediate memory. *Quarterly Journal of Experimental Psychology, 10,* 12–21.

Cermak, L. S., & Butters, N. (1972). The role of interference and encoding in the short–term memory of Korsakoff patients. *Neuropsychologia, 10,* 89–95.

Connor, P. D., Sampson, P. D., Bookstein, F. L., Barr, H. M., & Streissguth, A. P., (2000). Direct and indirect effects of prenatal alcohol damage on executive function. *Developmental Neuropsychology, 18,* 331–354.

Corkin, S. (1982). Some relationships between global amnesias and the memory impairments in Alzheimer's disease. In S. Corkin, K. L. Davis, J. H. Groudin, E. Usdin, & R. J. Wurtman (Eds.), *Alzheimer's disease: A report of progress in research.* Hillsdale, N. J.: Lawrence Erlbaum Associates.

Crowder, R. G. (1982). The demise of short-term memory. *Acta Psychologia, 50,* 291–323.

Dannenbaum, S. E., Parkinson, S. R., & Inman, V. W. (1988). Short-term forgetting: Comparisons between patients with dementia of the Alzheimer type, depressed, and normal elderly. *Cognitive Neuropsychology, 5,* 213–234.

DeLuca, J., & Diamond, B. J. (1995). Aneurysm of the anterior communicating artery: A review of neuroanatomical and neuropsychological sequelae. *Journal of Clinical and Experimental Neuropsychology, 17,* 100–121.

Fleming, K., Goldberg, T. E., Gold, J. M., & Weinberger, D. R. (1995). Verbal working memory dysfunction in schizophrenia: Use of a Brown-Peterson paradigm. *Psychiatry Research, 56,* 155–161.

Floden, D., Stuss, D. T., & Craik, F. I. M. (2000). Age differences in performance on two versions of the Brown-Peterson task. *Aging, Neuropsychology, and Cognition, 7,* 247–259.

Forest, G., & Godbout, R. (2000). Effects of sleep deprivation on performance and EEG spectral analysis in young adults. *Brain and Cognition, 43,* 195–200.

Frisk, V., & Milner, B. (1990). The relationship of working memory to the immediate recall of stories following unilateral temporal or frontal lobectomy. *Neuropsychologia, 28,* 121–135.

Gansler, D. A., Fucetola, R., Krengel, M., Stetson, S., Zimering, R., & Makary, C. (1998). Are there cognitive subtypes in adult attention deficit/ hyperactivity disorder? *The Journal of Nervous and Mental Disease, 186,* 776–781.

Graceffa, A. M. S., Carlesimo, A. A., Peppe, A., & Caltagirone, C. (1999). Verbal working memory deficit in Parkinson's disease subjects. *European Neurology, 42,* 90–94.

Johnson, S. K., deLuca, J., Diamond, B. J., & Natelson, B. H. (1998). Memory dysfunction in fatiguing illness: Examining interference and distraction in short-term memory. *Cognitive Neuropsychiatry, 3,* 269–285.

Kopelman, M. D. (1985). Rates of forgetting in Alzheimer type dementia and Korsakoff's syndrome. *Neuropsychologia, 23,* 623–638.

Kopelman, M. D., & Stanhope, N. (1997). Rates of forgetting in organic amnesia following temporal lobe, diencephalic, or frontal lobe lesions. *Neuropsychology, 11,* 343–356.

Leng, N. R. C., & Parkin, A. J. (1989). Aetiological variation in the amnestic syndrome: Comparisons using the Brown-Peterson task. *Cortex, 25,* 251–259.

Mitrushina, M. N., Boone, K. B., Razani, J., & D'Elia, L. F. (2005). *Handbook of normative data for neuropsychological assessment* (2nd ed.). New York: Oxford University Press.

Morris, R. G. (1986). Short-term forgetting in senile dementia of the Alzheimer's type. *Cognitive Neuropsychology, 3,* 77–97.

Morrow, L. A., & Ryan, C. (2002). Normative data for a working memory test: The Four Word Short-Term Memory Test. *The Clinical Neuropsychologist, 16,* 373–380.

Paniak, C. E., Millar, H. B., Murphy, D., & Keizer, J. (1997). A Consonant Trigrams test for children: Development and norms. *The Clinical Neuropsychologist, 11,* 198–200.

Parkin, A. J. (1984). Amnesic syndrome: A lesion specific disorder? *Cortex, 20,* 478–508.

Parkin, A. J., Leng, N. R., Stanhope, N., & Smith, A. P. (1988). Memory impairment following ruptured aneurysm of the anterior communicating artery. *Brain and Cognition, 7,* 231–243.

Peterson, L. R., & Peterson, M. J. (1959). Short-term retention of individual verbal items. *Journal of Experimental Psychology, 58,* 193–198.

Sebastian, M. V., Menor, J., & Elosua, R. (2001). Patterns of errors in short-term forgetting in AD and ageing. *Memory, 9,* 223–231.

Stuss, D. T., Kaplan, E. F., Benson, D. F., Weir, W. S., Chuilli, S., & Sarazin, F. (1982). Evidence for the involvement of orbitofrontal cortex in memory functions: An interference effect. *Journal of Comparative and Physiological Psychology, 5,* 913–925.

Stuss, D. T., Stethem, L. L., Hugenholtz, H., & Richard, M. T. (1989). Traumatic brain injury: A comparison of three clinical tests, and analysis of recovery. *The Clinical Neuropsychologist, 3,* 145–156.

Stuss, D. T., Stethem, L. L., & Pelchat, G. (1988). Three tests of attention and rapid information processing: An extension. *The Clinical Neuropsychologist, 2,* 246–250.

Stuss, D. T., Stethem, L. L., & Poirier, C. A. (1987). Comparison of three tests of attention and rapid information processing across six age groups. *The Clinical Neuropsychologist, 1,* 139–152.

Vallar, G., & Baddeley, A. D. (1984). Fractionation of working memory: Neuropsychological evidence for a phonological short-term store. *Journal of Verbal Learning and Verbal Behavior, 23,* 151–161.

Winocur, G., Oxbury, S., Roberts, R., Agnetti, V., & Davis, C. (1984). Amnesia in a patient with bilateral lesions to the thalamus. *Neuropsychologia, 22,* 123–144.

Buschke Selective Reminding Test (SRT)

OTHER TEST NAMES

Other names for the Buschke Selective Reminding Test are the Selective Reminding Test (SRT) and the Verbal Selective Reminding Test (VSRT).

PURPOSE

The SRT measures verbal learning and memory using a multiple-trial list-learning paradigm.

SOURCE

There is no commercial source. Users may refer to this text to design their own material. The materials include a list of words, index cards containing the first two to three letters of each list word, and index cards containing the multiple-choice recognition items.

AGE RANGE

Adult norms are available for ages 18 to 91 years; children's norms range from ages 5 to 15 years.

DESCRIPTION

The SRT (Buschke, 1973; Buschke & Fuld, 1974) is an interesting procedure because it purports to parcel verbal memory into distinct component processes. It involves reading to the subject a list of words and then having the subject recall as many of these words as possible. Each subsequent learning trial involves the selective presentation of only those items that were not recalled on the immediately preceding trial. The SRT distinguishes between short-term and long-term components of memory by measuring recall of items that were not presented on a given trial. The rate at which subjects learn can also be evaluated.

A number of different versions of the test exist. For adults, the version described here is the same as that developed by Hannay and Levin (1985; Hannay, 1986). Briefly, the test consists of a series of 12 unrelated words presented over 12 selective reminding (SR) trials, or until the subject is able to recall the entire list on three consecutive trials. A cued-recall trial is presented after the 12th or last selective-reminding trial. The first two or three letters of each word are presented on an index card, and the subject is asked to recall the corresponding list word. After the cued-recall

Figure 10–11 Word list for Forms 1 through 4 of the adult version of the SRT. *Source:* From Hannay & Levin, 1985. Reprinted with the kind permission of Psychology Press.

Form 1	Form 2	Form 3	Form 4
Bowl	Shine	Throw	Egg
Passion	Disagree	Lily	Runway
Dawn	Fat	Film	Fort
Judgement	Wealthy	Discreet	Toothache
Grant	Drunk	Loft	Drown
Bee	Pin	Beef	Baby
Plane	Grass	Street	Lava
County	Moon	Helmet	Damp
Choice	Prepare	Snake	Pure
Seed	Prize	Dug	Vote
Wool	Duck	Pack	Strip
Meal	Leaf	Tin	Truth

trial, the examiner presents a multiple-choice recognition trial. Here, the examiner presents a series of 12 index cards, each consisting of a list word, a synonym, a homonym, and an unrelated distractor word. Finally, a delayed-recall trial is given without forewarning 30 min after the multiple-choice recognition trial. Therefore, several trials allow the examiner to identify the conditions that promote otherwise impaired memory (e.g., cueing, multiple-choice recognition) or disclose forgetting (e.g., delayed recall; Hannay & Levin, 1985).

Four different forms of the test are available. Figure 10–11 provides the word lists, and Figure 10–12 gives the multiple-choice and cued-recall items for the versions of the test used with adults. A Spanish version has recently been developed (Campo & Morales, 2004; Campo et al., 2000, 2003), as has a Hebrew version (Gigi et al., 1999).

For adolescents, aged 13 to 15 years, the test has been modified by reducing the number of learning trials to eight (Miller et al., personal communication, September 1996). Modifications of the test have also been developed for use with younger children. Clodfelter et al. (1987) developed two alternate forms for children aged 9 to 12 years, and these are shown in Figure 10–13. A list of 12 words is presented for

eight trials or until the child recalls all 12 words on two consecutive trials. Morgan (1982) developed alternate forms for children aged 5 to 8 years, and these are shown in Figure 10–14. The examiner presents a list of eight words that the subject must recall, in any order. The test continues for six SR trials or until the subject is able to recall correctly the entire list in two consecutive trials.

ADMINISTRATION

See Figure 10–15 for specific instructions on administering the SRT.

ADMINISTRATION TIME

The adult version requires 30 min; the children's version takes 10 min.

SCORING

See sample score sheets shown in Figures 10–16 through 10–18. A number of different scores are calculated (Buschke,

Figure 10–12 Multiple-choice and cued-recall items for Forms 1 through 4 of the SRT. *Source:* From Hannay, 1996, and Hannay & Levin, 1985.

Form 1   *Multiple-Choice Words*

1. bowl	dish	bell	view
2. love	poison	conform	passion
3. dawn	sunrise	bet	down
4. pasteboard	verdict	judgement	fudge
5. grand	grant	give	jazz
6. see	sting	fold	bee
7. pain	plane	pulled	jet
8. county	state	tasted	counter
9. voice	select	choice	cheese
10. flower	seed	herd	seek
11. date	sheep	wool	would
12. mill	queen	food	meal

Form 2

1. shine	glow	chime	cast
2. dispute	disappear	contour	disagree
3. fat	oil	trail	fit
4. stopwatch	affluent	wealthy	worthy
5. trunk	drunk	stoned	blunt
6. fin	peg	wake	pin
7. glass	grass	plan	lawn
8. moon	beam	spark	noon
9. propose	ready	prepare	husband
10. award	prize	pot	size
11. bark	bird	duck	luck
12. leap	ranch	blade	leaf

Form 3

1. throw	toss	through	plate
2. flower	lilt	intent	lily
3. film	movie	slave	kiln
4. waver	cautious	discreet	distinct
5. soft	loft	attic	tack
6. beet	meat	clue	beef
7. stream	street	speed	road
8. helmet	armor	bacon	velvet
9. smoke	serpent	snake	pool
10. hoed	dug	hay	dog
11. blank	bundle	pack	puck
12. ton	shirt	foil	tin

Form 4

1. egg	shell	beg	source
2. airline	runner	darling	runway
3. fort	castle	sink	fork
4. boldness	dentist	toothache	headache
5. blown	drown	float	rib
6. body	infant	middle	baby
7. larva	lava	echo	rock
8. damp	moist	hook	stamp
9. purse	clean	pure	bare
10. ballot	vote	dish	note
11. chain	peal	strip	slip
12. trust	rise	fact	truth

Cued-Recall Words

Form 1	*Form 2*	*Form 3*	*Form 4*
BO	SH	TH	RU
PA	DI	LI	FO
DA	FA	FI	TO
JUD	WEA	DI	DR
GR	DR	LO	BA
PL	GR	BE	LA
COU	MO	ST	DA
CH	PRE	HE	PU
SE	PR	DU	VO
WO	DU	PA	ST
ME	LE	SN	TR
—	—	—	—

Figure 10–13 Alternate forms of SRT for children, aged 9 to 12 years. *Source:* From Clodfelter et al., 1985. Reprinted with the kind permission of Psychology Press.

List 1	List 2
Garden	Market
Doctor	Palace
Metal	Flower
City	Picture
Money	Dollar
Cattle	River
Prison	Cotton
Clothing	Sugar
Water	College
Cabin	Baby
Tower	Temple
Bottle	Butter

1973; Buschke & Fuld, 1974; Hannay & Levin, 1985). These are shown in Figure 10–19. If a word is recalled on two consecutive trials, it is assumed to have entered long-term storage (LTS) on the first of these trials. Once a word enters LTS, it is considered to be in permanent storage, and it is scored as LTS on all following trials, regardless of the subject's subsequent recall. When a subject recalls a word that has entered LTS, it is scored as long-term retrieval (LTR). When a subject begins to recall a word in LTS consistently on all subsequent trials, it is also scored as consistent long-term retrieval (CLTR) or list-learning, beginning on the first of the uninterrupted successful recall trials. Inconsistent LTR refers to recall of a word in LTS followed by subsequent failure to recall the word. It is scored as random long-term retrieval (RLTR) until it is recalled consistently. Short-term recall (STR) refers to recall of a word that has not entered LTS. The total recall (Sum Recall) on each trial is the sum of STR and LTR. The number of reminders given by the examiner before the next recall attempt is equal to 12 – Sum Recall (for young children, 8 – Sum Recall) of the previous trial.

Record by number the order of the subject's recall on each trial. Intrusions of extra-list words are also recorded on each trial. The reader is directed to Levin et al. (1982, pp.110–111) for two completely scored examples.

DEMOGRAPHIC EFFECTS

Adults

Age. There is a decline on most SRT measures with advancing age (Campo & Morales, 2004; Larrabee et al., 1988; Sliwinski et al., 1997; Stricks et al., 1998; Wiederholt et al., 1993). Recognition scores tend to be less affected by aging, pointing to this measure as a potential marker of abnormality (Campo & Morales, 2004).

Gender. Gender also affects scores, with females performing better than males (Bishop et al., 1990; Campo & Morales, 2004; Larrabee et al., 1988; Trahan & Quintana, 1990; Wiederholt et al., 1993). Further, with increasing age, the performance of men declines more rapidly than that of women (Wiederholt et al., 1993). Age, however, is a more salient factor than gender. Larrabee et al. (1988) noted that age accounted for up to 10 times the variance in SRT performance predicted by gender alone.

IQ. Psychometric intelligence is moderately related to SRT performance (Bishop et al., 1990; Goldberg et al., 1989; Sherman et al., 1995). Therefore, use of SRT normative data that does not consider intellectual level may put clinicians at risk of overestimating memory deficits in individuals with low-average IQs (Bishop et al., 1990).

Education. The influence of education is inconsistent, with some studies finding it to be relatively unimportant (Goldberg et al., 1989; Larrabee et al., 1988; Petersen et al., 1992; Ruff et al., 1989; Trahan & Quintana, 1990), whereas others (Campo & Morales, 2004; Scherl et al., 2004; Sliwinski et al., 1997; Stricks et al., 1998; Wiederholt et al., 1993) note significantly better performance for those with more education on all indices except the short-term memory index.

Ethnicity. Stricks et al. (1998) found that English-speakers tended to score slightly higher than Spanish-speakers, although any performance differences might have been related to translation issues or other factors (e.g., cultural differences, quality of education).

Children

Age. Performance improves during childhood (Miller et al., 1996), with no significant changes occurring between the ages of 13 and 18 years (Levin & Grossman, 1976; Levin et al., 1982).

Figure 10–14 Word lists for three forms of SRT for children, aged 5 to 8 years. *Source:* From Morgan, 1982. Reprinted with the kind permission of Psychology Press.

List 1	*List 2*	*List 3*
Dog	Balloon	Apple
Horse	Crayons	Meat
Turtle	Doll	Egg
Lion	Bicycle	Candy
Squirrel	Paints	Carrot
Bear	Baseball	Cereal
Elephant	Clay	Bread
Rabbit	Book	Banana

Figure 10–15 Instructions for administering the SRT. Adapted from Hannay & Levin, 1985, Clodfolter et al., 1985, and Morgan, 1982.

Say to the subject: *This test is to see how quickly you can learn a list of words. I am going to read you a list of 12* (for young children, 8) *words. I want you to listen carefully, because when I stop, I want you to tell me as many of the words as you can recall. The words do not have to be in any particular order. When you have given me all the words that you can recall, I will tell you the words that you didn't give me from the list; then I want you to give me the entire list all over again. We do this 12* (for older children, 8; for younger children, 6) *times, and each time I want you to try to give me all 12* (for younger children, 8) *words.*

Read the list of words at a rate of one word every 2 s, and always present the words in order, beginning with the top of the list and working to the bottom. The presentation of words will, of course, skip over the words that were recalled correctly on the preceding trial. If the subject is able to recall correctly all 12 (for younger children, 8) words on three (for children, two) consecutive trials, discontinue, but score as if all trials had been given. If the subject recalls words not on the list, inform the subject, and note the extra words. The total number of words on the list is not disclosed.

For the cued-recall trial, the first two to three letters of each list word are presented on an index card and the subject is asked to say the word from the list that would begin with the first two letters on the card (see Figure 10–12). The cue cards are presented one at a time in the same order as the words on the list. There is no time limit, and the subject is allowed to return to a previous card if he or she wishes. Because one word on Form 1 (*bee*) can be clearly identified by the first two letters, it is omitted from cued recall, as are pin, tin, and egg on Forms 2, 3, and 4, respectively. Cues that fail initially to evoke the list word are presented a second time, after each cue has been given once. For the multiple-choice recognition trial, the subject is shown each of the 12 index cards and is asked to identify the list word. Give the cued-recall and multiple-choice trials even if the subject has recalled the entire list on the selective reminding trials. After a 30-min delay, ask the subject to recall all 12 words. During the 30-min delay, the subject should be given nonverbal tasks to perform.

Figure 10–16 Sample SRT Score Sheet—Form 1 (Adult).

Name _____ Date _____ Examiner _____

	1	2	3	4	5	6	7	8	9	10	11	12	CR	MC	30 min
Bowl															
Passion															
Dawn															
Judgement															
Grant															
Bee															
Plane															
County															
Choice															
Seed															
Wool															
Meal															

Total Recall _____

LTR _____

STR _____

LTS _____

CLTR _____

RLTR _____

Reminders _____

Intrusions _____

Trial 1 _____

Total Recall _____ (Number recalled over 12 trials)

LTS _____ (Number recalled twice in a row, assumed to be in LTS from that point on. Mark with red underliner, counting blanks. Compute sum over the 12 trials.)

STR _____ (Words that are not underlined. Compute sum over the 12 trials.)

CLTR _____ (Words that are continuously recalled. Mark with highlighter. Compute sum across the 12 trials.)

RLTR _____ (Words that are underlined but NOT CLTR. Do not count blanks. Compute sum across 12 trials.)

Reminders _____ (Compute sum over 12 trials. Maximum = 144)

Intrusions _____ (Compute sum over 12 trials.)

Cued Recall _____ (Maximum = 11)

Mult. Choice _____ (Maximum = 12)

30-Min Recall _____ (Maximum = 12)

Figure 10–17 Sample SRT Score Sheet—Form 1 (for children 9–12 years of age).

Name _____ Date _____ Examiner _____

	1	2	3	4	5	6	7	8
Garden								
Doctor								
Metal								
City								
Money								
Cattle								
Prison								
Clothing								
Water								
Cabin								
Tower								
Bottle								

Total Recall _____

LTR _____

STR _____

LTS _____

CLTR _____

RLTR _____

Reminders _____

Intrusions _____

Total Recall	_____	(Number recalled over 8 trials)
LTS	_____	(Words recalled twice in a row, assumed to be in LTS from that point on. Mark with red underliner, counting blanks. Compute sum over the 8 trials.)
STR	_____	(Words that are not underlined. Compute sum over the 8 trials.)
CLTR	_____	(Words that are continuously recalled. Mark with highlighter. Compute sum across the 8 trials.)
RLTR	_____	(Words that are underlined but NOT CLTR. Do not count blanks. Compute sum across 8 trials.)
Reminders	_____	(Compute sum over 8 trials. Maximum = 96)
Intrusions	_____	(Compute sum over 8 trials.)

Figure 10–18 Sample SRT Score Sheet—Form 1 (for children 5–8 years of age).

Name _____ Date _____ Examiner _____

	1	2	3	4	5	6
Dog						
Horse						
Turtle						
Lion						
Squirrel						
Bear						
Elephant						
Rabbit						

Total Recall _____

LTR _____

STR _____

LTS _____

CLTR _____

RLTR _____

Reminders _____

Intrusions _____

Total Recall _____ (Number recalled over 6 trials)

LTS _____ (Number recalled twice in a row, assumed to be in LTS from that point on. Mark with red underliner, counting blanks. Compute sum over the 6 trials.)

STR _____ (Words that are not underlined. Compute sum over the 6 trials.)

CLTR _____ (Words that are continuously recalled. Mark with highlighter. Compute sum across the 6 trials.)

RLTR _____ (Words that are underlined but NOT CLTR. Do not count blanks. Compute sum across 6 trials.)

Reminders _____ (Compute sum over 6 trials. Maximum = 48)

Intrusions _____ (Compute sum over 6 trials.)

Figure 10–19 Abbreviations and definitions of scores.

LTS	If a word is recalled on two consecutive trials, it is assumed to have entered long-term storage (LTS) on the first of these trials.
LTR	When a subject recalls a word that has entered LTS, it is scored as long-term retrieval (LTR).
CLTR	When a subject begins to recall a word in LTS consistently on all subsequent trials, it is also scored as consistent long-term retrieval (CLTR) or list-learning, beginning on the first of the uninterrupted successful recall trials.
RLTR	Inconsistent LTR refers to recall of a word in LTS followed by subsequent failure to recall the word. It is scored as random long-term retrieval (RLTR) until it is recalled consistently.
STR	Short-term recall refers to recall of a word that has not entered LTS.
Sum Recall	The total recall on each trial is the sum of STR and LTR.
Reminders	The number of reminders given by the examiner before the next recall attempt is equal to 12—Sum Recall (for young children, 8 or 6—Sum Recall) of the previous trial.

Gender. Females tend to outperform males (Levin et al., 1982; Miller et al., 1996).

IQ. Scores improve with increasing verbal IQ (Miller et al., 1996).

NORMATIVE DATA

Adults

Larrabee et al. (1988) provided norms for the adult version (Form 1) of the SRT, organized by age and gender, shown in Table 10–16. The reader should note that corrections need to be made for gender (see Note 2 on Table 10–16). In addition, note that the mean values for LTR and STR do not sum to the exact value of the total correct score. The same is true for the relationship of the mean values for CLTR and RLTR to LTR. These small discrepancies appeared because different gender corrections were used for these respective scores. Note too that various indices of acquisition (LTS, CLTR) decline with age, particularly after age 50 years. There are also age-related differences in rate of forgetting, but the effects tend to be quite modest and depend on the particular index used to measure what was stored in acquisition (Petersen et al., 1992; Trahan & Larrabee, 1993). To measure forgetting, Trahan and Larrabee (1993) recommended use of the acquisition score (defined as the Trial 12 LTS) minus the Delayed Recall score.

Table 10–16 Norms (Mean and *SD*) for Verbal Selective Reminding Test—12 Items

Variables	Age Groups (Years) and No. of Subjects						
	18–28 (57)	30–39 (29)	40–49 (31)	50–59 (24)	60–69 (50)	70–79 (59)	80–91 (27)
Age (years)	22.55 (3.30)	34.62 (2.69)	43.71 (2.91)	54.17 (2.74)	66.00 (2.47)	74.49 (2.92)	83.48 (3.10)
Education (years)	12.88 (1.73)	14.90 (2.47)	14.71 (2.72)	12.92 (1.98)	13.40 (3.57)	13.46 (3.78)	13.22 (3.76)
Female/Male	23/28	15/14	19/12	22/2	33/17	38/21	23/4
Total Score	128.18 (9.16)	124.59 (13.40)	125.03 (12.00)	121.62 (10.46)	114.82 (15.77)	105.27 (16.67)	97.96 (17.49)
LTR	122.16 (13.12)	118.14 (20.64)	118.55 (17.96)	112.71 (16.10)	101.52 (24.68)	89.95 (29.23)	77.22 (26.26)
STR	6.14 (4.82)	6.72 (7.59)	6.48 (6.72)	8.96 (6.40)	13.52 (9.52)	17.47 (10.41)	20.74 (9.62)
LTS	124.00 (10.47)	121.62 (18.36)	122.45 (15.64)	116.67 (14.52)	107.00 (21.79)	95.54 (24.86)	87.48 (25.26)
CLTR	115.12 (19.67)	107.93 (27.62)	107.10 (26.62)	101.50 (22.39)	88.92 (35.85)	69.68 (35.96)	54.96 (29.04)
RLTR	8.12 (9.42)	10.12 (9.73)	11.19 (11.34)	10.79 (9.25)	14.66 (11.83)	20.71 (14.37)	22.19 (10.70)
Reminders	16.0 (8.42)	18.10 (13.12)	19.03 (11.26)	22.25 (10.06)	28.12 (15.16)	36.95 (15.17)	43.96 (15.77)
Intrusions	0.84 (1.29)	0.97 (1.43)	1.81 (3.10)	1.17 (1.49)	3.90 (7.29)	4.22 (5.76)	3.30 (5.09)
Cued Recall	—	—	—	—	9.58[a] (1.93)	8.95[b] (2.12)	8.16[c] (2.22)
Multiple Choice	12.0 (0.0)	12.0 (0.0)	12.0 (0.0)	12.0 (0.0)	11.96 (0.20)	11.85 (0.58)	11.93 (0.27)
Delayed Recall	11.53 (0.83)	10.66 (1.97)	11.03 (1.43)	10.83 (1.40)	9.58 (2.46)	9.05 (2.62)	8.37 (2.45)

Note: Correction values for raw scores of males (calculate before entering normative tables): Total = +5; LTR = +9; STR = −4; LTS = +7; CLTR = +13; RLTR = −5; Reminders = −5; Intrusions = 0: Cued Recall = 0; Multiple Choice = 0; Delayed Recall = +1. Caution: Do not correct LTS or CLTR if raw score is 0. See text for definitions of Total, LTR, STR, LTS, CLTR, RLTR, Reminders by examiner, Intrusions, Cued Recall, Multiple Choice, and Delayed Recall.

[a] *n* = 31

[b] *n* = 38

[c] *n* = 19

Source: From Larrabee et al., 1988. Reprinted with permission of the American Psychological Association.

Table 10–17 Normative Data (Mean and *SD*) for SRT, Ages 9 to 15 Years

	Age (Years) and No. of Subjects						
	9 (81)	10 (140)	11 (132)	12 (122)	13 (96)	14 (116)	15 (52)
Total Recall	72.86 (9.14)	75.46 (8.37)	73.73 (8.39)	78.12 (7.88)	76.56 (7.42)	79.13 (7.76)	77.10 (8.18)
CLTR	52.81 (17.96)	58.01 (18.31)	52.88 (18.17)	61.37 (17.23)	58.33 (16.44)	64.59 (17.37)	60.31 (17.25)
STR	5.70 (3.83)	6.22 (4.68)	6.78 (5.03)	5.00 (4.15)	6.94 (4.80)	5.93 (4.37)	6.37 (5.25)
LTS	72.81 (10.41)	73.36 (10.73)	71.90 (11.92)	77.16 (9.84)	73.50 (10.58)	76.02 (10.24)	74.46 (11.09)
Cued Recall	9.80 (1.61)	10.31 (1.77)	9.97 (1.73)	10.57 (1.37)	9.30 (1.74)	0.72 (1.47)	9.60 (1.62)
RECG	10.96 (0.19)	11.94 (0.27)	11.95 (0.27)	12.00 —	11.80 (0.38)	11.90 (0.33)	11.90 (0.36)
30" DEL	9.95 (1.87)	10.21 (1.66)	10.14 (1.71)	10.72 (1.40)	9.82 (1.95)	10.57 (1.47)	10.27 (2.20)
SAV	95.00 (16.76)	92.44 (12.47)	95.66 (15.33)	96.09 (11.87)	89.71 (16.00)	94.10 (11.58)	92.82 (16.51)

Note: Children aged 9 to 12 years received Form 1 developed by Clodfelter et al. (1987), whereas those aged 13–16 years received Levin's Form I (8 trials).

Source: From Miller et al., 1996. Reprinted with permission (C. Paniak, personal communication, April 10, 2004).

Similar data have been reported for middle-aged adults by Ruff et al. (1989). Masur et al. (1989) also provided normative data for a large sample of elderly subjects. Their sample, however, contained a large number of non-native English speakers. This may account for the fact that their scores were somewhat lower than those reported here. Wiederholt et al. (1993) also gave data for a large sample of community-dwelling elderly individuals. However, these data were based on a somewhat different version of the SRT than that presented here, one in which 10 (not 12) items are presented for 6 (not 12) trials.

Children

Levin used Form 1 with adolescents, aged 13 to 18 years (Levin & Grossman, 1976; Levin et al., 1982) and provided data based on small samples of males ($n = 23$) and females ($n = 27$) for two measures, LTS and CLTR. Miller et al. (1996) modified the adult form by reducing the number of trials to eight. Table 10–17 provides data for students, aged 13 to 15 years, stratified on the basis of age. The savings score is calculated as a ratio of the number of words recalled on delay divided by the number recalled on the eighth and last learning trial.

Clodfelter et al. (1987) provided normative data for alternate forms of the SRT based on 58 children, aged 9 to 12 years. However, they provided data on only a few variables and did not address retention after delay. Miller et al. (1996) used Form 1 (List 1) developed by Clodfelter et al. (1987) and provided more extensive norms, based on 475 schoolchildren (see Table 10–17). The exclusion criteria for the sample studied by Miller et al. included failure of one or more grades, enrollment in an English as a second language program, a history of hospitalization for brain injury or behavioral problems, or participation in a self-contained special education program. In this age group, differences between the sexes (favoring girls) were small (about 0.3 *SD*), and the data are presented for both sexes combined. The sample had a WISC-III

Vocabulary scaled score of about 10 with a standard deviation (*SD*) close to 3 (C. Paniak, personal communication, April 10, 2004).

Normative data for parallel forms of the SRT for children aged 5 to 8 years were provided by Morgan (1982). The children were of average intelligence, based on their combined performance on WISC Information and Similarities subtests. Table 10–18 presents the means and standard deviations by age for four SRT variables (Recall per trial, LTS, LTR, and CLTR). The table shows that children's performance increases substantially with age. It should be noted that the data presented are of limited value because the sample sizes are quite small.

Short Form. Smith et al. (1995) pointed out that there is no theoretical rationale for choosing 12 as the requisite number of trials. They found that as few as 6 trials provided information highly consistent with that provided by 12 trials. The only score with consistently lower correlations with 12-trial scores was RLTR, a not surprising finding since it is a measure of random long-term recall and is not expected to be consistent across trials (see also Larrabee et al., 2000). Drane et al. (1998) also reported high (>.90) correlations between 6- and 12-trial LTS and CLTR in a sample of patients

Table 10–18 Normative Data (Mean and *SD*) for SRT, Ages 5 to 8

	Age 5–6 Years ($n = 16$)	Age 7–8 Years ($n = 14$)
Recall/trial	5.3 (1.2)	6.1 (1.1)
LTS	28.6 (10.1)	35.7 (9.1)
LTR	25.7 (9.9)	33.4 (10.2)
CLTR	18.9 (11.3)	27.7 (13.2)

Note: Scores are derived from a small group of healthy schoolchildren, of average intelligence.

Source: Adapted from Morgan, 1982.

Table 10–19 SRT Normative Data (Mean and *SD*) for 6-Trial Administration

Variables	Age Groups (Years) and No. of Subjects						
	18–29 (49)	30–39 (28)	40–49 (31)	50–59 (23)	60–69 (50)	70–79 (59)	80–91 (27)
Age	22.53 (3.36)	34.54 (2.70)	43.71 (2.91)	54.00 (2.68)	66.00 (2.47)	74.49 (2.91)	83.48 (3.11)
Education	12.92 (1.75)	14.96 (2.49)	14.71 (2.72)	13.09 (1.83)	13.43 (3.54)	13.46 (3.78)	13.22 (3.76)
Female/Male	23/26	15/13	19/12	21/2	33/17	38/21	23/4
Total Recall	55.35 (5.01)	54.48 (8.58)	54.26 (7.90)	53.13 (5.99)	49.74 (8.11)	45.36 (8.62)	41.93 (7.71)
STR	7.29 (4.50)	6.18 (5.25)	7.16 (5.84)	8.26 (5.20)	10.96 (5.79)	13.07 (5.24)	14.70 (5.43)
LTR	49.12 (8.80)	49.18 (12.93)	47.84 (12.88)	44.96 (10.00)	39.44 (13.10)	33.02 (12.45)	27.48 (12.46)
LTS	50.86 (8.71)	51.46 (12.51)	50.48 (12.83)	47.35 (10.10)	41.54 (12.93)	35.02 (12.40)	30.67 (13.32)
RLTR	4.43 (3.74)	5.89 (5.17)	7.00 (5.45)	6.57 (4.45)	5.44 (4.76)	5.32 (3.93)	7.74 (4.74)
CLTR	44.65 (9.85)	43.29 (15.20)	40.84 (14.65)	38.30 (11.18)	33.98 (14.01)	27.83 (12.94)	19.70 (10.84)
Intrusions	0.65 (.99)	0.82 (1.25)	1.29 (2.18)	0.83 (1.03)	1.38 (2.81)	1.85 (2.41)	1.38 (1.81)
Delayed Recall[a]	11.53 (0.83)	10.66 (1.97)	10.03 (1.43)	10.83 (1.40)	9.58 (2.46)	9.05 (2.62)	8.37 (2.45)

Note: Correction values for raw scores of males (calculate before entering normative tables: LTR = +4; STR = −2; LTS = +4, CLTR = +4. Caution: do not correct LTS or CLTR if raw score is 0. See text for definition of Total Recall, STR, LTR, LTS, RLTR, CLTR, and Intrusions.

[a]Delayed recall data are based on a 12-trial administration from data reported by Larrabee et al. (1988). These norms should be used only after the regression procedure described in the norms section. The delayed recall correction for males is +1.

Source: Larrabee et al., 2000. Reprinted with the kind permission of Psychology Press.

with temporal lobe epilepsy. Moreover, the 6- and 12-trial SRT administrations demonstrated comparable sensitivity and discrimination in patients with left versus right temporal lobe seizure focus, unless the 6-trial score fell in the range between 1 and 2 *SD*s below the age peer-appropriate mean. A 6- or 8-trial SRT would significantly reduce administration time and patient fatigue.

Wiederholt et al. (1993) provided normative data for a 6-trial, 10-item form, but only for elderly individuals. More recently, Larrabee et al. (2000) published normative data based on 267 neurologically normal adults (172 females, 95 males; age range, 18–91 years) for a 6-trial administration of Form 1 of the Hannay-Levin SRT. The data were constructed by rescoring SRT protocols of the normal subjects upon whom the 12-trial normative data were based (Larrabee et al., 1988). All subjects were interviewed before testing to exclude those with neurological or psychiatric disorders, a history of drug abuse, or evidence of mental deficiency based on educational and occupational attainment. Further, subjects aged 60 years and older had to achieve a passing score on a measure of temporal orientation. The data are shown in Table 10–19.

A regression-based procedure is also provided (Larrabee et al., 2000) so that existing delayed recall norms, based on a 12-item administration, can be used after a 6-trial administration. The regression equation for predicting 30-min delayed recall by 6-trial LTS is

Estimated 30-min delayed recall = 0.124(6-trial LTS) + 4.676

SE_E = 1.595. Once the predicted score is obtained, a confidence interval (CI) should be constructed around the predicted score, based on the SE_E, multiplied by the *z* scores for the desired CI (e.g., for a 90% CI, the range would be

±2.624). If the patient's actual 30-min delayed score falls within the CI, then the 30-min delay norms presented by Larrabee et al. (1998) can be used. These norms require a gender correction, whereby 1 point is added to the delayed recall scores of male subjects. If the patient's 30 min delayed free recall score falls outside the CI, this suggests either (a) acceleration of forgetting if the score is below the CI cutoff or (b) motivational factors if the score is above the CI cutoff, in a pattern suggesting better memory than learning. In either case, the 30-min delay norms cannot be used if performance falls outside the CI predicted on the basis of the 6-trial LTS.

Six-trial SRT scores generally show comparable classification of normal versus abnormal classification in most clinical settings, unless the 6-trial score falls in the range of 1 to 2 *SD*s below the age-appropriate mean (Drane et al., 1998; Larrabee et al., 2000). Accordingly, Larrabee et al. (2000) cautioned that, for scores in this range in clinical settings, the clinician should consider a 12-trial SRT administration, particularly if the SRT is the only measure of verbal learning and memory. Alternatively, if other measures of verbal memory have also been administered, they can be used in conjunction with the 6-trial SRT to more reliably assess the construct of verbal learning and memory.

The data provided by Larrabee et al. (2000) represent a fairly well-educated sample and are derived from the 12-trial version. Others have developed norms for the 12-word, 6-trial version. For example, Scherl et al. (2004) recruited a random sample of community-dwelling participants in New York and reported slightly lower scores than those reported by Larrabee et al. (2000). However, their sample was small (*N* = 75) and was limited to those aged 30 to 59 years. For individuals with more limited levels of education, the norms provided by Stricks et al. (1998) appear to be more appropriate. These authors used the 6-trial SRT, with a 15-min delayed recall trial followed by a multiple-choice recognition task. They provided norms based on a sample of 557 older, English-speaking adults living in the New York city area who were screened as nondemented by a physician. Individuals with neurological conditions that might affect cognition were also excluded. Approximately 4% of the subjects were Hispanic, and 60% were African American. About 68% were female. The normative data are shown in Table 10–20. In addition, a group of 412 nondemented, disease-free Spanish-speakers (largely of Caribbean origin) were tested in Spanish. These data are also provided in Table 10–20.

RELIABILITY

Test-Retest Reliability

Information regarding test-retest reliability using the same form is not available.

Alternate Form Reliability and Practice Effects

It has been difficult to develop lists of equal difficulty and reliability for repeated testing of individuals (Hannay & Levin, 1985; Kraemer et al., 1983; Loring & Papanicolaou, 1987; Said et al., 1990). For adults, we use the forms developed by Hannay and Levin (1985; Hannay, 1986) although other forms are available (e.g., Coen et al., 1990; Deptula et al., 1990; Dikmen et al., 1999). For college students, Forms 2 to 4 are of equivalent difficulty, whereas Form 1 is about 10% harder than Forms 3, 4, and 5 (Hannay & Levin, 1985). However, the four forms appear to be of equivalent difficulty for elderly subjects (Masur et al., 1989) and for patients with clinical memory disorders, at least for those with medically refractory epilepsy (Westerveld et al., 1994). The separate forms for the children's version are roughly of equivalent difficulty (Clodfelter et al., 1987; Morgan, 1982).

Alternate form reliability coefficients tend to be variable ($r = .48$ to $.85$) in magnitude for both normal and neurological samples (Clodfelter et al., 1987; Hannay & Levin, 1985; Morgan, 1982; Ruff et al., 1989; Westerveld et al., 1994), although values of .92 (for consistent retrieval) have been reported for patients with Alzheimer's disease (Masur et al., 1989). Total Recall scores are the most stable, and STM scores are the least stable (Westerveld et al., 1994). Westerveld et al. (1994) suggested that use of the mean or the better of two baseline assessments minimizes error variance, thereby enhancing interpretation of change. Alternatively, given that Total Recall scores generally are less variable and that SRT scores appear to measure a single construct, examiners may choose to rely on Total Recall scores (Westerveld et al., 1994).

There was no significant practice effect when patients with seizures underwent multiple administrations of alternate forms on four consecutive days (Westerveld et al., 1994). With normal individuals, however, there appears to be a nonspecific practice effect with repeated administration of alternate forms (Clodfelter et al., 1987; Hannay & Levin, 1985; Loring & Papanicolaou, 1987). Therefore, the ability to learn how to perform a complex task, as well as the ability to form associations between stimuli, may be accounting for group differences in research involving some populations (Loring & Papanicolaou, 1987; Sass et al., 1994).

Practice effects are also noted when healthy individuals are given alternate forms of the 6-trial SRT over a 12- to 16-week retest interval. Salinsky et al. (2001) tested a sample of 62 adults (age $M = 34$ years, range = 19–62; education $M = 13.8$ years, range 10–19) and reported Spearman correlations ranging from .55 (30-min recall) to .71 (CLTR). Practice effects were most pronounced for CLTR, Total Recall, and LTS but not 30-min recall. Salinsky et al. (2001) used a regression approach to derive estimates of change. Table 10–21 can be used to calculate a test-retest z score for individuals tested twice over a 12- to 16-week interval. The score on second testing (T2) can be predicted from the score measured at the first testing (T1) by using the table and the following equation

$$\text{T2 predicted} = \text{T1} \times (\beta_1) + \text{Constant}$$

An individual's z score can then be calculated as follows:

$$z = (\text{T2 measured} - \text{T2 predicted}) \div (|95\% \text{ CI}|/1.96)$$

Individuals whose scores exceed the extremes are considered to have significant changes. Dikmen et al. (1999) reported test-retest data for a 10-item, 10-trial version in a large group of neurologically normal adults. Most were tested over an 11-month interval. Their findings were similar to those reported by Salinsky et al. (2001).

VALIDITY

Relations within Test

The SRT is popular because it purports to parcel verbal memory into distinct component processes (e.g., LTS, LTR, CLTR, STR). In support of this notion, Beatty et al. (1996a) reported that, in patients with multiple sclerosis and controls, the probability of recall or recognition varied in a consistent manner as a function of the status of the words (CLTR, RLTR, or STR) in the subject's memory at the conclusion of training. For example, words that were being retrieved from CLTR at the end of acquisition were more likely to be recalled after delay than were words that

Table 10–20 Normative Data (Mean and *SD*) for English and Spanish Speakers on the 6-Trial Version of the SRT, Followed by a 15-min Delayed Recall Trial and a Recognition Trial, by Age and Education

	Age 60–69 Years		Age 70–79 Years		Age 80+ Years		Grand Mean
	<9 Years	9+ Years	<9 (n = 91)	9+ (n = 198)	<9 (n = 56)	9+ (n = 99)	
English Speakers[a] (n)	21	93	91	198	56	99	557
Total Recall	39.8 (10.3)	43.5 (9.3)	31.8 (9.5)	39.8 (9.8)	27.7 (10.7)	34.2 (11.9)	36.9 (11.3)
LTR	26.6 (13.3)	31.7 (13.3)	18.6 (10.7)	25.9 (13.3)	14.1 (10.6)	20.2 (14.1)	23.5 (13.8)
LTS	29.5 (14.2)	35.2 (13.6)	22.1 (11.9)	29.3 (14.0)	17.1 (11.5)	23.0 (14.7)	26.8 (14.5)
CLTR	19.1 (12.1)	23.4 (12.8)	11.3 (9.7)	18.2 (12.5)	7.1 (8.0)	13.8 (12.5)	16.1 (12.7)
Intrusions	1.6 (2.7)	0.9 (1.7)	1.3 (2.7)	0.6 (1.3)	1.3 (2.1)	1.1 (1.7)	1.0 (1.9)
Delayed Recall	5.3 (2.8)	6.7 (2.8)	4.5 (2.6)	5.8 (2.7)	2.8 (2.5)	4.9 (2.9)[b]	5.3[c] (2.9)
Delayed Recognition	10.9 (1.9)	11.4 (1.2)	10.2 (2.0)	11.2 (1.4)	9.1 (2.3)	10.8 (2.1)[b]	10.7[c] (1.8)
Spanish Speakers[d] (n)	74	21	179	47	66	25	412
Total Recall	36.2 (7.7)	40.5 (7.7)	34.1 (8.3)	39.1 (9.8)	27.6 (7.4)	30.6 (9.2)	34.1 (9.0)
LTR	22.8 (9.5)	27.2 (11.4)	21.3 (9.5)	26.0 (12.1)	14.8 (7.4)	16.1 (11.1)	21.0 (10.3)
LTS	25.5 (10.6)	30.5 (12.0)	24.5 (10.2)	28.9 (12.6)	18.4 (8.6)	18.9 (11.7)	24.2 (11.0)
CLTR	15.6 (8.9)	19.6 (11.8)	13.5 (8.9)	19.0 (11.0)	7.8 (8.6)	9.7 (9.5)	13.7 (9.9)
Intrusions	1.2 (1.8)	0.7 (1.4)	1.3 (2.1)	1.3 (1.7)	1.8 (2.6)	0.9 (1.7)	1.3 (2.1)
Delayed Recall	4.9 (2.1)	5.9[e] (2.3)	4.6[f] (1.9)	5.5 (2.5)	3.5 (2.1)	4.4 (2.2)	4.6[g] (2.2)
Delayed Recognition	10.8 (1.7)[k]	11.3[e] (1.1)	10.4[h] (1.8)	10.9 (1.8)	9.8[i] (2.6)	10.7 (1.7)	10.5[j] (1.9)

[a]<9 years of education: age *M* = 77.5, *SD* = 6.8; education *M* = 6.1, *SD* = 2.1; 75% Black, 3.5% Hispanic; 9+ years of education: age *M* = 75.1, *SD* = 6.6; education *M* = 12.7, *SD* = 2.6; 52.8% Black, 4.7% Hispanic.

[b] n = 98.

[c] n = 555.

[d]<9 years of education: age *M* = 74.5, *SD* = 6.9; education *M* = 4.5, *SD* = 2.7; 8% Black, 99.3% Hispanic; 9+ years of education: age *M* = 75.4, *SD* = 7.0; education *M* = 12.0, *SD* = 3.0; 5.9% Black, 66.9% Hispanic.

[e] n = 20.

[f] n = 178.

[g] n = 409.

[h] n = 177.

[i] n = 65.

[j] n = 406.

[k] n = 73.

Source: Adapted from Stricks et al., 1998.

Table 10–21 Test-Retest Regression Statistics for 6-Trial SRT

Measure	R^2	Constant	β_1	95% CI (+/−)	Average Standard Error
CLTR	.47	19.6	.69	18.0	9.18
Total Recall	.50	19.8	.7	9.1	4.64
LTS	.44	23.8	.6	24.6	7.45
30-min recall	.42	3.5	.67	3	1.53

Note: Average Standard Error = (|95% CI|/1.96).

Souce: Adapted from Salinsky et al., 2001.

not being consistently retrieved from LTS. Words that were being retrieved from STR were the least likely to be recalled after delay. On the other hand, there is evidence that the numerous scores that can be derived from the test tend to be highly intercorrelated, suggesting that these measures are assessing similar constructs (Kenisten, cited in Kraemer et al., 1983; Larrabee et al., 1988; Loring & Papanicolaou, 1987; Paniak et al., 1989; Smith et al., 1995; Westerveld et al., 1994). Further, although the SR procedure offers information regarding short- and long-term memory, the operational distinction between LTS and LTR is problematic (Loring & Papanicolaou, 1987). According to Bushke's definition, a word has entered LTS if it has been successfully recalled on two successive trials. By definition, failure to recall is due to a retrieval difficulty. However, the item may have been stored in a weak or degraded form, after which, through the process of additional repetition by the examiner, the word is encoded more deeply and efficiently (Loring & Papanicolaou, 1987). Therefore, operationally defined retrieval may have little to do with retrieval itself (e.g., it may reflect storage functions).

A single index from among those obtained using standard scoring methods may adequately convey the SRT result, given the redundancy of the scores. The total number of words recalled on all trials throughout the test, a fairly reliable measure, is recommended by Westerveld et al. (1994) as a measure of learning. To measure forgetting, Trahan and Larrabee (1993) recommend computing a score based on the number of words in LTS on the final learning trial (Trial 12 LTS) minus the 30-min delayed recall score.

Relations With Other Tests

Modest correlations have been demonstrated among the SRT and other tests of verbal learning and memory, such as the CVLT, RAVLT, and WMS (McCartney-Filgate & Vriezen, 1988; Shear & Craft, 1989). Larrabee and Curtiss (1995) evaluated the factor structure of several tests of memory and information-processing ability in a mixed clinical group and found that the SRT loaded on a general verbal visual memory factor (along with the Expanded Paired Associates Test, Continuous Recognition Memory Test, and Continuous

Visual Memory Test). By contrast, Allen and Ruff (1999) found that, in a healthy sample, the SRT loaded on a verbal memory factor along with WMS-R Logical Memory; visual memory tasks (RULIT, Rey Complex Figure) loaded on a separate factor.

Clinical Studies

The SRT has been used in a wide variety of patient populations. For example, it has been used effectively to assess memory functioning after head injury (e.g., Levin & Grossman, 1976; Paniak et al., 1989), with the severity of the injury (e.g., determined by length of unconsciousness) related to the level of memory performance.

Impairment has been noted in the context of left temporal lobe abnormality (e.g., Bell et al., 2005; Breier et al., 1997; Drane et al., 1998; Lee et al., 1989, 1990; Lencz et al., 1992; Levin et al., 1982; Loring et al., 1991; Martin et al., 1988; Snow et al., 1992). For example, Sass et al. (1990) showed that SRT scores correlated significantly with hippocampal pyramidal cell density obtained from pathologic analysis of excised tissue from the left, but not the right, hippocampus of left-speech dominant adults. Further, left-speech dominant patients with severe hippocampal neuron loss experienced no significant decrement in SRT performance after total excision of the left hippocampus (Sass et al., 1994), whereas patients with mild or moderate neuron loss had significant decline. It is important to note, however, that patients with diffuse cerebral lesions perform about the same as patients with focal involvement of the left temporal lobe on the SRT (Levin et al., 1982). Further, patients with left frontal lesions show lower overall recall than those with right frontal involvement; however, impairment is also evident in those with right hemisphere damage (Vilkki et al., 1998). Therefore, the SRT should not be used by itself to predict left temporal lobe abnormality.

In the SRT, as in many other memory tests (e.g., RAVLT, CVLT-II), retention is typically evaluated after a 30-min interval. The question arises whether impairment in consolidation over this relatively short delay is a good predictor of memory function after a longer delay period. Bell et al. (2005) examined patients with temporal lobe epilepsy with delays of 30 min and 24 hours. At the individual level, there was no difference in the percentage of patients versus controls who demonstrated isolated memory impairment after a 24-hour delay. That is, in the absence of overt seizure activity, accelerated forgetting over 24 hours appears to be uncommon in patients with temporal lobe epilepsy.

The test is useful in distinguishing normal adults from demented elderly individuals (Campo et al., 2003; Kuzis et al., 1999; Larrabee et al., 1985; Masur et al., 1989; Sabe et al., 1995). For instance, patients with dementia of the Alzheimer type (AD) recalled fewer words on Trial 1; they also recalled fewer words overall and entered fewer items into long-term memory, and they were more likely to show inconsistent recall from long-term memory as well as increased forgetting rates (Campo et al., 2003). Masur et al. (1989) noted that the measures LTR and CLTR were most valuable in distinguishing mild dementia from normal aging.

Scores from the SRT may also be useful as preclinical indicators of the development of dementia. Masur et al. (1990), using a modified SRT procedure (6 trials, delayed recall and recognition after a 5-min period of distraction), reported that the total recall and delayed recall scores obtained 1 to 2 years before diagnosis were the measures best able to predict dementia, with sensitivities of 47% and 44%, respectively. The predictive values were 37% and 40%, respectively, or better than 2.5 times the base rate. Krinsky-McHale et al. (2002) noted that a modified version of the SRT is useful in detecting early dementia even in adults with Down syndrome.

In patients with multiple sclerosis, the SRT has served to emphasize the heterogeneity of the memory disturbances. Beatty et al. (1996b) found evidence of three distinct patterns of SRT performance in these patients: unimpaired, mildly impaired with mainly retrieval problems, and more severely impaired with encoding as well as retrieval difficulties. Patients with Parkinson's disease also show difficulty on the SRT (Kuzis et al, 1999), likely due to an impairment in retrieval (Faglioni et al., 2000; Stern et al., 1998).

There is also evidence that individuals with mood or thought disorders (e.g., combat-related posttraumatic stress disorder, schizophrenia, depression) perform poorly on the SRT (Bremner et al., 1993; Goldberg et al., 1989; Ruchinskas et al., 2000; Sabe et al., 1995; but see Gass, 1996).

Ecological Validity

Levin et al. (1979) have reported that the degree of SRT long-term memory impairment 1 year after severe head injury corresponds to the overall level of disability in survivors. Patients who attained good recovery (i.e., resumption of work and normal social functioning) consistently recalled words without further reminding at a level comparable to that of normal adults. In contrast, consistent recall was grossly impaired in patients who were moderately or severely disabled at the time of the study.

COMMENT

The SRT has a number of positive features. The test is sensitive, but not specific, to side of seizure onset and degree of hippocampal neuron loss. In addition, the task allows the assessment of different aspects of memory (e.g., retrieval from short-term and long-term memory). It also distinguishes two qualitative aspects of retrieval from long-term memory, an inconsistent type (RLTR) and a consistent type (CLTR), providing information not obtainable from more global measures. These various measures have proved useful in characterizing memory disorders in a number of clinical conditions.

Further, the literature suggests an absence of practice effects in patients with neurological disorders, even if test sessions are on successive days. Therefore, the SRT has special merit when changes in memory function need to be evaluated. However, there are practice effects in normal subjects, and there is extreme variability in some scores in clinical groups, suggesting caution in interpreting retest data in some circumstances (e.g., relatively intact individuals, scores other than the Total Recall score).

Despite the positive evidence for retesting with alternate forms, users should be aware that SRT norms are based almost exclusively on Form 1 data, and alternate form reliabilities are not always high. Ideally, Form 1 should be used preferentially over other forms of the test if possible.

The abbreviated 6-item version has demonstrated generally acceptable reliability and validity across many settings and patient populations, unless the score falls between 1 and 2 SDs below normal. In such cases (e.g., subjects with mild deficits), the 12-item version or additional verbal memory tests should be given to increase diagnostic accuracy.

Performance on the SRT is sensitive to dementia. However, Sliwinski et al. (1997, 2003) argued that age-corrected norms are not optimal for detecting the presence of dementia. They found that age- and education-corrected SRT scores have a sensitivity for detecting dementia that is 28% lower than that of uncorrected scores. They suggested that such corrected norms (for this and possibly other memory tests) may be suboptimal for diagnosing dementia in elderly individuals, because the norms are likely to be contaminated by results from individuals with preclinical dementia. In addition, age corrections ignore the dramatic increase in the base rate of dementia that occurs with age. They recommended that norms should be weighted so as to provide information about the likelihood of cognitive impairment caused by probable dementia, given a specific test score, and risk factors, such as a person's age.

Finally, it should be noted that much of the work has focussed on adult populations. More research on the test's sensitivity to pediatric conditions involving memory would be useful.

REFERENCES

Allen, C. C., & Ruff, R. M. (1999). Factorial validation of the Ruff-Light Trail Learning Test. *Assessment, 6,* 43–50.

Beatty, W. W., Krull, K. R., Wilbanks, S. L., Blanco, C. R., Hames, K. A., & Paul, R. H. (1996a). Further validation of constructs from the Selective Reminding Test. *Journal of Clinical and Experimental Neuropsychology, 18,* 52–55.

Beatty, W. W., Krull, K. R., Wilbanks, S. L., Blanco, C. R., Hames, K. A., Tivis, R., & Paul, R. H. (1996b). Memory disturbance in multiple sclerosis: Reconsideration of patterns of performance on the Selective Reminding Test. *Journal of Clinical and Experimental Neuropsychology, 18,* 56–62.

Bell, B. D., Fine, J., Dow, C., Seidenberg, M., & Hermann, B. P. (2005). Temporal lobe epilepsy and the Selective Reminding Test: The conventional 30-minute delay suffices. *Psychological Assessment, 17*, 103–109.

Bishop, E. G., Dickson, A. L., & Allen, M. T. (1990). Psychometric intelligence and performance on Selective Reminding. *The Clinical Neuropsychologist, 4*, 141–150.

Breier, J. I., Brookshire, B. L., Fletcher, J. M., Thomas, A. B., Plenger, P. M., Wheless, J. W., Willmore, L. J., & Papanicolaou, A. (1997). Identification of side of seizure onset in temporal lobe epilepsy using memory tests in the context of reading deficits. *Journal of Clinical and Experimental Neuropsychology, 19*, 161–171.

Bremner, J. D., Scott, T. M., Delaney, R. C., Southwick, S. M., Mason, J. W., Johnson, D. R., Innis, R. B., McCarthy, G., Charney, D. S. (1993). Deficits in short-term memory in posttraumatic stress disorder. *American Journal of Psychiatry, 150*, 1015–1019.

Buschke, H. (1973). Selective reminding for analysis of memory and learning. *Journal of Verbal Learning and Verbal Behavior, 12*, 543–550.

Buschke, H., & Fuld, P. A. (1974). Evaluating storage, retention, and retrieval in disordered memory and learning. *Neurology, 24*, 1019–1025.

Campo, P., & Morales, M. (2004). Normative data and reliability for a Spanish version of the verbal Selective Reminding Test. *Archives of Clinical Neuropsychology, 19*, 421–435.

Campo, P., Morales, M., & Juan-Malpartida, M. (2000). Development of two Spanish versions of the verbal Selective Reminding Test. *Journal of Clinical and Experimental Neuropsychology, 22*, 279–285.

Campo, P., Morales, M., & Martinez-Castillo, E. (2003). Discrimination of normal from demented elderly on a Spanish version of the Verbal Selective Reminding Test. *Journal of Clinical and Experimental Neuropsychology, 25*, 991–999.

Clodfelter, C. J., Dickson, A. L., Newton Wilkes, C., & Johnson, R. B. (1987). Alternate forms of selective reminding for children. *The Clinical Neuropsychologist, 1*, 243–249.

Coen, R. F., Kinsella, A., Lambe, R., Kenny, M., Darragh, A. (1990). Creating equivalent word lists for the Buschke Selective Reminding Test. *Human Psychopharmacology: Clinical and Experimental, 5*, 47–51.

Deptula, D., Singh, R., Goldsmith, S., Block, R., Bagne, C. A., Pomara, N. (1990). Equivalence of five forms of the Selective Reminding Test in young and elderly subjects. *Psychological Reports, 3*, 1287–1295.

Dikmen, S. S., Heaton, R. K., Grant, I., & Temkin, N. R. (1999). Test-retest reliability and practice effects of expanded Halstead-Reitan neuropsychological test battery. *Journal of the International Neuropsychological Society, 5*, 346–356.

Drane, D. L., Loring, D. W., Lee, G. P., & Meador, K. J. (1998). Trial-length sensitivity of the Verbal Selective Reminding Test to lateralized temporal lobe impairment. *The Clinical Neuropsychologist, 12*, 68–73.

Faglioni, P., Saetti, M. C., & Botti, C. (2000). Verbal learning strategies in Parkinson's disease. *Neuropsychology, 14*, 456–479.

Gass, C. S. (1996). MMPI-2 variables in attention and memory test performance. *Psychological Assessment, 8*, 135–138.

Gigi, A., Schnaider-Beeri, M., Davidson, M., & Prohovnik, I. (1999). Validation of a Hebrew selective reminding test. *Israel Journal of Psychiatry and Related Sciences, 36*, 11–17.

Goldberg, T. E., Weinberger, D. R., Pliskin, N. H., Berman, K. F., & Podd, M. H. (1989). Recall memory deficit in schizophrenia. *Schizophrenia Research, 2*, 251–257.

Hannay, H. J. (1986). *Experimental techniques in human neuropsychology*. New York: Oxford University Press.

Hannay, J. H., & Levin, H. S. (1985). Selective reminding test: An examination of the equivalence of four forms. *Journal of Clinical and Experimental Neuropsychology, 7*, 251–263.

Kraemer, H. C., Peabody, C. A., Tinklenberg, J. R., & Yesavage, J. A. (1983). Mathematical and empirical development of a test of memory for clinical and research use. *Psychological Bulletin, 94*, 367–380.

Krinsky-McHale, S. J., Devenny, D. A., & Silverman, W. P. (2002). Changes in explicit memory associated with early dementia in adults with Down's syndrome. *Journal of Intellectual Disability Research, 46*, 198–208.

Kuzis, G., Sabe, L., Tiberti, C., Merello, M., Leiguarda, R., & Starkstein, S. E. (1999). Explicit and implicit learning in patients with Alzheimer disease and Parkinson disease with dementia. *Neuropsychiatry, Neuropsychology, and Behavioral Neurology, 12*, 265–269.

Larrabee, G. J., and Curtiss, G. (1995). Construct validity of various verbal and visual memory tests. *Journal of Clinical and Experimental Neuropsychology, 17*, 536–547.

Larrabee, G. J., Largen, J. W., & Levin, H. S. (1985). Sensitivity of age-decline resistant ("Hold") WAIS subtests to Alzheimer's disease. *Journal of Clinical and Experimental Neuropsychology, 7*, 497–504.

Larrabee, G. L., Trahan, D. E., Curtiss, G., & Levin, H. S. (1988). Normative data for the Verbal Selective Reminding Test. *Neuropsychology, 2*, 173–182.

Larrabee, G. J., Trahan, D. E., & Levin, H. S. (2000). Normative data for a six-trial administration of the Verbal Selective Reminding Test. *The Clinical Neuropsychologist, 14*, 110–118.

Lee, G. P., Loring, D. W., & Thompson, J. L. (1989). Construct validity of material-specific memory measures following unilateral temporal lobe ablations. *Psychological Assessment, 1*, 192–197.

Lee, G. P., Meador, K. J., Loring, D. W., Smith., J. R. et al. (1990). Behavioral activation of human hippocampal EEG: Relationship to recent memory. *Journal of Epilepsy, 3*, 137–142.

Lencz, T., McCarthy, G., Bronen, R. A., Scott, T. M., Insemi, J. A., Sass, K. J., Novelly, R. A., Kim, J. H., & Spencer, D. D. (1992). Quantitative magnetic resonance imaging in temporal lobe epilepsy: Relationship to neuropathology and neuropsychological function. *Annals of Neurology, 31*, 629–637.

Levin, H. S., & Grossman, R. G. (1976). Storage and retrieval. *Journal of Pediatric Psychology, 1*, 38–42.

Levin, H. S., Benton, A. L., & Grossman, R. G. (1982). *Neurobehavioral consequences of closed head injury*. New York: Oxford University Press.

Levin, H. S., Grossman, R. G., Rose, J. E., & Teasdale, G. (1979). Long-term neuropsychological outcome of closed head injury. *Journal of Neurosurgery, 50*, 412–422.

Loring, D. W., & Papanicolaou, A. C. (1987). Memory assessment in neuropsychology: Theoretical considerations and practical utility. *Journal of Clinical and Experimental Neuropsychology, 9*, 340–358.

Loring, D. W., Lee, G. P., Meador, K. J., Smith, J. R., Martin, R. C., Ackell, A. B., & Flanigin, H. F. (1991). Hippocampal contribution to verbal recent memory following dominant-hemisphere temporal lobectomy. *Journal of Clinical and Experimental Neuropsychology, 13*, 575–586.

Macartney-Filgate, M. S., & Vriezen, E. R. (1988). Intercorrelation of clinical tests of verbal memory. *Archives of Clinical Neuropsychology, 3,* 121–126.

Martin, R. C., Loring, D. W., Meador, K. J., & Lee, G. P. (1988). Differential forgetting in patients with temporal lobe dysfunction. *Archives of Clinical Neuropsychology, 3,* 351–358.

Masur, D. A., Fuld, P. A., Blau, A. D., Crystal, H., & Aronson, M. K. (1990). Predicting development of dementia in the elderly with the Selective Reminding Test. *Journal of Clinical and Experimental Neuropsychology, 12,* 529–538.

Masur, D. M., Fuld, P. A., Blau, A. D., Thal, L. J., Levin, H. S., & Aronson, M. K. (1989). Distinguishing normal and demented elderly with the Selective Reminding Test. *Journal of Clinical and Experimental Neuropsychology, 11,* 615–630.

Miller, H. B., Murphy, D., Paniak, C., & Spackman, L., & LaBonte, M. (1996). Selective Reminding Test: Norms for children ages 9 to 15. Unpublished data.

Morgan, S. F. (1982). Measuring long-term memory, storage and retrieval in children. *Journal of Clinical Neuropsychology, 4,* 77–85.

Paniak, C. E., Shore, D. L., & Rourke, B. P. (1989). Recovery of memory after severe closed head injury: Dissociations in recovery of memory parameters and predictors of outcome. *Journal of Clinical and Experimental Neuropsychology, 11,* 631–644.

Petersen, R. C., Smith, G., Kokmen, E., Ivnik, R. J., & Tangalos, E. G. (1992). Memory function in normal aging. *Neurology, 42,* 396–401.

Ruchinskas, R. A., Brishek, D. K., Crews, W. D., Barth, J. T., Francis, J. P., & Robbins, M. K. (2000). A neuropsychological normative database for lung transplant candidates. *Journal of Clinical Psychology in Medical Settings, 7,* 107–112.

Ruff, R. M., Quayhagen, M., & Light, R. H. (1989). Selective reminding tests: A normative study of verbal learning in adults. *Journal of Clinical and Experimental Neuropsychology, 11,* 539–550.

Sabe, L., Jason, L., Juejati, M., Leiguarda, R., & Strakstein, S. E. (1995). Dissociation between declarative and procedural learning in dementia and depression. *Journal of Clinical and Experimental Neuropsychology, 17,* 841–848.

Said, J. A., Shores, A., Batchelor, J., Thomas, D., et al. (1990). The children's Auditory-Verbal Selective Reminding Test: Equivalence and test-retest reliability of two forms with boys and girls. *Developmental Neuropsychology, 6,* 225–230.

Salinsky, M. C., Storzbach, D., Dodrill, C. B., & Binder, L. M. (2001). Test-retest bias, reliability, and regression equations for neuropsychological measures repeated over a 12-16-week period. *Journal of the International Neuropsychological Society, 7,* 597–605.

Sass, K. J., Spencer, D. D., Kim, J. H., Westerveld, M., Novelly, R. A., & Lencz, T. (1990). Verbal memory impairment correlates with hippocampal pyramidal cell density. *Neurology, 40,* 1694–1697.

Sass, K. J., Westerveld, M., Buchanan, C. P., Spencer, S. S., Kim, J. H., & Spencer, D. D. (1994). Degree of hippocampal neuron loss determines verbal memory decline following left anteromedial temporal lobectomy. *Epilepsia, 35,* 1179–1186.

Scherl, W. F., Krupp, L. B., Christodoulou, C., Morgan, T. M., Hyman, L., Chandler, B., Coyle, P. K., MacAllister, W. S., & Lyme Study Group. (2004). Normative data for the Selective Reminding Test: A random digit dialing sample. *Psychological Reports, 95,* 593–603.

Shear, J. M., & Craft, R. B. (1989). Examination of the concurrent validity of the California Verbal Learning Test. *The Clinical Neuropsychologist, 3,* 162–168.

Sherman, E. M. S., Strauss, E., Spellacy, F., & Hunter, M. (1995). Construct validity of WAIS-R factors: Neuropsychological test correlates in adults referred for possible head injury. *Psychological Assessment, 7,* 440–444.

Sliwinski, M., Buschke, H., Stewart, W. F., Masur, D., & Lipton, R. B. (1997). The effect of dementia risk factors on comparative diagnostic selective reminding norms. *Journal of the International Neuropsychological Society, 3,* 317–326.

Sliwinski, M., Lipton, R., & Buschke, H. (2003). Optimizing cognitive test norms for detection. In R. C. Petersen (Ed.), *Mild cognitive impairment: Aging to Alzheimer's disease* (pp. 89–104). London: Oxford University Press.

Smith, R. L., Goode, K. T., la Marche, J. A., & Boll, T. J. (1995). Selective reminding test short form administration: A comparison of two through twelve trials. *Psychological Assessment, 7,* 177–182.

Snow, J. H., English, R., & Lange, B. (1992). Clinical utility of the Selective Reminding Test—children's version. *Journal of Psychoeducational Assessment, 10,* 153–160.

Stern, Y., Tang, M. X., Jacobs, D. M., Sano, M., Marder, K., Bell, K., Doneief, G., Schofield, P., & Cote, L. (1998). Prospective comparative study of the evolution of probable Alzheimer's disease and Parkinson's disease dementia. *Journal of the International Neuropsychological Society, 4,* 279–284.

Stricks, L., Pittman, J., Jacobs, D. M., Sano, M., & Stern, Y. (1998). Normative data for a brief neuropsychological battery administered to English- and Spanish-speaking community-dwelling elders. *Journal of the International Neuropsychological Society, 4,* 311–318.

Trahan, D. E., & Larrabee, G. J. (1993). Clinical and methodological issues in measuring rate of forgetting with the Verbal Selective Reminding Test. *Psychological Assessment, 5,* 67–71.

Trahan, D. E., & Quintana, J. W. (1990). Analysis of gender effects upon verbal and visual memory performance in adults. *Archives of Clinical Neuropsychology, 5,* 325–334.

Vilkki, J., Servo, A., & Surma-aho, O. (1998). Word list learning and prediction of recall after frontal lobe lesions. *Neuropsychology, 12,* 268–277.

Westerveld, M., Sass, K .J., Sass, A., & Henry, H. G. (1994). Assessment of verbal memory in temporal lobe epilepsy using the Selective Reminding Test: Equivalence and reliability of alternate forms. *Journal of Epilepsy, 7,* 57–63.

Wiederholt, W. C., Cahn, D., Butters, N. M., Salmon, D. P., Kritz-Silverstein, D., & Barrett-Connor, E. (1993). Effects of age, gender, and education on selected neuropsychological tests in an elderly community cohort. *Journal of the American Geriatrics Society, 41,* 639–647.

California Verbal Learning Test-II (CVLT-II)

PURPOSE

The purpose of the California Verbal Learning Test-II (CVLT-II) is to measure verbal learning and memory using a multiple-trial list-learning task.

SOURCE

The test (software, manual, 25 Standard Record Forms, 1 Alternate Record Form and 25 Short Record Forms) can be ordered from The Psychological Corporation, 19500 Bulverde Road, San Antonio, TX 78259, 1-800-211-8378 (http://www.harcourtassessment.com) at a cost of $499 US.

AGE RANGE

The test can be given to individuals aged 16 to 89 years.

DESCRIPTION

As the authors (Delis et al., 2000) note, there are many tests available that assess the amount of verbal material remembered; however, few also measure how the information is learned and retrieved. The original version (Delis et al., 1987) was developed using this process-oriented approach and proved very popular because of its ability to parse multiple components of learning and memory and to characterize distinct memory profiles associated with different disorders. The CVLT was revised to accommodate new developments in the field and concerns raised about the first edition. The revised version, the CVLT-II, includes new word lists that are easier to understand than those in the first edition, a larger normative database, new measures to analyze aspects of learning and memory (see also Stricker et al., 2002), an optional forced-choice recognition task, alternate and short forms, and updated scoring software.

The Standard Form of the CVLT-II assesses both recall and recognition of two word lists over immediate and delayed memory trials. In the first five trials, the patient is asked to recall words from List A immediately after presentation of the list. List A is composed of 16 words, four from each of four semantic categories (furniture, vegetables, ways of traveling, and animals). Words from the same semantic category are never presented consecutively. A 16-word interference list (List B, which includes vegetables and animals and introduces two additional categories: musical instruments and parts of a house) is then presented for one trial, followed by short-delay free-recall and short-delay cued-recall trials of List A. A 20-min delay occurs next, during which nonverbal testing takes place. After the nonverbal testing, long-delay free-recall, long-delay cued-recall, and yes/no recognition trials of list A are administered. Finally, an optional forced-choice recognition trail is given about 10 min after the yes/no recognition trial. An Alternate Form is also available.

The CVLT-II Short Form (CVLT-SF) is designed for patients with severe cognitive dysfunction or as a screening instrument for memory impairment. Like the long form, it requires the person to learn and remember a list of words under various testing conditions, including free recall, cued recall, and recognition. It differs from the CVLT-II in several ways: a shorter list (9 words instead of 16), only one list of words instead of two, shorter delay intervals (10 and 5 min), and fewer recall trials (e.g., four instead of five learning trials).

ADMINISTRATION

See *Source*. The examiner reads the word list (at a rate slightly slower than 1 second per word) and records the patient's oral responses verbatim in the order in which they are given. The test should be given in one session.

ADMINISTRATION TIME

For the Standard version, the presentation and response recording time is about 20 min. Including the 20- and 10-min delay intervals, about 50 min is needed in total.

SCORING

Hand-scoring of the CVLT-II is possible. However, the CVLT-II (Standard Form) yields raw scores and standardized scores for more than 50 learning and memory variables. The depth of analysis provided by the software is superior and faster to that which can be computed practically by hand. The authors recommend that the test results be scored using the CVLT-II scoring software. About 10 to 15 min is required to score the CVLT-II using the software.

The software can be used to score the Standard Form, the Alternate Form, or the Short Form. It computes all raw and standardized scores, corrected for the examinee's age and gender. The examiner can choose to print one or any combination of three different reports: the Core Report, the Expanded Report, or the Research Report. The Core Report provides raw and standardized scores for 27 of the most commonly used CVLT-II measures. The Expanded Report generates the same information plus raw and standardized scores for 66 normed variables of the CVLT-II (51 for the Short Form), offering more in-depth analysis of an individual's verbal learning and memory performance. Finally, the Research Report provides raw scores for more than 260 non-normed variables that may be useful to researchers.

The following parameters are quantified:

- Levels of total recall and recognition on all trials
- Learning strategies (e.g., semantic clustering, serial clustering, subjective clustering)
- Primacy-recency effects in recall
- Rate of new learning per trial

- Consistency of item recall across trials
- Degree of vulnerability to proactive and retroactive interference
- Retention of information over short and longer delays
- Enhancement of recall performance by category cueing and recognition testing
- Breakdown of recognition performance (discriminability and response bias) derived from signal-detection theory
- Indices reflecting the relative integrity of encoding, storage, and retrieval processes
- Analysis of intrusion-error types in recall (e.g., semantically related, semantically unrelated, across-list intrusions)
- Repetition errors in recall
- Analysis of false-positive types in recognition testing
- Indices of test-taking effort

DEMOGRAPHIC EFFECTS

Age

According to the test manual, test scores are affected by age ($r = -.51$), with performance declining with advancing age.

Gender

As in the previous edition of the test, gender also affects most scores, with women tending to score an average of 5 words more than men across the five learning trials of List A. For some variables (e.g., Forced-Choice Recognition Accuracy), gender differences are not significant.

Education/IQ

Education also correlates with memory performance ($r = .29$ for CVLT-II Total). As might be expected, IQ shows a moderate relationship with CVLT-II performance (e.g., $r = .40$ between FSIQ and Trials 1–5 Correct).

Relative Contributions

According to the test authors, age accounts for 25.9% of the variance, followed by gender (5.1%), and education (4.5%). Race has a negligible impact, explaining 0.3% of the variance. The authors decided to correct for age and gender but not to stratify by education, because doing so would have resulted in cell sizes as low as 10 subjects per cell for some age groups.

NORMATIVE DATA

Standardization Sample

The sample consisted of 1087 normal volunteers, ranging in age from 16 to 89 years and in education from less than 9 to

Table 10–22 Characteristics of the CVLT-II Test Normative Sample

Number	1087
Age (years)	16 to 89[a]
Geographic location (%)	
California	65
Michigan	30
Eastern Seaboard—USA	5
Sample type	Recruited to match the 1999 U.S. Census in terms of race/ethnicity, education, and region
Education	<9 years: 6.5%, 9–11 years: 11.2%, 12 years: 34.15%, 13–15 years: 27.8%, >16 years: 20.3%
Gender	
Men	522
Women	565
Race/Ethnicity (approx. %)	
Caucasian	75
African American	11
Hispanic	9
Other	5
Screening	Screened for self-reported neurologic, psychiatric, or debilitating medical disorder

[a]Broken down into seven age groups: 16–19 ($n = 150$), 20–29 ($n = 190$), 30–44 ($n = 200$), 45–59 ($n = 150$), 60–69 ($n = 145$), 70–79 ($n = 145$), and 80–89 years ($n = 107$).

more than 16 years, matched to 1999 US Census data in terms of race/ethnicity, education, and region (see Table 10–22).

Norms were developed by converting raw scores on the List A Trials 1–5 Total measure to age- and gender-corrected T scores, with a mean of 50 and a standard deviation of 10. Raw scores on the other CVLT-II measures varied in the extent to which they reflected normal distributions, so they were converted to age- and gender-corrected z scores, with a mean of 0 and a standard deviation of 1. The range of z scores is +5 to −5, reported in increments of 0.5.

For most of the CVLT-II z scores, higher values indicate better performance; however, there are exceptions, including the various error measures (i.e., repetitions, intrusions, and false positives) and the recency-recall index, for which higher z scores reflect greater deficits. For a few variables, higher positive z scores tend to reflect deficient performances but not always (e.g., serial clustering index).

The forced-choice recognition variable was designed to yield a high ceiling effect, precluding z-score transformation. For this reason, normative results are reported in frequency and cumulative frequency values by age only. In addition, three intrusion error types (non-category, across-list, and synonym/subordinate) were rare in the normative sample and therefore were also normed in terms of frequency and cumulative-frequency values by age only.

Raw scores on the Alternate Form were calibrated to the Standard Form using linear equating. The equating study was based on a sample of 288 nonclinical adults (106 men, 182 women) who were given both forms in counterbalanced order. Raw scores on the Short Form were calibrated to raw scores on the Standard Form using equipercentile equating due to skewness of some variables on the Short Form. This equating study was based on a sample of 278 subjects who were given both forms in counterbalanced order.

RELIABILITY

Internal Consistency

The authors note that tests of recall ability pose special difficulties for the estimation of internal consistency because of problems with item interdependence within and between trials. First, because of limitations in learning and memory capacity, recall of any one word on a trial decreases the likelihood that other items will be recalled on that same trial. Second, the process of recalling a word on one trial tends to increase the probability that the same word will be recalled on subsequent trials. Accordingly, the authors used three approaches to estimate the internal consistency for the CVLT-II (see test manual).

The first approach analyzed total trial scores by splitting the immediate recall trials (trials 1 + 3 versus trials 2 + 4, and trials 2 + 4 versus trials 3 + 5) and then applying the Spearman-Brown formula to the average of these correlations, with a lengthening factor of 2.5. Split-half reliability was very high for the total normative sample ($r = .94$), as well as for a mixed clinical sample ($r = .96$). The second method involved examination of the subjects' performance in the four categories of words on List A across the five immediate-recall trials. Coefficient alphas calculated on word category scores across trials were high for the standardization sample ($r = .82$) and for the mixed clinical sample ($r = .83$). The third approach involved examining the number of times each of the 16 words on List A were recalled across the five immediate-recall trials. Reliability (split-half) was .79 for the standardization sample and .83 for the clinical sample. Similar values were obtained when coefficient alphas were computed. In short, these three approaches suggest that internal consistency is high for the five immediate-recall trials.

Test-Retest Reliability and Practice Effect

According to the test authors (see manual), the stability of scores was assessed by giving the Standard Form of the CVLT-II twice to a sample of 78 subjects (health status not reported), ranging in age from 16 to 88 years (mean = 46.9 years). The median retest interval was 21 days (range 9–49 days). As shown in Table 10–23, reliability coefficients for some of the measures, in particular those measuring overall level of achievement (e.g., Total Trials 1–5, Short- and Long-Delay Free Recall, Total Recognition Discrimination) are high; however, those measur-

Table 10–23 CVLT-II Test-Retest Correlations

Magnitude of Coefficient	Measure
Very high ($\geq$.90)	—
High (.80 to .89)	Trial 4 Correct
	Trials 1–5 Correct
	Short Delay Free Recall Correct
	Long Delay Free Recall Correct
	Total Recognition Discrimination
Adequate (.70 to .79)	Trial 5 Correct
	Semantic Clustering (Chance-Adjusted) Trials 1–5
	Long-Delay Yes/No Recognition Hits
	Long-Delay Yes/No Recognition False Positives
Marginal (.60 to .69)	Trial 2 Correct
	Trial B Correct
	Total Intrusions (all recall trials, all types)
Low ($\leq$.59)	Trial 1 Correct
	Trial 3 Correct
	Total Learning Slope, Trials 1–5
	Percent Recall Primacy Region
	Percent Recall Middle Region
	Percent Recall Recency Region
	Total Repetitions (all recall trials)
	Total Response Bias

Source: Adapted from Delis et al., 2000.

ing process/strategy aspects (e.g., Percent Recall, Total Learning Slope, Trial 1, Total Repetitions) are poor. On average, subjects recalled about 8 more words across the five learning trials on retesting. Whether these patterns apply equally for all age groups is not reported. Nor are data reported for the Short Form.

Alternate Form Reliability

Both the Standard Form and the Alternate Form were given to 288 nonclinical adults (106 men, 182 women; age $M = 47.77$, $SD = 23.51$). The median interval between administrations was 21 days (range, 0–77 days). A total of 155 subjects received the Standard Form first, followed by the Alternate Form; the remainder were given the tests in the reverse order. Reliability coefficients were adequate for the key CVLT-II overall achievement variables (e.g., List A Trials 1–5 Total, Short- and Long-Delay Free Recall and Recognition Discriminability). Coefficients were low for variables that assess efficiency of learning characteristics and error types (see Table 10–24). The authors suggest that exposure to the first form may alert the patients to other, potentially more efficient strategies at retest. Mean raw scores between the two forms were, however, quite similar and there were no order effects, suggesting that performance changed in unsystematic ways across subjects. That is, some individuals may have

Table 10–24 CVLT-II Alternate Form Reliability

Magnitude of Coefficient	Measure
Very High (≥.90)	—
High (.80 to .89)	—
Adequate (.70 to .79)	Trial 3 Correct
	Trial 4 Correct
	Trial 5 Correct
	Trials 1–5 Correct
	Short-Delay Free Recall Correct
	Long-Delay Free Recall Correct
Marginal (.60 to .69)	Trial 2 Correct
	Semantic Clustering (Chance-Adjusted) Trials 1–5
	Long Delay Yes/No Recognition Hits
	Forced-Choice Recognition Percent Total Accuracy
Low (≤.59)	Trial 1 Correct
	Trial B Correct
	Serial Clustering forward (Chance-Adjusted) Trials 1—5
	Percent Recall Primacy Region
	Percent Recall Middle Region
	Percent Recall Recency Region
	Total Intrusions (all recall trials, all types)
	Total Repetitions (all recall trials)
	Long-Delay Yes/No Recognition Hits
	Total Response Bias

Source: Adapted from Delis et al., 2000.

discovered an optimal strategy, but others improved less, or may even have deteriorated if a sub-optimal strategy was attempted.

Short-Form

Reliability estimates of this form are not reported.

VALIDITY

Relationship to CVLT

The CVLT-II correlates well with its predecessor. According to the test authors (see manual), a group of 62 nonclinical adults were given the CVLT and the CVLT-II in counterbalanced order, with 35 people receiving the CVLT first, and 27 receiving the CVLT-II first. The median interval between administrations was 7 days (range, 0–11 days). Correlation coefficients between variables ranged from marginal (Free-Recall Intrusions) to high (Long-Delay Yes/No Recognition False Positives). Most of the coefficients were adequate to high. The correlation for Total Recall of Trials 1–5 was .76.

The CVLT normative data were too stringent, probably because of the high level of education of the sample. The CVLT-II normative sample is more representative of the educational level of the U.S. population, resulting in less stringent norms and more accurate classification of an individual's performance (Delis et al., 2000). However, differences in CVLT and CVLT-II raw scores are negligible; therefore, the authors suggest that the best method for comparing a person's relative performance on the two tasks is to examine changes in raw scores rather than in standardized scores.

Factor Analysis

When 19 scores on the test were factor analyzed in the standardization sample, six factors emerged (Delis et al., 2000), similar to what was found in normal individuals for the first edition of the CVLT (Spreen & Strauss, 1998). The six factors were labeled general verbal learning (consisting of multiple measures of the level of immediate and delayed recall and recognition), response discrimination (consisting of intrusion errors and recognition response bias), primacy-recency effects, organization strategies (consisting of semantic and serial clustering), recall efficiency (consisting of repetition errors and subjective clustering), and acquisition rate (total learning slope).

A second exploratory factor analysis, carried out on a mixed clinical sample of 128 individuals, yielded roughly similar results. Only 16 of the CVLT-II variables were included. This analysis yielded a five-factor solution, similar to what was reported for the CVLT. The five-factor solution for the clinical sample contained components representing general verbal learning, response discrimination, recall efficiency, organizational strategies, and primacy-recency effects.

Clinical Studies

At this time, there have been few studies of the CVLT-II with clinical populations. The CVLT-II has been used to examine memory performance in patients with focal frontal lesions (Baldo et al., 2002). In comparison to age- and education-matched controls, such patients showed poorer overall recall, an increased tendency to make intrusions, reduced semantic clustering, and impaired yes/no recognition but normal forced-choice recognition. Further analysis of the error rates in the yes/no recognition task revealed that patients with focal frontal lesions were most likely to mistakenly endorse two types of distractors: semantically related words and words from the interference list. The findings were interpreted as being consistent with the role of the frontal lobes in the selection of relevant activations and the inhibition of irrelevant activations. As Baldo et al. (2002) noted, however, in the absence of a neurological control group, the specificity of their findings to frontal dysfunction alone cannot be determined.

The relation between mood and test performance was recently examined. Self-reported depression and anxiety had only a small impact on CVLT-II scores (O'Jile et al., 2005).

Malingering

Moore and Donders (2004) examined patients referred to a rehabilitation facility for traumatic brain injury and found the Forced Choice trial of the CVLT-II and the TOMM to be equally sensitive to invalid test performance. There was strong but not perfect agreement between the two instruments. Given the nonredundancy of the information obtained from these instruments, clinicians should not rely solely on the results of a single measure.

There is evidence that financial compensation-seeking and a prior psychiatric history increase the risk of invalid test performance on the CVLT-II (Moore & Donders, 2004). Individuals with long-standing emotional difficulties may be more likely to make reattribution errors, associated with underestimation of their premorbid problems and selective augmentation of cognitive and somatic symptoms; this may be the result of a perception that dysfunction caused by physical trauma is more socially acceptable (Moore & Donders, 2004).

COMMENT

The CVLT/CVLT-II is among the top three memory assessment instruments used by neuropsychologists (Rabin et al., 2005). The original version generated a wealth of research that has both theoretical and clinical relevance (see test manual for an excellent review of literature bearing on the CVLT). The new CVLT-II is also likely to play a prominent role in neuropsychology, and preliminary work (Baldo et al., 2002) suggests that it too will prove valuable in characterizing the unique learning and memory profiles of various neurological and psychiatric disorders.

The normative sample for the CVLT-II is clearly superior to that of the first edition: it is large (1087 adults) and is representative of the U.S. population. However, education and IQ do affect test scores, and age- and education/IQ-corrected normative data are needed to more accurately interpret an individual's performance. Further, clinical interpretation is hindered by the lack of actuarial data (e.g., base rates of specific discrepancies) to facilitate comparisons of variables (e.g., difference between number of words recalled on Trial 1 of List A and List B). Donders (1999) raised this issue with respect to the CVLT-C (children's version).

Interpretation of some of the test scores can be confusing. In most cases, a positive z score indicates intact performance; however, in other cases (e.g., error scores), higher z scores reflect greater deficits.

In contrast to other verbal memory tests, the authors have thoroughly investigated the internal consistency of the CVLT-II and found it to be excellent. Test-retest and alternate form reliability estimates appear reasonable for the various measures tapping overall level of achievement (e.g., Trials 1–5 Correct, Short- and Long-Delay Free Recall). However, reliability coefficients tend to be poor for process-oriented variables, suggesting that users should be cautious in drawing inferences regarding the strategic aspects of an individual's learning and memory abilities. Further, given the lack of information regarding reliability or validity for the Short Form, this version should be regarded as experimental at present.

Finally, it is important to bear in mind that the CVLT-II, although related conceptually and structurally to its predecessor, is a new measure. Therefore, clinicians cannot rely on algorithms derived from the CVLT to make inferences about a patient's performance on the CVLT-II.

REFERENCES

Baldo, J. V., Delis, D., Kramer, J., & Shimamura, A. P. (2002). Memory performance on the California Verbal Learning Test-II: Findings from patients with focal frontal lesions. *Journal of the International Neuropsychological Society, 8,* 539–546.

Delis, D. C., Kramer, J. H., Kaplan, E., & Ober, B. A. (1987). *California Verbal Learning Test.* San Antonio, Tex.: The Psychological Corporation.

Delis, D. C., Kramer, J. H., Kaplan, E., & Ober, B. A. (2000). *California Verbal Learning Test— Second Edition, Adult Version.* San Antonio, TX: The Psychological Corporation.

Donders, J. (1999). Performance discrepancies on the California Verbal Learning Test—Children's Version in the standardization sample. *Journal of the International Neuropsychological Society, 5,* 26–31.

Moore, B. A., & Donders, J. (2004). Predictors of invalid neuropsychological test performance after traumatic brain injury. *Brain Injury, 18,* 975–984.

O'Jile, J. R., Schrimsher, G. W., & O'Bryant, S. E. (2005). The relation of self-report of mood and anxiety to CVLT-C, CVLT, and CVLT-2 in a psychiatric sample. *Archives of Clinical Neuropsychology, 20,* 547–553.

Rabin, L. A., Barr, W. B., & Burton, L. A. (2005). Assessment practices of clinical neuropsychologists in the United States and Canada: A survey of INS, NAN, and APA Division 40 members. *Archives of Clinical Neuropsychology, 20,* 33–65.

Spreen, O., & Strauss, E. (1998). *A compendium of neuropsychological tests: Administration, norms and commentary.* New York: Oxford University Press.

Stricker, J. L., Brown, G. G., Wixted, J., Baldo, J. V., & Delis, D. C. (2002). New semantic and serial clustering indices for the California Verbal Learning Test-Second Edition: Background, rationale, and formulae. *Journal of the International Neuropsychological Society, 8,* 425–435.

California Verbal Learning Test—Children's Version (CVLT-C)

PURPOSE

The California Verbal Learning Test—Children's Version (CVLT-C) measures verbal learning and memory using a multiple-trial list-learning paradigm.

SOURCE

The test (manual and 25 Record Forms) can be ordered from The Psychological Corporation (www.harcourtassessment.com) at a cost of $260 US. Scoring software is also available (CVLT-C Scoring Assistant with Report Writer, Version 2.0) at a cost of $540 US. A Spanish version has also been developed (Rosselli et al., 2001).

AGE RANGE

The test can be given to individuals aged 5 years to 16 years, 11 months. Additional norms are also available for 4-year-olds (Goodman et al., 1999; see later discussion).

DESCRIPTION

Background and Overview

As Delis et al. (2000) noted, many tests assess the amount of verbal material remembered; however, few measure *how* the information is learned and retrieved. The original CVLT (Delis et al. 1987, 2000) was developed to measure memory and learning in adults using a process-oriented approach. It proved popular because of its ability to parse multiple components of learning and memory and to identify distinct memory profiles associated with different clinical disorders. The CVLT-C (Delis et al., 1994) was subsequently developed for use in children; it also measures quantitative (i.e., performance level) and qualitative (i.e., strategy use) aspects of learning and memory. In addition, like its predecessor, it is designed to assess memory within the context of an "everyday memory task" (Delis et al., 1994, p. 1) consisting of remembering items from a shopping list. The CVLT-C uses words from highly imageable, familiar categories such as fruits, clothing, and toys.

Test Paradigm

The CVLT-C requires the examinee to recall two word lists over immediate and delayed memory trials. In the first five trials, the patient is asked to recall words from List A (the "Monday" list). List A includes 15 words—five each from three semantic categories: fruit, clothing, and toys. A second 15-word interference list is then introduced (List B or "Tuesday" list), which must be recalled once. List B includes new words from a category introduced in List A (fruits), in addition to words from two new categories with different degrees of

semantic overlap—furniture, a nonshared category, and sweets, a category that is partially related to fruits through the superordinate "food" category. Words from List A and B were chosen to be of equal word-frequency value in English and of equivalent ranking as exemplars within a semantic category (see p. 77 of the manual for details). List B recall is immediately followed by short-delay free-recall and short-delay cued-recall trials of List A. A 20-min delay occurs next, during which unrelated, noninterfering tasks take place (i.e., nonverbal testing). Long-delay free-recall, long-delay cued-recall, and yes/no recognition trials of List A are then administered. CVLT-C variable definitions are shown in Table 10–25.

Learning Strategy Variables

The test allows a detailed examination of learning strategy. This includes scores for semantic clustering, defined as the ability to semantically organize information during recall. This capacity exhibits developmental trends as children increasingly use active strategies to increase recall with age. In contrast, a less effective strategy, serial clustering (recalling words in the same order in which they were presented) is usually associated with poorer recall but may also reflect an attempt by the subject to make the task more challenging. Serial clustering can therefore be found in both low and high memory scorers. Primacy/recency recall reflects the extent to which words are recalled from the beginning or the end of the list rather than from the middle; words in the middle of the list are the most difficult to recall due to proactive interference from earlier items in the list and retroactive interference from later items in the list. According to the authors, because these words are assumed to be in long-term storage, average to high primacy and middle region performance reflect strong learning skills. The easiest words to remember are those from the last part of the list, because they can be repeated from short-term memory without being encoded into long-term memory. Therefore, individuals with memory problems may show their best performance on the recency region of the word list (Delis et al., 1994).

The learning slope is also of interest; this score reflects the average number of new words recalled per learning trial. Different clinical populations may perform differently on this variable, depending on whether their primary problem is one of learning (normal Trial 1 score but flat learning curve), intact learning despite poor initial encoding (poor Trial 1 performance but normal learning curve), or inability to sustain focus over trials (good recall on initial trials but poor recall on later trials—an "inverted V pattern"; Delis et al., 1994). The first pattern is found, for example, in children with Williams syndrome, the second in children with Down syndrome or fetal alcohol syndrome, and the third pattern in those with attention-deficit hyperactivity disorder (ADHD; see p. 37 of manual for discussion and references; also see *Validity*). The

Table 10–25 CVLT-C Variable Definitions

Variable	
List A Total	Total number of words recalled across the five learning trials
List A1	Number of words recalled from the first trial
List A5	Number of words recalled from the fifth trial
List B	Number of words recalled from the interference list (List B)
List A Short-Delay Free Recall	Number of words recalled from List A immediately after exposure to the interference trial (List B)
List A Short-Delay Cued Recall	Number of words recalled from List A immediately after exposure to the interference trial (List B), with semantic cueing
List A Long-Delay Free Recall	Number of words recalled from List A after the long delay (20 min)
List A Long-Delay Cued Recall	Number of words recalled from List A after the long delay (20 min), with semantic cueing
Semantic Clustering	Number of word pairs recalled in a semantic cluster (i.e., consecutive words from the same semantic category), which reflects the extent to which the child has actively imposed a semantic organization on the word list
Serial Clustering	Number of word pairs recalled in a serial cluster (i.e., in the same order in which they were presented)
Primacy %[a]	Percentage of words correctly recalled from the beginning of List A
Middle %[a]	Percentage of words correctly recalled from the middle of List A
Recency %[a]	Percentage of words correctly recalled from the end of List A
Learning Slope	Average number of new words learned per trial (e.g., a score of 1 means that the child learned approximately one new word per trial)
Consistency %	Percentage of words recalled once on each of the four learning trials that were also recalled on the very next trial; reflects the consistency of learning over trials
Perseverations	Number of correct words repeated within a trial
Free Intrusions	Number of extra-list intrusions on all the free-recall trials
Cued Intrusions	Number of extra-list intrusions on all the cued-recall trials
Total Intrusions	Number of extra-list intrusions made on all recall trials (free and cued)
Recognition Hits	Total number of words identified as belonging to List A on recognition testing (yes/no format)
Discriminability	Accuracy of distinguishing target from distracter words on recognition testing
False Positives	Number of words incorrectly identified as List A targets during recognition testing
Response Bias	Response style during recognition testing, with positive scores indicating a liberal response bias (i.e., tendency to identify words as correct)

[a]Primacy and Recency regions on the CVLT-C are defined as the first and last four words of the list, respectively, and the Middle region is the middle seven words.

learning slope therefore has potential for helping characterize specific memory problems that would not be evident by examination of total recall summary scores alone. Other process variables, such as recall consistency, may also be differentially affected in populations with difficulty sustaining a consistent learning strategy over trials (e.g., ADHD). For an extended discussion of CVLT-C scores and their interpretation, see pages 32 to 37 in the test manual.

ADMINISTRATION

Standard Version

See *Source.* Instructions are printed on the record form and are detailed in the manual. The examiner reads the word list at a rate of one word per second, in an even tone of voice, and records the examinee's oral responses verbatim, in the order in which they are given. The test should be given in one uninterrupted session. Additionally, the examiner should not give any feedback to the child, including whether answers were correct or whether any responses have already been provided. A single prompt is given after the child has given his last response to ensure that he or she has performed to the best of his ability (i.e., "See if you can think of any more").

Modified Spanish Version

Tables 10–26 and 10–27 show the stimuli for a modified Spanish version, developed by Rosselli et al. (2001). Note that this version does not employ an interference trial. Rather, after presentation of the five recall trials and a 20-min delay, cued-recall and free recall trials are conducted, followed by a 45-word recognition trial.

APPROXIMATE TIME FOR ADMINISTRATION

The test takes 15 to 20 min. An additional 20 min must be provided to accommodate the delayed-recall interval, during which nonverbal, unrelated tasks are given.

SCORING

Scoring the CVLT-C

Hand-scoring of the CVLT-C is possible using tables provided in the manual. However, because of the sheer number of CVLT-C scores and the depth of analysis provided by the software, use of the CVLT-C scoring software is recommended over hand scoring. About 10 min is required to computer-score the CVLT-C.

Table 10–26 Modified Spanish CVLT-C "Monday" List

Bananos	Lápices
Camisas	Duraznos
Dados	Pelotas
Abrigos	Sombreros
Uvas	Fresas
Muñecas	Cinturones
Melones	Patines
Pantalones	

Note: This version does not use an interference trial.

Source: From Rosselli et al., 2001, p. 359. Reproduced by permission. Copyright 2001 by Lawrence Erlbaum Associates, Publishers. Mahwah, NJ. All rights reserved.

Table 10–27 Modified Spanish CVLT-C Recognition Words

Pantalones	Revistas
Anteojos	Muñecas
Mesas	Mangos
Lápices	Camisas
Blusas	Helados
Ciruelas	Cunas
Escobas	Naranjas
Bananos	Abrigos
Talones	Fresas
Patines	Pelotas
Galletas	Piñas
Manzanas	Títeres
Escritorios	Rosas
Presas	Peras
Llaves	Tapices
Sombreros	Dados
Uvas	Pasteles
Dulces	Lámparas
Raquetas	Peinillas
Alfombras	Duraznos
Melones	Cinturones
Cojines	Vestidos
	Relojes

Source: From Rosselli et al., 2001, p. 372. Reproduced by permission. Copyright 2001 by Lawrence Erlbaum Associates, Publishers. Mahwah, NJ. All rights reserved.

Scores

The CVLT-C provides over 20 normed-based scores (see Table 10–25 for definitions). The Total Recall score (i.e., words recalled from List A Trials 1–5) is presented as a T score ($M = 50$, $SD = 10$) with a range of 20 to 80. All other scores are presented as z scores ($M = 0$, $SD = 1$), with a range of −5 to +5, provided in increments of 0.50.

Interpretation

For most of the CVLT-C z scores, higher values indicate better performance; however, there are exceptions, including the various error measures (i.e., repetitions, intrusions, and false positives) and the recency-recall index, for which higher z scores reflect greater deficits. For a few variables (e.g., serial clustering index), higher positive z scores tend to reflect deficient performance, but not in every case (see *Description* and *Demographic Effects*).

Contrast Variables

Donders (1999b) provided data on four additional contrast variables that can be computed for the CVLT-C: (a) Proactive Interference, (b) Retroactive Interference, (c) Rapid Forgetting, and (d) Retrieval Problems. These are presented in Figure 10–20.

Proactive Interference = List B Recall — List A Trial 1 Recall

Retroactive Interference = List A Short-Delay Free Recall — List A Trial 5

Rapid Forgetting = List A Long-Delay Free Recall — List A Short-Delay Free Recall

Retrieval Problems = Discriminability — List A Long-Delay Free Recall

DEMOGRAPHIC EFFECTS

Age

There are clear developmental trends for learning on the CVLT-C. For instance, teenagers in the normative sample showed steeper learning curves than preadolescents, who in turn had steeper learning curves than younger children. Developmental trends are also observed for a number of other variables, including recall consistency and performance scores such as immediate recall (Trial 1, Trial 5, and Total Recall).

The ability to use semantic clustering as a learning strategy usually emerges between 9 and 12 years of age (see test manual for details). In the normative sample, semantic clustering showed a developmental curve across age (Delis et al., 1994). In contrast, serial clustering (i.e., remembering words in the order in which they were presented), a strategy that is usually less effective, was higher in the adolescents in the normative group than at other ages, which may reflect an attempt to make the task more challenging (Delis et al., 1994). In the normative sample, the youngest age group recalled fewer words from the middle region of the list than the other two age groups, but they recalled a higher number of words from the primacy region. Younger children also recalled more words from the recency region of the list than the adolescents (Delis et al., 1994). CVLT-C perseverations displays minimal improvement with age, whereas improvements in intrusions and false-positive rates are found with age (Beebe et al., 2000; Delis et al., 1994).

Gender

According to the authors, gender effects were minimal in the standardization sample (Delis et al., 1994). Likewise, no gender effects were found in a sample of 4-year-olds (Goodman et al., 1999). However, gender effects have been reported by others in the standardization sample (Kramer et al., 1997), in clinical groups such as ADHD patients (Cutting et al., 2003), and in some age groups such as adolescents, where girls outperformed boys (e.g., Beebe et al., 2000). Gender explains an additional 5% to 14% of variance in CVLT-C performance among children with head injury (Donders & Hoffman, 2002; Hoffman et al., 2000).

Education

As would be expected, parental education levels are linked to children's learning scores. Donders (1999a) found that more than 30% of children in the normative sample with below-average performance were from families with less than 12 years of parental education, whereas approximately 22% of the highest-performing children came from families with a college education.

IQ

Limited association with IQ subtests such as Block Design or Vocabulary have been reported (Beebe et al., 2000; see *Validity*).

NORMATIVE DATA

Standardization Sample

The normative sample consists of 920 children in 12 age groups, ranging in age from 5 years to 16 years 11 months. Norms were stratified based on 1988 U.S. Census data. Demographic information for the normative group is provided in Table 10–28.

Additional norms for 4-year-olds are provided by Goodman et al. (1999). These are shown in Table 10–29. The sample included 80 children (40 girls and 40 boys). Each month in the 4-year age range was represented, and approximately 14% of subjects were non-Caucasian or of mixed ethnicity; the mean Hollingshead score was 50.7. All children were screened via maternal questionnaire. Overall, a pattern of performance was obtained similar to that found in children from the CVLT-C normative sample. However, some differences were found. For example, 4-year-olds made a higher number of extra-list intrusions relative to correct responses on cued but not free recall. They also endorsed approximately one third of distracter items on recognition testing, even though they correctly identified more words than on free or cued recall

Table 10–28 Characteristics of the CVLT-C Normative Sample

Sample type	National, stratified random sample[a]
Number	920
Age	5 to 16 years 11 months[b]
Geographic location	Proportional representation from public and private schools in the western, north central, northeast, and southern USA
Years of education, parental (%)	
≤11	14.1%
12	34.8%
13–15	28.8%
≥16	22.3%
Gender	
Boys	461
Girls	459
Race/Ethnicity (%)	
White	69.7%
African American	14.7%
Hispanic	11.9%
Other	3.7%
Screening	English fluency; children receiving special education were not excluded (7% of the sample); 5% of sample was in gifted programs.

[a]Stratified according to 1988 U.S. Census data.
[b]Provided in the form of 12 one-year age bands, with 70 to 80 children per age band.

Table 10–29 Normative Data for 4-Year-Olds on the CVLT-C

Variable	Mean	SD	Median
List A Total	24.24	9.69	23.0
List A Trial 1	3.59	1.85	4.0
List A Trial 5	5.16	2.81	4.5
List B	2.98	2.01	3.0
List A Short-Delay Free Recall	3.13	2.68	3.0
List A Short-Delay Cued Recall	3.83	2.28	4.0
List A Long-Delay Free Recall	3.46	2.73	3.0
List A Long-Delay Cued Recall	3.41	2.44	3.0
Semantic Cluster	1.39	0.58	1.4
Serial Cluster	1.56	1.72	1.2
Primacy	29.08	12.68	28.0
Middle	37.84	13.93	38.5
Recency	33.05	14.65	30.0
Slope	0.37	0.69	0.35
Consistency	61.06	19.95	62.5
Perseverations	6.58	7.20	5.0
Free Intrusions	14.41	21.79	7.0
Cued Intrusions	12.74	10.69	11.5
Total Intrusions	27.15	29.08	19.0
Recognition Hits	10.04	4.39	12.0
Discriminability	63.56	17.59	64.44
False Positives	11.44	9.01	9.5
Response Bias	0.27	0.60	0.44

Source: From Goodman et al., 1999. Reprinted with the kind permission of Psychology Press.

trials. However, according to the authors, the children did not have a strong "yes" bias; their discriminability index of 63.6% indicated that they were not responding at chance levels (50%). Extra-list intrusion errors were much more common than perseverations. Notably, four children in the group made an extremely high number of intrusions (>100). Compared to free recall trials, in which correct responses were more common than intrusions, 4-year-olds made more extra-list intrusions than correct responses on the cued-recall trials. This tendency was found to decline sharply with age. Semantic and serial cluster scores were slightly above chance levels, consistent with developmental trends in strategy use.

Score Derivations/Conversions

For the Total Recall score, standardized scores were derived from normative data based on cumulative frequency of raw scores per age, normalization of distributions, derivation of standard scores for each age, and elimination of minor irregularities by smoothing. For the remaining scores, regression techniques were used (see Delis et al., 1994, p. 83, for details).

CVLT-C/Children's Category Test (CCT) Discrepancies

The CVLT-C is conormed with the Children's Category Test (CCT; Boll, 1993). Although both tasks involve learning, the CVLT-C is verbal and involves learning by repetition, whereas the CCT is nonverbal and involves learning by explicit feedback (Donders, 1998). Comparison between scores on the two tasks can therefore be of clinical interest. Donders (1998) provides tables including the magnitude of differences required between the two tests for statistical significance, as well as cumulative percentages of the standardization sample for CVLT-C/CCT discrepancies. These are presented in Tables 10–30 and 10–31, respectively. Large discrepancies are uncommon in the standardization sample. Discrepancies of more than 18 T-score points in children aged 5 to 8 years, and more than 16 T-score points in children 9 to 16 years of age, may be of clinical significance.

Contrast Variables

Donders (1999b) provided data on four contrast variables that can be computed for the CVLT-C: (a) Proactive Interference, (b) Retroactive Interference, (c) Rapid Forgetting, and (d) Retrieval Problems. Computational formulas for these variables are provided in Figure 10–20. Tables 10–32 and 10–33 show base rates of these specific CVLT-C contrast variables based on data from the standardization sample and the level of discrepancy required for statistical significance, as provided by Donders (1999b).

The direction of the difference is important in determining the presence of an effect on these variables: Proactive Interference, Retroactive Interference, and Rapid Forgetting must be negative, but Retrieval Problems must be positive to be of clinical significance. Donders (1999b) provided a simple rule

Table 10–30 Differences in T Scores Between Children's Category Test (CCT) Total and CVLT-C Total Indices Required for Statistical Significance, by Age

Age (Years)	Level of Significance	Difference Required
5	.10	6.14
	.05	7.92
6	.10	7.36
	.05	9.49
7	.10	6.77
	.05	8.73
8	.10	6.53
	.05	8.42
9	.10	6.39
	.05	8.23
10	.10	7.01
	.05	9.03
11	.10	6.66
	.05	8.58
12	.10	6.26
	.05	8.07
13	.10	7.00
	.05	9.03
14	.10	7.13
	.05	9.19
15	.10	6.89
	.05	8.88
16	.10	7.00
	.05	9.03
All Ages 5–8	.10	6.72
	.05	8.66
All Ages 9–16	.01	6.79
	.05	8.76

Source: From Donders, 1998. Reprinted with the permission of Cambridge University Press.

Table 10–31 Cumulative Percentages of the Standardization Sample Obtaining Various Discrepancies Between Children's Category Test (CCT) Total and CVLT-C Total T Scores

	Age (Years)			Age (Years)	
Difference	5–8	9–16	Difference	5–8	9–16
0	4	2	18	82	87
1	11	8	19	85	89
2	16	15	20	88	91
3	20	21	21	90	94
4	26	27	22	91	95
5	30	33	23	93	95
6	35	39	24	94	96
7	41	45	25	95	97
8	46	51	26	96	97
9	50	55	27	97	97
10	55	60	28	98	98
11	59	63	29	98	98
12	64	67	30	98	99
13	66	71	31	98	99
14	68	74	32	98	99
15	72	77	≥33	100	100
16	76	80	M	10.85	10.06
17	78	84	SD	7.99	7.33

Source: From Donders, 1998. Reprinted with the permission of Cambridge University Press. *Standardization Sample* from the *Children's Category Test*[R]. Copyright ©1993 by Harcourt Assessment, Inc. Reproduced with permission. All rights reserved. *Standardization Sample* from the *California Verbal Learning Test*[R]—*Children's Version*. Copyright © 1994 by Harcourt Assessment, Inc. Reproduced with permission. All rights reserved.

of thumb for interpreting contrasts. Contrast effects can be invoked for Proactive Interference at −1.5 or less, for Retroactive Interference at −1.5 or less, for Rapid Forgetting at −1 or less, and for Retrieval Problems a 1.5 or higher.

Modified Spanish Version

Data for the Modified Spanish Version, which was administered to 260 schoolage children (6–11 years of age) in Bogota, Columbia, are presented in Table 10–34. These data are slightly higher than the standardization norms.

RELIABILITY

Internal Consistency

The authors note that recall tests pose special difficulties for the estimation of internal consistency because of problems with item interdependence within and between trials. First, because of limitations in learning and memory capacity, recall of any one word on a trial decreases the likelihood that

other items will be recalled on that same trial. Second, item interdependence occurs across trials, because recall of a particular word on one trial increases the probability that it will be recalled on subsequent trials (Delis et al., 1994, 2000). Accordingly, the authors used three approaches to estimate the internal consistency for the CVLT-C, based on the Total Recall score on each of the List A learning trials: across-trial consistency, across-semantic-category consistency, and across-word consistency (see test manual for details). These analyses indicated good internal consistency of the total recall scores for the CVLT-C trials.

Standard Error of Measurement (SEM)

Across age, SEMs are on average about 4 T-score points for the total number of words recalled. The manual provides SEMs for the total words recalled (List A Trials 1–5) by age. These are reproduced in Table 10–35, for purposes of constructing confidence intervals. SEMs for other variables are not presented in the manual.

Test-Retest Reliability

Reliability coefficients for CVLT-C scores reported in the test manual range from adequate to high. However, many variables are associated with very low reliabilities (see Table 10–36). In addition, stability data are not presented for many

Table 10–32 Magnitude of CVLT-C Contrast Variables Required for Statistical Significance (in *Z*-Score Units)

Age (Years)	Level of Significance	Proactive Interference	Retroactive Interference	Rapid Forgetting	Retrieval Problems
5	.10	1.36	1.56	1.25	1.46
	.05	1.75	2.01	1.62	1.88
	.01	2.47	2.84	2.28	2.66
6	.10	1.55	1.31	1.18	1.37
	.05	2.00	1.68	1.52	1.77
	.01	2.82	2.38	2.14	2.49
7	.10	1.43	1.17	1.17	1.14
	.05	1.85	1.60	1.50	1.47
	.01	2.61	2.12	2.12	2.07
8	.10	1.51	1.28	0.88	1.34
	.05	1.95	1.65	1.14	1.73
	.01	2.75	2.33	1.61	2.45
9	.10	1.34	1.06	0.91	1.19
	.05	1.73	1.37	1.17	1.54
	.01	2.45	1.93	1.65	2.17
10	.10	1.41	1.00	0.85	1.19
	.05	1.82	1.29	1.09	1.54
	.01	2.56	1.82	1.54	2.17
11	.10	1.41	1.09	1.08	1.02
	.05	1.82	1.40	1.39	1.32
	.01	2.56	1.98	1.96	1.86
12	.10	1.34	0.95	0.85	0.96
	.05	1.73	1.22	1.09	1.24
	.01	2.45	1.72	1.54	1.75
13	.10	1.54	1.25	0.91	1.29
	.05	1.98	1.62	1.17	1.67
	.01	2.80	2.28	1.65	2.35
14	.10	1.45	0.91	0.79	1.14
	.05	1.87	1.17	1.02	1.47
	.01	2.63	1.65	1.45	2.07
15	.10	1.42	1.00	1.11	0.95
	.05	1.83	1.29	1.44	1.22
	.01	2.59	1.82	2.03	1.72
16	.10	1.43	1.28	0.83	0.95
	.05	1.85	1.65	1.07	1.22
	.01	2.61	2.33	1.52	1.72
All Ages	.10	1.43	1.18	1.00	1.23
	.05	1.85	1.52	1.29	1.58
	.01	2.61	2.14	1.82	2.24

Source: From Donders, 1999b. Reprinted with the permission of Cambridge University Press.

learning strategy/process variables. Stability data are based on a group of 106 children from three age groups (8-, 12-, and 16-year-olds) who were tested twice over an interval of approximately 1 month (Delis et al., 1994).

Practice Effects

Practice effects on the CVLT-C, based on the test-retest sample, appear considerable. For example, 8-year-olds recalled 5 more words, 12-year-olds recalled 6 more words, and 16-year-olds recalled 9 more words across trials at retest, one month af-

ter baseline. However, recognition hits and intrusion rates were not significantly changed at retest, and perseveration rate increased slightly, by only 1 point (Delis et al., 1994). Practice effects on Recognition may be mitigated by a ceiling effect.

VALIDITY

Factor Analysis and Cluster Analysis

Factor analyses of the performance measures (i.e., nonprocess variables) of the CVLT-C appear to support its construct

Table 10–33 Cumulative Percentages of the CVLT-C Standardization Sample for Contrast Variables

Value	Proactive Interference	Retroactive Interference	Rapid Forgetting	Retrieval Problems
≤ −3.0	1	1	1	1
−2.5	3	1	1	2
−2.0	5	3	1	3
−1.5	11	7	3	6
−1.0	24	17	10	15
−0.5	41	36	32	32
0.0	61	63	65	55
+0.5	77	85	86	75
+1.0	87	95	96	88
+1.5	94	98	99	97
+2.0	98	99	99	99
+2.5	99	100	100	100
≥ +3.0	100	100	100	100

Source: From Donders, 1999b. Reprinted with the permission of Cambridge University Press.

validity. An exploratory principal component analysis was performed by the authors and is described in the manual as yielding a six-component solution similar to that obtained for the adult CVLT (Delis et al., 1994). The standardization sample was reanalyzed using confirmatory factor analysis by Donders (1999c), who found a five-factor solution for the CVLT-C. The Attention Span factor included recall of information presented only once and recall relatively unconfounded by intralist interference effects (List A, Trial 1; List B; Middle Region Recall). The Learning Efficiency factor included overall memory performance along with qualitative variables thought to improve recall over trials (List A, Trial 5; Semantic Clustering; Recall Consistency). The Free Delayed Recall factor (Short-Delay Free Recall, Long-Delay Free Recall) and Cued Delayed Recall factors (Short-Delay Cued Recall, Long-Delay Cued Recall) also emerged separately, providing empirical support for the two separate dimensions of free and cued recall. The Inaccurate Recall factor appeared to support a separate ability allowing the discrimination of relevant from irrelevant information during learning (Total Intrusions, Recognition False Positives).

Using cluster analysis, Donders (1999a) also found five reliable clusters reflecting different patterns of performance across children. These included three clusters representing level of performance (below average, average, and above average) and two clusters representing pattern of performance. Of the pattern of performance clusters, the first was composed of children who had a below-average span of attention on List A, Trial 1 but who improved their performance to above-average levels over trials without endorsing many false-positives on recognition testing. The second cluster comprised children who also encoded poorly on the first trial of List A but whose performance did not improve substantially over time, although they also did not confuse learned information with distracters. In sum, the first group simply needed repeated exposure to the material to learn it well, whereas the second had a limited learning capacity that did not improve despite additional exposure to the material (Donders, 1999a). Donders cautioned that both of these subtypes are relatively common among normal children (together they represent >40% of the standardization sample) and therefore do not necessarily represent pathology when found in clinical samples.

Relationship to Other Memory Tests

There is scant literature on the relation between the CVLT-C and other list-learning tests in children. In terms of correlations with nonverbal learning paradigms, correlations between the conormed CCT and CVLT-C are low to moderate, indicating that the two tests measure different dimensions of learning ability (Donders, 1998). The CCT is thought to involve a considerable reasoning/executive functioning component that may not be as prominent in the CVLT-C, at least in terms of the performance (i.e., nonprocess) variables. See *CMS* and *WRAML2* in this volume for information on the test's correlation with other memory tests.

Correlation With Other Neuropsychological Tests

Correlations with tests of basic reading and reading comprehension are generally low (Cutting et al., 2003). The CVLT-C is supposed to differentiate between performance outcome

Table 10–34 Normative Data (Mean and *SD*) for the Modified Spanish CVLT-C

	Age (Years)		
	6–7 (*N* = 83)	8–9 (*N* = 121)	10–11 (*N* = 86)
CVLT-C, first trial	6.75 (1.84)	7.28 (1.79)	7.44 (1.66)
CVLT-C, fifth trial	10.51 (2.23)	11.86 (1.91)	12.24 (1.25)
CVLT-C, delayed cue recall	10.30 (2.75)	11.40 (1.93)	12.01 (1.69)
CVLT-C, delayed recall	9.79 (2.33)	11.12 (2.02)	11.70 (1.78)
CVLT-C, recognition	14.35 (1.02)	14.55 (0.71)	14.73 (0.60)

Source: From Rosselli et al., 2001, p. 363. Reproduced by permission. Copyright 2001 by Lawrence Erlbaum Associates, Publishers. Mahwah, NJ. All rights reserved.

Table 10–35 Confidence Interval (CI) Magnitudes for List A Trials 1–5 Total Score, by Age

Age (Years)	90% CI	95% CI
5	6	7
6	6	7
7	6	7
8	6	7
9	5	6
10	6	7
11	6	7
12	6	7
13	6	7
14	6	7
15	6	7
16	7	8

Note: Expressed in T-score format. To use the table, add the corresponding value to the child's obtained T score to yield the upper limit of the CI within which the child's true score is likely to lie; the lower limit is obtained by subtracting the value from the child's obtained score.

Source: Adapted from Delis et al., 1994, p. 122.

CPT correlate poorly with CVLT-C measures of learning process (Beebe et al., 2000).

Correlations With IQ

The CVLT-C is strongly correlated with the Processing Speed Index of the WISC-III in head-injured children ($r = .60$ to $.68$; Donders & Hoffman, 2002; Hoffman et al., 2000). This may relate to the fact that words on the CVLT-C are read at the fairly rapid pace of one word per second (Hoffman et al., 2000). In comparison, correlations with verbal ability are weaker ($r = .32$ to 40 with WISC-R Vocabulary; Delis et al., 1994).

Clinical Studies

The CVLT-C has been used in a number of clinical investigations to study verbal learning in children, including those with head injury (Donders & Hoffman, 2002; Hoffman et al., 2000; Roman et al., 1998; Yeates et al., 1995a), myelomeningocele (Yeates et al., 1995b), fetal alcohol syndrome (Mattson et al., 1996), dyslexia (Kramer et al., 1999), leukemia (Précourt et al., 2002), epilepsy (Hernandez et al., 2003; Williams et al., 2001), PKU (White et al., 2001), ADHD (Cutting et al., 2003; Loge et al., 1990), childhood stroke (Lansing et al., 2004), and low birthweight (Taylor et al., 2000).

With regard to pediatric head injury, CVLT-C performance is strongly related to length of coma ($r = -.52$ to $-.72$; Donders & Hoffman, 2002; Hoffman et al., 2000). CVLT-C performance has also been found to account for as much as 27% of

(e.g., total words recalled, discriminability) and performance process (e.g., recall consistency, semantic clustering). As noted by Beebe et al. (2000), most of the process variables relate to abilities subsumed under executive processing—for example, the use of organizational strategies during encoding (e.g., semantic clustering) or the use of self-monitoring (e.g., perseverations). Executive functioning tests such as the WCST and

Table 10–36 CVLT-C Test-Retest Reliabilities

	Age (Years)		
Magnitude of Coefficient	8	12	16
Very High (≥.90)	Perseverations	—	—
High (.80 to .89)	—	—	Free Recall Intrusions Cued Recall Intrusions Recognition Hits
Adequate (.70 to .79)	List A Trials 1–5 Short-Delay Cued Recall Free Recall Intrusions	List A Trials 1–5 Short-Delay Free Recall	Cued Recall Intrusions Discriminability False Positives
Marginal (.60 to .69)	Long-Delay Cued Recall False Positives	Long-Delay Free Recall Long-Delay Cued Recall	List A Trials 1–5 List B Free Recall Long-Delay Free Recall
Low (≤ .59)	List B Free Recall Short-Delay Free Recall Long-Delay Free Recall Semantic Cluster Ratio Cued Recall Intrusions Recognition Hits Discriminability	List B Free Recall Short-Delay Cued Recall Semantic Cluster Ratio Perseverations Free Recall Intrusions Cued Recall Intrusions Recognition Hits Discriminability False Positives	Short-Delay Free Recall Short-Delay Cued Recall Long-Delay Cued Recall Semantic Cluster Ratio Perseverations

the variance in coma duration (Hoffman et al., 2000; see also Donders & Nesbit-Greene, 2004). Longer length of coma, presence of an intracranial lesion on imaging, younger age, and male gender are associated with worse performance on the CVLT-C in children with head injury (Donders & Hoffman, 2002). In terms of impact of severity on performance, children with severe head injury showed significant impairments on the CVLT-C, whereas those with minor head injury had normal performance; neither group showed deficits in attentional span variables such as recall of List A Trial 1 or List B (Hoffman et al., 2000).

Children with head injury showed a greater decline in free recall from short- to long-delay trials, as well as relatively better performance under a recognition format (Yeates et al., 1995a). Head injury was also associated with higher rates of intrusions and false-positives on recognition trials (Roman et al., 1998; Yeates et al., 1995a). Compared with the CCT, the CVLT-C appears to be a superior measure in terms of sensitivity to cognitive sequelae and in terms of correlation with severity indicators such as length of coma in pediatric head injury (Hoffman et al., 1999, 2000).

There is also considerable research on the use of the CVLT-C test in other clinical groups. Most of these groups appear to show syndrome-specific patterns of performance on CVLT-C variables. For example, children with phenylketonuria (PKU) show poorer learning across trials and less use of semantic clustering than other children (White et al., 2001). Children with frontal lobe epilepsy reportedly make more intrusion errors and are more prone to interference than children with other epilepsy subtypes; in terms of overall learning, all groups with epilepsy perform below healthy controls (Hernandez et al., 2003), but children with well-controlled epilepsy perform well on the CVLT-C (Williams et al., 2001). Children with myelomeningocele and hydrocephalus do not show deficits in process variables despite poorer learning than controls (Yeates et al., 1995b). The same pattern is found in children with traumatic brain injury (TBI; Hoffman et al., 2000; Roman et al., 1998; Yeates et al., 1995a) and in those with ADHD (Cutting et al., 2003). On the other hand, children with PKU make less use of semantic clustering; this is particularly evident in older children with the disorder (White et al., 2001). Children with dyslexia have less efficient rehearsal and encoding than normal children, as evidenced by differences in serial position effects (Kramer et al., 1999), and they make twice as many semantically related false-positive errors as do controls. Children with ADHD, although not significantly impaired compared with normal subjects, are less efficient learners; they encode as many words as other children initially, but they show relative weaknesses in recalling words after delays on both free recall and recognition trials. In addition, children with ADHD tend to show a negative response bias on recognition testing but do not show impairments on strategic variables measured by the CVLT-C (Cutting et al., 2003).

The test has also demonstrated sensitivity to disease and treatment effects in childhood cancer. For example, girls with acute lymphoblastic leukemia treated with a combination of chemotherapy and cranial irradiation had worse performance on the CVLT-C than those treated with chemotherapy alone (Précourt et al., 2002).

Overall, there are few studies on the neuroanatomic correlates of the CVLT-C. However, a number of studies have examined performance in children with disorders associated with dysfunction in particular brain systems, including those involving prefrontal areas (i.e., PKU, ADHD, frontal lobe epilepsy, and TBI; see earlier discussion). No differences in performance between children with left or right hemisphere foci were reported in a group of children with epilepsy (Williams et al., 2001), although the sample included only children with well-controlled seizures who did not have abnormalities on neuroimaging. Similarly, after pediatric stroke, no differences between left- and right-hemisphere groups were found; both groups showed deficits in verbal learning (Lansing et al., 2004). Finally, unlike adults, children with TBI who have anterior lesions do not have an increased risk of proactive interference on the test; instead, they demonstrate an inefficient use of learning resources (Donders & Minnema, 2004).

Ecological Validity

The test is strongly predictive of long-term educational outcome after head injury and accounts for more variance in the prediction of special education needs than do demographic or neurological variables such as injury severity; it accounts for approximately 30% of the variance in long-term educational outcome. Additionally, children who obtain Total Recall scores of less than 45 on initial assessment are eight times more likely to be placed in special education at 1 year after injury and about 13 times more likely at 2-year assessment (Miller & Donders, 2003).

COMMENT

The CVLT-C is a well-designed, sophisticated tool for measuring verbal memory in children. A number of studies have examined CVLT-C performance across a wide variety of clinical syndromes of childhood, supporting its sensitivity and utility in both clinical and research settings. The strong predictive power of the CVLT-C in predicting special education placement after brain injury is also an asset (Miller & Donders, 2003), suggesting that the test may be of potential utility in predicting outcome in other patient groups as well. Further, with the addition of norms for 4-year-olds (Goodman et al., 1999), the test can be used across a wide range of ages.

The test provides a wealth of scores, but their psychometric properties are not necessarily equally strong. In contrast to many other available verbal memory tests, the authors have thoroughly investigated the internal consistency of the CVLT-C and found it to be excellent. However, stability coefficients for many CVLT-C variables are below acceptable standards for clinical use; many are even too low to be suitable for research. Although memory tests often suffer from practice effects, and the CVLT-C is no exception, practice effects cannot completely account for these low stability coefficients. Low reliability coefficients can also mean that performance improves or decreases in a nonsystematic way across subjects or that some subtests suffer from ceiling effect, which makes interpretation of retest scores problematic at best. Additionally, except for semantic clustering (which has poor test-retest reliability), stability information is not reported in the manual for many of the process variables. In the adult version (CVLT-II), reliability coefficients tend to be poor for process-oriented variables, suggesting that users should be cautious in drawing inferences regarding the strategic aspects of an individual's learning and memory abilities (see *CVLT-II*). There are also some questions about whether CVLT-C process variables truly reflect executive functioning (Beebe et al., 2000).

One recommendation for interpretation is to start with the main performance variables (e.g., one score for each factor domain, as done by Donders, 1999b), followed by contrast measures (see Figure 10–20). Qualitative or strategy use variables can then be used as a secondary level of analysis; they should be interpreted with caution, because they are interdependent or have poor sampling characteristics or both (Donders, 1999a). Our recommendation is that the total number of words recalled across the five learning trials is probably the most reliable score for clinical interpretation, given the psychometric properties of test scores provided in the manual and the validity information provided by researchers such as Donders (1999a, 1999b). Process variables are not recommended for use in clinical diagnosis, and interpretation of recognition and error scores (i.e., intrusions, perseverations) is not recommended for very young children (see later discussion).

Of note for users, clinical interpretation of some of the test scores can be confusing. In most cases a positive *z* score indicates good performance, but in others higher *z* scores reflect greater deficits. Users should take care to familiarize themselves with these aspects of scoring before interpreting CVLT-C scores. Additionally, clinicians should not infer pathology if all the *z* scores are not in the same range, both because of variation in patterns of performance in the normative sample and because of chance factors secondary to the high number of available CVLT-C variables (Donders, 1999a).

Some points should also be highlighted with regard to interpretation of scores in a developmental context. Cued recall does not appear to be effective in younger children (aged 4 to 8 years), because they may provide more intrusions than correct responses. A ratio of correct responses to intrusions can be computed in young children to verify a child's response style, because cueing may elicit disinhibited responses in this age group (Goodman et al., 1999). There are also floor effects on some variables in 4-year-olds, which would make it difficult to detect memory deficits on such variables as individual

recall trials, serial clustering, and discriminability (Goodman et al., 1999). Therefore, the total correct responses over the five learning trials is also probably the best single variable for interpretation in this age group.

REFERENCES

Beebe, D. W., Ris, M. D., & Dietrich, K. N. (2000). The relationship between CVLT-C process scores and measures of executive functioning: Lack of support among community-dwelling adolescents. *Journal of Clinical and Experimental Neuropsychology, 22*(6), 779–792.

Boll, T. (1993). *Children's Category Test.* San Antonio, Tex.: The Psychological Corporation.

Cutting, L. E., Koth, C. W., Mahone, M., & Denckla, M. (2003). Evidence for unexpected weaknesses in learning in children with attention-deficit/hyperactivity disorder without reading disabilities. *Journal of Learning Disabilities, 36*(3), 259–269.

Delis, D. C., Kramer, J. H., Kaplan, E., & Ober, B. A. (1987). *California Verbal Learning Test.* San Antonio, Tex.: The Psychological Corporation.

Delis, D. C., Kramer, J. H., Kaplan, E., & Ober, B. A. (1994). *California Verbal Learning Test—Children's Version.* San Antonio, Tex.: The Psychological Corporation.

Delis, D. C., Kramer, J. H., Kaplan, E., & Ober, B. A. (2000). *California Verbal Learning Test—Second Edition, Adult Version.* San Antonio, Tex.: The Psychological Corporation.

Donders, J. (1998). Performance discrepancies between the Children's Category Test (CCT) and the California Verbal Learning Test—Children's (CVLT-C) Version in the standardization sample. *Journal of the International Neuropsychological Society, 4,* 242–246.

Donders, J. (1999a). Cluster subtypes in the standardization sample of the California Verbal Learning Test—Children's Version. *Developmental Neuropsychology, 16*(2), 163–175.

Donders, J. (1999b). Performance discrepancies on the California Verbal Learning Test—Children's Version in the standardization sample. *Journal of the International Neuropsychological Society, 5,* 26–31.

Donders, J. (1999c). Structural equation analysis of the California Verbal Learning Test—Children's Version in the standardization sample. *Developmental Neuropsychology, 15*(3), 395–406.

Donders, J., & Hoffman, N. M. (2002). Gender differences in learning and memory after pediatric traumatic brain injury. *Neuropsychology, 16*(4), 491–499.

Donders, J., & Minnema, M. T. (2004). Performance discrepancies on the California Verbal Learning Test—Children's Version (CVLT-C) in children with traumatic brain injury. *Journal of the International Neuropsychological Society, 10,* 482–488.

Donders, J., & Nesbitt-Greene, K. (2004). Predictors of neuropsychological test performance after pediatric traumatic brain injury. *Assessment, 11*(4), 275–284.

Goodman, A. M., Delis, D. C., & Mattson, S. N. (1999). Normative data for 4-year-old children on the California Verbal Learning Test—Children's Version. *The Clinical Neuropsychologist, 13*(3), 274–282.

Hernandez, M. T., Sauerwein, H. C., Jambaqué, I., de Guise, E., Lussier, F., Lortie, A., Dulac, O., & Lassonde, M. (2003). Attention, memory, and behavioral adjustment in children with frontal lobe epilepsy. *Epilepsy and Behavior, 4,* 522–536.

Hoffman, N., Donders, J., & Thompson, E. H. (2000). Novel learning abilities after traumatic head injury in children. *Archives of Clinical Neuropsychology, 15*(1), 47–58.

Kramer, J. H., Delis, D. C., Kaplan, E., O'Donnell, L., & Prifitera, A. (1997). Developmental sex differences in verbal learning. *Neuropsychology, 11,* 577–584.

Kramer, J. H., Knee, K., & Delis, D. C. (1999). Verbal memory impairments in dyslexia. *Archives of Clinical Neuropsychology, 15*(1), 83–93.

Lansing, A. E., Max, J. E., Delis, D. C., Fox, P. T., Lancaster, J., Manes, F. F., & Schatz, A. (2004). Verbal learning and memory after childhood stroke. *Journal of the International Neuropsychological Society, 10,* 742–752.

Loge, D. V., Staton, R. D., & Beatty, W. W. (1990). Performance of children with ADHD on tests of sensitivity to frontal lobe dysfunction. *Journal of the American Academy of Child and Adolescent Psychiatry, 29,* 540–545.

Mattson, S. N., Riley, E. P., Delis, D. C., Stern, C., & Jones, K. L. (1996). Verbal learning and memory in children with Fetal Alcohol Syndrome. *Alcoholism: Clinical and Experimental Research, 20,* 810–816.

Miller, L. J., & Donders, J. (2003). Prediction of educational outcome after pediatric traumatic brain injury. *Rehabilitation Psychology, 48*(4), 237–241.

Précourt, S., Robaey, P., Lamothe, I., Lassonde, M., Sauerwein, H. C., & Moghrabi, A. (2002). Verbal cognitive functioning and learning in girls treated for acute lymphoblastic leukemia by chemother-apy with or without cranial irradiation. *Developmental Neuropsychology, 21*(2), 173–195.

Roman, M. J., Delis, D. C., Willerman, L., Magulac, M., Demadura, T. L., de la Pena, J. L., Loftis, C., Walsh, J., & Kracun, M. (1998). Impact of pediatric traumatic brain injury on components of verbal memory. *Journal of Clinical and Experimental Neuropsychology, 20,* 245–258.

Rosselli, M., Ardila, A., Bateman, J. R., & Guzman, M. (2001). Neuropsychological test scores, academic performance, and developmental disorders in Spanish-speaking children. *Developmental Neuropsychology, 20*(1), 355–373.

Taylor, H. G., Klien, N., Minich, N. M., & Hack, M. (2000). Verbal memory deficits in children with less than 750g birth weight. *Child Neuropsychology, 16,* 49–63.

White, D. A.., Nortz, M. J., Mandernach, T., & Huntington, K. (2001). Deficits in memory strategy use related to prefrontal dysfunction during early development: Evidence from children with phenylketonuria. *Neuropsychology, 15*(2), 221–229.

Williams, J., Phillips, T., Griebel, M. L., Sharp, G. B., Lange, B., Edgar, T. & Simpson, P. (2001). Patterns of memory performance in children with controlled epilepsy on the CVLT-C. *Child Neuropsychology, 7*(1), 15–20.

Yeates, K. O., Blumenstein, E., Patterson, C. M., & Delis, D. C. (1995a). Verbal learning and memory following pediatric closed-head injury. *Journal of the International Neuropsychological Society, 1,* 78–87.

Yeates, K. O., Enrile, B. G., Loss, N., & Blumenstein, E. (1995b). Verbal learning and memory in children with myelomeningocele. *Journal of Pediatric Psychology, 20,* 801–815.

Children's Memory Scale (CMS)

PURPOSE

The Children's Memory Scale (CMS) assesses learning and memory in children and adolescents.

SOURCE

The test can be obtained from The Psychological Corporation (http://www.harcourtassessment.com). The scale costs about $650 US, including scoring software. The CMS includes two Stimulus Booklets, Stimulus Cards for Family Pictures and Dot Location, and Dot Location Response Chips.

AGE RANGE

The CMS can be given to children aged 5 to 16 years.

DESCRIPTION

The CMS (Cohen, 1997) is a test battery designed to assess learning and memory in children and adolescents. Although it is not technically associated with the Wechsler name, it is similar in content and format to the WMS-III (see *Wechsler Memory Scale—III*). Like the WMS-III, it allows memory-IQ comparisons via a linked sample to other Wechsler scales (WISC-IV, WISC-III, and WPPSI-R).

According to the test manual, the CMS was designed with five primary goals: (a) consistency with current conceptualizations and research on learning and memory, (b) sensitivity to developmental changes, (c) capability for comparison between memory and intelligence, (d) inclusion of clinically and educationally relevant tasks, and (e) inclusion of motivating, child-friendly tasks within the context of a standardized assessment tool. As such, the test is intended to enable clinicians to identify learning and memory disorders, to isolate deficits in learning and recall strategy, and to serve an important role in the design of remedial programs for memory problems in children and adolescents (Cohen, 1997).

Because there currently exists no single, universally accepted memory theory, the CMS is based on currently accepted models of memory and learning, which are schematically presented in the manual as the "milkjug of memory" (Cohen, 1997, p. 7; see Figure 10–22; also see *Comments*). Core constructs are that attention is the foundation of learning and memory, that both auditory-verbal and visual-nonverbal aspects can be measured, that long-term memory is constructed of both declarative and procedural aspects, and that retrieval can be assessed via free recall and recognition. Note that procedural memory is not assessed with the CMS.

The CMS assesses memory in three ways: according to temporal dimension (immediate versus delayed), modality

Table 10–37 Structure of Primary Index Scores for the CMS

CMS Index Scores	Subtests
Verbal Immediate	Stories Immediate Word Pairs Total
Verbal Delayed	Stories Delayed Word Pairs Delayed
Visual Immediate	Faces Immediate Dot Locations Total
Visual Delayed	Faces Delayed Dot Locations Delayed
Attention/Concentration	Sequences Numbers
Delayed Recognition	Stories Delayed Recognition Word Pairs Delayed Recognition
Learning	Word Pairs, Trials 1–3 Total Score Dot Locations, Trials 1–3 Total Score

Note: The *General Memory Index* is derived from the sum of the *Verbal Immediate, Verbal Delayed, Visual Immediate,* and *Visual Delayed* Index Scores.

(verbal versus visual) and testing format (recall versus recognition; Flanagan et al., 2000). In addition, attention/concentration and learning (performance across trials) are measured. The test provides a General Memory score, which is a single composite score reflecting average memory performance across verbal and visual domains. The CMS consists of nine main subtests, six of which are core subtests that

Figure 10–21 CMS Test Structure. *Source:* Reprinted with permission from Cohen, 1997, p. 2.

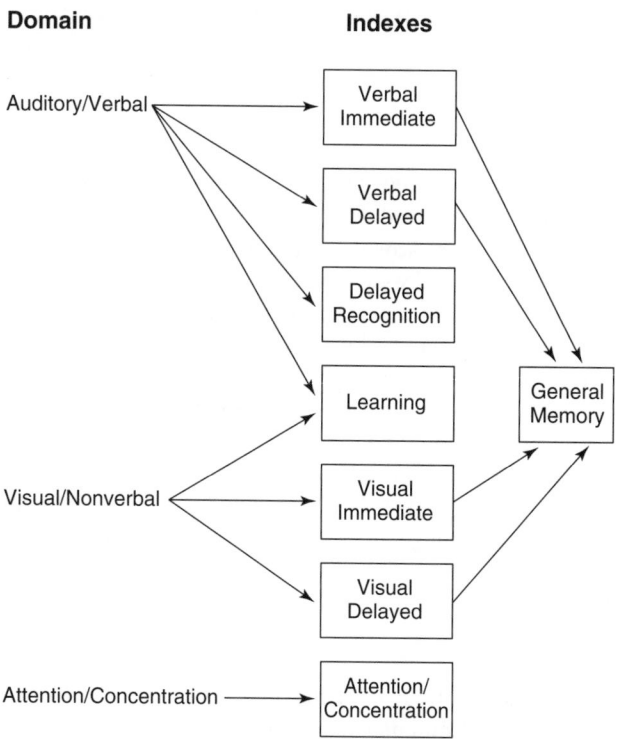

Figure 10–22 The Milkjug of Memory. *Source:* Reprinted with permission from Cohen, 1997, p. 7.

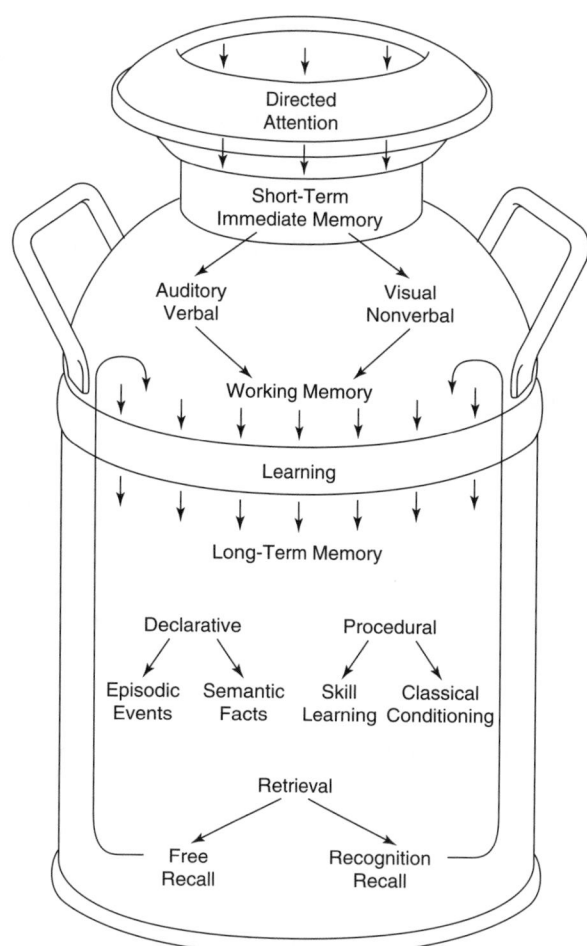

contribute to index scores. The remaining three subtests are supplemental. The test provides eight index scores (see Table 10–37 and Figure 10–21). CMS subtest descriptions are provided in Table 10–38.

ADMINISTRATION TIME

The test takes 30 to 45 min, not counting the 30-min delay interval. Thus, a full hour or more is required to administer the test (see *Comment*). Administration of supplemental subtests takes an additional 10 to 15 min of testing time; these can be administered during the delay interval.

ADMINISTRATION

See test manual. The test is relatively simple to administer; instructions are clearly printed on the easel-stimulus booklets, and start point, discontinuation, and scoring information are available on test protocols. Examiners should note that slightly different materials or administration procedures are used, depending on whether the child falls in the younger (5–8 years) or older (≥9 years) age group. Administration and

Table 10–38 Summary of CMS Scores

Index	Subtest	Description
Auditory/Verbal	Stories	Assesses recall for meaningful/semantically related information (prose passages); the subject must recall two stories that were read by the examiner; includes recall and recognition (yes/no) trials.
	Word Pairs	Assesses recall for semantically unrelated information (word pairs); the subject must recall a list of word pairs over three learning trials; the examiner provides the first word of each pair, and the subject must provide the matching word; includes recall and recognition (yes/no) trials.
	Word Lists[a]	Assesses recall for semantically unrelated information (word list); the subject must recall a list of words read over four learning trials, using a selective reminding procedure (i.e., only words that were not recalled are presented after the initial learning trial); a distractor list is also read; includes recall and recognition (yes/no) trials.
Visual/Nonverbal	Dot Locations	Assesses recall for spatial location; the subject must learn the location of an array of blue chips on a grid, over three learning trials; the subtest includes a distractor trial, along with a delayed recall procedure.
	Faces	Assesses recognition of human faces; the subject is asked to remember a series of faces, and then to recognize them among a series of distractor faces; immediate and delayed recall are assessed.
	Family Pictures[a]	Assesses recall of pictured scenes; the subject is shown four illustrated scenes of a family engaged in everyday activities; the subject is then presented with similar illustrations with the family members missing; the subject must tell the examiner which characters were missing and what activities they were engaged in; immediate and delayed recall are assessed.
Attention/Concentration	Numbers	This is the classic Digit Span paradigm, which assesses auditory working memory and attention; the subject must recall strings of random digits of increasing length in forward and backward order. Separate scores are provided for Forward and Backward digit recall.
	Sequences	Assesses verbal working memory; includes a series of short tasks involving sequential recall and working memory (e.g., backward recall of the days of the week).
	Picture Locations[a]	Assesses immediate visual memory; the examinee is presented with pictures in various locations on a page and then must recall their locations on a blank page.

[a]Supplemental subtests.

content differ for some subtests, depending on age (e.g., Dot Location, Stories, Faces, Picture Locations, Word Lists 2).

Subtests should be administered in standard order. There should be a 30-min delay between Dot Locations and Dot Locations 2. Note that, during the standardization of the test, supplemental subtests were administered during the delay interval, which is how they appear in the test booklet. If not administering supplemental subtests, the examiner should follow the order of the subtests as shown in the record form but ensure that the 30-min delay is maintained, using other noninterfering tasks.

SCORING

Scores

Subtest scores are provided in scaled score format ($M = 10$, $SD = 3$, range 1–19), and index scores are provided in standard score format ($M = 100$, $SD = 15$, range 50–150). Percentiles are also provided, and 90% and 95% confidence intervals are given for index scores. Information on the statistical differences among index scores and among subtests and the frequency of such differences in the standardization sample are provided on the standard printout. These can also be derived by using tables in the manual. Memory/IQ differences, including statistical significance and frequency, are also provided on the scoring printout and can be derived from information in the manual and from tables provided in this volume (see WISC-IV). The predicted-actual method is recommended by the author, although the simple-difference method is also provided.

Scoring

Scoring the test by hand, although possible, can be lengthy and complex. Computer scoring is therefore recommended.

Rules are provided in the manual for scoring subtests requiring a degree of subjective evaluation of examinee responses (i.e., Stories, Family Pictures, and Sequences).

DEMOGRAPHIC EFFECTS

Age

CMS scores increase with age (see test manual for details).

Gender

Gender effects on the test are unknown.

Ethnicity

To our knowledge, there are no independent studies on the effects of ethnicity on test scores.

IQ

See *Validity*.

NORMATIVE DATA

Standardization Sample

The CMS was normed using a random sample of 1000 American children aged 5 to 16 years. Norms were stratified according to 1995 U.S. Census data based on age, race/ethnicity, geographic region, and parental education. Norms are based on 10 age groups, with equal representation of boys and girls. See Table 10–39 for additional details. Note that some case-weighting was used to adjust race/ethnicity and parental level composition to match 1995 U.S. Census data.

RELIABILITY

Internal Consistency

The manual shows split-half reliabilities for most subtests and generalizeability coefficients for others, across age. In the latter case, generalizeability coefficients were used because of the "uniqueness of some subtests and item presentation formats, and inter-item dependency" (test manual, p. 97). As shown in Table 10–40, most CMS subtests have adequate to high internal reliability; this is particularly true for verbal subtests. Reliability for Family Pictures is questionable, as is that of Dot Locations Short Delay. Of the indices, the Visual Index scores have the lowest reliability ($r = .76$) and, as expected, General Memory has the highest ($r = .91$).

Standard Error of Measurement (*SEM*)

*SEM*s for CMS subtests are presented on page 107 of the manual. With regard to index scores, *SEM*s are smallest for

Table 10–39 Characteristics of the CMS Normative Sample

Sample type	National, stratified random sample[a]
Number	1000
Age	5 to 16 years[b]
Geographic location[c]	
Northeast	
North Central	
South	
West	
Parental Education[c]	
≤ 8th grade	
9th–11th grade	
high school	
1–3 years of college	
≥ 4 years of college	
Gender	
Boys	500
Girls	500
Race/Ethnicity (%)	
Caucasian	68.4%
African American	16.1%
Hispanic	11.6%
Other	3.9%
Screening	Exclusion criteria included below-level reading skills, grade repetition, referral for special education or remedial services, neurological diagnosis, and head injury.

[a]Based on 1995 U.S. Census data; participants were from public and private schools; 3.5% of the overall sample represents case-weighted data, in order to adjust ethnicity/parental education proportions to match Census proportions.
[b]Based on 10 age groupings: 5, 6, 7, 8, 9, 10, 11, 12, 13–14, and 15–16 years.
[c]Provided in graphical format only in the manual (see source), for the overall sample.

Adapted from Cohen, 1997.

the General Memory index (4.5) and largest for the Visual index (7.4), concomitant with the size of their estimated reliabilities. In the latter case, this would mean that for a child who obtains a standard score of 100, the 95% confidence interval would range from about 86 to 115, which is a sizable range.

Test-Retest Reliability

Test-retest reliability coefficients for the General Memory, Attention/Concentration, and Verbal Immediate indices are uniformly high across age (see Table 10–41). Test-retest reliability of the index scores was evaluated on a subsample of 125 children from the standardization sample, tested twice over a mean interval of about 60 days (Cohen, 1997). Three age groups were evaluated: 5 to 8 years ($n = 52$), 9 to 12 years ($n = 45$), and 13 to 16 years ($n = 28$). Note that in the older age group, these data show very poor test-retest reliability for the Visual Immediate and Visual Delayed indices ($r = .29$ and .38, respectively), as well as poor reliability for the Delayed

Table 10–40 Internal Reliability Coefficients for the CMS

Magnitude of Coefficient	Internal Reliability CMS Indexes	Internal Reliability CMS Subtests
Very High (≥.90)	General Memory Index	Word Pairs Learning
High (.80 to .89)	Verbal Immediate Index Verbal Delayed Index Attention/Concentration Index Learning Index Delayed Recognition Index	Word Pairs Total Score Word Pairs Long Delay[a] Numbers Total Score Sequences Total Score Word Lists Learning
Adequate (.70 to .79)	Visual Immediate Index Visual Delayed Index	Dot Locations Learning Dot Locations Total Score Dot Locations Long Delay[a] Stories Immediate Stories Delayed Stories Delayed Recognition[a] Stories Immediate Thematic Stories Delayed Thematic Faces Immediate Faces Delayed Word Pairs Delayed Recognition Word Pairs Immediate[a] Word Lists Delayed[a] Word Lists Delayed Recognition Numbers Forward Numbers Backward Picture Location Total Score
Marginal (.60 to .69)		Family Pictures Immediate Family Pictures Delayed
Low (≤.59)		Dot Locations Short Delay[a]

Note: Values represent mean reliabilities across age.
[a]Based on generalizeability coefficient.

Table 10–41 Test-Retest Reliability Coefficients for the CMS Indexes

Magnitude of Coefficient	Test-Retest Stability		
	5–8 Years	9–12 Years	13–16 Years
Very High (≥.90)	—	—	—
High (.80 to .89)	Verbal Immediate Index General Memory Index Attention/Concentration Index	Verbal Immediate Index General Memory Index Attention/Concentration Index	Verbal Immediate Index Verbal Delayed Index General Memory Index Attention/Concentration Index
Adequate (.70 to .79)	Visual Delayed Index Learning Index	Verbal Delayed Index	Learning Index
Marginal (.60 to .69)	Visual Immediate Index	Visual Immediate Index Visual Delayed Index Learning Index	—
Low (≤.59)	Verbal Delayed Index Delayed Recognition Index	Delayed Recognition Index	Visual Immediate Index Visual Delayed Index Delayed Recognition Index

Note: Correlations were corrected for variability.

Recognition Index ($r = .52$). Users should bear in mind that some recognition paradigms suffer from ceiling effects, which can affect reliability estimates. Subtest reliabilities are not provided in the manual.

The test manual also presents decision consistency coefficients for index scores and core battery subtests (i.e., percentage agreement) which reflect the likelihood that an examinee would obtain scores in the same general range at retest, when scores are divided into three broad classifications (impaired, borderline to low-average, and average to above-average). With regard to General Memory, coefficients for the three age groups were .71, .76 and .61, respectively. Although the manual states that "important classification decisions based on level of memory functioning are relatively consistent over time as measured by CMS dimensions" (p. 102), in the case of General Memory, according to these coefficients, anywhere from one-fourth to one-third of the group would be misclassified at retest. Classifications for the four Visual and Verbal indices varied from a low of .68 to a high of .93. See pages 102 to 103 of the manual for further details.

Practice Effects

On some index scores, practice effects are substantial. This is especially true for General Memory; for example, scores increased by 20 standard score points at retest in the adolescent subgroup described in the manual (see *Test-Retest Reliability* for sample details). Most other indices increased by 10 points or more. For the most part, practice effects are minimal (≤ 5 standard score points) on Attention/Concentration and Delayed Recognition indices. (Note that ceiling effects on recognition paradigms in normal subjects tend to attenuate estimates of practice effects.) The manual notes that practice effects are more likely to be small with longer test-retest durations; however, no data are presented to support this statement.

Interrater Reliability

Interrater reliability of core subtest scores and indexes is very high, as measured by intraclass correlations (all >.98; see test manual for details).

VALIDITY

Content

CMS content development appears to have been comprehensive. The test has been in development since 1986, and after some early studies on clinical subjects (Cohen, 1992), it was reviewed by a panel of experts in 1992 and modified. A national tryout occurred in 1993 and led to additional modifications. Additional subtests were deleted after the standardization itself. The manual indicates that items were evaluated for bias, but no details are provided. No information is provided on why certain subtests make up certain indices; presumably, this was determined based on theoretical grounds.

Subtest and Index Intercorrelations and Factor Structure

Although test structure appears reasonable at face value, empirical validation for some aspects remains somewhat weak, particularly as it pertains to the Visual indices. For instance, although the correlation matrix provided in the manual generally supports the composition of other index scores, the subtests making up the Visual indices are very poorly correlated (e.g., $r = .06$ to .16 between Dot Locations and Faces). In comparison, Verbal index subtests (Stories and Word Pairs) are moderately correlated with each other ($r = .30$ to .40 for Total scores), as are the Attention/Concentration subtests (Numbers and Sequences; $r = .47$). Correlations among supplementary subtests appear weak, and no information is provided on the relationship between core and supplementary subtests.

With regard to index scores, Visual and Verbal indices appear to measure relatively different aspects of memory, in accordance with the aims of the test, with all correlations between these indices being in the modest range ($r = .21$ to .27). Notably, the Attention/Concentration index is more highly correlated with the Verbal indices than with the Visual indices, underlining the fact that it is largely administered via the verbal modality ($r = .41$, versus $r = .20$ to .27). A large verbal component to the Attention/Concentration index is also suggested by the validity studies reviewed later.

According to the manual, confirmatory factor analysis in the standardization sample supports a three-factor solution for the CMS, comprised of Attention/Concentration, Visual Delayed, and Verbal Delayed subtests. Users should note that the analysis was restricted to models containing three factors or less. Importantly, Immediate Memory subtests do not appear to have been included, even though they make up a major part of the test. Therefore, a model paralleling the actual test structure, consisting of five memory indices—four indices and a supraordinal index for General Memory—and three additional factors to represent Attention/Concentration, Delayed Recognition, and Learning, was not tested in these analyses and awaits validation.

Correlations With Other Memory Tests

WMS-III. Sixteen-year-olds can be administered either the CMS or the WMS-III. Because these tests employ very similar paradigms, similar performance on the two tests is expected in this age group. The manual presents data on 86 16-year-olds tested with both tests (Cohen, 1997). Although mean scores for General Memory and attention index scores (i.e., CMS Attention/Concentration and WMS-III Working Memory) were very similar between the two measures (i.e., within 1 standard score point), 16-year-olds performed 3 to 4 points lower on the WMS-III verbal memory indices (Auditory Immediate and Auditory Delayed) and 2 to 4 points higher on the WMS-III visual memory indices (Visual Immediate and Visual Delayed), compared with their CMS scores.

Correlations between indices for the two versions support the convergent validity of the CMS, with high correlations between CMS Verbal Memory indices and WMS-III Auditory Memory indices ($r = .63$ to .74). However, convergent and divergent validity for the visual index scores is not as strong, with only modest correlation between the Visual Delayed indices of both measures ($r = .26$) and substantial correlations between verbal and visual indices. This suggests that the visual memory indices of the CMS and WMS-III may be difficult to compare in a clinical context, as is necessary when an individual has been administered both tests over time. Note that correlations for General Memory scores for the two tests, as well as those for the verbal indices, are fairly high ($r = .63$ to .67). However, the tests are clearly not interchangeable in this age group. Note too that the General Memory index of the WMS-III comprises only delayed memory tasks, whereas in the CMS, the index comprises both immediate and delayed tasks.

WRAML and WRAML2. Comparison to the WRAML, described in the manual for data from 33 children administered both instruments, indicates a substantial amount of construct overlap between the General Memory indices from both tests ($r = .64$). Evidence of convergent and divergent validity for the verbal indices of both tests is relatively strong, with large correlations between the CMS Verbal indices and the WRAML verbal domain ($r = .60, .51$) and lesser correlations for visual indices. Correlations involving the visual domain again suggest a lack of clear divergent validity, with moderately high correlations with WRAML verbal subtests ($r = .40$ to .41). Correlations supporting convergent validity are not consistent: Although correlations between the CMS Visual Immediate index and the WRAML Visual domain are relatively low ($r = .26$), the CMS Visual Delayed index is highly correlated with the WRAML Visual score ($r = .50$). Paradigm differences and differences in the composition of index scores may account for some of the inconsistencies between visual indices on the two tests.

Very high correlation with the WRAML Verbal score ($r = .70$) indicates additional evidence for a substantial verbal component in the CMS Attention/Concentration index. Notably, mean scores on the CMS General Memory index are about 5 points higher on the CMS than on the WRAML. For information on the relationship between the CMS and WRAML2, see *WRAML2*, in this volume.

CVLT-C. Comparisons with the CVLT-C are particularly helpful in determining the extent of overlap between verbal and visual domains on the CMS, because the CVLT-C is administered entirely in the auditory-verbal modality and represents a well-known and well-validated paradigm for assessing verbal memory. The manual describes data on a small sample of children administered both measures ($N = 22$). Surprisingly, the CMS Visual Immediate index was highly correlated with the main recall measure of the CVLT-C ($r = .50$, Total words recalled over Trials 1–5). A similar pattern occurred for

the CMS Attention/Concentration Index ($r = .55$), although it was also highly correlated with Trial 1 from the CVLT, a measure thought to reflect verbal working memory and encoding ($r = .55$). The Verbal indices were inconsistently correlated with total words recalled on the CVLT-C (Verbal Immediate, $r = .18$; Verbal Delayed, $r = .49$). Overall, evidence for convergent and divergent validity of the CMS indexes using the CVLT-C is conflicting; this may relate in part to the small sample size employed. As noted by the author, the CVLT-C provides somewhat different information than the verbal indices of the CMS. In fact, correlations between the CVLT-C and the CMS Word Lists, a supplemental subtest that also employs a word-list paradigm, are quite high (see test manual, p. 133). Note that, in contrast to the CVLT-C, Word Lists uses a selective reminding paradigm and semantically unrelated items.

Correlations With Intellectual Ability

The CMS correlates highly with IQ as measured by the WISC-III ($r = .58$ between General Memory and FSIQ, based on a sample of 413 children described in the manual). Although the WISC-III VCI correlates more highly with Verbal Memory index scores than Visual Memory index scores ($r = .52$ to .57 versus $r = .20$ to .44), the reverse is not true: WISC-III POI is actually more highly correlated with Verbal Memory than with Visual Memory index scores ($r = .28$ to .29 versus $r = .38$ to .41). As expected, the WISC-III Freedom-From-Distractibility Index correlates very highly with the CMS Attention/Concentration Index ($r = .73$), and, although the WISC-III Processing Speed Index (PSI) correlates well with Attention/Concentration ($r = .47$), it also correlates moderately well with most CMS indices. For information on correlations with the WISC-IV, see *WISC-IV* in this volume.

A similar pattern is also apparent with the Differential Abilities Scale (DAS). Although general cognitive and general memory indices from the two tests correlate highly ($r = .65$), CMS verbal memory does not appear to correlate more highly with DAS verbal measures than visual-spatial measures, and CMS visual memory shows an inconsistent pattern with regard to correlations with these domains (see test manual for details).

In younger children, FSIQ as measured by the WPPSI-R is highly correlated with General Memory ($r = .56$), and especially with Attention/Concentration ($r = .66$; $N = 38$; see manual for details). WPPSI-R VIQ and PIQ do not appear to selectively correlate with either verbal or visual memory as measured by the CMS. Information on correlations with the WPPSI-III can be found in the WPPSI-III review, in this volume.

Correlations With Academic Achievement

On the whole, the CMS is moderately correlated with academic achievement as measured by the WIAT; CMS verbal memory measures also correlate strongly with language-based academic skills. Specifically, CMS General Memory is highly correlated with the WIAT Total Score ($r = .56$, $N = 208$; see manual for further details). CMS verbal memory scores and language-based academic achievement are highly related ($>.50$), whereas correlations between CMS visual memory scores and language-based academic achievement are much lower ($<.30$).

Correlations with school grades, based on a large sample ($N = 744$; see test manual), indicate that the General Memory Index, Verbal indices, and Attention/Concentration Index are all moderately related to school performance. These same indices are also moderately to strongly related to standardized, group-administered achievement tests such as the SAT (data on other similar tests are also reviewed in the manual). In all cases, the Visual Memory indices were poor predictors of academic performance (whether defined as school grades or standardized test scores), including "nonverbal" areas such as mathematics. Interestingly, Attention/Concentration appears to be at least as strong as the General Memory or Verbal index scores in predicting academic achievement (and in some cases, it was a stronger predictor; see manual).

Relationship to Executive Functioning

Performance on the CMS is not independent of performance on executive functioning measures. Correlations with the WCST are for the most part in the moderate range (i.e., with few exceptions, in the .30 to .50 range; $N = 46$; Cohen, 1997). However, there does not appear to be a clear pattern emerging across verbal, visual, or attention/concentration domains, although correlations with the Visual indices are slightly weaker. This most likely reflects the multifactorial nature of the WCST, as well as the role of executive functioning and problem solving in memory performance. In contrast, correlations with the Children's Category Test (CCT) in older children (ages 9–15 years) indicate that the CMS Verbal and General Memory indices (but not the Visual or Attention/Concentration indices) are highly related with CCT performance ($r \geq .59$). (Note that the sample size in younger children is too small for interpretation.)

Relationship to Language Skills

The CMS General Memory index is highly correlated with the Total Language composite of the CELF-3 ($r = .52$), based on data presented in the test manual. This suggests a strong language-based component to successful performance on the test. Whereas correlations between Visual memory indices and CELF-3 expressive language scores are very small, other correlations involving receptive language are difficult to interpret because of the small sample size and limited power. However, the CMS Verbal Immediate index appears to correlate moderately well with receptive language

($r = .42$). Attention/Concentration again shows a moderate relationship to both expressive and receptive language scores on the CELF-3 ($r = .37$ to 47), which again underscores that this index primarily measures aspects of verbal rather than visual attention.

Clinical Studies

Clinical utility of the CMS rests on two factors: (a) the ability to discriminate between individuals with memory dysfunction and normal controls, and (b) the ability to differentiate between clinical groups. An additional consideration is whether the test provides strong evidence of clinical utility as shown by sensitivity/specificity data, or whether clinical utility is based on group studies alone. The manual presents preliminary data on a number of clinical groups in which memory or attentional dysfunction would be expected. These include children with epilepsy, traumatic brain injury, brain tumors, learning disabilities, attention-deficit/hyperactivity disorder (ADHD), and speech-language impairment. Although some of the group sizes are too small for interpretation, the general trend indicates that the CMS is sensitive to memory and attentional dysfunction occurring in a clinical context. Its ability to distinguish among clinical groups remains to be determined.

Overall, there is a surprising lack of clinical studies involving the test, even though it has been in circulation since 1997. One study indicated that the CMS is sensitive to the long-term effects of light to moderate prenatal alcohol exposure in the first trimester. Among subtests, the relationship was especially strong for Word Pairs (Willford et al., 2004). A study by the author involving an earlier version of the test showed that children with seizures originating in the left hemisphere performed worse on auditory-verbal memory subtests than did those with right-temporal seizures; the reverse pattern was obtained on visual-spatial memory subtests (Cohen, 1992). However, until further research is conducted, interpretation of test results with regard to neuroanatomical correlates is not recommended (see *Comments*).

COMMENT

There exist very few standardized memory batteries for children; as a result, most pediatric neuropsychologists welcomed the arrival of the CMS when it was published in 1997, and many added it to their list of standard testing tools for clinical evaluation. This occurred largely because the test is a "descendent" of the well-known WMS tests and because it is linked to Wechsler intelligence scales. The test certainly has several strengths, but users should be aware of its limitations, as outlined in the following paragraphs.

The test allows a broad, comprehensive assessment of most aspects of memory and learning. CMS materials are well designed and user-friendly, and the standardization sample is large and well constructed. The test was some years in development and was reviewed and revised several times before publication. Additionally, even though at present there is an almost complete lack of research studies on the CMS, the author has constructed a comprehensive manual. Data on the test's relationship to other important memory measures such as WMS-III, WRAML, and CVLT-C, as well as preliminary data on its administration to a number of clinical groups, are presented in detail. This is a definite asset that compensates somewhat for the lack of independent validation studies. The test also rests on a theoretical foundation, although the specifics are not entirely well detailed in the manual. However, most users, particularly those familiar with the WMS-III, will recognize the constructs and testing paradigms employed as those found in most current, validated memory batteries. Another asset is its linking with the WISC-IV to allow calculation of ability-memory discrepancies (see *WISC-IV*, in this volume).

Vaupel (2001) has thoroughly reviewed the CMS and noted some limitations. For instance, the test is moderately child-friendly but suffers from few manipulatives and ecologically relevant tasks. We also find that the use of different materials for different ages complicates longitudinal research, as well as comparison of retesting data in a clinical setting. Vaupel (2001) also indicated that, although the CMS is easy to administer, it is difficult to score by hand. Further, the test is relatively long, which can be difficult for some children with limited stamina or behavioral issues. The word-list task uses a selective reminding procedure that may be unpleasant for children (Vaupel, 2001). Further, additional research on the test's usefulness and validity in a cross-cultural context is needed.

Validation of the five-factor structure as it appears in the test has not yet been conducted. In addition, the Visual index scores, as separate and distinct dimensions of memory, suffer from several shortcomings, including poor reliability, low intercorrelations between index subtests, and inconsistent convergent and divergent validity. Based on correlations presented in the manual, Family Pictures, a supplemental visual subtest, has a substantial language component, as is the case for the WMS-III (Dulay et al., 2002). Developing reliable and valid tests of visual memory has proven challenging for neuropsychology. Thus, although these criticisms are hardly specific to the CMS, interpretation of the visual index scores should be done with caution in clinical diagnostic settings.

Users should note that the test does not provide adequate coverage of visual attention and visual working memory. Validity data from the manual indicate that the Attention/Concentration Index, comprising two largely auditory-verbal tasks, is highly related to verbal functioning. Because the supplemental task, Picture Location, has scant supportive validity evidence, additional visual attention tasks should be supplemented when evaluating individual patients.

Of note, several of the subtests suffer from floor and ceiling effects. Floor effects are evident on Word Pairs, Dot Locations, Stories Thematic, Word Pairs, Word Lists, and particularly Numbers Backward (e.g., a 5-year-old with a raw score of 0 on Numbers Backward obtains a standard score of 7). Ceilings are evident on Dot Locations, Word Pairs, Family Pictures, and Word Lists. Users should also note that in some children (i.e., 5- and 9-year-olds), it is possible to obtain an average score on certain Dot Locations trials, such as Short Delay and Long Delay, for chance performance. This is a result of the small number of possible item choices; for example, the child has six chips to place on a 12-position grid, and a chance-level score of three correct chip placements at age 5 yields a scaled score of 9.

As noted by the author, index scores continue to provide the most reliable and clinically useful aspect of the test. Interpretation at the subtest level is not recommended, and caution is recommended in interpreting changes on index scores at retest, given the substantial practice effects.

Authors of memory tests often note that interpreting test-retest reliability coefficients of memory measures can be difficult because of practice effects and other factors (e.g., ceiling effects) that may attenuate correlations between test and retest scores. However, an adequate demonstration of reliability is crucial to clinicians who use tests for clinical diagnosis. Further, memory measures with adequate test-retest reliability clearly exist (e.g., CVLT-C). The test-retest reliability of the CMS Visual index scores is inadequate and certainly falls short for use of this index in clinical diagnosis. This limitation raises questions about the accuracy and utility of the verbal-visual memory comparisons provided by the test manual, and it may pose a major problem in situations where comparisons between verbal and visual memory are of clinical importance (e.g., preoperative evaluation of children with intractable temporal lobe epilepsy), although this problem is not unique to the CMS (e.g., see *Wechsler Memory Scale—III*). In addition, from a construct validity standpoint, the two subtests making up the Visual indices (Faces and Dot Locations) correlate poorly with each other, which raises questions about the homogeneity of this index and whether the two subtests comprising it are actually measuring a similar domain (again, the same problem occurs with the WMS-III). Inclusion of several additional visual memory tests is recommended in situations in which visual memory must be adequately assessed. Note that correlations between Visual index scores for the CMS and WMS-III in adolescents are poor, as reviewed earlier. This should be taken into account when interpreting results for adolescents or young adults tested with both measures over time.

As noted previously, Delayed Recognition has poor test-retest reliability, which may relate to the non-normal distribution of scores that often occurs with testing of normal subjects on recognition paradigms. However, this may also pose problems when recall-recognition comparisons are sought for purposes of clinical diagnosis.

Interpretation of index scores and subtests with regard to brain localization is not recommended, despite the lengthy interpretive discussion presented in the test manual. To date, no adequate validation studies exist to support the proposed neuroanatomic correlates of the CMS index scores, and studies presented in the manual in support of these associations are based on adults, using memory paradigms that have not necessarily been evaluated in children.

REFERENCES

Cohen, M. J. (1992). Auditory/verbal and visual/spatial memory in children with complex partial epilepsy of temporal lobe origin. *Brain and Cognition, 20*(2), 315–326.

Cohen, M. J. (1997). *Children's Memory Scale.* San Antonio, Tex.: The Psychological Corporation.

Dulay, M. F., Schefft, B. K., Testa, S. M., Fargo, J. D., Privitera, M., & Yeh, H. (2002). What does the Family Pictures subtest of the Wechsler Memory Scale-III measure? Insight gained from patients evaluated for epilepsy surgery. *The Clinical Neuropsychologist, 16*(4), 452–462.

Flanagan, D. P., McGrew, K. S., & Ortiz, S. O. (2000). *The Wechsler Intelligence Scales and Gf-Gc Theory: A contemporary approach to interpretation.* Boston: Allyn & Bacon.

Vaupel, C. A. (2001). Children's Memory Scale. *Journal of Psychoeducational Assessment, 19,* 392–400.

Willford, J. A., Richardson, G. A., Leech, S. L., & Day, N. L. (2004). Verbal and visuospatial learning and memory function in children with moderate prenatal alcohol exposure. *Alcoholism: Clinical and Experimental Research, 28*(3), 497–507.

Doors and People Test (DPT)

PURPOSE

The purpose of the Doors and People Test (DPT) is to assess visual and verbal recall and recognition.

SOURCE

The test can be ordered from Harcourt Assessment (http://www.harcourt-uk.com) at a cost of £241.50 or about $454 US.

AGE RANGE

The test can be used with individuals aged 16 to 80+ years.

DESCRIPTION

The test (Baddeley et al., 1994) was developed to evaluate visual and verbal episodic memory, including both recall and recognition. Further goals were to ensure that the test would be reasonably short, yet acceptable to a wide range of patients with disorders of varying severity. It should avoid floor and ceiling effects, include both learning and forgetting measures, and include a check to ensure that deficits are not caused by perceptual problems. To meet these goals, the authors devised four subtests, which can be given separately (see Table 10–42). An overall score can also be obtained.

Visual recognition is tested with the Doors Test. The doors are from different types of buildings (e.g., houses, garages, sheds, barns, churches, public buildings) that vary in age from medieval to late 20th century, and their condition ranges from pristine to dilapidated. There are 24 target doors and 72 distractors. The patient is presented with a series of colored photographs of doors, presented one at a time (see Figure 10–23). After presentation of the target items, the patient is given the recognition test, which consists of groups of four doors, the target and three distractors, in a 2 × 2 array (see Figure 10–24). The target and distractors are from the same category; for example, if the target is a church door, the three distractors are also church doors. The targets are in two

sets of 12, an easy set (A) and a harder set (B). The recognition test for the easier set is given before the harder test is begun. The harder set is not given if performance on set A is poor (score < 9). Three practice trials are provided before administration of set A. One point is given for each correct response.

Visual recall is evaluated by the Shapes Test. The patient is asked to copy four cross shapes and then draw them from memory (Trial 1). If the patient obtains less than a perfect recall score, the drawings are shown again (but not copied) for 3 s, and the patient is asked to reproduce the figures from memory (Trial 2). If necessary, a third trial (Trial 3) is given if a perfect score is not attained on the previous trial. The maximum score for each drawing is 3, and the combined score over three trials is used to obtain the scaled score. After a delay of 10 to 15 min, delayed recall is tested.

Verbal recognition is assessed with the Names Test. Here the test stimuli consist of first/last name pairs. There are 24

Table 10–42 Description of Doors and People Tests

Task	Test	Description
Visual recognition	Doors	Subject is presented with a series of colored doors and then asked to recognize each target door from a set of four.
Visual recall	Shapes	Subject copies four shapes and then draws them from memory. Delayed recall is also tested.
Verbal recognition	Names	Subject reads out a series of names and is subsequently asked to recognize each of them from a set of four.
Verbal recall	People	Subject is required to learn the names of three people paired with an occupation and, after a delay, to recall the name associated with each occupation.

Figure 10–23 Example of target door. Reprinted with the permission of Harcourt Assessment.

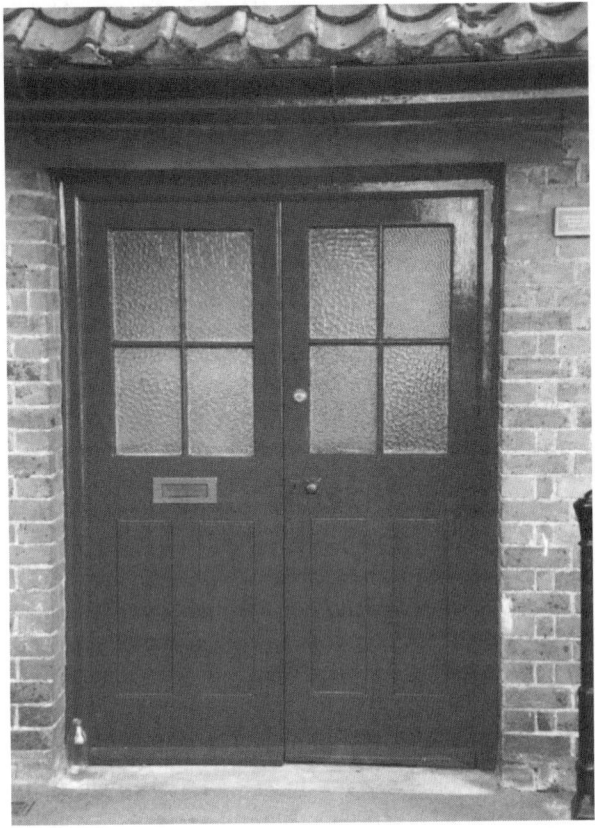

target names, each presented singly on a white card. After presentation of all the names, the recognition trial is given. For the recognition test, the targets are each presented with three distractors (all of which share the same first name) in a vertical list with the position of the target in the list counterbalanced. As in the Doors Test, the targets comprise two sets of 12, an easier set (A), which has female first names (e.g., Diane Nabney, Diane Neeson, Diane Norfar, Diane Nussey), and a harder set (B), which has male first names (e.g., David Robinson, David Robertson, David Richardson, David Rogerson). In this harder set, the foils and the names from the study list differ only in one syllable of the surname. The recognition test for the easier set is given before the harder test is begun. The harder test can be omitted if the patient scores less than 9 on set A. Three practice trials are given before set A is administered. One point is given for each correct name selected.

Verbal recall is tested via the People Test. The stimuli consist of names paired with occupations; there are three high-frequency names (e.g., Jim Green—Doctor) and one low-frequency (Cuthbert Cattermole—Minister) name. Each name-occupation pair is presented as a caption below a colored photograph of an individual. After presentation of the pictures, the patient is asked to recall the names associated with each occupation (e.g., "What was the Doctor's name?"). If the patient correctly recalls all four name pairs, the test is terminated. If

there are any errors, a second and, if necessary, a third trial is administered. After a delay of 10 to 15 min, recall is again tested. One point is given for each first name and surname correctly recalled, plus an extra mark for a correct pairing of name and occupation. Scores from the three trials are combined and used to derive a scaled score. If the test is terminated early, maximum marks are given for the remaining trials.

ADMINISTRATION

The instructions are provided in the test manual and also on the score sheet. There is a specified order when the full battery is given:

1. People Test (Immediate, with maximum of three learning trials)
2. Doors Test
3. People Test (Delayed)
4. Shapes Test (Immediate, with maximum of three learning trials)
5. Names Test
6. Shapes Test (Delayed)

ADMINISTRATION TIME

The time required is about 35 to 40 min.

SCORING

Details of how to mark the Shapes Test drawings are provided in an appendix in the manual. A number of different scores can be obtained from the battery, as shown in Table 10–43. Raw scores for each task are converted to age-scaled scores ($M = 10 \pm 3$) and percentiles according to age-based tables provided in the manual. In addition, an overall score can be derived by adding the scaled scores from the four (non-delayed) subtests and recording an overall scaled score from a table in the manual. The authors suggest that this is likely to be the most reliable and sensitive index of episodic memory, because it is based on data from all the tasks.

The overall score can be broken down in order to contrast verbal and visual scores, or recall and recognition scores. For example, a visual-verbal discrepancy score is obtained by subtracting the scaled score composite derived from the two verbal scaled scores (People and Names) from that based on the two visual scaled scores (Doors and Shapes).

Recall performance can be evaluated by a composite derived from age-scaled scores for the Shapes and People Tests, and recognition can be evaluated by combining scaled score from the Doors and Names Tests. A recall-recognition discrepancy is evaluated by taking the difference between the scaled scores derived from these two combined scores and consulting a table in the manual. Forgetting scores can also be derived by calculating the difference in performance on the final learning trial of each of the two recall subtests (People, Shapes) and the two delayed recall scores.

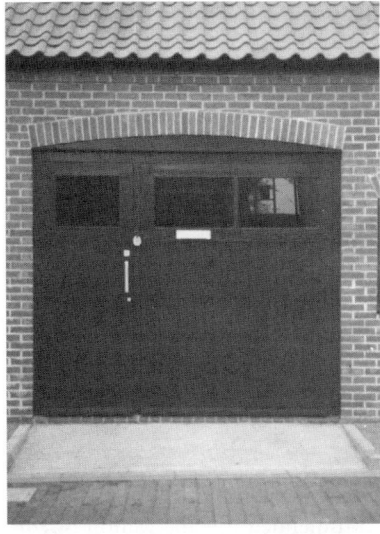
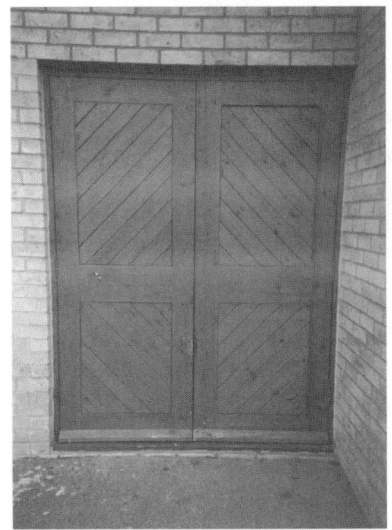
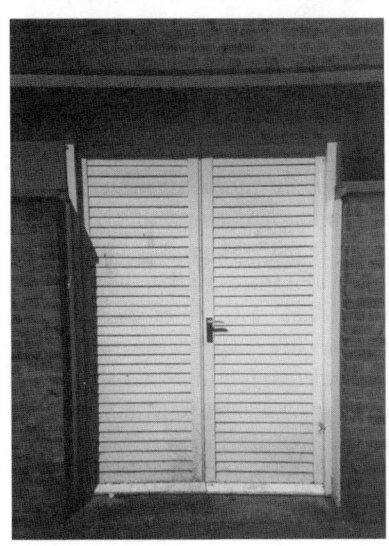
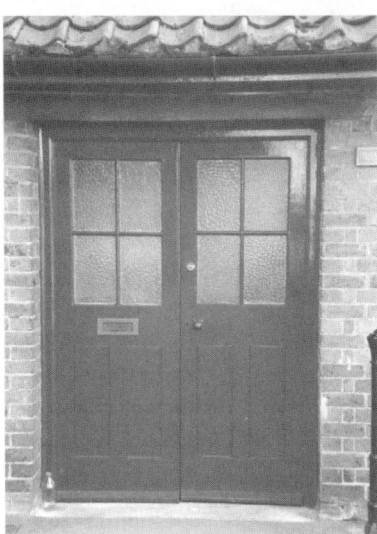

Figure 10–24 Example of target door and three distractors. Reprinted with the permission of Harcourt Assessment.

DEMOGRAPHIC EFFECTS

Age

In normal individuals, aging-related declines are evident for each test (Baddeley et al., 1994; Davis et al., 1999).

Gender

The influence of gender is not reported.

IQ/Education

Total Memory, Combined Visual, Combined Verbal, and Overall Forgetting scaled scores are all related to intellectual status (defined by the NART error score; Nelson & Willison, 1991). The influence of educational achievement is not reported (Davis et al., 1999).

NORMATIVE DATA

Standardization Sample

The authors collected a sample in the United Kingdom of 238 individuals, comprising equal numbers of subjects from each of six social class categories and balanced to have approximately equal numbers of men and women in each category in the age bands (16–31, 32–47, 48–63, 64–79, and 80–97 years; see Table 10–44). The sample size within each age group is not reported. No information on intellectual status, educational status, or race/ethnicity is provided.

Other Normative Data

The standardization data were cross-validated (Davis et al., 1999) in a sample of 281 normal individuals, ranging in age from 16 to 75 years ($M = 42.7$, $SD = 18.4$) living in the United

Table 10–43 Description of Scores on the Doors and People Test

Scores	Description
Verbal Recall (People)	Scores of Trials 1–3 combined
Visual Recognition (Doors)	Norms for set A, set B, and combined
Visual Recall (Shapes)	Scores of Trials 1–3 combined
Verbal Recognition (Names)	Norms for set A, set B, and combined
Overall	Based on sum of age-scaled scores of four nondelay subtests
Combined Visual	Combined scaled scores of Doors and Shapes
Combined Verbal	Combined scaled scores of People and Names
Visual-Verbal Discrepancy	Difference between scaled scores
Combined Recall	Combined scaled scores of People and Shapes
Combined Recognition	Combined scaled scores of Doors and Names
Recall-Recognition Discrepancy	Difference between scaled scores
Forgetting Score (Verbal)	Difference between Trial 3 and delayed recall on People
Forgetting Score (Visual)	Difference between Trial 3 and delayed recall on Shapes
Overall Forgetting Score	Combined scaled scores of Verbal and Visual Forgetting

Source: From Baddeley et al., 1994.

Kingdom. However, Davis et al. (1999) did note that for the Visual-Verbal index, an age-scaled score of 5 or less, corresponding approximately to the 5th percentile ($z \leq -1.67$) based on test manual norms, may be unduly conservative to use as a cutoff score to determine abnormality. Their own data suggested that a Visual-Verbal Discrepancy score of 7 or less may be regarded as abnormal.

Table 10–44 Characteristics of the Doors and People Test Normative Sample

Number	238
Age (years)	16 to 97[a]
Geographic location	United Kingdom
Sample type	Sampled from six social class categories
Education	Not reported
Gender	
Men	Approximately equal numbers of
Women	men and women in each age band
Race/Ethnicity	Not reported
Screening	Not reported

[a]Broken down into five age groups: 16–31, 32–47, 48–63, 64–79, and 80–97 years.

Table 10–45 Parameters for Linear Regression Equations Used to Predict Door and People Memory Indices on the Basis of NART Error Scores

Index	a	c	SD of Discrepancy Between Predicted and Obtained Scores
Total Memory	−.1676	13.38	2.82
Combined Visual	−.1215	12.73	2.68
Combined Verbal	−.1448	12.68	3.10
Overall Forgetting	−.0679	11.34	2.72

Note: y = a (NART error score) + c

Source: Reprinted with permission from Davis et al., 1999.

These authors also recommended the application of correction factors based on the regression of memory scores on premorbid intellectual status (NART errors) to improve diagnostic efficiency.

Davis et al. (1999) found that DPT scores correlate well with performance on the NART, a measure of premorbid intellectual status. Therefore, reliance on the DPT test manual norms is likely to underdiagnose memory impairment in patients of high premorbid IQ and overdiagnose impairment in less-able patients. Regression equations provided by Davies et al. (1999) may help to correct for this error (see Table 10–45). The equations allow an individual's score on each index to be predicted on the basis of his or her NART performance. The discrepancy between the predicted and obtained scores can then be converted into a *z* score by dividing it by the standard deviation of the discrepancy scores.

RELIABILITY

Test-Retest Reliability

No information is provided in the manual. Wilson et al. (2000) studied the performance of normal subjects and patients with severe head injury on the verbal recognition (Names) and visual recognition (Doors) tests across 20 successive test sessions. On each occasion, 12 items were selected for subsequent recognition from a total set of 24. Normal subjects showed a decline in performance on the verbal recognition task, probably due to an interference effect (a buildup of proactive interference). The brain-injured group showed no change over time. On the visual recognition task, both groups showed an average increase of 1 item over the 20 occasions.

Interrater Reliability

The test authors provide detailed instructions for scoring the drawings in the Shapes Test. They report that use of these instructions resulted in excellent agreement ($r = .98$) between two independent markers of the 237 subjects in the normative sample.

VALIDITY

Relations With Other Measures

Factor analysis of the DPT along with the Warrington Recognition Memory Test (RMT) and the Wechsler Memory Scale—Revised (WMS-R) in a heterogenous sample of neurologically impaired patients suggested three factors: a general recall factor (with loadings from DPT People and Shapes as well as WMS-R verbal, visual, and delay indices) and separate visual recognition (DPT Doors, WRMT Faces) and verbal recognition (DPT Names, WRMT Words) factors (Hunkin et al., 2000).

Wechsler Performance IQ showed moderately strong correlations with visual recognition memory ($r^2 \cong .60$); poorer nonverbal reasoning (Performance IQ) was associated with worse visual memory, at least in patients who had undergone temporal lobectomies (Morris et al., 1995).

Clinical Studies

The literature suggests that the test is useful in describing memory deficits in a variety of conditions. It is sensitive to the memory impairment that occurs in the early stage of Alzheimer-type dementia and reflects a deficit primarily in learning rather than accelerated forgetting or disrupted retrieval (Greene et al., 1996). In addition, Vargha-Khadem et al. (1997, 1998) described a young adult patient who developed memory impairment early in life as the result of damage apparently limited to the hippocampal region. He scored at the 50th percentile for recognition but below the 1st percentile for recall. Somewhat different findings emerge when the damage occurs later in life. Manns and Squire (1999) tested six patients with adult-onset amnesia, three of whom had damage limited to the hippocampal region. All patients, including the ones with damage limited to the hippocampal region, were found to be markedly impaired on the recall and recognition subtests of the DPT. Manns and Squire (1999) suggested that the spared recognition performance observed in the patient described by Vargha-Khadem et al. (1997, 1998) may reflect the capacity of the brain to reorganize early in life.

The test is also sensitive to laterality of impairment. Patients who had undergone unilateral left temporal lobectomy showed more impairment in verbal recall and recognition tasks, whereas patients who had undergone right temporal lobectomy showed impairment in visual recognition memory (Morris et al., 1995). In this study, sensitivity of the visual tasks in classifying the patients with right temporal lobectomy was slightly higher (70%) than that of the verbal tasks in classifying the left temporal cases (63%). Specificity however, was poor (54% and 43%, respectively).

COMMENT

The DPT is a test of episodic memory that appears to tap important mnemonic functions (recall, visual and verbal recognition). It is relatively simple to administer and is well tolerated by patients.

The normative sample is reasonable in size, although cell sizes are not reported. Of note, the data were cross-validated in a sample of 281 normal individuals aged 16 to 75 years (Davis et al., 1999). In neither study, however, were the effects of education, gender, or ethnicity reported. DPT scores are correlated with general intellectual status, and reliance on the DPT test manual norms may lead to systematic error in the interpretation of scores from patients who deviate from the average IQ range. Regression equations provided by Davies et al. (1999) may help in this regard.

Users should also note that ceiling effects are present for some of the tasks at some of the age ranges (e.g., Doors Set A, Names Set A, Shapes). For example, a 20-year-old who obtains a perfect score of 12 on the Shapes Test can obtain a scaled score of only 12. Therefore, users should evaluate the maximum scores that can be obtained in specific age bands to avoid interpretation errors.

Although there is some evidence of construct validity, use of this test is limited by the lack of data on reliability (e.g., test-retest reliability, practice effects). Further, although the materials and situations (e.g., associating a name with a face) appear analogous to those met in real life, the ability of the tests to predict everyday memory problems remains to be determined.

REFERENCES

Baddeley, A., Emslie, H., & Nimmo-Smith, I. (1994). *Doors and People.* Bury St. Edmunds, England: Thames Valley Test Company.

Davis, C., Bradshaw, C. M., & Szabadi, E. (1999). The Doors and People memory test: Validation of norms and some new correction formulae. *British Journal of Psychology, 38,* 305–314.

Greene, J. D. W., Baddeley, A. D., & Hodges, J. R. (1996). Analysis of the episodic memory deficit in early Alzheimer disease: Evidence from the Doors and People test. *Neuropsychologia, 34,* 537–551.

Hunkin, N. M., Stone, J. V., Isaac, C. L., Holdstock, J. S., Butterfield, R., Wallis, L. I., & Mayes, A. R. (2000). Factor analysis of three standardized tests of memory in a clinical population. *British Journal of Psychology, 39,* 169–180.

Manns, J. R., & Squire, L. R. (1999). Impaired recognition memory on the Doors and People Test after damage limited to the hippocampal region. *Hippocampus, 9,* 495–499.

Morris, R. G., Abrahams, S., Baddeley, A. D., & Polkey, C. E. (1995). Doors and People: Visual and verbal memory after unilateral temporal lobectomy. *Neuropsychology, 9,* 464–469.

Nelson, H., & Willison, J. (1991). National Adult Reading Test (NART): Test manual (Part II). Windsor, U.K.: NFER-Nelson.

Vargha-Khadem, F., Gadian, K. E., Connelly, A., Van Paesschen, W., & Mishkin, M. (1997). Differential effect of early hippocampal pathology on episodic and semantic memory. *Science, 277,* 376.

Vargha-Khadem, F., Watkins, K., Baddeley, A. D., et al. (1998). Dissociation between recognition and recall after early hippocampal damage. *S. Neurosci Abstracts, 24,* 1523.

Wilson, B. A., Watson, P. C., Baddeley, A. D., Emslie, H., & Evans, J. J. (2000). Improvement or simply practice? The effects of twenty repeated assessments on people with and without brain injury. *Journal of the International Neuropsychological Society, 6,* 469–479.

Hopkins Verbal Learning Test—Revised (HVLT-R)

PURPOSE

The Hopkins Verbal Learning Test—Revised (HVLT-R) is used to provide a brief assessment of verbal learning and memory.

SOURCE

The test (including manual and 25 test booklets) can be ordered from Psychological Assessment Resources (http://www.parinc.com), at a cost of $247 US.

AGE RANGE

The test can be given to individuals aged 13 to 80+ years.

DESCRIPTION

This test was devised by Brandt and Benedict (2001) and was designed to be methodologically similar to the BVMT-R (Benedict, 1997; see *Brief Visuospatial Memory Test—Revised*). It was intended for use with even moderately demented patients. It comprises six alternate forms, each consisting of a list of 12 nouns with four words drawn from each of three semantic categories (e.g., four-legged animals, precious stones, human dwellings). The semantic categories differ across the six forms. The HVLT-R includes three learning trials, a delayed recall trial (given without forewarning after a delay of 20–25 min), and a yes/no delayed recognition trial. This last trial consists of a randomized list of 12 target and 12 nontarget words, 6 of which are drawn from the same semantic categories as the targets.

The original version, the HVLT, was published by Brandt in 1991. It is identical to the HVLT-R, except that the original version had no Delayed Recall trial and the Recognition trial was given immediately after the three learning trials. The test was modeled after other word-list learning tasks (e.g., RAVLT, CVLT), but the list was shorter. When the Delayed Recall trial was introduced, the modified test was named the HVLT-R.

ADMINISTRATION

The instructions for administering the HVLT-R are provided in the test manual. Briefly, the examiner reads the word list and asks the patient to verbally repeat the list of words (immediately and after a delay) in any order, and to identify the words from a list that is presented orally. The interstimulus interval is 2 s. Recall performance is recorded verbatim on a scoring sheet for each of the immediate recall trials (Trials 1–3) and for the delayed recall and recognition trials. Subjects are not warned that delayed recall will be tested later. For selection of alternate forms when repeat testing is needed, see *Reliability*.

A slightly modified administration, which allows derivation of cued-recall and learning scores, has also been used in older African Americans (Friedman et al., 2002; also see *Normative Data*.)

ADMINISTRATION TIME

About 15 min is required for the test, excluding the delay interval.

SCORING

Minor errors in pronunciation (e.g., "cimmonim" for "cinnamon") or pluralization (e.g., "rubies" for "ruby") are corrected and are counted as correct. The maximum total for each recall trial (Learning Trials 1–3, Delayed Recall Trial 4) is 12. The recall scores are combined to form three additional measures of learning and memory. The Total Recall score is the sum of Learning Trials 1 to 3. The percent retained after the delay (% Retention) is calculated as Trial 4 recall divided by the best of Trials 2 and 3 ($\times$100). Finally, the Recognition Discrimination Index is the number of true positives minus the number of false positives.

Raw scores for four HVLT-R measures (Total Recall, Delayed Recall, % Retention, and the Recognition Discrimination Index) are converted to T scores by means of age-based tables provided in the test manual. These four variables constitute the primary measures for the test, although four other scores are recorded on the score sheet (total number of true-positive hits, semantically related false-positive errors, semantically unrelated false-positive errors, and total number of false-positive errors).

DEMOGRAPHIC EFFECTS

Age

The test authors report that age has the largest effect on every variable, accounting for a high of 19% of the variance on Total Recall and a low of 3% on % Retention.

Education/IQ

According to the test authors, education (highest grade completed) accounts for an additional 5% of the remaining variance on Total Recall (beyond age), and less on the other variables. Others (Friedman et al., 2002; Hester et al. 2004) have also reported that education has a significant impact on test scores. However, Vanderploeg et al. (2000) found that educational attainment did not affect HVLT-R performance in a predominantly white, community-dwelling sample. IQ affected recall but not recognition discrimination scores (Diaz-Asper et al., 2004).

Gender

Brandt and Benedict (2001) report that, in adults, gender makes a statistically significant contribution to every variable. However, it accounts, at most, for only 1.7% of the remaining variance (on Total Recall). Barr (2003) reported no gender differences in adolescents' scores, and Hester et al. (2004) found no gender effects in an Australian sample of older adults. By contrast, in community-dwelling older African Americans (Friedman et al. 2002) and in Caucasians (Vanderploeg et al., 2000), gender was found to account for modest amounts of test score variance (<10%) in addition to other variables (age, education). According to Vanderploeg et al. (2000), women tended to outperform men by about 3 points in Total Recall.

Ethnicity

The normative sample was predominantly Caucasian (J. Brandt, personal communication, February 18, 2005), and the impact of ethnicity is not reported.

NORMATIVE DATA

Standardization Sample

The description of the standardization sample is provided in Table 10–46. The sample included 1179 community-dwelling individuals who reported being free of neurological or psychiatric disorders. Their ages ranged from 16 to 92 years, with a mean age of 59 years ($SD = 18.62$). They had between 2 and 20 years of education, with a mean of 13.47 years ($SD = 2.88$). The majority ($n = 798$) were also given the MMSE, and their scores ranged from 22 to 30 ($M = 28.31$, $SD = +1.65$). Note that the inclusion of individuals with MMSE scores as low as 22 raises the concern that some cognitively compromised individuals may have been included in the normative base (G. Larrabee, personal communication, June 16, 2004). Race/ethnicity of participants was not reported.

As part of their participation in six different research protocols, the normal respondents were given one form of

Table 10–46 Characteristics of the HVLT-R Test Normative Sample

Number	1,179
Age (years)	16 to 92[a]
Geographic location	Not reported
Sample type	Community-dwelling residents
Education (years)	2–20, $M = 13.47$, $SD = 2.88$
Gender	
Men	300
Women	879
Race/Ethnicity	Not reported[b]
Screening	Self-reported as being free of neurological and psychiatric disorders

[a]Broken down into 13 age groups using the method of overlapping cells: (16–19, 20–29, 25–34, 30–39, 35–44, 45–54, 50–59, 55–64, 60–69, 65–74, 70–79, 75–84, and 80+ years).
[b]Predominantly Caucasian (J. Brandt, personal communication, February 18, 2005).

Source: Adapted from Brandt & Benedict, 2001.

the HVLT-R. Normative data, subdivided according to age, are provided in the manual for use with any of the six forms. Normative tables were constructed using the method of overlapping-midpoint age cells. The authors note that, for most age groups, the distributions of the four primary scores (Total Recall, Delayed Recall, % Retention, and Recognition Discrimination Index) are restricted in range or significantly skewed or both. There are ceiling effects for some variables (e.g., Delayed Recall, Recognition), especially for the younger age groups. Accordingly, the authors recommend caution in assigning T scores in these cases. Rather, it may be more appropriate to report either T-score ranges (e.g., "T ≥ 70") or descriptive categories (e.g., "recognition discrimination was errorless") in these instances.

Means and standard deviations (SDs) for a variety of other scores, including each of the three learning trials, total number of true-positive hits, semantically related false-positive errors, and semantically unrelated false-positive errors, are provided in the test manual and are stratified by age group.

Other Normative Data

Vanderploeg et al. (2000) provided age- and gender-adjusted normative data based on a community-dwelling sample of 394 older adults (ages 60 to 84, mean education = 14.1 years) in Florida; Hester et al. (2004) provided age- and education-adjusted normative data for 203 older Australian adults (91 males, 112 females), aged 60 to 89 years. Comparison between the Florida and Australian samples indicates a generally comparable profile of performance, although scores were slightly lower than those reported by Brandt and Benedict (2001). The Australian sample had a lower level of education ($M = 11.07$ years, $SD = 3.10$), and therefore this study extends the clinical utility of the HVLT-R to those with lower levels of education. Participants with a history of psychiatric illness, neurological disorder or drug abuse were excluded, as were those who were not fluent in English or who had an MMSE score of less than 25. The data for Form 1 are shown in Table 10–47. Note, however, that the cell sizes are quite small, particularly for the oldest age group (80–89 years).

For older African-American subjects, the data provided by Friedman et al. (2002) are preferred. These authors tested a population-based sample of 237 healthy African-American individuals (108 men, 129 women), living in Tampa, Florida, for Form 1 of the HVLT-R. Individuals who self-reported a history of neurological disorder were excluded from study. The data were stratified by age (60–71 years, $n = 111$; 72–80 years, $n = 126$), and score adjustments were given for education (<12 years, 12 years, >12 years) and gender. In addition to providing data on the standard indices, they also reported data for the Delayed Cued Recall and Learning measures. After delayed free recall, subjects were given memory cues and asked, one subcategory at a time, to recall all words from the subcategories. The Learning measure is calculated as the higher of Trial 2 or Trial 3 recall, minus Trial 1 recall. The data are provided in Tables 10–48 (ages 60–71) and 10–49 (ages

Table 10–47 Normative Data for HVLT-R Performance of an Australian Sample, Subdivided by Education

Measure	Age 60–69 Years						Age 70–79 Years						Age 80–89 Years					
	≤10			≥11			≤10			≥11			≤10			≥11		
	N	M	SD	N	M	SD	N	M	SD	N	M	SD	N	M	SD	N	M	SD
Trial 1	29	5.2	1.5	35	6.4	1.7	63	4.7	1.9	45	5.3	1.5	15	4.2	1.5	16	5.1	1.3
Trial 2	29	6.7	2.2	35	8.5	2.0	63	6.8	2.0	45	6.7	1.9	15	6.1	1.8	16	7.4	1.6
Trial 3	29	8.1	2.3	35	9.8	1.6	63	7.8	2.5	45	8.2	2.0	15	7.1	2.5	16	8.6	2.1
Learning	29	2.9	1.8	35	3.5	1.5	63	3.2	1.8	45	3.1	1.8	15	3.2	1.6	16	3.8	1.3
Total	29	20.0	5.5	35	24.6	4.8	63	19.4	5.8	45	20.2	4.6	15	17.4	5.2	16	21.1	4.6
Delayed Recall	16	6.3	3.3	25	8.4	2.9	43	6.4	3.5	32	7.3	2.7	10	5.4	3.1	10	5.4	2.6
% Retained	16	73.7	34.8	25	82.9	23.3	43	80.4	36.3	32	83.6	23.9	10	78.3	48.8	10	57.9	23.6
Discrimination Index	16	8.4	2.3	25	9.9	1.8	43	8.9	2.2	32	9.4	2.0	10	9.0	2.3	10	8.6	3.1

Source: Adapted from Hester et al., 2004.

72–84). Raw score adjustments (Table 10–50) are applied for the effects of education and gender before the standardized performance associated with the score is obtained.

Users should bear in mind, however, that the number of participants with greater than 12 years of education was relatively small ($n = 39$), possibly affecting the reliability and generalizeability of the normative values in this education group. Further, only Form 1 was used, and the version differed from the standard protocol in that a cued-recall trial was included between the Delayed Free Recall and the Delayed Recognition trials. Therefore, recognition data with this version are not comparable to scores from the standard administration.

Barr (2003) tested a group of 100 high school athletes (60 males, 40 females; aged 13–17 years, $M = 15.9$, $SD = .98$). The ethnic composition of the sample was 88% Caucasian. All spoke English as their native language and were in good academic standing at their school. Three reported a history of ADHD, and three reported a history of dyslexia or learning disability. Means and *SD*s are shown in Table 10–51. Performance appeared comparable to that of adults.

RELIABILITY

Test-Retest Reliability

Benedict et al. (1998) reported that 40 older adults completed different forms of the test on two occasions, with a mean test-retest interval of 6 weeks. Reliability coefficients for the four primary HVLT-R variables were .74 for Total Recall, .66 for Delayed Recall, .39 for % Retention, and .40 for the Recognition Discrimination Index (see Table 10–52). They noted that the restricted and non-normal distribution of some of the test variables may have limited the range of possible reliability coefficients.

Others have reported noticeably lower reliability coefficients. In high school athletes (32 males, 16 females; aged 13–17

years, $M = 15.96$, $SD = .94$), retested with an alternate form about 60 days after baseline testing, test-retest reliability coefficients were low (<.55; Barr, 2003; see Tables 10–53 and 10–54). Barr (2003) noted that variable motivation might play a role in the performance of subjects (e.g., some may not have taken the tests seriously).

Similarly, Woods et al. (2005) examined the reliability of standard as well as process measures of encoding (e.g., semantic and serial clustering), retrieval, and error rates in healthy young adults retested with an alternate form after an interval of about 1 year. Reliability coefficients were low for the various measures, with total recall showing the highest coefficient ($r = .49$). Woods et al. (2005) suggested that the low temporal stability of these measures (particularly component process variables) might relate in part to the low number of trials and list items on the HVLT. It should be noted, however, that the same pattern emerges when the 16-item version of the CVLT-II is used (see *California Verbal Learning Test—II*).

Alternate Form Reliability

The test manual (Brandt and Benedict, 2001) reports two studies of interform reliability. In the first (Benedict et al., 1998), 432 college students were given one form of the test selected at random. In the second study (Benedict et al., 1998), 18 students were administered a different form of the HVLT-R each week for 6 weeks. Results revealed that the six forms are equivalent for the recall trials. However, there were slight differences in the degree to which they elicited false-positive responses on the Delayed Recognition trial. More specifically, there were small but statistically significant differences among the 6 test forms on three of the HVLT-R variables: semantically related false-positive errors, semantically unrelated false-positive errors, and the Recognition Discrimination Index. Forms 1, 2, and 4 make a homogeneous subgroup, as do Forms 3, 5, and 6. Therefore, separate T-score conversion columns

Table 10–48 Normative Data for HVLT-R Performance for African American Individuals 60–71 Years of Age

Raw Score	Cumulative Percentile										% Retained Percentile
	Trial 1	Trial 2	Trial 3	Learning	Sum (Trials 1–3)	Delayed Recall	Cued Recall	True Positive	False Positive[a]	Discrimination	
30					99						
29											
28											
27					97						
26					96						
25					96						
24					94						
23					90						
22					86						
21					79						
20					72						
19					61						
18					52						
17					38						
16					26						
15					16						
14					7						
13					5						
12					1		99			87	
11		99	98		<1	99	98			63	
10		98	95			96	95			47	
9		95	83			87	78			32	
8	97	88	64			72	59	44		16	
7	92	60	32			50	32	27		7	
6	84	29	9	99		29	14	15		2	
5	59	5	1	95		8	3	5		1	
4	23	<5	<1	74		2	1	1	95	<1	
3	5			38		<2	<1	<1	79		
2	<5			7					48		
1				2					15		
0				<2					<15		

% Retained

140											99
117											96
114											95
113											93
111											91
100											53
89											51
88											45
86											30
83											21
82											20
80											16
78											14
71											9
67											5
63											3
50											<3
Mean	4.4	6.3	7.2	2.9	17.9	6.6	7.2	11.1	1.6	9.4	90.5
SD	1.3	1.3	1.4	1.1	3.5	1.6	1.6	1.3	1.1	1.9	15.0
Range	2–8	4–11	4–11	0–6	11–30	3–11	3–12	7–12	0–4	3–12	50–140

[a]Related false positives only. In this sample, there was only one unrelated false-positive response across groups. Also, reverse scored for example, more false positives is an indication of poor performance.

Source: From Friedman et al., 2002. Reprinted with the kind permission of Psychology Press.

Table 10–49 Normative Data for HVLT-R Performance for African American Individuals 72–84 Years of Age

Raw Score					Cumulative Percentile						% Retained Percentile
	Trial 1	Trial 2	Trial 3	Learning	Sum (Trials 1–3)	Delayed Recall	Cued Recall	True Positive	False Positive[a]	Discrimination	
28					99						
27											
26											
25					98						
24					96						
23					94						
22					90						
21					85						
20					81						
19					75						
18					70						
17					64						
16					57						
15					44						
14					29						
13					25						
12					21			55		89	
11			99		14		98	47		71	
10			96		8	98	96	38		60	
9		98	90		5	88	81	26		48	
8	98	91	78		2	79	69	13		37	
7	95	75	53		<2	65	52	5		25	
6	84	60	33			47	33	2	99	17	
5	75	29	15	97		27	18	1	98	10	
4	48	9	4	79		14	8	<1	90	5	
3	18	2	<4	39		6	2		71	2	
2	2	<2		17		1	<2		45	1	
1	2			3		<1			20	<1	
0	<2			2					<20		
−1				1							
−2				<1							
% Retained											
133											99
129											98
125											97
114											96
113											94
100											53
91											52
90											51
89											49
88											44
86											34
83											23
80											17
75											12
71											11
67											9
60											6
50											2
40											2
29											1
17											<1
Mean	3.8	5.4	6.3	1.2	15.5	5.8	6.4	10.1	1.8	8.4	88.8
SD	1.5	1.5	1.7	2.6	4.3	2	2	2.1	1.3	2.7	17.9
Range	0–8	2–9	3–11	−2–5	7–28	1–10	2–11	4–12	0–6	0–12	17–133

[a]Related false positives only. In this sample, there was only one unrelated false-positive response across groups. Also, reverse scored for example, more false positives is an indication of poor performance.

Source: From Friedman et al., 2002. Reprinted with the kind permission of Psychology Press.

Table 10–50 Education and Gender Adjustments to HVLT-R Raw Scores to Estimate Education and Gender-Based Level of Performance

HVLT-R Index	Education (Years)	Age 60–71 Years		Age 72–84 Years	
		Male	Female	Male	Female
Trial 1	<12	0	0	1	0
	12	0	0	0	−1
	>12	−1	−1	−1	−1
Trial 2	<12	0	0	1	0
	12	0	−1	1	−1
	>12	0	−1	1	−1
Trial 3	<12	0	0	1	0
	12	0	−1	1	−2
	>12	0	−1	0	−1
Learning	<12	0	0	0	0
	12	0	0	1	0
	>12	1	0	2	0
Sum of Trials 1–3	<12	1	1	2	−1
	12	1	−2	1	−5
	>12	0	−4	0	−3
Delayed Recall	<12	0	0	1	0
	12	1	−1	1	−2
	>12	1	−1	3	0
Cued Recall	<12	0	0	1	0
	12	1	0	0	−2
	>12	0	−1	0	−1
Percent Retained	<12	−1	−2	0	−1
	12	5	−5	8	−8
	>12	10	6	39	17
True Positives	<12	0	0	0	0
	12	0	0	1	−2
	>12	0	0	−1	−1
False Positives[a]	<12	0	0	−1	0
	12	0	0	1	0
	>12	0	1	0	1
Discrimination Index	<12	1	0	1	0
	12	0	0	0	−3
	>12	0	−1	−1	−2

Note: The values in the table can be added to or subtracted from a raw score before looking up level of performance information in Tables 10–48 and 10–49. This would result in an education- and gender-adjusted score.
[a]Correction provided applies only to the Related False Positive score.

Source: From Friedman et al., 2002. Reprinted with the kind permission of Psychology Press.

Table 10–51 Performance by 100 High School Athletes on the HVLT-R

Variable	Mean	SD
Total Learning (Trials 1–3)	25.8	4.8
Delayed Recall	9.4	1.9
Discrimination Index	11.7	0.7

Note: There were no gender differences.

Source: Adapted from Barr, 2003.

for the Recognition Discrimination Index for Forms 1, 2, and 4 and Forms 3, 5, and 6 are provided in each normative table in the test manual. The authors recommend that, when the HVLT-R is used in repeated examination, Forms 1, 2, and 4 be considered equivalent, and slightly more difficult on the Delayed Recognition trial than Forms 3, 5, and 6, which are equivalent.

Practice Effects and Measurement of Change

Practice effects did emerge when normal individuals were given the same form after a 2-week interval (Benedict & Zgaljardic, 1998). Scores improved in the second test session (with gains of about 3 points in total recall), and less learning occurred in the subsequent two test sessions. However, when alternate forms were used, practice effects were minimal (less than 1 point in total recall on the second test session; Barr,

Table 10–52 HVLT-R Test-Retest Correlations

Magnitude of Coefficient	Measure	
	Adults (Benedict et al., 1998)	Adolescents (Barr, 2003)
Very high (≥.90)		
High (.80 to .89)		
Adequate (.70 to .79)	Total Recall	
Marginal (.60 to .69)	Delayed Recall	
Low (≤.59)	Retention %	Total Recall
	Recognition Discrimination Index	Delayed Recall
		Discrimination Index

2003; Benedict & Zgaljardic, 1998), and the slopes of the learning curves appeared similar (Benedict & Zgaljardic, 1998).

As noted previously, Barr (2003) retested high school athletes with an alternate form after an interval of about 60 days. Reliable change indices (RCIs) are shown in Table 10–54. Each RCI value is followed by the percentage of adolescents with change scores exceeding the lower limit. This value represents the level of raw score decline that is required to exceed what might be expected on the basis of normal error variance and the effects of practice. Upper limits are also listed to aid in interpretation of possible improvements. As an example of the use of this table, suppose an athlete obtains a baseline score of 27 Total Learning. Repeat testing within 48 hours of a concussion reveals a score of 20. Table 10–54 shows that a drop of 7 points exceeds the lower limit (–6) of the 90% confidence interval.

Woods et al. (2005) retested healthy individuals (24 men, 17 women; age range, 20–55 years, $M = 35.20$, $SD = 11.64$; education range, 8–18 years, $M = 12.71$, $SD = 1.95$; WRAT-3 reading score, 75–118, $M = 101.10$, $SD = 10.26$) after an interval of about 1 year. Form 1 was given at the first test session and Form 2 at the second. The SDs of the mean difference scores on Forms 1 and 2 and RCIs were derived for a number of HVLT-R variables (including process ones). These are shown in Table 10–55.

VALIDITY

Relations With Other Tests

The test has shown evidence of convergent validity with similar measures such as the CVLT. In a sample of patients with dementia of the Alzheimer type (AD), Lacritz et al. (2001) found that total learning ($r = .36$), delayed recall ($r = .62$), intrusion errors ($r = .34$) and recognition hits ($r = .48$) were moderately related across tests. Learning curves and retention rates were quite similar, although patients recalled less information from the HVLT-R than from the CVLT on delayed recall. Both tasks were similarly related to severity of dementia ($r \cong .4$).

There also is evidence that the test correlates more strongly with verbal memory (e.g., WMS-R Logical Memory, $r = .65$ to .77) than with visual memory (WMS-R Visual Reproduction, $r = .54$ to .69; Shapiro et al., 1999). Correlations between Total Recall and VIQ ($r = .52$) and PIQ ($r = .49$) are moderate in size.

Benedict et al. (1996) evaluated patients with either non-lateralized cerebral pathology or psychiatric disease and performed factor analysis on scores from the HVLT-R along with the Trail Making Test, Controlled Oral Word Association Test, VMI, and BVMT-R. The HVLT-R recall and recognition scores loaded on a separate factor, suggesting that, in a mixed clinical sample, the test does measure something distinct (Benedict et al., 1996). Similar findings were reported by Shapiro et al. (1999) in a heterogeneous group of older neuropsychiatric patients and normal adults. However, support for this view is weakened because of the distortion introduced by using multiple scores from the same test (method variance problem; Larrabee, 2003).

Clinical Studies

Impaired performance has been noted in patients with AD (Brandt & Benedict, 2001). In addition to producing few correct

Table 10–53 Test Scores (Mean and SD) in 48 Adolescents at Baseline and at Retesting About 60 Days Later

	T1	T2	T2 – T1	r	SEM	S_{diff}
Total Learning (Trials 1–3)	27.0 (3.4)	27.3 (4.3)	0.27 (3.9)	.536	2.63	3.72
Delayed Recall	9.6 (1.8)	9.8 (2.1)	0.19 (1.9)	.563	1.21	1.71
Discrimination Index	11.6 (0.9)	11.7 (0.7)	–0.01 (0.9)	.389	0.73	1.03

Source: Adapted from Barr, 2003.

Table 10–54 Adjusted RCIs calculated for 90%, 80%, and 70% Confidence Interval (CI), Followed by the Percentage of the Sample of Adolescents With Scores Falling Below the Lower Limit

	90% CI	80% CI	70% CI
Total Learning (Trials 1–3)	−6, +6 (2.1)	−4, +5 (18.8)	−4, +4 (18.8)
Delayed Recall	−3, +3 (8.3)	−2, +2 (14.6)	−2, +2 (14.6)
Discrimination Index	−2, +2 (8.3)	−1, +1 (14.6)	−1, +1 (14.6)

Source: Adapted from Barr, 2003.

responses, AD patients, including those in the early stages of the disease, tend to make false-positive identifications on recognition testing, particularly of nontarget words that are semantically related to the targets. This is presumed to reflect the deterioration of semantic memory or impaired access to semantic representations.

Others have also reported that the test is useful in screening for dementia (Hogervorst et al., 2002; Shapiro et al., 1999; see also Kuslansky et al., 2004 with regard to the original HVLT). For example, Hogervorst et al. (2002) found that a combined memory score (sum of Total Recall and Discrimination Index) was more sensitive than the MMSE to the presence of dementia. Shapiro et al. (1999) reported that use of a Total Recall criterion of 1 *SD* below the normative value resulted in 95% sensitivity and 83% specificity. In a population with roughly equal numbers of AD patients and nondemented persons, the positive predictive value (PPV) of Total Recall was .84 (i.e., 84% of those who perform below the 1 *SD* criterion value have dementia), and the negative predictive value (NPV) was .94 (i.e., 94% of those who score at or above the criterion do not have dementia). In patients with vascular dementia (VaD), a 1 *SD* criterion score on Total Recall resulted in 85% sensitivity and 76% specificity (PPV = .76, NPV = .85). The authors cautioned that the predictive power indices are highly dependent on estimated base rates. Therefore, in settings where the prevalence of dementia is low, a more stringent cutoff score of 2 or 3 *SD*s should be used to limit the number of false-positive results.

In short, the HVLT-R appears to be a valid test for detecting dementia. However, it is less valid in discriminating AD from VaD. Shapiro et al. (1999) found that a classification rate of only 64% was obtained for discriminating such patients using only measures from the HVLT-R. Nonetheless, the HVLT-R may be useful in differentiating various other patterns of memory impairment. For example, individuals with Huntington's disease show impaired free recall and delayed recall performance, like patients with AD (Brandt & Benedict, 2001). However, recognition performance is relatively impaired in AD but intact in Huntington's disease.

Most research on the HVLT-R has evaluated its validity as a screening test for dementia. Recently, Carey et al. (2004) provided some support for use of the HVLT-R to detect neuropsychological impairment in persons with HIV infection, a disorder considered to produce a pattern of verbal learning and retrieval deficits consistent with prominent prefrontal-striatal pathophysiology. The HVLT-R Total Recall measure (especially in combination with the Grooved Pegboard Test nondominant hand or WAIS-III Digit Symbol score) demonstrated reasonably high degrees of diagnostic accuracy.

The availability of multiple, equivalent test forms is a particular strength. For example, the test has proved useful in clinical studies requiring serial assessment, such as evaluations of the cognitive effects associated with closed head in-

Table 10–55 HVLT-R Descriptive Statistics (Mean and *SD*), Reliability Data, and Reliability[e] Change Indices in Healthy Adults Retested After About 12 Months

Variable	Time 1	Time 2	r	M_{Diff}	SD^a	90% CI	95% CI
Total Recall	27.49 (4.12)	27.95 (4.05)	.49	.46	4.13	±6.77	±8.09
Delayed Recall	10.24 (1.20)	10.07 (1.81)	.36	.17	1.77	±2.90	±3.47
% Retained	95.24 (7.25)	91.46 (11.47)	0.14[d]	−3.78	12.49	±20.48	±24.48
Learning[c]	1.55 (.91)	1.46 (.88)	.15	−.09	1.16	±1.90	±2.27
Semantic clustering	2.12 (1.72)	1.82 (1.64)	.31	−.30	1.98	±3.25	±3.88
Serial clustering	.32 (.88)	1.63 (1.29)	−.25	1.31	1.74	±2.85	±3.41
Pair frequency	4.68 (3.63)	4.39 (4.10)	.17	−.29	4.98	±8.17	±9.76
Intrusions	.46 (.89)	.66 (1.30)	.15[d]	.20	1.40	±2.30	±2.74
Repetitions	1.39 (1.52)	1.63 (2.20)	.14[d]	.24	2.67	±4.38	±5.23
Recog. Discrim.	11.15 (.73)	11.12 (1.10)	.27[d]	−.02	1.11	±1.82	±2.18
Recog. SFP[b]	.63 (.66)	.66 (1.01)	.35[d]	.02	1.01	±1.66	±1.98
Retrieval index[e]	.90 (1.04)	1.05 (1.97)	.32[d]	.15	1.93	±3.17	±3.78

[a]The *SD* also serves as the 68% reliable change index (RCI) confidence interval.
[b]Semantic false positive errors
[c]Average new correct words per trial.
[d]Spearman's rho
[e]Delayed free recall vs. recognition discrimination.

Source: From Woods et al., 2005. Reprinted with the permission of Sage Publications, Inc.

jury (Bruce & Echemendia, 2003), changes in mood (Benedict et al., 1999), nutritional deficits (Lambert et al., 2002), and drug treatments (Womack & Heilman, 2003).

Kuslansky et al. (2004) reported that HVLT performance is compromised in persons with low reading ability, and clinicians needed to take reading performance into account when interpreting HVLT scores. This likely also holds for the HVLT-R.

Finally, there is some evidence that time of testing can affect performance in older adults. Older individuals evaluated at their nonpreferred time of day obtained slightly lower HVLT-R Total scores than when tested at their preferred time of day (Pardee et al., 2005). Therefore, testing at the nonoptimal time may increase the relative difficulty of the task for older adults.

COMMENT

This test is relatively brief and appears well suited for use with difficult-to-test or more severely impaired individuals. The availability of alternate forms facilitates serial or multiple testing (but see Lineweaver & Chelune, 2003, for a different view of alternate forms in serial assessment). Existing research suggests that Form 3 is less likely to produce false-positive recognition errors than Forms 1, 2, or 4. Although the degree of difference appears modest, the authors recommend that, when the HVLT-R is used in repeated examination, Forms 1, 2, and 4 or Forms 3, 5, and 6 be used together. Analyses of the recall trials data indicated that all six forms are interchangeable (Benedict et al., 1998).

The diagnostic validity of the HVLT-R has received support in the context of detecting dementia (Hogervorst et al., 2002; Shapiro et al., 1999), although the addition of other tests, such as reading ability, may improve discrimination of dementia subtypes (Kuslansky et al., 2004). Further, the inclusion of learning, delayed recall, and recognition components allows characterization of the unique learning and memory deficits associated with various disorders (e.g., Brandt & Benedict, 2001). However, a lengthier or more complex test, such as the CVLT-II, is necessary for the finer assessment of memory performance (i.e., to elicit errors) in patients with mild and/or more complex disorders (Lacritz et al., 2001). For example, the presence of false-positive errors may be accentuated when there are more distractor items on recognition testing and therefore more opportunity to make such errors. Note too that young and middle-aged well-educated adults achieve ceiling scores on the test, and older well-educated adults approach ceiling by the last learning trial.

Further, the user should note that women were overrepresented in the standardization sample, and the number of men in some of the cells was small (e.g., the 80+ age group included only 18 men). In addition, individuals with MMSE scores as low as 22 were included, raising concerns that some cognitively compromised individuals may have been included in the normative base. The availability of additional norms for older adults (Hester et al., 2004; Vanderploeg et al., 2000) and adolescents (Barr, 2003) is a positive feature.

It is also important to note that test-retest reliabilities for some of the variables (e.g., % Retention, Recognition Discrimination) are very low in adults (most likely as a reflection of their restricted range and non-normal distribution), rendering interpretation of some scores difficult. Greater confidence can be had with the Total Recall score, although, even here, rather large gains or declines in performance may be needed before change can be reliably detected. In adolescents, test-retest reliabilities of scores are disappointingly low.

REFERENCES

Barr, W. B. (2003). Neuropsychological testing of high school athletes: preliminary norms and test-retest indices. *Archives of Clinical Neuropsychology, 18,* 91–101.

Benedict, R. H. B., & Zgaljardic, D. J. (1998). Practice effects during repeated administrations of memory tests with and without alternate forms. *Journal of Clinical and Experimental Neuropsychology, 20,* 339–352.

Benedict, R. H. B., Dobraski, M., & Goldstein, M. Z. (1999). A preliminary study of the association between changes in mood and cognition in a mixed geriatric psychiatry sample. *Journal of Gerontology: Psychological Sciences, 54B,* P94–P99.

Benedict, R. H. B., Schretlen, D., Groninger, L., & Brandt, J. (1998). The Hopkins Verbal Learning Test-Revised: Normative data and analysis of interform and test-retest reliability. *The Clinical Neuropsychologist, 12,* 43–55.

Benedict, R. H. B., Schretlen, D., Groninger, L., Dobraski, M., & Shritz, B. (1996). Revision of the Brief Visuospatial Memory Test: Studies of normal performance, reliability, and validity. *Psychological Assessment, 8,* 145–153.

Brandt, J. (1991). The Hopkins Verbal Learning Test: Development of a new memory test with six equivalent forms. *The Clinical Neuropsychologist, 5,* 125–142.

Brandt, J., & Benedict, R. H. B. (2001). Hopkins Verbal Learning Test–Revised. Odessa, Fla.: PAR.

Bruce, J. M., & Echemendia, R. J. (2003). Delayed-onset deficits in verbal encoding strategies among patients with mild traumatic brain injury. *Neuropsychology, 17,* 622–629.

Carey, C. L., Woods, S. P., Rippeth, J. D., Gonzalez, R., Moore, D. J., Marcotte, T. D., Grant, I., Heaton, R. K., & the HNRC Group. (2004). Initial validation of a screening battery for the detection of HIV-associated cognitive impairment. *The Clinical Neuropsychologist, 18,* 234–248.

Diaz-Asper, C., Schretlen, D. J., & Pearlson, G. D. (2004). How well does IQ predict neuropsychological test performance in normal adults. *Journal of the International Neuropsychological Society, 10,* 82–90.

Friedman, M. A., Schinka, J. A., Mortimer, J. A., & Graves, A. B. (2002). Hopkins Verbal Learning Test—Revised: Norms for elderly African Americans. *The Clinical Neuropsychologist, 16,* 356–373.

Hester, R. L., Kinsella, G. J., Ong, B., & Turner, M. (2004). Hopkins Verbal Learning Test: Normative data for older Australian adults. *Australian Psychologist, 39,* 251–255.

Hogervorst, E., Combrinck, M., Lapuerta, P., Rue, J., Swales, K., & Budge, M. (2002). The Hopkins Verbal Learning Test and screening for dementia. *Dementia and Geriatric Cognitive Disorders, 13,* 13–20.

Kuslansky, G., Katz, M., Verghese, J., Hall, C. B., Lapuerta, P., LaRuffa, G., & Lipton, R. B. (2004). Detecting dementia with the Hopkins Verbal Learning Test and the Mini-Mental State examination. *Archives of Clinical Neuropsychology, 19,* 89–104.

Lacritz, L. H., Cullum, M. C., & Weiner, M. F. (2001). Comparison of the Hopkins Verbal Learning Test-Revised to the California Verbal Learning Test in Alzheimer's disease. *Applied Neuropsychology, 8,* 180–184.

Lambert, A., Knaggs, K., Scragg, R., Metcalf, P., & Schaaf, D. (2002). Effects of iron treatment on cognitive performance and working memory in non-anaemic, iron deficient girls. *New Zealand Journal of Psychology, 31,* 19–28.

Larrabee, G. J. (2003). Lessons on measuring construct validity: A commentary on Delis, Jacobson, Bondi, Hamilton, and Salmon. *Journal of the International Neuropsychological Society, 9,* 947–954.

Lineweaver, T. T., & Chelune, G. J., (2003). Use of the WAIS-III and WMS-III in the context of serial assessments: Interpreting reliable and meaningful change. In D. S. Tulsky, D. H. Saklofske, G. J.

Chelune, R. K. Heaton, R. J. Ivnik, R. Bornstein, A. Prifitera, & M. Ledbetter (Eds.), *Clinical interpretation of the WAIS-III and WMS-III.* New York: Academic Press.

Paradee, C. V., Rapport, L. J., Hanks, R. A., & Levy, J. A. (2005). Circadian preference and cognitive functioning among rehabilitation inpatients. *The Clinical Neuropsychologist, 19,* 55–72.

Shapiro, A. M., Benedict, R. H. B., Schretlen, D., & Brandt, J. (1999). Construct and concurrent validity of the Hopkins Verbal Learning Test-Revised. *The Clinical Neuropsychologist, 13,* 348–358.

Vanderploeg, R. D., Schinka, J. A., Jones, T., Small, B. J., Graves, A. B., & Mortimer, J. A. (2000). Elderly norms for the Hopkins Verbal Learning Test-Revised. *The Clinical Neuropsychologist, 14,* 318–334.

Womack, K. B., & Heilman, K. B. (2003). Tolterodine and memory: Dry but forgetful. *Archives of Neurology, 60,* 771–773.

Woods, S. P., Scott, J. C., Conover, E., Marcotte, T. D., Heaton, R. K., Grant, I., & HIV Neurobehavioral Research Center (HNRC) Group. (2005). Test-retest reliability of component process variables within the Hopkins Verbal Learning Test-Revised. *Assessment, 12,* 96–100.

Recognition Memory Test (RMT)

PURPOSE

The purpose of the Recognition Memory Test (RMT) is to assess recognition memory for printed words and photographs of faces. It is also useful for symptom validity testing.

SOURCE

The test (manual, test booklet and Word Card, 25 record forms) can be ordered from Western Psychological Services, 12031 Wilshire Boulevard, Los Angeles, CA 900025-1251, 1-800-648-8857 (http://www.wpspublish.com) at a cost of $168 US.

AGE RANGE

Normative data are available for ages 18–70 years for the Words subtest; for the Faces subtest, norms are available for ages 18–93 years.

DESCRIPTION

The RMT (Warrington, 1984) was developed to detect material-specific memory deficits, even of a subtle nature, across a wide age range. A recognition memory paradigm was chosen to provide comparable techniques for the assessment of verbal and nonverbal memory. Recognition memory tests have the advantage of being less vulnerable than recall tests to the effects of anxiety and depression. In addition, they lend themselves to the assessment of memory in patients with language deficits.

The RMT is a brief, easily administered test that measures recognition of words and faces. The test consists of a target list of 50 stimulus pictures (50 words or 50 unfamiliar male faces) that are shown to the patient one at a time. Immediately after presentation of the 50 items, the patient is given a two-alternative forced-choice recognition task and must select the item that was previously presented as a target.

ADMINISTRATION

The instructions are provided in the RMT test manual. The patient is told at the outset that this is a test of memory. He or she is then presented with 50 stimulus pictures (words or unfamiliar male faces) at intervals of 3 s and is required to respond "yes" or "no" to each item according to whether it is judged as pleasant or not pleasant. This ensures that the individual attends to each item. Memory for words (or faces) is tested immediately after the presentation. For both words and faces, retention is tested by a two-choice recognition task, each of the 50 stimuli being represented with one distractor item. The patient is required to point to the stimulus item (or to read the item aloud, in the case of the word list). The examiner records recognition memory responses on the answer sheet.

ADMINISTRATION TIME

The time required is about 15 min.

SCORING

The raw score is the number of items correctly recognized on each task. Raw scores are converted to standard scores ($M = 10$, $SD = 3$) and percentiles. One can also calculate a Words/Faces Discrepancy score to provide an estimate of material-specific memory impairment.

DEMOGRAPHIC EFFECTS

Age

Age is negatively correlated with performance (Bird et al., 2003; Diesfeldt & Vink, 1989; Harvey & Siegert, 1999; Warrington, 1984; but see Diesfeldt, 1990). The effect of age appears negligible up to the age of 40 years, at which point a decrement in scores emerges.

Gender

Gender has no impact on test scores (Diesfeldt, 1990; Diesfeldt & Vink, 1989; Soukop et al., 1999).

IQ

Intelligence (e.g., NART, Raven's Progressive Matrices, Mill Hill Vocabulary Test) shows modest to moderate correlations with performance on both the Words and Faces tasks ($r = .18$ to .56; Diesfeldt, 1990; Diesfeldt & Vink, 1989; Harvey & Siegert, 1999; Warrington, 1984). Some authors, however, have found that the relation between the NART and the Faces task is not significant (Bird et al., 2003; Harvey & Siegert, 1999).

Education

The effect of education is not certain. Among Dutch subjects, education did not affect performance (Diesfeldt, 1990; Diesfeldt & Vink, 1989). By contrast, Soukop et al. (1999) found a moderate relationship between the Faces task and education ($r = .39$). Harvey and Siegert (1999) reported a positive relation between years of education and scores on the Words task ($r = .39$); the correlation was not significant for the Faces task ($r = 13$).

Ethnicity

Race of the examinee (Caucasian, African American) does not affect performance on the Faces task, despite the fact that this subtest consists of White male faces only (O'Bryant et al., 2003).

NORMATIVE DATA

Standardization Sample

According to Warrington (1984), data were collected from 310 inpatients with extracerebral disease, ranging in age from 18 to 70 years (see Table 10–56). The norms for each task are presented in the test manual for three age groups: 18 to 39, 40 to 54, and 55 to 70 years. Users should note that test scores tend to be skewed toward the upper limits, particularly among young and middle-aged adults.

Table 10–56 Characteristics of the RMT Normative Sample

Number	310
Age (years)	18 to 70[a]
Geographic location	United Kingdom
Sample type	Mostly inpatients at three hospitals in England
Education	2–20 years ($M = 13.47$, $SD = 2.88$)
Gender	
Men	136
Women	134
Race/Ethnicity	Not reported
Screening	Any subject with a past history of cerebral disease was rejected, and only subjects educated in the normal English system were included

[a]Broken down into three age groups: 18–39 ($n = 98$), 40–54 ($n = 107$), and 55–70 ($n = 105$) years.

Source: Adapted from Warrington, 1984.

The frequency of occurrence of various Word/Face discrepancies is also provided in the manual. A Words/Faces Discrepancy score is considered significant (i.e., a selective deficit) if it occurs in fewer than 5% of the standardization sample. For Words to be significantly greater than Faces, correct identification of 10 or more words than faces is required; for Faces to be significantly greater, 6 or more faces than words must be identified.

Other Normative Reports

Harvey and Siegert (1999) tested a sample of 139 older adults (94 women, 45 men) in New Zealand, aged 70 to 90 years ($M = 77.24$, $SD = 4.8$). Most were living independently, although some (14%) were receiving some community support (e.g., Meals on Wheels). The sample was of average to above-average intelligence (males, NART IQ = 110, $SD = 11.2$; females, NART IQ = 106.72, $SD = 12.7$). Table 10–57 presents the scores for three age groups (70–74, 75–79, and 80+ years) for the Words and Faces tasks as cumulative frequency tables. Because intellectual level affects performance, these authors also provided means (and standard deviations) for the RMT tasks for the three age groups by NART score. However, some of the cell sizes are too small (e.g., $n = 2$) to be used for clinical purposes. They are provided here (see Table 10–58) to illustrate that there is a decline in performance with decreasing NART IQ score.

Diesfeldt and Vink (1989) provided normative data for subjects aged 69 to 93 years for the Faces task. The data appear very similar to those provided by Harvey and Siegert (1999). Healthy elderly individuals required about 4.3 min ($SD = 1.3$) to complete the word recognition task and about 5.4 min ($SD = 1.7$) minutes for recognition of the faces (Diesfeldt, 1990).

Table 10–57 Cumulative Frequencies (%) for the RMT, by Age (Years)

Score	RMT-Words			RMT-Faces		
	70–74 (n = 45)	75–79 (n = 48)	80+ (n = 45)	70–74 (n = 45)	75–79 (n = 49)	80+ (n = 45)
22					2	
26		2				
29	2				4	
30	4					4
31					8	7
32			2			9
33					10	18
34	7	4	7	7	12	24
35			11			31
36		8	16		20	36
37	11			16		42
38		14	18	24	22	49
39			22	36	33	53
40	20		24	40	39	64
41	24	21	27	42	43	67
42		25	36	47	49	69
43	27	31	42	53	67	78
44	36	40	44	67	74	84
45	40	48	47	76	82	87
46	47	60	58	84	88	91
47	56	75	67	89	96	98
48	64	79	80	98	98	100
49	82	92	91	100	100	
50	100	100	100			

Source: From Harvey & Seigert, 1999. Reprinted with permission of the New Zealand Journal of Psychology.

Of note, O'Bryant et al. (2003) recently tested a sample of 60 undergraduates at a large southern American university on the Faces subtest of the RMT and found that the mean score fell at about the 10th percentile according to norms provided in the test manual, despite average performance on other cognitive tasks. They urged re-examination of the norms for the RMT Faces subtest.

RELIABILITY

Internal Consistency

The RMT subtests were reported to have adequate internal consistency in a sample of 72 patients with traumatic brain injury (TBI), with Cronbach's alpha of .86 for Words and .77 for Faces (Malina et al., 1998).

Table 10–58 RMT Means and SDs for Each Age Group, by NART IQ Score

Age Group (Years)	Test	<100	100–110	111–120	>120
70–74 (n)		10	15	13	7
	Words	39.90 (5.8)	44.4 (5.0)	48.54 (2.5)	47.43 (3.1)
	Faces	40.5 (3.3)	43.27 (3.4)	41.39 (5.4)	43.14 (4.1)
75–79 (n)		12	9	19	9
	Words	41.46 (4.8)	43.89 (2.0)	44.79 (5.8)	47.78 (1.6)
	Faces	38.59 (5.2)	38.89 (5.9)	42.63 (5.7)	42.67 (2.7)
80+ (n)		9	17	17	2
	Words	39.56 (5.3)	43.47 (5.1)	46.24 (4.0)	47.50 (.7)
	Faces	37.78 (4.4)	39.65 (6.0)	38.41 (4.8)	41.50 (2.1)

Source: Adapted from Harvey & Siegert, 1999.

Test-Retest and Practice Effects

In young adults, test-retest reliability tends to be marginal ($r = .63$ and $.64$ for Words and Faces, respectively) after a retest interval of 2 weeks (O'Bryant et al. 2003), perhaps a reflection of the truncation in scores. In older adults and individuals with neurological disorders, coefficients are somewhat higher. Bird et al. (2003) gave either the same or two different versions of the RMT to 206 normal adults (aged 40–70 years, $M = 56.1$; $SD = 8.6$; education $M = 13.1$ years, $SD = 3.7$), with a 1-month interval between assessments. Test-retest reliabilities were higher when using the same version of the test ($r = .69$ for Words, $.76$ for Faces), as opposed to different versions ($r = .53$ for Words, $.41$ for Faces). In line with these findings, Soukop et al. (1999) reported a test-reliability of $.81$ in a small sample of patients with neurological conditions who were retested with the Faces subtest after an interval ranging from 2 to 20 months (mean, 7 months).

There are no practice effects when different versions of the RMT are used (Bird et al., 2003). Soukop et al. (1999) studied patients with neurological disorders and found no practice effects when the same version of the Faces subtest was repeated after an interval of about 7 months. A change in the difference score of greater than 6 points occurred in only 4 (10%) of the 40 patients. In contrast, practice effects (gains of about 3 to 4 raw score points) were present on retest with the same version of the Faces subtest in both young and older healthy adults (Bird et al., 2003; O'Bryant et al., 2003). On the Words task, gains of about 1 point have been noted (Bird et al., 2003; O'Bryant et al., 2003), although, in young and middle-aged adults, practice effects may be masked by ceiling effects. IQ (as indexed by the NART) does not play a significant role in determining practice effects on this test (Bird et al., 2003).

Bird et al. (2003) calculated 90% reliable change indices (RCIs) corrected for practice for use when the same version of the RMT is repeated (see Table 10–59). Overall, RCIs were larger for the Faces than for the Words subtest. In addition, RCIs were larger for older adults (55–70 years). Therefore, in this older group, large changes in raw test scores are needed to detect improvement on the Faces subtest, and relatively smaller changes in scores are needed to detect a decline in performance.

Table 10–59 90% Reliable Change Indices (RCIs) for the RMT Corrected for Practice Effects

	Words RCI	Faces RCI
Young group (40–54 years)	−4.4, +4.4	−1.5, +7.1
Old group (55–70 years)	−3.6, +5.4	−2.6, +7.2

Source: From Bird et al., 2003. Reprinted with permission of the British Psychological Society.

VALIDITY

Relations Between Words and Faces Subtests

The Words subtest shows a moderate correlation with the Faces subtest ($r = .30$ to $.57$; Compton et al., 1992; Diesfeldt, 1990; Harvey & Siegert, 1999; Hunkin et al., 2000).

Relations With Other Measures

Moderately strong correlations ($r = .42$ to $.51$) have been reported between the Faces subtest and other measures of visuospatial function (e.g., Block Design, Benton Face Recognition Test, Rey Complex Figure Test) (Soukop et al., 1999). The test does not appear to be significantly correlated with measures of verbal fluency, verbal reasoning (Similarities), or problem-solving (WCST; Soukop et al., 1999).

Further, the recognition memory scores appear to be dissociable from traditional recall measures. Sweet et al. (2000) found that the RMT Words/Faces Discrepancy score was not related to recall subtests of the WMS-R (Logical Memory and Visual Reproduction). Compton et al. (1992) evaluated clinic referrals with both the RMT and the Wechsler Memory Scale (WMS Logical Memory Immediate and Delayed; WMS Visual Reproduction Immediate and Delayed, WMS Digits). Factor analysis of the scores suggested that the tests (RMT, WMS) measure relatively independent aspects of memory function. However, contrary to expectation given the material specificity of the Words and Faces subtests, both tasks loaded together on a separate recognition memory factor.

The verbal and visual recognition components can, however, be differentiated. Factor analysis of the RMT along with the Doors and People Test (DPT) and the Wechsler Memory Scale—Revised (WMS-R) in a heterogenous sample of neurologically impaired patients suggested three factors: a general recall factor (with loadings from DPT People and Shapes as well as WMS-R verbal, visual, and delay indices) and separate visual recognition (DPT Doors, RMT Faces) and verbal recognition (DPT Names, RMT Words) factors (Hunkin et al., 2000).

Clinical Studies

The RMT has been used extensively in studies of amnesic syndromes (e.g., Aggleton & Shaw, 1996; Baddeley et al., 2001; Reed & Squire, 1997). Baddeley et al. (2001) described a young adult patient, Jon, who developed memory impairment early in life as a result of damage to the hippocampal region. He scored at the 25th percentile for recognition of words and faces on the RMT but below the 5th percentile on tests of recall. The relatively preserved recognition as opposed to recall performance of some amnesics (perhaps those, like Jon, with early onset damage) on forced-choice tasks such as the RMT may reflect the fact that such a procedure relies less on recollection and more on assessment of familiarity, a process that may be relatively preserved in patients whose brains have reorganized early in life.

Of note, some amnesics perform within normal limits on the RMT but poorly on other recognition tasks (Reed & Squire, 1997). Accordingly, examiners should be cautious in interpreting scores in the normal range.

There is also evidence that substantial brain dysfunction is required to disrupt RMT performance. For example, the RMT's sensitivity to the effects of TBI is low (Millis, 2002). Millis and Dijkers (1993) reported that the sensitivity of the Words subtest to brain injury in a sample of patients with mild to severe traumatic head injury was .63. Squire and Shimamura (1986) gave the RMT to a group of 10 amnestic patients; the median scores were 36.5 for the Words task and 38 for the Faces test, and no patients performed below chance. The patients were also retested with a parallel form after a 24-hour delay interval. None of the patients performed below chance after 24 hours; the median scores were 28.5 for the Words task and 33.5 for the Faces task.

The RMT does appear sensitive to the presence of brain impairment in older adults. Warrington (1984) reported that patients with mild brain atrophy showed impairment on the RMT. The test is also sensitive to the memory impairment associated with dementia of the Alzheimer type (AD) or with Lewy bodies (DLB; Calderon et al., 2001). Diesfeldt (1990) found that the test (especially the Faces subtest) is effective in identifying memory impairment in individuals with AD, particularly those younger than 80 years of age. At the 95% specificity level, the sensitivities of the Words and Faces subtests for the detection of memory impairment were 81% and 100%, respectively, for subjects younger than 80 years of age and less satisfactory, 59% and 76%, for those older than 80 years. Words/Faces Discrepancy scores did not differentiate between demented and nondemented adults. Fox et al. (1998) found that, in familial AD, verbal memory deficits on the RMT precede by 2 to 3 years more widespread deterioration and predate by 4 to 5 years the fulfillment of criteria for probable AD.

Sensitivity to Laterality of Disturbance

Warrington (1984) suggested that the discrepancy between Words and Faces scores could be used to detect laterality of disturbance. She reported that patients with left hemisphere damage performed significantly worse than patients with right hemisphere damage on the Words task; conversely, patients with right-hemisphere lesions scored significantly worse than the left-hemisphere group on the Faces task.

Other studies have been less supportive of the test's sensitivity to lateralized impairment (Baxendale, 1997; Bigler et al., 1996; Cahn et al., 1998; Hermann et al., 1995; Kneebone et al., 1997; Millis & Dijkers, 1993; Sweet et al., 2000). For example, Hermann et al. (1995) found that only 15% of patients with left temporal lobe epilepsy and 10% of patients with right-sided disturbance were correctly classified based on the Words/Faces Discrepancy score. These rates improved to 42% and 31%, respectively, 6 to 8 months after anterior temporal lobectomy. Specificity (true negatives) was high at about 90%.

Similarly, Sweet et al. (2000) examined a large sample of neurological patients and found that the sensitivity of the Words/Faces Discrepancy score for right and left hemisphere damage (10% and 48%, respectively) was too low to use confidently in a clinical setting. They also found that the RMT discrepancy score did not show the expected pattern of relationships with WMS-R subtests of similar material specificity. Finally, Cahn et al. (1998) found that, in patients with AD, scores on the Faces subtest correlated with right hemisphere volume, whereas scores on the Words task correlated with left hippocampal volume, but only in women.

There is some evidence that diagnostic capabilities of the test improve when patient IQ is taken into account; ceiling effects are less likely to mask any relationships in those with low IQ. Testa et al. (2004) examined presurgical candidates for temporal lobe surgery and found a strong degree of diagnostic utility for the Faces task among patients with lower but not higher IQ levels. They found that a person in the average to high-average IQ range who scored at or below the 5th percentile on the Faces tasks was 3.3 times as likely to have a right-sided disturbance than a person who scored above this level on the task. The odds ratios among persons with borderline or low-average FSIQ indicated that a person who scored below the 5th percentile on the Faces task was 12.4 times more likely to have right-sided dysfunction than a person who scored above this level on the task.

Perceptual Abilities

Perceptual abilities affect performance on the Faces subtest. Diesfeldt (1990) reported that performance on those items of Raven's Colored Progressive Matrices that require perceptual discrimination (more so than abstract reasoning) strongly predicted performance on the Faces subtest of the RMT. It is worth noting in this context that the photographs in the RMT include many noninternal facial features by which they can be recognized. The photographs consist of shots that display each model's hair, face, and approximately one third of the upper body. The hair, clothing, head postures, and body positions vary greatly among the models. In addition, some photographs contain missing corners, low brightness levels, or developmental imperfections (Duchaine & Weidenfeld, 2003). In fact, examinees can score in the normal range without using internal facial features (e.g., eyes, nose, mouth regions). Therefore, normal scores on the Faces subtest of the RMT do not demonstrate normal unfamiliar face recognition abilities (Duchaine & Weidenfeld, 2003).

Psychiatric Disorder

Whether psychological distress affects performance is uncertain. Boone et al. (1995) reported that, in elderly individuals, depression was associated with a subtle weakness on the Faces task. Contradictory findings were reported by Kalska et al. (1999), who noted no differences between patients with major depression and controls on the Words and Faces tasks.

Malingering

Although not originally designed as a test of motivation, the RMT has promise in the detection of exaggerated memory impairment, because substantial brain damage is required to disrupt test performance (Cato et al., 2003; Iverson & Franzen, 1994; 1998; Millis, 1992, 1994, 2002; Millis and Putnam, 1994). The test's forced two-choice procedure provides a known chance level of correct performance (i.e., 50%). Scores at or below chance (<19 correct on either task) suggest the possibility of poor effort. However, use of this criterion may be too stringent and may result in a high false-negative rate.

Other cutoff values have been proposed (for review, see Bianchini et al., 2001). Based on studies of patients with head injuries, Millis (2002) suggested that a score of 32 correct or less on the Words task in a patient with a mild head injury should raise the issue of poor motivation. Iverson and Franzen (1994) reported that individuals instructed to malinger could be effectively discriminated from patients with moderate-to-severe head injury using cutoff scores of 33 on the Words task and 30 on the Faces task. Subsequently, Iverson and Franzen (1998) refined their cutoff values based on scores of individuals who were memory-impaired, non-memory-impaired, or instructed to malinger. They suggested that a score lower than 38 on the Words task is questionable; a score less than 32 is suspicious, less than 28 is highly suspicious, and less than 20 is invalid. In the case of the Faces test, they proposed that a score less than 30 is questionable, less than 28 is suspicious, less than 26 is highly suspicious, and less than 20 is invalid. However, these values may be of limited utility, because others (Johnson & van den Brock, 2001) have reported that an unusually high proportion of nonlitigating neurological patients obtain scores of dubious validity (i.e., less than 38 and 30 on Words and Faces subtests, respectively; see also Barrash et al., 2004). Diesfeldt (1990) also found that some patients with severe memory disorders (e.g., patients with AD) may perform at chance level on the RMT. Therefore, poor performance may be considered suggestive, but not diagnostic, of poor motivation.

There is some evidence that the Words task is a better procedure than the Faces task for detecting exaggerated memory impairment (Cato et al., 2003; Millis, 1992). However, use of both tasks is recommended (Millis, 1994).

Modest to moderate correlations have been reported between the RMT-Words test and other measures often employed to assess suspect effort (Nelson et al., 2003). In no case, however, did the amount of shared variance exceed 50%. The implication is that the RMT offers nonredundant information regarding the validity of neuropsychological test results and supports the recommendation that examiners should use multiple effort measures within forensic examinations (Nelson et al., 2003).

To date, much of the attention given to the use of the RMT for the detection of response bias has focused on the overall correct score. Millis (2002) noted the possibility that other indices may also be useful. For example, based on his examination of patients with TBI of varying levels of severity (mild complicated to severe), the longest run of incorrect responses was 4 on the Words task and 5 on the Faces test. With regard to infrequently missed items on the Words task, the following items (on the answer sheet) were passed by more than 90% of the TBI sample: items 2, 5, 6, 8, 14, 16, 19, 23, 26, and 29. Whether these indices have favorable diagnostic properties remains to be determined.

COMMENT

The RMT has a number of positive characteristics. It appears to measure a distinct aspect of memory function, namely recognition memory, and can be further fractionated into verbal and visual components. The test is useful for patients with motor problems, and it lends itself to symptom validity testing. Further, the recognition paradigm is less psychologically taxing to a patient than a free-recall procedure and therefore may be more resistant to psychiatric conditions such as depression (Bird et al., 2003; Warrington, 1984).

On the other hand, there are some weaknesses (Adams, 1989; Kapur, 1987; Tyler et al., 1989; Warrington, 1984). The Words task has a relatively low ceiling, whereas the norms for the Faces task for young adults provided in the test manual may be too high (O'Bryant et al., 2003). It is possible that the cues offered by the faces stimuli (clothing, hair, posture) are more relevant to individuals in the United Kingdom than to those in the United States, making it easier for the U.K. participants to remember the faces.

Test-retest reliability coefficients are modest (Bird et al., 2003), and large changes in test scores are needed to detect a significant improvement or decline in an individual's performance. Therefore, the test may have limited use for monitoring of subtle changes in scores.

The test appears to be useful for detecting dementia, particularly in individuals younger than 80 years of age, but it may be insufficient for measurement of mild memory deficits or in subjects in this group who have a propensity for false-positive responding. In addition, the test's ability to classify individual patients with regard to laterality of disturbance is poor, although classification rates appear to improve substantially in those with lower levels of IQ (i.e., when the ceiling effects are less likely to be operating).

It is also important to bear in mind that a single administration of the RMT may not always record impaired recognition memory in a patient who is nevertheless amnesic on other tests (Reed & Squire, 1997). Therefore, it would be incorrect to assume that recognition memory is intact based on satisfactory performance on a single test such as the RMT; rather, performance on several different recognition tests must be considered together (Reed & Squire, 1997). Clinicians should also note that normal scores on the Faces subtest do not imply intact face recognition abilities, because noninternal feature information provided in the photographs is rich enough to support scores in the normal range (Duchaine & Weidenfeld, 2003).

Finally, the test has some value in detecting suboptimal effort. The face validity possessed by the RMT as a challenging memory test lessens the transparency of its dual role and probably contributes to its sensitivity (Barrash et al., 2004). Substantial brain dysfunction is required to disrupt RMT performance, and low scores (e.g., ≤32 on the Words task) in cases of mild TBI should raise the index of suspicion (Millis, 2002). However, concerns regarding the normative values in young adults for the Faces subtest suggest that considerable caution is needed in interpreting poor scores as necessarily indicative of poor effort.

REFERENCES

Adams, R. (1989). Review of the recognition memory test. In J. L. Connoley & J. J. Kramer (Eds.), *The tenth mental measurements yearbook* (pp. 693–694). Lincoln, Neb.: Buros Institute of Mental Measurements.

Aggleton, J. P., & Shaw, C. (1996). Amnesia and recognition memory: A reanalysis of psychometric data. *Neuropsychologia, 34,* 51–62.

Baddeley, A., Vargha-Khadem, F., & Mishkin, M. (2001). Preserved recognition in a case of developmental amnesia: Implications for the acquisition of semantic memory? *Journal of Cognitive Neuroscience, 13,* 357–369.

Barrash, J., Suhr, J., & Manzel, K. (2004). Detecting poor effort and malingering with an expanded version of the Auditory Verbal Learning Test (AVLTX): Validation with clinical samples. *Journal of Clinical and Experimental Neuropsychology, 26,* 125–140.

Baxendale, S. A. (1997). The role of the hippocampus in recognition memory. *Neuropsychologia, 35,* 591–598.

Bianchini, K. J., Mathias, C. W., & Greve, K. W. (2001). Symptom validity testing: A critical review. *The Clinical Neuropsychologist, 15,* 19–45.

Bigler, E. D., Johnson, S. C., Anderson, C. V., Blatter, D. D., Gale, S. D., Russo, A. A., Ryser, D. K., Macnamara, S. E., & Abildskov, T. J. (1996). Traumatic brain injury and memory: The role of hippocampal atrophy. *Neuropsychology, 10,* 333–342.

Bird, C. M., Papadopoulou, K., Ricciardelli, P., Rossor, M. N., & Cipolotti, L. (2003). Test-retest reliability, practice effects and reliable change indices for the recognition memory test. *British Journal of Clinical Psychology, 42,* 407–425.

Boone, K. B., Lesser, I. M., Miller, B. L., Wohl, M., Berman, N., Lee, A., Palmer, B., & Back, C. (1995). Cognitive functioning in older depressed outpatients: Relationship of presence and severity of depression to neuropsychological test scores. *Neuropsychology, 9,* 390–398.

Cahn, D. A., Sullivan, E. V., Shear, P. K., Marsh, L., Fama, R., Lim, K. O., Yesavage, J. A., Tinklenberg, J. A., & Pfefferbaum, A. (1998). Structural MRI correlates of recognition memory in Alzheimer's disease. *Journal of the International Neuropsychological Society, 4,* 106–114.

Calderon, J., Perry, R. J., Erzinclioglu, S. W., Berrios, G. E., Dening, T. R., Hodges, J. R. (2001). Perception, attention, and working memory are disproportionately impaired in dementia with Lewy bodies compared with Alzheimer's disease. *Journal of Neurology, Neurosurgery and Psychiatry, 70,* 157–164.

Cato, M. A., Brewster, J., Ryan, T., & Giuliano, A. J. (2003). Coaching and the ability to simulate mild traumatic brain injury symptoms. [Erratum.] *The Clinical Neuropsychologist, 17,* 285–286.

Compton, J. M., Sherer, M., & Adams, R. L. (1992). Factor analysis of the Wechsler Memory Scale and the Warrington Recognition Memory Test. *Archives of Clinical Neuropsychology, 7,* 165–173.

Diesfeldt, H. F. A. (1990). Recognition memory for Words and Faces in primary degenerative dementia of the Alzheimer type and normal old age. *Journal of Clinical and Experimental Neuropsychology, 12,* 931–945.

Diesfeldt, H., & Vink, M. (1989). Recognition memory for Words and Faces in the very old. *British Journal of Clinical Psychology, 28,* 247–253.

Duchaine, B. C., & Weidenfeld, A. (2003). An evaluation of two commonly used tests of unfamiliar face recognition. *Neuropsychologia, 41,* 713–720.

Fox, N. C., Warrington, E. K., Seiffer, A. L., Agnew, S. K., & Rossor, M. N. (1998). Presymptomatic cognitive deficits in individuals at risk of familial Alzheimer's disease: A longitudinal prospective study. *Brain, 121,* 1631–1639.

Harvey, J. A., & Siegert, R. J. (1999). Normative data for New Zealand elders on the Controlled Oral Word Association Test, Graded Naming Test, and the Recognition Memory Test. *New Zealand Journal of Psychology, 28,* 124–132.

Hermann, B. P., Connell, B., Barr, W. B., & Wyler, A. R. (1995). The utility of the Warrington Recognition Memory Test for temporal lobe epilepsy: Pre- and postoperative results. *Journal of Epilepsy, 8,* 139–145.

Hunkin, N. M., Stone, J. V., Isaac, C. L., Holdstock, J. S., Butterfield, R., Wallis, L. I., & Mayes, A. R. (2000). Factor analysis of three standardized tests of memory in a clinical population. *British Journal of Psychology, 39,* 169–180.

Iverson, G. L., & Franzen, M. D. (1994). The Recognition Memory Test, Digit Span, and Knox Cube Test as markers of malingered memory impairment. *Assessment, 1,* 323–334.

Iverson, G. L., & Franzen, M. D. (1998). Detecting malingered memory deficits with the recognition memory test. *Brain Injury, 12,* 275–282.

Johnson, Z., & van den Brock, M. D. (2001). Letter to the editor. *Brain Injury, 15,* 187–188.

Kalska, H., Punamaki, R. L., Makinen-Pelli, T., & Saarinen, M. (1999). Memory and metamemory functioning among depressed patients. *Applied Neuropsychology, 6,* 96–107.

Kapur, N. (1987). Some comments on the technical acceptability of Warrington's Recognition Memory Test. *The British Journal of Clinical Psychology, 26,* 144–146.

Kneebone, A. C., Chelune, G. J., & Lüders, H. O. (1997). Individual patient prediction of seizure lateralization in temporal lobe epilepsy: A comparison between neuropsychological memory measures and the intracarotid amobarbital procedure. *Journal of the International Neuropsychological Society, 3,* 159–168.

Malina, A. C., Bowers, D. A., Millis, S. R., & Uekert, S. (1998). Internal consistency of the Warrington recognition memory test. *Perceptual and Motor Skills, 86,* 1320–1322.

Millis, S. R. (1992). The Recognition Memory Test in the detection of malingered and exaggerated memory deficits. *The Clinical Neuropsychologist, 6,* 404–414.

Millis, S. R. (1994). Assessment of motivation and memory with the Recognition Memory Test after financially compensable mild head injury. *Journal of Clinical Psychology, 50,* 601–605.

Millis, S. R. (2002). Warrington's Recognition Memory Test in the detection of response bias. *Journal of Forensic Neuropsychology, 2*, 147–166.

Millis, S. R., & Dijkers, M. (1993). Use of the Recognition Memory Test in traumatic brain injury. *Brain Injury, 7*, 53–58.

Millis, S. R., & Putnam, S. H. (1994). The Recognition Memory Test in the assessment of memory impairment after financially compensable mild head injury: A replication. *Perceptual and Motor Skills, 79*, 384–386.

Nelson, N. W., Boone, K., Dueck, A., Wagener, L., Lu, P., & Grills, C. (2003). Relationships between eight measures of suspect effort. *The Clinical Neuropsychologist, 17*, 263–272.

O'Bryant, S. E., Hilsabeck, R. C., McCaffrey, R. J., & Gouvrier, W. D. (2003). The Recognition Memory Test: Examination of ethnic differences and norm validity. *Archives of Clinical Neuropsychology, 18*, 135–143.

Reed, J. M., & Squire, L. R. (1997). Impaired recognition memory in patients with lesions restricted to the hippocampal formation. *Behavioral Neuroscience, 111*, 667–675.

Soukop, V. M., Bimbela, A., & Scheiss, M. C. (1999). Recognition memory for Faces: Reliability and validity of the Warrington Recognition Memory Test (RMT) in a neurological sample. *Journal of Clinical Psychology in Medical Settings, 6*, 287–293.

Squire, L. R., & Shimamura, A. P. (1986). Characterizing amnestic patients for neurobehavioral study. *Behavioral Neuroscience, 100*, 866–877.

Sweet, J. J., Demakis, G. J., Ricker, J. H., & Millis, S. R. (2000). Diagnostic efficiency and material specificity of the Warrington Recognition Memory Test: A collaborative multisite investigation. *Archives of Clinical Neuropsychology, 15*, 301–309.

Testa, S. M., Schefft, B. K., Privatera, M. D., & Yeh, H. S. (2004). Warrington's recognition memory for faces: Interpretive strategy and diagnostic utility in temporal lobe epilepsy. *Epilepsy and Behavior, 5*, 236–243.

Tyler, P., Eastmond, K., & Davies, J. (1989). Why forget the false positives? *British Journal of Clinical Psychology, 28*, 377–378.

Warrington, E. K. (1984). *Recognition Memory Test manual*. Windsor, England: NFER-Nelson.

Rey Auditory Verbal Learning Test (RAVLT)

OTHER TEST NAMES

The other test name for the Rey Auditory-Verbal Learning Test (RAVLT) is the Auditory Verbal Learning Test (AVLT).

PURPOSE

The purpose of this test is to assess verbal learning and memory.

SOURCE

Users may refer to this text to design their material for use with English-speaking populations. The original French version of the test can be ordered from Etablissements d'Applications Psychotechniques (EAP), 6 bis, rue Andre-Chenier, F-92130 ISSY-Les-Moulineaux, France. Schmidt (1996) summarized literature on the RAVLT and provided metanorms. The kit (handbook, 25 record sheets, and score summaries) is available through Western Psychological Services, 12031 Wilshire Boulevard, Los Angeles, CA 90025-1251, tel. 1-800-648-8857 (http://www.wpspublish.com) at a cost of $79.95 US. Geffen has developed a computerized scoring program (to score individual trials and calculate derived indices, and including her norms) that is available through ACER, 19 Prospect Hill Road, Private Bag 55, Camberwell, Victoria 3124, Australia, tel. +61 3 9277 5555, fax +61 3 9277 5500 (http://www.acerpress.com.au). The cost of the CD-ROM is $99.95 Australian Dollars.

Alternate Language Versions

The test has been adapted for use in a number of other languages including Chinese (Lee, 2003), Spanish (Miranda & Valencia, 1997), Hebrew (Vakil & Blachstein, 1994; Vakil et al., 1998), German (Helmstaedter & Durwen, 1990), Flemish (Lannoo & Vingerhoets, 1997) and Dutch (Van den Burg & Kingma, 1999).

AGE RANGE

The test can be used with individuals aged 6 to 89 years.

DESCRIPTION

The RAVLT is a brief, easily administered, pencil-and-paper measure that assesses immediate memory span, new learning, susceptibility to interference, and recognition memory. The original version, a one-trial word-list memory test, was developed by the Swiss psychologist, Edouard Claparede, in the early 1900s, making it one of the oldest mental tests in continuous use, albeit in modified form (Boake, 2000). Another Swiss psychologist, Andre Rey (1958), one of Claparede's doctoral students, modified the task by introducing five recall trials followed by a recognition trial in which the subject was to identify the list words in a story that also contained an equal number of concrete nouns as distractors (Boake, 2000). Taylor (1959) and Lezak (1976, 1983) further altered the test and adapted it for use with English-speaking subjects.

There are many variants of the RAVLT (see Lezak et al., 2004; Mitrushina et al., 2005). The most commonly used version (see Figure 10–25) consists of 15 nouns (List A—almost identical to one of the word lists used by Claparede) that are read aloud (with a 1-s interval between words) for five consecutive trials, each trial followed by a free-recall test. The order of presentation of words remains fixed across trials. Instructions are repeated before each trial to minimize forgetting. On

Figure 10–25 RAVLT Sample Scoring Sheet. On the recognition list, A-words from List A; B-words from List B; S-words with a semantic association to a word on List A or B as indicated; P-words phonemically similar to a word on List A or B as indicated. *Source:* From Lezak, 1983.

Name _____

Date _____

Examiner _____

(Note: Do not re-read List A for Recall Trial A6 or A7)

List A	A1	A2	A3	A4	A5	List B	B1	A6	A7	
Drum						Desk				Drum
Curtain						Ranger				Curtain
Bell						Bird				Bell
Coffee						Shoe				Coffee
School						Stove				School
Parent						Mountain				Parent
Moon						Glasses				Moon
Garden						Towel				Garden
Hat						Cloud				Hat
Farmer						Boat				Farmer
Nose						Lamb				Nose
Turkey						Gun				Turkey
Color						Pencil				Color
House						Church				House
River						Fist				River
# Correct										

Total   A1 to A5 _____

Trial   A6–A5 _____

(continued)

Figure 10–25 *(continued)*

Word List for Testing RAVLT Recognition

Bell (A)	Home (SA)	Towel (B)	Boat (B)	Glasses (B)
Window (SA)	Fish (B)	Curtain (A)	Hot (PA)	Stocking (SB)
Hat (A)	Moon (A)	Flower (SA)	Parent (A)	Shoe (B)
Barn (SA)	Tree (PA)	Color (A)	Water (SA)	Teacher (SA)
Ranger (B)	Balloon (PA)	Desk (B)	Farmer (A)	Stove (B)
Nose (A)	Bird (B)	Gun (B)	Rose (SPA)	Nest (SPB)
Weather (SB)	Mountain (B)	Crayon (SA)	Cloud (B)	Children (SA)
School (A)	Coffee (A)	Church (B)	House (A)	Drum (A)
Hand (PA)	Mouse (PA)	Turkey (A)	Stranger (PB)	Toffee (PA)
Pencil (B)	River (A)	Fountain (PB)	Garden (A)	Lamb (B)

---

completion of Trial 5, an interference list of 15 words (List B) is presented, followed by a free-recall test of that list. Immediately after this, delayed recall of the first list is tested (Trial 6) without further presentation of those words. After a 20-min delay period, the examinee is again required to recall words from List A (Trial 7). Finally, a story that uses all the words from List A is presented, either orally or in written form (depending on the patient's reading ability), and the person must identify words recognized from List A. Alternatively, recognition can be tested with the use of a matrix array, in which the individual must identify List A words from a list of 50 words containing all items from Lists A and B and 20 words that are phonemically or semantically similar to those in Lists A and B. The list format is the more popular format, and there are good normative data for this version.

Scores

Analysis of task performance yields considerable information, including acquisition, learning rate, susceptibility to proactive and retroactive interference, and retention/forgetting. Learning is operationalized by changes in the number of words recalled across the five trials (Woodard et al., 1999). Acquisition is typically evaluated by summing the total number of words recalled across the first five recall trials, and learning rate is examined by comparing the number of words recalled on the first trial with the number of words recalled on the fifth recall trial. In this way, the examiner can determine whether repeated presentations of the word list contribute to gains in recall performance. Aspects of retention can be examined because the fifth trial is followed by the distractor list (List B), which in turn is followed by immediate (Trial 6) and delayed recall trials of the primary list; therefore, susceptibility to proactive interference (Trial 1 recall versus List B recall) and retroactive interference (Trial 5 versus Trial 6) can be assessed. Forgetting is typically assessed by comparing the number of words recalled on the fifth recall trial with the number of words recalled after the 20-minute delay (that is, by calculating a "savings" score).

A more complete characterization of memory can be had by evaluating performance across various serial positions of the presentation items, including primacy (performance is collapsed across serial positions 1–3); middle (performance is collapsed across serial positions 5–11); and recency (performance is collapsed across serial position 13–15). Finer-grained analysis of trial-by-trial performance can also be done by measuring the gains in access to items from one trial to the next ("gained access") and losses in access to items from one trial to the next ("lost access"); in this way deficits in intertrial acquisition and consolidation can be revealed (Woodard et al., 1999).

The addition of a recognition trial permits the identification of individuals with suspected retrieval problems, who may score better on this trial than on free recall. A person with a generalized memory deficit will perform poorly on both free recall and recognition trials (Bleecker et al., 1988). In addition, comparison of recognition of the two lists permits the evaluation of words that have been studied five times (List A) versus words that were studied once only (List B), as well as source monitoring for which list contained the words (Schmidt, 1996).

Various studies suggest that recollection of the temporal order of events may be more impaired than recall of the events themselves (e.g., Janowsky et al., 1989). Vakil and Blachstein (1994) introduced a supplementary measure of temporal order. After the standard administration of the RAVLT, without any warning, subjects are presented with the 15 words from List A in random order and asked to rewrite them in their original order. The temporal order score shows weak-to-modest relationships with other RAVLT measures, suggesting that this score may assess unique aspects of memory.

Other Forms

In addition to the standard form (Lists A and B), Lezak (1983) and Taylor (1959) provided an alternate list (List C) to be used as a substitute for either List A or List B. However, List C contains more low-frequency words and is more difficult than List A (Crawford et al., 1989; Ryan et al., 1986). Word frequencies also differ between lists B and C, with list B containing more low-frequency words. The substitution of List C for B may lead to elevated interference trial scores and to superior recognition performance for list A relative to that expected when List B is used (Fuller et al., 1997). Several other investigators have provided alternate forms of the test (e.g., Crawford et al., 1989; Geffen et al., 1994b; Lannoo & Vingerhoets, 1997; Majdan et al., 1996; Ryan et al., 1986; Shapiro & Harrison, 1990; Van den Burg & Kingma, 1999). The versions by Geffen et al. (1994b) and Majdan et al. (1996) seem to produce comparable scores and are presented in Figures 10–26 and 10–27.

In order to reduce cultural bias, the World Health Organization/University of California Los Angeles (WHO/UCLA) version of the AVLT was developed (Maj et al., 1993; Ponton et al., 1996, 2000). All test items were selected from five categories (body parts, animals, tools, household objects, and transportation vehicles) and presumably have universal familiarity. There are 15 items, including three examples from each category (see Figure 10–28). Note that this version differs from the standard one in that it does not consist of unrelated words.

ADMINISTRATION

For specific instructions, see Figure 10–29. Administration of the WHO/UCLA form (see Figure 10–28) is in the language of the examinee.

ADMINISTRATION TIME

The time required is 10 to 15 min.

SCORING

See sample scoring sheet (for recording correct answers) in Figure 10–25. Words that are repeated can be marked R;

words that are repeated and self-corrected can be marked RC. If the patient questions whether he or she has repeated a word but remains unsure, the word can be marked RQ. Words that are not on the list are errors and are marked E.

A number of different measures can be derived (see also Schmidt, 1996). Geffen et al. (1990) provided extensive indices of aspects of memory function, only some of which are reported here. The score for each trial is the number of words correctly recalled. In addition to scores on Trials 1 through 5, which may be used to plot a learning curve, the RAVLT yields scores for the total number of words recalled after interference (postdistractor trial or Trial 6), the number of words recalled after the 20-min delay, and the total number of words recognized from each list. Other scores, including a total score (the sum of Trials 1–5), the number of repetitions and extralist intrusions, and the amount of loss from Trial 5 to the postdistraction recall trial (Trial 6) can also be calculated. The percentage of words lost from Trial 5 to Trial 6 may be a particularly sensitive indicator of retroactive interference (i.e., the decremental effect of subsequent learning on retention of previously learned material). Conversely, if learning List A significantly interferes with learning List B, then an unusually high degree of proactive interference may be occurring.

Ivnik et al. (1992) introduced a number of other measures to summarize the learning and retrieval processes, and these are shown in Table 10–60. In order to use norms provided by Ivnik et al. (1992) for adults aged 55 to 97 years, the examiner must convert RAVLT component scores to age-corrected and normalized MOANS Scaled Scores ($M = 10$, $SD = 3$). MOANS Scaled Scores are then grouped, and summed within groups, to allow derivation of three summary indices: the Mayo Auditory-Verbal Learning Efficiency Index (MAVLEI), the Mayo Auditory-Verbal Delayed Recall Index (MAVDRI), and the Mayo Auditory-Verbal Percent Retention Index (MAVPRI). These MAYO summary indices have means equal to 100 and standard deviations (SDs) equal to 15. Note, however, that Ivnik et al. (1992) used a 30-word list, as opposed to a 50-word list, for their recognition trial (see Figure 10–30).

Vakil and Blachstein (1994) and Vakil et al. (1998) provided several different measures of temporal order (see *Normative Data*). These measures are highly correlated with one another. Pearson product moment correlations between the original order in which the word list is presented and the sequence in which the individual arranges the words can be used as a score of temporal order. The absolute deviation refers to the deviation of each word from its original position. The easiest to score is the number of hits; that is, the number of words correctly placed at their original serial position. See *Description* for additional discussion of RAVLT scores.

DEMOGRAPHIC EFFECTS

Effects of Demographic Variables

Age affects performance on the RAVLT; the influence of gender and intellectual/educational level is less consistent across

Figure 10–26 Alternate form of the RAVLT by Geffen et al., 1994. Abbreviations for the recognition list are the same as in Figure 10–25. *Source*: Adapted from Geffen, et al. 1994.

List A	Interference List B			
Pipe	Bench			
Wall	Officer			
Alarm	Cage			
Sugar	Sock			
Student	Fridge			
Mother	Cliff			
Star	Bottle			
Painting	Soap			
Bag	Sky			
Wheat	Ship			
Mouth	Goat			
Chicken	Bullet			
Sound	Paper			
Door	Chapel			
Stream	Crab			

Recognition List

Alarm (A)	Eye (SA)	Soap (B)	Ship (B)	Bottle (B)
Aunt (SA)	Crab (B)	Wall (A)	Car (PA)	Seat (SB)
Bag (A)	Star (A)	Clock (SA)	Mother (A)	Sock (B)
Creek (SA)	Rag (PA)	Sound (A)	Duck (SA)	Tone (SA)
Officer (B)	Bun (PA)	Bench (B)	Wheat (A)	Fridge (B)
Mouth (A)	Cage (B)	Bullet (B)	Floor (SPA)	Rock (SPB)
Arrow (SB)	Cliff (B)	Night (SA)	Sky (B)	Bread (SA)
Student (A)	Sugar (A)	Chapel (B)	Door (A)	Pipe (A)
Hail (PA)	Cream (PA)	Chicken (A)	Bridge (PB)	Ball (PA)
Paper (B)	Stream (A)	Coat (PB)	Painting (A)	Goat (B)

Figure 10–27 Two alternate forms of the RAVLT by Majdan et al., 1996. Words from principal list are in bold face; words from interference list are in italics. Reprinted with the kind permission of Psychology Press.

Form 1 — Recognition List

List A	List B	Buffers:	Bottle	Calendar	
Violin	Orange	**Scarf**	*Toad*	*Donkey*	Train
Tree	Table	Leaf	*Chin*	Pear	Uncle
Scarf	Toad	**Stairs**	**Ham**	**Cousin**	**Violin**
Ham	Corn	Frog	Piano	Grass	Stars
Suitcase	Bus	*Table*	**Field**	**Dog**	*Spider*
Cousin	Chin	**Banana**	*Soap*	Gloves	
Earth	Beach	Hospital	**Tree**	*Hotel*	
Stairs	Soap	**Suitcase**	City	**Bucket**	
Dog	Hotel	Peel	**Hunter**	Sofa	
Banana	Donkey	*Book*	*Orange*	**Town**	
Town	Spider	Blanket	*Money*	*Beach*	
Radio	Monkey	*Padlock*	Doctor	Cork	
Hunter	Book	**Earth**	*Soldier*	*Corn*	
Bucket	Soldier	Television	**Radio**	Lunchbox	
Field	Padlock	Rock	Chest	*Bus*	

Form 2 — Recognition List

List A	List B	Buffers:	TELEPHONE	ZOO	
Doll	Dish	**Nail**	*Hill*	Foot	*Fly*
Mirror	Jester	Stall	*Forest*	Bread	Dart
Nail	Hill	**Bed**	**Sailor**	**Desert**	**Doll**
Sailor	Coat	Engine	Pony	Street	Captain
Heart	Tool	*Jester*	**Road**	**Machine**	*Shield*
Desert	Forest	**Milk**	*Ladder*	Jail	
Face	Perfume	Soot	**Mirror**	*Girl*	

(continued)

781

Figure 10–27 *(continued)*

List A	List B	*Buffers:*	TELEPHONE	ZOO	
Letter	Ladder	Heart	Envelope	**Horse**	
Bed	Girl	Silk	**Music**	Joker	
Machine	Foot	*Insect*	*Dish*	**Letter**	
Milk	Shield	Screw	*Pie*	*Perfume*	
Helmet	Pie	*Car*	Song	Plate	
Music	Insect	**Face**	*Ball*	*Coat*	
Horse	Ball	Armour	**Helmet**	Sand	
Road	Car	Head	Pool	*Tool*	

studies (Anderson & Lajoie, 1996; Graf & Uttl, 1995; Kurlyo et al., 2001; Lannoo & Vingerhoetts, 1997; Ponton et al., 1996; Salthouse et al., 1996; Vakil et al., 1997, 1998; Van den Burg & Kingma, 1999; Van der Elst et al., 2005; also see Schmidt, 1996, and Mitrushina et al., 2005 for reviews).

Age

The evidence indicates that certain RAVLT scores improve as a function of age in children and tend to decrease in adults with advancing age. In the 8- 17-year-old range, the age effect is nonlinear: the younger age groups (8–10 years) are more distinguishable from each other than are the older age groups (11–17), suggesting that the capabilities required to cope optimally with the demands of the RAVLT (e.g., storage capacities, strategy utilization) are stabilized by about the age of 11 years (Vakil et al., 1998). In adults, two distinct segments can be distinguished as well: the age group 20 to 59 years is less distinguishable from each other than is the 60- to 90-year-old age range (Vakil & Blachstein, 1997).

In children, rates of learning, proactive interference, forgetting, recognition, and temporal order are less sensitive to age, whereas the number of words recalled on immediate and delayed trials is more age sensitive, increasing with older age (Vakil et al., 1998).

In adults, rates of learning, proactive interference, temporal order, and recognition show less change with age (Antonelli Incalzi et al., 1995; Mitrushina et al., 1991; Vakil & Blachstein, 1997), whereas the number of free-recall words on the learning and delay trials show greater decline with advancing age (Antonelli Incalzi et al., 1995; Dunlosky & Salthouse, 1996; Mitrushina et al., 1991, 2005; Vakil & Blachstein, 1997). How-

ever, Uttl (2005) has argued that, when ceiling effects on preceding recall trials are minimized by administering only three study-test trials, age-related declines on the RAVLT long-delay recall and recognition tests are comparable.

Most authors (Antonelli Incalzi et al., 1995, Dunlosky and Salthouse, 1996; Vakil and Blachstein, 1997) have found that forgetting increases with advancing age. However, contrary results were reported by Mitrushina et al. (1991). Some have observed an age-related decline in the primacy and middle portions, but not in the recency component, of free recall (Graf & Uttl, 1995); others (Antonelli Incalzi et al., 1995, Dunlosky & Salthouse, 1996) have reported a decline in the primacy component only; and Mitrushina et al. (1991) noted that age has no significant influence on primacy/recency effects. The lack of a serial position effect in the study by Mitrushina et al. (1991) may have been due in part to a restricted age range (the youngest participant was 57 years old). Graf and Uttl (1995) suggested that the age change in free recall reflects age changes in processing rate and capacity, whereas Mitrushina et al. (1991) suggested that they are caused by faulty retrieval mechanisms (see also Antonelli Incalzi et al., 1995). Findings from studies by Salthouse et al. (1996) and Dunlosky and Salthouse (1996) indicate that speed of processing plays a central role in mediating age-related effects on free-recall performance, but that it is not the only factor contributing to those effects.

Gender

Some authors have found that gender has no impact on test scores (e.g., Bishop et al., 1990; Forrester & Geffen, 1991; Kurlyo et al., 2001; Mitrushina et al., 2005; Ponton et al., 1996;

Figure 10–28 WHO/UCLA version of the RAVLT. On the recognition list, bold-face items are words from the principal list. *Source:* Courtesy of P. Satz.

List A	List B
Arm	Boot
Cat	Monkey
Axe	Bowl
Bed	Cow
Place	Finger
Ear	Dress
Dog	Spider
Hammer	Cup
Chair	Bee
Car	Foot
Eye	Hat
Horse	Butterfly
Knife	Kettle
Clock	Mouse
Bike	Hand

Recognition Items

Mirror	**Horse**	Truck
Hammer	Leg	**Eye**
Knife	**Dog**	Fish
Candle	Table	**Ear**
Motorcycle	**Cat**	**Bike**
Axe	Lips	Snake
Clock	Tree	Stool
Chair	**Arm**	Bus
Plane	Nose	**Bed**
Turtle	Sun	**Car**

Savage & Gouvier, 1992; Van den Burg & Kingma, 1999). When gender differences do emerge, females outperform males on the recall trials (by about one word per trial), but not on the recognition trials (Anderson & Lajoie, 1996; Bleecker et al., 1988; Geffen et al., 1990; Lannoo & Vingerhoets, 1997; Miatton et al., 2004; Vakil & Blachstein, 1994; Vakil et al., 1998; but see Harris et al., 2002, and Van der Elst et al., 2005, who found that females outperformed males on recognition as well). The female advantage is observed in adults as well as children.

IQ and Education

Recall tends to be better at higher IQ levels (Bolla-Wilson & Bleeker, 1986; Query & Megran, 1983; Vakil et al., 1997; Wiens et al., 1988). It should be noted that relations with FSIQ are not uniform across scores within the test. For example, correlations between intelligence and RAVLT recognition tend to be about half as strong as those between intelligence and various indices of learning and recall (Schmidt, 1996; Steinberg et al., 2005). Furthermore, the strength of the RAVLT-FSIQ correlations appears greatest at moderate levels of intelligence (Steinberg et al., 2005). Some have reported that performance is better at higher educational levels (Kurlyo et al., 2001; Query & Berger, 1980; Lannoo & Vingerhoets, 1997; Miatton et al., 2004; Query & Megran, 1983; Van der Elst et al., 2005), although others have not observed such an effect (Mitrushina et al., 1991; Wiens et al., 1988). Bolla-Wilson and Bleecker (1986) as well as Steinberg et al. (2005) argued that education does not account for RAVLT test score variance beyond that accounted for by IQ. In their recent meta-analysis, Mitrushina et al. (2005) reported that education did not make a significant contribution. They could not evaluate the impact of intelligence level because of the scarcity of data points.

Ethnicity/Acculturation

Among African Americans, lower levels of acculturation are linked to significantly poorer scores (Kennepohl et al., 2004). Comparison among normal individuals in Thailand, Zaire, Germany, and Italy suggested that the WHO/UCLA AVLT is freer of cultural influences than the traditional RAVLT (Maj et al., 1993).

NORMATIVE DATA

Overview

Trial 1 may be considered an indication of immediate memory, with normal young adults recalling seven words on average. Note, however, that it is not identical to Digit Span (Talley, 1986). The first trial of the RAVLT is essentially a supraspan task, whereas Digit Span is a subspan task (Moses, 1986; Schmidt, 1996). In general, normal people learn about five words from Trial 1 to Trial 5, and they recall one to two fewer

Figure 10–29 Administration Instructions for the RAVLT. *Source:* Adapted from Geffen et al.,
1990; Lezak, 1976, 1983; Schmidt, 1996; and Vakil and Blachstein, 1994.

For Trial 1, the examiner gives the following instructions: *I am going to read a list of words. Listen carefully, for when I stop you are to repeat back as many words as you can remember. It doesn't matter in what order you repeat them. Just try to remember as many as you can.*

The examiner reads the 15 words on List A, with a 1-s interval between words. Check off the words recalled, using numbers to keep track of the patient's order of word recall. No feedback should be given regarding the number of correct responses, repetitions, or errors.

After the patient indicates that he or she can recall no more words, the examiner rereads the list after giving a second set of instructions: *Now I am going to read the same words again, and once again when I stop I want you to tell me as many words as you can remember, including words you said the first time. It doesn't matter in what order you say them. Just say as many words as you can remember whether or not you said them before.*

The list is reread for Trials 3 through 5, using Trial 2 instructions each time. The examiner may praise the patient as he or she recalls more words; the examiner may tell the patient the number of words already recalled, particularly if the patient is able to use the information for reassurance or as a challenge.

After Trial 5, the examiner reads List B with instructions to perform as on the first (A) list trial: *Now I'm going to read a second list of words. Listen carefully, for when I stop you are to repeat back as many words as you can remember. It doesn't matter in what order you repeat them. Just try to remember as many as you can.*

Immediately after the List B trial, the examiner asks the patient to recall as many words from the first list (List A) as he or she can (Trial 6) without further presentation of those words: *Now tell me all the words that you can remember from the first list.*

After a 20-min delay period filled with other activity, the subject is asked to recall the words from List A: *A while ago, I read a list of words to you several times, and you had to repeat back the words. Tell me the words from that list.*

On completion of the delay trial, the recognition test should be given. The recognition task requires the patient to identify as many of the list words as he or she can and, if possible, the specific list of origin. If the patient can read at least at grade 7 level, ask the patient to read the list and circle the correct words. If the patient has difficulty with reading, the examiner should read the list to the patient: *I will say some words that were on the word lists that I read to you, and some other words that were not on those lists. Tell me each time I say a word that was read to you. If you can remember that the word was from the word lists, tell me if the word was from the first or second list.*

Optional Procedure. In order to assess temporal order judgment, present the patient with a sheet of paper containing the 15 List A words arranged in random order. Ask the patient to rewrite the word list to match the order of words in the original list as she/he heard them. (Note that administration of the temporal order judgement procedure may invalidate future test administrations, because the patient is exposed to the specific test list.)

Table 10–60 MOANS Summary Scores for the RAVLT

Score	Description	Procedure
Learning Over Trials Score (LOT)	Sum of words learned across Trials 1–5, corrected for immediate word span	Total Learning over five trials − (5 × Trial 1 score)
Short-Term Percent Retention (STPR)	Trial 6 Recall expressed as a proportion of Trial 5 Recall	100 × (Trial 6 Recall ÷ Trial 5 Recall)
Long-Term Percent Retention (LTPR)	Delayed Recall score expressed a proportion of Trial 5 recall	100 × (Delayed Recall Score ÷ Trial 5 Recall)
MAYO Auditory Verbal Learning Efficiency Index (MAVLEI or LEI)	Sum of MOANS Scaled Score for Trial 1 and LOT scores; reflects learning process	Sum MOANS Trial 1 and LOT
Mayo Auditory-Verbal Delayed Recall Index (MAVDRI or DRI)	Sum of Trial 6 and 30-min Delayed Recall score; reflects absolute amount remembered	Sum MOANS Trial 6 and 30-min Delayed Recall
Mayo Auditory-Verbal Percent Retention Index (MAVPRI or PRI)	Sum of Trials A6 and A7 expressed as percent retention scores; reflects recall after a delay as a function of amount originally learned	Sum of STPR and LTPR

Figure 10–30 MOANS 30-Word Recognition List. *Source:* Adapted from Ferman et al., 2005, with permission of the Mayo Foundation for Medical Education and Research.

Teacher	Coffee
River	Road
Bridge	Hat
Farmer	Turkey
Pen	Minute
Forehead	Nose
Kerchief	School
House	Bell
Moon	Face
Color	Garden
Beat	Classroom
Curtain	Parent
Floor	Children
Soldier	Broomstick
Drum	Gun

Recognition instructions: "Sometimes people can remember more of the words if they see them. Read all these words, and circle the ones that you think were on that first list that I read . . . the list I read five times to you."

Recognition hits (REC) = _____
False-positive errors (ERR) = _____
$RPC = [REC + (15 - ERR)] \times 100 =$ _____

words on the Recall Trial (Trial 6) than on Trial 5. There is little forgetting over a 30-min delay. Forgetting does, however, occur after lengthier delay periods. Geffen et al. (1997) reported that adults lose about one word after a 24-hour delay, and over a period of 7 days one additional word is forgotten. A proactive interference effect is observed for all adult groups (but not for children); recall for the second word list is inferior to initial recall of the first word list. Finally, a high incidence of false positives on the recognition task is quite unusual in normal adults.

There are a number of normative studies based on large samples of healthy people. The norms for Swiss people (Rey, 1958, reported in Lezak, 1976, 1983, and Taylor, 1959) cannot be used (see Wiens et al., 1988), for the following reasons:

1. The English translations for some of the words differ from the original words.
2. The current administration differs from that used by Rey (1964), in that feedback regarding correct and incorrect words was provided, no distraction trial was given, and a different presentation rate was used.
3. Educational and cultural differences invalidate comparison of current North American samples with those collected by Rey 60 years ago.

Table 10–61 Metanorms (Mean and *SD*) for RAVLT by Age

Age (Years)	n	Trial 1	Trial 2	Trial 3	Trial 4	Trial 5	Trial B	Trial 6	Trials 7 Delayed Recall	Recognition Memory	Trial 1–5 Total
16–19	78	6.8 (1.6)	9.2 (2.0)	11.4 (1.7)	12.3 (1.8)	12.8 (1.4)	6.5 (1.7)	11.4 (2.4)	11.7 (2.2)	14.2 (1.2)	53.9 (6.7)
20–29	498	7.0 (1.8)	9.9 (2.2)	11.5 (2.1)	12.4 (1.9)	12.9 (1.8)	6.7 (2.0)	11.5 (2.3)	11.3 (2.5)	14.3 (1.1)	56.7 (7.3)
30–39	1081	6.7 (1.8)	9.9 (2.2)	11.4 (2.2)	12.2 (2.0)	12.7 (1.9)	6.5 (2.0)	11.2 (2.7)	11.1 (2.8)	14.2 (1.2)	53.6 (8.3)
40–49	522	6.6 (1.7)	9.3 (1.9)	10.8 (2.1)	11.7 (2.10)	12.3 (1.9)	6.1 (1.9)	10.4 (2.6)	10.2 (2.8)	14.0 (1.4)	51.1 (8.6)
50–59	161	6.2 (1.6)	9.0 (1.9)	10.5 (1.9)	11.4 (1.9)	12.1 (2.1)	5.7 (2.2)	9.9 (2.8)	9.9 (3.2)	13.9 (1.4)	47.6 (8.1)
57–69	166	5.9 (1.6)	8.4 (2.0)	9.8 (2.3)	10.9 (2.3)	11.3 (2.3)	5.1 (1.3)	9.3 (2.9)	8.8 (3.0)	13.5 (1.3)	43.4 (7.7)
70–79	143	5.5 (1.6)	7.7 (2.1)	8.8 (2.1)	9.8 (2.4)	10.3 (2.40)	3.9 (1.6)	8.1 (3.0)	7.0 (2.4)	13.3 (1.5)	37.1 (7.5)
76–89	50	5.2 (1.5)	7.2 (1.8)	8.6 (2.3)	9.7 (2.3)	10.0 (2.3)	—	7.7 (3.4)	—	13.0 (2.3)	—

Source: Adapted from Schmidt, 1996.

ADULTS

In 1996, Schmidt provided a review of the literature and developed metanorms by which to gauge RAVLT performance for individuals aged 13 to 89 years (see *Source*; also see table 10–61). The norms were derived by calculating a pooled (weighted average) mean and *SD*. The advantage of these norms is that they provide a more stable score estimate. This does not necessarily mean that they are the most appropriate reference group for a given individual (Schmidt, 1996). Most of the studies included in the metanorms were conducted with high-functioning individuals who were well-educated and of high average intelligence, suggesting that the metanorms may be biased toward being too high (Schmidt, 1996). The norms are based on both story and list-recognition formats.

Mitrushina et al. (2005) recently compiled data from four to eight studies, comprising 453 to 1910 participants, ages 20 to 79 years, for Trial 1, Trial 5, recall after interference, recognition, and total recall. The values match closely the metanorms provided by Schmidt (1996) for most variables (Trial 1, Trial 5, recall after interference) and are similar in the rate of age-related changes for most of the variables. As with Schmidt (1996), mean education levels were quite high (about 14 years), and the metanorms may overestimate expected scores for individuals with lower educational or intellectual levels. Therefore, the examiner can refer to specific reference studies recommended for various groups (see Mitrushina et al., 2005 and later discussion here).

Geffen et al. (1990) published normative data for 153 healthy adults, aged 16 to 84 years, of above-average IQ. Subsequently, she compiled additional data (G. M. Geffen, personal communication, May, 1995) for healthy Australian adults (*N* = 437) whose estimated IQ (from the NART) fell within the average range (about 105). The updated mean recall and recognition data are shown in Tables 10–62a and 10–62b for men and women separately, in each of seven age groups. It is important to note, however, that the sample was not represen-

Table 10–62a RAVLT Scores for Adult Males: Mean Number and *SD* of Words Recalled and Recognized According to Age (years) and Trial

	16–19 (n = 13)	20–29 (n = 52)	30–39 (n = 50)	40–49 (n = 41)	50–59 (n = 32)	60–69 (n = 12)	70+ (n = 11)
Trial 1 List A	6.9 (1.8)	7.1 (1.4)	6.3 (1.7)	6.2 (1.6)	6.3 (1.5)	5.2 (1.6)	3.6 (0.8)
Trial 2 List A	9.7 (1.7)	9.7 (1.9)	9.0 (2.5)	8.9 (2.1)	8.4 (1.8)	6.8 (1.9)	5.7 (1.7)
Trial 3 List A	11.5 (1.2)	11.4 (1.8)	10.4 (2.5)	10.0 (2.5)	9.9 (1.8)	7.9 (2.8)	6.8 (1.6)
Trial 4 List A	12.8 (1.6)	11.8 (1.9)	11.3 (2.5)	11.0 (2.6)	10.7 (2.0)	8.7 (2.6)	8.3 (2.7)
Trial 5 List A	12.5 (1.3)	12.2 (2.0)	11.6 (2.5)	11.3 (1.9)	11.1 (2.2)	9.0 (2.3)	8.2 (2.5)
Total	53.4 (5.4)	52.2 (7.3)	48.6 (10.3)	47.4 (8.8)	46.4 (7.6)	37.6 (9.8)	32.6 (8.3)
Distractor List B	6.9 (1.9)	6.6 (1.8)	5.8 (1.8)	5.9 (1.7)	5.4 (1.8)	4.7 (1.5)	3.5 (1.2)
Trial A6 (Retention)	11.2 (1.6)	11.0 (2.4)	9.8 (3.3)	9.6 (3.0)	9.0 (2.8)	7.0 (2.9)	6.4 (1.7)
Trial A7 (Delayed Recall)	11.3 (1.7)	11.1 (2.4)	10.0 (3.4)	9.4 (3.3)	8.7 (3.0)	6.8 (3.7)	5.6 (2.6)
List A Recognition	14.4 (0.9)	12.8 (2.2)	12.7 (2.5)	12.2 (2.6)	11.4 (2.7)	10.1 (3.3)	11.5 (2.6)
List B Recognition	8.4 (3.8)	7.6 (3.7)	5.7 (3.2)	6.5 (3.7)	5.1 (3.5)	3.9 (2.5)	3.0 (2.5)
P (A) List A	0.95 (0.09)	0.9 (0.1)	0.9 (0.1)	0.9 (0.1)	0.9 (0.1)	0.8 (0.1)	0.8 (0.1)
P (B) List A	0.8 (0.1)	0.7 (0.1)	0.7 (0.1)	0.7 (0.1)	0.7 (0.1)	0.7 (0.1)	0.6 (0.8)

Note: p(A) = 0.5(1 + hit rate − false-positive rate).

Source: G. M. Geffen, personal communication, May, 1995.

Table 10–62b RAVLT Scores for Adult Females: Mean Number and *SD* of Words Recalled and Recognized According to Age (years) and Trial

	16–19 (*n* = 14)	20–29 (*n* = 48)	30–39 (*n* = 58)	40–49 (*n* = 45)	50–59 (*n* = 31)	60–69 (*n* = 18)	70+ (*n* = 10)
Trial 1 List A	8.0 (1.8)	7.2 (1.6)	7.3 (1.9)	6.6 (1.5)	6.3 (2.0)	6.3 (2.1)	5.6 (1.4)
Trial 2 List A	10.8 (2.1)	9.8 (2.0)	10.0 (2.2)	9.1 (1.9)	8.7 (2.1)	9.4 (2.0)	6.9 (2.1)
Trial 3 List A	12.6 (1.3)	11.3 (2.1)	11.5 (2.1)	10.9 (1.7)	10.5 (2.2)	10.6 (2.1)	8.9 (1.8)
Trial 4 List A	12.6 (1.6)	11.7 (2.0)	12.4 (2.1)	11.6 (2.2)	11.2 (2.2)	11.2 (1.7)	10.1 (1.9)
Trial 5 List A	13.3 (1.4)	12.3 (2.2)	12.4 (2.0)	12.4 (1.6)	11.8 (2.0)	11.9 (1.6)	10.1 (1.2)
Total	57.4 (5.9)	52.3 (8.0)	53.6 (8.3)	50.6 (7.1)	48.5 (8.4)	49.4 (7.5)	41.6 (6.6)
Distractor List B	7.5 (1.6)	6.5 (1.9)	6.6 (2.1)	5.9 (1.9)	5.2 (1.8)	5.6 (1.2)	4.2 (1.9)
Trial A6 (Retention)	12.1 (1.4)	11.2 (2.5)	11.4 (2.4)	10.4 (2.7)	10.0 (3.4)	9.4 (2.3)	7.8 (1.8)
Trial A7 (Delayed Recall)	11.8 (2.5)	11.1 (2.7)	11.2 (2.8)	10.6 (2.5)	10.0 (3.4)	10.2 (2.5)	8.3 (2.1)
List A Recognition	13.6 (2.1)	13.5 (1.6)	13.6 (1.9)	13.0 (2.2)	12.1 (2.7)	11.3 (2.8)	13.6 (2.0)
List B Recognition	7.9 (3.2)	7.8 (3.1)	8.5 (3.8)	7.4 (3.3)	6.0 (3.3)	6.2 (3.5)	7.5 (3.7)
P (A) List A	0.9 (0.01)	0.9 (0.1)	0.9 (0.1)	0.9 (0.1)	0.9 (0.1)	0.9 (0.1)	0.8 (0.1)
P (B) List A	0.7 (0.1)	0.7 (0.1)	0.8 (0.1)	0.7 (0.1)	0.7 (0.1)	0.7 (0.1)	0.7 (0.1)

Note: p(A) = 0.5(1 + hit rate − false-positive rate).

Source: G. M. Geffen, personal communication, May, 1995.

tative of the general population, because subjects were of average but mostly above-average intelligence and had more than an average number of years of education. Note too that subjects tested before 1990 had a 20-min delay (Trial A7), whereas those tested and added later had a 30-min delay. It is unlikely that there was an appreciable difference in performance after a 20-min versus a 30-min delay, because the amount forgotten tends to be minimal.

Bleecker et al. (1988), Mitrushina et al. (1991), Nielsen et al. (1989), Read (1986), Savage & Gouvier (1992), Selnes et al. (1991), Uchiyama et al. (1995), Vakil & Blachstein (1997), Van der Elst (2005), and Wiens et al. (1988) also provided normative data for healthy adults. The values are similar, but not identical, to those reported here, although in some cases their administration differs from Geffen's (e.g., no 20-min delayed-recall trial is given, or the story recognition procedure is used), applies to only a segment of the population (e.g., young and middle-aged adults [Nielsen et al., 1989; Wiens et al., 1988], males [Selnes et al., 1991; Uchiyama et al., 1995], highly educated individuals [Bleeker et al., 1988; Savage & Gouvier, 1992; Mitrushina et al., 1991; Vakil & Blachstein, 1997]), or derives from non-English-speaking individuals (Vakil & Blachstein, 1997; Van der Elst et al., 2005).

There is evidence that norm sets are not interchangeable and that set selection determines the likelihood of a patient being classed as memory-impaired. Stallings et al. (1995) showed that selection of the Savage and Gouvier (1992) norms results in a significantly lower rate of classification of impairment than would other norms, such as those by Wiens et al. (1988). The Wiens and Geffen sets appear to produce relatively similar results (Stallings et al., 1995).

Norms for older adults also exist. Ivnik et al. (1990) provided normative data based on 47 healthy subjects, aged 85 and older. Ivnik et al. (1992) extended their normative database to a sample of 530 healthy persons (62.3% female),

mostly well-educated (82.7% ≥grade 12) Caucasians (99.6%), aged 56 to 97 years. Tables 10–63 through 10–73 convert AVLT scores to age-corrected MOANS Scaled Scores (*M* = 10, *SD* = 3) and summary Mayo Auditory-Verbal Indices (*M* = 100, *SD* = 15). It is important to note that Ivnik et al. (1992) used a list with 30, not 50, words for their recognition trial. The list is shown in Figure 10–30.

Since completing their report, Harris et al. (2002) augmented their sample by an additional 311 subjects, for a total of 836 subjects. The subjects were of average IQ (MAYO FSIQ = 105.5, *SD* = 10.4), aged 58 to 98 years, predominantly female (63.8%), and overwhelmingly Caucasian. A recognition percent correct (RPC) score was calculated using the following formula: (True positives + True negatives)/30. Because RPC is an algebraic transformation of true-positives (TP) minus false-positive errors (FP), Table 10–74 can be used to conveniently calculate RPC for the difference score, TP − FP. In this study, gender differences were sufficiently pronounced (favoring women) to suggest the desirability of separated RPC norms for males and females. Tables 10–75 and 10–76 show age- and gender-specific RPC data for the 30-item recognition form. Similar data were provided by Tuokko and Woodward (1996).

Given that IQ is more strongly related to performance than education, Steinberg et al. (2005) have reanalyzed data from the Mayo Clinic's Older Americans Normative Studies (MOANS) and provided age- (55+) and IQ-adjusted percentile equivalents of MOANS age-adjusted RAVLT scores. Readers should note that all FSIQs are MAYO age-adjusted scores, which are based on the WAIS-R, not the WAIS-III. Given the upward shift in scores (Flynn effect) with the passage of time, use of the WAIS-R FSIQ, rather than the WAIS-III, might result in a given RAVLT appearing less favorable. The interested reader is referred to their article for the relevant tables.

Ferman et al. (2005) recently provided age- and education-adjusted normative data based on 306 African American

Table 10–63 MOANS Scaled Scores (Midpoint Age = 61 Years, Range = 56–66, N = 143)

MOANS Scaled Score	Learning Efficiency Index Measures			Delayed Recall Index Measures			Percent Retention Index Measures		Percentile Ranges
	Trial 1	LOT	List B	Trial 6	30-min Recall	Recognition	STPR	LTPR	
2	0–2	0	0	0–2	0	0–5	0–30	0–10	<1
3	—	1	1	3	—	6–7	31–42	11–13	1
4	—	2–3	2	—	—	—	43–44	14–15	2
5	3	4–6	—	4	1–3	8–9	45–50	16–37	3–5
6	—	7–8	—	5	4	10	51–58	38–53	6–10
7	4	9–11	3	6	5–6	11	59–69	54–58	11–18
8	—	12–13	—	7	7	12–13	70–75	59–64	19–28
9	5	14–16	—	8–9	8	—	76–80	65–75	29–40
10	6	17–19	4	10	9	14	81–87	76–83	41–59
11	—	20–21	5	11	10–11	—	88–91	84–88	60–71
12	7	22–23	—	12	12	15	92–93	89–93	72–81
13	8	24–26	6	13	13	—	94–95	94+	82–89
14	—	27	7	14	14	—	96+	—	90–94
15	9	28–29	8	15	15	—	—	—	95–97
16	—	—	9	—	—	—	—	—	98
17	10–12	30–32	—	—	—	—	—	—	99
18	13–15	33+	10–15	—	—	—	—	—	>99

Note: MOANS Scaled Scores are corrected for age influences. LOT = Leaning Over Trials; LTPR = Long-Term Percent Retention; MOANS = Mayo's Older Americans Normative Studies; STPR = Short-Term Percent Retention.

Source: Ivnik et al., 1992. Reprinted with the permission of the Mayo Foundation for Medical Education and Research.

Table 10–64 MOANS Scaled Scores (Midpoint Age = 64 Years, Range = 59–69, N = 168)

MOANS Scaled Score	Learning Efficiency Index Measures			Delayed Recall Index Measures			Percent Retention Index Measures		Percentile Ranges
	Trial 1	LOT	List B	Trial 6	30-min Recall	Recognition	STPR	LTPR	
2	0–1	0	0	0–1	0	0–5	0–20	0–10	<1
3	2	1	—	2	—	6	21–25	11–13	1
4	—	2–3	1	3	—	7	26–33	14–15	2
5	3	4–5	2	4	1–2	8	34–40	16–30	3–5
6	—	6–7	—	5	3	9–10	41–57	31–45	6–10
7	—	8–9	3	6	4	11	58–63	46–54	11–18
8	4	10–12	—	7	5–6	12	64–72	55–62	19–28
9	5	13–15	—	8	7	13	73–76	63–71	29–40
10	—	16–18	4	9	8–9	14	77–86	72–82	41–59
11	6	19–20	5	10	10	—	87–91	83–88	60–71
12	—	21–23	—	11–12	11	15	92–93	89–92	72–81
13	7	24–25	6	—	12	—	94–95	93–95	82–89
14	8	26	—	13	13	—	96+	96+	90–94
15	9	27	7	14	14	—	—	—	95–97
16	—	28–29	8	15	—	—	—	—	98
17	10–12	30–32	9	—	15	—	—	—	99
18	13–15	33+	10–15	—	—	—	—	—	>99

Note: MOANS Scaled Scores are corrected for age influences. LOT = Leaning Over Trials; LTPR = Long-Term Percent Retention; MOANS = Mayo's Older Americans Normative Studies; STPR = Short-Term Percent Retention.

Source: Ivnik et al., 1992. Reprinted with the permission of the Mayo Foundation for Medical Education and Research.

Table 10–65 MOANS Scaled Scores (Midpoint Age = 67 Years, Range = 62–72, N = 182)

MOANS Scaled Score	Learning Efficiency Index Measures			Delayed Recall Index Measures			Percent Retention Index Measures		Percentile Ranges
	Trial 1	LOT	List B	Trial 6	30-min Recall	Recognition	STPR	LTPR	
2	0–1	0	0	0	—	0–5	0–20	—	<1
3	—	1	—	1	0	6	21–25	0–5	1
4	2	2–3	1	2	—	7	26–33	6–12	2
5	—	4–5	—	3	1	8	34–40	13–21	3–5
6	3	6–7	2	4	2–3	9	41–57	22–42	6–10
7	—	8–9	—	5	4	10	58–63	43–53	11–18
8	4	10–11	3	6	5	11	64–71	54–60	19–28
9	—	12–13	—	7	6–7	12	72–76	61–70	29–40
10	5	14–18	4	8–9	8	13	77–86	71–80	41–59
11	6	19–20	—	10	9	14	87–91	81–84	60–71
12	—	21–22	5	11	10	15	92–93	85–90	72–81
13	7	23–25	—	12	11–12	—	94–95	91–94	82–89
14	—	26	6	13	13	—	96+	95+	90–94
15	8	27	7	—	—	—	—	—	95–97
16	—	28–29	8	14	14	—	—	—	98
17	9–10	30–32	9	15	15	—	—	—	99
18	11–15	33+	10–15	—	—	—	—	—	>99

Note: MOANS Scaled Scores are corrected for age influences. LOT = Leaning Over Trials; LTPR = Long-Term Percent Retention; MOANS = Mayo's Older Americans Normative Studies; STPR = Short-Term Percent Retention.

Source: Ivnik et al., 1992. Reprinted with the permission of the Mayo Foundation for Medical Education and Research.

Table 10–66 MOANS Scaled Scores (Midpoint Age = 70 Years, Range = 65–75, N = 194)

MOANS Scaled Score	Learning Efficiency Index Measures			Delayed Recall Index Measures			Percent Retention Index Measures		Percentile Ranges
	Trial 1	LOT	List B	Trial 6	30-min Recall	Recognition	STPR	LTPR	
2	0–1	0	0	0	—	0–5	0–20	—	<1
3	—	1	—	1	0	6	21–25	0–5	1
4	2	—	—	—	—	7	26–33	6–12	2
5	—	2–4	1	2–3	1	8	34–40	13–21	3–5
6	3	5–6	—	4	2–3	9	41–54	22–38	6–10
7	—	7–8	2	5	4	10	55–62	39–49	11–18
8	4	9–10	—	6	5	11	63–69	50–59	19–28
9	—	11–13	3	7	6	12	70–73	60–65	29–40
10	5	14–16	4	8	7	13	74–83	66–76	41–59
11	—	17–19	—	9	8	14	84–88	77–83	60–71
12	6	20–21	5	10	9	—	89–93	84–89	72–81
13	—	22–23	—	11	10–11	15	94–95	90–92	82–89
14	7	24–26	6	12	12	—	96+	93–94	90–94
15	—	27	7	13	13	—	—	95+	95–97
16	8	28–29	8	14	—	—	—	—	98
17	9	30–32	9	—	14	—	—	—	99
18	10–15	33+	10–15	15	15	—	—	—	>99

Note: MOANS Scaled Scores are corrected for age influences. LOT = Leaning Over Trials; LTPR = Long-Term Percent Retention; MOANS = Mayo's Older Americans Normative Studies; STPR = Short-Term Percent Retention.

Source: Ivnik et al., 1992. Reprinted with the permission of the Mayo Foundation for Medical Education and Research.

Table 10–67 MOANS Scaled Scores (Midpoint Age = 73 Years, Range = 68–78, N = 214)

MOANS Scaled Score	Learning Efficiency Index Measures			Delayed Recall Index Measures			Percent Retention Index Measures		Percentile Ranges
	Trial 1	LOT	List B	Trial 6	30-min Recall	Recognition	STPR	LTPR	
2	0	0	0	0	—	0–5	0–20	—	<1
3	1	1	—	1	—	—	21–25	—	1
4	—	—	—	—	0	—	26–33	0–10	2
5	2	2–4	1	2	1	6–7	34–40	11–19	3–5
6	—	5–6	—	3–4	2	8–9	41–54	20–36	6–10
7	3	7–8	2	5	3	10	55–61	37–49	11–18
8	—	9–10	—	—	4	11	62–66	50–56	19–28
9	4	11–12	3	6	5	12	67–71	57–63	29–40
10	5	13–16	—	7	6–7	13	72–80	64–74	41–59
11	—	17–18	4	8	8	—	81–86	75–80	60–71
12	—	19–20	5	9	9	14	87–92	81–86	72–81
13	6	21–23	—	10	10	15	93–95	87–90	82–89
14	7	24–26	6	11–12	11	—	96+	91–94	90–94
15	—	27	7	13	12	—	—	95+	95–97
16	8	28–29	8	14	13	—	—	—	98
17	—	30–32	9	—	14	—	—	—	99
18	9–15	33+	10–15	15	15	—	—	—	>99

Note: MOANS Scaled Scores are corrected for age influences. LOT = Leaning Over Trials; LTPR = Long-Term Percent Retention; MOANS = Mayo's Older Americans Normative Studies; STPR = Short-Term Percent Retention.

Source: Ivnik et al., 1992. Reprinted with the permission of the Mayo Foundation for Medical Education and Research.

Table 10–68 MOANS Scaled Scores (Midpoint Age = 76 Years, Range = 71–81, N = 203)

MOANS Scaled Score	Learning Efficiency Index Measures			Delayed Recall Index Measures			Percent Retention Index Measures		Percentile Ranges
	Trial 1	LOT	List B	Trial 6	30-min Recall	Recognition	STPR	LTPR	
2	0	0	—	0	—	0–5	0–20	—	<1
3	1	1	0	1	—	—	21–25	—	1
4	—	—	—	—	0	—	26–33	0–5	2
5	2	2–4	1	2	1	6–7	34–40	6–20	3–5
6	—	5–6	—	3–4	2	8–9	41–54	21–36	6–10
7	3	7–8	2	—	3	10	55–61	37–49	11–18
8	—	9	—	5	4	11	62–63	50–56	19–28
9	4	10–11	3	6	5	12	64–71	57–62	29–40
10	—	12–15	—	7	6	13	72–80	63–74	41–59
11	5	16–18	4	8	7–8	—	81–86	75–80	60–71
12	—	19–20	—	9	9	14	87–90	81–86	72–81
13	6	21–23	5	10	—	15	91–95	87–90	82–89
14	7	24–26	6	11–12	10–11	—	96+	91–94	90–94
15	—	27	7	13	—	—	—	95+	95–97
16	8	28–29	8	14	12	—	—	—	98
17	—	30–32	9	—	13	—	—	—	99
18	9–15	33+	10–15	15	14–15	—	—	—	>99

Note: MOANS Scaled Scores are corrected for age influences. LOT = Leaning Over Trials; LTPR = Long-Term Percent Retention; MOANS = Mayo's Older Americans Normative Studies; STPR = Short-Term Percent Retention.

Source: Ivnik et al., 1992. Reprinted with the permission of the Mayo Foundation for Medical Education and Research.

Table 10–69 MOANS Scaled Scores (Midpoint Age = 79 Years, Range = 74–84, *N* = 196).

MOANS Scaled Score	Learning Efficiency Index Measures			Delayed Recall Index Measures			Percent Retention Index Measures		Percentile Ranges
	Trial 1	LOT	List B	Trial 6	30-min Recall	Recognition	STPR	LTPR	
2	0	0	—	0	—	0–4	0–20	—	<1
3	1	1	—	1	—	5	21–25	—	1
4	—	—	—	—	—	—	26–33	—	2
5	2	2–3	0	2	0	6–7	34–38	0–7	3–5
6	—	4–5	1	3	1	8	39–46	8–27	6–10
7	3	6–7	2	4	2–3	9–10	47–58	28–44	11–18
8	—	8	—	5	4	11	59–63	45–56	19–28
9	—	9–10	—	—	5	—	64–70	57–61	29–40
10	4	11–14	3	6–7	6	12–13	71–78	62–71	41–59
11	5	15–17	4	8	7	—	79–84	72–79	60–71
12	—	18–19	—	—	8	14	85–89	80–86	72–81
13	6	20–22	5	9	9	15	90–93	87–90	82–89
14	—	23–25	6	10	10	—	94+	91–94	90–94
15	7	26–27	7	11–13	11	—	—	95+	95–97
16	8	28–29	8	14	12	—	—	—	98
17	—	30–32	9	—	13	—	—	—	99
18	9–15	33+	10–15	15	14–15	—	—	—	>99

Note: MOANS Scaled Scores are corrected for age influences. LOT = Leaning Over Trials; LTPR = Long-Term Percent Retention; MOANS = Mayo's Older Americans Normative Studies; STPR = Short-Term Percent Retention.

Source: Ivnik et al., 1992. Reprinted with the permission of the Mayo Foundation for Medical Education and Research.

Table 10–70 MOANS Scaled Scores (Midpoint Age = 82 Years, Range = 77–87, *N* = 168)

MOANS Scaled Score	Learning Efficiency Index Measures			Delayed Recall Index Measures			Percent Retention Index Measures		Percentile Ranges
	Trial 1	LOT	List B	Trial 6	30-min Recall	Recognition	STPR	LTPR	
2	—	—	—	0	—	0–2	0–10	—	<1
3	0	0	—	1	—	3–4	11–20	—	1
4	1	1	—	—	—	5	21–30	—	2
5	—	2–3	0	2	—	—	31–36	—	3–5
6	2	4–5	1	—	0–1	6–8	37–40	0–24	6–10
7	—	6–7	—	3–4	2	9–10	41–50	25–36	11–18
8	3	8	2	—	3	11	51–61	37–49	19–28
9	—	9–10	—	5	4	—	62–69	50–60	29–40
10	4	11–14	3	6	5	12–13	70–78	61–69	41–59
11	—	15–17	—	7	6	—	79–84	70–75	60–71
12	5	18–19	4	8	7–8	14	85–89	76–84	72–81
13	—	20–22	5	9	—	—	90–93	85–90	82–89
14	6	23–25	6	10	9–10	15	94+	91–94	90–94
15	7	26–27	7	11–13	11	—	—	95+	95–97
16	8	28–29	8	14	12	—	—	—	98
17	—	30–32	9	—	13	—	—	—	99
18	9–15	33+	10–15	15	14–15	—	—	—	>99

Note: MOANS Scaled Scores are corrected for age influences. LOT = Leaning Over Trials; LTPR = Long-Term Percent Retention; MOANS = Mayo's Older American Normative Studies; STPR = Short-Term Percent Retention.

Source: Ivnik et al., 1992. Reprinted with the permission of the Mayo Foundation for Medical Education and Research.

Table 10–71 MOANS Scaled Scores (Midpoint Age = 85 Years, Range = 80–90, N = 131)

MOANS Scaled Score	Learning Efficiency Index Measures			Delayed Recall Index Measures			Percent Retention Index Measures		Percentile Ranges
	Trial 1	LOT	List B	Trial 6	30-min Recall	Recognition	STPR	LTPR	
2	—	—	—	—	—	0–2	0–10	—	<1
3	0	—	—	0	—	3–4	11–20	—	1
4	1	0–1	—	1	—	5	21–25	—	2
5	—	2–3	—	2	—	—	26–33	—	3–5
6	2	4–5	0–1	—	0	6–8	34–40	0–24	6–10
7	—	6–7	—	3	1–2	9	41–44	25–32	11–18
8	—	8	2	4	3	10	45–58	33–49	19–28
9	3	9–10	—	5	4	11	59–66	50–59	29–40
10	4	11–14	3	6	5	12	67–78	60–69	41–59
11	—	15–17	—	7	6	13	79–84	70–75	60–71
12	5	18–19	4	8	7–8	—	85–89	76–84	72–81
13	—	20–22	—	9	—	14	90–93	85–90	82–89
14	6	23–25	5	10	9–10	15	94+	91–94	90–94
15	7	26–27	6	11–13	11	—	—	95+	95–97
16	—	28–29	7	14	12	—	—	—	98
17	8	30–31	8	—	13	—	—	—	99
18	9–15	32+	9–15	15	14–15	—	—	—	>99

Note: MOANS Scaled Scores are corrected for age influences. LOT = Leaning Over Trials; LTPR = Long-Term Percent Retention; MOANS = Mayo's Older Americans Normative Studies; STPR = Short-Term Percent Retention.

Source: Ivnik et al., 1992. Reprinted with the permission of the Mayo Foundation for Medical Education and Research.

Table 10–72 MOANS Scaled Scores (Midpoint Age = 88 Years, Range = 83, N = 98)

MOANS Scaled Score	Learning Efficiency Index Measures			Delayed Recall Index Measures			Percent Retention Index Measures		Percentile Ranges
	Trial 1	LOT	List B	Trial 6	30-min Recall	Recognition	STPR	LTPR	
2	—	—	—	—	—	0–2	—	—	<1
3	0	—	—	0	—	3–4	0–10	—	1
4	—	0	—	1	—	5	11–25	—	2
5	1	1–3	—	2	—	—	26–30	—	3–5
6	2	4–5	0	—	0	6–8	31–38	0–19	6–10
7	—	6–7	1	3	1–2	9	39–44	20–32	11–18
8	—	8	2	4	3	10	45–55	33–45	19–28
9	3	9–10	—	—	4	11	56–64	46–54	29–40
10	4	11–14	3	5–6	5	12	65–77	55–65	41–59
11	—	15–16	—	7	6	13	78–81	66–70	60–71
12	5	17–18	—	8	7	—	82–87	71–80	72–81
13	—	19–20	4	9	8	14	88–92	81–86	82–89
14	6	21–22	5	10	9–10	15	93+	87–92	90–94
15	7	23–25	—	11–13	11	—	—	93+	95–97
16	—	26	6	14	12	—	—	—	98
17	8	27	7	—	13	—	—	—	99
18	9–15	28+	8–15	15	14–15	—	—	—	>99

Note: MOANS Scaled Scores are corrected for age influences. LOT = Leaning Over Trials; LTPR = Long-Term Percent Retention; MOANS = Mayo's Older Americans Normative Studies; STPR = Short-Term Percent Retention.

Source: Ivnik et al., 1992. Reprinted with the permission of the Mayo Foundation for Medical Education and Research.

Table 10–73 RAVLT Norms: Table for Converting RAVLT MOANS Scaled Score Sums to MAYO Indices

RAVLT MOANS Scaled Score Sums				RAVLT MOANS Scaled Score Sums			
Learning Efficiency Sum	Delayed Recall Sum	Percent Retention Sum	MAYO Index Score	Learning Efficiency Sum	Delayed Recall Sum	Percent Retention Sum	MAYO Index Score
≤13	≤8	≤9	<65				101
	9		65			21	102
			66		22		103
14		10	67	22			104
	10		68				105
			69		23	22	106
		11	70				107
	11		71	23			108
15			72		24	23	109
	12	12	73				110
			74				111
			75		25	24	112
16	13	13	76	24			113
			77				114
			78		26	25	115
	14		79				116
		14	80	25			117
17			81		27		118
	15		82			26	119
		15	83				120
			84		28		121
	16		85	26		27	122
18		16	86		29		123
			87				124
	17		88			28	125
		17	89		30		126
19			90	27			127
	18		91			29	128
		18	92		31		129
			93				130
	19		94	28			131
20			95		32	30	132
		19	96				133
	20		97				134
			98		33	31	135
21		20	99	≥29	≥34	≥32	>135
	21		100				

Source: Ivnik et al., 1992. Reprinted with the permission of the Mayo Foundation for Medical Education and Research.

community-dwelling participants from the MOAANS project in Jacksonville, Florida. Participants ranged in age from 56 to 94 years and varied in education from 0 to 20 years of formal education. They were screened to exclude those with active neurological, psychiatric, or other conditions that might affect cognition. The test administration procedure was identical to that used in the MOAANS (see Ivnik et al., 1992) project and included the 30-item recognition task. Tables 10–77 through 10–83 convert AVLT scores to age-corrected MOAANS Scaled Scores ($M = 10$, $SD = 3$) and summary Mayo Auditory-Verbal Indices ($M = 100$, $SD = 15$; Table 10–84). Note that the number of recognition hits (REC) and false positive errors (ERR) are also provided in Tables 10–77 through 10–83. As

with the original MOAANS project, the cells are based on the method of overlapping age intervals.

Age- and education-adjusted adult MOAANS (MAE) scaled scores are obtained by applying the algorithms in Table 10–85 to each age-adjusted scaled score. Age- and education-corrected indices for learning (LEI), delayed recall (DRI), and percent retention (PRI) are computed in a two-step process. The MOAANS age- and education-adjusted scaled scores replace the MOAANS age-adjusted scaled scores. Once the appropriate sums are calculated, they can be transformed to their respective index scores by locating the values under the appropriate column in Table 10–86. The authors noted that one of the strengths of their normative sample is its inclusion

Table 10–74 Computation of MOANS RAVLT Recognition Percent Correct (RPC) from the True Positive minus False Positive Difference Score

TP – FP	RPC	TP – FP	RPC (Rounded)
15	100	–1	47
14	97	–2	43
13	93	–3	40
12	90	–4	37
11	87	–5	33
10	83	–6	30
9	80	–7	27
8	77	–8	23
7	73	–9	20
6	70	–10	17
5	67	–11	13
4	63	–12	10
3	60	–13	7
2	57	–14	3
1	53	–15	0
0	50		

Source: From Harris et al., 2002. Reprinted with the kind permission of Psychology Press.

of a wide range of educational levels; however, they cautioned that African Americans with qualitatively different educational backgrounds (e.g., those educated outside the segregated South) may perform differently. They also noted the presence of floor effects on the 30-min delayed recall trial, raising concerns regarding the utility of this measure with

regard to the information that it can provide about retention of information over time in this population. The RPC index appears to be more resistant to floor effects.

For Hispanic individuals living in the United States, Ponton et al. (1996) provided normative data from a sample of 300 Spanish-speaking individuals (mostly monolingual), using the WHO/UCLA version. The data, stratified by age, education, and gender are shown in Table 10–87.

Vakil and Blachstein (1994, 1997) provided normative data for evaluating temporal order judgments. Three measures were provided: (a) Hits—the number of words correctly placed at their original serial position; (b) Correlation—Pearson product moment correlation calculated for each subject, between the listed order and the true order; and (c) Absolute Deviation—the sum of the absolute deviation of each word from its original position, with the score for each deviation ranging from 0 to 14. The data, shown in Table 10–88, are based on administration of the RAVLT in Hebrew.

CHILDREN

A number of normative reports have appeared in recent years. Bishop et al. (1990) tested 252 children, aged 5 to 16 years, who were referred for neuropsychological assessment. These data, however, should not be used because (a) they are based on referrals to a hospital clinic of patients with conditions known to affect memory performance and (b) a non-standard administration procedure was used.

Forrester and Geffen (1991) tested 80 Australian schoolchildren, aged 7 to 15 years. The main drawback of the study was its small sample size. More recently, larger-scale studies

Table 10–75 MOANS Age- and Gender-Corrected Scaled Scores: RAVLT Recognition Trial (% Correct) for Males, by 10-Year Age-Range Midpoints (N = 310)

MOANS Scaled Score	61 (n = 60)	64 (n = 88)	67 (n = 113)	70 (n = 135)	73 (n = 156)	76 (n = 139)	79 (n = 125)	82 (n = 101)	85 (n = 70)	88+ (n = 49)	Percentile Range
2	<67	<67	<67	<63	<63	<60	<60	—	—	—	<1
3	67	67	—	63	63	60	60	<60	<60	<60	1
4	70	70	67	—	—	—	—	60	60	60	2
5	—	—	—	67	67	63	63	63	63	63	3–5
6	77–73	77–73	70	70	70	70–67	70–67	67	67	67	6–10
7	83–80	80	73	73	73	73	73	70	70	—	11–18
8	87	83	80–77	80–77	77	77	77	77–73	73	70	19–28
9	—	87	83	83	83–80	83–80	80	80	77	73	29–40
10	93–90	90	87	87	87	87	87–83	87–83	83–80	80–77	41–59
11	—	93	93–90	90	90	90	90	90	87	87–83	60–71
12	97	97	—	93	93	93	—	—	90	90	72–81
13	—	—	—	—	—	—	93	93	93	—	82–89
14	100	100	97	97	97	97	—	—	—	93	90–94
15	—	—	100	—	—	—	97	97	97	97	95–97
16	—	—	—	100	100	100	—	—	—	—	98
17	—	—	—	—	—	—	100	100	100	100	99
18	—	—	—	—	—	—	—	—	—	—	>99

Source: From Harris et al., 2002. Reprinted with the kind permission of Psychology Press.

Table 10–76 MOANS Age- and Gender-Corrected Scaled Scores: RAVLT Recognition Trail (% Correct) for Females, by 10-Year Age-Range Midpoint (*N* = 526)

MOANS Scaled Score	61 (*n* = 91)	64 (*n* = 99)	67 (*n* = 118)	70 (*n* = 138)	73 (*n* = 170)	76 (*n* = 221)	79 (*n* = 262)	82 (*n* = 256)	85 (*n* = 218)	88+ (*n* = 141)	Percentile Range
2	<73	<67	<67	<67	<67	<67	<67	<63	<63	<63	<1
3	73	67	67	67	67	67	—	<63	63	63	1
4	77	70	70	70	70	70	67	67	67	67	2
5	83–80	77–73	73	73	—	—	70	70	70	70	3–5
6	87	83–80	80–77	80–77	77–73	73	73	73	73	73	6–10
7	90	87	83	83	80	80–77	80–77	77	77	77	11–18
8	93	93–90	87	87	83	83	83	80	80	80	19–28
9	—	—	90	90	87	87	87	83	83	83	29–40
10	97	97	97–93	93	90	90	90	90–87	90–87	87	41–59
11	—	—	—	97	93	93	93	—	—	90	60–71
12	100	100	—	—	97	—	—	93	93	93	72–81
13	—	—	100	100	—	97	97	97	97	—	82–89
14	—	—	—	—	100	—	—	—	—	97	90–94
15	—	—	—	—	—	100	100	100	100	—	95–97
16	—	—	—	—	—	—	—	—	—	100	98
17	—	—	—	—	—	—	—	—	—	—	99
18	—	—	—	—	—	—	—	—	—	—	>99

Source: From Harris et al., 2002. Reprinted with the kind permission of Psychology Press.

have appeared. Anderson and Lajoie (1996) used an Australian normative sample of 376 children, aged 7 to 13.11 years, with approximately equal numbers of boys and girls in each age group. Van den Burg and Kingma (1999) reported data for a sample of 225 Dutch children, aged 6 to 12 years, and Vakil et al. (1998) administered a Hebrew translation of the standard form to 943 children, aged 8 to 17 years. In all cases, the values were similar. These findings suggest that the ability to memorize common, concrete nouns, as tapped by the RAVLT, develops at a similar rate during childhood in Western countries. The data provided by Vakil et al. (1998) appear appropriate for English-speaking children and are

Table 10–77 MOAANS AVLT Scaled Scores for Ages 56–62 Years (Midpoint Age = 61, Age Range for Norms = 56–66)

Scaled Score	Trial 1	List B	Trial 6	30-min Delay	REC	ERR	RPC	LOT	STPR	LTPR	Percentile Range
2	0	0	0–1	—	0–6	7+	—	<1	0–21	—	<1
3	1	—	—	—	7	—	<66	1	22–27	—	1
4	2	1	2	0	—	6	66–67	2	28–29	—	2
5	—	—	—	—	8	5	68–70	3–4	30–36	0	3–5
6	3	2	3	1	9	4	71–75	5–7	37–44	1–20	6–10
7	—	—	4	2–3	10	3	76–80	8–9	45–55	21–40	11–18
8	4	3	5	4	11–12	2	81–85	10	56–63	41–47	19–28
9	—	—	6	5	13	—	86–88	11–12	64–68	48–59	29–40
10	5	4	7	6–7	14	1	89–93	13–15	69–77	60–73	41–59
11	6	5	8	8	—	—	94–95	16–17	78–84	74–81	60–71
12	—	—	9	9	—	0	96–99	18–20	85–90	82–89	72–81
13	7	6	10–11	10	15	—	—	21–23	91–93	90–92	82–89
14	—	7	12	11	—	—	100	24–26	94+	93+	90–94
15	8	8	13	12	—	—	—	27–29	—	—	95–97
16	9	—	14	13	—	—	—	30–32	—	—	98
17	10+	9+	15	—	—	—	—	33+	—	—	99
18	—	—	—	14–15	—	—	—	—	—	—	>99

Note: The following abbreviations are used in Tables 10–77 through 10–83. ERR = false-positive errors; LOT = learning over trials; LTPR = long-term percent retention; REC = recognition bits; RPC = recognition percent correct; STPR = short-term percent retention.

Source: From Ferman et al., 2005. Reprinted with the permission of the Mayo Foundation for Medical Education and Research.

Table 10–78 MOAANS AVLT Scaled Scores for Age 63–65 Years (Midpoint Age = 64, Age Range for Norms = 59–69)

Scaled Score	Trial 1	List B	Trial 6	30-min Delay	REC	ERR	RPC	LOT	STPR	LTPR	Percentile Range
2	0	0	0–1	—	0–6	7+	—	<1	0–21	—	<1
3	1	—	—	—	7	—	<64	—	22–27	—	1
4	2	1	2	0	—	6	64–66	1	28–29	—	2
5	—	—	—	—	8	5	67–70	2–4	30–36	0	3–5
6	3	2	3	1	9	4	71–75	5–6	37–44	1–20	6–10
7	—	—	4	2–3	10–11	3	76–80	7–9	45–55	21–40	11–18
8	4	3	5	4	—	2	81–84	10	56–61	41–47	19–28
9	—	—	6	5	12	—	85–88	11–12	62–67	48–59	29–40
10	5	4	7	6–7	13–14	1	89–92	13–15	68–77	60–73	41–59
11	—	—	8	8	—	—	93–94	16–17	78–83	74–81	60–71
12	6	5	9	9	—	0	95–99	18–20	84–90	82–89	72–81
13	—	6	10	10	15	—	—	21–23	91–92	90–92	82–89
14	7	—	11	11	—	—	100	24–26	93+	93+	90–94
15	—	7–8	12	12	—	—	—	27–29	—	—	95–97
16	8	—	13	—	—	—	—	30–32	—	—	98
17	9	9+	14–15	13	—	—	—	33	—	—	99
18	10+	—	—	14–15	—	—	—	34+	—	—	>99

Source: From Ferman et al., 2005. Reprinted with the permission of the Mayo Foundation for Medical Education and Research.

shown separately for males and females (see Tables 10–89a and 10–89b, respectively). In this study, children with learning disabilities, those with attention disorders, and those requiring special academic assistance were excluded, as were those with very high or very low academic achievement. The administration was standard; however, after the recognition trial, the ability to remember temporal order was also assessed.

Data for 6-year-olds (Van den Burg & Kingma, 1999) and 7-year-olds (Forrester & Geffen, 1991) are shown in Table 10–90.

Note that no interference or recognition trials were given for the 6-year-olds. The delayed recall trial was given 20 to 30 min after the fifth learning trial.

RELIABILITY

Internal Reliability

Internal reliability (coefficient alpha) of the total score is high (about .90; Van den Burg & Kingma, 1999).

Table 10–79 MOAANS AVLT Scaled Scores for Age 66–68 Years (Midpoint Age = 67, Age Range for Norms = 62–72)

Scaled Score	Trial 1	List B	Trial 6	30-min Delay	REC	ERR	RPC	LOT	STPR	LTPR	Percentile Range
2	0	—	0	—	0–3	7+	—	<1	0–17	—	<1
3	1	0	1	—	4–6	—	<63	—	18–21	—	1
4	—	—	2	—	7	6	63–66	1	22–27	—	2
5	2	1	—	0	8	5	67–70	2–3	28–32	0	3–5
6	3	2	3	1	9	4	71–75	4–6	33–43	1–16	6–10
7	—	—	4	2–3	10	3	76–79	6–7	44–53	17–39	11–18
8	—	3	5	4	11	2	80–82	8–10	54–59	40–46	19–28
9	4	—	6	—	12	—	83–87	11–12	60–67	47–56	29–40
10	5	4	7	5–6	13	1	88–92	13–15	68–77	57–69	41–59
11	—	—	8	7–8	14	—	93–94	16–17	78–83	70–80	60–71
12	6	5	9	9	—	0	95–99	18–19	84–90	81–89	72–81
13	—	—	10	10	15	—	—	20–22	91–92	90–92	82–89
14	7	6	11	11	—	—	—	23–26	93+	93+	90–94
15	—	7	—	—	—	—	100	27–29	—	—	95–97
16	8	8	12	12	—	—	—	30–31	—	—	98
17	9	9+	13–14	13	—	—	—	32–33	—	—	99
18	10+	—	15	14–15	—	—	—	34+	—	—	>99

Source: From Ferman et al., 2005. Reprinted with the permission of the Mayo Foundation for Medical Education and Research.

Table 10–80 MOAANS AVLT Scaled Scores for Age 69–71 Years (Midpoint Age = 70, Age Range for Norms = 65–75)

Scaled Score	Trial 1	List B	Trial 6	30-min Delay	REC	ERR	RPC	LOT	STPR	LTPR	Percentile range
2	0	—	—	—	0–3	9+	—	<1	—	—	<1
3	1	0	0	—	4–6	7–8	<61	—	0–11	—	1
4	—	—	1	—	—	—	61–66	1	12–20	—	2
5	2	1	2	0	7	5–6	67–70	2	21–28	0	3–5
6	3	2	3	1	8–9	4	71–74	3–5	29–40	1–14	6–10
7	—	—	—	2–3	—	3	75–78	6–7	41–46	15–38	11–18
8	—	3	4	—	10–11	2	79–82	8–9	47–56	39–44	19–28
9	4	—	5	4	12	—	83–86	10–12	57–65	45–55	29–40
10	5	4	6–7	5–6	13	1	87–92	13–15	66–76	56–68	41–59
11	—	—	—	7	14	—	93–94	16–17	77–82	69–77	60–71
12	6	5	8	8	—	0	95	18–19	83–88	78–86	72–81
13	—	—	9	9–10	—	—	96–99	20–22	89–92	87–91	82–89
14	7	6	10	—	15	—	—	23	93+	92+	90–94
15	—	7	11	11	—	—	100	24–27	—	—	95–97
16	8	—	12	12	—	—	—	28–30	—	—	98
17	9	8	—	13	—	—	—	31–33	—	—	99
18	10+	9+	13+	14–15	—	—	—	34+	—	—	>99

Source: From Ferman et al., 2005. Reprinted with the permission of the Mayo Foundation for Medical Education and Research.

Test-Retest Reliability

Over 1-year intervals, the test has marginal/adequate test-retest reliability. Trial 5 and delayed-recall trials were among the more reliable scores (*r* values about .60 to .70; Mitrushina & Satz, 1991b; Snow et al., 1988; Uchiyama et al., 1995).

Alternate Form Reliability

Different studies yield a wide variety of reliability coefficients but generally fall above the marginal range (>.60; see *Practice* *Effects*). As noted earlier (see *Other Forms*), a number of authors have provided alternate forms of the test. The versions by Geffen et al. (1994b) and Majdan et al. (1996) appear to produce comparable scores.

Practice Effects

Small, but significant, improvements (on average 1 to 2 words per trial) can be expected on successive administrations of the same form of the RAVLT (Crawford et al., 1989; Lezak, 1982;

Table 10–81 MOAANS AVLT Scaled Scores for Age 72–74 Years (Midpoint Age = 73, Age Range for Norms = 68–78)

Scaled Score	Trial 1	List B	Trial 6	30-min Delay	REC	ERR	RPC	LOT	STPR	LTPR	Percentile Range
2	0	—	—	—	0–2	9+	—	<1	—	—	<1
3	1	0	0	—	3–5	8	<61	—	0–5	—	1
4	—	—	—	—	6	7	61–66	1	6–11	—	2
5	2	1	1	0	7	5–6	67–70	2	12–28	0	3–5
6	—	2	2–3	1	8–9	4	71–74	3–5	29–40	1–14	6–10
7	3	—	—	2–3	10	3	75–78	6–7	41–46	15–38	11–18
8	—	3	4	—	11	2	79–82	8–9	47–56	39–44	19–28
9	4	—	5	4	12	—	83–86	10–12	57–65	45–55	29–40
10	5	4	6–7	5–6	13	1	87–92	13–15	66–74	56–68	41–59
11	—	—	—	7	14	—	93–94	16–17	75–81	69–77	60–71
12	—	5	8	8	—	0	95	18–19	82–88	78–86	72–81
13	6	—	9	9–10	—	—	96–99	20–22	89–92	87–91	82–89
14	7	6	10	—	15	—	—	23	93+	92+	90–94
15	—	7	11	11	—	—	100	24–26	—	—	95–97
16	8	—	12	12	—	—	—	27	—	—	98
17	9	8	—	13	—	—	—	28–30	—	—	99
18	10+	9+	13+	14–15	—	—	—	31+	—	—	>99

Source: From Ferman et al., 2005. Reprinted with the permission of the Mayo Foundation for Medical Education and Research.

Table 10–82 MOAANS AVLT Scaled Scores for Age 75–77 Years (Midpoint Age = 76, Age Range for Norms = 71–81)

Scaled Score	Trial 1	List B	Trial 6	30-min Delay	REC	ERR	RPC	LOT	STPR	LTPR	Percentile Range
2	0	—	—	—	0–2	9+	—	<1	—	—	<1
3	1	0	0	—	3–5	8	<60	—	0–5	—	1
4	—	—	—	—	6	7	60–65	1	6–10	—	2
5	—	1	1	0	7	5–6	66–69	2	11–22	0	3–5
6	2	—	2	1	8	4	70–72	3–5	23–33	1–14	6–10
7	3	2	3	2	9	3	73–76	6–7	34–43	15–36	11–18
8	—	—	4	3	10–11	2	77–80	8	44–55	37–44	19–28
9	4	3	5	4	12	—	81–84	9–11	56–63	45–54	29–40
10	—	4	6	5	13	1	85–89	12–14	64–72	55–63	41–59
11	5	—	7	6	—	—	90–92	15–17	73–79	64–70	60–71
12	—	5	8	7–8	14	0	93–95	18–19	80–87	71–85	72–81
13	6	—	9	9	—	—	96–97	20–22	88–92	86–91	82–89
14	—	6	10	10	15	—	98–99	23	93+	92+	90–94
15	7	—	11	11	—	—	100	24–25	—	—	95–97
16	8	7	12	12	—	—	—	26	—	—	98
17	9	8	—	13	—	—	—	27–30	—	—	99
18	10+	9+	13+	14–15	—	—	—	31+	—	—	>99

Source: From Ferman et al., 2005. Reprinted with the permission of the Mayo Foundation for Medical Education and Research.

Uchiyama et al., 1995), although in older adults (aged 57–85 years) tested yearly for 3 years, the gains on Trials 5 and 7 tended to be negligible (Mitrushina & Satz, 1991a).

The literature suggests that practice effects are reduced when people are retested with a different RAVLT version (Crawford et al., 1989; Delaney et al., 1992; Geffen et al., 1994b; Lemay et al., 2004; Moritz et al., 2003; Van den Burg & Kingma, 1999).

Geffen et al. (1994b) tested healthy individuals (age *M* = 31.3 years, *SD* =12.7) on two forms (the original form and their alternate form) on two separate occasions, 6 to 14 days apart. They found that mean performance on the various trials was no different on the two forms. Further, the measures of total recall on Trial 5 and the post-distractor trial (A6) yielded reliability coefficients sufficiently high (≥.70) for clinical use. Reliability of Trial 1, recognition, and derived scores was low. They suggested that these scores may have diagnostic significance in a single test session but not in comparison across sessions.

Others have reported comparable findings (e.g., Delaney et al., 1992; Lemay et al., 2004; Moritz et al., 2003; Ryan et al., 1986; Uchiyama et al., 1995). For example, Lemay et al. (2004)

Table 10–83 MOAANS AVLT Scaled Scores for Age 78+ Years (Midpoint Age = 79, Age Range for Norms = 74–94)

Scaled Score	Trial 1	List B	Trial 6	30-min Delay	REC	ERR	RPC	LOT	STPR	LTPR	Percentile Range
2	0	—	—	—	—	—	—	<1	—	—	<1
3	1	0	0	—	0–5	—	<60	—	0	—	1
4	—	—	—	—	6	9+	61–61	1	1–6	—	2
5	—	1	1	—	7	6–8	62–66	2	7–11	—	3–5
6	2	—	2	0	8	4–5	67–70	3–4	12–31	0–9	6–10
7	—	2	3	1	9	3	71–73	5–6	32–42	10–20	11–18
8	3	—	4	2–3	10	2	74–78	7–8	43–50	21–40	19–28
9	—	3	—	4	11	—	79–83	9–11	51–59	41–52	29–40
10	4	—	5–6	5	12–13	1	84–88	12–14	60–71	53–63	41–59
11	5	4	7	6	—	—	89–91	15–16	72–76	64–70	60–71
12	—	—	—	7	14	0	92–94	17–18	77–86	71–82	72–81
13	6	5	8–9	8–9	—	—	95	19–21	87–91	83–90	82–89
14	—	—	10	10	15	—	96–99	22–23	—	91+	90–94
15	—	6	11	—	—	—	100	24	92+	—	95–97
16	7	—	—	11	—	—	—	25	—	—	98
17	—	7+	12	12	—	—	—	26	—	—	99
18	8+	—	13+	13–15	—	—	—	27+	—	—	>99

Source: From Ferman et al., 2005. Reprinted with the permission of the Mayo Foundation for Medical Education and Research.

Table 10–84 MOAANS AVLT Age-Adjusted Index Score Conversions

Index Score	MOAANS Learning Efficiency Index (LEI)	MOAANS Auditory-Verbal Delayed Recall Index (DRI)	MOAANS Auditory-Verbal Percent Retention Index (PRI)	Index Score
<65	<13	<9	<10	≤65
66		9		66
67			10	67
69	13	10		69
71			11	71
73	14	11	12	73
76	15		13	76
77		12		77
80		13		80
81			14	81
82	16			82
84		14		84
86		15	15	86
87	17			87
89		16	16	89
91	18			91
92		17	17	92
94		18	18	94
96	19			96
97		19	19	97
100	20	20	20	100
103		21	21	103
105	21	22		105
107			22	107
108		23		108
109	22		23	109
111		24		111
112			24	112
114	23	25		114
115			25	115
117		26		117
119	24	27	26	119
121		28		121
123			27	123
124	25			124
125		29		125
129	26	30		129
130			28	130
132		31		132
133	27			133
>135	<27	>31	>28	>135

Source: From Ferman et al., 2005. Reprinted with the permission of the Mayo Foundation for Medical Education and Research.

Table 10–85 Computational Algorithm for Age- and Education-Corrected MOAANS Scores

AVLT variable	K	W_1	W_2
Trial 1	1.06	1.11	0.17
List B	0.49	1.10	0.13
Trial 6	1.08	1.09	0.16
30-min delay	1.07	1.09	0.16
Recognition	0.40	1.10	0.11
False-positive errors	−1.43	1.30	0.09
Recognition percent correct (RPC)	0.77	1.10	0.15
Learning over trials (LOC)	−0.11	1.07	0.04
Short-term percent retention (STPR)	−0.10	1.13	0.09
Long-term percent retention (LTPR)	−0.08	1.17	0.12

Age- and education-corrected MOAANS scaled scores ($MSS_{A\&E}$) are calculated using the age-corrected scaled score derived from Tables 10–77 through 10–83 (MSS_A) and the patient's years of education using the formula:

$$MSS_{A\&E} = K + (W_2 \times MSS_A) - (W_2 \times Educ)$$

where K = a constant, W_1 = a regression-derived weight to be applied to MSS_A and W_2 = a regression-derived weight to be applied to education.

Source: From Ferman et al., 2005. Reprinted with the permission of the Mayo Foundation for Medical Education and Research.

Moritz et al. (2003) tested 31 patients (20 males, 11 females) with schizophrenia (age $M = 33.03$ years, $SD = 11.26$; education $M = 11.77$ years, $SD = 1.45$) and 38 healthy controls (26 males, 12 females; age $M = 32.45$ years, $SD = 9.98$; education $M = 11.47$ years, $SD = 1.48$) on two occasions, spaced 2 weeks apart. The standard form was given at baseline and an alternate version (B) at retest. In both samples, reliability coefficients were generally higher for the total score (healthy subjects, $r = .72$; schizophrenic patients, $r = .69$) than for the individual learning trials, and practice effects were absent. Reliable change estimates for the RAVLT total score were derived for each sample, and these are shown in Table 10–91. Therefore, when using alternate forms with patients with schizophrenia, clinicians can be 90% confident that a change of 16 or more points in the total score is not the result of measure error (for healthy participants, the corresponding value is 9). The authors stressed that it is clearly possible for patients to experience real change even if their scores do not exceed the criterion. Clinicians simply should have less confidence in clinical inferences based on changes that fall within the probable range of measurement error, and they need to seek additional evidence to support such an opinion.

In children, reliabilities appear similar to those noted in adults. Van den Burg and Kingma (1999) used the standard Dutch version and constructed two additional test forms. A sample of 225 children was tested twice (with a 3-month interval between test sessions), with alternate versions being given on the two test sessions. Means and variances of the three test versions were similar, and there were no practice effects on any of the measures. The most reliable measures were the total number of words recalled ($r = .70$), followed by the 20-min delayed recall score ($r = .62$) and Trial 5 ($r = .61$).

evaluated middle-aged and older adults on three test occasions with intersession intervals of 14 days, using the standard and two alternate forms. The total and delayed recall trials had acceptable reliability (r values >.70). Acquisition trials, recognition trials, and derived scores (except retrieval efficiency) showed unacceptably low reliabilities.

Table 10–86 MOAANS AVLT Age- and Education-Adjusted Index Score Conversions

Index Score	MOAANS Learning Efficiency Index (LEI)	MOAANS Auditory-Verbal Delayed Recall Index (DRI)	MOAANS Auditory-Verbal Percent Retention Index (PRI)	Index Score
≤65	<12	<9	<9	≤65
66	12		9	66
67		9		67
69	13			69
70			10	70
71		10		71
72	14			72
73			11	73
75		11		75
76			12	76
78	15	12		78
80			13	80
81	16	13		81
83			14	83
84		14		84
86	17		15	86
87		15		87
89			16	89
90	18	16		90
91			17	91
92		17		92
93		18		93
94			18	94
96	19	19	19	96
99		20	20	99
100	20			100
102		21	21	102
105	21	22	22	105
107			23	107
108	22	23		108
110		24	24	110
112	23	25	25	112
115	24	26	26	115
117		27		117
118			27	118
119		28		119
120	25			120
121		29		121
122			28	122
125		30	29	125
126	26			126
128		31		128
131	27	32	30	131
≥135	>27	>32	>30	≥135

Source: From Ferman et al., 2005. Reprinted with the permission of the Mayo Foundation for Medical Education and Research.

These authors suggested that variables related to the child (e.g., fluctuations in attention) and the examiner (e.g., persistence in encouraging the child to produce words) may account in part for the modest test-retest reliabilities.

VALIDITY

Relations Within the Test

Delayed-recall scores correlate highly with total scores ($r > .75$; Van den Burg & Kingma, 1999). Other indices (e.g., percent recall from primacy, middle, and recency regions) also have significant correlations ($r > .8$) with the total number of words recalled and therefore are not pure measures of the qualitative traits that they purportedly assess (Schmidt, 1997). However, an index based on recency minus primacy (Gainotti & Marra, 1994) seems not to be substantially confounded with number of words recalled and therefore appears promising (Schmidt, 1997). The index of temporal order may also provide some unique information. Correlations between temporal order and various RAVLT scores are weak to high: learning rate, .12; proactive interference, −.10; total words, .54; delayed recall, .64. The strongest relations are with indexes that represent total amount of words learned and delayed recall (Vakil & Blachstein, 1994).

With regard to the internal structure of the test, either one factor (Salthouse et al., 1996; Vakil & Blachstein, 1993), or two or three factors (Vakil & Blachstein, 1993) emerge in normal adults, depending on the particular combination of scores included in the analyses and the criteria used to determine the number of factors. Vakil and Blachstein (1993) identified two basic factors that they interpreted as reflecting acquisition (defined by variables such as Trial 1, List B trial, and Total score) and retention. The latter can be further subdivided into a storage component (defined primarily by recognition memory) and a retrieval component (defined by Trial 5, delayed-recall trials, temporal order). By contrast, Mueller et al. (1997) examined two heterogeneous clinical samples, one comprised mostly of people with probable dementia of the Alzheimer type (AD) or major depression and the other of patients with seizures, using a German version of the RAVLT. Structural equation modelling suggested that short-term memory (STM) and long-term latent memory (LTM) variables provided a good explanation of the test in both clinical samples.

Relations With Other Measures

The RAVLT correlates moderately well with other measures of learning and memory such as the WMS-R Logical Memory and Visual Reproduction subtests (Johnstone et al., 2000), and the CVLT (Crossen & Wiens, 1994; Stallings et al., 1995). Slightly lower raw scores are obtained on the RAVLT than on the CVLT, probably reflecting in part the slightly shorter RAVLT list. The RAVLT may also be somewhat harder than the CVLT, requiring more effortful strategies for encoding and retrieval. The CVLT consists of words that can be categorized, with semantic clustering becoming the strategy of choice for normal adults. The RAVLT words do not show a clear semantic relationship, and temporal tagging may become a more important strategy (Vakil & Blachstein, 1994; Vakil et al., 2004). When standard, as opposed to raw, scores

Table 10–87 Mean and *SD*s for Hispanic Persons on the Spanish Version of the WHO/UCLA AVLT, by Age and Number of Years of Education

| | Age 16–29 | | Age 30–39 | | Age 40–49 | | Age 50–75 | |
	<10 Years	>10 Years	<10 Years	>10 Years	<10 Years	>10 Years	<10 Years	>10 Years
Females (n)	12	30	22	44	16	11	25	20
Trial 5	13.3 (1.6)	13.5 (1.9)	12.8 (2.2)	13.8 (1.4)	12.6 (1.0)	13.3 (2.1)	11.5 (1.9)	13.2 (1.3)
Trial A6 (Retention)	11.6 (1.7)	12.4 (2.3)	11.6 (2.7)	12.1 (2.1)	10.6 (1.6)	12.1 (1.9)	10.2 (2.6)	10.8 (2.6)
Trial A7 (20-min delay)	11.8 (2.2)	12.9 (2.5)	11.9 (2.6)	12.9 (2.0)	11.1 (1.6)	12.5 (1.9)	10.6 (2.4)	12.5 (2.0)
Males (n)	11	25	13	18	12	17	18	6
Trial A5	12.7 (1.6)	13.1 (1.9)	12.2 (1.6)	13.3 (1.3)	12.9 (1.8)	13.5 (1.4)	12.1 (1.7)	12.7 (1.5)
Trial A6 (Retention)	11.7 (1.4)	12.2 (2.7)	11.5 (2.2)	11.6 (2.1)	10.5 (3.0)	13.0 (2.0)	10.5 (2.1)	11.0 (1.7)
Trial A7 (20-min delay)	12.4 (1.9)	12.5 (2.1)	11.2 (2.4)	12.6 (1.6)	11.4 (2.4)	13.2 (1.8)	10.8 (2.2)	11.8 (1.6)

Source: From Ponton et al., 1996. Reprinted with permission of Cambridge University Press.

are considered, CVLT scores are considerably lower than those of the RAVLT in head-injured patients (Stallings et al., 1995). The discrepancies may reflect differences in the composition of the standardization samples, or the greater sensitivity of the CVLT to memory impairment (perhaps related to the requirement of semantic clustering), or both. Stallings et al. (1995) noted that use of the CVLT, as opposed to the RAVLT, results in a higher frequency of head-injury patients' being classed as memory-impaired, and their memory impairments appear greater. If both tests are given within a few days of one another, there are no significant effects for order of presentation (Crossen & Wiens, 1994; Stallings et al., 1995). It will be informative to compare the RAVLT with the CVLT-II, which reportedly does not suffer from inflated norms.

Factor analytic studies indicate that the RAVLT loads primarily with other verbal memory tests, such as those found on the WMS (Anderson & Lajoie, 1996; Johnstone et al., 2000; Mitrushina & Satz, 1991b; Ryan et al., 1984; Salthouse et al.,

1996; Strauss et al., 1995). The RAVLT, however, may measure a construct that is not singularly verbal in nature. Factor analyses of variable sets that include the RAVLT indicate that memory variables load together regardless of whether they are verbal or nonverbal measures (Malec et al., 1991; Moses, 1986; Smith et al., 1992; but see Johnstone et al., 2000, who found that the RAVLT loaded with measures of verbal but not nonverbal memory).

Clinical Studies

The RAVLT is sensitive to neurological impairment (Powell et al., 1991), laterality of brain damage (Kilpatrick et al., 1997; Malec et al., 1991; Miceli et al., 1981), and memory deficits in a variety of patient groups, including those with left temporal lobe dysfunction (Majdan et al., 1996; Malec et al., 1991), ruptured aneurysm of the anterior communicating artery (Simard et al., 2003; Stefanova et al., 2002), specific language

Table 10–88 Means and *SD*s of Measures Assessing Temporal Order

| | Age Group (Years) | | | | | |
Measure	20–29	30–39	40–49	50–59	60–69	70–79
Males (n)	57	39	42	27	48	44
Total trials 1–5	56.68 (6.12)	54.51 (8.85)	54.29 (9.23)	50.81 (5.82)	46.79 (8.93)	41.48 (7.24)
Hits	6.16 (3.69)	5.82 (3.28)	4.50 (3.01)	4.22 (3.08)	3.56 (2.78)	3.16 (1.74)
Absolute Deviation	26.32 (15.62)	27.00 (17.49)	34.33 (17.87)	35.15 (15.19)	39.94 (14.34)	45.73 (14.47)
Correlation score	0.79 (0.18)	0.77 (0.22)	0.69 (0.25)	0.66 (0.20)	0.60 (0.20)	0.53 (0.23)
Females (n)	60	24	44	28	67	48
Total trials 1–5	59.48 (6.29)	58.04 (5.86)	55.41 (7.83)	55.86 (6.38)	50.21 (8.92)	42.29 (9.50)
Hits	7.05 (3.60)	6.08 (3.15)	4.55 (3.24)	4.82 (2.42)	3.85 (2.78)	3.48 (2.09)
Absolute Deviation	22.17 (16.04)	23.67 (14.80)	34.68 (17.88)	31.29 (10.98)	40.30 (18.79)	44.46 (14.84)
Correlation score	0.83 (0.19)	0.82 (0.19)	0.67 (0.26)	0.73 (0.15)	0.61 (0.25)	0.55 (0.23)

Note: The sample is based on a group of 528 highly educated Israelis. Total scores (Trials 1–5) are also provided (Vakil, Personal communication, January 13, 2004).

Source: Adapted from Vakil et al., 1997.

Table 10–89a Boys: RAVLT Means and (SDs) of the Raw Memory Scores for Each Age Group

| | Age Group (Years) | | | | | | | | | |
Trial	8 (n = 51)	9 (n = 51)	10 (n = 56)	11 (n = 55)	12 (n = 45)	13 (n = 42)	14 (n = 42)	15 (n = 61)	16 (n = 47)	17 (n = 37)
T1 (List A)	6.10 (1.98)	5.69 (1.48)	6.30 (1.49)	6.80 (1.71)	6.80 (1.89)	7.29 (1.50)	7.12 (1.53)	7.46 (2.01)	7.17 (1.49)	6.97 (1.36)
T2	7.84 (2.18)	8.43 (1.71)	9.29 (2.08)	9.76 (2.08)	9.44 (2.15)	10.00 (2.37)	10.04 (2.15)	10.54 (2.20)	10.02 (2.04)	9.83 (2.15)
T3	9.04 (2.61)	10.12 (2.16)	10.66 (1.78)	11.54 (1.80)	11.53 (1.73)	11.71 (2.03)	11.59 (1.97)	12.00 (1.77)	11.40 (1.71)	11.43 (1.86)
T4	10.00 (2.36)	10.82 (2.40)	11.23 (1.81)	12.27 (1.70)	12.20 (1.47)	12.16 (1.75)	12.30 (1.77)	12.42 (1.67)	12.19 (1.51)	12.48 (1.60)
T5	10.61 (2.05)	11.71 (1.89)	11.78 (1.70)	12.38 (1.81)	12.91 (1.47)	12.28 (1.81)	12.80 (1.56)	12.96 (1.73)	12.63 (1.55)	12.27 (1.72)
Total	43.59 (7.92)	46.76 (7.33)	49.27 (7.11)	52.76 (6.92)	52.89 (6.65)	53.45 (7.74)	53.88 (7.06)	55.39 (7.61)	53.43 (6.46)	53.00 (6.73)
List B	5.06 (1.58)	5.35 (1.76)	5.59 (1.56)	6.09 (1.76)	6.40 (2.08)	6.02 (1.88)	6.67 (2.09)	6.93 (2.35)	6.32 (2.18)	6.40 (1.82)
T6 (List A)	8.92 (2.78)	9.47 (2.52)	9.89 (2.17)	11.31 (2.03)	11.24 (2.25)	11.17 (2.73)	10.95 (2.28)	11.72 (2.33)	11.34 (2.03)	11.08 (2.26)
T7 (DR)	8.98 (2.63)	9.86 (2.31)	10.20 (2.49)	11.29 (2.43)	11.71 (2.12)	11.48 (2.52)	10.95 (2.56)	11.57 (2.35)	11.34 (2.30)	10.81 (2.50)
T8 (RC)[a]	13.75 (1.65)	13.27 (3.03)	13.84 (1.04)	14.07 (1.03)	14.40 (0.81)	14.24 (1.10)	14.26 (1.36)	13.93 (1.48)	13.98 (1.36)	14.14 (1.05)
T9 (AD)	37.17 (18.59)	32.92 (15.27)	29.71 (16.50)	28.40 (17.48)	26.18 (16.22)	28.86 (17.44)	27.56 (15.44)	28.51 (14.97)	31.37 (14.98)	28.69 (14.25)
T9 (CO)	0.63 (0.27)	0.70 (0.21)	0.77 (0.16)	0.75 (0.23)	0.78 (0.20)	0.75 (0.23)	0.77 (0.19)	0.76 (0.17)	0.73 (0.21)	0.75 (0.19)

Note: AD = absolute deviation; CO = correlation score; DR = delayed recall; RC = recognition (hit rate).
[a]Because the distribution of this measure was found not to be normal, medians are presented for the age groups in ascending order (15, 14, 15, 14, 13, 13).

Source: From Vakil et al., 1998, and Vakil, personal communication, January 13, 2004.

Table 10–89b Girls: RAVLT Means and SDs of the Raw Memory Scores for Each Age Group

Trial	Age Group (Years)									
	8 (n = 49)	9 (n = 49)	10 (n = 54)	11 (n = 48)	12 (n = 45)	13 (n = 41)	14 (n = 45)	15 (n = 43)	16 (n = 43)	17 (n = 39)
T1 (List A)	5.82 (1.54)	5.96 (1.57)	6.85 (1.62)	7.33 (1.73)	7.27 (1.70)	7.10 (1.73)	7.56 (1.42)	8.14 (2.14)	7.56 (1.87)	7.67 (1.59)
T2	8.04 (1.98)	8.80 (2.25)	9.70 (1.10)	10.44 (2.07)	10.44 (1.73)	10.10 (2.07)	10.53 (1.96)	10.77 (2.23)	10.00 (2.30)	10.72 (2.13)
T3	9.51 (2.41)	10.45 (2.33)	11.48 (2.07)	11.92 (2.06)	12.13 (1.63)	11.61 (1.77)	11.98 (1.30)	12.53 (2.03)	11.79 (1.74)	12.41 (1.63)
T4	10.08 (2.90)	11.61 (1.62)	12.00 (1.85)	12.46 (1.76)	12.36 (1.43)	12.17 (1.91)	12.42 (1.56)	13.00 (1.48)	12.16 (2.03)	12.54 (1.54)
T5	11.08 (2.53)	12.29 (1.59)	12.56 (1.66)	12.90 (1.74)	12.96 (1.35)	12.80 (1.49)	13.13 (1.29)	13.14 (1.68)	13.09 (1.23)	13.03 (1.44)
Total	44.53 (9.22)	49.10 (7.19)	52.59 (7.07)	55.04 (7.20)	55.16 (5.66)	53.78 (7.18)	55.62 (5.65)	57.58 (8.11)	54.60 (7.41)	56.36 (6.03)
List B	4.69 (1.79)	5.59 (1.50)	6.33 (2.11)	6.19 (1.54)	6.64 (1.54)	6.41 (2.17)	6.51 (1.42)	7.32 (2.92)	6.42 (1.99)	6.54 (1.80)
T6 (List A)	9.18 (3.29)	10.69 (2.13)	11.11 (1.93)	11.54 (1.98)	11.22 (1.96)	11.02 (1.85)	11.89 (1.67)	12.02 (2.56)	11.39 (2.17)	11.87 (2.04)
T7 (DR)	9.45 (3.00)	10.75 (2.22)	11.09 (2.36)	11.69 (1.99)	11.60 (1.90)	11.49 (2.27)	12.24 (1.77)	12.16 (2.40)	11.88 (1.90)	12.10 (2.11)
T8 (RC)[a]	13.59 (2.45)	14.10 (2.30)	14.05 (2.18)	14.67 (0.59)	14.15 (2.36)	14.17 (1.11)	14.00 (2.32)	14.16 (1.53)	14.16 (1.02)	14.20 (2.46)
T9 (AD)	31.23 (16.10)	26.96 (12.67)	27.04 (14.06)	24.65 (15.10)	23.12 (15.76)	30.52 (16.27)	24.66 (10.20)	28.79 (18.00)	30.37 (16.76)	26.21 (11.64)
T9 (CO)	0.72 (0.20)	0.79 (0.17)	0.79 (0.18)	0.80 (0.21)	0.79 (0.21)	0.73 (0.22)	0.81 (0.12)	0.76 (0.22)	0.72 (0.23)	0.79 (0.15)

Note: AD = absolute deviation; CO = correlation score; DR = delayed recall; RC = recognition (hit rate).

[a]Because the distribution of this measure was found not to be normal, medians are presented for the age groups in ascending order (15, 14, 15, 14, 13, 13).

Source: Vakil et al., 1998, and Vakil, personal communication, January 13, 2004.

Table 10–90 RAVLT Scores (*M* and *SD*) for Children Aged
6 and 7 Years

	Age 6 Years[a] (N = 41)	Age 7 Years[b] (N = 20)
Trial 1	4.1 (1.0)	4.5 (1.3)
Trial 2	6.1 (1.6)	6.7 (1.8)
Trial 3	6.8 (1.7)	8.1 (2.2)
Trial 4	8.1 (2.3)	9.4 (2.3)
Trial 5	8.0 (2.3)	10.2 (2.6)
Total	33.1 (7.3)	38.9 (7.9)
List B		4.5 (1.6)
Trial A6		8.0 (2.8)
Trial A7 (Delay)	7.5 (2.2)	8.4 (2.6)
List A Recognition		14.5 (0.7)
List B Recognition		6.1 (2.2)
False Positives		1.1 (0.7)

[a]Adapted from Van den Burg & Kingma, 1999.
[b]Adapted from Forrester & Geffen, 1991.

impairment (Records et al., 1995), AD (Bigler et al., 1989; Mitrushina et al., 1994; Mungas, 1983; Shimamura et al., 1987; Tierney et al., 1994, 1996; Woodard et al., 1999), Parkinson's disease (Alegret et al., 2001), Huntington's disease (Shimamura et al., 1987), Koraskoff's (Shimamura et al., 1987), closed-head injury (CHI) in adults (Bigler et al., 1989; Geffen et al., 1994a; Potter et al., 2002; Shum et al., 2000; Vakil et al., 1991), CHI in children (Vakil et al., 2004), AIDS (Ryan et al., 1992), childhood diabetes (Fox et al., 2003), childhood learning disabilities (Van Strien, 1999), intellectual deficiency (Vakil et al., 1997); chronic fatigue syndrome (Crowe & Casey, 1999), lead exposure (Stewart et al., 1999), and psychiatric disorders including depression and schizophrenia (Moritz et al., 2001; Mungas, 1983; Rosenberg et al., 1984; Seltzer et al., 1997; Torres et al., 2001).

Information from the test can be used to differentiate clinically among various conditions (but see Crockett et al., 1992). For example, normal aging appears to be associated with deficits in acquisition more than in consolidation (Dunlosky & Salthouse, 1996), whereas both deficient acquisition and consolidation appear to be involved in AD (Woodard et al., 1999). Patients with AD show more impairment on the RAVLT than do patients with CHI or AIDS, along with a flat learning curve that demonstrates negligible improvement with repeated trials, recency effects only, and an excessive number of word intrusions (confabulation) on the recognition trial (Antonelli Incalzi et al., 1995; Bigler et al., 1989; Mitrushina et al., 1994).

CHI patients, by contrast, show both a recency and a primacy effect (Bigler et al., 1989), although the primacy effect is impaired in children with CHI (Vakil et al., 2004). Both adults and children with CHI show improvement over repeated trials (positive-slope learning curve; Bigler et al., 1989; Shum et al., 2000; Vakil et al., 2004). Although general impairment of verbal memory is a feature of CHI, exaggerated retroactive interference effects are characteristic (Geffen et al., 1994a; Vakil et al., 2004); however, this problem with retroactive interference may resolve after the first year of injury in adults (Shum et al., 2000). Moreover, retention of the learning list after the distractor trial appears to vary with severity of the CHI in adults: the more severe the injury (the longer the duration of posttraumatic amnesia), the fewer words are recalled after interference (Geffen et al., 1994a). In children, the longer the coma, the lower the number of total words recalled and the stronger the retroactive interference effect (Trial 5 versus Trial A6; Vakil et al., 2004). Temporal order judgments are also impaired in CHI (Vakil et al., 1991, 2004).

AIDS patients show relatively intact learning and recognition; however, their forgetting rates (comparing Trial 5 to Trial 6) are impaired (Mitrushina et al., 1991). Patients with Parkinson's disease, AD, or frontal lobe dementia tend to produce an increased number of intrusion errors on the recall trials; however, the nature of the intrusions differs. Intrusions unrelated to words on the list are more commonly observed in patients with AD or frontal lobe dementia, perhaps reflecting a deficit in self-regulatory mechanisms (Rouleau et al., 2001).

Acute mental stress typical of everyday life appears to have little measurable effect on test performance (Hoffman & al'Absi, 2004). Various authors have noted that psychological distress, in the form of depression, posttraumatic stress, and other anxiety disorders, has some effect on RAVLT performance (Bleecker et al., 1988; Gainotti & Marra, 1994; Hinkin et al., 1992; Query & Megran, 1983; Uddo et al., 1993), although others have failed to observe a correlation (Gibbs et al., 1990; Vingerhoets et al., 1995; Wiens et al., 1988). The weight of evidence suggests, however, that caution is needed in interpreting RAVLT performance in patients with a past history or clinical suspicion of depression, posttraumatic stress disorder, or anxiety. Qualitative indices may prove useful in this regard. Uddo et al. (1993) found that veterans diagnosed with posttraumatic stress disorder exhibited less facile acquisition, were more sensitive to proactive interference, and

Table 10–91 Total Score (Trials T1–T5) in Normal Adults (Mean Age, About 33 Years) and Individuals with Schizophrenia (Mean Age, About 33 Years) Retested with a RAVLT Alternate Form After 2 Weeks

Measure	T1 Mean and SD	T1 SEM	T2 Mean and SD	T2 SEM	r	S_diff	90%CI	80%CI
Healthy	59.2 (6.1)	3.22	57.8 (8.5)	4.50	.72	5.54	9.08	7.09
Patients	46.3	12.3	45.7	12.1	.69	9.58	15.70	12.26

Source: Adapted from Moritz et al., 2003.

showed greater perseveration on the RAVLT, compared with control subjects. Despite differences in learning, the two groups did not differ in the proportion of information recalled after a delay. Gainotti and Marra (1994) reported that preservation of the recency effect and attenuation of the primacy effect, as well as extralist intrusions on delayed recall, point to a diagnosis of depressive pseudodementia. On the other hand, the presence of several false-positive errors on delayed recognition tends to be specific to AD patients and is rarely found in patients with depressive pseudodementia.

Ecological Validity

The test has some ecological validity. For example, patients with schizophrenia who have better verbal memory on the RAVLT are more likely to perform better on tasks of independent living (e.g., shopping; Remfer et al., 2003). Scores on the RAVLT also appear to offer some predictive utility. AD patients who show a positive learning curve are more likely to benefit from rehabilitative group therapy than are patients who show little learning (Haddad & Nussbaum, 1989). In adult patients with traumatic brain injury, performance on the RAVLT is predictive of psychosocial outcome (community integration) at 1 year after injury (Millis et al., 1994). Kinsella et al. (1997) reported that verbal learning and memory indices from the RAVLT at 3-months after traumatic brain injury are good predictors of subsequent needs for special education in children.

Malingering

Claparede and Rey used the task to detect invalid responding (Boake, 2000). Subsequent work has shown that poorly motivated individuals often exhibit a pattern of excessive impairment on the RAVLT. In particular, there is evidence that severe RAVLT recognition memory impairment (e.g., scores <7) most likely reflects motivation to exaggerate deficits in patients with CHI (Binder et al., 1993, 2003; Chouinard & Rouleau, 1997; Greiffenstein et al., 1994; King et al., 1998; Meyers et al., 2001; Sherman et al., 2002). The recognition memory measure exhibits a high degree of specificity for motivation to perform poorly, but only modest sensitivity. For example, Binder et al. (2003) reported that 92% of patients with moderate to severe head injury obtained scores of more than 5 correct responses, whereas only 38% of poorly motivated patients (classed according to performance on the Portland Digit Recognition Test) obtained such scores.

Abnormal serial position effects (absence of primacy effects in recall) have also been explored. Bernard (1991) found that individuals attempting to fake injury tended to do so by suppressing recall of words from the first third of the list (absence of primacy but not recency effect), behaving like patients with severe amnesia. However, subsequent studies have yielded contradictory results. Suhr (2002) reported that simulators (including those who had been warned about the possibility of detection) showed a suppressed primacy effect during learning trials, whereas normal subjects and patients

with moderate to severe head injury tended to have normal serial position curves. She noted that a flattened primacy index was not commonly seen in head-injured individuals; however, a minority of simulators showed such a pattern; her primacy index correctly identified only 13% of malingerers, with a false-positive rate of only 3%). That is, a suppressed primacy effect appears to be relatively specific, but not particularly sensitive, to malingering. Further, others have found that indices based on serial position effects failed to reliably distinguish between simulators and controls (Bernard et al., 1993; Powell et al., 2004; Sullivan et al., 2002).

Other indicators (e.g., Trial 5, total of Trials 1–5, number of false positives on the recognition trial, discrepancies in recall-recognition scores; failure to recognize words recalled at least three times on the learning trials) are of some utility but are not very effective in identifying deliberate attempts to perform poorly on the RAVLT (Boone et al., 2005; Suhr & Gunstad, 2000; Sullivan et al., 2002). Similarly, inclusion of measures of implicit memory (e.g., word stems completed with RAVLT items) and of temporal order (an index more of automatic than of explicit memory) result in only modest sensitivity and do not appear to justify the added administration time of these additional trials (Boone et al., 2005).

Recent evidence suggests that indices that incorporate recognition performance are most useful, with some recognition parameters (e.g., location of words in the original list presentation) more sensitive than others. Boone et al. (2005) reported that a cutoff of 12 or less for true recognition (recognition minus false positives) plus primacy recognition (i.e., number of words recognized from the first third of the test) was associated with 73.8% sensitivity at 90% specificity. This combination score was modestly superior to the sensitivity obtained with the standard recognition score (59%–67%, depending on the cutoff value). With a base rate of malingering of 30%, the positive and negative predictive values were 75% and 88.6%, respectively, for the RAVLT combination score (true recognition plus primacy recognition), compared with 81.1% and 86.6% for simple recognition correct (≤9).

The addition of a second delayed recall and recognition trial at 60 min (referred to as the expanded AVLT or AVLTX) may also enhance diagnostic accuracy. Barrash et al. (2004) constructed an exaggeration index (EI) based on the notion that malingerers would have difficulty estimating their 30-min performance, keeping track of the words that they reported and those that they feigned forgetting. The EI is a composite index reflecting the extent to which memory performance is characterized by inconsistencies that are atypical of brain-damaged individuals. It comprises seven aspects of improbable performance: exceedingly poor learning, lack of primacy effect, worsening recall, worsening recognition, failure to recognize learned words, and exceedingly poor recognition (see Table 10–92). The EI demonstrated good sensitivity, identifying two thirds of the probable malingerers as such, and positive predictive accuracy was .84 (with a base rate of malingering of 30%). In comparison to the EI, the Recognition Memory Test demonstrated a higher level of sensitivity but

Table 10–92 Exaggeration Index for the Expanded Auditory Verbal Learning Test

Inconsistency	Scaled Score			
	0	1	2	3
1. Exceedingly poor learning—Immediate recall of 15-word list, summed across learning Trials 1–5	≥28	23–27	18–22	0–17
2. Lack of primacy effect—Immediate recall of words 1–3, summed across learning Trials 1–5	≥4	1–3	0	—
3. Worsening recall—Delayed recall at 30-min minus delayed recall at 60 min	0–2	3	4	≥5
4. Worsening recognition—Delayed recognition at 30 min minus delayed recognition at 60 min	0–2	—	3	≥4
5. Learned words not recognized (scored only if made ≥2 false positive responses)—Words recalled on ≥4 learning trials but not recognized at 30 min plus words recalled on ≥4 learning trials but not recognized at 60 min	0–2	3–4	5–8	≥9
6. Recalled words not recognized—Words recalled at 30 min but not recognized at 60 min	0–4	5–6	7–8	≥9
7. Exceedingly poor recognition—Recognition of target words summed across 30- and 60-min delays	>20	14–19	11–13	0–10

Note: Total score for the index is calculated by summing the scaled scores for the seven inconsistencies.

Source: Suhr et al., 2004. Reprinted with the kind permission of Psychology Press.

lower positive predictive accuracy (.67). Initial development of the EI-AVLTX was based on patient groups (brain-damaged, psychiatric, probable malingerers) referred for neuropsychological assessment. Subsequent studies by these authors (Suhr et al., 2004), using a simulation paradigm, found the EI-AVLTX to be modestly sensitive and relatively specific to malingering, as well as robust to the effects of a warning about malingering detection. Scores of 2 are considered consistent with "probable malingering," and scores of 3 are "highly probable" (Barrash et al., 2004; Suhr et al., 2004).

Measures derived from the RAVLT (e.g., recognition trial score, delayed recall score) show modest to moderate relations with other indices of motivational status (e.g., Warrington Recognition Memory Test, Rey 15-Item), although the amount of shared variance is less than 50% (Nelson et al., 2003). The implication is that the RAVLT provides nonredundant information and can serve as a relatively independent source of information regarding the validity of neuropsychological test performance.

COMMENT

The RAVLT has a very long history in the field (Boake, 2000) and was one of the first standard tests of multitrial list learning to achieve widespread clinical use (Woodard et al., 1999). It is commonly used in the assessment of memory disorders and appears able to provide a wealth of information to characterize memory functioning (e.g., learning rate, susceptibility to proactive and retroactive interference). The test has been administered in various languages (e.g., French, German, Chinese, Dutch, Spanish, and Hebrew) and cultures, and the convergence of findings contributes to the validity of the test.

Some authors use a presentation rate of one word per second (e.g., Forrester & Geffen, 1991), whereas others (e.g., Van den Burg & Kingma, 1999) use a 1-second interval between words. However, the various studies yield similar results, suggesting little effect in the range of rates considered here. Further, in testing recognition, some authors use story formats and others use word list formats. The word list formats also differ from the study formats, in terms of, for example, word list length, delay intervals, and whether an intervening delayed recall trial was administered. Based on his review of the available literature, Schmidt (1996) suggested that the recognition memory scores are quite robust with regard to these procedural permutations, with no systematic differences occurring for different recognition procedures.

The most reliable measures are the total score, the delayed recall score, and the Trial 5 score. Although other measures are interesting from a research perspective, their reliabilities tend to be low and suggest caution in interpreting other features (e.g., flatness of the learning curve, number of errors, number of repetitions), including those that rely on differences between scores. In view of the moderate-to-low test-retest reliabilities, the clinician is encouraged to include additional tests of verbal memory to confirm diagnostic impressions.

The normative data appear fairly robust for use in Western countries. However, estimates of memory function based on norms derived from individuals of average to above-average intellect may suggest a deficit, when none is present, in individuals of below-average intellectual attainment. Norms adjusted for premorbid IQ would therefore be useful.

It is important to note that ceiling effects appear to be present on the later recall trials (group mean less than about 1.5 *SD*s from the maximum score), with many young adults unable to demonstrate their true memory ability. Uttl (2005) noted that ceiling effects can negatively affect test reliability and validity because of attenuated variability in test scores. Such ceiling effects restrict use of the test for both clinical and research applications. Therefore, in clinical settings, inferences about the degree of memory deficits based on these norms may be incorrect, skewed by artificially lowered means and attenuated *SD*s. Similarly, inferences about normal age-related changes in specific memory processes may be misleading. Ceiling effects can be minimized by administering fewer learning trials (e.g., three trials).

Indices from the test (e.g., performance on the recognition trial, inconsistencies across trials) appear to be useful in the evaluation of motivational status. If extremely poor performance is obtained, the index of suspicion is high. However, the lack of high sensitivity argues against using these indices as effective screens in medicolegal situations, because many potential cases of motivation to perform poorly would escape detection (Binder et al., 2003).

REFERENCES

Anderson, V. A., & Lajoie, G. (1996). Development of memory and learning skills in school-aged children: A neuropsychological perspective. *Applied Neuropsychology, 3/4,* 128–139.

Antonelli Incalzi, R., Capparella, O., Gemma, A., Marra, C., & Carbonin, P. U. (1995). Effects of aging and Alzheimer's disease on verbal memory. *Journal of Clinical and Experimental Neuropsychology, 17,* 580–589.

Alegret, M., Junque, C., Valleoriola, F., Vendrell, P., Pilleri, M., Rumia, J., & Tolosa, E. (2001). Effects of bilateral subthalamic stimulation on cognitive function in Parkinson disease. *Archives of Neurology, 58,* 1223–1227.

Barrash, J., Suhr, J., & Manzel, K. (2004). Detecting poor effort and malingering with an expanded version of the Auditory Verbal Learning Test (AVLTX): Validation with clinical samples. *Journal of Clinical and Experimental Neuropsychology, 26,* 125–140.

Bernard, L. C. (1991). The detection of faked deficits on the Rey Auditory Verbal Learning Test. *Archives of Clinical Neuropsychology, 6,* 81–88.

Bernard, L. C., Houston, W., & Natoli, L. (1993). Malingering on neuropsychological memory tests: Potential objective indicators. *Journal of Clinical Psychology, 49,* 45–53.

Bigler, E. D., Rosa, L., Schultz, F., Hall, S., & Harris, J. (1989). Rey-Auditory Verbal Learning and Rey-Osterrieth Complex Figure Design Test Performance in Alzheimer's Disease and closed head injury. *Journal of Clinical Psychology, 45,* 277–280.

Binder, L. M., Kelly, M. P., Villanueva, M. R., & Winslow, M. M. (2003). Motivation and neuropsychological test performance following mild head injury. *Journal of Clinical and Experimental Neuropsychology, 25,* 420–430.

Binder, L. M., Villanueva, M. R., Howieson, D., & Moore, R. T. (1993). The Rey AVLT Recognition memory task measures motivational impairment after mild head trauma. *Archives of Clinical Neuropsychology, 7,* 137–147.

Bishop, J., Knights, R. M., & Stoddart, C. (1990). Rey Auditory-Verbal Learning Test: Performance of English and French children aged 5 to 16. *The Clinical Neuropsychologist, 4,* 133–140.

Bleecker, M. L., Bolla-Wilson, K., Agnew, J., & Meyers, D. A. (1988). Age-related sex differences in verbal memory. *Journal of Clinical Psychology, 44,* 403–411.

Boake, C. (2000). Edouard Claparede and the Auditory Verbal Learning Test. *Journal of Clinical and Experimental Neuropsychology, 22,* 286–292.

Bolla-Wilson, K., & Bleecker, M. L. (1986). Influence of verbal intelligence, sex, age, and education on the Rey Auditory Verbal Learning Test. *Developmental Neuropsychology, 2,* 203–211.

Boone, K. B., Lu, P., & Wen, J. (2005). Comparison of various RAVLT scores in the detection of noncredible memory performance. *Archives of Clinical Neuropsychology, 20,* 301–319.

Chouinard, M. J., & Rouleau, I. (1997). The 48-Pictures Test: A two-alternative forced-choice recognition test for the detection of malingering. *Journal of the International Neuropsychological Society, 3,* 545–552.

Crawford, J. R., Stewart, L. E., & Moore, J. W. (1989). Demonstration of savings on the AVLT and development of a parallel form. *Journal of Clinical and Experimental Neuropsychology, 11,* 975–981.

Crockett, D. J., Hadjistavropoulos, T., & Hurwitz, T. (1992). Primacy and recency effects in the assessment of memory using the Rey Auditory Verbal Learning Test. *Archives of Clinical Neuropsychology, 7,* 97–107.

Crossen, J. R., & Wiens, A. N. (1994). Comparison of the auditory-verbal learning test (AVLT) and California Verbal Learning Test (CVLT) in a sample of normal subjects. *Journal of Clinical and Experimental Neuropsychology, 16,* 190–194.

Crowe, S. F., & Casey, A. (1999). A neuropsychological study of the chronic fatigue syndrome: Support for a deficit in memory function independent of depression. *Australian Psychologist, 34,* 70–75.

Delaney, R. C., Prevey, M. L., Cramer, J., Mattson, R. H., & VA Epilepsy Cooperative Study 264 Research Group. (1992). Test-retest comparability and control subject data for the Rey-Auditory Verbal Learning Test and Rey-Osterrieth/Taylor Complex Figures. *Archives of Clinical Neuropsychology, 7,* 523–528.

Dunlosky, J., & Salthouse, T. A. (1996). A decomposition of age-related differences in multitrial free recall. *Aging, Neuropsychology, and Cognition, 3,* 2–14.

Ferman, T. J., Lucas, J. A., Ivnik, R. J., Smith, G. E., Willis, F. B., Petersen, R. C., & Graff-Radford, N. R. (2005). Mayo's Older African American Normative Studies: Auditory-Verbal Learning Test norms for African American elders. *The Clinical Neuropsychologist, 19,* 214–228.

Forrester, G., & Geffen, G. (1991). Performance measure of 7- to 15-year-old children on the Auditory Verbal Learning Test. *The Clinical Neuropsychologist, 5,* 345–359.

Fox, M. A., Chen, R. S., & Holmes, C. S. (2003). Gender differences in memory and learning in children with insulin-dependent diabetes (IDDM) over a 4-year follow-up interval. *Journal of Pediatric Psychology, 28,* 569–578.

Fuller, K. H., Gouvier, W. D., & Savage, R. M. (1997). Comparison of List B and List C of the Rey Auditory Verbal Learning Test. *The Clinical Neuropsychologist, 11,* 201–204.

Gainotti, G., & Marra, C. (1994). Some aspects of memory disorders clearly distinguish dementia of the Alzheimer's type from depressive pseudodementia. *Journal of Clinical and Experimental Neuropsychology, 16,* 65–74.

Geffen, G. M., Butterworth, P., Forrester, G. M., & Geffen, L. B. (1994a). Auditory verbal learning test components as measures of the severity of closed head injury. *Brain Injury, 8,* 405–411.

Geffen, G. M., Butterworth, P., & Geffen, L. B. (1994b). Test-retest reliability of a new form of the Auditory Verbal Learning Test (AVLT). *Archives of Clinical Neuropsychology, 9,* 303–316.

Geffen, G. M., Geffen, L., & Bishop, K. (1997). Extended delayed recall of AVLT word lists: Effects of age and sex on adult performance. *Australian Journal of Psychology, 49,* 78–84.

Geffen, G., Moar, K. J., O'Hanlon, A. P., Clark, C. R., & Geffen, L. B. (1990). Performance measures of 16- to 86-year-old males and females on the Auditory Verbal Learning Test. *The Clinical Neuropsychologist, 4,* 45–63.

Gibbs, A., Andrewes, D. G., Szmuckler, G., Mulhall, B., & Bowden, S. C. (1990). Early HIV-related neuropsychological impairment: Relationship to stage of viral infection. *Journal of Clinical and Experimental Neuropsychology, 12,* 766–780.

Graf, P., & Uttl, B. (1995). Component processes of memory: Changes across the adult lifespan. *Swiss Journal of Psychology, 54,* 113–130.

Greiffenstein, M., Baker, W., & Gola, T. (1994). Validation of malingered amnesia measures with a large clinical sample. *Psychological Assessment, 6,* 218–224.

Haddad, L. B., & Nussbaum, P. (1989). Predictive utility of the Rey Auditory-Verbal Learning Test with Alzheimer's patients. *The Clinical Gerontologist, 9,* 53–59.

Harris, M. E., Ivnik, R. J., & Smith, G. E. (2002). Mayo's Older Americans Normative Studies: Expanded AVLT recognition troal norms for ages 57 to 98. *Journal of Clinical and Experimental Neuropsychology, 24,* 214–220.

Helmstaedter, C., & Durwen, H. F. (1990). VLMT: Verbaler Lern- und Merkfahigkeitstest (VLMT: Verbal Learning and Memory Test). *Schwietzer Archiv fur Nurologie und Psychiatrie, 141,* 21–30.

Hinkin, C. H., Van Gorp, W. G., Satz, P. Weisman, J. D., Thommes, J., & Buckingham, S. (1992). Depressed mood and its relationship to neuropsychological test performance in HIV-1 seropositive individuals. *Journal of Clinical and Experimental Neuropsychology, 14,* 289–297.

Hoffman, R., & al'Absi, M. (2004). The effects of acute stress on subsequent neuropsychological test performance. *Archives of Clinical Neuropsychology, 19,* 497–506.

Ivnik, R. J., Malec, J. F., Tangalos, E. G., Petersen, R. C., Kokmen, S., & Kurland, L. T. (1990). The Auditory-Verbal Learning Test (AVLT): Norms for ages 55 years and older. *Psychological Assessment, 2,* 304–312.

Ivnik, R. J., Malec, J. F., Tangalos, E. G., Petersen, R. C., Kokmen, E., & Kurland, L. T. (1992). Mayo's Older Americans Normative Studies: Updated AVLT norms for ages 56 to 97. *The Clinical Neuropsychologist, 6,* 83–104.

Janowsky, J. S., Shimamura, A. P., & Squire, L. R. (1989). Source memory impairment in patients with frontal lobe lesions. *Neuropsychologia, 27,* 1043–1056.

Johnstone, B., Vieth, A. Z., Johnson, J. C., & Shaw, J. A. (2000). Recall as a function of single versus multiple trials: Implications for rehabilitation. *Rehabiliation Psychology, 45,* 3–19.

Kennepohl, S., Shore, D., Nabors, N., & Hanks, R. (2004). African American acculturation and neuropsychological test performance following traumatic brain injury. *Journal of the International Neuropsychological Society, 10,* 566–577.

Kilpatrick, C., Murrie, V., Cook, M., Andrewes, D., Desmond, P., & Hopper, J. (1997). Degree of left hippocampal atrophy correlates with severity of neuropsychological deficits. *Seizure, 6,* 213–218.

King, J. H., Gfeller, J. D., & Davis, H. P. (1998). Detecting simulated memory impairment with the Rey Auditory Verbal Learning Test: Implications of base rates and study generalizeability. *Journal of Clinical and Experimental Neuropsychology, 20,* 603–612.

Kinsella, G. J., Prior, M., Sawyer, M., Ong, B., Murtagh, D., Eisenmajer, R., Bryan, D., Anderson, V., & Klug, G. (1997). Predictors and indicators of academic outcome in children 2 years following traumatic brain injury. *Journal of the International Neuropsychological Society, 3,* 608–616.

Kurlyo, M., Temple, R. O., Elliott, T. R., & Crawford, D. (2001). Rey Auditory Verbal Learning Test (AVLT) performance in individuals with recent-onset spinal cord injury. *Rehabilitation Psychology, 46,* 247–261.

Lannoo, E., & Vingerhoets, G. (1997). Flemish normative data on common neuropsychological test: Influence of age, education, and gender. *Psychologica Belgica, 37,* 141–155.

Lee, T. M. C. (2003). *Normative data: Neuropsychological measures for Hong Kong Chinese.* Neuropsychology Laboratory, The University of Hong Kong, Hong Kong.

Lemay, S., Bedard, M. A., Rouleau, I., & Tremblay, P. L. G. (2004). Practice effect and test-retest reliability of attentional and executive tests in middle-aged to elderly subjects. *The Clinical Neuropsychologist, 18,* 284–302.

Lezak, M. D. (1976). *Neuropsychological assessment.* New York: Oxford University Press.

Lezak, M. D. (1982). The test-retest stability of some tests commonly used in neuropsychological assessment. Paper presented to the Fifth European Conference of the International Neuropsychological Society. Deauville, France.

Lezak, M. D. (1983). *Neuropsychological assessment* (2nd ed.). New York: Oxford University Press.

Lezak, M. D., Howieson, D. B., Loring, D. W., Hannay, H. J., & Fischer, J. S. (2004). *Neuropsychological assessment* (4th ed.). New York: Oxford University Press.

Maj, M., D'Elia, L., Satz, P., Janssen, R., Zaudig, M., Uchiyama, C., Starace, F., Galderisi, S., & Chervinsky, A. (1993). Evaluation of two new neuropsychological tests designed to minimize cultural bias in the assessment of HIV-1 seropositive persons: A WHO study. *Archives of Clinical Neuropsychology, 8,* 123–135.

Majdan, A., Sziklas, V., & Jones-Gotman, M. (1996). Performance of healthy subjects and patients with resection from the anterior temporal lobe on matched tests of verbal and visuoperceptual learning. *Journal of Clinical and Experimental Neuropsychology, 18,* 416–430.

Malec, J. F., Ivnik, R. J., & Hinkeldey, N. S. (1991). Visual Spatial Learning Test. *Psychological Assessment, 3,* 82–88.

Meyers, J. E., Morrison, A. L., & Miller, J. C. (2001). How low is too low, revisited: Sentence repetition and AVLT-recognition in the detection of malingering. *Applied Neuropsychology, 4,* 234–241.

Miatton, M., Wolters, M., Lannoo, E., & Vingerhoets, G. (2004). Updated and extended normative data of commonly used neuropsychological tests. *Psychologica Belgica, 44,* 189–216.

Miceli, G., Caltagirone, C., Gainotti, G., Masullo, C., & Silveri, M. C. (1981). Neuropsychological correlates of localized cerebral lesions in nonaphasic brain-damaged patients. *Journal of Clinical Neuropsychology, 3,* 53–63.

Millis, S. R., Rosenthal, M., & Lourie, I. F. (1994). Predicting community integration after traumatic brain injury with neuropsychological measures. *International Journal of Neuroscience, 79,* 165–167.

Miranda, J. P., & Valencia, R. R. (1997). English and Spanish versions of a memory test: Word-length effects versus spoken-duration effects. *Hispanic Journal of Behavioral Sciences, 19,* 171–181.

Mitrushina, M., & Satz, P. (1991a). Changes in cognitive functioning associated with normal aging. *Archives of Clinical Neuropsychology, 6,* 49–60.

Mitrushina, M., & Satz, P. (1991b). Effect of repeated administration of a neuropsychological battery in the elderly. *Journal of Clinical Psychology, 47,* 790–801.

Mitrushina, M. N., Boone, K. B., Razani, J., & D'Elia, L. F. (2005). *Handbook of normative data for neuropsychological assessment* (2nd ed.). New York: Oxford University Press.

Mitrushina, M., Satz, P., Chervinsky, A., & D'Elia, L. (1991). Performance of four age groups of normal elderly on the Rey Auditory-Verbal Learning Test. *Journal of Clinical Psychology, 47,* 351–357.

Mitrushina, M., Satz, P., Drebing, C., & Van Gorp, W. (1994). The differential pattern of memory deficit in normal aging and dementias of different etiology. *Journal of Clinical Psychology, 50,* 246–252.

Moses, J. A. (1986). Factor structure of Benton's test of visual retention, visual construction, and visual form discrimination. *Archives of Clinical Neuropsychology, 1,* 147–156.

Moritz, S., Heeren, D., Andresen, B., & Krausz, M. (2001). An analysis of the specificity and the syndromal correlates of verbal memory impairments in schizophrenia. *Psychiatry Research, 101,* 23–31.

Moritz, S., Iverson, G. L., & Woodward, T. S. (2003). Reliable change indexes for memory performance in schizophrenia as a means to determine drug-induced cognitive decline. *Applied Neuropsychology, 10,* 115–120.

Mueller, H., Hasse-Sander, R., Horn, C., Helmstaedter, C., & Elger, C. E. (1997). Rey-Auditory Verbal Learning Test: Structure of a modified German version. *Journal of Clinical Psychology, 53,* 663–671.

Mungas, D. (1983). Differential clinical sensitivity of specific parameters of the Rey Auditory-Verbal Learning Test. *Journal of Consulting and Clinical Psychology, 51,* 848–855.

Nelson, N. W., Boone, K., Dueck, A., Wagener, L., Lu, P., & Grills, C. (2003). Relationships between eight measures of suspect effort. *The Clinical Neuropsychologist, 17,* 263–272.

Nielsen, H., Knudsen, L., & Daugbjerg, O. (1989). Normative data for eight neuropsychological tests based on a Danish sample. *Scandinavian Journal of Psychology, 30,* 37–45.

Ponton, M. O., Gonzalez, J. J., Hernandez, I., Herrera, L., & Higareda, I. (2000). Factor analysis of the Neuropsychological Screening Battery for Hispanics (NeSBHIS). *Applied Neuropsychology, 7,* 32–39.

Ponton, M. O., Satz, P., Herrera, L., Ortiz, F., Urrutia, C. P., Young, R., D'Elia, L. F., Furst, C. J., & Namerow, N. (1996). Normative data stratified by age and education for the Neuropsychological Screening Battery for Hispanics (NeSBHIS): Initial report. *Journal of the International Neuropsychological Society, 2,* 96–104.

Potter, D. D., Jory, S. H., Bassett, M. R. A., Barrett, K., & Mychalkiw, W. (2002). Effect of mild head injury on event-related potential correlates of Stroop task performance. *Journal of the International Neuropsychological Society, 8,* 828–837.

Powell, J. B., Cripe, L. I., & Dodrill, C. B. (1991). Assessment of brain impairment with the Rey Auditory-Verbal Learning Test: A comparison with other neuropsychological measures. *Archives of Clinical Neuropsychology, 6,* 241–249.

Powell, M. R., Gfeller, J. D., Oliveri, M. V., Stanton, S., & Hendricks, B. (2004). The Rey AVLT serial position effect: A useful indicator of symptom exaggeration? *The Clinical Neuropsychologist, 18,* 465–476.

Query, W. T., & Berger, R. A. (1980). AVLT memory scores as a function of age among general medical, neurological, and alcoholic patients. *Journal of Clinical Psychology, 36,* 1009–1012.

Query, W. T., & Megran, J. (1983). Age-related norms for the AVLT in a male patient population. *Journal of Clinical Psychology, 39,* 136–138.

Read, D. E. (1986). Unpublished data, University of Victoria.

Records, N. L., Tomblin, J. B., & Buckwalter, P. R. (1995). Auditory verbal learning and memory in young adults with specific language impairment. *The Clinical Neuropsychologist, 9,* 187–193.

Remfer, M. V., Hamera, E. K., Brown, C. E., Cromwell, R. L. (2003). The relations between cognition and the independent living skill of shopping in people with schizophrenia. *Psychiatry Research, 117,* 103–112.

Rey, A. (1958). *L'examen clinique en psychologie.* Paris: Presse Universitaire de France.

Rouleau, I., Imbault, H., Laframboise, M., & Bedard, M. A. (2001). Patterns of intrusions in verbal recall: Comparison of Alzheimer's disease, Parkinson's disease, and frontal lobe dementia. *Brain and Cognition, 46,* 244–249.

Rosenberg, S. J., Ryan, J. J., & Prifiteria, A. (1984). Rey Auditory-Verbal Learning Test performance of patients with and without memory impairment. *Journal of Clinical Psychology, 40,* 785–787.

Ryan, J. J., Geisser, M. E., Randall, D. M., & Georgemiller, R. J. (1986). Alternate form reliability and equivancy of the Rey Auditory Verbal Learning Test. *Journal of Clinical and Experimental Neuropsychology, 8,* 611–616.

Ryan, J. J., Paolo, A. M., & Skrade, M. (1992). Rey Auditory Verbal Learning Test performance of a federal corrections sample with acquired immunodeficiency syndrome. *International Journal of Neuroscience, 64,* 177–181.

Ryan, J. J., Rosenberg, S. J., & Mittenberg, W. (1984). Factor analysis of the Rey Auditory-Verbal Learning Test. *International Journal of Clinical Neuropsychology, 6,* 239–241.

Salthouse, T. A., Fristoe, N., & Rhee, S. H. (1996). How localized are age-related effects on neuropsychological measures? *Neuropsychology, 10,* 272–285.

Savage, R. M., & Gouvier, W. D. (1992). Rey Auditory-Verbal Learning Test: The effects of age and gender, and norms for delayed recall and story recognition trials. *Archives of Clinical Neuropsychology, 7,* 407–414.

Schmidt, M. (1996). *Rey Auditory-Verbal Learning Test.* Los Angeles: Western Psychological Services.

Schmidt, M. (1997). Some cautions on interpreting qualitative indices for word-list learning tests. *The Clinical Neuropsychologist, 11,* 81–86.

Selnes, O. A., Jacobson, I., Machado, A. M., Becker, J. T., Wesch, J., Miller, E. N., Visscher, B., & McArthur, B. (1991). Normative data for a brief neuropsychological screening battery. *Perceptual and Motor Skills, 73,* 539–550.

Seltzer, J., Conrad, C., & Cassens, G. (1997). Neuropsychological profiles in schizophrenia: Paranoid versus undifferentiated distinctions. *Schizophrenia Research, 23,* 131–138.

Shapiro, D. M., and Harrison, D. (1990). Alternate forms of the AVLT: A procedure and test of form equivalency. *Archives of Clinical Neuropsychology, 5,* 405–410.

Sherman, D. S., Boone, K. B., Lu, P., & Razani, J. (2002). Reexamination of a Rey Auditory Verbal Learning Test/Rey Complex Figure discriminant function to detect suspect effort. *The Clinical Neuropsychologist, 16,* 242–250.

Shimamura, A. P., Salmon, D. P., Squire, L. R., & Butters, N. (1987). Memory dysfunction and word priming in dementia and amnesia. *Behavioral Neuroscience, 101,* 347–351.

Shum, D. H. K., Harris, D., & O'Gorman, J. G. (2000). Effects of severe traumatic brain injury on visual memory. *Journal of Clinical and Experimental Neuropsychology, 22,* 25–39.

Simard, S., Rouleauu, I., Brosseau, J., Laframboise, M., & Bojanowsky, M. (2003). Impact of executive dysfunctions on episodic memory abilities in patients with ruptured aneurysm of the anterior communicating artery. *Brain and Cognition, 53*, 354–358.

Smith, G. E., Malec, J. F., & Ivnik, R. J. (1992). Validity of the construct of nonverbal memory: A factor-analytic study in a normal elderly sample. *Journal of Clinical and Experimental Neuropsychology, 14*, 211–221.

Snow, W. G., Tierney, M. C., Zorzitto, M. L., Fisher, R. H., & Reid, D. W. (1988). One-year test-retest reliability of selected neuropsychological tests in older adults. Paper presented to the International Neuropsychological Society, New Orleans.

Stallings, G., Boake, C., & Sherer, M. (1995). Comparison of the California Verbal Learning Test and the Rey Auditory-Verbal Learning Test in head-injured patients. *Journal of Clinical and Experimental Neuropsychology, 17*, 706–712.

Stefanova, E. D., Kostic, V. S., Ziropadja, L., Markovic, M., & Ocic, G. (2002). Serial position learning effects in patients with aneurysms of the anterior communicating artery. *Journal of Clinical and Experimental Neuropsychology, 24*, 687–694.

Steinberg, B. A., Bieliauskas, L. A., Smith, G. E., Ivnik, R. J., & Malec, J. F. (2005). MAYO's Older Americans Normative Studies: Age- and IQ-adjusted norms for the Auditory Verbal Learning Test and Visual Spatial Learning Test. *The Clinical Neuropsychologist, 19*, 464–523.

Stewart, W. F., Schwartz, B. S., Simon, D., Bola, K. I., Todd, A. C., & Links, J. (1999). Neurobehavioral function and tibial and chelatable lead levels in 543 former organolead workers. *Neurology, 52*, 1610–1617.

Strauss, E., Hunter, M., & Wada, J. (1995). Risk factors for cognitive impairment in epilepsy. *Neuropsychology, 9*, 457–464.

Suhr, J. A. (2002). Malingering, coaching, and the serial position effect. *Archives of Clinical Neuropsychology, 17*, 69–78.

Suhr, J. A., & Gunstad, J. (2000). The effects of coaching on the sensitivity and specificity of malingering measures. *Archives of Clinical Neuropsychology, 15*, 415–424.

Suhr, J., Gunstad, J., Greub, B., & Barrash, J. (2004). Exaggeration Index for an expanded version of the Auditory Verbal Learning Test: Robustness to coaching. *Journal of Clinical and Experimental Neuropsychology, 26*, 416–427.

Sullivan, K., Deffenti, C., & Keane, B. (2002). Malingering on the RAVLT Part II: Detection strategies. *Archives of Clinical Neuropsychology, 17*, 223–233.

Talley, J. L. (1986). Memory in learning disabled children: Digit span and the Rey Auditory Verbal Learning Test. *Archives of Clinical Neuropsychology, 1*, 315–322.

Taylor, E. M. (1959). *The appraisal of children with cerebral deficits.* Cambridge, Mass.: Harvard University Press.

Tierney, M. C., Nores, A., Snow, W. G., et al. (1994). Use of the Rey Auditory Verbal Learning Test in differentiating normal aging from Alzheimer's and Parkinson's dementia. *Psychological Assessment, 6*, 129–134.

Tierney, M. C., Snow, W. G., Szalai, J. P., Fisher, R. H., & Zorzitto, M. L. (1996). A brief neuropsychological battery for the differential diagnosis of probable Alzheimer's disease. *The Clinical Neuropsychologist, 10*, 96–103.

Torres, I. J., Flashman, L. A., O'Leary, D. S., & Andreasen, N. C. (2001). Effects of retroactive and proactive interference on word list recall in schizophrenia. *Journal of the International Neuropsychological Society, 7*, 481–490.

Tuokko, H., & Woodward, T. S. (1996). Development and validation of a demographic correction system for neuropsychological measures used in the Canadian Study of Health and Aging. *Journal of Clinical and Experimental Neuropsychology, 18*, 479–616.

Uchiyama, C. L., D'Elia, L. F., Dellinger, A. M., Becker, J. T., Selnes, O. A., Wesch, J. E., Chen, B. B., Satz, P., van Gorp, W., & Miller, E. N. (1995). Alternate forms of the Auditory-Verbal Learning Test: Issues of test comparability, longitudinal reliability, and moderating demographic variables. *Archives of Clinical Neuropsychology, 10*, 133–146.

Uddo, M., Vasterling, J. J., Brailey, K., & Sutker, P. (1993). Memory and attention in combat-related post-traumatic stress disorder. *Journal of Psychopathology and Behavioral Assessment, 15*, 43–51.

Uttl, B. (2005). Measurement of individual differences. *Psychological Science, 16*, 460–467.

Vakil, E., & Blachstein, H. (1993). Rey Auditory Verbal Learning Test: Structure analysis. *Journal of Clinical Psychology, 49*, 883–890.

Vakil, E., & Blachstein, H. (1994). A supplementary measure in the Rey AVLT for assessing incidental learning of temporal order. *Journal of Clinical Psychology, 50*, 241–245.

Vakil, E., & Blachstein, H. (1997). Rey AVLT: Developmental norms for adults and the sensitivity of different memory measures to age. *The Clinical Neuropsychologist, 11*, 356–369.

Vakil, E., Blachstein, H., & Hoofien, D. (1991). Automatic temporal order judgement: The effect of intentionality of retrieval on closed-head injured patients. *Journal of Clinical and Experimental Neuropsychology, 13*, 291–298.

Vakil, E., Blachstein, H., Rochberg, J., & Vardi, M. (2004). Characterization of memory impairment following closed-head injury in children using the Rey Auditory Verbal Learning Test. *Child Neuropsychology, 10*, 57–66.

Vakil, E., Blachstein, H., & Sheinman, M. (1998). Rey AVLT: Developmental norms for children and the sensitivity of different memory measures to age. *Child Neuropsychology, 4*, 161–177.

Vakil, E., Shelef-Reshef, E., & Levy-Shiff, R. (1997). Procedural and declarative memory processes: Individuals with and without mental retardation. *American Journal on Mental Retardation, 102*, 147–160.

Van den Burg, W., & Kingma, A. (1999). Performance of 225 Dutch school children on Rey's Auditory Verbal Learning Test: Parallel test-retest reliabilities with an interval of 3 months and normative data. *Archives of Clinical Neuropsychology, 14*, 545–559.

Van der Elst, W., van Boxtel, P. J., van Breukelen, J. P., & Jolles, J. (2005). Rey's Verbal Learning Test: Normative data for 1855 healthy participants aged 24–81 years and the influence of age, sex, education, and mode of presentation. *Journal of the International Neuropsychological Society, 11*, 290–302.

Van Strien, J. W. (1999). Verbal learning in boys with P-type dyslexia, L-type dyslexia, and boys without learning disabilities: Differences in learning curves and in serial position curves. *Child Neuropsychology, 5*, 145–153.

Vingerhoets, G., De Soete, G., & Jannes, C. (1995). Relationship between emotional variables and cognitive test performance before and after open-heart surgery. *The Clinical Neuropsychologist, 9*, 198–202.

Wiens, A. N., McMinn, M. R., & Crossen, J. R. (1988). Rey Auditory-Verbal Learning Test: Development of norms for healthy young adults. *The Clinical Neuropsychologist, 2*, 67–87.

Woodard, J. L., Dunlosky, J., & Salthouse, T. A. (1999). Task decomposition analysis of intertrial free recall performance on the Rey Auditory Verbal Learning Test in normal aging and Alzheimer's disease. *Journal of Clinical and Experimental Neuropsychology, 21*, 666–676.

Rey-Osterrieth Complex Figure Test (ROCF)

OTHER TEST NAMES

Other names for the Rey-Osterrieth Complex Figure Test (ROCF) are the Rey Complex Figure Test (RCTF), the Complex Figure Test (CFT), and Rey Figure (RF).

PURPOSE

The purpose of this test is to assess visual-spatial constructional ability and visual memory.

SOURCE

The test (stimuli for the copy, recall, and recognition subtests; manual; manual supplement; and 50 test booklets; Meyers & Meyers, 1995b, 1996) can be ordered from Psychological Assessment Resources (http://www.parinc.com), at a cost of $244 US. Alternatively, the reader can refer to information provided here to design materials.

PAR also offers two qualitative scoring systems: the Boston Qualitative Scoring System (BQSS) for the Rey-Osterrieth Complex Figure, by Stern et al. (1999), at a cost of $196 US, and the Developmental Scoring System for the Rey-Osterrieth Complex Figure (DSS-ROCF), by Bernstein and Waber (1996), at a cost of $155 US.

The Extended Complex Figure Test (ECTF) by Fastenau (2002) is available through Western Psychological Services, (http://www.wpspublish.com) at a cost of $145 US.

AGE RANGE

The test can be given to individuals aged 6 to 93 years.

DESCRIPTION

The ROCF has a long history in the field of neuropsychology. It was developed by Rey (1941) and elaborated by Osterrieth (1944). These two key French papers have been translated into English by Corwin and Bylsma (1993). The ROCF is one of the most commonly used tests in the field (Camara et al., 2000), ranking among the top 10 tests used by neuropsychologists (Rabin et al., 2005). Its popularity derives from the fact that it permits assessment of a variety of cognitive processes, including planning, organizational skills, and problem-solving strategies, as well as perceptual, motor, and episodic memory functions (Meyers & Meyers, 1995a, Waber & Holmes, 1986). The materials consist of blank pieces of paper and the Rey-Osterrieth figure (Figure 10–31).

The test developed by Rey (1941) consisted of a copy trial followed by a recall trial 3 min later. Current administration procedures vary considerably (see Table 10–93). Some investigators (Loring et al., 1988a; Chiulli et al., 1989; Meyers & Meyers, 1995b) give both immediate and delayed-recall trials of the CFT, whereas others (Bennett-Levy, 1984; Denman,

1987; King, 1981; Kolb & Whishaw, 1985; L. B. Taylor, 1969, 1979) measure only delayed recall. Further, the amount of delay varies from 3 min (Bigler et al., 1989; Boone et al., 1993; Rey, 1941) to 45 minutes (L. B. Taylor, 1969, 1979). There is little difference in performance between immediate and 3-min delayed recall scores (Meyers & Meyers, 1995a). The length of delay chosen (15, 30, 45, or 60 min) does not affect overall recall performance, provided the delay is no longer than 1 hour (Berry & Carpenter, 1992). Most forgetting tends to occur very quickly, within the first few minutes after copying (Berry & Carpenter, 1992; Chiulli et al., 1995; Delaney et al., 1992; Lezak et al., 2004). Because very little difference is observed in normal subjects between immediate and delayed-recall trials (e.g., Chiulli et al., 1989, 1995, Loring et al., 1990; Mitrushina et al., 2005), a decline between the immediate and delayed-recall trials is of clinical significance.

After the 30-min recall, a recognition subtest (Meyers & Lange, 1994; Meyers & Meyers, 1995a) can be given (see *Source*). The recognition subtest was developed from elements of the Rey and Taylor figures. Twenty-four figures are randomly placed on four pages in two columns per page. The subject is required to circle the 12 figures that were part of the original design drawn.

In a survey of members of the International Neuropsychology Society (INS) by Knight et al. (2003), the largest percentage of respondents (57%) reported typically administering a protocol that included a copy trial, an immediate recall trial, and a delayed recall trial. The most frequently endorsed interval between the copy and the immediate trial was 0 to 5 s. The average interval between the immediate and delayed recall trials was 27 min (SD = 14 min), with the 16- to 30-min range most frequently endorsed. The average interval between the copy trial and the delayed trials was also 27 min (SD = 14 min), and 30 min was the most frequently reported delay interval.

Scores

The measures of performance that are typically derived include a copy score (which reflects the accuracy of the original copy and is a measure of visual-constructional ability), the time required to copy the figure; immediate or 3-min and 30-min delayed-recall scores (which assess the amount of information retained over time); and the number of items correctly and incorrectly identified on the recognition task.

Other Versions and Variants

There are a number of alternate figures, such as the Taylor Figure (L. B. Taylor, 1969, 1979; Figure 10–32), the modified Taylor Figure (Hubley & Tremblay, 2002; Figure 10–33), and the four Medical College of Georgia (MCG) complex figures (Loring & Meador, 2003; Meador et al., 1991, 1993; Figures 10–34 through 10–37).

Figure 10–31 Rey-Osterrieth Complex Figure Test: Form A (Rey figure) and legend.
Source: Osterrieth (1944).

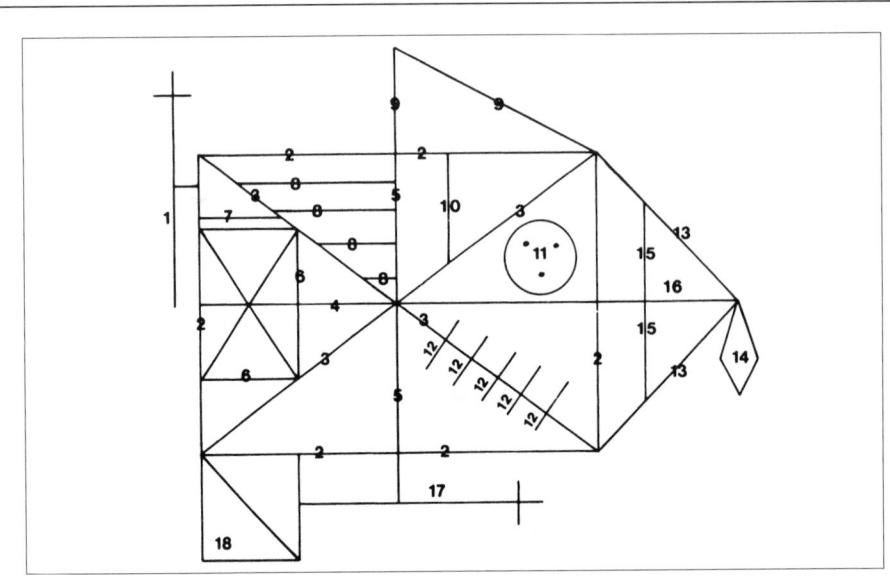

REY-OSTERRIETH COMPLEX FIGURE TEST
FORM A (Rey Figure)

Details: COPY   DELAY

1. Cross upper left corner, outside of rectangle   _____   _____
2. Large rectangle   _____   _____
3. Diagonal cross   _____   _____
4. Horizontal midline of 2   _____   _____
5. Vertical midline   _____   _____
6. Small rectangle, within 2 to the left   _____   _____
7. Small segment above 6   _____   _____
8. Four parallel lines within 2, upper left   _____   _____
9. Triangle above 2 upper right   _____   _____
10. Small vertical line within 2, below 9   _____   _____
11. Circle with three dots within 2   _____   _____
12. Five parallel lines with 2 crossing 3, lower right   _____   _____
13. Sides of triangle attached to 2 on right   _____   _____
14. Diamond attached to 13   _____   _____
15. Vertical line within triangle 13 parallel to right
    vertical of 2   _____   _____
16. Horizontal line within 13, continuing 4 to right   _____   _____
17. Cross attached to low center   _____   _____
18. Square attached to 2, lower left   _____   _____

                        TOTAL SCORE   _____   _____

Scoring:
Consider each of the eighteen units separately, and appraise accuracy of each unit and relative position within the whole of the design. For each unit count as follows:

Correct	{ placed properly	2 points
	{ placed poorly	1 point
Distorted or incomplete	{ placed properly	1 point
but recognizable	{ placed poorly	½ point
Absent or not recognizable		0 points
Maximum		36 points

812

Table 10–93 Selection of Norms Grouped by Copy-Recall Interval and Scoring Criteria

	Interval	Source	Scoring Criteria for Accuracy	Age Range (Years)	Qualitative Scoring Norms
Administration A	Copy and 30-min delayed recall	Kolb & Whishaw (1985); & Spreen & Strauss (1991)	L. B. Taylor	6–70+	
Administration B	Copy, immediate recall, & 30-min delayed recall	Chiulli et al. (1989) Chiulli et al. (1995)	E. M. Taylor L. B. Taylor	65–93 70–91	% adopting configurational approach
Administration C	Copy and 3-minute recall	Boone et al. 1993 Anderson et al., 2001	E. M. Taylor E. M. Taylor	45–83 7–13 years & months	1. Waber & Holmes Level of Organization 2. RCF-OSS
Administration D	Copy, 3-min recall, 30-min recall, and recognition	Meyers & Meyers (1995b)	Meyers & Meyers	6–89	

Fastenau (1996) developed recognition and matching trials (the Extended Complex Figure Test, ECFT) to clarify contributions of perception and memory retrieval to defective memory recall performance. He has also provided norms for this extended version (Fastenau, 2002; Fastenau et al., 1999).

In the standard procedure, the task is essentially an incidental learning test: There is no warning of the memory component until the patient is asked to recall the figure from memory. Tombaugh et al. (1992) used the Taylor Figure in an intentional learning paradigm. Individuals were told that they would be shown a design and then would have to draw it from memory, that they would be given four tries at this, and that they would be asked to recall the design later. On each of the four trials, individuals observed the Taylor Figure for 30 s. The figure was then removed, and the subject had a maximum of 2 min to reproduce the figure from memory. A retention trial was given about 15 min after the last acquisition trial. This was followed by a copy trial in which subjects were given 4 min to draw the figure with the model present. Tombaugh et al. (1992) provided specific scoring criteria (maximum score = 69 points) and normative data for people aged 20 to 79 years.

ADMINISTRATION

For instructions, see Meyers and Meyers (1995b). Alternatively, the examiner can use the instructions shown in Figure 10–38 or refer to Knight (2003) for a more extensive listing of administration procedures. Bush and Marthin (2004) found no significant differences between dominant and nondominant hand performance on the copy portion of the task in a sample of adults without neurological compromise. The implication is that use of the nondominant hand to complete the copy portion may be an acceptable alternative if the dominant hand is nonfunctional.

Copy

There are two methods for recording a patient's strategy: the colored pencil method and the flowchart method. One can use a system of colored pencils (pens) to record the patient's strategy while copying the figure. Each time the person completes a section of the drawing, the examiner hands the patient a different colored pencil and notes the order of the colors. The examiner uses three or four different colored pencils and switches pencils at approximately equal points in the construction of the figure. The examiner should not switch pencils while the patient is in the middle of drawing one of the standard 18 elements.

Alternatively, to use the flowchart method, the examiner can reproduce the patient's drawing on a separate sheet, noting the order (by numbering) and directionality (by an arrow) of each line as it is drawn. The latter system is preferred by some authors (Meyers & Meyers, 1995b). When figures are scored using the traditional 36-point scoring system, the amount and quality (i.e., accuracy, placement) of information copied and recalled is not affected by the administration procedure (pen-switching versus flowchart; Ruffolo et al., 2001). There is also no difference in administration time between the two procedures using the traditional 36-point system. However, when assessing *qualitative* aspects (see *Scoring*), there is evidence that pen-switching results in better performance on qualitative scores, and the productions drawn with pen switching are also significantly faster to score (Ruffolo et al., 2001). In short, when scoring qualitative aspects, the pen-switching method is preferred.

The card and the subject's copy are exposed for a maximum of 5 min and a minimum of 2½ min.

Three-Minute Recall

There is no time limit on the 3-min recall task. As in the copy trial, the order of approach may be recorded by using the sys-

Figure 10–32 Rey-Osterrieth Complex Figure Test: Form B (Taylor alternate version) and legend. *Source:* Courtesy of L. Taylor.

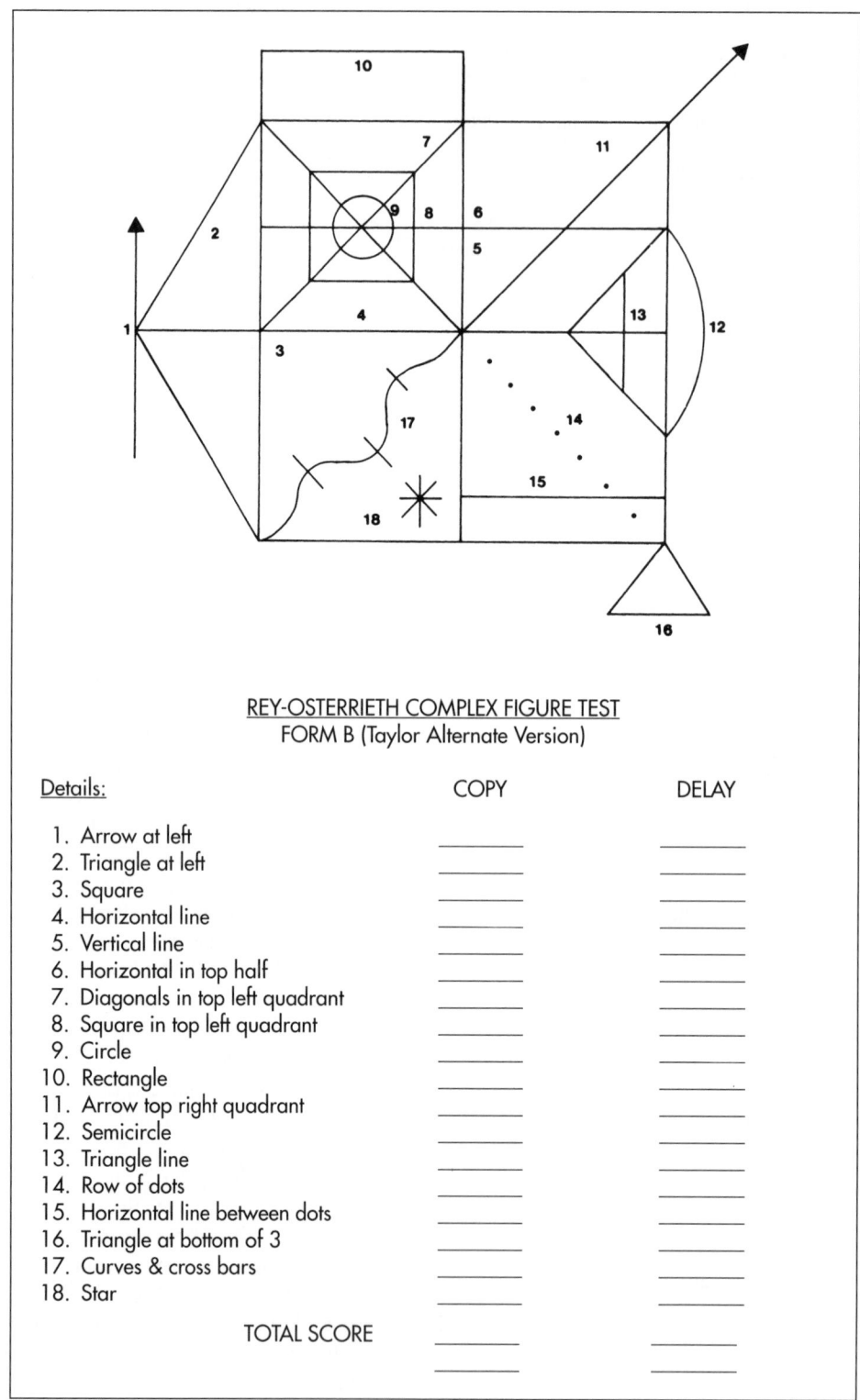

REY-OSTERRIETH COMPLEX FIGURE TEST
FORM B (Taylor Alternate Version)

Details:	COPY	DELAY
1. Arrow at left	_____	_____
2. Triangle at left	_____	_____
3. Square	_____	_____
4. Horizontal line	_____	_____
5. Vertical line	_____	_____
6. Horizontal in top half	_____	_____
7. Diagonals in top left quadrant	_____	_____
8. Square in top left quadrant	_____	_____
9. Circle	_____	_____
10. Rectangle	_____	_____
11. Arrow top right quadrant	_____	_____
12. Semicircle	_____	_____
13. Triangle line	_____	_____
14. Row of dots	_____	_____
15. Horizontal line between dots	_____	_____
16. Triangle at bottom of 3	_____	_____
17. Curves & cross bars	_____	_____
18. Star	_____	_____
TOTAL SCORE	_____	_____
	_____	_____

Figure 10–33 Modified Taylor Complex Figure (MTCF) showing scoring components. © 1996, 1998: A. M. Hubley. Reproduced by permission.

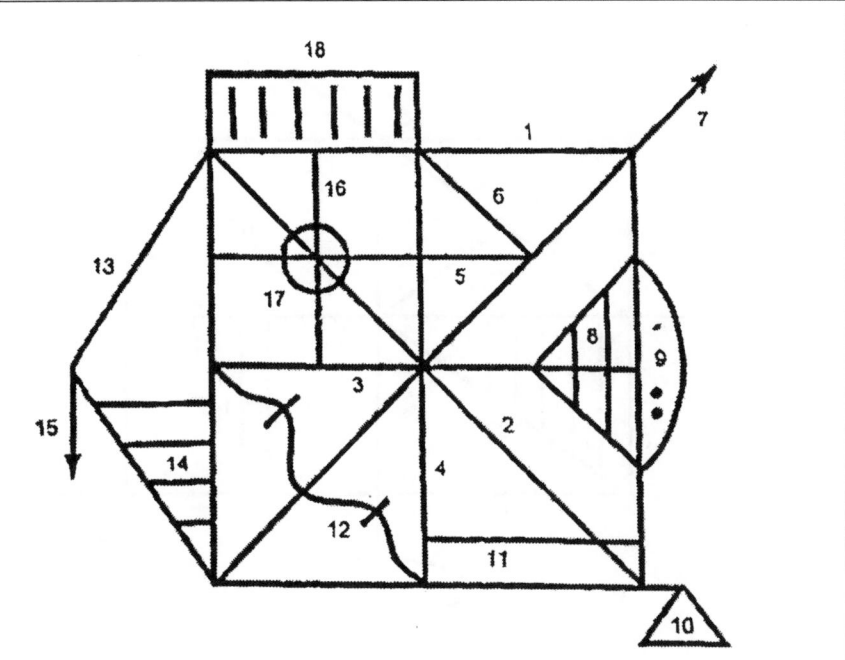

Component:
 1. Large square
 2. Crossed diagonal lines in 1
 3. Horizontal midline of 1
 4. Vertical midline of 1
 5. Short horizontal line in upper right quadrant
 6. Short diagonal line in upper right quadrant
 7. Diagonal arrow attached to corner of 1
 8. Triangle in 1 on right, two vertical lines included
 9. Semicircle attached to right side of 1, two dots included
10. Triangle attached to 1 by horizontal line
11. Horizontal line in lower right quadrant
12. Wavy line, includes two short lines
13. Large triangle attached to left of 1
14. Four horizontal lines within 13
15. Arrow attached to apex of 13
16. Horizontal and vertical lines in upper left quadrant
17. Circle in upper left quadrant
18. Small rectangle above 1 on left, six lines included

Scoring:
Consider each of the eighteen units separately. Appraise accuracy of each unit and relative position within the whole of the design. For each unit count as follows:

Correct, placed properly	2 points
Correct, placed poorly	1 point
Distorted or incomplete but recognizable, placed properly	1 point
Distorted or incomplete but recognizable, placed poorly	½ point
Absent or not recognizable	0 points
Maximum	36 points

Figure 10–34 Medical College of Georgia Complex Figure 1 and legend. *Source:* Courtesy of D. W. Loring. Reproduced with permission.

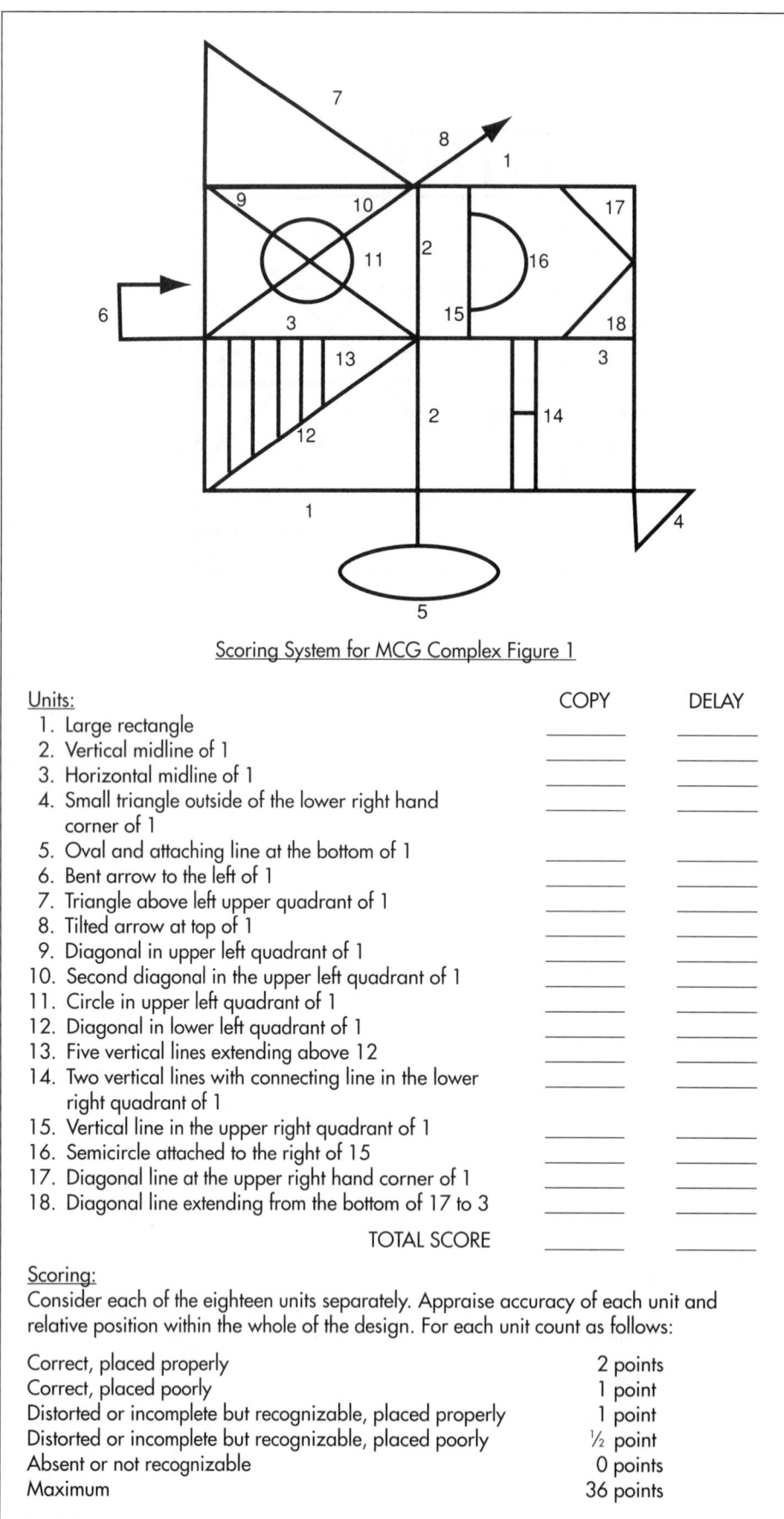

Scoring System for MCG Complex Figure 1

Units:	COPY	DELAY
1. Large rectangle	_____	_____
2. Vertical midline of 1	_____	_____
3. Horizontal midline of 1	_____	_____
4. Small triangle outside of the lower right hand corner of 1	_____	_____
5. Oval and attaching line at the bottom of 1	_____	_____
6. Bent arrow to the left of 1	_____	_____
7. Triangle above left upper quadrant of 1	_____	_____
8. Tilted arrow at top of 1	_____	_____
9. Diagonal in upper left quadrant of 1	_____	_____
10. Second diagonal in the upper left quadrant of 1	_____	_____
11. Circle in upper left quadrant of 1	_____	_____
12. Diagonal in lower left quadrant of 1	_____	_____
13. Five vertical lines extending above 12	_____	_____
14. Two vertical lines with connecting line in the lower right quadrant of 1	_____	_____
15. Vertical line in the upper right quadrant of 1	_____	_____
16. Semicircle attached to the right of 15	_____	_____
17. Diagonal line at the upper right hand corner of 1	_____	_____
18. Diagonal line extending from the bottom of 17 to 3	_____	_____
TOTAL SCORE	_____	_____

Scoring:
Consider each of the eighteen units separately. Appraise accuracy of each unit and relative position within the whole of the design. For each unit count as follows:

Correct, placed properly	2 points
Correct, placed poorly	1 point
Distorted or incomplete but recognizable, placed properly	1 point
Distorted or incomplete but recognizable, placed poorly	½ point
Absent or not recognizable	0 points
Maximum	36 points

Figure 10–35 Medical College of Georgia Complex Figure 2 and legend. *Source:* Courtesy of D. W. Loring. Reproduced with permission.

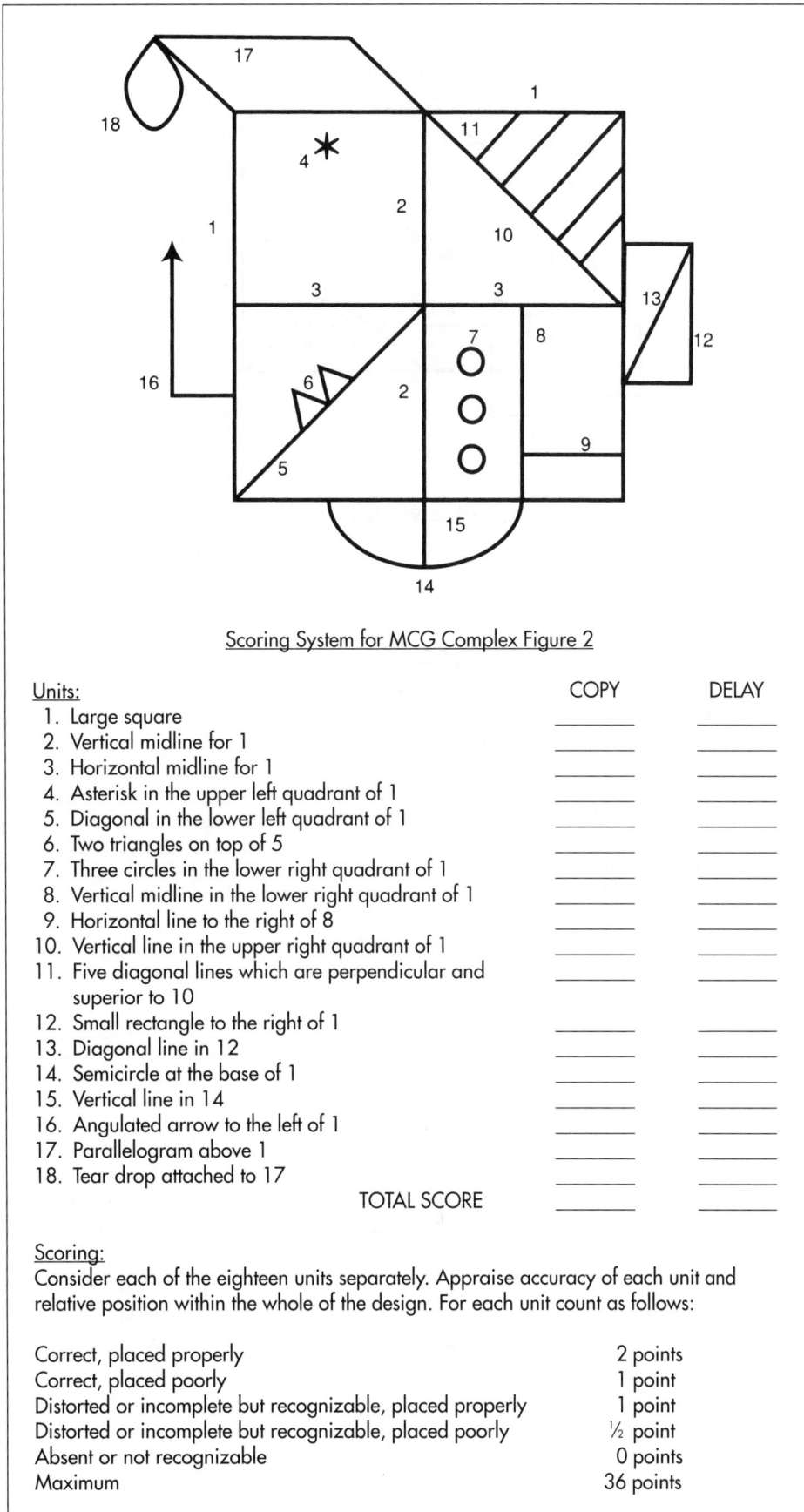

Scoring System for MCG Complex Figure 2

Units:	COPY	DELAY
1. Large square	_____	_____
2. Vertical midline for 1	_____	_____
3. Horizontal midline for 1	_____	_____
4. Asterisk in the upper left quadrant of 1	_____	_____
5. Diagonal in the lower left quadrant of 1	_____	_____
6. Two triangles on top of 5	_____	_____
7. Three circles in the lower right quadrant of 1	_____	_____
8. Vertical midline in the lower right quadrant of 1	_____	_____
9. Horizontal line to the right of 8	_____	_____
10. Vertical line in the upper right quadrant of 1	_____	_____
11. Five diagonal lines which are perpendicular and superior to 10	_____	_____
12. Small rectangle to the right of 1	_____	_____
13. Diagonal line in 12	_____	_____
14. Semicircle at the base of 1	_____	_____
15. Vertical line in 14	_____	_____
16. Angulated arrow to the left of 1	_____	_____
17. Parallelogram above 1	_____	_____
18. Tear drop attached to 17	_____	_____
TOTAL SCORE	_____	_____

Scoring:
Consider each of the eighteen units separately. Appraise accuracy of each unit and relative position within the whole of the design. For each unit count as follows:

Correct, placed properly	2 points
Correct, placed poorly	1 point
Distorted or incomplete but recognizable, placed properly	1 point
Distorted or incomplete but recognizable, placed poorly	½ point
Absent or not recognizable	0 points
Maximum	36 points

Figure 10–36 Medical College of Georgia Complex Figure 3 and legend. *Source:* Courtesy of D. W. Loring. Reproduced with permission.

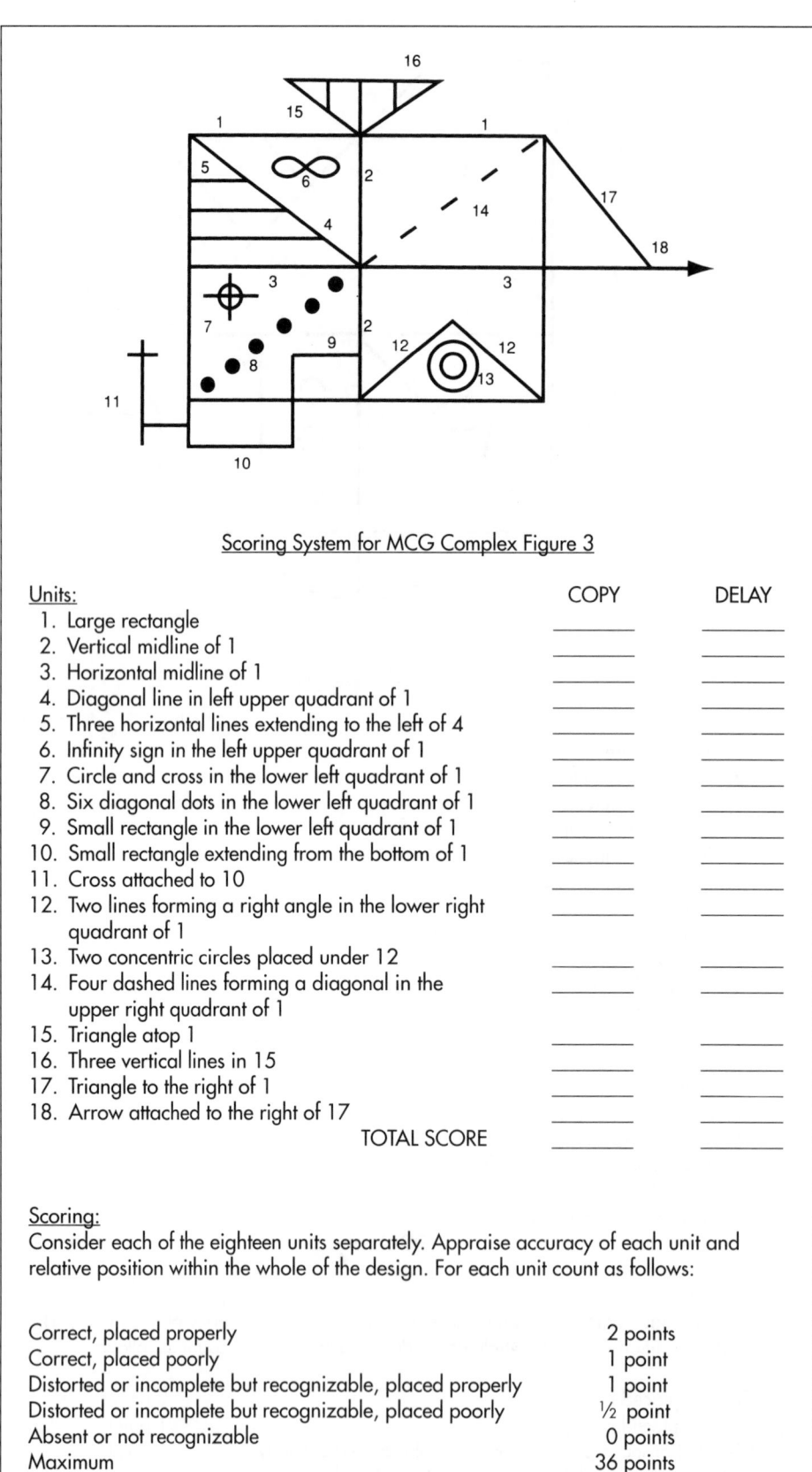

Scoring System for MCG Complex Figure 3

Units:	COPY	DELAY
1. Large rectangle	_____	_____
2. Vertical midline of 1	_____	_____
3. Horizontal midline of 1	_____	_____
4. Diagonal line in left upper quadrant of 1	_____	_____
5. Three horizontal lines extending to the left of 4	_____	_____
6. Infinity sign in the left upper quadrant of 1	_____	_____
7. Circle and cross in the lower left quadrant of 1	_____	_____
8. Six diagonal dots in the lower left quadrant of 1	_____	_____
9. Small rectangle in the lower left quadrant of 1	_____	_____
10. Small rectangle extending from the bottom of 1	_____	_____
11. Cross attached to 10	_____	_____
12. Two lines forming a right angle in the lower right quadrant of 1	_____	_____
13. Two concentric circles placed under 12	_____	_____
14. Four dashed lines forming a diagonal in the upper right quadrant of 1	_____	_____
15. Triangle atop 1	_____	_____
16. Three vertical lines in 15	_____	_____
17. Triangle to the right of 1	_____	_____
18. Arrow attached to the right of 17	_____	_____
TOTAL SCORE	_____	_____

Scoring:
Consider each of the eighteen units separately. Appraise accuracy of each unit and relative position within the whole of the design. For each unit count as follows:

Correct, placed properly	2 points
Correct, placed poorly	1 point
Distorted or incomplete but recognizable, placed properly	1 point
Distorted or incomplete but recognizable, placed poorly	½ point
Absent or not recognizable	0 points
Maximum	36 points

Figure 10–37 Medical College of Georgia Complex Figure 4 and legend. *Source:* Courtesy of D. W. Loring. Reproduced with permission.

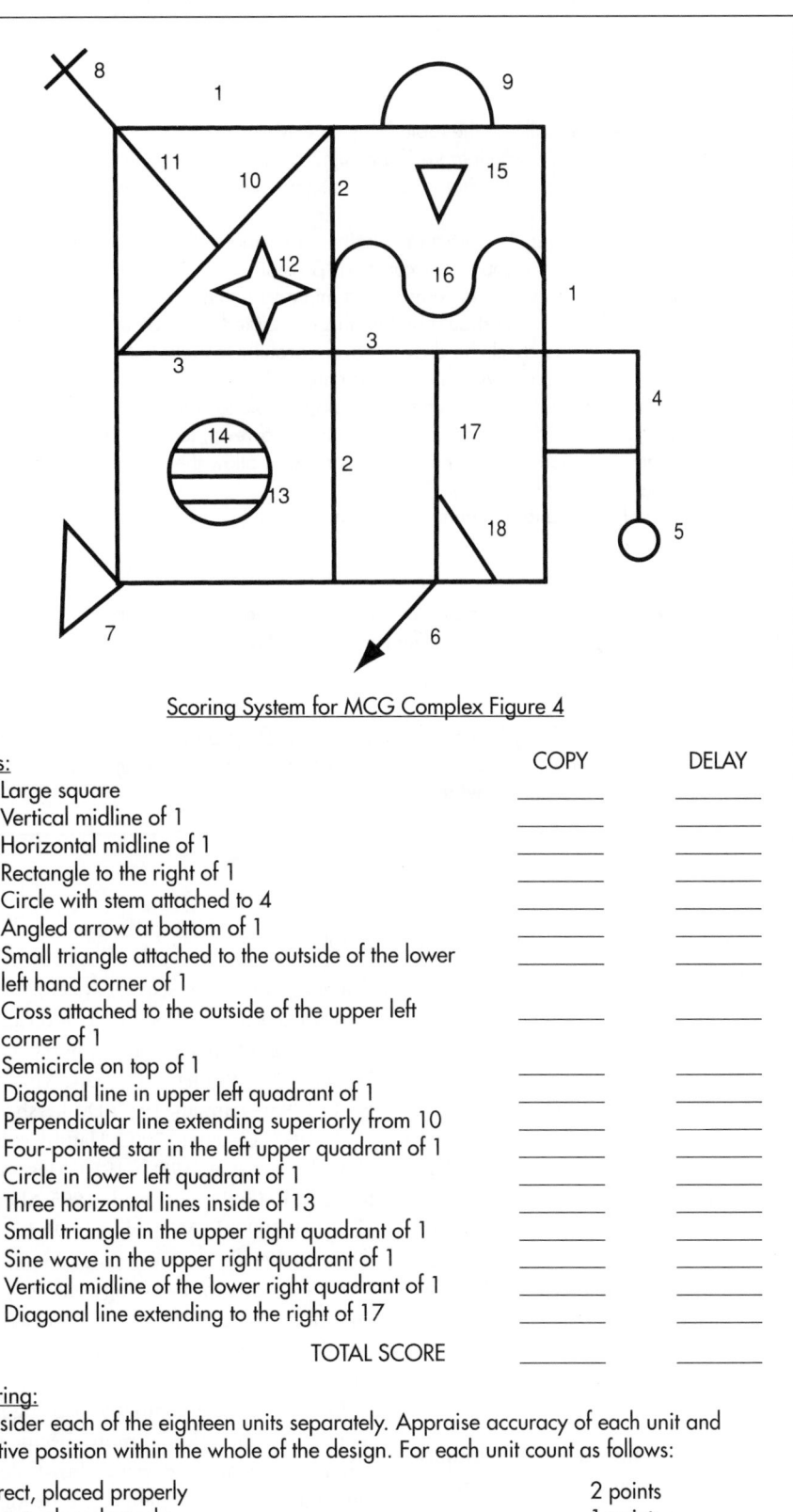

Scoring System for MCG Complex Figure 4

Units:	COPY	DELAY
1. Large square	_____	_____
2. Vertical midline of 1	_____	_____
3. Horizontal midline of 1	_____	_____
4. Rectangle to the right of 1	_____	_____
5. Circle with stem attached to 4	_____	_____
6. Angled arrow at bottom of 1	_____	_____
7. Small triangle attached to the outside of the lower left hand corner of 1	_____	_____
8. Cross attached to the outside of the upper left corner of 1	_____	_____
9. Semicircle on top of 1	_____	_____
10. Diagonal line in upper left quadrant of 1	_____	_____
11. Perpendicular line extending superiorly from 10	_____	_____
12. Four-pointed star in the left upper quadrant of 1	_____	_____
13. Circle in lower left quadrant of 1	_____	_____
14. Three horizontal lines inside of 13	_____	_____
15. Small triangle in the upper right quadrant of 1	_____	_____
16. Sine wave in the upper right quadrant of 1	_____	_____
17. Vertical midline of the lower right quadrant of 1	_____	_____
18. Diagonal line extending to the right of 17	_____	_____
TOTAL SCORE	_____	_____

Scoring:
Consider each of the eighteen units separately. Appraise accuracy of each unit and relative position within the whole of the design. For each unit count as follows:

Correct, placed properly	2 points
Correct, placed poorly	1 point
Distorted or incomplete but recognizable, placed properly	1 point
Distorted or incomplete but recognizable, placed poorly	½ point
Absent or not recognizable	0 points
Maximum	36 points

Figure 10–38 Instructions for Administration of the ROCF.

Copy:

Put a plain sheet of 8½ × 11-inch paper vertically on the table (Meyers & Meyers, 1995b).

Then say: *I am going to show you a card on which there is a design that I would like you to copy on this sheet of paper. Please copy the figure as carefully as you can.* Begin timing as soon as you expose the drawing. Note that Meyers and Meyers (1995b) allow erasing.

It is important to supervise the drawing carefully, particularly in the early stages. If the drawing is careless, the patient should be reminded that he or she is to make the copy as accurate as possible.

The card and the subject's copy are exposed for a maximum of 5 min and a minimum of 2½ min. If by 2½ min it is obvious that the patient is drawing too slowly, he or she should be told this and asked to speed up. If the patient is finished drawing before 2½ min, he or she should be told to check the drawing over carefully to make sure it is complete. After the drawing is finished, it is removed from sight along with the stimulus card.

Record the *total* time taken to complete the drawing. Subjects should be able to complete the drawing in no more than 5 min, unless they have considerable motor difficulty. It is more important, however, for a subject to complete the drawing as well as he or she can than it is to get it finished within 5 min. For this reason, allow the subject as much time as needed to make the best copy that he or she is capable of drawing.

Expose the card for a maximum of 5 min and a minimum of 2½ min.

3-Minute Recall

After a 3-min delay filled with talking or some other verbal task, provide a clean sheet of paper and say to the patient: *Remember a short time ago I had you copy a figure. I would like you to draw that figure again.* There is no time limit.

Delayed Recall

After a 30-min delay filled with interfering activity (not constructional), say: *Do you remember the design I had you copy a while ago? Now I would like you to draw the figure from memory as carefully and completely as you can on this sheet of paper. If you make a mistake, do not erase; just correct whatever you think is wrong.*

---

tem of colored pencils or by drawing along with the patient on a separate sheet, noting the sequence and organization of the reproduction.

Delayed Recall

The examiner waits about 30 min after the first administration of the ROCF and then requests recall of the figure. The interposed tests should be quite different from the ROCF, to avoid interference. One should especially not give any tests of drawing. There is no time limit, and the order of approach may be recorded by using the system of colored pencils or by drawing along on a separate sheet.

Recognition

After the 30-min recall, the patient is provided with stimulus sheets and is instructed to circle the figures that were part of the design that was copied and drawn.

ADMINISTRATION TIME

The time required is about 10-15 min (excluding delays).

SCORING

There are numerous scoring systems that provide various criteria for scoring the Rey-Osterrieth Complex Figure (Awad et al., 2004; Bennett-Levy, 1984; Berry et al., 1991; Bernstein & Waber, 1996; Binder, 1982; Chervinsky et al., 1992; Chiulli et al., 1995; Denman, 1987; Deckersbach et al., 2000a; Duley et al., 1993; Fastenau, 2002; Hamby et al., 1993; Kirk & Kelly, 1986; Loring et al., 1988b, 1990; Meyers & Meyers, 1995a; Osterrieth, 1944; Rapport et al., 1995; Shorr et al., 1992; Stern et al., 1994, 1999; E. M. Taylor, 1959; L. B. Taylor, 1991; Visser, 1973; Waber & Holmes, 1985, 1986). Most of the systems provide criteria for assessing accuracy of copy and recall (i.e., quantity). Some of the systems also assess quality (e.g., organization, fragmentation, symmetry, inattention) of the construction.

Over time, the quantitative scoring systems have changed, mainly by elaboration of more specific scoring criteria for the original 18 elements developed by Osterrieth (Knight, 2003). Qualitative scoring systems have steadily evolved from single measures with a limited focus (e.g., segmentation/fragmentation, discontinuity/disjunction) to more comprehensive, multivariate measures of strategy and organization with established psychometric properties (Knight, 2003). The most extensive quantitative scoring systems are the RCFT (Meyers

& Meyers, 1995b), the Denman (1987) system, and the ECTF (Fasteneau, 2000). Each scoring system is available with a manual covering administration, scoring, and age-stratified norms for children and adults. The BQSS (Stern et al., 1999) and DSS-ROCF (Bernstein & Waber, 1996) are the most comprehensive qualitative scoring systems. The DSS-ROCF norms focus more on children, whereas the BQSS is normed for adults.

Accuracy

Copy and Memory Trials. These are generally scored in the same manner in terms of accuracy. According to the survey of INS members (Knight et al., 2003), the majority (76%) reported using the Rey-Osterrieth 36-point system described by Lezak (1976, 1983, 1995; Lezak et al., 2004), proposed by Osterrieth (1944), and adapted by E. M. Taylor (1959). The figure is broken down into 18 scorable elements: between 0.5 and 2.0 points are awarded for each element, depending on the accuracy, distortion, and location of its reproduction. Two points are awarded if the unit is correct and is placed properly, 1 point if the unit is correct but placed poorly, 1 point if the unit is distorted but placed correctly, 0.5 points if the unit is distorted and placed poorly, and no points if the unit is absent or not recognizable. The highest possible score on each figure is 36.

These criteria are clear as to the specific elements that are to be scored; they leave considerable latitude, however, in deciding what constitutes a scorable distortion or misplacement (Duley et al., 1993). More explicit criteria have been proposed by others (e.g., Denman, 1987; Duley et al., 1993; Meyers & Meyers, 1995a; L. B. Taylor, 1991). In order to use the normative data appropriately, it is important to be attentive to both the method of administration (e.g., whether an immediate-recall trial is interposed between the copy and 30-min delayed-recall trials) and the particular scoring criteria used to generate the norms. We generally use the normative data (ages 6–89 years) provided by Meyers and Meyers (1995b) for copy, 3-min recall, 30-min recall, and recognition trials of the Rey Figure, and their explicit scoring guidelines are used for protocols within this age range. The scoring criteria developed by L. B. Taylor (1991) are stricter than those of E. M. Taylor and are provided in Figures 10–39 and 10–40.

One can also calculate a percent recall score, (CFT recall/CFT copy) × 100), to remove the effects of level of performance on copy administration from the memory performance (Snow, 1979). Brooks (1972) developed a percent forgetting score, (CFT immediate recall − CFT delayed recall) ÷ (CF immediate recall) × 100. Lezak (1995) noted, however, that these scores should be interpreted cautiously, because very defective copy and recall scores (immediate or delayed) can look good if copy (or immediate recall) is so low that recall (or delayed recall) cannot go much lower.

Recognition. A correct response on the recognition subtest (Meyers & Meyers, 1995b) is credited if the patient correctly circles a figure as having been part of the ROCF; a correct response is also awarded if the figure was not part of the ROCF and was not circled. The maximum correct score is 24. False positives (if a figure that was not part of the ROCF was circled) and false negatives (if a figure that should have been circled was not) are also noted.

Quality

Interpretation of the ROCF should consider not only the actual score but also qualitative aspects of performance. For example, some patients have difficulty with the organizational processes that are crucial for efficient encoding and retrieval of information, whereas others have trouble with the consolidation and storage of new memories. The ROCF is suited to address such distinctions.

Osterrieth (1944) was the first to draw attention to the fact that both children and adults vary in their approach to construction of the figure. He delineated four qualitatively different strategies used by adults and six used by children. He also recognized that a relationship exists between strategy used at copy, strategy at recall, and quality of recall; however, he did not specify the nature of this relationship in any detail (Bennett-Levy, 1984). A number of subsequent investigators have devised quantitative scoring systems that assess item distortion and misplacement, approach, or style and level of organization (Anderson et al., 2001; Bennett-Levy, 1984; Bernstein & Waber, 1996; Binder, 1982; Chervinsky et al., 1992; Chiulli et al., 1995; Hamby et al., 1993; Kirk & Kelly, 1986; Loring et al., 1988b; Rapport et al., 1995, 1996; Savage et al., 1999; Shorr et al., 1992; Stern et al., 1994, 1999; Visser, 1973; Waber & Holmes, 1985, 1986) and have suggested ways in which a strategy used at copy may affect recall performance.

Developmental Scoring System for the Rey-Osterrieth Complex Figure (DSS-ROCF). Waber and Holmes (1985, 1986; see also Bernstein & Waber, 1996) devised the DSS-ROCF, a system that assesses organization and style in addition to accuracy. The organizational parameter, yielding an ordinal scale, was designed to capture the "goodness" of the overall structure and focuses on such features as the integrity of the base rectangle and the integration of other structures with the base rectangle. The style parameter, yielding a categorical scale, assesses the manner in which the design is executed, independent of its organizational quality; it ranges from part-oriented to configurational. The system shows a gradual increase in organizational scores and configural strategies between the ages of 5 and 14 years and has demonstrated utility with regard to developmental issues. The criteria for the organizational parameter are shown in Table 10–94.

Rey Complex Figure Organizational Strategy Score (RCF-OSS)

Another system developed for use with children is the RCF-OSS (Anderson et al., 2001). The system rates drawings on a seven-point scale by level of organizational strategy, from

Figure 10–39 Taylor Scoring Criteria for the Rey Complex Figure. *Source:* L. B. Taylor, personal communication, May 1989.

Detail 1: The cross at the upper left corner, outside of the rectangle. The cross must come down to the horizontal midline of the rectangle and must extend above the rectangle. The line that joins the cross to the rectangle must be approximately in the middle of the cross and must come between Detail 7 and the top of the rectangle.

Detail 2: The large rectangle. The horizontal dimensions of the rectangle must not be greater than twice the vertical dimensions of the rectangle, nor must the rectangle resemble a square. Because there are so many possibilities of distorting the rectangle and it is not possible to score for position, a score of ½ point is given if the rectangle is incomplete or distorted in any way.

Detail 3: The diagonal cross must touch each of the four corners of the rectangle and must intersect in the middle of the rectangle.

Detail 4: The horizontal midline of the rectangle must go clearly across from the midpoint of the left side of the rectangle to the midpoint of the right side of the rectangle in one unbroken line.

Detail 5: The vertical midline must start at the midpoint of the bottom of the rectangle and go through in one unbroken line to the midpoint at the top of the rectangle. In scoring for position of details 4, 5, and 6, they should intersect at the midpoint of the rectangle. Usually, if they do not, only one of them is scored as incorrect for position. Very seldom are all three scored as incorrect for not being in position.

Detail 6: The small rectangle within the large rectangle and to the left side of it. The boundaries of Detail 6 are defined by the top of the rectangle falling between lines 2 and 3 of the parallel lines that make up Detail 8, and the width of the small rectangle must be approximately one-quarter of the width of the large rectangle; that is, it should come to the midpoint between the left side of the large rectangle and the vertical midpoint of the rectangle. The cross within Detail 6 must come from the four corners of the rectangle and should intersect at the midpoint of the rectangle (i.e., words intersecting on Detail 4).

Detail 7: The straight line above Detail 6 must be shorter than the horizontal aspect of Detail 6 and must fall between the top of Detail 6 and the second line of Detail 8.

Detail 8: The four parallel lines within the rectangle in the upper left corner should be parallel, with the spaces between them approximately equal. If the lines are unduly slanted or, of course, if there are more or less than four of them, then the scoring is penalized.

Detail 9: The triangle above the rectangle on the upper right, with the height less than the base.

Detail 10: The small vertical line within the rectangle just below Detail 9. The line should be clearly shifted to the left within the upper right quadrangle in the rectangle.

Detail 11: The circle with three dots must be in the lower right half of the upper right quadrangle. It must not touch any of the three sides of the triangular area in which it is placed, and the positioning of the dots should be such that there are two above and one below, so that it resembles a face.

Detail 12: The five parallel lines that are crossing the lower right aspect of Detail 3 must all be within the lower right quadrangle. They must not touch any sides of the quadrangle, and they should be approximately equidistant from one another.

Detail 13: The triangle on the right end of the large rectangle. The height of the triangle must not be greater than half of the horizontal midline of the rectangle and, as already mentioned, the slope of the sides of the triangle must not be a continuation of the slope of Detail 9.

Detail 14: The diamond attached to the end of Detail 13 should be diamond-shaped and must be attached to the end of Detail 13; it must not extend down below the bottom of the large rectangle, Detail 2.

Detail 15: The vertical line within triangle 13 must be parallel to the right vertical of Detail 2, the large rectangle, and it must be shifted to the left within Detail 13.

Detail 16: The horizontal line within Detail 13, which is a continuation of Detail 4 to the right, must come from the midpoint of the right side of the large rectangle and extend to the top of triangle 13. If triangle 13 is slightly askew, or if Detail 4 does not meet the midpoint of the right side of the rectangle, Detail 16 should still be scored as a full 2 points if it went to the top of the triangle from the midpoint of the right side of the rectangle.

Detail 17: The cross attached to the lower center area of the rectangle. The right side of the cross must be clearly longer than the left side of the cross but must not extend beyond the right end of the large rectangle. It should also, at its left end, commence at the midpoint of the right side of the square, which is Detail 18.

Detail 18: The square on the lower left corner of Detail 2. It must clearly be a square, as opposed to the rectangular shape of Detail 6, and its sides should be the same size as the vertical aspect of Detail 6, extending halfway between the left side of the rectangle and the vertical midline of the rectangle.

Figure 10–40 Scoring Guidelines of the Taylor (Alternate) Form of Rey Complex Figure. *Source:* L. B. Taylor, personal communication, May, 1989.

Detail 1: Vertical arrow at the left of the figure, extending above and below the midpoints of the upper and lower quadrants of the large square, but not extending beyond the upper and lower limits of the square, and with its midpoint meeting Detail 4.

Detail 2: Triangle whose base is the left side of the large square, with the altitude of the triangle less than half of the width of the large square.

Detail 3: Large square, which is the basic element of the figure, and which must look like a square and not a rectangle.

Detail 4: Horizontal midline of the large square, which extends outside the large square to midpoint of Detail 1.

Detail 5: Vertical midline of the large square.

Detail 6: Horizontal line bisecting the top half of the large square.

Detail 7: Diagonal lines bisecting one another from the corners of the top left quadrant of the large square.

Detail 8: Small square, situated in the center of the top left quadrant, one-fourth the size of the quadrant, and with the corners of the square located on the diagonals (Detail 7).

Detail 9: Circle in the center of Detail 8, in the top left quadrant.

Detail 10: Rectangle above the top left quadrant, with its height less than one-fourth of the height of the large square.

Detail 11: Arrow extending from the center of the large square through the top right corner of the right upper quadrant, with not more than one-third of its length outside the large square.

Detail 12: Semicircle at the right of the figure, extending from the horizontal bisector of the top half of the base square (Detail 6) to the equivalent point in the lower half of the base square.

Detail 13: Triangle in the right half of the base square, with the same base as the semicircle (Detail 12), and with an altitude that is one-fourth the width of the large square.

Detail 14: Row of seven dots (not circles) in the lower right quadrant, evenly spaced in a straight line from the center of the large square to the lower right corner of the quadrant.

Detail 15: Horizontal line in the lower right quadrant, between the sixth and seventh dots of Detail 14.

Detail 16: Equilateral triangle whose apex is at the lower right corner of the large square and whose altitude is not more than one-fourth of the height of the large square.

Detail 17: Curved line with a cross-bar at the center of each of three sinusoids in the lower left quadrant, extending from the bottom left corner to the top right corner of the quadrant.

Detail 18: Star, composed of eight lines radiating from a center point, and situated in the lower left quadrant, near its lower right corner.

Level 1 (unrecognizable or substitution) to Level 7 (excellent organization). Like other qualitative scoring systems, it places importance on the base rectangle and the vertical and horizontal midlines (often referred to as the "configural components") and also assesses the sequence of elements drawn. Interrater reliability is high (>.80), as is temporal stability (.79 to .94). In terms of construct validity, the scores correlate modestly with traditional measures of executive function (.12 to .35) and memory (.16 to .26). In support of the diagnostic utility of the system, Mathews et al. (2001) report that children with focal frontal lesions show reduced organizational strategy scores, with productions being fragmented and poorly planned. By contrast, children with temporal lobe lesions use the same strategy as controls, although their recall is impaired.

Table 10–94 Criteria for Five Levels of Organization

Level I:	Any design that does not satisfy criteria for Level II
Level II:	(1) Upper and lower left corner of base rectangle;
	(2) Left side of base rectangle aligned;
	(3) Lower horizontal of base rectangle aligned at the middle;
	(4) Lower horizontal aligned at lower left box *or* middle horizontal aligned at left center box *or* upper horizontal aligned;
Level III:	(1) Upper and lower left corner of base rectangle;
	(2) Lower right corner of base rectangle;
	(3) Four sides of base rectangle-aligned;
	(4) Middle vertical aligned at center *or* middle horizontal aligned at left center box *or* main horizontal and vertical intersect *or* main diagonals intersect
Level IV:	(1) Upper and lower left corner of base rectangle;
	(2) Lower right corner of base rectangle;
	(3) Four sides of base rectangle aligned;
	(4) Diagonals of base rectangle intersect;
	(5) Main horizontal and vertical intersect *or* middle vertical aligned at center *or* middle horizontal aligned at left center box
Level V:	(1) Four corners of base rectangle aligned;
	(2) Four sides of base rectangle aligned;
	(3) Main horizontal and vertical aligned;
	(4) Diagonals aligned;
	(5) Horizantal, vertical, and diagonals intersect.

Source: From Waber & Holmes, 1985, 1986. Reprinted with the kind permission of Psychology Press.

Boston Qualitative Scoring System (BQSS)

The most comprehensive system, the BQSS, was developed by Stern et al. (1994, 1999). It was normed on 433 adults, ages 18 to 94 years, but has been used with children as well (e.g., Akshoomoff et al., 2002). The BQSS divides the figure into three hierarchically arranged elements (i.e., Configurals, Clusters, and Details), each of which is scored according to its presence, accuracy (for Configurals and Clusters), and placement (for Clusters and Details). Scores range from 0 (poor) to 4 (good). In addition, several other scores based on the entire production (Fragmentation, Planning, Neatness, and Perseveration) and the Organization Summary Score (sum of Planning and Fragmentation) were developed to be sensitive to executive dysfunction. Scores for the Fragmentation, Planning, Neatness, and Perseveration variables range from 0 (poor) to 4 (good), whereas the Organization Summary Score ranges from 0 (poor) to 8 (good). The criteria for the Planning score are shown in Table 10–95.

Interrater reliability is high for most scores (>.80) but poor for others, such as asymmetry and confabulation (Folbrecht et al., 1999) or cluster placement and detail placement (Stern et al., 1999). Reliability coefficients are higher for two or more raters. Accordingly, it is recommended that more than one rater score the Rey Figure and that their average score be used for interpretation (Folbrecht et al., 1999). Internal consistency reliabilities are also high (>.70) (Folbrecht et al., 1999).

Some support for the validity of the BQSS executive scores derives from studies of patient populations with known executive dysfunction (Schreiber et al., 1999; Somerville et al., 2000; Troyer & Wishart, 1997) and from the pattern of correlations with other executive and nonexecutive measures. For example, Sommerville et al. (2000) reported that the executive BQSS variables were more highly correlated with executive measures (e.g., WCST perseverative responses, COWA; average correlation = .26) than with nonexecutive measures (e.g., Digit Span, LM and VR retention; average correlation = .16). In addition, the BQSS Organization Summary Score significantly differentiated patients with either no, mild, or severe executive dysfunction (defined according to performance on other tests of executive function).

The advantage of the BQSS lies in its ability to characterize unique differences among patients that are not evident in the traditional 36-point scoring system. For example, the BQSS is more sensitive to aging effects than the traditional system is (Hartman & Potter, 1998), and it appears useful in determining whether poor organization could account for recall difficulties. Similarly, Elderkin-Thompson et al. (2004a, 2004b) found that the Planning score was particularly useful in understanding visual-spatial memory impairment in depressed elderly patients. These patients appear not to encode the figure in an organized manner, and this lack of structure seems to account for their poor memory.

According to the authors, scoring takes 5 to 15 min for a single reproduction and decreases to about 5 min once the examiner is familiar with the method. However, others (Folbrecht et al. 1999; Hartman & Potter, 1998) have noted average scoring times of about 13 to 20 min per figure. Although scoring time decreased with experience, the scorers were never able to decrease scoring time to 5 min or less. One

Table 10–95 Criteria for Scoring Planning on the BQSS

Score	Meaning
4	Configural or large structural elements are drawn before clusters or details
3	Only the large rectangle and triangle are completed before clusters and details are started, although the design is systematic and overall shape is maintained
2	Large rectangle and most elements are present, and there is some systematic order to the drawing
1	Rectangle is recognizable, and the drawing is somewhat logical

Source: Adapted from Stern et al., 1999.

possibility might be to supplement more traditional scoring systems with the Organization Summary Score and/or the Planning score from the BQSS, because these values can be calculated independently of the rest of the system and offer excellent reliability (Elderkin-Thompson et al., 2004a; Hartman & Potter, 1998).

Boone (2000) also noted that empirical evidence is lacking for some of the clinical interpretations of scores (e.g., regarding the presence of right or left hemisphere damage). She also recommended that a computer scoring program be provided to make the BQSS more user-friendly.

Hamby Scoring System

The system provided by Hamby et al. (1993) is simpler and focuses on one aspect of production: organizational quality. It employs a five-point Likert scale (higher ratings indicating better organization) and can be applied to both the Rey and the Taylor Figures. The authors reported that the system is easy to learn, is quick to score (<1 min per protocol), shows very good interrater reliability, and appears to have clinical utility. Organizational quality, but not copy and delay scores, on the Rey Figure distinguished between symptomatic and asymptomatic HIV-positive subjects.

Bennett-Levy and Bylsma Scoring Systems

Both the Bennett-Levy (1984) and the Bylsma et al. (1995) systems are based on the premise that perceptual organization is reflected by the order in which the examinee copies segments and the degree of fragmentation of lines or elements. Interrater reliabilities are high for both systems (>.90), and both require about 1 min to score (see also Troyer & Wishart, 1997).

Chiulli Scoring System

A relatively gross approach, employed by Chiulli et al. (1995), involves categorizing the drawings as configural if examinees begin with construction of the base rectangle; all other approaches are scored as nonconfigural. Reliability data, however, are not reported.

Savage Scoring System

The system developed by Savage et al. (1999) evaluates five organizational units (the large rectangle, the diagonal cross, the vertical midline, the horizontal midline, and the vertex of the triangle on the right), each of which must be drawn as an unfragmented piece to receive credit for organization. Support for the validity of this system has been established in patients with obsessive-compulsive disorder (for review, see Deckersbach et al., 2000a). Interrater reliability is also high ($r = .94$; Deckersbach et al., 2000a).

Rapport Scoring System

Rapport et al. (1995, 1996) adapted the standard and Denman scoring systems to evaluate hemispatial deficits on the Rey Figure. The measures evaluated include (a) percent of omitted items on the left or right halves of the figure; (b) attentional bias to right space, as indicated when the patient begins the figure copy by drawing any portion that is rightward of the vertical midline of the large rectangle; and (c) accuracy of reproduction of the two sides of the figure. Rapport et al. (1996) noted that, when the standard scoring system is used, an asymmetric error profile of two or more left-sided omissions indicates a strong likelihood of neglect.

Comparison Among Systems

A few authors have compared the various scoring systems to one another (see Knight, 2003). Fastenau et al. (1996) reported that their scoring system was no better than that designed by Osterrieth in terms of reliability and validity and that their system took about six times longer to apply. Rapport et al. (1997) reported that interrater and internal consistency reliabilities for both the Osterrieth and the Denman scoring systems were high and equivalent. Troyer and Wishart (1996) compared a number of qualitative scoring systems (Bennett-Levy, 1984; Binder, 1982; Bylsma et al., 1995; Hamby et al., 1993; Osterrieth, 1944; Shorr et al., 1992; Stern et al., 1994; Visser, 1973; Waber & Holmes, 1985) and found that most systems were intercorrelated ($r = .34$ to $.84$), with the exception of the system by Waber and Holmes ($r = .25$ to $.32$). Two of the qualitative scoring systems (Bennet-Levy 1984; Bylsma et al., 1995) had particularly favorable characteristics (Troyer & Wishart, 1997). Both showed approximately normally distributed scores, moderate variability between subjects, and average scores falling within the upper-middle change. Further, scores from both systems were moderately related to recall scores, indicating that recall and qualitative copy performance are related yet distinct constructs. Correlations with tests of executive function were moderate, providing evidence of convergent validity, and correlations with tests of general cognitive ability were low, providing evidence of discriminant validity. Interrater reliabilities were high, and scoring required only 1 to 2 min per protocol.

Using the DSS-ROCF and the BQSS, Harris et al. (1999, cited in Knight, 2003) scored the Copy protocols from a sample of 7- to 11-year-old children. Although the DSS-ROCF has a developmental focus and the BQSS was designed for assessing adults, both systems proved sensitive to age-related improvements in visual-spatial organization, analysis, and accuracy. In addition, factor analysis suggested that comparable dimensions were being measured. The reader is referred to Knight (2003) for more extensive commentary on ROCF scoring approaches.

DEMOGRAPHIC EFFECTS

Age

Age contributes to performance on the ROCF. Copy scores increase with age, the rate of increase slowing between ages 12 and 16 years, with adult levels being reached at about age 17 years (Meyers & Meyers, 1996). Some suggest little decrement in copy scores with advancing age (see also Chervinsky et al., 1992; Mitrushina et al., 1990). Others, however, have found that age influences copy performance, particularly after age 70 years, although the changes are quite subtle (Boone et al., 1993; Chiulli et al., 1995; Denman, 1987; Meyers & Meyers, 1995b; Miatton et al., 2004; Ponton et al., 1996; Ostrosky-Solis et al., 1998; Rosselli and Ardila, 1991; Tombaugh et al., 1992). Mitrushina et al. (2005) in their recent meta-analysis, documented an age-related decline in copy scores as well as an increase in variability with advancing age. Drawings are not less organized in older adults (aged 60+ years), although they are messier, reflecting minor inaccuracies in drawing (e.g., curved lines, rounded corners, gaps, overshoots) that are perhaps due to either mild visual-spatial deficiencies or motor problems (Hartman & Potter, 1998).

Scores on the immediate- and delayed-recall trials also increase significantly between 6 and 12 years of age, with slowing across the age range of 12 to 17 years and showing a decline with advancing age (Anderson & Lajoie, 1996; Boone et al., 1993; Caffarra et al., 2002; Chervinsky et al., 1992; Chiulli et al., 1995; Denman, 1987; Hartman & Potter, 1998; Kramer & Wells, 2004; Meyers & Meyers, 1995b, 1996; Miatton et al., 2004; Mitrushina et al., 1990, 2005; Ostrosky-Solis et al., 1998; Ponton et al., 1996; Rosselli & Ardila, 1991). Advancing age is primarily associated with an increase in the number of omitted elements of the drawing, rather than distortion of the elements (Hartman & Potter, 1998; Mitrushina et al., 1990). Not only do mean scores decrease with aging, but also standard deviations (*SD*s) increase with advancing age; that is, there is greater heterogeneity in the older age groups (Mitrushina et al., 2005; Ostrosky-Solis et al., 1998).

Rates of forgetting (copy score minus delay score) also show some relation with age (Ostrosky-Solis et al., 1998; but see Mitrushina & Satz, 1989), suggesting that memory declines in the elderly may be attributable, at least in part, to impaired storage. Young adults (aged 20–30 years) retain about 65% of the information they acquired on the copy trial; individuals aged 70+ retain less than 40% of the information. Recognition performance shows a slight decline with advancing age (Meyers & Meyers, 1995b).

Gender

The importance of gender is controversial. Some have reported that males outperform females (Ardila & Rosselli, 1989; Ardila et al., 1989; Bennett-Levy, 1984; Caffarra et al., 2002; King, 1981; Kramer & Wells, 2004), but the differences in performance have generally been small (about 2 points) or nonexistent (Berry et al., 1991; Boone et al., 1993; Chiulli et al., 1995; Demsky et al., 2000; Loring et al., 1990; Meyers & Meyers, 1995b, 1996; Ponton et al., 1996; Poulton & Moffitt, 1995; Tombaugh & Hubley, 1991; Tombaugh et al., 1992). Some suggest that the ambiguous and contradictory data may reflect the fact that there is considerable variability within the sexes. They argue that, in addition to gender, handedness (Karapetsas & Vlachos, 1997; Weinstein et al., 1990), familial handedness (Weinstein et al., 1990), and academic concentration (e.g., mathematics/science or other; Vlachos et al., 2003; Weinstein et al., 1990) need to be taken into consideration.

IQ

Scores on the ROCF show a modest correlation with measures of general intellectual ability (Boone et al., 1993; Chiulli et al., 1989, 1995; Diaz-Asper et al., 2004), particularly with nonverbal reasoning ability (Chervinsky et al., 1992; Sherman et al., 1995; Tombaugh et al., 1992). The higher the IQ, the higher the ROCF scores. The fact that the correlations with IQ are only modest indicates that the ROCF provides a large amount of information not accounted for by IQ (Chervinsky et al., 1992).

Education

The influence of education is less certain. A few authors (Ardila & Rosselli, 1989; Ardila et al., 1989; Berry et al., 1991; Caffarra et al., 2002; Miatton et al., 2004; Ponton et al., 1996; Rosselli & Ardila, 1991) have reported poorer scores in individuals with lower educational levels. Some, however, have found that ROCF measures are relatively unaffected by education (Chervinsky et al., 1992; Delaney et al., 1992; Meyers & Meyers, 1995b; Tombaugh et al., 1992) if the influence of IQ is partialled out (Boone et al., 1993). Ashton et al. (2005) reported that level of education did not affect recall and recognition above and beyond perceptual organization skills.

Ethnicity

In children, ethnicity has no impact on copy performance (Demsky et al., 2000). However, in adults, minority status shows modest correlations (.27 to .36) with copy and recall scores (Cornell et al., 1997). Cross-cultural differences have been reported (Rosselli & Ardila, 1991).

Table 10–96 Normative Data (Mean and *SD*) for ROCF—Administration A, Ages 6–85 Years, Copy and 30-Min Delay; (L. B. Taylor Scoring Criteria)

Trials	6 (*n* = 192)	7 (*n* = 353)	8 (*n* = 347)	9 (*n* = 329)	10 (*n* = 301)	11 (*n* = 280)	12 (*n* = 225)	13 (*n* = 237)
Copy	16.66 (7.97)	21.29 (7.67)	23.64 (8.00)	24.46 (6.94)	27.20 (7.58)	28.61 (7.31)	30.21 (6.69)	32.63 (4.35)
30-min Recall	10.53 (5.80)	13.57 (6.28)	16.34 (6.77)	18.71 (6.61)	19.73 (6.71)	22.59 (6.65)	23.20 (6.38)	24.59 (6.29)
% Recall								
Copy-Recall								

	14 (*n* = 180)	15 (*n* = 116)	20–29 (*n* = 20)	30–39 (*n* = 20)	40–49 (*n* = 18)	50–59 (*n* = 21)	60–69 (*n* = 21)	70+ (*n* = 23)
Copy	33.53 (3.18)	33.60 (2.98)	33.70 (1.59)	31.75 (3.21)	32.31 (2.67)	31.19 (3.68)	30.79 (4.21)	29.57 (3.37)
30-min Recall	26.24 (5.40)	26.00 (6.35)	21.80 (6.56)	17.20 (7.08)	16.56 (6.69)	14.88 (6.95)	14.21 (7.50)	11.74 (6.11)
% Recall			64.12 (18.39)	53.45 (20.13)	50.61 (18.77)	47.16 (20.59)	46.19 (22.91)	38.57 (18.22)
Copy-Recall			11.95 (5.72)	14.58 (6.12)	15.75 (5.58)	16.31 (6.41)	16.57 (7.53)	17.83 (14.58)

Note: Subjects aged 6–15 years were healthy school children in Lethbridge, Alberta, Canada. Subjects aged 21–84 years are well-educated adults.

Source: From Kolb & Whishaw, 1985, for ages 6–15 years; Spreen & Strauss, 1991, for ages 21–84 years.

NORMATIVE DATA

With respect to norms for evaluating the accuracy of the figure, wide variability exists with regard to the type of administration (i.e., number and timing of recall trials; Corwin & Bylsma, 1993; Lezak et al., 2004; Mitrushina et al., 2005; Tombaugh et al., 1992). As a consequence, one cannot assume that normative data for immediate recall can be used to evaluate delayed recall. There is some evidence (Loring et al., 1990; Meyers & Meyers, 1995a) that inclusion of an immediate-recall trial increases delayed-recall performance by about 2 to 6 points in healthy young adults. Further, diverse scoring systems complicate attempts to compile norms from different sources.

Mitrushina et al. (2005) recently compiled metanorms for adults aged 22 to 79 years, based on the standard 36-point scoring system on the copy, immediate recall, and delayed recall conditions. Data for 3-min delayed recall was not examined. The delayed-recall trial included studies varying in delay interval between 15 and 60 min and was preceded by an immediate or a 3-min delayed recall trial but not both. Nine studies, comprising 1340 participants, were analyzed for the copy condition, and seven studies, based on a total of 1056 participants, were analyzed for the delayed-recall condition. Mitrushina et al. (2005) noted that the mean education of their sample was relatively high (about 14 years) and that their normative values may overestimate expected scores for individuals with lower educational levels. The values match closely the normative data provided in the manual by Meyers and Meyers (1995b). It should be noted that the educational achievement of the normative sample provided by Meyers and Meyers was similarly high.

Several sets of normative data based on the copy-recall interval or intervals used and the scoring criteria applied are discussed here (see Table 10–93).

Administration A

This administration comprises a copy trial and a 30-min recall trial with no interposed immediate-recall trial; it is scored ac-

cording to L. B. Taylor's criteria. The data for healthy children aged 6 to 15 years (Kolb & Whishaw, 1985), and adults aged 20 to 70+ years (Spreen & Strauss, 1991) are given in Table 10–96.

Demsky et al. (2000) provided normative data, based on a sample of 432 children, aged 6 to 11 years, for the copy portion only, using the scoring approach of E. M. Taylor (1959). Note that the data were based on a group administration procedure, with the figure presented via overhead transparency. The values were slightly lower (about 2 points) than those reported by Kolb and Whishaw (1990), probably reflecting differences in test administration.

Administration B

This administration comprises a copy trial followed by an immediate-recall trial and a 30-min delayed-recall trial; it is scored according to the criteria of E. M. Taylor (1959, in Lezak et al., 2004). Data for healthy adults, aged 65 to 93 years, of above-average IQ (Shipley estimated FSIQ = 112) are shown in Table 10–97. These elderly subjects required on average 212 s (*SD* = 81 s) to copy the figure (S. J. Chiulli, personal communication, 1990).

Chiulli et al. (1995) also provided data on a sample of healthy, highly educated (mean >13 years), Caucasian, elderly individuals using L. B. Taylor's scoring criteria. In addition, they evaluated the approach to the drawing; that is, the drawing was classed as configural or not, depending on whether the construction began with the base rectangle. Data for accuracy and approach are shown in Table 10–98.

Denman (1987) also provided data for individuals aged 10 to 89 years for copy, immediate-recall, and delayed-recall trials of the Rey Figure. His scoring criteria were based on a maximum score of 72 for each condition, and the raw scores must be converted to scaled scores (1–19) by means of age-based normative tables.

Rosselli and Ardila (1991) gave normative data for copy (both accuracy and time to complete the task) and immediate

Table 10–97 Normative Data ROCF–Administration B, Ages 65–93 Years With Copy, Immediate, and 30-Minute Delay Trials (E. M. Taylor Scoring Criteria, as Described by Lezak et al., 2004)

Trial	65–69	70–74	75–79	80–84	85–93
Copy					
Mean (*SD*)	31.10 (3.59)	32.03 (3.27)	30.49 (4.48)	30.76 (4.06)	30.80 (2.60)
n	10	50	57	35	10
Immediate					
Mean (*SD*)	15.50 (5.54)	15.44 (6.51)	15.39 (6.75)	14.47 (6.31)	9.45 (3.92)
n	10	49	57	35	10
30-min Recall					
Mean (*SD*)	15.30 (4.98)	15.35 (6.37)	15.12 (6.34)	13.76 (6.07)	9.39 (4.93)
n	9	50	57	35	10

Note: Data are for healthy adults, aged 65–93 years, of above-average IQ (Shipley estimated FSIQ = 112).

Source: From Chiulli et al., 1989. Reprinted with permission.

memory conditions, derived from a large sample of people aged 56 and older from Bogota, Colombia. Scoring criteria were those of E. M. Taylor (1959, in Lezak et al., 2004). The scores for both copy and recall conditions were considerably lower than those reported by investigators working with North American populations and probably reflect cultural and educational differences.

Administration C

This administration comprises a copy trial followed by a 3-min recall trial; it is scored according to the criteria of E. M. Taylor (1959). Osterrieth's (1944) normative data should not be used because (a) the data were based on 60 adults in the 16- to 60-year-old age range and no breakdown by age was presented,

and (b) educational and cultural differences invalidate comparison of current North American samples with those collected by Osterrieth in Europe more than 60 years ago.

Boone et al. (1993) obtained normative data for healthy North American adults, and these data are shown in Table 10–99. Anderson et al. (1997, 2001) provided data based on a sample of 376 children, aged 7 years to 13 years 11 months, with approximately equal numbers of boys and girls in each age group. Children with a history of neurological, developmental, or psychiatric disorders and those requiring special educational assistance were excluded. Scoring of copy and recall accuracy was done using E. M. Taylor's criteria (see Table 10–100). Scores for five levels of organization (Waber & Holmes, 1986; see Table 10–94) were also calculated for each copy drawing.

Administration D

This administration comprises a copy trial followed by 3-min and 30-min recall trials as well as a recognition trial. Meyers and Meyers (1995b) provided normative data (see Table 10–101) based on a sample of 601 healthy adults, aged 18 to 89 years,

Table 10–98 Administration B: Accuracy (Mean and *SD*) and Number (Percentage) of Subjects Adopting a Configural Approach on the ROCF, by Age in Years (L.B. Taylor's Scoring Criteria for Accuracy.)

Trial	70–74 (*n* = 46)	75–79 (*n* = 58)	80–91 (*n* = 49)
Copy			
Accuracy	32.6 (2.8)	31.0 (4.0)	29.8 (4.6)
Approach	18 (39%)	21 (36%)	17 (35%)
Immediate			
Accuracy	17.2 (6.2)	14.2 (6.6)	12.9 (6.4)
Approach	24 (55%)	23 (41%)	19 (40%)
30-min delay			
Accuracy	16.9(6.3)	14.2 (6.2)	12.4 (6.0)
Approach	24 (55%)	29 (52%)	19 (41%)

Note: Data are based on 153 healthy, highly educated, noninstitutionalized elderly. The approach used to complete the drawing was classed as configural if the drawing began with construction of the large rectangle.

Source: From Chiulli et al., 1995. Reprinted with the kind permission of Psychology Press.

Table 10–99 Administration C: Normative Data (Mean and *SD*) for Ages 45–83 Years on the ROCF for Copy and 3-min Delayed Recall Trials (E.M. Taylor's Scoring Criteria, as Described in Lezak et al., 2004)

Trial	45–59 (*n* = 38)	60–69 (*n* = 31)	70–83 (*n* = 22)
Copy	34.18 (1.8)	33.76 (2.8)	31.25 (4.7)
3-min Recall	18.88 (6.1)	17.33 (5.2)	13.77 (5.0)
% Retention	55.03 (17.1)	51.16 (13.6)	43.77 (14.8)

Note: Data for healthy adults of above-average education (*M* = 14.5 years) and intelligence (mean WAIS-R IQ = 115.89), with permission of Swets & Zeitlinger.

Source: Adapted from Boone et al., 1993.

Table 10–100 Administration C—Developmental Trends (Mean and SD) for Accuracy on the ROCF (E. M. Taylor Scoring Criteria) and Levels of Organization (Waber & Holmes, 1986).

	Age (Years)						
	7 ($n = 56$)	8 ($n = 56$)	9 ($n = 61$)	10 ($n = 62$)	11 ($n = 51$)	12 ($n = 54$)	13 ($n = 51$)
Accuracy	21.95 (6.9)	23.96 (5.9)	27.57 (3.5)	29.11 (3.9)	28.89 (4.9)	31.06 (5.2)	31.41 (2.9)
Memory	11.12 (5.5)	11.61 (6.0)	13.71 (5.0)	16.25 (5.9)	17.71 (4.9)	17.93 (6.6)	19.7 (6.1)
Organization							
Score	1.63 (0.8)	1.89 (0.9)	2.07 (0.8)	2.37 (1.0)	2.59 (0.9)	3.3 (1.0)	3.47 (0.9)

Source: From Anderson et al., 1997, 2001.

and a sample of 505 normal children and adolescents, aged 6 to 17 years. Their explicit scoring guidelines must be used (see source). Caution should be used when interpreting ROCF performance for patients aged 80 to 89 years because of the small number of normative subjects in this age range ($n = 15$). Age-corrected T scores and percentile equivalents are provided for 3-min (called "Immediate") Recall, Delayed

Table 10–101 Characteristics of the Normative Sample for Administration D of the ROCF

Number	601 adults, 505 children
Age (years)	6–89[a]
Geographic location	Majority of adults recruited from the north central and western areas of the United States; a subset of the adult normative sample $n = (394)$ matched U.S. Census data for age distribution for the year 2000
Sample type	University students, volunteers from suburban communities
Education	Approximately 14 years for adults
Gender	
Males	Adults, not reported; children, 50.3%
Females	Adults, not reported; children, 49.7%
Race/Ethnicity	Not reported for adults; in children, about 86% White, 3.6% African American, 3.4% Asian American, 5.0% Hispanic American, and 1.8% Other
Screening	Adults, no history of neurological dysfunction, psychiatric disorder, learning disability, on alcohol or drug abuse or dependence; children, no history of neurological dysfunction, learning disorder, emotional disorder, or attention disorder

[a]Data are grouped into half-year intervals for ages 6–10 years and into yearly intervals for ages 10 years to 17 years 11 months. Normative tables are grouped into a 2-year age span for 18- to 19-year-olds, 5-year spans for ages 20–79 years, and a 10-year span for ages 80–89 years.

Source: From Meyers & Meyers, 1995b.

Recall, and Recognition Total Correct. Normative data for Copy, Time to Copy, Recognition True Positives, Recognition True and False Positives, and Recognition True and False Negatives are presented in five categories (e.g., scores greater than the 16th percentile, scores within the 16th to 11th percentile).

The frequency of occurrence of different scores for each scoring unit was examined in a heterogeneous sample of brain-damaged patients ($n = 100$) and in a matched normative sample. This base-rate information is provided in the test manual for the various drawing and recognition trials.

RELIABILITY

Internal Reliability

The internal consistency of the Rey Figure was evaluated by treating each detail as an item and computing split-half and alpha coefficients (Berry et al., 1991; Fasteneau et al., 1996). Both split-half and coefficient alpha reliabilities were greater than .60 for the copy condition and greater than .80 for recall conditions (immediate recall and 20- or 30-min delayed recall) in adults, suggesting that all of the details tap into a single factor.

Test-Retest Reliability

Meyers and Meyers (1995b) noted that ranges for some of the scores (e.g., copy, recognition) are restricted due to the maximum- or near-maximum level performance attained by most normal subjects, artificially reducing the magnitude of the test-retest correlation coefficients (see also Levine et al., 2004). Moreover, the incidental learning paradigm is contaminated when a subject is retested after the original administration. Based on these considerations, Meyers and Meyers (1995b) evaluated test-retest reliability only for scores with sufficient range (Immediate Recall, $r = .76$; Delayed Recall, $r = .89$; Recognition Total Correct, $r = .87$) in a sample of 12 normal subjects after a retest interval of about 6 months. To measure the temporal stability of clinical interpretation, age-corrected T scores for these measures were classified according to the system of Heaton et al. (1991; e.g., average = T score 45–54, below average = T score 40–44, mildly impaired = T

Table 10–102 Change Scores, Standard Deviations, and Reliability Coefficients

Measure	Time 1 (T1)		Time 2 (T2)		T2 – T1		
	Mean	SD	Mean	SD	Mean	SD	R
Copy	34.8	1.83	34.7	1.59	−.03	1.76	.47
Immediate Recall	22.8	6.25	25.3	6.0	2.48	4.51	.73
Delayed Recall	22.5	6.2	24.8	6.01	2.30	4.32	.79

Note: Based on a sample of 478 well-educated (*M* = 16.4 years, *SD* = 2.3), mostly Caucasian men (age *M* = 42.2 years, *SD* = 8.6).

Source: Adapted from Levine et al., 2004.

score 35–39). The percentage agreement in the clinical interpretation between the first and second testing sessions was high (91.7) for these same three measures (Immediate Recall, Delayed Recall, and Recognition Total Correct). Meyers and Meyers (1995b) also reported no significant differences for other ROCF variables (Copy, Time to Copy, Recognition True Positives, False Positives, True Negatives, False Negatives) across the retest interval.

Berry et al. (1991) retested elderly individuals after 1 year and found that the copy condition was not reliable across this interval (*r* = .18). Reliabilities of the immediate-recall and 30-min delayed-recall trials were also low (.47 to .59). Somewhat better values have been reported by others. Mitrushina and Satz (1991) reported that, in older adults assessed over three annual probes, the coefficients ranged from 0.56 to 0.68 for copy and 0.57 to 0.77 for 3-min delayed recall. Similar findings were reported by Levine et al. (2004; see *Practice Effects*).

Practice Effects

Levine et al. (2004) reported gains for immediate and delayed recall Rey trials for 478 healthy men (age *M* = 42.2, *SD* = 8.6; education *M* = 16.4, *SD* = 2.3; mostly Caucasians) who were reassessed across a wide time interval, 4 to 24 months (*M* = 251 days, *SD* = 129). Table 10–102 shows change scores, *SD*s of the change scores, and test-retest reliability coefficients for use in Reliable Change Index (RCI) formulas. Table 10–103 shows the regression formulas that can be used to estimate Time 2 scores. The residual *SD*s for the regression formulas are also shown and can be used to establish the normal range for retest scores. For example, a 90% confidence interval can be created

around the scores by multiplying the residual *SD* by 1.645, which allows for 5% of people to fall outside of the upper and lower extremes. Individuals whose scores exceed the extremes are considered to have significant changes. Neither the length of the retest interval nor educational level contributed significantly to the regression equation.

Interrater Reliability

Scoring according to the criteria of Osterrieth (1944) and E. M. Taylor (1959), or variants of these criteria, yield adequate to high interrater and intrarater reliability for total scores (>.8; Berry et al., 1991; Boone et al., 1993; Caffarra et al., 2002; Casey et al., 1991; Delaney et al., 1992; Fastenau et al., 1996; Tupler et al., 1995). Reliabilities for the 18 individual items, however, ranged from poor (.14) to excellent (.96), suggesting that the Osterrieth system would benefit from more detailed specification of quantitative decision rules (e.g., minimal angle size required for 1 point; Tupler et al., 1995). The strict scoring criteria described by others (Bennett-Levy, 1984; Duley et al., 1993; Fastenau et al., 1996; Hubley & Tremblay, 2002; Loring et al., 1990; Meyers & Meyers, 1995a; Shorr et al., 1992; Stern et al., 1994, 1999; Strauss and Spreen, 1990; L.B. Taylor, 1991; Tombaugh et al., 1992) also show high (>.90) interrater reliability for total scores.

Alternate Forms

Another issue concerns the comparability of the Rey and its alternate versions. Reliability coefficients are in the moderate range when the Rey and Taylor figures are evaluated (Berry et al., 1991; Delaney et al., 1992). In children aged 8 to 10 years, with and without attention-deficit/hyperactivity disorder (ADHD), there is no difference between designs, both for copying and for remembering (Sadeh et al., 1996). In healthy young adults, the copy administrations of the various figures (Rey, Taylor, MCG) are of equivalent difficulty; however, recall of the Rey Figure is somewhat harder (about 2 points lower in normal people) compared with the Taylor and MCG figures (Delaney et al., 1992; Duley et al., 1993; Hamby et al., 1993; Kuehn & Snow, 1992; Meador et al., 1993; Miatton et al., 2004; Peirson & Jansen, 1997; Strauss & Spreen, 1990; Tombaugh & Hubley, 1991; Vingerhoets et al., 1998). Recall

Table 10–103 Regression Equations for Estimating Retest Scores

Measure	Regression Equation	Residual SD
Rey Copy	20.57 + (.407 × Time 1 score)	1.41
Immediate Delay	9.32 + (.701 × Time 1 score)	4.11
Delay Recall	8.27 + (.735 × Time 1 score)	3.99

Note: Based on a sample of 478 well-educated (*M* = 16.4 years, *SD* = 2.3), mostly Caucasian men (age *M* = 42.2 years, *SD* = 8.6).

Source: Adapted from Levine et al., 2004.

of the figures is differentially influenced by demographic factors; age affects recall of both the Rey and Taylor figures; but Rey recall is also influenced by education (a higher educational level results in higher Rey recall; Vingerhoets et al., 1998). Gender also contributes differently. Women perform better than men on the Taylor Figure copy trial, whereas men outperform women on the Rey delayed-recall trial (Vingerhoets et al., 1998). The Rey Figure also takes more time to both copy and reproduce from memory than does the Taylor Figure (Peirson & Jansen, 1997; Tombaugh & Hubley, 1991). The Rey Figure appears to have a more complex organizational structure (Hamby et al., 1993), it contains a greater number and variety of lines (Hubley & Tombaugh, 2002), and it does not lend itself readily to a verbal strategy (Casey et al., 1991). As a result, individuals with visual imagery problems cannot compensate by using a verbal strategy. With the Taylor Figure, in contrast, deficits in visual imagery may be circumvented and therefore obscured by the use of verbal strategies.

The greater recall difficulty of the Rey Figure suggests that this measure may be more sensitive than the alternate versions to the presence of memory deficits, particularly nonverbal ones (Strauss & Spreen, 1990; see also Hamby et al., 1993). Even though the Taylor Figure is easier to remember than the Rey Figure, parallel forgetting functions occur for both figures, indicating that both reflect comparable degrees of sensitivity when they are used to measure rates of forgetting (Tombaugh & Hubley, 1991).

Of note, the newly developed modified version of the Taylor Figure (Modified Taylor Complex Figure, MTCF) appears to yield copy and memory scores that are comparable to those for the Rey Figure; however, when both forms were given to the same individuals spaced 1 week apart, alternate form reliability was adequate on all trials (>.65) except the copy trial (Hubley & Tombaugh, 2002), suggesting that their use as matched forms to measure constructional ability requires some caution. There are no significant differences in test scores between the Taylor Figure and the four MCG figures (Meador et al., 1993).

VALIDITY

The precise cognitive operations required for adequate performance are thought to include visual perception, visual-spatial organization, motor functioning, and, on the recall condition, memory (Chervinsky et al., 1992). Overall, the data from correlational and factor analytic studies support the validity of the CFT as a measure of visual-constructional ability (copy) and memory (recall and recognition). There is less evidence concerning the specific executive functions contributing to task performance.

Relations Among Test Measures

Meyers and Meyers (1995b) correlated ROCF scores from 601 normal individuals and found that the largest correlation was between Immediate (3-min) Recall and Delayed Recall ($r = .88$). The recall measures demonstrated lower but still significant correlations ($r = .15$) with Recognition Total Correct, suggesting that they are assessing different aspects of memory. Time to Copy had minimal relations to the accuracy of the copy or the recall. Moderate correlations were noted between Copy raw score and Immediate (3-min) Recall ($r = .33$) and Delayed Recall ($r = .38$) scores, suggesting a relationship between the ability to copy the complex figure and the ability to later recall and draw the figure from memory (also *Relation Between Copy Strategy and Recall*). Similar findings emerged in a heterogeneous sample of patients with documented neurological dysfunction (Meyers & Meyers, 1995b).

Meyers and Meyers (1995b) also conducted a principal-components factor analysis of the data for normal individuals. The analysis suggested a five-factor solution. The first factor was termed a Visuospatial Recall factor due to high loading from the 3- and 30-min delay trials. Factor 2 reflected a Visuospatial Recognition factor. Factor 3, labeled a Response Bias factor, demonstrated a high loading of Recognition False Positives. Factor 4 was interpreted as a Processing Speed factor because of a high loading of Time to Copy. Finally, Factor 5 reflected Visuospatial Constructional Ability, with a high loading of the Copy score. Analysis of data from brain-damaged patients ($n = 100$) revealed the same five factors, supporting the notion that the test measures different dimensions, not a unitary visual memory construct.

Relations With Other Test Measures

Memory and visuomotor ability contribute to performance. In a heterogeneous sample of patients with neurological disorders, Meyers and Meyers (1995b) found that the Copy, 3-min Recall, and 30-min Recall, and Recognition Total Correct scores were significantly correlated with tasks requiring memory and constructional ability (BVRT Total Correct, RAVLT Trial 5, Form Discrimination, Hooper, Trails B, and the Token Test). Language measures (FAS, Sentence Repetition) had no significant relationships with any ROCF measures. Modest correlations were reported between ROCF recall and total recall on the RAVLT ($r = .36$; Anderson & Lajoie, 1996).

In adults and children, correlational analyses indicate that scores on the ROCF are moderately related to performance on visual-spatial subtests (Block Design and Object Assembly) of the Wechsler Intelligence Test (e.g., Poulton & Moffitt, 1995; Tombaugh et al., 1992; Wood et al., 1982). Similarly, Sherman et al. (1995) found that scores on the ROCF (both copy and 30-min delay) were moderately related to the Perceptual Organization factor of the WAIS-R. Scores on the ROCF were not related to the Verbal Comprehension and Freedom from Distractibility factors of the WAIS-R. Meyers and Meyers (1995b) also reported that, in a mixed sample of patients with neurological disorders, ROCF measures correlated more strongly with Performance subtests than with Verbal subtests.

In children, there is some overlap in the content of the copy portion of the ROCF and the Beery Developmental Test of Visual Motor Integration (VMI), the shared variance ranging from 7% to 13% depending on the age of the child (Demsky et al., 2000). The differences between the tests may reflect, at least in part, the greater planning involved in copying the Rey Figure, compared with the VMI (Demsky et al., 2000).

Factor analytic findings of the ROCF and other neuropsychological tests suggest that ROCF scores load heavily on what appears to be a visual-spatial perceptual/memory factor, based on common loadings with the WMS Visual Reproduction (Berry et al., 1991; Ostrosky-Solis et al., 1998), Line Orientation (Berry et al., 1991), Hooper (Johnstone & Wilhelm, 1997), and Raven's Standard Progressive Matrices scores (Ponton et al., 2000).

Working memory also plays a role, at least in the copying of the figure. In patients with dementia, copy scores were most consistently correlated with tasks requiring patients to monitor their behavior and sustain a complex mental set while performing mental manipulations; by contrast, no relationship was found to measures of response selection/inhibition, suggesting some selectivity with respect to the types of executive functions underlying competent copying of the complex figure (Freeman et al., 2000).

Relation Between Copy Strategy and Recall

Qualitative copy scores tend to be correlated with both copy and recall accuracy scores. A strategy that involves clustering the elements into meaningful units is more effective than one that relies on the recall of isolated elements (e.g., Akshoomoff & Stiles, 1995b; Anderson et al., 2001; Bennett-Levy, 1984; Chiulli et al., 1995; Deckersbach et al., 2000a; Hamby et al., 1993; Shorr et al., 1992). Consequently, it is important to consider organizational strategy when assessing visual memory of the figure.

In this context, it is worth noting that perceptual bias (the tendency to allocate more attentional or perceptual resources to either the global or the local features of a stimulus) also affect performance. In healthy individuals, the tendency to view a stimulus from a global (as opposed to a local) vantage point is associated with better recall (Kramer & Wells, 2004).

Developmental Patterns—Copy

The copy portion of the test is sensitive to developmental changes. Usually, older children (age 13 years) and literate adults copy the design from left to right (Ardila et al., 1989; Poulton & Moffitt, 1995; Waber & Holmes, 1985). Children as young as 6 years of age are able to draw most of the items in the complex figure, and by 9 years of age the majority of details are included and placed correctly (Akshoomoff & Stiles, 1995a; Waber & Holmes, 1985). The designs are most commonly copied in a piecemeal fashion by younger children; with increasing age, they use a more integrated approach (Akshoomoff & Stiles, 1995a; Anderson et al., 2001), with the design becoming more configurational. At about age 13 years, a shift to the base rectangle strategy occurs, wherein the large central rectangle is drawn first and details are added on in relation to it. However, about one third of 13-year-olds use a fragmented approach, with additional changes most likely occurring in later adolescence (Anderson et al., 2001).

According to Osterrieth (1944), 83% of adults adopt a conceptual or part-configurational approach, and only 15% use a piecemeal approach. Use of a configural approach shows little decline with advancing age (Chiulli et al., 1995). However, the role of organization differs between young and old adults. Hartman and Potter (1998) noted that, in comparison to young adults (aged 18–32 years), older adults (aged 60–81 years) appear to rely more on the hierarchical structure of the figure to maintain accuracy of individual elements, with failures to organize resulting in reduced copy scores. In contrast, younger adults are able to draw individual elements accurately even in the absence of a well-organized production. Therefore, the organizational abilities of older adults are not only well preserved but also appear important for maintaining a high level of performance.

Developmental Patterns—Memory

In the memory production, a piecemeal strategy is rare after age 9 years. In older children and adults, errors (typically in the form of omissions) are common in the memory condition but rare in the copy condition (Hartman & Potter, 1998; Mitrushina et al., 1990).

In short, age-related differences in adults on the copy condition are relatively minor. On the memory trial, errors of omission are prominent with advancing age. Therefore, marked distortion or disorganization of the drawing elements in either the copy or recall condition may signify abnormality rather than normal aging (Hartman & Potter, 1998).

Clinical Studies

The test is sensitive to individuals with a history of central nervous system health problems known to affect memory and executive function, such as head injury (Berry et al., 1991; Poulton & Moffitt, 1995), medial temporal lobe damage (Kixmiller et al., 2000), seizure disorders (Poulton & Moffitt, 1995), Alzheimer's disease (Ardila et al., 2000; Berry et al., 1991; Bigler et al. 1989; Freeman et al., 2000; Tei et al., 1997), Parkinson's disease (Cooper et al., 1991; Freeman et al., 2000; Ogden et al., 1990), ischemic vascular dementia (Freeman et al., 2000), Korsakoff's disease (Kixmiller et al., 2000), Huntington's disease (Fedio et al., 1979), cocaine and polydrug abuse (Rosselli & Ardila, 1996), and anterior communicating artery aneurysm (Diamond & DeLuca, 1996;

Diamond et al., 1997; Kixmiller et al., 2000). Detoxified alcoholics also showed impaired recall and recognition performance, most likely because of inefficient learning (poor organizational and problem-solving skills) and retrieval strategies (Dawson & Grant, 2000). Bigler et al. (1996) reported that the degree of hippocampal atrophy in patients with moderate to severe head injury was related to percent recall on the test.

The task is also sensitive to disorders occurring in childhood, including frontal lobe epilepsy (Hernandez et al., 2003), very low birth weight (Taylor et al., 2004), congenital syndromes (Poulton & Moffitt, 1995), Turner's syndrome (Romans et al., 1997), traumatic brain injury (TBI; Garth et al., 1997), ADHD (Seidman et al., 1997), and learning disabilities (Kirkwood et al., 2001; Waber & Bernstein, 1995). Functional imaging studies in normal children suggest that indices of frontal lobe maturation (frontal lobe grey matter thinning bilaterally) and mesial temporal lobe grey matter volume are predictive of recall performance, even when age is controlled (Sowell et al., 2001).

Further, information from the copy portion of the test may be useful in differentiating different disorders. For example, a piecemeal approach to the copying of the ROCF is characteristic of patients (adults as well as children) with either left-or right-hemisphere lesions (Akshoomoff et al., 2002; Binder, 1982; Trojano et al., 2004; Visser, 1973). However, the drawings by patients with right-brain lesions tend to be less accurate (but see Rapport et al., 1995 and 1996, who found that this might apply only to patients who show neglect) and more distorted than those of their left-sided counterparts (Binder, 1982). However, patients with left hemisphere damage exhibited more difficulty copying right-sided local elements (Poreh & Shye, 1998). Differences between patients with parietal-occipital lesions and patients with frontal lobe lesions were also noted on the copy trial (Lezak, 1995; Pillon, 1981; L. B. Taylor, cited in Kolb & Whishaw, 1985). Adult patients with posterior lesions are more likely to have difficulty with the spatial organization of the figure. Patients with frontal lobe lesions are more likely to have difficulty planning their approach to the task. Children with frontal lesions also have difficulty copying and planning their drawings, tending to use a piecemeal, fragmented approach (Matthews et al., 2001). Patients with schizophrenia, a disorder involving prominent executive dysfunction, are also impaired on copy accuracy, using a detail-oriented style as opposed to a gestalt approach (Seidman et al., 2003). The copy task is also sensitive to hemispatial neglect. Patients with right cerebrovascular accident who were identified as having neglect on a letter-cancellation task showed an increased incidence of omission of items on the left side of the figure, a rightward attentional bias (reflected in their starting point on the task), and a poorer accuracy of reproduction on the left side (Rapport et al., 1995, 1996).

With regard to the memory trials, there is a tendency for adult patients with right-hemisphere lesions to perform more

poorly than patients with left-hemisphere disturbances on the recall trial (Loring et al., 1988b). The test, however, is not a perfect predictor of side of lesion (Lee et al., 1989; Loring et al., 1988b), and others have found the task to be insensitive to right-hemisphere lesions (Ashton et al., 2005; Barr et al., 1997; King, 1981). Analysis of qualitative features (e.g., distortion of overall configuration, major mislocation, location of element) may be helpful in distinguishing laterality of dysfunction (Breir et al., 1996; Loring et al., 1988b; Poreh & Shye, 1998). If the initial copy is performed satisfactorily, misplacement and distortion on the recall trial tend to be characteristic of patients with right-, as opposed to left-hemisphere dysfunction (Breir et al., 1996; Loring et al., 1988b). Poreh and Shye (1998) found that patients with left-hemisphere damage randomly recalled the local elements of the right side of the figure, whereas the left side and middle (global) portions were copied and recalled as a separate class. Patients with right-hemisphere damage, on the other hand, showed no evidence of a tendency to exhibit either a left- or right-hemifield superiority.

Prenatal or perinatal injury may result in selective deficits depending on the laterality of the dysfunction. Akshoomoff et al. (2002) reported that children (aged 12 or 13 years) with early right-hemisphere injury (mostly stroke) were more likely to reproduce the figure in a piecemeal manner; by contrast, children with early left-hemisphere injury were more likely to organize their memory reproductions around the core rectangle but included few additional details. Matthews et al. (2001), however, failed to observe laterality differences in children with temporal lobe pathology (most with epilepsy), although the age at onset of the disorder was not reported in this study.

Poor performance on the memory trials may also occur in individuals with various psychiatric disorders. Meyers and Meyers (1995b) found that patients with diffuse brain injury performed more poorly than those with chronic psychiatric disorders (schizophrenia, bipolar disorder, major depression), and the psychiatric group performed significantly more poorly than the normal group on both 3- and 30-min recall trials. For other ROCF variables (e.g., Copy, Copy Time, Recognition), brain-injured patients performed significantly more poorly than psychiatric or normal groups, but the latter two groups did not differ significantly from one another (see also Rosenstein, 1999, who noted no relation between ROCF copy scores and BDI or GDS scores in a heterogeneous clinical sample).

Seidman et al. (2003) reported that patients with schizophrenia were impaired on copy, recall, and recognition components and that recall accuracy deficits remained significant after controlling for organizational approach on the copy portion. The implication is that initial organizational processing impairments are an important component of retention difficulties in schizophrenia but do not fully account for recall difficulty. Patients with bipolar disorder performed at a level intermediate between that of controls and that of patients with schizophrenia. Poor recall performance was also reported in patients with obsessive-compulsive disorder, probably due in part to inefficient organizational strategies during the copy condition (Deckersbach et al., 2000a; Mataix-Cols et al., 2003; Savage et al., 2000; Shin et al., 2004). Similar problems have been reported in patients with body dysmorphic disorder (Deckersbach et al., 2000b).

Patients with borderline personality disorder also exhibited deficits on immediate and delayed recall of the CFT (Harris et al., 2002). Some authors have reported that anxiety (e.g., posttraumatic stress disorder) or depression negatively affects recall (Boone et al., 1995; Uddo et al., 1993; Wishart et al., 1993). For example, in a sample of volunteers with no history of neurological disorder, Meyers and Meyers (1995b) found moderate correlations between Beck Depression Inventory scores and Recognition Total Correct ($r = -.39$). Individuals classed as depressed (Beck score ≥ 14) scored on average 4.7 T scores lower on 3-min recall, 6.5 T scores lower on 30-min delayed recall, and 8.8 T scores lower on Recognition Total Correct. However, other authors (Chiulli et al., 1995; Suhr & Gunstad, 2005; Vingerhoets et al., 1995) have noted that psychological distress (anxiety, depression) has no effect on recall of the ROCF. Acute mental stress, typical of everyday life, appears to have little impact on test performance (Hoffman & al'Absi, 2004).

Recently, the question of the test's sensitivity to TBI has been questioned. Ashton et al. (2005) found that higher levels of (WAIS-III) perceptual organization skills and, to a lesser extent, the absence of a diffuse intracranial injury were predictive of better performance on the recall and recognition trials. Measures of injury severity proved unrelated to performance. Further, a large proportion of the sample improved by at least 1 SD from delayed recall to recognition, and this was mediated by perceptual organization skills but not by injury parameters. Given the limited sensitivity of the recall and recognition trials to injury severity, these authors concluded that performance on the ROCF after TBI was more affected by perceptual organization skills and that clinicians should supplement the ROCF with other measures of learning and memory.

Expectations regarding diagnosis (diagnosis threat) may negatively influence recall performance. Suhr and Gunstad (2005) reported that head-injured individuals exposed to diagnosis threat performed more poorly than matched controls on the Rey recall portion, despite no differences in effort (Word Memory Test), anxiety, or depression. The findings suggest that a person's knowledge and expectancies about neurological insult (e.g., head injury) and its cognitive consequences can affect performance, perhaps due to distractibility and poor cognitive efficiency.

There is evidence (Berry & Carpenter, 1992; Delaney et al., 1992) that most forgetting tends to occur very quickly, within the first few minutes after copying, perhaps as a result of an overloading of working memory. Although virtually no forgetting occurs in normal subjects between immediate recall and 20- or 30-min delay intervals, a substantial decline (of about 10 points) does occur after intervals of about 1 month (Tombaugh & Hubley, 1991).

With regard to the recognition trial, Meyers and Lange (1994) reported that the task is effective in discriminating brain-injured individuals from normal subjects and from persons with psychiatric disorders.

Ecological Validity

Hemispatial deficits noted on the ROCF copy trial are related to inpatient falls (Rapport et al., 1995). Recall of the complex figure shows a moderate relation to functional memory, assessed via the Rivermead Behavioral Memory Test (Ostrosky-Solis et al., 1998). In psychiatric patients, recognition scores correlated with overall functional ability better than recall scores did (Meyers & Lange, 1994). The higher the recognition trial score, the more independently functioning were the subjects.

In criminal offenders, organizational quality is linked to self-reported impulsivity (Cornell et al., 1997). More impulsive individuals were less likely to follow a well-organized plan; however, self-reported impulsivity did not affect copy or recall accuracy.

Malingering

The ROCF may also be useful in the detection of malingering. For example, Knight and Meyers (1995) found that individuals instructed to malinger could be distinguished from brain-damaged individuals by a pattern of poorer level of accuracy, slower production speed, and poorer delayed and recognition memory (see also Meyers & Meyers, 1995b). Meyers and Volbrecht (1999) examined memory error patterns (MEPs) in litigants, nonlitigants, suspected malingerers (based on litigation status and failure on effort measures), and simulators. They reported that all of the malingerers and most (80%) of the simulators produced either a "storage" MEP (defined as a decline of more than 3 T scores from the 3-min delayed recall trial to the recognition trial) or an "attention" MEP (achieved when 3-min delayed recall, 30-min delayed recall, and recognition scores all fall below a T score of 24).

Lu et al. (2003) examined patients with suspect effort (based on litigation status, noncredible cognitive performance on other tasks, and behavioral indicators of suspect effort) and patients with various neurological and psychiatric disorders who had or did not have memory impairment. They found that patients suspected of poor effort displayed significantly lower recognition scores than did patients with bona fide visual memory impairment. The presence of one or more atypical recognition errors (items 1, 4, 6, 10, 11, 16, 18, and 21, which are rarely answered incorrectly by normal subjects or brain-damaged patients) was also more common among the patients with suspect effort. However, individual ROCF scores (copy, immediate recall, true-positive recognition, false-positive errors) were not very sensitive in capturing suspect effort. Nor were particular configurations on the various test

Table 10–104 Positive Predictive Values (PPV) and Negative Predictive Values (NPV) for ROCF Scores at Base Rates of 15%, 30%, and 45%

Scores	15%		30%		45%	
	PPV%	NPV%	PPV%	NPV%	PPV%	NPV%
Copy						
≤27	52.6	91.7	70.4	81.2	82.9	68.8
≤25	64.3	91.2	81.0	80.4	89.7	67.7
Immediate Recall						
≤10	36.0	90.3	56.7	78.6	72.2	65.2
≤9	43.8	89.3	63.6	77.4	77.8	63.4
True-Positive Recognition						
≤5	55.6	91.8	76.9	82.4	85.7	69.9
≤4	58.3	89.7	77.8	78.2	88.0	65.0
≤3	71.4	88.4	90.0	75.4	93.3	61.1
False-Positive Errors						
>3	33.3	86.6	54.5	72.6	69.2	57.4
>4	100.0	85.8	100.0	72.0	100.0	56.5
Combination Score						
≤47	60.9	95.2	78.4	90.1	88.0	82.1
≤45	70.0	95.4	84.8	89.5	91.5	81.5
≤43	68.4	94.5	83.9	87.6	90.7	77.6
≤42	68.8	92.9	84.6	84.3	91.7	72.8

Note: The recognition trial was given after the immediate-recall trial. Combination score = copy score + [(true-positive recognition − atypical recognition score) × 3]

Source: Adapted from Lu et al., 2003.

trials identified by Meyers and Volbrecht (1999) sensitive to noncredible performance.

Positive and negative predictive values for various ROCF scores, at differing base rates, are shown in Table 10–104. A cutoff score of 25 or less for the copy trial resulted in a PPV of 90% and an NPV of 68% at the estimated study base rate of 45%. For the true-positive recognition score, a cutoff point of 5 or less yielded a PPV of 86% and an NPV of 70% at a similar base rate. To improve classification accuracy, a combination score incorporating the copy, true-positive recognition, and atypical recognition error scores was constructed. A cutoff score of 45 or less yielded a sensitivity of 74% while misclassifying about 4% of patients with verbal memory impairment, 12% of those without visual memory impairment, and 3% of those with memory impairment. This same cutoff resulted in PPVs of 70% to 91.5% and NPVs of 81.5% to 95.4% at the estimated study base rate of 45% and alternative base rates of 15% and 30%. The equation for the combination score is as follows:

$$\text{Combination score} = \text{Copy score} + [(\text{true-positive recognition} - \text{Atypical recognition errors}) \times 3]$$

Even though individual test scores are not particularly sensitive to suspect effort, examination of individual scores

may alert the clinical to the possibility of suspect effort (Lu et al., 2003). Therefore, when abnormal scores are obtained (e.g., true-positive recognition score ≤3, >4 false positive errors), they may be considered pathognomonic for suspect effort.

Indices derived from the ROCF show moderate correlations with other measures of suspect effort; however, none exceeds 50% shared score variance (Nelson et al., 2003). The implication is that the information provided by the ROCF contributes additional information that is helpful in evaluating effort.

COMMENT

Overall, the ROCF provides a rich source of information about a variety of cognitive processes, including visual-spatial skills, visual-construction ability, visual memory, and executive dysfunction in adults as well as children. The inclusion of the recognition trial appears to be a useful addition to recall testing. Analysis of the profile or pattern of test scores on the various components (copy, recall, and recognition trials) is recommended (e.g., Meyers & Meyers, 1995b) and may help to distinguish among disorders. For example, Kixmiller et al. (2000) noted that three amnesic patient groups (anterior communicating artery, Korsakoff's disease, medial temporal lobe) displayed different profiles of visual-perceptual accuracy, organization, and recall performance on the ROCF.

It should be noted that the distribution of scores for the copy and recognition conditions are not normally distributed. The majority of healthy individuals are able to draw the figure without major distortions and obtain high scores on the recognition trial. Therefore, a label of "superior" given to a high copy or recognition score is meaningless; on the other hand, low performance has clinical significance (see also Mitrushina et al., 2005). Further, interpretation of the recall scores (see also Meyers & Meyers, 1995b) must consider whether the initial copy is performed adequately. Disrupted encoding (e.g., due to visual-perceptual or organizational difficulties) might be suggested if initial copy is poor. Disrupted storage may be suggested if recall trials are low. One may raise the question of a retrieval problem if the Recognition Total Correct score is higher than the 3- and 30-min recall scores. These hypotheses, however, need to be evaluated further with additional instruments.

The ROCF affords the examinee multiple approaches and strategies. As Seidman et al. (2003) pointed out, there is no obvious beginning or end; there are many ways (more or less efficient) in which a person can arrive at an accurate rendition, and there are built-in visual components that lend themselves to being perceived as large-scale organization features or small details. These features allow measurement of strategic processes such as planning and monitoring because some approaches are more common and more efficient than others, thus providing sensitivity to unusual performance (Akshoomoff et al., 2002).

Numerous systems have been developed to assess accuracy and qualitative (e.g., planning, organizational) aspects. The most extensive quantitative systems are those developed by Meyers and Meyers (RCTF; 1995b), Denman (1987), and Fastenau (ECTF; 2002), whereas the most comprehensive qualitative systems are those of Bernstein and Waber (DSS-ROCF; 1996) and Stern (BQSS; 1999). In general, the literature shows that qualitative copy scores are correlated significantly with both copy accuracy and recall scores. Additionally, most of these qualitative copy scores correlate moderately with measures of executive ability and appear to be useful in characterizing developmental patterns and distinguishing patients from controls. As yet, no procedure has been uniformly accepted (Troyer & Wishart, 1997), although our impression is that some, such as those of Bernstein and Waber (1996) and Stern et al. (1994, 1999) are gaining popularity in the literature. The DSS-ROCF norms (Bernstein & Waber, 1996) focus on children, and the BQSS is normed for young to older adults. In each case, the logic of the scores generated could be extended across the lifespan (Knight, 2003). Their advantage lies in their ability to characterize unique differences among patients that are not evident when using the traditional 36-point scoring system.

A number of alternate figures have been proposed, with the Taylor Figure the most commonly reported. It is important to bear in mind that the Rey Figure is harder to recall than the Taylor Figure (or MCG figures), and it may be more sensitive to the presence of visual memory deficits. Memory performance on the Taylor Figure should be evaluated against normative data that are specific to this figure and should never be compared against normative data for the Rey Figure.

The test can do "double duty" (Meyers & Volbrecht, 2003). Not only can it be used to assess cognitive function, but it also shows potential for detection of suspect effort. In particular, inclusion of the recognition trial increases the test's effectiveness for detection of noncredible performance. The scores derived from the test appear to provide relatively independent sources of information regarding the validity of test results. However, sensitivity of the various measures derived from the ROCF is modest, suggesting that other sources of information are important.

REFERENCES

Akshoomoff, N. A., & Stiles, J. (1995a). Developmental trends in visuospatial analysis and planning: I. Copying a complex figure. *Neuropsychology, 9*, 364–377.

Akshoomoff, N. A., & Stiles, J. (1995b). Developmental trends in visuospatial analysis and planning: II. Memory for a complex figure. *Neuropsychology, 9*, 378–389.

Akshoomoff, N. A., Feroleto, C. C., Doyle, R. E., & Stiles, J. (2002). The impact of early unilateral brain injury on perceptual organization and visual memory. *Neuropsychologia, 40*, 539–561.

Anderson, V. A., & Lajoie, G. (1996). Development of memory and learning skills in school-aged children: A neuropsychological perspective. *Applied Neuropsychology, 3/4*, 128–139.

Anderson, P., Anderson, V., & Garth, J. (2001). Assessment and development of organizational ability: The Rey Complex Figure Organizational Strategy Score (RCF-OSS). *The Clinical Neuropsychologist, 15*, 81–94.

Anderson, V., Lajoie, G., & Bell, R. (1997). *Neuropsychology assessment of the school-aged child.* Department of Psychology, Royal Children's Hospital, Melbourne, Australia.

Ardila, A., & Rosselli, M. (1989). Neuropsychological characteristics of normal aging. *Developmental Neuropsychology, 5*, 307–320.

Ardila, A., & Rosselli, M., & Rosas, P. (1989). Neuropsychological assessment in illiterates: Visuospatial and memory abilities. *Brain and Cognition, 11*, 147–166.

Ardila, A., Lopera, F., Rosselli, M., Moreno, S., Madrigal, L., Arango-Lasprilla, J. C., Arcos, M., Murcia, C., Arango-Viana, J. C., & Ossa, J. (2000). Neuropsychological profile of a large kindred with familial Alzheimer's disease caused by the E280A single presenilin-1 mutation. *Archives of Clinical Neuropsychology, 15*, 515–528.

Ashton, V. L., Donders, J., & Hoffman, N. M. (2005). Rey Complex Figure test performance after traumatic brain injury. *Journal of Clinical and Experimental Neuropsychology, 27*, 55–64.

Awad, N., Tsiakas, M., Gagnon, M., Mertens, V. B., Hill, E., & Messier, C. (2004). Explicit and objective scoring criteria for the Taylor Complex Figure Test. *Journal of Clinical and Experimental Neuropsychology, 26*, 405–415.

Barr, W. B., Chelune, G. J., Hermann, B. P., Loring, D., Perrine, K., Strauss, E., Trenerry, M. R., & Westerveld, M. (1997). The use of figural reproduction tests as measures of nonverbal memory in epilepsy surgery candidates. *Journal of the International Neuropsychological Society, 3*, 435–443.

Bennett-Levy, J. (1984). Determinants of performance on the Rey-Osterrieth Complex-Figure Test: An analysis, and a new technique for single-case measurement. *British Journal of Psychology, 23*, 109–119.

Bernstein, J. H., & Waber, D. P. (1996). *Developmental Scoring System for the Rey-Osterrieth Complex Figure.* Odessa, Fla.: Psychological Assessment Resources.

Berry, D. T. R., & Carpenter, G. S. (1992). Effect of four different delay periods on recall of the Rey-Osterrieth Complex Figure by older persons. *The Clinical Neuropsychologist, 6*, 80–84.

Berry, D. T. R., Allen, R. S., & Schmitt, F. A. (1991). Rey-Osterrieth Figure: Psychometric characteristics in a geriatric sample. *The Clinical Neuropsychologist, 5*, 143–153.

Bigler, E. D., Johnson, S. C., Anderson, C. V., Blatter, D. D., Gale, S. D., Russo, A. A., Ryser, D. K., Macnamara, S. E., & Abildskov, T. J. (1996). Traumatic brain injury and memory: The role of hippocampal atrophy. *Neuropsychology, 10*, 333–342.

Bigler, E. D., Rosa, L., Schultz, F., Hall, S., and Harris, J. (1989). Rey-Auditory Verbal Learning and Rey-Osterrieth Complex Figure Design test performance in Alzheimer's disease and closed head injury. *Journal of Clinical Psychology, 45*, 277–280.

Binder, L. M. (1982). Constructional strategies on complex figure drawing after unilateral brain damage. *Journal of Clinical Neuropsychology, 4*, 51–58.

Blysma, F. W., Bobhole, J. H., Schretlen, D., & Carreo, D. (1995). *A brief reliable approach to coding how subjects copy the Rey-Osterrieth Complex Figure.* Paper presented at the meeting of the International Neuropsychological Society, Seattle, Washington.

Boone, K. B. (2000). The Boston Qualitative Scoring System for the Rey-Osterrieth Complex Figure. *Journal of Clinical and Experimental Neuropsychology, 22*, 430–432.

Boone, K. B., Lesser, I. M., Hill-Gutierrez, E., Berman, N. G., & D'Elia, L. F. (1993). Rey-Osterrieth Complex Figure performance in healthy, older adults: Relationship to age, education, sex, and IQ. *The Clinical Neuropsychologist, 7*, 22–28.

Boone, K. B., Lesser, I. M., Miller, B. L., Wohl, M., Berman, N., Lee, A., Palmer, B., & Back, C. (1995). Cognitive functioning in older depressed outpatients: Relationship of presence and severity of depression to neuropsychological test scores. *Neuropsychology, 9*, 390–398.

Breier, J. I., Plenger, P. M., Castillo, R., Fuchs, K., Wheloss, J. W., Thomas, A. B., et al. (1996). Effects of temporal lobe epilepsy on spatial and figural aspects of memory for a complex geometric figure. *Journal of the International Neuropsychological Society, 2*, 535–540.

Brooks, D. (1972). Memory and head injury. *Journal of Nervous and Mental Disease, 155*, 350–355.

Bush, S., & Marthin, T. A. (2004). Intermanual differences on the Rey Complex Figure Test. *Rehabilitation Psychology, 49*, 76–78.

Caffarra, P., Vezzadini, G., Dieci, F., Zonato, F., & Venneri, A. (2002). Rey-Osterrieth complex figure: Normative values in an Italian population sample. *Neurological Science, 22*, 443–447.

Camara, W. J., Nathan, J. S., & Puente, A. E. (2000). Psychological test usage: Implications in professional psychology. *Professional Psychology: Research and Practice, 31*, 141–154.

Casey, M. B., Winner, E., Hurwitz, I., & DaSilva, D. (1991). Does processing style affect recall of the Rey-Osterrieth or Taylor Complex Figures? *Journal of Clinical and Experimental Neuropsychology, 13*, 600–606.

Chervinsky, A., Mitrushina, M., & Satz, P. (1992). Comparison of four methods of scoring the Rey-Osterrieth Complex Figure Drawing Test on four age groups of normal elderly. *Brain Dysfunction, 5*, 267–287.

Chiulli, S. J., Haaland, K. Y., LaRue, A., & Garry, P. J. (1995). Impact of age on drawing the Rey-Osterrieth figure. *The Clinical Neuropsychologist, 9*, 219–224.

Chiulli, S. J., Yeo, R. A., Haaland, K. Y., & Garry, P. J. (1989). *Complex figure copy and recall in the elderly.* Paper presented at the meeting of the International Neuropsychological Society, Vancouver, Canada.

Cooper, J. A., Sagar, H. J., Jordan, N., Harvey, N. S., & Sullivan, E. V. (1991). Cognitive impairment in early, untreated Parkinson's disease and its relationship to motor disability. *Brain, 114*, 2095–2122.

Cornell, D. G., Roberts, M., & Oram, G. (1997). The Rey-Osterrieth Complex Figure Test as a neuropsychological measure in criminal offenders. *Archives of Clinical Neuropsychology, 12*, 47–56.

Corwin, J., & Bylsma, F. W. (1993). "Psychological Examination of Traumatic Encephalopathy" by A. Rey and "The Complex Figure Copy Test" by P. A. Osterrieth. *The Clinical Neuropsychologist, 7*, 3–21.

Dawson, L. K., & Grant, I. (2000). Alcoholics' initial organizational and problem-solving skills predict learning and memory performance on the Rey-Osterrieth Complex Figure. *Journal of International Neuropsychological Society, 6*, 12–19.

Deckersbach, T., Savage, C. R., Henin, A., Mataix-Cols, D., Otto, M. W., Wilhelm, S., Rauch, S. L., Baer, L., & Jenike, M. A. (2000a). Reliability and validity of a scoring system for measuring organizational approach in the Complex Figure Test. *Journal of Clinical and Experimental Neuropsychology, 22*, 640–648.

Deckersbach, T., Savage, C. R., Phillips, K. A., Wilhelm, S., Buhlmann, U., Rauch, S. L., Baer, L., & Jenike, M. A. (2000b). Characteristics of memory dysfunction in body dysmorphic disorder. *Journal of the International Neuropsychological Society, 6*, 673–681.

Delaney, R. C., Prevey, M. L., Cramer, J., Mattson, R. H., & VA Epilepsy Cooperative Study 264 Research Group. (1992). Test-retest comparability and control subject data for the Rey-Auditory Verbal Learning Test and Rey-Osterrieth/Taylor Complex Figures. *Archives of Clinical Neuropsychology, 7*, 523–528.

Demsky, Y., Carone, D. A., Burns, W. J., & Sellers, A. (2000). Assessment of visual-motor coordination in 6- to 11-yr-olds. *Perceptual and Motor Skills, 91*, 311–321.

Denman, S. B. (1987). *Denman Neuropsychology Memory Scale.* Charleston: S. C.: S. B. Denman.

Diamond, B. J., & DeLuca, J. (1996). Rey-Osterrieth Complex Figure Test performance following anterior communicating artery aneurysm. *Archives of Clinical Neuropsychology, 11*, 21–28.

Diamond, B. J., DeLuca, J., & Kelley, S. M. (1997). Memory and executive functions in amnesic and non-amnesic patients with aneurysms of the anterior communicating artery. *Brain, 120*, 1015–1025.

Diaz-Asper, C., Schretlen, D. J., & Pearlson, G. D. (2004). How well does IQ predict neuropsychological test performance in normal adults. *Journal of the International Neuropsychological Society, 10*, 82–90.

Duley, J. F., Wilkins, J. W., Hamby, S. L., Hopkins, D. G., Burwell, R. D., & Barry, N. S. (1993). Explicit scoring criteria for the Rey-Osterrieth and Taylor Complex figures. *The Clinical Neuropsychologist, 7*, 29–38.

Elderkin-Thompson, V., Boone, K. B., Kumar, A., & Minz, J. (2004a). Validity of the Boston Qualitative Scoring System for the Rey-Osterrieth Complex Figure among depressed elderly patients. *Journal of Clinical and Experimental Neuropsychology, 26*, 598–607.

Elderkin-Thompson, V., Kumar, A., Mintz, J., Boone, K., Bahng, E., & Lavretsky, H. (2004b). Executive dysfunction and visuospatial ability among depressed elders in a community setting. *Archives of Clinical Neuropsychology, 19*, 597–611.

Fastenau, P. S. (1996). Developmental and preliminary standardization of the "Extended Complex Figure Test" (ECFT). *Journal of Clinical and Experimental Neuropsychology, 18*, 63–76.

Fastenau, P. S. (2002). The Extended Complex Figure Test (ECTF). Los Angeles: Western Psychological Services.

Fastenau, P. S., Bennett, J. M., & Denburg, N. L. (1996). Application of psychometric standards to scoring system evaluation: Is "new" necessarily "improved"? *Journal of Clinical and Experimental Neuropsychology, 18*, 462–472.

Fastenau, P. S., Denburg, N. L., & Hufford, B. J. (1999). Adult norms for the Rey-Osterrieth Complex Figure Test and for supplemental recognition and matching trials from the Extended Complex Figure Test. *The Clinical Neuropsychologist, 13*, 30–47.

Fedio, P., Cox, C. S., Neophytides, A., Canal-Frederick, G., et al. (1979). Neuropsychological profile of Huntington's disease: Patients and those at risk. In T. N. Chase, N. S., Wexler, & A. Barbeau (Eds.), *Advances in Neurology* (Vol. 23). New York: Raven Press.

Folbrecht, J. R., Charter, R. A., Walden, D. K., & Dobbs, S. M. (1999). Psychometric properties of the Boston Qualitative Scoring System for the Rey-Osterrieth Complex Figure. *The Clinical Neuropsychologist, 13,* 442–449.

Freeman, R. Q., Giovannetti, T., Lamar, M., Cloud, B. S., Stern, R. A., Kaplan, E., & Libon, D. J. (2000). Visuoconstructional problems in dementia: Contribution of executive systems functions. *Neuropsychology, 14,* 415–426.

Garth, J., Anderson, V., & Wrennall, J. (1997). Executive functions following moderate-to-severe frontal lobe injury: Impact of injury and age at injury. *Pediatric Rehabilitation, 1,* 99–108.

Hamby, S. L., Wilkins, J. W., & Barry, N. S. (1993). Organizational quality on the Rey-Osterrieth and Taylor Complex Figure tests: A new scoring system. *Psychological Assessment, 5,* 27–33.

Harris, C. L., Dinn, W. M., & Marcinkiewicz, J. A. (2002). Partial seizure-like symptoms in borderline personality disorder. *Epilepsy and Behavior, 3,* 433–438.

Hartman, M., & Potter, G. (1998). Sources of age differences on the Rey-Osterrieth Complex Figure Test. *The Clinical Neuropsychologist, 12,* 513–524.

Heaton, R. K., Grant, I., & Mathews, C. G. (1991). *Comprehensive norms for an expanded Halsted-Reitan battery: Demographic corrections, research findings, and clinical applications.* Odessa, Fla.: Psychological Assessment Resources.

Hernandez, M. T., Sauerwein, H. C., Jambaque, I., de Guise, E., Lussier, F., Lortie, A., Dulac, O., & Lassonde, M. (2003). Attention, memory, and behavioural adjustment in children with frontal lobe epilepsy. *Epilepsy and Behavior, 4,* 522–536.

Hoffman, R., & al'Absi, M. (2004). The effects of acute stress on subsequent neuropsychological test performance. *Archives of Clinical Neuropsychology, 19,* 497–506.

Hubley, A. M., & Tremblay, D. (2002). Comparability of total score performance on the Rey-Osterrieth Complex Figure and a modified Taylor Complex Figure. *Journal of Clinical and Experimental Neuropsychology, 24,* 370–382.

Johnstone, B., & Wilhelm, K. L. (1997). The construct validity of the Hooper Visual Organization Test. *Assessment, 4,* 243–248.

Karapetsas, A. N., & Vlachos, F. M. (1997). Sex and handedness in development of visuomotor skills. *Perceptual and Motor Skills, 85,* 131–140.

King, M. C. (1981). Effects of non-focal brain dysfunction on visual memory. *Journal of Clinical Psychology, 37,* 638–643.

Kirk, U., & Kelly, M. S. (1986). *Scoring scale for the Rey-Osterrieth Complex Figure.* Paper presented at the meeting of the International Neuropsychological Society, Denver, Colorado.

Kirkwood, M. W., Weiler, M. D., Holmes Bernstein, J., Forbes, P. W., & Waber, D. P. (2001). Sources of poor performance on the Rey-Osterrieth Complex Figure Test among children with learning difficulties: A dynamic assessment approach. *The Clinical Neuropsychologist, 15,* 345–356.

Kixmiller, J. S., Verfaellie, M., Mather, M. M., & Cermak, L. S. (2000). Role of perceptual and organizational factors in amnesics' recall of the Rey-Osterrieth Complex Figure: A comparison of three amnesic groups. *Journal of Clinical and Experimental Neuropsychology, 22,* 198–207.

Knight, J. A.(2003). ROCF administration procedures and scoring systems. In J. A. Knight (Ed.), *The handbook of Rey-Osterrieth Complex Figure usage: Clinical and research application.* Lutz, Fla.: PAR.

Knight, J. A., & Meyers, J. E. (1995). *Comparison of malingered and brain-injured productions on the Rey-Osterrieth Complex Figure*

Test. Paper presented at the meeting of the International Neuropsychological Society, Seattle, Washington.

Knight, J. A., Kaplan, E., & Ireland, L. D. (2003). Survey findings of Rey-Osterrieth Complex Figure usage. In J. A. Knight (Ed.), *The handbook of Rey-Osterrieth Complex Figure usage: Clinical and research application.* Lutz, Fla.: PAR.

Kolb, B., & Whishaw, I. (1985). *Fundamentals of human neuropsychology* (2nd ed.). New York: W. H. Freeman.

Kramer, J. H., & Wells, A. M. (2004). The role of perceptual bias in complex figure recall. *Journal of Clinical and Experimental Neuropsychology, 26,* 838–845.

Kuehn, S. M., & Snow, W. G. (1992). Are the Rey and Taylor figures equivalent? *Archives of Clinical Neuropsychology, 7,* 445–448.

Lee, G. P., Loring, D. W., & Thompson, J. L. (1989). Construct validity of material-specific memory measures following unilateral temporal lobe ablations. *Psychological Assessment, 1,* 192–197.

Levine, A. J., Miller, E. N., Becker, J. T., Selnes, O. A., & Cohen, B. A. (2004). Normative data for determining significance of test-retest differences on eight common neuropsychological instruments. *The Clinical Neuropsychologist, 18,* 373–384.

Lezak, M. D. (1976, 1983, 1995). *Neuropsychological assessment..* New York: Oxford University Press.

Lezak, M. D., Howieson, D. B., & Loring, D. W. (2004). *Neuropsychological assessment* (4th ed.). New York: Oxford University Press.

Loring, D. W., & Meador, K. J. (2003). The Medical College of Georgia (MCG) complex Figures: Four forms for follow-up. In J. A. Knight (Ed.), *The handbook of Rey-Osterrieth Complex Figure usage: Clinical and research application.* Lutz, Fla.: PAR.

Loring, D. W., Lee, G. P., Martin, R. C., & Meador, K. J. (1988a). Material-specific learning in patients with partial complex seizures of temporal lobe origin: Convergent validation of memory constructs. *Journal of Epilepsy, 1,* 53–59.

Loring, D. W., Lee, G. P., & Meador, K. J. (1988b). Revising the Rey-Osterrieth: Rating right hemisphere recall. *Archives of Clinical Neuropsychology, 3,* 239–247.

Loring, D. W., Martin, R. C., Meador, K. J., & Lee, G. P. (1990). Psychometric construction of the Rey-Osterrieth Complex Figure: Methodological considerations and interrater reliability. *Archives of Clinical Neuropsychology, 5,* 1–14.

Lu, P. H., Boone, K. B., Cozolino, L., & Mitchell, E. (2003). Effectiveness of the Rey-Osterrieth Complex Figure Test and the Meyers and Meyers Recognition Trial in the detection of suspect effort. *The Clinical Neuropsychologist, 17,* 426–440.

Mataix-Cols, D., Alonso, P., Hernandez, R., Deckersbach, T., Savage, C. R., Menchon, J. M., & Vellejo, J. (2003). Relation of neurological soft signs to nonverbal memory performance in obsessive-compulsive disorder. *Journal of Clinical and Experimental Neuropsychology, 25,* 842–851.

Mathews, L. K., Anderson, V., & Anderson, P. (2001). Assessing the validity of the Rey complex figure as a diagnostic tool: Accuracy, recall and organization strategy scores in children with brain insult. *Clinical Neuropsychological Assessment, 2,* 85–99.

Meador, K. J., Loring, D. W., Allen, M. E., Zamrini, E. Y., Moore, E. E., Abney, O. L., & King, D. W. (1991). Comparative cognitive effects of carbamazepine and phenytoin in healthy adults. *Neurology, 41,* 1537–1540.

Meador, K. J., Moore, E. E., Nichols, M. E., Abney, O. L., Taylor, H. S., Zamrini, E. Y., & Loring, D. W. (1993). The role of cholinergic systems in visuospatial processing and memory. *Journal of Clinical and Experimental Neuropsychology, 15,* 832–842.

Meyers, J. E., & Lange, D. (1994). Recognition subtest for the Complex Figure. *The Clinical Neuropsychologist, 8,* 153–166.

Meyers, J. E., & Meyers, K. R. (1995a). Rey Complex Figure Test under four different administration procedures. *The Clinical Neuropsychologist, 9,* 63–67.

Meyers, J., & Meyers, K. (1995b). *The Meyers Scoring System for the Rey Complex Figure and the Recognition Trial: Professional manual.* Odessa, Fla.: Psychological Assessment Resources.

Meyers, J., & Meyers, K. (1996). *Rey Complex Figure and the Recognition Trial: Professional manual. Supplemental norms for children and adolescents.* Odessa, Fla.: Psychological Assessment Resources.

Meyers, J. E., & Volbrecht, M. (1999). Detection of malingerers using the Rey Complex Figure and Recognition Trial. *Applied Neuropsychology, 6,* 201–207.

Meyers, J. E., & Volbrecht, M. E. (2003). A validation of multiple malingering detection methods in a large clinical sample. *Archives of Clinical Neuropsychology, 18,* 261–276.

Miatton, M., Wolters, M., Lannoo, E., & Vingerhoets, G. (2004). Updated and extended normative data of commonly used neuropsychological tests. *Psychologica Belgica, 44,* 189–216.

Mitrushina, M., & Satz, P. (1989). Differential decline of specific memory components in normal aging. *Brain Dysfunction, 2,* 330–335.

Mitrushina, M. & Satz, P. (1991). Effect of repeated administration of a neuropsychological battery in the elderly. *Journal of Clinical Psychology, 47,* 790–801.

Mitrushina, M. M., Boone, K. B., Razani, J., & D'Elia, L. F. (2005). *Handbook of normative data for neuropsychological assessment* (2nd ed.). New York: Oxford University Press.

Mitrushina, M., Satz, P., & Chervinsky, A. B. (1990). Efficiency of recall on the Rey-Osterrieth Complex Figure in normal aging. *Brain Dysfunction, 3,* 148–150.

Nelson, N. W., Boone, K., Dueck, A., Wagener, L., Lu, P., & Grills, C. (2003). Relationships between eight measures of suspect effort. *The Clinical Neuropsychologist, 17,* 263–272.

Ogden, J. A., Growdon, J. H., & Corkin, S. (1990). Deficits on visuospatial tasks involving forward planning in high-functioning Parkinsonians. *Neuropsychiatry, Neuropsychology, and Behavioral Neurology, 3,* 125–139.

Osterrieth, P. A. (1944). Le test de copie d'une figure complex: Contribution a l'étude de la perception et de la mémoire. *Archives de Psychologie, 30,* 286–356.

Ostrosky-Solis, F., & Jaine, R. M., & Ardila, A. (1998). Memory abilities during normal aging. *International Journal of Neuroscience, 93,* 151–162.

Peirson, A. R., & Jansen, P. (1997). Comparability of the Rey-Osterrieth and Taylor forms of the Complex Figure Test. *The Clinical Neuropsychologist, 11,* 244–248.

Pillon, B. (1981). Troubles visuo-constructifs et méthodes de compensation: Résultats de 85 patients atteints de lésions cérébrales. *Neuropsychologia, 19,* 375–383.

Ponton, M. O., Gonzalez, J. J., Hernandez, I., Herrera, L., & Higareda, I. (2000). Factor analysis of the Neuropsychological Screening Battery for Hispanics (NeSBHIS). *Applied Neuropsychology, 7,* 32–39.

Ponton, M. O., Satz, P., Herrera, L., Ortiz, F., Urrutia, C. P., Young, R., D'Elia, L. F., Furst, C. J., & Namerow, N. (1996). Normative data stratified by age and education for the Neuropsychological Screening Battery for Hispanics (NeSBHIS): Initial report. *Journal of the International Neuropsychological Society, 2,* 96–104.

Poreh, A., & Shye, S. (1998). Examination of the global and local features of the Rey Osterrieth Complex Figure using faceted smallest space analysis. *The Clinical Neuropsychologist, 12,* 453–467.

Poulton, R. G., & Moffitt, T. E. (1995). The Rey-Osterrieth Complex Figure Test: Norms for young adolescents and an examination of validity. *Archives of Clinical Neuropsychology, 10,* 47–56.

Rabin, L. A., Barr, W. B., & Burton, L. A. (2005). Assessment practices of clinical neuropsychologists in the United States and Canada: A survey of INS, NAN, and APA Division 40 members. *Archives of Clinical Neuropsychology, 20,* 33–65.

Rapport, L. J., Charter, R. A., Dutra, R., Farchione, T. J., & Kingsley, J. L. (1997). Psychometric properties of the Rey-Osterrieth Complex Figure: Lezak-Osterrieth versus Denman scoring systems. *The Clinical Neuropsychologist, 11,* 46–53.

Rapport, L. J., Dutra, R. L., Webster, J. S., Charter, R., & Morrill, B. (1995). Hemispatial deficits on the Rey-Osterrieth Complex Figure drawing. *The Clinical Neuropsychologist, 9,* 169–179.

Rapport, L. J., Farchione, T. J., Dutra, R. L., Webster, J. S., & Charter, R. (1996). Measures of hemi-inattention on the Rey Figure copy by the Lezak-Osterrieth scoring method. *The Clinical Neuropsychologist, 10,* 450–454.

Rey, A. (1941). L'examen psychologique dans les cas d'encephalopathie traumatique. *Archives de Psychologie, 28,* 286–340.

Romans, S. M., Roeltgen, D. P., Kushner, H., & Ross, J. L. (1997). Executive function in girls with Turner's syndrome. *Developmental Neuropsychology, 13,* 23–40.

Rosenstein, L. D. (1999). Visuoconstructional drawing ability in the differential diagnosis of neurologic compromise versus depression. *Archives of Clinical Neuropsychology, 14,* 359–372.

Rosselli, M., & Ardila, A. (1991). Effects of age, education, and gender on the Rey-Osterrieth Complex Figure. *The Clinical Neuropsychologist, 5,* 370–376.

Rosselli, M., & Ardila, A. (1996). Cognitive effects of cocaine and polydrug abuse. *Journal of Clinical and Experimental Neuropsychology, 18,* 122–135.

Ruffolo, J. S., Javorsky, D. J., Tremont, G., Westervelt, H. J., & Stern, R. A. (2001). A comparison of administration procedures for the Rey-Osterrieth Complex Figure: Flowcharts versus pen switching. *Psychological Assessment, 13,* 299–305.

Sadeh, M., Ariel, R., & Inbar, D. (1996). Rey-Osterrieth and Taylor complex figures: Equivalent measures of visual organization and visual memory in ADHD and normal children. *Child Neuropsychology, 2,* 63–71.

Savage, C. R., Baer, L., Keuthen, N. J., Brown, H. D., Rauch, S. L., & Jenike, M. A. (1999). Organizational strategies mediate nonverbal memory impairment in obsessive-compulsive disorder. *Biological Psychiatry, 45,* 905–916.

Savage, C. R., Deckersbach, T., Wilhelm, S., Rauch, S. L., Baer, L., Reid, T., & Jenicke, M. A. (2000). Strategic processing and episodic memory impairment in obsessive compulsive disorder. *Neuropsychology, 14,* 141–151.

Schreiber, H. E., Javorsky, D. J., Robinson, J., & Stern, R. A. (1999). Rey-Osterrieth Complex Figure performance in adults with attention deficit hyperactivity disorder: A validation study of the Boston Qualitative Scoring System. *The Clinical Neuropsychologist, 13,* 509–520.

Seidman, L. J., Beiderman, J., Faraone, S. V., Weber, W., & Ouellete, C. (1997). Toward defining a neuropsychology of attention deficit-hyperactivity disorder: Performance of children and adolescents from a large clinically referred sample. *Journal of Consulting and Clinical Psychology, 65,* 150–160.

Seidman, L. J., Lanca, M., Kremen, W. S., Faraone, S. V., & Tsuang, M. T. (2003). Organizational and visual memory deficits in schizophrenia and bipolar psychoses using the Rey-Osterrieth Complex Figure: Effects of duration of illness. *Journal of Clinical and Experimental Neuropsychology, 25,* 949–964.

Sherman, E. M. S., Strauss, E., Spellacy, F., & Hunter, M. (1995). Construct validity of WAIS-R factors: Neuropsychological test correlates in adults referred for possible head injury. *Psychological Assessment, 7,* 440–444.

Shin, M. S., Park, S. J., Kim, M. S., Lee, Y. H., Ha, T. H., & Kwon, J. S. (2004). Deficits in organizational strategy and visual memory in obsessive-compulsive disorder. *Neuropsychology, 18,* 665–672.

Shorr, J. S., Delis, D. C., & Massman, P. J. (1992). Memory for the Rey-Osterrieth Figure: Perceptual clustering, encoding, and storage. *Neuropsychologia, 6,* 43–50.

Snow, W. (1979). *The Rey-Osterrieth Complex Figure Test as a measure of visual recall.* Paper presented at the seventh annual meeting of the International Neuropsychological Society, New York.

Somerville, J., Tremont, J., & Stern, R. A. (2000). The Boston Qualitative Scoring System as a measure of executive functioning in Rey-Osterrieth Complex Figure performance. *Journal of Clinical and Experimental Neuropsychology, 22,* 613–621.

Sowell, E. R., Delis, D., Stiles, J., & Jernigan, T. L. (2001). Improved memory functioning and frontal lobe maturation between childhood and adolescence: A structural MRI study. *Journal of the International Neuropsychological Society, 7,* 312–322.

Spreen, O., & Strauss, E. (1991). *A compendium of neuropsychological tests: Administration, norms and commentary.* New York: Oxford University Press.

Stern, R. A., Javorsky, D. J., Singer, E. A., Singer Harris, N. G., Somerville, J. A., Duke, L. M., Thompson, J., & Kaplan, E. (1999). *The Boston Qualitative Scoring System for the Rey-Osterrieth Complex Figure.* Odessa, Fla.: Psychological Assessment Resources.

Stern, R. A., Singer, E. A., Duke, L. M., Singer, N. G., Morey, C. E., Daughtrey, E. W., & Kaplan, E. (1994). The Boston qualitative scoring system for the Rey-Osterrieth Complex Figure: Description and interrater reliability. *The Clinical Neuropsychologist, 8,* 309–322.

Strauss, E., & Spreen, O. (1990). A comparison of the Rey and Taylor figures. *Archives of Clinical Neuropsychology, 5,* 417–420.

Suhr, J. A., & Gunstad, J. (2005). Further exploration of the effect of "diagnosis threat" on cognitive performance in individuals with mild head injury. *Journal of the International Neuropsychological Society, 11,* 23–29.

Taylor, E. M. (1959). *Psychological appraisal of children with cerebral defects.* Cambridge, Mass.: Harvard University Press.

Taylor, H. G., Minich, N. M., Klein, N., & Hack, M (2004). Longitudinal outcomes of very low birth weight: Neuropsychological findings. *Journal of the International Neuropsychological Society, 10,* 149–163.

Taylor, L. B. (1969). Localization of cerebral lesions by psychological testing. *Clinical Neurosurgery, 16,* 269–287.

Taylor, L. B. (1979). Psychological assessment of neurosurgical patients. In T. Rasmussen & R. Marino (Eds.), *Functional neurosurgery.* New York: Raven Press.

Taylor, L. B. (1991). Scoring criteria for the ROCF. In Spreen, O., & Strauss, E. *A compendium of neuropsychological tests: Administration, norms, and commentary.* New York: Oxford University Press.

Tei, H., Miyazaki, A., Iwata, M., Osawa, M., Nagata, Y.,& Maruyama, S. (1997). Early-stage Alzheimer's disease and multiple subcortical infarction with mild cognitive impairment: Neuropsychological comparison using an easily applicable test battery. *Dementia & Geriatric Cognitive Disorders, 8,* 355–358.

Tombaugh, T. N., & Hubley, A. M. (1991). Four studies comparing the Rey-Osterrieth and Taylor complex figures. *Journal of Clinical and Experimental Neuropsychology, 13,* 587–599.

Tombaugh, T. N., Schmidt, J. P., & Faulkner, P. (1992). A new procedure for administering the Taylor Complex Figure: Normative data over a 60-year age span. *The Clinical Neuropsychologist, 6,* 63–79.

Trojano, L., Fragassi, N. A., Chiacchio, L., Izzo, O., Izzo, G., Di Cesare, G., Cristinzio, C., & Grossi, D. (2004). Relationships between constructional and visuospatial abilities in normal subjects and in focal brain-damaged patients. *Journal of Clinical and Experimental Neuropsychology, 26,* 1103–1112.

Troyer, A. K., & Wishart, H. (1996). *A comparison of qualitative scoring systems for the Rey Osterrieth Complex Figure test.* Paper presented at the meeting of the International Neuropsychological Society, Chicago.

Troyer, A. K., & Wishart, H. (1997). A comparison of qualitative scoring systems for the Rey-Osterrieth Complex Figure test. *The Clinical Neuropsychologist, 11,* 381–390.

Tupler, L. A., Welsh, K. A., Asare-Aboagye, Y., & Dawson, D. V. (1995). Reliability of the Rey-Osterrieth Complex Figure in use with memory-impaired patients. *Journal of Clinical and Experimental Neuropsychology, 17,* 566–579.

Uddo, M., Vasterling, J. J., Brailey, K., & Sutker, P. B. (1993). Memory and attention in combat-related post-traumatic stress disorder (PTSD). *Journal of Psychopathology and Behavioral Assessment, 15,* 43–52.

Vingerhoets, G., De Soete, G., & Jannes, C. (1995). Relationship between emotional variables and cognitive test performance before and after open-heart surgery. *The Clinical Neuropsychologist, 9,* 198–202.

Vingerhoets, G., Lannoo, E., & Wolters, M. (1998). Comparing the Rey-Osterrieth and Taylor complex figures: Empirical data and meta-analysis. *Psychologica Belgica, 38-2,* 109–119.

Visser, R. S. H. (1973). *Manual of the Complex Figure Test.* Lisse, Netherlands: Swets & Zeitlinger.

Vlachos, F., Andeou, G., & Andreou, E. (2003). Biological and environmental influences in visuospatial abilities. *Learning and Individual Differences, 13,* 339–347.

Waber, D. P., & Bernstein, J. H. (1995). Performance of learning-disabled and non-learning disabled on the Rey-Osterrieth Complex Figure: Validation of the Developmental Scoring System. *Developmental Neuropsychology, 11,* 237–252.

Waber, D. P., & Holmes, J. M. (1985). Assessing children's copy productions of the Rey-Osterrieth Complex Figure. *Journal of Clinical and Experimental Neuropsychology, 7,* 264–280.

Waber, D. P., & Holmes, J. M. (1986). Assessing children's memory productions of the Rey-Osterrieth Complex Figure. *Journal of Clinical and Experimental Neuropsychology, 8,* 565–580.

Weinstein, C. S., Kaplan, E., Casey, M. B., & Hurwitz, I. (1990). Delineation of female performance on the Rey-Osterrieth Complex Figure. *Neuropsychology, 4,* 117–127.

Wishart, H., Strauss, E., Hunter, M., Pinch, D., & Wada, J. (1993). Cognitive correlates of interictal affective and behavioral disturbances in people with epilepsy. *Journal of Epilepsy, 6,* 98–104.

Wood, F. B., Ebert, V., & Kinsbourne, M. (1982). The episodic-semantic memory distinction in memory and amnesia: Clinical and experimental observations. In L. Cermak (Ed.), *Memory and amnesia.* Hillsdale, N. J.: Lawrence Erlbaum.

Rivermead Behavioural Memory Test–Second Edition (RBMT-II)

PURPOSE

The purpose of the Rivermead Behavioural Memory Test—Second Edition (RBMT-II) is to detect impairment of everyday memory functioning and monitor change over time.

SOURCE

The kit for the RBMT-II includes a manual, two supplements, four test books, 25 scoring sheets, an audiotape, and a timer and costs $437 US. The kit for the Extended Version (RBME-E) includes two stimulus books, two picture cards, a timer, 25 score sheets, and a manual and costs about $558 US. The kit for children (RBMT-C) includes a manual, a supplementary book, 25 scoring sheets, stimulus materials, a packet of gold stars, an audiotape, and a timer and costs about $335 US. All can be ordered from Harcourt Assessment (http://www.harcourt-uk.com).

Other Versions

The RBMT has been translated into a number of languages, including Dutch (Van Balen & Groot Zwaaftink, 1987), German (Markowitsch et al., 1993), Spanish (Perez & Godoy, 1998) and Chinese (Man & Li, 2001).

AGE RANGE

Norms for individuals aged 11 to 94 years are currently available. The children's version (RBMT-C) is appropriate for use with 5- to 10 year-olds.

DESCRIPTION

RBMT/RBMT-II

The RBMT (Wilson et al., 1985) was originally designed to detect memory problems that might interfere with rehabilitation of adults with acquired neurological damage (Cockburn & Keene, 2001; Wilson et al., 1989c). The test does not adhere to any particular theoretical model of memory; instead, it attempts to mimic the demands made on memory by normal daily life (Aldrich & Wilson, 1991). It does this through the use of items that involve either remembering to carry out some everyday task or retaining the type of information needed for adequate everyday functioning. The second edition (RBMT-II) (Wilson et al., 2003b) involves only minor changes to the original: it includes an updated set of photographs that are more representative of the multiracial nature of society, a slight change in the scoring procedure for the Route task, and packaging in a plastic as opposed to the previous cardboard box.

The RBMT (i.e., RBMT-II) consists of 11 subtests that were chosen after a study of memory problems typically experienced by head-injured people (Sunderland et al., 1983; see Table 10–105). The tasks include remembering a person's first and last name, remembering a hidden belonging, remembering an appointment, picture recognition, remembering the gist of a short passage, face recognition, remembering a new route, delivering a message, answering orientation questions, and remembering the date. Two items, remembering a short passage and remembering a route around the room, have both an immediate and a delayed recall component.

Memory for common objects and for faces is assessed using a recognition paradigm in which subjects must identify the original items among distractors. Prospective memory is assessed on three measures: (a) remembering at the end of the session to ask for a personal possession that was put away at the beginning of the session; (b) remembering when an alarm rings to ask a specific question that was assigned when the alarm was set 20 minutes earlier; and (c) remembering to take a message on the route around the room and deliver it at a specific point along the route. Orientation items assess knowledge of time, place, and person. There are four parallel versions of the RBMT/RBMT-II (Versions A through D), so that some of the practice effects caused by repeated testing with the same test can be minimized.

RBMT-C

The childrens' version (RBMT-C; Adrich & Wilson, 1991; Wilson et al., 1991c) is identical to the adult version except that two subtests—remembering a story and the orientation questions—are modified (e.g., prompt questions are included after free recall). In addition, subtests 1 and 2 (Name Learning) and subtest 4 (Remembering an Appointment) are not scored for children younger than 8 years of age.

RBMT-E

The RBMT was designed as a screening test and is not sufficiently sensitive to detect mild deficits. To enhance the test's sensitivity, Wilson and her colleagues decided to devise a more sensitive measure by increasing the level of difficulty through doubling the amount of material to be remembered. Versions A and B of the original test were combined to make

Table 10–105 RBMT, RBMT-E, and RBMT-C Tasks

Subtests 1 and 2	First and Second Names	Subject is shown photographic portraits and asked to recall first and last names of people in the photographs after a delay
Subtest 3	Belonging	A possession of the subject is borrowed and secreted; the subject is requested to ask for the belonging at the end of the test session and remember where it is hidden
Subtest 4	Appointment	An alarm is set, and the examinee is required to ask a particular question when the alarm sounds
Subtest 5	Picture Recognition	Line drawings are shown, and the subject must recognize them from distractors after a delay
Subtest 6	Story (Immediate, Delay)	Subject listens to a story and then recalls it
Subtest 7	Face Recognition	Subject is shown a set of faces and must recognize them from distractors after a delay
Subtest 8	Route (Immediate, Delay)	Subject must retrace a route shown by the examiner
Subtest 9	Messages (Immediate, Delay)	Subject must remember to retrieve a message left on the route
Subtests 10 and 11	Orientation and Date	Subject is asked a set of questions

Version 1 of the RBMT-E, and Versions C and D of the original test were combined to make Version 2 of the RBMT-E (Wilson et al., 1999). Doubling was not considered necessary for the Story subtest, because it does not show ceiling effects in normal individuals. Some additional modifications were made (e.g., adding a third name to the name learning subtest together with a photograph of a person of African-Caribbean or Asian descent; adding extra faces to the face recognition subtest) to avoid ceiling and floor effects. Because of its increased sensitivity, Dr. Wilson tends to use the RBMT-E more often than the RBMT unless dealing with a severely impaired person whose morale might suffer with anything too difficult (B. Wilson, personal communication, January 3, 2004).

ADMINISTRATION

Instructions for administration are given in the manuals (see *Source*). Briefly, the examiner presents stimuli, asks questions, traces a route, and records responses. Abbreviated versions (with some subtests omitted) are suggested in the RBMT manual for individuals with expressive language or perceptual disorders. For patients with expressive language difficulties, the Name, Orientation, and Story subtests are excluded. For perceptually impaired patients, the Route, Orientation, Date, and Faces subtests are excluded. Tables are provided in the RBMT manual for evaluating individuals with language or perceptual problems. This reduces the likelihood of overestimating the severity of memory impairment. If patients are unable to attempt a specific RBMT item (e.g., Story Recall), a filter task needs to be introduced to retain the time sequence of other items (Cockburn et al., 1990a).

The Route Recall task may be difficult to administer to immobile patients. For the standard RBMT, this limitation has been addressed in various ways. For example, patients may be asked to move a small figure around a line drawing of a room (Towle & Wilsher, 1989) or to move a model car around a ground plan of an area laid out with model trees, houses, bridge, and garage (Evans et al., 1996). A similar set of substitute tasks has been proposed for the two versions of the RBMT-E. Clare et al. (2000) suggested that the Route and Message subtests could be replaced by other versions of the tasks (Model Route Immediate, Newspaper Immediate, Model Route Delayed, and Newspaper Delayed) in which small figures are moved around mockups of the tasks (examiners are referred to Clare et al., 2000, to set up their own display). Normative data have been provided for these tasks (see *Normative Data*). As with the standard version, the route is first demonstrated by the tester, and the patient is then asked to demonstrate it both immediately and after a delay.

ADMINISTRATION TIME

The RBMT can be given in about 25 min.

SCORING

Scoring guidelines are found in the manuals.

RBMT/RBMT-II

Two scoring systems are used: a Screening Score of 0 (fail) or 1 (pass) for each item and a more detailed Profile Score of 0 (abnormal), 1 (borderline), or 2 (normal) depending on the raw score for each item, yielding maximum scores of 12 and 24, respectively. The Screening Score indicates whether the patient has memory problems sufficient to interfere with daily functioning, whereas the Standardized Profile Score (SPS) gives an indication of the severity and nature of the difficulty (Wills et al., 2000). The latter is preferred because it uses more of the available information (Cockburn & Smith, 2003).

Scoring of the Immediate and Delayed Routes is slightly different on the RBMT-II (e.g., maximum raw score is now 11 as opposed to 5). The authors (Wilson et al., 2003b) provide some data showing that the new scoring system yields results comparable to those of the original method. The percentage of patients obtaining full, borderline, or failing scores was found to be similar with both methods.

RBMT-C

For the RBMT-C, raw scores on each item are converted to SPSs, corresponding to normal (2 points), borderline (1) and impaired (0). The maximum SPS is 22 for 8- to 10-year-olds, 20 for 7-year-olds, and 18 for 5- and 6-year-olds.

RBMT-E

For the RBMT-E, raw scores for each subtest are converted to Profile Scores, ranging from 0 to 4. For some subtests, the Profile Score depends on age or premorbid IQ (below average, average, above average). The latter can be obtained from tests such as the NART, SCOLP, or WTAR. An overall profile score is also obtained by summing the score from subtests 1 through 11 (maximum possible score, 48) and then converting this total to a score ranging from 0 (impaired) to 4 (exceptionally good memory).

If the model versions of the Route and Messages task are used with the RBMT-E, the Route task is scored with a possible total of 19 points, following the same system as for the standard Route subtest (Clare et al., 2000). One point is scored for each correct location visited, regardless of position in the sequence (a maximum of 9 points). Next, 1 point is scored for starting in the correct place and 1 point for finishing in the correct place (a maximum of 2 points). Next, each location is considered in turn, together with the location following it, and 1 point is scored if both are correct and in the correct order (a maximum of 8 points). Finally, 1 point is deducted for every incorrect or repeated stage. The Newspaper subtest is scored with a maximum of 6 points: For each item, 2 points are awarded for picking the item up spontaneously or 1 point if a prompt is given, and a further 1 point is given if the item is left at the correct location.

DEMOGRAPHIC EFFECTS

Age

RBMT/RBMT-II scores increase with age and reach adult levels at about age 8 years. Some have reported that middle-aged adults show a decline in performance (Fraser et al., 1999; Martin et al., 2000), whereas others have reported that decline emerges only after age 70 years (see *Source*; Elfkides et al., 2002; Van Balen et al., 1996).

On the RBMT-E, age affects performance on Story (delayed), Route (immediate and delayed), Messages (delayed), Appointment, and Belonging subtests, with younger adults performing better than older ones (Wilson et al., 1999).

IQ

Modest-to-moderate correlations of the RBMT with intelligence are reported ($r = .21$ to $.58$; Cockburn & Smith, 1989b, 2003; Fennig et al., 2002; Wilson et al., 1989; Wilson et al., 1990; Wilson et al., 2003b). On the RBMT/ RBMT-II, the influence of intelligence operates primarily through performance on the Orientation and Story recall components of the test (Wilson et al., 1989b). In children, IQ scores correlate with RBMT-C scores in the younger age groups (5–6 years) but not older groups (7+ years; Aldrich & Wilson, 1991; Moradi et al., 1999). IQ affects scores on most RBMT-E subtests (Story, Picture Recognition, Route, Orientation, First and Second Names; Wilson et al., 1999).

Education

Education also affects RBMT performance (Elfkides et al., 2002; Fennig et al., 2002).

Gender

Gender has little influence on performance in adolescents or adults (Aldrich & Wilson, 1991; Man & Li, 2001; Wilson et al., 1990, 1991b), although Elfkides et al. (2002) noted that men performed better than women on the Belonging and Immediate Route tasks.

On the RBMT-E, gender affects scores on some subtests (Route delayed, Messages immediate and delayed, First Names, Appointment, and Belonging), with women performing better than men (Wilson et al., 1999).

Ethnicity

On the RBMT-E, subjects of European, African-Caribbean, and Asian origin were evaluated, with no systematic differences reported (Wilson et al., 1999).

NORMATIVE DATA

RBMT/RBMT-II

Standardization Sample—Adult. The RBMT/RBMT-II was initially standardized on a sample of brain-damaged patients ($N = 176$, mean age = 44.4 years) and a sample of 118 healthy subjects aged 16 to 69 years ($M = 41.17$) with a mean IQ of 106 (range = 68–136; see *Source*). Percentile tables for

Table 10–106 Cutoff points for RBMT-II for Subjects Aged 11–69 Years

Level of Memory Function	Adults and Adolescents of Average Intelligence		Adolescents of Below-Average Intelligence	
	Screening Score	Standardized Profile Score	Screening Score	Standardized Profile Score
Abnormal	<10	<22	<9	<20

Source: Adapted from Wilson et al., 2003b. The reader is referred to Wilson et al. for more precise information.

these groups can be found in the RBMT/RBMT-II manual. These are of minimal use, however, because most of the patients scored below the 5th percentile relative to the normal control group. Accordingly, the authors suggest cutoff points for severity of memory impairment (normal, poor memory, moderately impaired, severely impaired) based on their clinical experience. Screening Scores lower than 10 and Profile Scores lower than 22 are considered abnormal (Wilson et al., 1991b; see Table 10–106). RBMT/RBMT-II scores should be interpreted with caution in individuals with low IQs, because low RBMT/RBMT-II scores may reflect intellectual limitation rather than impaired memory function.

The RBMT was subsequently standardized with community-dwelling elderly people ($N = 119$) aged 70 years and older (Cockburn & Smith, 1989; see Table 10–107). For people older than 70 years of age, a table is provided in the RBMT supplement (Cockburn & Smith, 1989, 2003) so that an individual's profile score can be compared with that expected for a person of similar age and premorbid IQ (measured by the NART). Note that 34 of the older participants were recruited from hospitals, and 4 were unable to complete all of the RBMT tasks due to vision or speech problems. A further 15 were unable to complete the additional tests in the validation study. It is likely, therefore, that the norms provided by Cockburn and Smith (1989) overrepresent the performance of unwell older adults. In addition, no mention is made that participants were screened for dementia.

Other Normative Data for Adults. Scores were higher for a New Zealand sample (Fraser et al., 1999) of 131 well, independently living older adults, aged 60 to 89 years ($M = 72.71$ years) and ranging in education from 6 to 18 years ($M = 10.46$). The participants were reported to be healthy (no history of cerebrovascular accident, cardiac disease, or respiratory illness) and to have no concerns about their memory. All scored above a cutoff point on a modified version of the MMSE. The 70- to 89-year-old volunteers in the New Zealand study scored an average of about 4 points higher on the overall Profile Score than did the participants in the study by Cockburn and Smith (1989). However, the scores of the 60- to 69-year-old group of New Zealanders were lower than those of the 16- to 69-year-old group studied by Wilson et al. (1989b). That is, the standard RBMT norms appear to overestimate the performance of people in the age range 60 to 69 years. Given the better health status of the New Zealand sample, the fact that a cognitive screen for dementia was given, and the provision of separate norms for the 60- to 69-year-old age group, the New Zealand data (shown in Table 10–108) are preferred over those provided by Cockburn & Smith (1989).

Table 10–107 Characteristics of the Older Adults in the Normative Sample for the RBMT

Number	119[a]
Age (years)	70–94
Geographic location	United Kingdom
Sample type	85 randomly selected from records of attending general practitioners; 34 recruited from geriatric day hospital and from occupants of floating beds in a community hospital
Education (years)	Approximately 10
Gender	
Men	44
Women	75
Race/Ethnicity	Not reported
Screening	Not reported

[a]Four people could not complete the RBMT because of poor vision, and one could not complete it because of dysphasia following a stroke.

Source: Adapted from Cockburn & Smith, 1989.

RBMT/RBMT-C

Standardization Sample—Children and Adolescents. Data for healthy adolescents ($N = 85$) aged 11 to 14 years (Wilson et al., 1990) and children ($N = 335$) aged 5 years to 10 years 11 months (Aldrich & Wilson 1991; Wilson et al., 1991c) are also provided (see *Source*). The characteristics of the sample are shown in Tables 10–109, and 10–110 shows the cutoff values for suspect performance according to age. The reader is referred to the test manual for more precise information regarding performance (normal, borderline, impaired).

Adolescents performed like adults, and within the age group 11 to 14 years there were no significant differences (Wilson et al., 1990). The authors suggested that the cutoff points applied to adults can be used with children of average or above-average ability. For those adolescents whose intellectual

Table 10–108 RBMT Subtest and Summary Profile Scores (Mean and *SD*) in a New Zealand Sample, aged 60–89 years

Subtest	60–69 (*n* = 41)		70–79 (*n* = 64)		80–89 (*n* = 64)	
	Raw	Profile	Raw	Profile	Raw	Profile
Names	3.37 (0.99)	1.44 (0.81)	2.89 (1.38)	1.11 (0.96)	2.96 (1.28)	1.23 (0.91)
Belonging	3.49 (0.71)	1.51 (0.71)	3.39 (1.14)	1.53 (0.78)	3.08 (1.35)	1.34 (0.75)
Appointment	1.68 (0.61)	1.71 (0.60)	1.55 (0.71)	1.55 (0.71)	1.23 (0.86)	1.27 (0.83)
Pictures	9.93 (0.26)	1.90 (0.30)	9.91 (0.39)	1.89 (0.40)	9.88 (0.33)	1.92 (0.27)
Story Immediate	6.63 (2.55)	1.59 (0.67)	6.76 (2.36)	1.55 (0.67)	6.58 (1.90)	1.77 (0.43)
Story Delayed	5.70 (2.43)	1.83 (0.44)	5.67 (2.06)	1.80 (0.48)	5.21 (1.95)	1.92 (0.27)
Faces	4.78 (0.48)	1.80 (0.46)	4.66 (0.76)	1.73 (0.54)	4.73 (0.72)	1.69 (0.62)
Route Immediate	4.76 (0.49)	1.76 (0.49)	4.58 (0.66)	1.56 (0.69)	4.77 (0.43)	1.73 (0.53)
Route Delayed	4.73 (0.55)	1.73 (0.55)	4.56 (0.73)	1.56 (0.73)	4.65 (0.63)	1.65 (0.69)
Message	5.63 (0.66)	1.51 (0.78)	5.39 (0.97)	1.45 (0.83)	5.12 (1.31)	1.35 (0.80)
Orientation	8.88 (0.40)	1.88 (0.40)	8.83 (0.42)	1.83 (0.42)	8.92 (0.27)	1.92 (0.27)
Date	1.90 (0.37)	1.90 (0.37)	1.84 (0.51)	1.88 (0.45)	1.92 (0.39)	1.96 (0.20)
Profile Total		20.61 (2.62)		19.55 (3.18)		19.62 (2.47)

Source: Dr. J. Leathem, personal communication, February 17, 2004.

Table 10–109 Characteristics of the Children and Adolescents in the Normative Sample for the RBMT and RBMT-C

Number	Children, 335; adolescents, 85
Age (years)	Children, 5–10; Adolescents, 11–14
Geographic location	United Kingdom
Sample type	Children: Pupils from nine schools, urban and rural; Adolescents: Pupils from three schools, urban, suburban, and rural
Parental education	Not reported
Gender (%)	
Male	About 50
Female	About 50
Race/Ethnicity	Not reported
Screening	Asked for pupils of average, above-average, and below-average IQ; pupils with learning difficulties excluded

Note: Ages 5–6 years, *n* = 63; ages 6–7, *n* = 63; ages 7–8, *n* = 57; ages 8–9, *n* = 50; ages 9–10, *n* = 53; ages 10–11, *n* = 49; age 11, *n* = 20; age 12, *n* = 22; age 13, *n* = 21; age 14, *n* = 22.

Table 10–110 Ranges of Standardized Profile Score for Suspect Functioning for Subjects Aged 5–11 Years on the RBMT-C

Age Group	Suspect
5 years to 6 years 11 months	<16
7 years to 7 years 11 months	<18
8 years to 10 years 11 months	<20

Source: Adapted from Wilson et al., 1991c. The reader is referred to Wilson et al. for more precise information.

functioning is below average, they suggested dropping 1 point from the Screening Score cutoff and 2 points from the SPS cutoff (see Table 10–106).

RBMT-E and Model Versions

Standardization Sample. The test was standardized on a sample of 191 individuals, aged 16 to 76 years (*M* = 39.4, *SD* = 15.45), in England and Australia (see Table 10–111). The sample size was rather small given the wide age range covered and inclusion/exclusion criteria were not specified. The authors suggested that overall Profile Scores of 2 to 4, corresponding to Profile Score totals of 28 to 48, indicate average or better memory. Note that, based on this classification scheme, a significant proportion (25%) of the normative sample obtained scores in the abnormal ranges.

Other Normative Data. The model versions of the Route and Newspaper tasks were given to 111 healthy adults (72 women, 39 men), ranging in age from 16 to 76 years (*M* = 41.1, *SD* = 15.5) with a mean NART score of 113 (*SD* = 7.35, range = 90–127; Clare et al., 2000). The participants were part of the standardization sample for the RBMT-E in Sydney and Cambridge, and the tasks were administered as part of the longer test session in which the full RBMT-E was given. The normative data are reported in Table 10–112.

RELIABILITY

Internal Consistency

A high value of Cronbach's alpha (.86) was demonstrated for the Chinese version of the RBMT (Man & Li, 2001). No information on other versions is available.

Table 10–111 Characteristics of the Adults in the Normative Sample for the RBMT-E

Number	191
Age (years)	16–76 ($M = 39.4$, $SD = 15.45$)[a]
Geographic location	From three cities: Cambridge, UK; London, UK; Sydney, Australia
Sample type	Participants were tested from three ability bands based on either the NART or Spot the Word from the SCOLP (below average, average, above average); within each band, people were assessed from three age levels: 16–19, 30–50, and 51 + years; number within each cell not reported; subjects from Cambridge and Sydney were of European origin; subjects from London were of African–Caribbean and Asian origin
Education	Not reported
Gender	
Male	82
Female	109
Race/Ethnicity	No systematic differences noted
Screening	Not reported

[a]Age ranges: 16–29 years, $n = 70$; 30–50 years, $n = 68$; 51 + years, $n = 53$.

Test-Retest Reliability

Man and Li (2001) administered the same form of the RBMT to stroke patients twice within a 2-week period and reported high test-retest reliability ($r = .89$).

Alternate Form Reliability

RBMT/RBMT-II. Parallel-form reliability was determined by giving two versions of the RBMT to 118 patients (Wilson et al., 1989b, 1991b). All four parallel forms were used, and the order of presentation was random. The interval between test administrations was not reported. Correlations between performances on the various versions ranged from .67 to .88, with all but one higher than .80. Not surprisingly, the finer-grained Profile Score gave a more reliable estimate of the patient's abilities. Considering data from all 118 patients who were tested twice, the correlations between the two scores were .78 for the Screening Score and .85 for the Profile Score. Performance on the second test administration tended to be slightly better than on the first administration, principally due to one item, remembering a belonging. Whether the four forms were of comparable difficulty is not reported. Fraser et al. (1999) gave Version A to 26 older adults and Version B to 105 adults. They found no differences in SPS or subtest raw scores between Versions A and B. The SPSs for the two versions correlated at .94. Man and Li (2001) reported that correlations between raw scores of different versions ranged from .38 to .92. Wilson et al. (2003b) reported that 85 adolescents were given two versions of the RBMT with the order of presentation counterbalanced (interval not reported). Mean scores (Screening, SPS) were the same on both assessments.

RBMT-C. Aldrich and Wilson (1991) reported that children took two versions of the test (AB, BC, CD, or DA) about 48 hours apart. Correlation coefficients were somewhat low for the children's version (RBMT-C) and fell in the range of .44 to .73, depending on age. The lower correlations may reflect ceiling effects in the older age groups (Aldrich & Wilson, 1991). There were no learning effects from first to second administration of different versions of the RBMT-C.

RBMT-E. With regard to the RBMT-E, the two versions were given to 191 control subjects aged 16 to 76 years (see *Source*). A further 6 individuals were administered one version only. The mean age for the 197 subjects was 39.4 years ($SD = 15.45$). Roughly half of the subjects were given Version 1 followed, at least 1 week later, by Version 2; the remainder

Table 10–112 Conversion of Raw Scores to Profile Scores for the Modified Administration of the RBMT-E Model Route and Newspaper Tasks

Task	Subgroups (Age in Years)	Profile Score				
		0	1	2	3	4
Model Route Immediate	Version 1 (<30, 30–50)	0–10	11–13	14–17	18	19
	Version 1 (>50)	0–8	9–11	12–15	16–18	19
	Version 2 (all ages)	0–7	8–11	12–16	17–18	19
Model Route Delayed	Version1 (<30, 30–50)	0–8	9–12	13–16	17–18	19
	Version 1 (>50)	0–7	8–9	10–15	16–18	19
	Version 2 (all ages)	0–8	9–11	12–15	16–18	19
Newspaper Immediate	All	0–2	3	4	5	6
Newspaper Delayed	All	0–2	3	4	5	6

Source: From Clare et al., 2000. Reprinted with the permission of the British Psychological Society.

were given Version 2 followed by Version 1. There were significant differences between the two versions on immediate story recall, immediate and delayed recall of the route and recall of surnames. These differences (<1 raw score point) are taken into account in the scaled scoring.

Interrater Reliability

High interrater agreement (100%) was reported for both scoring procedures on the RBMT (Wilson et al., 1989b, 1991b). Man and Li (2001) also reported high interrater reliability (.74 to .95) when two raters evaluated stroke patients on the Chinese version of the RBMT.

VALIDITY

Relations With Other Measures

The RBMT shows moderate correlations with various laboratory measures of memory, including the Warrington Recognition Memory Test, Wechsler Memory Scale (WMS), Luria Nebraska Memory Scale, recall of the Rey Figure, and the Rey Auditory Verbal Learning Test (Goldstein & Polkey, 1992; Fennig et al., 2002; Makatura et al., 1999; Malec et al., 1990; Wilson et al., 1989c). RBMT scores are less strongly correlated with measures of attention (e.g., Digit Span Forward or Backward) in adults (Makatura et al., 1999; Wilson et al., 1990). However, in children aged 7 to 9 years, a moderate relationship was observed (Aldrich & Wilson, 1991).

The RBMT shows a strong correlation with the MMSE ($r > .85$; Cockburn & Keene, 2001; Man & Li, 2001) and with a short form of the WAIS-R ($r = .57$; Fennig et al., 2002). Malec et al. (1990) reported that the test was not significantly correlated with the Verbal Comprehension factor of the WAIS-R, nor with measures that are thought to tap executive dysfunction (e.g., Trails B, Stroop, Mazes). It did, however, show a moderate correlation with the Perceptual Organization factor of the WAIS-R.

The implication is that the RBMT does assess specific memory processes tapped by conventional laboratory memory tests (immediate learning and delayed recall of new information) but is not entirely redundant with these tasks. Further, in adults, the RBMT does not depend on remotely acquired, well-established memories. However, performance may be confounded by general conceptual status and visual-spatial deficits.

Factor Analytic Findings

Efklides et al. (2002) reported that confirmatory factor analysis of the RBMT along with the WMS and the Everyday Memory Questionnaire (EMQ, consisting of subjective metamemory reports) in a sample of healthy adults, as well as in patients with dementia of the Alzheimer type (AD), suggested a verbal memory factor (RBMT Story subtests, WMS Logical Memory), a new learning factor (RBMT Names and Appointment subtests, WMS Associate Learning), and an orientation factor (RBMT Orientation/Date, WMS Information/Orientation). RBMT visual recognition tasks did not load with the visual reproduction subtest of the WMS. In neither the healthy adults nor the patients with AD was a purely prospective memory component identified (influencing Belonging, Appointment, and Message subtests). Some have also questioned the interpretation of the Message subtest as measure of prospective memory. Maylor (1995) pointed out that this test is not self-initiated, in that the examinee is asked to repeat what the examiner does during the observational component of both the Route and Message subtests.

Clinical Studies

Poor RBMT performance has been noted in patients with a variety of disorders known to affect memory, including dementia (Huppert & Beardsall, 1993), diencephalic damage (Markowitsch et al., 1993), exposure to neurotoxins (Koltai et al., 1996), alcohol-related disorders (Van Balen et al., 1996), stroke (Lincoln & Tinson, 1989; Van Balen et al., 1996; Wilson et al., 1989b, 1991b), schizophrenia (Kelly et al., 2000; Fennig et al., 2002), temporal lobectomy (Goldstein & Polkey, 1992), and traumatic brain injury (TBI; Schwartz & McMillan, 1989; Van Balen et al., 1996; Wilson et al., 1989b, 1991b). There is also evidence that RBMT scores correlate moderately with length of coma (Van Balen et al., 1996) and duration of posttraumatic amnesia (Geffen et al., 1991; Schwartz & McMillan, 1989). Users of MDMA (Ecstasy) who were abstinent for at least 2 weeks before testing also showed impaired prospective memory (Appointment and Message subtests; Zakzanis et al., 2003), and continued use of the drug (over the course of 1 year) was associated with a progressive decline in terms of immediate and delayed Story Recall (Zakzanis & Young, 2001). Adults with mild/moderate intellectual disabilities have particular difficulty with items that rely primarily on the recall of verbal information (e.g., Story recall, Names; Martin et al., 2000).

As might be expected, patients with AD are impaired on the RBMT (Cockburn & Kenne, 2001; Efklides et al., 2002; Van Balen et al., 1996). A modified version (e.g., incorporating additional scores for correct naming of pictures, addition of questions to elicit cued recall after immediate and delayed story recall) proved useful in tracking change in AD patients over a 3-year interval (Cockburn & Keene, 2001). The RBMT may also be of some use in distinguishing vascular from nonvascular forms of dementia. In addition to the overall Profile and Screening scores, Glass (1998) found that groups differed on the Appointment, Story (Immediate), and Route (Immediate, Delayed) subtests, with vascular dementia patients showing more intact ability. The RBMT-C has been used administered to children (Wilson & Ivani-Chalian, 1995) and adults (Hon et al., 1998) with Down syndrome, although individuals with severe or profound disability are untestable on this task (Hon et al., 1998).

Of note, the RBMT appears to be as effective as the WMS-R in discriminating among patient groups. Perez and Godoy

(1998) showed that the RBMT correctly classified 80% of AD patients, 75% of older adults with complaints of memory problems, 75% of patients diagnosed with complex partial epilepsy, and 60% of controls, resulting in a mean of 72.5% correctly classified (compared with 66.3% for the WMS-R).

Expressive language disorders impair performance on some of the RBMT items (memory for the Name, delayed Story Recall, and Orientation items), whereas perceptual problems impair scores on other items (the immediate and delayed Route, Orientation, Date, and Faces items; see also Malec et al., 1990). Wilson et al. (1989b) recommended that, when assessing patients with language or perceptual disturbances, the examiner should omit these items and evaluate performance on the remaining individual items. Some normative data for such modified versions are provided in the RBMT manual (see also Cockburn et al., 1990a, 1990b), allowing the clinician to detect sparing or impairment of memory despite the presence of other neuropsychological impairment (e.g., word-finding difficulties). Wilson and her colleagues (see *Source*; Cockburn et al., 1990a) reported that similar patterns of performance were shown by patients with left-hemisphere strokes without language loss and by those with right-hemisphere strokes. The implication is that side of lesion per se may be a relatively minor factor in the measurement of preserved everyday memory ability (see also Goldstein & Polkey, 1992).

According to the test authors, the RBMT is not influenced by self-reported anxiety or depression (Wilson et al., 1989c). There is evidence however, that anxiety can activate monitoring/checking procedures that may impede task performance (e.g., on the Appointment task), perhaps by interfering with working memory capacity (Cockburn & Smith, 1994). Patients with major depressive disorder are impaired on the test (Fennig et al., 2002). Tarbuck and Paykel (1995) reported improvement after recovery; however, in the absence of a control group, the confounding effect of practice must also be considered. There is also evidence that children and adolescents (aged 11–17 years) with posttraumatic stress disorder show poorer memory performance compared with controls (Moradi et al., 1999).

RBMT-E. There is evidence showing that those brain-injured individuals who score in the normal or near-normal range on the original RBMT have deficits on the RBMT-E (Wills et al., 2000; Wilson et al., 1999). These patients also score below matched controls on the test, particularly on the Route and Message subtests (Wills et al., 2000). There is additional evidence that the test is sensitive to mild forms of memory impairment. Stephens et al. (2003) reported that women who use hormone replacement therapy score higher than nonusers on the RBMT-E, in particular on the Story (immediate and delayed) and Message (delayed) subtests.

Ecological/Predictive Validity

The RBMT correlates moderately well with therapist-observed rates of memory lapses and subjective ratings of memory problems by patients and relatives (Aldrich & Wilson, 1991;

Cockburn & Keene, 2001; Davis et al., 1995; Goldstein & Polkey, 1992; Koltai et al., 1996; Lincoln & Tinson, 1989; Malec et al., 1990; Schwartz & McMillan, 1989; Wilson et al., 1989b, 1991b). When premorbid ability is taken into account, a positive relationship between memory complaints and RBMT performance is also demonstrated (Levy-Cushman & Abeles, 1998). Some have suggested that the RBMT is more closely related to subjective ratings of everyday memory problems than are standard psychological measures (Lincoln and Tinson, 1989; Van der Feen et al., 1988; Makatura et al., 1999; but see Koltai et al., 1996, who reported that, for individuals exposed to neurotoxins, the RBMT and other tests such as the WMS-R did not differ significantly in their relation to estimates of everyday memory functioning).

Scores on the RBMT correlate moderately with employment status (Geffen et al., 1991: Schwartz & McMillan, 1989), the ability to learn a new technological skill (Wilson et al., 1989a), community integration/functioning (Colantonio et al., 2000; Kelly et al., 2000), everyday psychosocial functioning (Fennig et al., 2002), general physical activity (Cockburn & Smith, 1989), activities of daily living (Cockburn & Smith, 1989) and the ability to live independently (Goldstein et al., 1992; Man & Li, 2001; Wilson, 1991a; Wilson et al., 1990). For example, Wilson and colleagues (1990; 1991a) reported that people who scored below 12 on the SPS were unlikely to be living alone, or in paid employment, or in full-time education, whereas most of those scoring higher than 12 were likely to be engaged in one or more of these activities.

The RBMT may be better able to distinguish the independent from the dependent individuals than standard psychological measures are (Fennig et al., 2002; Wilson, 1991a), although this may hold only for certain patient populations (e.g., demented patients, Goldstein et al., 1992; patients with schizophrenia, Fennig et al., 2002). There is some evidence that prediction of everyday adaptive abilities can be improved by the use of additional tests of executive function, in particular Trails B (Malec et al., 1990).

The RBMT is also predictive of long-term memory outcome after TBI. Wiseman et al. (2000) reported that baseline RBMT scores obtained before hospital discharge were predictive of informant reports (but not self-reports) of memory impairment, as well as performance on tests of memory, about 10 years after injury. Baseline RBMT scores were also predictive of long-term social functioning among patients with schizophrenia (Guaiana et al., 2004).

COMMENT

The literature suggests that the RBMT is a useful complement to more traditional memory-assessment techniques, sampling memory behaviors characteristic of everyday life. It can be used across various age groups and cultures. The test has reasonable convergent and divergent validity, has been used with a wide selection of patient populations, has impressive evidence of ecological validity, and may be better than standard memory tests in predicting everyday memory problems.

The inclusion of prospective memory tasks (remembering to carry out actions) is unique among memory tests. This feature may make it a particularly useful measure in populations such as the elderly, because such tasks may be especially susceptible to the early stages of dementia (Huppert and Beardsall, 1993). One should bear in mind, however, that the interpretation of the Message subtest as a measure of prospective memory is not universally accepted.

Of note, no guidelines are provided for speed of presentation of the story subtest. There is evidence that speed of presentation can substantially alter story recall in a wide range of individuals, with better recall in slow versus fast presentation conditions (Arnett, 2004). Relatedly, when alternate forms of the test were used for repeat testing, different speeds of administration at the various points in time could result in incorrect inferences about any changes in performance (Arnett, 2004). It is important to standardize speed of presentation to ensure that erroneous conclusions are not drawn (Arnett, 2004).

The RBMT/RBMT-II has a low ceiling and is not suitable for detecting mild forms of impairment (Wilson et al., 1989c). Other tests, including the RBMT-E, are preferred in such cases. Therefore, the RBMT is most suitable for patients with moderate to severe impairment. Further, although the RBMT can indicate specific memory deficits, it does not appear to be particularly sensitive to such disorders (Goldstein & Polkey, 1992; Wilson et al., 1989b). More traditional laboratory methods are needed to identify the nature of the memory impairment.

The RBMT/RBMT-II correlates highly with the MMSE, suggesting that there may be little benefit in routinely giving the longer RBMT for screening purposes in cases of suspected dementia; however, performance on individual items may provide useful information about preserved abilities as the overall MMSE score drops (Cockburn & Keene, 2001).

The RBMT/RBMT-II can be given to children, although scores should be interpreted with caution in those with below-average intellectual functioning (Aldrich & Wilson, 1991; Wilson et al., 1990). For individuals aged 60 years and older, normative data provided by Fraser et al. (1999) should be used. The norms included with the test manual appear to overestimate performance of individuals aged 60 to 69 years and to underestimate performance of people older than 70 years of age. The description of the RBMT-E normative sample is somewhat sparse. In addition, the classification scheme may require some adjustment, because use of this scheme results in a significant proportion (about 25%) of the standardization sample obtaining abnormal scores.

A modified version of the RBMT is recommended (see *Source*, Cockburn et al., 1990a, 1990b) for patients younger than 70 years of age who are experiencing expressive language deficits or perceptual problems. Unfortunately, tables are not provided for elderly individuals with language or perceptual difficulties. In such cases, a total score should not be calculated, but comparisons of individual item scores can be made.

Modifications are also available for mobility-impaired individuals. However, a task based on remembering a route traced by a model figure may well tap somewhat different aspects of memory than one that requires the individual to navigate around the room, because in the latter case the person's own position is changing relative to the environment, whereas this does not occur in the model version (Clare et al., 2000).

Further, additional research is needed regarding the test's psychometric properties. Although interrater reliability is high, information regarding internal consistency and test-retest reliability is meager for the standard form and the RBMT-C and nonexistent for the RBMT-E. Additional validity information is needed for the RBMT-C.

REFERENCES

Aldrich, F. K., & Wilson, B. (1991). Rivermead Behavioural Memory Test for Children (RBMT-C): A preliminary evaluation. *British Journal of Clinical Psychology, 30,* 161–168.

Arnett, P. A. (2004). Speed of presentation influences story recall in college students and persons with multiple sclerosis. *Archives of Clinical Neuropsychology, 19,* 507–523.

Clare, L., Wilson, B. A., Emslie, H., Tate, R., & Watson, P. (2000). Adapting the Rivermead Behavioral Memory Test Extended Version (RBMT-E) for people with restricted mobility. *British Journal of Psychology, 39,* 363–369.

Cockburn, J., & Keene, J. (2001). Are changes in everyday memory over time in autopsy-confirmed Alzheimer's disease related to changes in reported behavior? *Neuropsychological Rehabilitation, 11,* 201–271.

Cockburn, J., & Smith, P. T. (1989, 2003). *The Rivermead Behavioural Memory Test. Supplement 3: Elderly People.* Bury St. Edmunds, England: Thames Valley Test Company.

Cockburn, J., & Smith, P. T. (1994). Anxiety and errors of prospective memory among elderly people. *British Journal of Psychology, 85,* 273–282.

Cockburn, J., Wilson, B., Baddeley, A., & Hiorns, R. (1990a). Assessing everyday memory in patients with dysphasia. *British Journal of Clinical Psychology, 29,* 353–360.

Cockburn, J., Wilson, B. A., Baddeley, A., & Hiorns, R. (1990b). Assessing everyday memory in patients with perceptual problems. *Clinical Rehabilitation, 4,* 129–135.

Colantonio, A., Ratcliff, G., Chase, S., & Escobar, M. (2000). Is cognitive performance related to level of community integration many years after traumatic brain injury? *Brain and Cognition, 44,* 19–20.

Davis, A. M., Cockburn, J. M., & Wade, D. T. (1995). A subjective memory assessment questionnaire for use with elderly people after stroke. *Clinical Rehabilitation, 9,* 238–244.

Efklides, A., Yiultsi, E., Kangellidou, T., Kounti, F., Dina, F., & Tsolaki, M. (2002). Wechsler Memory Scale, Rivermead Behavioral Memory Test, and Everyday Memory questionnaire in healthy adults and Alzheimer patients. *European Journal of Psychological Assessment, 18,* 63–77.

Evans, J. J., Wilson, B. A., & Emslie, H. (1996). Selecting, administering and interpreting cognitive tests. Bury St. Edmunds: Thames Valley Test Company.

Fennig, S., Mottes, A., Ricter-Levin, G., Treves, I., & Levkovitz, Y. (2002). Everyday memory and laboratory memory tests: General function prediction in schizophrenia and remitted depression. *Journal of Nervous & Mental Disease, 190,* 677–682.

Fraser, S., Glass. J. N., & Leathem, J. M. (1999). Everyday memory in an elderly New Zealand population: Performance on the Rivermead

Behavioral Memory Test. *New Zealand Journal of Psychology, 28,* 118–123.

Geffen, G. M., Encel, J. S., & Forrester, G. M. (1991). Stages of recovery during post-traumatic amnesia and subsequent everyday deficits. *Cognitive Neuroscience and Neuropsychology, 2,* 105–108.

Glass, J. N. (1998). Differential subtest scores on the Rivermead Behavioral Memory Test (RBMT) in an elderly population with diagnosis of vascular or nonvascular dementia. *Applied Neuropsychology, 5,* 57–64.

Goldstein, G., McCue, M., Rogers, J., & Nussbaum, P. D. (1992). Diagnostic differences in memory test based predictions of functional capacity in the elderly. *Neuropsychological Rehabilitation, 2,* 307–317.

Goldstein, L. H., & Polkey, C. E. (1992). Behavioural memory after temporal lobectomy or amygdalo-hippocampectomy. *British Journal of Clinical Psychology, 31,* 75–81.

Guiaiana, G., Tyson, P., & Mortimer, A. M. (2004). The Rivermead Behavioral Memory Test can predict social functioning among schizophrenic patients treated with clozapine. *International Journal of Psychiatry in Clinical Practice, 8,* 245–249.

Hon, J., Huppert, F. A., Holland, A. J., & Watson, P. (1998). The value of the Rivermead Behavioral Test (Children's Version) in an epidemiological study of older adults with Down syndrome. *British Journal of Clinical Psychology, 37,* 15–29.

Huppert, F. A., & Beardsall, L. (1993). Prospective memory impairment as an early indicator of dementia. *Journal of Clinical and Experimental Neuropsychology, 15,* 805–821.

Kelly, C., Sharkey, V., Morrison, G., Allardyce, J., McReadie, R. G. (2000). Assessing subtle memory impairments in a catchment-area-based population of patients with schizophrenia. *British Journal of Psychiatry, 177,* 348–353.

Koltai, D. C., Bowler, R. M., & Shore, M. D. (1996). Rivermead Behavioural Memory Test and Wechsler Memory Scale-Revised: Relationship to everyday memory impairment. *Assessment, 3,* 443–448.

Levy-Cushman, J., & Abeles, N. (1998). Memory complaints in the able elderly. *Clinical Gerontologist, 19,* 3–24.

Lincoln, N. B., & Tinson, D. (1989). The relation between subjective and objective memory impairment after stroke. *British Journal of Clinical Psychology, 27,* 61–65.

Makatura, T. J., Lam, C. S., Leahy, B. J., Castillo, M. T., & Kalpakjian, C. Z. (1999). Standardized memory tests and the appraisal of everyday memory. *Brain Injury, 13,* 355–367.

Malec, J., Zweber, B., & DePompolo, R. (1990). The Rivermead Behavioural Memory Test, laboratory neurocognitive measures, and everyday functioning. *Journal of Head Trauma Rehabilitation, 5,* 60–68.

Man, D. W. K., & Li, R. (2001). Assessing Chinese adults' memory abilities: Validation of the Chinese version of the Rivermead Behavioral Memory Test. *The Clinical Gerontologist, 24,* 27–36.

Markowitsch, H. J., von Cramon, Y., & Schuri, U. (1993). Mnestic performance profile of a bilateral diencephalic infarct patient with preserved intelligence and severe amnestic disturbances. *Journal of Clinical and Experimental Neuropsychology, 15,* 627–652.

Martin, C., West, J., Cull, C., & Adams, M. (2000). A preliminary study investigating how people with mild intellectual disabilities perform on the Rivermead Behavioral Memory Test. *Journal of Applied Research in Intellectual Disabilities, 13,* 186–193.

Maylor, E. A., (1995). Prospective memory in normal ageing and dementia. *Neurocase, 1,* 285–289.

Moradi, A. R., Doost, H. T. N., Taghavi, M. R., Yule, W., & Dalgleish, T. (1999). Everyday memory deficits in children and adolescents with PTSD: Performance on the Rivermead Behavioral Memory Test. *Journal of Child Psychology & Psychiatry and Allied Disciplines, 40,* 357–361.

Perez, M., & Godoy, J. (1998). Comparison between a "traditional" memory test and a "behavioral" memory battery in Spanish patients. *Journal of Clinical and Experimental Neuropsychology, 20,* 496–502.

Schwartz, A. F., & McMillan, T. M. (1989). Assessment of everyday memory after severe head injury. *Cortex, 25,* 665–671.

Stephens, C. V., Hamilton, Y. M., & Pachana, N. A. (2003). Hormone replacement therapy and everyday memory in mid-aged New Zealand women. *New Zealand Journal of Psychology, 32,* 13–21.

Sunderland, A., Harris, B., & Baddeley, A. D. (1983). Do laboratory tests predict everyday behavior? A neuropsychological study. *Journal of Verbal Learning and Verbal Behavior, 22,* 341–357.

Tarbuck, A. F., & Paykel, E. S. (1995). Effects of major depression on the cognitive function of younger and older subjects. *Psychological Medicine, 25,* 285–296.

Towle, D., & Wilsher, C. R. (1989). The Rivermead Behavioural Memory Test: Remembering a short route. *British Journal of Clinical Psychology, 28,* 287–288.

Van Balen, H. G. G., & Groot Zwaftink, A. J. M. (1987). The Rivermead Behavioral Memory Test. Handleiding (The Rivermead Behavioral Memory Test Manual). Reading, England: Thames Valley Test Company.

Van Balen, H. G. G., Westzaan, P. S. H., & Mulder, T. (1996). Stratified norms for the Rivermead Behavioral Memory Test. *Neuropsychological Rehabilitation, 6,* 203–217.

Van der Feen, van Balen, H. G. G., & Eling, P. (1988). Assessing everyday memory in rehabilitation: A validation study. *International Journal of Rehabilitation Research, 11,* 406.

Wills, P., Clare, L., Shiel, A., & Wilson, B. A. (2000). Assessing subtle memory impairment in the everyday memory performance of brain injured people: Exploring the potential of the Extended Rivermead Behavioural Memory Test. *Brain Injury, 14,* 693–704.

Wilson, B. A. (1991a). Long-term prognosis of patients with severe memory disorders. *Neuropsychological Rehabilitation, 1,* 117–134.

Wilson, B., & Ivani-Chalian, R. (1995). Performance of adults with Down's syndrome on the Children's Version of the Rivermead Behavioral Memory Test: A brief report. *British Journal of Clinical Psychology, 34,* 85–88.

Wilson, B. A., Baddeley, A. D., & Cockburn, J. M. (1989a). How do old dogs learn new tricks: Teaching a technological skill to brain-injured people. *Cortex, 25,* 115–119.

Wilson, B. A., Baddeley, A., Cockburn, J., & Hiorns, R. (1989b, 1991b). *Rivermead Behavioural Memory Test: Supplement Two.* Bury St. Edmunds, England: Thames Valley Test Company.

Wilson, B. A., Baddeley, A., Cockburn, J., & Hiorns, R. (1989c). The development and validation of a test battery for detecting and monitoring everyday memory problems. *Journal of Clinical and Experimental Neuropsychology, 11,* 855–870.

Wilson, B. A., Clare, L., Cockburn, J. M., Baddeley, A. D., Tate, R., & Watson, P. (1999). *The Rivermead Behavioural Memory Test—Extended Version.* Bury St. Edmunds, England: Thames Valley Test Company.

Wilson, B. A., Cockburn, J., & Baddeley, A. (1985, 2003a). *The Rivermead Behavioural Memory Test.* Bury St. Edmunds, England: Thames Valley Test Company.

Wilson, B. A., Cockburn, J., Baddeley, A., & Hiorns, R. (2003b). The Rivermead Behavioral Memory Test-II Supplement Two. Bury St. Edmunds: Thames Valley Test Company.

Wilson, B. A., Forester, S., Bryant, T., & Cockburn, J. (1990). Performance of 11–14 year olds on the Rivermead Behavioural Memory Test. *Clinical Psychology Forum, December 30*, 8–10.

Wilson, B. A., Ivani-Chalian, R., & Aldrich, F. (1991c). *The Rivermead Behavioural Memory Test for children aged 5 to 10 years.* Bury St. Edmunds, England: Thames Valley Test Company.

Wiseman, K. A., Ratcliff, G., Chase, S., Laporte, D. L., Robertson, D. U., & Colantonio, A. (2000). Does a test of functional memory during the post-acute period predict long-term outcome of traumatic brain injury? *Brain and Cognition, 44*, 14–18.

Zakzanis, K. K., & Young, D. A. (2001). Memory impairment in abstinent MDMA ("Ecstasy") users: A longitudinal investigation. *Neurology, 56*, 966–969.

Zakzanis, K. K., Young, D. A., & Campbell, Z. (2003). Prospective memory impairment in abstinent MDMA ("Ecstasy") users. *Cognitive Neuropsychiatry, 8*, 141–153.

Ruff-Light Trail Learning Test (RULIT)

PURPOSE

The purpose of the Ruff-Light Trail Learning Test (RULIT) is to measure visuospatial learning and memory during a multiple-trial learning task.

SOURCE

The test (manual, 50 test booklets, and stimulus cards) can be ordered from Psychological Assessment Resources (http://www.parinc.com), tel. 1-800-331-TEST (8378) at a cost of $130 US.

AGE RANGE

The test can be used with individuals aged 16 to 70 years.

DESCRIPTION

There are numerous tasks to evaluate verbal learning and memory but few that assess visuospatial learning. The RULIT (Ruff & Allen, 1999) was developed as a visuospatial alternative to tests of verbal learning. In addition, the RULIT was developed to avoid a paradigm that would require drawing skills, keen eyesight, good motor control, refined visuospatial integration, and the evaluation of learning predicated mostly on recognition. Moreover, the RULIT was designed to correlate with measures of visuospatial skill and visual memory and to be sensitive to right-hemisphere dysfunction.

The RULIT stimulus card contains a complex configuration of circles interconnected by lines (see Figure 10–41). The examinee is asked to learn a specific trail by tracing with an index finger (of either hand) a line connecting 17 circles from a START circle to an END circle. From each circle along the way, the person has two to five choices for the next circle. At each point (step) along the trail, the examiner informs the person whether a correct or incorrect choice has been made. If the choice was correct, the individual can proceed to the next step. If an incorrect choice was made, the respondent goes back to the preceding position on the trail and tries again until the correct choice is made. Therefore, it is possible for patients to make numerous errors at any given step along the trail. Administration proceeds until the patient has traversed the entire 15-step trail. Successive trials are given until the

Figure 10–41 Example of RULIT Stimulus Card. *Source:* Reprinted with permission from Ruff, 1999.

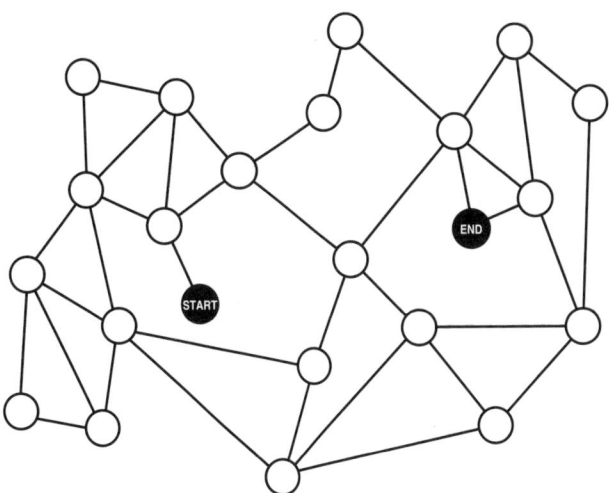

respondent has gone through the 15-step trail 10 times, or until the trail is recalled without error on two consecutive trials. Long-term recall is evaluated by having the respondent retrace the trail after a 60-min delay. There are two alternate versions (cards) of the test.

ADMINISTRATION

See *Source.* Briefly, the correct sequence for each trail is provided in the test manual and booklet. After each step in the trail, the examiner tells the examinee whether his or her selection was correct. The examiner records the number correct and the number of errors.

APPROXIMATE TIME FOR ADMINISTRATION

The test takes about 20 min.

SCORING

There are three main components: Learning, Immediate Memory, and Delayed Memory (see Table 10–113).

Table 10–113 RULIT Test Measures

Component	Measure	Description
Learning	Total Correct	Total number of correct choices for Trials 2 through 10
	Trials to Completion	Total number of trials administered before task is mastered
	Trial Errors	Number of errors made for each trial
	Step Errors	Number of errors committed across each step of each trial, excluding Trial 1, summed horizontally
	Total Step Errors	Total errors for all steps summed vertically
Immediate Memory	Trial 2 Correct	Number correct on Trial 2
	Trial 2 Errors	Number of errors on Trial 2
Delayed Memory	Delayed Correct	Number correct on 60-min delayed-recall trial
	Delayed Errors	Number of errors on 60-min delayed-recall trial

Learning Component Measures

At each step, a correct response is recorded (by marking a "C" or checkmark in the test booklet) if the initial response is correct. If the respondent makes one or more errors at any particular step before making the correct choice, this is noted in the test booklet by marking the number of errors for each step on each trial in the appropriate box. Moreover, because Step 0 is a forced choice, the correct choice made on the first step (i.e., Step 0) is not recorded or counted. The maximum correct responses per trial is 15. Total Correct represent the number of correct responses for Steps 1 though 15 summed across Trials 2 through 10. Examinees who master the trail (i.e., two consecutive trials with no errors) before Trial 10 receive full credit (i.e., 15 correct responses) for all remaining trials.

Trials to Completion is recorded for those individuals who master the trail without error on two consecutive trials on or before Trial 10. The number of errors at each step in Trials 2 through 10 are also summed and noted.

Immediate Memory Component

The number of correctly completed steps in Trial 2 is used to evaluate immediate memory. The rationale is that the examinee has just been exposed to the trail in Trial 1, and therefore Trial 2 represents the initial capacity to remember a 15-step trail without repetition. The number of errors on Trial 2 is also recorded.

Delayed Memory Component

The Delayed Correct Score represents the number of correct choices on the 15-step trail after a 60-min delay. The number of errors is also recorded.

DEMOGRAPHIC EFFECTS

Age

According to the test manual, test scores are affected by age, with performance declining in the oldest age group (55+ years).

Gender

Gender has a small impact on total correct scores (1.2%; Ruff & Allen, 1999).

Education

Education also affects total correct scores; however, the magnitude of the effect is considered to be very small (1.3%) and therefore not clinically meaningful (Ruff & Allen, 1999).

IQ

Full Scale and Performance IQ, but not Verbal IQ, correlate weakly (about .20) with RULIT scores (Ruff & Allen, 1999; Ruff et al., 1996).

Ethnicity

The impact of ethnicity/acculturation is not reported.

NORMATIVE DATA

Standardization Sample

The characteristics of the standardization sample are shown in Table 10–114. The sample consists of 307 normal volunteers, ranging in age between 16 and 70 years and in education from 7 to 22 years. Note that the subjects are largely from California; the method of recruitment and ethnicity are not specified in the manual.

Norms were developed by converting raw scores to normalized z scores, which were subsequently transformed to T scores, with a mean of 50 and a standard deviation of 10. Because age, but not gender or education, had substantial effects on test scores, normative tables were developed for two age groups: 16 to 54 years and 55 to 70 years. T-score values are reported only for Trial 2 Correct, Total Correct, and Total Step

Table 10–114 Characteristics of the RULIT Normative Sample

Number	307
Age (years)	16 to 70[a]
Geographic location	65% California, 30% Michigan, 5% Eastern Seaboard—USA
Sample type	Unknown
Education (years)	7 to 22[b]
Gender	
Men	155
Women	152
Race/Ethnicity	Details not provided
Screening	Self-reported as having no psychiatric, significant substance abuse, or neurological disorder

[a]Broken down into four age groups: 16–24 years, $n = 72$; 25–39 years, $n = 69$; 40–54 years, $n = 83$; and 55–70 years, $n = 83$.
[b]Broken down into three educational bands: ≤12 years, $n = 104$; 13–15 years, $n = 96$; and ≥16 years, $n = 107$.

errors. Most normal individuals made very few errors on delayed recall. Because of concerns regarding the normality of underlying distributions, raw score cutoffs for Delayed Correct and Delayed Errors are provided for each age group at the end of the appropriate table.

Learning curves can also be evaluated. For each age group, scores at the 5th, 25th, 50th, and 75th percentile levels are plotted in figures provided in the test manual and on the response booklet. The examiner can plot an individual's performance and compare that learning curve with those found in the manual for each age group.

The examiner can also analyze the step error distribution across trials by comparing it with that found in the standardization sample at the 1st, 5th, 25th, and 50th percentile rank on Stimulus Card 1 (Figure 5 in the test manual). Because errors tended to occur at just a few steps within the trial, the authors suggested that the profile of step errors may inform the examiner about the patient's motivational status. However, data supporting this proposal remain to be provided.

RELIABILITY

Test-Retest Reliability and Practice Effects

These are not reported.

Alternate Form Reliability

The authors (Ruff and Allen, 1999) report that 64 normal individuals were divided into two groups, matched by age ($M = 32.6$ and 34.2 years) and education ($M = 14.9$ and 15.5 years). One group was given Stimulus Card 1 followed by Stimulus Card 2, and the other group was given the cards in reverse order (interval not reported). The correlation coefficient for Total Correct was reported to be high, $r = .77$. The

test authors state that the forms were balanced for difficulty, although data supporting this claim are not provided in the test manual.

VALIDITY

Correlations With Other Neuropsychological Tests

Total correct scores are weakly or modestly related to a range of other measures of attention and memory (e.g., Ruff 2 and 7, Rey Complex Figure Delayed, Verbal Selective Reminding Test, Block Span Immediate Recall) in normal adults (Ruff & Allen, 1996; Ruff et al., 1996). The magnitude of the correlations appears slightly higher for visual than for verbal memory measures. The highest correlations are with the Rey Complex Delayed scores ($r \cong .47$). RULIT scores are modestly correlated with measures of psychomotor speed (e.g., Total Correct and Digit Symbol are correlated at .29); however, measures of executive function (COWA, Ruff Figural Fluency, WCST) are largely unrelated to RULIT measures. As noted earlier (see *Demographic Effects*), Full Scale and Performance IQ, but not Verbal IQ, are weakly correlated ($r \cong .20$) with RULIT scores.

Factor Analytic Findings

When scores on the test were subjected to factor analysis along with other measures of verbal and visual learning and memory (Selective Reminding Test, Rey Complex Figure, WMS-R Logical Memory Immediate and Delayed) in the standardization sample, two factors emerged (Allen & Ruff, 1999). The first, labeled visual memory, included the RULIT and the Rey Complex Figure delay scores. The second, labeled verbal learning and memory, included the Selective Reminding and Logical Memory test scores.

The test authors report that, when additional tests of verbal and visuospatial ability were added (Block Design, Block Span, Ruff 2 and 7, Letter Span, WAIS-R Vocabulary, Seashore Rhythm), four components were identified; these were labeled visuospatial processing and memory, verbal learning and memory, visual attention, and verbal auditory attention. RULIT measures loaded with the other visual memory task (Rey Complex Figure) and with the WAIS-R Block Design subtest. In short, the RULIT scores appeared to be associated primarily with a visuospatial or visuospatial memory factor, as distinct from a factor including verbal memory measures.

Clinical Studies

The authors (Mahalick et al., 1991; Ruff & Allen, 1999) reported that patients with right-hemisphere, but not left-hemisphere, lesions are impaired on this task. Using impairment cutoff scores equal to the 16th percentile (i.e., a T score of 40) for Total Step Errors, a specificity of 89% and a sensitivity of 74% were achieved for capturing right-hemisphere damage. The overall hit rate was

83%. The authors noted that additional studies are needed to further define the differential roles of anterior versus posterior regions with regard to the various components of the RULIT.

COMMENT

The RULIT has a number of strengths. The test was developed to eliminate many confounds that could interfere with visuospatial learning (e.g., poor motor control, poor drawing ability). Therefore, it may be particularly appropriate for those patients with motor or constructional problems. It is also quite portable for bedside evaluations. The relatively low correlations with other domains (e.g., Wechsler IQ, Block Design) suggest that the level of reasoning required (spatial analysis, in particular) is quite small. Further, few subjects master the task by the third trial, suggesting that it is a challenging task even for young adults. There is also evidence of convergent and divergent validity, and the diagnostic utility of the test in distinguishing patients with right- versus left-hemisphere damage is supported by data provided in the test manual.

The test was designed to provide a visual analog of verbal learning measures, and it appears to measure a construct similar to that of other visuospatial tasks (e.g., Rey Figure). However, the various tasks are clearly not identical. For example, in contrast to the Rey Figure, the RULIT is an intentional (not incidental) learning task and provides greater opportunity for learning (due to repeated presentation). Further, recall is cued and may involve a combination of declarative and procedural memory (Ruff et al., 1996). The possibility that the RULIT assesses both declarative and procedural aspects of memory suggests that there may be different reasons why patients pass (or fail) the test. Its use in diverse clinical populations is needed to more clearly delineate the components of memory underlying the task.

The RULIT purports to parcel visuospatial memory into distinct processes (e.g., Learning, Immediate Memory, Delayed Memory). However, there is no evidence that the various scores that can be derived from the test are in fact assessing different aspects or that these distinctions are clinically meaningful. A single index (e.g., Total Correct) may be sufficient to convey the results of the test.

The normative sample is described with regard to age, education, and gender. However, information regarding recruitment strategy is not provided, and the influence of ethnicity or cultural factors is not known. Additional normative studies are needed to more clearly confirm the suitability of the data for clinical use across a wide range of examinees.

Further, information on reliability is limited. Although alternate form reliability appears good, test-retest reliability and practice effects are not reported. Finally, additional research is needed by investigators other than the authors to demonstrate the test's utility in diverse clinical populations.

REFERENCES

Allen, C. C., & Ruff, R. M. (1999). Factorial validation of the Ruff-Light Trail Learning Test. *Assessment, 6*, 43–50.

Mahalick, D. M., Ruff, R. M., & Sang, H. S. (1991). Neuropsychological sequelae of arteriovenous malformations. *Neurosurgery, 29*, 351–357.

Ruff, R. M., & Allen, C. C. (1999). *Ruff-Light Trail Learning Test.* Odessa, Fla.: PAR.

Ruff, R. M., Light, R., & Parker, S. (1996). Visuospatial learning: Ruff Light Trail Learning Test. *Archives of Clinical Neuropsychology, 11*, 313–327.

Sentence Repetition Test

OTHER TEST NAME

Another test name for the Sentence Repetition Test is Sentence Memory.

PURPOSE

The purpose of this test is to assess immediate memory for sentences of increasing length.

SOURCE

An audiotape, a manual, and scoring forms can be ordered from the Test Material Sales Office, Department of Psychology, University of Victoria, P.O. Box 3050, Victoria, BC, V8W 2Y2, Canada at a cost of $40 US. Other versions of the test can also be found as part of several standardized batteries (see Description).

AGE RANGE

The test can be given to individuals aged 3 to 86 years.

DESCRIPTION

The Sentence Repetition Test taps linguistic knowledge and working memory, making it a useful tool for assessing impairments in language as well as phonological working memory systems. Our version consists of two equivalent forms (Forms A and B; Figure 10–42) of 22 (tape-recorded) sentences, increasing in length from 1 syllable ("Look") to 26 syllables ("Riding his black horse, the general came to the scene of the battle and began shouting at his brave men"). To allow for sufficient material at low and high levels of performance, the sentence length increases in one-syllable steps for the first 12 and the last 6 sentences; sentences 13 to 16 increase in two-syllable steps. Grammatical structure and

Figure 10–42 Sentence Repetition Test, Forms A and B, sample scoring sheets. *Source:* Spreen & Benton, 1969, 1977.

Sentence Repetition—Form A—Sample Score Sheet	Name _____

1. Look

2. Come here.

3. Help yourself.

4. Bring the table.

5. Summer is coming.

6. The iron was quite hot.

7. The birds were singing all day.

8. The paper was under the chair.

9. The sun was shining throughout the day.

10. He entered about eight o'clock that night.

11. The pretty house on the mountain seemed empty.

12. The lady followed the path down the hill toward home.

13. The island in the ocean was first noticed by the young boy.

14. The distance between these two cities is too far to travel by car.

15. A judge here knows the law better than those people who must appear before him.

16. There is a new method in making steel which is far better than that used before.

17. This nation has a good government which gives us many freedoms not known in times past.

18. The friendly man told us the directions to the modern building where we could find the club.

19. The king knew how to rule his country so that his people would show respect for his government.

20. Yesterday he said he would be near the village station before it was time for the train to come.

21. His interest in the problem increased each time that he looked at the report which lay on the table.

22. Riding his black horse, the general came to the scene of the battle and began shouting at his brave men.

TOTAL SCORE

(continued)

Figure 10–42 (*continued*)

Sentence Repetition—Form B—Sample Score Sheet	Name _____	
1. See		
2. Go there.		
3. Come along.		
4. Sing the music.		
5. Winter is over.		
6. The trees began to grow.		
7. The weather can be nice here.		
8. The table was painted dark blue.		
9. The new green dress was very pretty.		
10. She washed her hair before eating supper.		
11. The boy ran quickly into that red building.		
12. He seemed happy to pay the artist for the picture.		
13. He was asked to come to their dinner party in the country.		
14. The famous doctor lived in this city for quite a number of years.		
15. The meeting of the parties took place in the famous field near the mountain pass.		
16. The valley was so dry that storms could not supply enough water to grow the wheat.		
17. The industry really needs men who are prepared to give good service for their high pay.		
18. Yesterday the clerk of the town bank opened the safe and counted the money that was there.		
19. He probably did not notice that the price of corn in the market increased much since last week.		
20. Sometimes he went down to the village to buy various supplies and hear some of the news from home.		
21. He was required to come to the late dinner even though he had some other plans for that evening.		
22. After seeing the map, we realized that we took a wrong turn when going past the college in that town.		
	TOTAL SCORE	

Figure 10–43 Instructions for Sentence Repetition Test.

Auditotape Administration

Playback volume should be set at a comfortable hearing level (approximately 70 db) and may be increased for hard-of-hearing patients. Say: *I am going to play some sentences.* (Point to tape recorder.) *Listen carefully, and after you have heard each sentence, repeat it as well as you can. Remember, listen carefully, and repeat the sentence right after you hear it.*

Repeat the instructions if necessary, and start tape recorder with Sentence Repetition Form A. Occasionally, a patient will not respond after hearing the first sentence. In this case, stop the tape and say, *Would you repeat what you heard?* If the patient responds, say, *That's right. Do the same with each sentence you hear.* If the patient does not respond, say, *Listen carefully. Then repeat what you heard.*

Sentences should not be repeated during the test, although the basic instructions may be repeated.

Discontinue after five consecutive failures.

Oral Administration

Say: *I will say some sentences. Listen carefully, and when I have finished, repeat the sentence back exactly as I have said it. Remember, do not begin until I have given you the whose sentence.*

Read the sentences slowly.

Discontinue after five consecutive failures.

---

vocabulary have been held deliberately to simple, declarative sentences.

The Sentence Repetition Test is part (test 5) of the Neurosensory Center Comprehensive Examination for Aphasia (Spreen & Benton, 1969, 1977). There are several other versions of the test. Benton et al., (1994) used a similar test with two parallel forms of only 14 items and with varying grammatical complexity. The CELF-4 contains a similar subtest with 32 items, designed for children and adolescents aged 5 to 21 years. Sentence repetition subtests can also be found in the BDAE-3, WJ-III and WRAML-2.

ADMINISTRATION

The examinee is seated about 2 m from a tape recorder and is asked to recall sentences presented via the tape recorder (see Figure 10–43 for instructions). Alternatively, the examiner can read the sentences out loud to the clients (see Figure 10–42). Note that norms are available for the oral version. With either the audiotape or the oral version, the test is discontinued after five consecutive failures.

ADMINISTRATION TIME

The test takes between 10 and 15 min.

SCORING

A score of 1 is given for each sentence repeated correctly. Note that since "toward" in item 12, Form A, is often repeated as "towards," "towards" is accepted as correct. On sentences 1 through 10, failure on a single sentence is disregarded if the next five sentences are correctly repeated. Scores are approximations of syllable length. For example, a score of 16 indicates

that the individual was able to recall sentences to a maximum length of about 16 syllables. Poor articulation, if intelligible, should be noted but not scored as an error. Record errors verbatim. The maximum raw score is 22.

DEMOGRAPHIC EFFECTS

Age

Children make gains with increasing age (Gaddes & Crockett, 1975; Spreen & Gaddes, 1969) until about age 12, when adult performance is reached (Carmichael & MacDonald, 1984). In adults, Spreen and Benton (1977) reported that age affected test scores. However, other authors (Meyers et al., 2000; Vargo & Black, 1984) have reported that age has no effect.

Gender

Gender does not affect scores (Carmichael & MacDonald, 1984; Meyers et al., 2000; Vargo & Black, 1984).

Education/IQ

Education is correlated with performance ($r = .37$ for Form A and $r = .38$ for Form B; Meyers et al., 2000; Spreen & Benton, 1977), although the effects of education do not appear to be significant until high levels of education (>16 years) are encountered (Meyers et al., 2000). IQ is also positively related to performance (Klonoff et al., 1970; Lawriw, 1976; Vargo & Black, 1984).

Hand Preference

Handedness does not affect test scores (Meyers et al., 2000).

Table 10–115 Means, Standard Deviations, and 5th Percentile Scores for Adults on the Sentence Repetition (SR) Test

Education Group (Years)	Age	Education	SR Score	Percentile
≤12 (n = 42)	37.4 (20.89)	11.71 (0.81)	14.45 (1.23)	12
13–15 yrs (n = 35)	39.06 (18.84)	13.97 (0.82)	15.00 (1.81)	13
≥16 (n = 27)	44.67 (15.15)	17.67 (1.94)	15.81 (1.71)	13
Total (N = 104)	39.98 (18.89)	14.02 (2.66)	14.99 (1.65)	13

Note: Based on a sample of 104 adults, aged 16–86 years, ranging in education from 8 to 22 years. Except for 1 Asian individual, the sample was Caucasian.

Source: Adapted from Meyers et al., 2000.

NORMATIVE DATA

The original scoring (Spreen and Benton, 1977) made corrections for age and education in adults. Spreen and Benton (1977) noted that patients seemed to attend better if the examiner spoke the sentences. Accordingly, they suggested that 1 point should be subtracted if the test is administered orally without the audiotape. More updated norms are now available for the oral version (Meyers et al., 2000), and these establish a slightly higher standard of performance (by about 1 point). The data are stratified by education but not by age. The means and standard deviations are provided in Table 10–115, along with the 5th percentile scores of performance on Form A.

Table 10–116 provides norms obtained from 1081 children, ranging in age from 3 to 13 years (Carmichael & MacDonald, 1984), from British Columbia, Canada. The oral presentation of the test was used.

RELIABILITY

Internal Consistency

This is not reported.

Table 10–116 Means and Standard Deviations for Children on the Sentence Repetition Test, by Age

Mean Age (Years)	Mean	SD
3.0 (n = 43)	5.8	2.9
4.0 (n = 56)	8.8	1.9
5.4 (n = 114)	9.0	2.7
6.5 (n = 114)	10.9	2.8
7.5 (n = 102)	12.3	2.8
8.5 (n = 117)	13.3	3.0
9.5 (n = 101)	14.6	2.4
10.5 (n = 94)	14.5	3.2
11.5 (n = 110)	15.8	2.5
12.5 (n = 98)	16.8	3.2

Note: Based on a sample of 1081 children, aged 3 to 13 years, living in Kamloops, B.C., Canada.

Source: Adapted from Carmichael & MacDonald, 1984.

Test-Retest Reliability

Brown et al. (1989) reported a test-retest correlation of .71 in 248 children (mean age = 8 years) with mixed diagnoses after an interval of 2 years, 6 months. Klonoff et al. (1970) reported a test-retest reliability of .84 in patients with chronic schizophrenia who were retested after a 1-year interval.

Alternate Form Reliability

Forms A and B appear roughly equivalent in difficulty. Correlation between Forms A and B in an unselected group of 47 subjects was .79, and in a mentally retarded population (N = 25), it was .81 (Spreen & Benton, 1966). In a group of 50 healthy adults, the correlation between Forms A and B was reported to be .84, and there were no significant differences in average scores between test forms (Meyers et al., 2000).

VALIDITY

Relations With Other Measures

The test correlates with the repetition of words, phrases, and sentences of the Western Aphasia Battery (r = .88; Shewan & Kertesz, 1980). The correlation in adults with Digit Repetition Forward is .75, and that with Digit Repetition Reversed is .66 (Lawriw, 1976). In 353 schoolage children, the Sentence Repetition Test formed a separate dimension in a factor analysis of the 20 subtests of the NCCEA, accounting for 81% of the total variance of this factor, and was relatively independent of digit repetition (Crockett, 1974).

Intellectual level contributes to performance. Correlations with Wechsler FSIQ range from .33 to .62 (Lawriw, 1976; Vargo & Black, 1984). As might be expected, the test correlates more strongly with VIQ (.61) than with PIQ (.42; Meyers et al., 2000). The test also shows a moderate correlation with the overall Memory Quotient of the Wechsler Memory Scale (r = .38; Vargo & Black, 1984).

Clinical Studies

The test has been given to a number of different patient populations. Children with learning disabilities have difficulty on this task (Epstein, 1982; Spreen, 1988). Further, the test is sensitive to severity of head injury in children and adolescents (Ewing-Cobbs et al., 1987), as well as in adults (Meyers et al., 2000; Peck et al., 1992). Therefore, the longer the loss of consciousness, the lower the performance, and the more individuals fail the task (i.e., obtain scores below the 5th percentile; Meyers et al., 2000). However, performance does not appear to be impaired in patients with schizophrenia (Klonoff et al., 1970).

The test is more sensitive to left- than right-hemisphere injury (but see Vargo & Black, 1984). Meyers et al. (2000) noted that no patient with a right cerebrovascular accident (CVA) failed the test, whereas about 18% of those with left CVA obtained scores below the 5th percentile. The test is also particularly sensitive to aphasic disturbances (Lawriw, 1976; Sarno, 1986). For example, Lawriw (1976) found that 56% of aphasic patients scored below the lowest score of the normal controls with low average intelligence. Crockett (1977) reported that the test contributed to the discrimination of four empirically derived subtypes of aphasia in adults; impairment of sentence repetition was especially characteristic of individuals classed as "Type A" (good comprehension with poor attention, memory, and reproduction of speech).

COMMENT

The test is fairly simple and brief to administer. Although performance does not decline with advancing age in adults, a person's educational or intellectual level must be considered when interpreting test results. Therefore, although poor performance may represent a specific language disturbance, such a performance may also reflect more global factors, such as low intellectual level. The presence of updated norms should assist clinicians in diagnosing and making recommendations (Meyers et al., 2000). However, the effects of race/ethnicity and acculturation on performance are not known. Further, at present there is no way to evaluate subtypes of errors (e.g., omissions, substitutions of tense).

In addition, the comparability of the administration procedures (oral versus audiotape) remains to be evaluated. Test-retest and alternate form reliability appear satisfactory, although information on internal consistency and magnitude of practice effects is lacking. In terms of its diagnostic utility, the test shows excellent specificity (normal versus neurologically impaired), although sensitivity to impairment has ranged from 7% to 34%, depending on the severity and location of the injury (Meyers et al., 2000).

REFERENCES

Benton, A. L., Hamsher, K. deS., & Sivan, A. B. (1994). *Multilingual aphasia examination.* San Antonio, Tex. Psychological Corporation.

Brown, S. J., Rourke, B. P., & Cicchetti, D. V. (1989). Reliability of tests and measures used in the neuropsychological assessment of children. *The Clinical Neuropsychologist, 3,* 353–368.

Carmichael, J., & McDonald, J. (1984). Developmental norms for neuropsychological tests. *Journal of Clinical and Consulting Psychology, 52,* 476–477.

Crockett, D. J. (1974). Component analysis within correlations of language skill tests in normal children. *Journal of Special Education, 8,* 361–375.

Crockett, D. J. (1977). A comparison of empirically derived groups of aphasic patients on the Neurosensory Center Comprehensive Examination for Aphasia. *Journal of Clinical Psychology, 33,* 194–198.

Epstein, A. G. (1982). Mastery of language measured by means of a sentence span test. Unpublished manuscript, Lyngby, Denmark.

Ewing-Cobbs, L., Levin, H. S., Eisenberg, H. M., & Fletcher, J. M. (1987). Language functions following closed-head injury in children and adolescents. *Journal of Clinical and Experimental Neuropsychology, 9,* 575–592.

Gaddes, W. H., & Crockett, D. J. (1975). The Spreen-Benton aphasia tests, normative data as a measure of normal language development. *Brain and Language, 2,* 257–280.

Klonoff, H., Fibiger, C. H., & Hutton, G. H. (1970). Neuropsychological patterns in chronic schizophrenia. *Journal of Nervous and Mental Disease, 150,* 291–300.

Lawriw, I. (1976). A test of the predictive validity and a cross-validation of the Neurosensory Center Comprehensive Examination for Aphasia. M. A. thesis, University of Victoria, Victoria, B.C., Canada.

Meyers, J. E., Volkert, K., & Diep. A. (2000). Sentence Repetition Test: Updated norms and clinical utility. *Applied Neuropsychology, 7,* 154–159.

Murdoch, B. E., Chenery, H. J., Wilks, V., & Boyle, R. S. (1987). Language disorders in dementia of the Alzheimer type. *Brain and Language, 31,* 122–137.

Peck, E. A., Mitchell, S. A., Burke, E. A., & Schwartz, S. M. (1992). *Post head injury normative data for selected Benton neuropsychological tests.* Paper presented at the annual meeting of the American Psychological Association, Washington, D.C.

Sarno, M. T. (1986). Verbal impairment in head injury. *Archives of Physical and Medical Rehabilitation, 67,* 399–405.

Shewan, C. M., & Kertesz, A. (1980). Reliability and validity characteristics of the Western Aphasia Battery (WAB). *Journal of Speech and Hearing Disorders, 45,* 308–324.

Spreen, O. (1988). *Learning Disabled Children Growing Up.* New York: Oxford University Press.

Spreen, O., & Benton, A. L. (1966). *Reliability of the Sentence Repetition Test.* Unpublished paper, Iowa City, Ia.

Spreen, O., & Benton, A. L. (1969, 1977). *Neurosensory Center Comprehensive Examination for Aphasia.* Victoria, B.C.: University of Victoria, Neuropsychology Laboratory.

Spreen, O., & Gaddes, W. H. (1969). Developmental norms for 15 neuropsychological tests age 6 to 15. *Cortex, 5,* 171–191.

Vargo, M. E. & Black, F. W. (1984). Normative data for the Spreen-Benton Sentence Repetition Test: Its relationship to age, intelligence, and memory. *Cortex, 20,* 585–590.

Wechsler Memory Scale–Third Edition (WMS-III)

PURPOSE

The Wechsler Memory Scale—Third Edition (WMS-III) was designed to assess auditory and visual declarative memory and auditory and visual working memory abilities in adults and adolescents.

SOURCE

The WMS-III Complete Kit (including the Administration Manual, the Technical Manual, 25 record forms, 25 visual reproduction response booklets, Stimulus Booklets 1 and 2, and the Spatial Span Board) can be obtained from Harcourt Assessment (http://www.harcourtassessment.com) for about $525 US. The company also provides a computer scoring system (WAIS-III/WMS-III/WIAT-III) that gives demographically corrected norms (United States normative data only); the cost is $225 US. The Six-Factor Model (Tulsky et al., 2003b) is an alternative method for creating composites. Examiners can download the WAIS-III/WMS-III Demographically Adjusted Norms Six-Factor Model Analysis Tool from the Harcourt Assessment web page (http://harcourtassessment.com/haiweb/Cultures/en-US/dotCom/6factormodel/6+Factor+Model.htm). The tool calculates demographically adjusted T scores and base rate discrepancies.

A short form, the WMS-III Abbreviated, is also available. It consists of four subtests (Logical Memory I and II and Family Pictures I and II) that are used to derive composite scores (Immediate Memory, Delayed Memory, and Total memory), which can be compared with WAIS-III FSIQ. The technical manual, stimulus book, and 25 record forms cost $168 US.

AGE RANGE

The age range is 16 to 89 years.

DESCRIPTION

The WMS-III is the latest version in the family of Wechsler Memory Scales (see Tulsky et al., 2003a, for a detailed account of the origins and modifications made to the scales). It and its predecessor (WMS-R) rank first among tests of memory functioning in neuropsychological evaluations (Borum & Grisso, 1995; Camara et al., 2000; Lees-Haley et al., 1995; Rabin et al., 2005).

The original WMS (Wechsler, 1945) contained seven subtests: Personal and Current Information, Mental Control, Logical Memory, Digits Forward and Backward, Visual Reproduction, and Associate Learning. There were two forms, Form I (Wechsler, 1945) and Form II (Stone & Wechsler, 1946), although most of the published studies deal with Form I. The validity and psychometric properties of the WMS were extensively criticized. These included inadequate norms, scores combined into a summary score (the MQ) that did not differ-

entiate various facets of memory, overreliance on immediate as opposed to delayed recall, imprecise scoring criteria, and overreliance on verbal tasks (Butters et al., 1988; Erickson & Scott, 1977; Larrabee et al., 1985; Loring & Papanicolaou, 1987; Prigatano, 1977, 1978), prompting several variations (e.g., Milberg et al., 1986; Russell, 1975) and a revision.

In 1987, the test was revised (WMS-R; Wechsler, 1987), broadening its coverage of nonverbal and visual memory and incorporating delayed recall procedures. The WMS-R was a significant improvement over its predecessor. However, it too had limitations (for review, see Lezak et al, 2004; Lichtenberger et al., 2002; Spreen & Strauss, 1998). Among the most noteworthy were the limited age range of norms (e.g., no data beyond age 74 years), reliance on verbal memory, delayed memory not separated into verbal and nonverbal components, absence of recognition tasks, limited reliability of the subtests and some of the index scores, and lack of support for the construct validity of some of the indices (e.g., verbal memory, visual memory).

Based on the published literature, solicited reviews of the WMS-R, and recommendations from an advisory panel, the Psychological Corporation developed the WMS-III (The Psychological Corporation, 1997, 2002). Among the improvements were the increase in sample size, broadening of the age range (16–89 years), sampling of individuals in each age range (as opposed to the use of interpolated norms for some age groups), improved reliability coefficients, changes in content of stimuli (particularly visual material), the inclusion of new measures of attention/concentration and working memory, the addition of recognition measures to attempt to identify retrieval problems, and an emphasis on the construct of delayed memory. The test was also co-developed with the WAIS-III and WTAR, allowing for more precise and meaningful comparisons between memory and intellectual ability.

The WMS-III includes 11 subtests, 6 of which are considered primary and 5 optional (see Table 10–117). Table 10–118 provides a brief description of each of the subtests. Primary subtests must be given to obtain index scores. Optional subtests can be given to obtain supplementary information. Table 10–119 shows the subtest composition of the eight primary indices of

Table 10–117 Subtests of the WMS-III

	Auditory Presentation	Visual Presentation
Primary	Logical Memory I and II Verbal Paired Associates I and II	Faces I and II Family Pictures I and II
Optional	Letter-Number Sequencing Information and Orientation Word Lists I and II Mental Control Digit Span	Spatial Span Visual Reproduction I and II

Table 10–118 Description of WMS-III Subtests

Subtest	Description
Information and Orientation (Optional)	Subject responds to questions regarding personal and general knowledge (e.g., birthdate, name of President, day of the week)
Logical Memory I and II (LM I and II)	Subject recalls two paragraphs read aloud by the examiner, both immediately and after a delay; a yes/no recognition test follows the delay
Faces I and II	Subject must recognize faces, both immediately after presentation and after a delay
Verbal Paired Associated I and II (VPA I and II)	Examiner presents a list of word pairs; then the subject hears one word and must provide the word that went with it. There are four trials of the list. The pairs are also tested after a delay. A recognition trial is also included; the subject must identify the word pairs from a list of distractors.
Family Pictures I and II	The subject is shown four scenes one at a time and then must recall the characters in the scene and what they were doing. Recall is also tested after a delay.
Word List I and II (Optional)	A 12-item list-learning task in which the subject must recall the list after each of four learning trials. Recall of the word list is also tested after presentation of a new list and after a delay. Finally, the subject is read a list of 24 words and must identify the list I words.
Visual Reproduction I and II (VRI and II) (Optional)	The subject must reproduce figures both immediately after presentation and following a delay. Recognition, copying and matching conditions are also provided.
Letter-Number Sequencing	The examiner reads a list consisting of a combination of numbers and letters, and the subject must recite them back, the numbers first in ascending order, and then the letters in alphabetic order.
Spatial Span	The examiner touches a sequence of blocks that the subject must repeat in the same order. In the second task, the subject must point to the same blocks in the reverse order.
Mental Control (Optional)	The subject must recite sequences (e.g., days of the week) as well as manipulate sequences (e.g., recite days backward)
Digit Span	The subject repeats strings of digits of increasing length said by the examiner in the same (forward) and in reverse (backward) order.

Table 10–119 Structure of Primary Index Scores

Immediate Memory	Auditory Immediate	Logical Memory I Recall Verbal Paired Associates I Recall
	Visual Immediate	Faces I Recognition Family Pictures I Recall
General Memory	Auditory (Delayed Recall)	Logical Memory II Recall Verbal Paired Associates II Recall
	Auditory Recognition Delayed	Logical Memory II Recognition Verbal Paired Associates II Recognition
	Visual (Delayed)	Faces II Recognition Family Pictures II Recall
Working Memory	Auditory Visual	Letter-Number Sequencing Spatial Span

the WMS-III. As in the WAIS-III, Index scores have a mean of 100 and a standard deviation (SD) of 15; subtest scores have a mean of 10 and an SD of 3.

In addition to the eight primary indices, the WMS-III includes four Auditory Process Composites: Single-Trial Learning (a measure of recall capacity after a single exposure), Learning Slope (a measure of ability to acquire information after repeated exposures—the relative increase from first to last trial for Logical Memory I [LM I] Story B and Verbal Paired Associates I [VPA I]), Retention (a measure of delayed free recall as a function of immediate recall, based on LM and VPA), and Retrieval (a measure of the extent to which cueing increases information retrieval beyond that available though free recall, based on LM and VPA). A variety of other supplemental scores based on individual subtests can also be computed, including a thematic total score for Logical Memory, scores to determine the contribution of visual perceptual, constructional, and memory processes to Visual Reproduction, and a number of indices (e.g., recognition, learning slope, percent retention) from a word list learning task.

The reader is referred to the important volume by Tulsky et al. (2003a), which serves as an interpretive guide to the WAIS-III/WMS-III. Also included are chapters on accommodating clients who are non-native English speakers or who have specific disabilities (e.g., hearing impairment). Other practical issues (e.g., what to do if a subtest or response is spoiled, when and how to query) are also considered.

ADMINISTRATION

See *Source.* Briefly, the examiner asks test questions, displays items to the patient, and records the patient's responses in an individual response booklet (Wechsler, 1997). Discontinuation and scoring rules as well as time limits are noted in the test manual and on the record form. There is a suggested order of subtest administration.

The WMS-III standardization sample group also completed the WAIS-III. Order of administration did not significantly affect scores (Zhu & Tulsky, 2000). The authors cautioned that, despite this overall effect at the group level, test-order effects may affect some individuals.

The Letter-Number Sequencing task is included in both the WAIS-III and the WMS-III; however, in the standardization sample, the task was given only once, during the WMS-III. Even though there is not a very large practice effect on this subtest (see the WAIS-/WMS-III Technical Manual), it should be given only once in the testing session (Tulsky & Ledbetter, 2000). There is no significant difference in Letter-Number Sequencing test scores if the task was given as part of the WAIS-III or in the WMS-III (Tulsky & Ledbetter, 2000).

Short Forms

To reduce administration time, Immediate Memory and General Memory summary indices can be predicted from equations developed by Axelrod and Woodard (2000) by leaving out one

Table 10–120 Equations to Obtain Prorated Versions of the WMS-III

Index	Equation	SEE
Immediate Memory	$LMI \times 1.381 + VPAI \times 1.148 + FacesI \times 1.264 + 0.113$	2.33
	$LMI \times 1.135 + VPAI \times 1.102 + FPI \times 1.216 + 4.758$	2.11
General Memory	$LMII \times 1.359 + VPAII \times 1.117 + FacesII \times 1.149 + ARD \times 1.186 - 0.114$	2.33
	$LMII \times 1.128 + VPAII \times 1.112 + FPII \times 1.166 + ARD \times 1.178 + 4.344$	2.46

Note: Subtest age-scaled scores are entered into each formula, and the final Immediate and General Memory index scores are converted from the sum of scaled scores via Table E1 in the *WMS-III Administration and Scoring Manual.*

Source: From Axelrod & Woodard, 2000. Reprinted with permission of APA.

of the two visual memory subtests (Faces or Family Pictures). The equations were derived from a sample of subjects, primarily male, with a variety of clinical conditions. The equations for the three-subtest prorated forms are shown in Table 10–120. Subtest age-scaled scores are entered into each formula, and the final Immediate and General Memory index scores are converted from the sum of scaled scores via Table E1 in the WMS-III Administration and Scoring Manual.

Cross-validation of these equations in another predominantly male clinical sample (Axelrod et al., 2001) revealed that the three-subtest equations correlated with full WMS-III Immediate and General Memory (r = .97 and .96, respectively). In addition, at least 95% of the predicted scores were within two SEMs (that is, ±9 points) of obtained Immediate and General Memory scores. Eliminating either Faces or Family Pictures results in a time savings of about 5 min for Immediate Memory and 3 to 4 min for General Memory. These short forms may be useful when there is a need to minimize fatigue or frustration, or in cases of reduced level of cooperation.

In low-functioning individuals, it may be possible to reduce the 48 response items on the Faces task to the first 32 items. In a mixed clinical sample, Migoya et al. (2002) reported that total raw scores predicted from the 32-item version (by multiplying the 32-item score by 1.5) correlate highly (>.85) with the raw scores obtained on 48 items. Using the 32-item version, 100% (Faces I) and 94% (Faces II) of the predicted raw scores were less than 4 points away from the actual total raw score. In most individuals, however, little time would likely be saved by such a modification.

ADMINISTRATION TIME

According to the test authors, the primary subtests take about 30 to 35 min to administer. There should be a 15- to 35-min delay interval between the completion of LMI and the beginning of LMII. The test authors indicate that administration of the optional subtests adds about 15 to 20 min to the actual testing time.

These numbers, however, appear optimistic. One study with a clinical sample found administration time of the basic subtests to average 42 min, with 88% of the administrations taking longer than 34 min (Axelrod, 2001).The addition of Orientation and Word List learning added an additional 10 min. There was little relationship between administration time and performance. Together, the WAIS-III/WMS-III battery, including all of the supplemental tasks, required at least 2 hours (Axelrod, 2001). Note that these times refer to administration only; scoring time is not included.

SCORING

See *Source*. The Record Form provides space to record and score the subject's responses, to draw a profile of subtest scores, and to summarize information about the patient's behavior in the test situation. Much of the scoring is straightforward, but there are a few subtests (e.g., Logical Memory, Family Pictures, Visual Reproduction) in which subjectivity intrudes. Appendices are provided in the Administration and Scoring Manual, which provides examples of scoring criteria. A detailed recording should be provided, so that scoring can be reviewed later.

Subtest and Index Scores

The raw scores of subtests (primary and supplemental) and Auditory Process Composite subtest scores are converted to age-scaled scores, which range from 1 to 19 ($M = 10$, $SD = 3$), using tables D1 through D3 provided in the Administration and Scoring Manual. The Index scores are obtained by summing the scaled scores that comprise the specific Index, using table E1. Index scores range from the mid-40s to 155 ($M = 100$, $SD = 15$), except in the case of the Auditory Recognition Delayed Index, which ranges from 55 to 145.

Discrepancy Data

Considerable discrepancy base-rate data (including IQ-Memory discrepancy information) are available via the test manuals (Administration and Scoring Manual, Technical Manual), the recent text by Tulsky et al. (2003a), and the scoring software (see also *Normative Data*).

Software

Computer software is available from the test publisher so that raw scores can be automatically converted to appropriate age-scaled scores, index scores, percentiles, confidence intervals, and corresponding graphs. The program also generates Primary Index Differences and Ability-Memory Differences (and indicates whether they are significant), as well as cumulative percentages of the normative group that received scores greater than or equal to the amount of the difference. Comparisons between Digits Forward and Digits Backward are also provided. The advantage of using the scoring program is that it significantly reduces scoring time and examiner error. In addition to correcting for age, computer software is also available (see *Source*) for use in the United States that takes into account other demographic influences (i.e., education, gender, and ethnicity). Users can also download a program to compute demographically adjusted index scores derived from a six-factor model of the WAIS-III/WMS-III (see *Source*).

DEMOGRAPHIC EFFECTS

Age

Age has moderately strong relationships with a visual memory factor defined by Family Pictures I and II and Visual Reproductions I and II ($r^2 = .45$), whereas more moderate associations with age are seen for Working Memory ($r^2 = .24$), Auditory Memory ($r^2 = .20$), and an alternate visual memory factor defined by Family Pictures I and II and Faces I and II ($r^2 = .38$; Heaton et al., 2003).

Education

Heaton et al. (2003) pointed out that specificity (the likelihood of being correctly classed as normal) on the memory factors (which, it should be noted, do not always correspond with the standard Index scores) varies greatly with educational level. Therefore, using only age-corrected norms, the likelihood of normal individuals being classed as "impaired" is excessively high (25%–45%) if they have not completed high school. By contrast, few at the highest education level are similarly classified (2%–6%). What this means is that highly educated people would need to show a much greater decrement in test performance to be correctly classed as "impaired" using norms that are corrected only for age.

Gender

Gender effects are generally small: The largest differences favor women and occur on the Auditory and Visual Memory factors, although they translate into specificity differences of only about 5% (Heaton et al., 2003). Basso et al. (2000) reported that, with regard to the VPA subtest, the discrepancy favoring women approximated 2 scaled score points, a difference of about two-thirds of a standard deviation.

Ethnicity

In general, Caucasians score highest, followed by Hispanics and then African Americans (Heaton et al., 2003). Failure to correct for ethnicity means that African Americans would be twice as likely to be misclassified as impaired, compared with Caucasians. Accordingly, normative adjustments are required (see *Source*).

Table 10–121 Characteristics of the WMS-III Normative Sample.

Number	A total of 1032 adults were tested. This sample was weighted to match 1995 U.S. Census data and each age group was required to have an average FSIQ of 100. This weighting method yielded a sample of 1250 subjects.
Age (years)	16 to 89[a]
Geographic location	From geographic regions in proportions consistent with US census data
Sample type	Based on a representative sample of the U.S. population stratified on the basis of age, sex, race/ethnicity, educational level, and geographic region with concurrent collection of intellectual ability
Education	<8 to >16 years and consistent with U.S. Census proportions; for examinees aged 16–19 years, parent education was used.
Gender	An equal number of males and females in each age group from 16 to 64 years; the older age groups included more women than men, in proportions consistent with 1995 U.S. Census data
Race/Ethnicity	The proportions of Whites, African Americans, Hispanics, and other racial/ethnic groups were based on racial/ethnic proportions within each age band according to 1995 U.S. Census data
Screening	Screened via self-report for sensory, substance abuse, medical, psychiatric, or motor condition that could potentially affect performance

[a]Broken down into 13 age groups: 16–17, 18–19, 20–24, 25–29, 30–34, 35–44, 45–54, 55–64, 65–69, 70–74, 75–79, 80–84, and 85–89 years; 100 subjects were included in each age group except the two oldest groups, which consisted of 75 participants each.

NORMATIVE DATA

Standardization Sample

The characteristics of the sample are shown in Table 10–121. The standardization group was based on a weighted sample of 1250 individuals aged 16 to 89 years, selected to match 1995 U.S. Census data on the basis of age, sex, race/ethnicity, education level, and geographic region.

Three sets of normative scores have been derived. The first is based on age-corrected subtest scores and should be used when clinical questions dictate comparison of an individual's performance with that of his or her age peers.

The second set is based on the performance of a reference group consisting of individuals in the standardization sample between the ages of 20 and 34 years who were considered to be representative of the U.S. Census data for this age range. The reference-group subtest scaled scores should not be summed to derive Index scores.

For the third set, Heaton et al. (2003) developed regression-based demographic corrections that adjust for the influences of age, education, gender, and certain ethnicities (non-Hispanic White, African American, and Hispanic). The corrected norms (T scores with a mean of 50 and an SD of 10) are available through Harcourt Assessment (see Source) and are described in detail by Heaton et al. (2003) and Taylor and Heaton (2001). The demographically adjusted norms allow the clinician to determine whether the examinee's current performance is below expectations, given their age, education, gender, and ethnicity (The Psychological Corporation, 2002). They propose a 1 SD cutoff of demographically corrected factor scores (T scores <40) to define cognitive impairment. This results in an 85% specificity rate (i.e., percentage of normal subjects correctly designated as normal) that is constant for the three ethnicity groups and is not affected by differences in age, education, or gender. Note that demographically adjusted norms are not intended to make judgments for the individual patient about intellectual capacity, expected functional capacity, or predicted academic abilities (The Psychological Corporation, 2002).

Discrepancy Data—Indices

Discrepancies between Primary Index scores can be evaluated to determine whether differences are significant and unusual by referring to Tables F1 and F2 in the Administration and Scoring Manual. The WMS-III Administration and Scoring Manual presents cumulative frequencies for composite-score discrepancies irrespective of the direction of the difference. For example, if the Auditory Immediate score minus the Visual Immediate score equals −20, the value reported in the frequency table is 20. It is not possible to determine how often the Auditory Immediate memory score will be greater than the Visual Immediate score or vice versa; however, it is possible to know how often the Auditory and Visual Immediate memory scores differ by 20. Table D7 in the WAIS-III/WMS-III Technical Manual provides directional discrepancy-score base rates for the WMS-III Index scores.

The WMS-III allows for comparison between the Immediate Memory Index and the delayed memory index, called the General Memory Index. However, Tulsky et al., (2004) noted that the Immediate and General Memory indices are not parallel in structure. The former is composed of four immediate subtests (LM I, VPA I, Faces I, and Family Pictures I), whereas the latter is composed of the sum of the scaled scores for the delayed trials of these four subtests as well as the scaled score of the Auditory Recognition Delayed total score. Inclusion of Auditory Recognition Delayed in the General Memory Index is also highly problematic, because it is skewed and limited by extreme ceiling effects (Tulsky et al., 2003a). To remedy these problems, Tulsky et al. (2004) presented a new index score, the Delayed Memory Index, that does not include auditory recognition. They provided normative tables for the new index based on inclusion of the Faces subtest or, alternatively, the Visual Reproduction subtest, and also for a new Immediate Memory Index that includes the Visual Reproduction subtest in place of Faces. They also provided base rate information for discrepancy scores between the Immediate and Delayed Memory indices.

Ability-memory discrepancies can be evaluated for significance and frequency of occurrence using either the simple-difference method (WMS-III index score subtracted from WAIS-III FSIQ, VIQ, or PIQ score) or the predicted-actual method (obtained WMS-III index score subtracted from FSIQ, VIQ, or PIQ predicted index score) by referring to tables in Appendix B (Predicted-Difference Method) or Appendix C (Simple-Difference Method) of the WAIS-III/WMS-III Technical Manual. The predicted difference method is preferred, because it takes into account score reliability and offers greater protection against errors arising from regression to the mean effects (The Psychological Corporation, 1997, 2002); however, it should be supplemented by estimates of premorbid functioning (e.g., reading-based measures; Skeel et al., 2004). The accuracy of memory performance estimates based on the WAIS-III FSIQ scores does not appear to be influenced by the amount of inter-subtest scatter in the WAIS-III (Ryan et al., 2002).

It is important to note that frequency data for WMS-III discrepancies are based on total sample data and therefore fail to account for the effects of ability level on either discrepancy size or direction. Dori and Chelune (2004) presented educationally stratified, directional prevalence rates of discrepancy scores for the WMS-III and between the WAIS-III and the WMS-III. In addition, they provided unidirectional cutoff scores that define simple-difference prevalence rates at various decision points (i.e., 5%, 10%, and 15%). Table 10–122 presents within-test base-rate information for the WMS-III, and Table 10–123 provides base-rate data for discrepancy scores between the WAIS-III and the WMS-III. To illustrate how these tables can be used, assume that a patient with less than 12 years of education obtains a VIQ-GM discrepancy score of 18, where VIQ (V1) is greater than GM (V2); the clinician would discover that this discrepancy is quite rare, occurring in 5% or less of the general population. However, a discrepancy of 28 points would be needed for VIQ to be less than GM.

Tulsky et al. (2003b) suggested an alternate model for creating composites from WAIS-III/WMS-III subtests (see Table 10–124). Three indices are from the WAIS-III (VCI, POI, PSI). The WMI and Auditory Memory Index are from the WMS-III, along with two Visual Memory Indices: one a new combi-nation consisting of VR I and II and Family Pictures I and II; the other, a combination of the WMS-III original primary visual subtests, Faces I and II and Family Pictures I and II. As noted earlier, the new visual memory indices were constructed because of concern regarding the construct validity of the Faces subtest. Faces and Family Pictures correlate weakly, and the resulting index scores correlate at best modestly with other WAIS-III/WMS-III indices. As a consequence, differences between scores on the visual memory indices and other indices within the battery must be very large before they can be considered unusual, rendering discrepancy analysis ineffectual. Hawkins and Tulsky (2004) showed that the new visual memory indices (combining Visual Reproductions and Family Pictures) enhance the efficacy of discrepancy analysis because, for any given discrepancy, greater numbers of patients will be identified as showing an abnormal depression on the visual index when the index is formed by the new rather than the original subtest combination. Hawkins and Tulsky (2003, 2004) provided discrepancy data, stratified by FSIQ, for contrasts derived from the six-factor model of the WAIS-III/WMS-III (see also *Validity*).

The development of demographically adjusted scores (see *Normative Data*) reduces but does not eliminate the need for discrepancy analysis. Demographic factors account for significant amounts of variance in ability but imperfectly estimate the scores of individuals. Accordingly, Hawkins and Tulsky (2003) also provided discrepancy base rates for demographically adjusted T scores based on scores derived from the alternate six-factor model from WAIS-III/WMS-III subtests. The scaled-score to T-score conversions for these index scores and base rate data for index contrasts can be obtained by accessing the WAIS-III/WMS-III Demographically Adjusted Six-Factor Model Analysis Tool from Harcourt Assessment (see *Source*).

Discrepancy Data—Subtests

The discussion thus far has considered the global scores. Differences between subtest Scaled scores can be evaluated for significance by referring to Tables F3 and F4 in the Administration and Scoring Manual. When interpreting the WMS-III, examiners may wish to identify strengths and weaknesses across the 11 primary subtests and/or for subtests that contribute only to Auditory, Visual, Immediate or General Memory Indices. Table 10–125 (Ryan et al., 2000) can be used to evaluate differences between subtest scores and the mean of the corresponding primary subtests. Also included are the frequencies of differences obtained by 1%, 2%, 5%, 10%, and 25% of the WMS-III standardization sample. To use the table, the examiner must calculate the average age-adjusted score for the relevant primary subtests and subtract this value from each of the individual subtest scores. Deviations from the overall mean are then compared with the values in the table with regard to level of confidence and frequency of occurrence. Ryan et al. (2000) provided cutoff values based on the total sample statistics. Cole et al. (2003) extended their work and provided tables (at confidence intervals of .01 and .05) for

Table 10–122 Unidirectional Base-Rate Information for WMS-III Discrepancy Scores

WMS-III Indexes	Education <12[a]						Education = 12[b]						Education = 13–15[c]						Education ≥16[d]					
	V1 > V2			V1 < V2			V1 > V2			V1 < V2			V1 > V2			V1 < V2			V1 > V2			V1 < V2		
(V1)–(V2)	5%	10%	15%	15%	10%	5%	5%	10%	15%	15%	10%	5%	5%	10%	15%	15%	10%	5%	5%	10%	15%	15%	10%	5%
WM-IM	27	20	17	18	21	28	26	22	19	16	20	26	32	26	20	17	22	26	33	20	16	21	24	27
IM-GM	11	10	8	8	9	12	12	10	8	8	10	11	12	8	8	8	9	12	13	9	8	9	11	13
WM-GM	25	20	16	18	21	27	26	21	17	17	20	25	31	26	18	18	23	26	27	21	18	17	22	26
WM-AudI	29	23	18	18	22	27	29	23	18	16	21	27	29	24	20	16	22	30	27	20	17	19	22	26
WM-AudD	27	22	17	20	24	30	30	23	20	14	19	25	31	23	18	18	21	30	26	18	14	17	21	25
WM-VisI	28	22	18	22	26	36	28	22	18	19	22	28	36	31	25	17	19	25	37	25	21	20	25	35
WM-VisD	22	19	15	22	26	31	28	21	16	19	24	30	34	28	25	17	19	26	36	25	19	18	21	28
AudI-AudD	14	10	8	10	13	15	14	11	9	8	10	12	13	10	7	7	10	11	11	10	9	8	10	12
VisI-VisD	15	11	10	10	12	14	13	10	7	10	11	15	16	10	8	10	11	16	16	13	10	10	13	17
AudI-VisI	24	19	15	24	30	33	27	21	18	18	24	30	34	24	21	14	19	24	30	26	23	18	22	27
AudD-VisD	24	17	13	18	22	26	25	19	15	21	24	30	33	25	21	14	17	22	33	25	21	17	21	26

Note: WMS-III = Wechsler Memory Scale—Third Edition; V1 = first variable listed; V2 = second variable listed; WM = Working Memory; IM = Immediate Memory; GM = General Memory; AudI = Auditory Immediate; AudD = Auditory Delayed; VisI = Visual Immediate; VisD = Visual Delayed.

[a]Weighted *N* = 309 for all comparisons.

[b]Weighted *N* = 423 for all comparisons.

[c]Weighted *N* = 294 for all comparisons.

[d]Weighted *N* = 294 for all comparisons.

Source: From Dori & Chelune, 2004, *Wechsler Memory Scale—Third Edition.* Copyright © 1997 by Harcourt Assessment, Inc. Reproduced by permission. All rights reserved.

Table 10-123 Unidirectional Base-Rate Information for WAIS-III and WMS-III Discrepancy Scores

WAIS-III and WMS-III Indexes	Education <12[a]						Education = 12[b]						Education = 13–15[c]						Education ≥16[d]					
	V1 > V2			V1 < V2			V1 > V2			V1 < V2			V1 > V2			V1 < V2			V1 > V2			V1 < V2		
(V1)–(V2)	5%	10%	15%	15%	10%	5%	5%	10%	15%	15%	10%	5%	5%	10%	15%	15%	10%	5%	5%	10%	15%	15%	10%	5%
VIQ-WM	18	13	10	16	21	24	19	15	13	15	19	23	23	16	14	14	18	20	30	24	21	7	10	15
VIQ-IM	19	14	11	20	24	27	25	18	16	16	20	25	25	22	16	13	18	21	36	28	23	10	13	19
VIQ-GM	18	14	11	19	21	28	24	16	14	18	20	23	24	21	15	13	16	20	38	27	21	9	13	17
PIQ-WM	19	14	11	15	19	21	21	16	14	14	17	20	20	15	14	14	18	23	22	20	17	8	11	16
PIQ-IM	23	17	13	18	22	29	24	19	15	15	18	23	24	20	18	16	19	25	29	23	17	13	16	20
PIQ-GM	21	16	14	18	21	27	22	17	15	15	17	22	25	18	15	15	18	22	28	21	18	12	14	19
VCI-WM	28	14	12	13	16	21	20	16	14	15	18	21	25	20	16	16	20	22	24	21	19	10	13	17
VCI-IM	21	16	13	19	23	27	28	19	16	17	20	25	25	20	18	18	18	21	33	28	22	9	13	15
VCI-GM	19	16	11	19	22	27	24	19	15	18	21	24	24	20	16	16	17	20	37	27	23	9	12	15
POI-WM	24	19	12	12	15	17	22	16	13	13	16	21	22	19	13	13	23	29	20	14	12	14	18	21
POI-IM	27	20	16	17	24	31	26	20	15	15	18	24	26	20	15	15	20	24	27	23	19	16	20	24
POI-GM	25	19	15	18	22	28	25	19	16	16	19	25	27	20	15	15	22	27	30	21	17	15	17	22
WMI-WM	14	11	9	11	14	19	15	11	10	10	13	16	16	12	11	10	12	14	21	16	7	7	10	12
WMI-IM	27	20	17	18	21	28	25	21	16	18	21	25	32	26	17	17	22	26	33	20	21	21	24	27
WMI-GM	25	20	16	17	21	27	26	21	17	17	21	26	32	26	18	18	23	26	27	21	17	17	22	26
PSI-WM	24	17	14	12	14	20	20	20	14	16	17	26	28	23	19	19	19	29	20	16	14	19	23	28
PSI-IM	27	19	15	17	20	26	22	22	17	18	21	27	33	26	17	17	19	27	26	22	17	16	20	26
PSI-GM	25	18	14	17	20	27	20	20	18	18	21	25	28	25	17	17	20	27	25	21	18	17	20	25
VIQ-AudI	20	15	12	17	23	27	20	18	15	15	17	22	22	19	13	13	16	21	31	27	20	8	10	13
VIQ-AudD	23	15	12	17	24	29	24	18	16	16	19	23	24	19	14	14	18	23	33	25	21	7	10	12
PIQ-VisI	23	16	12	21	28	32	27	20	17	16	21	27	32	24	20	20	18	23	34	31	24	15	19	27
PIQ-VisD	21	16	12	22	25	28	23	20	18	17	21	26	29	22	19	19	18	23	32	28	23	14	18	22
VCI-AudI	20	16	13	18	21	28	25	18	16	16	19	23	23	18	14	14	16	18	29	26	22	7	9	12
VCI-AudD	24	16	13	18	25	29	26	20	15	15	20	22	24	19	15	14	17	21	33	26	22	6	10	14
POI-VisI	26	16	14	23	28	36	28	22	17	17	19	29	35	25	18	18	22	28	35	31	24	18	21	28
POI-VisD	23	17	12	21	26	30	26	21	19	18	21	28	30	25	21	19	25	28	34	27	22	15	20	26

Note: WAIS-III = Wechsler Adult Intelligence Scale—Third Edition; WMS-III = Wechsler Memory Scale—Third Edition; V1 = first variable listed; V2 = second variable listed; VIQ = Verbal IQ; WM = Working Memory (from WMS); IM = Immediate Memory; GM = General Memory; PIQ = Performance IQ; VCI = Verbal Comprehension Index; POI = Perceptual Organization Index; WMI = Working Memory Index (from WAIS); PSI = Processing Speed Index; AudI = Auditory Immediate; AudD = Auditory Delayed; VisI = Visual Immediate; VisD = Visual Delayed.

[a]Weighted *N* = 309 for all comparisons.
[b]Weighted *N* = 423 for all comparisons.
[c]Weighted *N* = 294 for all comparisons.
[d]Weighted *N* = 224 for all comparisons.

Table 10–124 WAIS-III & WMS-III Six-Factor Model and Contributing Subtests

Factors	Subtests
Verbal Comprehension	Vocabulary
	Information
	Similarities
Perceptual Organization	Block Design
	Matrix Reasoning
	Picture Arrangement
Working Memory	Letter-Number Sequencing
	Spatial Span
Processing Speed	Digit Symbol–coding
	Symbol Search
Auditory Memory	Logical Memory I and II
	Paired Associates I and II
Visual Memory	Family Pictures I and II
	Visual Reproduction I and II

Source: From Tulsky et al., 2003a.

multiple age groups. They also provided a table of critical scores for the supplementary subtests compared with the mean of the 11 primary subtests. Although the examiner can use the exact values that are specific for particular age groups, the rounded values (at the .05 level) across all ages are probably sufficient to suggest strengths and weaknesses (Lichtenberger et al., 2002).

Users should note that ipsative analysis of subtest scaled scores is controversial. Some researchers have promoted ipsative profile analysis (e.g., Lichtenberger et al., 2002), whereas others have argued that the reliability (McMann & Barnett, 1997; McDermott et al. 1990) and validity (Watkins & Glutting, 2000) of profile interpretation at this level is poor. Lichtenberger et al. (2002) believe that it is a justifiable means by which to gather more clinical information and to develop additional hypotheses about a person's memory. These hypotheses, however, must then be supported by additional sources of data.

RELIABILITY

Internal Consistency/Generalizeability Coefficients

The reliability of WMS-III subtests and indices (see Table 10–126) tends to be adequate to high (see WAIS-III/WMS-III Technical Manual, 1997, 2002). The median reliability of subtests is .81, and .87 for Indices; that for supplemental subtest scores is somewhat lower, at .77, although still adequate.

Reliabilities of Primary Index discrepancy scores range from .00 to .89 (Charter, 2002). Some of the discrepancy scores have reliabilities too low for clinical use (e.g., Auditory Immediate/Auditory Delayed, Visual Immediate/Visual Delayed, Immediate Memory/General Memory, Auditory Delayed/Auditory Recognition Delayed). Reliability coefficients for the discrepancy scores based on the Primary Index subtest scores are also generally quite low. Charter (2002) reported that Ability/Memory discrepancy reliability coefficients for the Simple-Difference Method were all greater than .70.

Standard Errors of Measurement (*SEMs*)

SEMs for each subtest average about 1 to 1.5 age-scaled score points; for the primary indices, *SEMs* averaged across age groups range from 3.88 points (Auditory Immediate) to 7.71 points (Auditory Recognition Delayed).

Test-Retest Reliability and Practice Effects

According to the WAIS-III/WMS-III Technical Manual (1997, 2002), 297 individuals (10 to 30 in each of the 13 age groups) were retested after an interval ranging from 2 to 12 weeks (M = 35.6 days). Stability coefficients for Primary subtest scores ranged from .62 to .82 (median = .71), and those for the Primary indices ranged from .70 to .88 (median = .82). Although the Auditory Recognition Delayed Index had marginal reliability for ages 16 to 54 years, reliabilities of other Primary indices were acceptable to high (see Table 10–125). Mean Primary subtest scaled scores increased by about 1 to 3 points, except for subtests making up the Working Memory Index (Letter-Number Sequencing, Spatial Span), which showed gains of less than 0.5 points. In general, the older age group (55–89 years) showed smaller gains than the younger age group (16–54 years).

Two methods were used to assess stability for the supplementary subtest scores: test-retest correlations and, in those tasks with relatively small raw-score ranges (e.g., Information, Orientation), decision-consistency coefficients (i.e., the concordance of the decisions in terms of percent correct classification into scaled score ranges). The decision-consistency coefficients range from 50% to 100%, and it is clear from Table 10–127 that the reliabilities of some scores were too low for clinical decision making (e.g., VRII % Retention, Spatial Span Backward). In general, reliabilities tended to be somewhat higher for the older age group (55–89 years). Gains of about 1 to 2 scaled score points were evident on most tasks, with the older age group (55–89 years) tending to show slightly smaller gains than the younger age group (16–54 years).

Iverson (1999, 2001) provided preliminary data, based on reliable change methodology (e.g., Jacobson & Truax, 1991; Chelune et al., 1993), to assist with determinations of improvement or decline on the WMS-III in various clinical samples, including patients with Alzheimer's disease (AD), chronic alcohol use, schizophrenia, or moderate to severe traumatic brain injury (TBI) sustained 6 to 18 months previous to testing. Table 10–128 shows the 90% confidence intervals for measurement error in these groups. Change scores outside these intervals are most likely not a result of measurement error. Note that large retest-difference scores are required to exceed the 90% confidence interval for measurement error. It is also

Table 10–125 Differences Between Individual Subtest Scaled Scores and Mean Scaled Score at Various Levels of Confidence and Frequencies of Differences

Subtest	Level of Confidence			Cumulative %				
	.01	.05	.15	1%	2%	5%	10%	25%
Primary Subtests								
Logical Memory I	3.16	2.62	2.18	5.22	4.71	3.97	3.34	2.33
Faces I	4.78	4.12	3.58	6.88	6.22	5.23	4.50	3.07
Verbal Paired Associates I	2.68	2.30	2.00	5.60	5.06	4.26	3.58	2.50
Family Pictures I	4.21	3.62	3.15	5.63	5.09	4.28	3.60	2.51
Letter-Number Sequencing	4.10	3.53	3.07	6.24	5.64	4.74	3.99	2.78
Spatial Span	4.35	3.75	3.26	6.89	6.22	5.23	4.41	3.07
Logical Memory II	4.38	3.77	3.28	5.01	4.52	3.80	3.20	2.23
Faces II	4.78	4.12	3.58	6.72	6.07	5.10	4.30	2.99
Verbal Paired Associates II	3.96	3.41	2.96	5.71	5.16	4.34	3.65	2.55
Family Pictures II	3.93	3.38	2.94	5.46	4.93	4.15	3.49	2.44
Auditory Recognition Delay	4.78	4.12	3.58	5.46	4.93	4.15	3.49	2.43
Auditory Memory Subtests								
Logical Memory I	3.17	2.68	2.26	4.26	3.85	3.24	2.73	1.90
Logical Memory II	3.93	3.31	2.80	4.24	3.83	3.22	2.71	1.89
Verbal Paired Associates I	2.56	2.16	1.83	4.85	4.38	3.68	3.10	2.16
Verbal Paired Associates II	3.36	2.84	2.40	5.08	4.59	3.86	3.25	2.27
Letter-Number Sequencing	3.71	3.13	2.64	6.17	5.57	4.68	3.94	2.75
Auditory Recognition Delay	4.27	3.60	3.05	4.75	4.29	3.61	3.04	2.12
Visual Memory Subtests								
Faces I	4.17	3.48	2.93	5.60	5.06	4.25	3.58	2.50
Faces II	4.17	3.48	2.93	5.60	5.06	4.25	3.58	2.50
Family Pictures I	3.77	3.15	2.65	4.82	4.36	3.67	3.09	2.15
Family Pictures II	3.55	2.97	2.50	4.77	4.31	3.63	3.05	2.13
Spatial Span	3.86	3.23	2.71	6.79	6.13	5.15	4.34	3.02
Immediate Memory Subtests								
Logical Memory I	2.93	2.43	2.02	5.31	4.80	4.04	3.40	2.37
Faces I	3.77	3.12	2.59	6.35	5.73	4.82	4.06	2.83
Verbal Paired Associates I	2.48	2.05	1.71	5.37	4.85	4.08	3.43	2.39
Family Pictures I	3.40	2.81	2.34	5.24	4.73	3.98	3.35	2.33
Delayed Memory Subtests								
Logical Memory II	3.87	3.23	2.72	4.70	4.24	3.57	3.00	2.09
Faces II	4.16	3.48	2.92	6.58	5.94	5.00	4.21	2.93
Verbal Paired Associates II	3.56	2.97	2.50	5.52	4.99	4.19	3.53	2.46
Family Pictures II	3.54	2.96	2.49	5.52	4.99	4.19	3.53	2.46
Auditory Recognition Delay	4.16	3.48	2.92	4.95	4.47	3.76	3.17	2.21

Source: Adapted from Ryan et al., 2000.

important to bear in mind that these data are crude estimates, because the clinical subjects were not tested twice, and no adjustments were made for practice effects. Rather, the reliability coefficients from the normal population with the *SD*s from the clinical populations were used to calculate *SEM*s, and the *SEM* from time 1 was used twice in the formula for the standard error of the difference.

In unoperated seizure patients tested on two occasions, with a mean intertest interval of 7 months, reliability coefficients tended to be lower, ranging from .56 (Auditory Recog-

nition Delay, Spatial Span) to .88 (Immediate Memory; Martin et al., 2002). Mean score change was usually in a positive direction, with the exception of Working Memory and Auditory Delayed Memory, which both displayed a modest decline (about 2 points) at retesting. Martin et al. (2002) also determined reliable change index (RCI) scores and standardized regression-based (SRB) change score norms in these patients. These methods are useful for determining the effects of epilepsy surgery on cognitive functioning independent of test-retest artifacts including practice effects. Table 10–129 presents the

Table 10–126 Magnitude of Reliability Coefficients of WMS-III Primary Subtests and Indices

Magnitude of Coefficient	Internal Consistency	Generalizeability Coefficients	Test-Retest
Very High (≥.90)	VPA I Auditory Immediate Immediate Memory General Memory		
High (.80 to .89)	LM I Family Pictures I and II Letter-Number Sequence VPA II Visual Immediate Visual Delayed Auditory Delayed Working Memory	Mental Control Digit Span Total Word List II Recall Total	VPA I Auditory Immediate Immediate Memory Auditory Delayed General Memory Working Memory (age group 55–89 years)
Adequate (.70 to .79)	Faces I Spatial Span LM II Faces II Auditory Recognition Delayed	Logical Memory I & II Word List I Recall Total VRI Spatial Span Word List II Recognition VR II Recall Total VRII Recognition VR Copy Total	LM I and II Faces I (age group 16–54 years) Letter-Number Sequence Spatial Span VPA II Visual Immediate Visual Delayed Auditory Recognition Delayed (age group 55–89 years) Working Memory (age group 16–54 years)
Marginal (.60 to .69)			Family Pictures I Family Pictures II (age group 16–54 years) Faces I (age group 55–89 years) Faces II (age group 16–54 years) Audit Recognition Delayed (age group 16–54 years)
Low (≤.59)			

RCI values across the Index scores and the individual subtest scores. Table 10–130 shows the SRB equations that are predictive of postoperative performance. Preoperative performance was the single largest contributor to each predictive regression equation.

Interrater Reliability

According to the WAIS-III/WMS-III Technical Manual (1997, 2002), 10 protocols from each age group were randomly selected from the standardization sample and were independently scored twice. The interscorer reliability coefficients for the subtests requiring the most scoring judgment (LM I and II, Family Pictures I and II, and VR I and II) were all greater than .90, most likely as a result of the explicit scoring criteria provided in the WMS-III Administration and Scoring Manual.

VALIDITY

Index/Subtest Intercorrelations

As might be expected, intercorrelations between the immediate and delayed conditions of the Primary subtests show the highest degree of association. Subtests thought to tap working memory (Letter-Number Sequencing and Spatial Span) correlate moderately well with one another (but see Wilde & Strauss, 2002) and generally show low correlations with other memory subtests. Consistent with expectation, auditorily presented subtests show moderate correlations with other auditorily presented subtests (e.g., LM I Recall/VPA I Recall $r = .48$); however, visually presented subtests correlate only modestly with one another (e.g., Faces I Recall/Family Pictures I Recall $r = .30$), and in some cases they show stronger relations with auditorily presented subtests (e.g., Family Pictures I Recall/ LM I Recall $r = .40$; see WAIS-III/WMS-III Technical Manual), suggesting the role of verbal mediation in the Family Pictures subtest (see also Dulay et al., 2002). These findings raise questions about the validity of summing Faces with Family Pictures to form the Visual Memory Indices.

The Auditory Immediate Index correlates highly with the Auditory Delayed Index ($r = .88$), whereas the Visual Immediate Index shows a strong association with the Visual Delayed Index ($r = .84$). The WAIS-III/WMS-III Technical Manual also includes the intercorrelations of the Primary Indices with the Auditory Process Composites. The Single-Trial Learning Composite correlates highly (.90) with the Auditory Immediate Index. Surprisingly, the Learning Slope composite has relatively low correlations with all indices. The Retention Composite cor-

Table 10–127 Test-Retest and Decision-Consistency Reliabilities for WMS-III Supplemental Subtest Scores

Magnitude of Coefficient and Percentage Decision Consistency	Test-Retest Coefficient	Percentage Decision Consistency
Very High (≥.90, ≥.90%)		Information and Orientation VPA % Retention (age group 16–54 years) VR II Discrimination Total Score
High (.80–.89, 80–90%)	Mental Control (age group 55–89 years)	Word Lists I Learning Slope (age group 55–89 years) Faces II % Retention Family Pix % Retention Word List II % Retention (age group 55–89 years)
Adequate (.70–.79, 70–79%)	Word Lists I Recall Total (age group 55–89 years) VRI Recall Total (age group 55–89 years) Mental Control (age group 16–54 years) VRII Recall Total (age group 16–54 years) VRII Recognition (age group 55–89 years)	LM I First Recall Total Score (age group 55–89 years) LM Learning Slope VPA I First Recall Total VPA I Learning Slope Word Lists First Recall Total (age group 55–89 years) Word Lists I Learning Slope (age group 16–54 years) Word List I Contrast 2 (age group 55–89 years) VPA % Retention (age group 55–89 years)
Marginal (.60–.69, 60–69%)	Word Lists I Recall Total (age group 16–54 years) Word List II Recall Total Word List II Recognition Total VRI Recall Total (age group 16–54 years) Spatial Span Forward Spatial Span Backward (age group 55–89 years) LM II Thematic Total VRII Recall Total (age group 16–54 years) VR copy (age group 16–54 years)	LM I First Recall Total Score (age group 15–64 years) LM I Thematic Total Word Lists First Recall Total (age group 16–54 years) Word List I Contrast 2 (age group 16–54 years) LM II % Retention VRII % Retention (age group 55–89 years)
Low (≤.59, ≤59%)	Spatial Span Backward (age group 16–54 years) VRII Recognition (age group 16–54 years) VR Copy (age group 55–89 years)	Word Lists I Contrast 1 Word List II % Retention (age group 16–54 years) VRII % Retention (age group 16–54 years)

relates most highly ($r = .78$) with the Auditory Delayed Index, whereas the Retrieval index has generally low correlations with Recall indices ($p < .30$) and a correspondingly higher positive relationship ($r = .45$) with the Auditory Recognition Delayed Index. This positive relationship is expected because the Retrieval composite represents the difference between auditory recognition and auditory recall, with positive scores indicating that recognition is higher relative to recall and negative scores indicating the opposite pattern.

Factor Structure of WMS-III

The original publication of the technical manual reported that results of confirmatory factor analytic studies on the standardization sample with the primary subtests supported a five-factor model (working memory, auditory immediate memory, auditory delayed memory, visual immediate memory, and visual delayed memory factors). However, Millis et al. (1999) failed to replicate the results in the standardization

Table 10–128 Confidence Interval (90%) for Reliable Change in Clinical Groups

WMS-III	Alzheimer's Disease	Chronic Alcoholism	Schizophrenia	Traumatic Brain Injury
Auditory Immediate	9.95	14.28	14.46	17.91
Visual Immediate	12.38	17.17	16.91	16.45
Immediate Memory	10.58	15.30	14.56	16.42
Auditory Delayed	8.91	15.10	14.50	21.24
Visual Delayed	9.20	15.97	17.52	16.45
Auditory Recognition Delayed	10.76	18.99	21.78	24.26
General Memory	7.23	11.86	13.20	13.78
Working Memory	17.65	11.87	17.25	15.19

Source: Adapted from Iverson, 1999, 2001.

Table 10-129 Reliable Change Index (RCI) Values in Patients with Complex Partial Seizures

Variable	Correction for Practice	Adjusted RCI (90%)	Adjusted RCI (80%)
Auditory Immediate	+1	≤ − 14, ≥ + 16	≤ − 11, ≥ + 13
Visual Immediate	+3	≤ − 15, ≥ + 21	≤ − 11, ≥ + 17
Immediate Memory	+2	≤ − 12, ≥ + 16	≤ − 9, ≥ + 13
Auditory Delayed	−2	≤ − 19, ≥ + 15	≤ − 15, ≥ + 11
Visual Delayed	+5	≤ − 13, ≥ + 23	≤ − 9, ≥ + 19
Auditory Recognition	−1	≤ − 22, ≥ + 20	≤ − 18, ≥ + 16
General Memory	+1	≤ − 16, ≥ + 18	≤ − 13, ≥ + 15
Working Memory	−2	≤ − 22, ≥ + 18	≤ − 18, ≥ + 14
LM Immediate	0	≤ − 3, ≥ + 3	≤ − 3, ≥ + 3
LM Delayed	0	≤ − 4, ≥ + 4	≤ − 3, ≥ + 3
Faces Immediate	+1	≤ − 3, ≥ + 5	≤ − 2, ≥ + 4
Faces Delayed	+1	≤ − 3, ≥ + 5	≤ − 2, ≥ + 4
VPA Immediate	0	≤ − 3, ≥ + 3	≤ − 3, ≥ + 3
VPA Delayed	0	≤ − 4, ≥ + 4	≤ − 3, ≥ + 3
Family Pictures Immediate	0	≤ − 3, ≥ + 3	≤ − 3, ≥ + 3
Family Pictures Delayed	0	≤ − 4, ≥ + 4	≤ − 3, ≥ + 3
Letter-Number Sequencing	0	≤ − 4, ≥ + 4	≤ − 3, ≥ + 3
Spatial Span	+1	≤ − 4, ≥ + 6	≤ − 3, ≥ + 5

Source: Adapted from Martin et al., 2002.

Table 10-130 Regression Equations for WMS-III Measures

Variable	R	SEE	Constant	β For Baseline	β For Age	β For Education	β For Age at Seizure Onset/Age at Seizure First Risk	β For Gender
Auditory Immediate	0.81	8.90	3.75	0.82		1.00		
Visual Immediate	0.78	10.98	12.97	0.89				
Immediate Memory	0.88	8.93	−.46	1.03				
Auditory Delayed	0.79	8.61	19.00	0.60		1.28		
Visual Delayed	0.81	12.18	−2.17	1.09				
Auditory Recognition	0.66	11.00	48.13	0.55				
General Memory	0.79	10.53	13.91	0.86				
Working Memory	0.70	10.49	33.12	0.60				
LM Immediate	0.72	2.00	2.41	0.72				
LM Delayed	0.67	2.17	.90	0.47		0.25	1.27	
Faces Immediate	0.60	2.32	2.99	0.74				
Faces Delayed	0.67	2.48	1.62	0.88				1.68
VPA Immediate	0.81	1.93	−2.74	0.87		0.28		
VPA Delayed	0.75	2.14	−.73	0.67		0.26		
Family Pictures Immediate	0.81	1.94	4.33	0.73	−0.05			
Family Pictures Delayed	0.78	2.52	0.97	0.93				
Letter-Number Sequencing	0.69	2.27	2.66	0.66				
Spatial Span	0.56	2.61	2.93	0.54				

Note: The WMS-III values are standard scores.

β = unstandardized Beta (slope); SEE = standard error of the estimate. Example: A patient's preoperative Auditory Immediate Memory Index (AMI) = 86, and the postoperative AMI (Y_o) = 80; the predicted postoperative AMI score (Y_p) = 3.75 + [0.82 × (baseline score)] + [1.0 × (years of education)] = 88.3. After calculation, the z-score change value = $(Y_o − Y_p)/SE_{regression\ equation}$ = − 0.93. This is within the ± 1.64 (90%) confidence interval and therefore is not considered to be significant change because it does not extend beyond the lower 5% of the distribution of the control sample change scores.

Source: Adapted from Martin et al., 2002.

sample and reported that models specifying separate immediate and delayed memory factors were hampered by inadmissible solutions signaling model specification error. They concluded that a three-factor model including the dimensions of working memory, visual memory, and auditory memory provided the best fit for the standardization sample (see also Price et al., 2002). In a sample of patients with intractable temporal lobe epilepsy, a three-factor model (working memory, visual memory, auditory memory) and a nested, more parsimonious two-factor model of working memory and general memory provided the best fit of the data (Wilde et al., 2003). In short, the results suggested that specification of a separate visual memory factor provided little advantage for this sample, an unexpected finding in a population with lateralized dysfunction, for which one might have predicted separate auditory and visual memory dimensions.

However, when selected Word List subtests were included with the primary subtests, findings in both the standardization sample and a mixed clinical sample supported a four-factor model comprising auditory memory (LM I and II, VPA I and II, Auditory Recognition Delayed), visual memory (Faces I and II, Family Pictures I and II), working memory (Letter-Number Sequence, Spatial Span), and learning (Word List I and II recall, Word List II Recognition; Burton et al., 2003).

In short, the available data provide no statistical support for separate immediate and delayed indices in either normal or clinical samples. This may be a result of the high correlation between immediate and delayed conditions of the same memory tasks. Tulsky and his colleagues (Tulsky & Price, 2003; Tulsky et al., 2003) have developed norms based on collapsing of the immediate and delayed recall indices. The interpretation of separate auditory and visual dimensions (as well as differences between scores) should also be made with caution, at least in patients with temporal lobe epilepsy (Bell et al., 2004; Wilde et al., 2003).

Relationship With WAIS-III

IQ is moderately related to memory scores (e.g., FSIQ/General Memory $r = .60$), supporting the association between intelligence and memory and the potential utility of discrepancy analyses for determining weaknesses in memory relative to general intellectual ability.

As expected, auditory memory measures show higher correlations with WAIS-III verbal measures (VCI $r = .54$ to .57) compared with nonverbal measures (POI $r = .44$ to .46) measures; however, contrary to expectation, the WMS-III Delayed Visual Memory Index correlates equally with WAIS-III VCI and POI ($r = .36$). The high correlation between the WMS-III and WAIS-III Working Memory Indices ($r = .82$) is expected, because they measure a similar construct in addition to sharing one subtest.

Although the two tests are moderately related to one another, the WMS-III measures areas of functioning not tapped by the WAIS-III. Tulsky and his colleagues (Tulsky & Price, 2003; Tulsky et al., 2003) have concluded that a six-factor model demonstrates the best fit with the WMS-III/WAIS-III

data. The factors are verbal comprehension, visual-perceptual organization, working memory, processing speed, auditory memory, and visual memory. As noted earlier, Tulsky's group (see *Normative Data*) have developed norms to parallel the six-factor structure. They have also developed an alternate visual memory index, substituting Visual Reproduction for Faces, given the relatively low loading of Faces on the Visual Memory factor. In addition, they have removed the recognition index from the core battery and presented it as an optional score. Whether the six-factor model, and corresponding index scores, will prove to be useful in making clinical decisions remains to be determined.

Relationship With Other Measures

There is some evidence of convergent and divergent validity, at least for the auditory memory and working memory dimensions. At present, there is not sufficient support for the indices derived from visually presented material.

For example, a sample of 207 healthy adults (age $M = 44.7$ years, $SD = 20.6$) were given both the WMS-R and the WMS-III in counterbalanced order, with the interval between testings sessions ranging from 2 to 12 weeks (median = 32 days; WAIS-III/WMS-III Technical Manual, 1997, 2002). The correlations of the WMS-III Auditory Immediate Index with the WMS-R Verbal Memory Index ($r = .72$), the WMS-III Visual Immediate Memory Index with the WMS-R Visual Memory Index ($r = .36$), and the WMS-III Immediate Memory Index with the WMS-R General Memory Index ($r = .62$) were in the moderate-high range, with auditory memory tasks showing stronger correlations than those based on visually presented material. As expected, the WMS-III Working Memory Index correlated highest with the WMS-R Attention/Concentration Index ($r = .64$). A similar picture emerged in adolescents, aged 16 years, given the Children's Memory Scale (CMS) and the WMS-III.

In a heterogenous sample of individuals with neurological and developmental disorders, the WMS-III Working Memory Index correlated higher with other measures of attention/concentration (e.g., r values ranged from .48 to .85 for WAIS-R Digit Span, WMS-R Attention-Concentration Index, MicroCog Attention/Mental Control Index, Trails B) than with the other WMS-III memory indices (WAIS-III/WMS-III Technical Manual, 1997, 2002). The WMS-III Working Memory Index had relatively lower correlation with other measures of auditory and visual episodic memory (e.g., R values ranged from .11 to .42 for CVLT, MicroCog, ROCF). The WMS-III Auditory Memory Indices had somewhat stronger correlations with verbal memory tasks (e.g., Auditory Immediate/CVLT Total $r = .71$) than with visual memory tasks (e.g., Auditory Immediate/ROCF Immediate Memory $r = .55$; WAIS-III/WMS-III Technical Manual, 1997, 2002). However, the WMS-III Visual Delayed Memory Index showed a stronger correlation with CVLT Total ($r = .40$) than with delayed memory of the Rey Figure ($r = .22$).

The WMS-III memory indices show modest correlations with language measures such as the BNT (r values ranging from .25 to .39). Correlations of similar magnitude occur with the COWA (FAS), ranging from .21 (Visual Immediate Memory Index) to .50 (Working Memory Index; WAIS-III/WMS-III Technical Manual, 1997, 2002).

Correlations between the WMS-III and measures of spatial processing (MicroCog, Judgment of Line Orientation, ROCF Copy) are mixed. As might be expected, the WMS-III visual memory indices correlate more highly with the Spatial Processing Index of MicroCog ($r = .47$ to .71) than do the auditory memory indices ($r = .31$ to .57). However, correlations with JOLO appear to be equivalent for auditory and visual indices ($r = .30$ to .50 and $r = .35$ to .37, respectively) and become nonsignificant when the effects of general intellectual status (FSIQ) are controlled. Except for the Working Memory Index ($r = .28$), correlations with the Copy trial of the ROCF are very low. The WMS-III Working Memory Index has the highest correlation with the WCST, but only with total correct ($r = .60$), not with perseverative errors ($r = -.01$; WAIS-III/WMS-III Technical Manual, 1997, 2002). Correlations with measures of manual speed and dexterity (Finger Tapping, Grooved Pegboard) tend to be low; however, those who score higher on visual memory indices tend to demonstrate faster performance on the Grooved Pegboard dominant hand measure ($r = -.41$ to $-.53$).

Clinical Studies

The WMS-III appears sensitive to verbal memory deficits that occur in developmental disorders such as attention-deficit/hyperactivity disorder (ADHD) and reading disability (WAIS-III/WMS-III Technical Manual, 1997, 2002). According to the WAIS-III/WMS-III Technical Manual (1997, 2002), the WMS-III also appears sensitive to memory difficulties associated with various neurological conditions, such as AD, Huntington's disease (HD), Parkinson's disease (PD), TBI (Fisher et al., 2000; Langeluddecke & Lucas, 2005), and multiple sclerosis (MS).

The WAIS-III/WMS-III Technical Manual (1999, 2002) provides data based on small samples of selected neurological disorders. In general, memory scores tend to be lower than IQ scores after brain damage; however, the magnitude of the IQ/Memory Index discrepancies is not sufficiently large to serve as "red flags" for brain dysfunction per se (Hawkins, 1998). Further, compared with the Immediate Memory Index, the WMS-III General Memory Index (measuring delayed recall and recognition) does not exhibit greater sensitivity to memory deficits (Hawkins, 1998; Heaton et al., 2003; Langeluddecke & Lucas, 2005). This may be because Faces I Recognition incorporates a delay between stimulus presentation and recognition and one LM I story is presented twice. VPA, consisting of novel unrelated pairs, runs over four trials. In addition, as noted earlier, immediate and delayed conditions are highly correlated with one another, and factor analytic findings do not suggest separable dimensions. In short, Immediate Memory may be a misnomer in this case, and the Immediate and General (Delayed) Indices may be redundant.

Examination of clinical data provided in the technical manual as well as other reports suggests that visual memory is particularly vulnerable to brain disorders (see also Hawkins, 1998; Hawkins & Tulsky, 2003; Langeluddecke & Lucas, 2005; Taylor & Heaton, 2001), perhaps because of its timed presentation format.

Although firm conclusions are difficult because of the small numbers involved, information from the test may be useful in differentiating patterns of memory impairment associated with diverse conditions (see also Dori & Chelune, 2004; Heaton et al., 2003; Taylor & Heaton, 2001). For example, patients with Korsakoff's syndrome showed significant impairment on the WMS-III measures of episodic memory (visual and auditory memory indices) despite relatively intact working memory and general intellectual level (FSIQ $M = 92.8$, $SD = 13.6$). Patients with mild AD also showed impaired episodic memory performance (i.e., scores of 70 or less on the Auditory and Visual Memory Indices), whereas performance on the Working Memory Index appeared less affected. By contrast, patients with HD tended to have more difficulty on the visual as opposed to the auditory subtests. The extent of memory impairment evident in patients with PD appeared much less than that observed in patients with AD, despite similar FSIQ scores (AD $M = 86.6$, $SD = 13.1$; PD $M = 88.2$, $SD = 10.1$). Patients with moderate to severe head injuries showed an unexpected pattern of memory performance, with lower scores on the visual as opposed to the auditory memory indices, a pattern also seen in patients with HD and a small group ($n = 25$) of patients with MS. These trends are promising, and additional, larger-scale studies reporting relevant data such as sensitivity, specificity, and diagnosis-specific odds ratios are required.

Laterality

The test is sensitive to laterality of disturbance. Patients with left temporal lobe epilepsy tended to perform better on the visual than the auditory tasks, whereas patients with right temporal lobe epilepsy showed the opposite pattern (Doss et al., 2000; Heaton et al., 2003; WAIS-III/WMS-III Technical Manual 1997, 2002); however, the utility of the WMS-III in detecting laterality of disturbance (e.g., using Auditory-Visual Delayed Index difference scores) appears very limited, at least in preoperative cases (Dulay et al., 2002; Wilde et al., 2001; but see Chiaravalloti et al., 2004). In postsurgical cases, material-specific effects do emerge (Doss et al., 2004). Interestingly, the differences between left- and right-sided temporal lobectomy groups was more pronounced in the immediate than in the delayed conditions. VPA I, Faces I, and, to a lesser extent, Family Pictures II best discriminated left- and right-hemisphere groups, with almost 50% of the variance accounted for.

Aging

Age-related declines are evident on both recall and recognition of LM and VR. Haaland and her colleagues (Haaland et al., 2003; Price et al., 2004) examined the standardization sample and found that decreases in recall and recognition performance emerged in the fifth decade. However, delayed recall and recognition, when adjusted for immediate recall, showed only minimal age-associated deterioration (Price et al., 2004). These findings led the authors to conclude that the aging effect is due largely to deterioration in encoding during acquisition, rather than problems with retrieval or storage of new information (Haaland et al., 2003; Price et al., 2004; but see Uttl et al., 2002, who cautioned against using various WMS-III subtests to inform about aging). In other words, normal aging does not commonly produce more rapid forgetting, because most of the information that is initially encoded is recalled on delay; rather, information is not stored at all or is not stored well enough to be retrieved after a delay, perhaps because of superficial encoding. From a clinical standpoint, the sensitivity of the WMS-III to subtle deficits in delayed recall and recognition is decreased by the large influence of immediate recall, particularly with advancing age. Accordingly, impaired retention may serve as a useful marker of abnormality (Price et al., 2004).

Base Rates of Impairment

Tulsky and his colleagues (Tulsky & Price, 2003; Tulsky et al., 2003) suggested that the WAIS/WMS battery together measures six basic constructs: verbal comprehension, visual-perceptual organization, working memory, processing speed, auditory memory, and visual memory (Table 10–124). Clinicians need to be aware that about 46% of normal subjects obtain at least one "impaired" factor score (using a 1 SD cutoff) on the six-factor WAIS/WMS battery (Taylor & Heaton, 2001). Few, however, are impaired on more than two factor scores (about 10%). With a three-factor (auditory memory, processing speed, visual memory) or a four-factor (perceptual organization, auditory memory, processing speed, visual memory) battery, the criterion for diagnosing abnormality would be more than one impaired score, whereas, for a two-factor battery (processing speed, visual memory), the criterion is one impaired score.

Additional Issues Related to Subtests

Faces. The Faces subtest has been the subject of recent criticism. It appears to function in a different manner from the Family Pictures subtest (see *Relationship to WAIS-III*), and its correlation with the Visual Reproduction subtest of the WMS-III is quite low (about .20; WAIS-III/WMS-III Technical Manual).

There are additional concerns with this subtest. Levy (2003) pointed out that the administration and scoring formats of the test result in considerable overlap between the ranges of raw scores expected under chance performance (17–31) and the scaled scores that represent normal functioning. As a consequence, older clients with severe impairment would rarely obtain a scaled score within the severely impaired range and often perform within normal limits if they

guess on the trials. For example, in the age group 65 to 69 years, scaled scores of 7 and 8, which indicate performance within the low-average range, correspond to raw scores between 29 and 31 (i.e., within the chance interval). The use of signal detection methodology to take into account response patterns may increase the utility of this task (Chiaravalloti et al., 2004; Holdnack & Delis, 2004).

Family Pictures. This subtest relies heavily on verbal abilities (Dulay et al., 2002; Wilde et al., 2003). For example, Dulay et al. (2002) reported that Logical Memory is the best predictor of Family Pictures, accounting for about 27% to 31% of the variance. Tests such as the Faces subtest of the Warrington RMT and the BVRT account for less than 10% additional variance. There is also evidence from both normal and clinical samples that Family Pictures and Faces subtests do not form a coherent factor, rendering the visual indices suspect (Millis et al., 1999; Wilde et al., 2003). Whether breaking the scores into subcomponents (character, location, activity) would improve diagnostic utility is not certain. Dulay et al. (2002) reported that the location score did not differentiate patients with right temporal lobe epilepsy from other epilepsy patients. By contrast, Holley et al. (2000) reported that the location score differentiated right from left temporal lobectomy patients when verbal mediation strategies were taken into account.

Digit Span and Spatial Span. The WAIS-III/WMS-III Technical Manual (2002) states that Spatial Span is a visual analog of Digit Span. However, recent findings in both healthy subjects and clinical samples have suggested that Digit Span and Spatial Span operate in different ways (Hester et al., 2004; Myerson et al., 2003; Wilde & Strauss, 2002; Wilde et al., 2004). For example, Digit Span Forward scores tend to be greater than Digit Span Backward scores, but in Spatial Span, there is a much higher incidence of backward scores being greater than forward scores. There are also methodological differences between the tasks. For example, in Digit Span, the sequences are different in forward and backward conditions; in Spatial Span, they are identical, providing additional exposure of the sequence. Therefore, clinicians should be cautious about making direct comparisons between Digit Span and Spatial Span. Suggestions regarding laterality of disturbance based on Digit Span and Spatial Span performance are also discouraged in the absence of validity studies on this topic (Wilde & Strauss, 2002). Of note, Wilde et al. (2001) failed to find a meaningful difference in Spatial Span scores in patients with lateralized temporal lobe disturbance, casting doubt on the utility of such a discrepancy approach in detecting lateralized dysfunction.

Clinical lore suggests that the backward conditions of both span tasks are more demanding of working memory processing than the forward conditions and that, consequently, the backward conditions are more sensitive to advancing age and clinical conditions. However, recent findings contradict this belief. Age-related declines appear to be similar in forward and backward conditions in both tasks (Hester et al.,

2004; Myerson et al., 2003; Wilde et al., 2004). Although backward span conditions tend to be lower in those conditions for which working memory deficits are generally well established (e.g., AD, HD), forward span is generally affected whenever backward span is impaired, lessening the unique value of poor backward span performance (Wilde et al., 2004).

From a clinical point of view, these findings minimize concerns about combining forward and backward values into a single score; in fact, inclusion of both conditions increases the reliability of the measure. The findings also suggest that backward span is not a clinically sensitive measure of working memory. Abnormally large discrepancies may well signify working memory deficits; however, problems with working memory can be present even in the absence of such a discrepancy (Wilde et al., 2004).

Finally, research is needed to evaluate the task's validity as a measure of visual-spatial working memory. In a mixed clinical sample, Spatial Span showed a modest relation with Digit Span ($r = .34$), but not with Letter-Number Sequence ($r = .03$), raising concerns about the meaning of this subtest (Wilde & Strauss, 2002).

Word Lists.   Measures from the Word List test tend to correlate highly with those from the CVLT (Recognition $r = .50$; Total Immediate Recall $r = .76$); however, the level of concordance is less than optimal (McDowell et al., 2004). In a heterogeneous clinical sample, McDowell et al. (2004) reported that test agreement for recognition memory impairment was just above chance; for recall measures, test agreement was 76% to 80%. Almost all disagreements were composed of an impairment on the CVLT that was not present on the Word List task, suggesting that the latter task is less sensitive to dysfunction than the CVLT.

Prediction of Premorbid Memory Functioning.   With the demographically adjusted norms (WAIS-III/WMS-III/WIAT-II software), the clinician can estimate memory performance relative to a homogeneous subgroup similar in age, education level, gender, and race/ethnicity. In this way, the clinician can determine whether the patient's current performance is below expectations, given specific background variables.

Another approach incorporates a performance-based measure, the WTAR (see *Wechsler Test of Adult Reading*), a test of reading of irregularly spelled words, that was conormed with the WAIS-III and WMS-III and is available for use in the United States and the United Kingdom. The WTAR may be particularly useful in estimating premorbid status in light of recent research suggesting that reliance on years of education may not be sufficient to account for quality of educational experience (Manly et al., 2002). Tables in the WTAR manual allow WMS-III scores to be predicted by WTAR performance only or by a combination of WTAR performance and demographics (age, education, gender, race/ethnicity). Additional tables allow the examiner to evaluate the significance and rarity of the discrepancy between predicted and obtained values. Users should bear in mind, however, that correlations between the WTAR and WMS-III memory performance are only moderate (for the U.S. standardization sample, Working Memory $r = .51$; General Memory $r = .49$; and Immediate Memory $r = .47$), and in a clinical sample, the correlations were even smaller ($r = .32$ to .33). With regard to accuracy of classification based on the WTAR alone, estimates for WMS-III memory performance were low (about 55% within ±10 points). In short, WTAR performance should be considered only as a modest predictor of premorbid memory ability.

Ecological Validity

There is some evidence that performance on the WMS-III (especially delayed verbal recall) can predict motor learning (e.g., a procedure using a walker) in older adults (Tunney et al., 2002). Total recall of Word List I, but not Working Memory, was highly related ($r = .67$) to prospective memory performance in neurological patients seen in a rehabilitation setting (Titov & Knight, 2000).

Malingering

A number of measures derived from the WMS-III may facilitate detection of suboptimal performance. Probable malingerers tend to suppress their performance on all WMS-III subtests and indices (Langeluddecke & Lucas, 2003). The delayed recognition tasks appear particularly useful. Langeluddecke & Lucas (2003) reported that 80% of probable malingerers obtained raw scores below 43/54 on the Auditory Recognition Delayed Total Score, whereas only 8.2% of patients with severe TBI performed below this cutoff. For Word List II recognition, 81% of probable malingerers obtained scores below the cutoff (18/24), compared with 4.4% of subjects with severe TBI.

Killgore & DellaPietra (2000) suggested that an index (Rarely Missed Index, RMI) based on a weighted combination of six rarely missed items on the LM Delayed Recognition task may enhance detection, adding predictive utility beyond that provided by examination of the total score on this subtest. These six items (items 12, 16, 18, 22, 24, and 29) are endorsed at frequencies exceeding chance even by individuals with no prior knowledge of the story content. Each of the six rarely missed items is assigned a weighted point value, as listed in Table 10–131. Calculation of the RMI is achieved by summing the weighted point values for each of the six items endorsed correctly by the patient. Wrong answers receive no points. The RMI scores can range from −22 to 226. Using a cutoff score of 136, the RMI demonstrated high sensitivity (97%) and specificity (100%) in discriminating between analog malingerers and patients with neurological impairment. Miller et al. (2004) found high specificity (95% correct classification) for the RMI cut-score of 136 among individuals diagnosed with alcohol or polysubstance abuse who were not in litigation or seeking compensation/gain. However, less favorable results were reported in a personal injury setting. Lange et al. (2005) evaluated litigating and nonlitigating patients and found the RMI

Table 10–131 RMI Point Values for Each of the Six Rarely Missed Logical Memory Delayed Recognition Items.

LMDR Item Number	RMI Point Value
12	−22
16	55
18	84
22	67
24	13
29	7

Source: Adapted from Killgore & DellaPietra, 2000.

to display low sensitivity (.25), very high specificity (range = .91 to .95), moderate positive predictive power (range = .50 to .71), and moderate to high negative predictive power (range = .68 to .83). In short, the RMI does not reliably detect symptom exaggeration, at least in the context of personal injury, and appears to be of limited value. Positive RMI scores are obtained infrequently, and the clinician can have only a moderate degree of confidence that the subject's performance is reflective of exaggeration.

The Faces I subtest can also provide information with regard to motivational status, because it appears to be less influenced by TBI than by malingering. Glassmire et al. (2003) studied nonlitigating TBI patients and controls (mean age about 33 years) under standard and instructed malingering conditions. They found that the total raw score provided a stronger classification accuracy than an empirically weighted combination of the five easiest items (i.e., floor effect items 10, 17, 39, 43, and 45). A raw score cutoff of 31/48 (corresponding to chance-level performance) yielded the maximum classification accuracy, with 93.3% sensitivity and 80% specificity. Differences between indices (e.g., Immediate Memory/Working Memory; FSIQ/General Memory) and "easy" tasks such as Digit Span, Spatial Span, and Mental Control were not very sensitive to suboptimal effort.

COMMENT

The WMS-III has undergone extensive revision and may measure different constructs than its predecessor. Whereas the WMS-R tended to support either a two-factor model (general memory and attention concentration) or three-factor models (attention-concentration, immediate memory, and delayed memory constructs; see Spreen & Strauss, 1998, for review), the WMS-III yields the dimensions of working memory, visual memory, and auditory memory or a more parsimonious two-factor model of working memory and general memory. Such differences between tests likely have clinical relevance in the examination of specific disorders.

The WMS-III has a number of significant strengths. The standardization sample is substantial, covers a wide age range, and is closely matched to U.S. Census data. The test was conormed with the WAIS-III, allowing for more accurate and sophisticated interpretation of IQ-memory discrepancies (Franzen & Iverson, 2000; Lichtenberger et al., 2002). The availability of demographically corrected norms is also a major strength. Reliability tends to be adequate to high. The Auditory Immediate Index, Immediate Memory Index, Auditory Delayed Index, and General Memory Index are the most reliable in terms of both internal consistency and test-retest reliability. Accordingly, the psychologist should have greatest confidence in the precision of these scores. At the subtest level, LM I and VPA I are the most reliable. However, the Auditory Recognition Delayed Index, Faces, Family Pictures, and some supplemental as well as discrepancy scores show marginal to low reliability, and the clinician needs to interpret these scores with considerable caution.

Some subtests have truncated floors and ceilings depending on the age group (Flanagan et al., 2000; Lichtenberger et al., 2002; Uttl, 2005). For example, an 80 year-old who recalls none of the word pairs on VPA still earns a scaled score of 7, reflecting low-average performance. By the same token, a 50-year-old who retains 100% of learned word pairs only achieves a scaled score of 12. Accordingly, scores from these tests must be interpreted with caution (Lacrtiz & Cullum, 2003); for additional commentary on ceiling effects of VPA and the development of longer (15-, 16-, and 28-item) tests see Uttl et al., 2002 and Uttl, 2005. In a similar vein, the distribution of scores for the Auditory Recognition Index is quite restricted and negatively skewed, because most of the standardization sample obtained perfect scores on recognition variables. As a consequence, the Auditory Recognition Delayed Index is more of a deficit than an ability index: it is most useful as an indication of deficiency when someone does poorly. Normal or even near-perfect scores on the LM and VPA recognition subtests do not necessarily indicate intact performance in this area. Uttl (2005; Uttl et al., 2002) warned that the WMS-III norms for these subtests (as well as the Word List test, which also suffers from ceiling effects for young adults) cannot be used to make decisions about the memory ability of most adults and are not appropriate for research with healthy adults.

Tulsky et al. (2003a) advise against computing an index score for the Auditory Recognition Delayed Index; rather, they present an alternate way to determine whether an individual has scored as poorly as the lowest performers in the WMS-III standardization sample, using cumulative percentages associated with raw scores for each of the Auditory Recognition variables. They provide a table for this purpose in their book (page 129).

Woodard et al. (2004) also noted that the Auditory Recognition Delayed index reflects a composite of two verbal recognition measures (LM Recognition and VPA Recognition) and that such a composite does not adequately capture the pattern of performance on either of these two measures (i.e., the same Auditory Recognition Delayed Index could be obtained by different performances on the two components). They recommended examination of each of these components (consistent with Tulsky et al., 2003a).

The Faces subtest appears to have insufficient commonality with Family Pictures, raising concerns about interpretation of the Visual Memory factor (Millis et al., 1999; Wilde et al., 2003). In addition, concerns have been raised about the ability of the Faces subtest to detect impairment, particularly in the elderly (Levy, 2003). Other tests (e.g., Warrington's Recognition Memory Test—Faces) may have more power to detect impairment in elderly subjects. Levy (2003) suggested that the Faces subtest should not be used with individuals older than 65 years of age.

Further research is necessary in clinical populations to determine how best to use these recognition subtests and of what benefit they can be (Lacritz & Cullum, 2003). Given the forced-choice testing format associated with each of the recognition subtests, examination of a variety of performance indices using signal detection theory (e.g., focusing on hits as well as false alarms, tendency to produce more yes or more no responses) may enhance their clinical utility, particularly in patients with dementia or depression (e.g., Holdnack & Delis, 2004; Woodard et al., 2004). Some of the tasks (e.g., Faces, LM Recognition) may also be of value in the assessment of motivational status.

The continued use of the immediate and delayed indices does not appear to be supported in normal or clinical populations (e.g., Bell et al., 2004; Burton et al., 2003; Doss et al., 2004; Langeluddecke & Lucas, 2005; Wilde et al., 2003). Each subtest on the WMS-III requires retention of material for the immediate task beyond that which would be possible based on models of working memory; therefore, it seems likely that, to perform adequately on the immediate memory measures, multiple memory components (including encoding, storage, and retrieval) would be required. Whether the immediate-delayed distinction is useful in particular patient groups (e.g., AD) awaits further research. Exclusion of the delayed components would save about 10 to 15 min in administration time. However, administration of the delayed trials may be useful in some cases. Some patients do much better on the delayed trials, perhaps because anxiety undermined earlier efforts. Therefore, the delay trial may allow the clinician to rule out an amnestic condition otherwise suggested by low immediate subtest scores (Hawkins, 1998).

The literature does not support the notion that Spatial Span is an analog of Digit Span. The tasks operate in somewhat different ways, and clinicians should be cautious in making direct comparisons between these span tasks. Nor does the literature support the conceptual distinction between forward and backward Digit or Spatial Span. If backward span is low, forward span is also likely to be low. It is also worth noting that some researchers have suggested that backward span tasks require relatively little working memory processing (e.g., Dobbs & Rule, 1989; Engle et al., 1999).

Larrabee (2004) questioned the advisability of basing the Working Memory Index on Letter-Number Sequence and Spatial Span. In part, his hesitation stemmed from factor analytic findings suggesting that Spatial Span has little to do with Attention/Working Memory and more to do with visual-spatial processes of the sort tapped by the Wechsler Perceptual Organization factor. In addition, he noted that, by making Digit Span an optional subtest, one potentially loses the added value of Digit Span as a measure of motivation.

The published version of the WMS-III is not equivalent on a number of parameters with the final version published by The Psychological Corporation (Doss et al., 2000). Specifically, the standardization protocol included additional subtests and delayed trials, and the subtests included in the WMS-III Primary Indices were administered in a different order. However, comparable WMS-III index scores were obtained between the standardization and published versions in patients with seizure disorders (Doss et al., 2000), suggesting that the norms derived from administration of the standardization version are applicable to data derived from the published version of the WMS-III. It is possible, however, that systematic differences between versions could emerge in populations in which factors such as fatigue or increased susceptibility to interference are prominent (Doss et al., 2000).

The available evidence suggests that the test has clinical utility, showing sensitivity to memory disturbances in a variety of patient populations. Users should bear in mind that the WMS-III assesses only limited aspects of memory (auditory, visual, and working memory). There are many areas that are not evaluated by this test, such as olfactory, kinesthetic, procedural, and prospective memory. Information on its relation to everyday memory performance is also limited. In short, it may be necessary to supplement the WMS-III with other tests or to use entirely different instruments (Lichtenberger et al., 2002).

REFERENCES

Axelrod, B. N. (2001). Administration duration for the Wechsler Adult Intelligence Scale-III. *Archives of Clinical Neuropsychology, 16*, 293–301.

Axelrod, B. N., & Woodard, J. L. (2000). Parsimonious prediction of Wechsler Memory Scale-III memory indexes. *Psychological Assessment, 12*, 431–435.

Axelrod, B. N., Ryan, J. J., & Woodard, J. L. (2001). Cross-validation of prediction equations for Wechsler Memory Scale-III indexes. *Assessment, 8*, 367–372.

Basso, M. R., Harrington, K., Matson, M., & Lowery, N. (2000). Sex differences on the WMS-III: Findings concerning Verbal Paired Associated and Faces. *The Clinical Neuropsychologist, 14*, 231–235.

Bell, B. D., Hermann, B. P., & Seidenberg, M. (2004). Significant discrepancies between immediate and delayed WMS-III indices are rare in temporal lobe epilepsy patients. *The Clinical Neuropsychologist, 18*, 303–311.

Borum, R., & Grisso, T. (1995). Psychological test use in criminal forensic evaluations. *Professional Psychology: Research and Practice, 26*, 465–473.

Burton, D. B., Ryan, J. J., Axelrod, B. N., Schellenberger, T., & Richards, H. M. (2003). A confirmatory factor analysis of the WMS-III in a clinical sample with crossvalidation in the standardization sample. *Archives of Clinical Neuropsychology, 18*, 629–641.

Butters, N., Salmon, D. P., Cullum, C. M., Cairns, P., Tröster, A. I., Jacobs, D., et al. (1988). Differentiation of amnestic and demented patients with the Wechsler Memory Scale-Revised. *The Clinical Neuropsychologist, 2,* 133–148.

Camara, W. J., Nathan, J. S., & Puente, A. E. (2000). Psychological test usage: Implications in professional psychology. *Professional Psychology: Research and Practice, 31,* 141–154.

Charter, R. A. (2002). Reliability of the WMS-III discrepancy comparisons. *Perceptual and Motor Skills, 94,* 387–390.

Chelune, G. I., Nangle, R. I., Luders, H., Sedlak, J., & Awad, I. A. (1993). Individual change after epilepsy surgery: Practice effects and base-rate information. *Neuropsychology, 7,* 41–52.

Chiaravalloti, N., Tulsky, D. S., & Glosser, G. (2004). Validation of the WMS-III facial memory subtest with the Graduate Hospital Facial Memory Test in a sample of right and left anterior temporal lobectomy patients. *Journal of Clinical and Experimental Neuropsychology, 26,* 484–497.

Cole, J. C., Lopez, B. R., & McLeod, J. S. (2003). Comprehensive tables for determination of strengths and weakness on the WMS-III. *Journal of Psychoeducational Assessment, 21,* 79–88.

Dobbs, A. R., & Rule, B. G. (1989). Adult age differences in working memory. *Psychology and Aging, 4,* 500–503.

Dori, G. A., & Chelune, G. J. (2004). Education-stratified base-rate information on discrepancy scores within and between the Wechsler Adult Intelligence Scale-Third Edition and the Wechsler Memory Scale-Third Edition. *Psychological Assessment, 16,* 146–154.

Doss, R. C., Chelune, G. J., & Naugle, R. I. (2000). Comparability of the expanded WMS-III standardization protocol to the published WMS-III among right and left temporal lobectomy patients. *Clinical Neuropsychologist, 14,* 468–473.

Doss, R. C., Chelune, G. J., & Naugle, R. I. (2004). WMS-III performance in epilepsy patients following temporal lobectomy. *Journal of the International Neuropsychological Society, 10,* 173–179.

Dulay, M. F., Schefft, B. K., Test, S. M., Fargo, J. D., Prifitera, M., & Yeh, H. (2002). What does the Family Pictures subtest of the Wechsler Memory Scale-III measure? Insight gained from patients evaluated for surgery. *The Clinical Neuropsychologist, 16,* 452–462.

Engle, R. W., Laughlin, J. E., Tuholski, S. W., & Conway, A. R. A. (1999). Working memory, short-term memory, and general fluid intelligence: A latent variable approach. *Journal of Experimental Psychology: General, 128,* 309–331.

Erickson, R. A., & Scott, M. L. (1977). Clinical memory testing: A review. *Psychological Bulletin, 84,* 1130–1149.

Fisher, D. C., Ledbetter, M. F., Cohen, N. J., Marmor, D., & Tulsky, D. S. (2000). WAIS-III and WMS-III profiles of mildly to severely brain-injured patients. *Applied Neuropsychology, 7,* 126–132.

Flanagan, D. P., McGrew, K. S., & Ortiz, S. O. (2000). *The Wechsler intelligence scales and Gf-Gc theory.* Boston: Allyn & Bacon.

Franzen, M. D., & Iverson, G. L. (2000). The Wechsler Scales. In Groth-Marnat, G. (Ed.), *Neuropsychological assessment in clinical practice: A guide to test interpretation and integration.* New York: Wiley.

Glassmire, D. M., Bierley, R. A., Wieniewski, A. M., Greene, R. L., Kennedy, J. E., & Date, E. (2003). Using the WMS-III Faces subtest to detect malingered memory impairment. *Journal of Clinical and Experimental Neuropsychology, 25,* 465–481.

Haaland, K. Y., Price, L., & Larue, A. (2003). What does the WMS-III tell us about memory changes with normal aging. *Journal of the International Neuropsychological Society, 9,* 89–96.

Hawkins, K. A. (1998). Indicators of brain dysfunction derived from graphic representations of the WAIS-III/WMS-III Technical Manual clinical samples data: A preliminary approach to clinical utility. *The Clinical Neuropsychologist, 12,* 535–551.

Hawkins, K. A., & Tulsky, D. S. (2003). WAIS-III WMS-III discrepancy analysis: Six factor model index discrepancy base rates, implications, and a preliminary consideration of utility. In D. S. Tulsky, D. H. Saklofske, G. J. Chelune, R. K. Heaton, R. J. Ivnik, R. Bornstein, A. Prifitera, & M. F. Ledbetter (Eds.), *Clinical interpretation of the WAIS-III and WMS-III* (pp. 211–272). Orlando, Fla.: Academic Press.

Hawkins, K. A., & Tulsky, D. S. (2004). Replacement of the Faces subtest by Visual Reproductions within Wechsler Memory Scale-Third Edition (WMS-III) Visual Memory Indexes: Implications for discrepancy analysis. *Journal of Clinical and Experimental Neuropsychology, 26,* 498–510.

Heaton, R. K., Taylor, M. J., & Manly, J. J. (2003). Demographic effects and use of demographically corrected norms with the WAIS-III and WMS-III. In D. S. Tulsky, D. H. Saklofske, G. J. Chelune, R. K. Heaton, R. J. Ivnik, R. Bornstein, A. Prifitera, & M. F. Ledbetter (Eds.), *Clinical interpretation of the WAIS-III and WMS-III* (pp. 183–210). Orlando, Fla.: Academic Press.

Hester, R. L., Kinsella, G. J., & Ong, B. (2004). Effect of age on forward and backward span tasks. *Journal of the International Neuropsychological Society, 10,* 475–481.

Holdnack, J. A., & Delis, D. C. (2004). Parsing the recognition memory components of the WMS-III Face memory subtest: Normative data and clinical findings in dementia groups. *Journal of Clinical and Experimental Neuropsychology, 26,* 459–483.

Holley, F. K., Lineweaver, T. T., & Chelune, G. J. (2000). Performance differences on three components of the Family Pictures subtest among right and left temporal lobectomy patients. *Archives of Clinical Neuropsychology, 15,* 679.

Iverson, G. (1999). Interpreting change on the WAIS-III/WMS-III following traumatic brain injury. *The Journal of Cognitive Rehabilitation, 17,* 16–20.

Iverson, G. L. (2001). Interpreting change on the WAIS-III/WMS-III in clinical samples. *Archives of Clinical Neuropsychology, 16,* 183–191.

Jacobson, N. S., & Truax, P. (1991). Clinical significance: A statistical approach to defining meaningful change in psychotherapy research. *J. Consult. Clin. Psychol., 59,* 12–19.

Killgore, W. D. S., & DellaPietra, L. (2000). Using the WMS-III to detect malingering: Empirical validation of the Rarely Missed Index (RMI). *Journal of Clinical and Experimental Neuropsychology, 22,* 761–771.

Lacritz, L. H., & Cullum, C. M. (2003). The WAIS-III and WME-III: Practical issues and frequently asked questions. In D. S. Tulsky, D. H. Saklofske, G. J. Chelune, R. K. Heaton, R. J. Ivnik, R. Bornstein, A. Prifitera, & M. F. Ledbetter (Eds.), *Clinical interpretation of the WAIS-III and WMS-III* (pp. 491–532). Orlando, Fla.: Academic Press.

Lange, R. T., Sullivan, K., & Anderson, D. (2005). Ecological validity of the WMS-III Rarely Missed Index in personal injury litigation. *Journal of Clinical and Experimental Neuropsychology, 27,* 412–424.

Langeluddecke, P. M., & Lucas, S. K. (2003). Quantitative measures of memory malingering on the Wechsler Memory Scale—Third Edition in mild head injury litigants. *Archives of Clinical Neuropsychology, 18,* 181–198.

Langeluddecke, P. M., & Lucas, S. K. (2005). WMS-III findings in litigants following moderate to extremely severe brain trauma. *Journal of Clinical and Experimental Neuropsychology, 27,* 576–590.

Larrabee, G. J. (2004). A review of Clinical Interpretation of the WAIS-III and WMS-III: Where do we go from here and what should we do with WAIS-IV and WMS-IV? *Journal of Clinical and Experimental Neuropsychology, 26,* 706–717.

Larrabee, G. J., Kane, R. L., Schuck, J. R., & Francis, D. J. (1985). Construct validity of various memory test procedures. *Journal of Clinical and Experimental Neuropsychology, 7,* 497–504.

Lees-Haley, P. R., Smith, H. H., Williams, C. W., & Dunn, J. T. (1995). Forensic neuropsychological test usage: An empirical survey. *Archives of Clinical Neuropsychology, 11,* 45–51.

Levy, B. (2003). About the power for detecting severe impairment in older adults with the Faces test from the Wechsler Memory Scale-III: Simply guess and save face. *Journal of Clinical and Experimental Neuropsychology, 25,* 376–381.

Lezak, M. D., Howieson, D. B., & Loring, D. W. (2004). *Neuropsychological assessment* (4th ed.). New York: Oxford University Press.

Lichtenberger, E. O., Kaufman, A. S., & Lai, Z. C. (2002). *Essentials of WMS-III assessment.* New York: Wiley.

Loring, D. W., & Papanicolaou, A. C. (1987). Memory assessment in neuropsychology: Theoretical considerations and practical utility. *Journal of Clinical and Experimental Neuropsychology, 9,* 340–358.

MacMann, G. M., & Barnett, D. W. (1997). Myth of the master detective: Reliability of interpretations for Kaufman's "intelligent testing" approach to the WISC-III. *School Psychology Quarterly, 12,* 197–234.

Manly, J. J., Jacobs, D. M., Touradji, P., Small, S. A., & Stern, Y. (2002). Reading level attenuates differences in neuropsychological test performance between African American and White elders. *Journal of the International Neuropsychological Society, 8,* 341–348.

Martin, R., Sawrie, S., Gilliam, F., Mackey, M., Faught, E., Knowlton, R., & Kuzniekcy, R. (2002). Determining reliable cognitive change after epilepsy surgery: Development of reliable change indices and standarized regression-based change norms for the WMS-III and WAIS-III. *Epilepsia, 43*(12), 1551–1558.

McDermott, P. A., Fantuzzo, J. W., & Glutting, J. J. (1990). Just say no to subtest analysis: A critique of Wechsler theory and practice. *Journal of Psychoeducational Assessment, 8,* 290–302.

McDowell, B. D., Bayless, J. D., Moser, D. J., Meyers, J. E., & Paulsen, J. S. (2004). Concordance between the CVLT and the WMS-III word lists test. *Archives of Clinical Neuropsychology, 19,* 319–324.

Meyerson, J., Emery, L., White, D. A., & Hale, S. (2003). Effects of age, domain, and processing demands on memory span: Evidence and differential decline. *Aging, Neuropsychology and Cognition, 10,* 20–27.

Migoya, J., Zimmerman, S. W., & Golden, C. J. (2002). Abbreviated form of the Wechsler Memory Scale-III Faces subtest. *Assessment, 9,* 142–144.

Milberg, W. P., Hebben, N., & Kaplan, E. (1986). The Boston process approach to neuropsychological assessment. In I. Grant & K. M. Adams (Eds.), *Neuropsychiatric disorders.* New York: Oxford University Press.

Miller, L. J., Ryan, J. J., Carruthers, C. A., & Cluff, R. B. (2004). Brief screening indexes for malingering: A confirmation of Vocabulary minus Digit Span from the WAIS-III and the Rarely Missed Index from the WMS-III. *The Clinical Neuropsychologist, 18,* 327–333.

Millis, S. R., Malina, A. C., Bowers, D. A., & Ricker, J. H. (1999). Confirmatory factor analysis of the Wechsler Memory Scale-III. *Journal of Clinical and Experimental Neuropsychology, 21,* 87–93.

Price, L., Said, K., & Haaland, K. Y. (2004). Age-associated memory impairment of Logical Memory and Visual Reproduction. *Journal of Clinical and Experimental Neuropsychology, 26,* 531–538.

Price, L. R., Tulsky, D., Millis, S., & Weiss, L. (2002). Redefining the factor structure of the Wechsler Memory Scale-III: Confirmatory factor analysis with cross-validation. *Journal of Clinical and Experimental Neuropsychology, 24,* 574–585.

Prigitano, G. P. (1977). Wechsler Memory Scale is a poor screening test for brain dysfunction. *Journal of Clinical Psychology, 33,* 772–777.

Prigitano, G. P. (1978). Wechsler Memory Scale: A selective review of the literature. *Journal of Clinical Psychology, 34,* 816–832.

Rabin, L. A., Barr, W. B., & Burton, L. A. (2005). Assessment practices of clinical neuropsychologists in the United States and Canada: A survey of INS, NAN, and APA Division 40 members. *Archives of Clinical Neuropsychology, 20,* 33–65.

Ryan, J. J., Arb, J. D., & Ament, P. A. (2000). Supplementary WMS-III tables for determining primary subtest strengths and weaknesses. *Psychological Assessment, 12,* 193–196.

Ryan, J. J., Kreiner, D. S., & Burton, D. B. (2002). Does high scatter affect the predictive validity of WAIS-III IQs? *Applied Neuropsychology, 9,* 173–178.

Russell, E. W. (1975). A multiple scoring method for the assessment of complex memory functions. *Journal of Consulting and Clinical Psychology, 43,* 800–809.

Skeel, R. L., Sitzer, D., Fogal, T., Wells, J., & Johnstone, B. (2004). Comparison of predicted-difference, simple-difference and premorbid-estimation methodologies for evaluating IQ and memory score discrepancies. *Archives of Clinical Neuropsychology, 19,* 363–374.

Spreen, O., & Strauss, E. (1998). *A compendium of neuropsychological tests: Administration, norms and commentary.* New York: Oxford University Press.

Stone, C., & Wechsler, D. (1946). *Wechsler Memory Scale form II.* San Antonio, Tex.: The Psychological Corporation.

Taylor, M. J., & Heaton, R. K. (2001). Sensitivity and specificity of WAIS-III/WMS-III demographically corrected factor scores in neuropsychological assessment. *Journal of the International Neuropsychological Society, 7,* 867–874.

The Psychological Corporation (1997, 2002). *WAIS-III/WMS-III Technical Manual.* San Antonio, Tex.: The Psychological Corporation.

Titov, N., & Knight, R.G. (2000). A procedure for testing prospective remembering in persons with neurological impairments. *Brain Injury, 14,* 877–886.

Tulsky, D. S., & Ledbetter, M. F. (2000). Updating to the WAIS-III and WMS-III: Considerations for research and clinical practice. *Psychological Assessment, 12,* 253–262.

Tulsky, D. S., & Price, L. R. (2003). The joint WAIS-III and WMS-III factor structure: Development and cross-validation of a six-factor model of cognitive functioning. *Psychological Assessment, 15,* 149–162.

Tulsky, D. S., Chelune, G. J., & Price, L. R. (2004). Development of a new Delayed Memory Index for the WMS-III. *Journal of Clinical and Experimental Neuropsychology, 26,* 563–576.

Tulsky, D. S., Chiaravalloti, N. D., Palmer, B. W., & Chelune, G. J. (2003a). The Wechsler Memory Scale, Third Edition: A new perspective. In D. S. Tulsky, D. H. Saklofske, G. J. Chelune, R. K. Heaton, R. J. Ivnik, R. Bornstein, A. Prifitera, & M. F. Ledbetter (Eds.), *Clinical interpretation of the WAIS-III and WMS-III* (pp. 93–139). Orlando, Fla.: Academic Press.

Tulsky, D. S., Ivnik, R. J., Price, L. R., & Wilkins, C. (2003b). Assessment of cognitive functioning with the WAIS-III and WMS-III: Development of a six-factor model. In D. S. Tulsky, D. H. Saklofske, G. J. Chelune, R. K. Heaton, R. J. Ivnik, R. Bornstein, A. Prifitera, & M. F. Ledbetter (Eds.), *Clinical interpretation of the WAIS-III and WMS-III* (pp. 147–179). Orlando, Fla.: Academic Press.

Tunney, N., Taylor, L. F., Higbie, E. J., & Haist, F. (2002). Declarative memory and motor learning in the older adult. *Physical and Occupational Therapy in Geriatrics, 20,* 21–42.

Uttl, B. (2005). Measurement of individual differences. *Psychological Science, 16,* 460–467.

Uttl, B., Graf, P., & Richter, L. K. (2002). Verbal Paired Associates tests limits on validity and reliability. *Archives of Clinical Neuropsychology, 17,* 567–581.

Watkins, M. W., & Glutting, J. J. (2000). Incremental validity of the WISC-III profile elevation, scatter, and shape information for predicting reading and math achievement. *Psychological Assessment, 12,* 402–408.

Wechsler, D. (1945). A standardized memory scale for clinical use. *Journal of Psychology, 19,* 87–95.

Wechsler, D. (1987). *Wechsler Memory Scale-Revised.* San Antonio, Tex.: The Psychological Corporation.

Wechsler, D. (1997). *WMS-III Administration and Scoring Manual.* San Antonio, Tex.: The Psychological Corporation.

Wilde, N., Strauss, E., Chelune, G. J., Loring, D. W., Martin, R. C., Hermann, B. P., Sherman, E. M. S., & Hunter, M. (2001). WMS-III performance in patients with temporal lobe epilepsy: Group differences and individual classification. *Journal of the International Neuropsychological Society, 7,* 881–891.

Wilde, N., & Strauss, E. (2002). Functional equivalence of WAIS-III/WMS-III Digit and Spatial Span under forward and backward recall conditions. *The Clinical Neuropsychologist, 16,* 322–330.

Wilde, N. J., Strauss, E., Chelune, G. J., Hermann, B. P., Hunter, M., Loring, D. W., Martin, R. C., & Sherman, E. M. S. (2003). Confirmatory factor analysis of the WMS-III in patients with temporal lobe epilepsy. *Psychological Assessment, 15,* 56–63.

Wilde, N. J., Strauss, E., & Tulsky, D. S. (2004). Memory span on the Wechsler Scales. *Journal of Clinical and Experimental Neuropsychology, 26,* 539–549.

Woodard, J. L., Axelrod, B. N., Mordecai, K., & Shannon, K. D. (2004). Value of signal detection theory Indexes for Wechsler Memory Scale-III recognition measures. *Journal of Clinical and Experimental Neuropsychology, 26,* 577–586.

Zhu, J., & Tulsky, D. S. (2000). Co-norming the WAIS-III and WMS-III: Is there a test-order effect on IQ and memory scores? *The Clinical Neuropsychologist, 14,* 461–467.

Wide Range Assessment of Memory and Learning–Second Edition (WRAML2)

PURPOSE

This battery is designed to assess memory skills in children and adults.

SOURCE

The Wide Range Assessment of Memory and Learning—Second Edition (WRAML2) can be ordered from Psychological Assessment Resources (www.parinc.com) at a cost of $475 US. Scoring software is also available (for Windows 98 or later) for $195 US.

The WRAML2 kit contains a manual, 25 Examiner Forms, 25 Picture Memory Response Forms, 25 Picture Recognition Forms, 25 Design Memory Response Forms, 25 Design Memory Recognition Forms, 4 Picture Memory Scenes, 5 Design Memory Cards, a Finger Windows Card, a Sound Symbol Booklet, 2 Symbolic Working Memory Cards, and a carrying case. The test includes five forms: Examiner Form, Picture Memory Response Form, Design Memory Response Form, Picture Memory Recognition Form, and Design Memory Recognition Form.

AGE RANGE

The WRAML2 is normed from ages 5 to 90 years.

DESCRIPTION

The WRAML2 (Sheslow & Adams, 2003) is the second edition of the WRAML (Sheslow & Adams, 1990). Although the general format remains, the new edition has several new features. In addition to changes in index composition (most importantly the addition of the Attention/Concentration Index and the removal of the Learning Index), the test was restandardized and the age range was extended to adulthood. The Visual Learning subtest was dropped from the new edition, and additional Optional subtests were added, as well as new subtests comprising the Attention/Concentration Index. Further, the test now has various Delay Recall and Recognition subtests and indices that were not included in the first edition. The test itself was recalibrated in terms of item difficulty, and the testing materials were updated. Story Memory includes new stories, and Picture Memory includes colored scenes. The designs on the Design Memory Cards were changed, and an additional Design Card was added. The manual is also much more detailed than its predecessor. The Verbal Learning and Sound-Symbol subtests remain virtually unchanged from the previous edition.

Although the authors note that the test is not bound to a specific model of memory functioning, the revision was undertaken with contemporary memory assessment theories in mind, including consideration of (a) the role of executive processes in memory (by including the new Working Memory and Attention/Concentration Index scores), (b) the distinction between recall and recognition (by adding new Recognition Index scores), and (c) the distinctions between different types of memory representations (by including "Gist" and "Verbatim" scores for Story Memory). Expanded error analyses (i.e., semantic versus phonological errors on Verbal Learning and commission errors on Picture Memory) were also provided (Sheslow & Adams, 2003).

Test Structure

The test's overall structure is shown in Figure 10–44. The WRAML2 Core Battery consists of two verbal, two visual and

Figure 10–44 WRAML2 test structure. *Source:* Reprinted with permission from Sheslow & Adams, 2003, p. 19.

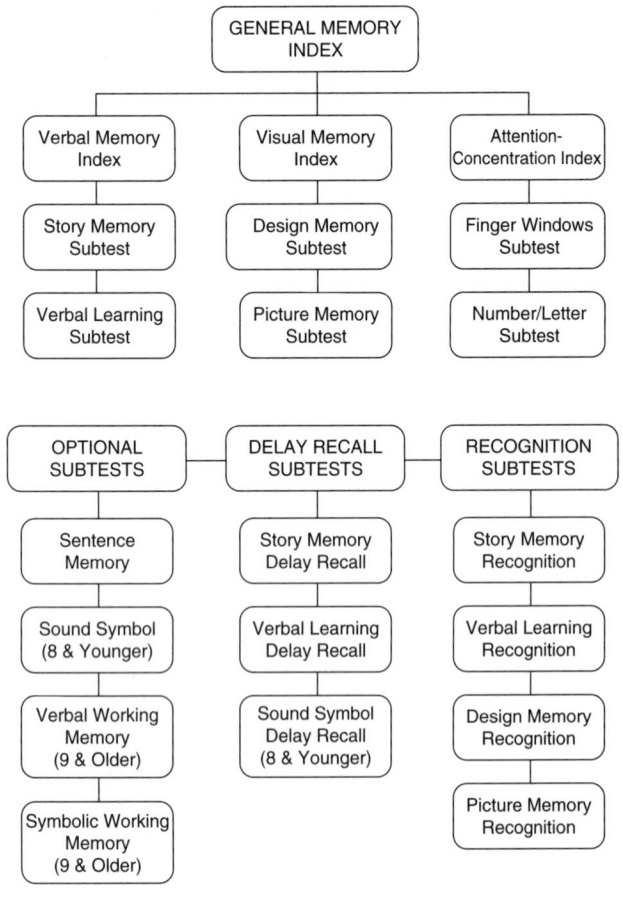

two attention/concentration subtests. These provide a Verbal Memory Index, a Visual Memory Index, and an Attention/Concentration Index, which together form the General Memory Index (GMI). (See Table 10–132 for index composition.) An additional index, the Working Memory Index, is based on two subtests that do not contribute to the GMI (Symbolic Working Memory and Verbal Working Memory). A Screening Battery can also be administered, which consists of the four Core Battery subtests that assess verbal and visual memory (see Table 10–132). This yields the Screening Battery Index. The General Recognition Index is based on the Verbal Recog-

nition Index and Visual Recognition Index, which are derived from recognition paradigms for the four memory subtests from the Core Battery. Delay Recall scores are not provided as an index but are presented as scaled scores for the separate subtests that allow this format (i.e., verbal subtests only). The WRAML2 also includes Optional subtests that are not included in the composite scores; these may be administered if additional testing is required. (See Table 10–133 for Optional subtests and Table 10–134 for subtest descriptions.) Notably, the WRAML2 Verbal Learning subtest does not contain semantically related words that can be grouped into meaningful categories to aid recall, as is the case for tests such as the CVLT-C.

ADMINISTRATION TIME

According to the manual, the Core Battery takes less than 1 hour to administer, and the Screening Battery takes approximately 20 min.

ADMINISTRATION

See the test administration manual.

SCORING

Scores

Raw scores for subtests are converted to scaled scores ($M = 10$, $SD = 3$), and composite scores are presented in standard score format ($M = 100$, $SD = 15$). Percentiles and confidence intervals are also provided, as are age equivalents for the child and adolescent age groups. Standard scores range from 55 to 145. Statistical significance and baserate data for index score discrepancies and for discrepancies between Core subtests and corresponding Recognition subtests are also provided in the manual.

Qualitative Analyses

The test also provides a number of Qualitative Analyses scores, including scores for Story Memory (Story A versus B versus C, Verbatim and Gist), Picture Memory (commission

Table 10–132 Core Index Composition for the WRAML2

General Memory Index (GMI)	Verbal Memory Index	*Story Memory*
		Verbal Learning
	Visual Memory Index	*Design Memory*
		Picture Memory
	Attention/Concentration Index	Finger Windows
		Number/Letter

Note: Subtests in italics comprise the Screening Memory Index (SMI). Recognition subtests for the Verbal Memory Index and Visual Memory Index form the General Recognition Index (GRI).

Table 10–133 Optional Subtests and Index Score Composition for the WRAML2

Working Memory Index	Verbal Working Memory (for subjects ≥9 years of age)
	Symbolic Working Memory (≥9 years)
Other Optional Subtests	Sentence Memory
	Sound-Symbol (≤8 years)
Delay Recall Subtests	Story Memory Recall
	Verbal Learning Recall
	Sound Symbol Recall (≤8 years)
Recognition Subtests	Story Recognition
	Design Recognition
	Picture Memory Recognition
	Verbal Learning Recognition

errors), Verbal Learning (trial-by-trial performance, slope, and intrusion errors; semantic and phonological errors on recognition) and Sound Symbol (trial-by-trial performance, slope, and retention). These are listed in Table 10–135. Many of these have restricted range or other psychometric properties that preclude the use of scaled scores. However, the manual provides descriptive statistics (means and standard deviations) along with percentile cutoffs (raw score equivalents for the 15th and 5th percentiles) for these scores.

DEMOGRAPHIC EFFECTS

Age

The WRAML2 age-related growth curve is steepest from age 5 to 9 years, changes little during adulthood (25 to 64 years), and declines after 65 years of age (Sheslow & Adams, 2003).

Gender

Item bias and factor analyses indicate no effects of gender on WRAML2 performance (Sheslow & Adams, 2003). However, in the previous edition of the test, gender was related to WRAML performance in children after traumatic brain injury (TBI), with girls outperforming boys. When injury severity variables and age were accounted for, gender contributed 9% of additional variance to the prediction of WRAML performance. However, the relationship between gender and WRAML performance after TBI may be mediated by processing speed; when this variable was used as a covariate, gender differences disappeared (Donders & Woodward, 2003).

Education

Item bias and factor analyses indicate no effects of education on WRAML2 scores (Sheslow & Adams, 2003).

IQ

The WRAML2 shows a higher correlation with IQ in adults than in children, as shown by correlations with the WAIS-III and WISC-III presented in the manual ($r = .67$ versus $r = .44$; Sheslow & Adams, 2003; see *Validity*).

Ethnicity

To date, there are no published studies on the utility of the test in minority populations. However, elimination of bias was taken into account in the construction of the WRAML using item bias analysis of Core subtests, and factor analyses described in the manual indicate no effects of ethnicity on test structure.

NORMATIVE DATA

Standardization Sample

Norms are based on a national stratified sampling technique encompassing 1200 individuals. Norms were collected between 2002 and 2003, and were designed to match the 2001 U.S. Census in terms of gender, race/ethnicity, education, and geographic region. Weighting procedures were used to correct the sample for slight variations in composition to make it consistent with Census data. For each of the 15 age groups, 80 individuals were selected. Age bands were constructed based on growth curve data, with intervals of 6 months from 5 to 9 years, 1 year for ages 10 and 11, 2 years for ages 12 to 19, 5 years for ages 20 to 24, 10 years for ages 25 to 64, and 5 years for ages 65 to 89 (see manual for further details). Sample characteristics are shown in Table 10–136.

RELIABILITY

Internal Consistency

Internal reliability of the index scores is high ($r = .86$ to .93; see Table 10–137). Alpha reliabilities for the GMI and for the Screening Memory Index are both .93., and median reliabilities across age for Core subtests are also strong (range = .83 to .92; Sheslow & Adams, 2003). Reliabilities are less optimal for some of the recognition subtests (e.g., $r = .40$ for Design Recognition; see Table 10–137); this is a common occurrence when a large proportion of normal subjects perform at ceiling on recognition paradigms. The manual clearly states that interpretation of the Recognition subtests, and particularly of the Visual Recognition Index, must be done with caution.

The manual also presents Rasch analysis data for each subtest, with person separation reliabilities for core subtests ranging from .85 to .94, and for Optional subtests from .56 to .93. As expected, values are lower on those subtests with ceilings or fewer items (e.g., Verbal Learning Delay, Sounds Symbol Delay, recognition subtests). Item separation reliabilities for

Table 10–134 Description of WRAML2 Subtests

Verbal Index Subtests

Story Memory | Two stories are read to the examinee, who must then repeat them from memory; delayed recall is assessed after 15 min; a multiple-choice recognition paradigm follows; Story Memory can be scored according to exact recall (Verbatim score) or according to thematic recall (Gist score), as well as Delay, Memory Retention (difference between Story Memory Delay and Core Story Memory scores), comparison between individual stories, and recognition score.

Verbal Learning | This is a standard word list-learning task, with four learning trials and either 13 words (ages 8 and under) or 16 words (≥9 years); a delay trial is administered after 10 min, followed by a recognition trial; scores are provided for each trial, as well as a retention score (difference between Delay Recall and Trial 4), Verbal Learning Slope (Trial 4 – Trial 1), intrusion errors, and two-choice recognition score (yes/no).

Visual Index Subtests

Design Memory | The examinee is shown five cards with geometric designs; each is presented for 5s; after a 10-s delay, the examinee must draw the design from memory; a multiple-item recognition paradigm (yes/no format) follows, in which the examinee must state whether a particular design was seen before (there is no free-recall delay subtest).

Picture Memory | The examinee is shown a pictured scene (colored line drawings) for 10s, then is presented with a similar scene in which he or she must identify any items that have been altered or added; four different scenes are presented; a recognition trial follows, in which the examinee must state whether a particular component of the scene was previously presented (yes/no format). Commission errors can be scored for this subtest (there is no free-recall delay subtest).

Attention/Concentration Index Subtests

Finger Windows | The examiner executes a series of movements using a vertically presented card with holes in which to place the fingers; the examinee must reproduce the sequence; increasingly long sequences are presented.

Number-Letter | The examinee must repeat a sequence of numbers and letters presented orally by the examiner.

Optional Subtests

Sentence Memory | This is a standard sentence repetition task in which the examinee repeats sentences of increasing length and complexity.

Sound-Symbol | This is a cross-modal paired-associates task in which the examinee must remember the abstract designs that went with a sound; it provides scores for delay, Trials 1–4, retention, and learning slope.

Working Memory Subtests (Ages 9+ only)

Verbal Working Memory | The examinee hears a list of words composed of animal names and objects and then repeats the list, placing all the animal names first; on later trials, the examinee must recall the animals according to their size (i.e., from small to large), followed by all the nonanimal words; at the highest level (≥14 years), the examinee must repeat both sets of stimuli in order of size.

Symbolic Working Memory | The examiner dictates a number series (e.g,. "8-2-4"), and the examinee reproduces the series in correct numerical order by pointing to numbers on a card; in the second part of the test, the examinee hears a random number-letter series (e.g., "3-B-1-A") which must then be reproduced by pointing on a number-letter card, with the numbers in correct order first, followed by the letters.

the Core subtests are either .99 or 1.00, and the range for subtests is .90 to 1.00.

Standard Error of Measurement (*SEM*)

*SEM*s for the WRAML2 index scores are for the most part respectable, with most falling between 4 and 6 points (i.e., GMI, Verbal Memory Index, Attention/Concentration Index, Memory Screening Index, Verbal Recognition Index, Working Memory Index). The *SEM* for the Visual Recognition Index is about 10 points, which translates into a very large confidence interval; for example, an individual with an obtained score of 100 would have a 95% confidence interval ranging from 80 to 120. Note that this problem is also evident on other scales (e.g., WMS-III,

Table 10–135 WRAML2 Qualitative Analyses Scores

Subtest	Qualitative measure
Story Memory	Individual Story Comparison Vebatim and Gist Measures Retention (Delay–Immediate Recall)
Verbal Learning	Learning Curve Learning Slope Retention (Delay Recall-Trial 4) Intrusion Errors
Picture Memory	Commission Errors
Sound-Symbol	Retention (Delay Recall-Trial 4) Learning Curve Learning Slope

Table 10–136 Characteristics of the WRAML2 Normative Sample

Sample type	Randomized stratified standardization sample
Number	1200
Age (years)	5 to 90 years[a]
Geographic location[b] (%)	
Northeast	18
South	35
North Central	22
West	25
Education[b] (%)	
College and more	18
Some college	27
High school graduation	34
Less than high school	20
Socio economic status (SES)	Education was used as a marker of SES
Gender (%)	
Males	48
Females	52
Race/Ethnicity[b] (%)	
Caucasian	71
African American	12
Hispanic	12
Other	5
Screening	None[c]

[a] Based on several age groupings, with 80 individuals in each group: 5 years 0 months (5:0) to 5:11, 6:0 to 6:11, 7:0 to 7:11, 8:0 to 8:11, 9:0 to 10:11, 11:0 to 13:11, 14:0 to 17:11, 18:0 to 24:11, 25:0 to 39:11, 40:0 to 54:11, 55:0 to 64:11, 65:0 to 69:11, 70:0 to 74:11, 75:0 to 79:11, and 80:0 to 90:0.

[b] Reflects weighted percentages.

[c] Quality-control checks were conducted in the final norming sample to ensure that individuals with disabilities were not overrepresented in the final sample (G. Robertson, personal communication, October, 2004).

Source: Adapted from Sheslow & Adams, 2003.

CMS). Core subtest *SEMs* are less than 1.7 scaled score points, with the exception of Design Memory Recognition and Picture Memory Recognition, which exceed 2 scaled score points (2.3 and 2.1 points, respectively; Sheslow & Adams, 2003).

Test-Retest Reliability

Although test-retest reliability is strong for some indexes (i.e., GMI, Verbal Memory Index, Working Memory Index), others fall below standards for clinical decision making (i.e., Visual Memory Index). The same holds true for subtests. See Table 10–137 for reliability classifications based on data presented in the manual for 142 individuals (age range = 5 to 84 years), equated for gender, education, ethnicity, and geographic location from the standardization sample. Note that, although the median retest interval was 49 days, the actual range was between 2 weeks and more than 1 year (i.e., 14 to 401 days; Sheslow & Adams, 2003).

Practice Effects

As one would expect for a memory test, there is a practice effect on WRAML2 scores, with an average gain of 6 to 7 points on most index scores. The largest increase is for the Memory Screening Index (gain = 8.1), and the smallest is for Attention/Concentration (gain = 1.7). Scaled score increases range between negligible practice effects (Symbolic Working Memory gain = 0.2) to almost 2 scaled score point gains at retest (i.e., Design Memory, Design Memory Recognition; Sheslow & Adams, 2003).

Interscorer Reliability

For the subtest requiring subjective judgment, interscorer reliability is high (e.g., Design Memory *r* = .98; Sheslow & Adams, 2003).

VALIDITY

Content Validity

The WRAML2 was developed after an exhaustive test revision process, including review by expert users, creation of a "try-out" battery, administration of this battery to several hundred children and adults, analysis and refinement, and a full standardization process. Core subtests were also statistically evaluated for item bias with regard to gender and ethnicity (see manual for full details).

Screener Versus Core Battery

The correlation between the GMI and the Screening Battery Index is very high (*r* = .91), with less than 1 standard score point difference between index scores in the standardization sample (Sheslow & Adams, 2003). Note that, in the previous version, the screening index tended to overestimate the GMI

Table 10–137 Magnitude of Internal Reliability and Test-Retest Reliability Coefficients for the WRAML2

Magnitude of Coefficient	Internal Reliability	Test-Retest Reliability
Very High (≥.90)	*General Memory Index* *Screening Memory Index* *Verbal Memory Index* *Working Memory Index* Story Memory Story Memory Delay Recall Story Memory: Retention	—
High (.80 to .89)	*Visual Memory Index* *Attention/Concentration Index* *Verbal Recognition Index* Design Memory Verbal Learning Picture Memory Finger Windows Number-Letter Verbal Working Memory Symbolic Working Memory Sound-Symbol Sentence Memory Story Memory: Story A Story Memory: Story B Story Memory: Story C Story Memory: Verbatim	*Verbal Memory Index* *General Memory Index* *Working Memory Index*
Adequate (.70 to .79)	*General Recognition Index* Verbal Learning Delay Recall Story Memory Recognition Verbal Learning Recognition Story Memory: Gist	*Memory Screening Index* *General Recognition Index* Story Memory Verbal Learning Verbal Working Memory Sentence Memory Story Memory Delay Recall Verbal Learning Delay Recall Sound Symbol Delay Recall Story Memory: Story C
Marginal (.60 to .69)	Sound Symbol Delay Recall	*Visual Memory Index* *Attention/Concentration Index* *Verbal Recognition Index* *Visual Recognition Index* Picture Memory Finger Windows Number Letter Symbolic Working Memory Sound Symbol Story Memory Recognition Story Memory: Story B Story Memory: Verbatim Story Memory: Gist
Low (≤.59)	*Visual Recognition Index* Design Recognition Picture Recognition	Design Memory Design Memory Recognition Picture Memory Recognition Verbal Learning Recognition Story Memory: Story A Story Memory: Retention

Note: Index scores are in italics; internal reliability coefficients represent coefficient alpha; test-retest coefficients represent corrected r's.

Source: Reprinted with permission from Sheslow & Adams, 2003.

by almost 5 points and thus provided a false-negative bias (Kennedy & Guilmette, 1997).

Subtest Intercorrelations

Intercorrelations between subtests making up the various WRAML2 index scores appear to vary by age. In younger children (ages 5–8 years), subtest intercorrelations presented in the manual generally support the Verbal Memory Index, with verbal subtests moderately intercorrelated ($r = .42$). However, intercorrelations between subtests making up the Attention/Concentration and between those of the Visual Memory Index are modest in this age group ($r = .26$ and $r = .19$, respectively). In older subjects (9 years to adult), there appears to be more homogeneity to the index scores. Verbal subtests correlate highly ($r = .51$), as do subtests making up the Working Memory Index ($r = .62$). Note that correlations between subtests belonging to the Attention/Concentration Index and those belonging to the Working Memory Index are also in the moderate to high range ($r = .39$ to $.57$), which suggests that these two indexes may not represent distinct cognitive domains. The correlation for the visual subtests making up the Visual Memory Index in older subjects is also quite respectable (e.g., $r = .41$ between Design Memory and Picture Memory).

Factor Structure

Exploratory and confirmatory factor analyses of the six Core subtests in the standardization data reveal three factors: Verbal Memory, Visual Memory, and Attention/Concentration, consistent with the index composition of the WRAML2. Of the six Core subtests, Picture Memory and Number-Letter have the largest unique variances, suggesting high subtest specificity (Sheslow & Adams, 2003). Factor analyses across age, gender, ethnicity, and education indicate consistency of the three-factor solution across demographic subgroups (Sheslow & Adams, 2003). Addition of the Working Memory subtests yields a four-factor solution; however, this solution shows a high degree of redundancy between the Attention/Concentration and Working Memory subtests, as is suggested by the WRAML2 subtest intercorrelation matrix for these subtests. A three-factor solution is also found for the Optional subtests, supporting the three Optional index scores (Working Memory, Verbal Recognition Index, and Visual Recognition Index; Sheslow & Adams, 2003).

Correlations With Other Memory Scales

Correlations between the WRAML2 and CMS in 29 healthy children are reported in the manual (Sheslow & Adams, 2003). These indicate that the tests generally measure similar constructs, but that there are important differences between the two measures. First, although the WRAML2 GMI correlates moderately with the corresponding score from the CMS ($r = .49$), the WRAML2 GMI actually appears to correlate more highly with the CMS Attention/Concentration Index ($r = .64$). This may have to do with an important distinction between the tests: unlike the CMS, the WRAML2 includes the Attention/Concentration subtests in its calculation of the GMI. Verbal index scores from the two tests are moderately correlated ($r = .36$, for WRAML2 Verbal Memory and CMS Verbal Immediate), and the attention/concentration factors from the two tests have significant overlap ($r = .58$). However, visual index scores from the two tests are only moderately correlated. Specifically, WRAML2 Visual Index scores appear to correlate more highly with the CMS Verbal Immediate Index and Attention/Concentration factors than with the CMS Visual Index ($r = .55$ and $r = .52$, versus $r = .37$, respectively).

In terms of mean score differences, the WRAML2 Verbal Memory Index and the WRAML2 Attention/Concentration Index are about 4 to 5 points higher than the corresponding index scores from the CMS (Verbal Immediate and Attention/Concentration); visual index scores are within 1 point of each other. GMI mean scores are less than 1 standard score point from each other (Cheslow & Adams, 2003).

Comparisons with the TOMAL in a small group of children with attention-deficit/hyperactivity disorder (ADHD) are also presented in the test manual. In contrast to the CMS results, visual index scores from the two tests are highly correlated ($r = .58$), and WRAML2 Visual Memory scores show only modest overlap with TOMAL Verbal Memory scores ($r = .26$). General Memory composite scores are also highly related ($r = .69$), although the TOMAL composite score is about 6 points higher than the GMI (Sheslow & Adams, 2003).

In adults, the GMI scores from the WRAML2 and WMS-III are highly correlated, as are the Working Memory Index scores from the two tests ($r = .60$ for both), based on a sample of 79 healthy adults presented in the manual (Sheslow & Adams, 2003). The WRAML2 Attention/Concentration Index is also highly related to the WMS-III Working Memory Index, again suggesting that Attention/Concentration and Working Memory measure a similar construct ($r = .65$). Correlations involving the verbal indexes are also high ($r = .66$ for WRAML Verbal Memory and WMS-III Auditory Immediate). Correlations involving the visual scales are less clearly indicative of a distinct visual memory domain; the WRAML2 Visual Memory Index correlates moderately with the corresponding index from the WMS-III (Visual Immediate $r = .42$) but also demonstrates a moderate degree of overlap with verbal index scores from the WMS-III ($r = .33$ to $.42$). Mean scores for the WMS-III are generally higher than WRAML2 scores (e.g., 4.7 points for the GMI, 3.7 points for the verbal scales; 3.1 points for Working Memory; see p. 131 of Sheslow & Adams, 2003, for more details).

Correlations between the WRAML2 and CVLT/CVLT-II show a high degree of association in terms of overlap between the WRAML2 Verbal Memory score and CVLT Trial 1–5 score. As expected, the Visual Memory Index is only moderately correlated with the CVLT in healthy subjects, which provides some evidence for the construct validity of the verbal/visual dichotomy in WRAML2 index scores ($r = .64$ and $r = .36$, respectively; Sheslow & Adams, 2003).

Correlations With Intellectual Ability

In children, the WRAML2 GMI and the WISC-III IQ are moderately correlated ($r = .44$), and mean scores are relatively similar, albeit slightly higher for the GMI compared with the FSIQ (106.6 versus 108.6; $N = 29$; Sheslow & Adams, 2003). VIQ is modestly related to Verbal Memory and Visual Memory ($r = .29$ and $r = .36$). PIQ is related to Visual Memory but not to Verbal Memory ($r = .30$ versus $r = .14$; Sheslow & Adams, 2003). The test's relationship to the WISC-IV is not yet known.

In adults, the correlation between the GMI and FSIQ, based on WAIS-III, is higher ($r = .67$; $N = 68$). The Verbal Comprehension Index is more highly correlated with Verbal Memory than with Visual Memory ($r = .58$ versus $r = .31$), but the Perceptual Organization Index is equally related to Verbal Memory and Visual Memory ($r = .55$ versus $r = .49$). Working Memory Index scores from the two tests are highly correlated ($r = .69$). The WAIS-III FSIQ score is about 5 points higher than the GMI (Sheslow & Adams, 2003).

Correlations With Achievement

With regard to achievement, the WRAML2 GMI appears to be a very good predictor of Reading Fluency and Math Fluency ($r = .60$ and $r = .58$), whereas the Attention/Concentration Index appears to be a good predictor of Spelling ($r = .59$) as measured by the WJ-III ($N = 29$; Sheslow & Adams, 2003). The GMI score also appears to be moderately associated with performance on the WRAT3 ($r = .39$ to .49). The authors noted that Attention/Concentration is one of the best predictor of scores on the WJ-III and WRAT3 (exceeding the GMI in some cases) and has high correlations with reading fluency and math (Sheslow & Adams, 2003). Apart from the correlation between Verbal Memory and Reading Fluency ($r = .33$), correlations between WJ-III scores and WRAML2 Verbal/Visual index scores are generally low ($r = .09$ to .23). Therefore, when the individual components are considered, Attention/Concentration appears to be the main predictor of academic achievement (as measured by the WJ-III).

Clinical Studies

Because the test was only recently released, there are as yet no independent published studies on its validity. However, the test manual presents data on several clinical groups compared with matched controls. Significant differences in memory functioning were obtained between controls and individuals with Alzheimer's disease (GMI difference = −21.6), children with learning disability (GMI difference = −21.4), adults with TBI (GMI difference = −17.4), adults with alcohol abuse (Verbal Memory difference = −14.6), and patients with Parkinson's disease (no difference). Note that in the patients with Alzheimer's disease, significant differences were not obtained on some of the Optional subtests. In TBI patients, the smallest difference was obtained on Attention/Concentration, and Number-Letter performance was not different from that of the matched controls. Effect sizes for these differences are presented in the manual (Sheslow & Adams, 2003, pp. 143–148).

The previous version of the WRAML has been used in several clinical populations, including children with ADHD (Dewey et al., 1998; Mealer et al., 1996; Phelps, 1996), lymphoblastic leukemia (Hill et al., 1997), learning disability (Dewey et al., 1998; Phelps, 1996), epilepsy (Williams & Haut, 1995), diabetes (Lynch et al., 2004), prenatal alcohol exposure (Roebuck-Spencer & Mattson, 2004), and pediatric TBI (Donders & Woodward, 2003; Farmer et al., 1999; Woodward & Donders, 1998). The memory screening index was found to be related to length of coma in pediatric TBI ($r = −.50$; Woodward & Donders, 1998) and proved able to discriminate those with severe TBI from those with mild/moderate injuries. However, the authors of this study expressed strong reservations about using the WRAML memory screening index as the exclusive memory measure in clinical assessment, in part because of inadequate information on delayed recall and recognition. Donders and Woodward (2003) concluded that performance on the WRAML may depend in part on processing speed adequacy in children with TBI, as measured by WISC-III Processing Speed. In a study of children exposed to heavy prenatal alcohol use, children reached a learning plateau earlier on the CVLT-C than on the WRAML Verbal Learning subtest, probably because of their ability to use semantic clustering strategies on the CVLT-C but not on the WRAML (Roebuck-Spencer & Mattson, 2004). Further research will help determine whether these findings also apply to the WRAML2.

COMMENT

The original WRAML was, according to its authors, the first well-normed memory battery for children (Sheslow & Adams, 2003). Although it was used by many pediatric neuropsychologists, the WRAML suffered from some technical and methodological limitations. These included a lack of separate scaled scores for delay and recognition memory, and criticism for not being derived from any clear model of memory (Clark & Medway, 1992). In addition, the factor solution presented in the manual was not replicated in other studies, including clinical populations (Aylward et al., 1995; Burton et al., 1999; Dewey et al., 1997; Phelps, 1995; Woodward & Donders, 1998), and in the standardization sample itself (Burton et al., 1996; Woodward & Donders, 1998). Most studies indicated that the WRAML had an attention/concentration factor in addition to distinct verbal and visual memory factors (Dewey et al., 1997) and that the presence of a Learning Index factor was not supported. All of these criticisms have been rectified in the new edition, and the correct factor structure is reflected in the WRAML2 composites (see Table 10–132).

The WRAML2 manual provides a good review of the history of memory assessment, along with a rationale for the theoretical underpinnings of the test. The manual itself is well written and provides an exhaustive review of the test's psychometric properties, including information that is not always readily available in test manuals, such as data on internal reliability by age, stability coefficients for almost all scores including optional scores and subtests, factor analyses across demographic characteristics (age, gender, ethnicity, and education), item bias analyses for gender and ethnicity, and effect sizes for group differences in clinical studies of sensitivity. From a practical perspective, the test stands out among memory batteries in that it allows continuity between assessments for children and adults, an asset in longitudinal studies or in clinical settings where retesting frequently occurs. Although most of the subtests follow familiar memory testing paradigms (e.g., list-learning, design memory), some new subtests may be of interest. For example, Verbal Working Memory may be useful for young children because of the use of real objects and animals instead of letters and numbers. Also, Symbolic Working Memory, an analog to Number-Letter, does not require an oral response and therefore may have some utility in assessing working memory in individuals with language difficulties.

WRAML2 floors seem adequate, with the possible exception of Design Memory, in which, for 5-year-olds, a score of 0 yields a scaled score of 5, and a score of 2 yields a scaled score of 6. Users should be aware of this, given the possibility of obtaining points for random design production. The remainder of the subtests appear to have adequate floors and ceilings. However, many of the recognition subtests and some delay subtests (e.g., Verbal Learning, Sound-Symbol) should be interpreted with caution because of restricted range. This is discussed in detail in the manual (Sheslow & Adams, 2003).

Because Qualitative Analyses and Optional subtests are designed to "enhance the diagnostic value of the Core Subtests" (Sheslow & Adams, 2003, p. 73), a discussion of the utility of comparing these scores with Core subtest scores is provided in Chapter 5 of the manual. The authors clearly state the limitations inherent in comparisons involving scores with restricted ranges or formats (e.g., yes/no recognition leading to reduced variability) and provide general guidelines for interpretation, keeping these caveats in mind. Although these interpretations are potentially of clinical utility, interpretation of Qualitative Analyses scores is not recommended in a clinical context, regardless of any caveats provided by the test authors. The reason is the low reliability of some scores (e.g., Story Memory Verbatim, Gist, Story A, Story B, Retention) and the lack of reliability information on others (e.g., Picture Memory commissions, Verbal Learning trial-by-trial, slope, intrusion errors, semantic and phonological errors; Symbol Search trial-by-trial, slope).

Some criticism leveled at the previous edition may still need to be addressed, including the lack of a clear rationale for selection of subtests in the Screening Battery (Woodward & Donders, 1998).

Factor analyses of the previous version of the battery in various populations indicated that some factor solutions did not account for large amounts of variance, leading researchers such as Gioia to conclude that the subtests should be interpreted "as unique entities rather than within the existing composite scales" (Gioia, 1998, p. 134). In the case of the WRAML2, factor analyses involving the entire set of subtests would be of interest, given the overlap between Attention/Concentration and Working Memory, as suggested by the subtest intercorrelation matrix. In addition, research on the previous edition of the test indicated that, in the standardization sample, correlations between subtests tended to be low across age (most often between

.20 and .40) and were not accounted for by statistical artifacts such as restriction of range or poor reliability (Putzke et al., 2001). However, there was some evidence of developmental increase in intertask consistency with age on the WRAML, translating into higher subtest intercorrelations with age. This pattern may be due to increased self-regulatory mechanisms and increased knowledge-base connections that occur as children mature (Putzke et al., 2001). Therefore, one interpretation is that low correlations between subtest scores on the WRAML, which appear to also occur to some degree on the WRAML2 (see in particular the discussion on visual subtests in *Validity*), may in part be due to developmental changes in memory functioning (or, alternatively, in attention or motivation). Of note, however, are the low correlations between the WRAML2 subtests making up the Visual Index, paired with the less-than-optimal reliabilities for the visual subtests, which suggests that these scores should not form the basis of clinical decision making for younger children. Note that the low reliability of visual subtests and lack of homogeneity in visual index scores are not specific to the WRAML2 (see *CMS* and *WMS-III*) and may be a general, inherent problem in assessing visual memory.

Earlier studies suggested that there was a risk of inconsistent score classification with the previous version of the test, with relatively low overlap between subtests on the WRAML (Putzke et al., 1998) as well as considerable individual variability across WRAML memory subtests (Putzke et al., 2001). The result was that a substantial proportion of nonclinical children obtained clinical-level discrepancies across subtests. For example, Putzke et al. (2001) found that 80% of normal children had at least one scaled score discrepancy of 6 scaled score points on the WRAML (i.e., ≥2 SDs), with about one fourth of the sample having at least one discrepancy of 9 points or more (i.e., ≥3 SDs). Between 15% and 19% of normal children also had at least one subtest score in the impaired range, defined as one scaled score of 4 or less, on the WRAML (Putzke et al., 2001). Further research is needed to determine whether these findings apply to the WRAML2. Note that Taylor and Heaton (2001) pointed out that it is not uncommon in adults to find impairment on one WAIS/WMS factor, but impairments on more than two factor scores is rare.

Finally, although the test does appear sensitive to memory impairment, there is as yet no evidence that it can distinguish among disorders in children or adults. Information on this topic is likely to be forthcoming as more research involving the WRAML2 emerges. Evidence of its ability to track change, and information on ecological validity would also help increase its clinical utility.

REFERENCES

Aylward, G. P., Gioia, G., Verhulst, S. J., & Bell, S. (1995). Factor structure of the Wide Range Assessment of Memory and Learning in a clinical population. *Journal of Psychoeducational Assessment, 13* (2), 132–142.

Burton, D. B., Donders, J., & Mittenberg, W. (1996). A structural equation modeling of the Wide Range Assessment of Memory and Learning in the standardization sample. *Child Neuropsychology, 2*(1), 39–47.

Burton, D. B., Mittenberg, W., Gold, S., & Drabman, R. (1999). A structural equation analysis of the Wide Range Assessment of Memory and Learning in a clinical sample. *Child Neuropsychology, 5*(1), 34–40.

Clark, R. M., & Medway, F. J. (1992). Review of the Wide Range Assessment of Memory and Learning. In J. J. Kramer & J. Close Conoley (Eds.), *The Eleventh Mental Measurements Yearbook.* Lincoln, Neb.: Buros Institute.

Dewey, D., Kaplan, B. J., & Crawford, S. G. (1997). Factor structure of the WRAML in children with ADHD or reading disabilities: Further evidence of an attention/concentration factor. *Developmental Neuropsychology, 13*(4), 501–506.

Dewey, D., Kaplan, B. J., Crawford, S. G., & Fisher, G. C. (1998). Predictive accuracy of the Wide Range Assessment of Memory and Learning in children with Attention Deficit Hyperactivity Disorder and reading disorder. *Developmental Neuropsychology, 19*(2), 173–189.

Donders, J., & Woodward, H. R. (2003). Gender as a moderator of memory after traumatic brain injury in children. *Journal of Head Trauma Rehabilitation, 18*(2), 106–115.

Farmer, J. E., Haut, J. S., Williams, J., Kapila, C., Johnstone, B., & Kirk, K. S. (1999). Comprehensive assessment of memory functioning following traumatic brain injury in children. *Developmental Neuropsychology, 15*(2), 269–289.

Gioia, G. A. (1998). Re-examining the factor structure of the Wide Range Assessment of Memory and Learning: Implications for clinical interpretation. *Assessment, 5*(2), 127–139.

Kennedy, M. L., & Guilmette, T. J. (1997). The relationship between the WRAML memory screening and general memory indices in a clinical population. *Assessment, 4*(1), 69–72.

Hill, D. E., Ciesielski, K. T., Sethre-Hofstad, L., Duncan, M. H., & Lorenzi, M. (1997). Visual and verbal short-term memory deficits in childhood leukemia survivors after intrathecal chemotherapy. *Journal of Pediatric Psychology, 22*(6), 861–870.

Luo, X., & Li, X. (2003). Memory and learning ability of children with ADHD. *Chinese Mental Health Journal, 17*(3), 188–190.

Lynch, P. A., Chen, R., & Holmes, C. S. (2004). Factor structure of the Wide Range Assessment of Memory and Learning (WRAML) in children with insulin dependent diabetes mellitus (IDDM). *Child Neuropsychology, 10*(4), 306–317.

Mealer, C., Morgan, S., & Luscomb, R. (1996). Cognitive functioning of ADHD and non-ADHD boys on the WISC-III and WRAML: An analysis within a memory model. *Journal of Attention Disorders, 1*(3), 133–145.

Phelps, L. (1995). Exploratory factor analysis of the WRAML with academically at-risk students. *Journal of Psychoeducational Assessment, 13*(4), 384–390.

Phelps, L. (1996). Discriminative validity of the WRAML with ADHD and LD children. *Psychology in the Schools, 33*(1), 5–12.

Putzke, J. D., Williams, M. A., Adams, W., & Boll, T. J. (1998). Does memory test performance in children become more consistent with age? Cross-sectional comparisons using the WRAML. *Journal of Clinical and Experimental Neuropsychology, 20*(6), 835–845.

Putzke, J. D., Williams, M. A., Glutting, J. J., Konold, T. R., & Boll, T. J. (2001). Developmental memory performance: Inter-task consistency and base-rate variability on the WRAML. *Journal of Clinical and Experimental Neuropsychology, 23*(3), 253–264.

Roebuck-Spencer, T. M., & Mattson, S. N. (2004). Implicit strategy affects learning in children with heavy prenatal alcohol exposure. *Alcoholism: Clinical and Experimental Research, 28*(9), 1424–1431.

Sheslow, D., & Adams, W. (1990). *Wide Range Assessment of Memory and Learning.* Wilmington, Del.: Wide Range.

Sheslow, D., & Adams, W. (2003). *Wide Range Assessment of Memory and Learning, Second Edition administration and technical manual.* Wilmington, Del.: Wide Range.

Taylor, M. J., & Heaton, R. K. (2001). Sensitivity and specificity of WAIS-III/WMS-III demographically corrected factor scores in neuropsychological assessment. *Journal of the International Neuropsychological Society, 7*, 867–874.

Williams, J., & Haut, J. S. (1995). Differential performances on the WRAML in children and adolescents diagnosed with epilepsy, head injury, and substance abuse. *Developmental Neuropsychology, 11*(2), 201–213.

Woodward, H., & Donders, J. (1998). The performance of children with traumatic head injury on the Wide Range Assessment of Memory and Learning-Screening. *Applied Neuropsychology, 5*(3), 113–119.

11

Language Tests

Because of the central importance of verbal communication deficits after brain damage, as well as delays in language development in children, numerous tests of language function have been developed (see Spreen & Risser, 2003, for a recent review). Brief screening tests such as the one included in the Halstead-Reitan test battery (Reitan, 1991; Wheeler & Reitan, 1962) arose in the 1950s for the purpose of screening for the presence of "organicity." However, such cursory examination is rarely necessary today, because most patients are referred with an established clinical impression of aphasia. Further, the accuracy of screening devices is limited because specificity is poor. That is, there are many reasons why a nonaphasic patient might fail an aphasia screening test. Therefore, screening tests, per se, have fallen out of use (Rabin et al., 2005) in favor of other approaches (Spreen & Risser, 2003).

Comprehensive batteries are used for diagnostic purposes, to describe cognitive strengths and weaknesses, and to provide information for treatment purposes. There are a variety of batteries to choose from (see Spreen & Risser, 2003). We present here the relatively brief Multilingual Aphasia Examination (MAE) and the more detailed Boston Diagnostic Aphasia Examination (BDAE) because these are two of the more popular language measures in neuropsychological contexts. Both offer a wide variety of subtests that allow the examiner to assess diverse language disorders with considerable flexibility. Because the subtests are relatively brief, they can be used in the acute phase (e.g., after cerebrovascular accident) and with low-functioning (e.g., demented) patients.

We also review a selection of commonly used specific-function tests (see Table 11–1). The Token Test (De Renzi & Vignola, 1962) and its variants have proved most durable as an index of language comprehension. The Boston Naming Test (BNT2) is one of the most commonly employed measures of naming ability (Camara et al., 2000; Rabin et al., 2005). The EOWPVT3 and the EVT also assess lexical retrieval ability and have strong psychometric properties. The fact that they are conormed with receptive vocabulary tests (ROWVT, PPVT-III) makes them particularly useful for evaluating receptive/expressive discrepancies. In general, examiners should always administer expressive tests before other vocabulary tests, to avoid score inflation (see reviews for more information). It is also important to bear in mind that performance on these vocabulary tests may convey little about performance in other language areas, such as social communication. Tests directed at the functional ability of the patient to communicate in daily life are detailed in Spreen & Risser (2003). Approaches often go beyond the patients themselves to examine the effectiveness of communication in social settings via rating scales given to family members or caregivers (see, for example, *Scales of Independent Behavior—Revised*).

Finally, we also describe a dichotic listening task. Such tools appear useful with regard to lateralized cognitive processes. Their utility in cases of white matter disturbance is also noteworthy, because they may detect abnormality when other standard tasks do not.

REFERENCES

Camara, W. J., Nathan, J. S., & Puente, A. E. (2000). Psychological test usage: Implications in professional psychology. *Professional Psychology: Research and Practice, 31,* 141–154.

De Renzi, E., & Vignolo, L. (1962). The Token Test. A sensitive test to detect receptive disturbances in aphasics. *Brain, 85,* 665–678.

Rabin, L. A., Barr, W. B., & Burton, L. A. (2005). Assessment practices of clinical neuropsychologists in the United States and Canada: A survey of INS, NAN, and APA Division 40 members. *Archives of Clinical Neuropsychology, 20,* 33–66.

Reitan, R. M. (1991). *Aphasia Screening Test.* Tucson, Ariz.: Reitan Neuropsychology Laboratory.

Spreen, O., & Risser, A. H. (2003). *Assessment of aphasia.* New York: Oxford University Press.

Wheeler, L., & Reitan, R. M. (1962). The presence and laterality of brain damage predicted from responses to a short aphasia screening test. *Perceptual and Motor Skills, 15,* 783–799.

Table 11–1 Some Measures of Language Abilities

Test	Age Range (Years)	Administration Time (Min)	Key Processes	Test-Retest Reliability	Other Versions	Co-normed
BDAE	≥16	90; 40–60 for short form	Conversational speech, auditory comprehension, oral expression, reading, writing, praxis, constructional ability, calculations, finger gnosis Right-Left orientation	NA	Short, Standard, and Extended formats	
BNT	5–13; ≥18	10–20	Visual object naming	High over short intervals; mixed over long	Standard and Short Forms	
Dichotic Listening	2–30	10–20	Language processing, language lateralization, inattention, motivational status	Mixed		
EOWPVT3	2–18	10–15	Retrieval of names of pictured objects, actions, or concepts	High over short intervals	NA	ROWPVT
EVT	2½–90+	10–25	Word retrieval	Adequate to high	NA	PPVT-III
MAE	2–12, 16–97	20–40	Naming, sentence repetition, verbal fluency, comprehension, reading comprehension, spelling	NA	Alternate versions of Sentence Repetition, COWA, Spelling, and Token Test	COWA and Token are conormed with other tests as part of the MOANS project
PPVT-III	2½–90+	10–15	Receptive vocabulary	High	PPVTIIIA and B	EVT
Token Test	≥6	10	Comprehension of commands, motivational status	High for neurologically impaired patients	NA	

Boston Diagnostic Aphasia Examination—Third Edition (BDAE-3)

PURPOSE

The purpose of the Boston Diagnostic Aphasia Examination (BDAE) is to provide a full assessment of an aphasic patient's language functioning with specific reference to the classic, anatomically based aphasia syndromes.

SOURCE

The test kit, including a test manual, stimulus cards for Standard and Short Forms, 25 BDAE Standard Form and 25 Short Form booklets, and the 60-item Boston Naming Test (described later in this chapter) with 25 record booklets, is available through Psychological Assessment Resources (http://www.parinc.com), at a cost of $219 US. Note that the manual is provided as part of Goodglass' book, *Assessment of Aphasia and Related Disorders, Third Edition* (2001a), which is provided with the test kit. Also available is a 90-min video to instruct the test user. The test is also available from The Psychological Corporation (http://www.harcourtassessment.com), at a cost of $200 US.

Other Versions

Spanish (Goodglass & Kaplan, 1986), French (Mazaux & Orgogozo, 1985), Hindi (Kacker et al., 1991), and Finnish (Laine et al., 1993) versions are available, although they do not yet employ the newest BDAE-3 format.

AGE RANGE

The age range is 16 years to old age.

APPROXIMATE TIME FOR ADMINISTRATION

The test takes about 90 min (40–60 min for the Short Form).

DESCRIPTION

The BDAE is a battery of tests designed to meet three goals: to enable diagnosis of aphasia syndromes, to measure the breadth and severity of aphasic disturbance, and to provide a comprehensive assessment of language to guide therapy (Goodglass et al., 2001a). The BDAE was initially published by Goodglass and Kaplan in 1972; it was revised in 1983 (Goodglass & Kaplan, 1983b) and again in 2001 (third edition, BDAE-3; Goodglass et al., 2001a, 2001b).

The test has been substantially revised. Changes from the previous edition include the addition of abbreviated and expanded testing formats, the incorporation of the Boston Naming Test (Kaplan et al., 1983) as a subtest, the addition of a Language Competence Index, and clarification of scoring procedures and definitions. The revision was also designed to integrate recent advances in neurolinguistics research, including methods to assess narrative and discourse complexity, category-specific dissociations in lexical production/comprehension, syntax comprehension, and analysis of grapheme-phoneme conversion during reading. However, the ultimate goal of the authors in developing the test was clinical utility (Goodglass et al., 2001a). The authors note that, like all methods for evaluating aphasia, the test has limitations. For instance, the score profile does not automatically produce a diagnosis, nor does it indicate the most suitable therapy. Examiners should use the test as a framework for sampling language performance and should feel free to build on this framework to further explore the patient's abilities (Goodglass et al., 2001a).

The BDAE-3 includes more than 50 subtests and can be administered in three different formats: Standard, Short, and Extended. The Standard format is most closely related to earlier versions of the BDAE. The new Short Form of the test provides "a brief, no-frills assessment," whereas the Extended version offers a fuller neurolinguistic assessment that includes evaluation of free narrative, processing of word categories, syntax comprehension, and reading/writing (Goodglass et al., 2001a). The BDAE-3 allows both a quantitative and a qualitative evaluation of language. For example, although several scores are based on pass/fail criteria, rating scales allow a qualitative evaluation of language aspects such as speech melody, fluency, anomia, syntactic organization, and paraphasia types.

Like earlier versions, the standard BDAE-3 is divided into five language-related sections and an additional section on praxis. The five language domains include conversational and expository speech, auditory comprehension, oral expression, reading, and writing. These are assessed by a number of different subtests, which are shown in Table 11–2, along with the specific subtests from the Standard and Extended Battery. In addition to individual subtest scores, the test also provides three main scoring methods (see *Scoring*): the Severity Rating Scale (a rating of the severity of observed language/speech disturbance), the Rating Scale Profile of Speech Characteristics (a rating of observed speech characteristics and of scores in two main language domains), and the Language Competency Index (a composite score of language performance on BDAE-3 subtests).

The extended version of the BDAE-3 includes a sixth section, "Praxis," which examines natural and conventional gestures, use of pretended objects, and bucco-facial and respiratory movements (Table 11–2).

Supplementary nonlanguage tests (previously called the Boston Parietal Lobe Battery, but now referred to as the Spatial-Quantitative Battery) were included as a separate adjunct in earlier versions of the BDAE and remain an option for the BDAE-3 (Table 11–3).

ADMINISTRATION

See *Source*. The 44-page test booklet serves as the guide for administration. Subtests appear in the same order in the booklet and in the stimulus card book. Short Form items are presented in bold typeface, and Extended Form items appear in italics. The abbreviated administration can also be given using a separate Short Form test booklet. For the Standard administration, all the Short Form items in boldface are administered, in addition to items in regular typeface.

SCORING

See *Source*. Scoring instructions are provided in the manual and answer booklet. The profile summary automatically translates raw scores into percentile ranks. The Score Summary Sheet provides a visual profile of performance across all the BDAE-3 subtests grouped by domain.

The Severity Rating Scale (p. 9 of the test booklet) is designed to provide an estimate of the severity of impairment; this need not be specific to aphasia but can also include other speech disorders, such as dysarthria. The rating ranges from 0 (neither useful comprehension nor speech output is possible) to 5 (normal comprehension and speech output).

The Rating Scale Profile of Speech Characteristics is a profile form that includes aspects of speech that are not easily objectively quantified: articulatory agility, phrase length, grammatical facility, melodic line (prosody), and extent of word finding difficulties. Each dimension is rated on a seven-point scale by the examiner. In addition, the profile includes mean percentile scores from two objective domains considered crucial to diagnostic differentiation (Sentence Repetition and Auditory Comprehension). At the bottom of the profile, the examiner may also provide ratings for rate, volume, and voice quality.

Table 11–2 BDAE-3 Domains and Subtests for the Standard and Extended Battery

Domain	Standard Battery	Extended Battery
Conversational and Expository Speech	Simple Social Responses[a] Free Conversation[a] Picture Description (Cookie Theft)[a]	Aesop's Fables[a]
Auditory Comprehension	Basic Word Discrimination Commands Complex Ideational Material	Word Comprehension by Categories—Tools/Implements Word Comprehension by Categories—Foods Word Comprehension by Categories—Animals Word Comprehension by Categories—Body Parts Word Comprehension by Categories—Comprehension Word Comprehension by Categories—Map Locations Semantic Probe Syntactic Processing—Touch A with B Reversible Possessives Embedded Sentences
Oral Expression	Nonverbal Agility Verbal Agility Automatized Sequences Recitation Melody Rhythm Single Word Repetition Repetition of Sentences Responsive Naming Boston Naming Test Screening for Naming of Special Categories (Letters, Numbers, Colors)	Repetition of Nonsense Words Naming in Categories—Colors Naming in Categories—Actions Naming in Categories—Animals Naming in Categories—Tools/Implements
Reading	Matching Across Cases and Scripts[b] Number Matching (three subtasks) Picture-Word Match Lexical Decision[b] Homophone Matching[b] Free Grammatical Morphemes[b] Basic Oral Word Reading Oral Reading of Sentences with Comprehension Reading Comprehension—Sentences and Paragraphs	Advanced Phonic Analysis—Pseudohomophone Matching Bound Grammatical Morphemes Derivational Morphemes Oral Reading of Special Word Lists—Mixed Morphological Types Oral Reading of Special Word Lists—Semantic Paralexia Prone Words
Writing	Mechanics of Writing Primer Word Vocabulary Regular Phonics Common Irregular Forms Written Picture Naming (Objects, Actions, Animals) Narrative Writing (Cookie Theft)[b]	Uncommon Irregularities Oral Spelling Nonsense Words Cognitive/Grammatical Influences—Part of Speech (Functors, Derivational Affixes, Verb Forms) Loaded Sentences
Praxis	—	Natural Gestures Conventional Gestures Use of Pretended Objects Bucco-Facial Respiratory Movements

Note: Extended subtests are administered in addition to Standard subtests.

[a] Provide basis for the Severity Rating and the Profile of Speech Characteristics.

[b] Includes an Extended testing option.

Table 11–3 The Spatial-Quantitative Battery

Constructional Deficits	Drawing To Command
	Stick Constuction Memory
	Three-Dimensional Blocks
Finger Agnosia	Verbal: Comprehension
	Visual: Finger Naming
	Verbal-Visual: Paired-Finger Identification
	Visual-Visual: Matching Two Finger Positions
	Tactile-Visual
Acalculia	Arithmetic
	Clock Setting
Right-Left Orientation	Double-Other Person
	Double-Own Body
	Single-Other Person
	Single-Self

The Language Competency Index provides a percentile-based global measure of aphasia severity, based on a combination of fluency, auditory comprehension, and naming subtest scores (according to the authors, reading and writing performance are not included because they can be disproportionally affected, compared with spoken language). The formula for calculating this index is presented on the last page of the test booklet and is computed as shown in Figure 11–1.

DEMOGRAPHIC EFFECTS

Age

The influence of age is controversial. Some authors (Heaton et al., 2004) have found little impact of age on performance, whereas others have reported that age affects performance on at least some of the BDAE and Parietal Lobe Battery tasks (Borod et al., 1980; Farver & Farver, 1982; Pineda et al., 2000; Radanovic & Mansur, 2002; Rosselli et al., 1990). The younger the participants, the better the performance.

Gender

The influence of gender appears to be small (Pineda et al., 2000; Rosselli et al., 1990) or nonexistent on the BDAE (Heaton et al., 2004; Radamovic & Mansur, 2002) and on the Parietal Lobe Battery (Farver & Farver, 1982).

Education

Education has a stronger effect on test scores, with lower academic achievement associated with lower scores (Borod et al., 1980; Heaton et al., 1991; Jacobs et al., 1997; Pineda et al., 2000; Radanovic & Mansur, 2002; Rosselli et al., 1990). For example, Heaton et al. (2004) examined the Complex Ideational subtest in 326 normal individuals and found that 7% of the variance in test scores was accounted for by education. Rosselli et al. (1990) gave the Spanish version to 180 normal Colombian participants, aged 16 to 65 years, and found marked differences according to educational achievement. More recently, Pineda et al. (2000) examined 156 individuals, ages 19 to 60 years in Columbia and noted that education was a low (<15%) to modest (>17%) predictor of variance in BDAE scores.

Socioeconomic Status and Ethnicity

Pineda et al. (2000) found that occupational status and socioeconomic status were low but significant predictors of performance on some subtests (Comprehension of Commands, Body-Part Naming).

For most expressive subtests of the BDAE, there are no significant differences in scores obtained by upper- and middle-status African American and Caucasian individuals (Molrine & Pierce, 2002). Ethnicity, however, can affect performance. Jacobs et al. (1997) compared the performance of English- and Spanish-speaking older adults (matched for age and education) on two of the tasks of the BDAE (repetition of high frequency phrases and an abbreviated version of the Complex Ideational Material subtest). Spanish-speakers obtained lower scores on the auditory comprehension task. Level of acculturation was an important determinant of test performance, because subjects tested in Spanish who reported that they could speak English well did not differ from participants tested in English.

Figure 11–1 Computation of Language Competency Index for the BDAE-3.

Language Competence Index: (*Expression Component* + *Auditory Comprehension Component*)/2

Expression Component = mean of percentiles for two expression subtests (Boston Naming Test and Grammatical Form rating from the Severity Rating)

Auditory Comprehension Component = mean of the percentiles for three auditory comprehension subtests (Word Discrimination, Commands, and Complex Ideational Material)

NORMATIVE DATA

Standardization Sample

Unlike norms for previous test versions, which originated from inpatient data accumulated over time at the Boston Veterans Administration Medical Center, the aphasic subjects for the BDAE-3 were referred concurrently by field examiners at different testing sites; they also represented a wider range of severity because they came from inpatient, outpatient, and private practice sources. The normative data are therefore less skewed toward severely impaired subjects compared with previous editions of the test; specifically, they are evenly distributed across severity ratings on the Aphasia Severity Rating Scale. As a result, a given BDAE-3 score corresponds to a lower percentile than it would have in previous editions. Tables to convert 1983 edition scores to 1999 scores are provided in the manual.

The test manual provides means and standard deviations for the BDAE-3 subtests for aphasic subjects. The number of subjects varies from a maximum of 85 to a low of 31, depending on the subtest. Means are also provided for 15 normal subjects. In most cases, normal subjects, on average, failed less than one item per subtest. One exception was the "Touch A with B" subtest, on which one normal individual failed more than half of the items.

Normative data for the Spatial-Quantitative Battery are provided in the manual based on data collected by Borod et al. (1980) on 147 neurologically normal men (ages 25 to 85 years, education ranging from < 8 years to college-level). These are provided because ceiling scores are not necessarily obtained for normal subjects on these subtests, as is the case for the language subtests of the BDAE-3.

Other Normative Data

Norms for the Complex Ideational Material subtest are provided by Heaton et al. (2004) for individuals aged 20 to 85 years. They are based on a sample of 326 Caucasian individuals with a mean age of 52.0 years ($SD = 18.6$). Pineda et al. (2000) provided normative data, broken down by age (19–35 and 36–50 years) and education (1–9, 10–15, and > 16 years) on the Spanish version of the BDAE (Goodglass & Kaplan, 1986), based on a sample of 156 healthy participants living in Medellin, Columbia. These are reproduced in Table 11–4. Norms for Spanish-speaking individuals are also provided by Rosselli et al. (1990).

Norms (means but no standard deviations) for the Parietal Lobe Battery in older subjects (aged 40 to 89 years) are presented by Farver and Farver (1982).

RELIABILITY

Internal Reliability

Although reliability coefficients are for the most part acceptable to high, there is variability across subtests (Goodglass

et al., 2001a). For example, alpha coefficients presented in the manual range from very high for Sentence Repetition and the Boston Naming Test (> .95) to low for Auditory Comprehension—Foods—Extended and Reading—Picture-Word Match (< .65). No information is provided on the internal consistency of the rating scores, language competency index, praxis assessment, or Spatial-Quantitative Battery.

Test-Retest Reliability

Stability coefficients are not presented in the manual. The authors state that repeatability varies among aphasics to a greater degree than among other populations, but that once recovery has stabilized, retest performance should fairly closely approximate baseline performance. No data are provided to support these claims. No stability information is provided for ratings, language competency index, praxis assessment, or Spatial-Quantitative Battery.

Alternate Form Reliability

For most subtests, correlations between the Short and Standard Forms are very high (> .90; Goodglass et al., 2001a). Two exceptions are the Word Discrimination and Matching Numbers subtests, which have slightly lower correlations between Standard and Short Forms ($r = .77$ and .76, respectively). No information is provided for ratings, language competency index, praxis assessment, or Spatial-Quantitative Battery.

Interrater Reliability

The reliability of the Speech Characteristics Profile (melodic line, phrase length, articulatory agility, grammatical form, paraphasias, word-finding, auditory comprehension) was first examined for the original BDAE, employing three judges who rated the tape-recorded speech samples of 99 patients. The lowest interjudge correlations were .78 and .79 for word-finding difficulties and paraphasias, respectively; the other dimensions had coefficients of at least .85. Other interrater agreement studies have also shown satisfactory results (Davis, 1993; Molrine & Pierce, 2002). In contrast, Gordon (1998) investigated fluency-nonfluency judgments of 24 experienced speech therapists listening to spontaneous speech and sentence repetition of 10 aphasic patients. She found only two-thirds agreement among raters for half of the patients even though the therapists reported that they used such ratings all the time. High variability was also found for individual subjects, especially on articulation and paraphasia ratings.

VALIDITY

Internal Structure

The authors provide a partial correlation matrix showing intercorrelations between BDAE-3 subtests for the standardization sample (Goodglass et al., 2001a). Only subtests with

Table 11–4 Age- and Education-Corrected Normative Data (Mean and *SD*) for the BDAE—Spanish Version.

	Age 19–35 Years			Age 36–50 Years		
	Education			Education		
	1–9	10–15	>16	1–9	10–15	>16
Comprehension						
Word Discrimination	70.1 (2.0)	70.7 (2.5)	71.1 (1.9)	68.9 (3.8)	71.1 (1.3)	71.4 (1.3)
Body-Part Identification	18.1 (1.5)	18.6 (1.5)	19.3 (1.2)	18.4 (1.3)	19.0 (0.9)	19.3 (1.7)
Commands	14.0 (1.1)	14.5 (1.0)	14.3 (1.0)	14.0 (1.4)	14.6 (1.0)	14.6 (0.7)
Complex Material	8.3 (2.3)	8.9 (1.4)	9.2 (1.5)	7.9 (2.0)	9.4 (1.4)	9.5 (1.7)
Automatic Speech						
Automated Sentences	13.8 (0.7)	13.8 (0.4)	13.8 (0.4)	13.0 (1.5)	13.8 (0.6)	13.8 (0.8)
Singing and Rhyming	1.8 (0.7)	1.9 (0.3)	1.9 (0.4)	1.8 (0.6)	1.9 (0.5)	1.8 (0.6)
Repetition						
Words	10.0 (0)	9.9 (0.2)	10.0 (0)	10.0 (0)	10.0 (0)	30.0 (0)
High Probability	7.6 (0.7)	7.9 (0.4)	8.0 (0)	7.5 (0.9)	7.9 (0.3)	7.9 (0.3)
Low Probability	7.7 (0.7)	9.9 (0.3)	8.0 (0)	7.6 (0.5)	7.9 (0.4)	7.9 (0.4)
Oral Reading						
Words	28.2 (5.0)	30.0 (0)	30.0 (0)	29.9 (0.4)	30.0 (0)	30.0 (0)
Oral Sentences	8.8 (3.0)	10.0 (0)	9.9 (0.2)	10.0 (0)	10.0 (0)	9.9 (0.2)
Naming						
Responsive Naming	27.8 (6.0)	29.9 (0.4)	29.1 (4.2)	30.0 (0)	29.2 (3.8)	29.9 (0.6)
Confrontation Naming	93.8 (3.2)	95.7 (0.9)	95.8 (0.7)	91.1 (5.5)	94.7 (3.0)	95.5 (2.3)
Body-Part Naming	26.6 (2.4)	27.1 (2.5)	28.1 (1.9)	26.4 (2.7)	28.0 (2.2)	28.5 (2.2)
Animal Naming	21.3 (6.0)	26.4 (5.8)	29.6 (4.8)	21.0 (4.2)	24.0 (6.9)	28.5 (2.2)
Reading Comprehension						
Symbol Discrimination	8.8 (2.9)	9.9 (0.2)	10.0 (0)	9.4 (1.1)	9.7 (1.0)	9.9 (0.4)
Word Recognition	7.9 (0.3)	7.8 (1.2)	7.9 (0.3)	8.0 (0)	8.0 (0)	7.9 (0.2)
Oral Spelling	5.6 (2.1)	6.6 (1.6)	7.3 (1.1)	5.3 (2.1)	6.5 (1.5)	7.2 (1.0)
Word-Picture Matching	9.9 (0.3)	10.0 (0)	10.0 (0)	10.0 (0)	10.0 (0)	10.0 (0)
Sentences—Paragraphs	8.3 (1.3)	9.4 (0.9)	9.7 (0.5)	9.1 (1.3)	9.6 (0.8)	9.6 (0.5)
Writing						
Mechanics	5.0 (0)	5.0 (0)	4.9 (0.3)	5.0 (0)	4.9 (0.2)	4.9 (0.2)
Serial Writing	44.7 (7.2)	47.2 (1.5)	47.6 (0.9)	42.3 (6.8)	47.8 (1.5)	47.4 (1.2)
Primer-Level Dictation	13.3 (1.1)	13.7 (1.7)	14.0 (0)	13.5 (0.9)	13.9 (0.3)	13.6 (1.9)
Written Confrontation Naming	8.9 (2.6)	9.9 (0.2)	10.0 (0)	9.8 (0.5)	9.9 (0.2)	9.9 (0.4)
Spelling to Dictation	9.2 (2.3)	9.9 (0.2)	9.9 (0.2)	9.4 (1.0)	9.9 (0.3)	9.9 (0.2)
Sentences to Dictation	10.7 (3.6)	12.0 (0)	12.0 (0)	12.0 (0)	12.0 (0)	11.8 (0.7)
Narrative Writing	4.8 (0.7)	4.9 (0.3)	4.9 (0.3)	5.0 (0)	5.0 (0)	4.8 (0.7)

Source: Pineda et al., 2000.

correlations of .60 or greater are presented, with severity partialled out. These are interpreted by the authors as indicating "a number of sharply defined clusters" (p. 16). However, without actual data on the entire correlation matrix, it is difficult to estimate convergent and discriminant validity within and across the BDAE-3 clusters, particularly when one considers the less-than-optimal subject-to-variable ratio (i.e., 31 to 85 subjects and more than 50 subtests).

Currently, no studies have examined the factor structure of the BDAE-3. However, data exist for earlier versions. Goodglass and Kaplan (1972) found a strong general language factor, along with other factors covering spatial-quantitative-somatagnostic, articulation-grammatical fluency, auditory-comprehension, and paraphasia domains. Goodglass and Kaplan (1983a) also described a second factor analysis using a sample of 242 aphasic patients and concluded that auditory comprehension, repetition-recitation, reading, and writing were factors of equal importance, followed by fluency and paraphasia. Pineda et al. (2000) reported similar (although not identical) findings in normal individuals. A seven-factor solution was obtained, representing oral reading, writing, semantic knowledge, lexical graphic attention, semantic fluency, repetition, and motor performance.

With regard to the Parietal Lobe Battery, Borod et al. (1984) applied the battery to 163 right-handed male aphasics and found four factors: construction, visual schemata, verbal components of the Gerstmann syndrome, and visual finger recognition.

Correlations With Other Tests

With regard to relations with other measures, Love and Oster (2002) supported the validity of syntactic auditory comprehension by examining correlations with a specific test assessing syntactic complexity (SOAP—subject-relative, object-relative, active, and passive). The BDAE oral apraxia task specifically was related to other articulation tasks (Sussman et al., 1986). Divenyi and Robinson (1989) reported correlations of .86 and .93 for the auditory comprehension measure in the BDAE with the Token Test and with the respective part of the Porch Index of Communicative Ability (PICA). However, the BDAE auditory comprehension subtest was not an adequate predictor of auditory paragraph comprehension when independent standardized material was used (Brookshire & Nicholas, 1984). With regard to the reading test items, Nicholas et al. (1986) showed that both aphasic and healthy subjects were able to answer a similar number of questions about the items without having actually read the passage, suggesting a high passage dependency of this test. This dependency applied not only to the BDAE but also to similar tasks in aphasia batteries such as the WAB.

Neuroanatomic Correlates

Goodglass and Kaplan (1972) based the design of their instrument on the observation that various components of language function may be selectively damaged by CNS lesions. This selectivity is an indication of the neuroanatomical organization of language, the localization of the lesion causing the observed deficit, and the functional interactions of various parts of the language system. A number of studies have validated this stated purpose (e.g., Naeser & Hayward, 1978; Naeser et al., 1981, 1987). In a recent exploration of the role of subcortical structures in cognition, Radanovic and Scaff (2003) found that naming and auditory comprehension were specifically impaired in patients with thalamic lesions, whereas motor-articulatory problems predominated in patients with basal ganglia lesions.

On the Parietal Lobe Battery, impairment is strongest in patients with lesions in both left parietal and frontal areas (Borod et al., 1984). The Spatial-Quantitative tests (formerly called the Parietal Lobe Battery), together with the WAIS,

were applied to right- and left-handed aphasics: left-handed aphasics performed significantly more poorly on both, especially on tasks involving visual-spatial construction, suggesting that, in left-handers, the left hemisphere is typically dominant for tasks usually considered as right-hemisphere specific (Borod et al., 1985).

Clinical Studies

Aphasia.   According to Goodglass and Kaplan (1983a), discriminant validity between cases of Broca's, Wernicke's, conduction, and anomic aphasia is optimal if the following tests are entered into the equation: body-part identification, repetition of high-probability sentences, paraphasia rating, word-finding rating, phrase-length rating, and verbal paraphasias. Li and Williams (1990) showed that, in the Repeating Phrases and Sentences subtest, conduction aphasics showed a greater number of phonemic attempts, word revisions, and word and phrase repetitions; Broca's aphasics showed more phonemic errors and omissions; and Wernicke's aphasics produced more unrelated words and jargon.

It is important to note that decision rules for the "diagnosis" of the individual subtypes are not always clearly defined, although Reinvang and Graves (1975) attempted such clarification. Crary et al. (1992) tried to isolate subtypes of aphasia empirically by means of a Q-type factor analysis for the BDAE and the closely related WAB. The resulting seven patient clusters (labeled Broca, anomic, global, Wernicke, conduction, and two unclassified clusters) agreed only poorly (in 38% of 47 patients), using the classification rules of the test itself; the results were even worse for the WAB. The study, although based on a limited subject population and the use of a somewhat dated cluster-analysis technique, suggested that BDAE classification rules are based on clinical rather than construct validity. Similarly, Naeser and Hayward (1978) and Reinvang (1985) pointed out that scale profiles can aid in the classification but do not firmly classify patients into subtypes of aphasia. The test authors acknowledge that 30% to 80% of aphasic patients are not classifiable; this is also consistent with the clinical experience that a majority of aphasic patients show mixed rather than pure symptomatology.

Dementia.   The sensitivity of earlier versions of the test has been explored in dementia patients. In persons with dementia of the Alzheimer type (AD), Kirshner (1982) found language to be fluent, with normal prosody, syntax, and phrase length; few paraphasias were found, but word-finding problems and poor repetition of low-probability phrases were present. Sentence comprehension, but not letter or word reading, were found to be related to severity of AD (Cummings et al., 1986). Whitworth and Larson (1989) compared 25 AD patients, 25 patients with other dementias, and 58 age-matched controls: They found significant differences compared with controls on all but 4 of 38 BDAE scores (the exceptions were paraphasia, articulation, primer dictation, and word reading). Discriminant function analysis produced correct classification for 95% of the three patient groups. Nineteen test scores contributed to the discrimination of four levels ("stages") of severity of dementia, resulting in correct classification of 100% of 22 patients with dementia. Gorelick et al. (1993) found also that scores on the BDAE Commands and Responsive Naming subtests were lower in 66 patients with multi-infarct dementia, compared with a group of 86 patients who had infarcts without dementia. In a comparison of patients with multi-infarct dementia, AD patients, and normal control subjects, Mendez and Ashla-Mendez (1991) found that the unstructured Cookie Theft card description discriminated better between groups than structured tests. In this study, the multi-infarct group produced fewer words per minute and fewer constructional assemblages.

Head Injury.   Using an earlier version of the test, 218 patients with closed head injury showed significantly poorer word fluency skills than normal subjects. Although their strategies were similar to those used by the normal examinees, some qualitative differences in semantic associations were found, which were related to severity of cognitive disruption (Gruen et al., 1990).

Ecological Validity

Predictive validity has also been examined with earlier BDAE versions. The BDAE appears to predict progress in speech therapy (Davidoff & Katz, 1985; Helm-Estabrooks & Ramsberger, 1989). Additionally, Marshall and Neuberger (1994) found that measured pretreatment effort in self-correction (but not success of self-correction) and good auditory comprehension were related to improvement during treatment as measured by the BDAE.

COMMENT

The BDAE is one of the most popular batteries for use in aphasia settings. It also ranks among the top five language tests used by speech-language pathologists who provide services to patients with traumatic head injuries (Frank & Barrineau, 1996). However, the test is lengthy (90 min), and it is probably more useful for assessments in the context of detailed studies of aphasia and aphasia rehabilitation than as a routine language test. However, the BDAE-3 now includes a Short Form, which reduces administration time. The Extended format, in turn, provides an even more extensive examination than the Standard administration. In addition, the BDAE has always included useful directions for observing and recording many specific types of errors (e.g., paraphasias) found in individuals with aphasia, reflecting the Boston Process Approach (see chapter on *Test Selection*). Consequently, knowledge of the "Boston school" approach to aphasia classification is necessary to interpret the BDAE (e.g., Benson, 1979a). This applies to both the Speech Characteristics Profile and the Aphasia Severity Rating Scale, which are central to diagnostic decision making with the

BDAE—especially its fluency-nonfluency dimension. More detailed diagnoses may incorporate corroborative information from the profile sheet delineating subtest performances. The test manual provides profiles for classic and rarer aphasic subtypes. Note, however, that despite the term "diagnostic" in the title of the test, the classification of aphasia subtypes has so far shown only limited success, mostly because aphasic disorders are typically of a mixed rather than a pure type.

The detailed examination of conversational and expository speech has always been an important and relatively unique aspect of the BDAE; the BDAE-3 offers an even more extensive procedure for this assessment than earlier versions of the test. With its wealth of subtests, the BDAE-3 allows examiners to assess a wide variety of types of language disorders, including very specific deficits, with a great deal of flexibility. The use of short subtests comprised of few items makes it ideal for assessing deficits in the acute phase (e.g., after cerebrovascular accident, inpatient head injury) and in low-functioning patients (e.g., those with dementia), particularly when the Short Form is used.

Nevertheless, the test suffers from a number of psychometric limitations. The aphasic sample on which percentiles are based is not well described, particularly with regard to basic demographic information such as age, gender, and education. The same can be said for the very small normal sample ($N = 15$). This is a major limitation, given that educational and ethnicity/acculturation effects were reported for previous editions. For example, there is a risk of overdiagnosis of impairment in individuals with low education (Borod et al., 1990; Rosselli et al., 1990; Pineda et al., 2000). Users who assess Spanish-speaking individuals may want to continue using the earlier version (BDAE—Spanish Version; Goodglass & Kaplan, 1986), with the age- and education-corrected norms shown in Table 11–4.

No reliability information is provided for the praxis or Spatial-Quantitative subtests or for the new Language Competency Index. Furthermore, the manual does not include any information on test-retest reliabilities of any of its scores, despite the test's obvious potential in tracking language disorders in patients over time. Additionally, some studies have documented limited interrater reliability (e.g., Gordon, 1998). Finally, much of the existing research on the BDAE is based on previous editions of the tests. Given the number of new subtests in the new edition, studies evaluating the construct validity and clinical utility of the new version are needed.

REFERENCES

Bayles, K. A., & Tomoeda, C. K. (1990). *Arizona Battery for Communication Disorders of Dementia (ABCD)*. Tucson, Ariz.: Canyonlands Publishing.

Benson, D. F. (1979). *Aphasia, alexia, and agraphia.* New York: Churchill Livingstone.

Benton, A. L., Hamsher, K. deS., & Sivan, A. B. (1994). *Multilingual Aphasia Examination* (3rd ed.). San Antonio, Tex.: Psychological Corporation.

Borod, J. C., Goodglass, H., & Kaplan, E. (1980). Normative data on the Boston Diagnostic Aphasia Examination, Parietal Lobe Battery, and the Boston Naming Test. *Journal of Clinical Neuropsychology, 2,* 209–15.

Borod, J. C., Carper, M., Goodglass, H., & Naeser, M. (1984). Aphasic performance on a battery of constructional, visuo-spatial, and qualitative tasks: factorial structure and CT scan localization. *Journal of Clinical Neuropsychology, 6,* 189–204.

Borod, J. C., Carper, M., & Naeser, M. (1985). Left-handed and right-handed aphasics with left hemisphere lesions compared on non-verbal performance measures. *Cortex, 21,* 81–90.

Brookshire, R. H., & Nicholas, L. E. (1984). Comprehension of directly and indirectly stated main ideas and details in discourse by brain-damaged and non-brain-damaged listeners. *Brain and Language, 21,* 21–36.

Crary, M. A., Wertz, R. T., & Deal, J. L. (1992). Classifying aphasias: Cluster analysis of Western Aphasia Battery and Boston Diagnostic Aphasia Examination. *Aphasiology, 6,* 29–36.

Cummings, J. L., Houlihan, J. P., & Hill, M. A. (1986). The pattern of reading deterioration in dementia of the Alzheimer type: Observations and implications. *Brain and Language, 29,* 315–323.

Davis, A. G. (1993). *A survey of adult aphasia* (2nd ed.). Englewood Cliffs, N.J.: Prentice-Hall.

Divenyl, P. L., & Robinson, A. J. (1989). Nonlinguistic auditory capabilities in aphasia. *Brain and Language, 37,* 290–326.

Eisenson, J. (1994). *Examining for aphasia* (3rd ed.). Austin, Tex.: Pro-Ed.

Farver, P. F. & Farver, T. B. (1982). Performance of normal older adults on tests designed to measure parietal lobe function (constructional apraxia, Gerstmann syndrome, visuospatial organization). *American Journal of Occupational Therapy, 36,* 444–449.

Fitch-West, J., & Sands, E. S. (1986). *Bedside evaluation and screening test of aphasia.* Austin, Tex.: Pro-Ed.

Frank, E. M., & Barrineau, S. (1996). Current speech-language assessment protocols for adults with traumatic brain injury. *Journal of Medical Speech-Language Pathology, 4*(2), 81–101.

Goodglass, H., & Kaplan, E. (1972). *Boston Diagnostic Aphasia Examination (BDAE).* Philadelphia: Lea & Febiger.

Goodglass, H., & Kaplan, E. (1983a). *The assessment of aphasia and related disorders* (2nd ed.). Philadelphia: Lea & Febiger.

Goodglass, H., & Kaplan, E. (1983b). *Boston Diagnostic Aphasia Examination (BDAE).* Philadelphia: Lea & Febiger. Distributed by Psychological Assessment Resources, Odessa, Fla.

Goodglass, H., & Kaplan, E. (1986). *La evaluacion de la afasia y de transfornos relacionados* (2nd ed.). Madrid: Editorial Medica Panamericana.

Goodglass, H., Kaplan, E., & Barresi, B. (2001a). *The assessment of aphasia and related disorders* (3rd ed.). Philadelphia: Lippincott Williams & Wilkins.

Goodglass, H., Kaplan, E., & Barresi, B. (2001b). *Boston Diagnostic Aphasia Examination* (3rd ed.). Philadelphia: Lippincott Williams & Wilkins.

Gordon, J. K. (1998). The fluency dimension in aphasia. *Aphasiology, 12,* 673–688.

Gorelick, P. B., Brody, J., Cohen, D., & Freels, S. (1993). Risk factors for dementia associated with multiple cerebral infarcts: A case-control analysis in predominantly African-American hospital-based patients. *Archives of Neurology, 50,* 714–720.

Gruen, A. K., Frankle, B. C., & Schwartz, R. (1990). Word fluency generation skills of head-injured patients in an acute trauma center. *Journal of Communication Disorders, 23,* 163–170.

Heaton, R. K., Miller, S. W., Taylor, M. J., & Grant, I. (2004). *Revised comprehensive norms for an expanded Halstead-Reitan battery: Demographically adjusted neuropsychological norms for African American and Caucasian adults.* Lutz, Fla.: PAR.

Helm-Estabrooks, N., Ramsberger, G., Morgan, A. R., & Nicholas, M. (1989). *BASA: Boston Assessment of Severe Aphasia.* Chicago: Riverside Publishing Company.

Holland, A. L. (1980). *Communicative abilities of daily living: Manual.* Baltimore, Md.: University Park Press.

Huber, W., Poeck, K., & Willmes, K. (1984). The Aachen Aphasia Test. In F. C. Rose (Ed.), *Advances in neurology: Progress in aphasiology* (Vol. 42, pp. 291–303). New York: Raven Press.

Jacobs, D. M., Sano, M., Albert, S. Schofield, P. (1997). Cross-cultural neuropsychological assessment: A comparison of randomly selected demographically matched cohorts of English- and Spanish-speaking older adults. *Journal of Clinical and Experimental Neuropsychology, 19,* 331–339.

Kacker, S. K., Pandit, R., & Dua, D. (1991). Reliability and validity studies of examination for aphasia test in Hindi. *Indian Journal of Disability and Rehabilitation, 5,* 13–19.

Kaplan, E., Goodglass, H., Weintraub, S. (1983). *The Boston Naming Test.* Philadelphia: Lea & Febiger.

Kertesz, A. (1982). *Western Aphasia Battery.* San Antonio, Tex.: Psychological Corporation.

Kertesz, A. (1993). *Western Aphasia Battery Scoring Assistant.* San Antonio, Tex.: Psychological Corporation.

Kirk, S. A., McCarthy, J., & Kirk, W. (1968). *The Illinois Test of Psycholinguistic Abilities.* Urbana, Ill.: Illinois University Press.

Kirshner, H. S. (1982). Language disorders in dementia. In F. Freeman & H. S. Kirshner (Eds.), *Neurolinguistics,* Vol. 12. *Neurology of Aphasia.* Amsterdam: Swets & Zeitlinger.

Laine, M., Koivuselka-Dallinen, P., Hanninen, R., & Niemi, J. (1993). *Bostonin Nimentestestin Suomenmkielinen.* Helsinki: Psykologien Kusannus.

Li, E. C., & Williams, S. E. (1990). Repetition deficits in three aphasic syndromes. *Journal of Communication Disorders, 23,* 77–88.

Love, T. & Oster, E. (2002). On the categorization of aphasic typologies: The SOAP (a test of syntactic complexity). *Journal of Psycholinguistic Research, 31,* 503–529.

Lyon, J. G., Cariski, D., Keisler, L., Rosenbeck, J., Levine, R., Kumpula, J., et al. (1997). Communication partners: Enhancing participation in life and communication for adults with aphasia in natural settings. *Aphasiology, 11,* 693–708.

Mazaux, J. M., & Orgogozo, J. M. (1985). *Echelle d'évaluation de l'aphasie.* Issy-les-moulineaux, France: EAP.

Mendez, M. F., & Ashla-Mendez, M. (1991). Differences between multi-infarct dementia and Alzheimer's disease on unstructured neuropsychological tasks. *Journal of Clinical and Experimental Neuropsychology, 13,* 923–932.

Mesulam, M. M. (2001). Primary progressive aphasia. *Annals of Neurology, 49,* 425–432.

Molrine, C. J., & Pierce, R. S. (2002). Black and White adults' expressive language in three tests of aphasia. *Journal of Speech-Language Pathology, 11,* 139–150.

Naeser, M. A., & Hayward, R. W. (1978). Lesion localization in aphasia with cranial computed tomography and the Boston Diagnostic Aphasia Exam. *Neurology, 28,* 545–551.

Naeser, M. A., Hayward, R. W., Laughlin, S. A., & Zatz, L. M. (1981). Quantitative CT scan studies in aphasia 1: Infarct size and CT numbers. *Brain and Language, 12,* 140–164.

Naeser, M. A., Mazurski, P., Goodglass, H., & Peraino, M. (1987). Auditory syntactic comprehension in nine aphasia groups (with CT scans) and children: Differences in degree but not order of difficulty observed. *Cortex, 23,* 359–380.

Newcomer, P. L., & Hammill, D. D. (1988). *Tests of language development* (2nd ed.). Austin, Tex.: Pro-Ed.

Nicholas, L. E., MacLennan, D. L., & Brookshire, R. H. (1986). Validity of multiple-sentence reading comprehension tests for aphasic adults. *Journal of Speech and Hearing Disorders, 51,* 83–87.

Pineda, D. A., Rosselli, M., Ardila, A., Mejia, S. E., Romero, M. G., & Perez, C. (2000). The Boston Diagnostic Aphasia Examination-Spanish Version: The influence of demographic variables. *Journal of the International Neuropsychological Society, 6,* 802–814.

Porch, B. (1971). *The Porch Index of Communicative Ability. Vol. 2: Administration and scoring.* Palo Alto, Calif.: Consulting Psychologists Press.

Radanovic, M. & Mansur, L. L. (2002). Performance of a Brazilian population sample on the Boston Diagnostic Aphasia Examination: A pilot study. *Brazilian Journal of Medical and Biological Research, 35,* 305–317.

Radanovic, M., & Scaff, M. (2003). Speech and language disturbances due to subcortical lesions. *Brain and Language, 84,* 337–352.

Radanovic, M., Sehana, M. L. H., Mansur, L. L., Mitrini, R., et al. (2001). Primary progressive aphasia: Analysis of 16 cases. *Arquivos de Neuro-Psiquiatria, 59,* 512–520.

Reinvang, L. (1985). *Aphasia and brain organization.* New York: Plenum Press.

Reinvang, I., & Graves, R. (1975). A basic aphasia examination: Description with discussion of first results. *Scandinavian Journal of Rehabilitation Medicine, 7,* 129–135.

Reitan, R. M. (1984). *Aphasia and sensory-perceptual deficits in adults.* Tucson, Ariz.: Reitan Neuropsychology Laboratory.

Reitan, R. M., & Wolfson, D. (1992). A short screening examination for impaired brain functions in early school-age children. *Clinical Neuropsychologist, 6,* 287–294.

Rosselli, M., Ardila, A., Florez, A., & Castro, C. (1990). Normative data on the Boston Diagnostic Aphasia Evaluation in a Spanish-speaking population. *Journal of Clinical and Experimental Neuropsychology, 12,* 313–322.

Sarno, M. T. (1969). *The Functional Communication Profile: Manual of directions.* New York: New York University Medical Center, Institute of Rehabilitation Medicine.

Schuell, H. (1973). *Differential diagnosis of aphasia with the Minnesota Test* (2nd ed.). Minneapolis: University of Minnesota Press.

Semel, E., Wiig, E. H., & Secord, W. (1987). *Clinical evaluation of language fundamentals.* San Antonio, Tex.: Psychological Corporation.

Spreen, O., & Benton, A. L. (1977). *Neurosensory Center Comprehensive Examination for Aphasia (NCCEA).* Victoria, B.C.: Neuropsychology Laboratory, University of Victoria.

Spreen, O., & Risser, A. (1990). Assessment of aphasia. In M. T. Sarno (Ed.), *Acquired aphasia* (2nd ed.). New York: Academic Press.

Sussman, H., Marquardt, T., Hutchinson, J., & MacNeilage, P. (1986). Compensatory articulation in Broca's aphasia. *Brain and Language, 27,* 56–74.

Wallace, G., & Hammill, D. D. (1994). *Comprehensive Receptive and Expressive Vocabulary Test (CREVT).* Austin, Tex.: Pro-Ed.

Whitworth, R. H., & Larson, C. M. (1989). Differential diagnosis and staging of Alzheimer's disease with an aphasia battery. *Neuropsychiatry, Neuropsychology, and Behavioral Neurology, 1,* 255–265.

Boston Naming Test—2 (BNT-2)

PURPOSE

The purpose of the Boston Naming Test—2 (BNT-2) is to assess visual naming ability using black and white drawings of common objects.

SOURCE

The BNT-2 is available separately (Kaplan et al., 2001) and as part of the revised BDAE-2 (Goodglass et al., 2000) from Pro-Ed, 8700 Shoal Creek Blvd, Austin, TX 78757-6897 (http://www.proedinc.com), at a cost of about $52 US.

Other Languages

The BNT (i.e., the BNT-2) and its short forms have been used with various foreign populations and languages including Chinese (Cheung et al., 2004; Tsang & Lee, 2003), Italian (Riva et al., 2000), Jamaican (Unverzagt et al., 1999), Dutch (Marien et al., 1998; Storms et al., 2004), Korean (Kim & Na, 1999), and French-Canadian (Morrison et al., 1996). A 30-item adaptation is available for Spanish-speaking people in the United States (Ponton et al., 1996).

AGE RANGE

The age range is 5 to 13 years and 18 years and older.

DESCRIPTION

This popular test, originally published by Kaplan et al. (1978) as an experimental version with 85 items, was revised to a 60-item test (Kaplan et al., 1983). The current version (BNT-2) retains the same 60 items and includes a short 15-item version as well as a multiple-choice version (see later discussion). The stimuli to be named for the BNT-2 are line drawings of objects with increasing difficulty, ranging from simple, high-frequency vocabulary words (e.g., *comb*) to rare words (e.g., *abacus*) (see Figure 11–2).

Short Forms

Short forms have been developed (e.g., Fastenau et al., 1998; Graves et al., 2004; Lansing et al., 1999; Mack et al., 1992; Saxton et al., 2000; Teng et al., 1989; Williams et al., 1989) in order to reduce test time for patients. One 15-item version,

Figure 11–2 Example of BNT item. *Source:* Reprinted with permission from PRO-ED.

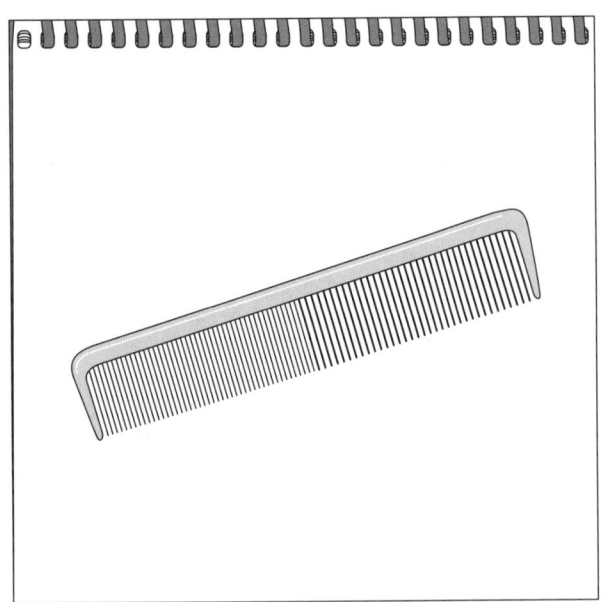

developed by Mack et al. (1992), known as short-form 4 (Mack SF4), was adopted by the authors of the BNT-2 (see Table 11–5). This short form precedes the standard 60 items in both the stimulus booklet and the answer sheet. The new BNT-2 also includes a multiple-choice version to better assess the integrity of the lexicon. Following the standard presentation, the examiner returns to those items initially failed. The patient chooses one of four choices read aloud by the examiner.

A different 15-item version is currently in use by participants of the Consortium to Establish a Registry for Alzheimer Disease (CERAD; Morris et al., 1989). The items are stratified into three groups of five items each, representing objects of high (easy to name), medium, and low (hard to name) frequency of occurrence in the English language.

The Williams (1989) 30-item test is also a popular version. It has demonstrated good reliability, high correlation with the full BNT60, and high agreement accuracy (Franzen et al., 1995; Graves et al., 2004; Lansing et al., 1999).

More recently, Graves et al. (2004) used item response theory to develop two new 15- and 30-item short forms that have high internal reliability (alphas of .84 for the 15-item form and .90 for the 30-item form), high correlations with the long form, and high classification agreement with the full BNT on abnormal AD/vascular dementia patient classification. The authors also developed an adaptive form: The examiner gives the 15-item version and stops there if the score is outside a specific confidence interval, otherwise continuing to give the full 30-item short form (see *Administration*). The various items in these short forms are shown in Table 11–5.

ADMINISTRATION

Long Form (BNT-2, BNT 60)

For children and all aphasic patients, begin with item 1 and discontinue after eight successive failures (in previous versions of this test, the discontinuation rule was six consecutive errors). For all other adult subjects, begin with item 30 (*harmonica*). If any of the next eight items is failed, proceed backward from item 29 until eight consecutive preceding items are passed without assistance (i.e., without provision of a stimulus or phonemic cue); then resume in a forward direction, and discontinue the test when the patient makes eight consecutive errors.

Credit is given if the item is correctly named within 20 s. If (and only if) the patient clearly misperceived the picture, he or she is told that the picture represents something else and is supplied with the bracketed stimulus cues on the record form. A phonemic cue is given after every failure to respond correctly, whether spontaneously or after a stimulus cue. For example, if the response given for *mushroom* is "umbrella," the patient is given the stimulus cue ("something to eat") and is given an additional 20 s to name the picture. If the client then correctly names the item within 20 s, a check is entered in the stimulus cue correct column. If the patient is unable to name the picture correctly within 20 s after the stimulus cue is given, a second (phonemic) cue is offered (i.e., the underlined initial phoneme of the name of the item, "m").

The rules for discontinuation and for entry into the test at an advanced level save considerable time for subjects without obvious impairment. However, the rules for discontinuation are not clearly stated in the test manual. Correct responses provided after a phonemic cue are not included in the total score. However, the manual is not clear as to whether such responses should be used to determine test discontinuation. S. Weintraub (personal communication, April 9, 2003) uses a rigorous interpretation that includes correct responses to phonemic cues in the count of errors. Nonetheless, some clinicians do not include such responses in the failure tally for the discontinuation decision. Ferman et al. (1998) reported that use of a "lenient" discontinuation method (excluding phonemically correct responses in the count of errors for the "six consecutive failures" tally) led to score changes in 3% of the total population of 655 normal elderly subjects and in 31% of 140 AD patients. Among normal examinees, discrepant scores were most often found in persons aged 80 years and older, and scores differed by up to 16 points. Because different interpretations of the discontinuation rule may alter test scores, it is important that authors clearly describe the manner in which published normative data were collected. Note too that the normative data provided by Ferman et al. (1998) were collected using a discontinuation rule of six, not eight, items.

Short Form (Mack SF4)

The Mack SF4 form always begins with item 1 and is discontinued after eight consecutive failures.

Table 11–5 BNT Short-Form items in the Mack SF4, CERAD, Williams et al. (1989), and Graves et al. (2004) versions

Mack SF4 BNT 15	CERAD	Williams et al. BNT 30	Graves et al. BNT 30	Graves et al.
4 house	1 bed	11 helicopter	13 octopus	19 bench
7 comb	2 tree	13 octopus	17 camel	24 seahorse
10 toothbrush	4 house	18 mask	19 pretzel	31 rhinoceros
13 octopus	5 whistle	19 pretzel	21 racquet	32 acorn
20 bench	7 flower	23 volcano	22 snail	35 dominoes
23 volcano	10 toothbrush	24 seahorse	23 volcano	41 pelican
26 canoe	17 camel	28 wreath	24 seahorse	42 stethoscope
29 beaver	18 mask	30 harmonica	25 dart	44 muzzle
36 cactus	23 volcano	31 rhinoceros	28 wreath	45 unicorn
39 hammock	26 canoe	32 acorn	29 beaver	48 accordion
42 stethoscope	30 harmonica	33 igloo	31 rhinoceros	53 scroll
45 unicorn	35 dominoes	34 stilts	32 acorn	54 tongs
52 tripod	39 hammock	35 dominoes	33 igloo	55 sphinx
55 sphinx	46 funnel	37 escalator	34 stilts	57 trellis
58 palette	54 tongs	39 hammock	35 dominoes	58 palette
		40 knocker	36 cactus	
		41 pelican	38 harp	
		43 pyramid	41 pelican	
		44 muzzle	42 stethoscope	
		48 noose	43 pyramid	
		49 asparagus	44 muzzle	
		50 compass	45 unicorn	
		51 latch	48 noose	
		52 tripod	53 scroll	
		53 scroll	54 tongs	
		54 tongs	55 sphinx	
		55 sphinx	57 trellis	
		57 trellis	58 palette	
		58 palette	59 protractor	
		60 abacus	60 abacus	

Note: Numbers refer to the item numbers in the published 60-item BNT.

Multiple-Choice Form

After the test is completed, the examiner returns to each item not correctly named after a phonemic cue and presents the card with that item and four printed choices. The examiner reads each word and asks the patient to indicate the correct choice.

Adaptive 30/15 Version

Graves et al. (2004) developed an adaptive 30/15 item version of the BNT in which the examiner first administers their 15-item short form. If the score is 12 or greater, the patient is given credit for 13 additional items; if the score is 3 or less, the examiner stops and uses the score obtained. Otherwise, the examiner administers the remaining items to complete their 30-item test.

TIME FOR ADMINISTRATION

The complete test takes about 10 to 20 min.

SCORING

Scores include the number of spontaneously produced correct responses, the number of cues given, the number of correct responses given after semantic cueing, and the number given after phonemic cueing. The total correct is the sum of the number of spontaneously given correct responses and the number of correct responses given after a stimulus cue.

Certain responses scored as incorrect on the BNT are in fact commonly used synonyms in certain geographical regions. In the United States, examples include "snake," "worm," or "rope" for *pretzel*, "Tom (or Tommy) Walkers," "walkers," "walking sticks," or "sticks" for *stilts*, "face" or "falseface" for *mask*, and "harp," "French harp," "Jew's harp," "mouth organ," or "organ" for *harmonica*. Goldstein et al. (in press) found that these synonyms were used by 13% of their sample of 1387 participants, most frequently by elderly, poorly educated persons living in southern (as opposed to midwestern) U.S. states, although "mouth harp" and "mouth organ" also occurred in the Midwest. Patients with AD also used more synonyms. Adjustment of scores for these variants led to minimal changes which, according to the authors, were "unlikely to change quantitative interpretations"; however, they warned that clinicians should be careful to avoid labeling such synonyms as paraphasias. Tombaugh and Hubley (1997) also noted that "mouth organ" and other incorrect responses ("lock" or "bolt" for *latch,* "dice" for *dominoes,* "toadstool" for *mushroom*) often occur in Canada and suggested that, in these and similar cases, a follow-up question should be asked: "What is another name for this?"

Some centers still use the older 85-item version. Heaton et al. (1999) provided a method to convert the 85-item BNT to the BNT60 metric, and vice versa. Raw scores are first converted to scaled scores ($M = 10$, $SD = 3$). A prediction equation is then used to convert the scaled scores into demographically (age, education, and gender) corrected T scores.

DEMOGRAPHIC EFFECTS

Age

Cross-sectional studies suggest that age affects performance on the long form. According to Heaton et al. (2004), in adults ranging in age from 20 to 85 years, age accounted for 9% of the variance in test scores in Caucasians (3% in African Americans). Scores increase in childhood, improve up to about the fourth decade of life, and subsequently decline, particularly after about 70 years of age (Albert et al., 1988; Goldstein et al., in press; Ivnik et al., 1996; MacKay et al., 2005; Marien et al., 1998; Mitrushina & Satz, 1989; Mitrushina et al., 2005; Randolph et al., 1999; Riva et al., 2000; Saxton et al., 2000; Storms et al., 2004; Tombaugh & Hubley, 1997; Tsang & Lee, 2003; also see *Source*). There is also an increase in the standard deviations (*SD*s) for older groups, suggesting that some people maintain high BNT performance with advancing age while others decline (Mitrushina & Satz, 1995; Mitrushina et al., 2005).

Longitudinal analyses produce lesser estimates of change than cross-sectional analyses do (Connor et al., 2004). A recent longitudinal study revealed no age-related change in normal elderly individuals (aged 59–96 years) over a 4-year period (Cruice et al., 2000), although with longer intervals such as 7 years (Au et al., 1995) or 20 years (Connor et al., 2004), subtle decline has been reported (about 2% per decade between ages 30 and 94 years), accelerating with advancing age (Connor et al., 2004). Individuals who have high levels of performance show less decline over time (Connor et al., 2004), consistent with the cognitive reserve hypothesis (Satz, 1993) that some combination of high level of intelligence, education, and a cognitively active lifestyle offers a neuroprotective effect.

Naming ability declines with increasing age on short forms as well (Fastenau et al., 1998; Graves et al., 2004; Kent & Luszcz, 2002). Longitudinal analyses suggest that the decline is greatest for individuals aged 80 years and older (Kent & Luszcz, 2002).

Gender

Some authors have reported that gender is unrelated to BNT performance (e.g., Henderson et al., 1998; Ivnik et al., 1996; Lucas et al., 2005; Riva et al., 2000). Others, however, have found that men outperform women in older samples (Connor et al., 2004; Goldstein et al., in press; Heaton et al., 1999; Marien et al., 1998; Randolph et al., 1999; Ripich et al., 1995; Ross & Lichtenberg, 1998; Welch et al., 1996), perhaps because of a preponderance of male-biased items (e.g., compass, tripod, yoke; Randolph et al., 1999). Heaton et al. (2004) noted that about 1% of the variance in test scores of African Americans was accounted for by gender; in Caucasians, the amount was nil.

The effect of gender is inconsequential on short versions (Kent & Luszcz, 2002).

IQ/Education

Verbal intelligence affects BNT scores (Killgore & Adams, 1999; Thompson & Heaton, 1989; Steinberg et al., 2005; Tombaugh & Hubley, 1997) as does full-scale IQ (Diaz-Asper et al., 2004). Educational achievement also affects scores (Axelrod et al., 1994; Goldstein et al., in press; Heaton et al., 1999; Henderson et al., 1998; Ivnik et al., 1996; Lucas et al., 2005; Marien et al., 1998; Neils et al., 1995; Randolph et al., 1999; Ross et al., 1995; Ross & Lichtenberg, 1998; Saxton et al., 2000; Thompson & Heaton, 1989; Tombaugh & Hubley, 1997; Welch et al., 1996), although less so than does IQ (Steinberg et al., 2005). Whereas IQ accounts for about 37% of the variance in test scores (Steinberg et al., 2005), education accounts for about 10% to 11% of the variance in test scores in Caucasians (13% in African Americans; Heaton et al., 2004; Steinberg et al., 2005). Steinberg et al. (2005) have recently reported that education was wholly redundant with the larger contributions of intelligence to test scores. Individuals with higher IQ (more years of education) are likely to have had exposure to a wider vocabulary, resulting in higher test scores. There is also an interaction of age and education, such that there is less of an age effect in more highly educated individuals (Connor et al., 2004; Neils et al., 1995; Welch et al., 1996).

Education also affects naming ability on the short forms, with higher education associated with better naming ability (Fasteau et al., 1998; Kent & Luszcz, 2002).

Vocabulary

Reading vocabulary (from the Spot-the-Word or Gates-Mcginitie Reading Tests) is strongly correlated ($r = .61$ to $.81$) with BNT performance (Graves & Carswell, 2003; Hawkins et al., 1993; Senior et al., 2001). Therefore, limited vocabulary may represent a substantial risk for misdiagnosis of anomia (see later discussion).

Geographical Region, Ethnicity, and Acculturation

Geographic region, ethnicity, and level of acculturation can affect performance (Azrin et al., 1996; Fillenbaum et al., 1997; Goldstein et al., in press; Heaton et al., 2004; Lucas et al., 2005; Manly et al., 1998; Roberts et al., 2002; Ross & Lichtenberg, 1998; Welsh et al., 1995; but see Henderson et al., 1998; Manly et al., 2002). In general, Caucasians scored higher than African Americans, and midwesterners outperformed people from the south, particularly African Americans in the south (Goldstein et al., in press). Even within a particular ethnic group, those who were more familiar with the dominant American culture scored higher than those who were less acculturated (Manly et al., 1998; Touradji et al., 2001).

Not all minority groups perform poorly on the BNT. Native Americans apparently performed as well as non-Native-American elderly (Ferraro et al., 2002). With regard to other populations, Canadians (Tombaugh & Hubley, 1997) scored slightly higher than Americans (e.g., Ivnik et al., 1996; Mitrushina & Satz, 1995; Van Gorp et al., 1986), and both tended to score higher than Australians (Cruice et al., 2000; Worrall et al., 1995), New Zealanders (Barker-Collo, 2002), or Dutch-speaking Belgians (Storms et al., 2004; also see Marien et al., 1998, who showed that the percentages correct per item differed in Dutch-speaking and Australian-English-speaking populations), suggesting that norms for the BNT may differ considerably over populations, languages, and cultural relevance.

Linguistic Background

Linguistic background also affects test scores. Roberts et al. (2002) compared 42 unilingual English individuals, 32 Spanish/English bilinguals, and 49 French/English bilinguals and found that BNT scores were similar for both sets of bilingual participants; however, both groups scored far lower than the English unilinguals. They concluded that English language norms cannot be used for bilingual speakers, even proficient ones.

NORMATIVE DATA

Long Form (BNT 60)

Standardization Sample. The norms accompanying the 60-item test (see Table 11–6) were based on small groups of adults (cell sizes of 11 to 56 individuals, depending on the age group), aged 18 to 79 years ($N = 178$), who were of above-average education (M = about 14 years). No information is provided regarding geographical region or ethnicity of the sample or in what year these data were collected. This is important given the general rise in ability over time (e.g., Flynn effect) and because norms may change over time as some

Table 11–6 Characteristics of the BNT Normative Sample Provided by Kaplan et al., 2001

Number	178
Age (years)	18–79[a]
Geographic location	NA
Sample type	NA
Education (years)	Mean, about 14
Gender	NA
Race/Ethnicity	NA
Screening	NA

[a]18–39 $N = 21$; 40–49 $N = 11$; 50–59 $N = 49$; 60–69 $N = 56$; 70–79 $N = 41$.

objects represented come into disuse or change in form (Storms et al., 2004).

Other Normative Data. A variety of normative reports have appeared in the literature for English speakers (Boone et al., 1995; Heaton et al., 2004; Ivnik et al., 1996; Mitrushina & Satz, 1995; Neils et al., 1995; Ross et al., 1995, 1998; Saxton et al., 2000; Tombaugh & Hubley, 1997; Van Gorp et al., 1986). Given the importance of age, geographical region, ethnicity, and education, several larger-scale normative sets are discussed here (see *Source* for use with other language communities).

United States. Heaton et al. (2004) compiled data from studies conducted over a period of about 25 years and presented norms separately for two ethnicity groups (Caucasians, African Americans) organized by age, gender, and education. The samples were large and covered a wide range in terms of age and education; exclusion criteria were specified (see Table 11–7). T scores lower than 40 were classed as impaired. Note that regionally correct answers, such as "tom walkers" for *stilts*, were not given credit in the norms.

Mitrushina et al. (2005) compiled data for the 60-item version from 14 studies, comprising a total of 1684 participants. The data are presented in 5-year increments, from ages 25 to 84 years. Note that their sample was highly educated (M = 13.79 years, SD = 1.5) and of above-average IQ (M = 116.1, SD = 2.6). The data are very similar to those provided by Kaplan et al. (2001); the educational achievement of their sample was also above average. Given the influence of education and IQ on test scores, the values provided by both Mitrushina et al. (2005) and Kaplan et al. (2001) are likely to overestimate expected performance for individuals with lower educational/intellectual levels.

Ivnik et al. (1996) provided age-corrected norms for the BNT derived from the Mayo Older Americans Normative Studies (the MOANS projects). Raw scores are converted to age-corrected scaled scores having a mean of 10 and an SD of 3. These data are shown in Table 11–8. The sample consisted of 663 individuals (almost all Caucasians) older than 55 years of age. These authors also provided a computational formula

Table 11–7 Characteristics of the BNT Normative Sample Provided by Heaton et al., 2004

Number	1000
Age (years)	20–85[a]
Geographic location	Various states in United States and Manitoba, Canada
Sample type	Individuals recruited as part of multicenter studies
Education (years)	0–20[b]
Gender (%)	
Male	53.3
Female	47.7
Race/Ethnicity	
Caucasian	350
African American	650
Screening	No reported history of learning disability, neurological disorder, serious psychiatric disorder, or alcohol or drug abuse

[a]Age groups: 20–34, 35–39, 40–44, 45–49, 50–54, 55–59, 60–64, 65–69, 70–74, 75–79, and 80–89 years.
[b]Education groups: 7–8, 9–11, 12, 13–15, 16–17, and 18–20.

to derive MOANS scaled scores corrected for age and education (years of formal school completed). The formula is as follows:

$$\text{Age- and Education-Corrected MOANS Scaled Score} = 3.32 + (1.07 \times \text{Age-Corrected MOANS Scaled Score}) - (0.34 \times \text{Years of formal education})$$

Ivnik et al. (1996) noted that the MOANS sample was derived from a population of almost exclusively Caucasian older

adults who lived in an economically stable region of the United States and were relatively well-educated (e.g., more than 25% had completed ≥ 16 years of education). They cautioned against use of these norms for persons of other ethnic, cultural, social, or economic backgrounds.

Steinberg et al. (2005) have recently expanded the utility of the MOANS project by providing age- and IQ-adjusted percentile equivalents of MOANS Age-adjusted BNT scores, for use with individuals aged 55+. Users should note that all FSIQs are MAYO age-adjusted scores that are based on the WAIS-R, not the WAIS-III. Given the upward shift in scores (Flynn effect) with the passage of time, use of the WAIS-R FSIQ as opposed to the WAIS-III may result in a given BNT score appearing less favorable.

Recently, Lucas et al. (2005) provided age- and education-adjusted normative data based on 304 African American, community-dwelling participants from the Mayo Older African American Normative Studies (MOAANS) project in Jacksonville, Florida. Participants were predominantly female (75%), ranged in age from 56 to 94 years ($M = 69.6$, $SD = 6.87$), and varied in education from 0 to 20 years of formal education ($M = 12.2$, $SD = 3.48$). Examinees were screened to exclude those with active neurological, psychiatric, or other conditions that might affect cognition. These authors administered the BNT using the lenient interpretation of the discontinuation rule (i.e., items correctly named after presentation of phonemic cues were not counted as failures), making it possible to score and derive normative data for both the rigorous administration (counting items named correctly with a phonemic cue as errors) and the lenient administration. They accepted "Tom Walkers" or "Tommy Walkers" as correct for *stilts* and "mouth harp" as a correct response for *harmonica*.

Table 11–8 MOANS Age-Based BNT Norms in Well-Educated Caucasian Adults

Scaled Score	57–62	63–65	66–68	69–71	72–74	75–77	78–80	81–83	84–86	87–89	90–97	Percentile Ranges
N	171	243	187	197	220	247	309	255	209	138	78	
2	<41	<39	<39	<38	<25	<25	<25	<25	<25	<25	<22	<1
3	41–42	39–42	39	38	25–32	25–27	25–27	25	25	25	22	1
4	43–44	43	40–43	39	33–37	28–33	28–33	26–30	26–29	26–27	23–24	2
5	45–48	44–46	44–46	40–43	38–41	34–38	34–37	31–35	30–33	28–33	25–30	3–5
6	49–50	47–49	47–48	44–47	42–45	39–42	38–40	36–38	34–37	34–36	31–33	6–10
7	51	50–51	49–51	48–50	46–48	43–46	41–44	39–42	38–41	37–39	34–36	11–18
8	52–53	52	52	51–52	49–50	47–48	45–48	43–45	42–43	40–42	37–40	19–28
9	54	53–54	53–54	53	51–52	49–51	49–50	46–48	44–48	43–46	41–42	29–40
10	55–56	55	55	54–55	53–54	52–53	51–53	49–52	49–52	47–51	43–48	41–59
11	—	56	56	56	55	54–55	54	53	53	52	49–50	60–71
12	57	57	57	57	56	56	55	54	54	53–54	51–52	71–81
13	58	58	58	58	57	57	56	55–56	55–56	55–56	53–55	82–89
14	—	—	—	—	58	58	57–58	57	57	57	56	90–94
15	59	59	—	—	—	—	—	58	58	58	57	95–97
16	60	60	59–60	59	59	59	59	59	59	59	58	98
17	—	—	—	60	60	60	60	60	60	60	59	99
18	—	—	—	—	—	—	—	—	—	—	60	>99

Source: Adapted from Ivnik et al., 1996. Reprinted with the kind permission of Psychology Press.

Table 11–9a MOAANS Age-based BNT Norms in African American Adults Using Rigorous (R) and Lenient (L) Administration Rules

Scaled Score	56–62		63–65		66–68		69–71		72–74		75–77		78+		Percentile Ranges
	R	L	R	L	R	L	R	L	R	L	R	L	R	L	
N	108	105	130	127	165	162	180	177	156	154	119	117	78	76	
2	0–16	0–17	0–16	0–14	0–15	0–14	0–15	0–14	0–14	0–14	0–14	0–14	0–14	0–14	<1
3	17–18	18–21	17	15–17	16	15–17	16	15–17	15–16	15–17	15–16	15–17	15–16	15–17	1
4	19–21	22	18–19	18–19	17–19	18	17–18	18	17–18	18	17–18	18	17–18	18	2
5	22–23	23–27	20–21	20–23	20–21	19–23	19–20	19–23	19–20	19–23	19–20	19–23	19–20	19–23	3–5
6	24–30	28–34	22–24	24–28	22–24	24–28	21–24	24–27	21–24	24–27	21–24	24–27	21–22	—	6–10
7	31–37	35–38	25–33	29–35	25–32	29–34	25–32	28–33	25–32	28–32	25–32	28–32	23–29	24–30	11–18
8	38–40	39–41	34–39	36–40	33–37	35–38	33–36	34–36	33–36	33–36	33–36	33–36	30–32	31–33	19–28
9	41–44	42–45	40–43	41–43	38–42	39–43	37–41	37–41	37–41	37–40	37–41	37–40	33–37	34–38	29–40
10	45–50	46–50	44–48	44–49	43–47	44–47	42–47	42–47	42–47	41–44	42–47	41–47	38–44	39–45	41–59
11	51–52	51–52	49–51	50–51	48–50	48–50	48–50	48–50	48–50	48–50	48–50	48–50	45–49	46–50	60–71
12	53–54	53–54	52–53	52–54	51–52	51–52	51–52	51–52	51–52	51–52	51–52	51–52	50–52	51–52	72–81
13	55	55	54–55	55	53–54	53–54	53–54	53–54	53–54	53–54	53–54	53–54	53–54	53–54	82–89
14	56–57	56–57	56–57	56–57	55–56	55–56	55–56	55–56	55–56	55	55–56	55	55	55	90–94
15	58	58	58	58	57	57	57	57	57	56–57	57	56–57	56	56	95–97
16	—	—	—	—	58	58	58	58	—	—	—	—	—	—	98
17	59	59	59	—	59	—	59	—	58	58	58	58	57–58	57	99
18	60	60	60	59–60	60	59–60	60	59–60	59–60	59–60	59–60	59–60	59–60	58–60	>99

Source: Adapted from Lucas et al., 2005. Reprinted with the permission of the Mayo Foundation for Medical Education and Research.

Mispronunciations of words (e.g., "stedascope" for *stethoscope*, "spinx" for *sphinx*, "tressle" for *trellis*) were considered incorrect. Age-corrected MOAANS scaled scores and percentile ranks for BNT data scored using both the lenient and the rigorous interpretation are presented in Table 11–9a. Age- and education-corrected MOAANS scaled scores can also be computed using the formula provided in Table 11–9b.

Lucas et al. (2005) also provided cumulative frequency data for the number of correct responses to phonemic cues administered under each discontinuation rule. They reported that it was fairly common for African American elders to get eight additional BNT items correct with phonemic cueing under both rigorous (frequency = 28%) and lenient (frequency = 32%) administrations. They also noted that, depending on which discontinuation rule was used, 20% to 28% of the sample were administered 20 or more phonemic cues, indicating incorrect spontaneous responses to items and failure of stimulus cues (when given) to facilitate naming on at least one third of the test items. These findings raise concerns regarding the equivalence of BNT item familiarity across ethnic groups and geographic regions and suggest caution in the interpretation of BNT performance in African Americans (see also *Demographic Effects*).

Canada. Tombaugh and Hubley (1997) presented age- and education-stratified norms based on a sample of 219 healthy, relatively well-educated (*M* = 12.9 years) volunteers residing in Ottawa, Canada. None of the individuals had less than 9 years of education. The data are shown in Table 11–10.

Norms for Children. Norms for ages 5 years 0 months through 12 years 5 months are provided by the test authors (Kaplan et al., 2001) and are based on small groups of participants (cell sizes of 14 to 35 individuals, depending on the age group). The data were collected in 1987. Geographical region and ethnicity of the sample are not reported. Nor is it clear which discontinuation rule (six or eight items) was used.

A meta-analysis of five normative studies by Yeates (1994) provided norms for ages 5 to 13 years, weighted for number of subjects and *SD* (see Table 11–11). Yeates (1994) noted that, beyond age range and sample size, the descriptions of the samples were often incomplete, lacking even the most basic demographic information (e.g., gender). Based on the available information, he thought the normative data were collected largely from Caucasian children, both boys and girls, who were attending public and private schools and living with

Table 11–9b Computational Formula for Age- and Education-Corrected MOAANS Scaled Scores

	K	W$_1$	W$_2$
BNT "rigorous" administration	3.53	1.20	0.44
BNT "lenient" administration	3.49	1.21	0.46

Note: Age- and education-corrected MOAANS Scaled Scores (MSS$_{A\&E}$) can be calculated for BNT scores by using age-corrected MOAANS Scaled Scores (MSS$_A$) and education (years completed) in the following formula: MSS$_{A\&E}$ = K + (W$_1$ * MSS$_A$) − (W$_2$ * EDUC).

Source: Adapted from Lucas et al., 2005. Reprinted with the permission of the Mayo Foundation for Medical Education and Research.

Table 11–10 BNT Normative Data Expressed as Percentiles for Age and Education Based on a Canadian Sample

| Percentile | Age 25–69 | | Age 70–88 | | Total |
	9–12 (N = 78)	13–21 (N = 70)	9–12 (N = 45)	13–21 (N = 26)	(N = 219)
90	59	60	59	59	60
75	58	60	58	58	58
50	56	58	55	56	57
25	54	56	52	53	54
10	51	53	47	49	51
Mean education (years)	11.3	15.1	11.2	14.9	12.9

Source: Adapted from Tombaugh & Hubley, 1997.

primarily middle-class families in suburban or urban areas of the northeastern United States. These observations highlight the need for the collection of large-scale, more representative normative samples. There is also a gap in the BNT norms for adolescents between the ages of 14 and 17 years.

Error Types. Verbal semantic paraphasias and "don't know" responses are the most common types of errors in children (Storms et al., 2004) as well as adults (Marien et al., 1998; Tombaugh & Hubley, 1997). Neologisms, delayed responses, empty words, and phonemic paraphasias are rare in normal individuals.

BNT Scores Estimated From Premorbid Indicators. The distribution of BNT scores for normal people deviates from the normal bell curve in that BNT scores are skewed toward the high end of the range, and most scores cluster very closely around this ceiling (Hawkins & Bender, 2002). These properties of negative skew (asymmetry) and extreme kurtosis (peakedness) mean that the test does not discriminate well at the average and higher levels. Further, normal individuals with limited vocabularies do score substantially below the mean. Because small *SD*s are associated with extreme kurtosis, even a small deviation will suggest pathology if correc-

tions for vocabulary and education are inadequate (Hawkins & Bender, 2002).

In fact, studies generating BNT norms have generally not been adequately representative of the population, with most featuring a disproportionate representation of highly educated subjects. Hawkins and Bender (2002) recommended that BNT norms should be finely stratified by education (the norms presented by Heaton et al., 2004, are an important contribution) and that, whenever possible, the clinical interpretation of BNT scores should be further moderated by estimations of premorbid verbal ability that are fairly resistant to cerebral damage. Table 11–12 shows performance expectations based on non-age-corrected WAIS-R Vocabulary scores (Killgore & Adams, 1999), and Table 11–13 gives some performance expectations based on Gates-MacGinitie reading level (Hawkins et al., 1993).

Table 11–11 Norms for Schoolchildren on the BNT

Age (Years)	n	Mean	Standard Deviation
5	62	27.76	5.9
6	150	33.56	4.9
7	153	36.87	5.2
8	147	38.99	4.6
9	152	41.74	4.6
10	167	45.10	4.5
11	146	46.84	4.8
12	80	48.55	3.9
13	22	49.55	4.7

Source: From Yeates, 1994. Reprinted with the kind permission of Psychology Press.

Table 11–12 BNT Performance Expectations Predicted from WAIS-R Vocabulary Scores (N = 62)

| WAIS-R Vocabulary Score | Predicted BNT Score | | |
	Predicted	1SE Below	2SE Below
14+	60	55.6	50.8
13	58.8	54.0	49.2
12	57.2	52.4	47.6
11	55.5	50.7	45.9
10	53.9	49.1	44.3
9	52.3	47.5	42.7
8	50.7	45.9	41.1
7	49.1	44.3	39.5
6	47.4	42.6	37.9
5	45.8	41.0	36.2
4	44.2	39.4	34.6
3	42.6	37.8	33.0
2	41.0	36.2	31.4
1	39.4	34.6	29.8

Note: WAIS-R Vocabulary scores are not age-corrected. Predicted BNT = (1.6 × Vocabulary) + 37.7; standard error of the estimate = 4.8.

Source: From Killgore & Adams, 1999. *Perceptual and Motor Skills, 83,* 327–337. © Perceptual and Motor Skills 1999.

Table 11–13 Adult Norms Corrected for Reading Vocabulary Level

Reading Level[a]	Percentile Rank[b]	Estimated BNT Total
4.1	01	34.4
5.0	03	37.2
6.1	05	39.9
7.0	08	42.0
8.0	13	44.7
9.2	21	47.5
10.1	29	49.6
11.1	40	51.6
12.2	45	52.3
Post high school	58	53.7
	66	54.3
	82	55.7
	90	56.4

Note: Based on a mixed psychiatric and normal sample (*N* = 88).
[a]Estimated on the basis of Gates-McGinite Reading Vocabulary.
[b]Based on Gates-McGinite Reading Vocabulary, Level 7–9, Form K.

Source: Adapted from Hawkins et al., 1993, with permission of the authors and Elsevier Science Ltd.

Recently, Graves and Carswell (2003) used a sample of 98 normal older Canadians (age *M* = 71.9 years) to develop a regression equation to predict BNT scores from the Spot-the-Word Test of the SCOLP (see *The Speed and Capacity of Language Processing Test*). The predicted premorbid BNT score is determined as follows (*r* = .61, *SEE* = 2.72 items):

Predicted BNT = 33.668 + 0.423(STW Raw Score)

Table 11–14 shows the discrepancy score distributions. Discrepancies below a chosen cutoff point (which establishes the specificity for normal subjects) can be considered abnormal (e.g., below the 5th percentile). Senior et al. (2001) also developed a regression equation to predict BNT scores using the Spot-the-Word Test in a normal sample of individuals living in Australia. The equation is similar to the one provided by Graves et al. (2003) (see *The Speed and Capacity of Language Processing Test*).

Short Form

Fastenau et al. (1998) provided normative data for the short form (Mack SF4) based on a sample of 108 healthy individuals, aged 57 to 85 years (*M* = 72.2, *SD* = 7.0), in the United States. The sample was predominantly Caucasian (95%) and well-educated (97% had at least 12 years of education). The data are shown in Table 11–15. Slightly lower scores were obtained in a slightly older (*M* = 76.19 years, *SD* = 5.72) Australian sample of average IQ (NART estimate = 102.9, *SD* = 9.1; Kent & Luszcz, 2002). Their data are shown in Table 11–16.

Normative information for the CERAD form is shown in Table 11–17 (Welsh et al., 1994). The data are based on a sample of healthy Caucasian individuals, aged 50 to 89 years, who

Table 11–14 Actual Minus Predicted BNT Discrepancy Based on the SCOLP Spot-the-Word Test

Discrepancy	Percentile	Discrepancy	Percentile
−10.71	1	.219	49.0
−7.94	2	.334	50.0
−6.67	3.1	.373	54.1
−5.24	4.1	.642	56.1
−4.51	5.1	.796	60.2
−4.36	6.1	.911	62.2
−4.13	7.1	.950	63.3
−3.94	8.2	1.03	65.3
−3.24	9.2	1.07	66.3
−3.20	10.2	1.22	68.4
−2.59	11.2	1.30	69.4
−2.51	13.3	1.33	70.4
−2.36	16.3	1.37	73.5
−2.21	18.4	1.49	74.5
−2.13	19.4	1.60	75.5
−2.09	21.4	1.80	76.5
−2.01	22.4	1.91	77.6
−1.67	23.5	2.07	80.6
−1.63	24.5	2.22	83.7
−1.51	25.5	2.33	84.7
−1.40	26.5	2.60	85.7
−1.36	30.6	2.64	88.8
−1.01	31.6	2.76	89.8
−.78	32.7	2.91	91.8
−.71	33.7	2.99	92.9
−.67	34.7	3.30	93.9
−.55	35.7	3.49	94.9
−.20	38.8	3.76	95.9
−.09	41.8	4.18	96.9
−.050	42.9	4.26	98.0
.065	43.9	6.03	100.0

Source: Graves & Carswell, personal communication, R. Graves, January 2003.

were for the most part well-educated. Participants with lower education were few, and therefore the norms for this subgroup must be regarded as preliminary. Both age and education, but not gender, affected performance.

Graves et al. (2004) recommend a cutoff of less than 25 on their own 30-item version, and 11 on their 15-item form. These cutoff points represent values set at the 20th percentile of 62 normal patients, aged 38 to 83 years (*M* = 59.2, *SD* = 10.5) attending a memory disorders clinic who were

Table 11–15 15-Item BNT Short-Form (Mack SF4) Data (Mean and *SD*) for Primarily Caucasian, Well-Educated, Healthy Adults in the United States, by Age

	57–68 Years	69–76 Years	77–85 Years	Total
No. of subjects	35	38	35	108
SF4 score	14.0 (1.2)	13.1 (1.7)	13.1 (2.3)	13.4 (1.8)

Source: Adapted from Fastenau et al., 1998.

Table 11–16 15-Item BNT Short Form (Mack SF4) Data (Mean and *SD*) for Healthy Adults in Australia With MMSE Scores Within the Normal Range, Using Overlapping Age Groups

	Age Group (Midpoint) in Years					
	65–70 (70)	68–78 (73)	71–81 (76)	74–84 (79)	77–87 (82)	80–93 (87)
No. of subjects	95	122	119	96	77	54
	12.78 (1.96)	12.66 (1.94)	12.50 (2.21)	12.36 (2.30)	11.88 (2.58)	11.65 (2.72)

Source: Adapted from Kent & Luszcz, 2002.

found to have no significant medical or neurological complications. Using a value set at the 10th percentile, the cutoff points would be less than 21 on the Williams form, 22 on their 30-item form, and 10 on their 15-item forms (Table 11–18).

Multiple-Choice Form

No data are provided for this version.

RELIABILITY

Internal Consistency

Internal consistency (coefficient alpha) for the 60-item form has been reported to range between .78 and .96 (Graves et al., 2004; Fastenau et al., 1998; Franzen et al., 1995; Saxton et al., 2000; Tombaugh & Hubley, 1997; Storms et al., 2004; Williams et al., 1989).

Table 11–17 CERAD Short Form Data (Mean and *SD*) Based on a Sample of Well-Educated, Healthy Caucasian Adults, by Age and Education

	Age 50–69 Years		Age 70–89 Years	
	No.	Score	No.	Score
≥12 years				
Men	61	14.7 (0.7)	66	14.6 (0.7)
Women	151	14.7 (0.6)	89	14.5 (0.7)
<12 years (total)	23	14.4 (1.1)	23	14.3 (3.7)

Source: Adapted from Welsh et al., 1994.

Table 11–18 Recommended Cutoff Scores for BNT Short Forms by Williams et al. (1989) and by Graves et al. (2004)

	20th Percentile	10th Percentile
Williams BNT30		<21
Graves et al. BNT30	<25	<22
Graves et al. BNT15	<11	<10

Source: Adapted from Graves et al., 2004.

Reliability coefficients tend to be lower for the abbreviated versions, including the Mack SF4 version (.49 to .84) and the CERAD version (.36 to .83; Fastenau et al., 1998; Franzen et al., 1995; Graves et al., 2004; Tombaugh & Hubley, 1997). Reliability is high (Graves et al., 2004; Tombaugh & Hubley, 1997) for the versions developed by Williams et al. (1989) and Graves et al. (2004).

Test-Retest Reliability and Practice Effects

Over short intervals, reliability is high. For example, Flanagan and Jackson (1997) reported that the test exhibits acceptable score stability in older, healthy, right-handed adults (aged 50–76 years) when administered with an interval of approximately 1 to 2 weeks ($r = .91$; $SEM = 1.02$). A gain of about 1 point was noted on the second test session. The standard error of measurement (SEM) of 1.02 indicates that the chances are 95 in 100 that a non-brain-injured older adult would score, on the second administration, within ± 2.04 points of his or her first score.

Over longer intervals, findings are mixed. Mitrushina and Satz (1995) tested 122 healthy, elderly Caucasian adults between the ages of 57 and 85 years on three occasions, each spaced about 1 year apart. Test-retest reliability coefficients were marginal to high (.62 to .89), depending on the interval, with good consistency in mean scores over the three probes. Low correlations (.59) were reported by Kent and Luszcz (2002) in a community sample of older adults ($N = 326$) in Australia tested over 8 years. On the other hand, Dikmen et al. (1999) found high retest reliability (.92) and modest practice effects in 55 normal or neurologically stable adults on repeat testing with the older, 85-item version after an average interval of 11 months.

Stability has also been investigated in patients with epilepsy. A test-retest reliability of .94 was found by Sawrie et al. (1996) after 8 months in 51 adults with intractable epilepsy (age $M = 31.53$, $SD = 8.09$; FSIQ $M = 90.9$, $SD = 11.25$). To detect meaningful change after epilepsy surgery, Sawrie et al. (1996) provided 90% confidence intervals (± 5 points), adjusted for expected practice effects. This interval represents a statistically derived cutoff value within which 90% of the BNT change scores theoretically reside. Therefore, any change score equaling or exceeding this cutoff value at either end of the distribution would constitute significant change. They also derived a regression equation to predict a patient's retest score ($SEE = 2.63$):

$$Y_{predicted} = 7.61 + 0.87 \text{ (Baseline Score)}$$

The predicted value can be compared to the patient's observed score to quantify the magnitude and direction of change. The difference between the predicted score and the observed retest score is transformed into a standardized z score using the following equation:

$$z \text{ score} = (Y_{observed} - Y_{predicted})/SEE$$

Statically meaningful and significant change ($p < .05$) can be identified when the standardized change score exceeds ± 1.64 SDs.

Reliability data are not available for children.

VALIDITY

Relations With Other Measures

Several studies have related scores on the BNT with those on other language-related measures. For example, the BNT correlates highly ($r = .76$ to $.86$) with the Visual Naming Test of the Multilingual Aphasia Examination (Axelrod et al., 1994; Schefft et al., 2003). Riva et al. (2000) reported a closer link between an Italian version of the BNT and semantic fluency tasks (food = .57, animals = .64) than between the BNT and phonemic fluency tests (S = .44, B = .43) in healthy children aged 5 to 11 years. Nonetheless, BNT and fluency tasks loaded on one factor.

The BNT is also related to measures of intelligence. Axelrod et al. (1994) reported that, in their mixed clinical sample, the BNT was highly dependent on verbal intellectual ability (Verbal Comprehension Factor of the WAIS-R) and negligibly influenced by perceptual organization skills and distractibility. Schefft et al. (2003) reported that, in patients with seizures, the BNT showed stronger relations with VIQ ($r = .61$) than with PIQ ($r = .43$). However, in normal, healthy, older adults, BNT scores showed moderate relations (.41) with both verbal (VIQ) and nonverbal (PIQ) ability (Mitrushina & Satz, 1995). In children aged 6 to 12 years, BNT scores were found to correlate strongly with general intelligence ($r = .62$) as measured by the Standard Raven Progressive Matrices (Storms et al., 2004).

There is some suggestion that the strategies older individuals use to retrieve names may change with time, with predominantly verbal processing on the first occasion shifting to predominantly visual-spatial processing later on (Mitrushina & Satz, 1995). Visual acuity was shown to be negatively correlated with BNT performance (Worrall et al., 1995), but only to a small extent (Kent & Luszcz, 2002).

Clinical Findings

Poor performance on the BNT can occur in a variety of clinical conditions, including left-hemisphere cerebrovascular accidents (CVAs; e.g., Kohn & Goodglass, 1985), anoxia (Tweedy & Schulman, 1982), subcortical disease (multiple sclerosis and Parkinson's disease; Beatty & Monson, 1989; Henry & Crawford, 2004; Lezak et al., 1990; Locascio et al., 2003), and small white matter infarcts in the brainstem (van Zandvoort et al., 2003).

The presence of anomia in AD is well documented. Patients with AD tend to show impairment on the BNT (Henry et al., 2004; Lansing et al., 1999; Mack et al., 1992; Testa et al., 2004; Williams et al., 1989), more so than patients with vascular dementia (Barr et al., 1992; Lukatela et al., 1998). BNT impairment occurs regardless of disease severity in AD; however, it is ubiquitous only in moderate to severe dementia (Testa et al., 2004). Therefore, impairment does not appear to be necessary for a diagnosis of AD. Further, BNT impairment is not particularly useful in discriminating individuals at baseline who are subsequently diagnosed with AD, and measures of delayed recall (e.g., percent retention on the RAVLT) prove more useful in predicting conversion to AD (Testa et al., 2004). Finally, BNT scores are not especially useful in predicting rates of cognitive deterioration in AD. Beatty et al. (2002) found that poor performance on the BNT and young age identified AD patients at greater risk for cognitive decline (as measured with the Dementia Rating Scale 1 year later), although they accounted for only 6% of the variance.

The mechanism underlying naming deficits in AD is controversial. Most recent investigations rule out disruption in the perceptual stage as a primary cause of this breakdown; however, the relative contributions of disturbance in lexical retrieval and content and organization of the semantic system are issues of debate (Mitrushina et al., 2005). Similar controversy surrounds the nature of the age-related decline in BNT performance (Mitrushina et al., 2005).

Scores tends to be reduced in patients with temporal lobe epilepsy but are better than for patients with AD (Randolph et al., 1999). The BNT is more sensitive than the Visual Naming subtest of the Multilingual Aphasia Examination (MAE) in identifying left temporal lobe dysfunction (77.5% versus 17.5%), particularly in those with full-scale IQs of 90 or higher (Schefft et al., 2003). Within this FSIQ group, a person scoring at or below the 5th percentile on the BNT was 4.1 times as likely to have left temporal lobe epilepsy than someone who scored above the 5th percentile. The presence of phonemic paraphasias (which tended to be elicited by the BNT but not the MAE) was also useful in lateralizing the side of seizure origin. The differential patterns of classification rates in lateralizing side of dysfunction probably reflect the more demanding nature of the BNT, compared with the Visual Naming subtest of the MAE (Schefft et al., 2003).

Decline in visual confrontation naming may also occur as a postacute complication of left anterior temporal lobectomy (Bell et al., 2000; Hermann et al., 1999). Among those patients who demonstrated statistically meaningful decline, age at acquisition of a word was a significant predictor of performance;

that is, words acquired early in childhood were less affected than words acquired late (Bell et al., 2000).

Impairment has also been reported in patients with psychiatric conditions, including schizophrenia (Landre et al. 1992) and depression (Hill et al., 1992; Ferraro et al., 1997; but see Boone et al., 1995).

Children with severe closed head injury demonstrate significant impairment on the BNT; however, children with mild head injury and children treated for posterior fossa tumor or acute lymphoblastic leukemia do not (Jordan et al., 1992, 1996). Deficits on the BNT have also been reported in children exposed prenatally to polychlorinated biphenyls (PCBs; Grandjean et al., 2001).

Short Forms

Correlations among the various short forms tend to be moderate to high (e.g., $r = .42$ to $.62$ for the 15-item Mack SF4 [Mack et al., 1992]) when the various short forms are given in counterbalanced order (rather than extrapolating data for shortened versions after the entire 60-item test is given; Fastenau et al., 1998; Kent & Luszcz, 2002). Correlations between the Mack SF4 and CERAD versions and the full BNT60 tend to be high ($r = .62$ to $.98$; (Mack et al., 1992; Graves et al., 2004; Fastenau et al., 1998; Franzen et al., 1995), although agreement between the tests regarding abnormality is not guaranteed (Franzen et al., 1995; Graves et al., 2004). The CERAD short form appears particularly easy for individuals and tends to misclassify, as normal, people who would otherwise be classed as experiencing naming difficulty. Better agreement with the full BNT is obtained with the 30-item versions developed by Graves et al. (2004) and the empirical version devised by Williams et al. (1989; Tombaugh & Hubley, 1997). The new 15-item short form developed by Graves et al. (2004) also shows high internal consistency, and it agrees well with the classifications made by the full BNT60 (e.g., kappa > .80). However, additional cross-validation studies are needed for the forms developed by Graves and colleagues.

COMMENT

The BNT has emerged as a popular test of visual confrontation naming. With the exception perhaps of the COWA, there is no test of verbal function that has received as much use in neuropsychology as the BNT (Franzen, 2000). In fact, a recent survey of assessment practices of neuropsychologists revealed that the BNT ranked fourth in terms of frequency of use (Rabin et al., 2005).

Phonemic cueing does not differentially benefit normal subjects or patient groups (AD, temporal lobe epilepsy; Randolph et al., 1999), suggesting that this technique is not diagnostically useful. Randolph et al. (1999) recommended that it might be dispensed with, particularly because its inclusion can lead to variability in scoring criteria (Ferman et al., 1998).

Most healthy adults obtain high scores on the BNT. That is, the test does not discriminate well among high-scoring individuals, and any inferences regarding sparing or impairment must be made with caution. The test is most valuable in identifying low performers. However, interpretation must be moderated by estimations of premorbid ability, a variable that appears to be more important than age in evaluating BNT performance. Hawkins and Bender (2002) recommended that premorbid vocabulary or verbal IQ provides the best basis for BNT performance expectations. In the absence of such data, reading vocabulary tests (e.g., Gates-MacGinitie, Spot-the-Word) may provide guidance for BNT expectations. The alternative measure, years of education completed, bears a lesser relationship to BNT performance but should also be considered.

A variety of other individual difference variables (e.g., ethnicity, level of acculturation, regional differences, linguistic background) have a significant impact on BNT performance, arguing for the need of language- and culture-specific normative data. Accordingly, considerable caution is needed when interpreting results for individuals from a population that is inadequately represented in the normative data. Caution should also be used when a translated version of the test is employed in non-English-speaking populations, because item difficulty may vary in different languages. The "aging" of the norms should also be considered, given the general rise in ability (Flynn effect) and the possibility that some of the items represented in the tasks may have fallen into disuse (Storms et al., 2004). As with other tests relying on pictorial material (e.g., PPVT-III), visual-perceptual integrity should be checked if errors occur.

A number of short forms have been developed. Although they tend to provide relatively homogeneous tests of naming ability, the forms are not interchangeable. In addition, differences in classification arise between short (particularly 15-item) and long forms of the test. The CERAD version appears to be the least desirable in terms of its psychometric properties (e.g., inferior internal reliability, lower agreement with full BNT, inclusion of easy items; Franzen et al., 1995; Larrain & Cimino, 1998; Tombaugh & Hubley, 1997). Reliability is mixed for the Mack SF4. The Williams version has shown excellent results in a variety of cross-validation studies. The new BNT15 and BNT30 forms developed by Graves et al. (2004) appear very promising with regard to reliability and classification agreement accuracy with the full BNT. However, users should exercise caution in basing clinical judgments on these new forms until cross-validation studies are available.

Although some norms for children exist, the data are poorly described and there is a gap for adolescents aged 14 to 17 years. In addition, no corresponding information on test-retest reliability and stability is available. Consequently, the clinician or researcher might consider other measures with stronger psychometric properties for evaluating naming deficits in children (e.g., EOWPVT-3, EVT, WJ ACH III Picture Vocabulary, CELF-3, WPPSI-III).

REFERENCES

Albert, M. S., Heller, H. S., & Milberg, W. (1988). Changes in naming ability with age. *Psychology and Aging, 3,* 173–178.

Au, R., Joung, P. C., Nicholas, M., Obler, L. K., Kass, R., & Albert, M. L. (1995). Naming ability across the adult life span. *Aging and Cognition, 2,* 300–311.

Axelrod, B. N., Ricker, J. H., & Cherry, S. A. (1994). Concurrent validity of the MAE visual naming test. *Archives of Clinical Neuropsychology, 9,* 317–321.

Azrin, R. L., Mercury, M. G., Millsaps, C., Goldstein, D., Trejo, T., & Pliskin, N. H. (1996). Cautionary note on the Boston Naming Test: Cultural considerations [Abstract]. *Archives of Clinical Neuropsychology, 11,* 365–366.

Barker-Collo, S. L. (2002). The 60-item Boston Naming Test: Cultural bias and possible adaptations for New Zealand. *Aphasiology, 15,* 85–92.

Barr, A., Benedict, R., Tune, L., & Brandt, J. (1992). Neuropsychological differentiation of Alzheimer's disease from vascular dementia. *International Journal of Geriatric Psychiatry, 7,* 621–627.

Beatty, W. W., & Monson, N. (1989). Lexical processing in Parkinson's disease and multiple sclerosis. *Journal of Geriatric Psychiatry and Neurology, 2,* 145–152.

Beatty, W. W., Salmon, D. P., Troester, A. I., & Tivis, R. D. (2002). Do primary and supplementary measures of semantic memory predict cognitive decline by patients with Alzheimer's disease? *Aging, Neuropsychology, and Cognition, 9,* 1–10.

Bell, B. D., Davies, K. G., Hermann, B. P., & Walters, G. (2000). Confrontation naming after anterior temporal lobectomy is related to age of acquisition of the object names. *Neuropsychologia, 38,* 83–92.

Boone, K. B., Lesser, I. M., Miller, B. L., Wohl, M., Berman, N., Lee, A., Palmer, B., & Back, C. (1995). Cognitive functioning in older depressed outpatients: Relationship of presence and severity of depression to neuropsychological test scores. *Neuropsychology, 9,* 390–398.

Cheung, R. W., Cheung, M. C., & Chan, A. S. (2004). Confrontation naming in Chinese patients with left, right, or bilateral brain damage. *Journal of the International Neuropsychological Society, 10,* 46–53.

Connor, L. T., Spiro III, A., Oberm L. K., & Albert, M. L. (2004). Change in object naming ability during adulthood. *Journal of Gerontology: Psychological Sciences, 59B,* P203–P209.

Cruice, M. N., Worrall, L. E., & Hickson, L. M. H. (2000). Boston Naming Test results for healthy older Australians: A longitudinal and cross-sectional study. *Aphasiology, 14,* 143–155.

Diaz-Asper, C., Schretlen, D. J., & Pearlson, G. D. (2004). How well does IQ predict neuropsychological test performance in normal adults. *Journal of the International Neuropsychological Society, 10,* 82–90.

Dikmen, S. S., Heaton, R. K., Grant, I., & Temkin, N. R. (1999). Test-retest reliability and practice effects of expanded Halstead-Reitan neuropsychological test battery. *Journal of the International Neuropsychological Society, 5,* 346–356.

Fastenau, P. S., Denburg, N. L., & Mauer, B. A. (1998). Parallel short forms for the Boston Naming Test: Psychometric properties and norms for older adults. *Journal of Clinical and Experimental Neuropsychology, 20,* 828–834.

Ferman, T. J., Ivnik, R. J., & Lucas, J. A. (1998). Boston Naming Test discontinuation rule: rigorous versus lenient interpretations. *Assessment, 5,* 13–18.

Ferraro, F. R., Bercier, B., & Chelminski, I. (1997). Geriatric Depression Scale—Short Form in Native American elderly adults. *Clinical Gerontologist, 17,* 58–60.

Ferraro, F. R., Bercier, B. J., Holm, J., & McDonald, J. D. (2002). Preliminary normative data from a brief neuropsychological test battery in a sample of Native American elderly. In F. R. Ferraro (Ed.), *Minority and cross-cultural aspects of neuropsychological assessment: Studies on neuropsychology, development, and cognition.* Bristol, Pa.: Swets & Zeitlinger.

Fillenbaum, G. G., Huber, M., & Taussig, I. M. (1997). Performance of elderly white and African American community residents on the abbreviated CERAD Boston Naming Test. *Journal of Clinical and Experimental Neuropsychology, 19,* 204–210.

Flanagan, J. L., & Jackson, S. T. (1997). Test-retest reliability of three aphasia tests: Performance of non-brain-damaged older adults. *Journal of Communication Disorders, 30,* 33–43.

Franzen, M. D. (2000). *Reliability and validity in neuropsychological assessment* (2nd ed.). New York: Kluwer Academic/Plenum Publishers.

Franzen, M. D., Haut, M. W., Rankin, E., & Keefover, R. (1995). Empirical comparison of alternate forms of the Boston Naming Test. *Clinical Neuropsychologist, 9,* 225–229.

Goldstein, D. S., Ventura, T., & Pliskin, N. (in press). Demographics, dementia, and the Boston Naming Test. *The Clinical Neuropsychologist.*

Goodglass, H., Kaplan, E., & Barresi, B. (2000). *The assessment of aphasia and related disorders* (3rd ed.). Philadelphia: Lea & Febiger.

Grandjean, P., Weihe, P., Burse, V. W., Needham, L. L., Storr-Hansen, E., Heinzow, B., Debes, F., Murata, K., Simonsen, H., Ellefsen, P., Budtz-Jorgensen, E., Keiding, N., & White, R. F. (2001). Neurobehavioral deficits associated with PCB in 7-year-old children prenatally exposed to seafood neurotoxicants. *Neurotoxicology and Teratology, 23,* 305–317.

Graves, R. E., Bezeau, S. C., Fogarty, J., & Blair, R., (2004). Boston Naming Test Short Forms: A comparison of previous forms with new item response theory based forms. *Journal of Clinical and Experimental Neuropsychology, 26,* 891–902.

Graves, R. E., & Carswell, L. (2003). *Prediction of premorbid Boston Naming and California Verbal Learning Test scores.* Paper presented to the International Neuropsychological Society, Honolulu, Hawaii.

Hawkins, K. A., & Bender, S. (2002). Norms and the relationship of Boston Naming Test performance to vocabulary and education: A review. *Aphasiology, 16,* 1143–1153.

Hawkins, K. A., Sledge, W. H., Orleans, J. F., Quinland, D. M., Rakfeldt, J., & Hoffman, R. E. (1993). Normative implications of the relationship between reading vocabulary and Boston Naming Test performance. *Archives of Clinical Neuropsychology, 8,* 525–537.

Heaton, R. K., Avitable, N., Grant, I., & Mathews, C. G. (1999). Further crossvalidation of regression-based neuropsychological norms with an update for the Boston Naming Test. *Journal of Clinical and Experimental Neuropsychology, 21,* 572–582.

Heaton, R. K., Miller, S. W., Taylor, M. J., & Grant, I. (1991, 1992, 2004). *Revised comprehensive norms for an expanded Halstead-Reitan battery: Demographically adjusted neuropsychological norms for African American and Caucasian adults.* Lutz, Fla.: PAR.

Henderson, L. W., Frank, E. W., Pigatt, T., Abramson, R. K., & Houston, M. (1998). Race, gender and educational level effects on Boston Naming Test scores. *Aphasiology, 12,* 901–911.

Henry, J. D., & Crawford, J. R. (2004). Verbal fluency deficits in Parkinson's disease: A meta-analysis. *Journal of the International Neuropsychological Society, 10,* 608–622.

Henry, J. D., Crawford, J. R., & Phillips, L. H. (2004). Verbal fluency performance in dementia of the Alzheimer's type: a meta-analysis. *Neuropsychologia, 42,* 1212–1224.

Hermann, B. P., Perrine, K., Chelune, G. J., Barr, W., Loring, D. W., Strauss, E., Trenerry, M. R., & Westerveld, M. (1999). Visual confrontation naming following left anterior temporal lobectomy: A comparison of surgical approaches. *Neuropsychology, 13,* 3–9.

Hill, C. D., Stoudemire, A., Morris, R., Martino-Saltzman, D., Markwalter, H. R., & Lewison, B. J. (1992). Dysnomia in the differential diagnosis of major depression, depression-related cognitive dysfunction, and dementia. *Journal of Neuropsychiatry and Clinical Neuroscience, 4,* 64–69.

Ivnik, R. J., Malec, J. F., Smith, G. E., Tangalos, E. G., & Peterson, R. C. (1996). Neuropsychological test norms above age 55: COWAT, BNT, MAE Token, WRAT-R Reading, AMNART, Stroop, TMT, and JLO. *The Clinical Neuropsychologist, 10,* 262–278.

Jordan, F. M., Cannon, A., & Murdoch, B. E. (1992). Language abilities of mildly closed head injured (CHI) children 10 years postinjury. *Brain Injury, 6,* 39–44.

Jordan, F. M., Murdoch, B. E., Hudson-Tennent, L. J., & Boon, D. L. (1996). Naming performance of brain-injured children. *Aphasiology, 10,* 755–766.

Kaplan, E. F., Goodglass, H., & Weintraub, S. (1978, 1983). *The Boston Naming Test: Experimental edition (1978).* Boston: Kaplan & Goodglass. (2nd ed., Philadelphia: Lea & Febiger.)

Kaplan, E. F., Goodglass, H., & Weintraub, S. (2001). *The Boston Naming Test* (2nd ed.). Philadelphia: Lippincott Williams & Wilkins.

Kent, P. S., & Luszcz, M. A. (2002). Review of the Boston Naming test and multiple-occasion normative data for older adults on 15-item versions. *The Clinical Neuropsychologist, 16,* 555–574.

Killgore, W. D. S., & Adams, R. L. (1999). Prediction of Boston Naming Test performance from vocabulary scores: Preliminary guidelines for interpretation. *Perceptual and Motor Skills, 89,* 327–337.

Kim, H. L., & Na, D. L. (1999). Normative data on the Korean version of the Boston Naming Test. *Journal of Clinical and Experimental Neuropsychology, 21,* 127–133.

Kohn, S. E., & Goodglass, H. (1985). Picture-naming in aphasia. *Brain and Language, 24,* 266–283.

Landre, N. A., Taylor, M. A., & Kearns, K. P. (1992). Language functioning in schizophrenic and aphasic patients. *Neuropsychiatry, Neuropsychology, and Behavioral Neurology, 5,* 7–14.

Lansing, A. E., Ivnik, R. J., Cullum, C. M., & Randolph, C. (1999). An empirically derived short form of the Boston Naming Test. *Archives of Clinical Neuropsychology, 14,* 481–487.

Larrain, C. M., & Cimino, C. R. (1998). Alternate forms of the Boston Naming Test in Alzheimer's disease. *The Clinical Neuropsychologist, 12,* 525–530.

Lezak, M. D., Whitham, R., & Bourdette, D. (1990). Emotional impact of cognitive insufficiencies in multiple sclerosis (MS) [Abstract]. *Journal of Clinical and Experimental Neuropsychology, 12,* 50.

Locascio, J. J., Corkin, S., & Growde, J. H. (2003). Relation between clinical characteristics of Parkinson's disease and cognitive decline. *Journal of Clinical and Experimental Neuropsychology, 25,* 94–109.

Lucas, J. A., Ivnik, R. J., Smith, G. E., Ferman, T. J., Willis, F. B., Petersen, R. C., & Graff-Radford, N. R. (2005). Mayo's Older African Americans Normative Studies: Norms for Boston Naming Test, Controlled Oral Word Association, Category Fluency, Animal Naming, Token Test, WRAT-3 Reading, Trail Making Test, Stroop Test, and Judgment of Line Orientation. *The Clinical Neuropsychologist, 19,* 243–269.

Lukatela, K., Malloy, P., Jenkins, M., & Cohen, R. (1998). The naming deficit in early Alzheimer's and vascular dementia. *Neuropsychology, 12,* 565–572.

Mack, W. J., Freed, D. M., Williams, B. W., & Henderson, V. W. (1992). Boston Naming Test: Shortened version for use in Alzheimer's disease. *Journal of Gerontology, 47,* 164–168.

MacKay, A., Connor, L. T., & Storandt, M. (2005). Dementia does not explain correlation between age and scores on Boston Naming Test. *Archives of Clinical Neuropsychology, 20,* 129–133.

Manly, J. J., Jacobs, D. M., Touradji, P., Small, S. A., & Stern, Y. (2002). Reading level attenuates differences in neuropsychological test performance between African American and White elders. *Journal of the International Neuropsychological Society, 8,* 314–348.

Manly, J. J., Miller, S. W., Heaton, R. K., Byrd, D., Reilly, J., Velasquez, R. J., Saccuzzo, D. P., Grant, I., & the HIV Neurobehavioral Research Center (HNRC) group (1998). The effect of African American acculturation on neuropsychological test performance in normal and HIV-positive individuals. *Journal of the International Neuropsychological Society, 4,* 291–302.

Marien, P., Mampaey, E., Vervaet, A., Saerens, J., & De Deyn, P. P. (1998). Normative data for the Boston Naming Test in native Dutch-speaking Belgian elderly. *Brain and Language, 65,* 447–467.

Mitrushina, M. M., Boone, K. B., Razani, J., & D'Elia, L. F. (2005). *Handbook of Normative Data for Neuropsychological Assessment* (2nd ed.) New York: Oxford University Press.

Mitrushina, M., & Satz, P. (1989). Differential decline of specific memory components in normal aging. *Brain Dysfunction, 2,* 330–335.

Mitrushina, M., & Satz, P. (1995). Repeated testing of normal elderly with the Boston Naming Test. *Aging Clinical and Experimental Research, 7,* 123–127.

Morris, J. C., Heyman, A., Mohs, R. C., Hughes, J. P., vam Belle, G., Fillenbaum, G., Mellits, E. D., Clark, C., & the CERAD Investigators. (1989). The Consortium to Establish a Registry for Alzheimer's Disease (CERAD). Part 1: Clinical and neuropsychological assessment of Alzheimer's disease. *Neurology, 39,* 1159–1165.

Morrison, L. E., Smith, L. A., & Sarazin, F. F. A. (1996). Boston Naming Test: A French-Canadian normative study (preliminary analyses) [Abstract]. *Journal of the International Neuropsychological Society, 2,* 4.

Neils, J., Baris, J. M., Carter, C., Dell'aira, A. L., Nordloh, S. J., Weiler, E., & Weisiger, B. (1995). Effects of age, education, and living environment on BNT performance. *Journal of Speech and Hearing Research, 38,* 1143–1149.

Ponton, M. O., Satz, P., Herrera Ortiz, F., Urrutia, C. P., Young, R., D'Elia, L. F., Furst, C. J., & Namerow, N. (1996). Normative data stratified by age and education for the Neuropsychological Screening Battery for Hispanics (NESBHIS): Initial Report. *Journal of the International Neuropsychological Society, 2,* 96–104.

Rabin, L. A., Barr, W. B., & Burton, L. A. (2005). Assessment practices of clinical neuropsychologists in the United States and Canada: A survey of INS, NAN, and APA Division 40 members. *Archives of Clinical Neuropsychology, 20,* 33–65.

Randolph, C., Lansing, A., Ivnick, R. J., Cullum, C. M., & Hermann, B. P. (1999). Determinants of confrontation naming performance. *Archives of Clinical Neuropsychology, 14,* 489–496.

Ripich, D. N., Petrill, S. A., Whitehouse, P. J., & Ziol, E. W. (1995). Gender differences in language of AD patients: A longitudinal study. *Neurology, 45,* 299–302.

Riva, D., Nichelli, F., & Devoti, M. (2000). Developmental aspects of verbal fluency and confrontation naming in children. *Brain and Language, 71,* 267–284.

Roberts, P. M., Garcia, L. J., Desrochers, A., & Hernandez, D. (2002) English performance of proficient bilingual adults on the Boston Naming Test. *Aphasiology, 16,* 635–645.

Ross, T. P., & Lichtenberg, P. A. (1998). Expanded normative data for the Boston Naming Test with urban, elderly medical patients. *The Clinical Neuropsychologist, 12,* 475–481.

Ross, T. P., Lichtenberg, P. A., & Christensen, K. (1995). Normative data on the Boston Naming Test for elderly adults in a demographically diverse medical sample. *The Clinical Neuropsychologist, 9,* 321–325.

Satz, P. (1993). Brain reserve capacity on symptom onset after brain injury: A formulation and review of evidence for threshold theory. *Neuropsychology, 7,* 273–295.

Sawrie, S. M., Chelune, G. J., Naugle, R. I., & Luders, H. O. (1996). Empirical methods for assessing meaningful change following epilepsy surgery. *Journal of the International Neuropsychological Association, 2,* 556–564.

Saxton, J., Ratcliff, G., Munro, C. A., Coffey, C. E., Becker, J. E., Fried, L., & Kuller, L. (2000). Normative data on the Boston Naming Test and two equivalent 30-item short-forms. *The Clinical Neuropsychologist, 14,* 526–534.

Schefft, B. K., Testa, S. M., Dulay, M. F., Privitera, M. D., & Yeh, H. S. (2003). Preoperative assessment of confrontation naming ability and interictal paraphasia production in unilateral temporal lobe epilepsy. *Epilepsy and Behavior, 4,* 161–168.

Senior, G., Douglas, L., & Dawes, S. (2001). *Discrepancy analysis: A new/old approach to psychological test data interpretation.* Presentation at the 21st annual conference of the National Academy of Neuropsychology, San Francisco, California.

Steinberg, B. A., Bieliauskas, L. A., Smith, G. E., Langellotti, C., & Ivnik, R. J. (2005). MAYO's Older Americans Normative Studies: Age- and IQ-adjusted norms for the Boston Naming Test, the MAE Token Test, and the Judgement of Line Orientation Test. *The Clinical Neuropsychologist, 19,* 280–328.

Storms, G., Saerens, J., & De Deyn, P. P. (2004). Normative data for the Boston Naming Test in native Dutch-speaking Belgian children and the relation with intelligence. *Brain and Language, 91,* 274–281.

Teng, E. L., Wimer, C., Roberts, E., Damasio, A. R., Eslinger, P. J., Folstein, M. F., Tune, L. E., Whitehouse, P. J., Bardolph, E. L., Hui, H. C., & Henderson, V. W. (1989). Alzheimer dementia: Performance on parallel forms of the Dementia Assessment Battery. *Journal of Clinical and Experimental Neuropsychology, 11,* 899–912.

Testa, J. A., Ivnik, R. J., Boeve, B., Pedersen, R. C., Pankratz, V. S., Knopman, D., Tangalos, E., & Smith, G. E. (2004). Confrontation naming does not add incremental diagnostic utility in MCI and Alzheimer's disease. *Journal of the International Neuropsychological Society, 10,* 504–512.

Thompson, L. L., & Heaton, R. K. (1989). Comparison of different versions of the Boston Naming Test. *The Clinical Neuropsychologist, 3,* 184–192.

Tombaugh, T. N., & Hubley, A. (1997). The 60-item Boston Naming Test: Norms for cognitively intact adults aged 25 to 88 years. *Journal of Clinical and Experimental Neuropsychology, 19,* 922–932.

Touradji, P., Manly, J. J., Jacobs, D. M., & Stern, Y. (2001). Neuropsychological test performance: A study of non-Hispanic white elderly. *Journal of Clinical and Experimental Neuropsychology, 23,* 643–649.

Tsang, H. L., & Lee, T. M. C. (2003). The effect of aging on confrontational naming ability. *Archives of Clinical Neuropsychology, 18,* 81–89.

Tweedy, J. R., & Schulman, P. D. (1982). Toward a functional classification of naming impairment. *Brain and Language, 15,* 193–206.

Unverzagt, F. W., Morgan, O. S., Thesiger, C. H. (1999). Clinical utility of CERAD neuropsychological battery in elderly Jamaicans. *Journal of International Neuropsychological Society, 5,* 255–259.

Van Gorp, W. G., Satz, P., Kiersch, M. E., & Henry, R. (1986). Normative data on the Boston Naming Test for a group of normal older adults. *Journal of Clinical and Experimental Neuropsychology, 8,* 702–705.

Van Zandvoort, M., de Haan, E., van Gijn, J., & Kappelle, L. J. (2003). Cognitive functioning in patients with a small infarct in the brainstem. *Journal of the International Neuropsychological Society, 9,* 490–494.

Welch, L. W., Doineau, D., Johnson, S., & King, D. (1996). Education and gender normative data for the Boston Naming Test in a group of older adults. *Brain and Language, 53,* 260–266.

Welsh, K. A., Butters, N., Mohs, R. C., Beekly, D., Edland, S., Fillenbaum, G., & Heyman, A. (1994). The Consortium to Establish a Registry for Alzheimer's Disease (CERAD). Part V: A normative study of the neuropsychological battery. *Neurology, 44,* 609–614.

Welsh, K. A., Fillenbaum, G., Wilkinson, W., Heyman, A., Mohs, R. C., Stern, Y., Harrell, L., Edland, S. D., & Beekly, D. (1995). Neuropsychological test performance in African-American and white patients with Alzheimer's disease. *Neurology, 45,* 2207–2211.

Williams, B. W., Mack, W., & Henderson, V. W. (1989). Boston naming test in Alzheimer's disease. *Neuropsychologia, 27,* 1073–1079.

Worrall, L. E., Yiu, E. M. L., Hickson, L. M. H., & Barnett, H. M. (1995). Normative data for the Boston Naming test for Australian elderly. *Aphasiology, 9,* 541–551.

Yeates, K. O. (1994). Comparison of developmental norms for the Boston Naming Test. *The Clinical Neuropsychologist, 8,* 91–98.

Dichotic Listening—Words

PURPOSE

The Dichotic Listening—Words test can provide an indication of language processing and lateralization. It is also a measure of divided attention.

SOURCE

The cassette tape with dichotic words, instructions, and recording sheets can be obtained from the Psychology Clinic, University of Victoria, Victoria, B.C. V8W 3P5, Canada (http://www.uvic.ca/psyc/testsale) for $50 US.

AGE RANGE

The test can be given to children, beginning at age 2 years, and to adults aged 18 to 30 years.

DESCRIPTION

The dichotic listening (DL) test was originally developed by Broadbent (1958) to investigate the ability to attend to two signals simultaneously, one to each ear. Kimura (1961) modified the task by using spoken one-syllable numbers in sets of three pairs, with the subject required to repeat as many numbers as possible. Kimura noted that, in patients with epilepsy with documented left-hemisphere speech dominance, right-ear recall was better than recall from the left ear. Patients with right-hemisphere speech dominance showed the reverse pattern.

The ear advantage (right ear advantage or REA, left-ear advantage or LEA) is thought to reflect hemisphere dominance for processing stimuli, based on suppression of the ipsilateral and enhancement of the contralateral auditory pathways (Kimura, 1967; see Kinsbourne, 1970 for an attentional model). Thus, DL can serve as a functional test of hemispheric speech dominance. It can also be used to evaluate the integrity of the central auditory pathway. For example, abnormally low scores in one ear may suggest a lesion in the contralateral hemisphere (Meyers et al., 2002; Sparks et al., 1970) or in the corpus callosum (Sidtis, 1988). The test has also been used clinically as a measure of divided attention and stimulus processing speed (Meyers et al., 2002; Spellacy & Ehle, 1990).

We describe here a verbal DL test using a free-recall technique similar to the one used by Kimura (1961), although other similar tasks are available (e.g., Meyers et al., 2002). Others have employed a focused-attention technique, in which participants attend to only one ear for a series of trials, or according to an exogenous cue before each dichotic trial (Geffen et al., 1978; Hugdahl et al., 2003a,b,c; Voyer & Flight, 2001), to control for attentional biases on the part of the participants.

Our free-recall technique involves presentation of six one-syllable words, three to each ear. The tape prepared in our laboratory is synchronized for stimulus onset and calibrated for equal loudness in both ears. Both right- and left-ear stimuli begin with the same consonant, to control for voice-onset time.

The apparatus consists of a high-quality stereo audiotape player and amplifier, a pair of earphones plugged into the appropriate outlets, and the DL tape. The right and left channels on the tape may be connected to the right or left earphones of the subject. They can be used alternately, or they can be reversed after half of the test is completed to avoid bias due to poor earphone calibration. Care should be taken to indicate on the answer sheet which channel was signaling into which ear.

A sound-level meter (Scott or similar product) should be used to calibrate and balance the earphones before the test is started. The earphones should be calibrated to produce exactly equal loudness of 65 to 70 dB for both ears, the "most comfortable loudness level" suggested by Riegler (1980).

Before administering the test, the examiner should check the examinee for adequate hearing in both ears. DL effects are fairly robust in the presence of minor hearing impairment (discrepancy of 5–10 dB between right and left ear), but with higher discrepancies the results should be interpreted with caution. If the discrepancy is beyond 20 dB, the test should not be given.

ADMINISTRATION

The subject is seated with earphones on, with the earphone marked "right" on the right ear and the one marked "left" on the left ear. Instruct the client to report the words heard after each trial (see Figure 11–3).

After each set of three word-pairs, stop the tape and wait for the subject to respond. Reverse the earphones halfway through the test. Circle the words the subject remembered on the answer sheet (Figure 11–4). Dubious responses should be written above the word they resemble, but only the words on the answer sheet are accepted as correct.

If the subject responds with only one or two words, you may say, "Is that all?" or, "Are those all the words you can remember?" before proceeding to the next set.

APPROXIMATE TIME FOR ADMINISTRATION

About 10 to 20 min is required.

SCORING

Count 1 point for each word that is listed on the answer sheet. Total each side.

DEMOGRAPHIC EFFECTS

Age

Children of kindergarten age already show right-ear superiority, and right-left differences reach adult levels by grade 3 (see

Figure 11–3 Instructions for administration of Dichotic Listening—Words.

Say: *You are going to hear some words, and I want you to repeat as many of these words as possible.*

On the tape are two three-word sets of single words. The first set is heard on the right ear. After the subject repeats these words correctly, play the second set, which is heard on the left ear. These practice sets can be repeated if the subject fails to understand the instructions. If the subject completes the practice trials correctly, say:

You will now hear words which will come to both ears at the same time. I want you to repeat all the words you hear. Each time you will hear three sets of words, and when I stop the tape, you must start repeating the words immediately, as many as you can remember.

Table 11–19). Overall recall scores in school-age children in fact exceed those of normal adults, possibly owing to the lack of tape clarity as well as differences in attention. Whether advancing age affects performance on this particular task is not known, although there is evidence of such effects on similar DL tasks (Meyers et al., 2002; Rodriguez et al., 1990). An expanded normative base, with age-stratified norms, is needed.

Gender

Gender differences, suggesting a stronger left hemisphere lateralization for males, have been reported in some experimental studies. However, a meta-analysis of 49 experiments by Hiscock et al. (1994) confirmed Bryden's (1988) conclusion that "there are sex differences in DL performance, although they are small and of marginal significance" (Hiscock et al., 1994, pp. 31–32).

NORMATIVE DATA

In general, the total recall on the full-length tape is approximately 40 words. Normative data for children from preschool to regular kindergarten ages up to grade 6 are provided in Table 11–19. The data provided for adults are derived from university students and therefore should be used only with young adults.

RELIABILITY

Test-Retest Reliability

Test-retest reliability coefficients vary depending on the number of trials, the type of stimuli, and type of procedure (e.g., free recall, focused attention; Bruder, 1988; Gadea et al., 2000; Hugdahl & Hammar, 1997). For the task described here, test-retest reliabilities of the ear and ear difference scores are reported to be good in patients with medically refractory seizures tested twice in one day ($r = .75$ to .92; Strauss et al., 1987).

Hiscock et al. (2000) reported that, in university students, the retest reliability of the ear difference score of the Victoria version was only .45. Neither the incidence nor the strength of the REA increased significantly when the number of word pairs was increased to 528.

VALIDITY

The Victoria version of the test agrees reasonably well with speech lateralization as determined by the sodium amytal test (Wada test; Strauss et al., 1987). In that study, patients with left-hemisphere speech lateralization obtained scores of 29.03 for the right ear and 12.95 for the left ear; the corresponding scores were 15.20 and 21.48 for patients with right-hemisphere speech and 19.88 and 13.24 for patients with bilateral speech. However, the percentage of patients with REA in each of the three groups was 86%, 50%, and 71%, respectively. Therefore, failure to obtain a right-left ear difference suggests that language lateralization may not be following the normal pattern but should not be used as definite evidence regarding hemispheric dominance. Based on a study of 106 patients for whom hemisphere dominance was determined by the intracarotid amobarbital test, Lee et al. (1994) warned that DL is not an indicator of language dominance in the individual case and that even group differences between left, right, and bilateral language dominant patients may not be statistically significant. Hence, firm statements about language lateralization cannot be made; the test provides clues only.

About 80% of normal right-handers show an REA on this and other DL tests (Hiscock et al., 2000); this seems to underestimate the incidence of left-hemisphere language lateralization (about 65%–75% REA; Lake & Bryden, 1976; Lee et al. 1994). In a sample of 126 children aged 6 to 9 years, Hugdahl and Andersson (1989) found an REA in 65%, an LEA in 25.4%, and no ear advantage in 9.6%. According to Mondor and Bryden (1992), the failure of dichotic tests to categorize all subjects correctly is caused by confounding factors (e.g., attentional biases). Alternative explanations are available, including certain experiential factors (e.g., familiarity with the

Figure 11-4 Dichotic Listening—Words Sample Score Sheet.

Name _____

DOB _____

Date Tested _____

Examiner _____

Trials	Right Ear (Right Headphone)			Left Ear (Left Headphone)		
Practice	Dig	Boy	Feed	Numb	Pad	Hope
1	Pack	Tent	Hat	Port	Tea	Cow
2	Fame	Sum	Bond	Fur	Sale	Bee
3	Duck	Ship	Gas	Deck	Shoe	Gun
4	Vine	Zone	Mob	Vane	Zoo	Meal
5	Nose	Pride	Track	Name	Plate	Trail
6	Coast	Flight	Sake	Corn	Fleet	Sunk
7	Bowl	Damp	Good	Bell	Deed	Game
8	Shine	Vent	Zest	Sheep	Vast	Zeal
9	Mass	Nine	Pin	Mill	Nail	Pace
10	Tin	Cloth	Faith	Torn	Clock	Fresh
11	Spit	Belt	Night	Speak	Bark	Need

REVERSE HEADPHONES

	Right Ear (Left Headphone)			Left Ear (Right Headphone)		
12	Shore	Quest	Vault	Shell	Guard	Vote
13	Though	Map	Note	There	Mad	Nick
14	Pal	Tongue	Cream	Pig	Teeth	Crust
15	Flag	Send	Blown	Fault	Sand	Brain
16	Dawn	Give	Shift	Ditch	Glow	Shirt
17	Vim	Then	Mink	View	This	Mouth
18	Noun	Pan	Top	Noon	Pork	Tan
19	Coop	Fog	Style	Cord	Fit	Stamp
20	Birth	Neck	Grain	Band	Noise	Glove
21	Shame	Verb	That	Shoot	Voice	Than
22	Male	Nudge	Coop	Mine	Nice	Cord

Right Total _____   Left Total _____

Grand Total _____

Table 11–19 Verbal Dichotic Listening: Norms for Children and Adults

Grade/Age	Sex	n	Right Ear	Left Ear	Total
Age 2	F	2	13.0	5.0	18.0
	M	3	12.0	2.0	14.0
Age 3	F	9	19.1	5.6	24.7
	M	5	15.3	4.8	20.0
Age 4	F	7	24.1	8.0	31.9
	M	7	25.3	9.8	35.2
Kindergarten					
Age 5	F	10	19.6	13.1	32.7
	M	9	20.2	16.9	37.1
Elementary					
Grade 1	F	15	24.7	12.7	37.4
	M	12	26.8	16.0	42.8
Grade 2	F	29	29.0	12.4	41.3
	M	16	30.4	13.2	43.6
Grade 3	F	19	29.6	16.9	46.5
	M	11	29.1	19.2	48.3
Grade 4	F	15	32.5	16.9	48.7
	M	16	30.0	22.6	52.6
Grade 5	F	23	33.3	20.0	53.3
	M	15	31.0	20.6	51.5
Grade 6	F	12	30.5	19.6	50.1
	M	18	32.5	20.2	52.9
Adult					
Right-handers		175	$M = 24.95$	$M = 16.23$	$M = 41.18$
			$SD = 9.60$	$SD = 8.30$	$SD = 10.12$

Note: Kosaka and Kolb used the Victoria tape for adults, reversing the headphones after half the trials.

Source: Children's norms from Kosaka & Kolb (unpublished data, 1977); adult right-hander norms from Strauss et al., 1987.

stimuli), anomalies in the auditory pathways, and contributions of right hemispheric processing (e.g., perceptual) that are typically not revealed by clinical methods such as the Wada test (Kinsbourne et al., 2000).

Overall, the majority of individuals exhibit an REA for the recognition of verbal material. Abnormal DL test results have been documented in numerous conditions. For example, impairment has been reported in patients who present with head injury (Evitts et al., 2003; Meyers et al., 2002; Richardson et al. 1990), and the more severe the injury (i.e., longer loss of consciousness), the more impaired the performance (Meyers et al., 2002). Abnormality has also been reported in patients with Parkinson's disease (Richardson et al., 1990), malaria encephalitis (Richardson et al., 1990), exposure to organic solvents (Hallgren et al., 1998), and damage to the anterior communicating artery (Evitts et al., 2003). Studies of patients with documented white matter disease (e.g., multiple sclerosis [MS]) have shown impairment on DL tasks (Jerger & Jerger, 1975; Levin et al., 1989; Pujol et al., 1991; Rao et al., 1989). Deficits in DL have also been found in patients with Alzheimer's disease (Mohr et al., 1990) and in patients who

had experienced high fever (hyperpyrexia) without direct brain involvement (Varney et al., 1994).

Early damage produces effects similar to those reported in adults, with poor performance in the ear contralateral to the lesion. For example, in children with acquired epileptic aphasia or Landau-Kleffner syndrome, unilateral ear extinction contralateral to the affected temporal cortex has been reported (Metz-Lutz et al., 1997). Similarly, a left ear advantage for dichotic digits and impairment in right hand function was reported in some individuals with congenital left hemisphere lesions (Isaacs et al., 1996). The implication is that, in this group, early hemispheric damage was extensive enough to encroach on motor and language areas, perhaps shifting language representation to the right.

Dyslexic children have difficulties with speech perception, and some researchers have explored whether such children show reduced or reversed ear asymmetry in a DL situation. The literature suggests that dyslexic children show an REA using consonant-vowel (CV) syllables, although their right ear scores are slightly reduced compared with those of controls (Hugdahl et al., 2003b). Asbjornsen et al. (2003) compared 43 reading-impaired children with 20 normal reading children, aged 11 to 13 years, with both the free-recall and the directed-attention procedure. Both procedures produced significant group differences, but only 42% of the samples could be correctly classified based on DL difference scores only. Adding measures of the WCST and Stroop scores to the discriminant function analysis produced a 90.74% correct classification.

The DL test is somewhat sensitive to lateralized deficits. For example, Meyers et al. (2002) examined stroke patients. They noted left-ear suppression with right-hemisphere strokes; with left-hemisphere lesions, performance could be affected in either the left or the right channels, or both. By contrast, Grote et al. (1995) reported that, in patients with epilepsy and left-hemisphere speech dominance, a reduced right-ear score was always predictive of a left-hemisphere seizure focus, but left-ear extinction could be associated with unilateral lesions in either hemisphere. Hugdahl et al. (2003a) found that patients with right frontal lesions had a normal REA, like the controls, but patients with left frontal lesions failed to show an REA. A shift to left-ear advantage in aphasics (Papanicolaou et al., 1987) has been interpreted as evidence of increased right-hemisphere involvement during recovery from aphasia, or of attentional factors, or of a lesion effect in the left hemisphere (Moore & Papanicolaou, 1991; Niccum & Speaks, 1991).

Springer et al. (1991) found that DL distinguishes between dysphoric patients with complaints of seizure-like phenomena and other depressives, and that DL scores improve after carbamazepine treatment. By contrast, Hugdahl et al. (2003c) found no impairment in depressive patients compared with healthy controls; however, patients with schizophrenia did show impairment. Others (e.g., Bruder et al., 1999) have also reported abnormal results in patients with chronic schizophrenia.

Frontotemporal networks appear to be important in the generation of the typical ear asymmetry. For example, a study by Niccum et al. (1983) indicated that integrity of the left posterior superior area is essential for the perception of right-ear stimuli. Strauss et al. (1985) reported that patients with epilepsy who showed an REA on a verbal DL test were likely to have a wider left posterior sylvian region (as measured on carotid arteriograms); patients who showed a left ear advantage were more likely to have a wider right posterior sylvian region. Some individuals with dyslexia show altered planum asymmetry, and performance on DL tasks may reflect this unusual pattern (Foster et al., 2002; Hugdahl et al., 2003b).

Jancke et al. (2003) used functional magnetic resonance imaging (fMRI) to trace the hemodynamic response to DL and found that the presupplementary motor area and the left planum temporale were primarily involved. Roberts et al. (1990) demonstrated generally reduced DL scores in a series of 24 patients with complex partial seizures due to electrophysiological dysfunction that interfered with normal signal transmission from the left or right ear to the perisylvian language zone. The scores improved significantly after antiepileptic medication was instituted.

With regard to the role of the corpus callosum, the splenium appears to be needed for auditory transfer, because splenial lesions result in left-ear suppression (Pollmann et al., 2002; Sugishita et al., 1995). Reinvang et al. (1994) found reduced left-ear scores in MS patients with left-hemisphere dominance and narrowing of the corpus callosum, presumably because of a lessening of interhemispheric transfer. Wishart et al. (1995) found in MS patients a pattern of left-sided suppression and/or right-sided enhancement, consistent with impairment of interhemispheric transfer. Lassonde and collaborators (Lassonde & Bryden, 1990; Lassonde et al., 1981) found enhanced rather than reduced lateral differences in acallosal children, and they suggested that the corpus callosum inhibits rather than promotes interhemispheric transfer. Peru et al. (2003) described a single patient who showed complete left-ear suppression after a callosal lesion but recovered almost completely with the passage of 4 years. The authors concluded that functional recovery of interhemispheric interaction had occurred.

Malingering

Meyers et al. (1999) found that litigants (but not nonlitigants) and analog malingerers tended to perform poorly on a DL test, resembling individuals who had sustained severe traumatic brain injuries. Therefore, low scores in litigants who suffer mild injuries to the head may signify suboptimal effort.

COMMENT

The DL task described here appears to be a reasonably reliable and noninvasive tool that can be used when issues of lateralized cognitive processing are of importance. However, different DL tests may well yield different results with regard to issues of hemispheric lateralization. Free-recall listening conditions (as in the test described here) allow for significant attentional bias on the part of the examinee (e.g., the patient may bias attention toward the easier or toward the more difficult ear), possibly altering laterality effects. Whether directed response procedures produce more reliable results is uncertain (Hiscock et al., 2000). The Fused Dichotic Words Test (FDWT; Wexler & Hawles, 1983) provides a higher level of classification accuracy in patients with known language lateralization (Zatorre, 1989), although the proportion of right-handers who show an REA is similar for the FDWT and the Victoria Test (Hiscock et al., 2000).

The DL test is sensitive to a wide variety of disorders and is well tolerated by patients. Its utility in cases of white matter disturbance is noteworthy, and it may indicate abnormality when other more standard tests do not (Varney et al., 1998).

Individual differences (e.g., gender, age) affect performance. In the absence of appropriate normative data, the task described here should not be used with individuals older than 30 years of age.

REFERENCES

Asbjornsen, A. E., Helland, T., Obrzut, J. E., & Bolick, C. A. (2003). The role of dichotic listening performance and tasks of executive functions in reading impairment: A discriminant function analysis. *Child Neuropsychology, 9*, 277–288.

Broadbent, D. E. (1958). *Perception and communication.* Oxford, U.K.: Pergamon Press.

Bruder, C. F. (1988). Dichotic listening in psychiatric patients. In K. Hugdahl (Ed.), *Handbook of dichotic listening: Theory, methods, and research.* New York: Wiley.

Bruder, G., Kayser, J., Tenke, C., Amador, X., Friedman, M., Sharif, Z., & Gorman, J. (1999). Left temporal lobe dysfunction in schizophrenia: Event-related potential and behavioural evidence from phonetic and tonal dichotic listening tasks. *Archives of General Psychiatry, 56*, 267–276.

Bryden, M. P. (1988). An overview of the dichotic listening procedure and its relation to cerebral organization. In K. Hugdahl (Ed.), *Handbook of dichotic listening: Theory, methods, and research.* New York: Wiley.

Evitts, P. M., Nelson, L. L., & McGuire, R. A. (2003). Impairments in dichotic listening in patients presenting anterior communicating artery aneurysm. *Applied Neuropsychology, 10*, 89–95.

Foster, L. M., Hynd, G. W., Morgan, A. E., & Hugdahl, K. (2002). Planum temporale asymmetry and ear advantage in developmental dyslexia and attention-deficit/hyperactivity disorder (ADHD). *Journal of the International Neuropsychological Society, 8*, 22–36.

Gadea, M., Gomez, C., & Espert, R. (2000). Test-retest performance for the consonant–vowel dichotic listening test with and without attentional manipulations. *Journal of Clinical and Experimental Neuropsychology, 22*, 793–803.

Geffen, G., Traub, E., & Stierman, I. (1978). Language laterality assessed by unilateral ECT and dichotic monitoring. *Journal of Neurology, Neurosurgery, and Psychiatry, 41*, 354–360.

Graves, R. E., & Allen, T. (1995). *Utilizing the sound blaster 16 board for dichotic listening studies.* Unpublished manuscript. Department of Psychology, University of Victoria, British Columbia, Canada.

Grote, C. L., Pierre-Louis, S. J. C., Smith, M. C., Roberts, R. J., & Varney, N. R. (1995). Significance of unilateral ear extinction on the dichotic listening test. *Journal of Clinical and Experimental Neuropsychology, 17*, 1–8.

Hallgren, M., Johansson, M., Larsby, B., & Arlinger, S. (1998). Dichotic speech tests. *Scand Audiol Suppl., 49*, 35–39.

Hiscock, M., Cole, L. C., Benthall, J. G., Carlson, V. L., & Ricketts, J. M. (2000). Toward solving the inferential problem in laterality research: Effects of increased reliability on the validity of the dichotic listening right-ear advantage. *Journal of the International Neuropsychological Society, 6*, 539–547.

Hiscock, M., Inch, R., Jacek, C., Hiscock-Kalil, C., & Kalil, K. M. (1994). Is there a sex difference in human laterality: I. An exhaustive survey of laterality studies from six neuropsychological journals. *Journal of Clinical and Experimental Neuropsychology, 16*, 423–435.

Hugdahl, K., & Andersson, N. (1989). Dichotic listening in 126 left-handed children: Ear advantage, familial sinistrality, and sex differences. *Neuropsychologia, 27*, 999–1006.

Hugdahl, K., Bodner, T., Weiss, E., & Benke, T. (2003a). Dichotic listening performance and frontal lobe function. *Cognitive Brain Research, 16*, 58–65.

Hugdahl, K., & Hammar, A. (1997). Test-retest reliability for the consonant-vowel syllables dichotic listening paradigm. *Journal of Clinical and Experimental Neuropsychology, 19*, 667–675.

Hugdahl, K., Heiervang, E., Ersland, L., Lundervold, A., Steinmetz, H., & Smievoll, A. I. (2003b). Significant relation between MR measures of planum temporale area and dichotic listening processing of syllables in dyslexic children. *Neuropsychologia, 41*, 666–675.

Hugdahl, K., Rund, B. R., Lund, A., Asbjornsen, A., Egeland, J., Landro, N. I., Roness, A., Stordal, K. I., & Sundet K. (2003c). Attentional and executive dysfunctions in schizophrenia and depression: Evidence from dichotic listening performance. *Biological Psychiatry, 53*, 609–616.

Isaacs, E., Christie, D., Vargha-Khadem, F., & Mishkin, M. (1996). Effects of hemispheric side of injury, age at injury, and presence of seizure disorder on functional ear and hand asymmetries in hemiplegic children. *Neuropsychologia, 34*, 127–137.

Jaenke, L., Specht, K., Shah, J. N., & Hugdahl, K. (2003). Focused attention in a simple dichotic listening task: An fMRI experiment. *Cognitive Brain Research, 16*, 257–266.

Jerger, J., & Jerger, S. (1975). Clinical validity of central auditory tests. *Scandinavian Audiology, 4*, 147–163.

Johnson, B. H., Laberg, J. C., Eid, J., & Hugdahl, K. (2002). Dichotic listening and sleep deprivation: Vigilance effects. *Scandinavian Journal of Psychology, 43*, 413–417.

Kimura, D. (1961). Cerebral dominance and the perception of verbal stimuli. *Canadian Journal of Psychology, 15*, 166–171.

Kimura, D. (1967). Functional asymmetry of the brain in dichotic listening. *Cortex, 3*, 163–168.

Kinsbourne, M. (1970). The cerebral basis of lateral asymmetries in attention. *Acta Psychologica, 33*, 193–201.

Lake, D. A., & Bryden, M. P. (1976). Handedness and sex differences in hemispheric asymmetry. *Brain and Language, 3*, 266–282.

Lassonde, M., & Bryden, M. P. (1990). Dichotic listening, callosal agenesis, and cerebral laterality. *Brain and Language, 39*, 475–481.

Lassonde, M., Lortie, J., Ptito, M., & Geoffroy, G. (1981). Hemispheric asymmetry in callosal agenesis as revealed by dichotic listening performance. *Neuropsychologia, 19*, 455–458.

Lee, G. P., Loring, D. W., Newell, J. R., & Meador, E. J. (1994). Is dichotic listening a valid predictor of cerebral language dominance? *The Clinical Neuropsychologist, 8*, 429–438.

Levin, H. S., High, W. M., Williams, D. H., Eisenberg, H. M., Amparo, E. G., Guinto, F. C. Jr., & Ewert, J. (1989). Dichotic listening and manual performance in relation to magnetic resonance imaging after closed head injury. *Journal of Neurology, Neurosurgery and Psychiatry, 52*, 1162–1169.

Metz-Lutz, M. N., Hirsch, E., Maquet, P., de Saint Martin, A., Rudolf, G., Wioland, N., & Marescaux, C. (1997). Dichotic listening performance in the follow-up of Landau and Kleffner syndrome. *Child Neuropsychology, 3*, 47–60.

Meyers, J. E., Galinsky, A. M., & Volbrecht, M. (1999). Malingering and mild brain injury: How low is too low. *Applied Neuropsychology, 6*, 208–216.

Meyers, J. E., Roberts, R. J., Bayless, J. D., Volkert, K., & Evitts, P. E. (2002). Dichotic listening: Expanded norms and clinical application. *Archives of Clinical Neuropsychology, 17*, 79–90.

Mohr, E., Cox, C., Williams, J., Chase, T. N., & Fedio, P. (1990). Impairment of central auditory function in Alzheimer's disease. *Journal of Clinical and Experimental Neuropsychology, 12*, 235–246.

Mondor, T. A., & Bryden, M. P. (1992). On the relation between auditory spatial attention and auditory perceptual asymmetries. *Perception and Psychophysics, 52*, 393–402.

Moore, B. D., & Papanicolaou, A. C. (1991). Dichotic listening in aphasics: Response to Niccum and Speaks. *Journal of Clinical and Experimental Neuropsychology, 14*, 641–645.

Niccum, N., Rubens, A. D., & Selnes, O. A. (1983). Dichotic listening performance, language impairment, and lesion localization in aphasic listeners. *Journal of Speech and Hearing Research, 26,* 42–49.

Niccum, N., & Speaks, C. (1991). Interpretation of outcome on dichotic listening tests following stroke. *Journal of Clinical and Experimental Neuropsychology, 13,* 614–628.

Papanicolaou, A. C., Moore, B. D., Levin, H. S., & Eisenberg, H. M. (1987). Evoked potential correlates of right-hemisphere involvement in language recovery following stroke. *Archives of Neurology, 44,* 521–524.

Peru, A., Beltramello, A., Moro, V., Sattibaldi, L., & Bertolucchi, G. (2003). Temporary and permanent signs of interhemispheric disconnection after traumatic brain injury. *Neuropsychologia, 41,* 634–643.

Pollmann, S., Maertens, M., von Cramon, D. Y., Lepsien, J., & Hugdahl, K. (2002). Dichotic listening in patients with splenial and non-splenial callosal lesions. *Neuropsychology, 16,* 56–64.

Pujol, J. J., Junque, C., Vendrell, P., Garcia, P., Capdevila, A., & Marti-Vilalta, J. L. (1991). Left-ear extinction in patients with MRI periventricular lesions. *Neuropsychologia, 29,* 177–184.

Rao, S. M., Bernadin, L., Leo, G. J., Ellington, L., Ryan, S. B., & Burg, L. S. (1989). Cerebral disconnection in multiple sclerosis: Relationship to atrophy of the corpus callosum. *Archives of Neurology, 46,* 918–920.

Reinvang, I., Bakke, S. J., Hugdahl, K., Karlsen, N. R., et al. (1994). Dichotic listening performance in relation to callosal area on the MRI scan. *Neuropsychology, 8,* 445–450.

Richardson, E. D., Springer, J. A., Varney, N. R., Struchen, M. A., & Roberts, R. J. (1990). Dichotic listening in the clinic: New neuropsychological applications. *The Clinical Neuropsychologist, 8,* 416–428.

Riegler, J. (1980). Most comfortable loudness level of geriatric patients as a function of Seashore Loudness Discrimination scores, detection threshold, age, sex, setting, and musical background. *Journal of Music Therapy, 17,* 214–222.

Roberts, R. J., Varney, N. R., Paulsen, J. S., & Dickinson, E. D. (1990). Dichotic listening and complex partial seizures. *Journal of Clinical and Experimental Neuropsychology, 12,* 448–458.

Rodriguez, G. F., DiSarno, N. J., & Hardiman, C. J. (1990). Central auditory processing in normal-hearing elderly adults. *Audiology, 29,* 85–92.

Sidtis, J. J. (1988). Dichotic listening after commissurotomy. In K. Hugdahl (Ed.). *Handbook of dichotic listening* (pp. 161–184). Chichester, England: Wiley.

Sparks, R., Goodglass, H., & Nickel, B. (1970). Ipsilateral vs. contralateral extinction in dichotic listening resulting from hemisphere lesions. *Cortex, 6,* 249–260.

Spellacy, F., & Ehle, D. L. (1990). *The dichotic listening test as a measure of stimulus processing speed following mild to moderate concussion.* Unpublished manuscript, University of Victoria, Victoria, B.C., Canada.

Springer, J. A., Garvey, M. J., Varney, N. R., & Roberts, H. J. (1991). Dichotic listening failure in dysphoric neuropsychiatric patients who endorse multiple seizure symptoms. *Journal of Nervous and Mental Disease, 179,* 459–467.

Strauss, E., Gaddes, W. H., & Wada, J. (1987). Performance on a free-recall verbal dichotic listening task and cerebral dominance determined by the carotid amytal test. *Neuropsychologia, 25,* 747–753.

Strauss, E., Lapointe, J. S., Wada, J. A., Gaddes, W., & Kosaka, B. (1985). Language dominance: Correlation of radiological and functional data. *Neuropsychologia, 23,* 415–420.

Sugishita, M., Otomo, K. Yamasaki, K., & Yoshioka, M. (1995). Dichotic listening in patients with partial section of the corpus callosum. *Brain, 118,* 417–427.

Varney, N. R., Campbell, D., & Roberts, H. J. (1994). Long-term neuropsychological sequelae of fever associated with amnesia. *Archives of Clinical Neuropsychology, 9,* 347–352.

Varney, N. R., Kubu, C. S., & Morrow, L. A. (1998). Dichotic listening performances of patients with chronic exposure to organic solvents. *The Clinical Neuropsychologist, 12,* 107–112.

Voyer, D., & Flight, J. I. (2001). Reliability and magnitude of auditory laterality effects: The influence of attention. *Brain and Cognition, 46,* 397–413.

Wexler, B. E., & Halwes, R. K. (1983). Increasing power of dichotic methods: The fused rhymed word test. *Neuropsychologia, 21,* 59–66.

Wishart, H. A., Strauss, E., Hunter, M., & Moll, A. (1995). Interhemispheric transfer in multiple sclerosis. *Journal of Clinical and Experimental Neuropsychology, 17,* 937–940.

Zatorre, R. J. (1989). Perceptual asymmetry on the Dichotic Fused Rhymed Words Test and cerebral speech lateralization determined by carotid sodium Amytal test. *Neuropsychologia, 6,* 539–547.

Expressive One-Word Picture Vocabulary Test—Third Edition (EOWPVT3)

PURPOSE

The Expressive One-Word Picture Vocabulary Test—Third Edition (EOWPVT3) is designed to assess expressive vocabulary in children and adolescents.

SOURCE

The test can be ordered from Academic Therapy Publications (http://www.academictherapy.com) for $140 US. The test includes a manual, 170 test plates bound in a spiral stimulus booklet with fold-out easel, and 25 record forms. A parallel, co-normed version assessing receptive vocabulary is available (Receptive One-Word Picture Vocabulary Test; ROWPVT3). A bilingual edition for testing individuals in Spanish and English, the EOWPVT: Spanish-Bilingual Edition (EOWPVT-SBE), is available from the same source for $140 (US). Test forms and manuals can also be ordered separately, because the same test plates are used in both versions.

AGE RANGE

The EOWPVT3 is normed from age 2 years 0 months to 18 years 11 months. The EOWPVT-SBE can be used from ages 4 to 12 years.

DESCRIPTION

The EOWPVT3 (Brownell, 2000a), also known as the EOW-PVT, 2000 Edition, is a standard expressive vocabulary test that requires the child to name a picture depicting an object, action, or concept. It is the third revision of the test, which was originally published in 1979 (EOWPVT; Gardner, 1979) and revised in 1990 (EOWPVT-R; Gardner, 1990). An Upper Extension of the test was also published in 1983, for adolescents (Gardner, 1983). The new test combines the EOWPT-R and the EOWPVT Upper Extension into one test and extends the age level up to 18 years 11 months. The previous regional norms were replaced by national U.S. norms stratified according to several demographic variables (see *Normative Data*). Several items were added or replaced, and the administration was modified to allow prompting and cueing from the examiner according to specific rules. All test items now consist of full-color drawings. The test is conormed with the Receptive One-Word Picture Vocabulary Test—Third Edition (ROWPVT3; Brownell, 2000b). Sample items are shown in Figure 11–5.

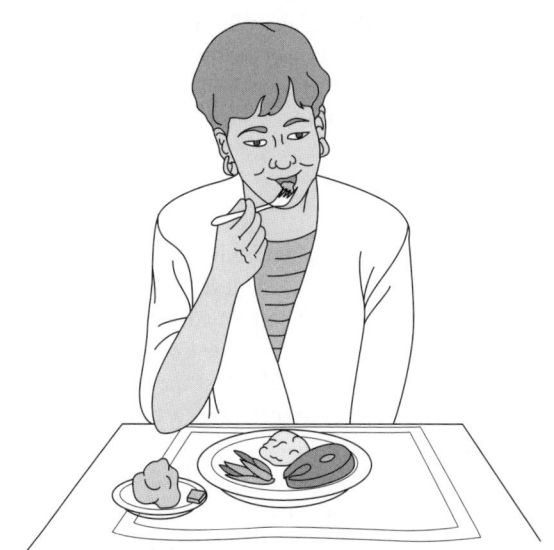

Figure 11–5 EOWPVT3 sample items. Top: Examiner prompt is, "What's she doing?" Bottom: Examiner prompt is, "What are these?" Originals presented in color. *Source:* Reprinted with permission from Brownell, 2001a.

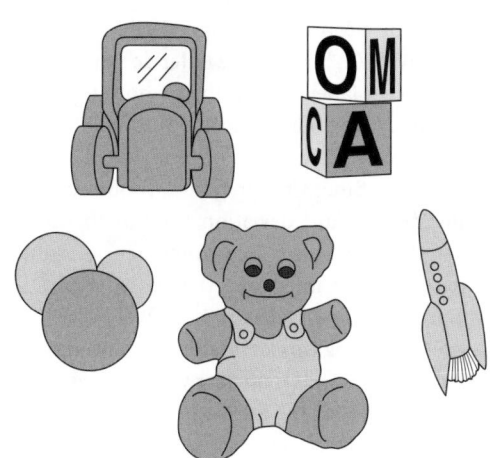

ADMINISTRATION TIME

The test takes approximately 10 to 15 min to administer and about 5 min to score.

ADMINISTRATION

See the administration manual. Testing occurs according to entry levels based on age or ability. A basal level of eight consecutive correct responses must be attained before proceeding, and a ceiling of six consecutive incorrect responses is required before discontinuing the test. Start points based on chronological age are shown on the record form.

During testing, the examiner is allowed to use specific prompts and cues to clarify examinee responses. These are listed on pages 23 to 27 of the administration manual. General instructions are also reprinted on the record form.

SCORING

Raw scores are converted to standard scores ($M = 100$, $SD = 15$), percentiles, and age equivalents. Confidence intervals, normal curve equivalents (NCEs), scaled scores, T scores, and stanines are also provided. Significance levels for difference scores comparing performance on the EOWPVT3 with that on the conormed ROWPVT3 are also provided in the manual, as are data on the frequency of occurrence of different discrepancy values. Brief interpretation guidelines for discrepancy patterns between the two tests are also provided.

Scores can be tabulated in a variety of ways, such as Correct first responses, Correct cued responses, or Incorrect first or cued responses. However, only Total correct responses (cued and noncued) are norm-referenced.

DEMOGRAPHIC EFFECTS

Age

According to information presented in the manual, smoothed raw score medians increase with age; the correlation of raw scores with age is also very high ($r = .84$; Brownell, 2000a).

Gender

Although there are no published studies on gender effects on the EOWPVT3, test development ensured that there would be no differential performance based on gender in the standardization group (see *Content Validity*). No gender differences were found on previous versions of the test (Stoner & Spencer, 1983; Wiesner & Beer, 1991).

IQ

The EOWPVT3 is reportedly highly related to IQ ($r = .88$ with Verbal, and $r = .71$ with Nonverbal), based on correlation with the Otis-Lennon School Ability Test—Seventh Edition; these data are presented in the manual (Brownell, 2000a). The previous version of the test was also highly correlated with Wechsler IQ in children ($r = .61$ to $.78$; Gardner, 1990; Kutsick et al., 1988; Wiesner & Beer, 1991).

Ethnicity

Although there are no published studies on the relationship of the EOWPVT3 to ethnicity, test development ensured that there would be no differential performance based on ethnicity/race in the standardization group (see *Content Validity*). The author is also careful to emphasize that the test measures English language vocabulary rather than a broader language-based domain.

In the previous version, ethnicity and cultural background did influence scores to some degree. For example, Peña et al. (1992) concluded that, in primarily Puerto Rican and African American children enrolled in Head Start programs, poor scores on expressive vocabulary tests requiring description (e.g., the Stanford Binet-IV Comprehension subtest) were a better indicator of probable learning disability (LD) than scores on the EOWPVT, because the latter demanded only the production of object labels, a skill that is not emphasized in all cultural groups. As a result, minority children obtained low scores on the EOWPVT, regardless of probable LD status, but not on the Stanford-Binet Comprehension subtest: only 18% scored within ± 1 standard deviation (*SD*) of the EOWPVT mean, compared with 60% for the Comprehension subtest.

In children with HIV infection, African Americans scored lower than European Americans on the EOWPVT-R, even after correction for demographic, intellectual, and disease factors (Llorente et al., 2004). It is unclear whether this difference was wholly attributable to the test or to some interaction between ethnicity and HIV status.

NORMATIVE DATA

Standardization Sample

Norms are based on the performance of 2327 individuals who were selected from a larger sample to meet demographic criteria based on 1998 U.S. Census data. Data were stratified by age, geographic region, ethnicity, level of parent education, community size, and gender. Testing was conducted in 1999 at 220 sites in 32 U.S. states. Individuals with disabilities were not excluded; a percentage of these individuals was included in the norms, and data were used for validity studies. See Table 11–20 for characteristics of the normative sample. Data are presented in intervals of 1 month (for ages 2 to 4 years), 2 months (5 to 10 years), 3 months (11 to 13 years), or 4 months (14 to 18 years).

Table 11–20 Characteristics of the EOWPVT3 Normative Sample

Sample type	National, stratified random sample
Number	2,327
Age (years)	2 years 0 months to 18 years 11 months[a]
Geographic location (%)	
Northeast	19
South	24
North Central	35
West	22
Parental education (%)	
Grade 11 or less	12
High school	33
1–3 years of college	27
4 + years of college	29
Socioeconomic status (SES)	Not specified
Gender (%)	
Males	52
Females	48
Race/Ethnicity (%)	
White	73
Black	14
Hispanic	10
Asian	2
Other	1
Screening	None[b]

[a]Based on several age groupings: 1-month intervals for ages 2–4 years, 2 months for ages 5–10 years, 3 months for ages 11–13 years, and 4 months for ages 14–18 years.
[b]90% of the sample had no disability, consistent with US Census rates for the schoolage population; the remainder had learning disability (2%), speech-language disorder (6%), mental retardation (1%), or other conditions (1%).

During standardization, the EOWPVT3 was administered first, followed by the ROWPVT3. Note that most of the standardization subjects were administered black-and-white test items, not the color items that appear in the final test version. Based on work by Hayden (1996, cited in Brownell, 2000a) and comparisons with a matched group using the color sample, stimulus type did not appear to differentially affect test scores.

Characteristics of the EOWPVT-SBE are shown in Table 11–21. Readers are referred to Brownell (2001a) for further information on the test and its conormed receptive equivalent (ROWPVT-SBE; Brownell, 2001b).

Score Derivations

Standard scores were derived by smoothing raw score distributions to remove sampling irregularities (see manual). Scores were interpolated between each of the age groups. In addition, standard score distributions for 1 year below the youngest age group and 1 year above the oldest age group in the standardization sample were extrapolated. As a result, scores from the extrapolated age bands should be used with

Table 11–21 Characteristics of the EOWPVT-Spanish-Bilingual Edition (SBE) Normative Sample

Sample type	National, stratified random sample[a]
Number	1050
Age (years)	4 to 12
Geographic location (%)	
Northeast	5
South	11
North Central	19
West	65
Hispanic Origin (%)	
Mexican	85
Puerto Rican	5
Cuban	3
Central/South American	7
Other Hispanic	1
Parental education (%)	
Grade 11 or Less	52
High school	29
1–3 Years of college	13
4+ Years of college	7
Residence (%)	
Urban	84
Rural	17
Socioeconomic status (SES)	Not specified
Gender (%)	
Males	51
Females	49
Race/Ethnicity	Not specified
Disability Status (%)	
No Disability	91
Learning Disability	4
Speech-Language Disability	3
Mentally Retarded	1
Other	<1
Screening	None

[a]Norms composition designed to reflect the U.S. Hispanic population, based on U.S. Census data from 2001.

Source: Adapted from Brownell, 2001a.

caution, because they are not based on actual data; this presumably affects age equivalents, which range all the way down to 1 year 0 months (i.e., even though 1-year-olds were not actually included in the standardization).

RELIABILITY

Internal Reliability

Coefficient alphas and split half coefficients, computed for the whole group and by age group, are uniformly high (i.e., alphas of .93 to .98, split half coefficients from .96 to .99).

Standard Error of Measurement (SEM)

The median SEM across age for the EOWPVT3 is 3.00 standard score points. SEMs by age vary from about 2 points in younger adolescents to almost 3 points in the youngest age group (age 2 years SEM = 2.97; Brownell, 2000a). Associated values for constructing confidence intervals are presented in the manual and also appear on the record form.

Test-Retest Reliability

Temporal stability was assessed using 226 subjects retested over an average interval of 20 days (Brownell, 2000a). Corrected test-retest correlations are quite high, ranging from .88 to .97 across age, with an overall coefficient of .90.

Practice Effects

The average standard score gain is about 3 points, based on a test interval of 20 days (see manual). Gains were largest in the youngest age band (e.g., almost 6 points in 2- to 4-year-olds). Additional analyses examining reliability of administration indicate that when the test is readministered to the same subject by a different examiner after a very short interval (i.e., immediately after the initial administration), scores are very highly correlated ($r = .93$) and produce the same level of practice effect (about 3 points; Brownell, 2000a).

Interscorer Reliability

Reliability of scoring, reliability of response evaluation, and reliability of administration were all found to be uniformly good (see Brownell, 2000a, for details).

VALIDITY

Content Validity

The test revision was undertaken with considerable attention to detail. This included item selection (via parent feedback and several vocabulary sources), pilot testing, initial item analysis based on classical test theory and item response theory, second testing analysis, item bias studies (i.e., item review by examiners in the standardization study, review by cultural review panel, and differential item functional analysis based on gender, residence, and race/ethnicity groups), item selection, and final item analysis of standardization data.

Comparison With Previous Editions

Correlations of the EOWPVT3 with previous editions of the EOWPVT are high, ranging from .85 (1990 edition) to .86 (1979 edition). Based on means presented in the manual, standard scores for the current version appear to be about 6 points lower than scores for both prior versions (Brownell, 2000a).

Correlations With Other Language Tests

The manual summarizes data on the test's correlations (corrected for variability) with several other vocabulary tests, including EVT ($r = .72$), PPVT-III ($r = .76$), ROWPVT3 ($r = .72$ to .75), WISC-III Vocabulary ($r = .86$), Stanford Binet-IV Vocabulary ($r = .83$), and SAT9 Vocabulary ($r = .67$), along with several others. These are based on scores of individuals in the standardization sample who were also administered these tests ($n = 19$ to 67, excluding ROWPVT3 correlations that include the entire sample). The median corrected correlation for these tests was .79; correlations with expressive vocabulary tests were not much different than those with receptive tests (e.g., median $r = .81$ versus .76; Brownell, 2000a). Of note, 56% of the variance is shared between the EOWPVT3 and the ROWPVT3 (Brownell, 2000a).

Correlations with broader language measures such as the CELF-3 Expressive, Receptive, and Total Language scores are also high ($r = .85$ to .87; Brownell, 2000a). Correlations with other language batteries (e.g., TACL-R, TOLD-P) are also presented in the manual and are generally strong (median correlation for total scores = .76). However, using the previous version of the test, others have found that the EOWPVT is not necessarily a good predictor of conversational language performance measured by specific scores such as mean length of utterance (Ukrainetz & Blomquist, 2002). Similarly, the previous version showed moderate correlations with measures of lexical diversity in children (Silverman & Ratner, 2002). Notably, the expressive and receptive tests show approximately equivalent associations with expressive speech sample variables, with correlations being mostly in the moderate range ($r = .32$ to .46; Ukrainetz & Blomquist, 2002).

Correlations With Achievement

Correlations with academic achievement indicate a high degree of association between EOWPVT3 and reading and language composite scores. For example, the test is highly correlated with the WJ-R Reading composite ($r = .85$, corrected), with a median correlation of .64 to .75 for other achievement batteries (see Brownell, 2000a, for additional details). Data on the test's relationship to other achievement domains are lacking.

Correlations With IQ

In healthy children, the test is highly related to IQ ($r = .88$ with Verbal, $r = .71$ with Nonverbal), based on correlation to the Otis-Lennon School Ability Test—Seventh Edition presented in the manual (Brownell, 2000a).

The previous version of the test was also highly correlated with IQ in young children ($r = .69$, WPPSI-R; Gardner, 1990). In special education students, the previous version of the test was highly correlated with FSIQ as measured by the WISC-R ($r = .61$; Wiesner & Beer, 1991). In younger children with language delay, the EOWPVT was also highly correlated with WPPSI FSIQ ($r = .78$; Kutsick et al., 1988).

Clinical Studies

The manual presents means and SDs on the EOWPVT3 for a large clinical sample ($N = 1,023$) consisting of children with mental retardation, autism, language delay, expressive/receptive language disorder, behavior disorder, LD, hearing loss, auditory processing deficit, attention-deficit/hyperactivity disorder (ADHD), articulation disorder, and fluency disorder. Compared with the standardization mean, all groups had significantly lower EOWPVT3 scores, with the exception of those with ADHD, articulation, or fluency disorders. Because naming problems are not expected in ADHD and the latter two groups represent children with speech production deficits (not language disorders per se) this finding provides evidence of construct validity for the test (Brownell, 2000a).

Given its recent publication date, there are as yet no independent published studies on clinical groups. However, prior versions of the test have demonstrated clinical sensitivity and have shown evidence of ecological validity. This includes sensitivity to effects of cholinergic medications in autistic children (Chez et al., 2004) and to growth in vocabulary development in children with cochlear implants (El-Hakim et al., 2001). It has also been used in studies of the effects of amino acid supplementation in autism (Chez et al., 2002), speech and language outcome after hemispherectomy (Eisele & Aram, 1993; Stark et al., 1995), and in children with psychiatric and behavior disorders (Giddan et al., 1996; Ruhl et al., 1992). The test has also provided evidence of subtle language dysfunction in children who stutter (Silverman & Ratner, 2002), to which receptive language measures such as the PPVT-R are less sensitive, and it has served to differentiate minority children with probable LD from non-LD children using dynamic therapy (i.e., test-teach-retest methodology) aimed at increasing exposure to labeling strategies (Peña et al., 2002).

Because environments with limited language exposure have been linked to later language delays, the test has also been used in studies tracking language development in at-risk children of teen mothers, where the EOWPVT has been found to correlate moderately with home ratings and other markers of effective caregiving ($r = .38$ to .42). In a study of minority children enrolled in Head Start, the test, combined with dynamic assessment, has been used to help differentiate children who are unable to meet classroom demands (academically at-risk) from those with bona fide language disorders (Peña et al., 1992). In the early literacy intervention program Reach Out and Read (ROR), which provides books to disadvantaged children during inner-city pediatric clinic visits, EOWPVT-R scores were related to the number of visits and books given (Theriot et al., 2003; but see Sharif et al., 2002). ROR benefits also appear to be "dose related," in that each additional ROR visit was associated with a 0.2-point increase in EOWPVT scores (Mendelsohn et al., 2001). Using the EOWPVT-R, researchers have also found that mothers of language-impaired preschoolers accurately predict their performance on the test, but that mothers of normally developing children overestimate their child's performance (Evans & Wodar, 1997).

COMMENT

The EOWPVT3 is a well-designed, well-standardized test that is much improved compared to its predecessor. The norms, in particular, are comprehensive and are described in considerable detail. (The previous version was associated with possible score inflation [Ukrainetz & Blomquist, 2002]). The manual is well written and includes a useful discussion of vocabulary testing and its inherent limitations. The revised methodology, which allows the examiner to give prompts and cues according to set rules, is a definite improvement over the previous version, which at times tended to confuse some children—for instance, when a single word was required for items comprising multiple pictures. The record form is also well designed and is more sophisticated than that of the previous version; it now includes test instructions, examiner cues/prompts, and values for constructing confidence intervals.

The test is of considerable utility to neuropsychologists, and it is preferred for assessing children over other naming tests constructed with less psychometric rigor and less comprehensive norms (e.g., Boston Naming Test). Although studies on the new test are yet to be published, prior versions were used in a number of studies documenting its sensitivity and utility in the clinical evaluation of expressive vocabulary in children. Many of these also provide impressive evidence of the test's ecological validity.

Traditionally, the test was also used to predict verbal intelligence (Gardner, 1979). For example, regression equations to this effect were published by Vance et al. (1989) for predicting WPPSI scores from a combination of EOWPVT and PPVT-R scores. However, little mention of this use is apparent in the more recent literature. Given its high correlation with IQ-based verbal subtests such as WISC Vocabulary, it would be helpful to have additional evidence that the test adds unique information to the assessment of language disorders. Additionally, more evidence is needed that the test (either by itself or in combination with other tests) can distinguish between childhood disorders involving language. The fact that it is conormed with the ROWPVT3 confers an advantage over other expressive vocabulary tests; however, evidence concerning the utility of expressive/receptive test score comparisons in diagnostic evaluations is mixed.

Users should always administer the EOWPVT3 test before any receptive or other vocabulary test, to avoid score inflation by exposure to similar items (Llorente et al., 2000). Indeed, tests such as the PPVT-III, although conceptually similar and possibly requiring similar strategies and similar activation of language abilities, also share a number of identical items with the EOWPVT-R. Llorente et al. (2000) noted that some items also employ almost identical drawings.

Use of age equivalents to describe performance is not recommended, given the psychometric limitations of this metric and evidence of a lack of agreement among vocabulary tests when this score type is used (Howlin et al., 1994).

Users should be aware that individuals from various cultures who perform below normative standards on the test may simply be "language-different" rather than language-disordered (Peña et al., 1992). In findings reviewed by Peña et al. (1992), certain ethnic/cultural groups may differ in terms of the extent to which they (1) use factual questions or rehearsal when interacting with children; (2) use commands, nonspecific labels, and object functions rather than object labels; (3) talk about babies rather than at babies; or (4) show low demand for use of object labels compared with descriptions of objects. Overall, some cultures may de-emphasize labeling, the main functional language skill measured by the EOWPVT3. As a result, minority children tested with the EOWPVT3 (or other similar tests) may be inappropriately identified as being at risk for language or learning problems, even if modifications are made to allow for cultural/linguistic differences (e.g., bilingual examiners, response coding in either language, use of alternate acceptable responses based on the cultural group; Peña et al., 2002).

Similarly, Ukrainetz and Blomquist (2002) cautioned that scores on vocabulary tests such as the EOWPVT might be expected to be associated with specific functional aspects of daily language use in children, such as performance on worksheet assignments, but would not necessarily predict performance in other areas, such as social communicative exchanges or written imaginative narrative. Finally, it is important to note that the EOWPVT3, by definition, includes only the subset of words that can be illustrated.

REFERENCES

Brownell, R. (2000a). *Expressive One-Word Picture Vocabulary Test—Third Edition manual.* Novato, Calif.: Academic Therapy Publications.

Brownell, R. (2000b). *Receptive One-Word Picture Vocabulary Test—Third Edition manual.* Novato, Calif.: Academic Therapy Publications.

Brownell, R. (2001a). *Expressive One-Word Picture Vocabulary Test Spanish-Bilingual Edition manual.* Novato, Calif.: Academic Therapy Publications.

Brownell, R. (2001b). *Receptive One-Word Picture Vocabulary Test Spanish-Bilingual Edition manual.* Novato, Calif.: Academic Therapy Publications.

El-Hakim, H., Levasseur, J., Papsin, B. C., Panesar, J., Mount, R. J., Stevens, D., & Harrison, R. V. (2001). Assessment of vocabulary development in children after cochlear implantation. *Archives of Otolaryngology and Head and Neck Surgery, 127,* 1053–1059.

Eisele, J. A., & Aram, D. M. (1993). Differential effects of early left hemisphere damage on lexical comprehension and production. *Aphasiology, 7*(5), 513–523.

Evans, M. A., & Wodar, S. (1997). Maternal sensitivity to vocabulary development in specific language-impaired and language-normal preschoolers. *Applied Psycholinguistics, 18*(3), 243–256.

Gardner, M. F. (1979). *Expressive One-Word Picture Vocabulary Test.* Novato, Calif.: Academic Therapy Publications.

Gardner, M. F. (1983). *Expressive One-Word Picture Vocabulary Test Upper Extension manual.* Navato, Calif.: Academic Therapy Publications.

Gardner, M. F. (1990). *Expressive One-Word Picture Vocabulary Test— Revised.* Novato, Calif.: Academic Therapy Publications.

Giddan, J. J., Milling, L., & Campbell, N. B. (1996). Unrecognized language and speech deficits in preadolescent psychiatric inpatients. *American Journal of Orthopsychiatry, 66*(1), 85–92.

Howlin, P., & Cross, P. (1994). The variability of language test scores in 3- and 4-year-old children of normal non-verbal intelligence: A brief research report. *European Journal of Disorders of Communication, 29*(3), 279–288.

Kutsick, K., Vance, B., Schwarting, F., & West, R. (1988). A comparison of three different measures of intelligence with preschool children identified at-risk. *Psychology in the Schools, 25*(3), 270–275.

Llorente, A. M., Sines, M. C., Rozelle, J. C., Turcich, M. R., & Casatta, A. (2000). Effects of test administration order on children's neuropsychological performance: Emerging one-word expressive and receptive language skills. *The Clinical Neuropsychologist, 14*(2), 162–172.

Llorente, A. M., Turcich, M., & Lawrence, K. A. (2004). Differences in neuropsychological performance associated with ethnicity in children with HIV-1 infection: Preliminary findings. *Applied Neuropsychology, 11*(1), 47–53.

Luster, T., & Vandenbelt, M. (1999). Caregiving by low-income adolescent mothers and the language abilities of their 30-month old children. *Infant Mental Health Journal, 20*(2), 148–165.

Mendelsohn, A. L., Mogilner, L. N., Dreyer, B. P., Forman, J. A., Weinstein, S. C., Broderick, M., Cheng, K. J., Magloire, T., Moore, T., & Napier, C. (2001). The impact of a clinic-based literacy intervention on language development in inner-city preschool children. *Pediatrics, 107*(1), 130–134.

Peña, E. Quinn, R., & Iglesias, A. (1992). The application of dynamic methods to language assessment: A nonbiased procedure. *The Journal of Special Education, 26*(3), 269–280.

Ruhl, K. L., Hughes, C. A., & Camarata, S. M. (1992). Analysis of the expressive and receptive language characteristics of emotionally handicapped students served in public school settings. *Journal of Childhood Communication Disorders, 14*(2), 165–176.

Sharif, I., Reiber, S., Ozuah, P. O., & Reiber, S. (2002). Exposure to Reach Out and Read and vocabulary outcomes in inner-city preschoolers. *Journal of the National Medical Association, 94*(3), 171–177.

Silverman, S., & Ratner, N. B. (2002). Measuring lexical diversity in children who stutter: Application of *vocd. Journal of Fluency Disorders, 5222*, 1–16.

Stoner, S., & Spencer, W. (1983). Sex differences in expressive vocabulary of Head Start children. *Perceptual and Motor Skills, 56*(3), 1008.

Theriot, J. A., Franco, S. M., Sisson, B. A., Metcalf, S. C., Kennedy, M. A., & Bada, H. S. (2003). The impact of early literacy guidance on language skills of 3-year-olds. *Clinical Pediatrics, 42*, 165–172.

Ukrainetz, T. A., & Blomquist, C. (2002). The criterion validity of four vocabulary tests compared with a language sample. *Child language teaching and therapy, 18*(1), 59–78.

Vance, B., West, R., & Kutsick, K. (1989). Prediction of Wechsler Preschool and Primary Scale of Intelligence IQ scores for preschool children using the Peabody Picture Vocabulary Test-R and the Expressive One-Word Picture Vocabulary Test. *Journal of Clinical Psychology, 45*(4), 642–644.

Wiesner, M., & Beer, J. (1991). Correlations among WISC-R IQs and several measures of receptive and expressive language for children referred for special education. *Psychology Reports, 69*(3), 1009–1010.

Expressive Vocabulary Test (EVT)

PURPOSE

The Expressive Vocabulary Test (EVT) is designed to assess expressive vocabulary.

SOURCE

The test kit can be ordered from American Guidance Services (http://www.agsnet.com) for $170 US. This includes forms, stimulus booklet, and examiner's manual. The test can also be purchased in combination with the PPVT-III, with which it is conormed. Scoring software (ASSIST) costs $200 US.

AGE RANGE

EVT norms extend from ages 2½ to 90 + years.

DESCRIPTION

Overview

The EVT (Williams, 1997) is an individually administered, untimed, standardized test that assesses vocabulary via two tasks: (a) labeling and (b) synonyms. Word retrieval can be evaluated by comparing EVT performance with that on the PPVT-III (Dunn & Dunn, 1997), a receptive vocabulary test with which it is conormed.

According to the author, the EVT serves several purposes, but its primary goals are to serve as a screening test for expressive language difficulties and to measure English proficiency in persons for whom English is a second language (the latter usage should be noted on the test form; Williams, 1997). Traditionally, single-word, expressive vocabulary tests such as the EVT have been considered of considerable utility in the assessment of language difficulties. Unlike vocabulary tests found in most IQ batteries, which require lengthy explanations of word meanings, these tests allow examiners to assess vocabulary skills relatively uncontaminated by broader deficits in expressive language (Williams, 1997). Moreover, in contrast to receptive vocabulary tests, they may also be considered useful for evaluating word-finding difficulties in neuropsychological evaluations. Receptive vocabulary tests such as the PPVT-III employ recognition formats that provide information on an individual's lexical store but shed no light on whether the individual can actually retrieve the word from the lexical store

(Williams, 1997). Failure on the EVT in the context of adequate PPVT-III performance therefore suggests an inability to retrieve words from the lexical store (Williams, 1997).

Test Structure

The test consists of 4 practice items and 190 test items requiring knowledge of either a noun, a verb, or an adjective. The first 38 items require labeling; the examiner points to a picture and the examinee must provide a one-word response. The next 52 items are synonym items; the examinee is presented with either a word or a spoken phrase and must provide the corresponding word. Synonym items are also presented with pictures in order to provide contextual cues. See Figure 11–6 for a sample item. According to the author, the synonym task was included because of ceiling effects associated

Figure 11–6 Sample item from the Expressive Vocabulary Test (EVT). *Source:* Reprinted with permission from Williams, 1997.

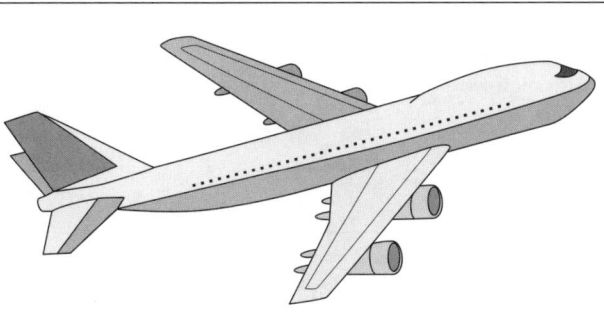

FOR AGES 5 TO ADULT

Example 3

Say: *I am going to show you a picture and say a word. You are to tell me another word that means the same thing and goes with the picture. Your answer must be only one word.*

Or, because of the examinee's age or level of understanding, you may say: *I am going to show you a picture and say a name for it. You are to tell me another name for the picture. You must say only one thing.*

Point to the picture of the jet and say: *Jet. Tell me another word* [name] *for jet.*

Teach:
If the examinee responds correctly with "airplane" or "plane," reinforce the correct response by saying: *That's right. Plane* [airplane] *is another word for jet.*

If the examinee responds incorrectly or does not respond, teach the correct response by saying: *Plane is another word for jet.*

Continue with Example 4.

with labeling tasks and because synonyms allow a range of possible correct answers instead of a single correct response (Williams, 1997).

ADMINISTRATION TIME

According to the manual, the test takes 10 to 25 min to administer.

ADMINISTRATION

See manual. Testing starts according to entry levels based on age or ability and continues until a basal and a ceiling are established. A basal is established with five consecutive correct items; a ceiling is obtained with five consecutive incorrect items (the "five and five rule"; Williams, 1997).

Although the test is not timed, individuals should be encouraged to respond after 10 s. The examiner may use specific prompts (see manual) to encourage responding. Items may also be repeated. To facilitate the transition from labeling to synonym items, low-level synonym items are actually easier than high-level labeling items (Williams, 1997). When both tests are given, the EVT should be administered after the PPVT-III, as was done during the standardization [see *Comment*].

SCORING

To score the test, examiners can refer to a list of the most common correct and incorrect responses for each item, listed on the record form (in blue and orange, respectively), and to the manual for a complete listing of correct and incorrect responses by item. Poor pronunciation and articulation errors are not penalized.

Raw scores are converted to standard scores ($M = 100$, $SD = 15$), percentiles, and age equivalents. Confidence intervals, normal curve equivalents (NCEs), and stanines are also provided. Significance levels for difference scores comparing performance on the EVT with that on the PPVT-III are provided in the EVT manual (Williams, 1997), as are data on the frequency of occurrence of various discrepancy values. Standard scores range from 40 to 160. Procedures taken to derive standard scores are described in detail on page 63 of the manual. Age equivalents are available for ages 1 year 9 months to 22 years. Note that age equivalents below age 2 years 6 months are based on extrapolation and should be used with caution (Dunn & Dunn, 1997).

DEMOGRAPHIC EFFECTS

Age

EVT performance increases steadily with age, with the most rapid growth in the early years, a more gradual change in later years, and a slight decrease after age 50 (Williams, 1997).

Gender

There are no reported gender effects on the test (Williams, 1997).

IQ

Like most vocabulary tests, the EVT correlates highly with IQ across the age range (Williams, 1997; see *Validity*).

Education

EVT scores were not related to maternal education in a group of New Zealand preschoolers (Reese & Read, 2000) or in a group of preschoolers in Wyoming that included normal and language-impaired children (Gray et al., 1999). However, more research is needed in this area, given large effects of maternal education on vocabulary tests such as the PPVT-III (see *PPVT-III* review in this volume).

Ethnicity

Apart from small studies with limited power that found few effects (e.g., Gray et al., 1999), there have been no studies on the effect of ethnicity on test scores. Specific steps to avoid bias in test items were taken during standardization (see *Validity*).

NORMATIVE DATA

Standardization Sample

The test was normed on a stratified sample of 2725 individuals, selected to match 1994 U.S. Census data, at 240 testing sites in the United States. Standardization occurred in 1995 to 1996. Norms were stratified according to gender, education level, race/ethnicity, geographic location, and percentage of subjects with disabilities (Williams, 1997). See Table 11–22 for sample characteristics.

RELIABILITY

Internal Consistency

Split-half coefficients for each age band, derived from a Rasch ability estimate based on the actual items taken by each examinee, are uniformly high (median $r = .91$, range = .83 to .97; Williams, 1997). Coefficient alphas, also derived by Rasch simulation, are also very high (median = .95, range = .90 to .98; Williams, 1997).

Standard Error of Measurement (*SEM*)

The median *SEM* across age is 4.6, with a range of 2.6 (ages 41–50 years, 61 + years) to 6.2 (age 5 years; Williams, 1997). Therefore, as expected, confidence intervals would be larger for younger children than for adults.

Table 11–22 Characteristics of the EVT Normative Sample

Sample type	National stratified randomized sample
Number	2725[a]
Age	2 years 6 months to 90+ years
Geographic location (%)	
Northeast	19
South	33
North Central	29
West	20
Parent or Examinee Education[b] (%)	
Grade 11 or Less	17
High School	31
1–3 Years of College	31
4+ Years of College	20
Socioeconomic status (SES)	Education was used as an SES marker
Gender (%)	
Males	47
Females	53
Race/Ethnicity (%)	
African American	18
Hispanic	13
White	64
Other	5
Screening	None[c]

[a]Based on several age groupings: 2-month intervals for ages 2 years 6 months to 6 years, 3 months for ages 7–18 years, 2 years for ages 19–24 years, and multiyear intervals for adults (25–30, 31–40, 41–50, 51–60, and 61–90+ years).
[b]Parental education was used for persons 24 years of age and younger; the examinee's education level was used for ages 25 years and older.
[c]Individuals in special education categories were included in the standardization sample as follows (14.2% of sample): learning disability (6%), speech impairment (2%), mental retardation (1%), hearing impairment (<1%), gifted/talented (3%), adults with mental retardation 25 years of age or older (2%).

Test-Retest Reliability

All coefficients reported in the manual, corrected for restriction of range, are in the adequate to very high range. Specifically, temporal stability was assessed using 226 subjects in four age groups, with retesting after a mean of 42 days (range, 8–203 days). Reliabilities were .77, .84, .90, and .96, respectively, for the four age groups: 67 preschoolers (ages 2 years 6 months to 5 years 11 months), 70 schoolage children (ages 6 years to 10 years 11 months), 51 adolescents (ages 12 years to 17 years 11 months), and 38 adults (26 years to 57 years 11 months (Williams, 1997).

Reese and Read (2000) explored long-term reliability in New Zealand preschoolers who were tested at ages 2 years 8 months and 3 years 4 months. Test-retest reliability of EVT raw scores was strong, given the age at testing and the time interval ($r = .79$; Reese & Read, 2000). Note that at testing EVT preceded PPVT-III, whereas at retest, PPVT-III preceded EVT, with a 1-week interval between EVT and PPVT-III.

Practice Effects

Practice effects are relatively small on the EVT, at least after intervals of about 42 days. Preschoolers and adolescents gain less than 3 standard score points at retesting, whereas schoolaged children and adults gain between 3 and 4 points (Williams, 1997).

Interscorer Reliability

Gray et al. (1999) reported 99.1% agreement for EVT scoring in preschoolers.

VALIDITY

Content Validity

Test development of EVT content was rigorous and extensive, and care was taken to eliminate sources of bias in test items. Words in common usage reflecting typical life experiences were chosen from several sources—among them, spoken word frequency counts, reading vocabulary sources, and *Merriam-Webster's Collegiate Thesaurus* (Williams, 1997). Two pilot studies in 1993 were used to develop an item pool and evaluate the assessment approach; a national tryout occurred in 1994, simultaneously with the PPVT-III (including item analysis and bias review), and standardization was completed in 1996. Rational item analysis was provided by a panel of independent consultants representing African Americans, Asian Americans, Hispanic Americans, Native Americans, and women.

Correlations With Other Language Tests

In every study reviewed, the EVT is highly correlated with its co-normed companion test, the PPVT-III. In the standardization sample, correlations with the PPVT-III at each age level are generally high, with a range of .61 to .88 (median correlations of .79 and .77 for PPVT forms IIIA and IIIB; Williams, 1997), with the highest correlations tending to occur in adults. Reese and Read (2000) reported an EVT/PPVT-IIIA correlation of .60 at age 2 years 8 months in New Zealand preschoolers and EVT/PPVT-IIIB correlation of .69 at age 3 years 4 months. Similar values have been reported in North American preschoolers ($r = .75$, Ukrainetz & Blomquist, 2002; $r = .54$, Gray et al., 1999) and in clinical groups such as children with autism ($r = .51$, Condouris et al., 2003) and preschoolers with speech and language impairments ($r = .57$, Gray et al., 1999).

The EVT appears to be highly correlated with a variety of vocabulary tests, regardless of modality (expressive versus receptive), norm base (conormed versus separately normed), or age. The manual reports that correlations with expressive language tasks are higher than those with receptive language tasks in normal children on the Oral and Written Language Scales (OWLS; $r = .47$ to .86; Williams, 1997). However, others have reported similarly high correlations with both receptive and expressive vocabulary tests such as the ROWPVT and EOWPVT-R ($r = .66$

and .79, respectively; Ukrainetz & Blomquist, 2002) and with the PPVT-III (discussed earlier). Correlations with language subtests and composites from the CELF are also moderately high in children with autism (.40 to .58; Condouris et al., 2003).

Correlations with other kinds of measures of language competence also support the EVT's construct validity. This includes moderate correlations with natural language samples in typically developing children (Ukrainetz & Blomquist, 2002) and in children with autism (Condouris et al., 2003) and with a parent-reported scale of vocabulary level for preschoolers ($r = .50$; Reese & Read, 2000).

Correlations With Non-Language Domains (Discriminant Validity)

Although the test is presumed to measure primarily language competence, studies on the contribution of non-language cognitive domains to performance are lacking, apart from data presented in the manual that suggests a lesser (but not negligible) association of nonverbal intelligence with test performance compared to verbal intelligence (Williams, 1997; see later discussion).

Correlations With IQ

Correlations with FSIQ were high across age in a subset of the standardization sample including children ($r = .68$, WISC-III), adolescents ($r = .66$, KAIT), and adults ($r = .84$, K-BIT; Williams, 1997). In children, correlation with VIQ are higher than with PIQ ($r = .72$ versus .56, WISC-IIII), but in adults and adolescents, correlations with KAIT and K-BIT do not necessarily support a verbal/nonverbal dichotomy (Williams, 1997).

Correlations With Achievement

To our knowledge, there is as yet no information on the test's correlation with tests of achievement or with markers of achievement such as school grades.

Clinical Studies

As evidence of further validity, the manual describes EVT performance for a number of clinical groups compared with matched controls (Williams, 1997). Lower EVT performance was found in groups of children defined as having either language delay, language impairment, or reading disability. Speech-impaired children (i.e., with stuttering or articulation problems) did not score significantly lower on the EVT than matched controls. Gifted children obtained significantly higher scores than controls ($M = 118.7$, $SD = 10.4$), with similarly high scores on the PPVT-III. Children and adolescents with mental retardation scored significantly lower than matched controls (64.8 versus 101.9), as did adults with mental retardation (47.0 versus 99.2). In children and adults with mental retardation, PPVT-III scores tended to be about 10 to 11 points higher than EVT scores (Williams, 1997).

The author concludes, based on significant group differences for groups with language difficulties (delay or impairment), that the EVT is "therefore a good screening device for language impairment" (Williams, 1997, p. 78). However, the means obtained by the clinical groups with language difficulties are not low from any clinical standard, which makes it difficult to see how the test could be used clinically to identify language impairments in children unless an extremely high (i.e., normal) clinical cutoff score was used to define impairment. For instance, the mean performance for children with language delay was 92.7 (compared with 100.8 for the control subjects). Similarly, children with language impairment obtained a mean score of 94.7 (versus 104.2 for controls). The same problem occurs in children with reading disability, who, as a group, obtained a mean EVT score of 98.8 (versus 105.2 for controls); PPVT-IIIA scores were also well within normal (i.e., 104.7), albeit significantly lower than the control mean. The author concludes that "measuring an individual's vocabulary knowledge could contribute to the understanding and assessment of reading skills or difficulties" (Williams, 1997, p. 80). The data actually suggest otherwise—that, on average, children with reading disability obtain scores in the normal range on the EVT. These data raise questions about the test's sensitivity to language delay, language impairment, and reading disability.

Misgivings about the test's utility as a screening device for preschoolers were also noted by Gray et al. (1999), who reported similar values for a speech-language impairment group. In this study involving 62 children, half of whom had clinician-confirmed language impairments, most of the children with speech and language impairments scored within the normal range on vocabulary tests, including the EVT. The EVT's ability to detect speech-language impairments was not high; even though preschoolers with language impairment had an average mean that was lower than that of their normal-language peers, there was considerable overlap in the distribution of scores ($M = 92$ and 104, respectively). EVT sensitivity, specificity, positive predictive validity, false negative rate and false positive rate were 70%, 68%, 70%, 16%, and 15%, respectively. Adjusting the cutoff to obtain the best classification accuracy resulted in a cutoff value that far exceeded the standard for impairment used in clinical practice (i.e., < 1.5 SDs below the normative mean). The test with the highest identification rate was the EOWPVT-R; however, even its identification rate was not high (i.e., only 13/31 children with language impairment had scores < 1.5 SD below the mean).

Condouris et al. (2003) found that children with autism performed better on standardized measures such as the EVT and PPVT-III than on measures derived from natural language samples, due to deficits in pragmatic language use. The mean score of their autism group on the EVT was 84.02 ($SD = 19.19$).

Receptive-Expressive Discrepancies

The utility of using PPVT-III/EVT expressive/receptive discrepancies to detect word-finding difficulties, which are assumed to

be of higher frequency in language-impaired individuals, is not well supported by empirical research, at least in children. Gray et al. (1999) found that PPVT-III/EVT receptive > expressive discrepancies of greater than 1 SD were common in a normal language group (32%, compared with 19% in a language-impaired group). A low rate was also found for EOWPVT-R/ROWPVT discrepancy comparisons (i.e., 7/31 versus 2/31). Notably, the counterintuitive pattern of expressive > receptive was relatively rare with the PPVT-III/EVT combination in both normal and speech impaired children (3/31 and 2/31, respectively), but not with the ROWPVT/EOWPVT-R, on which 32% (10/31) of speech-impaired children showed the pattern. Note that, in another study using the PPVT-R, not a single child was found to have a receptive-only language deficit (Lahey et al., 1999). However, because early CNS injury/abnormality often results in global language impairments in young children, expressive/receptive discrepancies may be of more clinical utility in adults with acquired language deficits. Actual research on the clinical utility of using discrepancies involving the EVT in adults is lacking.

COMMENT

Like the PPVT-III, the EVT is a well-constructed, psychometrically sound test for assessing expressive vocabulary. It has several assets: careful construction and standardization; a large, representative normative group including individuals of various ethnic backgrounds and a subset of individuals with disabilities (see McFadden, 1996, for a discussion of this broader issue), good reliability; adequate ceilings and floors despite the broad age range; and strong criterion validity, at least with regard to correlations with other language tests.

Despite these obvious strengths, it is not clear that the EVT is especially sensitive to language difficulties (whether defined as delay or impairment), at least in the populations in which this question has been studied (i.e., preschoolers and children). Although significant differences have been demonstrated in comparisons with controls, group means for clinical conditions affecting language are not unduly low in studies published to date; in fact, most are within normal limits. Although this does not exclude the possibility that a subset of children with language difficulties does very poorly on the test, difficulties arise when the test is used as a screening instrument, because the EVT, like the PPVT-III and other vocabulary tests, does not show high sensitivity or positive predictive power. Although better results are expected in older children and adults, there is no research yet supporting this proposal.

Comparing EVT and PPVT-III performance to assess word retrieval may be problematic, at least in children, in whom the question has been studied [see *Validity*]. Gray et al. (1999) concluded that comparing receptive and expressive vocabulary scores in children can be misleading because discrepancies are relatively frequent in normal children; consequently, supporting data must be provided for any test that claims to identify word-finding problems using a discrepancy method. Such data have not yet been provided for the EVT/PPVT-III or for any other test combination professing to assess word retrieval (e.g., EOWPVT/ROWPVT). Further, Gray et al. (1999) concluded that, in preschoolers, interpretation of vocabulary competence may depend on the test used.

According to the EVT manual, the PPVT-III was administered before the EVT during standardization of both instruments; to be precise, both forms of the PPVT-III (IIIA and IIIB) were administered to each subject before the EVT was administered. Note that Llorente et al. (2000) found carryover effects when a receptive test (PPVT-R) was administered before an expressive vocabulary test (EOWPVT). How changes to the standard procedure (such as administering the EVT in isolation or preceded by a receptive vocabulary test other than the PPVT-III) might affect scores is unknown.

The EVT is an interesting test in that, unlike standard vocabulary tests requiring single-word answers (e.g., BNT), there is a range of possible correct answers that can be given for items. Although this has not yet been studied, it is possible that this response format confers an advantage when assessing ethnically diverse populations, given research suggesting that different ethnic and linguistic communities may not place high value on "labeling" skills per se (see PPVT-III and EOWPVT3 reviews, in this volume). More research on the clinical sensitivity and rationale for synonym items would be beneficial.

REFERENCES

Condouris, K., Meyer, E., & Tager-Flusberg, H. (2003). The relationship between standardized measures of language and measures of spontaneous speech in children with autism. *American Journal of Speech-Language Pathology, 12,* 349–358.

Dunn, L. M., & Dunn, L. M. (1997). *Examiner's manual for the Peabody Picture Vocabulary Test Third Edition.* Circle Pines, Minn.: American Guidance Service.

Gray, S., Plante, E., Vance, R., & Henrichsen, M. (1999). The diagnostic accuracy of four vocabulary tests administered to preschool-age children. *Language, Speech, and Hearing Services in Schools, 30,* 196–206.

Lahey, M., & Edwards, J. (1999). Naming errors of children with specific language impairment. *Journal of Speech, Language, and Hearing Research, 42,* 195–205.

Llorente, A. M., Sines, M. C., Rozelle, J. C., Turcich, M. R., & Casatta, A. (2000). Effects of test administration order on children's neuropsychological performance: Emerging one-word expressive and receptive language skills. *The Clinical Neuropsychologist, 14*(2), 162–172.

McFadden, T. U. (1996). Creating language impairments in typically achieving children: The pitfalls of "normal" normative sampling. *Language, Speech, and Hearing Services in Schools, 27,* 3–9.

Reese, E., & Read, S. (2000). Predictive validity of the New Zealand MacArthur Communicative Development Inventory: Words and sentences. *Journal of Child Language, 27,* 255–266.

Ukrainetz, T. A., & Blomquist, C. (2002). The criterion validity of four vocabulary tests compared with a language sample. *Child Language Teaching and Therapy, 18*(1), 59–78.

Williams, K. T. (1997). *Expressive Vocabulary Test.* Circle Pines, Minn.: American Guidance Service.

Multilingual Aphasia Examination (MAE)

PURPOSE

The Multilingual Aphasia Examination (MAE) provides a relatively brief examination of the presence, severity, and qualitative aspects of aphasic language disorders.

SOURCE

The MAE (Third Edition) is available from Psychological Assessment Resources, P.O. Box 998, Odessa, FL 33556 (http://www.parinc.com), at a price of $379 US for the complete set, including manual, picture books, set of tokens and letter, and 100 record forms. A Spanish version (Examen de afasiia multilingue-S or MAE-S) is available from the same source for $249 US. There are French, Spanish and German translations of the MAE (Second Edition). These are available from AJA Associates, 504 Manor Drive, Iowa City, IA 52246.

AGE RANGE

The test can be used with children aged 6 to 12 years and with adults aged 16 to 97 years.

DESCRIPTION

The MAE does not claim to follow a specific model of language function, although it covers the most common aspects of language function affected in aphasia. It includes nine subtests and two rating scales (see Table 11–23). There are three tasks that assess different aspects of oral expression—visual naming, sentence repetition, and verbal fluency (the Controlled Oral Word Association or COWA); one that assesses verbal comprehension of commands (the Token Test—an abbreviated version of the DeRenzi-Vignolo 1962 version); two that assess aural and written comprehension; and three that evaluate oral, written, and block spelling. Speech articulation and the fluency-nonfluency dimension of expressive speech are rated. Oral, written, and block spelling tasks use three interchangeable lists of 11 words. An alternate version of Sentence Repetition, COWA, and the Token Test is available for repeat assessment.

Two MAE subtests (COWA and the Token Test) have generated considerable literature in their own right and have also been incorporated into other cognitive batteries (e.g., Mayo norms; Ivnik et al., 1996). The reader is referred to descriptions of the COWA elsewhere in this volume (see *Verbal Fluency*).

Table 11–23 Description of MAE Subtests and Rating Scales

Subtest/Scale	Description
Visual Naming	Requires naming of line drawings or parts thereof (e.g., telephone, telephone dial; 30 items, each scored as 0, 1 or 2 points
Sentence Repetition	Requires the repetition of 14 sentences of increasing length up to 22 syllables; vocabulary and syntax are deliberately simple, but interrogative, negative, and other forms are included
Controlled Oral Word Association	Word generation to three letters (CFL, PRW, see *Verbal Fluency* for a detailed discussion of this subtest)
Oral Spelling	The word is presented, then presented again in a sentence, and the patient must spell it orally (11 words)
Written Spelling (to dictation)	The word is presented, then presented again in a sentence, and the patient must write it (11 words)
Block Letter Spelling	Plastic letters are spread in front of the patient, who then must use these letters to spell the word (11 words)
Token Test	Consists of 22 commands at two levels of complexity (e.g., "Point to a large yellow square"), each scored as 0, 1 or 2 points.
Aural Comprehension of Words and Phrases	The patient must point to one of four choices of line drawings on six plates corresponding to the word or phrase (e.g., "dog under the table");18 items
Reading Comprehension of Words and Phrases	Reading Comprehension is also administered in a multiple-choice format: A set of words and phrases is presented in written form (capital block letters), the patient must point to the appropriate choice on the same six plates used in the previous test.
Rating of Articulation	Articulation is rated immediately on completion of the other tests on a 9-point scale, ranging from 0 ("speechless or usually unintelligible speech") to 8 ("normal speech").
Rating of Praxis Features of Writing	Praxis features of writing are rated after completion of the written spelling test for imprecision, distortion, and legibility on a 9-point scale; scores range from 0 ("illegible scrawl") to 8 ("good penmanship").

Initially, standardization data were available for the English version (Benton & Hamsher, 1978). Subsequent revisions included additional data on the performances of elderly subjects and patients with brain disease (Benton & Hamsher, 1989; Benton et al., 1994). As its name implies, the MAE was conceived as a test battery consisting of functionally equivalent forms in different languages.

The Spanish version (Rey & Benton, 1991, Rey et al., 1999) contains the same subtests, but items and wordings are rephrased appropriately for individuals of Cuban, Mexican, and Puerto Rican origin. For example, COWA uses the letters P, T, and M, reflecting similar levels of difficulty in Spanish. Hence, performance of the task in each language is functionally equivalent; that is, the different language versions of the MAE are functionally equivalent in content rather than being simple translations.

ADMINISTRATION

See *Source.*

ADMINISTRATION TIME

Approximately 40 min or less is required. The Spanish manual suggests an administration time of 20 min in nonaphasic individuals.

SCORING

Scoring is fully described in the source and is relatively simple and straightforward. Of the nine tests, two (Sentence Repetition, COWA) require corrections for age and educational level and six require correction for education only. The MAE Token

Table 11–24 MAE Scoring Adjustments

Subtest	Education (Years)	Score Adjustment
Visual Naming	<9	+8
	9–11	+6
	12–13	+4
	14–15	+2
Sentence Repetition		
Age 25–59 years	6–8	+3
	9–11	+2
	12–1	—
	16+	—
Age 60–69 years	6–8	+4
	9–11	+3
	12–15	+1
	16+	—
COWA		
Age 25–54 years	<9	+9
	9–11	+5
	12–15	+3
	16+	—
Age 55–59 years	<9	+10
	9–11	+7
	12–15	+4
	16+	+1
Age 60–69 years	<9	+12
	9–11	+9
	12–15	+6
	16+	+3
Spelling		
Male	8–11	+2
	12+	—
Female	8–11	+1
	12+	—
Aural Comprehension	8–11	+1
	12+	—
Reading Comprehension	8–11	+1
	12+	—

Source: Adapted from Benton et al., 1994.

Test does not require corrections, according to the authors. The scoring adjustments are shown in Table 11–24. The test comes with scoring sheets for each subtest and a summary sheet that provides space for percentiles (compared to healthy controls and to patients with aphasia).

DEMOGRAPHIC EFFECTS

Age

Borderline adult performance is reached at about age 12 years 3 months, although values for the Token Test and COWA approach plateau values starting at age 10 years (Schum et al., 1989). The test manual discusses studies of norms for elderly subjects and concludes that no noteworthy decline in performance has been found up to age 79 years, but that subnormal performance, especially on the Sentence Repetition and the Token Test, is "not rare" for subjects 80 to 89 years of age, perhaps because of the demands of these tests on memory (see also Schum & Sivan, 1997). In older adults, correlations with age tend to be small (< .30) for both COWA and the Token Test (Ivnik et al., 1996; Lucas et al., 2005).

Education

Education has a stronger effect than age on COWA scores ($r = .38$ to .42) and Token Test scores ($r = .24$ to .32; Elias et al., 1997; Ivnik et al., 1996; Lucas et al., 2005; Steinberg et al., 2005), with performance improving at higher educational levels. For the Token Test, education becomes redundant when IQ is taken into account (Steinberg et al., 2005). IQ and test scores are less strongly associated at the higher ends of the IQ continuum (Steinberg et al., 2005).

Gender

Schum and Sivan (1997) found no gender differences among older adults on the MAE. Similarly, Ivnik et al. (1996) and Lucas et al. (2005) reported little effect of gender on COWA and Token Test scores. Elias et al. (1997) found that gender accounted for only 1% of the variance for COWA in a sample of 1893 community residents. In this sample, the oldest participants with the fewest years of education had the lowest performance on COWA, with lower levels for men than for women.

Ethnicity/Acculturation

Ethnicity affects test scores. Roberts and Hamsher (1984) found lower norm values for Visual Naming in an urban inner-city black population. They argued that Visual Naming may be especially sensitive to cultural experience, and that separate normative data should be obtained for this population. Kennepohl et al. (2004) found that lower levels of acculturation were linked to lower scores on the Token Test among African Americans who had sustained a traumatic brain injury (TBI).

There do not appear to be nationality effects (i.e., Puerto Rican versus Mexican) on the Spanish version of the test (MAE-S; Rey et al., 1999).

NORMATIVE DATA

Standardization Sample

The MAE manual provides normative data (in the form of percentiles) based on a sample of 360 normal Iowa adults (aged 16–69 years) whose native language was English and who were without evidence or history of neurological disability (see Table 11–25). A second sample of 50 aphasic patients is included and may be used to discern aphasic subtypes.

Table 11–25 Characteristics of the MAE Standardization Samples

Number	Adults: 360 Children: 229
Age (years)	Adults: 16–69 (mean age not reported) Children: 6–12
Geographic location	Iowa
Sample type	Adults: not reported Children: attending three schools in Iowa
Education	Adults: Not reported
Gender	Adults: not reported Children: 98 males, 131 females
Race/Ethnicity	Not reported
Screening	Adults: no evidence or history of neurological disease, mental retardation, or hospitalization for psychiatric disorder
	Children: screened to exclude those receiving special education or diagnosed with a learning disability; included only those with PPVT-R standard scores between 80 and 120

The manual also includes normative information for 229 children (98 males, 131 females), aged 6 to 12 years, drawn from three Iowa elementary schools, and based on a study by Schum et al., (1989). All children were from rural areas or small towns. Intelligence was assessed with the PPVT-R, and only those with standard scores between 80 and 120 were included. Children receiving special education services and those diagnosed as learning disabled were excluded.

The MAE-S manual includes normative information from a sample of 234 normal Spanish-speaking adults from Texas and Puerto Rico (aged 18 to 70 years) without history or evidence of neurological or psychiatric disability. Cutoff values based on this normative group are reported to be quite comparable to those of the English version (Rey et al., 1999).

Other Normative Data

Schum and Sivan (1997) examined 54 older adult volunteers, residing in a college community in Iowa, who had above-average education (about 15 years) and self-ratings of good or very good health. Table 11–26 presents the mean performance on the MAE subtests, subdivided by age group. Individual MAE subtest scores were adjusted for education levels when necessary, in accordance with specifications in the MAE manual (Benton et al., 1994). For Sentence Repetition and COWA, adjustments were made using the highest available age category (60–69 years) and educational level. Only Sentence Repetition showed a significant decline across the four age groups. There was also a slight, but not statistically significant, decline in performance on the Token Test. Note, however, that the cell sizes were very small and the participants reflected a highly selected group of older adults.

More extensive normative data are available for the COWA and the Token Test. The reader is referred to *Verbal Fluency* with regard to the COWA. Ivnik et al. (1996) provided age- and education-corrected scores for the Token Test for use with older adults, aged 56 to 95 + years. Note that these norms were derived from a large sample (399) of Caucasian individuals living in an economically advantaged region of the United States. Their data are shown in Table 11–27, along with an equation to adjust scores for education level. Midpoint intervals were used to maximize the available information. The MOANS norms have a mean of 10 and an *SD* of 3. The authors cautioned that the validity of these norms for persons of other ethnic/cultural or socioeconomic backgrounds is questionable.

Steinberg et al. (2005) have expanded the utility of the MOANS project by providing age- and IQ-adjusted percentile equivalents of MOANS Age-adjusted Token Test scores, for use with individuals aged 55+. Users should note that all FSIQs are MAYO age-adjusted scores, which are based on the WAIS-R, not the WAIS-III. Given the upward shift in scores (Flynn effect) with the passage of time, use of the WAIS-R

Table 11–26 MAE Tests and Descriptive Data (Mean and *SD*) by Age Group

Test	70–74 (*n* = 15)	75–79 (*n* = 22)	80–84 (*n* = 10)	85–90 (*n* = 7)	Total (*N* = 54)
Visual Naming	53.9 (4.7)	53.6 (4.3)	51.6 (5.8)	52.6 (6.0)	53.2 (4.9)
Sentence Repetition	12.7 (1.2)	12.1 (1.2)	11.0 (1.7)	10.3 (1.8)	11.9 (1.6)
COWA	47.7 (10.8)	42.4 (12.1)	43.3 (14.3)	44.4 (13.5)	44.3 (12.2)
Oral Spelling	10.6 (0.6)	10.5 (1.2)	10.7 (0.7)	10.7 (0.8)	10.6 (0.9)
Written Spelling	10.9 (0.3)	10.5 (0.6)	10.8 (0.4)	10.9 (0.4)	10.7 (0.5)
Block Spelling	10.7 (0.6)	10.1 (1.3)	10.4 (1.1)	10.4 (1.0)	10.3 (1.1)
Token Test	42.9 (1.7)	42.4 (1.6)	41.6 (2.8)	40.3 (3.3)	42.1 (2.2)
Aural Comprehension	17.9 (0.3)	17.6 (0.7)	17.8 (0.4)	17.6 (0.8)	17.7 (0.6)
Written Comprehension	17.9 (0.4)	17.9 (0.3)	17.9 (0.3)	18.0 (0.0)	17.9 (0.3)
Articulation	7.9 (0.3)	7.9 (0.5)	8.0 (0.0)	7.9 (0.4)	7.9 (0.4)
Writing	7.9 (0.4)	7.6 (0.7)	7.9 (0.3)	7.6 (0.8)	7.7 (0.6)

Source: Adapted from Schum & Sivan, 1997.

Table 11–27 Token Test MOANS Norms for Persons (Predominantly Caucasian) Aged 56–97 Years

Percentile Ranges	56–62	63–65	66–68	69–71	72–74	75–77	78–80	81–83	84–86	87–89	90–97	Scaled Score
n	94	94	94	94	130	178	227	230	204	140	88	
<1	<29	<29	<29	<29	<29	<29	<24	<19	<18	<18	<17	2
1	29–30	29–30	29–30	29–30	29–30	29–30	24–28	19–23	18–22	18–20	17	3
2	31–32	31–32	31–32	31–32	31	31	29	24–28	23–27	21–27	18–19	4
3–5	33–35	33–35	33–35	33–35	32–35	32–34	30–33	29–31	28–30	28–29	20–25	5
6–10	36	36	36	36	36	35	34	32–33	31–33	30–32	26–32	6
11–18	37–38	37–38	37–38	37–38	37	36–37	35–36	34–35	34–35	33–34	33–34	7
19–28	39	39	39	39	38–39	38	37	36–37	36	35–36	35–36	8
29–40	40–41	40–41	40–41	40–41	40	39–40	38	38	37	37	37	9
41–59	42	42	42	42	41–42	41–42	39–41	39–41	38–41	38–40	38–40	10
60–71	43	43	43	43	43		42	42	42	41–42	41	11
72–81	44	44	44	44	44	43–44	43	43	43	—	42	12
82–89							44	44	44	43	43	13
90–94										44	44	14
95–97												15
98												16
99												17
>99												18

Note: Based on Mayo's Older Normative Studies (MOANS). Age- and Education-corrected MOANS Scaled Score ($\text{MSS}_{\text{A\&E}}$) is calculated from a person's age-corrected MOANS Scaled Score (MSS_A) and that person's education expressed in years of formal schooling completed as follows: $\text{MSS}_{\text{A\&E}} = 0.47 + (1.33 \times \text{MSS}_A) - (0.31 \times \text{Education})$. Mean FSIQ about 106, range: 76–138.

Source: Adapted from Ivnik et al., 1996. Reprinted with the kind permission of Psychology Press.

FSIQ rather than the WAIS-III might result in a given Token Test score appearing less favorable.

Lucas et al. (2005) recently provided age- and education-adjusted normative data based on 289 African American, community-dwelling participants from the MOAANS (Mayo Older African Americans Normative Studies) project in Jacksonville, Florida. Participants were predominantly female (74%), ranged in age from 56 to 94 years ($M = 69.6$, $SD = 6.87$), and varied in education from 0 to 20 years of formal education ($M = 12.2$, $SD = 3.48$). They were screened to exclude those with active neurological, psychiatric, or other conditions that might affect cognition. Table 11–28a presents their data, and Table 11–28b provides the computational formula used to calculate age- and education-adjusted MOAANS scaled scores. The authors urged that their data be used with caution, because the number of very old adults is somewhat small and they used a sample of convenience that may not represent the full range of cultural and educational experiences of the African American community.

RELIABILITY

Internal Consistency

This is not reported.

Test-Retest Reliability

This is not reported.

Alternate-Form Reliability

There are no differences between Forms A and B for Sentence Repetition, COWA, or the Token Test (Schum & Sivan, 1997). There are also no differences for the three alternate spelling lists for the Oral, Written, and Block Spelling tests (Benton & Hamsher, 1989; Schum et al., 1989; Schum & Sivan, 1997).

VALIDITY

Correlations With Other Tests

The Visual Naming subtest correlates highly with the 60-item BNT ($r = .76$ to $.86$; Axelrod et al., 1994; Schefft et al., 2004) and moderately with the language domain of the NEPSY ($r = .42$; Korkman et al., 1998). Axelrod et al. (1994) reported that Visual Naming showed strong relations to the WAIS-R verbal-comprehension factor but only minimal relations to the perceptual-organization and distractibility factors. Lincoln et al. (1994) used test performances on the MAE to better understand performances on the WAIS-R in a sample of patients with closed-head injury. WAIS-R Verbal subtests were correlated most strongly with MAE Visual Naming, with the exception of Digit Span and Arithmetic, which were correlated more closely with performance on MAE Sentence Repetition. As might be anticipated, WAIS-R Performance subtests showed lesser degrees of correlation with the MAE, but they showed modest correlations with the MAE Token Test and COWA.

Table 11-28a MOAANS Age-Based Norms for Token Test in African American Adults

Scaled Score	56–62	63–65	66–68	69–71	72–74	75–77	78+	Percentile Ranges
2	0–19	0–19	0–19	0–19	0–19	0–19	0–19	<1
3	20–26	20–25	20–25	20–25	20–25	20–25	20–25	1
4	27–29	26–27	26–27	26–27	26–27	26–27	26–27	2
5	30–32	28–30	28–30	28–30	28–30	28–30	28–30	3–5
6	33–36	31–35	31–35	31–34	31–34	31–34	31–34	6–10
7	37–38	36–38	36–37	35–37	35–37	35–37	35–37	11–18
8	39–40	39–40	38–39	38–39	38	38	38	19–28
9	41	41	40–41	40	39–40	39–40	39	29–40
10	42–43	42	42	41–42	41–42	41	40	41–59
11	—	43	43	43	43	42	41–42	60–71
12	—	—	—	—	—	43	43	72–81
13	44	44	44	44	44	—	—	82–89
14	—	—	—	—	—	44	44	90–94
15	—	—	—	—	—	—	—	95–97
16	—	—	—	—	—	—	—	98
17	—	—	—	—	—	—	—	99
18	—	—	—	—	—	—	—	>99
n	101	121	157	172	147	113	76	

Source: Adapted from Lucas et al., 2005. Reprinted with the permission of the Mayo Foundation for Medical Education and Research.

Factor Structure

A factor analysis of 16 aphasia battery subtests (including subtests of the MAE, NCCEA, and the WAB), given to healthy Taiwanese volunteers (Hua et al., 1997), suggested a major factor of verbal comprehension (including Token Test, Sentence Repetition, Digit Repetition, Visual Naming, Reading, and Aural Comprehension). A second factor was labeled effortful writing. A third factor involved mainly verbal expression and word production.

Clinical Studies

The MAE (particularly the Token Test) is sensitive to language disorders. Jones and Benton (1995) evaluated the sensitivity of the MAE in aphasics with focal left-hemisphere lesions and normal controls. The aphasic group performed poorly on all subtests of the MAE relative to the controls. Using the suggested cutoffs, between 2.6% and 7.0% of normal subjects and between 14.4% and 64.6% of aphasics were misclassified by individual subtests. All aphasics and 15% of controls performed poorly on at least one MAE subtest. Using a cutoff of two defective performances, 96% of aphasics, but only 3% of controls, performed poorly. The implication is that diagnosis should not be based on individual subtests. Other research has examined the use of both MAE performance and clinical features of aphasics' language (e.g., paraphasias in conversational speech, *conduite d'approche*) to provide an MAE differential diagnosis of aphasic subtypes (K. Hamsher, personal communication, 1988).

As might be expected, patients with left temporal lobe epilepsy (TLE) showed significant impairment on the MAE (and on tests of verbal learning) compared with those with right TLE (Hermann & Wyler, 1988; Hermann et al., 1992). However, the Boston Naming Test (BNT) is diagnostically more sensitive than the Visual Naming subtest of the MAE in identifying left TLE (Schefft et al., 2003), perhaps because it is considerably easier than the BNT and also tends not to elicit paraphasias. O'Shea et al. (1996) found that self-report of memory problems in patients with TLE compared with controls was related only to COWA, but not to other MAE subtests.

The MAE Token Test has been shown to be a sensitive indicator of acute confusional states (delirium) in nonaphasic medical patients (Lee & Hamsher, 1988). Whether low verbal fluency forecasts a diagnosis of probable Alzheimer's disease is uncertain (Elias et al., 2000). Measures of retention of information (e.g., Logical Memory retained) and abstract reasoning (WAIS Similarities) are more powerful predictors (Elias et al., 2000).

Patients who have sustained head injuries also show language difficulties on the MAE. Levin et al. (1976, 1981) examined the linguistic performance of patients with closed-head injuries, reporting a high frequency of naming errors, defective

Table 11–28b Computational Formula for Age- and Education-corrected MOAANS Scaled Scores

	K	W_1	W_2
Token Test	0.67	1.23	0.23

Note: Age- and education-corrected MOAANS Scaled Scores (MSS$_{A\&E}$) can be calculated for Token Test scores by using age-corrected MOAANS Scaled Scores (MSS$_A$) and education (expressed in years completed) in the following formula: MSS$_{A\&E}$ = K + ($W_1 \times$ MSS$_A$) – ($W_2 \times$ EDUC).

Source: From Lucas et al., 2005.

associative word-finding, and impaired comprehension on the Token Test; these findings were correlated with severity of head injury. Millis et al. (2001) described similar findings in a longitudinal study of persons with TBI who received inpatient rehabilitation, and Rey et al. (2001) reported similar findings in Hispanics after TBI using the Spanish version of the MAE. Articulatory difficulties were also noted after TBI (Levin, 1981; Rey et al., 2001).

Language-related difficulties evident on the MAE may affect memory performance. Crosson et al. (1993) reported that, in patients who sustained head injury, visual object naming (Visual Naming) and auditory comprehension (Token Test) were predictive of total number of words recalled (but not percent retained) on the California Verbal Learning Test. The implication is that examiners should explore language deficits as a cause of performance deficits on verbal memory tasks.

In a study of 26 children (Schum et al., 1989), 13 of 15 children with dyslexia performed defectively on the reading and spelling tests, and 6 performed poorly on the COWA; 1 of 4 stutterers had defective performance on Visual Naming, and 2 of them performed poorly on Controlled Word Association and the MAE Token Test. Six of seven children with expressive language disorder performed defectively on the MAE.

COMMENT

The MAE is a relatively short aphasia battery. One strength of the MAE is the availability of a carefully constructed Spanish version. Further, measures of naming and auditory comprehension may be particularly useful in the evaluation of head-injured individuals in an attempt to understand verbal memory measures (Crosson et al., 1993). For example, when language deficits do emerge, indexing delayed recall to initial learning (e.g., percent recall) may give an estimate of verbal memory ability that is less influenced by language abilities.

Unfortunately, the MAE normative group is poorly described, and the information is dated (see *Verbal Fluency* for additional COWA normative data). The availability of more recent norms for elderly subjects is a positive sign; however, for most of the tasks, the normative sample was small, very well educated, and from the midwestern United States. Accordingly, caution is advised in applying these norms, particularly to individuals whose characteristics differ. Baron (2004) presented some additional, previously unpublished normative data for children; however, the characteristics of these samples were not reported. Clinicians and researchers are referred to other measures (e.g., CELF-4), which have better psychometric properties, including a more extensive and more current normative base.

Further, the lack of reliability information presents a serious obstacle for use of the MAE in clinical diagnosis. In addition, there are ceiling effects for most of the tasks, and misclassifications regarding the presence or absence of language disturbance do occur when using individual subtests. Greater confidence is justified when the tests are used in combination or along with clinical features of aphasic speech (e.g., paraphasias).

Comments on the clinical interpretation of each subtest can be found at the end of each section in the test manual, but validity information is not fully explained. For instance, we learn that Controlled Word Association is most impaired in patients with left frontal lobe lesions (no documentation given); that Visual Naming and Sentence Repetition showed a correlation of .39 in a patient group otherwise undefined; and that Visual Naming and Controlled Word Association showed a correlation of .56 in 42 patients. The question as to whether Aural Comprehension adds significantly to the information provided by the Token Test is raised and argued but is not answered with documentation.

REFERENCES

Axelrod, B. N., Ricker, J. H., & Cherry, S. A. (1994). Concurrent validity of the MAE Visual Naming Test. *Archives of Clinical Neuropsychology, 9,* 317–321.

Baron, I. S. (2004). *Neuropsychological evaluation of the child.* New York: Oxford University Press.

Benton, A. L., & Hamsher, K. (1978). *Multilingual Aphasia Examination: Manual of instructions.* Iowa City, Ia.: AJA Associates.

Benton, A. L., & Hamsher, K. (1989). *Multilingual Aphasia Examination—Second Edition.* Iowa City, Ia.: AJA Associates.

Benton, A. L., Hamsher, K. de S., Rey, G. J., & Sivan, A. B. (1994). *Multilingual Aphasia Examination* (3rd ed.). Iowa City, IA: AJA Associates.

Crosson, B., Cooper, P. V., Lincoln, R. K. & Bauer, R. M. (1993). Relationship between verbal memory and language performance after blunt head injury. *Clinical Neuropsychologist, 7,* 250–267.

De Renzi, E., & Vignolo, L. (1962). The Token Test: A sensitive test to detect receptive disturbances in aphasics. *Brain, 85,* 665–678.

Elias, M. F., Beiser, A., Wolf, P. A., Au, R., White, R. F., & D'Agostino, R. B. (2000). The preclinical phase of Alzheimer disease: A 22-year prospective study of the Framingham cohort. *Archives of Neurology, 57,* 808–813.

Elias, M. F., Elias, P. K., D'Agostino, R. B., Silbershatz, H., & Wolf, P. A. (1997). Role of age, education, and gender on cognitive performance in the Framingham Heart Study: Community-based norms. *Experimental Aging Research, 23,* 201–235.

Hermann, B. P., Seidenberg, M., Haltiner, A., & Wyler, A. R. (1992). Adequacy of language function and verbal memory performance in unilateral temporal lobe epilepsy. *Cortex, 28,* 423–433.

Hermann, B. P., & Wyler, A. R. (1988). Effects of anterior temporal lobectomy on language function. *Annals of Neurology, 23,* 585–588.

Hua, M. S., Chang, S. H., & Chen, S. T. (1997). Factor structure and age effects with an aphasia test battery in normal Taiwanese adults. *Neuropsychology, 11,* 156–162.

Ivnik, R. J., Malec, J. F., & Smith, G. E. (1996). Neuropsychological tests' norms above age 55: COWAT, BNT, MAE, WRAT-R Reading, AMNART, STROOP, TMT and JLO. *Clinical Neuropsychologist, 10,* 262–278.

Jones, R. D., & Benton, A. L. (1995). Use of the Multilingual Aphasia Examination in the detection of language disorders [Abstract]. *Journal of the International Neuropsychological Society, 1,* 364.

Kennepohl, S., Shore, D., Nobors, N., & Hanks, R. (2004). African American acculturation and neuropsychological test performance following traumatic brain injury. *Journal of the International Neuropsychological Society, 10,* 566–577.

Korkman, M., Kirk, U., & Kemp, S. (1998). *NEPSY: A Developmental Neuropsychological Assessment manual.* San Antonio, Tex.: The Psychological Corporation.

Lee, G. P., & Hamsher, K. (1988). Neuropsychological findings in toxicometabolic confusional states. *Journal of Clinical and Experimental Neuropsychology, 10,* 769–778.

Levin, H., Grossman, R. G., & Kelly, P. J. (1976). Aphasic disorders in patients with closed-head injury. *Journal of Neurology, Neurosurgery, and Psychiatry, 39,* 1062–1070.

Levin, H., Grossman, R. G., Sarwar, M., & Meyers, C. A. (1981). Linguistic recovery after closed head injury. *Brain and Language, 12,* 360–374.

Lincoln, R. K., Crosson, B., Bauer, R. M., Cooper, P. V., & Velozo, C. A. (1994). Relationship between WAIS-R subtests and language measures after blunt head injury. *The Clinical Neuropsychologist, 8,* 140–152.

Lucas, J. A., Ivnik, R. J., Smith, G. E., Ferman, T. J., Willis, F. B., Petersen, R. C., & Graff-Radford, N. R. (2005). Mayo's Older African Americans Normative Studies: Norms for Boston Naming Test, Controlled Oral Word Association, Category Fluency, Animal Naming, Token Test, WRAT-3 Reading, Trail Making Test, Stroop Test, and Judgment of Line Orientation. *The Clinical Neuropsychologist, 19,* 243–269.

O'Shea, M. F., Saling, M. M., Bladin, P. F., & Berkovic, S. F. (1996). Does naming contribute to memory self-report in temporal lobe epilepsy? *Journal of Clinical and Experimental Neuropsychology, 18,* 98–109.

Millis, S. R., Rosenthal, M., Novack, T. A., Sherer, M., Nick, T. G., Kreutzer, J. S., High, W. M., & Ricker, J. H. (2001). Long-term neuropsychological outcome after traumatic brain injury. *Journal of Head Trauma Rehabilitation, 16,* 343–355.

Rey, G. J., & Benton, A. L. (1991). Examen de Afasia Multilingue. Iowa City, Ia.: AJA Associates.

Rey, G. J., Feldman, E., Hernandez, D., Levin, B. E., Rivas-Vasques, R., Nedd, K. J., & Benton, A. L. (2001). Application of the Multilingual Aphasia Examination—Spanish in the evaluation of Hispanic patients post closed-head trauma. *Clinical Neuropsychologist, 15,* 13–18.

Rey, G. J., Feldman, E., Rivas-Vasques, R., Levin, B. E., & Benton, A. (1999). Neuropsychological test development and normative data on Hispanics. *Archives of Clinical Neuropsychology, 14,* 593–601.

Roberts, R. J., & Hamsher, K. (1984). Effects of minority status on facial recognition and naming performance. *Journal of Clinical Psychology, 40,* 539–545.

Schefft, B. K., Testa, S. M., Dulay, M. F., Privitera, M. D., & Yeh, H. S. (2003). Preoperative assessment of confrontation naming ability and interictal paraphasia in unilateral temporal lobe epilepsy. *Epilepsy and Behavior, 4,* 161–168.

Schum, R. L., & Sivan, A. B. (1997). Verbal abilities in healthy elderly adults. *Applied Neuropsychology, 4,* 130–134.

Schum, R. L., Sivan, A. B., & Benton, A. L. (1989). Multilingual Aphasia Examination: Norms for children. *The Clinical Neuropsychologist, 3,* 375–383.

Steinberg, B. A., Bieliauskas, L. A., Smith, G. E., Langellotti, C., & Ivnik, R. J. (2005). MAYO's Older Americans Normative Studies: Age- and IQ-adjusted norms for the Boston Naming Test, the MAE Token Test, and the Judgement of Line Orientation Test. *The Clinical Neuropsychologist, 19,* 280–328.

Peabody Picture Vocabulary Test—Third Edition (PPVT-III)

PURPOSE

The Peabody Picture Vocabulary Test—Third Edition (PPVT-III) is designed to assess receptive vocabulary.

SOURCE

The test kit can be ordered from American Guidance Services (http://www.agsnet.com) for $300 US. This includes two sets of forms (IIIA and IIIB), stimulus booklets, norms booklets, and examiner's manuals. The test can also be purchased in combination with the Expressive Vocabulary Test (EVT), with which it is conormed. Scoring software (ASSIST) can be obtained for $200 US. The Technical References manual, which outlines test development and psychometrics in further detail, can be obtained from the publishers at an extra cost of about $50 US.

A Spanish version of the previous, revised edition (i.e., PPTV-R), the Test de Vocabulario en Imagenes Peabody (TVIP), is also available for assessing Spanish-speaking and bilingual children and adolescents (Dunn et al., 1986).

AGE RANGE

PPVT-III norms extend from ages 2½ to 90 + years; TVIP norms extend to age 17 years 11 months.

DESCRIPTION

Background

The PPVT-III (Dunn & Dunn, 1997) is the third edition of the PPVT, one of the oldest and most commonly used standardized tests (Stockman, 2000), originally published in 1959 (Dunn, 1959) and revised in 1981 (PPVT-R; Dunn & Dunn, 1981). The original PPVT had two forms comprising 150 items each and had limited norms. The PPVT-R contained 175 items per form and was nationally normed. Compared with the PPVT-R, the PPVT-III differs in several ways, including more test items per form, extended age norms, and updated illustrations. Additionally, it is conormed with the EVT (Williams, 1997). Despite these improvements, the PPVT-R continues to be used frequently, particularly in longitudinal, large-scale studies in the United States and Canada (e.g., Brooks-Gunn et al., 2003; Padilla et al., 2002; To et al., 2004).

Test Overview

Like its predecessors, the PPVT-III is an individually administered, untimed, norm-referenced test of receptive vocabulary that employs a multiple-choice, nonverbal response format. Specifically, the examiner says a word and the examinee must

Figure 11–7 Sample item from the PPVT-III. *Source:* Reprinted with permission from Dunn et al., 1997.

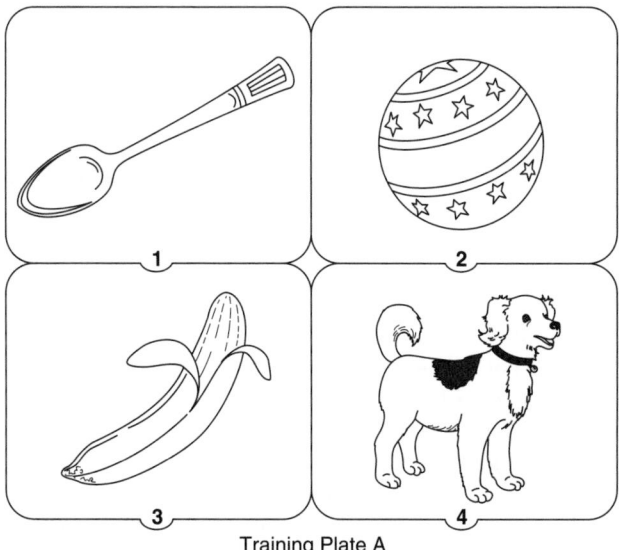

Training Plate A

select, by pointing, the corresponding picture in an array of four black-and-white illustrations (see Figure 11–7 for a sample item). The test consists of 4 practice items and 204 test items grouped into 17 sets of 12 items, arranged in order of difficulty. Each item within a 12-item set is arranged with the three easiest items first, and the next three easiest items last, so as not to begin or end item sets with failures. The test is available in two alternate forms of equivalent difficulty (IIIA and IIIB). Items for the PPVT-III were selected to represent gerunds, nouns, and adjectives, using 20 categories such as actions, animals, body parts, school/office equipment, buildings and outdoor structures, clothing, emotions, foods, workers, household objects.

Uses of the Test

According to the authors, the PPVT-III serves several purposes. Its primary goals are to serve as an achievement test of receptive vocabulary attainment for standard English and as a screening test of verbal ability. It is also considered a screening test of intellectual functioning (Dunn & Dunn, 1997). According to the test authors, it can be used to test preschool children because it is easy to administer and "highly reliable," even at the youngest ages, to screen for verbal ability when English is the primary language, to screen for giftedness and mental retardation in English speakers, and to measure English proficiency in persons for whom English is a second language. It also can be used for establishing and restoring rapport, because it is appealing and does not expose the examinee to failure. Because of its nonverbal aspect and limited requirement for examiner interaction, it is also appropriate for nonreaders, individuals with written output problems, those with severe expressive language impairments, and those who have difficulty interacting with others (e.g., autism, withdrawal, psychosis). Other advantages are that formal training in psychometrics is

not required to administer the test, which is an asset for large-scale research studies. At the same time, the authors caution that the test is a screening device only; a more comprehensive evaluation is required for diagnostic purposes.

The PPVT-R has also been computerized for use during neurophysiological testing involving ERPs (Connolly et al., 1995; D'Arcy et al., 2003; Marchand et al., 2002) to assess individuals with left-hemisphere stroke and other neurological conditions.

PPVT-III Versus PPVT-R

About 54% of words were retained from the PPVT-R in the PPVT-III, and 46% are new. However, because many illustrations were also updated, only about 30 items are actually identical in both instruments (i.e., 7%). The PPVT-III also contains more action words than its predecessors, with almost half the items representing people or body parts (Dunn & Dunn, 1997). Artwork is designed to include representations of different races and a balanced gender representation, as well as persons with physical differences. See *Comment* for further discussion of PPVT-III/PPVT-R differences based on normative composition.

Stockman (2000) noted that more words are sampled at each age with the PPVT-III than with the PPVT-R. The PPVT-III samples a minimum of 12 words per age level, with an average of almost 26 words per age level; in comparison, there are as few as 5 words at some PPVT-R age levels. At times, the same word is sampled at different ages, but usually at an older age on the PPVT-III (e.g., "pedal" is found at age 6 years 5 months in the PPVT-R, but at age 10 to 11 years in PPVT-III; Stockman, 2000). In addition, words in the PPVT-III tend, on average, to have a higher frequency of usage than those in the PPVT-R (Stockman, 2000). Even when the same word is used in both tests, different picture stimuli, or different foils, may be presented; out of 97 identical words, only 6 use the same picture in both the PPVT-III and PPVT-R). Additionally, as noted earlier, there is a different lexical composition in the two tests, with many more verbs in the PPVT-III.

There are also differences in how the two alternate PPVT-III forms relate to the PPVT-R. Form IIIA has the largest overlap with PPVT-R items (97 items in common, compared with only 3 items for Form IIIB; Stockman, 2000). Therefore, the PPVT-III Form IIIA shares a 47% overlap with PPVT-R, but IIIB overlaps only 1.5% (Stockman, 2000).

ADMINISTRATION TIME

According to the authors, the test takes 11 to 12 min to administer. Testing time ranged from 8 to 16 min for two thirds of the standardization sample (Dunn & Dunn, 1997).

ADMINISTRATION

Standard Administration Procedure

See the Administration Manual. Testing occurs according to entry levels based on age or ability and continues until a basal set and a ceiling set are established. A basal set is established with the lowest set of consecutive items containing one or no errors; a ceiling set is established with a set containing eight incorrect responses. All items within a set are administered before moving on to the next set. Most individuals require about five sets or 60 items (Dunn & Dunn, 1997) before discontinuation.

According to the manual, the PPVT-III was administered before the EVT during standardization of both instruments. Test order should be maintained when using these tests clinically (see *Comment* for further discussion).

Although a pronunciation guide is provided on the record form, examiners are urged to become familiar with the pronunciations of all the words employed before initiating testing, particularly of upper-level words. Although the test is not timed, individuals should be encouraged to choose a response after 15 s.

Modified Administrations

The standard administration can be modified for use in special populations. For example, the authors note that persons with severe cerebral palsy can signal "yes" or "no" as the examiner points to each picture (Dunn & Dunn, 1997). Use of eye gaze as an alternate response mode may be an acceptable alternative in patients with severe motor or language impairments (Spillane et al, 1996).

SCORING

Raw scores are converted to standard scores ($M = 100$, $SD = 15$), percentiles, and age equivalents. Confidence intervals, normal curve equivalents (NCEs), and stanines are also provided. Significance levels for difference scores comparing performance on the PPVT-III with that on the EVT are provided in the EVT manual (Williams, 1997), as are data on the frequency of occurrence of various discrepancy values. Standard scores range from 40 to 160. Age equivalents are available for ages 1 year 9 months to 22 years. Age equivalents below age 2 years 6 months are based on extrapolation and should be used with caution (Dunn & Dunn, 1997). Ideally, confidence intervals should be constructed around obtained scores and used to interpret test performance (see *Standard Error of Measurement (SEM)*).

Because of inherent differences in test format, the manual presents a correction factor for transforming raw PPVT-R scores to raw PPVT-III scores. However, PPVT-III standard scores tend to remain higher even after the correction factor is applied (see *Validity*).

DEMOGRAPHIC EFFECTS

Age

PPVT-III performance increases steeply in the preschool and elementary school years, grows steadily but at a lesser rate until age 22, and remains stable until age 56, after which it begins to decline slightly (Dunn & Dunn, 1997). Note that these trends are based on cross-sectional analyses; longitudinal studies are needed to confirm them, particularly with regard to age-related declines.

Gender

There are no reported gender effects on the test (Dunn & Dunn, 1997; Washington & Craig, 1999).

IQ

Like most vocabulary tests, the PPVT-III correlates highly with IQ. For example, data presented in the manual on 41 children administered the WISC-III indicate very high correlations between the tests (FSIQ = .90, VIQ = .91, PIQ = .82 for form IIIA, with the PPVT-III mean about 3 points higher). High correlations with the WISC-III are also reported in students referred for academic difficulties ($r = .82$, .88, and .87 for FSIQ, VIQ, and VCI, respectively; Hodapp & Gerken, 1999). Among index scores, the highest correlation is obtained with Verbal Comprehension ($r = .88$) and the lowest—although still substantial—with Processing Speed ($r = .56$). Correlations with other IQ tests such as KAIT and K-BIT are also quite high ($r = .85$ and $r = .78$ between PPVT-IIIA and full-scale composites for each scale; Dunn & Dunn, 1997). The test is also highly correlated with the K-BIT in individuals with developmental disabilities ($r = .92$; Powell et al., 2002). Somewhat lower correlations are reported between PPVT-III and WAIS-III ($r = .46$, .40, and .26, for VIQ, FSIQ, and PIQ, respectively; Bell et al., 2001). In one study, the PPVT-III correlated highly with the K-ABC Mental Processing Composite ($r = .58$) in at-risk African American children (i.e., those whose mothers were unmarried, had < 12 years of education, and were unemployed; Campbell et al., 2001).

Education

In children, PPVT-R scores are linearly related to maternal education, one of the strongest predictors of language development in children (Dolloghan et al., 1999; Padilla et al., 2002). In one study, mothers with less than high school, high school, and college educations had children with average PPVT-R scores of 90, 101, and 110, respectively (Dolloghan et al., 1999). Similar findings have been reported with the PPVT-III (Washington & Craig, 1999), although maternal education effects have not been found in all samples (e.g., Reese & Read, 2000). In adult neurological patients, education effects have been reported on the PPVT-R (Snitz et al., 2000; see *Utility in Premorbid Estimation*).

Ethnicity

One of the proposed advantages of the test in assessing disadvantaged individuals and those from minority groups is that

Table 11–29 PPVT-III Performance for Low SES African American and Spanish American Children

Study	Demographic Group	Location	N	Age (Years)	Mean PPVT-III Score (SD)
Washington & Craig (1999)	Low SES African American preschoolers	Detroit, Mich.	59	3–4	91.0 (11.0)
Campbell et al. (2001)	Low SES African American children	Memphis, Tenn.	416	5–7	82.3 (12.2)
Wasik & Bond (2001)	Low SES African American preschoolers	Baltimore, Md.	127	4	72.5–74.4[a]
Champion et al. (2003)	Low SES African American preschoolers	Tampa Bay, Fla.	49	3–5	86.8 (11.0)
Dickinson et al. (2004)	Low SES Spanish/English bilingual preschoolers	Northeast and Southeast United States	123	2–5	77.4 (13.1)[b]

[a]range of means for four classrooms; SDs not presented.
[b]the TVIP score for this group was higher (i.e., $M = 86.1$, $SD = 14.4$).

it does not require reading or writing and does not require verbal fluency (Chase-Landsdale et al., 1991; Padilla et al., 2002). However, there were concerns about racial bias with regard to the prior version of the test. Large-scale studies involving longitudinal assessment of Head Start children administered the PPVT-R are particularly useful in providing clues to the sociodemographic variables affecting test performance. For example, in Mexican American children, maternal education, poverty, and immigrant status are all significant predictors of performance on the test (Padilla et al., 2002). Padilla et al. (2002) found that scores for African American children and Mexican American children were 31 and 26 percentile points lower than those of White children, respectively. PPVT-R scores in Mexican American children were also positively related to household characteristics such as lower number of siblings, married parents, and maternal age greater than 20 years. Health care factors also predicted performance; children with no health insurance or Medicaid scored lower than did children with private health insurance. However, even when all sociodemographic factors were accounted for, a substantial percentage of the variance in score differences between African American and Mexican American children and White children remained unexplained.

In other studies, African American children tended to score 4 to 13 points lower than White children on the PPVT-R, even after demographic conditions and home environment variables were accounted for. Additionally, discrepancies were 1.5 to 3 times greater than with other instruments such as the Stanford-Binet and WPPSI (Brooks-Gunn et al., 2003). Accordingly, some researchers conclude that the PPVT-R should not be used in African American preschoolers or in children from impoverished backgrounds (Washington & Craig, 1992). Interestingly, Washington and Craig (1999) reported that the PPVT-R was originally developed to address some of the biases inherent in the 1959 edition of the test, but that it was largely unsuccessful in doing so.

It is unclear whether these concerns have been completely eliminated with the PPVT-III. As indicated earlier, the PPVT-III standardization sample includes a substantial proportion of individuals of various ethnic/racial backgrounds (i.e., 36%). Washington and Craig (1999) found higher means in African American preschoolers administered the PPVT-III than in a previous study using the PPVT-R (Washington & Craig, 1992). However, this has not been the case for several other studies, which have continued to report low means in at-risk but normally developing African American children (see Table 11–29). Additionally, there is some indication that the test may yield lower scores in some minority groups than other testing instruments, notably full-length IQ tests. For example, Campbell et al. (2001) found that PPVT-III scores were about 8 points lower than K-ABC composite scores in African American children.

One of the standards for assessing a test's comparability in different populations is to determine whether it shows similar score distributions across groups. Ideally, score distribution should approximate the normal curve. Although most of the group scored below the normative mean on the PPVT-R, Washington & Craig (1999) found that about 62% of African American at-risk preschoolers performed within 1 SD of the mean on the PPVT-III, which was similar to the expected rate of 68% within 1 SD for the normative sample. This finding has not been replicated by other groups, who instead have reported that significant numbers of poor, African American preschoolers fall below the normative mean when assessed with the PPVT-III. For example, Champion et al. (2003) found that 40% of normally developing African American preschoolers enrolled in Head Start scored more than 1 SD below the mean and 22% scored in the impaired range (< 1.5 SDs). The authors listed a number of PPVT-III items that were missed by the children and were thought to have salient alternate meanings for African Americans, including "fly," "digging," and "wrapping." However, apart from three items that were missed by more than 50% of the sample (i.e., "porcupine," "camper," and "furry"), misses were unsystematic across items. Therefore, adjusting scores or removing items would not have increased scores for these children.

Means obtained by Wasik and Bond (2001) for an economically disadvantaged, at-risk sample of primarily African American children in Baltimore, Maryland, were even lower (see Table 11–29). Note that the group mean increased from 72.5 to 81.3 after a 15-week interactive book reading program, underlining the fact that low scores in economically disadvantaged preschoolers may reflect lack of experience with vocabulary rather than language delay.

In one study, White children from Great Britain and the United States given the PPVT-R had equivalent scores despite an extra year of formal education due to earlier school entry age in the British children; however, at ages 10 to 14 years, White U.S. children outperformed their British counterparts (Michael, 2003). When all ethnicities were included, U.S. children performed more poorly than British children in some age groups.

NORMATIVE DATA

Standardization Sample

The test was normed on a stratified sample of 2725 individuals (2000 children/adolescents and 725 persons older than 19 years of age; see Table 11–30). They were selected from a larger

Table 11–30 Characteristics of the PPVT-III Normative Sample

Sample type	National stratified, randomized sample
Number	2725
Age	2 years 6 months to 90+ years[a]
Geographic location (%)	
Northeast	19
South	28
North Central	33
West	20
Parental Education/Education[b] (%)	
Grade 11 or less	17
High school	31
1–3 Years of College	31
4+ Years of College	20
Socioeconomic Status (SES)	Education was used as an SES marker
Gender (%)	
Males	47
Females	53
Race/Ethnicity (%)	
African American	18
Hispanic	13
White	64
Other	5
Screening	None[c]

[a]Based on several age groupings: 2-month intervals for ages 2 years 6 months to 6 years, 3-months for 7–18, 2 years for 19–24, and multiyear intervals for adults (25–30, 31–40, 41–50, 51–60, and 61–90+ years).
[b]Parental education was used for persons ≤24 years of age; examinee's education level was used for ages 25+.
[c]Individuals in special education categories were included in the standardization sample as follows: learning disability (6%), speech impairment (2%), mental retardation (1%), hearing impairment (<1%), gifted/talented (3%), and adults ≥25 years of age with mental retardation (2%).

sample of more than 3700 persons to match 1994 U.S. Census data, at 268 testing sites in the United States. Standardization occurred between 1995 and 1996. Norms were stratified according to gender, education level, race/ethnicity, geographic location, and percentage of people with disabilities. Detailed procedures on standardization and score construction can be found in the Technical Manual (Williams & Wang, 1997), and on page 46 of the Examiner's Manual. Interestingly, the authors note that there is an argument not to normalize scores on tests such as the PPVT (i.e., by adjusting raw scores to fit the normal distribution), because hearing vocabulary is not normally distributed but is positively skewed at the lower end of the distribution (Dunn & Dunn, 1997).

Other Normative Datasets

Mean scores obtained by different investigators for normally developing but at-risk African American and Mexican American children are presented in Table 11–29. These means can be used as a benchmark when assessing African American and Mexican American children from disadvantaged backgrounds, to avoid overdiagnosis of language impairments in these groups. (See *Demographic Effects* and *Comments*.)

RELIABILITY

Internal Consistency

Alpha coefficients and split-half coefficients, computed for forms IIIA and IIIB, are uniformly high (median alpha = .95 for both forms, range = .92 to .98; split-half coefficient median = .94 for both forms, range = .86 to .97). These reliabilities are higher than those for the PPVT-R, for which the median split-half reliability is reported as .81 (Dunn & Dunn, 1997).

Standard Error of Measurement (*SEM*)

*SEM*s for the PPVT-III are based on alternate form reliabilities. The authors note that, because content for forms IIIA and IIIB were from the same item pool and were subjected to the same rigorous item analysis, examination of alternate form reliability provides an acceptable internal reliability estimate. The median *SEM* across age for the PPVT-III is 3.7 standard score points. *SEM*s by age vary from a low of about 3.4 points in school-age children to a high of 5.2 points in 2-year-olds (Dunn & Dunn, 1997). These values can be used to construct confidence intervals around obtained scores, as outlined in Chapter 1.

Test-Retest Reliability

Temporal stability was assessed using 226 subjects in four age groups retested after a 1-month interval. Both forms were given both times (see Technical Manual). All correlations, corrected for restriction of range, were very high (≥ 90 at every age; range = .91 to .94). Groups included 67 preschoolers (ages 2 years 6 months to 5 years 11 months), 70 school-age children (6 years to 10 years 11 months), 51 adolescents (12 years to 17 years 11 months), and 38 adults (26 years to 57 years 11 months).

Reese and Read (2000) explored the long-term reliability of the test in New Zealand preschoolers and found considerably lower values. When alternate forms were administered at age 2 years 8 months and then again at age 3 years 4 months, reliability was relatively marginal from an absolute standard of reliability ($r = .61$; Reese & Read, 2000), but it was within broadly expected limits given the age of the sample (i.e., as in most cognitive tests, reliabilities are lower in younger age groups).

Practice Effects

At retest, gains are relatively small. Preschoolers and school-aged children gained less than 2 points at retesting, whereas adults and adolescents gained between 1 and almost 4 points after a 1-month interval (Dunn & Dunn, 1997).

Alternate Forms Reliability

Alternate form reliability is high (median coefficient of .94). Correlations between forms IIIA and IIIB are lowest in the youngest age band ($r = .88$ at age 2 years 6 months).

Interscorer Reliability

Gray et al. (1999) reported 99.5% agreement for PPVT-III scoring in preschoolers.

VALIDITY

Content Validity

Test development of PPVT-III content, including bias review, was rigorous and extensive. The initial PPVT item pool was based on almost 4000 illustratable words from the 1953 *Webster's New Collegiate Dictionary*; the PPVT-R based its items on the 1967 edition of this dictionary, along with other sources. This word pool was further expanded for the PPVT-III using word frequency sources, vocabulary sources, picture dictionaries, and the 1981 Webster's dictionary. Item review was conducted using both classic and Rasch analyses. Rational item analysis was provided by panel review and a national user survey. The former included review by a panel of independent consultants representing African Americans, Asian Americans, Hispanic Americans, Native Americans, and women. Following this, a national tryout was conducted, after which additional classic and Rasch analyses were conducted to identify items with bias against subgroups based on demographic variables. Two parallel forms were then created and used in the final standardization.

Comparison With Previous Editions

The PPVT-III and PPVT-R are not equivalent tests, despite high correlations between versions ($r = .97$, Williams & Wang, 1997; $r = .76$, Pankratz et al., 2004). High correlations between two tests do not mean that standard scores for individuals will necessarily be equivalent, or that the tests assess identical domains. Additionally, despite high intercorrelations, the tests differ in several ways (see *Description*). One major difference is that there are more items on the PPVT-III to allow age extensions at both ends of the age distribution, and more items are sampled at each age level, which means that raw scores are typically greater with the PPVT-III. Average raw score differences can reach as high as 23 points (Stockman, 2000), depending on age. A method to convert PPVT-R scores to PPVT-III scores is provided on page 63 of the Examiner's Manual (and presented in detail in the Technical Manual); the method involves adding an age-dependent correction factor to the PPVT-R raw score. However, as Stockman (2000) demonstrated, the score conversion method presented in the manual does not eliminate standard score differences between the two tests. At almost all ages, PPVT-III standard scores are higher than corresponding PPVT-R scores, even after the correction factor is applied. (e.g., there is an average difference of 12.5 points, ranging from 1 to 24 standard score points, for the example provided by Stockman, 2000). Only in the youngest age groups are scores relatively equivalent. At older ages, use of one test instead of the other could significantly affect clinical decision making regarding impairment. Ukrainetz and Duncan (2000) also report that there may be as much as a 10-point standard score difference in young children.

PPVT-III and PPVT-R scores may also differ in some adult subgroups. For example, Pankratz et al. (2004) reported that PPVT-III standard scores for groups of adults with poor language skills were significantly higher than PPVT-R scores, even though scores for normal-language controls were equivalent between versions. Specifically, students with learning disability and adults with familial speech and language impairment scored approximately 7 points higher on the PPVT-III than on the PPVT-R (Pankratz et al., 2004). The authors noted that, because of this selective upward shift in scores for language-impaired individuals, use of the PPVT-III for classification purposes at the individual level would result in fewer individuals being identified as having language impairment. Secondly, at a group level, selection of the PPVT-III would result in smaller differences between normal and language-impaired groups and, consequently, lesser sensitivity if the test were used for research or diagnosis of language impairment. Therefore, in addition to differences in raw scores, there may be additional differences in difficulty level that are not eliminated by conversion to standard scores. Whether the two tests yield equivalent score distributions in minorities is also an issue (see *Ethnicity*).

There have been few studies on the concordance of the PPVT-III and the TVIP, the Spanish version of the test. In bilingual, primarily Spanish-speaking American children, only a surprisingly modest correlation was obtained between scores on the PPVT-III and on the TVIP ($r = .23$; Dickinson et al., 2004). In addition, mean scores differ between versions, with higher scores obtained on the TVIP (see note at the bottom of Table 11–29). This underlines the need to assess bilingual children in both languages before using PPVT-III results for determining language impairment.

Score comparisons involving the original PPVT appear to be consistent with the Flynn effect. In a study comparing two age cohorts in a single school, a sample of schoolchildren was administered the original version (PPVT) and the current version (PPVT-III). Scores on the original PPVT were about 5 points higher than PPVT-III scores. Additionally, they were about 5 points higher than those of a previous age cohort who had been administered the PPVT 20 years earlier (Nettlebeck & Wilson, 2004).

Correlations With Other Language Tests

The construct validity of the test is well established, based on comparisons with several language tests. For example, in one study, the test was highly correlated with other vocabulary tests such as the EVT, EOWPVT, and ROWPVT in normally developing preschoolers ($r = .75$, .84, and .79, respectively; Ukrainetz & Blomquist, 2002). Note that cross-test correlations were uniformly high, regardless of the modality (expressive versus receptive) or the norms base (conormed versus separately normed) of the other tests. Other studies suggest moderate to strong correlations with language tests in normally developing and language-impaired preschoolers, including EVT, EOWPVT-R, and ROWPVT ($r = .33$ to .77; Gray et al., 1999).

In one study, PPVT-III and EVT correlated highly in children with autism ($r = .51$); however, the PPVT-III did not correlate highly with another receptive language measure, the CELF Concepts and Directions subtests (a task similar to the Token Test; Condouris et al., 2003). In Spanish American bilingual children enrolled in Head Start, both the PPVT-III and TVIP were moderately related to phonological awareness scores assessed in both English and Spanish ($r = .32$ to .48; Dickinson et al., 2004).

Correlations with natural samples of expressive speech are somewhat lower, as is the case for most standardized language tests. High correlations with spontaneous speech samples would not necessarily be expected from a vocabulary test such as the PPVT-III, which takes most of its items from written word sources (e.g., dictionaries, word frequency counts). In addition, most individuals use only a subsample of their known vocabulary when engaging in spoken language (Stockman, 2000). Compared with other language tests such as the EVT, EOWPVT and ROWPVT, the PPVT-III demonstrates some of the lowest correlations with scores based on samples of spontaneous language ($r = .12$ to .36; Ukrainetz & Blomquist, 2002), with the ROWPVT having better agreement with these measures. However, the test appears to be moderately

related to spontaneous language samples in African American preschoolers ($r = .42$; Washington & Craig, 1999) and in children with autism ($r = .37$ to .41; Condouris et al., 2003).

At the individual level, concordance with other language tests is not as strong. For instance, Gray et al. (1999) found that the ability of the PPVT-III to detect speech-language impairments was not high. Even though preschoolers with language impairment had an average score that was lower than their normal-language peers, there was considerable overlap in the distribution of scores, and the mean of the language-impaired group was within normal limits (97, versus 112 for the controls). PPVT-III sensitivity, specificity, positive predictive validity, false negative rate, and false positive rate were 74%, 71%, 73%, 15%, and 13%, respectively, in a sample of 62 children, half of whom had clinician-confirmed language impairments. Attaining the best classification accuracy resulted in cutoffs that far exceeded the standard cutoffs for impairment used in clinical practice (i.e., a standard score of 104 on PPVT-III). Using a more conventional clinical cutoff (< 1.5 SDs below the normative mean), only 4 of 31 children with language impairment obtained a low PPVT-III score. The test with the highest identification rate was the EOWPVT-R; however, even its identification rate was not high (i.e., only 13/31 children with language impairment had scores < 1.5 SD below the mean).

Receptive-Expressive Discrepancies

The utility of using PPVT-III/EVT expressive/receptive discrepancies to identify language-impaired individuals is not well supported by empirical research. Gray et al. (1999) found that PPVT-III/EVT receptive > expressive discrepancies were common in a normal language group (32%, compared with 19% in a language-impaired group). A low rate was also found for EOWPVT-R/ROWPVT comparisons (i.e., 7/31 versus 2/31). Notably, the counterintuitive pattern of expressive > receptive was relatively rare with the PPVT-III/EVT combination in both normal and speech-impaired children (3/31 and 2/31, respectively), but not with ROWPVT/EOWPVT-R, in which 32% (10/31) of speech impaired children showed the pattern. Note that, in another study using the PPVT-R, not a single child in a language-impaired group was found to have a receptive-only language deficit (Lahey & Edwards, 1999).

Correlations With Non-Language Domains (Discriminant Validity)

Although the items are presented visually and the response modality is motor, the PPVTR-III does not appear to depend heavily on visual processing or visual-motor skills. This is probably because examinees do not need to process small details, but rather need merely to grasp the gist/gestalt of the stimuli, which were specifically designed by the test authors to be salient. For example, the PPVT-III is only modestly related to nonverbal reasoning as measured by K-ABC Triangles ($r = .23$, Washington & Craig, 1999). Similarly, the PPVT-R is not related to the Porteus Maze Test (Levin et al., 2001), and it loads on a factor separate from nonverbal, visuomotor tasks such as the VMI and the Draw-A-Man test (Kastner et al., 2001). In adults, it is not highly correlated with nonverbal IQ (Bell et al., 2001).

However, PPVT-III performance appears to add to the prediction of working memory and inhibitory control in preschoolers, consistent with theories linking the parallel development of language and working memory/inhibition skills in young children (Wolfe & Bell, 2003). In line with these findings, the PPVT-III also appears to be moderately related to planning in preschoolers ($r = .32$ to .42) and to theory of mind ($r = .49$; Carlson et al., 2004). Izard et al. (2001) found that PPVT-R performance in at-risk preschoolers was a significant predictor of later emotional knowledge, a skill necessary for social interaction ($r = .61$). Similarly, Harvey et al. (1999) found that children with extremely low birth weight who scored low on the PPVT-R were more likely to have low scores on a number of executive functioning tests at 5 years of age.

Correlations With IQ

In addition to addressing the usual questions about divergent/convergent validity and suitability in populations with different levels of cognitive functioning, understanding the test's relationship to IQ is important because the test itself, according to the authors, can be used as an IQ screener and has been used by others as a premorbid IQ estimator. The manual summarizes some of the previous findings regarding the high correlations between vocabulary tests and IQ, dating from the time of Binet and Simon (1916). This includes the fact that vocabulary subtests from a variety of IQ tests correlate more highly with FSIQ than other subtests, and the fact that they are usually the subtests with the highest g loadings (Dunn & Dunn, 1997). This rationale is presumably the reason the test is purported to measure IQ (see *Demographic Effects* for information on correlations with IQ in various populations).

Utility in IQ Estimation

To use a test as an IQ estimate, equivalence of standard scores at the individual level must be demonstrated, in addition to high test/IQ intercorrelations. Evidence for the PPVT-III as a strong IQ estimator is mixed, due to a limited concordance between scores among individuals. Although the test yields mean standard scores similar to WISC-III FSIQ scores in children referred for academic concerns (93 versus 92; Hodapp & Gerken, 1999; see also Examiner's Manual), and VIQ and VCI are within 3 points of PPVT-III, individual agreement rates between standard score classifications are not available. In low SES African American children, the test was a poor screening device when used to screen for intellectual deficits on the K-ABC. Campbell et al. (2001) reported that, even though sensitivity, specificity, and negative predictive validity were greater than .80 (i.e., .87, .83 and .99, respectively), the test had poor positive predictive validity (.16) when a standard

Table 11-31 Accuracy of Selected Cutoff Scores for the PPVT-III When Used for Screening Purposes in Low SES, African American Children

Cutoff Score	Sensitivity	Specificity	PPV	NPV	Hit Rate
Screening for Intellectual Deficits[a]					
51[b]	.20	.99	.60	.97	.96
67[c,d]	.80	.91	.25	.99	.91
68[c]	.80	.88	.20	.99	.88
69[c]	.80	.86	.17	.99	.86
70[c]	.87	.83	.16	.99	.83
71[c]	.87	.80	.14	.99	.80
Screening for Achievement Deficits[e]					
60[f]	.12	1.00	1.00	.84	.84
63[g]	.24	.99	.78	.85	.85
75[h]	.68	.81	.45	.92	.79

Note: PPV = positive predictive validity; NPV = negative predictive validity.
[a]Base rate of MPC scores at or below 70 = 3.6%.
[b]Cutoff score that yielded highest overall hit rate.
[c]Cutoff score that achieved sensitivity, specificity, and hit rate at or above .80 per Carran and Scott's (1992) guidelines.
[d]Cutoff score that yielded referral rate 3 times higher than base rate per Lichtenstein and Ireton's (1991) guidelines.
[e]Base rate of one or more achievement scores at or below 70 = 18.1%.
[f]Cutoff score that yielded highest PPV.
[g]Cutoff score that yielded highest overall hit rate.
[h]Cutoff score that yielded referral rate 1.5 times higher than base rate per Lichtenstein and Ireton's (1991) guidelines. No cutoff score achieved sensitivity, specificity, and hit rate at or above .80 per Carran and Scott's (1992) guidelines.

Source: From Campbell et al., 2001. Campbell, J. M., Bell, S. K., Keith, L. K. Assessment. 8(1) pp. 85–94, Copyright © 2001. Reprinted by Permission of Sage Publications Inc.

score of 70 was used as the screening cutoff point. Decreasing the PPVT-III cutoff to a score of 51 achieved a better positive predictive validity (.60) and increased both specificity and negative predictive validity (.99 and .97) but resulted in unacceptably low sensitivity (.20). However, the authors noted that, even though the PPVT-III failed to meet established criteria for screening in terms of cutoff scores, screening instruments for preschoolers typically achieve relatively low sensitivities (.48 to .60), better specificities (.90 range), and positive predictive values in the .40 to .65 range (Campbell et al., 2001, page 91). Part of the difficulty is the inherent problem of detecting low base rate disorders, which is the goal in large-scale screening programs. The authors provided a range of cutoff scores to guide cutoff selection, balancing the relative risks of false positives and false negatives, which may be specific to the situation in which the screening test is to be used (see Table 11–31).

In at-risk African American children (i.e., those whose mothers were unmarried, had < 12 years of education, and were unemployed; Campbell et al., 2001), PPVT-III standard scores were, on average, 8 points lower than those for the K-ABC Mental Composite. The authors noted that the Flynn effect may have contributed to score differences, because the K-ABC was normed more than a decade before the PPVT-III. However, given the literature showing lower vocabulary scores in low SES African American children (reviewed earlier), it is unlikely that the Flynn effect accounted entirely for the difference found.

Among university students, Bell et al. (2001) found that PPVT-III scores were significantly lower than WAIS-III VIQ scores (112.8 versus 116.4). In terms of individual concordance between the PPVT-III and IQ, more than one third of subjects had scores that differed by 10 points or more with regard to VIQ (33%) or FSIQ (35%). Discrepancies also varied by IQ level; in the average to high-average range, the PPVT-III mean was within 4 points of VIQ and FSIQ, but the PPVT-III tended to underestimate IQ by about 10 points in individuals in the superior IQ range. Bell et al. (2001) concluded that the test could have potential to predict IQ in those of average or high-average IQ, but that the test cannot replace the Wechsler scales because it may underestimate WAIS-III FSIQ scores by as much as 10 points (Bell et al., 2001).

Similar inconsistencies were reported for the previous edition of the test. Although the two tests are highly correlated, the PPVT-R tended to underestimate WAIS-R IQ by 4 to 12 points in various clinical groups (Carvajal et al., 1989; Craig & Olson, 1991; Prout & Schawartz, 1984; Stevenson, 1986). Other authors have reported that the test overestimates IQ (Price et al., 1990), or both underestimates and overestimates, depending on the IQ level (Alpeter & Johnson, 1989; Mangiaracina & Simon, 1986). As expected, the PPVT-R has demonstrated its highest correlations with the Verbal Comprehension factor of the WAIS-R and with the Vocabulary subtest (Ingram et al., 1998).

Based on differences in clinical classification between PPVT-R and WAIS-R in brain-injured adults, Ingram et al. (1998) concluded that the PPVT-R was not an adequate screener at the individual level but might be appropriate in group studies. Specifically, in comparing PPVT-R scores with scores on the Verbal Comprehension factor, there was categorization agreement in only 43% of the cases, with the Verbal Comprehension factor higher in 74% of cases.

Utility in Premorbid Estimation

Several premorbid IQ estimation techniques are based on word-reading, a skill that is assumed to be relatively resistant to cognitive insult (e.g., NART, WTAR). Snitz et al (2000) argued that receptive vocabulary measures may also serve the same purpose, with the added benefit that these measures do not require verbal output but only a pointing response.

Although there are as yet no published studies on the utility of the PPVT-III in this regard, the PPVT-R has been used for this purpose. Compared with the Barona equation, Snitz et al. (2000) found that the PPVT-R was less likely to overestimate WAIS-R IQ in cognitively intact, elderly patients. However, PPVT-R scores decreased with increasing levels of cognitive impairment, indicating that these scores were indeed vulnerable to cognitive decline. In addition, the PPVT-R was a poor estimator of IQ in patients with less than 12 years of education. In those with more than 12 years of education, it stayed stable across levels of impairment, whereas declines

were noted on the WAIS-R and MMSE, suggesting that the PPVT-R is more resistant to neurological compromise than these other cognitive tests. However, this study involved only a small number of subjects, and the absolute means were smaller as impairment level increased, even among those with 13 years or more of education.

Note that PPVT-R is also not immune to the effects of traumatic brain injury (TBI) in children. PPVT-R is related to TBI severity: In one study, mild TBI was associated with generally average scores, and lower scores were obtained in subjects with severe TBI (i.e., 99.5 versus 87.8; Levin et al., 2001).

Correlations With Achievement

The test appears to be moderately to highly related to academic achievement and predicts later achievement before or at school entry. For example, in at-risk African American children, the PPVT-III was moderately to highly related to achievement subtests of the K-ABC ($r = .64$, .55, and .48, for Riddles, Arithmetic, and Reading/Decoding, respectively; Campbell et al., 2001). In children with familial reading disability, PPVT-III performance at the beginning of the school year, before any formal reading instruction, was related to reading and spelling scores at the end of the school year ($r = .30$ and .31; Fielding-Barnsley & Purdie, 2003). In bilingual, primarily Spanish-speaking preschoolers enrolled in Head Start, both English (PPVT-III) and Spanish (TVIP) versions of the test were moderately related to emergent literacy awareness ($r = .30$ to .33; Dickinson et al., 2004). In adults with developmental delays, the PPVT-III correlated highly with WRAT-3 subtests ($r = .81$, .72, and .86, for Reading, Spelling, and Arithmetic, respectively; Powell et al., 2002). It is important to note that the literature reviewed to date provides correlations only, rather than agreement classifications between PPVT-III and achievement test scores. The latter would be of more utility in determining the significance of particular PPVT-III scores for later achievement. Nevertheless, these studies provide evidence that the test may be useful for predicting school achievement.

Similar research findings are available for the PPVT-R. Scores on the PPVT-R administered at the beginning of kindergarten were related to achievement at the end of first grade, as measured by the Stanford Achievement Test ($r = .55$; Kastner et al., 2001). In addition, in primarily African American, economically disadvantaged children, the PPVT-R at age 5 years was significantly correlated with teacher ratings of academic competence at age 9 years (Izard et al., 2001). Correlations between the PPVT-R and the PIAT appear to increase as children get older, with modest correlations in 5-year-olds ($r = .36$ to 40) and higher correlations in 14-year-olds ($r = .58$ to .71; Michael, 2003).

Clinical Studies

The PPVT-III has been used in a number of clinical research studies, and the PPVT-R continues to be actively used in several large longitudinal studies. The tests have also used in a variety of studies on various clinical conditions, in which it has demonstrated sensitivity to treatment and responsivity to change, as well as ecological validity.

In research on language, PPVT-III sensitivity to detection of language impairment was investigated in preschoolers (Gray et al., 1999), including its utility as a screening instrument for at-risk African American children (Campbell et al., 2001; see *Correlations With Language Tests*). PPVT-III scores were correlated with number of books given in early literacy intervention programs for at-risk African-American preschoolers (Theriot et al., 2003). In a study on the efficacy of a 15-week interactive book-reading program (e.g., involving open-ended questioning and dialogue during reading), PPVT-III scores were significantly increased in at-risk, primarily African American children by about 7 points, compared with classrooms in which this technique was not used but identical books were read aloud to the children (Wasik & Bond, 2001). A similar effect was demonstrated with regard to book reading by parents. Among children at risk for reading disability, those receiving an 8-week program to encourage interactive reading by parents to their children (i.e., dialogic reading) before formal reading instruction scored higher on the PPVT-III at the end of the school year than did untreated controls (Fielding-Barnsley & Purdie, 2003).

The test has also shown utility in identifying the specific strengths and weaknesses of children with various syndromes associated with mental retardation. For example, despite developmental delay and mental retardation associated with Costello syndrome, some children have preserved receptive vocabulary (Axelrad et al., 2004). The PPVT-R has also been used with other genetic syndromes associated with mental retardation, including Williams syndrome and Down syndrome (e.g., Klein & Mervis, 1999), and in research on functional literacy in Down syndrome (Bochner et al., 2001).

The PPVT-III has also been used successfully to study receptive vocabulary acquisition in children treated with hearing aids versus cochlear implants (Eisenberg et al., 2004). Condouris et al. (2003) found that measures derived from natural language samples yielded lower scores than did standardized language measures such as the PPVT-III and EVT in individuals with autism, due to deficits in pragmatic language use.

Previous versions, most notably the PPVT-R, are also frequently used in clinical studies. This includes research demonstrating increased receptive vocabulary after literacy intervention (Sharif et al., 2003), benefits of immersion in a second language on English vocabulary acquisition (Cunningham & Graham, 2000), and benefits of breast-feeding for 6 months or more on language development, especially in female babies, and in a dose-response pattern yielding increases of 4 to 8 points (Oddy et al., 2003; Quinn et al., 2001). The test has also been used in comparisons of different infant formulas in large, longitudinal studies (Auestad et al., 2003) and to show the utility of active storybook reading in increasing vocabulary acquisition (Ewers & Brownson, 1999). The PPVT-R is reportedly sensitive to the benefits of early intervention in

deaf and hard of hearing children (Moeller, 2000), and it was used in a large randomized clinical trial involving tympanostomy tube insertion in children with persistent middle-ear effusion (Paradise et al., 2003). The same test demonstrated no differences in ability between children who stutter and typically developing children (Silverman & Ratner, 2002) and in this group was not related to conversational vocabulary. In addition, longitudinal studies of persistent stutterers showed no long-term effects on PPVT-R scores (compared with recovered stutterers; Ryan, 2001). The PPVT has been used to determine the predictors of reading acquisition in children (Cronin, 2001). In another study, children from Head Start who liked school less also tended to have lower PPVT-R scores (Ramey et al., 1998).

In one study of pediatric TBI, PPVT-R performance was not related to the presence of frontal lesions (Levin et al., 2001). However, performance was related to TBI severity; mild TBI was associated with generally average scores, and lower scores were obtained in severe TBI (99.5 versus 87.8; Levin et al., 2001). The test has also been used to track developmental growth curves in language development in very low-birth-weight infants with intraventricular hemorrhage (Ment et al., 2003), in whom the presence of significant central nervous system injury was a predictor of decreasing scores over time.

Using the Spanish version, Kordas et al. (2004) found a strong linear association between blood lead levels and PPVT performance in Mexican schoolchildren living near a lead foundry. For every 10-unit rise in blood lead concentration, PPVT scores decreased by 3.7 points. Consistent with the expected effects of iron deficiency, a similar, although weaker, inverse relationship was found for iron: for every unit increase in iron, there was a 0.16 point increase in PPVT scores. In one large, nationally representative U.S. study, the test was used as a measure of intelligence, and scores were inversely related to sexual behavior in adolescents (Halpern et al., 2000).

COMMENT

The PPVT has a long history of use in psychology and language assessment. It is an excellent test from many perspectives, including test design, standardization, reliability, validity, and demonstrated utility in a variety of clinical disorders and conditions and in a number of sociodemographic groups. From a practical standpoint, the test is appealing for young children, is useful for patients with motor or verbal deficits, and elicits some degree of performance in almost all patients, including those who are extremely low functioning and those who have difficulty engaging in structured testing. The test also has appeal for screening programs and large-scale research projects because it is cost-effective in terms of materials, time, and expertise required for administration and scoring (Campbell et al., 2001).

In a comprehensive analysis of the PPVT-R and PPVT-III, Stockman (2000) reviewed differences between the two tests. These are important to note in order to improve interpretation of score comparisons, particularly because the PPVT-III has been suspected of being "easier" than the PPVT-R (Ukrainetz & Duncan, 2000). One of the most important differences between the tests is the ethnic and sociodemographic composition of the standardization samples. Whereas the original PPVT was normed on white children in Nashville, Tennessee, the PPVT-R was nationally normed and had a minority representation of almost 15%. In contrast, ethnic representation in the PPVT-III norms is now 36%, consistent with changing U.S. demographics, particularly in the younger age levels. There is also a larger percentage of children from low social classes (based on education). These norm differences have implications for score levels and impairment classifications, because, on average, children from minority backgrounds (whether due to poverty, low maternal education, or a combination of sociodemographic and economic factors) do more poorly on vocabulary tests than do groups within "the economic and ethnic mainstream" (Ramey et al., 1998; Stockman, 2000).

Further affecting norms is the fact that 14.2% of the PPVT-III standardization sample consisted of individuals with clinical conditions (see Table 11–30); the corresponding percentage for the PPVT-R is unknown (Stockman, 2000). As Stockman (2000) noted, the inclusion of clinical groups within norming samples is an asset, not a limitation (see also McFadden, 1996). When individuals with impairments are removed, the normal distribution is truncated, resulting in a distribution in which lower-functioning (but language-normal) individuals are placed in the lowest ranks, effectively shifting the entire distribution downward. When the test is used to screen for language difficulties, this raises the risk of misidentifying individuals who are normally functioning, but have lower language scores, as impaired.

Although there is controversy as to whether the test is as sensitive as its predecessor, the PPVT-III was standardized and developed with exacting, empirically based standards and surpasses the PPVT-R in many ways (e.g., normative sample, reliability, test content). There are several major differences between the versions, as reviewed earlier, including item overlap, age range, and standardization sample composition. The PPVT-R is still being used in several large-scale, longitudinal studies and will no doubt continue to appear in research studies for some time. However, scores from the two instruments may not be directly comparable (see previous discussion). In particular, there is evidence that the PPVT-R yields lower scores in some ethnic groups, particularly low SES African American and Mexican American children, and that it underestimates ability, compared with full-length IQ tests, even after demographic factors such as maternal education and home environment are controlled for (Brooks-Gunn et al., 2003; Washington & Craig, 1992). Accordingly, Brooks-Gunn et al. (2003) recommended caution in interpreting ethnic effects on the test, because it "accentuates the Black-White test gap" (p. 249). Given the limitations of the PPVT-R with regard to providing an unbiased assessment in ethnic groups, the PPVT-III is preferable for use in clinical assessment. In research, version selection

should also be done judiciously by evaluating how the choice of instrument might affect the goals of the research or diagnostic usage, given the possibility of differing sensitivity between the PPVT-III and PPVT-R (Pankratz et al., 2004).

Despite improvements, users should note that the PPVT-III is not necessarily completely unbiased (e.g., Campbell et al., 2001). After careful review, Washington and Craig (1999) concluded that it is not *unduly* racially/ethnically biased. At the same time, it is equally important to realize that the test has been unusually well scrutinized for racial/ethnic biases, which cannot be said for the majority of tests in current usage, and that group differences on language tests arise as a result of complex factors, including interactions of test characteristics and population characteristics. For example, Dolloghan et al. (1999) noted that "sociodemographic variables, such as socioeconomic status and ethnicity, have been associated with quantitative, qualitative, or stylistic difference in child-directed language" (p. 1440). As Stockman (2000) commented, the words known by an individual are, by definition, influenced by the cultural and linguistic experiences of that individual. Therefore, low scores can reflect different experiences with language rather than deficits. For example, Champion et al. (2003) noted that African Americans are known for using words creatively, in a way that is innovative and changeable and that places considerable value on novel figurative language instead of precision in labeling. Because "labeling" skills may be differentially reinforced in different linguistic communities, language assessment of African American children and of individuals from groups in which other features of language use might be differentially emphasized (see Pena et al., 2001) should not be based solely on the PPVT-III.

From a clinical perspective, the test should be used with a clear comprehension of its limitations. For example, it is a questionable predictor of speech/language impairment in preschoolers (Gray et al., 1999), and there is limited evidence that receptive > expressive discrepancies are indicative of word-finding problems, at least in preschoolers (Gray et al., 1999).

As noted earlier, users should also realize that PPVT-III scores may be higher than PPVT-R scores. In other words, it may be an "easier" test than its predecessor, or, more appropriately, its predecessor may have been unnecessarily difficult, particularly for minorities. This occurs in part because of lower performance expectations on the PPVT-III due to the inclusion of a higher percentage of minorities and persons with disabilities in the standardization sample (Stockman, 2000). The complexities inherent in determining sample composition in a test designed for use in a multicultural (and in some cases, multilingual) population were discussed by Stockman (2000). Although they are not provided in the test manual, demographically adjusted scores would be a useful addition to the test.

In assessing autistic individuals, the PPVT-III may provide information on linguistic capacity, whereas evaluation of natural language samples provide information on linguistic usage because autistic children may not spontaneously use the vocabulary they know due to pragmatic language deficits (Condouris et al., 2003). Therefore, the test provides information on structural language but not on functional language skills such as pragmatics and discourse (Condouris et al., 2003). Similarly, Ukrainetz and Blomquist (2002) caution that scores on vocabulary tests such as the PPVT-III, which consist of assessing knowledge of labels, might be expected to be associated with specific functional aspects of daily language (e.g., performance on school assignments) but would not necessarily predict performance in other areas (e.g., social communicative exchanges, written imaginative narrative). Finally, it is important to note that the PPVT-III, by definition, includes only the subset of words that can be illustrated, and that the test samples words that are most often used in written form rather than in everyday speech. Again, this word sampling bias (Stockman, 2000) puts those with limited access to books or other written media at a disadvantage.

There is evidence that administration of a receptive vocabulary test before an expressive vocabulary test (in this case, the PPVT-R before the EOWPVT-R) enhances performance on the latter (Llorente et al., 2000). PPVT-III/EVT norms were gathered with the PPVT-III administered first, followed by the EVT. Of interest is whether any enhancement effect occurred and carried over to the EVT, and whether any such effect is accounted for in the EVT norms. Until this issue is clarified, users planning on administering the EVT should follow normative procedures and administer the PPVT-III first. The issue of carryover effects deserves further study with regard to other expressive vocabulary tests that might be used in conjunction with the PPVT-III and with regard to possible effects of varying test order.

Although the PPVT-III is still used occasionally as an IQ estimate (Halpern et al., 2000; Mayer, 2001), its use in this way is not recommended. The test is simply "not an intelligence test and should not be used to make placement decisions" (Hodapp & Gerken, 1999, p. 1139). In the same vein, its utility as a premorbid IQ estimate deserves further study. However, despite less-than-perfect agreement with IQ, the test may still provide an estimate of residual capacity in severely impaired patients who cannot communicate verbally (Ingram et al., 1998). Further, it has proved useful in characterizing the strengths and weaknesses of a variety of populations, both adult and child. It is important to bear in mind, however, that receptive > expressive discrepancies may be common in healthy individuals, at least in the populations in which this test instrument has been studied (i.e., primarily young children).

Lastly, users should be aware that, although the Examiner's Manual contains abbreviated information on the test's psychometric properties, much of this information is provided in an additional manual (Williams & Wang, 1997), which must be purchased at extra cost. It would be preferable for future versions to make this information available as part of the standard test package.

REFERENCES

Alpeter, T. S., & Johnson, K. A. (1989). Use of the PPVT-R for intellectual screening with adults: A caution. *Journal of Psychoeducational Assessment, 7,* 39–45.

Auestad, N., Scott, D. T., Janowsky, J. S., Jacobsen, C., Carroll, R. E., Montalto, M. B., Halter, R., Qiu, W., Jacobs, J. R., Connor, W. E., Connor, S. L., Taylor, J. A., Neuringer, M., Fitzgerald, K. M., & Hall, R. T. (2003). Visual, cognitive, and language assessments at 39 months: A follow-up study of children fed formulas containing long-chain polyunsaturated fatty acids to 1 year of age. *Pediatrics, 112*(3), 177–188.

Axelrad, M. E., Glidden, R., Nicholson, L., & Gripp, K. W. (2004). Adaptive skills, cognitive, and behavioral characteristics of Costello syndrome. *American Journal of Medical Genetics, 128A,* 396–400.

Bell, N. L., Lassiter, K. S., Matthews, T. D., & Hutchinson, M. B. (2001). Comparison of the Peabody Picture Vocabulary Test—Third Edition and Wechsler Adult Intelligence Scale—Third Edition with university students. *Journal of Clinical Psychology, 57*(3), 417–422.

Binet, A., & Simon, T. (1916). *The development of intelligence in children* (E. S. Kite, Trans.). Baltimore: Williams & Williams.

Bochner, S., Outhred, L., & Pieterse, M. (2001). A study of functional literacy skills in young adults with Down syndrome. *International Journal of Disability, Development and Education, 48*(1), 67–90.

Brooks-Gunn, J., Klebanov, P. K., Smith, J., Duncan, G. J., & Lee, K. (2003). The Black-White test score gap in young children: Contributions of test and family characteristics. *Applied Developmental Science, 7*(4), 239–252.

Campbell, J. M., Bell, S. K., Keith, L. K. (2001). Concurrent validity of the Peabody Picture Vocabulary Test—Third Edition as an intelligence and achievement screener for low SES African American children. *Assessment, 8*(1), 85–94.

Carlson, S. M., Moses, L. J., & Claxton, L. J. (2004). Individual differences in executive functioning and theory of mind: An investigation of inhibitory control and planning ability. *Journal of Experimental Child Psychology, 87,* 299–319.

Carvajal, H., Shaffer, C., & Weaver, K. A. (1989). Correlations of scores of maximum security inmates on Wechsler Adult Intelligence Scale—Revised and Peabody Picture Vocabulary Test—Revised. *Psychological Reports, 65,* 268–270.

Champion, T. B., Hyter, Y. D., McCabe, A., & Bland-Stewart, L. M. (2003). "A matter of vocabulary": Performances of low-income African American Head Start children on the Peabody Picture Vocabulary Test–III. *Communication Disorders Quarterly, 24*(3), 121–127.

Chase-Lansdale, P., Lindsay, F. L., Mott, F. L., Brooks-Gunn, J., & Phillips, D. (1991). Children of the National Longitudinal Survey of Youth: A unique research opportunity. *Developmental Psychology, 27,* 919–931.

Condouris, K., Meyer, E., & Tager-Flusberg, H. (2003). The relationship between standardized measures of language and measures of spontaneous speech in children with autism. *American Journal of Speech-Language Pathology, 12,* 349–358.

Connolly, J. F., Byrne, J. M., Dywan, C. A. (1995). Assessing adult receptive vocabulary with event-related potentials: An investigation of cross-modal and cross-form priming. *Journal of Clinical and Experimental Neuropsychology, 17,* 548–565.

Craig, R. J., & Olson, R. E. (1991). Relationship between Wechsler scales and Peabody Picture Vocabulary Test–Revised scores among disability applicants. *Journal of Clinical Psychology, 47,* 420–429.

Cronin, V. S. (2001). The syntagmatic-paradigmatic shift and reading development. *Journal of Child Language, 29,* 189–204.

Cunningham, T. H., & Graham, C. R. (2000). Increasing native English vocabulary recognition through Spanish immersion: Cognate transfer from foreign to first language. *Journal of Educational Psychology, 92*(1), 37–49.

D'Arcy, R. C. N., Marchand, Y., Eskes, G. A., Harrison, E. R., Philips, S. J., Major, A., & Connolly, J. F. (2003). Electrophysiological assessment of language function following stroke. *Clinical Neurophysiology, 114,* 662–272.

Dickinson, D. K., McCabe, A., Clark-Chiarelli, N., & Wolf, A. (2004). Cross-language transfer of phonological awareness in low income Spanish and English bilingual preschool children. *Applied Psycholinguistics, 25,* 323–347.

Dolloghan, C. A., Campbell, T. F., Paradise, J. L., Feldman, H. M., Janosky, J. E., Pitcairn, D. N., Kurs-Lasky, M. (1999). Maternal education and measures of early speech and language. *Journal of Speech, Language, and Hearing Research, 42,* 1432–1443.

Dunn, L. M. (1959). *Peabody Picture Vocabulary Test—Revised.* Circle Pines, Minn.: American Guidance Service.

Dunn, L. M., & Dunn, L. M. (1981). *Peabody Picture Vocabulary Test—Revised.* Circle Pines, Minn.: American Guidance Service.

Dunn, L. M., & Dunn, L. M. (1997). *Examiner's manual for the Peabody Picture Vocabulary Test Third Edition.* Circle Pines, Minn.: American Guidance Service.

Dunn, L. M., Lugo, D. E., Padilla, E. R., & Dunn, L. M. (1986). *Test de Vocabulario en Imágenes Peabody.* Circle Pines, Minn.: American Guidance Service.

Eisenberg, L. S., Kirk, K. I., Martinez, A. S., Ying, E. A., & Miyamato, R. T. (2004). Communication abilities of children with aided residual hearing: Comparison with cochlear implant users. *Archives of Otolaryngology and Head and Neck Surgery, 130,* 563–569.

Ewers, C. A., & Brownson, S. M. (1999). Kindergarteners' vocabulary acquisition as a function of active vs. passive storybook reading, prior vocabulary, and working memory. *Journal of Reading Psychology, 20,* 11–20.

Fielding-Barnsley, R., & Purdie, N. (2003). Early intervention in the home for children at risk of reading failure. *Support for Learning, 18*(2), 77–82.

Gray, S., Plante, E., Vance, R., & Henrichsen, M. (1999). The diagnostic accuracy of four vocabulary tests administered to preschool-age children. *Language, Speech, and Hearing Services in Schools, 30,* 196–206.

Halpern, C. T., Joyner, K., Udry, R., & Suchindran, C. (2000). Smart teens don't have sex (or kiss much either). *Journal of Adolescent Health, 26,* 213–225.

Harvey, J. M., O'Callaghan, M. J., & Mohay, H. (1999). Executive function of children with extremely low birthweight: A case control study. *Developmental Medicine and Child Neurology, 41,* 292–297.

Hodapp, A. F., & Gerken, K. C. (1999). Correlations between scores for the Peabody Picture Vocabulary test–III and the Wechsler Intelligence Scale for Children–III. *Psychological Reports, 84*(3), 1139–1142.

Ingram, F., Caroselli, J., Robinson, H., Hetzel, R. D., Reed, K., & Masel, B. E. (1998). The PPVT-R: Validity as a quick screen of intelligence in a postacute rehabilitation setting for brain-injured adults. *Journal of Clinical Psychology, 54*(7), 877–884.

Izard, C., Fine, S., Schultz, D., Mostow, A., Ackerman, B., & Youngstrom, E. (2001). Emotion knowledge as a predictor of social behavior and academic competence in children at risk. *Psychological Science, 12*(1), 18–23.

Kastner, J. W., May, W., & Hildman, L. (2001). Relationship between language skills and academic achievement in first grade. *Perceptual and Motor Skills, 92*(2), 381–390.

Klein, B. P., & Mervis, C. B. (1999). Contrasting patterns of cognitive abilities of 9- and 10-year-olds with Williams syndrome or Down syndrome. *Developmental Neuropsychology, 16*(2), 177–196.

Kordas, K., Lopez, P., Rosado, J. L., Vargas, G. G., Rico, J. A., Ronquillo, D., Cebrian, M. E., & Stoltzfus, R. J. (2004). Blood lead, anemia, and short stature are independently associated with cognitive performance in Mexican school children. *Journal of Nutrition, 134,* 363–371.

Lahey, M., & Edwards, J. (1999). Naming errors of children with specific language impairment. *Journal of Speech, Language, and Hearing Research, 42,* 195–205.

Levin, H. S., Song, J., Ewing-Cobbs, L., & Robertson, G. (2001). Porteus Maze performance following traumatic brain injury in children. *Neuropsychology, 15*(4), 557–567.

Llorente, A. M., Sines, M. C., Rozelle, J. C., Turcich, M. R., & Casatta, A. (2000). Effects of test administration order on children's neuropsychological performance: Emerging one-word expressive and receptive language skills. *The Clinical Neuropsychologist, 14*(2), 162–172.

Mangiaracina, J., & Simon, M. J. (1986). Comparison of the PPVT-R and WAIS-R in state hospital psychiatric patients. *Journal of Clinical Psychology, 42,* 817–820.

Marchand, Y., D'Arcy, R. C. N., & Connolly, J. F. (2002). Linking neurophysiological and neuropsychological measures for aphasia assessment. *Clinical Neurophysiology, 113,* 1715–1722.

Mayer, J. D. (2001). Emotional intelligence and giftedness. *Roeper Review, 23*(3), 131.

McFadden, T. U. (1996). Creating language impairments in typically-achieving children: The pitfalls of "normal" normative sampling. *Language, Speech, and Hearing Services in the Schools, 27,* 3–9.

Ment, L. R., Vohr, B., Allan, W., Katz, K. H., Schneider, K. C., Westerveld, M., Duncan, C. C., Makuch, R. W. (2003). Change in cognitive function over time in very low-birth-weight infants. *Journal of the American Medical Association, 289*(6), 705–711.

Michael, R. T. (2003). Children's cognitive skill development in Britain and the United States. *International Journal of Behavioral Development, 27*(5), 369–408.

Moeller, M. P. (2000). Early intervention and language development in children who are deaf and hard of hearing. *Pediatrics, 106*(3), 1–9.

Nettelbeck, T., & Wilson, C. (2004). The Flynn effect: Smarter not faster. *Intelligence, 32,* 85–93.

Oddy, W. H., Kendall, G. E., Blair, E., de Klerk, N. H., Stanley, F. J., Landau, L. I., Silburn, L. I., & Zubrick, S. (2003). Breast feeding and cognitive development in childhood: A prospective birth study. *Paediatric and Perinatal Epidemiology, 17,* 81–90.

Padilla, Y. C., Boardman, J. D., Hummer, R. A., & Espitia, M. (2002). Is the Mexican American epidemiologic paradox advantage at birth maintained through early childhood? *Social Forces, 80*(3), 1101–1123.

Pankratz, M., Morrison, A., & Plante, E. (2004). Difference in standard scores of adults on the Peabody Picture Vocabulary Test (Revised and Third Edition). *Journal of Speech, Language, and Hearing Research, 47,* 714–718.

Paradise, J. L., Dollaghan, C. A., Campbell, T. F., Feldman, H. M., Bernard, B. S., Colborn, D. K., Rockette, H. E., Janosky, J. E., Pitcairn, D. L., Kurs-Lasky, M., Sabo, D. L., & Smith, C. G. (2003). Otitis media and tympanostomy tube insertion during the first three years of life: Developmental outcome at the age of four years. *Pediatrics, 112*(2), 265–277.

Pena, E., Quinn, R., & Iglesias, A. (1992). The application of dynamic methods to language assessment: A nonbiased procedure. *The Journal of Special Education, 26*(3), 269–280.

Powell, S., Plamondon, R., & Retzlaff, P. (2002). Screening cognitive abilities in adults with developmental disabilities: Correlations of the K-BIT, PPVT-3, WRAT-3, and CVLT. *Journal of Developmental and Physical Disabilities, 14*(3), 239–246.

Price, D. R., Herbert, D. A., Walsh, M. L., & Law, J. G. (1990). Study of WAIS-R, Quick Test and PPVT IQs for neuropsychiatric patients. *Perceptual and Motor Skills, 70,* 1320–1322.

Prout, H. T., & Schwartz, J. F. (1984). Validity of the Peabody Picture Vocabulary Test–Revised with mentally retarded adults. *Journal of Clinical Psychology, 40,* 584–587.

Quinn, P. J., O'Callaghan, M., Williams, G. M., Najman, J. M., Andersen, M. J., & Bor, W. (2001). The effect of breastfeeding on child development at 5 years: A cohort study. *Journal of Paediatric Child Health, 37,* 465–469.

Ramey, S. L., Lanzi, R. G., Philips, M. M., & Ramey, C. T. (1998). Perspectives of former Head Start children and their parents on school and the transition to school. *The Elementary School Journal, 98*(4), 311–327.

Reese, E., & Read, S. (2000). Predictive validity of the New Zealand MacArthur Communicative Development Inventory: Words and sentences. *Journal of Child Language, 27,* 255–266.

Ryan, B. P. (2001). A longitudinal study of articulation, language, rate, and fluency of 22 preschool children who stutter. *Journal of Fluency Disorders, 26,* 107–127.

Sharif, I., Ozuah, P. O., Dinkevich, E. I., & Mulvihill, M. (2003). Impact of a brief literacy intervention on urban preschoolers. *Early Childhood Education Journal, 30*(3), 177–180.

Silverman, S., & Ratner, N. B. (2002). Measuring lexical diversity in children who stutter: Application of *vocd. Journal of Fluency Disorders, 27,* 289–304.

Snitz, B. E., Bieliauskas, L. A., Crossland, A., Basso, M. R., & Roper, B. (2000). PPVT-R as an estimate of premorbid intelligence in older adults. *The Clinical Neuropsychologist, 14*(2), 181–186.

Spillane, M. M., Ross, K. K., & Vasa, S. F. (1996). A comparison of eye-gaze and standard response mode on the PPVT-R. *Psychology in the Schools, 33*(4), 265–271.

Stevenson, J. D. (1986). Alternate form reliability and concurrent validity of PPVT-R for referred rehabilitation agency adults. *Journal of Clinical Psychology, 42,* 650–653.

Stockman, I. J. (2000). The new Peabody Picture Vocabulary Test–III: An illusion of unbiased assessment? *Language, Speech, and Hearing Services in the Schools, 31,* 340–353.

Theriot, J. A., Franco, S. M., Sisson, B. A., Metcalf, S. C., Kennedy, M. A., & Bada, H. S. (2003). The impact of early literacy guidance on language skills of 3-year-olds. *Clinical Pediatrics, 42,* 165–172.

To, T., Guttman, S., Dick, P. T., Rosenfield, J. D., Parkin, P. C., Tassoudji, M., Vydykhan, T., Cao, H., & Harris, J. K. (2004). Risk markers for poor developmental attainment in young children: Results from a longitudinal national survey. *Archives of Pediatric and Adolescent Medicine, 158,* 643–649.

Ukrainetz, T. A., & Blomquist, C. (2002). The criterion validity of four vocabulary tests compared with a language sample. *Child Language Teaching and Therapy, 18*(1), 59–78.

Ukrainetz, T. A., & Duncan, D. S. (2000). From old to new: Examining score increases on the Peabody Picture Vocabulary Test–III. *Language, Speech, and Hearing Services in Schools, 31,* 336–339.

Washington, J. A., & Craig, H. K. (1992). Performances of low-income, African American preschool and kindergarten children on the Peabody Picture Vocabulary Test–Revised. *Language, Speech & Hearing Services in the Schools, 23,* 329–333.

Washington, J. A., & Craig, H. K. (1999). Performances of at-risk, African American preschoolers on the Peabody Picture Vocabulary Test–III. *Language, Speech & Hearing Services in the Schools, 30,* 75–82.

Wasik, B. A., & Bond, M. A. (2001). Beyond the pages of a book: Interactive book reading and language development in preschool classrooms. *Journal of Educational Psychology, 93*(2), 243–250.

Williams, K. T. (1997). *Expressive Vocabulary Test.* Circle Pines, Minn.: American Guidance Service.

Williams, K. T., & Wang, J. J. (1997). *Technical references to the Peabody Picture Vocabulary Test—Third Edition (PPVT-III).* Circle Pines, Minn.: American Guidance Service.

Wolfe, C. D., & Bell, M. A. (2003). Working memory and inhibitory control in early childhood: Contributions from physiology, temperament and language. *Developmental Psychobiology, 44,* 68–83.

Token Test (TT)

PURPOSE

The Token Test (TT) assesses comprehension of verbal commands of increasing complexity.

SOURCE

The manual for the 39-item form, answer sheets, and plastic tokens can be ordered from the Psychology Clinic, University of Victoria, Victoria, B.C., Canada, V8W 3P5 (http://www.uvic.ca/psyc/testsale), at a cost of $70 US. Other English-language versions are commercially available, for example as part of the Multilingual Aphasia Examination (MAE; Benton et al., 1994). Similar tasks are included in the NEPSY and the CELF-4.

Computer-generated versions of the TT have been created (e.g., D'Arcy & Connolly, 1999; D'Arcy et al., 2000). Translated versions of the TT are available in several languages, including German (Orgass, 1976) and Polish (Kosciesca, 1995). The German Aachen Aphasia Test (AAT) includes a version of the TT.

AGE RANGE

The test can be used with individuals ranging in age from 6 years to old age.

DESCRIPTION

The test was originally developed by De Renzi and Vignolo (1962) and by Boller and Vignolo (1966) and included 62

Figure 11–8 Token Arrangement in Front of Subject.

> Row 1: Large circles in order: red, blue, yellow, white, green
>
> Row 2: Large squares in order: blue, red, white, green, yellow
>
> Row 3: Small circles in order: white, blue, yellow, red, green
>
> Row 4: Small squares in order: yellow, green, red, blue, white

commands. A number of different versions have appeared, including short forms (De Renzi and Faglioni, 1978; Spellacy and Spreen, 1969; Van Harskamp and Van Dongen, 1977). A 22-item version is part of the MAE (Benton et. al., 1994; see *Multilingual Aphasia Examination*). This version has become a part of test batteries designed for purposes other than traditional aphasia assessment. For example, it is part of the Traumatic Brain Injury Model Systems neuropsychology battery (Millis et al., 2001), and it was one of the tests used to create the extended neuropsychological normative data set for elderly individuals used in the Mayo's Older Americans Normative Studies (MOANS) project (Ivnik et al., 1996).

The version presented here is part of the Neurosensory Center Comprehensive Examination for Aphasia (NCCEA, Test 11; Spreen and Benton, 1969, 1977) and can be used with children as well as adults. It has also been included as part of the Meyers Short Battery (MSB; Volbrecht et al., 2000). It uses 20 plastic tokens in five colors (red, white, yellow, blue, and green), two sizes (small, approximately 2 cm in diameter; large, approximately 3 cm in diameter), and two shapes (circles and squares—squares replacing the rectangles in the original De Renzi and Vignolo version), arranged in a fixed order in front of the patient (Figure 11–8). Thirty-nine commands of increasing length and complexity are listed on the answer sheet (Figure 11–9). The Spellacy and Spreen (1969) short form uses the following 16 items from Figure 11–9: items 6, 10, 12, 16, 17, 19, 20, 21, 22, 23, 24, 26, 27, 29, 33, and 35.

ADMINISTRATION

Present tokens in the order shown in Figure 11–8, and ask the first question: "Show me a circle." Pronounce the questions clearly and slowly, but take care not to deliberately stretch speech during the presentation of the test, because this may lead to improvement of test performance in aphasics (Poeck and Pietron, 1981). Instructions for parts A and B may be repeated once. No other instructions may be repeated. If the patient makes no response, he or she should be encouraged to give at least a partial response. For example, if the patient says that he or she does not remember or asks for repetition of instructions, say: "Do it as I said. Do as much as you remem-

ber." Discontinue after three consecutive failures (i.e., on sections A, B and C, if no part of the question received credit; on section D, if only one part received credit; and on sections E and F, if only two parts received credit).

The first section (questions 1 through 7) also provides a gross check on color blindness, which could affect performance on this test. If difficulties in color recognition are noticed, further examination with the Ishihara plates or a similar test of color blindness is necessary. If gross color blindness is established both on this test and by a color-vision test, the test should be discontinued.

ADMINISTRATION TIME

The test takes about 10 min.

SCORING

The questions are listed on the score sheet (Figure 11–9). Our version of the TT uses a scoring system that credits almost *every word* of each item, rather than assigning a score of 1 point for the *entire item*. Give 1-point credit for each part of a question correctly performed. For example, the correct performance of questions 1 through 7 receives 1 credit each, and the correct performance of questions 12 through 15 ("*small, white circle*") receives 3 credits each. For questions 24 to 39, the verb and the preposition as well as the correct token receive credit (e.g., "*Put the red circle on the green square*" = 6 credits). Occasionally a preposition may be interpreted in several ways, such as item 25, "*Put the white square behind the yellow circle*" (i.e., "behind" may be viewed as away from the patient or as to the right of the yellow circle). In these instances, any reasonable interpretation of the preposition is accepted and scored as correct. Similarly, if the patient puts the green circle behind the red square, he or she receives 5 points, because the performance shows that five parts of the command (i.e., put, red, green, circle, and square) were comprehended, but the relationship ("on") was not. If the test is discontinued, prorate the remaining items of that section on the basis of the person's performance on the administered items. For example, if the test is discontinued after item 26 (third item of part F), and items 24 through 26 received 2 points each, the remaining 13 items would also receive 2 points each, for a total of 32 points for part F. If all or most of the items of sections B, C, D, E, and/or F were not given because of earlier failures, add a score of 3 points for part B, 5 for Part C, 6 for Part D, 9 for Part E, and 18 for part F. No correction for age or educational level is necessary (but see later discussion of age effects). The maximum score is 163.

DEMOGRAPHIC EFFECTS

Age

Performance improves in childhood, reaching adult levels by about age 11 years, and shows little decline with advancing

Figure 11–9 NCCEA Subtest 11 (Token Test) Sample scoring sheet. The initial order of token presentation is shown in Figure 11–8.

Name _____ Date _____ Age _____ Examiner _____

Score Sheet
IDENTIFICATION BY SENTENCE (TOKEN TEST)

A. Present tokens as in Figure 11–8. Instructions may be repeated once	
1. Show me a circle	
2. Show me a square	
3. Show me a yellow one	
4. Show me a red one	
5. Show me a blue one	
6. Show me a green one	
7. Show me a white one	
TOTAL A(7)	

B. Present only large tokens. Instructions may be repeated once	
8. Show me the **yellow** **square**	
9. Show me the **blue** **circle**	
10. Show me the **green** **circle**	
11. Show me the **white** **square**	
TOTAL B(8)	

C. Present all tokens as in Figure 11–8. Do not repeat instructions	
12. Show me the **small** **white** **circle**	
13. Show me the **large** **yellow** **square**	
14. Show me the **large** **green** **square**	
15. Show me the **small** **blue** **square**	
TOTAL C(12)	

D. Present large tokens only. Do not repeat instructions	
16. Take the **red** **circle** and the **green** **square**	
17. Take the **yellow** **square** and the **blue** **square**	
18. Take the **white** **square** and the **green** **circle**	
19. Take the **white** **circle** and the **red** **circle**	
TOTAL D(16)	

(continued)

955

Figure 11–9 *(continued)*

E. Present all tokens as in Figure 11–8. Do not repeat instructions	
20. Take the **large white circle** and the **small green square**	
21. Take the **small blue circle** and the **large yellow square**	
22. Take the **large green square** and the **large red square**	
23. Take the **large white square** and the **small green circle**	
TOTAL E(24)	

F. Present large tokens only. Do not repeat instructions	
24. **Put** the **red circle on** the **green square.**	
25. **Put** the **white square behind** the **yellow circle.**	
26. **Touch** the **blue circle with** the **red square.**	
27. **Touch** the **blue circle and** the **red square.**	
28. **Pick up** the **blue circle OR** the **red square.**	
29. **Move** the **green square away from** the **yellow square.**	
30. **Put** the **white circle in front of** the **blue square.**	
31. **If** there is a **black circle, pick up** the **red square.**	
32. **Pick up all squares except** the **yellow** one.	
33. **Put** the **green square beside** the **red circle.**	
34. **Touch** the **squares slowly and** the **circles quickly.**	
35. **Put** the **red circle between** the **yellow square** and the **green square.**	
36. **Touch all circles, except** the **green** one.	
37. **Pick up** the **red circle—no—**the **white square.**	
38. **Instead of** the **white square, pick up** the **yellow circle.**	
39. **Together with** the **yellow circle, pick up** the **blue circle.**	
TOTAL F(96)	
TOTAL A–F (163)	

age (Rich, 1993). Others have also reported few age-related effects on other versions of the TT (De Renzi and Faglioni, 1978; Ivnik et al., 1996; Swisher and Sarno, 1969). However, using our version, Emery (1986) found an age-related decline in individuals age 30–93 years.

Gender

No information on gender effects is available.

IQ/Education

General conceptual ability plays a role. There is a high correlation between the TT and the MMSE ($r = .74$; Swihart et al.,

1989). In children, correlations with the WISC-R Verbal and Performance IQs were reported as .25 and .42, respectively (Kitson, 1985). De Renzi and Faglioni (1978) recommended a correction for education, $+2.36 - (.30 \times \text{Years of schooling})$, for an item-by-item scoring, but our experience has been that such a correction is not needed for our version with subjects who have a grade 8 education or higher.

Ethnicity/Acculturation

Ethnicity does not appear to affect performance. Ripich et al. (1997) used the Spellacy and Spreen short version of the TT to compare 11 African Americans and 32 white patients with

Table 11–32 Percentile Ranks for the Token Test
for Normal Adults (*N* = 82)

Score	Percentile Rank
162	70
161	50
158	30
157	18
156	14
154	10
153	6
151	—

early or midstage dementia of the Alzheimer type (AD); they found no differences based on ethnicity. However, differences in acculturation were reported for a similar measure, the MAE Token Test, among African Americans (Kennepohl et al., 2004).

NORMATIVE DATA

Adults

Table 11–32 provides our normative data for 82 adult volunteers residing in Victoria, British Columbia, Canada, aged 25 to 75 years. The mean score for adults (and adolescents ≥ 14 years) is 161. Scores lower than 157 are virtually absent in a normal adult population. Tuokko and Woodward (1996) reported that this cutoff value also holds for elderly subjects between 60 and 85 years of age.

Children

Normative data for children with the Victoria version, presented in Table 11–33, are based on studies by Hamsher (personal communication, 1981) and Gaddes and Crockett (1975). Zaidel (1977) reported mean scores of 143.7 for subjects aged 5 years 5 months and 125.4 for those aged 4 years 6 months with the Victoria version, suggesting a consistent downward extension of these norms. The progression of scores is quite similar to that reported for other versions of the TT (e.g., the NEPSY subtest Comprehension of Instructions, CELF-4 Concepts and Following Directions).

Lass et al. (1975), examining 240 healthy school children, found only minimal variability among age groups from 6 years (*M* = 13.9, *SD* = 1.6) to 12 years (*M* = 14.7, *SD* = 1.0), using the 16-item short form introduced by Spellacy and Spreen (1969).

RELIABILITY

Internal Consistency

The Kuder-Richardson internal reliability coefficient for our 39-item version was .92 (Spellacy and Spreen, 1969). Van Harskamp and Van Dongen (1977) reported an internal reliability of .90 for Part E scored on a pass-fail basis.

Test-Retest Reliability and Practice Effects

For normal children older than 11 years of age and for adults with average intelligence, ceiling scores can be expected. For this reason, 1-year retest reliability in healthy older adults has been reported as only .50 (Snow et al., 1988). In a general clinical sample of subjects screened for suboptimal effort, retest reliability was marginal (*r* = .68) after a retest interval of 6 months (Meyers & Rohling, 2004). Gains of about 2.75 points (*SD* = 11.29, *SEM* = 1.42) were noted on retest. Reliability coefficients are higher with more impaired populations. In 41 patients with dementia who were reassessed with our version of the TT after a 10-month interval, test-retest reliability was .85 for the 16-item Spreen and Spellacy short version (Taylor, 1998).

VALIDITY

Relations Within Test

There is evidence that the various parts of the TT do not measure the same general language factor. Solving the first four parts requires a single uniform mode of processing; the last part is different because it incorporates items of greater syntactic/semantic variability (Orgass, 1976; Willmes, 1981).

Relations With Other Measures

General cognitive ability appears to be important in task performance (McNeil, 1983; Riedel & Studdert-Kennedy, 1985). As might be expected, there is a high correlation between the TT and the MMSE (*r* = .74; Swihart et al., 1989). Coupar (1976) reported a moderate correlation between our version of the TT and the Raven Progressive Matrices for brain-damaged subjects (*r* = .35). It correlates highly with other measures of receptive ability, such as the Peabody Picture Vocabulary Test (*r* = .71; Lass & Golden, 1975).

The TT embodies a variety of cognitive processes in addition to auditory comprehension, including analysis of the whole into a series of elements, the ability to generate a visual image of the verbal information, short-term memory (Lesser, 1976), and the ability to effectively ignore the automatically evoked, distracting stimulus (Winer et al., 2004). Therefore, performance on the TT can be affected by difficulties other than "pure" deficits in auditory comprehension.

Correlations with the Western Aphasia Battery aphasia quotient was .55, but with the Functional Assessment of Communication Skills (ASHA), the correlation was only .14. Correlation with a measure of discourse quantity was − .30, and with a measure of discourse quality it was .46 (Ulatowska et al., 2003). In short, performance on the TT appears to be only a modest predictor of functional competence.

Table 11-33 Token Test Norms in Percentiles for Children

Score	Age (Years)							
	6	7	8	9	10	11	12	13
163	90	90	90	90	84	84	84	84
162	88	86	86	86	75	75	75	75
161	86	84	81	78	65	61	61	57
160	84	78	78	72	57	50	47	39
159	84	75	68	65	47	35	32	19
158	81	72	65	53	35	25	19	8
157	78	68	61	47	25	16	10	2
156	78	61	57	39	19	8	4	0.9
155	75	57	53	28	12	4	2	
154	72	53	43	22	7	2	1	
153	72	50	35	16	4	1	0.7	
152	68	47	28	10	2	0.8		
151	65	39	22	8	1	0.3		
150	61	35	16	4	0.9			
149	61	32	12	2	0.5			
148	57	28	7	1				
147	53	25	4	1				
146	53	19	3	0.8				
145	50	16	2	0.5				
144	47	14	1					
143	43	12	1					
142	43	10	0.7					
141	39	7						
140	35	5						
139	35	4						
138	32	4						
137	28	3						
136	25	2						
135	25	1						
134	22							
133	19							
132	19							
131	16							
130	14							
129	14							
128	12							
127	10							
126	8							
125	8							
124	7							
123	5							
122	5							
121	4							
120	4							
119	3							
118	3							
117	2							
116	2							
115	2							
114	1							

Source: Hamsher (personal communication, 1981) and Gaddes and Crockett, 1975.

Clinical Studies

Aphasia. The TT, in its original version by De Renzi and Vignolo (1962), as well as in various modifications, has proved useful for discriminating between aphasic and non-aphasic brain-damaged patients (Boller & Dennis, 1979; Gallaher, 1979; Orgass, 1976). For example, De Renzi and Faglioni (1978) reported correct classification rates of 93% for aphasics and 95% for patients without damage to the central nervous system. Good discrimination between aphasic and nonaphasic adults was also reported by Cohen et al. (1976), Orgass (1976), Orgass and Poeck (1966), Sarno (our version, 1986), and Woll et al. (the original De Renzi and Vignolo version, in a cross-validation study, 1976). Ulatowska et al. (2001) examined 30 African American aphasics with left-hemisphere stroke (mean age, 51 years) and 30 matched healthy African American controls with our version of the TT and found a highly significant difference ($M = 106.8$ and 152.3, respectively). Morley et al., (1979) found that the TT discriminated particularly well between normal subjects and aphasics with high levels of ability, in comparison with the discrimination offered by the BDAE comprehension section and the relevant section of the PICA.

The scoring on the Victoria version is sensitive to even minor impairments of receptive language. Spellacy and Spreen (1969) reported a correct classification rate of 89% for unselected aphasics and 72% for nonaphasic brain-damaged patients, using a cutoff score of 156. De Renzi and Faglioni (1978) and Cavalli et al. (1981) found virtually no difference between patients with right-hemisphere lesions and normal controls. Our own data do show a mild impairment in right-hemisphere nonaphasic patients. The difference between these two findings is probably our more sensitive scoring system. This contention was born out by the findings of Swisher and Sarno (1969, using our version) that patients with right-hemisphere lesions without aphasia had significantly poorer scores than controls on Parts E and F of the test, although left brain-damaged aphasics still showed the highest number of errors.

A study by Coupar (1976) used our version to compare the performances of 15 aphasic subjects, 9 patients with right-hemisphere lesion, 9 leukotomized patients, and 15 normal controls and found significant differences between all four groups ($M = 119.9$, 143.3, 158.11, and 160.1, respectively).

Head Injury. As noted earlier, the Victoria version of the TT is included as part of the MSB (Volbrecht et al., 2000). Meyers and Rohling (2004) recently reported that the battery distinguishes patients with traumatic brain injury (TBI) from those with mild TBI, with a 96% correct classification rate. Other versions of the TT also appear to be sensitive to head injury. For example, in a 5-year follow-up of 90 patients with traumatic head injury who received inpatient rehabilitation, the MAE version of the TT found impairment in 21.5% of cases and showed no significant improvement over time (5 years; Millis et al., 2001). The Spanish MAE version is also sensitive to language difficulties occurring after head injury. Further, scores decline with increasing severity of injury as determined by the Glasgow Coma Scale (GCS) score (Rey et al., 2001).

Dementia. Rich (1993) reported severe impairment in AD patients compared with elderly controls. For this patient group, the TT measures not only auditory comprehension but also severity of cognitive impairment (Swihart et al., 1989). In cases of dementia (probable AD and multiinfarct dementia), the Spreen and Spellacy 16-item short form proved to be one of the best indicators of overall level of cognitive functioning and was very sensitive to cognitive decline over a 10-month period (Taylor, 1998).

Validity Studies in Children

The test is sensitive to language impairment in children: Ewing-Cobbs et al. (1987) reported that about 25% of children and adolescents with closed head injury showed impaired scores on the TT. Jordan (1994) noted that such effects persist into adulthood. Stark et al. (1995) compared children and young adults who had undergone right or left hemispherectomy. The TT and other tests of language development showed syntactic comprehension and rapid-rate auditory processing deficits after left but not right hemispherectomy; speech production, on the other hand, was similar for the two groups.

Impairment on the TT was also reported in children with hyperbilirubinemia (Harris et al., 1983; Lenhard, 1983), low birth weight (Harris et al., 1983), developmental aphasia (Tallal et al., 1985), developmental delay (Cole & Fewell, 1983), and autism (Minshew et al., 1995).

Naeser et al. (1987) claimed that the TT performance of 3-year-old children resembled that of patients with severe Wernicke's aphasia, and the performance of 6-year-olds was similar to that of aphasics with mild comprehension deficits and frontal-parietal perisylvian lesions (i.e., the notion of comprehension deficit in aphasia as a regression to earlier developmental stages). A similar regression hypothesis was proposed in a comparison of pre-middle-aged, young-old, and old-old adults (Emery, 1986). Elliott et al. (1990) found a relationship between TT performance and fine-grained auditory discrimination of rapidly presented consonant-vowel stimuli (e.g., pa-da-ba) in younger children (aged 6 to 7 years, $r = .64$), but not in older children (aged 9 to 11 years, $r = .37$). This may be related to the developmental stage of the child, or, as the authors point out, to the increasing influence of the written mode of language learning.

A study by Whitehouse (1983) reported significant differences between dyslexic and normal-reading adolescents (grades 7 through 12), but emphasized that 55% of the dyslexics did not make any more errors than normal readers did. She concluded that errors on Part E of the original TT (De Renzi and Vignolo, 1962), where most errors occurred in dyslexics, reflected impaired ability to process cognitive information. In contrast, Slaghuis et al. (1993) compared 35 dyslexic boys, aged 7 to 14 years, with a matched control group and argued that TT performance indicated a phonological coding deficit present in 91% of the dyslexics but only 20% of the controls.

Examining 113 children who had had meningitis, Taylor and Schatschneider (1992) found that the test related significantly to sociobehavioral outcome measures (e.g., the Vineland Scales), as well as other neuropsychological tests.

Malingering

Meyers et al. (1999) suggested that standard neuropsychological measures such as the TT can do double duty, not only as clinically useful neuropsychological tests but also to detect malingering. They compared the TT (our version) in 27 patients with moderate/severe brain damage, 35 nonlitigating patients with mild brain damage, 49 litigating patients with mild brain damage, 20 malingering "actors," and 30 normal controls, all with a mean age of approximately 30 years. Based on this study, they recommended a cutoff score of 150, with scores at that level or lower raising the index of suspicion. They also noted that failure on two or more malingering indexes derived from standard neuropsychological tasks is very rare, even in those with lengthy loss of consciousness.

COMMENT

The TT and its variants have a long history in neuropsychology. The advantages of the TT lie in sound discriminative validity, reasonable reliability, and portability. It is also cost-effective in terms of material, time, and expertise required in administration and scoring. In addition, it is sensitive to all forms of aphasia, but especially to receptive aphasia. The latter parts of the test (parts E and F) have been shown to differ from the first four parts because they require complex auditory/cognitive processing as well as short-term memory, making the test useful in a variety of other conditions (e.g., dementia, head injury) as well.

On the other hand, there are a number of limitations. First, the normative samples are poorly described, and the data were collected more than 25 years ago. Therefore, caution is advised in relying on the norms provided here. Although the test can be used with children, the clinician/researcher might consider other measures with stronger psychometric properties (e.g., CELF-4; Semel et al., 2003). Second, there are different versions of the TT, and this can be confusing. However, it should be remembered that all are adaptations of the original test items and wordings by De Renzi and Vignolo (1962), and that only the number of items and the scoring differs; hence, validity studies with different versions tend to support the validity of others. In fact, even short versions tend to show discriminant validity similar to that of the long version (e.g., Taylor, 1998; van Harskamp & van Dongen, 1977).

Brookshire's (1973) early advice remains valid: The clinician should keep in mind that, although it is a sensitive indicator of comprehension deficits, the TT relies on a limited stimulus array. Other tests of auditory comprehension should be used to supplement the TT. Note that there are many reasons, other than simple comprehension per se, why patients may perform poorly on this task. Rao (1990) also pointed out that the test introduces a somewhat artificial test situation and therefore has less "ecovalidity" than other, functional communication measures.

REFERENCES

Benton, A. L., Hamsher, K. de S., & Sivan, A. B. (1994). *Multilingual Aphasia Examination* (3rd ed.). Iowa City, Ia.: AJA Associates.

Boller, F. & Dennis, M. (1979). *Auditory comprehension: Clinical and experimental studies with the Token Test.* New York: Academic Press.

Boller, F. & Vignolo, L. (1966). Latent sensory aphasia in hemisphere-damaged patients: An experimental study with the Token-Test. *Brain, 89,* 815–831.

Brookshire, R. H. (1973). The use of consequences in speech pathology: Incentive and feedback functions. *Journal of Communication Disorders, 6,* 88–92.

Cavalli, M., De Renzi, E., Faglioni, P. & Vitale, A. (1981). Impairment of right brain-damaged patients on a linguistic cognitive task. *Cortex, 17,* 545–556.

Cohen, R., Kelter, S., Engel, D. List, G., & Strohner, H.(1976). Zur Validitaet des Token-Tests. *Nervenarzt, 47,* 357–361.

Cole, K. N., & Fewell, R. R. (1983). A quick language screening test for young children. *Journal of Speech and Hearing Disorders, 48,* 149–153.

Coupar, M. (1976). Detection of mild aphasia: A study using the Token Test. *British Journal of Medical Psychology, 49,* 141–144.

D'Arcy, R. C. N., & Connolly, J. F. (1999). An event-related brain potential study of receptive speech comprehension using a modified Token Test. *Neuropsychologia, 37,* 1477–1489.

D'Arcy, R. C. N., Connolly, J. F., & Crocker, S. F. (2000). Latency shifts in the N2b component track phonological deviations in spoken words. *Clinical Neurophysiology, 111,* 40–44.

De Renzi, E., & Faglioni, P. (1978). Development of a shortened version of the Token Test. *Cortex, 14,* 41–49.

De Renzi, E., & Vignolo, L. (1962). The Token Test: A sensitive test to detect receptive disturbances in aphasics. *Brain, 85,* 665–678.

Elliott, L. L., Hammer, M. A., & Scholl, M. E. (1990). Fine-grained auditory discrimination and performance on tests of receptive vocabulary and receptive language. *Annals of Dyslexia, 40,* 170–179.

Emery, O. B. (1986). Linguistic decrement in normal aging. *Language and Communication, 6,* 47–64.

Ewing-Cobbs, L., Levin, H. S., Eisenberg, H. M., & Fletcher, J. M. (1987). Language functions allowing closed-head injury in children and adolescents. *Journal of Clinical and Experimental Neuropsychology, 9,* 575–592.

Gaddes, W. H., & Crockett, D. J. (1975). The Spreen-Benton aphasia test: Normative data as a measure of normal language development. *Brain and Language, 4,* 257–280.

Gallaher, A. J. (1979). Temporal reliability of aphasic performance on the Token Test. *Brain and Language, 7,* 34–41.

Harris, V. L., Keith, R. W., & Novak, K. K. (1983). Relationship between two dichotic listening tests and the Token Test for children. *Ear and Hearing, 6,* 278–282.

Ivnik, R. J., Malec, J. F., & Smith, G. E. (1996). Neuropsychological tests norms above age 55: COWAT, MAE Token, WRAT-R Reading, AMNART, Stroop, TMT and JLO. *The Clinical Neuropsychologist, 10,* 262–278.

Jordan, F. M. (1994). Severe closed-head injury in childhood: Linguistic outcomes in adulthood. *Brain Injury, 8,* 501–508.

Kennepohl, S., Shore, D., Nobors, N., & Hanks, R. (2004). African American acculturation and neuropsychological test performance following traumatic brain injury. *Journal of the International Neuropsychological Society, 10,* 566–577.

Kitson, D. L. (1985). Comparison of the Token Test of language development and the WISC-R. *Perceptual and Motor Skills, 61,* 532–534.

Kosciesza, M. (1995). Polish adaptation of the "Token Test" for children and its practical application. *Psychologia Wychowawcza, 38,* 350–358.

Lass, N. J., DePaolo, A. M., Simcoe, J. C., & Samuel, S. M. (1975). A normative study of children's performance on the short form of the Token Test. *Journal of Communication Disorders, 8,* 193–198.

Lass, N. J., & Golden, S. S. (1975). A comparative study of children's performance on three tests for receptive language abilities. *Journal of Auditory Research, 15,* 177–182.

Lenhard, M. L. (1983). Effects of neonatal hyperbilirubinemia on Token Test performance of six-year old children. *Journal of Auditory Research, 23,* 195–204.

Lesser, R. (1976). Verbal and non-verbal memory components in the Token Test. *Neuropsychologia, 14,* 79–85.

McNeil, M. R. (1983). Aphasia: Neurological considerations. *Topics in Language Disorders, 3,* 1–19.

Meyers, J. E., Galinsky, A. M., & Volbrecht, M. (1999). Malingering and mild brain injury: How low is too low? *Applied Neuropsychology, 6,* 208–216.

Meyers, J. E., & Rohling, M. L. (2004). Validation of the Meyers Short Battery on mild TBI patients. *Archives of Clinical Neuropsychology, 19,* 637–651.

Millis, S. R., Rosenthal, M., Novack, T. A., Sherer, M., Nick, T. G., Kreutzer, J. S., High, W. M., & Ricker, J. H. (2001). Long-term neuropsychological outcome after traumatic brain injury. *Journal of Head Trauma Rehabilitation, 16,* 343–355.

Minshew, N. J., Goldstein, G., & Siegel, D. J. (1995). Speech and language in high-functioning autistic individuals. *Neuropsychology, 9,* 255–261.

Morley, G. K., Lundgren, S., & Haxby, J. (1979). Comparison and clinical applicability of auditory comprehension scores on the behavioral neurologic deficit evaluation: Boston Diagnostic Aphasia Examination, Porch Index of Communicative Ability, and Token Test. *Journal of Clinical Neuropsychology, 1,* 249–258.

Naeser, M. A., Mazurski, P., Goodglass, H., & Peraino, M. (1987). Auditory syntactic comprehension in nine aphasic groups (with CT scan) and children: Differences in degree, but not order of difficulty observed. *Cortex, 23,* 359–380.

Orgass, B. (1976). Eine Revision des Token Tests II: Validitaetsnachweis, Normierung und Standardisierung. *Diagnostica, 22,* 141–156.

Orgass, B., & Poeck, K. (1966). Clinical validation of a new test for aphasia: An experimental study of the Token Test. *Cortex, 2,* 222–243.

Poeck, K., & Pietron, H. P. (1981). The influence of stretched speech presentation on Token Test performance in aphasic and right brain damaged patients. *Neuropsychologia, 19,* 133–136.

Rao, P. (1990). Functional communication assessment of the elderly. In E. Cherov (Ed.), *Proceedings of the Research Symposium on Communication Sciences and Disorders and Aging* (pp. 28–34). Rockville, Md.: American Speech and Hearing Association.

Rey, G. J., Feldman, E., Hernandez, D., Levin, B. E., Rivas-Vazquez, R., Nedd, K. J., & Benton, A. L. (2001). Application of the Multilingual Aphasia Examination–Spanish in the evaluation of Hispanic patients post closed-head trauma. *The Clinical Neuropsychologist, 15,* 13–18.

Rich, J. B. (1993). *Pictorial and verbal implicit and recognition memory in aging and Alzheimer's disease: A transfer-appropriate processing account.* Ph.D. dissertation, University of Victoria, Victoria, B.C., Canada.

Riedel, K., & Studdert-Kennedy, M. (1985). Extending formant transitions may not improve aphasic's perception of stop consonant place of articulation. *Brain and Language, 24,* 223–232.

Ripich, D. N., Carpenter, B., & Ziol, E. (1997). Comparison of African-American and white persons with Alzheimer's disease on language measures. *Neurology, 48,* 781–783.

Sarno, M. T.(1986) Verbal impairment in head injury. *Archives of Physical and Medical Rehabilitation, 67,* 399–404.

Semel, E., Wiig, E. H., & Secord, W. A. (2003). *CELF-4.* San Antonio, Tex.: The Psychological Corporation.

Slaghuis, W. L., Lovegrove, W. J., & Davidson, J. A. (1993). Visual and language processing deficits are concurrent in dyslexia. *Cortex, 29,* 601–615.

Snow, W. G., Tierney, M. C., Zorzitto, M. L., Fisher, R. H., & Reid, D. W. (1988). One-year test-retest reliability of selected neuropsychological tests in older adults. Paper presented at the International Neuropsychological Society Meeting, New Orleans [Abstract]. *Journal of Clinical and Experimental Neuropsychology, 10,* 60.

Spellacy, F., & Spreen, O. (1969). A short form of the Token Test. *Cortex, 5,* 390–397.

Spreen, O., & Benton, A. L. (1969, 1977), *The Neurosensory Center Comprehensive Examination for Aphasia.* Neuropsychology Laboratory, University of Victoria, Victoria, B.C., Canada.

Stark, R. E., Bleile, K., Brandt, J., & Freeman, J. (1995). Speech-language outcomes of hemispherectomy in children and young adults. *Brain and Language, 51,* 406–421.

Swihart, A. A., Panisset, M., Becker, J. T., Beyer, J. T., Beyer, J. R., & Boller, F. (1989). The Token Test: Validity and diagnostic power in Alzheimer's disease. *Developmental Neuropsychology, 5,* 71–80.

Swisher, L. P., & Sarno, M. T. (1969). Token Test scores of three matched patient groups: Left brain-damaged with aphasia; right brain-damaged without aphasia; non brain-damaged. *Cortex, 5,* 264–273.

Tallal, P., Stark, R. E., & Mellits, D. (1985). The relationship between auditory temporal analysis and receptive language development: Evidence from studies of developmental language disorder. *Neuropsychologia, 23,* 527–534.

Taylor, H. G., & Schatschneider, C. (1992). Child neuropsychological assessment: A test of basic assumptions. *The Clinical Neuropsychologist, 6,* 259–275.

Taylor, R. (1998). Indices of neuropsychological functioning and decline over time in dementia. *Archives of Gerontology and Geriatrics, 27,* 165–170.

Tuokko, H., & Woodward, T. S. (1996). Development and validation of a demographic system for neuropsychological measures used in the Canadian Study of Health and Aging. *Journal of Clinical and Experimental Neuropsychology, 18,* 479–616.

Ulatowska, H. K., Olness, G. S., Wertz, R. T., Samson, A. G., Keebler, M. W., & Goins, K. E. (2003). Relationship between discourse and

Western Aphasia Battery performance in African Americans with aphasia. *Aphasiology, 17,* 511–521.

Ulatowska, H. K., Olness, G. S., Wertz, R. T., Thompson, J., Keebler, M. W., Hill, C. L., & Auther, L. L. (2001). Comparison of language impairment, functional communication, and discourse measures in African-American aphasic and normal adults. *Aphasiology, 15,* 2007–2016.

Van Harskamp, F., & Van Dongen, H. R. (1977). Construction and validation of different short forms of the Token Test. *Neuropsychologia, 15,* 467–470.

Volbrecht, M., Meyers, J. E., & Kaster-Bundgaard, J. (2000). Neuropsychological outcome of head injury using a short battery. *Archives of Clinical Neuropsychology, 15,* 251–265.

Whitehouse, C. C. (1983). Token Test performance by dyslexic adolescents. *Brain and Language, 18,* 224–235.

Willmes, K. (1981). A new look at the Token Test using probabilistic test models. *Neuropsychologia, 19,* 631–645.

Winer, D. A., Connor, L. T., & Obler, L. K. (2004). Inhibition and auditory comprehension in Wernicke's aphasia. *Aphasiology, 18,* 599–609.

Woll, G., Naumann, E., Cohen, R., & Kelter, S. (1976). Kreuzvalidierung der Revision des Token Tests durch Orgass. *Diagnostica, 22,* 157–162.

Zaidel, E. (1977). Unilateral auditory language comprehension on the Token Test following cerebral commissurotomy and hemispherectomy. *Neuropsychologia, 15,* 1–18.

12

Tests of Visual Perception

Farah (2003) has observed that higher-level vision has two main goals: the identification of stimuli and their localization. These two goals, abbreviated as "what" and "where," are consistent with studies of animals as well as humans, suggesting that there are different cortical pathways for object and spatial vision, located in ventral and dorsal cortices, respectively. Based on experimental studies of animals, Mishkin and his colleagues (Mishkin et al., 1983; Ungerleider & Mishkin, 1982) proposed that identification of objects is associated with a pathway connecting the striate, prestriate, and inferior temporal areas, whereas spatial processing is linked to a pathway connecting striate, prestriate, and inferior parietal areas (see Figure 12–1).

Early evidence for the existence of two cortical visual streams in humans came from neurological case reports (Potzl, 1928; Lange, 1936) documenting that some patients had selectively impaired object recognition but retained good spatial abilities, whereas others showed the reverse pattern (Farah, 2003). The same dissociation is observed after posterior right hemisphere damage, but to a weaker extent. Although patients with right posterior damage are often impaired on both spatial analysis and object perception tasks, there appears to be little relationship between these problems (McCarthy & Warrington, 1990; Newcombe & Russell, 1969; Warrington & James, 1988; Warrington & Rabin, 1970). For example, Newcombe and Russell (1969) examined World War II veterans with missile injuries to the head on two tasks: face identification (closure) and maze learning. In the facial identification task, patients had to judge the age and gender of faces rendered as fragmentary regions of light and shadow. In the maze-learning task, patients had to learn, by trial and error, the correct path through an array. Newcombe and Russell (1969) reported evidence of dissociated deficits in patients with postrolandic lesions, with no overlap in scores of those most severely impaired in closure and those most severely impaired in maze learning, supporting the idea that "what" and "where" are processed independently (Farah, 2003). Furthermore, the men with poor facial identification

performance had posterior temporal lesions, whereas the men with poor maze performance had posterior parietal lesions.

Disorders of object perception (apperceptive agnosia—impairment of visual recognition not resulting from more elementary visual problems or more general intellectual difficulties) are observed on tasks that manipulate the perceptual dimensions of objects, such as using fragmented or degraded versions, altering the angle from which an object is viewed, and changing lighting conditions. Tests that use such techniques include Benton's Facial Recognition Test, the Hooper Visual Organization Test, and the four tasks included in the Visual Object and Space Perception Battery (VOSP): Incomplete Letters, Silhouettes, Object Decision, and Progressive Silhouettes (Warrington & James, 1991; see Table 12–1).

McCarthy and Warrington (1990) distinguished two main aspects of spatial processing. The first refers to impairments in locating single objects in space with intact visual acuity (visual disorientation). The critical lesion site is thought to be the occipital-parietal junction; in some cases, a unilateral form of the disorder is observed after damage to this area in either the left or right hemisphere alone. The ability to determine single-point localization is considered to be a prerequisite for higher-order functions of spatial perception. The second aspect of spatial processing goes beyond that tapped by single-point localization and refers to spatial processing in more complex tasks (spatial analysis). Faulty analysis of relative spatial information (visual-spatial agnosia) can be observed on measures of assembling (e.g., Block Design) and drawing (e.g., Clock Drawing), although it should be noted that disorganized arrangement of puzzles or poor drawing can be caused by other impairments as well (e.g., executive dysfunction). A number of simpler tasks are also used to examine spatial perception, including line orientation (Judgment of Line Orientation), position discrimination, stimulus orientation, and enumeration (see *Visual Object and Space Perception Battery*). In general, deficits

Figure 12–1 The two cortical visual systems: Dorsal areas thought to be important for spatial or "where" processing, and ventral areas are important for appearance or "what" processing.

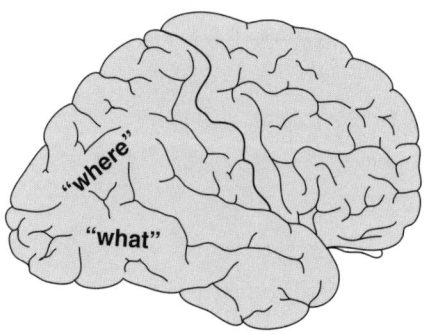

on these tasks are linked to posterior right hemisphere disturbance.

Visual-spatial disorders include hemispatial neglect—a deficit in awareness of stimuli contralateral to a lesion that does not involve sensory projection systems or the primary cortical sensory areas to which they project (Heilman et al., 2003). Most commonly, the neglect affects the left side of space, reflecting right hemisphere damage. Neglect is seen most frequently after temporoparietal lesions, although it can occur with lesions in other brain regions (Heilman et al., 2003).

There are many tests of spatial neglect (Heilman et al., 2003; Lezak et al., 2004), including line bisection, cancellation, and drawing tasks. In line bisection, the examiner draws the line for the patient or asks the patient to copy an already drawn horizontal line. The patient is instructed to divide the line by placing a mark (e.g., an "X") at the center point (see Figure 12–2). The score is the length by which the patient's estimated center deviates from the actual center. Patients with spatial neglect usually displace their mark to the ipsilesional side (contralateral neglect). In simple cancellation tests, such as that described by Albert (1973), the patient is asked to cancel or cross out lines scattered in a seemingly random pattern across a sheet of paper (see Figure 12–3). Patients may fail to cancel lines on the contralesional side of the page. The available evidence suggests that simple line-crossing tasks are likely to miss patients with mild forms of neglect. Tasks that require not only simple detection (e.g., line bisection, line cancellation) but also selection from distractors are more sensitive (e.g., Ferber & Karnath, 2001). This is the basis of the Bells Cancellation Test and the Balloons Test. Spatial neglect can also be assessed by asking patients to copy or make drawings spontaneously. For example, patients with neglect may write in only one side of the clock, include only the numbers that belong to that side, or write all 12 numbers on one side (Heilman et al., 2003).

In this section, we review the Balloons Test, Bells Test, Clock Drawing Test, Facial Recognition Test, Hooper Visual Organization Test, Judgment of Line Orientation Test, and the VOSP (see Table 12–1). Additional tasks can be found in

Table 12–1 Tests of Visual Perception

Test	Age Range (Years)	Administration Time (Min)	Processes	Test-Retest Reliability
Balloons Test	Adults	10	Visual inattention	Marginal to adequate
Bells Test	Teenage/adult	<5	Visual inattention	Marginal
Clock Drawing Test	6–12; adult	5	Visual-spatial ability Executive control Visual inattention	Adequate
Facial Recognition	6–14; 16+	Long: 10; Short: 7	Recognition of unfamiliar faces	Marginal to adequate
Hooper Visual Organization Test	5–91	10–15	Visual-perceptual ability	Marginal to high
Judgment of Line Orientation	7–96	15–20	Angular judgments; motivational status	High
Visual Object and Space Perception	20–70+	5–10 per test; 40–80 for entire battery	Object perception Incomplete Letters Silhouettes Object Decision Progressive Silhouettes Space perception Dot Counting Position Discrimination Number Location Cube Analysis	NA

Note: NA = not applicable.

Figure 12–2 Performance of patient with hemispatial neglect on the line bisection task. *Source:* Reprinted with permission from Heilman et al., 2003.

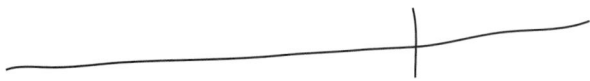

Figure 12–3 Performance by patient with hemispatial neglect on a crossing-out task. *Source:* Reprinted with permission from Heilman et al., 2003.

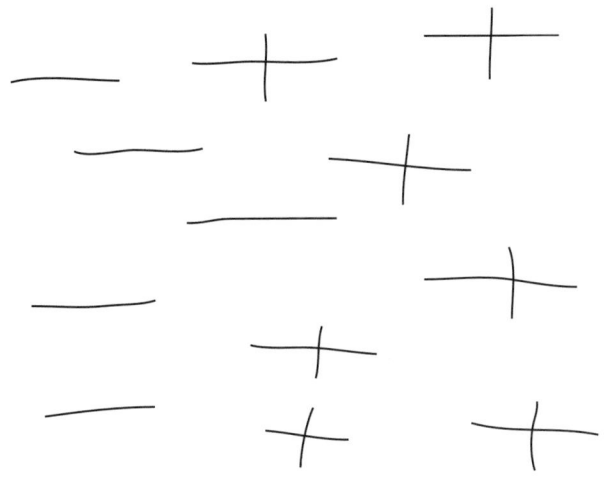

various batteries such as the KBNA, NAB, NEPSY, Wechsler Scales, and Woodcock-Johnson-III.

REFERENCES

Albert, M. D. (1973). A simple test of visual neglect. *Neurology, 23,* 658–664.

Farah, M. J. (2003). Disorders of visual-spatial perception and cognition. In K. M. Heilman & E. Valenstein (Eds.), *Clinical neuropsychology* (4th ed., pp. 146–160). New York: Oxford University Press.

Ferber, S., & Karnath, H. O. (2001). How to assess spatial neglect: Line bisection or cancellation tasks? *Journal of Clinical and Experimental Neuropsychology, 23,* 599–607.

Heilman, K. M., Watson, R. T., & Valenstein, E. (2003). Neglect and related disorders. In K. M. Heilman & E. Valenstein (Eds.), *Clinical neuropsychology* (4th ed., pp. 296–346). New York: Oxford University Press.

Lange, J. (1936). *Agrosien und Apraxien.* In O. Bunke & O. Foerster (Eds.), *Handbuch der Neurologie.* Berlin: Springer-Verlag.

Lezak, M. D., Howieson, D. B., Loring, D. W., Hannay, H. J., & Fischer, J. S. (2004). *Neuropsychological assessment* (4th ed.). New York: Oxford University Press.

McCarthy, R. A., & Warrington, E. K. (1990). *Cognitive neuropsychology.* San Diego, Calif.: Academic Press.

Mishkin, M., Ungerleider, L. G., & Macko, K. (1983). Object vision and spatial vision: Two cortical pathways. *Trends in Neuropsychology, 6,* 414–417.

Newcombe, F., & Russell, W. (1969). Dissociated visual perceptual and spatial deficits in focal lesions of the right hemisphere. *Journal of Neurology, Neurosurgery and Psychiatry, 32,* 73–81.

Potzl, O. (1928). *Die Aphasielehre vom Standpunkte der Klinishcen Psychiatrie.* Leipzig: Franz Deuticke.

Ungerleider, L. G., & Mishkin, M. (1982). Two cortical visual systems. In D. J. Engle, M. A. Goodale, & R. J. Mansfield (Eds.), *Analysis of visual behavior* (pp. 549–586). Cambridge, MA: MIT Press.

Warrington, E. K., & James, M. (1988). Visual apperceptive agnosia: A clinico-anatomical study of three cases. *Cortex, 24,* 13–32.

Warrington, E. K., & James, M. (1991). *The Visual Object and Space Perception Battery.* Bury St. Edmunds, England: Thames Valley Test Company.

Warrington, E. K., & Rabin, P. (1970). Perceptual matching in patients with cerebral lesions. *Neuropsychologia, 8,* 475–487.

Balloons Test

PURPOSE

The Balloons Test (Edgeworth et al., 1998) is designed to screen for visual inattention.

SOURCE

The test (containing a manual, test cards, and 25 scoring sheets) is available from Harcourt Assessment (http://www.harcourt-uk.com) at a cost of about $283 US.

AGE RANGE

No age range is specified. Data in the manual refer only to older subjects.

DESCRIPTION

The Balloons Test consists of two subtests, each containing 202 items. In subtest A, the control task, 22 of the 202 items are targets to be canceled. Targets are circles with a line adjoining (i.e., "balloons"). The other items are circles (see Figure 12–4). Patients are simply required to locate and put a line through each balloon in a fixed time limit of 3 min. Ten targets and 90 distractors are presented on either side of the midline, which is marked with an arrow, and two balloons that are located close to the midline are used to demonstrate the task. In subtest B, the number and position of balloons and circles is the reverse of subtest A, and the targets are now circles. Ninety balloons and 10 target circles are presented on either side of the midline, again with two central circles used to demonstrate the task.

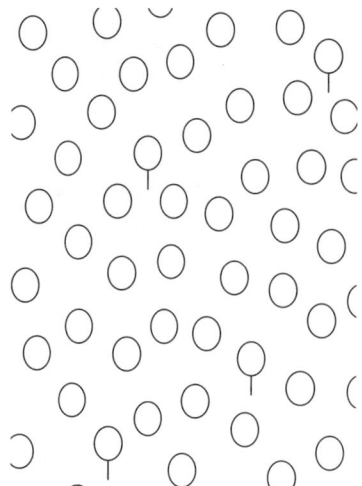 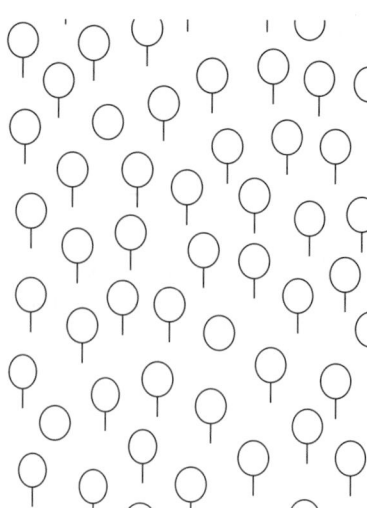

Figure 12–4 The Balloons Test. Left: Section of Subtest A. Right: Section of Subset B.

The test is based on the "pop-out" phenomenon described by Treisman and Gelade (1980), whereby the novel objects stand out against the repeated objects. Detection of balloons among circles (subtest A) reflects a relatively parallel process; that is, the time taken to detect targets does not increase significantly as the number of distractors increases. Therefore, subtest A is a control measure in which the attentional demands for serial search are kept to a minimum. By contrast, subtest B is a test of serial search that makes greater demands on attention. In this subtest, the targets do not "pop out"; rather, they must be searched for effortfully in a serial manner. A larger number of omissions on subtest B than A allows exclusion of the possibility that omissions are caused by visual field defects unrelated to attention. There must be an attentional deficit for the omissions to differ markedly, because the two arrays are visually similar but vary in attentional demand.

ADMINISTRATION

The examiner times the test and asks the subject to use a pen of a different color after 90 s. This is done to permit analysis of the search pattern.

Patients who incorrectly report that they have completed the task before the end of the time limit are encouraged to continue. The authors caution that, as with all visual perceptual tests, it is important that visual acuity and other oculomotor aspects of vision have been taken into account.

ADMINISTRATION TIME

A time limit of 3 min is set for each subtest. The total test takes about 10 min.

SCORING

Performance is evaluated by counting the number of targets canceled in each subtest (Total A and Total B). A Generalized

Inattention Index is noted (yes/no): Patients with a Total B score of less than 17 are classed as having generalized visual inattention. A laterality index is also computed (Laterality B); it consists of the number of targets canceled on the left, expressed as a percentage of the total number of targets canceled (Total B). Those with a Total B score of less than 17 and a Laterality B score of less than 45% are classed as having a unilateral visual attention deficit.

DEMOGRAPHIC EFFECTS

Demographic effects are not reported.

NORMATIVE DATA

Standardization Sample

The test was standardized on 72 patients with right cerebrovascular accidents (CVAs). All were right-handed and were tested at least 14 days after their stroke (on average about 6 months after stroke). A subgroup of 39 patients were classed as showing visual neglect according to another test (Star Cancellation Test of the Behavioral Inattention Test). A control group of 55 non-brain-damaged subjects were given subtest B. These subjects were recruited from an outpatient rheumatology clinic at a hospital in London. The characteristics of the samples are shown in Table 12–2. Norms for the test were established from the results of the rheumatology control subjects.

RELIABILITY

Test-Retest Reliability

The test authors report that subtest B was given to 29 subjects (presumably patients) on two separate occasions, with a mean retest interval of 7.7 days. For the Generalized Inattention

Table 12–2 Characteristics of Standardization Sample for Balloons Test

Number	72 patients with right CVA (39 with visual neglect according to Star Cancellation test of the Behavioral Inattention Test); 55 controls
Age	Patients with visual neglect: $M = 67.2$, $SD = 8.8$
	Patients without neglect: $M = 69.3$, $SD = 11.9$
	Controls: $M = 64.3$, $SD = 12.3$
Geographic location	United Kingdom
Sample type	Controls were from an outpatient rheumatology clinic at a hospital in London
Education	NA
Gender	Controls: 49% male, 51% female
	CVA patients: 56% male, 44% female
Race/Ethnicity	Not reported
Screening	Patients: no premorbid psychiatric or other neurologic condition; previous history of stroke was not an exclusion criterion; those with severe visual impairment, general cognitive deterioration, or language comprehension deficits were excluded
	Controls: Medical notes checked, and only those with no reported history of neurological or psychiatric disorder and those with normal or corrected-to-normal vision were included

Index, the two administrations yielded a correlation of .64. Using the Generalized Inattention Index, the numbers of visual neglect cases identified by test and retest were compared, and 83% agreement was found. The authors also report that the correlation for the Lateralized Inattention Index was .71.

VALIDITY

Relationships With Other Measures

The test authors report that the validity of the test as a measure of visual neglect was established in two ways. First, the relationships between the Balloons Test subtest B correlated highly ($r = .78$) with scores of the Star Cancellation subtest of the Behavioral Inattention Test. Second, scores on the Balloons Test were compared with a short questionnaire completed by a relative or caregiver that focused on functional difficulties associated with neglect (Catherine Berego Scale; Azouvi et al., 1996); this comparison resulted in a correlation of .67.

Clinical Findings

The authors evaluated 62 patients with right CVAs, 39 of whom had been diagnosed (via a different measure, the Star Cancellation Test) as showing visual neglect. As might be expected, the visual neglect group performed worse than the non-neglect group both on subtest A and subtest B. The effect was especially pronounced for the laterality index, confirming that visual neglect tends to affect the left side of space more than the right side.

Edgeworth et al. (1998) advocated the use of colored pens because they noted that the manner in which a patient approaches the task can offer insight into the location of the damage. That is, patients with right-hemisphere lesions show a strong tendency to initiate search on the right side of the stimulus sheet and to scan the sheet in an unsystematic manner, particularly if the stimulus array is random. By contrast, those with left-sided lesions usually begin the search in the upper left-hand corner and proceed with systematic, horizontal and vertical sweeps of the stimulus sheet (Weintraub & Mesulam, 1988). Unfortunately, Edgeworth et al. (1998) provided no confirmation of these patterns on their task.

COMMENT

This test is quick and simple to give. It uses the "pop-out" effect and a strict time limitation. The imposition of a time limit and the inclusion of the instruction to continue searching if the subject stops prematurely are positive features that reduce the possibility that deficits in sustained attention will affect performance.

Unfortunately, so far the test has produced no further independent studies. Users should also note that norms are available only for a group of older adults with a mean age of about 64 years. Further, test-retest correlations are marginal/adequate; however, because hemineglect is a fluctuating deficit, a perfect correspondence of results between two administrations of the test might not be expected. Although the authors offer guidelines for the diagnosis of left inattention, they do not provide data on patients with left-hemisphere damage and therefore cannot give guidance for the diagnosis of right inattention. These limitations restrict the clinical usefulness of the test, although it clearly deserves further study.

REFERENCES

Azouvi, P., Marchal, F., Samual, E., Morin, L., Renard, C., Louis-Dreyfus, A., et al. (1996). Functional consequences and awareness of unilateral neglect: Study of an evaluation scale. *Neuropsychological Rehabilitation, 6,* 81–160.

Edgeworth, J., Roberson, I., & McMillan, T. M. (1998). *The Balloons Test.* Bury St. Edmunds: Thames Valley Test Company.

Treisman, A., & Gelade, G. (1980). A feature-integration theory of attention. *Cognitive Psychology, 12,* 97–136.

Weintraub, S., & Mesulam, M. (1988). Visual hemispatial inattention: Stimulus parameters and exploratory strategies. *Journal of Neurology, Neurosurgery, and Psychiatry, 51,* 1481–1488.

Bells Cancellation Test

PURPOSE

The purpose of the Bells Cancellation Test (or Bells Test) is to detect visual inattention.

SOURCE

The test can be copied from the original publication or from this book.

AGE RANGE

The age range is teenage and adult.

DESCRIPTION

The Bells Test (Gauthier et al., 1989) consists of a 21.5 × 28 cm sheet of paper on which seven lines of 35 distractor figures (e.g., bird, key, apple, mushroom, car) and five target figures (bells) are presented (see Figures 12–5 through 12–7). The target figures are arranged so that five each appear in seven equal columns on the page. The number of distractor figures in each column also remains constant.

The test can be modified for use with children (Biancardi & Stoppa, 1997; Laurent-Vannier et al., 2001). For example, Laurent-Vannier et al. (2001) described an adaptation for children aged 2½ to 8 years using teddy bears instead of bells.

ADMINISTRATION

The patient is seated at a table across from the examiner with both forearms placed comfortably on the table. He or she is presented with a demonstration sheet that includes the target figure at the center and all distractors (see Figure 12–5). The subject is asked to name the items as the examiner points to them. If unable to name the items because of language problems, he or she is asked to place cards representing each object on top of the object to ensure proper object recognition. The examiner then presents the test copy (see Figure 12–6) and provides the following instructions: "*Your task consists of circling with the pencil all the bells that you can find on this sheet. Start when I say 'GO' and stop when you have circled all the bells*" (adapted from Gauthier et al., 1989, pp. 49–50). There is no time limit.

If the patient stops before all bells are circled, the examiner gives the following reminder only once: "*Are you sure that all bells are now circled? Please check again.*" The examiner continues to check bells circled after this admonition but marks them by underlining or circling the numbers for later identification.

Care should be taken that the sheet is placed in the center of the patient's view and that he or she does not lean to the right or left of the sheet.

ADMINISTRATION TIME

The test requires 1 to 5 min after instructions.

SCORING

The examiner keeps the score sheet (Figure 12–7) away from the view of the patient and records the results by successively numbering the circling of bells by the patient as well as the circling of other elements in the approximate location. This allows analysis of the scanning pattern of the patient after the

Figure 12–5 Demonstration Sheet for the Bells Test, used to familiarize the subject with the bell figure and distractor figures. *Source:* From Gauthier et al., 1989.

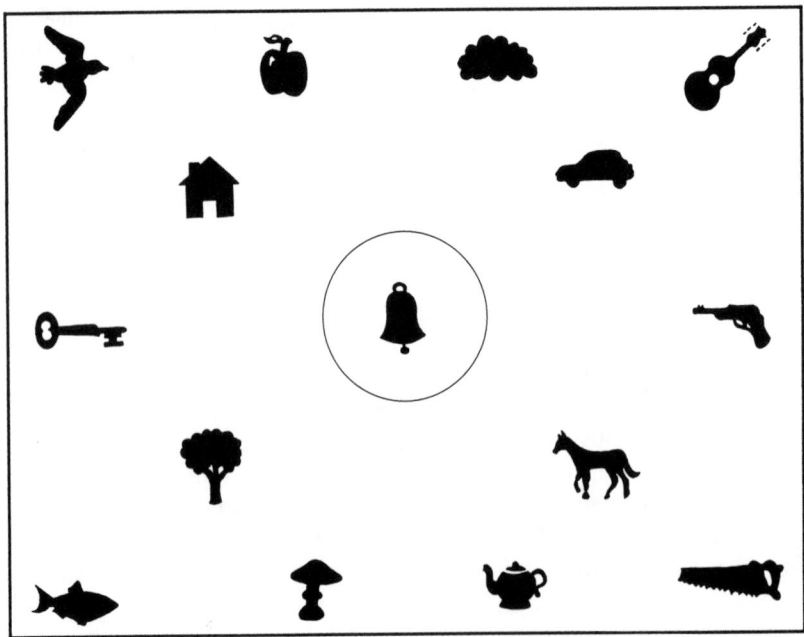

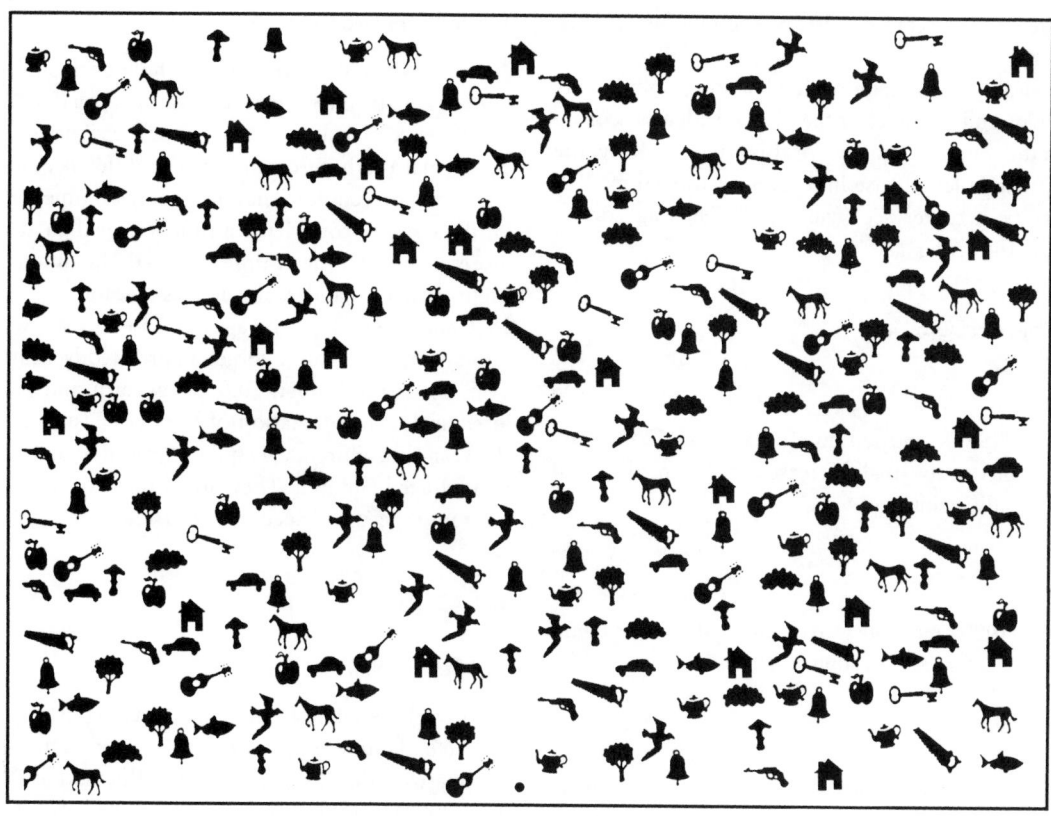

Figure 12–7 Scoring Sheet for the Bells Test, indicating bells in central location and in three left and three right sectors of the visual field. *Source:* From Gauthier et al., 1989.

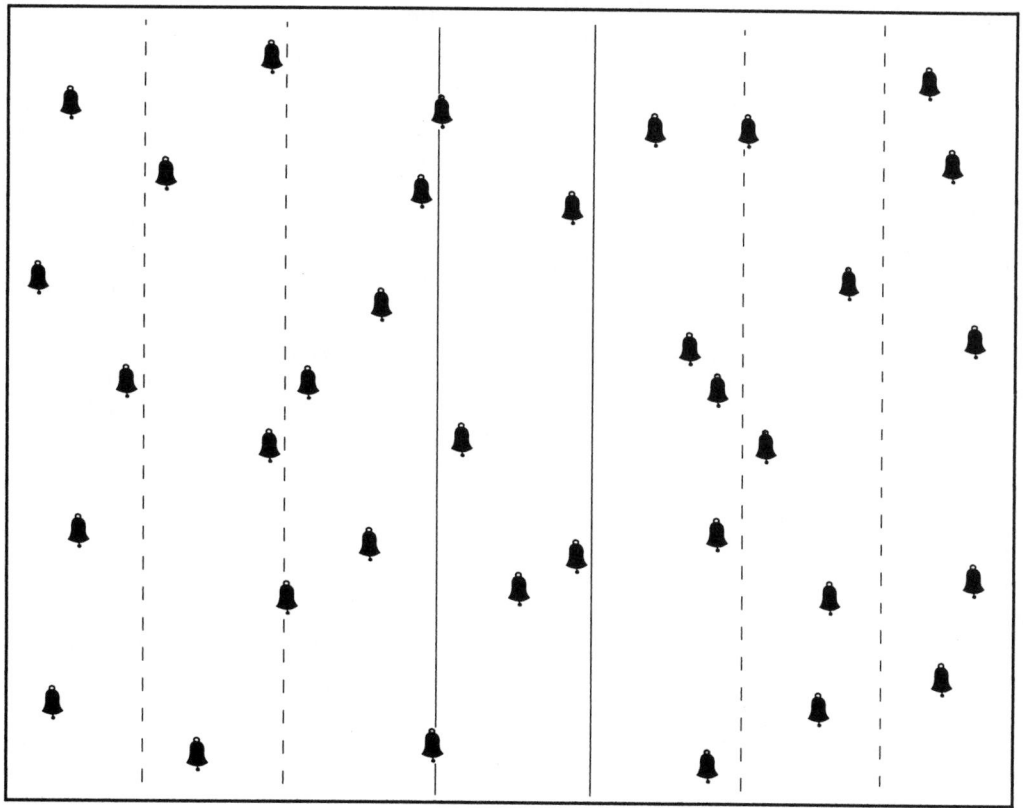

test is completed. The score consists of the number of bells correctly circled.

Gauthier et al. (1989) recommended scoring only the errors in the right and left sides of the visual field, and scoring omissions in the center separately. For this type of scoring, the test sheet is divided lengthwise into seven sectors (three left, three right, and one center; see Figure 12–7). The total correct is 30 (omitting the center).

DEMOGRAPHIC EFFECTS

Age

Gauthier et al. (1989) reported no effects of age. Rousseaux et al. (2001) noted only small increases in the incidence of omissions with advancing age.

Gender

Gauthier et al. (1989) and Rousseaux et al. (2002) reported no significant effects of gender in adult subjects.

Education

Education has only a small impact on scores, with increasing education linked to better performance (Rousseaux et al., 2002).

Ethnicity

Dawson (1997) noted that fewer adult Chinese subjects started their search with the left-top or left-middle orientation than was reported by Gauthier et al. (1989), and fewer used a systematic search pattern.

NORMATIVE DATA

Standardization Data

The number of errors in the three left and the three right segments of the Bells Test for older hospitalized controls (mean age = 71 years) without neurological deficit and for older right- and left-CVA patients (mean age = 68 years) are shown in Table 12–3. Based on these data, the authors recommended that more than 3 omissions on one or the other side indicates a lateralized inattention deficit. Young control subjects (aged 18–28 years) showed an organized scanning pattern, either vertical or horizontal, and made no more than two errors on either half of the test; normal subjects between the ages of 50 and 81 years omitted no more than three bells; in contrast, CVA patients tended to show a more disorganized scanning pattern and higher error scores.

The authors consider total time for completion of the test to be irrelevant to the measurement of neglect, although it may be of importance when test performances at different times during the recovery stage are compared.

Other Normative Data

Based on their study of 576 healthy French subjects between the ages of 20 and 80 years, Rousseaux et al. (2002) considered a difference of 1 omission between the right and the left side as normal (95th percentile), and a difference of 5 as pathologic (5th percentile). They also analyzed time for completion of the test and considered a time longer than 183 s to be abnormal (normal mean time = 105 s). The difference between right- and left-handers was not significant.

Children between the ages of 3 to 13 years were found to omit no more than 1 target figure (teddy bears instead of bells; Laurent-Vannier, 2001). Biancardi and Stoppa (1997) used an Italian adaptation of the Bells Test suitable for 4- to 14-year old children, which they applied to 350 preschool and school-aged children. They noted that no further increase in response speed and accuracy occurred after 8 years of age.

RELIABILITY

Test-Retest Reliability

Two-week test-retest reliability was reported as marginal ($r = .69$; Gauthier et al., 1989). However, Vanier et al. (1990) emphasized that hemineglect is a fluctuating deficit; therefore, a perfect correspondence of results between two performances on the tests should not be expected.

VALIDITY

Relationships With Other Measures

To establish concurrent validity, Vanier et al. (1990) compared the Bells Test with Albert's (1973) line-crossing task and found that the former identified a higher percentage of stroke patients with neglect. Similarly, in a recent evaluation of four different methods of assessing neglect (line bisection, letter cancellation, star cancellation, Bells Test) Ferber & Karnath (2001, 2002) concluded that line bisection missed 40% of a well-defined patient population with neglect, whereas the Bells Test and letter cancellation test missed only 6% (2/35 patients). The use of distractor items ("background noise") instead of line crossing, as in the Bells Test, tends to detect mild and moderate neglect more readily (Marsh & Kersel, 1993; Weintraub & Mesulam, 1985) perhaps because it is more demanding of selective attention (Ferber & Karnath, 2002).

Clinical Findings

The results by Gauthier et al. (1985) suggested that patients with right-hemisphere lesions are more likely to show neglect. This was demonstrated in other studies with other tests (Battersby et al., 1956; Costa et al., 1969; Friedland & Weinstein, 1977; Gainotti et al., 1972).

Azouvi et al. (2002) examined 206 consecutive patients with a right-hemisphere stroke with the Bells Test. They

Table 12–3 Distribution of Subjects According to the Number of Omitted Bells in Each Half of Visual Space

| | Controls (n = 20) | Brain Damaged Patients | |
		Right (n = 19)	Left (n = 20)
Left Omissions			
0	11	1	10
1–3	9	8	8
4–35	0	10	2
Right Omissions			
0	11	5	10
1–3	9	13	7
4–35	0	1	3

Source: From Gauthier et al., 1989. Reprinted with permission.

found an average of 8.4 omissions, with an average of 3.1 more omissions on the left compared with the right side; moreover, the starting point of the search tended to be in the fourth vector (from left to right). These three variables correlated significantly with omissions during the reading of 12 lines, writing (expanded left margin), omissions in the detection of overlapping figures, the tendency to omit figures on the left side, and, to a lesser extent, line bisection, figure copying, and clock drawing. The Bells Test variables loaded on a separate factor together with figure copying, reading, and writing. Behavioral neglect was assessed by 10 observations on grooming, dressing, eating, mouth cleaning, gaze orientation, and other activities in the Catherine Bergego scale (Bergego, 1995); this scale correlated with the total number of omissions (.77), with right minus left omissions (.62), and with the starting point (.57). The authors concluded that the Bells Test and the reading test were the most sensitive tests. They suggested a cutoff point of 6 omissions, 2 more omissions on the left side than the right side, and a starting point more to the left than sector 5. Sensitivity increased up to 85% when several measures of neglect were used. Hence, normal performance on a single measure does not rule out spatial neglect in a given patient. Personal and extrapersonal neglect were found to be significantly more severe in patients with lesions located posterior to the Rolandic sulcus. However, the authors also found a small number of patients with lesions in the prefrontal region.

Tant et al. (2002) recommended the Bells Test as a screening task for measuring driving behavior in patients with hemianopia.

COMMENT

The Bells Test has established itself as a highly sensitive measure of visual neglect. It is easy to administer and is well tolerated by patients. It is also suitable for children if appropriate changes (teddy bears instead of bells) are made. Because targets are embedded within numerous distractors (increasing the demands on visual selective attention), the task appears to be more useful for the detection of neglect than line-crossing tasks are. In line-crossing tasks, all given stimuli serve as targets, and the patients do not have to segregate distractors from target stimuli (Ferber & Karnath, 2002). As a consequence, the Bells Test is more likely than the simple cancellation task to reflect patients' visual exploratory deficits (Ferber & Karnath, 2002). Yet, it should not be used as a single method to measure visual neglect; other tests, especially behavioral inattention measures, should be used to confirm the results.

REFERENCES

Albert, M. C. (1973). A simple test of visual neglect. *Neurology, 23,* 558–664.

Azouvi, P., Samuel, C., Louis-Dreyfus, A., Bernati, T., Bartolomeo, P., Beis, J. M., Chokron, S., Leclercq, M., Marchal, F., Martin, Y., De Montety, G., Olivier, S., Perennou, D., Pradat-Diehl, P., Prairial, C., Rode, G., Sieroff, E., Wiart, L., Rousseaux, M., & French Collaborative Study Group on Assessment of Unilateral Neglect (GEREN/GRECO). (2002). Sensitivity of clinical and behavioral tests of spatial neglect after right hemisphere stroke. *Journal of Neurology, Neurosurgery and Psychiatry, 73,* 160–166.

Battersby, W. S., Bender, M. B., & Pollack, M. (1956). Unilateral spatial agnosia (inattention) in patients with cerebral lesions. *Brain, 79,* 68–93.

Bergego, C., Azouvi, P., Samuel, C., Marchal, F., Louis-Dreyfus, A., Jokic, C., et al. (1995). Validation d'une echelle d'evaluation fonctionelle de heminegligence dans la vie quotidienne: l'echelle CB. *Annales de Readaptation et de Medicine Physique, 38,* 183–189.

Biancardi, A., & Stoppa, E. (1997). Il test delle Campanelle modificato: Una proposta per lo studio dell'attenzione in eta evolutiva. *Psichiatria dell'infancia e dell'adolescenza, 64,* 73–84.

Costa, L. D., Vaughan, H. G., Horwitz, M., & Ritter, W. (1969). Patterns of behavior deficit associated with visual spatial neglect. *Cortex, 5,* 242–263.

Dawson, D. R. (1997). Visual scanning patterns in an adult Chinese population: Preliminary normative data. *Occupational Therapy Journal of Research, 17,* 264–279.

Ferber, S., & Karnath. H. O. (2001). How to assess spatial neglect: Line bisection or cancellation tasks? *Journal of Clinical and Experimental Neuropsychology, 23,* 599–607.

Ferber, S., & Karnath, H. O. (2002). Neglect-tests im Vergleich: Welche sind geeignet? *Zeitschrift fuer Neuropsychologie, 13,* 39–44.

Friedland, R. P., & Weinstein, E. A. (1977). Hemi-inattention and hemisphere specialization: Introduction and historical review. In E. A. Weinstein & R. P. Friedland (Eds.), *Advances in neurology, Vol. 18: Hemi-inattention and hemisphere specialization* (pp. 1–31). New York: Raven Press.

Gainotti, G., Messerli, P., & Tissot, R. (1972). Qualitative analysis of unilateral spatial neglect in relation to laterality of cerebral lesions. *Journal of Neurology, Neurosurgery, and Psychiatry, 35,* 545–550.

Gauthier, L., DeHaut, F., & Joanette, Y. (1989). The Bells Test: A quantitative and qualitative test for visual neglect. *International Journal of Clinical Neuropsychology, 11,* 49–54.

Gauthier, L., Gauthier, F., & Joanette, Y. (1985). Visual neglect in left, right and bilateral Parkinsonism [Abstract]. *Journal of Clinical and Experimental Neuropsychology, 7,* 145.

Laurent-Vannier, A., Pradat-Diehl, P., & Chevignard, M. (2001). Negligence spatiale unilaterale et motrice chez l'enfant. *Revue Neurologique, 157,* 414–422.

Marsh, N. V., & Kersel, D. A. (1993). Screening tests for visual neglect following stroke. *Neuropsychological Rehabilitation, 3,* 245–257.

Rousseaux, M., Beis, J. M., Pradat-Diehl, P., Martin, Y., Bartolomeo, P., Bernati, T., et al. (2001). Presentation d'une batterie de depistage de la negligence spatiale: Normes et effets de l'age, du niveau d'education, du sexe, de la main et de la lateralité. *Revue Neurologique, 157,* 1385–1400.

Tant, M. L. M., Brouwer, M. L. M., Cornelissen, F. W., & Koojman, A. C. (2002). Driving and visuospatial performance in people with hemianopia. *Neuropsychological Rehabilitation, 12,* 419–437.

Vanier, M., Gauthier, L., Lambert, J., Pepin, E. P., Robillard, A., Dubouloz, C. J., et al. (1990). Evaluation of left visuospatial neglect: Norms and discrimination power of two tests. *Neuropsychology, 4,* 87–96.

Weintraub, S., & Mesulam, M. M. (1985). Mental state assessment of young and elderly adults in behavioral neurology. In M. M. Mesulam (Ed.), *Contemporary neurology series, Vol. 26: Principles of behavioral neurology* (pp. 71–123). Philadelphia: F. A. Davis.

Clock Drawing Test (CDT)

PURPOSE

The Clock Drawing Test screens for dementia as well as for visual-spatial, constructional, and executive difficulties.

SOURCE

No specific test material is required. Tuokko et al. (1995) offer a commercial version, The Clock Test, published by Multi-Health Systems, 908 Niagara Falls Blvd., Tonawanda, NY 14120-2060 (http://www.mhs.com) for $195 US.

Other Sources

Clock drawing is part of the 7-Minute Screen (Solomon et al., 1998) and CAMCOG (Roth et al., 1986). Clock drawing and setting are also part of the parietal lobe battery (also called Spatial-Quantitative Battery) in the Boston Diagnostic Aphasia Examination (BDAE) (Goodglass & Kaplan, 1983, 2001) and the KBNA (Leach et al., 2000) described elsewhere in this volume.

AGE RANGE

Norms are available for ages 6 to 12 years and for adults.

DESCRIPTION

The simple freehand drawing of a clock face, together with the drawing of a daisy, a house, a person, and a bicycle, has been part of the brief mental status examination in neurology for a long time (Battersby et al., 1956; Critchley, 1953; Goodglass & Kaplan, 1972; Strub & Black, 1977) and is frequently recommended as a screening test for dementia. In contrast to the primarily verbal content of most dementia scales, clock drawing relies on visual-spatial, constructional, and higher-order cognitive abilities, including executive aspects. The test requires merely a sheet of paper and a pencil and can be given as part of a bedside examination or, in other instances, when lengthy neuropsychological testing is not possible.

More than a dozen different versions of the task have been published (see Table 12–4). Many of these are described by Shulman (2000), Lezak et al. (2004) and Tuokko and O'Connell (in press). Various authors assess freehand drawing although others provide a sheet with a printed empty circle (7–10 cm in diameter), representing the shape of the clock face asking the patient to write the numbers and draw the hands for a given time setting. Some prefer to use the predrawn circle because it focuses the clock drawing performance on number and hand placement, thereby circumventing some difficulties inherent in procedures in which the participant draws the circle as well (i.e., a poorly drawn circle confounds the remainder of the clock-drawing performance; Tuokko et al., 2000). Several authors (e.g., Libon et al., 1993, 1996; Rouleau et al., 1992; Royall et al., 1998; see also *Kaplan Baycrest Neurocognitive Assessment*) also include copying conditions to improve understanding of performance. A variety of times (see Table 12–4) have been used. A commonly used time setting is "10 after 11" (or "10 past 11"); this time setting may help in identifying the "pull" of executive dysfunction, because the 11 is right beside the 10, pulling the minute hand toward the 11, and because it requires recoding of 10 minutes into a 2-hour segment (i.e., setting the minute hand at 2 o'clock; Freedman et al., 1994). It also involves both visual fields. The identification of hemilateral neglect or hemianopia is facilitated if the two hands of the clock are in different halves of the clock face.

ADMINISTRATION

Adults

As noted in Table 12–4, there are many different administration systems. For the free-drawing version (e.g., Goodglass and Kaplan, 1983; Libon et al., 1993; Rouleau et al., 1992), place upright a standard, unlined letter-size sheet of paper and a pencil in front of the patient and say: "*I want you to draw the face of a clock with all the numbers on it. Make it large.*" After completion of the clock face, instruct as follows: "*Now, please set the time to 10 after 11 (or 20 to 4).*" Instructions may be repeated or rephrased if the patient does not

Table 12–4 Summary of Clock Drawing Tasks

Author	Circle	Time(hours:min)	Total Score	Participant Samples (in Addition to "Cognitively Normal" Older Adults)	Cutoff	Sensitivity[a]	Specificity[a]
Mendez et al., 1992 (CDIS)	Free-drawn	11:10	20	Dementia (mixed), Alzheimer's disease (AD), stroke, mood/anxiety disorders, schizophrenia	<18	88–94	26–65
Royall et al., 1998 (CLOX)	CLOX1: Free-drawn; CLOX2: Copying	1:45	15	AD	<10 (CLOX1) <12 (CLOX2)		
Rouleau et al., 1992	Free-drawn	11:10	Quantitative 10 Qualitative-errors	Dementia (mixed), AD, vascular dementia (VaD), diffuse Lewy body disease (DLBD), Huntington's disease (HD), Parkinson's disease (PD), stroke, schizophrenia AD, HD, VaD, & stroke	NA		
Freeman et al., 1994	Free-drawn	6:45	15	AD, PD, VaD, mood/anxiety disorders, stroke, schizophrenia, young/middle-aged adults	NA		
	Predrawn	6:05	13	AD, PD, schizophrenia, young/middle-aged adults			
Sunderland et al., 1989	Predrawn	2:45	10	AD	<6	56–79	58–91
Lin et al., 2003	Predrawn	10:10	16	AD	<23		
Wolf-Klein et al., 1989	Predrawn	11:10	10	AD	<7	39–79	72–95
Manos & Wu, 1994	Predrawn	11:10	10	Dementia (mixed), AD, VaD, Frontotemporal dementia (FTD), rehabilitation outpatients, surgical inpatients	<8	67	86
Tuokko et al., 1992	Predrawn	11:10	Error tally	Dementia (mixed), AD	>2 errors	91–92	50–86
Shulman et al., 1986 Shulman, 2000	Predrawn	11:10	5	Dementia, depression	<4	81–93	48–96
Cohen et al., 2000	Free-drawing; Predrawn	3:00 (Free); 9:30 and 10:20 (predrawn)	13: clock construction 5: clock setting	Normal children aged 6–12 years	Depends on age		

[a]Based on Schramm et al., 2002; Shulman, 2000; Storey et al., 2001.

Source: Adapted from Tuokko & O'Connell (in press).

Step 1: Turn this form over on a light-colored surface so that the circle below is visible. Have the subject draw a clock on the back. Instruct him or her as follows: **Draw me a clock that says 1:45. Set the hands and numbers on the face so that a child could read them.** Repeat the instructions until they are clearly understood. Once the subject begins to draw, no further assistance is allowed. Rate this clock (CLOX1).

Step 2: Return to this side and let the subject observe you draw a clock in the circle below. Place 12, 6, 3, and 9 first. Set the hands again to "1:45". Make the hands into arrows. Invite the subject to copy your clock in the lower right corner. Score this clock (CLOX2).

Organization Elements	Point Value	CLOX 1	CLOX 2
Does figure resemble a clock?	1		
Circular face present?	1		
Dimensions >1 inch?	1		
All numbers inside the perimeter?	1		
12, 6, 3, and 9 placed first?	1		
Spacing intact? (symmetry on either side of 12 and 6 o'clock)	1		
No sectoring or tic marks?	1		
Only Arab numerals?	1		
Only numbers 1–12 among the numerals present?	1		
Sequence 1–12 intact? (no omissions or intrusions)	1		
Only 2 hands present? (ignore sectoring/tic marks)	1		
All hands represented as arrows?	1		
Hour hand between 1 and 2 o'clock?	1		
Minute hand longer than hour hand?	1		
None of the following: (1) hand pointing to 4 or 5 o'clock?	1		
(2) "1:45" present?			
(3) intrusions from "hand" or "face" present?			
(4) any letters, words or pictures?			
(5) any intrusion from circle below?			

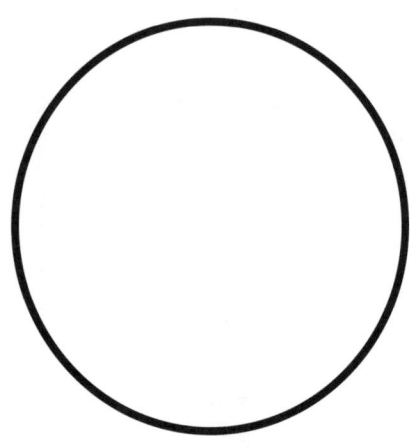

understand, but no other help should be given. The time taken to complete the task may be noted.

If using a predrawn circle, provide a sheet with a circle about 4 in (10 cm) in diameter (Shulman, 2000) and say: *"This circle represents a clock face. Please put in the numbers so that it looks like a clock and then set the time to 10 minutes past 11."* Shulman (2000) recommended that the tester should not use the word "hands" in the instructions.

The instructions for administering the CLOX test (Royall et al., 1998) are provided in Figure 12–8.

Children

According to Cohen et al. (2000), the child is provided with a piece of paper and instructed to "draw the face of a clock and make the clock say 3:00." After this, the child is presented with two predrawn clocks and is asked to indicate the times of 9:30 and 10:20 (Cohen et al., 2000).

ADMINISTRATION TIME

Approximately 5 min is required.

SCORING

Quantitative Systems

Scoring systems range from a 3-point system (Goodglass & Kaplan, 1983, 2001) to more complex systems (e.g., a 20-point scale by Mendez et al., 1992). The 10-point scoring system, adapted from Sunderland et al. (1989) and Libon et al (1993) is commonly used for the freehand version and is shown in Table 12–5. The Shulman scoring system is simple and appears to be quite useful (see *Validity*); it is shown in Table 12–6. The system (CLOX) proposed by Royall et al. (1998) is presented in Figure 12–8.

For children, Cohen et al. (2000) recommend scoring clock construction and clock setting separately (see Table 12–7). Clock construction has a maximum score of 13, and clock setting is measured on a 5-point scale.

Qualitative Systems

In addition to the quantitative score, a number of authors (e.g., Cosentino et al., 2004; Libon et al., 1996; Rouleau et al. 1992; Suhr et al., 1998; Tuokko et al., 1992) have developed qualitative scoring systems that include evaluation of clock size, omissions, graphic difficulties (e.g., numbers hard to read, distortions in the hands), stimulus-bound (e.g., setting the hands on 10 and 11), conceptual (e.g., writing the time on the clock rather than setting the hands, lack of numbers on the clock), perseverative (e.g., more than two hands, writing numbers beyond "12"), and spatial/planning (e.g., neglect, gaps in number spacing, numbers outside clockface or counterclockwise) types of errors.

Table 12–5 Criteria for Evaluating Free-Drawn Clock Drawing in Adults

10	Normal drawing, numbers and hands in approximately correct positions, hour hand distinctly different from minute hand and approaching 4 o'clock.
9	Slight errors in placement of hands—not exactly on 8 and 4 (or 10 and 11), but not on one of the adjoining numbers—or one missing number on clock face.
8	More noticeable errors in placement of hour and minute hand (off by one number); number spacing shows a gap.
7	Placement of hands significantly off course (more than one number); very inappropriate spacing of numbers (e.g., all on one side).
6	Inappropriate use of clock hands (use of digital display or circling of numbers despite repeated instructions); crowding of numbers at one end of the clock or reversal of numbers.
5	Perseverative or otherwise inappropriate arrangement of numbers (e.g., numbers indicated by dots). Hands may be represented but do not clearly point at a number.
4	Numbers absent, written outside of clock, or in distorted sequence. Integrity of clock face missing. Hands not clearly represented or drawn outside of clock face.
3	Numbers and clock face no longer connected in the drawing. Hands not recognizably present.
2	Drawing reveals some evidence of instructions received, but representation of clock is only vague; inappropriate spatial arrangement of numbers.
1	Irrelevant, uninterpretable figure or no attempt.

Note: Roman numerals and embellishments of the clock (clock feet, bells) are acceptable.

Source: Adapted from Sunderland et al., 1989, and Libon et al., 1993.

DEMOGRAPHIC EFFECTS

Age

Cross-sectional studies reveal that age affects clock drawing in adults (e.g., Freedman et al., 1994; Marcopulos et al., 1997; Tuokko et al., 1995) with performance declining particularly after age 70 years (Kozora & Cullum, 1994; Marcopulos et al., 1997; but see Cahn & Kaplan, 1997, who suggested that clock drawing remains fairly preserved from age 70 to 90 years). Longitudinal examination reveals slight decline with advancing age. Ratcliff et al. (2003) examined 1208 elderly community-living individuals in southern Pennsylvania, aged 65 to 74 years and greater than 74 years, drawn from the voters' list. The testing was repeated every 2 years. The results, based on an 8-point scoring system, showed a small but significant decline (from 7.55 to 6.94 points) for "survivors" who participated in all five tests over the 10-year period.

In children, the ability to draw a clock improves significantly with age (Cohen et al., 2000; Edmonds et al., 1994; Kirk et al., 1996). For example, Cohen et al. (2000) examined public school children between the ages of 6 and 12 years and

Table 12–6 Criteria for Evaluating Predrawn Clock Drawing in Adults—Shulman Method

5	Perfect clock
4	Minor visual-spatial errors
3	Inaccurate representation of 10 after 11 when the visual-spatial organization is well done
2	Moderate visual-spatial disorganization of numbers such that accurate denotation of "10 after 11" is impossible
1	Severe level of visual-spatial disorganization
0	Inability to make any reasonable representation of a clock

Source: Adapted from Shulman, 2000.

found that most 6-year-olds had a basic concept of a clock, most 8-year-olds were successfully able to set the time, and most 10-year olds could successfully construct a clock face. However, there was increasing skill development through age 12 years. With regard to specific error types, they found that by age 7 years, the vast majority of children no longer demonstrated number reversals, and by age 8, they no longer neglected entire quadrants of space. Number positioning (spacing) errors and erasures were still present at age 12 years.

Education

Education impacts performance (La Rue et al., 1999; Marcopulos et al., 1997; Ratcliff et al., 2003).

IQ

Clock drawing shows moderate/high correlations with measures of intellectual status (see *Validity*).

Ethnicity

Marcopulos et al (1997) reported no effect of race in an elderly rural U.S. sample. In contrast, La Rue et al. (1999) found small ethnic effects when comparing 797 Hispanic and white elderly subjects. English-only participants scored higher than Spanish-only participants.

Gender

La Rue et al. (1999) found a gender difference in performance, favoring males, among older adults. The effect became less robust when health-related factors were taken into account. No gender differences were noted in children for either drawing or copying tasks (Dilworth et al., 2004; Kirk et al., 1996).

NORMATIVE DATA

Adults

Cutoff values for a variety of administration/scoring systems are shown in Table 12–4. The reader may wish to refer

Table 12–7 Criteria for Evaluating Clock Drawing in Children

Points	Criteria
Criteria for Assessing Clock Face Construction/Form (maximum score = 13)	
1	Some indication of the concept of a clock
1	Hands present, regardless of location or size
1–4	1 point for each quadrant of clock face used
1	Equal spacing of all numbers (1–12)
0–2	2 points for all numbers (1–12) present and in correct sequence
	1 point if numbers are out of sequence, repeated, or sequence goes beyond 12
	0 points if any numbers (1–12) are missing
1	Numbers 3 and 9 directly opposite each other
1	Numbers 12 and 6 directly opposite each other
0–2	2 points if all numbers are in correct spatial orientation
	1 point if 1 or more numbers are rotated ≥45 degrees
	0 points if 1 or more numbers are reversed
Criteria for Assessing the Concept of Time (maximum score = 5)	
1	The hour hand is distinctly different from the minute hand; this should be sufficiently distinct so as not to require measurement (e.g., if the minute hand is 1 inch, then the hour hand should be 3/4 inch or less).
1–4	4 points if the placement of hands is pointing directly to the correct numbers
	3 points if the placement of hands is off by less than 1 number
	2 points if the placement of hands is off by 1 number
	1 point if the placement of hands is off by more than 1 number, or the hour/minute hands are reversed, or one of the hands is missing

Source: Adapted from Cohen et al., 2000.

to data (using the 10-point scale) provided by Marcopulos and McLain (2003) when assessing rural elderly individuals with very low levels of education (Table 12–8). The "robust" data are based on a study of older adults (about half African Americans) who had been assessed 4 years earlier. In this way, those who dropped out or who demonstrated significant decline (at least 1 SD) over the 4-year period on the MMSE, DRS, and Fuld Object Memory Evaluation could be excluded, in order to leave "robust" participants. Note that some of the cell sizes are very small (fewer than 20 subjects). These data are included to illustrate trends and should not be considered normative estimates.

Children

Cohen et al. (2000) provided data on a sample of 429 normal public school children, aged 6 to 12 years, attending grades 1 through 6 in two school districts in central Georgia. The mean age of the sample was 8.89 years (SD = 1.77), and there were

Table 12–8 Means and Standard Deviations for Clock-Drawing (Free-Drawn) by Age and Educational Level ($N = 79$)

Age (Years)	Education (Years)					
	0–6			7–10		
	N	M	SD	N	M	SD
55–74	9	8.7	1.1	26	8.7	1.4
75+	17	7.2	1.8	27	7.9	2.0

Note: Total sample $M = 8.1$, $SD = 1.7$. Subjects were asked to draw the face of a clock showing the numbers with the hands set to 10 min after 11. Clock drawing was rated on a 10-point scale (Libon et al., 1993).

Source: From Marcopulos & McLain, 2003. Reprinted with the kind permission of Psychology Press.

210 boys and 219 girls. The majority (393) wrote with the right hand, and 36 wrote with the left hand. Data from children who were not reading at grade level or who had a history of grade retention, behavior disorder, learning disorder, or stimulant medication use were not included in the analyses. Note that the children were tested in groups in their respective classrooms, with all clocks and watches removed from view. Mean scores for the clock setting and construction portions are shown in Table 12–9. About 90% of children 8 years of age received a score of 4 or 5 on time to the hour, 92% to the half-hour, and 80% to the minute. About 82% of the children 10 years of age were able to successfully construct a clock, having a score of 11 or greater. The age at which clock drawing reaches an asymptote is not known.

RELIABILITY

Test-Retest Reliability

Retest reliability for clock drawing after 12 weeks was .78 for patients with Alzheimer's disease (AD) (Mendez et al., 1992). Tuokko et al. (1995) found similar values when AD patients were retested after 4 days. A practice effect has not yet been reported.

Interrater Reliability

Interrater and intrarater reliability are high (> .80) for most methods used with adults (e.g., Lezak et al., 2004; Royall et al., 1998; Schramm et al., 2002; Storey et al., 2001; Suhr et al., 1998; Tuokko et al., 2000). For the version developed for children, Cohen et al. (2000) reported high interrater reliability for form ($r = .96$) and time ($r \geq .94$) scoring methods.

VALIDITY

Scoring Methods

The various scoring methods tend to be highly correlated with one another. For example, Kozora and Cullum (1994) found a moderately high correlation between 3-point (Goodglass & Kaplan, 1983), 10-point (Spreen & Strauss, 1991), and their own 16-point scoring systems (.67 to .70). Tuokko et al. (2000) reported a correlation of $-.72$ between the Tuokko and Wolf-Klein systems. Royall et al. (1999) compared six methods of clock drawing and found correlations ranging from -0.73 (CLOX1 with Shulman) to 0.95 (CLOX1 with Mendez). Finally, Heinik et al. (2004) reported correlations of .80 and higher among the CAMCOG, Shulman, and Freedman systems in patients with AD or vascular dementia.

Sensitivity and specificity with regard to a diagnosis of dementia vary with scoring method and sample composition (see Table 12–4). In general, however, the methods developed by Mendez, Tuokko, and Shulman appear to be the most sensitive, although specificity is often modest at best. For example, Tuokko et al. (2000) compared a number of scoring methods (Shulman et al., 1986; Tuokko et al., 1992; Watson et al., 1993; Wolf-Klein et al., 1989) in older adults diagnosed with or without dementia. The Tuokko and Shulman systems provided high sensitivities (91% and 93%, respectively) but low specificities (50% and 48%, respectively). The Wolf-Klein and Watson cutoff values produced relatively low sensitivities (74% and 59%, respectively) and specificities (72% and 67%, respectively). In a comparison of five scoring methods (Manos, 1997; Shulman et al., 1986; Sunderland et al., 1989;

Table 12–9 Means (and *SDs*) for Clock Drawing in Children

Age (Years)	n	Time Drawn to the Clock			
		Hour[a]	Half-hour[a]	Minute[a]	Construction[b]
6	40	3.20 (1.65)	3.20 (1.45)	2.15 (1.46)	8.65 (2.14)
7	79	3.97 (1.27)	3.86 (1.26)	3.03 (1.62)	9.46 (1.73)
8	70	4.59 (0.96)	4.35 (0.91)	4.30 (1.18)	10.84 (1.14)
9	69	4.68 (0.76)	4.55 (0.80)	4.57 (0.92)	10.81 (1.13)
10	91	4.56 (0.90)	4.35 (0.99)	4.38 (1.06)	11.34 (0.98)
11	54	4.62 (0.89)	4.51 (0.84)	4.47 (1.09)	11.39 (1.09)
12	26	4.54 (0.86)	4.69 (0.68)	4.65 (0.89)	11.62 (0.98)

[a]Scale ranges from 1 to 5, with higher scores indicating better performance.
[b]Scale ranges from 1 to 13, with higher scores indicating better performance.

Source: Adapted from Cohen et al., 2000.

Watson et al., 1993; Wolf-Klein et al., 1989), Schramm et al. (2002) found optimal results for distinguishing demented from normal individuals with the Shulman method. They reported a sensitivity of 81% and a specificity of 79%. Similarly, Brodaty and Moore (1997) found that, although three different scoring methods (Shulman, Sunderland, and Wolf-Klein) identified mild to moderate dementia reasonably well, the Shulman method performed best, and it was superior to the MMSE. Storey et al. (2001) compared scoring methods (Shulman, Sunderland, Wolf-Klein, Mendez, and Watson) in a sample of geriatric medical outpatients. They found that the methods used by Shulman (93% sensitivity, 55% specificity) and Mendez (96% sensitivity, 26% specificity) predicted dementia more accurately than did those by Sunderland (69% sensitivity, 44% specificity), Watson (69% sensitivity, 44% specificity), or Wolf-Klein (43% sensitivity, 86% specificity).

Scoring systems not only differ with regard to their sensitivity to dementia but also with respect to their ability to monitor progression of cognitive deterioration. A study of 26 mildly and 23 moderately impaired AD patients (Heinik et al., 2002b) found that the two groups performed at a similar level using the Shulman method, but patients with moderate AD performed significantly worse than those with mild AD using Freedman's method.

Relationships With Other Measures

Clock drawing shows moderate correlations with measures of temporal orientation (e.g., WMS-R Orientation; Suhr et al., 1998), visual-spatial/visual-constructional skill (e.g., Block Design, Hooper Visual Organization Test, Rey Complex Figure; Kibby et al., 2001; Libon et al., 1993, 1996; Suhr et al., 1998) and with measures of executive functioning such as the Competing Programs/Go–No-Go task (Libon et al., 1993), the verbal fluency task (COWA; Suhr et al., 1998), and the EXIT25 (Royall et al., 1999). Semantic memory is also implicated in clock drawing (e.g., BNT correlation = .43; Libon et al., 1996). In children, WISC-R Vocabulary and, to a lesser extent, Block Design are predictive of drawing scores 3 years later (Dilworth et al., 2004).

Clock drawing also provides an indication of general cognitive functioning, correlating moderately/highly with global measures such as the MMSE (.41 to .80; Adunsky et al., 2002; Heinik et al., 2004; Rai & Blackman, 1998; Royall et al., 1999; Shulman, 2000), CAMCOG (Heinik et al., 2004), the Mattis Dementia Rating Scale (.38 to .45), the Global Impression of Neuropsychological Impairment Scale (.49 to .60), and the Block Design test under extended time conditions (.41; Adunsky et al., 2002; Kozora & Cullum, 1994; Mendez et al., 1992; Nussbaum et al., 1992; Shulman et al., 1993), as well as subtests of the WAIS-R (information, similarities, digit span, and block design subtests; .41 to .57; Tuokko et al., 1995). Therefore, as a preliminary screen, clock drawing appears to provide a reasonable measure of cognitive functioning.

The CDT comprises two conditions: free drawing followed by a copy condition. The interpretation of clock drawings produced in the command versus copy conditions is in some dispute (see *Dementia*). Royall and his colleagues (Royall & Espino, 2002; Royall et al., 1998, 2004) argue that their CLOX1 (free drawing) task is sensitive to executive functioning, correlating highly with measures of executive ability (e.g., Wisconsin Card Sorting Test, Executive Interview Test [EXIT] 25), whereas CLOX2 (copying) is more dependent on visual-constructional skills. The correlation with MMSE was somewhat stronger for CLOX2 ($r = .44$) than for CLOX1 ($r = .31$) in a large, older, community-dwelling Mexican-American sample (Royall & Espino, 2002; Royall et al., 2004). Furthermore, the copy condition was able to discriminate between patients with gross constructional impairment (as measured with the MMSE pentagon task) and patients without such impairment.

By contrast, Libon et al. (1993, 1996) and Rouleau et al. (1992) found that, when the performance of patients with AD was compared with that of patients with subcortical deficits, such as Huntington's disease (HD) and vascular dementia, only the former group displayed marked improvement in the copy condition. They concluded that the copy condition may be particularly sensitive to executive dysfunction, such as impaired organization and planning. For Libon et al. (1993, 1996) and Rouleau et al. (1992), a main source of difficulty in the command condition for the AD group reflected deficient knowledge required to bring to mind an accurate representation of a clock. More recently, Libon and his colleagues (Cosentino et al., 2004) modified their position to suggest that the drawing-to-command condition places demands on both executive control and semantic knowledge systems; however, in contrast to Royall et al (1998), they suggested that the copy condition also places significant demands on executive functioning.

Dementia

The test is useful in distinguishing normal elderly from patients with dementia due to AD (e.g., Manos, 1999; Royall et al., 1998; Tuokko et al., 1992), Parkinson's disease (Freedman et al., 1994), and Huntington's disease (Rouleau et al., 1992), as well as from those with mild cognitive impairment (Cahn et al., 1994; Tuokko et al., 2000). The various CDT methods identify dementia better than chance (Storey et al., 2001). The CDT also appears useful in documenting severity of cognitive impairment (Dastoor et al., 1991; Manos & Wu, 1994; Royall et al., 1998; Sunderland et al., 1989; Tuokko et al., 2000) and of predicting subsequent cognitive decline (e.g., Ferrucci et al., 1996; O'Rourke et al., 1997) and rate of decline (Rouleau et al., 1996).

The ability of the CDT to distinguish among disorders is less clear. Some authors (Heinik et al., 2002a; Kitabayashi et al., 2002; Moretti et al., 2002) have reported that the CDT has some value in differentiating AD from vascular dementia. Others, however, have questioned its utility in this regard (Barr et al., 1992; Cosentino et al., 2004; Libon et al., 1993, 1996; Wolf-Klien et al., 1989). There is some evidence that inclusion of a copy condition (in addition to drawing to command) may improve diagnostic accuracy, although interpretation of clock drawings produced in the command versus the copy condition has engendered some debate.

Libon et al. (1993, 1996) noted that clock drawings improved from the command to the copy condition in patients with AD, whereas no such improvement occurred among patients with vascular dementia. In addition, Libon et al. (1996) found that patients with vascular dementia made more graphomotor errors (distortions in size or shape of the circle) in the drawing-on-command condition, and more executive control errors (e.g., turning the page while writing numbers, writing numbers counterclockwise, perseverations) in the copy condition than did AD patients. They suggested that their findings reflected greater deficits in semantic memory systems in patients with AD and greater deficits in frontal systems among the vascular dementia patients. They proposed that the first step in executing the command to "draw the face of a clock, put in all the numbers, and set the numbers to read 10 after 11" is to access all of the necessary associations and attributes associated with this proposition from semantic memory. By contrast, in the copy condition, there are fewer, if any, demands placed on semantic memory; rather, one must appreciate the visual-spatial attributes of the stimulus and then mentally plan and execute the task. This proposal is consistent with the results reported by Rouleau et al. (1992) who examined clock drawing performance in patients with AD and Huntington's disease (a disorder affecting frontal-striatal systems). They found that AD subjects made significant improvement from the command to the copy condition, whereas HD subjects did not.

By contrast, according to Royall et al. (1998), the command condition places high demands on executive control functioning, because patients are required to perform in a novel context; they are required to choose the form of the clock (analog, digital) and the size and formation of the clock features. In contrast, the copy condition provides a purer measure of visual-constructional ability. Royall et al. (2004) proposed that patients with cortical types of dementia (e.g., AD) show executive and nonexecutive deficits and, as a consequence, impairment on both free drawing (CLOX1) and copy (CLOX2) tasks. By contrast, in other types of dementias (e.g., frontocortical, subcortical) that result in only executive dysfunction, impairment is limited to the drawing portion of the task (CLOX1).

More recently, Liban and his colleagues (Cosentino et al., 2004) studied errors (e.g., gross motor, time, perseveration/pull to stimulus, spatial layout) made by patients with either AD, vascular dementia, or Parkinson's disease on both the command and copy conditions. They found that the drawing-to-command condition did not distinguish among the groups. Further, the kinds of errors made correlated with neuropsychological measures of both executive control and semantic memory. In contrast, the copy condition was able to distinguish among groups and appeared to elicit errors of executive control (e.g., spatial layout, perseveration/pull to stimulus). Therefore, in contrast to Royall et al. (1998), they found that the copy condition placed significant demands on executive control.

Depression

Whether depression affects performance remains controversial. Lee and Lawler (1995) found that clock drawing may be abnormal in geriatric populations because of depression, and that scores improve when the depression resolves (i.e., poor scores may be state dependent). Kirby et al. (2001) examined the utility of the CDT among older people in primary care (523 normal elderly, 41 with dementia, 84 with depression). They reported that the sensitivity of the CDT in the detection of dementia was 76%. The specificities of the CDT against normal elderly and depressed elderly were 81% and 77% respectively, which was below the values found for the MMSE. In contrast, Herrmann et al., (1998) found that, although patients with AD were impaired on clock drawing, patients with major affective disorder did not differ from age-matched controls. Others have also reported little impact of depression on clock drawing (Bodner et al., 2004; Brodaty & Moore, 1997; Manos, 1997).

Other Conditions

There has been less study of clock drawing in nondemented patients. Patients with schizophrenia performed significantly worse than matched healthy controls, even when matched on the MMSE (Bozikas et al., 2004; Herrmann et al., 1999).

Clock drawing can be affected by hemianopsia and visual neglect, which is apparent in corresponding unilateral errors (e.g., Ogden, 1985). Chokron et al (2004) found that suppressing visual control may improve left neglect patients' performance in clock drawing. Whereas control subjects drew clocks in the same manner whether their eyes were open or closed, neglect patients drew more complete and more symmetrical drawings when their eyes were closed. The authors proposed that a difficulty in disengaging attention from right-sided visual stimuli could play a critical role in clock drawing performance (and neglect of left hemispace) in these patients.

Clock drawing performance in children has received limited attention. A recent study (Kibby et al., 2001), however, indicated that children with ADHD perform worse than controls on both clock face construction and setting the hands to the requested time. They were more likely to demonstrate quadrant neglect and spacing errors later in childhood, when these features are no longer evident in normal children. Further, those ADHD children with poor performance on the WCST tended to perform worse during clock face construction, consistent with the notion that these children have deficits in executive functioning.

Neuroanatomical Correlates

The test is reported to be sensitive to visuospatial disorders or constructional apraxia, such as is found with right or bilateral temporoparietal lesions (Critchley, 1953). A functional magnetic resonance imaging (fMRI) study with normal subjects (Trojano et al., 2002) suggested that the task activates the superior parietal lobule, with the left hemisphere mainly activated with "categorical" clock stimuli and the right with "coordinate" spatial judgment tasks. A study with 26 patients satisfying criteria for probable AD (Ueda et al., 2002) suggested that reduced left posterior temporal regional cerebral blood flow correlated most closely with CDT scores and severity of AD. In contrast, a study of 29 AD patients showed a significant relationship between CDT scores and right, but not left, superior temporal grey matter volumes (Cahn-Weiner et al., 1999). The authors concluded that CDT performance in AD is attributable to multiple cognitive domains, but specifically to regional volume loss in the right temporal cortex.

Frontal lobe functioning has also been implicated. Based on case studies, Freedman et al. (1994) suggested that major spatial disorganization (sometimes with retention of the essential elements of the clock) can be expected in patients with focal right parietal lesions; those with frontal lesions often show difficulty in integrating the multiple task demands of clock drawing (number sequence and spatial layout); patients with left posterior lesions may show difficulty with numbers and time settings because of receptive aphasia; and similar problems may occur with left anterior lesions (e.g., setting the clock after instead of before). Jones (2000) noted that occasionally a patient may reverse the clock number placement from right to left without omitting numbers. This phenomenon was attributed to subcortical or cortical lesions in the right hemisphere.

Suhr et al. (1998) attempted to find differences between patients with respect to lesion location. They reported that clock drawing was able to differentiate normal elderly from CVA patients; however, none of six quantitative scoring systems was able to differentiate between seven different stroke groups (left, right, bilateral, cortical, subcortical, anterior, posterior) in the acute recovery period. On the other hand, qualitative features (e.g., number rotations, perseverations) were helpful in differentiating groups. In particular, right-hemisphere stroke patients displayed more graphic difficulty and worse spatial planning relative to left-hemisphere stroke patients. Patients with subcortical stroke showed more graphic difficulty relative to cortical patients, whereas cortical patients had more perseveration.

Predictive Validity

As noted earlier (see *Dementia*), the test has value in predicting cognitive decline in older adults (e.g., Ferrucci et al., 1996; O'Rourke et al., 1997; Rouleau et al., 1996). In addition, Adunsky et al. (2002) reported that the test was related to functional outcome of hip fracture in 143 elderly patients undergoing rehabilitation: The CDT correlated significantly with the MMSE and cognitive functional independence measures, but not with absolute outcome parameters (gain in

motor functions). In studies of community-dwelling older adults, Royall and colleagues (Royall & Espino, 2002; Royall et al., 2000, 2004) found that poor performance on the CLOX was related to functional impairment.

A Belgian study (De Raedt & Ponjaert-Kristofferen, 2001) compared results on the CDT, MMSE, TMT Part A, and a visual acuity test with the outcome of a "real world" 35-km road test of driving ability by independent instructors. They found a specificity of 85% and a sensitivity of 80% for the battery. Trails A and age were the best contributors, and CDT was the third-strongest variable. The MMSE did not contribute independently to the discrimination.

COMMENT

The CDT is quick to administer and is well tolerated by clients and clinicians. Not surprisingly, it has become one of the most frequently used screening instruments for dementing disorders (e.g., Reilly et al., 2004), and it compares favorably with other screening tools (e.g., MMSE; Cahn et al., 1996; Rai and Blackman, 1998; Shulman, 2000). However, the various screening tools are not interchangeable, and the CDT may prove more effective in certain groups, such as those with vascular dementia (e.g., Royall et al., 2004). Although education and cultural factors have some impact on performance, their influence may be less pronounced than other cognitive tasks. Accordingly, the CDT may prove particularly useful when language is a serious barrier to cognitive testing (Shulman, 2000). Further, the task appears useful in documenting the severity of cognitive impairment and in predicting subsequent cognitive decline.

Its success as a screening measure for dementia rests on the complexity of the task, which calls on visual-spatial, conceptual, memory, and executive functions to different degrees. This complexity, however, comes at a cost, making it difficult to determine the reasons for patient failure. Therefore, a positive result on the CDT simply signals the need for further inquiry (Shulman, 2000). The inclusion of additional conditions (e.g., copying, clock reading) and examination of the nature of the errors may provide important clues regarding spared and impaired processes.

There are a variety of different administration and scoring methods. All have good interrater and retest reliability, and most are highly correlated with one another. However, they are not equal in utility. With regard to sensitivity to dementia, the Mendez, Shulman, and Tuokko methods fare best, whereas the Wolf-Klein method appears least sensitive. Schramm et al. (2002) noted that, in contrast to the other methods, the Wolf-Klein method asks the respondent to merely "put the numbers on the clock"; the patient is not required to set the clock. Therefore, to detect dementia, it appears important to take into account the ability to position the hands. Bear in mind that, although sensitivity may be high with these techniques, specificity can be poor (particularly for the Mendez method), and additional testing will be needed to distinguish true from false positives. Further, it may be that particular methods (e.g., Royall et al., 1998; Cosentino et al., 2004) are better suited (e.g., more sensitive to executive dysfunction) than others to distinguish among different conditions.

Recent studies (e.g., Cohen et al., 2000; Dilworth et al. 2004) provide valuable data for children but need to be extended to adolescents. The utility of the CDT for studying disorders occurring in childhood populations, including those purported to affect executive functioning, also needs additional investigation.

REFERENCES

Adunsky, A., Fleissig, V., Levenkrohn, M., Arad, M., & Noy, S. (2002). A comparative study of Mini-Mental Test, Clock Drawing Task and Cognitive-FIM in evaluating functional outcome of elderly hip fracture patients. *Clinical Rehabilitation, 16*, 414–419.

Barr, A., Benedict, R., Tune, L., & Brandt, J. (1992). Neuropsychological differentiation of Alzheimer's disease from vascular dementia. *International Journal of Geriatric Psychiatry, 7*, 621–627.

Battersby, W. S., Bender, M. B., Pollack, M., & Kahn, R. L. (1956). Unilateral "spatial agnosia" ("inattention") in patients with cortical lesions. *Brain, 79*, 68–93.

Bodner, T., Delazer, M., Kemmler, G., Gurka, P., Marksteiner, J., & Fleischhacker, W. W. (2004). Clock drawing, clock reading, clock setting, and judgment of clock faces in elderly people with dementia and depression. *Journal of the American Geriatric Society, 52*, 1146–1150.

Bozikas, V. P., Kosmidis, M. H., Gamvrula, K., et al. (2004). Clock drawing test in patients with schizophrenia. *Psychiatry Research, 121*, 229–238.

Brodaty, H., & Moore, C. M. (1997). The Clock Drawing Test for dementia of the Alzheimer's type: A comparison of three scoring methods in a memory disorders clinic. *International Journal of Geriatric Psychiatry, 12*, 619–627.

Cahn, D. A., & Kaplan, E. (1997). Clock drawing in the oldest old. *The Clinical Neuropsychologist, 11*, 96–100.

Cahn, D. A., Salmon, D. P., Monsch, A. U., et al. (1996). Screening for dementia of the Alzheimer type in the community: The utility of the Clock Drawing Test. *Archives of Clinical Neuropsychology, 11*, 529–539.

Cahn, D. A., Wiederholt, W. C., Salmon, D. P., et al. (1994). Detection of cognitive impairment in Spanish-speaking elderly with the Clock Drawing Test [Abstract]. *Archives of Clinical Neuropsychology, 9*, 112.

Cahn-Weiner, D. A., Sullivan, E. V., Shear, P. K., Fama, R., Lim, K. O., Yesavage, J. A., Tinklenberg, J. R., & Pfefferbaum, A. (1999). Brain structural and cognitive correlates of clock drawing performance in Alzheimer's disease. *Journal of the International Neuropsychological Society, 5*, 502–509.

Chokron, S., Colliot, P., & Bartolomeo, P. (2004). The role of vision in spatial presentation. *Cortex, 40*, 281–290.

Cohen, M. J., Ricci, C. A., Kibby, M. Y., & Edmonds. J. E. (2000). Developmental progression of clock face drawing in children. *Child Neuropsychology, 6*, 64–76.

Cosentino, S., Jefferson, A., Chute, D. L., Kaplan, E., & Libon, D. J. (2004). Clock drawing errors in dementia. *Cognitive Behavioral Neurology, 17*, 74–84.

Critchley, M. ([1953] 1966). *The parietal lobes.* New York: Hafner.

Dastoor, D. P., Schwartz, G., & Kurzman, D. (1991). Clock-Drawing: An assessment technique in dementia. *Journal of Clinical and Experimental Gerontology, 13*, 69–85.

De Raedt, R., & Ponjaert-Kristofferen, I. (2001). Short cognitive/neuropsychological test battery for first-tier fitness-to-drive assessment of older adults. *Clinical Neuropsychologist, 15*, 329–336.

Dilworth, J. E., Greenberg, M. T., & Kusche, C. (2004). Early neuropsychological correlates of later clock drawing and clock copying abilities among school aged children. *Child Neuropsychology, 10*, 24–35.

Edmonds, J. E., Cohen, M. J., Riccio, C. A., et al. (1994). The development of clock face drawing in normal children [Abstract]. *Archives of Clinical Neuropsychology, 9*, 125.

Ferrucci, L., Cecchi, F., Guralnik, J. M., & Giampaoli, S. (1996). Does the clock drawing test predict cognitive decline in older persons independent of the Mini-Mental State Examination? *Journal of the American Geriatric Society, 44*, 1326–1331.

Freedman, M., Kaplan, E., Delis, D., & Morris, R. (1994). *Clock Drawing: A neuropsychological analysis.* New York: Oxford University Press.

Goodglass, H., & Kaplan, E. (1972). *The assessment of aphasia and related disorders.* Philadelphia: Lea & Febiger.

Goodglass, H., & Kaplan, E. (1983). *Assessment of aphasia and related disorders* (2nd ed.). Philadelphia: Lea & Febiger.

Goodglass, H., Kaplan, E., & Barresi, B. (2001). *The assessment of aphasia and related disorders* (3rd ed.). Philadelphia: Lippincott, Williams & Wilkins.

Heinik, J., Solomesh, I., & Beckman, P. (2004). Correlation between the CAMCOG, the MMSE, and three clock drawing tests in a specialized outpatient psychogeriatric service. *Archives of Gerontology and Geriatrics, 38*, 77–84.

Heinik, J., Solomesh, I., Raikher, B., & Lin, R. (2002a). Can Clock Drawing Test help to differentiate between dementia of the Alzheimer's type and vascular dementia? A preliminary study. *International Journal of Geriatric Psychiatry, 17*, 600–703.

Heinik, J., Solomesh, I., Shein, V., & Becker, D. (2002b). Clock Drawing Test in mild and moderate dementia of the Alzheimer's type: A comparative and correlational study. *International Journal of Geriatric Psychiatry, 17*, 480–485.

Herrmann, N., Kidron, D., Shulman, K. I., Kaplan, E., Binns, M., Leach, L., & Freedman, M. (1998). Clock tests in depression, Alzheimer's disease, and elderly controls. *International Journal of Psychiatry in Medicine, 28*, 437–447.

Herrmann, N., Kidron, D., Shulman, K. I.., Kaplan, E., Binns, M., Soni, J., Leach, L., & Freedman, M. (1999). The use of clock tests in schizophrenia. *General Hospital Psychiatry, 21*, 70–73.

Jones, D. S. (2000). Reversed clock phenomenon: A right-hemisphere syndrome. *Neurology, 55*, 1939–1942.

Kibby, M. Y., Cohen, M. J., & Hynd, G. W. (2001). Clock face drawing in children with attention-deficit/hyperactivity disorder. *Archives of Clinical Neuropsychology, 17*, 531–546.

Kirby, M., Denihan, A., Bruce, I., Xoakley, D., & Lawlor, B. A. (2001). The clock drawing test in primary care: Sensitivity in dementia detection, and specificity against normal and depressed elderly. *International Journal of Geriatric Psychiatry, 16*, 935–940.

Kirk, U., McCarthy, C., & Kaplan, E. (1996). The development of clock-drawing skills: Implications for neuropsychological assessment of children. Paper presented at the meeting of the International Neuropsychological Society, Chicago.

Kitabayashi, Y., Ueda, H., Narumoto, J., Nakamura, K., Kita, H., & Fukui, K. (2002). Qualitative analyses of clock drawings in Alzheimer's disease and vascular dementia. *Psychiatry and Clinical Neuroscience, 55*, 485–491.

Kozora, E., & Cullum, M. (1994). Qualitative features of clock drawing in normal aging and Alzheimer's disease. *Assessment, 1,* 179–187.

La Rue, A., Romero, L. J., Ortiz, I. E., Liang, H. C., & Lindeman, R. D. (1999). Neuropsychological performance of Hispanic and non-Hispanic older adults: An epidemiologic survey. *The Clinical Neuropsychologist, 13,* 474–486.

Leach, L., Kaplan, E., Rewilak, D., Richards, B., & Proulx, B-B. (2000). *Kaplan Baycrest Neurocognitive Assessment.* San Antonio, Tex.: The Psychological Corporation.

Lee, H., & Lawler, B. A. (1995). State-dependent nature of the Clock Drawing Test in geriatric depression. *Journal of the American Geriatric Society, 43,* 796–798.

Lezak, M. D., Howieson, D. B., & Loring, D. W. (2004). *Neuropsychological assessment* (4th Ed.). New York: Oxford University Press.

Libon, D. J., Malamut, B. L., Swenson, R., Sands, L. P., & Cloud, B. S. (1996). Further analyses of clock drawings among demented and non-demented older subjects. *Archives of Clinical Neuropsychology, 11,* 193–205.

Libon, D. J., Swenson, R. A., Barnoski, E. J., & Sands, L. P. (1993). Clock drawing as an assessment tool for dementia. *Archives of Clinical Neuropsychology, 8,* 405–415.

Manos, P. J. (1997). The utility of the 10-point clock test as a screen for cognitive impairment in general hospital patients. *General Hospital Psychiatry, 19,* 439–444.

Manos, P. J. (1999). Ten-point clock test sensitivity for Alzheimer's disease in patients with MMSE scores greater than 23. *International Journal of Geriatric Psychiatry, 14,* 454–458.

Manos, P. J., & Wu, R. (1994). The ten point clock test: A quick screen and grading method for cognitive impairment in medical and surgical patients. *International Journal of Psychiatry and Medicine, 24,* 229–244.

Marcopulos, B. A., & McLain, C. A. (2003). Are our norms "Normal"? A 4-year follow-up study of a biracial sample of rural elders with low education. *The Clinical Neuropsychologist, 17,* 19–33.

Marcopulos, B. A., McLain, C. A., & Giuliano, A. J. (1997). Cognitive impairment or inadequate norms? *The Clinical Neuropsychologist, 11,* 111–131.

Mendez, M. F., Ala, T., & Underwood, K. L. (1992). Development of scoring criteria for the clock drawing task in Alzheimer's disease. *Journal of the American Geriatrics Society, 40,* 1095–1099.

Moretti, R., Torre, P., Antonello, R. M., Gazzato, G. & Bava, A. (2002). Ten-point clock test: A correlation analysis with other neuropsychological tests in dementia. *International Journal of Geriatric Psychiatry, 17,* 347–353.

Nussbaum, P. D., Fields, R. B., & Starrat, C. (1992). Comparison of three scoring procedures for the clock drawing [Abstract]. *Journal of Clinical and Experimental Neuropsychology, 14,* 44.

Ogden, J. A. (1985). Anterior-posterior interhemispheric differences in the loci of lesions producing visual hemineglect. *Brain and Cognition, 4,* 59–75.

O'Rourke, N., Tuokko, H., Hayden, S., & Beattie, B. L. (1997). Early identification of dementia: Predictive validity of the clock test. *Archives of Clinical Neuropsychology, 12,* 257–267.

Rai, G. S., & Blackman, I. (1998). Dementia diagnosis: Usefulness of Mini Mental Status Examination and Clock Drawing Test. *Clinical Gerontologist, 19,* 68–70.

Ratcliff, G., Dodge, H., Birzescu, M., & Ganguli, M. (2003). Tracking cognitive functions over time: Ten-year longitudinal data from a community-based study. *Applied Neuropsychology, 10,* 76–88.

Reilly, S., Challis, D., Burns, A., & Hughes, J. (2004). The use of assessment scales in old age psychiatry services in England and Northern Ireland. *Aging and Mental Health, 8,* 249–255.

Roth, M., Tym, E., Mountjoy, C. Q., et al. (1986). CAMDEX: A standardized instrument for the diagnosis of mental disorder in the elderly with special reference to the early detection of dementia. *British Journal of Psychiatry, 149,* 698–709.

Rouleau, I., Salmon, D. P., & Butters, N. (1996). Longitudinal analysis of clock drawing in Alzheimer's disease patients. *Brain and Cognition, 18,* 79–87.

Rouleau, I., Salmon, D. P., Butters, N., Kennedy, C., & McGuire, K. (1992). Quantitative and qualitative analyses of clock face drawings in Alzheimer's and Huntington's diseases. *Brain and Cognition, 18,* 70–87.

Royall, D. R., & Espino, D. V. (2002). Not all clock-drawing tasks are the same. *Journal of the American Geriatric Society, 30,* 1166–1167.

Royall, D. R., Chiodo, L. K., & Polk, M. J. (2000). Correlates of disability among elderly retirees with "subcortical" cognitive impairment. *Journals of Gerontology: Series A: Biological Sciences and Medical Sciences, 55,* M541–M546.

Royall, D. R., Cordes, J. A., & Polk, M. (1998). CLOX: An executive clock drawing task. *Journal of Neurology, Neurosurgery, and Psychiatry, 64,* 588–594.

Royall, D. R., Espino, D. V., Polk, M. J., Palmer, R. F., & Markides, K. S. (2004). Prevalence and patterns of executive impairment in community dwelling Mexican Americans: Results from the Hispanic EPESE Study. *International Journal of Geriatric Psychiatry, 19,* 926–934.

Royall, D. R., Mulroy, A. R., Chiodo, L. K., & Polk, M. J. (1999). Clock drawing is sensitive to executive control: A comparison of six methods. *Journal of Gerontology: Psychological Sciences, 54B,* P328–P333.

Schramm, U., Berger, G., Mueller, R., Kratzsch, T., Peters, J., & Froelich, L. (2002). Psychometric properties of clock drawing test and MMSE or Short Performance Test (SKT) in dementia screening in a memory clinic population. *International Journal of Geriatric Psychiatry, 17,* 254–260.

Shulman, K. I. (2000). Clock-Drawing: Is it the ideal cognitive screening test? *International Journal of Geriatric Psychiatry, 15,* 548–561.

Shulman, K. I., Gold, D. P., Cohen, C. A., & Zucchero, C. A. (1993). Clock drawing and dementia in the community: A longitudinal study. *International Journal of Geriatric Psychiatry, 8,* 487–496.

Shulman, K. I., Shedletzky, R., & Silver, I. L. (1986). The challenge of time: Clock drawing and cognitive function in the elderly. *International Journal of Geriatric Psychiatry, 1,* 135–140.

Solomon, P. R., Hirschoff, A., Kelly, B., Relin, M., Brush, M., DeVeaux, R. D., & Pendlebury, W. W. (1998). A 7 minute neurocognitive screening battery highly sensitive to Alzheimer disease. *Archives of Neurology, 55,* 349–355.

Spreen, O., & Strauss, E. (1991). *A compendium of neuropsychological tests: Administration, norms and commentary.* New York: Oxford University Press.

Storey, J. E., Rowland, J. T. J., Basic, D., & Conforti, D. A. (2001). A comparison of five clock scoring methods using ROC (receiver operating characteristics) curve analysis. *International Journal of Geriatric Psychiatry, 16,* 394–399.

Strub, R. L., & Black, F. W. (1977). *The mental status examination in neurology.* Philadelphia: F. A. Davis.

Suhr, J., Grace, J., Allen, J., Nadler, J., & McKenna, M. (1998). Quantitative and qualitative performance of stroke versus normal elderly on six clock drawing systems. *Archives of Clinical Neuropsychology, 13,* 495–502.

Sunderland, T., Hill, J. L., Mellow, A. M., Lawlor, B. A., Gundersheimer, J., Newhouse, P. A., & Grafman, J. H. (1989). Clock drawing in Alzheimer's disease: A novel measure of dementia severity. *Journal of the American Geriatric Association, 37,* 725–729.

Trojano, L., Grossi, D., Linden, D., Formisano, E., Goebel, R., Girillo, S. F., Elefante, R., & Di Salle, F. (2002). Coordinate and categorical judgements in spatial imagery: An fMRI study. *Neuropsychologia, 40,* 1666–1674.

Tuokko, H., Hadjistavropoulos, T., Miller, J. A., & Beattie, B. L. (1992). The clock test: A sensitive measure to differentiate normal elderly from those with Alzheimer's disease. *Journal of the American Geriatrics Society, 40,* 579–584.

Tuokko, H., Hadjistavropoulos, T., Miller, J. A., Horton, A., & Beattie, B. L. (1995). *The Clock Test: Administration and scoring manual.* Toronto, Ont.: Multi-Health Systems.

Tuokko, H., Hadjistavropoulos, T., Rae, S., & O'Rourke, N. (2000). A comparison of alternative approaches to the scoring of clock drawing. *Archives of Clinical Neuropsychology, 15,* 137–148.

Tuokko, H., & O'Connell, M. (In press). A review of quantified approaches to the qualitative assessment of clock drawing. In A. Poreh (Ed.), *Quantified process approach.* Lisse: Swetts & Zeitlinger.

Ueda, H., Kitabayashi, Y., Narumoto, K., Kita, H., Kishikawa, Y., & Fukui, K. (2002). Relationship between clock drawing test performance and regional cerebral blood flow in Alzheimer's disease: A single photon emission computed tomography study. *Psychiatry and Clinical Neurosciences, 56,* 25–29.

Watson, Y. I., Arfken, C. L., & Birge, S. J. (1993). Clock completion: An objective screening test for dementia. *Journal of the American Geriatrics Society, 41,* 1235–1240.

Wolf-Klein, G. P., Silverstone, F. A., Levy, A. P., Brod, M. S., & Breuer, J. (1989). Screening for Alzheimer's disease by clock drawing. *Journal of the American Geriatric Association, 37,* 730–734.

Facial Recognition Test (FRT)

PURPOSE

The purpose of the Facial Recognition Test (FRT) test is to assess the ability to recognize unfamiliar human faces.

SOURCE

The test (book of photographs and 100 forms) can be ordered from PAR (http://www.parinc.com) at a cost of $95 US. The manual (available in English and Spanish) can be purchased separately at a cost of $39.

AGE RANGE

The age range is 6 to 90+ years; however, there are no norms for 15-year-olds.

DESCRIPTION

Loss of the ability to recognize the faces of familiar persons (prosopagnosia) was first described in a 54-year-old man by two Italian ophthalmologists, A. Quaglino and G. Borelli in 1867 (Benton et al., 1994). This patient's initial aphasia and left arm paresis disappeared and his blindness resolved into a left hemianopia over the course of 1 month. It was this association with signs of right hemisphere dysfunction that made facial agnosia particularly interesting in this and subsequent cases to neurologists and neuropsychologists. They (e.g., Benton & Van Allen, 1968; De Renzi et al., 1968; Tzavaras et al., 1970; Warrington & James, 1967) devised tests to assess the accuracy of perception and memory of unfamiliar faces with the aim of determining the anatomic and behavioral correlates of defective performance (Benton et al., 1994). Initial findings were that the impairment in recognition and memory of unfamiliar faces showed the same association with other signs of right-hemisphere disease as did prosopagnosia. However, subsequent case reports described severely prosopagnostic patients who seemed to show intact ability to recognize unfamiliar faces (but see Duchaine & Weidenfeld, 2003 and *Comments*). In addition, most patients with serious difficulties in the recognition of unfamiliar faces appeared able to recognize familiar faces (Benton et al., 1994). Moreover, it was noted that difficulty with recognition of unfamiliar faces was fairly common, particularly in patients with posterior right-hemisphere disease, whereas prosopagnosia was a fairly uncommon condition (Benton et al., 1994). Therefore, the impairment in facial recognition appeared to occur in at least two distinct forms: one represented by a failure to identify the faces of familiar persons and the other by a failure to identify unfamiliar faces. The FRT, developed by Benton and Van Allen (1968), provides a method to assess the ability to discriminate photographs of unfamiliar human faces.

In the FRT, clothing and hair are shaded out so that only facial features can be used. The full test (Long Form) consists of 54 items, whereas the Short Form (for use as a brief screening of face recognition; Levin et al., 1975) is an abbreviated version consisting of the first 27 items from the Long Form. A different short form was recently suggested by Christensen et al. (2002).

The FRT consists of three parts:

1. Matching of identical front-view photographs (see Figure 12–9). The patient is presented with a single front-view photograph of a single face (male or female) and is instructed to identify it (by pointing to it or providing the number that corresponds to it) in a display of six front-view photographs (the target and five distractors) that appears below the single photograph. There are six target faces, calling for a total of six responses.

2. Matching of front-view with three-quarter-view photographs (see Figure 12–10). The individual is presented with a single front-view photograph of a face

Figure 12–9 Example of Facial Recognition Test—identical front view. *Source:* Reproduced with special permission of Psychological Assessment Resources, PAR, Inc.

Figure 12–10 Example of Facial Recognition Test—three-quarter view. *Source:* Reproduced with special permission of Psychological Assessment Resources, PAR, Inc.

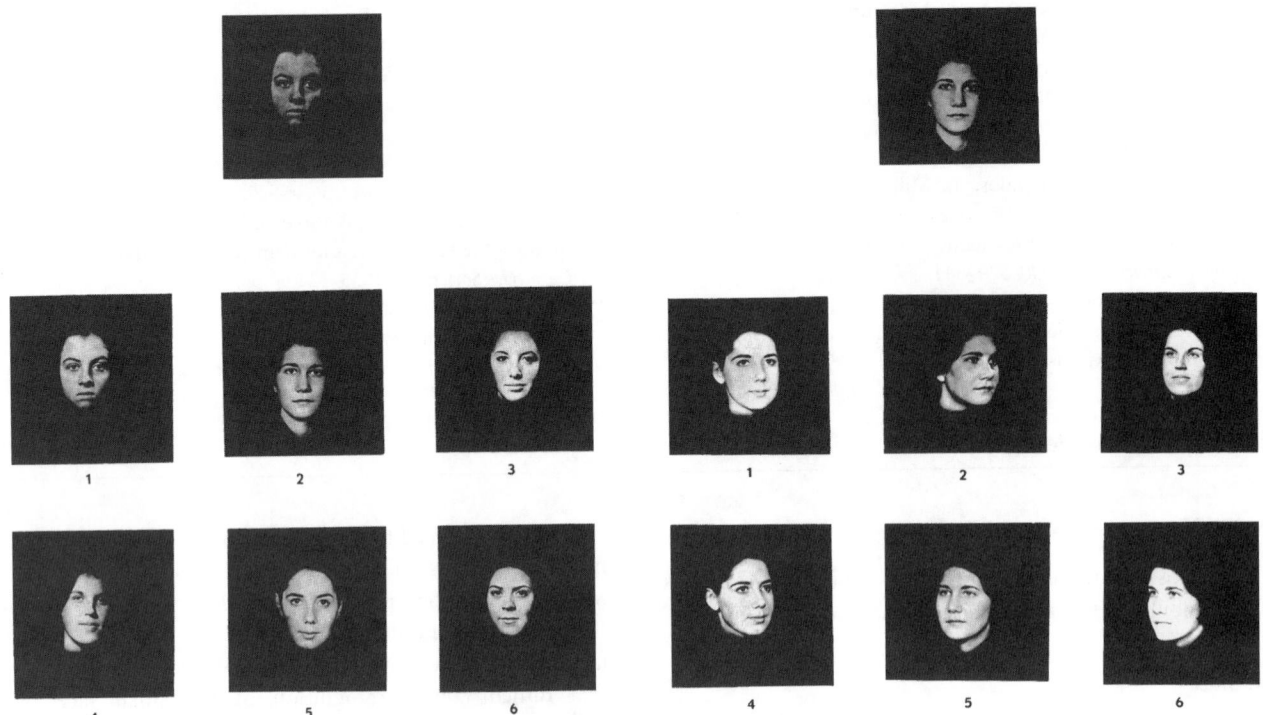

and is instructed to locate it three times in a display of six three-quarter views, three of which are views of the presented face and three views of other faces. There are 8 target faces, calling for a total of 24 responses.

3. Matching of front-view photographs under different lighting conditions (see Figure 12–11). The subject is presented with a single front-view photograph of a face taken under full lighting conditions and is instructed to locate it three times in a display of six front views taken under different lighting conditions; three photographs in the display are of the presented face, and three are of other faces. There are 8 target faces, calling for a total of 24 responses.

ADMINISTRATION

See *Source.* The test is assembled in a spiral-bound booklet. Each stimulus picture and its corresponding response choices are presented on two facing pages, with the single stimulus picture above the six response-choice pictures (*"Do you see this woman? Show me where she is on this picture"*). If they are able to do so, subjects are encouraged to hold and manipulate the test material to their best visual advantage.

The Long Form is administered by giving all of the test items. The Short Form is administered by giving only the first 13 pages. The Christensen short form consists of pages 7, 8, 10–12, 14–19, and 22 from the Long Form.

ADMINISTRATION TIME

In older adults, the median time to completion of the Long Form was 9 min, and 95% of the participants (aged 60 years and older) completed the test within 17 min (Christensen et al., 2002). According to Benton et al. (1994), the mean administration time for the Short Form in the setting of a neurology clinic was 7 min, with a range of 5 to 15 min.

SCORING

The total score reflects the number of correct responses for the three different item types. For the Long Form, the maximum score is 54. For the Short Form, the maximum score is 27. The maximum score for the Christensen short form is 36. On the Long Form, a minimum score of 25 may be expected on the basis of chance alone. Hence, the effective range of Long Form scores may be considered to be 25 to 54 points. For the Short Form, the effective range may be considered to be 11 to 27 points.

According to the test manual, if the Short Form is used, the number of correct responses on the record sheet needs to be converted to Long Form scores, following a conversion table in the manual. The test manual also provides age and education corrections for the Long Form and the converted Short Form scores. These corrections are based on performances of 286 subjects within the age range of 16 to 74 years (see *Standardization Sample*; Benton et al., 1994).

Figure 12-11 Example of Facial Recognition Test—different lighting conditions. *Source:* Reproduced with special permission of Psychological Assessment Resources, PAR, Inc.

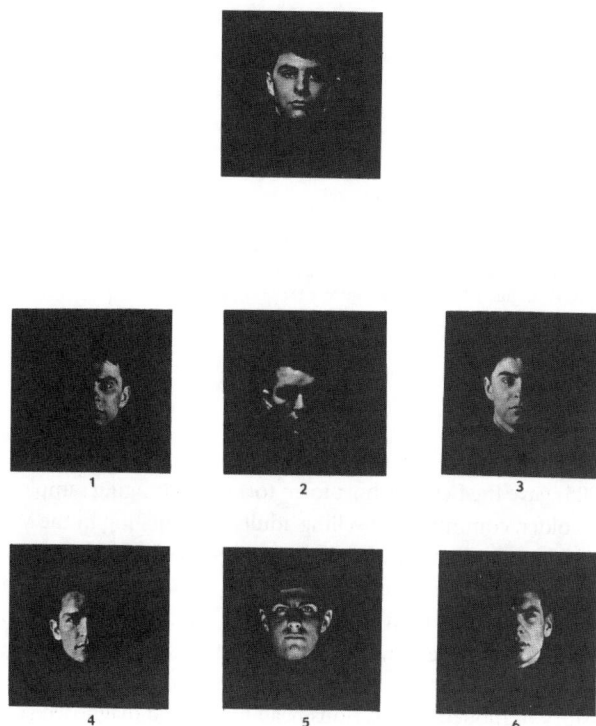

DEMOGRAPHIC EFFECTS

Age

Age affects performance (Benton et al., 1994; Christensen et al., 2002; Mittenberg et al., 1989; Schretlen et al., 2001). According to Benton et al. (1994), scores improve in childhood, with adult levels reached by about age 14 years. Test scores show some decline in old age.

Education/IQ

Education also affects performance (Benton et al., 1994; Christensen, 2002; but see Schretlen et al., 2001, who found no significant effect for education). Scores increase with increasing Full-Scale IQ (Diaz-Asper et al., 2004).

Gender

No gender-related differences have been reported (Benton et al., 1994; Christensen, 2002; Schretlen et al., 2001).

Ethnicity

Results for Hispanics appear to be equivalent to those obtained with English-speaking individuals (Rey et al., 1999). Similar test scores have also been obtained in Italian adults

(Ferracuti & Ferracuti, 1992) and in inner-city African Americans (Roberts & Hamsher, 1984), suggesting that the test is relatively independent of ethnic/cultural factors.

NORMATIVE DATA

Standardization Sample

Benton et al. (1994) provided score distributions for 286 adults (age range, 16–74 years). The characteristics of the sample are shown in Table 12–10. The standardization sample consisted of two groups. One group comprised 196 patients without evidence of neurological or psychiatric disease or evidence of mental deficiency. The other group consisted of 90 volunteers in a study of aging. Age and education corrections are provided for participants older than 54 years of age and are based on a division between participants with less than a 12th grade education and those with grade 12 or higher. Corrected scores of 40 or lower on the Long Form (20 or lower on the Short Form) raise the concern of abnormality.

Note that the data were collected more than 30 years ago from a restricted region of the United States.

Benton et al. (1994) also provided data from 266 children, aged 6 to 14 years, attending public schools in Iowa. Their IQ,

Table 12–10 Characteristics of the Facial Recognition Normative Sample

Number	Adults: 286
	Children: 229
Age (years)	Adults: 16–74 (mean age not reported)
	Children: 6–14
Geographic location	Iowa (USA)
Sample type	Adults: one sample (*N* = 196) consisted of patients from the neurological, neurosurgical, and medical services of the University of Iowa Hospital; a second sample consisted of 90 volunteers in a study of aging, aged 60–74 years
	Children: Attending public schools in Iowa
Education (years)	Adults: 6–12+
Gender	Adults: Males = 111, Females = 175
	Children: not reported
Race/Ethnicity	Not reported
Screening	Adults: Patients were included who showed no evidence or history of neurological disease, mental retardation, or hospitalization for psychiatric disorder
	Children: Screening not reported, although abbreviated WISC scores were between 85 and 116

Table 12–11 Normative Estimates for Facial Recognition Long Form

Age (Years)	60–69	70–79	80–89	90+	All
n	101	99	96	50	346
Mean (SD)	42.8 (4)	40.6 (4)	38.3 (4.3)	36.4 (4.5)	40 (4.7)
Coefficient alpha					.72
SEM					2.5
Cut scores derived from age-based means					
95% probability defective	30.7	28.5	25.6	23.3	
95% probability nondefective	38.9	36.7	33.8	31.5	

Note: Regression equation for estimated long form score = (−22) Age + (.12)Reading + (.12)Daughter's education + 48.31 (R = .60; SE = 3.78), where Age is in years. Reading is the WRAT-R Reading Level 2 Performance, and Daughter's education is in years, not including vocational school, (e.g., 8th grade = 8, bachelor's degree = 16, master's degree = 18, doctorate = 20 (maximum level).

Source: Adapted from Christensen et al., 2002.

based on a WISC short form, ranged from 85 to 116. It is worth noting that important information is lacking (e.g., sex distribution, SES, year data were collected) and standard deviations are not reported.

Other Normative Data

Long Form. Christensen et al. (2002) provided more extensive normative data on the Long Form, based on a sample of 346 healthy older adults, aged 60 to more than 90 years old (M = 74.8, SD = 8.9; education M = 11.6, SD = 2.6). Participants were recruited from Minneapolis and St. Paul, Minnesota, based on age, gender, and education according to 1990 U.S. Census characteristics for that geographical area. Participants were screened to exclude conditions that might affect cognition. The majority of the participants were Caucasian.

Application of Benton et al.'s (1994) age and education corrections to participants in the Christensen study who were aged 60 to 69 years yielded a mean score and variability consistent with those obtained in the Benton sample. However, scores for older participants were considerably lower than those suggested by Benton et al. (1994). The data of Christensen et al. (2002) are shown in Table 12–11 and are preferred for evaluation of older adults. The authors also found that other demographic data (highest education of daughter) and oral reading performance (WRAT-R Reading Level 2) improved prediction of an individual's score based on age alone. They provided a prediction equation to aid interpretation (see Table 12–11). Comparison of obtained versus predicted FRT scores may be useful in determining whether there has been significant decline.

Paquier et al. (1999) gave the FRT to 81 right-handed children who were attending regular schools. All had normal vision and no history of neurological problems. The mean age-related performance is shown in Table 12–12. The values were similar to those reported by Benton et al. (1994) except for children aged 13 and 14 years, for whom the Benton norms were slightly higher (means of 43.0 and 45.1, respectively). Note that the cell sizes were very small.

Short Forms. Dixon (personal communication, March 18, 2005) gave the Benton short form to a typically aging sample of 457 older, community-dwelling adults participating in the Victoria Longitudinal Study. Exclusion criteria included MMSE scores of 24 or lower, moderate or very serious visual or auditory impairment even with corrective aids, history of major neurological disease (e.g., stroke, Parkinson's disease, meningitis), history of severe depression, insulin-controlled diabetes, history of moderate or serious head injury, and diagnosed substance abuse within the past 5 years. The data are presented in Table 12–13. In order to maximize the amount of information available, overlapping-midpoint age ranges were used.

Christensen et al. (2002) provided normative data by age group for their short form, and these are shown in Table 12–14. The data are derived from the sample described earlier (see *Long Form*).

RELIABILITY

Internal Consistency

Coefficient alpha for the Long Form in 206 undergraduates was only .57 (Hoptman & Davidson, 1993); however, internal

Table 12–12 Mean FRT Performance in Children by Age

Age (Years)	n	Mean (SD)
7	10	35.0 (4.5)
8	10	37.0 (3.0)
9	11	38.9 (5.8)
10	11	41.2 (4.4)
11	9	39.8 (5.1)
12	9	41.5 (4.3)
13	10	41.9 (3.0)
14	11	41.4 (4.4)

Source: Adapted from Paquier et al. (1999).

Table 12–13 Benton Facial Recognition Short Form

Age Range (Midpoint)	53–60 (57)	55–65 (60)	60–70 (65)	65–75 (70)	70–80 (75)	75–85 (80)	80–90 (85)
n	92	180	172	145	135	112	58
Gender (F/M)	71/21	138/42	121/51	93/52	88/47	74/38	39/19
Mean education (SD)	15.72 (2.72)	15.68 (2.77)	15.50 (2.96)	15.13 (2.84)	14.95 (2.85)	14.66 (2.91)	14.34 (2.85)
Mean Benton score (SD)	22.90 (2.18)	22.87 (2.12)	22.65 (2.07)	22.20 (2.15)	21.84 (2.30)	21.40 (2.32)	20.57 (2.47)

Source: R. Dixon, personal communication, March 18, 2005.

Table 12–14 Mean Scores for Christensen et al. (2002) Short Form

Age (Years)	60–69	70–79	80–84	85–89	90+
Mean	28.8	27.3	26.0	25.7	24.4
SD	3.1	3.2	3.7	3.3	3.50

Note: Item numbers for this short form: 7,8,10,11,12,14,15,16,17,18,19,22.

Source: Adapted from Christensen et al., 2002.

reliability was higher when the first six items of the test (identity matches) were omitted (.66). In 346 healthy older adults, Christensen et al. (2002) found an internal consistency of .72 for the Long Form and .53 for the Short Form. In response to the poor internal consistency of the existing Short Form, Christensen et al. (2002) developed a new short form that yielded a coefficient alpha of .69 (item numbers 7, 8, 10–12, 14–19, and 22). The standard error of measurement was 2.0.

Test-Retest Reliability

Test-retest reliability after 1 year in older adults has been reported to be between .60 (Short Form) and .71 (Long Form; Christensen et al., 2002; Levin et al., 1991), with no significant change in mean scores. Scores on the modified short form by Christensen et al. (2002) did not change over a 1-year interval and had a stability coefficient of .71 (N = 100).

VALIDITY

Relations Between Long and Short Forms

Correlations between the Long and Short forms range from .88 in normal subjects to .92 in brain-damaged subjects (Benton et al., 1994). Christensen's (2002) modified short form correlated highly with the Long Form (> .90) in healthy older adults.

Relationships With Other Measures

As noted earlier (see *Demographic Effects*), performance improves with increasing Full-Scale IQ (Diaz-Asper et al., 2004). Correlations between FRT scores and VIQ are not significant in patients with CVAs (Trahan, 1997). However, PIQ and FRT are highly correlated in patients with right CVAs

with neglect (r = .60) and in those without neglect (r = .62; Trahan, 1997), suggesting a significant visual-perceptual component. Similarly, Larrabee and Curtiss (Larrabee, 2000) found that the FRT loaded on a visual-perceptual reasoning factor defined by tests such as WAIS Picture Completion, Picture Arrangement, Block Design, Object Assembly, and Digit Symbol, as well as WCST perseverative errors and Trails B. By contrast, Hermann et al. (1993) reported that the FRT loaded with the Hooper Visual Organization Test but not with WAIS-R subtests or the Judgment of Line Orientation Test, which loaded together, suggesting that the FRT is more sensitive to object recognition than to spatial localization abilities.

In children, the FRT is unrelated to memory for faces (r = .03, Korkman et al., 1998).

Clinical Findings

The test is sensitive to right posterior damage (e.g., Dricker et al., 1978; Egelko et al., 1988; Hamsher et al., 1979; Mulder et al., 1995; Trahan, 1997). For example, Trahan (1997) found that 53% of 85 patients with right-hemisphere CVA were impaired on the FRT, as opposed to only 27% of 45 patients with left-hemisphere CVA. In particular, patients with left visual neglect showed impaired FRT scores.

Although the FRT is sensitive to right posterior disturbance, poor FRT performance has been reported in patient groups with dysfunction in other brain areas. Some patients with left hemisphere lesions also have difficulty on this test. For example, Hamsher et al. (1979) noted a subgroup of aphasic patients with left hemisphere damage and impairment in language comprehension who performed defectively on the FRT, suggesting that language (perhaps a verbal analytic strategy) does play a role in FRT performance. Patients with left hemisphere damage who were not aphasic or whose aphasia was not characterized by substantial impairment in oral language comprehension performed within normal limits. Mattson et al. (2000) reported accurate but slow performance in a patient with a focal lesion confined to the left posterior hemisphere. Note too that Trahan (1997) found that about 25% of his cases with left-sided CVAs were impaired on the FRT, although their deficits tended to be milder than those with right-sided CVAs. Finally, Pueschel and Zaidel (1994) adapted the FRT to a tachistoscopic same/different task and found an advantage for the left hemifield only for the most difficult, shaded items, suggesting that each hemisphere may contribute to successful task performance.

Hermann et al. (1993) found that anterior temporal lobectomy (right or left) resulted in a decline of face recognition ability, but not of performance on the Judgment of Line Orientation Test, the Hooper, or the WAIS-R Performance subtests. The selective decline in facial recognition ability was thought to be caused by compromise of the occipitotemporal object recognition system leaving unaffected the occipitoparietal spatial localization system, as proposed by Mishkin and his colleagues (Mishkin et al., 1983; Ungerleider & Mishkin, 1982).

Memory does not appear to play a significant role in task performance. A case report by Botez-Marquand and Botez (1992) described a severely amnesic female patient who performed normally on the FRT.

In children with perinatal brain damage, impairment has been reported regardless of the side of the lesion (Ballantyne & Trauner, 1999; Strauss & Verity, 1983). Paquier et al. (1999) evaluated healthy children and children with acquired left or right cerebral lesions and found that the test did not predict the presence or laterality of cerebral lesions. In fact, most of the children performed within the normal range. Ballantyne and Trauner (1999) proposed that in children there is sufficient ability to reorganize such that residual effects are less pronounced and less lateralized.

Deficits in face recognition have been reported in patients with Parkinson's disease (Beatty et al., 1989; Bentin et al., 1981; Hovestadt et al., 1987; Levin et al., 1991), multiple sclerosis (Beatty et al., 1989), alcoholism (Schwartz et al., 2002), AD (Andrikopoulos, 1997), and moderate-to-severe closed head injury (Levin et al., 1977; Peck et al., 1992; Risser and Andrikopoulos, 1997). Matser et al. (1999) also found impairment on the FRT in amateur soccer players compared with a group of control athletes. In Williams syndrome, the trajectory of development appears to be atypical (delayed; Karmiloff-Smith et al., 2004).

Advancing age is also associated with a decline in face processing (Benton et al., 1994; Christensen et al., 2002; Mittenberg et al., 1989). The decline may reflect normal age-related decrements in processing speed as well as atrophic brain changes. In a study of healthy adults, aged 20 to 92 years, Schretlen et al. (2001) found that normal atrophic brain changes (MRI ventricle-to-brain ratios) and declines in processing speed contributed to individual differences in face recognition as measured by the FRT, even though in this task people are free to inspect pictures for as long as they want in order to make same/different judgments.

Some researchers (Levin and Benton, 1977; Risser and Andrikopulos, 1997) have reported that face recognition scores in psychiatric patients are indistinguishable from those of normal subjects, but others (e.g., Borod et al., 1993; Echternacht, 1986; Kuscharska-Pietura et al., 2002) have found more defective scores in such patients. For example, Kucharska-Pietura et al. (2002) reported a performance deficit on the FRT among patients with schizophrenia compared with controls. Similarly, Borod et al. (1993) evaluated adults with schizophrenia,

patients with right hemisphere damage, and normal controls on the FRT. Both of the patient groups were impaired relative to normal controls, but they were not different from each other. Hence, impaired performance on this test should not be interpreted, in and of itself, as evidence of focal neurological disturbance.

Relationship to Vision

Intact vision is important for this test. Kempen et al. (1994) reported significantly poorer scores on this test with patients whose Jaeger near-vision was J5 (equivalent to 20/50) or worse due to refractory error, compared with subjects with normal vision. For this reason, a standard vision test should be administered before an interpretation of the results is attempted in patients with suspected visual disturbance.

Visual field defects do not necessarily affect test scores. For example, Benton et al. (1994) evaluated 26 patients with right posterior lesions and visual field defects. Fifteen (58%) of them performed defectively on the FRT. Of 10 patients with right posterior lesions and no visual field defect, 4 (40%) performed defectively.

Feature-Matching Strategy

Subjects commonly rely on feature matching strategies using the hairline and eyebrows rather than recognizing the facial configuration. In fact, just the presence of the eyebrows and hairline is sufficient to support normal performance (Duchaine & Weidenfeld, 2003). Therefore, a normal score on the FRT does not demonstrate normal unfamiliar face recognition abilities.

COMMENT

The FRT is commonly used by neuropsychologists to assess face recognition abilities. The task has a number of positive features. First, it is relatively brief and portable and can be administered at the bedside. Further, it lends itself for use with a wide variety of patients, because it is untimed and requires little motor involvement, although adequate vision is important. Moreover, unlike tests such as the Warrington Recognition Memory for Faces (RMF), target faces and test items are presented simultaneously, so that patients are not required to rely on a memory trace.

Users should bear in mind, however, that much of the normative data stems from studies conducted by Benton and his colleagues more than 30 years ago. Norms provided for the child sample lack standard deviations as well as important demographic information. Current norms are preferred, although it should be noted that, in the case of adults, these cover a limited age range (the elderly) from restricted geographical regions, and, in the case of children, the sample size is quite small. In neither case do the norms derive from national, randomly stratified samples.

The Long Form has shown adequate internal consistency in some studies (i.e., Christensen et al., 2002) but not in others

(Hoptman & Davidson, 1993). Accordingly, use of the standard error of measurement for computation of confidence intervals is important (Christensen et al., 2002). The internal consistency of the Short Form is poor, and the form should not be used clinically. The Christensen modified short form has slightly better psychometric properties, although it too falls short of acceptable standards. Accordingly, diagnostic decisions using the FRT should be avoided unless supported by other measures with stronger psychometric properties.

The FRT appears to tap object recognition more so than spatial localization abilities. However, normal scores on this test may not reflect intact face recognition processes, because examinees may be able to score in the normal range without recognizing the facial configuration. That is, they may rely on feature-based procedures such as matching the eyebrows or hairlines, as opposed to configural processing (Duchaine & Weidenfeld, 2003). Therefore, impaired performance does indicate impaired face recognition and is informative, but examiners cannot rely on normal FRT performance to reflect intact face recognition processes. In a similar vein, models of face processing that are supported by dissociations involving normal performance on this task (i.e., normal unfamiliar face recognition and impaired familiar face recognition) must be questioned (Duchaine & Weidenfeld, 2003). Duchaine and Weidenfeld (2003) noted that reliance on a feature-based strategy requires more time. They suggested that it may be possible to test configural processing with the FRT by adding time norms or by limiting the amount of time allowed for each item.

REFERENCES

Andrikopoulos, J. (1997). Qualitative facial recognition test performance in Alzheimer's disease [Abstract]. *Archives of Clinical Neuropsychology, 12,* 282.

Ballantyne, A. O., & Trauner, D. A. (1999). Facial recognition in children after perinatal stroke. *Neuropsychiatry, Neuropsychology, and Behavioral Neurology, 12,* 82–87.

Beatty, W. W., Goodkin, D. E., & Weir, W. S. (1989). Affective judgements by patients with Parkinson's disease or chronic progressive multiple sclerosis. *Bulletin of the Psychonomic Society, 27,* 361–364.

Bentin, S., Silverberg, R., & Gordon, H. W. (1981). Asymmetrical cognitive deterioration in demented and Parkinsonian patients. *Cortex, 17,* 533–544.

Benton, A. L., Sivan, A. B., Hamsher, K. de S., Varney, N. R., & Spreen, O. (1994). *Contributions to neuropsychological assessment: A clinical manual* (2nd ed.). New York: Oxford University Press.

Benton, A.L., & Van Allen, M. W. (1968). Impairment in facial recognition in patients with cerebral disease. *Cortex, 4,* 344–358.

Borod, J. C., Martin, C. C., Alpert, M., & Brozgold, A. (1993). Perception of facial emotion in schizophrenic and right brain-damaged patients. *Journal of Nervous and Mental Disease, 181,* 494–502.

Botez-Marquand, T., & Botez, M. I. (1992). Visual memory deficits after damage to the anterior commissure and right fornix. *Archives of Neurology, 49,* 321–324.

Christensen, K. J., Riley, B. E., Hefferman, K. A., Love, S. B., & McLaughlin, M. E. (2002). Facial recognition test in the elderly: Norms, reliability and premorbid estimation. *Clinical Neuropsychologist, 16,* 51–56.

De Renzi, E., Faglioni, P., & Spinnler, H. (1968). The performance of patients with unilateral brain damage on facial recognition tasks. *Cortex, 4,* 17–34.

Diaz-Asper, C., Schretlen, D. J., & Pearlson, G. D. (2004). How well does IQ predict neuropsychological test performance in normal adults. *Journal of the International Neuropsychological Society, 10,* 82–90.

Dricker, J., Butters, N., Berman, G., Samuels, I., & Carey, S. (1978). The recognition and encoding of faces by alcoholic Korsakoff and right hemisphere patients. *Neuropsychologia, 16,* 683–695.

Duchaine, B. C., & Weidenfeld, A. (2003). An evaluation of two commonly used tests of unfamiliar face recognition. *Neuropsychologia, 41,* 713–720.

Echternacht, R. (1986). *The performance of pseudoneurological chronic psychiatric inpatients on the test of Facial Recognition. Judgment of Line Orientation, and Aphasia Screening Test.* Paper presented at the Seventh Annual Meeting of the Midwest Neuropsychology Group, Rochester, Minn.

Egelko, S., Gordon, W. A., Hibbard, M. R., Diller, L., Lieberman, A., Holliday, R., Ragnarsson, K., Shaver, M. S., & Orazem, J. (1988). Relationship among CT scans, neurologic exam, and neuropsychological test performance in right-brain-damaged stroke patients. *Journal of Clinical and Experimental Neuropsychology, 10,* 539–564.

Ferracuti, F., & Ferracuti, S. (1992). Taratura del campione Italiano. In *Test de Riconoscento di Volti Ignoti* (pp. 26–29). Florence: Organizzazione Speciali.

Hamsher, K. de S., Levin, H. S., & Benton, A. L. (1979). Facial recognition in patients with focal brain lesions. *Archives of Neurology, 36,* 837–839.

Hermann, B. P., Seidenberg, M., Wyler, A., & Haltiner, A. (1993). Dissociation of object recognition and spatial localization abilities following temporal lobe lesions in humans. *Neuropsychology, 7,* 343–350.

Hoptman, M. J., & Davidson, R. J. (1993). *Benton's Facial Recognition Task: A psychometric evaluation.* Paper presented at the meeting of the International Neuropsychological Society, Galveston, Tex.

Hovestadt, A., de Jong, G. J., & Meerwaldt, J. D. (1987). Spatial disorientation as an early symptom of Parkinson's disease. *Neurology, 37,* 485–487.

Karmiloff-Smith, A., Thomas, M., Annaz, D., Humphreys, K., Ewing, S., Brace, N., Duren, M., Pike, G., Grice, S., & Campbell, R. (2004). Exploring the Williams syndrome face-processing debate: The importance of building developmental trajectories. *Journal of Child Psychology and Psychiatry, 45,* 1258–1274.

Kempen, J. H., Kritchevsky, M., & Feldman, S. T. (1994). Effect of visual impairment on neuropsychological test performance. *Journal of Clinical and Experimental Neuropsychology, 16,* 223–231.

Korkman, M., Kirk, U., & Kemp, S. (1998). *NEPSY: A developmental neuropsychological assessment manual.* San Antonio, Tex.: The Psychological Corporation.

Kucharska-Pietura, K., David, A. S., Dropko, P., Klimkowski, M. (2002). The perception of emotional chimeric faces in schizophrenia: Further evidence of right hemisphere dysfunction. *Neuropsychiatry, Neuropsychology and Behavioral Neurology, 15,* 72–78.

Larrabee, G. J. (2000). Association between IQ and neuropsychological test performance: Commentary on Tremont, Hoffman, Scott, and Adams (1998). *The Clinical Neuropsychologist, 14,* 139–145.

Levin, B. E., Llabre, M. M., & Reisman, S. (1991). Visuospatial impairment in Parkinson's disease. *Neurology, 41,* 365–369.

Levin, H. S., & Benton, A. L. (1977). Facial recognition in "pseudoneurological" patients. *Journal of Nervous and Mental Disease, 164,* 135–138.

Levin, H. S., Grossman, R. G., & Kelly, J. (1977). Impairment in facial recognition after closed head injuries of varying severity. *Cortex, 13,* 119–130.

Levin, H. S., Hamsher, K. de S., & Benton, A. L. (1975). A short form of the test of facial recognition for clinical use. *Journal of Psychology, 91,* 223–228.

Matser, E. J. T., Kessels, A. G., Lezak, M. D., Jordan, B. D., & Troost, J. (1999). Neuropsychological impairment in amateur soccer players. *Journal of the American Medical Association, 282,* 971–973.

Mattson, A. J., Levin, H. S., & Grafman, J. (2000). A case of prosopagnosia following moderate closed head injury with left hemisphere focal lesion. *Cortex, 36,* 125–137.

Mishkin, M., Ungerleider, L. G., & Macko, K. A. (1983). Object vision and spatial vision: Two cortical pathways. *Trends in Neuroscience, 6,* 414–417.

Mittenberg, W., Seidenberg, M., O'Leary, D. S., & DiGiulio, D. V. (1989). Changes in cerebral functioning associated with normal aging. *Journal of Clinical and Experimental Neuropsychology, 11,* 918–932.

Mulder, J. L., Bouma, A., & Ansink, J. J. (1995). The role of visual discrimination disorders and neglect in perceptual categorization deficits in right and left hemisphere damaged patients. *Cortex, 31,* 487–501.

Paquier, P. F., van Mourik, M., Van Dongen, H. R., Gatsman-Berrevoets, C. E., Greten, V. L., & Stronks, D. L. (1999). Clinical utility of the Judgment of Line Orientation Test and Facial Recognition Test in children with acquired unilateral cerebral lesions. *Journal of Child Neurology, 14,* 243–248.

Peck, E. A., Mitchell, S. A., Burke, E. A., & Schwartz, S. M. (1992). *Post head injury normative data for selected Benton neuropsychological tests.* Paper presented at the meeting of the American Psychological Association, Washington, D. C.

Pueschel, J., & Zaidel, E. (1994). The Benton-Van Allen faces: A lateralized tachistoscopic study. *Neuropsychologia, 32,* 357–387.

Rey, G. J., Feldman, E., Rivas-Vazquez, R., Levin, B. E., & Benton, A. (1999). Neuropsychological test development and normative data on Hispanics. *Archives of Clinical Neuropsychology, 14,* 593–601.

Risser, A. H., & Andrikopoulos, J. (1997). *Facial Recognition Test performance in traumatic brain injury.* Paper presented at the meeting of the International Neuropsychological Society, Orlando, Fla.

Roberts, R. J., & Hamsher, K. (1984). Effects of minority status on facial recognition and naming performance. *Journal of Clinical Psychology, 40,* 539–545.

Schretlen, D. J., Pearlson, G. D., Anthony, J. C., & Yates, K. O. (2001). Determinants of Benton Facial Recognition Test performance in normal adults. *Neuropsychology, 15,* 405–410.

Schwartz, B. L., Parker, E. S., Deutsch, S. I., Rosse, R. B., Kaushik, M., & Isaac, A. (2002). Source monitoring in alcoholism. *Journal of Clinical and Experimental Neuropsychology, 24,* 806–817.

Strauss, E., & Verity, L. (1983). Effects of hemispherectomy in infantile hemiplegics. *Brain and Language, 20,* 1–11.

Trahan, D. E. (1997). Relationship between facial discrimination and visual neglect in patients with unilateral vascular lesions. *Archives of Clinical Neuropsychology, 12,* 57–62.

Tzavaras, A., Hecaen, H., & Le Bras, H. (1970). La probleme de la specifiteé du deficit de la reconnaisance du visage humain lors des lesions hemispherique unilaterales. *Neuropsychologia, 8,* 403–416.

Ungerleider, L. G., & Mishkin, M. (1982). Two cortical visual systems. In D. J. Ingle, M. A. Goodale, & R. J. W. Mansfield (Eds.), *Analysis of visual behaviour* (pp. 549–586). Cambridge, Mass.: MIT Press.

Warrington, E. K., & James, M. (1967). An experimental investigation of facial recognition in patients with unilateral cerebral lesions. *Cortex, 3,* 317–326.

Hooper Visual Organization Test (VOT)

PURPOSE

The Hooper Visual Organization Test (VOT) is a test of visual-spatial ability.

SOURCE

The Hooper VOT can be ordered from Western Psychological Services, 12031 Wilshire Blvd., Los Angeles, CA 90025 (http://www.wpspublish.com). The kit includes four reusable test picture booklets, a manual, 25 test booklets, 100 answer sheets, and a scoring key. It costs $188 US.

AGE RANGE

Norms are available for individuals aged 5 to 91 years.

DESCRIPTION

This test was originally designed to differentiate adults with and without brain damage (Hooper, 1958). It consists of 30 drawings of common objects on 4 × 4-inch cards in a ring binder (test booklet). Each object is cut into two or more parts and illogically arranged in the drawing (see Figure 12–12). The task is to name the object, either orally or in writing. The 1983 edition, developed by the staff of Western Psychological Services (no author credited), is based on Hooper's original studies but adds references to other studies, age- and education-corrected raw score tables, and a T-score conversion table.

The task can be time-consuming for some patients. Accordingly, Merten (2002, 2004a) presented a shortened 15-item version, based on an empirical and rational item analysis (Merten & Beal, 1999). Items with insufficient discriminant power, inappropriate cultural dependence, or questionable scoring rules and those otherwise maladaptive were eliminated. The short form was developed on a sample of 320 unselected neurological patients and a cross-validation sample of another 320 neurological patients. A practice item (horse) was also added, to assist understanding of the task demands.

Figure 12–12 This HVOT figure, properly integrated, depicts a "mouse" or "guinea pig." *Source:* Reprinted with permission of Western Psychological Services.

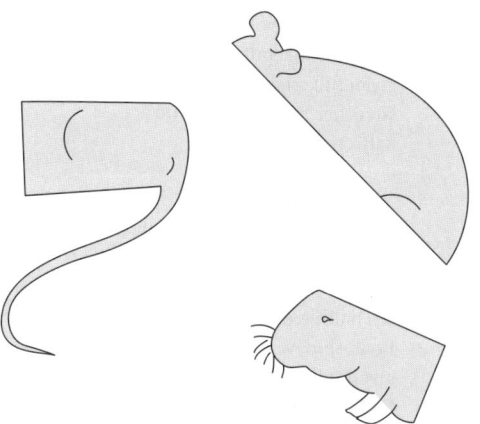

ADMINISTRATION

See *Source.* With individual administration, the correct naming of each object is required. Group administration relies on written responses.

Merten (2002) formulated clearer administration rules. He recommended that the examiner do the following:

1. Ask for specification if a category answer is given (e.g., if the examinee says "fruit" for number 3, say: "What fruit do you mean?"). Guessing is encouraged.
2. If necessary, remind patients of the task to be fulfilled.
3. If different answers are proposed, assist the testee to make a decision (e.g., if the examinee states, "This might be a rabbit or a horse," say: "Which one of the two do you think it is?").
4. Assist persons with anomic symptoms to name objects or animals if they seem to have recognized them.

ADMINISTRATION TIME

The time required is about 10 to 15 min; less than 10 min is required for the short form.

SCORING

Standard Version

The score is simply the total number of correct responses, although half-credit is given for some of the items for partially correct responses (e.g., "tower" or "castle" instead of light-house). At the examiner's discretion, other answers may be given full credit, but only if they are actual synonyms or closely resemble the correct answers.

Raw scores can be adjusted for age and education and raw or corrected scores can be transformed to a T score by means of tables provided in the test manual. Higher T scores imply lower raw scores. Qualitative scoring includes the distinction between isolate, perseverative, bizarre, and neologistic responses.

15-Item Short Form

Scoring rules for the short form are shown in Table 12–15 (Merten, 2002).

Merten (2002) proposed additional scoring rules for both the long and short forms. He recommended that the examiner do the following:

1. Allow subspecification (e.g., "Cheshire cat" for cat).
2. Allow colloquial, regional, or infantile expressions.
3. Not penalize answers such as "an apple, cut into slices."

Age

Performance follows a U-shaped function, with scores improving during childhood and declining with advancing age (e.g., Source; Kirk, 1992; Libon et al., 1994; Mason & Ganzler, 1964; Merten, 2002; Nabors et al., 1997; Seidel, 1994; Walsh et al., 1997). For example, Merten (2002) reported a correlation of − .50 in adults ranging in age from 15 to 87 years who were seen for neuropsychological examination.

Gender

There is no systematic relationship to gender (see *Source;* Merten & Beal, 1999; Nabors et al., 1997; Seidel, 1994), although Kirk (1992) found that boys performed better than girls.

Education/IQ

Examinees with more formal education obtain higher raw scores (see *Source;* Merten & Beal, 2000; Merton, 2002; Nabors et al., 1997; Richardson & Marottoli, 1996; Walsh et al., 1997). However, correlations with age tend to be larger than those for education (e.g., $r = .21$, Merten & Beal, 1999), and most of the shared variance with education is attributable to general intelligence (Mason & Ganzler, 1964; also see *Source).* The test manual recommends that the task not be used with individuals with IQs lower than about 75.

Ethnicity

There is little evidence of ethnic bias in U.S. samples (see *Source;* Lewis et al., 1997; Nabors et al., 1997), although the test manual does suggest that the examiner should be sensitive to cultural and regional variations in language.

NORMATIVE DATA

Standardization Sample

The norms published with the test manual rely on data collected about 40 years ago by Mason and Ganzler (1964) (see

Table 12–15 Modified Scoring Rules for the Hooper Short Form Items

No.	Content	Original Item No.	Modified or Specified Scoring Rules
1	Table/bench	3	
2	Teakettle	16	Teapot, coffeepot, and so on are given full credit
3	Apple	11	No other fruits allowed; no half-credits
4	Airplane	4	
5	Scissors	13	
6	Chair/sofa	17	Sofa, settee, couch, and so on are given full credit
7	Book	23	
8	Cat	20	No half-credits
9	Sailboat	15	Boat, ship, vessel, and so on are given full credit
10	Mouse/rat	22	Full credit is given for naming other rodents, such as rat or guinea pig; no half-credits
11	Cane/walking stick	14	Hockey stick is not accepted as correct
12	Rabbit/hare	24	No half-credits
13	Block	25	
14	Key	28	
15	Ring	29	

Source: Adapted from Merten, 2000.

Table 12–16) and are based on a sample of 231 males (mostly patients with pulmonary disease or general surgery patients) at a Veterans Administration hospital. Participants were screened to exclude those with a history of psychiatric or neurological disorders, alcoholism, or other factors that might suggest mental disorder. The sample spanned the adult age span (10% < 30 years, 6% > 70 years). The population was exclusively or primarily Caucasian (Lewis et al., 1997). Most of the testing was completed in small groups, but some was done individually, sometimes without supervision (see Mason & Ganzler, 1964; also see *Source*). There was no time limit. Note that the normative scores tend to be quite skewed, meaning that the VOT is not very sensitive to impairment at the upper score range.

Other Normative Data—Adults

In addition to using the T-score table, a number of different cutoff points have been proposed for the long form (see *Source*). Based on the high correlation ($r = .95$) between short and long forms in a large sample of neurological patients ($N = 640$), Merten (2002) used linear regression analysis to develop cutoffs for the short form. The cutoff values for the long and short forms are shown in Table 12–17.

Users should bear in mind, however, that no single cutoff point is appropriate for all individuals in all settings. For example, Nabors et al. (1997) reported that a lower cutoff value (15) may be needed when working with an elderly medical

Table 12–16 Characteristics of the Adult Normative Sample for the VOT

Number	231
Age (years)	
<30	22
30–39	59
40–49	59
50–59	38
60–69	40
70–75	13
Geographic Location	Long Beach, California
Sample type	Largely patients at a Veterans Administration hospital with pulmonary disease or requiring surgery for disorders such as fracture, infection, or hernia; also, a few (<15) nonprofessional hospital personnel and volunteer hospital workers were tested
Education	NA
Gender (%)	
Men	100
Women	0
Race/Ethnicity	Exlusively or predominantly Caucasian
Screening	Screened to exclude those with history of psychiatric or neurological disorder or alcoholism

Table 12–17 Selected Cutoff Values for the Long and Short Forms of the Hooper Test

Source	Description	Long Form	Short Form
Test manual (1983), Merten (2002)	Suggestion of further assessment	<24	<13
Test manual (1983), Merten (2002)	Probable visual-spatial deficits, minimizing false positives	<21	<11
Merten (2002)	Probable visual-spatial deficits in geriatric patients		<8

population in an urban setting, to avoid false-positive results. Similarly, Richardson and Marattoli (1996) evaluated elderly individuals and noted that the ability to adjust for education is particularly important when testing older adults, because their median educational attainment is less than 12 years. Failure to do so will result in false-positive findings, particularly for examinees who are poorly educated. They recruited 101 independently living, active drivers, aged 76 to 91 years, with educational levels ranging from grade 4 to college. Data were excluded for participants who reported a history of neurological disease or excessive use of alcohol or scored below education-adjusted cutoffs for dementia on the MMSE. The sample included slightly more males than females (47.5%) and was predominantly Caucasian. Data are presented in Table 12–18 for two age groups (76–80 and 81–91 years), each of which is broken down into two education groups (<12 years and ≥12 years of formal education). The older, more educated participants appeared to perform more poorly than the younger, similarly educated individuals. No obvious age effect was observed between the two less educated groups.

Other Normative Data—Children

Seidel (1994) provided norms for a sample of 211 children between the ages of 5 and 11 years (VIQ *M* = about 99.4, *SD* = 13.0). They were English-speaking, lived in an Eastern Canadian city, and were randomly selected from a pool of volunteers obtained from four public elementary schools chosen to represent a wide range of socioeconomic status. Attempts were made to equate the number of subjects by gender and age. Children with VIQs lower than 70 were excluded from

analysis. All participants were tested individually. The normative data are shown in Table 12–19.

Kirk (1992) also presented normative data for 434 English-speaking children, ages 5 to 13 years, who were attending private and parochial schools in the New York metropolitan area. None of the subjects was identified as learning disabled or language impaired. The values for 5- to 11-year-olds are similar to those provided by Seidel (1994). In Kirk's study, 13-year-old boys approached adult levels of performance, whereas scores for girls were significantly lower. The data for 12- and 13-year-old children are also shown in Table 12–18.

RELIABILITY

Internal Consistency

This is reported to be high ($r \geq .80$) in adults (see *Source*; Lopez et al., 2003; Merten & Beal, 1999) and adequate in children ($r = .72$; Seidel, 1994). The Merten 15-item short form was given in its own right to a sample of neurological patients. Estimates of internal consistency yielded coefficients of .84 (Cronbach's alpha) and .85 (split-half; Merten, 2004a).

The item order of the standard form appears to have been established a priori, without empirical testing. Several authors have found the item ranking to deviate from the order of difficulty (e.g., Kirk, 1992; Merten & Beal, 1999). In addition, some items do not possess sufficient discriminatory power. For example, Lopez et al. (2003) reported that items 1, 2, 15, and 27 provided poor discrimination between cognitively intact and cognitively impaired individuals.

Table 12–18 Means and *SD* for VOT in Older Adults, by Education

Age 76–80 Years		Age 81–91 Years	
<12 Years (*n* = 26)	≥12 Years (*n* = 24)	<12 Years (*n* = 18)	≥12 Years (*n* = 33)
17.90 (4.01)	21.69 (4.09)	17.62 (6.17)	19.71 (2.97)

Source: Adapted from Richardson & Marattoli, 1996.

Table 12–19 Normative Data for Children on the VOT

Age	n	Mean Correct (SD)
5	21	18.4 (3.1)
6	34	19.4 (3.8)
7	32	21.1 (3.1)
8	28	23.4 (2.0)
9	28	23.7 (2.9)
10	34	24.0 (2.5)
11	30	24.1 (2.9)
12 (boys)	21	25.74 (2.56)
12 (girls)	22	23.80 (2.54)
13 (boys)	18	25.94 (3.51)
13 (girls)	9	23.11 (3.30)

Source: Ages 5–11 years, from Seidel, 1994; ages 12–13 years, from Kirk, 1992.

Test-Retest Reliability

Lezak (1982; Lezak et al., 2004) reported a coefficient of concordance of .86, indicating good test-retest reliability after 6 months and again after 12 months (sample composition not reported). Similarly, reliability at 8 months in 51 adults with intractable epilepsy was .75 (Sawrie et al., 1996). However, 1-year retest reliability in healthy elderly subjects was only .68 using a shortened 10-item version (Levin et al., 1991).

Merten (2004a) used his 15-item short form and retested a sample of neurological patients after an interval of 203 days. The test-retest correlation was .93, and the mean increase was 0.6 points. Seven-day retest reliability for a subgroup of 36 patients was .93, with a mean increase of 1.1 points (Merten, 2004b).

Interrater Reliability

The scoring instructions allow the examiner to give credit (1 or 1½ points) for answers that are synonyms or closely resemble the correct answers. Nonetheless, interrater reliabilities are high (>.95) for three and two raters (Lopez et al., 2003).

VALIDITY

Relationships With Other Measures

Successful performance appears to depend primarily on visual-spatial abilities of the sort measured by the Wechsler test, and less so on the capacity to label objects. For example, a study by Paolo et al. (1996) found that performance subtests of the Wechsler test accounted for 44% of the variance, whereas the Boston Naming Test (BNT) accounted for only 5% of the VOT variance. Similarly, Ricker and Axelrod (1995) reported that object naming accounted for 11% of the variance in VOT performance, and WAIS-R perceptual organization accounted for 48%. Johnstone and Wilhelm (1997) conducted a principal component factor analysis of the VOT,

WAIS-R and other tasks (e.g., Rey-Osterrieth, BNT, COWA, WMS-R VR) in a heterogeneous sample of patients (15 to 69 years old) who were referred for neuropsychological evaluation. They found that the VOT loaded primarily on a global visual-spatial intelligence factor and had its highest correlates with PIQ subtests.

Hermann et al. (1993) gave the VOT along with a battery of other tests to patients with temporal lobe epilepsy preoperatively. The VOT loaded equally on two visual factors, one defined by the WAIS-R Performance subtests and the other by the Facial Recognition Test. Merten (2005) conducted a principal axis factor analysis of the VOT with 20 other tests based on 200 neurological patients in Berlin; he found that the VOT loaded primarily on a global nonverbal performance factor, together with the WAIS Block Design, Trails A and B, Ravens Progressive Matrices, the Line Orientation Test, and VOSP Silhouettes, among others. Similarly, Paul et al. (2001) reported that in patients with vascular dementia, more than 60% of the variance in VOT performance was accounted for by WAIS-R Block Design; performance on the BNT did not make a significant contribution.

Similar findings have been reported for children. In a clinical sample of children referred for neuropsychological examination, Seidel (1994) found the VOT to measure skills significantly related to the WISC-R Perceptual Organization factor but not to verbal processing (Verbal Comprehension) or attention (Freedom from Distractibility). The highest correlation was with Block Design ($r = .63$). Further, factor analytic findings suggested that the test loaded primarily on a visuospatial/visuomotor dimension.

Although perceptual organization skill is critical for success, object naming does play a role. Ricker and Axelrod (1995) gave the VOT along with a naming test consisting of the VOT figures to a group of 50 patients seen for neuropsychological evaluation. The ability to name the stimuli was unrelated to the ability to synthesize the fragmented parts. However, the extent of any language disorder in these patients was not described. To further explore the relationship between naming ability and VOT performance, Schultheis et al. (2000) examined 14 stroke or TBI patients (mean age, 35 years) with anomia, defined as scoring in the lower 10% of norms for the BNT. The standard VOT and a multiple-choice version of the VOT that required the patient to choose one of four words printed below each picture were administered. The patients obtained a significantly greater number of correct responses for the multiple-choice version compared with the standard VOT. This improvement applied equally to those with right- and those with left-hemisphere lesions, although the former group had a greater error score overall. The authors concluded that naming ability does play a role in VOT performance.

Clinical Studies

Impairment has been reported in a number of conditions, including autism (Jollife & Baron-Cohen, 2001), dementia

(Nabors et al., 1997; Paul et al., 2001; Walsh et al., 1997; Zec et al., 1992) and Parkinson's disease (Gollaher, 1996; Levin et al., 1991).

The validity of this test for "general screening for brain damage" has been hotly debated (Boyd, 1982a, 1982b; Rathbun & Smith, 1982; Woodward, 1982). For example, correct classification rates of 74% between unselected brain-damaged subjects and healthy controls with a cutoff score of 25 have been reported (Boyd, 1981). However, Wetzel and Murphy (1991) found that many brain-injured persons perform well on the VOT, raising the concern of a high rate of false-negative results. Such a screening function has become increasingly obsolete with the advent of other neuroimaging and neuropsychological tools. In a recent study of 305 neurological patients, Merten and Beal (1999) found that, although the contingency between the VOT and the MMSE and another German screening test was significant (contingency coefficient C = .40, Kendall's tau = .39, $p < .001$), discrepancies on the level of individual classification were considerable.

Given the high visual-spatial demands of the task, one might expect right posterior involvement. Although some authors (Boyd, 1981; Schultheis et al., 2000; Wang, 1977; Wetzel & Murphy, 1991; York & Cermak, 1995) have been unable to demonstrate performance differences between patients with left or right hemisphere damage, trends have often been evident (Fitz et al., 1992; Schultheis et al., 2000; York & Cermak, 1995) and suggest impairment in the context of right hemisphere disturbance. In a comparison of 44 geriatric patients with right-hemisphere CVA and 23 with left-hemisphere CVA, Nadler et al. (1996) found significantly poorer VOT performance in the former group. Also, in scoring this test for qualitative error types, right CVA patients made more partial and unformed/unassociated errors, whereas left-hemisphere CVA patients made more language-based errors. Lewis et al. (1997) examined 153 patients with focal lesions and 75 controls. Dividing locus of lesion into quadrants, they found that VOT performance of patients with right anterior lesions was significantly poorer than that of patients with lesions in the other three quadrants or controls. These findings, therefore, challenge suggestions of predominant right posterior involvement.

Farver and Farver (1982) and Tamkin and Hyer (1984) interpreted age-related decline on this test in normal subjects, aged 40 to 88 years, together with six other parietal lobe tests of the BDAE, as evidence of cognitive dysfunction related to right parietal lobe/right hemisphere functional decline with age. However, Libon et al. (1994) compared the performance of young-old (64–74 years) and old-old (75–94 years) normal, healthy subjects and found age-related decline on the test, which was strongly related to decline on other tests of executive function (e.g., semantic and phonemic controlled word association, Stroop). The authors concluded that age-related decline on the VOT is more likely associated with decline of frontal lobe rather than right-hemisphere functions.

A recent study (Moritz et al., 2004) adapted the task to functional magnetic resonance imaging (fMRI) analysis and suggested an extensive bilateral response across all brain lobes, predominantly in the posterior brain, in regions of superior parietal lobules, ventral temporooccipital cortex, posterior visual association areas, and, to a lesser extent, the frontal eye fields bilaterally and left dorsolateral prefrontal cortex. Presumably these clusters reflect brain regions subserving visual-spatial processes, object identification, and covert naming.

Psychiatric Disorders

Gerson (1974) concluded that the test is "not sensitive to . . . thought disorders" (p. 98) and that neologisms and bizarre responses did not occur in this population at all. However, others have reported that scores are lower in psychiatric inpatients (e.g., Tamkin & Jacobsen, 1984) and patients with schizophrenia. Lee and Cheung (2005) reported poor performance on the VOT in patients with schizophrenia, perhaps reflecting difficulties with attention. Zakzanis et al. (2001) noted that the VOT contributed significantly to the differentiation between patients with late-onset schizophrenia and those with frontotemporal dementia. Performance was more impaired in those with schizophrenia.

Ecological Validity

Whether the VOT predicts functional ability is uncertain. Richardson et al. (1995) found that it was the best of five neuropsychological tests in the prediction of performance-based ratings of activities of daily living in a geriatric population. In contrast, Greve et al. (2000) found that, in CVA patients, the relationship between VOT scores and functional independence measures (FIM) was not significant. Performance on the VOT appears somewhat related to driving performance in the elderly; however, other tasks (e.g., reaction time, useful field of view) are stronger predictors (Myers et al., 2000).

Short Form

Merten (2002) reported that the short form correlates highly with WAIS Block Design ($r = .71$), as does the long form ($r = .75$). Correlations with other screening instruments (e.g., MMSE, Raven's) were similar and high for both forms. Further, patients with lateralized right hemisphere damage scored significantly lower on this version than did those with left hemisphere damage (Merten, 2004b).

COMMENT

This test is still relatively popular with clinicians, more than 50 years since its original publication. It is brief and easy to administer. It can be given individually or in a group setting. In addition, it can be used with a variety of populations, adult or child, and may be particularly useful in those compromised by limited motor ability other than speech.

Although reliability appears satisfactory, other psychometric properties are not. In fact, Boyd (1981) stated that the test has never been properly validated. Users should note that normative information for adults is dated, deriving from a sample of individuals, most with medical disorders, by poorly standardized procedures. The task requires clearer administration rules to advise the examiner how to assist people with anomic disorders, when and how to demand response specification, how to treat multiple responses, and so on (Merten, 2002). Scoring rules also appear to be arbitrary and need to be revised (Merten, 2002; Seidel, 1994). Contemporary normative data, stratified by age and IQ, also need to be provided.

Wetzel and Murphy (1991) found that discontinuing the test after five consecutive failures did not significantly change the scoring of this test. However, Merten and Beal (1999) cautioned against such a procedure, because item ranking in the current form does not adequately reflect the order of item difficulty.

The VOT is not an adequate screening device of cognitive deficits, because of its high rate of false-negative classifications (Merten & Beal, 1999). Although it may serve as a screen for visual-perceptual dysfunction, its ability to contribute additional information to the diagnostic process beyond that provided by other visual-spatial tasks (e.g., Wechsler Performance subtests) is uncertain. In fact, Johnstone and Wilhelm (1997) considered the VOT to be another measure of visual-spatial intelligence, not distinct from abilities tapped by Wechsler Performance subtests. Further, the VOT lacks the capacity to provide differential diagnosis with respect to the location of functional deficits. Examination of error types, however, may prove useful in revealing the source and nature of the disturbance (Nadler et al., 1996).

Users should also note that, although the test mainly measures visual-spatial/perceptual ability, the task does require naming. Accordingly, results in even mildly aphasic patients may be questionable. Merten (Merten, 2002; Merten & Beal, 1999) recommended that anomic patients should be assisted to maximize their VOT scores as a measure of their visual-perceptual abilities.

The validity of the test requires additional study. Whether the task predicts functional outcome above and beyond that provided by other standard tests (e.g., Wechsler Performance subtests) also remains to be determined (Johnstone & Wilhelm, 1997).

Merten (2002) developed a short version and clarified instructions and scoring in an attempt to improve the internal consistency of the test. His 15-item version shows validity and reliability similar to the full-length version in neurological patients and may be a suitable substitute for the full VOT.

REFERENCES

Boyd, J. L. (1981). A validity study of the Hooper Visual Organization Test. *Journal of Consulting and Clinical Psychology, 49,* 15–19.

Boyd, J. L. (1982a). Reply to Rathbun and Smith: Who made the Hooper blooper? *Journal of Consulting and Clinical Psychology, 50,* 284–285.

Boyd, J. L. (1982b). Reply to Woodward. *Journal of Consulting and Clinical Psychology, 50,* 289–290.

Farver, P. F., & Farver, T. B. (1982). Performance of normal older adults on tests designed to measure parietal lobe functions. *American Journal of Occupational Therapy, 36,* 444–449.

Fitz, A. G., Conrad, P. M., Hom, D. L., & Sarff, P. L. (1992). Hooper Visual Organization Test performance in lateralized brain injury. *Archives of Clinical Neuropsychology, 7,* 243–250.

Gerson, A. (1974). Validity and reliability of the Hooper Visual Organization Test. *Perceptual and Motor Skills, 39,* 95–100.

Gollaher, K. K. (1996). Visuospatial and visuo-constructional functioning in Parkinson's disease. *Dissertation Abstracts International, 56*(11-B), 6427.

Greve, K. W., Lindberg, R. F., Bianchini, K. J., & Adams, D. (2000). Construct validity and predictive value of the Hooper Visual Organization Test in stroke rehabilitation. *Applied Neuropsychology, 7,* 515–522.

Hermann, B. P., Seidenberg, M., Wyler, A., & Haltiner, A. (1993). Dissociation of object recognition and spatial localization abilities following temporal lobe lesions in humans. *Neuropsychology, 7,* 343–350.

Hooper, H. E. (1958). *The Hooper Visual Organization Test: Manual.* Beverly Hills, Calif.: Western Psychological Services.

Johnstone, B., & Wilhelm, K. L. (1997). The construct validity of the Hooper Visual Organization Test. *Assessment, 4,* 243–248.

Joliffe, T., & Baron-Cohen, R. (2001). A test of central coherence theory: Can adults with high-functioning autism or Asperger syndrome integrate fragments of an object? *Cognitive Neuropsychiatry, 6,* 193–216.

Kirk, U. (1992). Evidence for early acquisition of visual organization ability: A developmental study. *The Clinical Neuropsychologist, 6,* 171–177.

Lee, T. M. C., & Cheung, P. P. Y. (2005). The relationship between visual-perception and attention in Chinese with schizophrenia. *Schizophrenia Research, 72,* 185–193.

Levin, B. E., Llabre, M. M., & Reisman, S. (1991). Visuospatial impairment in Parkinson's disease. *Neurology, 41,* 365–369.

Lewis, S., Campbell, A., & Takushi-Chinen, R., Brown, A., Dennis, G., Wood, D., & Weir, R. (1997). Visual Organization Test performance in an African-American population with acute unilateral cerebral lesions. *International Journal of Neuroscience, 91,* 295–302.

Lezak, M. D. (1982). *The test-retest stability and reliability of some tests commonly used in neuropsychological assessment.* Paper presented at the meeting of the International Neuropsychological Society, Deauville, France.

Lezak, M. D., Howieson, D. B., & Loring, D. W. (2004). *Neuropsychological assessment* (4th ed.). New York: Oxford University Press.

Libon, D. J., Glosser, G., Malamut, B. L., Kaplan, E., Goldberg, E., Swenson, R., & Sands, L. P. (1994). Age, executive functions, and visuospatial functioning in healthy older adults. *Neuropsychology, 8,* 38–43.

Lopez, M. N., Lazar, M. D., & Oh, S. (2003). Psychometric properties of the Hooper Visual Organization Test. *Assessment, 10,* 66–70.

Mason, C. F., & Ganzler, H. (1964). Adult norms for the Shipley Institute of Living Scale and Hooper Visual Organization test based on age and education. *Journal of Gerontology, 19,* 419–424.

Merten, T. (2002). A short version of the Hooper Visual Organization Test: Development and validation. *The Clinical Neuropsychologist, 16,* 136–144.

Merten, T. (2004a). A short version of the Hooper Visual Organization Test: Reliability and validity. *Applied Neuropsychology, 11*, 99–102.

Merten, T. (2004b). Eine kurzform des Hooper Visual Organization Test. *Zeitschrift fur Neuropsychologie, 15.*

Merten, T. (2005). Factor structure of the Hooper Visual Organization Test: A cross-cultural replication and extension. *Archives of Clinical Neuropsychology, 20*, 123–128.

Merten, T., & Beal, C. (1999). An analysis of the Hooper Visual Organization Test with neurological patients. *The Clinical Neuropsychologist, 13*, 521–529.

Moritz, C. H., Johnson, S. C., McMillan, K. M., Haughton, V. M., & Meyerand, M. E. (2004). Functional MRI neuroanatomic correlates of the Hooper Visual Organization Test. *Journal of the International Neuropsychological Society, 10*, 939–947.

Myers, R. S., Ball, K. K., Kalina, T. D., Roth, D. L., & Goode, K. T. (2000). Relation of useful field of view and other screening tests to on-road driving performance. *Perceptual and Motor Skills, 91*, 279–290.

Nabors, N. A., Vangel, S. J., Lichtenberg, P. A., & Walsh, P. (1997). Normative and clinical utility of the Hooper Visual Organization Test with geriatric medical inpatients. *Journal of Clinical Geropsychology, 3*, 191–198.

Nadler, J. D., Grace, J., White, D. A., Butters, M. A., & Malloy, P. F. (1996). Laterality differences in quantitative and qualitative Hooper performance. *Archives of Clinical Neuropsychology, 11*, 223–229.

Paolo, A. M., Cluff, R. B., & Ryan, J. J. (1996). Influence of perceptual organization and naming abilities on the Hooper Visual Organization Test. *Neuropsychiatry, Neuropsychology, and Behavioral Neurology, 9*, 254–257.

Paul, R., Cohen, R., Moser, D., Ott, B., Zawacki, T., & Gordon, N. (2001). Performance on the Hooper Visual Organization Test in patients diagnosed with subcortical vascular dementia: Relation to naming performance. *Neuropsychiatry, Neuropsychology and Behavioral Neurology, 14*, 93–97.

Rathbun, J., & Smith, A. (1982). Comment on the validity of Boyd's validation study of the Hooper Visual Organization Test. *Journal of Consulting and Clinical Psychology, 50*, 281–283.

Richardson, E. D., & Marottoli, R. A. (1996). Education-specific normative data on common neuropsychological indices for individuals older than 75 years. *The Clinical Neuropsychologist, 10*, 375–381.

Richardson, E. D., Nadler, J. D., & Malloy, P. F. (1995). Neuropsychologic prediction of performance measures of daily living skills in geriatric patients. *Neuropsychology, 9*, 565–572.

Ricker, J. H., & Axelrod, B. N. (1995). Hooper Visual Organization Test: Effects of object naming ability. *Clinical Neuropsychologist, 9*, 57–62.

Sawrie, S. M., Chelune, G. J., Naugle, R. I., & Luders, H. O. (1996). Empirical methods for assessing meaningful neuropsychological changes following epilepsy surgery. *Journal of the International Neuropsychological Society, 2*, 556–564.

Schultheis, M. T., Caplan, B., Ricker, J. H., & Woessner, R. (2000). Fractioning the Hooper: A multiple-choice response format. *The Clinical Neuropsychologist, 14*, 196–201.

Seidel, W. T. (1994). Applicability of the Hooper Visual Organization Test to pediatric populations: Preliminary findings. *Clinical Neuropsychologist, 8*, 59–68.

Tamkin, A. S., & Hyer, L. A. (1984). Testing for cognitive dysfunction in the aging population. *Military Medicine, 149*, 397–399.

Tamkin, A. S., & Jacobsen, R. (1984). Age-related norms for the Hooper Visual Organization Test. *Journal of Clinical Psychology, 40*, 1459–1463.

Walsh, P. F., Lichtenberg, P. A., & Rowe, R. J. (1997). Hooper Visual Organization Test performance in geriatric rehabilitation patients. *Clinical Gerontologist, 17*, 3–11.

Wang, P. L. (1977). Visual organization ability in brain-damaged adults. *Perceptual and Motor Skills, 45*, 723–728.

Wetzel, L., & Murphy, S. G. (1991). Validity of the use of a discontinuation rule and evaluation of discriminability of the Hooper Visual Organization Test. *Neuropsychology, 5*, 119–122.

Woodward, C. A. (1982). The Hooper Visual Organization Test: A case against its use in neuropsychological assessment. *Journal of Consulting and Clinical Psychology, 50*, 286–288.

York, C. D., & Cermak, S. A. (1995). Visual perception and praxis in adults after stroke. *American Journal of Occupational Therapy, 49*, 543–550.

Zakzanis, K. K., Kielar, A., Young, D., & Boulos, M. (2001). Neuropsychological differentiation of late onset schizophrenia and frontotemporal dementia. *Cognitive Neuropsychiatry, 6*, 63–77.

Zec, R. F., Vicari, S., Kocis, M., & Reynolds, T. (1992). Sensitivity of different neuropsychological tests to very mild DAT [Abstract]. *Clinical Neuropsychologist, 6*, 327.

Judgment of Line Orientation (JLO)

PURPOSE

The Judgment of Line Orientation (JLO) test measures spatial perception and orientation.

SOURCE

The test is available from Psychological Assessment Resources (http://www.parinc.com), at a price of $111 US. A set of 100 additional record forms cost $35 US. The manual (together with that for 11 other tests from the Benton Laboratory; Benton et al., 1994) is available from the same source for $39 US.

AGE RANGE

Norms are available for ages 7 to 96 years.

DESCRIPTION

A large number of tests have been devised to assess various aspects of spatial ability. The impetus for the development of the JLO task as a clinical instrument came in part from findings of a left visual field/right hemisphere (RH) superiority among right-handed university students in identifying the direction of lines presented tachistoscopically to the left and right visual fields (see Benton et al., 1994, for a history of the

Figure 12–13 Example of JLO item. *Source:* Reproduced by special permission of Psychological Assessment Resources, Inc.

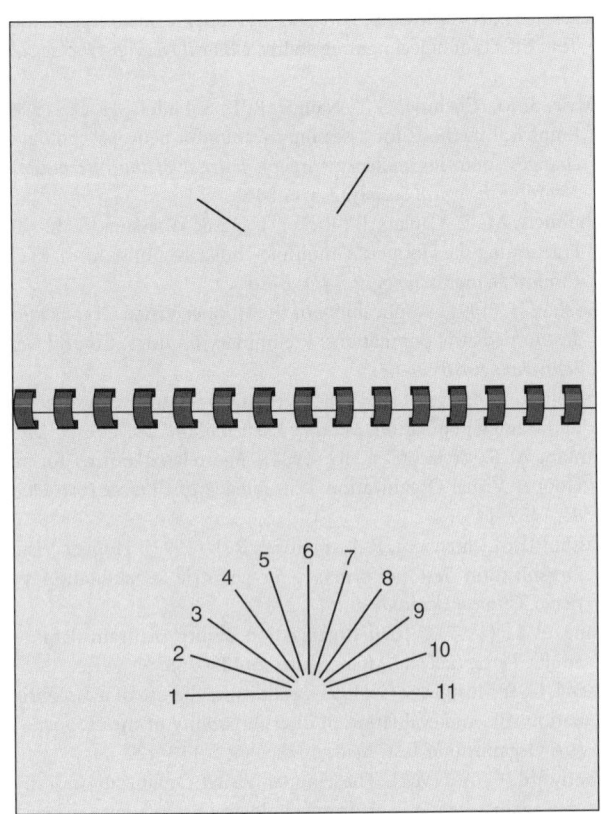

task). In addition, patients with RH pathology performed defectively on such tasks (Benton et al., 1994).

There are two forms of the task, Form H and Form V, each consisting of the same 30 items, presented in a somewhat different order. In each form, items are presented in a generally ascending order of difficulty (but see Qualls et al., 2000). The test materials for each form are spiral-bound in a single booklet and consist of 35 stimuli appearing in the upper part of the booklet and a multiple-choice card (the same for all stimuli) appearing in the lower part (see Figure 12–13). The first five items are practice items. The multiple-choice response card consists of an array of lines, labeled "1" through "11" and drawn at 18-degree intervals from the point of origin. The respondent is required to identify which two lines, from the multiple-choice array, match the directions of the lines on the stimulus card. The lines on the stimulus card are shorter than the ones on the response card.

Short Forms

A number of short forms have been presented: Odd (Form O) and Even (E) 15-item short forms (Vanderploeg et al., 1997; Woodard et al., 1996, 1998) have been proposed for Form V. Another pair of 15-item, internally consistent short forms (Forms Q and S) were developed by Qualls et al. (2000); they used an item analysis to ensure equivalence of the two forms.

Winegarden et al. (1998) described a 20-item short form consisting of items 11 through 30 from Form V.

ADMINISTRATION

See test manual. Briefly, the test booklet and the multiple-choice card are placed flat on the table in front of the patient and at a 45-degree angle to the multiple-choice array, in such a way that both are in an area of preserved vision. The patient is instructed to look at the two lines of the stimulus card and to find "which of the lines below are in exactly the same position and point in the same direction." "Tell me the number of the lines." If the patient has difficulty comprehending the instructions, the examiner may proceed by asking the patient to show the corresponding direction for just one line. Instructions and practice items may be repeated until the patient gives two correct responses for the practice items. If this criterion is not met, the test is discontinued. There is no time limit for responding.

ADMINISTRATION TIME

About 15 to 20 min is required.

SCORING

For the standard 30-item form, the score is the total number of correct responses. If the norms in the test manual are used, corrections for age and sex consist of adding 1 point to the obtained scores of subjects in the 50- to 64-year-old age bracket, 3 points to the obtained scores of subjects in the 65- to 74-year-old age bracket, and an additional 2 points to the obtained scores of women in all age brackets.

For the 15-item O and E short forms, the score is the total number correct. One point should be added to scores of females before the score is looked up in the table for the short form (Woodard et al., 1998).

Ska et al. (1990) introduced a qualitative scoring system that distinguishes four main error types: (a) misplacement of lines within the same quadrant (e.g., line confused with another from the same quadrant); (b) misperception of vertical and/or horizontal lines (e.g., incorrect identification of lines 1, 11, and 6); (c) displacement of a line from one quadrant to the other; and (d) displacement of a line to the opposite quadrant in combination with vertical or horizontal errors.

DEMOGRAPHIC EFFECTS

Age

Age shows a curvilinear relationship with test scores (Benton et al., 1994). Scores increase during childhood, reaching adult levels by about age 13 years in both girls and boys. In adults, beginning at about 50 years of age, scores decline slightly with advancing age on the long form (Benton et al., 1994; Ivnik et al., 1996; Monste et al., 2001) and on the 15-item short form (Woodard et al., 1996).

Gender

Male subjects tend to score about 2 points higher than females on the long form (Basso & Lowery, 2004; Basso et al., 2000; Benton et al., 1994; Ferracuti & Ferracuti, 1992; Glamser & Turner, 1995; Riva & Benton, 1993) and on the 15-item short form (Vanderploeg et al., 1997; Woodard et al., 1996). Sexual orientation has a strong effect on performance (Rahman and Wilson, 2003; Rahman et al., 2004). Although men perform better overall, there are large, significant differences between heterosexual and homosexual men, in favor of the heterosexual group; the scores of heterosexual and homosexual women do not differ (Rahman & Wilson, 2003).

Education

Benton et al. (1994) noted a trend for less well-educated individuals to score lower than the better-educated on the long form. Others (Ivnik et al., 1996; Lucas et al., 2005) have also observed a modest impact of education on test scores in older adults ($r = .21$ to .33). Higher scores are also associated with increasing levels of education on the 15-item short form (Woodard et al., 1996).

IQ

In adults, IQ has a moderate/large effect on performance (Rahman et al., 2004; Steinberg et al., 2005; Trahan, 1998; Woodard et al., 1996). In fact, education becomes redundant when IQ is taken into account (Steinberg et al., 2005). IQ and JLO test scores are less strongly associated at the higher ends of the IQ continuum (Steinberg et al., 2005). Benton et al. (1994) reported that that VIQ has little impact on JLO scores in children.

Culture/Ethnicity

Benton et al. (1994) concluded that Italian and North American children performed at the same level. Within-group variability was also equal. Trahan (1998) observed no score differences between Caucasian and African American adult stroke patients, although the sample was very small. Lucas et al. (2005), however, noted relatively poor performance in older African Americans. Rey et al. (1999) reported median scores and cutoff points for defective performance between Hispanic and English-speaking samples in the United States. The distribution for Hispanic participants (median JLO score = 24, cutoff = 17) was comparable to that reported by Benton et al. (1983) for English-speaking individuals (median JLO score = 25, cutoff = 15).

NORMATIVE DATA

Standardization Samples

The characteristics of the adult sample are shown in Table 12–20. Benton et al. (1994) noted that the test has a relatively

Table 12–20 JLO: Characteristics of the Adult Normative Sample

Number	137
Age (years)	
16–49	58
50–64	43
65–74	36
Geographic location	Iowa (USA)
Sample type	Normal subjects or control patients
Education	NA
Gender	
Men	65
Women	72
Race/Ethnicity	Not reported
Screening	Patients with neurological disease excluded

Source: Adapted from Benton et al., 1994.

low ceiling. In their sample of 137 "normal subjects or control patients," scores (corrected for age and gender) of 21 or higher were made by 93% of the sample. Accordingly, the authors recommended a cutoff of 19 to 20 points (after correction) as borderline.

The characteristics of the child sample are shown in Table 12–21. Norms were based on 221 children who were between 7 and 14 years of age and ranged from 81 to 127 in WISC-R Verbal IQ ($M = 107$, $SD = 11$; Lindgren & Benton, 1980). In the first phase of the study, 154 children in grades 1, 4, and 7 were tested. In the second phase, 1 year later, 94 of these children (then in grades 2 and 5) were retested, and an additional 67 children in grades 3 and 6 were tested. Therefore, normative values are based on 315 observations across the age ranges.

Table 12–21 JLO: Characteristics of the Child Normative Sample

Number	221
Age (years)	7–14
Geographic location	Iowa (USA)
Sample type	School children in grades 1 through 7
Socioeconomic status	NA
Gender	
Boys	NA
Girls	NA
Race/Ethnicity	NA
Screening	Prorated WISC-R Verbal IQs ranged from 81 to 127 with a mean of 107 ($SD = 11$); children whose age was not appropriate for grade placement or whose IQ was <80 or >130 were excluded.

Source: Adapted from Benton et al., 1994.

Table 12–22 JLO Scores (Mean and *SD*) by Gender for Young Adults, Aged 18–30 Years

Group	*n*	Mean (*SD*)
Women	109	22.80 (5.66)
Men	58	26.21 (4.37)

Note: Participants were administered the JLO in a group setting.

Source: Adapted from Glamser & Turner, 1995.

Other Normative Data

Glamser and Turner (1995) evaluated a sample of 167 college students (109 women, 58 men), ranging in age from 18 to 30 years, using a group-administered version of the JLO (via an overhead projector) with no time pressure. Approximately 23% of the sample were African Americans. The scores were very similar (see Table 12–22) to those reported by Benton et al. (1994) for adults aged 16 to 49 years (men, *M* = 26.6; women, *M* = 23.3).

Ivnik et al. (1996) provided normative information for use with persons aged 55 to 97 years (see Table 12–23). Midpoint age intervals were used to maximize the information available at each age. Note that MOANS aged-corrected scaled scores have a mean of 10 and a standard deviation of 3. A computational formula is also provided in Table 12–23 to derive age- and education-corrected MOANS scaled scores. Although the sample size was large (216), it consisted almost exclusively of Caucasian older adults living in an economically stable region of the United States. Accordingly, Ivnik et al. (1996) urged

caution in the use of these norms for persons of other ethnic, cultural, or socioeconomic backgrounds. Of note, scores for individuals aged 65 to 74 years appeared to be consistent with those reported by Benton et al. (1994).

Steinberg et al. (2005) have expanded the utility of the MOANS project by providing age- and IQ adjusted percentile equivalents of MOANS age-adjusted JLO scores, for use with individuals aged 55+. Users should note that all FSIQs are Mayo age-adjusted scores which are based on the WAIS-R, not the WAIS-III. Given the upward shift in scores (Flynn effect) with the passage of time, use of the WAIS-R FSIQ as opposed to the WAIS-III might result in a given JLO score appearing less favorable.

Lucas et al. (2005) have recently provided normative data derived from African American community-dwelling participants from the MOAANS (Mayo African American Normative Studies) project in Jacksonville, Florida. Participants were predominantly female (75%), ranged in age from 56 to 94 years (mean age = 69.6, *SD* = 6.87), and varied in education from 0 to 20 years of formal education (mean education = 12.2, *SD* = 3.48). They were screened to exclude those with active neurological, psychiatric, or other conditions that might affect cognition. The authors note that over 10% of the normative group failed the sample items which would result in discontinuation of the test and interpretation of severe visual impairment (Benton et al., 1994). To improve the clinical utility of the JLO, they provide separate MOAANS norms for the subsample of individuals who passed the sample items and were administered the 30 test items. These data are provided in addition to norms for the entire sample (i.e., including

Table 12–23 JLO MOANS Norms for Persons Aged 56–97 Years

Percentile Ranges	56–62	63–65	66–68	69–71	72–74	75–77	78–80	81–83	84–86	87–89	90–97	Scaled Score
n	119	119	119	119	119	119	119	127	113	82	82	
<1	—	—	—	—	—	—	—	—	—	—	—	2
1	—	—	—	—	—	—	—	—	—	—	—	3
2	0–7	0–7	0–7	0–7	0–7	0–7	—	—	—	—	—	4
3–5	8–11	8–11	8–11	8–11	8–11	8–11	0–10	0–10	0–8	—	—	5
6–10	12–14	12–14	12–14	12–14	12–14	12–14	11–13	11–13	9–12	0–9	0–9	6
11–18	15–17	15–17	15–17	15–17	15–17	15–17	14–16	14–16	13–15	10–14	10–14	7
19–28	18–19	18–19	18–19	18–19	18–19	18–19	17–18	17–18	16–17	15–16	15–16	8
29–40	20	20	20	20	20	20	19–20	19	18	17–18	17–18	9
41–50	21–22	21–22	21–22	21–22	21–22	21–22	21–22	20–21	19–21	19–21	19–21	10
60–71	23	23	23	23	23	23	—	22	22	22	22	11
72–81	24	24	24	24	24	24	23–24	23–24	23–24	23	23	12
82–89	25–26	25–26	25–26	25–26	25–26	25–26	25	—	—	24	24	13
90–94	27–28	27–28	27–28	27–28	27–28	27–28	26	25–26	25	25	25	14
95–97	29	29	29	29	29	29	27–28	27–28	26–28	26–27	26–27	15
98	30	30	30	30	30	30	29	29	29	28–29	28–29	16
99	—	—	—	—	—	—	30	30	30	30	30	17
>99	—	—	—	—	—	—	—	—	—	—	—	18

Note: Based on Mayo's Older Normative Studies (MOANS). Age- and education-corrected MOANS Scaled Score ($MSS_{A\&E}$) is calculated from a person's age-corrected MOANS Scaled Score (MSS_A) and that person's education expressed in years of formal schooling completed, as follows: $MSS_{A\&E} = 1.54 + (1.10 \times MSS_A) - (0.23 \times Education)$.

Source: Adapted from Ivnik et al., 1996. Reprinted with the kind permission of Psychology Press.

Table 12–24a MOAANS JLO Scaled Scores in African American Adults: Sample Failures Included and Sample Failures Excluded, by Age

Scaled Scores	56–62		63–65		66–68		69–71		72–74		75–77		78+		Percentile Ranges
	Incl	Excl	Incl	Excl	Incl	Excl	Incl	Excl	Incl	Excl	Incl	Excl	Incl	Excl	
n	108	98	130	114	166	144	181	158	157	139	119	105	79	71	
2	—	0–5	—	0–5	—	0–5	—	0–5	—	0–5	—	0–5	—	0–5	<1
3	—	—	—	—	—	—	—	—	—	—	—	—	—	—	<1
4	—	6	—	6	—	6	—	—	—	—	—	—	—	—	1
5	0	7–8	—	7–8	—	7–8	—	7–8	—	7–8	—	6	—	6	2
6	1–5	9–10	0–5	9–10	0–5	9–10	0–5	9–10	0–5	9–10	0–5	9	0–1	7–9	3–5
7	6–10	11–12	6–9	11–12	6–9	11–12	6–9	11–12	6–9	11–12	6–9	10–12	2–8	10–12	6–10
8	11–13	13–14	10–12	13–14	10–12	13–14	10–12	13–14	10–12	13–14	10–12	13–14	9–11	13	11–18
9	14–15	15–16	13–15	15–16	13–15	15–16	13–15	15–16	13–15	15–16	13–14	15	12–13	14–15	19–28
10	16–18	17–18	16–18	17–18	16–18	17–18	16–17	17–18	16–17	17–18	15–17	16–17	14–16	16–17	29–40
11	19–20	19–20	19–20	19–20	19	19–20	18–19	19	18	19	18	18	17	18	41–59
12	21	21–22	21	21–22	20–21	21	20	20–21	19–20	20	19	19–20	18–19	19	60–71
13	22–24	23–24	22–23	23–24	22–23	22–23	21–22	22	21	21–22	20	21	20	20	72–81
14	25	25	24–25	25	24	24	23	23	22–23	23	21	22	21	21	82–89
15	26	26–27	—	26	25	25	24–25	24–25	24–25	24	22–23	23	22	22	90–94
16	27	28	26	27	26	26	26	26	26	25–26	24–26	24–26	23	23	95–97
17	28+	29	27–28	28	27–28	27–28	27–28	27–28	27–28	27	27	27	24	24–25	98
18	—	30	29+	29+	29+	29+	29+	29+	29+	28+	28+	28+	25+	26+	99
															>99

Source: Adapted from Lucas et al., 2005. Reprinted with the kind permission of the Mayo Foundation for Medical Education and Research. All rights reserved.

those who received scores of zero due to failure of sample test items). Table 12–24a presents the age scaled scores and Table 12–24b provides the computational formula used to calculate age- and education-adjusted MOAANS scaled scores. The authors urge that their data should be used with caution since the number of very old adults is relatively small and they used a sample of convenience which may not represent the full range of cultural and educational experiences of the African American community.

The JLO has been given to samples of school children outside the United States. Children in the United States and Italy performed at the same level (Riva & Benton, 1993; Riva et al., 1986); however, scores in the Netherlands/Belgium appeared to be slightly higher (although cell sizes were very small; Paquier et al., 1999). The mean scores of the children in the three countries are shown in Table 12–25.

Short Form

Woodard et al. (1998) presented norms for the two short forms (O and E), based on a sample of 131 healthy, community-living geriatric individuals between 55 and 84 years of age ($M = 65.8$, $SD = 6.7$). The mean educational level was 14 years ($SD = 2.3$, range = 9–20), and the mean MMSE score was 27.5 ($SD = 2.0$, range = 21–30). The sample was predominantly female (87%), Caucasian (97.6%) and right-handed (93.9%). They also included a cross-validation sample of 49 similar participants between 55 and 79 years of age, predominantly Caucasian (98%), but more balanced with respect to gender (53.1% females). Scores lower than 8 were quite rare in either sample and for either form. Based on findings from both samples, they recommended that short form scores of 10 be considered as borderline, and those of 8 and 9 as indicating mild deficit; for female subjects, 1 point should be added to

Table 12–24b Computational Formula for Age- and Education-Corrected MOAANS Scaled Scores

	K	W_1	W_2
JLO (excl. failures)	2.11	1.14	0.28
JLO (incl. failures)	1.45	1.20	0.29

Note: Age- and education-corrected MOAANS Scaled Scores ($MSS_{A\&E}$) can be calculated for JLO scores by using age-corrected MOAANS Scaled Scores (MSS_A) and education (expressed in years completed) in the following formula: $MSS_{A\&E} = K + (W_1 \times MSS_A) - (W_2 \times EDUC)$.

Source: From Lucas et al., 2005. Reprinted with the kind permission of the Mayo Foundation for Medical Education and Research. All rights reserved.

the score. The interpretation of scores for JLO short forms O and E, the frequency of individuals obtaining each score in the derivation sample, and the percentile ranges encompassed by each score are shown in Table 12–26.

RELIABILITY

Internal Consistency

Split-half reliability for the standard 30-item version is high in children ($r = .84$) (Benton et al., 1994) and in adults ($r = .84$ to .91; Benton et al., 1994; Qualls et al., 2000; Vanderploeg et al., 1997; Winegarden et al., 1998; Woodard et al., 1996).

Reliability coefficients for the 15-item O and E short forms are lower ($r = .69$ to .75; Vanderploeg et al., 1997; Winegarden et al., 1998; Woodard et al., 1996), an expected effect given the decrease in the number of items (Woodard et al., 1996).

Winegarden et al. (1998) report an internal consistency of .80 for a 20-item short form. The two 15-item short forms

Table 12–25 Normative Data for Children in Three Different Countries

Age (Years)		Italy[a]		United States[b]		Netherlands[c]
		Boys	Girls	Boys	Girls	Combined
7	Mean (SD)			16.8 (4.5)	15.3 (5.4)	17.3 (3.1)
	n			24	23	10
8	Mean (SD)	18.3 (6.2)	18.1 (5.8)	19.0 (4.3)	17.6 (3.7)	21.8 (4.9)
	n	15	15	23	27	10
9	Mean (SD)	19.3 (5.0)	17.8 (6.2)	21.7 (4.1)	19.7 (4.2)	22.1 (3.4)
	n	13	17	18	19	11
10	Mean (SD)	20.6 (5.2)	21.3 (3.7)	20.6 (6.6)	19.3 (5.2)	23.1 (3.5)
	n	18	12	17	19	11
11	Mean (SD)	24.0 (5.3)	22.7 (3.5)	22.8 (5.3)	21.7 (5.1)	22.0 (4.9)
	n	15	15	20	24	9
12	Mean (SD)	23.1 (2.7)	20.6 (3.9)	24.7 (3.8)	22.7 (4.0)	24.6 (3.8)
	n	14	16	20	22	9
13	Mean (SD)			26.1 (3.5)	22.7 (4.2)	24.4 (2.9)
	n			18	18	10
14	Mean (SD)			26.3 (2.7)	23.1 (4.0)	24.8 (3.1)
	n			13	10	11

[a]Riva & Benton, 1993.
[b]Lindgren & Benton, 1980.
[c]Paquier et al., 1999.

developed by Qualls et al. (2000) achieved an internal consistency alpha of .82 and .81 in 100 neurological patients.

Test-Retest Reliability and Practice Effects

Woodard et al. (1996) argued that Forms V and H are not really alternate forms, because they use the same stimuli with only a subtle difference in the order of presentation. Benton et al. (1994) reported that a sample of 37 patients was given both forms of the test, with the test-retest interval ranging from 6 hours to 21 days. The reliability coefficient was .90 (SEM = 1.8 points) and there was no evidence of a systematic practice effect. Montse et al. (2001) gave form H twice, with a 20-min test-retest interval, to a sample of patients with Parkinson's disease and to controls. There were no effects of practice.

Levin et al. (1991) retested healthy elderly adults with a 15-item version (form not specified) after a 1-year interval and reported a correlation coefficient of only .59.

VALIDITY

Relationships With Other Measures

Correlations tend to be higher with WAIS-R visual-spatial subtests (Block Design $r = .68$; Object Assembly $r = .69$) compared to verbal ones (Information $r = .45$; Vocabulary $r = .28$; Trahan, 1998). Factor analytic findings in patients with temporal lobe epilepsy (Hermann et al., 1993) and outpatient neuropsychiatric patients (Larrabee, 2000) suggest that the test loads with the Wechsler performance subtests and taps abilities somewhat separate from that of facial recognition.

Global-local perceptual biases are associated with perception of visual-spatial orientation. Basso and Lowery (2004) found that scores on JLO increased with an increasing global (configural versus local/detail) perceptual bias.

Table 12–26 Normative Table for Short Forms O and E derived from JLO Form V

Score	Frequency	Cumulative %	Interpretation
0–5	0	0	Severe deficit
6	1	1	Moderate deficit
7	2	2	Moderate deficit
8	7	8	Mild deficit
9	6	12	Mild deficit
10	9	19	Borderline
11	20	34	Normal
12	19	49	Normal
13	25	68	Normal
14	16	80	Normal
15+	26	100	Normal

Note: Based on Total $N = 131$, overall Mean = 12.3, SD = 2.3, range 6–16. One point should be added to scores of females before looking up the score on this table, producing a maximum possible score of 16.

Source: From Woodard et al., 1998. Reprinted with the kind permission of Psychology Press.

Clinical Studies

Impairment on the JLO task has been reported in a variety of conditions known to affect visual-spatial ability, including left visual neglect (Trahan, 1998), dementia of the Alzheimer type (AD; Ska et al., 1990; but see Finton et al., 1998), Turner syndrome (Kesler et al., 2004), and Parkinson's disease (e.g., Finton et al., 1998; Levin et al., 1991; Montse et al., 2001).

Of note, most studies have examined the number correct. A few studies have evaluated error types. Whether patients with AD make specific types of errors is uncertain. Ska et al. (1990) found that several error types (e.g., judging a line to be in one quadrant when it was in the other) tended to occur in patients with AD but not in normal controls. By contrast, Finton et al. (1998) found no specific error that characterized patients with AD. Differences in severity of the disorder may explain these conflicting results. There is evidence that patients with Parkinson's disease tend to make a greater proportion of complex intraquadrant errors and horizontal line errors, but fewer simple intraquadrant errors, than controls, suggesting a visual-spatial deficit (Finton et al., 1998; Monste et al., 2001).

Benton's classic studies (Benton et al., 1994, 1978; Hamsher et al., 1992) demonstrated that patients with right posterior damage perform worse than those with left-hemisphere (LH) damage. More recent work (Trahan, 1998) has shown that patients with RH lesions, particularly those with visual neglect, have a much higher incidence of defective performance relative to their left-sided counterparts (Trahan, 1998; but see Qualls et al., 2000). Further, although impairment can occur in patients with left parietal dysfunction, right parietal damage is associated with the more severe deficit (Ng et al., 2000). These findings were corroborated by fMRI studies, which suggested a more dominant role of the right posterior hemisphere in this task (Gur et al., 2000; Ng et al., 2000, 2001), possibly leading the way and "kick-starting" the spatial processing. This may involve initial perception of lower spatial contrast frequencies, supporting global (gestalt, configural) features of the complex stimulus array before more local, detailed analysis by LH regions (Ng et al., 2000).

Additional hypotheses regarding the specialized contributions of each hemisphere to line orientation derive from an ingenious study by Mehta and Newcombe (1996). They attempted to break down the task requirements for JLO by presenting (a) a pure angle-matching task ("indicate whether two single lines are at the same angle"), (b) a task similar to the JLO except that a single line must be matched to the array, and (c) an angle-matching with distractors task (judge whether the middle line in a three-line display is in the same direction as the middle line in a similar display). Comparing the results of 15 veterans with penetrating head injury in the LH to 15 well-matched veterans with RH injury and 25 matched controls, they found that patients with LH injury made significantly more errors than the control group on the JLO task, but that the difference between RH patients and controls did not reach significance. The pure angle-matching task showed very few errors, but latencies were significantly longer for the RH group. Both latencies and errors for the distractor task

were significantly higher for the RH group compared with both LH and control groups. The authors concluded that both the RH and the LH contribute to JLO performance, speculating that the LH contributes by "keeping track of decisions and updating decisions in more complex aspects" (p. 338). That is, in the standard JLO, it is necessary to keep simultaneous account of decisions and update decisions arising from at least three comparisons: a comparison between the target angle and its matched counterpart in the array, and two further comparisons between the target angle and the two nearest alternative responses, on either side of the correct angle in the array.

Depression can affect test scores (Kronfol et al., 1978), as can psychotic disorder (e.g., schizophrenia; Hardoy et al., 2004; Lee & Cheung, 2004). A follow-up study of 39 schizophrenic inpatients in a nonacute period found significant improvement on JLO scores, in line with scores presented in normative samples (Sweeney et al., 1991).

Impact of Vision

Decreased visual acuity does not significantly affect performance (Kempen et al., 1994). The stimuli have a high degree of contrast without fine details. Blurring and loss of contrast sensitivity are expected to have little impact, because information about global configuration is still available. Other types of visual disorders (e.g., macular degeneration) may well affect test performance.

Time of Day

Time of testing may affect performance in older adults. Older individuals obtained slightly lower scores when tested at their nonpreferred, rather than their preferred, time of day (Paradee et al., 2005).

Children

The literature with adults suggests a close association between defective JLO performance and disturbance of the RH. However, in children, the situation appears to be different. Paquier et al. (1999) reported that JLO performance did not predict the presence of cerebral pathology. Nor did it contribute to the prediction of side of damage in children with acquired unilateral cerebral lesions. Therefore, in children the task is better used to assess adequacy of visual-spatial processes than to specify underlying pathology.

Short Forms

The 15-item short forms (O and E) have been shown to correlate highly with one another (r = .71 to .81), producing similar mean scores and distributions (Vanderploeg et al., 1997; Woodard et al., 1996, 1998). There appears to be no effect of administration order, suggesting that these forms are useful for serial examinations. The forms also were shown to be equivalent to the full 30-item version in heterogeneous samples of patients with psychiatric or neurological disease (Vanderploeg et al., 1997; Woodard et al., 1996), geriatric populations (Woodard et al., 1998), and patients with TBI (Mount et al., 2002). That is, the short forms correlated highly ($r = .90$ to $.95$) with the long form (Mount et al., 2002; Vanderploeg et al., 1997; Winegarden et al., 1998; Woodard et al., 1996).

Simple doubling of the score, so as to use standard long-form normative data, is not advised, because such a practice can produce erroneous results (Woodard et al., 1996); rather, appropriate normative data should be used (Woodard et al., 1998). The ability of these O and E short forms to distinguish individuals with focal RH and LH damage remains to be evaluated.

The 15-item short form developed by Qualls et al. (2000; Form Q, comprising Form V items 16, 9, 6, 2, 12, 30, 7, 17, 19, 28, 20, 21, 26, 24, and 22, administered in that order) correlated highly with the full test ($r = .94$) and agreed relatively well with the long form in detecting the presence of impairment (kappa = .85). However, agreement was not sufficiently high in classifying patients as normal, mild, moderate, or severely impaired. In addition, neither Form Q nor the long form discriminated between LH and RH stroke patients (Qualls et al., 2000).

Winegarden et al. (1998) reported a correlation of .97 between the full-length JLO and a 20-item short form. Short-form scores have been equated with long-form scores (Winegarden et al., 1998), although normative data remain to be provided.

Malingering

Meyers et al. (1999) suggested that a score of 12 or less on the standard JLO is sufficiently rare in patients with moderate to severe traumatic brain injuries to raise the concern of suboptimal effort. Iverson (2001) evaluated the utility of this cutoff point in a large sample of individuals involved in head injury litigation. Patients identified as biased in their responses on two other tests (WMT, CARB) also showed poor performance on the JLO. However, the cutoff on the JLO was not sufficiently sensitive to exaggeration in most cases. In this sample, 88% of those who obtained suspicious scores on either the CARB or the WMT scored higher than the cutoff for suspicion on the JLO. Iverson (2001) concluded that the JLO should not be used to assess motivational status; rather, it should be simply interpreted with caution if a patient's score falls in a range that does not make neuropsychological sense.

COMMENT

The JLO test has a number of advantages. It requires minimal motor skills, demands little or no verbal mediation, and appears to tap a relatively low-level skill (Collaer & Nelson, 2002). In addition, the test produces similar normative standards in North America and Europe, supporting its use in Western countries. Reliability generally appears high, and the test appears to be free of practice effects.

The literature suggests that age, gender, IQ, and education have an effect on test scores. Norms for younger adults (< 55 years) take age and gender into account, but not IQ or education. Norms for older adults (>55 years) take age and gender or age and education/IQ into account, but not age, gender, and IQ/education. Data for children are available, although information on socioeconomic status and parental education are lacking. Note too that the test has a low ceiling in the normal population, with many individuals earning perfect or near-perfect scores, restricting the range of performance. Therefore, a "normal" score may not reflect intact visual-spatial ability. By the same token, very low scores among elderly African Americans may not reflect cognitive dysfunction but rather culturally related factors such as test relevance, task familiarity, motivation/level of comfort in the test situation, and quality of educational experience (Lucas et al., 2005; Manly, 2005).

Despite its demonstrated validity and reliability, the test can be frustrating for elderly or severely impaired patients, who often take a considerable amount of time to make decisions about the slope of line angles. Short forms correlate highly with the long forms. However, the short forms do not categorize severity of impairment in the same way as the standard JLO (Qualls et al., 2000). In addition, information on test-retest reliability is limited, and further research is needed to determine their efficacy in detecting lateralized disturbance as well as perceptual impairments (defined by independent criteria; Qualls et al., 2000). Therefore, the short forms are probably most useful for screening purposes, when patient fatigue is a concern; if severity of impairment is an issue, the full form should be given. Further, users should not simply double the score and apply standard JLO normative data.

In adults, the test appears sensitive to RH pathology. Although the test may be useful in exploring visual-spatial ability in children, its utility in predicting pathology or side of lesion in children has been seriously questioned.

REFERENCES

Basso, M. R., Harrington, K., Matson, M., Lowery, N. (2000). Sex differences on the WMS-III: Findings concerning Verbal Paired Associates and Faces. *The Clinical Neuropsychologist, 14,* 231–245.

Basso, M. R., & Lowery, N. (2004). Global-local visual biases correspond with visual-spatial orientation. *Journal of Clinical and Experimental Neuropsychology, 26,* 24–30.

Benton, A. L., Sivan, A. B., Hamsher, K. deS., Varney, N. R., & Spreen, O. (1983). *Contributions to neuropsychological assessment.* Orlando, Fla.: Psychological Assessment Resources.

Benton, A. L., Sivan, A. B., Hamsher, K. deS., Varney, N. R., & Spreen, O. (1994). *Contributions to neuropsychological assessment* (2nd ed.). Orlando, Fla.: Psychological Assessment Resources.

Benton, A. L., Varney, N. R., & Hamsher, K. (1978). Visuospatial judgment: A clinical test. *Archives of Neurology, 35,* 364–367.

Collaer, M. L., & Nelson, J. D. (2002). Large visuospatial sex difference in line judgment: Possible role of attentional factors. *Brain and Cognition, 49,* 1–12.

Ferracuti, F., & Ferracuti, S. (1992). Taratura del compione italiano. In A. L. Benton, N. R. Varney, & K. Hamsher (Eds.) *Test di Guidatione di Orientamenta de Linee.* Firenze: Organizzioni Speciali.

Finton, M. J., Lucas, J. A., Graff-Radford, N. R., & Uitti, R. J. (1998). Analysis of visuospatial errors in patients with Alzheimer's disease or Parkinson's disease. *Journal of Clinical and Experimental Neuropsychology, 20,* 138–193.

Glamser, F. D., & Turner, R. W. (1995). Youth sport participation and associated sex differences on a measure of spatial ability. *Perceptual and Motor Skills, 81,* 1099–1105.

Gur, R. C., Aslop, D., Glahn, D., Petty, R., Swanson, C. L., Maldjian, J. A., Turetsky, B. I., Detre, J. A., Gee, J., & Gur, R. E. (2000). An fMRI study of sex differences in regional activation to a verbal and a spatial task. *Brain and Language, 74,* 157–170.

Hamsher, K., Capruso, D. X., & Benton, A. L. (1992). Visualspatial judgment and right hemisphere disease. *Cortex, 23,* 493–496.

Hardoy, M. C., Carta, M. G., Catena, M., Hardoy, M. J., Cadeddu, M., Dell'Osso, L., Hugdahl, K., & Carpiniello, B. (2004). Impairment in visual and spatial perception in schizophrenia and delusional disorders. *Psychiatry Research, 127,* 163–166.

Hermann, B. P., Seidenberg, M., Wyler, A., & Haltiner, A. (1993). Dissociation of object recognition and spatial localization abilities following temporal lobe lesions in humans. *Neuropsychology, 7,* 343–350.

Iverson, G. L. (2001). Can malingering be identified with the Judgment of Line Orientation Test? *Applied Neuropsychology, 8,* 167–173.

Ivnik, R. J., Malec, J. F., Smith, G. E., Tangalos, E. G., & Petersen, R. C. (1996). Neuropsychological tests' norms above age 55: COWAT, BNT, MAE Token, WRAT-R Reading, AMNART, Stoop, TMT, and JLO. *The Clinical Neuropsychologist, 10,* 262–278.

Kempen, J. H., Kritchevsky, M., & Feldman, S. T. (1994). Effect of visual impairment on neuropsychological test performance. *Journal of Clinical and Experimental Neuropsychology, 16,* 223–231.

Kesler, S. R., Haberecht, M. F., Menon, V., Warsofsky, I. S., Dyer-Friedman, J., Neely, E. K., & Reiss, A. L. (2004). Functional neuroanatomy of spatial orientation processing in Turner syndrome. *Cerebral Cortex, 14,* 174–180.

Kronfol, Z., Hamsher, K., Digre, K., & Waziri, R. (1978). Depression and hemispheric functions. *British Journal of Psychiatry, 132,* 560–567.

Larrabee, G. J. (2000). Association between IQ and neuropsychological test performance: Commentary on Tremont, Hoffman, Scott, and Adams (1998). *The Clinical Neuropsychologist, 14,* 139–145.

Lee, T. M. C., & Cheung, P. P. Y. (2005). The relationship between visual-perception and attention in Chinese with schizophrenia. *Schizophrenia Research, 72,* 185–193.

Levin, B. E., Llabre, M. M., Weiner, W. J., Sanchez-Ramos, J., Singer, C., & Brown, M. C. (1991). Visuospatial impairment in Parkinson's disease. *Neurology, 41,* 365–369.

Lindgren, S. D., & Benton, A. L. (1980). Developmental patterns of visuospatial judgment. *Journal of Pediatric Psychology, 5,* 217–225.

Lucas, J. A., Ivnik, R. J., Smith, G. E., Ferman, T. J., Willis, F. B., Petersen, R. C., & Graff-Radford, N. R. (2005). Mayo's Older African Americans Normative Studies: Norms for Boston Naming Test, Controlled Oral Word Association, Category Fluency, Animal Naming, Token Test, WRAT-3 Reading, Trail Making Test, Stroop

Test, and Judgement of Line Orientation. *The Clinical Neuropsychologist, 19,* 243–269.

Manly, J. J. (2005). Advantages and disadvantages of separate norms for African Americans. *The Clinical Neuropsychologist, 19,* 270–275.

Mehta, Z., & Newcombe, F. (1996). Dissociable contributions of the two hemispheres to judgments of line orientation. *Journal of the International Neuropsychological Society, 2,* 335–339.

Meyers, J. E., Galinsky, A. M., & Volbrecht, M. (1999). Malingering and mild brain injury: How low is low? *Applied Neuropsychology, 6,* 208–216.

Montse, A., Pere, V., Carme, J., Francesc, V., & Eduardo, T. (2001). Visuospatial deficits in Parkinson's disease assessed by Judgment of Line Orientation Test: Error analysis and practice effects. *Journal of Clinical and Experimental Neuropsychology, 23,* 592–598.

Mount, D. L., Hogg, J., & Johnstone, B. (2002). Applicability of the 15-item versions of the Judgment of Line Orientation Test for individuals with traumatic brain injury. *Brain Injury, 16,* 1051–1055.

Ng, V. W. K., Bullmore, E. T., de Zubicaray, G. I., Cooper, A., Suckling, J., & Williams, S. C. R. (2001). Identifying rate-limiting nodes in large-scale cortical networks for visuospatial processing: An illustration using fMRI. *Journal of Cognitive Neuroscience, 13,* 537–545.

Ng, V. W. K., Eslinger, P. J., Williams, S. C. R., Brammer, M. J., Bullmore, E. T., Andrew, C. M., Suckling, J., Morris, R. G., & Benton, A. L. (2000). Hemispheric preference in visuospatial processing: A complementary approach with fMRI and lesion studies. *Human Brain Mapping, 10,* 80–86.

Paquier, P. F., van Mourik, M., Van Dongen, H. R., Catsman-Berrevoets, C. E., Creten, W. L., & Stronks, D. L. (1999). Clinical utility of the Judgment of Line Orientation Test and Facial Recognition Test in children with acquired unilateral cerebral lesions. *Journal of Child Neurology, 14,* 243–248.

Paradee, C. V., Rapport, L. J., Hanks, R. A., & Levy, J. A. (2005). Circadian preference and cognitive functioning among rehabilitation inpatients. The Clinical Neuropsychologist, 19, 55–72.

Qualls, C. E., Bliwise, N. G., & Stringer, A. Y. (2000). Short forms of the Benton Judgment of Line Orientation Test: Development and psychometric properties. *Archives of Clinical Neuropsychology, 15,* 159–163.

Rahman, Q., & Wilson, G. D. (2003). Large sexual-orientation-related differences in performance on mental rotation and judgment of line orientation tasks. *Neuropsychology, 17,* 25–31.

Rahman, Q., Wilson, G. D., & Abrahams, S. (2004). Biosocial factors, sexual orientation and neurocognitive functioning. *Psychoneuroendocrinology, 29,* 867–881.

Rey, G. J., Feldman, E., Rivas-Vazquez, R., Levin, B. E., & Bentin, A. (1999). Neuropsychological test development and normative data on Hispanics. *Archives of Clinical Neuropsychology, 14,* 593–601.

Riva, D., & Benton, A. L. (1993). Visuospatial judgment: A crossnational comparison. *Cortex, 29,* 141–143.

Riva, D., Pecchini, M., & Cazzaniga, L. (1986). Lo sviluppo del giodizio visuo-spaziale nei bambini. *Giornale Neuropsichiatrica, 6,* 39–44.

Ska, B., Poissant, A., & Joanette, Y. (1990). Line orientation judgment in normal elderly and subjects with dementia of the Alzheimer's type. *Journal of Clinical and Experimental Neuropsychology, 12,* 695–702.

Steinberg, B. A., Bieliauskas, L. A., Smith, G. E., Langellotti, C., & Ivnik, R. J. (2005). MAYO's Older Americans Normative

Studies: Age- and IQ-adjusted norms for the Boston Naming Test, the MAE Token Test, and the Judgement of Line Orientation Test. *The Clinical Neuropsychologist, 19,* 280–328.

Sweeney, J. A., Haas, G. L., Keilp, J. G., & Long, M. (1991). Evaluation of the stability of neuropsychological functioning after acute episodes of schizophrenia: One-year followup study. *Psychiatry Research, 38,* 63–76.

Trahan, D. E. (1998). Judgment of line orientation in patients with unilateral cerebrovascular lesions. *Assessment, 5,* 227–235.

Vanderploeg, R. D., LaLone, L. V., Greblo, P., & Schinka, J. A. (1997). Odd-even short forms of the Judgment of Line Orientation Test. *Applied Neuropsychology, 4,* 244–246.

Winegarden, B. J., Yates, B. L., Moses, J. A., Benton, A. L., & Faustman, W. O. (1998). Development of an optimally reliable short form for Judgment of Line Orientation. *The Clinical Neuropsychologist, 12,* 311–314.

Woodard, J. L., Benedict, R. H. B., Roberts, V. J., Goldstein, F. C., Kinner, K. M., Caruso, D. X., & Clark, A. N. (1996). Short-form alternatives to the Judgment of Line Orientation test. *Journal of Clinical and Experimental Neuropsychology, 18,* 898–904.

Woodard, J. L., Benedict, R. H. B., Salthouse, T. A., Toth, J. P., Zgaljardic, D. J., & Hancock, H. E. (1998). Normative data for equivalent, parallel forms of the Judgment of Line Orientation Test. *Journal of Clinical and Experimental Neuropsychology, 20,* 457–462.

Visual Object and Space Perception Battery (VOSP)

PURPOSE

The Visual Object and Space Perception (VOSP) battery is designed to explore object and space perception.

SOURCE

The test (Warrington & James, 1991) is available from Harcourt Assessment (http://www.harcourt-uk.com), at a price of about $303 US. The price includes a manual, three-ring binder test booklets for the eight tests, and 25 scoring sheets.

AGE RANGE

The test can be given to individuals aged 20 to 84 years.

DESCRIPTION

The VOSP (Warrington & James, 1991) is a battery of eight tasks developed by Warrington and her colleagues (Taylor and Warrington, 1973; Warrington, 1982; Warrington & James, 1967, 1986, 1988, 1991; Warrington and Rabin, 1970; Warrington and Taylor, 1973) to assess those skills for which patients with right-hemisphere damage demonstrate selective deficits. Its theoretical base follows Warrington's proposal that object and space perception are functionally independent domains that may be dissociated in brain-damaged individuals and that relate to different anatomical locations. This resulted in the creation of four subtests for object perception (Tests 1 to 4: Incomplete Letters, Silhouettes, Object Decision, and Progressive Silhouettes) and four for space perception (Tests 5 to 8: Dot Counting, Position Discrimination, Number Location, and Cube Analysis). In addition, one test of visual shape detection was included to ensure that patients have adequate visual-sensory capacities. Descriptions of the subtests are provided in Table 12–27, and examples of each are shown in Figure 12–14. According to the test authors (Warrington & James, 1991), the particular tests were chosen because of their selectivity and sensitivity to right-hemisphere damage. Further, they were devised to require very simple responses: None requires significant praxic ability (e.g., copying, construction). All of the tasks are untimed.

ADMINISTRATION

Each test is preceded by two practice items. Discontinuation rules are described for each subtest in the manual (Warrington & James, 1991). Any number of tasks may be administered, and there is no prescribed order.

ADMINISTRATION TIME

Total administration time is not reported. We estimate that each subtest takes about 5 to 10 min, for a total testing time of approximately 40 to 80 min.

SCORING

See *Source*. For all subtests, the manual includes a 5% cutoff score for identifying a significant deficit (i.e., a score obtained by 5% or less of normal subjects in the same age band). For the Silhouettes and Progressive Silhouettes tests, the spread of scores permits allocation of performance to below the 5th percentile, as well as to 25%, below 50%, and above 50% cumulative frequency scores.

Test users should be alert to potential errors in the sequence of cards comprising the Position Discrimination test (Bonello et al., 1997). Two answers provided by the scoring sheet appeared to be incorrect, because measurement of the squares revealed that the correct responses should actually identify the opposite squares.

DEMOGRAPHIC EFFECTS

Age

Performance declines after age 50 years (Herrera-Guzman et al., 2004; Warrington & James, 1991). An additional decline in performance appears after age 70 years on some tasks (Number Location, Object Decision, Progressive Silhouettes, Silhouettes)

Table 12–27 Description of VOSP Tasks

Shape Detection Screening Test	This is a test of figure-ground perception, using 20 cards. The subject is asked to point out the random pattern figure that has a speckled X superimposed in the middle of the pattern. Number correct is scored. Patients scoring <15 points on this screening task should be considered inappropriate for the administration of the VOSP.
Test 1. Incomplete Letters	The individual is asked to identify by naming or tracing 20 stimulus letters degraded by 70% or 30%. The total number of correct identifications is counted.
Test 2. Silhouettes	The subtest consists of 15 animals and 15 common objects photographed from an unusual view and shown only as dark black silhouettes. The items are arranged in order of difficulty. The score is the total number of silhouettes correctly identified.
Test 3. Object Decision	Each card shows four silhouettes, containing the shape of one real object and three distractor items (nonsense shapes). The examinee is asked to point out the real one. The number of correct choices (maximum = 20) is recorded.
Test 4. Progressive Silhouettes	Objects (handgun and trumpet) are shown in various views and progressively more complete shapes. Each series has 10 progressively easier approximations of the target object. Subject is asked to identify the object. The number of trials on each item is scored (maximum 10 + 10 = 20).
Test 5. Dot Counting	The 10 cards contain a number of randomly arranged black dots. The individual is asked to indicate how many dots there are. The number of correctly identified cards is scored (maximum = 10).
Test 6. Position Discrimination	Each of 20 cards contains two square boxes with a dot in the center. One of the dots is slightly off-center. The subject is asked to indicate the dot that is exactly in the center of the box. The number of correct choices is scored (maximum = 20).
Test 7. Number Location	Each of 10 cards contains two squares. The upper square shows randomly arranged numbers; the lower square shows one black dot. The individual is asked to compare the two squares and indicate the number on the upper box that corresponds to the position of the dot in the lower box. The number correctly located is scored (maximum = 10).
Test 8. Cube Analysis	Each of 10 cards contains the outline drawing of bricks. The subject is asked how many "solid" bricks are shown on each card (i.e. not counting "hidden" bricks). The total number of correct counts is scored (maximum = 10).

but not others (Dot Counting, Incomplete Letters, Position Discrimination). The failure to observe age-related declines on these latter tasks is likely due to ceiling effects (Bonello et al., 1997; Herrera-Guzman et al., 2004). There is also some suggestion of a differential progression of the effects of aging, with object perception declining earlier than space perception (Bonello et al., 1997).

Gender

Bonello et al. (1997) reported that gender does not affect performance. However, Herrera-Guzman et al. (2004) found gender-related differences on five of the eight tasks: Silhouettes, Object Decision, Progressive Silhouettes, Position Discrimination, and Cube Analysis.

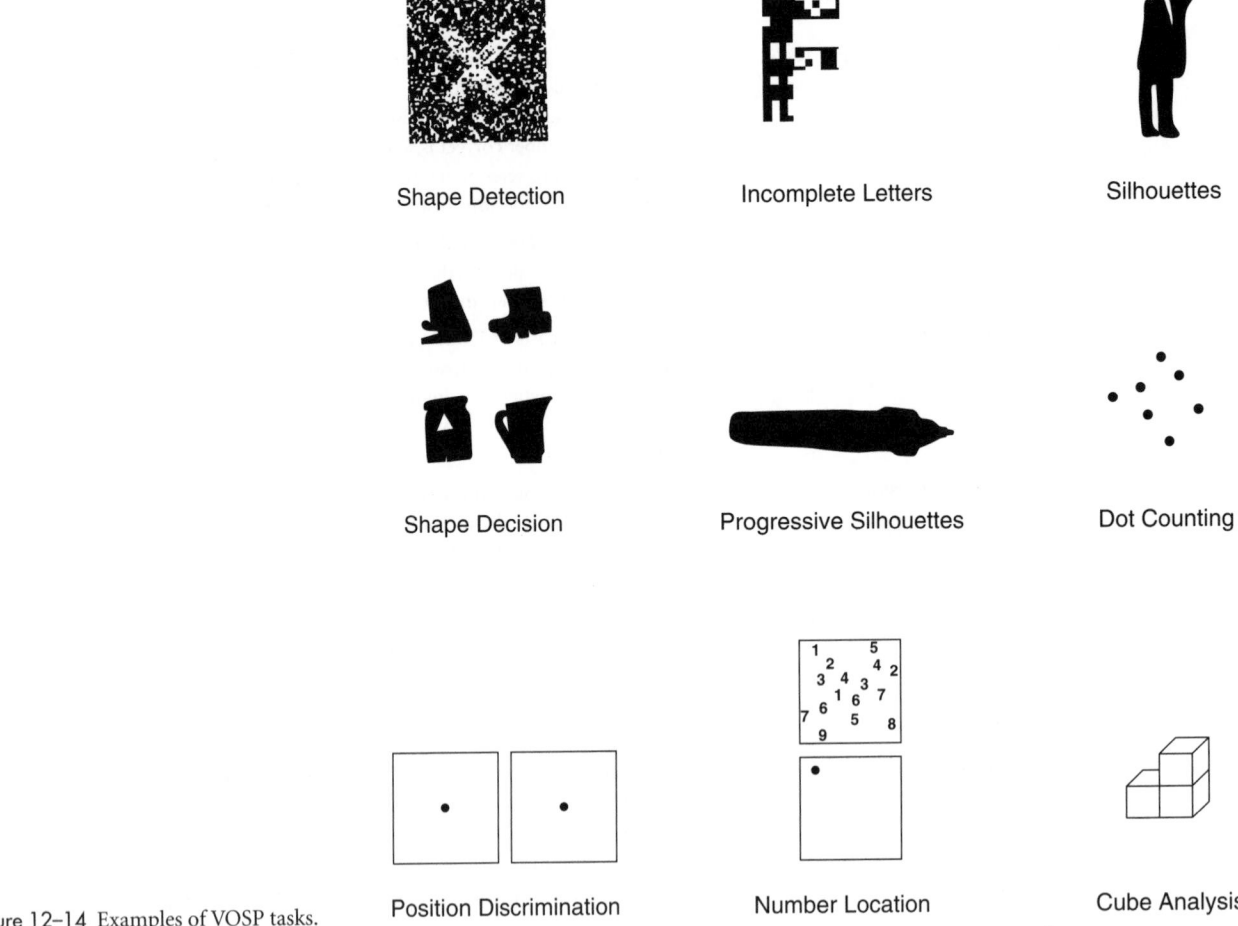

Shape Detection   Incomplete Letters   Silhouettes

Shape Decision   Progressive Silhouettes   Dot Counting

Position Discrimination   Number Location   Cube Analysis

Figure 12–14 Examples of VOSP tasks.

Education/ IQ

Weak but significant associations have been reported between education and performance on Number Location (Bonello et al., 1997), Object Decision (Bonello et al., 1997; Herrera-Guzman et al., 2004) and Silhouettes (Herrera-Guzman et al., 2004). Similarly, weak but significant associations have been reported between IQ (Shipley, NART) and performance on Silhouettes ($r = .29$ to .30; Bird et al., 2004; Bonello et al., 1997), Dot Counting ($r = .27$; Bonello et al., 1997), and Cube Analysis ($r = .29$; Bonello et al., 1997).

Ethnicity/Culture

Whether cultural factors affect performance is not clear. Bonello et al. (1997) reported differences between the British standardization sample and an American one, despite the fact that both groups were equivalent in intelligence. However, a variety of other differences existed between the samples (e.g., the use of medical patients versus healthy individuals), clouding interpretation. Herrera-Guzman et al. (2004) reported no differences between their sample (older adults in Spain) and the British and American samples.

NORMATIVE DATA

Standardization Sample

The characteristics of the VOSP normative sample are shown in Table 12–28. For each test, a standardization study and a validation study are reported in the test manual. The aim of the standardization study was to provide age-related norms for each test. The purpose of the validation study was to establish that the task difficulty was set at an appropriate level to ensure a significant "hit" rate (task sensitivity) in the critical right-hemisphere group and an insignificant "hit" rate (task selectivity) in the left-hemisphere group.

One standardization sample (109 males and 91 females; NART estimated IQ of 109.7, $SD = 8.5$) was used to develop norms for tests 1 and 5 through 8, and a second sample (72 males and 78 females; NART estimated IQ of 110.7, $SD = 9.3$) was used for tests 2 through 4. The range of ages appeared to be equivalent for both samples. All were medical patients in a London, U.K., hospital with extracerebral neurological conditions. Effects of age were negligible up to age 50 years, but a minor effect of age was noted for older individuals. For this reason, means and standard deviations

Table 12–28 Characteristics of the VOSP Normative Sample

Number	200 subjects given tests 1, 5, 6, 7, and 8; 150 subjects given tests 2, 3, and 4
Age (years)	20–69[a]
Geographic location	United Kingdom
Sample type	Hospital patients
Education	Not reported
Gender[b]	
Male	181
Female	169
Race/Ethnicity	Not reported
Screening	Only patients diagnosed with extracerebral neurological conditions were included.

[a]The cell size in each 10-year age grouping ranges from 23 to 55.
[b]Sample 1 was composed of 109 males and 91 females; sample 2 was composed of 72 males and 78 females. The gender composition of each age band was not reported.

(SDs) for all subtests were reported as two age bands (≤49 years and ≥50 years).

Other Normative Data

The normative data provided in the VOSP manual do not appear appropriate for use with older American individuals. Bonello et al. (1997) reported data (see Table 12–29) for a sample of 111 older healthy volunteers, aged 50 to 84 years ($M = 68.2$, $SD = 9.5$), in Michigan, USA, who passed a health screening. Education of the sample ranged from 4 to 18 years ($M = 13.3$, $SD = 2.2$) and had an estimated IQ (based on the Shipley Test) in the above-average range, 112.5 ($SD = 26.17$), similar to the British standardization sample. To investigate specificities of the VOSP tests, the number of participants in the sample who would have been misclassified as "impaired" was determined using the recommended cutoffs provided in the test manual. They found that the use of the cutoff scores in the manual would have led to an unacceptable rate of misclassification, particularly in the case of Silhouettes and Number Location. They also noted that, whereas the manual reports a mild decrement in performance after age 50, their results indicate an additional decrement in performance after age 70 years on five of the eight tests.

RELIABILITY

Internal Consistency

In general, these tend to be low for healthy individuals. Internal consistency reliabilities were reported for 111 Michigan individuals between the ages of 50 to 84 years (Bonello et al., 1997; Table 12–30). The highest estimates of internal consistency were observed on Cube Analysis, Silhouettes, and Number Location, whereas the alpha values for Incomplete Letters, Object Decision, Progressive Silhouettes, and Dot Counting were unacceptably low. The poor coefficient alpha for Progressive Silhouettes is probably due to the fact that this subtest has only two items.

Examination of the discriminant indices (i.e., corrected-item total correlations) revealed considerable variability in the value of the items comprising each test. Bonello et al. (1997), following Nunnally and Bernstein's (1994) recommendation for scale retention, found that only 7 of 20 Incomplete Letter items, 14 of 30 Silhouettes items, 0 of 2 Progressive Silhouettes items, 2 of 10 items in Dot Counting, 9 of 20 items in Position Discrimination, 9 of 10 items in Number Location, and 9 of 10 items of Cube Analysis would be useful for retention if the test were revised.

Test-Retest Reliability and Practice Effects

Bird et al. (2004) retested a sample of 99 healthy adults between 39 and 75 years of age ($M = $ about 57, $SD = $ about 8.3; education = about 13 years) on the Silhouette Test after an interval of

Table 12–29 Normative Data (Mean and SD) for the VOSP Tests in a U.S. Sample

Test	Age <70 Years (n = 52)	Age ≥70 Years (n = 59)	Specificity for Total Sample[b] (N = 111)
Incomplete Letters	19.46 (0.73)	19.12 (1.37)	98.2
Silhouettes	20.40 (3.77)	15.53 (3.87)	68.5
Object Decision	17.54 (1.89)	15.61 (2.43)	83.8
Progressive Silhouettes	9.62 (2.20)	12.03 (2.40)	92.8
Dot Counting	9.77 (0.61)	9.68 (0.68)	92.8
Position Discrimination[a]	19.48 (1.34)	19.27 (1.03)	84.7
Number Location	9.08 (1.31)	7.12 (2.88)	71.2
Cube Analysis	9.54 (0.80)	8.54 (2.05)	92.8

[a]Test as scored accurately; scoring sheet provided with the test contained errors.
[b]Specificities using recommended cutoffs provided in the test manual.

Source: From Bonello et al., 1997. Reprinted with the kind permission of Psychology Press.

Table 12–30 VOSP Internal Consistency

Magnitude of Coefficient	Measure
Very High (≥.90)	—
High (.80 to .89)	Number Location
Adequate (.70 to .79)	Cube Analysis
	Silhouettes
Marginal (.60 to .69)	Position
	Discrimination
Low (≤.59)	Incomplete Letters
	Object Decision
	Progressive Silhouettes
	Dot Counting

Note: Coefficient Alpha reported for the total sample ($N = 111$).

Source: From Bonello et al., 1997. Reprinted with the kind permission of Psychology Press.

approximately 1 month. Test-retest reliability was found to be high ($r = .88$). Practice effects were small, and reliable change indices (RCIs) corrected for practice were rather small, suggesting that the test is useful for monitoring change in perceptual functioning. Neither age nor IQ appeared to mediate practice effects. Table 12–31 shows the mean performance of participants at both time intervals as well as RCIs corrected for practice. The RCI was calculated as the *SD*s of the difference score, multiplied by 1.645 (where $1.645 = Z_{0.95}$), corrected for practice by adding the mean change in scores from time 1 to time 2. Therefore, in this sample, 10% of subjects had a change in score that fell outside the RCIs corrected for practice.

VALIDITY

Factor Analytic Findings

Rapport et al. (1998) conducted a factor analysis of the VOSP subtests in a sample of older individuals (Bonello et al., 1997), in order to find confirmation for a one- or two-factor theory of object and space perception. The analyses provided support for the two-factor model. However, the object perception measures were stronger and more reliable indicators of their respective latent construct than were the space perception measures. The authors emphasized that the model was confirmed only for older individuals and that an analysis of data of other groups (e.g., younger subjects) might provide different results.

Clinical Findings

Warrington and James (1991) presented data from two consecutive series of patients with unilateral brain lesions, documented with computed tomographic scans, angiography, or surgical findings. Series 1 patients were given tests 1 and 5 through 8, whereas tests 2 through 4 were given to patients in series 2. Patients in both groups were divided into right- and left-hemisphere lesion subgroups. For all subtests, patients in the right-hemisphere group showed more deficient scores than those in the left-hemisphere group. Of note, for Object Decision, Progressive Silhouettes, Dot Counting, Position Discrimination, Number Location, and Cube Analysis, the number of left-hemisphere patients obtaining a deficit score was no greater, and sometimes less (Progressive Silhouettes), than the number predicted by the performance of the standardization sample, suggesting few false positives.

In addition to patients with right-hemisphere disturbance, impairment on the VOSP has been reported in adults with velo-cardio-facial syndrome, a genetic disorder associated with deletions on the long arm of chromosome 22 (Henry et al., 2002). The authors speculated that the chromosomal defect causing the syndrome is also responsible for the cognitive defect. In addition, patients with dementia with Lewy bodies (DLB) had substantially greater impairment on the VOSP (on Fragmented Letters, Object Decision, and Cube Analysis) than patients with AD matched for overall dementia severity (Calderon et al., 2001). VOSP Silhouette Identification was found to be related to neuronal loss in the striatum of patients with Huntington's disease (Sanchez-Pemaute et al. 2000).

COMMENT

The VOSP exemplifies a theory-driven approach to assessment, because both object and space perception may manifest as selective deficits, even among patients with normal visual acuity (McCarthy & Warrington, 1990). There is also evidence for the anatomical separation of object and space perception (e.g., Mishkin et al., 1983).

From a psychometric perspective, internal consistency for some of the VOSP tests is poor, at least in healthy subjects. However, estimates of internal consistency reliability calculated using a homogeneous, healthy sample are likely to produce a restricted range of scores and to artificially lower correlation coefficients. This issue requires additional study in

Table 12–31 Test-Retest Reliability of the Silhouettes Subtest, Practice Effects, and 95% RCI Corrected for Practice

Test	N	Test-Retest Reliability	Time 1 Mean (SD)	Time 2 Mean (SD)	RCI Corrected for Practice Lower	RCI Corrected for Practice Upper
Silhouettes	99	.88	21.6 (4.1)	22.8 (4.1)	−2.3	+4.5

Source: Adapted from Bird et al., 2004.

clinical samples. Further, information on test-retest reliability is meager, although recent findings (Bird et al., 2004) suggest that the Silhouettes subtest is useful for monitoring changes in object perception.

The British norms published with the test do not seem to be appropriate for North American populations. Idiosyncrasies of the British standardization sample include an above-average level of intelligence (estimated VIQ $M = 110$), the use of medical patients as controls, and the fact that the VOSP battery was not given to the standardization sample in its entirety: 200 subjects were given five of the VOSP tasks, and 150 subjects were given the remaining three tests (Bonello et al., 1997). Therefore, as Bonello et al. (1997) pointed out, the effects of the dual-sample on performance-related factors such as fatigue, response set, and general task familiarity cannot be determined. The provision of data from other countries (United States, Bonello et al., 1997; Spain, Herrera-Guzman et al., 2004) is a positive feature. Research examining VOSP performance in American adults with specific neurological conditions would better facilitate the identification of cutting scores to identify impairment in North American samples (Bonello et al., 1997).

Factor analytic findings (Rapport et al., 1998) in healthy older adults provided confirmation for Warrington's two-factor theory. However, the object perception subtests appeared stronger than the space perception measures in measuring their latent constructs, suggesting that revision of the space perception measures (especially Position Discrimination) may be beneficial (Rapport et al., 1998). The validity of the VOSP in detecting right-hemisphere damage has also been demonstrated (see *Source*). However, ceiling effects are found on a number of tasks (e.g., Incomplete Letters, Dot Counting, Position Discrimination) in healthy individuals. Accordingly, the tests may have limited ability to detect subtle forms of impairment. Test users should also note potential scoring errors in the Position Discrimination test (Bonello et al., 1997).

REFERENCES

Bird, C. M., Papadopoulou, K., Ricciardelli, P., Rossor, M. N., & Cipolott, L. (2004). Monitoring cognitive changes: Psychometric properties of six cognitive tests. *British Journal of Clinical Psychology, 43,* 197–210.

Bonello, P. J., Rapport, L. J., & Millis, S. R. (1997). Psychometric properties of the Visual Object and Space Perception Battery in normal older adults. *The Clinical Neuropsychologist, 11,* 436–442.

Calderon, J., Perry, R. J., Erzinclioglu, S. W., Berrios, G. E., Dening, T. R., & Hodges, J. R. (2001). Perception, attention, and working memory are disproportionately impaired in dementia with Lewy bodies compared with Alzheimer's disease. *Journal of Neurology, Neurosurgery and Psychiatry, 70,* 157–164.

Henry, J. C., Amelsvort, T. van, Morris, R. G., Owen, M. J., Murphy, D. G. M., & Murphy, K. C. (2002). An investigation of the neuropsychological profile in adults with velo-cardio-facial syndrome. *Neuropsychologia, 40,* 471–478.

Herrera-Guzman, I., Pena-Casanova, J., Lara, J. P., Gudayol-Ferre, E., & Bohm, P. (2004). Influence of age, sex and education on the Visual Object and Space Perception Battery (VOSP) in a healthy normal elderly population. *The Clinical Neuropsychologist, 18,* 385–394.

McCarthy, R. A., & Warrington, E. K. (1990). *Cognitive neuropsychology.* San Diego: Academic Press.

Mishkin, M., Ungerleider, L. G., & Macko, K. (1983). Object vision and spatial vision: Two cortical pathways. *Trends in Neuropsychology, 6,* 414–417.

Nunnally, J. C., & Bernstein, I. H. (1994). *Psychometric theory* (3rd ed.). New York: McGraw-Hill.

Rapport, L. J., Millis, S. R., & Bonello, P. J. (1998). Validation of the Warrington theory of visual processing and the Visual Object and Space Perception Battery. *Journal of Clinical and Experimental Neuropsychology, 20,* 211–220.

Sanchez-Pemaute, R., Kuenig, G., Alba, A. del Barrio, de Yebenes, J. G., et al. (2000). Bradykinesia in early Huntington's disease. *Neurology, 54,* 119–125.

Taylor, A. M., & Warrington, E. K. (1973). Visual discrimination in patients with localized cerebral lesions. *Cortex, 9,* 82–93.

Warrington, E. K. (1982). Neuropsychological studies of object recognition. *Philosophical Transactions of the Royal Society of London, 298,* 15–33.

Warrington, E. K., & James, M. (1967). Disorders of visual perception in patients with localized cerebral lesions. *Neuropsychologia, 5,* 253–266.

Warrington, E. K., & James, M. (1986). Visual object recognition in patients with right-hemisphere lesions: Axes or features? *Perception, 15,* 355–366.

Warrington, E. K., & James, M. (1988). Visual apperceptive agnosia: A clinical-anatomical study of three cases. *Cortex, 24,* 13–32.

Warrington, E. K. & James, M. (1991). *The Visual Object and Space Perception Battery.* Bury St. Edmunds, Suffolk, England: Thames Valley Test Company.

Warrington, E. K. & Rabin, P. (1970). Perceptual matching in patients with cerebral lesions. *Neuropsychologia, 8,* 475–487.

Warrington, E. K., & Taylor, A. M. (1973). Contribution of the right parietal lobe to object recognition. *Cortex, 9,* 152–164.

13

Tests of Somatosensory Function, Olfactory Function, and Body Orientation

Assessment of somatosensory and olfactory functioning is often neglected in neuropsychological practice, despite the fact that such impairments are found routinely in neurological patients and may signify cognitive disturbance. In addition, unlike many other neuropsychological tests, they are relatively unaffected by education and deficits are not consistently observed in depression.

Tactile sensitivity is part of the routine examination in neurology; it is typically conducted with touch by gauze pad or pin prick. A small number of standardized techniques including calibrated stimulators have been developed since the studies by Bender et al. (1948) of extinction on double stimulation, Benton's (1959) work on right-left discrimination and finger

localization, and Teuber's (Semmes et al., 1960) investigations of somatosensory changes after penetrating head injury.

Neuropsychological examinations with standardized tests can and do surpass the accuracy of the clinical neurological examination. The main interest is usually on differences between the two sides (usually hands) of the body, although bilaterally raised thresholds may also be of significance. Our selection (see Table 13–1) includes the Rivermead Assessment of Somatosensory Performance (RASP), a task that is relatively new, is easy to administer, and provides a quantifiable assessment of a range of somatosensory functions. We also include tests of psychologically more complex functions: finger localization, right-left orientation, and the Tactual Performance Test (TPT). Of note,

Table 13–1 Some Measures of Somatosensory Function, Olfactory Function, and Body Orientation

Test	Age Range (Years)	Administration Time (Min)	Processes	Test-Retest Reliability
Finger Localization	6–13, 16–65	10	Identification of fingers Motivational status	NA (adequate for a slightly different form)
Right-Left Orientation	16–64	5	Discrimination of right from left	NA
RASP	24–80	25–35	Somatosensory function 　Sharp/dull discrimination 　Surface Pressure 　Surface localization 　Sensory extinction 　Two-point discrimination 　Temperature discrimination 　Proprioception movement 　and direction discrimination	High for all except Proprioceptive direction; no information regarding Extinction and Two-point discrimination
Smell Identification	5–99	40-items: 10, 3 and 12 items: < 5	Odor identification Motivational status	High for long form, adequate for brief form
TPT	5–85	15–50	Tactile form recognition, memory for shapes and spatial location	Adequate for time scores, low for memory

the TPT includes measures of location and memory and appears to be a useful diagnostic instrument with blind individuals (Bigler & Tucker, 1981). Additional tasks can be found in the NEPSY and the BDAE-3 (see reviews in this volume).

Olfactory disturbances can also affect the quality of life and may place the individual, as well as others, at risk. Further, impairments of smell are found in a variety of neurological disorders and may signal impending cognitive decline in otherwise healthy individuals. We present here the Smell Identification Test (also known as the University of Pennsylvania Smell Identification Test), which is the most widely used tool for measuring olfactory dysfunction.

REFERENCES

Bender, M. B., Wortis, S. B., & Cramer, J. (1948). Organic mental syndromes with phenomena of extinction and allesthesia. *Archives of Neurology and Psychiatry, 59,* 273–291.

Benton, A. L. (1959). *Right-left discrimination and finger localization.* New York: Hoeber.

Bigler, E. D., & Tucker, D. M. (1981). Comparison of Verbal IQ, Tactual Performance, Seashore Rhythm, and Finger Oscillation Tests in the blind and brain-damaged. *Journal of Clinical Psychology, 37,* 849–851.

Semmes, J., Weinstein, S., Ghent, L., & Teuber, H. L. (1960). *Somatosensory changes after penetrating brain wounds in man.* Cambridge, Mass.: Harvard University Press.

Finger Localization

PURPOSE

The Finger Localization test assesses the identification, naming, and localization of fingers.

SOURCE

The test is contained in *Contributions to Neuropsychological Assessment,* by Benton et al. (1994), published by Oxford University Press, 198 Madison Avenue, New York, NY, 10016-4308 (http://www.oup-usa.org), and can be purchased at a cost of $35 US. It can also be purchased from PAR (http://parinc.com) at a cost of $39 US.

AGE RANGE

Norms are available for individuals aged 6 to 13 years and 16 to 65 years.

DESCRIPTION

Attention to finger recognition and its pathological counterpart, finger agnosia, gained prominence after Gerstmann's (1924) and Head's (1920) descriptions. The finger agnosia described by Gerstmann involved a bilateral impairment in recognition that extended to the fingers of the examiner as well those of the patient's hands. He interpreted the performance failure as an expression of a limited disorder of body schema. He coined the term "finger agnosia" and ascribed its occurrence to focal disease in the territory of the left angular gyrus. However, Head (1920) described unilateral impairment as a form of sensory defect resulting from parietal lobe disease (Benton et al., 1994). This form of defective finger recognition is quite different in nature from the bilateral disturbances in naming and identifying by name to which Gerstmann called attention (Benton et al., 1994). Therefore, multiple tasks are required to probe for the presence of all the disabilities that have been designated by the term "finger agnosia."

Benton's 60-item test (Benton et al., 1994) consists of three parts (see Figure 13–1): Part A requires patients to identify their fingers when touched by the examiner; B requires patients to identify their fingers with the hand hidden from view; and C requires patients to identify pairs of their fingers touched simultaneously with their hands hidden from view.

The mode of response is left up to the patient. The patient may name the fingers, point to them on an outline (see Figure 13–2), or call out their numbers.

Other Versions

An abbreviated version (four items each for Parts A and B, six items for Part C) has been used with children (De Agostini & Dellatolas, 2001). Another version of finger gnosis is included as part of the Parietal Lobe Battery (see *Boston Diagnostic Aphasia Examination*). A shorter examination is offered by Reitan & Wolfson (1985) and Russell and Starkey (1993).

ADMINISTRATION

In all parts of the test, the patient's hand rests on the table, palms up, fingers extended and slightly separated. In patients with spastic hemiplegia who cannot assume this positioning, assessment of finger recognition is restricted to the unaffected hand. Instructions are provided in Figure 13–3.

ADMINISTRATION TIME

The task takes about 10 min to administer.

SCORING

Correct responses are checked, and incorrect responses should be recorded by number. Responses on Part C are counted as correct only if both fingers are accurately identified. A total

Name _____ No._____ Date _____

Age _____ Sex _____ Education _____ Handedness _____ Examiner _____

Finger localization (Form B)*

A. <u>Identification of Single Fingers—Hand Visible</u>
Tips of fingers are touched in the following order (1 = thumb; 5 = little finger):

Score
R_____   Right Hand   2____5____3____1____4____3____5____2____4____1____
L_____   Left Hand   1____4____2____5____3____4____1____3____5____2____

B. <u>Identification of Single Fingers—Hand Hidden</u>
Tips of fingers are touched in the following order:

Score
R_____   Right Hand   5____1____3____2____4____3____5____1____4____2____
L_____   Left Hand   2____4____1____5____3____4____2____3____1____5____

C. <u>Identification of Two Simultaneously Touched Fingers—Hand Hidden</u>

Score
R_____   Right Hand   1-4____2-3____2-4____3-5____3-4____2-3____2-5____1-2____3-4____1-3____
L_____   Left Hand   1-3____3-4____1-2____2-5____2-3____3-4____3-5____2-4____2-3____1-4____

Total Score_____   R Score_____   L Score_____

*Form A consists of the identical sequences of trials with the difference that the right hand sequences are presented to the left hand and vice versa.

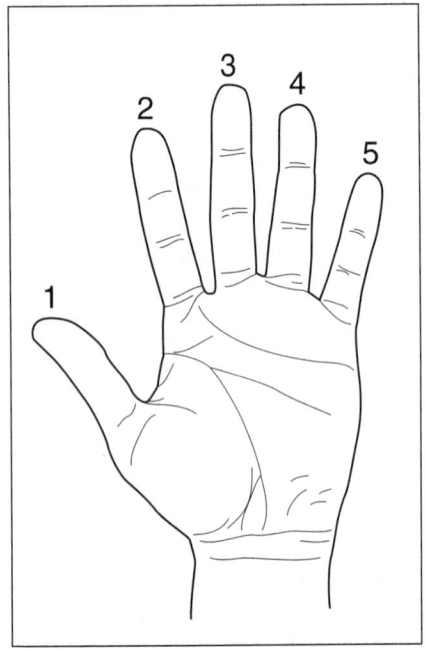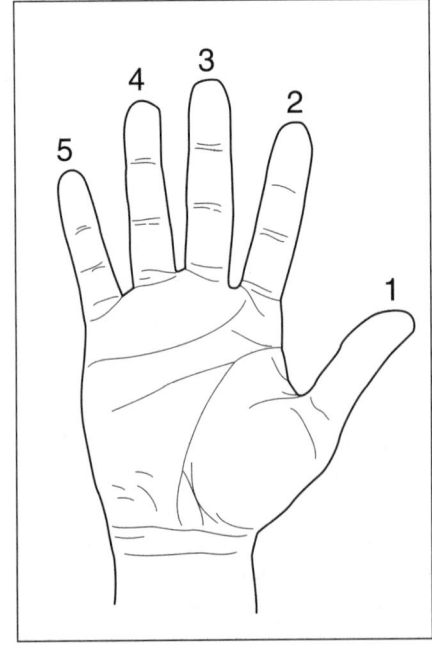

1014

Figure 13–3 Instructions for Finger Localization. *Source:*
Adapted from Benton et al., 1994.

Part A

*Say: I am going to touch different fingers on your hand;
you tell me which finger I touch. You can name the fingers, if you wish, or you can point on this card.*

The finger tip should be touched firmly with the
pointed end of a pencil for about 2 s. There should be no
question that the patient feels the stimulation. In patients
with sensory defect or disturbed attention, the stimulation
may be prolonged to 3–4 s to ensure adequate reception
of the stimulus. Some patients with severe sensory defect
cannot be tested on the affected hand.

Part B

*Say: Now put your (right, left) hand under this curtain.
You won't see me touching your finger but you will feel it.*

Guide the patient's hand, palm up, into the box; have
patient extend and slightly separate the fingers. *Say: Tell
me which finger I touch. You can name the finger or
point to it on this card or call the number of the card.*

Part C

*Say: Now I am going to touch two your fingers at the
same time. Tell me which fingers I touch. Again, either
name the fingers or point to them on the card or call
their numbers on the card.*

---

score for the whole test (maximum = 60) and separate scores
for the right and left hands (30 for each) are computed.

DEMOGRAPHIC EFFECTS

Age

Finger localization develops steadily and rapidly with age before age 6 and continues to develop up to age 12 years, when
adult levels are reached (Benton et al., 1994; De Agostini &
Dellatolas, 2001). Benton et al. (1994) found no effect of age in
hospitalized individuals without evidence of brain or psychiatric disorder, aged 16 to 65 years.

Education/IQ

Benton et al. (1994) reported that education did not influence
performance. In children, those with superior IQ performed
better than those with normal IQ (Benton et al., 1994).

Gender

No relationship with gender has been reported (Benton et al.,
1994; De Agostini & Dellatolas, 2001). However, gender effects

(favoring females) and gender by age effects were found on a
modified version (Yeudall et al., 1987).

Handedness

De Agostini & Dellatolas (2001) noted that increasing dextral-
ity was associated with slightly higher scores on an abbreviated version of the task.

NORMATIVE DATA

Standardization Sample

The test was given to 104 medical patients who had no evidence of brain disease or psychiatric illness (see Table 13–2).
Errors were few, with 60% of the sample making two or fewer
errors (Benton et al., 1994; see Table 13–3). When errors did
occur, they tended to be made on Part C of the test (localization of simultaneously touched fingers out of view).

The distributions of scores for the right and left hands
were very similar ($M = 28.65$ and 28.84, respectively). Differences between hands usually did not exceed one or two
points; in fact, a difference score of 2 points or less was shown
by 94% of the patients (Benton et al., 1994).

Benton et al. (1994) also provide some normative guidelines derived from studies of schoolchildren conducted more
than 50 years ago using an older and shorter version of the test
(Part C consisted of 5 trials on each hand instead of 10). In order to make the findings of children comparable to those of
adults, the children's scores were prorated by doubling the
number correct on Part C for each hand before computing the
total score. One of the sample groups (from Canada) was of
superior intellect and obtained higher scores than children in
the other groups, who appeared to be of average intellect.

Other Normative Data

Norms for children (Spreen, unpublished data; see Table
13–4) agreed closely with those presented by Wake (unpublished data, see *Source*) but were higher than those reported

Table 13–2 Characteristics of the Finger Localization
Standardization Sample

Number	104
Age (years)	16–65
Geographic location	United States
Sample type	Hospital patients
Education (years)	5–16+
Gender	
Male	64
Female	40
Race/Ethnicity	Not reported
Screening	No history or evidence of brain disease or psychiatric illness

Table 13–3 Finger Localization: Distribution of Scores in Right and Left Hands

Score	Right Hand		Left Hand		Classification
	n	Percentile	n	Percentile	
30	38	82+	45	78+	Normal
29	28	63	29	57	Normal
28	18	37	16	29	Normal
27	12	19	7	13	Normal
26	4	8	3	7	Borderline
25	2	4	2	4	Moderately defective
24	—	—	—	—	Moderately defective
23	2	2	—	—	Moderately defective
22	—	—	2	2	Moderately defective
< 22	—	—	—	—	

Source: From Benton et al., 1994. Used by permission of Oxford University Press.

Table 13–4 Finger Localization Normative Data for Children Aged 6–13 Years

Age (Years)	Normal Children				Superior-IQ Children			
	n	Right	Left	Total	n	Right	Left	Total
6	12	21	21	42	21	25	25	50
7	50	24	24	48	24	25	25	50
8	41	25	25	50	20	28	28	56
9	38	26	26	52	21	28	28	56
10	36	27	27	54	24	28	28	56
11	38	27	27	54	20	28	28	56
12	36	28	28	56	22	28	28	56
13	52	28	28	56				

Note: Standard deviations range from 3.0 at age 6, to 1.7 at age 13.

Source: Spreen, unpublished data.

by Benton et al. (1994) for both normal- and superior-IQ children. The data were collected about 30 years ago from schoolchildren in British Columbia.

RELIABILITY

Internal Consistency

This was evaluated in 158 children aged 5 to 9 years (IQ = 85–115) using the original, shortened version of the task (10 trials of each hand for Parts A and B; 5 trials each for Part C). Internal consistency of the total test was found to be high, .91.

Test-Retest Reliability

This was evaluated in children using equivalent forms of the original, shortened version of the task (Benton, 1955). Reliability coefficients were reported to be .70 for a 20-min interval in a sample of 46 children and .75 for a 10-week interval in a sample of 25 children.

Interrater Reliability

This is not reported.

VALIDITY

Clinical Studies

Benton et al. (1994) note that it is important to distinguish between bilateral and unilateral defects in finger localization. Gerstmann's bilateral "finger agnosia" and Head's unilateral impairment are different conditions, each with their own correlates and diagnostic implications.

Although bilateral impairment is generally associated with both aphasic disorders and general mental impairment, the deficit may also be shown by patients who are neither aphasic nor demented (Della Sala & Spinnler, 1994; Gainotti et al., 1972; see Benton et al., 1994, for review). Relatively small lesions in the left posterior perisylvian region have been identified as the pathological basis for the deficit (Benton et al., 1994).

Gainotti and Tiacci (1973) investigated unilateral impairment and reported that contralateral impairment was more frequent in those with right- as opposed to left-hemisphere lesions. However, Benton et al. (1994) did not find this difference in their small series.

With regard to predictive validity, performances of kindergarten children on finger localization tests were predictive of subsequent reading achievement (Badian et al., 1990). However, it is unclear why such a relationship exists (Benton et al., 1994).

In instances of isolated finger agnosia, the deficit does not affect the patient's everyday behavior and, therefore, may be easily overlooked (Della Sala & Spinnler, 1994).

Malingering

Simulators (nurses) performed well below brain-injured patients (Hayward et al., 1987). In addition, their performances included bizarre errors that were not made by patients.

COMMENT

Finger gnosis is an important aspect of various neurological disorders. It can occur as an isolated phenomenon and has also been described as one of the core features of Gerstmann's syndrome, along with right-left disorientation, dysgraphia, and dyscalculia. Benton's task recognizes that there may be different causes of finger recognition deficits. The availability of different response formats makes it unlikely that performance will be affected by even mild forms of aphasia. However, normative studies are dated and, in the case of adults, derive from samples of medical patients. The sample of children is poorly described. Additional studies of the psychometric properties of the task are needed. In particular, information regarding the various aspects of reliability is sparse. In addition, concurrent validity studies need to be conducted (Franzen, 2000).

Of note, the task can be adapted for use to detect callosal dysfunction, as in multiple sclerosis (Brown, 2003). The examiner may stimulate the finger on one hand and ask the patient to indicate the corresponding finger on the other hand. Interhemispheric transfer is implicated in crossed but not uncrossed localization, because tactile information from the stimulated hand must be transferred across the corpus callosum in order for the other hand to respond.

REFERENCES

Badian, N. A., McAnulty, G. B., Duffy, F. H., & Als, H. (1990). Prediction of dyslexia in kindergarten boys. *Annals of Dyslexia, 40*, 152–169.

Benton, A. L. (1955). Development of finger localization capacity in school children. *Child Development, 26*, 225–230.

Benton, A. L., Sivan, A. B., Hamsher, K. deS. Varney, & Spreen, O. (1994). *Contributions to neuropsychological assessment.* New York: Oxford University Press.

Brown, W. S. (2003). Clinical neuropsychological assessment of callosal dysfunction: Multiple sclerosis and dyslexia. In E. Zaidel & M. Iacoboni (Eds.). *The parallel brain: the cognitive neuroscience of the corpus callosum.* Cambridge, Mass.: MIT Press.

De Agostini, M., & Dellatoals, G. (2001). *Developmental Neuropsychology, 20,* 429–444.

Della Sala, S., & Spinnler, H. (1994). Finger agnosia: Fiction or reality. *Archives of Neurology, 51,* 448–449.

Franzen, M. D. (2000). *Reliability and validity in neuropsychological assessment* (2nd ed.). New York: Kluwer Academic/Plenum Publishers.

Gainotti, G., Cianchetti, C., & Tiacci, C. (1972). The influence of hemispheric side of lesions on non-verbal tasks of finger localization. *Cortex, 8,* 364–381.

Gainotti, G., & Tiacci, C. (1973). The unilateral forms of finger agnosia. *Confinia Neurologica, 35,* 271–284.

Gerstmann, J. (1924). Fingeragnosie: eine umschriebene Storung der Orientierung am eigener Korper. *Wiener klinische Wochenschrift, 37,* 1010–1012.

Hayward, L., Hall, W., Hunt, M., & Zubrick, S. R. (1987). Can localized brain impairment be simulated on neuropsychological test profiles? *Australian and New Zealand Journal of Psychiatry, 21,* 87–93.

Head, H. (1920). *Studies in neurology.* London: Oxford University.

Reitan, R. M., & Wolfson, D. (1985). *The Halstead-Reitan neuropsychological test battery: Theory and clinical interpretation.* Tuscon, Ariz.: Neuropsychology Press.

Russell, E. W., & Starkey, R. I. (1993). Halstead Russell Neuropsychological Evaluation System (HRNES-R). Los Angeles: Western Psychological Services.

Yeudall, L. T., Reddon, J. R., Gill, D. M., & Stefanyk, W. O. (1987). Normative data for the Haltead-Reitan neuropsychological tests stratified by age and sex. *Journal of Clinical Psychology, 43,* 346–367.

Right-Left Orientation (RLO)

PURPOSE

The Right-Left Orientation (RLO) test assesses the identification of left and right.

SOURCE

Benton's test is available from Psychological Assessment Resources (http://www.parinc.com) for $59 US. The manual (including 11 other tests) is published under the title *Contributions to Neuropsychological Assessment: A Clinical Manual* (Benton et al., 1994) and costs $39 US. Another version is included in the Parietal Lobe Battery of the Boston Diagnostic Aphasia Examination, described elsewhere in this volume.

AGE RANGE

Normative data are available for ages 16 to 64 years.

DESCRIPTION

The inability of some brain-damaged patients to discriminate the right and left sides of the body was first described in the 19th century and was thought to reflect an impairment in spatial thinking (Badal, 1988, Pick; 1908; Gerstmann, 1930; all cited in Benton et al., 1994). However, Head (1926, cited in Benton et al., 1994) regarded right-left disorientation as a form of defective symbolic thinking. Benton et al. (1994) consider both types of interpretation to be valid in the sense that both spatial and symbolic determinants enter into right-left discrimination performances.

Benton et al. (1994) described a 20-item form that requires the patient to point to lateral body parts on verbal command. The patient must point to body parts on the patient's own body and on the examiner's body (e.g., "Show me your left hand"; "Point to my right eye") and must perform double movements (e.g., "Touch your left ear with your right hand"; "Put your right hand on my left ear").

The task can be used with a wide variety of clients, because it makes no demands on naming ability and the motor skill required is minimal. An alternate form (Form B) is available, in which the commands in Form A are reversed (e.g., "Show me your right hand, . . . your left eye," and so on). In addition, modified versions for hemiplegic patients are also available (see Benton et al., 1994).

ADMINISTRATION

The patient is seated across a table from the examiner and given the instructions as laid out in the answer sheet. Emphasis should be given to the words "right" and "left."

Any item may be repeated once if the patient appears hesitant or requests the examiner to do so. No time limit is imposed.

APPROXIMATE TIME FOR ADMINISTRATION

The test requires about 5 min.

SCORING

Number Correct

A score of 1 is assigned to each item that is performed exactly as it appears on the answer sheet. Partially correct responses receive no credit. If the patient changes his or her answer before the next item is given, the changed answer is recorded. For erroneous responses, the patient's error is noted in the margin, next to the item.

Reversal Score

A reversal score of 1 is assigned to each item that is completely reversed in orientation. Reversal scores are given only if right and left are consistently reversed. The rationale for scoring re-

versals is that the examinee (especially a child) shows some consistent side discrimination, although the names ("right" and "left") are reversed. Dellatolas et al. (1998) confirmed the utility of reversal scores: in a sample of 294 schoolchildren aged 5 to 8 years who were given an abbreviated version of the task, those who made one to three errors (14% of the sample) scored significantly worse on a number of other tasks (e.g., word fluency, syntactic comprehension, number processing) than those who showed systematic reversal (30%) or those who made no errors.

Total Score

The total score is either the number of items performed correctly or the reversal score, whichever is higher.

DEMOGRAPHIC EFFECTS

Age

Usually, a child who answers correctly for single own-body commands also answers correctly for double own-body commands, a capacity that is acquired at about 6 to 7 years of age (Dellatolas et al., 1998); however, they usually make errors in identifying right and left on a confronting person (Benton et al., 1994; Dellatolas et al., 1998). The capacity to answer correctly for opposite-facing person commands usually is not acquired before 8 years of age (Dellatolas et al., 1998). Mastery of the confronting-person task is achieved by about the age of 12 to 13 years (Benton et al., 1994; Brito et al., 1998).

Gender

A number of authors (Benton et al. 1994; Brito et al., 1998; Dellatolas et al., 1998; Snyder, 1991) have reported no significant gender differences.

Education/IQ

Benton et al. (1994) reported no impact of educational level on this form. However, Kaszniak et al. (1979) reported a modest relation ($r = .33$) in patients with suspected dementia. The correlation with intelligence was only minimal in children (Clark & Klonoff, 1990; Brito et al., 1998). Brito et al. (1998) found that academic standing affected performance, with nonachieving Brazilian subjects performing worse than achievers.

Ethnicity/Other

Brito et al. (1998), using Benton's 20-item version with 398 5- to 14-year-old Brazilian children, reported that they showed a delay in the attainment of identification of single lateral parts of their own body and in executing uncrossed commands, when compared with North American children, but they caught up later, so that by age 11 their performance became indistinguishable from that of U.S. children. In this sample of

Table 13–5 Characteristics of Right-Left Orientation
Standardization Sample

Number	234
Age (years)	16-64 (mean age not reported)
Geographic location	Iowa (USA)
Sample type	Healthy persons or patients without a history or current evidence of brain disease
Education	NA
Gender	
Males	126
Females	108
Race/Ethnicity	Not reported
Screening	Patients with neurological disorders were excluded

children, ethnic group and an index of socioeconomic status (paternal occupation) had no impact on performance.

NORMATIVE DATA

Standardization Sample

The test was given to 234 people (126 men, 108 women) within the age range of 16 to 64 years who were either healthy or were patients without a history or current evidence of brain disease (Benton et al., 1994; see Table 13–5). The majority made perfect scores, and 96% made scores in the range of 17 to 20 points. A score of less than 17 was considered defective. Errors were few, and when they occurred they consisted mainly of misidentifications of a lateral body part of the confronting examiner (not of the self).

RELIABILITY

Test-Retest Reliability

Studies of reliability are scant. Sarazin and Spreen (1986) reported a 15-year (age 10–25) stability of .27 in learning-disabled subjects on an older, longer version of the Benton form. This low value, however, should be considered minimal, because it covers a large time span during development in an exceptional group.

VALIDITY

Relationships With Other Measures

The Benton form correlates highly (.63) with other measures that require identification of visually presented stimuli as right or left (Snyder, 1991).

Most authors point out that right-left discrimination is not a unitary function but involves conceptual abilities, spatial

orientation, and possibly hand preference (Benton et al., 1994). A relationship between the development of right-left orientation and handedness has been proposed on theoretical grounds, with the preferred hand acting as an internal reference point that the child uses to orient for right-left decision making (see Dellatolas et al., 1998, for review). However, the correlation between handedness and knowledge of right and left is low (Dellatolas et al., 1998; Snyder, 1991).

Correlation of the Benton form (this one and the earlier 32-item version) with intelligence was only minimal in children (Brito et al., 1998; Clark & Klonoff, 1990). However, in school-age children, nonachievers had significantly lower scores than achievers; in a principal component factor analysis, RLO performance was closely related to Human Figure Drawing, forming a factor of "human body representation" (Brito et al., 1998).

Clinical Findings

Right-left confusion is often affected by left parietal damage (McFie & Zangwill, 1960; Semmes et al., 1960; Sauguet et al., 1971). In line with these findings, Benton et al. (1994) noted that right-left disorientation with respect to one's own body is uncommon in patients who are not aphasic or demented. If one considers only the confronting-person parts of the test, 43% of aphasic and only 4% of nonaphasic left-hemisphere patients, but also 16% of nonaphasic right-hemisphere patients fail this part. Hence, the left parietal lobe hypothesis does not seem to apply to opposing-body parts of the test, which may require more mental rotation and spatial thinking.

Patients with dementia have difficulty with the task (Benton et al., 1994). Orientation on one's own body is not affected in the early stages of the disorder; but mild and moderately impaired patients make significantly more errors than controls when mental rotation is required (Kalman et al., 1995). Fischer et al. (1990) also found that right-left orientation (using Benton's 20-item version on a confronting doll instead of the drawing) was more impaired in elderly inpatients with dementia of the Alzheimer type, compared with 18 inpatients with multi-infarct dementia and 16 normal controls; impairment was also significantly related to the severity of dementia.

The close relationship of right-left orientation to the Gerstmann syndrome and to aphasia has been pointed out (Benton, 1979, 1984; Benton et al., 1994). However, impaired right-left orientation in combination with other components of the Gerstmann syndrome has also been reported in patients who were not aphasic. For example, Grigsby et al. (1987) reported the case of an 8-year-old boy with fragile X syndrome who showed the full syndrome (dyscalculia, poor right-left orientation, dysgraphia, finger agnosia, constructional dyspraxia) in the absence of aphasia.

Right-left orientation is also low in those with learning disorders (Spreen, 1988) and in children with attention disorders. In a study of Brazilian schoolchildren with a mean age of 9.4 years, Brito et al. (1999) contrasted a subgroup of hyperactive/impulsive children and one of inattentive children with normal classmates. On Benton's RLO, the groups showed means of 10.3, 9.9, and 12.3, respectively. Only the difference between normal subjects and inattentive children was significant for this test.

COMMENT

The task is brief and easy to administer and is suitable for individuals with language impairments. Further, the demands on motor skills are minimal, and many hemiparetic patients are able to execute the commands with the affected arm (Benton et al., 1994). However, norms are not available for adults aged 65 years and older. In addition, information on reliability is very limited. With regard to validity, the test appears sensitive to some developmental disorders. In adults, right-left disorientation is uncommon in patients who are not aphasic or demented.

REFERENCES

Benton, A. L. (1979). Body-schema disturbances: Right-left orientation and finger localization. In K. M. Heilman & E. Valenstein (Eds.), *Clinical neuropsychology.* New York: Oxford University Press.

Benton, A. L. (1984). Dyslexia and spatial thinking. *Annals of Dyslexia, 34,* 69–85.

Benton, A. L., Sivan, A. B., Hamsher, K. deS., Varney, N. R., & Spreen, O. (1994). *Contributions to neuropsychological assessment: A clinical manual* (2nd ed.). Orlando, Fla.: Psychological Assessment Resources.

Brito, G.N., Alfradique, G. M. N., Pereira, C. C. S., Porto, C. M. B., & Santos, T. R. (1998). Developmental norms for eight instruments used in the neuropsychological assessment of children: Studies in Brazil. *Brazilian Journal of Medical and Biological Research, 31,* 399–412.

Brito, G. N., Pereira, C., & Santos-Morales, T. R. (1999). Behavioral and neuropsychological correlates of hyperactivity and inattention in Brazilian school children. *Developmental Medicine and Child Neurology, 41,* 732–739.

Clark, C., & Klonoff, H. (1990). Right and left orientation in children aged five to thirteen years. *Journal of Clinical and Experimental Neuropsychology, 12,* 459–466.

Dellatolas, G., Viguier, D., Deloche, G., & De Agostini, M. (1998). Right-left orientation and significance of systematic reversal in children. *Cortex, 34,* 659–676.

Fischer, P., Marterer, A., & Danielczyk, W. (1990). Right-left disorientation in dementia of the Alzheimer type. *Neurology, 40,* 1619–1620.

Grigsby, J. P., Service, D., Kemper, M. B., & Hageman, R. J. (1987). Developmental Gerstmann syndrome without aphasia in fragile-X syndrome. *Neuropsychologia, 25,* 881–891.

Kalman, J., Magloczky, E., & Janka, Z. (1995). Disturbed visuo-spatial orientation in the early stage of Alzheimer's dementia. *Archives of Gerontology and Geriatrics, 21,* 27–34.

Kaszniak, A. W., Garron, D. C., Fox, J. H., Bergen, D., & Huckman, M.. (1979). Cerebral atrophy, EEG slowing, age, education, and cognitive functioning in suspected dementia. *Neurology, 29,* 1273–1279.

McFie, J., & Zangwill, O. L. (1960). Visual-constructive disabilities associated with lesions of the left hemisphere. *Brain, 83,* 243–260.

Sanders, R. D., Keshaven, M. S., Forman, S. D., Pieri, J. N., McLaughlin, N., Allen, D. N., van Kammen D. P., & Goldstein, G. (2000). Factor structure of neurologic examination abnormalities in unmedicated schizophrenia. *Psychiatry Research, 95,* 237–243.

Sarazin, F., & Spreen, O. (1986). Fifteen year reliability of some neuropsychological tests in learning disabled subjects with and without neurological impairment. *Journal of Clinical and Experimental Neuropsychology, 8,* 190–200.

Sauguet, J., Benton, A. L., & Hecaen, H. (1971). Disturbances of the body schema in relation to language impairment and hemispheric locus of lesion. *Journal of Neurology, Neurosurgery and Psychiatry, 34,* 496–501.

Semmes, J., Weinstein, S., Ghent, L., & Teuber, H. L. (1960). *Somatosensory changes after penetrating brain wounds in man.* Cambridge, Mass.: Harvard University Press.

Snyder, T. J. (1991). Self-rated right-left confusability and objectively measured right-left discrimination. *Developmental Neuropsychology, 7,* 219–230.

Spreen, O. (1988). *Learning disabled children growing up.* New York: Oxford University Press.

Rivermead Assessment of Somatosensory Performance (RASP)

PURPOSE

The purpose of the Rivermead Assessment of Somatosensory Performance (RASP) is to assess somatosensory loss associated with neurological disturbances.

SOURCE

The test can be ordered from Harcourt Assessment (http://www.harcourt-uk.com), at a cost of about $333 US.

AGE RANGE

Norms are based on adults, aged 24 to 80 years.

DESCRIPTION

The RASP (Winward et al., 2000) is a standardized procedure to assess a range of somatosensory functions traditionally considered important for clinical assessment. It covers a representative range of body areas, including the cheeks of the face, the palms, the backs of the hands, the top of the feet, and the bottom of each big toe. It consists of seven subtests (see Table 13–6), which can be divided into five primary ones (Sharp/Dull Discrimination, Surface Pressure Touch, Surface Localization, Temperature Discrimination, and Movement and Direction Proprioception Discrimination) and two secondary ones (Sensory Extinction and Two-Point Discrimination). The subtests are given with the

Table 13–6 RASP Subtests

Task	Description
1. Sharp/dull discrimination	Two Neurometers, one with a sharp and one with a dull end, are applied in a pseudorandom sequence over all 10 skin regions; the patient is asked whether the stimulus is sharp or dull
2. Surface pressure	The Neurometer is applied over all 10 regions, and the patient is asked whether he or she felt a touch.
3. Surface localization	The Neurometer is used to apply stimuli to all 10 regions; after each stimulus, the patient must identify where he or she was touched.
4. Sensory extinction (bilateral touch discrimination)	The regions tested include the face and the backs of both hands. On this subtest, patients are touched on one side or touched simultaneously on both sides. After each trial, the patient indicates whether he or she was touched once or twice.
5. Two-point discrimination	The Neurodisc is applied to the index fingertip: the subject must indicate whether one or two points were felt. The two-point stimulus of 3 mm is applied first. If the subject cannot feel two points reliably, discrimination is tested at 4 mm and then, if failed, at 5 mm.
6. Temperature discrimination	The hot and cold Neurotemps are placed on various body regions, and the patient indicates whether the touch was warm or cold
7. Proprioception movement and direction discrimination	The subtest is given on the following joints of the left and right sides: elbow, wrists, thumbs or fingers, ankles, and toes. The joint is passively moved, and the subject indicates whether movement was detected and in which direction, up or down.

patient's eyes closed. There is a preferred order of subtest administration. However, not all subtests need be given to a particular client.

In addition to providing a detailed procedure, the RASP includes several instruments (Neurometer, Neurotemp, and Two-Point Neurodisc) that are used to standardize test procedures. For example, the Neurometer (a pen-shaped device) is used to test sharp/dull discrimination, surface pressure touch, surface localization, and sensory extinction; it is calibrated so that it produces the same amount of pressure on each trial. The Neurotemps are two paddle-shaped instruments with plastic handles, one red (warm) and one blue (cold), encasing copper discs. The handles contain liquid crystal temperature displays that are kept within specific ranges (cold, 6–10 °C; warm, 44–49 °C). The Two-Point Neurodisc is a four-pointed, fixed-distance discriminator that is used to establish the extent of two-point discrimination. The three fixed two-point distances are 3, 4, and 5 mm; the Neurodisc also has a single point.

ADMINISTRATION

Administration requires the scoring sheet, the instruments, and knowledge of the 10 application areas (5 left and 5 right) displayed on the body reference chart in the appendix of the manual. The 10 regions represent areas on the face, hands, and feet. Note that four of the application areas require access to the feet. The Neurotemps should be prepared before the test session; the red Neurotemp must be immersed in hot water and the blue in cold water.

For each subtest, the examiner moves from the unaffected to the affected side, head to feet. There are six trials per test area. Patients may respond verbally, use hand signals, or point to descriptors on cards.

The authors include a series of "sham" trials on two of the five primary subtests (Sharp/Dull Discrimination and Surface Pressure Touch), in order to help identify (and possibly exclude) those patients whose performance may be unreliable (e.g., because of fatigue, confusion, or suggestibility). A "sham" or "catch" trial is one in which the examiner pretends to give a stimulus when in fact none is applied to the patient. There are two sham trials per region. The authors suggest that 2 or fewer responses to sham trials is normal, 3 to 5 sham responses is mild, 6 to 8 sham responses is moderate, and 8 to 10 sham responses is severe, suggesting that the patient's responding is unreliable.

APPROXIMATE TIME FOR ADMINISTRATION

The seven subtests take about 25 to 35 min to administer.

SCORING

Scores for each subtest are recorded on specific tables provided on the score sheet. For each stimulus correctly identified, the subject is awarded a score of 1; therefore, within each test area, the patient can score a maximum of 6 points. Most subtests have a possible total of 60 points; however, Sensory Extinction has a total of 12 possible points, and Two-Point Discrimination is recorded as pass/fail. Shams are scored separately. In the case of sham trials, false-positive responses are scored as 1, and the maximum for each test region is 2.

DEMOGRAPHIC EFFECTS

No information is provided regarding the influence of demographic variables such as age and gender.

NORMATIVE DATA

Standardization Sample

The test was standardized on 50 patients with left-hemisphere strokes and 50 with right-hemisphere strokes. The patients with left-sided damage (27 males, 23 females) were about 6 weeks post-stroke and ranged in age from 23 to 96 years ($M = 64$, $SD = 15.6$). The patients with right-hemisphere strokes (26 males, 24 females) were about 5 weeks post-injury and ranged in age from 35 to 85 years ($M = 64$, $SD = 15.4$). A control group of 50 non-brain-damaged individuals (age $M = 60.0$ years, $SD = 12.7$) was also included (see Table 13–7); they generally performed at about ceiling level on most tasks. Based on the performance of the patients and controls, the authors provided recommended cutoff values for inferring impairment of one side.

RELIABILITY

Test-Retest Reliability and Practice Effects

Winward et al. (2002) tested 12 stroke patients on two separate occasions with an average interval of 30 days. Test-retest reliability was high ($r > .80$) for all of the primary subtests except Proprioceptive Direction, which was low ($r = .50$; see Table 13–8). Information regarding the two secondary tasks (Extinction and Two-Point Discrimination) is not provided.

Table 13–7 Characteristics of the RASP Normative Sample

Number	50
Age (years)	24–80
Geographic location	United Kingdom
Sample type	Hospital employees and volunteers from the local community
Education	Not reported
Gender	
Male	21
Female	29
Race/Ethnicity	Not reported
Screening	Not reported

Table 13–8 RASP Test-Retest Correlations

Magnitude of Coefficient	Measure
Very High (≥.90)	Surface pressure touch
	Surface localization
High (.80 to .89)	Sharp/dull
	Temperature
	Proprioceptive movement
Adequate (.70 to .79)	
Marginal (.60 to .69)	
Low (≤.59)	Proprioceptive direction

Note: Sensory extinction was not reported.

Source: Adapted from Winward et al., 2002.

Nor is information provided regarding practice effects on any of the subtests.

Interrater Reliability

The performances of 15 patients were scored independently by two different raters and one of the test authors. Reliability was found to be high, .92 (Winward et al., 2000, 2002).

VALIDITY

In terms of face and content validity, the RASP appears acceptable because all the subtests were adapted from traditional tests. Further, scores on the subtests had moderately high correlations with each another ($r = .37$ to $.89$) in stroke cases, suggesting that the battery measures a range of related phenomena (Winward et al., 2002).

Criterion-related validity was established by evaluating patients with single right- or left-hemisphere strokes as well as age-matched normal controls (Winward et al., 2000; 2002). Patients scored significantly worse than controls, and the RASP detected somatosensory impairment on the side contralateral to the lesion. Based on these data, cutoff scores are presented in the manual.

In general, RASP scores (except for Proprioception Movement and Direction) show little relation with motoric ability or activities of daily living (Winward et al., 2002).

COMMENT

Winward et al. (2000, 2002) noted that somatosensory assessment is often neglected after stroke despite the fact that such impairments are found in more than 50% of stroke patients and can have a significant impact on everyday activities. The RASP is a new test that is relatively short, is easy to administer, and provides a quantifiable assessment of somatosensory functioning. The development of customized test instruments is also a positive feature.

The inclusion of sham trials is a novel feature to enhance reliability. Although the sham trials attempt to mimic real trials, the difference in the proximity of the sound of the Neurometer's depression is noticeable for the real versus the sham trials when applied to the face. That is, patients may use sound (and not somatosensory sensation) to differentiate real and sham trials.[1]

In addition, it is unfortunate that the Temperature Discrimination subtest is not the first task given, because of the difficulty involved in attaining and maintaining the correct temperature ranges. Administration may require a hot-water thermos and a glass of ice to maintain hot and cold temperatures of the Neurotemps.

With regard to psychometric properties, interrater reliability is good. Test-retest reliability appears high for all primary subtests except Proprioceptive Direction; however, the extent of any practice effects are not reported, nor is test-retest information presented for the two supplementary tasks. In the absence of such information, interpretation of change is difficult. Information regarding internal consistency is also lacking.

Users should note that no data are provided regarding the influence of variables (e.g., age, gender, cognitive dysfunction) that might affect performance. In addition, there are ceiling effects in normal adults on all tasks, which would make it difficult to detect subtle disturbances. The validity of summing scores across body parts also needs to be evaluated (Winward et al., 2002).

Although the battery is fairly comprehensive, it is important to bear in mind that not all dimensions of somatosensory function are assessed (e.g., form recognition is not evaluated). Depending on the diagnostic issue, users may need to supplement with other tasks. Finally, the test authors point out that it is not clear whether all tests are necessary or whether some are redundant (Winward et al., 2002). The high correlation between some test scores (e.g., Proprioceptive Movement and Direction) suggests that it may be possible to reduce the number of tests administered.

NOTE

1. We thank Megan O'Connell for alerting us to some of the issues outlined here.

REFERENCES

Winward, C. E., Halligan, P. W., & Wade, D. T. (2000). *Rivermead Assessment of Somatosensory Performance Manual.* Bury St. Edmunds, England: Thames Valley Test Company.

Winward, C. E., Halligan, P. W., & Wade, D. T. (2002). The Rivermead Assessment of Somatosensory Performance (RASP): Standardization and reliability data. *Clinical Rehabilitation, 16,* 523–533.

Smell Identification Test (SIT)

OTHER TEST NAME

The Smell Identification Test (SIT) is also known as the University of Pennsylvania Smell Identification Test (UPSIT).

PURPOSE

The purpose of this test is to measure olfaction.

SOURCE

The 40-item SIT, including a manual, a set of 7 single-administration test booklets, and a scoring key, is available through Sensonics (http://www.smelltest.com) at a cost of $26.45 US. The manual is also available in French, German, and Spanish. A 12-item Brief Smell Identification Test (B-SIT) and a 3-item Pocket Smell Test (PST) are also sold. The 40-item SIT can also be ordered from Psychological Assessment Resources (PAR), Inc., P.O. Box 998, Odessa, FL 33556 (http://www.parinc.com).

AGE RANGE

The normative base ranges in age from 5 to 99 years.

DESCRIPTION

Assessment of smell is important, because olfactory disturbances can affect quality of life (e.g., interest in and desire for food) and can place the individual, as well as others, at risk (e.g., from toxic fumes). Further, impaired smell may signal neurological compromise, serving as an early warning of further decline (e.g., Alzheimer's disease [AD]).

The SIT is the most widely used tool for measuring olfactory dysfunction. The 40-item standard version of the test (Doty, 1995) consists of a set of four envelope-sized booklets, each containing 10 "scratch and sniff" above-threshold odorants embedded on brown strips. The stimuli are released by scratching the strips with a pencil tip. Above each odorant is a multiple-choice array with four alternative responses. For example, one of the items reads: "This odor smells most like: (a) chocolate; (b) banana; (c) onion; or (d) fruit punch." The respondent marks one of the four alternatives, even if no smell sensation is perceived. The score is the number of items correctly answered.

According to Doty (1995), the standard version allows for detection of more extreme as well as subtle impairments. The 12-item B-SIT is useful for screening smell impairments when less than 5 min of time is available. The B-SIT was designed to include odors that are easily recognized by persons from a variety of cultures. Accordingly, it is also the version more appropriate for use outside North America. The 3-item PST provides for a very gross screen. Doty (1995) recommends that, if a patient fails one or more of the three PST items, the standard version should be given to more accurately quantify the degree of loss.

ADMINISTRATION

The test was designed to be self-administered. Instructions are printed on the face page of the first of four booklets and should be read by or to the examinee before beginning the test. In order to release stimuli, it is important to emphasize to the examinee that the strip should be marked with a few strong strokes of the pencil tip across the strip's entire width (e.g., wide letter "z") and that the label should be sniffed immediately after it has been scratched to ensure that the odor has not significantly dissipated. Individuals are allowed unlimited time to respond. The test booklets should be given in chronological order. Although the test is typically administered to both nostrils, unilateral olfactory testing may be of value, such as in the detection of some types of tumors or in temporal lobe epilespy (TLE). Normative data for such an administration are available (see *Normative Data*). For unirhinal SIT administration, one nostril is occluded using a suitably sized piece of tape (3M Company) across that nostril. Two books (20 items) are presented to each nostril, leading to two scores, each out of a possible 20.

ADMINISTRATION TIME

The complete version takes about 10 to 15 min; brief versions take less than 5 min.

SCORING

The maximum possible score is 40 on the standard SIT. A person's score is compared with those from normal individuals of equivalent age and gender. Test scores are converted to percentiles.

DEMOGRAPHIC EFFECTS

Age

Performance improves during childhood, with adult levels appearing at about age 15 years. Performance is generally stable through middle adulthood, with scores declining after about age 60 years on both the standard (Doty, 1995; Doty et al., 1984a, 1984b; Frank et al., 2003; Minor et al., 2004; Ship & Weiffenbach, 1993) and the B-SIT (Doty, 2001) versions. The age-related decline is more marked among males (Doty et al., 1984b).

Gender

Females perform better than males on both the standard and brief versions (Doty, 1995, 2001; Doty et al., 1984a, 1985; Ship & Weiffenbach, 1993; Ship et al., 1996; but see Frank et al., 2003). The gender effect transcends cultural differences. Gender does not affect unirhinal performance (Good et al., 2003).

Education

Education shows a small correlation with SIT scores (Good et al., 2003). Those with no secondary education identify about one odor less per nostril.

Race/Ethnicity

Korean Americans outperform African and Causasian Americans who, in turn, outperform Native Japanese on the SIT (Doty et al., 1985).

Smoking

Smoking does impair performance (Doty et al., 1984b; Frye et al., 1990; Good et al., 2003; McLean et al., 2004; Minor et al., 2004) although it may have a "normalizing" effect in some patients with psychosis (McLean et al., 2004). Smoking interacts with educational status. Among individuals with no secondary education, smokers on average identify one odor less per nostril (Good et al., 2003).

NORMATIVE DATA

Standard Version—Standardization Sample

Percentile norms are based on the administration of the SIT to 1819 men and 2109 women, ranging in age from 5 to 85+. The description of the normative sample is sparse (see Table 13–9).

In general, after the age of 15 years, raw test scores higher than 34 in men and 35 in women suggest normal smell functioning, scores between 30 and 33/34 indicate mild difficulties (mild microsmia), those between 26 and 29/30 suggest moderate difficulties (moderate microsmia), and those

Table 13–9 Characteristics of the 40-Item SIT Normative Sample

Number	3928
Age (years)	5 to 85+[a]
Geographic location	Not reported
Sample type	Not reported
Education	Not reported
Gender	
Male	1819
Female	2109
Race/Ethnicity	Not reported
Screening	Not reported

[a]Broken down by gender and age; there are 17 5-year age bands, with 60–232 individuals per age band.

between 6 and 25 suggest severe difficulties (severe microsmia–anosmia), whereas scores of 5 and lower raise the concern of malingering.

Other Normative Data

Lower scores emerge when the test is given unirhinally. Good et al. (2003) provided unirhinal norms based on a sample of 270 healthy individuals, aged 15 to 64. Approximately 60% were male, 90% were right-handed, and 17% were current smokers. The mean education level was 15 years. The data are

shown in Table 13–10. Because of the effects of education and smoking on performance, Good et al. (2003) recommended adding 1 point to raw scores for each nostril for nonsmokers with no postsecondary education, and 2 points for smokers with no postsecondary education, before classifying performance according to these norms.

Table 13–11 presents data summarizing the distribution of internostril discrepancies (left minus right) within each age group. No correction is necessary in employing these norms. A laterality quotient was also computed to examine nostril asymmetry in order to correct for baseline effects (Left SIT – Right SIT)/(Left SIT + Right SIT). Despite a right nostril/right hemisphere advantage for olfactory discrimination (Good et al., 2002; Zatorre & Jones-Gotman, 1991), no lateral asymmetry was observed in unirhinal SIT scores.

B-SIT—Standardization Sample

A group of 198 healthy adults (83 men, mean age about 41 years; 115 women, mean age about 44 years) were given the B-SIT. Their mean responses on the 12 B-SIT items were compared with the mean of the 12 analogous SIT scores. Because the means and distributions of test scores were comparable, Doty (2001) employed the SIT database to establish B-SIT norms. Percentile ranks are provided for males and females for each 5-year age category ranging from age 5 to more than 84 years. In general, scores lower than 9 suggest abnormality for individuals 10 years and older.

Table 13–10 Descriptive Statistics for Unirhinal Performance on the SIT, by Age

	15–24		25–34		35–44		45–54		55–64		All Subjects	
	Right	Left	Right	Left	Right	Left	Right	Left	Right	Left	Right	Left
Mean[a]	16.9	17.0	17.5	17.7	16.8	17.4	16.9	16.9	16.0	16.4	16.9	17.2
SEM	0.21	0.29	0.22	0.20	0.30	0.33	0.26	0.26	0.45	0.35	0.13	0.13
Median	17	18	18	18	17	18	17	17	16	17	17	18
SD	1.62	2.26	1.91	1.68	2.07	2.32	1.81	1.80	2.83	2.19	2.06	2.06
5%	14	13	13	15	13	12	13	14	10	12	13	13
10%	15	14	15	16	13	13	15	14	11	12	14	14
25%	16	16	17	17	15	16	16	16	14	16	16	16
50%	17	18	18	18	17	18	17	17	16	17	17	18
75%	18	19	19	19	18	19	18	18	18	18	18	19
90%	19	19	19	20	19	20	19	19	19	19	19	19
95%	19	19	20	20	20	20	19	20	20	19	20	20

Note: Adjustment formula for raw scores:

Education	Smoker	Nonsmoker
≤12 years	+2	+1
≥13 years	0	0

[a]Mean score out of a possible 20.

Source: Good et al., 2003. Reprinted with the kind permission of Psychology Press.

Table 13–11 Distribution of Internostril Discrepancy Scores With Recommended Cutoffs for the SIT, by Age

	15–24	25–34	35–44	45–54	55–64	All Subjects
Mean (L-R)	0.03	0.23	0.63	0	0.44	0.25
SE of mean	0.30	0.23	0.32	0.30	0.39	0.13
SD	2.32	2.00	2.27	2.12	2.49	2.22
LQ[a]	−0.019	0.007	0.017	0.0001	0.0168	0.0073
L > R, 5%	4	3	5	4	4	4
L > R, 10%	4	3	4	3	3	3
R > L, 5%	4	3	3	3	3	3
R > L, 10%	3	2	2	3	3	2

[a]LQ (Laterality Quotient) = [Left UPSIT − Right UPSIT]/[Left UPSIT + Right UPSIT].

Source: Good et al., 2003. Reprinted with the kind permission of Psychology Press.

RELIABILITY

Internal Consistency

According to the test author (Doty, 1995, 2001; Doty et al., 1989), split-half reliability coefficients are high for the standard version (about $r = .93$) and acceptable for the B-SIT ($r = .71$). The different booklets of the SIT correlate highly with one another (median $r = .92$) and with the overall SIT score (median $r = .85$), suggesting that they can be used, in appropriate instances, independently (Doty et al., 1989).

Recently, Minor et al. (2004), using item-response theory, found that the items of the SIT measured a single construct of olfactory ability in healthy controls and in chronically medicated outpatients with schizophrenia. Examination of item difficulty, however, revealed that the test did not incorporate enough difficult items to obtain accurate measurement in the upper range of olfactory identification. On the other hand, normal controls showed a highly skewed distribution, supporting the test's utility in detecting odor-identification deficits in otherwise healthy populations.

Test-Retest Reliability

For the standard version, this is reported to be high, both over short intervals of 2 weeks or less ($r = .91$ to .95; Doty, 1995; Frank et al., 2003) and for tests administered 6 or more months apart ($r = .92$; Doty, 1995). For the B-SIT, test-retest reliability is lower, though still adequate (.71), when the test is given on two test occasions separated by at least 1 week (Doty, 2001).

VALIDITY

Relationships With Other Measures

Correlations between scores on the SIT and detection threshold tests are on the order of .80 and higher (Doty, 1995; Doty et al., 1984b). Frank et al. (2003) reported that the test correlated moderately well with other olfactory detection measures. However, it should be noted that SIT impairment (i.e., identification deficits) can occur in the context of normal detection ability (e.g., Jones-Gotman & Zatorre, 1988).

Relationships Between the SIT and Short Forms

The short form (B-SIT) correlates highly with the long form in patients with schizophrenia (.85) and in comparison individuals (.83; Goudsmit et al., 2004).

Ability Levels

According to the SIT manual, scores can separate individuals into five levels: normosmia, mild microsmia, moderate microsmia, severe microsmia, and total anosmia (see *Normative Data*). However, Minor et al. (2004) evaluated normal subjects and patients with schizophrenia, using Rasch analysis, and found support for only three ability levels, roughly corresponding to Doty's normosmia (normal olfactory ability), microsmia (decreased olfactory ability), and anosmia (complete inability to perceive qualitative odors).

Neuroanatomical Correlates

The olfactory system is unique in that primary afferents from the olfactory bulb synapse directly on cortical processing areas within the pyriform and entorhinal cortices (Fulbright et al., 1998). The vast majority of the projections remain ipsilateral (Cinelli & Kauer, 1992; Doty & Snow, 1987). Secondary projections reach orbital frontal regions either directly or indirectly through the mediodorsal nucleus of the thalamus (Potter & Nauta, 1979; Qureshy et al., 2000). Other brain regions associated with olfactory processing include the anterior cingulate (Qureshy et al., 2000), the insula (Zatorre et al., 1992), the amygdala (Zald & Pardo, 1997), the cuneus (Royet et al., 1999), and possibly the cerebellum (Dade et al., 1998; Yousem et al., 1997). It should be noted that olfactory projections are not completely unilateral: smell information arriving at one hemisphere crosses to the other via the anterior commissure, the corpus callosum, and possibly the hippocampal commissure (Postolache et al., 1999).

Clinical Studies

Olfactory deficits, as measured by the SIT, have been found in a number of disorders known to affect these regions. Deficits have been reported in schizophrenia (e.g., Good et al., 2002; Goudsmit et al., 2004; Kohler et al., 2001; Kopala et al., 1994; Malaspina & Coleman, 2003; Minor et al., 2004; Moberg et al., 1997; Stedman & Clair, 1998), MS (Doty et al., 1984b, 1999), Kallman's syndrome (Doty et al., 1984b), Parkinson's disease (e.g., Busenbark et al., 1992; Doty et al., 1988, 1991, 1995; Hawkes et al., 1997; Wenning et al., 1995), cerebellar hereditary ataxia (Fernandez-Ruiz et al., 2004), essential tremor (Louis et al., 2002; but see Busenbark et al., 1992), Huntington's disease (Bylsma et al., 1997), Korsakoff's syndrome (Doty et al., 1984b; Mair et al., 1986), chronic alcohol use (Ditraglia et al., 1991), vascular dementia (Gray et al., 2001), Down's syndrome (Hemdal et al., 1993), ADHD-inattentive type (Gansler et al., 1998) and in HIV+ individuals (Brody et al., 1991; Westervelt et al., 1997).

Olfactory impairment is evident in patients who have undergone unilateral temporal or frontal lobectomy, but not after a frontal lobe excision sparing the orbital cortex nor after left parietal or central area lesions (Jones-Gotman & Zatorre, 1988). The impairment is greater after frontal versus temporal lobectomy, emphasizing the importance of the orbitofrontal cortex to complex olfactory processing (Jones-Gotman & Zatorre, 1988). In nonoperated cases, patients with right-sided (but not left-sided) TLE exhibit significant impairment on the SIT, consistent with the notion of greater reliance of olfactory processing on right hemisphere structures (Kohler et al., 2001).

Olfactory impairments are also prominent in patients with AD (e.g., Doty et al., 1987, 1988; Gray et al., 2001; Moberg et al., 1997; Morgan et al., 1995), as might be expected given the temporal-limbic involvement in this condition. The ability to identify odors is affected early in AD, whereas the ability to detect odors is affected later (Serby et al., 1991). Olfactory identification deficits are also evident in those with mild cognitive impairment and are predictive of the development of AD over a 2-year interval (Devanand et al., 2000; see also Royall et al., 2002). In such individuals, olfactory loss accompanied by lack of awareness of olfactory identification deficits predicts AD independent of measures of attention, memory, and general cognitive status (e.g., modified MMSE; Devanand et al., 2000).

Cross-sectional studies reveal age-related declines in olfactory identification (see *Demographic Effects*). Longitudinal studies also reveal decline with age. Over a 3-year period, scores begin to worsen significantly by age 55 (particularly in men), reaching an estimated decrease of 1 SIT point per year in both men and women in their 80s (Ship et al., 1996). The age-related declines occur even in the absence of overt medical conditions.

A number of authors have reported an increased incidence of anosmia after head trauma. For example, Callahan and Hinkebein (2002) gave the SIT to 122 adults diagnosed with traumatic brain injury (TBI; 49% severe, 16% moderate, 35% mild) and found that 56% exhibited impairment on the full SIT. The risk of postinjury anosmia increases with injury severity: The more severe the injury, the more severe the olfactory deficit. Further, about 40% of these subjects were unaware of their deficit.

Whether olfactory performance is affected by depression is uncertain. Some find no deficits in those diagnosed with depression (e.g., Kopala et al., 1994; Postolache et al., 1999). However, a negative relationship has been reported between severity of depression and right nostril olfactory performance (Postolache et al., 1999).

Odor identification may not only indicate olfactory function but may also signify cognitive disturbance, because individuals with olfactory deficits often demonstrate cognitive deficits, particularly memory deficits (e.g., Good et al., 2002; Gray et al., 2001; Royall et al., 2002; Stedman & Clair, 1998). For example, Good et al (2002) examined patients with schizophrenia and reported an association between SIT and memory test scores (e.g., RAVLT, BVRT). Similarly, Royall et al. (2002) examined elderly retirees and found that verbal memory impairment was associated with anosmia as defined by the SIT, consistent with a mesiotemporal disorder. A relationship between executive function and odor identification has been observed less consistently. Brewer et al. (1996) noted a relationship between SIT ability and performance on the modified WCST in patients with schizophrenia and controls. Others, however, have failed to find a relationship between olfactory deficits and executive dysfunction (verbal and design fluency; e.g., Good et al., 2002). Thus, odor identification may relate to certain executive processes and not others.

In addition to short-term memory, the SIT relies on lexical functioning, because the person must recognize and select the name of the previously smelled odor from a list—a task that requires semantic categorization (Nagy & Loveland, 2001). However, odor identification deficits do not appear to be entirely due to cognitive problems (Doty et al., 1984b; Frank et al., 2003; Mair et al., 1986). For example, Morgan et al. (1995) investigated the impact of lexical functioning on odor identification in patients with probable AD. They showed that patients obtained poorer scores on the SIT than on a Picture Identification Test, a task identical to the SIT except that the subject is required to match a picture instead of an odor to one of four verbal descriptors. Further, the odor identification deficit in patients was evident when a picture-based odor identification task was used; that is, odor identification continued to be poor even when lexical demands were eliminated.

Ecological Validity

Olfactory deficits on the SIT (as well as the B-SIT) are linked to social dysfunction in schizophrenia, suggesting that they may share a common pathophysiology (Goudsmit et al., 2004). There is also evidence that deficits in grooming and hygiene (including poor body odor) observed in patients experiencing a first-episode of schizophrenia are associated with an impairment in left-nostril (possibly left-hemisphere) olfactory processing (Szezko et al., 2004).

Although some (Martzke et al., 1991; Varney, 1988) have asserted that anosmia (tested coarsely) after TBI is predictive of vocational dysfunction, Correia et al. (2001) failed to confirm the claim. Only 7% of their sample of patients with mild to moderate TBI and SIT scores indicative of anosmia (and nonmalingering) were vocationally dysfunctional.

Short Forms

Impairment on the B-SIT has been reported in Parkinson's disease (Double et al., 2003). Disturbance has also been reported in those with mild cognitive impairment (MCI), particularly in individuals with the APOE ε4 allele (Wang et al., 2002). The implication is that the decreased olfactory functioning in MCI may be a marker for the early diagnosis of AD, and the APOE genotype may be part of the basis of olfactory identification decline.

In line with this proposal (and consistent with the literature for the full SIT), there is evidence that olfactory impairment assessed on the B-SIT increases the risk of future cognitive decline in healthy older adults. B-SIT scores predicted decline in verbal memory in nondemented older adults 2 to 4.5 years after initial testing (Graves et al., 1999; Swan & Carmelli, 2002). Those with a combination of being anosmic at testing and carrying the APOE ε4 allele appear to be at particularly high risk of cognitive decline. Normal elderly people who are anosmic at baseline and carry at least one ε4 allele have been shown to have almost five times greater risk of developing cognitive decline over 2 years, compared with controls without these risk factors (Graves et al., 1999). The B-SIT classified people with cognitive decline better than a global cognitive test did (Graves et al., 1999).

On the 3-item screening measure, missing even one item was associated with a 2:1 likelihood of being anosmic in a sample of individuals with TBI (Callahan & Hinkbein (2002). However, Callahan and Hinkebein advised caution in the use of this screening measure, because almost 20% of patients performing perfectly on the 3-item screen scored in the anosmic range on the full UPSIT.

Malingering

Doty et al. (1984b) asked 158 healthy individuals to feign "total" anosmia on the SIT. The modal number correct was zero. Because one fourth of the items should be correctly identified on the basis of chance alone, an anosmic should score on average 10/40 on the test. Therefore, based on simple probability, the chance of an anosmic obtaining a score of 5 or less is .05. Although such low scores may well characterize blatant

forms of malingering, the impact of more subtle forms of dissimulation remains to be determined.

Doty et al. (1998) suggested that the density of marking of the sandpaper may also prove useful in detecting malingerers. This proposal remains to be evaluated.

COMMENT

The SIT is a widely used tool for the assessment of olfactory function. It is portable, rapid, and easy to administer and to score and can be used with a wide spectrum of patients. The reagents are relatively stable and, as a result, the test booklets have a reasonably long shelf-life. Doty (1995) recommended that test booklets more than 2 years old not be used, in order to ensure that test validity is maintained. An additional feature of the SIT is that it provides a gross index of malingering. Further, the normative sample is large, although the description of the sample is sparse. Unirhinal normative data also exist (e.g., Good et al., 2003), allowing assessment of lateralized dysfunction.

Reliability is high for the standard version and adequate for the B-SIT. The SIT correlates well with other measures of olfactory function and appears to be useful in identifying impairments in a variety of populations. In neurodegenerative disorders such as Parkinson's disease and AD, research suggests early and significant olfactory dysfunction. Importantly, disturbance is not strongly related to education and is not observed consistently in patients with depression. However, ceiling effects are present, limiting the capacity of the SIT to distinguish average from superior olfactory ability. In addition, the test may only be able to separate individuals into three ability levels (normal, decreased, complete inability to identify smells), rather than the five suggested by Doty (1995).

The test also has predictive validity, at least in the elderly. Low scores may herald cognitive decline in otherwise healthy individuals and may serve as preclinical markers of diseases such as AD. Further, the test may be more useful than measures of global cognition to predict impending cognitive decline (e.g., Graves et al., 1999). However, anosmia in association with closed head injury does not appear to be a bleak prognostic indicator for vocational adjustment (Correia et al., 2001).

It should be noted that the test is sensitive to a wide number of clinical disorders. Disturbances can occur as a result of numerous causes, including upper respiratory tract infections, degenerative disorders, and neuropathological processes. Therefore, its utility in distinguishing among conditions is somewhat limited. In combination with other tests (e.g., APOE genotyping, neuropsychological assessment), however, specificity may be enhanced (Graves et al., 1999). Clinicians are also advised to consider the possible contribution of peripheral olfactory functioning when olfactory deficits emerge.

The sensitivity and reliability of the 12-item B-SIT are lower than those of the full SIT. In addition, missing data on the B-SIT has more of an impact than on the SIT, because of the SIT's greater range of possible scores (Graves et al., 1999). The 3-item screen provides a gross indication of olfactory ability; missing even one item on this test is suggestive of abnormality. However, caution is advised, because many patients perform normally on the screen yet poorly on the complete test (Callahan & Hinkebein, 2002). Accordingly the full or B-SIT version is recommended.

The task does make cognitive and linguistic demands. Poor performance by children appears to be related to age-related semantic features rather than poor odor function (Frank et al., 2003). Similarly, cognitive dysfunction in patient populations can affect SIT performance. Cultural factors also play a role. Although the SIT has been translated into several languages and the B-SIT appears very promising in this context, use of the task in diverse cultures should be approached with caution (Frank et al., 2003).

REFERENCES

Bylsma, F. W., Moberg, P. J., Doty, R. L., & Brandt, J. (1997). Odor identification in Huntington's disease patients and asymptomatic gene carriers. *Journal of Neuropsychiatry and Clinical Neurosciences, 9*, 598–600.

Brewer, W. J., Edwards, J., Anderson, V., Robinson, T., & Pantelis, C. (1996). Neuropsychological, olfactory, and hygiene deficits in men with negative symptom schizophrenia. *Biological Psychiatry, 40*, 1021–1031.

Brody, D., Serby, M., Etienne, N., & Kalkstein, D. (1991). Olfactory identification deficits in HIV infection. *American Journal of Psychiatry, 148*, 248–250.

Busenbark, K. L., Huber, S. J., Greer, G., Pahwa, R., et al. (1992). Olfactory function in essential tremor. *Neurology, 42*, 1631–1632.

Callahan, C. D., & Hinkebein, J. H. (2002). Assessment of anosmia after traumatic brain injury: Performance characteristics of the University of Pennsylvania Smell Identification Test. *Journal of Head Trauma Rehabilitation, 17*, 251–256.

Cinelli, A. R., & Kauer, J. S. (1992). Voltage-sensitive dyes and functional activity in the olfactory pathway. *Annual Review of Neuroscience, 15*, 321–351.

Correia, S., Faust, D., & Doty, R. L. (2001). A re-examination of the rate of vocational dysfunction among patients with anosmia and mild to moderate closed head injury. *Archives of Clinical Neuropsychology, 16*, 477–488.

Dade, L., Jones-Gotman, M., Zatorre, R., & Evans, A. (1998). Human brain function during odor encoding and recognition. *Annals of the New York Academy of Sciences, 855*, 572–574.

Devanand, D. P., Michaels-Marsten, K. S., Liu, X., Pelton, G. H., Padilla, M., Marder, K., Bell, K., Stern, Y., Mayeux, R., & Brook, J. S. (2000). Olfactory deficits in patients with mild cognitive impairment predict Alzheimer's disease at follow-up. *American Journal of Psychiatry, 157*, 1399–1405.

Ditraglia, G. M., Press, D. S., Butters, N., Jernigan, T. L., et al. (1991). Assessment of olfactory deficits in detoxified alcoholics. *Alcohol, 8*, 109–115.

Doty, R. L. (1995). *The Smell Identification Test administration manual* (3rd ed.). Haddon Heights, N.J.: Sensonics.

Doty, R. L. (2001). *The Brief Smell Identification Test administration manual.* Haddon Heights, N.J.: Sensonics.

Doty, R. L., Applebaum, S., Zusho, H., & Settle, G. (1985). Sex differences in odor identification ability: A cross-cultural analysis. *Neuropsychologia, 23*, 667–672.

Doty, R. L., Bromley, S. M., & Stern, M. B. (1995). Olfactory testing as an aid in the diagnosis of Parkinson's disease: Development of optimal discrimination criteria. *Neurodegeneration, 4*, 93–97.

Doty, R. L., Deems, D. A., & Stellar, S. (1988). Olfactory dysfunction in parkinsonism: A general deficit unrelated to neurologic signs, disease state, or disease duration. *Neurology, 38*, 1237–1244.

Doty, R. L., Frye, R. E., & Agrawal, U. (1989). Internal consistency reliability of the fractionated and whole University of Pensylvania Smell Identification Test. *Perception and Psychophysics, 45*, 381–384.

Doty, R. L., Genow, A., & Hummel, T. (1998). Scratch density differentiates microsmic from normosmic and anosmic subjects on the University of Pennsylvania Smell Identification Test. *Perceptual and Motor Skills, 86*, 211–216.

Doty, R. L., Li, C., Mannon, L. J., & Yousem, D. M. (1999). Olfactory dysfunction in multiple sclerosis: Relation to longitudinal changes in plaque numbers in central olfactory structures. *Neurology, 53*, 880–882.

Doty, R. L., Perl, D. P., Steele, J. C., Chen, K. M., et al. (1991). Odor identification deficit of the parkinsonism-dementia complex of Guam: Equivalence to that of Alzheimer's and idiopathic Parkinson's disease. *Neurology, 41*(Suppl. 2), 77–80.

Doty, R. L., & Snow, J. B. (1987). Olfaction. In J. Goldman, *The principles and practice of rhinology* (pp. 761–785). New York: Wiley.

Doty, R. L., Reyes, P. F., & Gregor, T. P. (1987). Presence of both odor identification and detection deficits in Alzheimer's disease. *Brain Research Bulletin, 18*, 597–600.

Doty, R. L., Shaman, P., Applebaum, S. L., Giberson, R., Siksorski, L., & Rosenberg, L. (1984a). Smell identification ablity: Changes with age. *Science, 226*, 1441–1443.

Doty, R. L., Shaman, P., & Dann, M. (1984b). Development of the University of Pennsylvania Smell Identification Test: A standardized microencapsulated test of olfactory function. *Physiology and Behavior, 32*, 489–502.

Double, K. L., Rowe, D. B., Hayes, M., Chan, D. K., Blackie, J., Corbett, A., Joffe, R., Fung, V. S., Morris, J., & Halliday, G. M. (2003). Identifying the pattern of olfactory deficits in Parkinson disease using the Brief Smell Identification Test. *Archives of Neurology, 60*, 545–549.

Fernandez-Ruiz, J., Diaz, R., Hall-Haro, C., et al. (2004). Olfactory dysfunction in hereditary ataxia and basal ganglia disorders. *Neuroreport: For Rapid Communication of Neuroscience Research, 14*, 1339–1341.

Frank, R. A., Dulay, M. F., & Gesteland, R. C. (2003). Assessment of the Sniff Magnitude Test as a clinical test of olfactory function. *Physiology and Behavior, 78*, 195–204.

Frye, R. E., Schwartz, B. S., & Doty, R. L. (1990). Dose-related effects of cigarette smoking on olfactory function. *JAMA, 263*, 1233–1236.

Fulbright, R., Skudlarski, P., Lacadie, C., Warrenburg, S., Bowers, A., Gore, J., & Wexler, B. (1998). Functional MR imaging of regional brain responses to pleasant and unpleasant odors. *American Journal of Neuroradiology, 19*, 1721–1726.

Gansler, D. A., Fucetola, R., Krengel, M., Stetson, S., Zimering, R., & Makary, C. (1998). Are there cognitive subtypes in adult attention deficit/hyperactivity disorder? *The Journal of Nervous and Mental Disease, 186*, 776–781.

Good, K. P., Martzke, J. S., Daoud, M. A., & Kopala, L. C. (2003). Unirhinal norms for the University of Pennsylvania Smell Identification Test. *The Clinical Neuropsychologist, 17,* 226–234.

Good, K. P., Martzke, J. S., Milliken, H. J., Honer, W. G., & Kopala, L. C. (2002). Unirhinal olfactory identification deficits in young male patients with schizophrenia and related disorders: Association with impaired memory function. *Schizophrenia Research, 56,* 211–223.

Goudsmit, N., Coleman, E., Seckinger, R. A., Wolitzky, R., Stanford, A. D., Corcoran, C., Goetz, R. R., & Malaspina, D. (2004). A brief smell identification test discriminates between deficit and nondeficit schizophrenia. *Psychiatry Research, 120,* 155–164.

Graves, A. B., Bowen, J. D., Rajaram, L., McCormick, W. C., McCurry, S. M., Schellenberg, G. D., & Larson, E. B. (1999). Impaired olfaction as a marker for cognitive decline. *Neurology, 53,* 1480–1487.

Gray, A. J., Staples, V., Murren, K., Dhariwal, A., & Bentham, P. (2001). Olfactory identification is impaired in clinic-based patients with vascular dementia and senile dementia of Alzheimer type. *International Journal of Geriatric Psychiatry, 16,* 513–517.

Hawkes, C. H., Shepard, B. C., & Daniel, S. E. (1997). Olfactory dysfunction in Parkinson's disease. *Journal of Neurology, Neurosurgery and Psychiatry, 62,* 436–446.

Hemdal, P., Corwin, J., and Oster, H. (1993). Olfactory identification deficits in Down's syndrome and idiopathic mental retardation. *Neuropsychologia, 31,* 977–984.

Jones-Gotman, M., & Zatorre, R. J. (1988). Olfactory identification deficits in patients with focal cerebral excision. *Neuropscyhologia, 26,* 387–400.

Kohler, C. G., Moberg, P. J., Gur, R. E., O'Connor, M. J., Sperling, M. R., & Doty, R. L. (2001). Olfactory dysfunction in schizophrenia and temporal lobe epilepsy. *Neuropsychiatry, Neuropsychology, and Behavioral Neurology, 14,* 83–88.

Kopala, L. C., Good, K. P., & Honer, W. G. (1994). Olfactory hallucinations and olfactory identification ability in patients with schizophrenia and other psychiatric disorders. *Schizophrenia Research, 12,* 205–211.

Louis, E. D., Bromley, S. M., Jurewicz, E. C., & Watner, D. (2002). Olfactory dysfunction in essential tremor: A deficit unrelated to disease duration or severity. *Neurology, 59,* 1631–1633.

Mair, R. G., Doty, R. L., Kelly, K. M., Wilson, C. S., Langlais, P. J., McEntee, W. J., & Vollmecke, T. A. (1986). Multimodal sensory discrimination deficits in Korsakoff's psychosis. *Neuropsychologia, 24,* 831–839.

Malaspina, D., & Coleman, E. (2003). Olfaction and social drive in schizophrenia. *Archives of General Psychiatry, 60,* 578–584.

Martzke, J. S., Swan, C. S., & Varney, N. R. (1991). Posttraumatic anosmia and orbital frontal damage: Neuropsychological and neuropsychiatric correlates. *Neuropsychology, 5,* 213–225.

McLean, D., Feron, F., MacKay-Sim, A., McCurdy, R., Chant, D., & McGrath, J. (2004). Paradoxical association between smoking and olfactory identification in psychosis versus controls. *Australian and New Zealand Journal of Psychiatry, 38,* 81–83.

Minor, K. L., Wright, B. D., & Park, S. (2004). The Smell Identification Test as a measure of olfactory identification ability in schizophrenia and healthy populations: A Rasch psychometric study. *Journal of Abnormal Psychology, 113,* 207–216.

Moberg, P. J., Doty, R. L., Mahr, R. N., Mesholam, R. I., Arnold, S. E., Turetsky, B. I., & Gur, R. E. (1997). Olfactory identification in elderly schizophrenia and Alzheimer's disease. *Neurobiology of Aging, 18,* 163–167.

Morgan, C. D., Nordin, S., & Murphy, C. (1995). Olfactory identification as an early marker for Alzheimer's disease: Impact of lexical functioning and detection sensitivity. *Journal of Clinical and Experimental Neuropsychology, 17,* 793–803.

Nagy, E., & Loveland, K. A. (2001). Olfactory deficit in Alzheimer's disease? *American Journal of Psychiatry, 158,* 1533.

Postolache, T. T., Doty, R. L., Wehr, T. A., et al. (1999). Monorhinal odor identification and depression scores in patients with seasonal affective disorder. *Journal of Affective Disorders, 56,* 27–35.

Potter, H., & Nauta, W. (1979). A note on the problem of olfactory associations of the orbitofrontal cortex in the monkey. *Neuroscience, 4,* 361–367.

Qureshy, A., Kawashima, R., Imran, M., et al. (2000). Functional mapping of human brain in olfactory processing: A PET study. *Journal of Neurophysiology, 84,* 1656–1666.

Royall, D. R., Chiodo, L. K., Polk, M. J., & Jaramillo, C. J. (2002). Severe dysosmia is specifically associated with Alzheimer-like memory deficits in nondemented elderly retirees. *Neuroepidemiology, 21,* 68–73.

Royet, J., Koenig, O., Gregoire, M., Cinotti, L., Larenne, F., Le Bars, D., et al. (1999). Functional anatomy of perceptual and semantic processing for odours. *Journal of Cognitive Neuroscience, 11,* 94–109.

Serby, M., Larson, P., & Kalkstein, D. (1991). The nature and course of olfactory deficits in Alzheimer's disease. *American Journal of Psychiatry, 148,* 357–360.

Ship, J. A., Pearson, J. D., Cruise, L. J., Brant, L. J., & Metter, E. J. (1996). Longitudinal changes in smell identification. *Journal of Gerontology, 51A,* M86–M91.

Ship, J. A., & Weiffenbach, J. M. (1993). Age, gender, medical treatment, and medication effects on smell identification. *Journals of Gerontology, 48,* M26–M32.

Stedman, T. J., & Clair, A. L. (1998). Neuropsychological, neurological and symptom correlates of impaired olfactory identification in schizophrenia. *Schizophrenia Research, 32,* 23–30.

Swan, G. E., & Carmelli, D. (2002). Impaired olfaction predicts cognitive decline in nondemented older adults. *Neuroepidemiology, 21,* 58–67.

Szeszko, P. R., Bates, J., Robinson, D., et al. (2004). Investigation of unirhinal olfactory identification in antipsychotic-free patients experiencing a first-episode schizophrenia. *Schizophrenia Research, 67,* 219–225.

Varney, N. (1988). Prognostic significance of anosmia in patients with closed-head trauma. *Journal of Clinical and Experimental Neuropsychology, 10,* 250–254.

Wang, Q-S., Tian, L., Huang, Y-L., Qin, S., He, L-Q., & Zhou, J-N. (2002). Olfactory identification and apolipoprotein E ε4 allele in mild cognitive impairment. *Brain Research, 951,* 77–81.

Wenning, G. K., Shephard, B., Hawkes, C., Petuckevitch, A., et al. (1995). Olfactory function in atypical parkinsonian syndromes. *Acata Neurologica Scandinavica, 91,* 247–250.

Westervelt, H. J., McCaffrey, R. J., Cousings, J. P., Wagle, W. A., & Haase, R. F. (1997). Longitudinal analysis of olfactory deficits in HIV infection. *Archives of Clinical Neuropsychology, 12,* 557–565.

Yousem, D., Williams, S., Howard, R., et al. (1997). Functional MR imaging during odor stimulation: Preliminary data. *Radiology, 204,* 833–838.

Zald, D., & Pardo, J. (1997). Emotion, olfaction, and the human amygdala: Amygdala activation during aversive olfactory stimulation. *Proceedings from the National Academy of Sciences, 94,* 4119–4124.

Zatorre, R. J., & Jones-Gotman, M. (1991). Human olfactory discrimination after unilateral frontal or temporal lobectomy. *Brain, 114,* 71–84.

Zatorre, R., Jones-Gotman, M., Evans, A., & Myer, E. (1992). Functional localization and lateralization of human olfactory cortex. *Nature, 360,* 339–340.

Tactual Performance Test (TPT)

OTHER TEST NAMES

Other names for the Tactual Performance Test (TPT) are Form Board Test and Seguin-Goddard Formboard.

PURPOSE

The purpose of this test is to assess tactile form recognition, incidental memory for shapes, and spatial location.

SOURCE

The test (10- and 6-hole boards, stand, and 10 blocks) can be ordered from Reitan Neuropsychology Laboratory, P.O. Box 66080, Tucson AZ 85728 (http://www.reitanlabs.com). The children's set costs $235 US, the adult set costs $280 US, and the composite set costs $340 US. Psychological Assessment Resources, Inc., 16204 N. Florida Ave, Lutz, FL 33549 (http://www.parinc.com) offers a portable version of both 6-hole and 10-hole boards, a P-TPT manual, an administration case, and 50 record forms for $399 US.

AGE RANGE

The test can be given to individuals aged 5 to 85 years.

DESCRIPTION

The material for this test, the Seguin Formboard, came from the Arthur (1947) battery of tests (Lezak et al., 2004). Although it was originally administered as a visual-spatial performance test, Halstead (1947) converted it into a tactile memory test by blindfolding subjects and adding a drawing recall trial (Lezak et al., 2004). It was subsequently incorporated by Reitan (1979) into his battery.

In this test of tactile memory, the patient is blindfolded and presented with blocks of differing shapes and a matching formboard with holes. The patient is instructed to insert the blocks into the board as quickly as possible, first with the preferred hand, then with the nonpreferred hand, and then using both hands together. After completion of these trials, the formboard is concealed, the blindfold is removed, and the patient is asked to draw from memory, indicating both the shapes of the blocks and their placement relative to each other. TPT performance is reported in terms of either time to complete the task or minutes per block, for (a) the preferred hand, (b) the nonpreferred hand, (c) both hands, and (d) the total time for the three tactile trials; in addition, (e) a memory score for the number of blocks correctly reproduced and (f) a location score for the number of blocks correctly located in the drawing are recorded.

There are two different formboards: The 10-hole formboard is used for patients aged 15 years and older, and the 6-hole formboard is used for children younger than 15 years of age. In addition to the formboard material, a clean, comfortably fitting blindfold (eye mask or gauze pads) and a stopwatch are required. Scoring forms (see Figure 13–4) can be easily produced. The material is sturdy and rarely needs replacement.

ADMINISTRATION

For persons 8 years old and younger, the 6-hole formboard is mounted horizontally in the stand with the cross in the upper left-hand corner. For individuals aged 9 years to 14 years 11 months, the 6-block formboard is mounted vertically in the stand with the cross in the upper right-hand corner. For patients 15 years and older, the 10-block board is mounted vertically in the stand with the cross in the upper right-hand corner.

The patient is seated, near and squarely facing the table. Two gauze pads are placed over the eyes, and a blindfold is tied over them. The examiner questions the patient about his or her ability to see, especially downward. After the examiner is certain the patient cannot see, the board is brought out. The blocks are placed in random sequence between the board and the patient. Blocks adjacent to each other on the board should not be placed next to each other on the table. For specific instructions, see Figure 13–5. Some examiners prefer to guide

Figure 13–4 TPT Sample scoring sheet.

Trial	Hand	Circle		Time
1	Dominant	R	L	_____
2	Nondominant	R	L	_____
3	Both			_____
Total Time	_____			
Memory	_____			
Location	_____			

Figure 13–5 Instructions for administering the TPT.

Dominant Hand

Ask the subject to give you the preferred (dominant) hand. Take the subject's wrist and move the hand over the board and the pieces on the table while giving the following instructions: *In front of you on the table is a board. This is the size and shape of it.* (Move the subject's hand around the edge of the board). *On the face of the board are holes of various shapes and sizes* (move subject's hand across the face of the board), *and here in front of you are blocks of various shapes and sizes* (pass the subject's hand over the blocks, then place the subject's hand in his or her lap). *You are to fit the blocks into the spaces on the board. There is a place for each block and a block for each opening. Now I want you to do your best using only your right hand* (or left if that is the dominant hand). *You may begin whenever you are ready.*

Start the stopwatch when the subject first touches the board or blocks, and stop it when the last piece has been placed. Record the time for each hand in minutes and seconds. It is helpful to praise the subject for correctly placed blocks and to encourage the subject if he or she is not doing well. As the blocks in front of the subject are used up, push over the others to keep a supply ready at hand. When the subject has finished, ask him or her not to remove the blindfold and suggest that the subject relax for a minute or two.

Some patients spend a very long time trying to complete the tasks. The trial can continue up to 15 min and then be discontinued unless the patient is about to complete the task.

Nondominant Hand

After laying out the blocks in random order, say: *Now I want you to do the test again, and this time you are to use only your left hand* (or right hand, if that is the nondominant hand). *Begin whenever you are ready.* Record the time needed for this hand.

Both Hands

Lay out the blocks again and say: *This time you may use both hands for the test.* When the subject is finished, ask him or her to leave the blindfold on for a few minutes and put the board out of sight. Say: *Please remove the blindfold.*

Memory

Place a sheet of white paper and pencil in front of the subject and say: *On this sheet of paper I want you to draw an outline of the shape of the board. On your drawing, put in the shapes of the blocks in the same place as you remember them on the board. Note that there are three parts to your task: the shape of the board, the shape of the blocks, and their location on the board. Be sure to label the top of your drawing. There is no time limit on this.*

the patient to each block presented in standardized order, whereas others allow the examinee to pick blocks in random order. Chavez et al. (1982) indicated that the two modes of presentation show no differences in results on the time trials of the test. However, a standardized block presentation was associated with higher memory scores, and a trend was noted for higher localization scores. See *Comments* for a discussion of rules for discontinuation.

APPROXIMATE TIME FOR ADMINISTRATION

The time required ranges from 15 to 50 min.

SCORING

There are a number of ways to score the test. It can be scored by calculating the total time for the three tactile placement trials (Time right, left, and both hands), by counting the number of blocks correctly drawn (Memory), and by counting the number of blocks properly located in the drawings (Location). Differences between right- and left-hand performance can also be noted.

Some authors have adopted the use of a minutes-per-block score (i.e., number of minutes divided by number of blocks correctly placed) for each of the three timed trials and for the total time score (Heaton et al., 1991, 1992, 2004). In this way, the examiner has a rate score that can be interpreted regardless of the number of blocks correctly placed. For example, if a patient places five blocks in 5 min., the rate is 5/5, or 1 block per minute.

In counting the blocks correctly reproduced, count only those that are fairly accurately drawn and indicate that the examinee had a true mental picture of the block. A star of four or five points is accepted as correct. The location score is obtained by counting the right place on the drawing in relation to the other blocks and the formboard.

Examinees who have difficulty reproducing a shape on the drawing part of the test are given credit if they can correctly name the shape. However, they should be urged to do their best at drawing the figures. If two figures on the drawing look very similar, the examiner should ask the patient if they are the same figure. For example, the square and the rectangle are often drawn very much alike. If the patient calls one a square and the other a rectangle (or a "long square"), the subject is given credit for both. If two identical figures are drawn, the examiner should give credit to the one most correctly localized, even if it is not the most accurate drawing.

In scoring location, the relationship of the figure to the board as well as to the other shapes drawn should be considered. For example, if the triangle is drawn near the top of the board and the cross and half-circle are placed on each side of it but another shape is drawn in above the triangle, then the triangle does not count as correctly localized. Reitan and Wolfson (1985) recommended dividing the page into nine segments for scoring. If the major portion of a block fits in its appropriate division, it is given credit for localization. No localization credit is given unless memory credit for the block has already been given. A scoring guide for TPT Location appears in an Appendix C of the HRNES Manual (Russell & Starkey, 1993).

DEMOGRAPHIC EFFECTS

Age

Age contributes significantly to performance, with scores improving in childhood and declining with advancing age (e.g., Bak & Greene, 1980; Cauthen, 1978; Fromm-Auch & Yeudall, 1983; Heaton et al., 2004; Knights & Norwood, 1980; Moore et al., 1984; Russell & Starkey, 1993; Spreen & Gaddes, 1969; Sweeney & Johnson, 2001). In children, there are fairly clear developmental trends for the time-related variables, with older children requiring less time to complete the TPT than younger ones. Developmental trends for the Memory and Location scores are less prominent (Leckliter et al., 1992), perhaps because of ceiling effects (at least on the Memory component). In adults aged 20 to 85 years, Heaton et al. (2004) reported that, in their Caucasian sample of adults, about 10% to 19% of the variance in scores on the TPT time trials was accounted for by age. In the African American sample, the values were 18% to 25%. For the Memory and Location trials,

age accounted for 21% and 26%, respectively, of the variance in test scores in the Caucasian sample, 27% and 21%, respectively, in the African American sample. The contribution of variables such as age is sufficiently large to invalidate the use of simple cutoff scores. Failure to take age into account results in an increased probability of misclassifying normal older adults as impaired. For example, Heaton et al. (2004) noted that application of a single set of norms for the Location score results in correct classification rate of 65% of Caucasians younger than 40 years of age but only 11% of those older than 60 years of age (see also Cauthen, 1978).

Education

The influence of education is less than that of age. Some authors (e.g., Ernst, 1987; Yeudall et al., 1987) found no relationship between educational level and TPT scores, whereas others reported better TPT performance with increasing levels of education (e.g., Alekoumbides et al., 1987; Heaton et al., 2004; Russell & Starkey, 2001). Heaton et al. (2004) documented in their large sample of neurologically normal individuals ($N = 1212$) that, in Caucasians, only about 1% to 4% of the variance in Time scores was accounted for by education; for Memory and Location, the percentages were somewhat greater, 10% and 6%, respectively.

IQ

IQ shows a moderate relationship with TPT scores (Cauthen, 1978; Dodrill, 1997; Heilbronner et al., 1991; Warner et al., 1987), with PIQ showing more of a correlation than VIQ (Wiens & Matarrazzo, 1977; Yeudall et al., 1987).

Gender

The effect of gender tends to be minimal, accounting for 1% or less of the variance in test scores (Heaton et al., 2004). Kupke (1983) reported an interaction effect of gender with Location and Memory scores; subjects in that study tended to show significantly better scores with examiners of the opposite sex (approximately 1 point on Memory, 1.5 points on Location).

Race/Ethnicity

A study comparing Anglo American, Mexican American, and Mexican subjects (Arnold et al., 1994) revealed an acculturation effect (faster performance in Anglo Americans) only for Time scores (dominant, nondominant, total), but not for Location or Memory scores. Because the amount of variance accounted for by age, education, and gender may differ in Caucasians and African Americans, Heaton et al. (2004) developed separate demographic corrections for these two groups.

Differences between North American and other children have been reported, but these may relate more to nutritional status than ethnicity (Boivin et al., 1995, 1996).

Hand Preference

There is no difference in test scores between right- and left-handed subjects (Gregory & Paul, 1980; Thompson et al., 1987).

NORMATIVE DATA

Adults

A number of authors have published or distributed normative data for use with adults (e.g., Alekoumbides et al., 1987; Cauthen, 1978; Dodrill, 1987; Ernst, 1987; Fromm-Auch & Yeudall, 1983; Harley et al., 1980; Heaton et al., 1991, 2004; Pauker, 1980; Russell & Starkey, 1993, 2001; Yeudall et al., 1987). Because of the effects of age, education, and ethnicity, we recommend the use of normative data provided by Heaton et al. (2004). As noted in Table 13–12, they provided norms separately for two ethnicity groups (Caucasians and African Americans) organized by age, gender, and education. The samples are large and cover a wide range in terms of age and education, and the exclusion criteria are specified. T scores lower than 40 are classed as impaired. If their manual is not available, Table 13–13 may be used as a rough guide. The data are from Fromm-Auch and Yeudall (1983) and represent a sample of healthy, well-educated ($M = 14.8$ years, $SD = 3.0$), bright (WAIS FSIQ $M = 119.1$, $SD = 8.8$) individuals residing in Canada. They were predominantly right-handed (83%). Note that the sample size of individuals aged 41 to 64 years is very small.

Table 13–12 Characteristics of the TPT Normative Sample provided by Heaton et al. (2004)

Number	1212
Age (years)	20–85[a]
Geographic location	Various states in United States and Manitoba, Canada
Sample type	Individuals recruited as part of multicenter studies
Education (years)	0–20[b]
Gender (%)	
Male	56.8
Female	43.2
Race/Ethnicity	
Caucasian	634
African American	578
Screening	No reported history of learning disability, neurological disorder, serious psychiatric disorder, or alcohol or drug abuse

[a]Age groups: 20–34, 35–39, 40–44, 45–49, 50–54, 55–59, 60–64, 65–69, 70–74, 75–79, and 80–89.
[b]Education groups: 7–8, 9–11, 12, 13–15, 16–17, and 18–20.

Table 13–13 Normative Data (Mean and *SD*) for Adults for the TPT by Age

	24–32 ($n = 56$)	33–40 ($n = 18$)	41–64 ($n = 10$)
DH (min)	4.5 (1.8)	4.9 (1.7)	5.6 (1.5)
NDH (min)	3.1 (1.1)	3.7 (1.0)	4.2 (1.6)
Both Hands (min)	1.8 (0.8)	2.3 (0.8)	2.5 (1.2)
Total Time (min)	9.4 (3.0)	10.9 (2.9)	12.2 (3.6)
Memory (no. Correct)	8.3 (1.1)	8.6 (1.1)	7.7 (1.3)
Location (no. Correct)	5.5 (1.8)	5.6 (2.2)	4.9 (1.8)

Source: Adapted from Fromm-Auch & Yeudall, 1983.

Children and Adolescents

Findeis and Weight (1994) developed meta-norms based on a series of articles published between 1969 and 1989. In addition to concerns regarding the outdated nature of the studies, users should note that the majority of the participants were Caucasian, came from middle- to upper-class socioeconomic backgrounds, and had above-average IQs (see Table 13–14). The data are shown in Table 13–15. The sizes of the standard deviations for the TPT Time variables indicate greater variability among younger children. For adolescents, the norms provided by Fromm-Auch and Yeudall (1983) may be used. These are shown in Table 13–16. The data for children aged 5 to 13 years are based on the 6-hole formboard, whereas those for adolescents aged 15 years and older are based on the 10-hole formboard.

Differences Between Hands

It has been reported that, on average, normal subjects show about 30% improvement in performance across the first two

Table 13–14 Characteristics of the TPT Meta-Norms provided by Findeis & Weight (1994)

Number	5–8 years: 515 9–14 years: 331
Age (years)	4–14
Geographic location	United States and Canada
Sample type	Subjects pooled from various articles published between 1969 and 1989; Full-Scale IQ = 112.87; from middle- and upper-class socioeconomic backgrounds
Education	Not Reported
Gender	
Male	Not Reported
Female	Not Reported
Race/Ethnicity	Mostly Caucasian
Screening	No history of neurological abnormalities

Table 13–15 Meta-Norms (Mean and *SD*) for TPT for Six-Hole Formboard Derived from Findeis & Weight (1994), by Age

	Age (Years)								
	5	6	7	8	9	10	11	12	13
DH (min)	6.46 (3.1)	5.93 (3.1)	5.17 (2.7)	4.15 (2.2)	4.36 (2.4)	3.67 (1.7)	3.15 (1.4)	3.20 (1.6)	2.44 (.8)
n	191	160	188	101	92	91	96	104	31
NDH (min)	5.24 (3.1)	4.74 (2.8)	3.66 (1.9)	3.13 (3.1)	3.08 (1.7)	2.73 (1.6)	2.17/(.9)	2.20 (1.4)	1.61 (.9)
n	191	160	188	166	92	91	96	104	32
Both Hands (min)	3.80 (2.6)	3.11 (2.1)	1.98 (1.2)	1.68 (1.1)	1.28 (.7)	1.27 (.7)	1.13 (.6)	1.03 (.5)	.80 (.3)
n	191	160	188	167	92	91	96	104	32
Total Time (min)	15.50 (5.6)	13.83 (6.8)	10.98 (4.5)	8.79 (3.8)	8.80 (4.1)	7.66 (3.3)	6.36 (2.3)	6.13 (2.6)	4.90 (1.5)
n	206	190	218	197	92	91	96	104	32
Memory (no. correct)	2.47 (1.8)	3.06 (1.5)	4.15 (1.2)	4.44 (1.2)	4.40 (1.2)	4.48 (1.2)	4.53 (1.1)	4.77 (.8)	5.04 (.9)
n	206	190	218	196	92	91	96	104	31
Location (no. correct)	1.10 (1.1)	1.80 (1.5)	2.69 (1.7)	3.22 (1.7)	3.00 (1.6)	3.07 (1.5)	3.07 (1.6)	3.75 (1.5)	3.00 (1.3)
n	206	190	218	196	57	49	58	71	10

Source: Findeis and Weight, 1994. Unpublished data.

Table 13–16 Normative Data for Adolescents and Young Adults for the TPT, by Age

	15–17 years ($n = 32$)		18–23 years ($n = 74$)	
	Mean (*SD*)	Range	Mean (*SD*)	Range
DH (min)	4.6 (1.2)	2.6–6.8	5.1 (2.2)	1.9–13.5
NDH (min)	3.3 (1.2)	1.1–6.4	3.5 (1.6)	1.1–10.8
Both Hands (min)	1.7 (0.5)	.8–3.3	2.1 (1.3)	0.4–9.3
Total Time (min)	9.5 (2.1)	4.7–14.1	11.4 (4.5)	4.2–29.1
Memory (no. correct)	8.9 (1.0)	6–10	8.2 (1.3)	4–10
Location (no. correct)	6.8 (2.5)	1–10	5.7 (2.1)	1–10

Source: Adapted from Fromm-Auch & Yeudall, 1983.

trials of the TPT (Boll, 1981). However, a reversal of this pattern (second trial with the nondominant hand and third trial with both hands slower than the first trial) is found not infrequently, especially in older normal subjects, perhaps because of a reduced rate of learning (Thompson et al., 1987). Thomson and Heaton (1991) warned that such reversals should not be interpreted as evidence of acquired right-hemisphere lesions unless the differences are large and other evidence supports such an interpretation.

In children, Finlayson (1978) showed that the Time score for the nonpreferred hand relative to the preferred hand Time score decreased significantly between the ages of 5 and 12 years, suggesting an increasing interhemispheric transfer effect of practice with age.

RELIABILITY

Internal Consistency

Internal reliability correlations, using either time in seconds to place each block or blocks-per-minute scores for the preferred hand, nonpreferred hand, both hands, and total time, have ranged from .61 to .90 in adults (Charter, 2000a; Charter et al., 1987, 2001). As shown in Table 13–17, the reliability of the preferred hand is of questionable clinical utility. The Memory score falls at the borderline/adequate range (.61 to .69), whereas the reliability coefficient for location is adequate (.69 to .79; Charter et al., 1987, 2000). Reliabilities of difference scores (e.g., nonpreferred minus preferred) are low (<.65; Charter, 2001). Therefore, the examiner can have little confi-

Table 13–17 TPT Internal Consistency

Magnitude of Coefficient	Measure
Very High (≥ .90)	Total Time
High (.80 to .89)	Nonpreferred Hand
	Both Hands
Adequate (.70 to .79)	Location
Marginal (.60 to .69)	Preferred Hand
	Memory
Low (≤ .59)	

dence that an examinee's obtained difference score is close to his or her hypothetical true difference score.

Test-Retest Reliability and Practice Effects

In adults, reliability coefficients tend to be adequate for the Time scores but lower than desirable for the Memory and Location scores. For example, Schludermann and Schludermann (1983) reported retest coefficients of .76 for Time, .60 for Memory, and .55 for Location scores in a sample of 174 executives retested after 2 years, and coefficients of .91, .72, and .53, respectively, for 86 subjects in the same sample who were tested again after 3 years. Goldstein and Watson (1989) reported retest reliabilities after 4 to 469 weeks for 150 neuropsychiatric patients; these ranged from .66 to .74 for Time, from .46 to .72 for Memory, and from .32 to .69 for Location, with similar values for alcoholics, trauma patients, and patients with vascular disorders, and somewhat lower coefficients for those with schizophrenia. However, in normal adults retested after an interval of 3 weeks, reliability coefficients were higher for Memory ($r = .80$) and Location ($r = .77$) than for Time ($r = .69$) scores (Bornstein et al., 1987). In children referred for neuropsychological evaluation, coefficients were unacceptably low (<.50) after an interval of about 2.6 years (Brown et al., 1989).

In normal adults (age $M = 32.3$, $SD = 10.3$; VIQ $M = 105.8$, $SD = 10.8$) who were retested after an interval of 3 weeks, improvement was evident on all scores (Bornstein et al., 1987). In patients with epilepsy who were evaluated on four occasions spaced 6 to 12 months apart, gains were evident only on the localization component (on average, <1 point per administration), although changes in drug regimen complicated interpretation (Dodrill & Troupin, 1975).

Dikmen et al. (1999) reported improvement in scores in a sample of 384 normal or neurologically stable individuals (aged 15–83 years, $M = 34.2$, $SD = 16.7$) who were retested about 9 months after initial testing. Table 13–18 provides information to determine whether there has been substantial change taking practice into account (but see Hinton-Bayre, 2000, and Maassen, 2004, who raised concerns about the RCI calculation procedure used by Dikmen et al. [1999] and suggested that the 90% prediction intervals should actually be

Table 13–18 TPT Test-Retest Effects in 384 Normal Individuals Assessed After Intervals 2–16 months

| | Time 1 | | Time 2 | | T2 – T1 | | T1, T2 |
| | (1) | | (2) | | (3) | (4) | |
Measure	Mean	SD	Mean	SD	Mean	SD	r
Total (time per block (min)	0.5	0.49	.43	0.33	−.09	.29	.83
Memory	7.71	1.59	7.97	1.56	.26	1.21	.71
Location	4.39	2.49	4.92	2.57	.53	2.27	.60

Note: Mean Age = 34.2, *SD* = 16.7, range = 15–83; Mean education = 12.1, *SD* = 2.6, range = 0–19; 66% male; retest interval mean = 9.1 months, *SD* = 3.0, range = 2.4–15.8. Hinton-Bayre (2000) has indicated that there is an error in these calculations. He notes that, using the Jacobson and Truax RCI formula, the 90% prediction interval (PI) for TPT total is ± 0.39.

Source: Adapted from Dikmen et al., 1999.

smaller). One first subtracts the mean T2 – T1 change (column 3) from the difference between the two testings for the individual and then compares the resulting value with 1.64 times the standard deviation of the difference (column 4). The 1.64 comes from the normal distribution and is exceeded in the positive or negative direction only 10% of the time if indeed there is no real change in clinical condition.

Interrater Reliability

Martin and Greene (1978; cited in Snow, 1987) reported that the percentage of agreement between judges on scoring of Memory ranged from 71% to 76.3 %. Localization was scored with 56% to 64% agreement. In some pairs of judges, the percentage of agreement in scoring Memory was as low as 36%; for Localization, it was as low as 29%. However, a more recent study comparing results from three scorers found excellent interscorer reliability coefficients for the Memory and Localization scores (both .98; Charter et al., 1998).

VALIDITY

Relations Within Test

In their review, Thompson and Parsons (1985) noted that the three different scores are related to one another. This is especially true for Memory and Location, with correlations ranging form .56 to .71. TPT Time and Memory correlations range from .32 to .72, and TPT Time and Location correlations range from .26 to .62. In general, those completing the timed tasks most rapidly are also those who most successfully recall the shapes and their locations (Dinkins & deFilippis, 1997; Goldstein & Shelly, 1972). In short, increasing exposure during the problem-solving component of the task does not necessarily translate into better performance on the memory component.

Relationships With Other Measures

Berger (1998) examined a heterogeneous clinical sample and reported moderate/high correlations (*r* = .48 to .63) between TPT Time, Memory, and Location scores and the Perceptual

Organization factor of the WAIS-R, suggesting that nonverbal reasoning is important for task performance. Correlations with the Verbal Comprehension and Freedom from Distractibility factors were minimal (*r* < .30).

Steese-Seda et al. (1995) administered the TPT and a visual-motor bimanual coordination task to a group of children and obtained significant positive correlations between performance on these two tasks, suggesting that they may share some common aspects.

Factor analytic findings point to considerable overlap in what the scores represent, although there is some individual contribution as well. For example, Bornstein (1990) found that all three TPT scores (Time, Memory, and Location) loaded on the same factor, with only minor loadings from a large number of other tests. However, Campbell et al. (1989) found that, in young adults, the Time scores loaded on a factor with other time-dependent scores (e.g., Picture Completion, Block Design); the Memory score loaded on an attention factor together with Digit Span, Digit Symbol, Seashore Rhythm, and Trails A; and the TPT Location scores loaded on all three of the extracted factors. The authors concluded that the test is multifactorial in nature (see also Johnstone et al., 2000).

Item Difficulty

Charter (2000b) reported that, on the time trials (preferred, nonpreferred, both hands), blocks at the top of the board are more difficult than blocks at the bottom of the board. They noted that subject strategy may contribute to item difficulty. If examinees try to fill the spaces on the top first, these spaces may be difficult because there are more block shapes to discriminate. There does not appear to be an easily discernible pattern of item difficulty in relation to block placement on the TPT board for Memory or Location trials (Charter & Dutra, 2001).

Clinical Studies

Discriminant validity for most Halstead-Reitan tests has traditionally been established by comparing scores for normal subjects, "pseudoneurological" patients (referred for evaluation but found not neurologically impaired), and "brain-damaged" individuals, using optimal cutoff scores. In studies examining the ability of individual measures to correctly classify subjects as brain-damaged or not (e.g., Dodrill, 1978; Goldstein & Shelly, 1972; Mutchnik et al., 1991; Reitan & Wolfson, 1996; Wheeler & Reitan, 1963; Wheeler et al., 1963), TPT Time was found to be one of the best predictors in the Halstead-Reitan battery. Some studies (Mutchnik et al., 1991; Wheeler et al., 1963) found Location to be more sensitive than the Memory scores, whereas others (Goldstein & Shelly, 1972) found the reverse. Of note, the TPT has also proved useful in differentiating brain-damaged from non-brain-damaged blind patients (Bigler & Tucker, 1981). In that study, the Memory and Location components were described orally by the subjects.

In general, time using the right hand is slower for patients with left-hemisphere brain damage, and left-hand time is slower for those with right-hemisphere damage (Dodrill, 1978; Reitan, 1959). Several studies have found that patients with right-hemisphere damage perform more slowly than do patients with left-hemisphere damage (Reitan, 1959, 1964), although Goldstein and Shelley (1972) reported that TPT Total time did not differentiate these two groups. The Memory and Location scores do not appear to discriminate reliably between right- and left-hemisphere deficits (Heilbronner et al., 1991; Thompson & Parsons, 1985).

Early studies found that patients with frontal lesions performed poorly on some or all TPT measures (Halstead, 1947; Shure & Halstead, 1958), but subsequent studies found more impairment in patients with posterior damage (Chapman & Wolff, 1959; Reitan, 1964). Chapman and Wolff (1959) suggested that patients with frontal damage performed more poorly in the early studies because they had larger lesions than did the patients with nonfrontal damage.

A number of studies have shown the TPT to be sensitive to the effects of various disorders, including multiple sclerosis (e.g., Ivnik, 1978), chronic obstructive pulmonary disease (Prigatano et al., 1983), Parkinson's disease (Reitan & Boll, 1971), Huntington's chorea (Boll et al., 1974), chronic alcoholism (e.g., Charter et al., 2001; Fabian et al., 1981; Gurling et al., 1991), and epilepsy (e.g., Dodrill, 1987). In a major study that compared adults 1 year after head injury with controls who had sustained damage to other parts of the body, Dikmen et al. (1995) found a highly significant difference between the two groups for Time scores. Although a dose-response relationship emerged, there was considerable overlap in scores across severity subgroups. Impairment has also been reported in neuropsychiatric conditions, including schizophrenia (e.g., Goldstein et al., 1998) and depression (Harris et al., 1981).

The TPT is also sensitive to developmental disturbances and the environmental milieu. For example, learning-disabled children have been reported to show impairment on the Memory and Localization subtests (McIntosh et al., 1995). With regard to the developmental milieu, Boivin et al. (1995) reported that 5- to 12-year-old children from rural parts of Zaire scored significantly lower than American and Canadian control groups on the TPT. They attributed this to poorer anthropomorphic indicators of nutritional well-being rather than to intercultural differences; that is, the test may be sensitive to the effects of malnutrition. In Lao children as well, TPT measures were related to physical (nutritional) development (Boivin et al., 1996).

Ecological and Predictive Validity

Driving performance is associated with TPT performance. Brain-damaged individuals who passed a driving evaluation required less time to complete the TPT (Rothke, 1989). In terms of predictive validity, Dodrill and Clemmons (1984) reported on a longitudinal investigation of measures, including the TPT, given during the high school years to individuals with epilepsy in order to predict outcome in adulthood. They found the TPT to be predictive for overall adjustment and independent living, but not for vocational adjustment.

Malingering

Goebel (1983) found that individuals instructed to feign brain damage underestimated the difficulty of the task for brain-damaged subjects and obtained scores more similar to those of normal controls than to scores of actual brain-damaged patients on all parts of the test.

COMMENT

Lezak et al. (2004) noted that the task is time-consuming to give and may provide very little new information in return. They also pointed to the considerable discomfort experienced by some patients while being blindfolded for as long as 10 min or more. They concluded that the test is "not worth the time and trouble." Some authors (e.g., Klonoff & Low, 1974; Clark & Klonoff, 1988; Russell, 1985) have recommended the use of the 6-block formboard with adults, arguing that this cuts administration time by about two-thirds and may alleviate some of the distress caused to the client. The TPT-6 correlates well with the TPT-10 (Russell, 1985), has high reliability (Clark & Klonoff, 1988), and demonstrates discriminative and construct validity (Clark & Klonoff, 1988). Unfortunately, adequate normative data are lacking.

Criticisms have also been raised regarding the lack of standardization of the procedure. Reitan (1979) suggested that termination is possible after 15 min if the patient is "getting discouraged and is making very slow progress" (p. 36) but recommended allowing the patient to continue if a correct performance appeared close. Others (e.g., Russell & Starkey, 1991) use a 10-min cutoff. Snow (1987) noted that, by reducing the time the patient spends on the test, one reduces the amount of exposure the patient has to the blocks and their locations on the board. Differing amounts of exposure duration may affect Memory and Location scores (but see Dinkins & deFilippis, 1997, *Relations Within Test*). Differences in block presentation (guided versus unstructured; Chavez et al., 1982) and type of formboard (Kupke, 1983) also affect performance. Kupke (1983) found better total Time scores in undergraduates with the use of a portable TPT as opposed to the standard version. Kupke noted that the holes proved to be "looser" on the portable version that he constructed. The scoring criteria for Memory and Location are also vague and may lead to differences in interpretations between examiners (but see Charter et al., 1998). The use of Russell and Starkey's (1993) system to score Location may help address some of the scoring problems. In short, standardization of the administration and scoring procedures is needed (Snow, 1987; Mitrushina et al., 2005). By addressing these issues, it may be possible to obtain a clearer understanding of the utility of this task.

Users should also bear in mind that age, education, and ethnicity/cultural factors influence performance and that reference to appropriate normative data is critical. The availability of the large normative data set for adults created by Heaton et al. (2004) is a strength, although it should be noted that the data were collected over a lengthy period (25 years). The norms for children have limited generalizability, because they are quite old and pertain to largely middle-upper-class Caucasian children. Therefore, restandardization is also needed, with an adequate representation of children.

Charter et al. (2000) pointed out that knowledge of internal consistency reliability is important, because it indicates how close an individual's obtained score would have come to the score he or she would have made had the test been a perfect measuring instrument. The low preferred-hand and Memory score reliabilities signify a wide range of possible true scores, lessening their clinical utility. Difference scores should also not be relied upon. Only limited reliability data are available for children and adolescents, and these suggest that interpretation of test scores should be approached with significant caution.

The precise meaning of the test scores is not certain. Nonverbal reasoning, attention, manual dexterity, and coordination appear to be important. TPT Time scores appear to be better indicators of brain dysfunction than Memory or Location scores although Time, Memory, and Location scores do not reliably identify laterality or location of damage.

Of note, the task appears to be a useful diagnostic instrument with blind individuals (Bigler & Tucker, 1981). It has also been used successfully in various cultural contexts, suggesting that it may be of value in assessing and monitoring at-risk adults, as well as children (e.g., Boivin et al., 1996). However, the task is not culture-fair, and direct intercultural comparisons should not be made.

REFERENCES

Alekoumbides, A., Charter, R. A., Adkins, T. G., & Seacat, G. F. (1987). The diagnosis of brain damage by the WAIS, WMS, and Reitan Battery utilizing standardized scores corrected for age and education. *International Journal of Clinical Neuropsychology, 9*, 11–28.

Arnold, B. R., Montgomery, G. T., Castaneda, I., & Longoria, R. (1994). Acculturation and performance of Hispanics on selected Halstead-Reitan neuropsychological tests. *Assessment, 1*, 239–248.

Arthur, G. (1947). *A Point Scale of Performance Tests* (Rev. Form II). New York: The Psychological Corporation.

Bak, J. S., & Greene, R. L. (1980). The effects of aging on a modified procedure for scoring localization and memory components of the Tactual Performance Test. *Clinical Neuropsychology, 2*, 114–117.

Benton, A. L., Sivan, A. B., Namsher, K. deS., et al. (1994). *Contributions to neuropsychologial assessment. A clinical manual* (2nd ed.) New York: Oxford University Press.

Berger, S. (1998). The WAIS-R factors: Usefulness and construct validity in neuropsychological assessments. *Applied Neuropsychology, 5*, 37–42.

Bigler, E. D., & Tucker, D. M. (1981). Comparison of Verbal IQ, Tactual Performance, Seashore Rhythm, and Finger Oscillation Tests in the blind and brain-damaged. *Journal of Clinical Psychology, 37*, 849–851.

Boivin, M. J., Chounramany, C., Giorani, B., Xaisida, S., Choulamountry, L., Phonethep, P., Crist, C. L., & Olness, K. (1996). Validating a cognitive ability testing protocol with Lao children for community development applications. *Neuropsychology, 10*, 588–599.

Boivin, M. J., Giorani, B., & Bornefeld, B. (1995). Use of the Tactual Performance Test for cognitive ability testing with African children. *Neuropsychology, 9*, 409–417.

Boll, T. J. (1981). The Halstead-Reitan Neuropsychology Battery. In S. B. Filskov & T. J. Boll (Eds.), *Handbook of clinical neuropsychology* (pp. 577–607). New York: Wiley.

Boll, T. J., Heaton, R. K., & Reitan, R. M. (1974). Neuropsychological and emotional correlates of Huntington's chorea. *Journal of Nervous and Mental Disease, 158*, 61–68.

Bornstein, R. A. (1990). Neuropsychological test batteries in neuropsychological assessment. In G. B. Baker & M. Hiscock (Eds.), *Neuromethods, Vol 17: Neuropsychology*. Clifton, N.J.: Humana Press.

Bornstein, R. A., Baker, G. B., & Douglas, A. B. (1987). Short-term retest reliability of the Halstead-Reitan Battery in a normal sample. *Journal of Nervous and Mental Disease, 175*, 229–232.

Brown, S. J., Rourke, B. P., & Cicchetti, D. V. (1989). Reliability of tests and measures used in the neuropsychological assessment of children. *The Clinical Neuropsychologist, 3*, 353–368.

Campbell, M. L., Drobes, D. J., & Horn, R. (1989). *Young adult norms, predictive validity, and relationship between Halstead-Reitan tests and WAIS-R scores.* Paper presented at the 9th meeting of the National Academy of Neuropsychology, Washington, D.C.

Cauthen, N. (1978). Normative data for the Tactual Performance Test. *Journal of Clinical Psychology, 34*, 456–460.

Chapman, L. F., & Wolff, H. G. (1959). The cerebral hemispheres and the highest integrative functions of man. *Archives of Neurology, 1*, 357–424.

Charter, R. A. (2000a). Internal consistency reliability of the Tactual Performance Test trials. *Perceptual & Motor Skills, 91*, 460–462.

Charter, R. A. (2000b). Item difficulty analysis of the Tactual Performance Test trials. *Perceptual and Motor Skills, 91*, 903–909.

Charter, R. A. (2001). Difference score reliability for Tactual Performance Test trials. *Perceptual and Motor Skills, 92*, 941–942.

Charter, R. A., Adkins, T. G., Alekoumbides, A., & Seacat, G. F. (1987). Reliability of the WAIS, WMS, and Reitan Battery: Raw scores and standardized scores corrected for age and education. *International Journal of Clinical Neuropsychology, 9*, 28–32.

Charter, R. A., & Dutra, R. L. (2001). Tactual Performance Test: Item analysis of the Memory and Location scores. *Perceptual and Motor Skills, 92,* 899–902.

Charter, R. A., Dutra, R. L., & Rapport, L. J. (2000). Tactual performance test: Internal consistency reliability of the memory and location scores. *Perceptual and Motor Skills, 91,* 143–146.

Charter, R. A., Lopez, M. N., Oh, S., & Lazar, M. D. (2001). Tactual performance test trials: Psychometric properties of the blocks-per-minute scores. *Perceptual and Motor Skills, 92,* 750–754.

Charter, R. A., Walden, D. K., & Hoffman, C. (1998). Interscorer reliabilities for Memory and Localization scores of the Tactual Performance Test. *The Clinical Neuropsychologist, 12,* 245–247.

Chavez, E. L., Schwartz, M. M., & Brandon, A. (1982). Effects of sex of subject and method of block presentation on the Tactual Performance Test. *Journal of Consulting and Clinical Psychology, 50,* 600–601.

Clark, S., & Klonoff, H. (1988). Reliability and construct validity of the six-block Tactual Performance Test in an adult sample. *Journal of Clinical and Experimental Neuropsychology, 10,* 175–184.

Dikmen, S. S., Heaton, R. K., Grant, I., & Temkin, N. R. (1999). Test-retest reliability and practice effects of expanded Halstead-Reitan neuropsychological test battery. *Journal of the International Neuropsychological Society, 5,* 346–356.

Dikmen, S. S., Machamer, J. E., Winn, H. R., & Temkin, N. R. (1995). Neuropsychological outcome at 1-year post head injury. *Neuropsychology, 9,* 80–90.

Dinkins, H. E., & DeFilippis, N. A. (1997). The effects of time of exposure on Tactual Performance Test Memory and Location scores. *Applied Neuropsychology, 4,* 247–248.

Dodrill, C. B. (1978). The hand dynamometer as a neuropsychological measure. *Journal of Consulting and Clinical Psychology, 46,* 1432–1435.

Dodrill, C. B. (1987). *What's normal?* Presidential Address. Seattle: Pacific Northwest Neuropsychological Association.

Dodrill, C. B. (1997). Myths of neuropsychology. *The Clinical Neuropsychologist, 11,* 1–17.

Dodrill, C. B., & Clemmons, D. (1984). Use of neuropsychological tests to identify high school students with epilepsy who later demonstrate inadequate performances in life. *Journal of Consulting and Clinical Psychology, 52,* 520–527.

Dodrill, C. B., & Troupin, A. S. (1975). Effects of repeated administrations of a comprehensive neuropsychological battery among chronic epileptics. *The Journal of Nervous and Mental Disease, 161,* 185–190.

Ernst, J. (1987). Neuropsychological problem-solving skills in the elderly. *Psychology and Aging, 2,* 363–365.

Fabian, M. S., Jenkins, R. L., & Parsons, O. A. (1981). Gender, alcoholism, and neuropsychological functioning. *Journal of Consulting and Clinical Psychology, 49,* 138–140.

Findeis, M. K., & Weight, D. K. (1994). *Meta-norms for two forms of neuropsychological test batteries for children.* Unpublished manuscript, Brigham Young University, Provo, Utah.

Finlayson, M. A. J. (1978). A behavioral manifestation of the development of interhemispheric transfer of learning in children. *Cortex, 14,* 290–295.

Fromm-Auch, D., & Yeudall, L. T. (1983). Normative data for the Halstead-Reitan neuropsychological tests. *Journal of Clinical Neuropsychology, 5,* 221–238.

Goebel, R. A. (1983). Detection of faking on the Halstead-Reitan neuropsychological test battery. *Journal of Clinical Psychology, 39,* 731–742.

Goldstein, G., Allen, D. N., & Seaton, B. E. (1998). A comparison of clustering solutions for cognitive heterogeneity in schizophrenia. *Journal of the International Neuropsychological Society, 4,* 353–362.

Goldstein, G., & Shelly, C. H. (1972). Statistical and normative studies of the Halstead Neuropsychological Test Battery relevant to a neuropsychiatric setting. *Perceptual and Motor Skills, 34,* 603–620.

Goldstein, G., & Watson, J. R. (1989). Test-retest reliability of the Halstead-Reitan battery and the WAIS in a neuropsychiatric population. *The Clinical Neuropsychologist, 3,* 265–273.

Gregory, R. J., & Paul, J. (1980). The effects of handedness and writing posture on neuropsychological test results. *Neuropsychologia, 18,* 231–235.

Gurling, H. M. D., Curtis, D., & Murray, R. M. (1991). Psychological deficit from excessive alcohol consumption: Evidence from a co-twin control study. *British Journal of Addiction, 86,* 151–155.

Halstead, W. (1947). *Brain and intelligence: A quantitative study of the frontal lobes.* Chicago: University of Chicago Press.

Harley, J. P., Leuthold, C. A., Matthews, C. G., & Bergs, L. E. (1980). *T-score norms: Wisconsin Neuropsychological Test Battery (CA 55-79).* Mimeo. Madison, Wisconsin.

Harris, M., Cross, H. J., & Van Nieuwkerk, R. (1981). The effects of state depression and sex on the Finger Tapping and Tactual Performance tests. *Clinical Neuropsychology, 3,* 28–34.

Heaton, R. K., Miller, S. W., Taylor, M. J., & Grant, I. (1991, 1992, 2004). *Revised comprehensive norms for an expanded Halstead-Reitan Battery: Demographically adjusted neuropsychological norms for African American and Caucasian adults.* Lutz, Fla.: PAR.

Heilbronner, R. L., Henry, G. K., Buck, P., Adams, R. L., & Fogle, T. (1991). Lateralized brain damage and performance on Trail Making A and B, Digit Span Forward and Backward, and TPT Memory and Location. *Archives of Clinical Neuropsychology, 6,* 252–258.

Hinton-Bayre, A. (2000). Reliable change formula query. *Journal of the International Neuropsychological Society, 6,* 362–363.

Ivnik, R. J. (1978). Neuropsychological test performance as a function of the duration of MS-related symptomatology. *Journal of Clinical Psychiatry, 39,* 304–312.

Johnstone, B., Vieth, A. Z., Johnson, J. C., & Shaw, J. A. (2000). Recall as a function of single versus multiple trials: Implications for rehabilitation. *Rehabilitation Psychology, 45,* 3–19.

Klonoff, H., & Low, M. (1974). Disordered brain function in young children and early adolescents: Neuropsychological and electrophysiological correlates. In R. M. Reitan & L. A. Davidson (Eds.). *Clinical neuropsychology: Current status and applications* (pp. 121–178). New York: Wiley.

Knights, R. M. & Norwood, J. A. (1980). *Revised smoothed normative data on the Neuropsychological Test Battery for Children.* Mimeo. Department of Psychology, Carleton University, Ottawa, Ontario, Canada.

Kupke, T. (1983). Effect of subject sex, examiner sex, and test apparatus on Halstead Category and Tactual Performance tests. *Journal of Consulting and Clinical Psychology, 51,* 624–626.

Leckliter, I. N., Forster, A. A., Klonoff, H., & Knights, R. M. (1992). A review of reference group data from normal children for the Halstead-Reitan Neuropsychological Test Battery for Older Children. *The Clinical Neuropsychologist, 6,* 201–229.

Lezak, M. D., Howieson, D. B., & Loring, D. W. (2004). *Neuropsychological assessment* (4th ed.). New York: Oxford University Press.

Maassen, G. H. (2004). The standard error in the Jacobson and Truax reliable change index: The classical approach to the assessment of reliable change. *Journal of the International Neuropsychological Society, 10,* 888–893.

McIntosh, D. E., Dunham, M. D., & Dean, R. (1995). Neuropsychological characteristics of learning disabled/gifted children. *International Journal of Neuroscience, 83,* 123–130.

Mitrushina, M. N., Boone, K. B., Razani, J. & D'Elia, L. F. (2005). *Handbook of normative data for neuropsychological assessment* (2nd ed.). New York: Oxford University Press.

Moore, T. E., Richards, B., & Hood, J. (1984). Aging and the coding of spatial information. *Journal of Gerontology, 39,* 210–212.

Mutchnik, M. G., Ross, L. K., & Long, C. J. (1991). Decision strategies for cerebral dysfunction IV: Determination of cerebral dysfunction. *Archives of Clinical Neuropsychology, 6,* 259–270.

Pauker, J. D. (1980). *Norms for the Halstead-Reitan Neuropsychological Test Battery based on a non-clinical adult sample.* Paper presented to the Canadian Psychological association, Calgary, Alberta, Canada.

Prigatano, G. P., Parsons, O. A., Wrigth, E., Levin, D. C., & Hawryluk, G. (1983). Neuropsychological test performance in mildly hypoxemic patients with chronic obstructive pulmonary disease. *Journal of Consulting and Clinical Psychology, 51,* 108–116.

Reitan, R. M. (1959). *The effects of brain lesions on adaptive abilities in human beings.* Unpublished manuscript, Indiana University Medical Center, Indianapolis, Indiana.

Reitan, R. M. (1964). Psychological deficits resulting from cerebral lesions in man. In J. M. Warren & K. A. Akert (Eds.), *The frontal granular cortex and behavior* (pp. 295–312). New York: McGraw-Hill.

Reitan, R. M. (1979). *Manual for administration of Neuropsychological Test Batteries for Adults and Children.* Tucson, Ariz.: Neuropsychology Laboratory.

Reitan, R. M., & Boll, T. J. (1971). Intellectual and cognitive functions in Parkinson's disease. *Journal of Consulting and Clinical Psychology, 37,* 364–369.

Reitan, R. M., & Wolfson, D. (1985). *The Halstead-Reitan Neuropsychological Test Battery.* Tucson, Arizona: Neuropsychology Press.

Reitan, R. M., & Wolfson, D. (1996). Relationships between specific and general tests of cerebral functioning. *The Clinical Neuropsychologist, 10,* 37–42.

Rothke, S. (1989). The relationship between neuropsychological test scores and performance on a driving evaluation. *International Journal of Clinical Neuropsychology, 11,* 134–136.

Russell, E. W. (1985). Comparison of the TPT-10- and 6-hole form board. *Journal of Clinical Psychology, 41,* 68–81.

Russell, E. W. & Starkey, R. I. (1993, 2001). *Halstead Russell Neuropsychological Evaluation System (HRNES) manual.* Los Angeles: Western Psychological Services.

Schludermann, E. H., & Schludermann, S. M. (1983). Halstead's studies in the neuropsychology of aging. *Archives of Gerontology and Geriatrics, 2,* 49–172.

Shure, G. H., & Halstead, W. C. (1958). Cerebral localization of intellectual processes. In N. L. Munn (Ed.), *Psychological Monographs General and Applied, 72*(12), No. 465.

Snow, W. G. (1987). Standardization of test administration and scoring criteria: Some shortcomings of current practice with the Halstead-Reitan Battery. *The Clinical Neuropsychologist, 1,* 250–262.

Spreen, O., & Gaddes, W. H. (1969). Developmental norms for 15 neuropsychological tests age 6 to 15. *Cortex, 5,* 171–191.

Steese-Seda, D., Brown, W. S., & Caetano, C. (1995). Development of visuomotor coordination in school aged children: The Bimanual Coordination Test. *Developmental Neuropsychology, 11,* 181–199.

Sweeney, J. E., & Johnson, A. M. (2001). Age and neuropsychological status following exposure to violent nonimpact acceleration forces in MVAs. *Journal of Forensic Neuropsychology, 2,* 31–40.

Thompson, L. L., & Heaton, R. K. (1991). Patterns of performance on the Tactual Performance Test. *The Clinical Neuropsychologist, 5,* 322–328.

Thompson, L. L., Heaton, R. K., Matthews, C. G., & Grant, I. (1987). Comparison of preferred and nonpreferred hand performance on four neuropsychological motor tasks. *The Clinical Neuropsychologist, 1,* 324–334.

Thompson, L. L. & Parsons, O. A. (1985). Contribution of the TPT to adult neuropsychological assessment. *Journal of Clinical and Experimental Neuropsychology, 7,* 430–444.

Warner, M. H., Ernst, J., Townes, B. D., & Peel, J. (1987). Relationship between IQ and neuropsychological measures in neuropsychiatric populations: Within-laboratory and cross-cultural replications using WAIS and WAIS-R. *Journal of Clinical and Experimental Neuropsychology, 9,* 549–562.

Wiens, A. M., & Matarazzo, J. D. (1977). WAIS and MMPI correlates of the Halstead-Reitan Neuropsychology Battery in normal male subjects. *The Journal of Nervous and Mental Disease, 164,* 112–121.

Wheeler, L., Burke, C. J., & Reitan, R. M. (1963). An application of discrimination functions to the problem of predicting brain damage using behavioral variables. *Perceptual and Motor Skills, 16,* 417–440.

Wheeler, L., & Reitan, R. M. (1963). Discriminant functions applied to the problem of predicting cerebral damage from behavior tests: A cross-validation study. *Perceptual and Motor Skills, 16,* 681–701.

Yeudall, L. T., Reddon, J. R., Gill, D. M., & Stefanyk, W. O. (1987). Normative data for the Halstead-Reitan neuropsychological tests stratified by age and sex. *Journal of Clinical Psychology, 43,* 346–367.

14

Tests of Motor Function

Tests of motor performance, usually of the hands, are an essential part of most neuropsychological examinations, because deficits are seen in numerous neurological disturbances. A number of measures are especially useful for identifying motor impairment and making inferences about the functional integrity of the two cerebral hemispheres. These include measures of somewhat separate aspects of handedness: preference (e.g., Annett, 1970), strength (e.g., Hand Dynamometer), speed (e.g., Finger Tapping), and dexterity (e.g., Grooved Pegboard, Purdue Pegboard; see Table 14–1. Aspects of motor function can also be measured by subtests included in batteries such as the BDAE-3, KBNA, and NEPSY (see reviews in this volume).

In general, performance with the preferred hand is slightly superior to that with the nonpreferred hand; however, there is considerable variability in the normal population, and the preferred hand is not necessarily the more proficient one (e.g., Benton et al., 1962; Satz et al., 1967). Patterns of performance indicating equal or better performance with the nonpreferred hand occur with considerable regularity in the normal population, and neurological disturbance should not be inferred from an isolated lack of concordance. Further, even fairly large intermanual discrepancies on one motor task are quite common in the normal population. On the other hand, discrepant performances that are consistent across several tests are quite rare in the normal population and therefore are more likely to suggest a lesion in the contralateral hemisphere (Bornstein, 1986; Thompson et al., 1987).

It is also worth bearing in mind that there can be reasons other than lateralized motor defect for a neurologically impaired individual to perform poorly on skilled motor tasks. These include peripheral injury, visual impairment, general cognitive slowing, deterioration of attentional processes, problems with task initiation and monitoring, and lack of effort.

Motor tasks are brief, are easy to give, and tend to be minimally affected by factors such as education and IQ, facilitating their use with a wide variety of individuals. In some populations (e.g., the elderly), task performance (e.g., strength) may correlate with cognitive functioning and provide clues regarding the general integrity of the central nervous system (e.g., Anstey & Smith, 1999). Performance may also help to predict subsequent cognitive change (Anstey et al., 2001) as well as the risk of mortality (MacDonald et al., 2004).

Table 14–1 Some Measures of Motor Function

Test	Age Range (Years)	Administration Time (Min)	Processes	Test-Retest Reliability
Finger Tapping	5–85	<10	Self-directed manual speed Motivational status	Variable (low to high)
Grip Strength	6–8 and 12–85	5	Manual strength Motivational status	Generally adequate
Grooved Pegboard	6–85	5	Manual dexterity Speed Motivational status	Marginal to high
Purdue Pegboard	5–89	5	Manual dexterity Bimanual coordination	Variable, depends on number of trials given

Adequate motor function is critical in the performance of almost all tasks of daily living. Not surprisingly, a number of studies have shown a relationship between motor problems (e.g., hemiplegia, dexterity) and functional outcome, including employment and social functioning, in a variety of neurological conditions (e.g., head injury, dementia). Accordingly, motor skills should be assessed routinely (Haaland et al., 1994). Performance of motor skills in everyday life can be assessed with some scales designed to measure everyday living (e.g., SIB-R, reviewed elsewhere in this volume).

REFERENCES

Annett, M. (1970). A classification of hand preference by association analysis. *British Journal of Psychology, 61,* 303–321.

Anstey, K. J., & Smith, G. A. (1999). Interrelationships among biological markers of aging, health, activity, acculturation, and cognitive performance in late adulthood. *Psychology and Aging, 14,* 605–618.

Anstey, K. J., Luszcz, M. A., Giles, L. C., & Andrews, G. R. (2001). Demographic, health, cognitive, and sensory variables as predictors of mortality in very old adults. *Psychology and Aging, 16,* 3–11.

Benton, A. L., Meyers, R., & Polder, G. J. (1962). Some aspects of handedness. *Psychiatrica et Neurologica Basel, 144,* 231–337.

Bornstein, R. A. (1986). Consistency of intermanual discrepancies in normal and unilateral brain lesion patients. *Journal of Consulting and Clinical Psychology, 54,* 719–723.

Haaland, K. Y., Temkin, N., Randahl, G., & Dikmen, S. (1994). Recovery of simple motor skills after head injury. *Journal of Clinical and Experimental Neuropsychology, 16,* 448–456.

MacDonald, S. W. S., Dixon, R. A., Cohen, A-L., & Hazlitt, J. E. (2004). Biological age and 12-year cognitive change in older adults: Findings from the Victoria Longitudinal Study. *Gerontology, 50,* 64–81.

Satz, P., Achenbach, K., & Fennell, E. (1967). Correlations between assessed manual laterality and predicted speech laterality in a normal population. *Neuropsychologia, 5,* 295–310.

Thompson, L. L., Heaton, R. K., Mathews, C. G., & Grant, I. (1987). Comparison of preferred and nonpreferred hand performance on four neuropsychological motor tasks. *The Clinical Neuropsychologist, 1,* 324–334.

Finger Tapping Test (FTT)

OTHER TEST NAME

The Finger Tapping Test (FTT)is also called the Finger Oscillation Test.

PURPOSE

The purpose of this test is to measure self-directed manual motor speed.

SOURCE

The manual finger tapper can be ordered from Reitan Neuropsychology Laboratory, P.O. Box 66080, Tucson AZ 85728 (http://www.reitanlabs.com), at a cost of $125 US. An electric finger tapper (for young children) costs $245 US. Psychological Assessment Resources, Inc., 16204 N. Florida Ave, Lutz, FL 33549 (http://www.parinc.com), offers a manual finger tapper at a cost of $155 US. However, different levels of performance may be obtained when subjects are tested with devices other than the Reitan apparatus (Snow, 1987; Whitfield & Newcomb, 1992). If another device is used (e.g., computer), the examiner should ensure that comparable results are obtained with the new finger tapping unit.

AGE RANGE

Norms are available for ages 5 to 85 years.

DESCRIPTION

Finger tapping measures are included in neuropsychological examinations in order to assess subtle motor and other cognitive impairment. The FTT (Reitan, 1969) was originally called the Finger Oscillation Test (FOT) and was part of Halstead's (1947) test battery. Despite its age, surveys have revealed that it ranks sixth among the top 20 tests used by neuropsychologists (Camara et al., (2000) and sixth in terms of use with regard to predicting an individual's ability to return to work (Rabin et al., 2005).

Using a specially adapted tapper and counter, the examinee is instructed to tap as rapidly as possible, using the index finger of the preferred hand. A comparable set of measurements is then obtained with the nonpreferred hand. The procedure calls for five consecutive trials within a 5-point range with each hand (Reitan & Wolfson, 1985). This procedure is used to avoid undue influence of single deviant scores on total performance. There are other variants of the procedure. For example, Russell & Starkey (1993) have the examinee perform six trials with each hand, in sets of three, alternating hands between sets. However, the most commonly used method is the one described by Reitan & Wolfson (1985), and it is the method considered here.

Note that an electric finger tapper is recommended for children aged 5 to 8 years, and the manual tapper is used for individuals aged 9 years and older. However, a recent report (Rosselli et al., 2001) that provides normative data for young children used the manual tapper.

ADMINISTRATION

The instructions derive from Reitan and Wolfson (1985). Have the individual place the preferred hand palm down, with fingers extended and the index finger placed on the key. Direct the subject to tap as quickly as he or she can, moving only the index finger, not the whole hand or arm. The subject is given five consecutive 10-s trials with the preferred hand. The procedure is then repeated with the nonpreferred hand. Five 10-s trials are given for each hand except when the results are too variable from one trial to another. Specifically, the test procedure requires that the five consecutive trials for each hand be within a 5-point range from fastest to slowest. If one or more of the trials exceed this range, additional trials are given and the scores of the deviant trials are discarded. A maximum of 10 trials with each hand is allowed. Do *not* alternate hand trials.

Fatigue may affect performance, and a brief rest period should be given after each trial. Even if no sign of fatigue is apparent, a rest period of 1 to 2 min is required after the third trial. A practice trial is given before the test begins so that the subject can get a "feel" for the apparatus.

Do not allow the subject to move the whole hand from the wrist. With young children and poorly coordinated adults, this requirement is difficult and may be relaxed as long as it is clear that the score is obtained by index finger oscillation and not by movement of the whole hand.

Begin timing when you hear the first "click" of the counter. In addition, listen for extra taps after you tell the subject to stop. Record the number on the counter when the examiner says stop, not when the subject in fact stops.

ADMINISTRATION TIME

The time required is 10 min.

SCORING

The finger tapping score is computed for each hand separately and is the mean of five consecutive 10-s trials within a range of 5 taps. A maximum of 10 trials with each hand is allowed, and if this criterion is not met, the score is the mean of the total number of trials.

DEMOGRAPHIC EFFECTS

When each hand is considered separately, several trends emerge from the normative data.

Age

In children, performance improves with increasing age (Finlayson & Reitan, 1976; Rosselli et al., 2001), whereas in adults, performance declines with advancing age (Bornstein, 1985; Goldstein & Braun, 1974; Heaton et al., 1991; Leckliter & Matarazzo, 1989; McCurry et al., 2001; Mitrushina et al., 2005; Ott et al., 1995; Shimoyama et al., 1990; Trahan et al., 1987; Ylikoski et al., 1998; but see Moehle & Long, 1989, who reported no age-related effect for 86 subjects aged 15 years and older) and variability increases with older age (Mitrushina et al., 2005). Heaton et al. (2004) reported that in their large normative sample (aged 20–85 years), about 12% to 18% of the variance in finger tapping scores was accounted for by age.

Gender

Rosselli et al. (2001) noted a gender effect in children, with boys performing better than girls. However, Finlayson & Reitan (1976) did not observe any gender-related differences. In adults, gender shows somewhat greater effect on finger tapping than age, with males outperforming females (Bornstein, 1985; Carlier et al., 1993; Fromm-Auch & Yeudall, 1983; Harris et al., 1981; Heaton et al., 1991; Leckliter & Matarazzo, 1989; Mitrushina et al., 2005; Nagasaki et al., 1988; Ruff & Parker, 1993; Shimoyama et al., 1990; Trahan et al., 1987; Ylikoski et al., 1998; but see McCurry et al., 2001 who failed to note a gender effect). Heaton et al. (2004) reported that, in adults, about 16% to 20% of the test scores were accounted for by gender. Dodrill (1979) suggested that the observed gender difference for finger tapping may be attributed to sexual dimorphism in body and hand size rather than a neuropsychological mechanism. However, Schmidt et al. (2000) noted that controlling for finger and hand size did not eliminate the main effect of gender on finger tapping.

Hand Preference

Scores tend to be higher with the preferred than with the nonpreferred hand in both children and adults (Finlayson & Reitan, 1976; Heaton et al., 2004; Shimoyama et al., 1990; but see Ruff & Parker, 1993).

IQ/Education

Performance tends to be better with increasing IQ (Leckliter & Matarazzo, 1989; but see Horton, 1999, who failed to note an association between increasing IQ and scores for the dominant hand) and with more years of education (Bornstein, 1985; Heaton et al., 1991; but see McCurry et al., 2001; Ruff & Parker, 1993; Ylikoski et al., 1998). However, age and gender have stronger effects than education on performance in adults (Bornstein, 1985). According to Heaton et al. (2004), education accounts for only about 2% to 4% of the variance in tapping scores.

Ethnicity

Performance tends to be somewhat better in Caucasians than in African Americans (Heaton et al., 2004). No differences were reported among Mexican American, Anglo American, and Mexican individuals on this task (Arnold et al., 1994).

Intermanual Differences

Age and years of education do not have a strong relationship with measures of intermanual difference in adults (Bornstein, 1986b; Heaton et al., 1991; Ruff & Parker, 1993; Thompson et al., 1987). The findings regarding gender differences in intermanual difference scores are inconsistent; some studies report greater between-hand differences for males than for females (Bornstein, 1986b; Fromm-Auch & Yeudall, 1983), and others do not (Ruff & Parker, 1993; Thompson et al., 1987). There is evidence that right-handers show larger intermanual differences than left-handers do (Thompson et al., 1987).

NORMATIVE DATA

Adults

Conventional cutoff scores (Reitan & Wolfson, 1985) should not be used, because high false-positive rates are likely to occur (Bernard, 1989; Bornstein, 1986c). These cutoffs were based on the performance of individuals who were largely middle-aged and above-average intellectually. For example, among Bornstein's sample of 365 healthy volunteers with a mean age of 43 years, use of conventional cutoff scores resulted in 80% of subjects being misclassified as impaired on preferred hand tapping scores.

Because of the effects of age, gender, education, and ethnicity, we recommend the use of normative data provided by Heaton et al. (2004). As noted in Table 14–2, they provided norms separately for two ethnicity groups (Caucasians and African Americans), organized by age, gender, and education. The sample is large and covers a wide range in terms of age (20–85 years) and education (0–20 years), and the exclusion criteria are specified. T scores lower than 40 are classed as impaired. According to Heaton et al. (2004), the procedure used was the one specified by Reitan and Wolfson (1985). Unfortunately, the method for determining hand preference was not described.

A number of other investigators have provided norms for segments of the adult population, including Bornstein, 1985

Table 14–2 Characteristics of the Finger Tapping Normative Sample provided by Heaton et al. (2004)

Number	1212
Age (years)	20–85[a]
Geographic location	Various states in the United States and Manitoba, Canada
Sample type	Individuals recruited as part of multicenter studies
Education (years)	0–20[b]
Gender (%)	
Male	56.8
Female	43.2
Race/Ethnicity	
Caucasian	634
African American	578
Screening	No reported history of learning disability, neurological disorder, serious psychiatric disorder, or alcohol or drug abuse

[a]Age groups: 20–34, 35–39, 40–44, 45–49, 50–54, 55–59, 60–64, 65–69, 70–74, 75–79, and 80–89 years.
[b]Education groups: 7–8, 9–11, 12, 13–15, 16–17, and 18–20 years.

(20–69 years); Fromm-Auch and Yeudall, 1983 (15–64 years); Goldstein and Braun, 1974 (20–79 years); Ruff & Parker, 1993 (16–70 years); and Trahan et al., 1987 (18–91 years). Recently, Mitrushina et al. (2005) compiled data from eight studies for males and four for females, comprising 530 to 963 participants (depending on hand preference and gender), aged 20 to 74 years. They noted that the integrity of their meta-analysis was undermined by the lack of consistency in reporting data regarding handedness. Their data appear fairly similar to those reported by Heaton et al. (2004).

Ruff and Parker (1993) provided cross-sectional normative data for 358 adult volunteers, aged 16 to 70 years. Their education level ranged from 7 to 22 years, and they resided in California (65%), Michigan (30%), and the U.S. Eastern seaboard (5%). All participants were screened to exclude those with a positive history of psychiatric hospitalization, chronic polydrug abuse, or neurological disorders. Hand preference was determined by both questionnaire and performance on a series of tasks. Note that the method of administration differed somewhat from that of Reitan and Wolfson (1985). That is, participants were given a brief opportunity to practice with either hand, after which five 10-s trials were alternatively given to the dominant and then the nondominant hand. If there was a spread of more than 5 taps between any two trials of one hand, then two additional trials were required for that hand. If seven trials were necessary, both the highest and lowest scores were eliminated, and the mean was calculated using the remaining five scores. Despite the differences, their data agree fairly well with those of Heaton et al. (2004) and Mitrushina et al. (2005). Table 14–3 provides their data (means and standard deviations) for both dominant and nondominant hands, stratified by age and gender.

McCurry et al. (2001) presented data based on a sample of Japanese American adults, aged 70 years and older, who were enrolled in a prospective study of aging and dementia in King County, Washington. None of the participants was classed as demented based on clinical and screening neuropsychological

Table 14–3 Mean Performance of Adults for Finger Tapping

	Dominant			Nondominant	
Age Group	N	M	SD	M	SD
Women					
16–24	45	49.5	5.1	45.6	5.1
25–39	45	49.0	4.1	44.6	4.6
40–54	44	47.0	5.6	43.5	5.2
55–70	45	45.7	5.5	40.4	5.2
Men					
16–24	45	52.9	5.1	48.2	4.4
25–39	44	52.7	6.8	48.7	5.7
40–54	45	54.3	5.7	48.9	5.8
55–70	45	53.5	6.4	48.3	5.0

Source: From Ruff & Parker, 1993. © Perceptual and Motor Skills 1993. Reprinted with permission.

Table 14-4 Finger Tapping Means, Standard Deviations, and Quartiles by Age for Japanese Americans

Age & Gender	n	Mean	SD	25th Percentile	Median	75th Percentile
Men 70–79 years						
Dominant	58	42.96	8.3	35	45	49
Nondominant	57	39.63	4.67	35	40	42
Female 70–79 years						
Dominant	44	42.77	7.88	40	42	47
Nondominant	43	39.27	7.01	36	40	42
Male 80–89 years						
Dominant	18	35.81	9.27	31	33	45
Nondominant	18	35.09	8.05	29	36	42
Female 80–89 years						
Dominant	37	36.62	9.28	30	36	44
Nondominant	35	33.78	7.63	28	37	41

Note: The sample consisted of 160 adults, Mean education about 11.0 ($SD = 3.0$); 72.9% born in the United States (94.9% in the age group 70–79; 35.7% in the age group 80+), 94% right-handed. Age but not gender, education, or language spoken significantly affected test scores.

Source: S. McCurry, personal communication, May 17, 2004.

examinations. The data are provided in Table 14–4 and represent an important source of information for this understudied segment of the U.S. population.

Children/Adolescents

Findeis and Weight (1994) developed meta-norms (Tables 14–5 and 14–6) based on a series of articles published between 1969 and 1989 (including those by Finlayson & Reitan, 1976; Klonoff & Low, 1974; Spreen & Gaddes, 1969). In addition to concerns regarding the outdated nature of the studies

and differences in administration across studies (e.g., type of tapper used, number of trials given), users should note that the majority of the participants were Caucasian, came from middle- to upper-class socioeconomic backgrounds, and had above-average IQs. Another limitation of the data is that the values are not provided separately for males and females, although Finlayson and Reitan (1976) noted no gender differences in children aged 6 to 14 years. Further, the method for determining hand preference is unknown.

Recently, Rosselli et al. (2001) provided data (see Table 14–7) on a sample of 290 Spanish-speaking children (141 boys, 149 girls), aged 6 to 11 years, in Bogota, Colombia. None of the subjects was mentally retarded. Based on the Waterloo

Table 14-5 Characteristics of the Finger Tapping Meta-Norms Provided by Findeis and Weight (1994)

Number	5–8 years: 515
	9–14 years: 331
Age (years)	4–14
Geographic location	United States and Canada
Sample Type	Subjects pooled from various articles published between 1969 and 1989; Full-Scale IQ = 112.87; from middle- and upper-class socioeconomic backgrounds
Education	Not reported
Gender	
Male	Not Reported
Female	Not Reported
Race/Ethnicity	Mostly Caucasian
Screening	No history of neurological abnormalities

Table 14-6 Meta-Norms for Finger Tapping Derived from Findeis and Weight (1994)

	Dominant Hand			Nondominant Hand		
Age	N	Mean	SD	N	Mean	SD
5	339	29.39	4.2	311	26.32	4.6
6	226	29.87	3.3	221	27.22	3.3
7	288	33.67	4.6	288	30.03	3.9
8	265	36.40	4.6	265	32.03	3.8
9	49	34.01	4.1	49	30.31	3.3
10	95	37.52	5.4	95	34.04	4.8
11	93	40.72	4.8	93	35.06	4.8
12	143	41.36	5.4	143	36.66	4.1
13	41	44.64	5.2	41	39.64	4.7
14	52	44.38	6.8	52	40.67	6.1

Source: Courtesy of the authors, August 18, 2003.

Table 14–7 Finger Tapping Normative Data for Spanish Speaking Boys and Girls Aged 6–11 Years

Hand	6–7 Years ($n = 83$)	8–9 Years ($n = 121$)	10–11 Years ($n = 86$)
Preferred	32.25 (4.96)	35.52 (5.35)	41.08 (5.08)
Nonpreferred	28.16 (3.81)	30.76 (4.65)	35.48 (4.99)

Note: The manual tapper was used with all children (Rosselli, personal communication, May 19, 2004).

Source: Adapted from Rosselli et al., 2001.

Handedness questionnaire, 268 children were right-handed and 22 were left-handed. In comparison with the meta-norms provided by Findeis and Weight (1994), the children in Colombia showed a greater increase in number of taps with both the preferred and the nonpreferred hand with age. In both studies, however, the improvement was more evident for the preferred hand.

RELIABILITY

Test-Retest Reliability and Practice Effects

Reliability coefficients ranging from .58 to .93 have been reported with both normal and patient samples (Bornstein et al., 1987; Dikmen et al., 1999; Dodrill & Troupin, 1975; Gill et al., 1986; Goldstein & Watson, 1989; Morrison et al., 1979; Provins & Cunliffe, 1972; Ruff & Parker, 1993; Sjogren et al., 2000; but see Matarazzo et al., 1974, for low values, <.50, in both normal subjects and patients with cerebrovascular disease retested after intervals of 3–5 months).

Some investigators have reported that the differences between hands are consistent ($r = >.70$; Massman & Doody, 1996; Provins & Cunliffe, 1972). Others, however, have indicated that the differences between hands are not highly reliable ($r = .50$; Morrison et al., 1979).

Practice effects tend to be minimal in both healthy (e.g., Bornstein et al., 1987; Salinsky et al., 2001) and impaired populations (e.g., Dodrill & Troupin, 1975). Haaland et al. (1994)

noted a slight improvement, two taps per 10 s, for both normal subjects and individuals with mild head injuries who were tested at 1 month and again at 1 year after injury. The similar, though subtle, improvement in finger tapping should alert clinicians to overinterpreting tapping improvement as evidence of recovery.

Dikmen et al. (1999) reported slight improvement in scores in a sample of 384 normal or neurologically stable individuals (aged 15–83 years, $M = 34.2$, $SD = 16.7$) who were retested about 9 months after initial testing. Table 14–8 provides information to determine whether there has been substantial change taking practice into account. One first subtracts the mean T2 – T1 change (column 3) from the difference between the two testings for the individual and then compares the resulting value with 1.64 times the standard deviation of the difference (column 4). The 1.64 comes from the normal distribution and is exceeded in the positive or negative direction only 10% of the time if indeed there is no real change in clinical condition. Dikmen et al. (1999) also noted that those with better initial scores have bigger improvements in test scores. Factors such as the length of retest interval, age, and education of the individual had little effect on change.

VALIDITY

Relationships With Other Measures

Factor analytic findings suggest that finger tapping and pegboard dexterity measure independent dimensions of manual proficiency (Fleishman & Hempel, 1954; Stanford & Barratt, 1996). However, when between-hand asymmetry is considered, finger-tapping correlates highly (.78) in normal adults with Purdue peg placement, a task that requires independent, precise finger movement. This suggests that both tasks depend at least in part on a common neural substrate; namely, asymmetry in the corticospinal system (Triggs et al., 2000). The correlation, however, is lower between finger tapping and grip strength asymmetry (.41); grip strength does not require independent or precise control of the fingers (Triggs et al., 2000).

Table 14–8 Finger Tapping Test-Retest Effects in 384 Normal or Neurologically Stable Individuals Assessed After Intervals of about 2–16 Months

Measure	Time 1		Time 2		T2 – T1		T1, T2
	(1) Mean	SD	(2) Mean	SD	(3) M	(4) SD	r
Dominant	50.88	6.59	51.36	6.46	.48	4.39	.77
Nondominant	47.02	6.39	47.87	6.47	.85	4.31	.78

Note: Mean Age = 34.2, $SD = 16$, 7, range = 15–83; Mean education = 12.1, $SD = 2.6$, range = 0–19; 66% male; retest interval mean = 9.1 months, $SD = 3.0$, range = 2.4–15.8.

Source: Adapted from Dikmen et al., 1999.

Finger tapping correlates moderately ($r = .46$ to $.51$) with the Perceptual Organization factor of the WAIS-R (Berger, 1998), suggesting that visual processing is important. It shows only a small correlation (.25) with the Processing Speed Index of the WAIS-III, suggesting that finger tapping involves only minimal amounts of the kind of central resources required in more complex measures of speeded perceptual processing (Kennedy et al., 2003). In adolescents, finger tapping loads on the same factor as various verbal skills (e.g., WRAT Reading, WISC-R VIQ), perhaps reflecting that both skills depend on precise timing and serial ordering of components (Stanford & Barratt, 1996).

Clinical Findings

The measure is sensitive to the presence and laterality of brain lesions (e.g., Barnes & Lucas, 1974; Bigler & Tucker, 1981; Dodrill, 1978; Dufouil et al., 2003; Finlayson & Reitan, 1980; Haaland & Delaney, 1981; Hom & Reitan, 1982, 1990; Reitan & Wolfson, 1994, 1996; Ylikoski et al., 1998). Given the crossed nature of the motor system, performance tends to be worse in the hand contralateral to the lesion.

Typically, the performances of the preferred and nonpreferred hands are compared on motor tasks to determine whether there is consistent evidence of poor performance with one hand relative to the other. In general, finger tapping performance with the preferred hand is superior to that with the nonpreferred hand (Bornstein, 1985, 1986a; Corey et al., 2001; Peters, 1990; Thompson, et al., 1987; Triggs et al., 2000). The most frequently reported guideline is that the preferred hand should perform about 10 percent better than the nonpreferred hand (Reitan & Wolfson, 1985). However, there is considerable variability in the normal population, and the preferred hand is not necessarily the faster one, especially when left-handed people are considered (Bornstein, 1986a; Corey et al., 2001; Thompson et al., 1987). Patterns of performance indicating equal or better performance with the nonpreferred hand occur with considerable regularity in the normal population (about 30%), and neurological involvement should not be inferred from an isolated lack of concordance. Fairly large discrepancies between the hands on the FTT alone also cannot be used to suggest unilateral impairment, because discrepancies of large magnitude are not uncommon (about 25%) in the normal population (Bornstein, 1986a; Thompson et al., 1987). Greater confidence in the clinical judgment of impaired motor function with one or the other hand can be gained from consideration of the consistency of intermanual discrepancies across several motor tasks, because truly consistent, deviant performances are quite rare in the normal population (Bornstein, 1986a, 1986b; Thompson et al., 1987).

It is also important to note that there could be reasons other than a lateralized motor defect for an individual with brain dysfunction to perform poorly with the nonpreferred hand on skilled motor tasks. For example, if intellectual efficiency is reduced, perhaps as a result of cortical and/or sub-cortical involvement in both hemispheres, then performance with the nonpreferred (less practiced) hand may be affected on tasks that require adaptation and skilled movement, such as finger tapping (Lewis & Kupke, 1992).

There is evidence that tapping speed is sensitive to a wide variety of conditions, including chronic alcoholism (Leckliter & Matarazzo, 1989), Korsakoff's syndrome (Welch et al., 1997), closed-head injury (Dikmen et al., 1995; Haaland et al., 1994; Prigatano & Borano, 2003), multiple sclerosis (Chipchase et al., 2003), chronic pain (Sjogren et al., 2000), and the mild stages of degenerative dementias (Muller et al., 1991; Ott et al., 1995; see also Massman & Doody, 1996, and Wefel et al., 1999), perhaps reflecting the involvement of other nonmotor processes. That is, in addition to direct motoric effects, the speed, coordination, and pacing requirements of finger tapping could be affected by variable levels of alertness, impaired ability to focus and maintain attention, problems with generating responses, or generalized slowing of responses.

Further, the test can distinguish patients with motor dysfunctions of cerebellar, basal ganglia, and cerebral origin from normal subjects (Shimoyama et al., 1990). However, tapping frequency cannot distinguish one abnormal group from another (Shimoyama et al., 1990). Other measures (e.g., intertap variability, time in flexion and extension in the tap cycle, time-sequential histograms of tapping intervals) may be able to distinguish among groups and to identify motor impairments that are not apparent in tapping rate (Roy et al., 1992; Shimoyama et al., 1990).

In a recent functional magnetic resonance imaging (fMRI) study with the right hand (Johnson & Prigatano, 2000), activations in regions of the contralateral and ipsilateral primary motor cortex, left lateral premotor cortex, left dorsolateral prefrontal cortex, and ipsilateral cerebellum were noted in normal individuals' performance on the FTT. Therefore, disturbances in a variety of brain regions and circuits may result in slow finger tapping.

Central dopamine plays a role in motor activity. Consistent with this notion, there is a relationship between performance on this fine motor task and striatal D_2 receptor density (Yang et al., 2003), suggesting that the Finger Tapping task may be a sensitive tool for monitoring various diseases (e.g., those affecting extrapyrapidal systems) and medication effects (e.g., detecting neuroleptic-induced motor impairments in patients with schizophrenia). Further, the sensitivity of the task to aging may be explained in part by a decline in dopamine D_2 density.

It is worth noting that, although most investigators evaluate speed of finger tapping, qualitative features of the task may also have diagnostic value. For example, Prigatano and Borgaro (2003) reported that abnormal finger-tapping patterns (e.g., failure to inhibit movement of fingers other than the index finger) are more common in individuals with traumatic brain injury than in normal subjects, and that the frequency of abnormal finger movements may relate to the severity of the injury.

Table 14–9 Positive Predictive Values (PPV) and Negative Predictive Values (NPV) for Dominant Hand Finger Tapping for Different Base Rates

Cutoff Value	15% Base Rate		30% Base Rate		50% Base Rate	
	PPV (%)	NPV (%)	PPV (%)	NPV (%)	PPV (%)	NPV (%)
Women						
15	75	87	86	74	91	55
28	63	93	80	85	87	70
32	48	94	68	87	83	73
35	39	94	60	87	78	85
38	28	94	48	86	69	73
Men						
21	80	88	89	74	93	55
33	53	90	76	79	87	62
35	50	91	68	80	84	64
38	45	91	67	82	83	65
40	35	92	58	82	77	67

Source: Arnold et al., 2005. Reprinted with the kind permission of Psychology Press.

Predictive Validity

Performance on the FTT is related to rehabilitation outcome after stroke (Prigatano & Wong, 1997) and also to employment status after various brain disorders (Dikmen & Morgan, 1980; Heaton et al., 1978). Those who tapped faster had better outcome. There is also evidence that performance on the test is moderately predictive of daily living skills in geriatric patients (Searight et al., 1989) and in traumatic brain-injury patients (Prigatano et al., 1990). In adolescents, the task appears to be related to cognitive tempo (impulsiveness and time judgment) (Stanford & Barratt, 1996).

Malingering

Whether the FTT is useful in identifying suboptimal performance is not certain. Using a simulation paradigm, some authors (Heaton et al., 1978; Rapport et al., 1998) found that malingerers performed worse than controls. Others (Greiffenstein et al., 1996; Trueblood & Schmidt, 1993), however, did not find the task to be a reliable index of malingering. Larrabee (2003) found that a score of less than 63 on combined (right plus left) finger tapping speed correctly identified 10/25 (40%) of individuals meeting criteria for definite malingered neurocognitive dysfunction and 29/31 (93.5%) of individuals with moderate/severe head injury.

This cutoff however, appears to require adjustment for gender. Arnold et al. (2005) evaluated finger-tapping performance in seven groups: (a) noncredible patients (as determined by failed psychometric and behavioral criteria); patients with (b) closed head injury, (c) dementia, (d) mental retardation, (e) psychosis, or (f) depression; and (g) healthy older adults. Dominant hand scores proved to be more sensitive to noncredible performance than other scores (nondominant, sum of both hands, difference between hands). With specificity set at

90% for the comparison groups combined, a dominant hand cutoff score of 35 for men yielded 50% sensitivity, and a cutoff of 28 yielded 61% sensitivity for women. However, specificity values for specific cutoffs varied considerably across the comparison groups, indicating that the cutoff should be selected based on gender and claimed diagnosis. Positive and negative predictive power for the dominant hand scores with the highest sensitivity/specificity rates at varying base rates of suspect performance are shown in Table 14–9. With a base rate of 30% noncredible subjects, a dominant-hand cutoff of ≤ 28 for women resulted in a positive predictive value (PPV) of 80% with a negative predictive value (NPV) of 85%. Using the same base rate of 30% for men, a cutoff score of ≤ 35 resulted in a PPV of 68% and a NPV of 80%. Therefore, the risk of false-positive results in males at base rates of 30% or less is quite high: more than 3 out of 10 individuals would be falsely identified as displaying suboptimal effort using this index. These data suggest that the FTT may be a more effective measure of motivational status in women than in men.

Greiffenstein et al. (1996) reported that compensation-seeking patients with postconcussion syndrome (PCS) demonstrated a nonphysiologic profile (grip strength < finger tapping <grooved pegboard). However, Rapport et al. (1998) observed that the presence of nonphysiologic configurations showed poor predictive accuracy among malingerers (coached, naïve) and controls.

COMMENT

Several authors (e.g., Baron, 2004; Snow, 1987) have noted problems of standardization in the FTT. Three different versions of the finger-tapping apparatus are available, and variations in test equipment may lead to different results. Further, administration rules vary with respect to number of trials, order of trials across hands, amount of practice provided, and scoring procedures. The method of determining hand preference frequently is not reported. Nonetheless, the finger-tapping procedure described by Reitan and Wolfson (1985) does often yield fairly reliable results. Although the demographically corrected norms for adults provided by Heaton et al. (1994) are an important contribution, normative data for children and adolescents in North America are quite old and rely on a restricted sample (e.g., Caucasian children of above-average IQ). Other normative sets, such as those presented in Table 14–7, are alternatives.

Reitan and Wolfson (1996) have suggested that finger tapping speed is a relatively pure measure of motor function. However, the task has significant cognitive contributions. Users should bear in mind that the speed, coordination, and pacing requirements of finger tapping can be affected by numerous factors, including variable levels of alertness, attention, problems with task initiation, or generalized slowing of responses. Visual processing also appears to be important. It is also worth noting that, although most investigators evaluate speed of finger tapping, qualitative features of the task may also have diagnostic value (Prigatano & Borgaro, 2003).

REFERENCES

Arnold, B. R., Montgomery, G. T., Castaneda, I., & Longoria, R. (1994). Acculturation and performance of hispanics on selected Halstead-Reitan neuropsychological tests. *Assessment, 1,* 239–248.

Arnold, G., Boone, K. B., Lu, P., Dean, A., Wen, J., Nitch, S., & McPherson, S. (2005). Sensitivity and specificity of Finger Tapping Test scores for the detection of suspect effort. *The Clinical Neuropsychologist, 19,* 105–120.

Barnes, G. W., & Lucas, G. J. (1974). Cerebral dysfunction vs. psychogenesis in Halstead-Reitan tests. *The Journal of Nervous and Mental Disease, 158,* 50–60.

Baron, I. S. (2004). *Neuropsychological evaluation of the child.* New York: Oxford University Press.

Berger, S. (1998). The WAIS-R factors: Usefulness and construct validity in neuropsychological assessment. *Applied Neuropsychology, 5,* 37–42.

Bernard, L. C. (1989). Halstead-Reitan neuropsychological test performance of black, hispanic, and white young adult males from poor academic backgrounds. *Archives of Clinical Neuropsychology, 4,* 267–274.

Bigler, E. D., & Tucker, D. M. (1981). Comparison of verbal IQ, tactual performance, Seashore rhythm and finger oscillation tests in the blind and brain damaged. *Journal of Clinical Psychology, 37,* 849–851.

Bornstein, R. A. (1985). Normative data on selected neuropsychological measures from a nonclinical sample. *Journal of Clinical Psychology, 41,* 651–659.

Bornstein, R. A. (1986a). Normative data on intermanual differences on three tests of motor performance. *Journal of Clinical and Experimental Neuropsychology, 8,* 12–20.

Bornstein, R. A. (1986b). Consistency of intermanual discrepancies in normal and unilateral brain lesion patients. *Journal of Consulting and Clinical Psychology, 54,* 719–723.

Bornstein, R. A. (1986c). Classification rates obtained with "standard" cut-off scores on selected neuropsychological measures. *Journal of Clinical and Experimental Neuropsychology, 8,* 413–420.

Bornstein, R. A., Baker, G. B., & Douglas, A. B. (1987). Short-term retest reliability of the Halstead-Reitan Battery in a normal sample. *Journal of Nervous and Mental Disease, 175,* 229–232.

Camara, W. J., Nathan, J. S., & Puente, A. E. (2000). Psychological test usage: Implications in professional psychology. *Professional Psychology: Research and Practice, 31,* 141–154.

Carlier, M., Dumont, A. M., Beau, J., & Michel, F. (1993). Hand performance of French children on a finger tapping test in relation to handedness, sex and age. *Perceptual and Motor Skills, 76,* 931–940.

Chipchase, S. Y., Lincoln, N. B., & Radford, K. A. (2003). Measuring fatigue in people with multiple sclerosis. *Disability and Rehabilitation: An International Multidisciplinary Journal, 25,* 778–784.

Corey, D. M., Hurley, M. M., & Foundas, A. L. (2001). Right and left handedness defined. *Neuropsychiatry, Neuropsychology, and Behavioral Neurology, 14,* 144–152.

Dikmen, S. S., Machamer, J. E., Winn, H. R., & Temkin, N. R. (1995). Neuropsychological outcome at 1-year post head injury. *Neuropsychology, 9,* 80–90.

Dikmen, S., & Morgan, S. F. (1980). Neuropsychological factors related to employability and occupational status in person with epilepsy. *Journal of Nervous and Mental Disease, 168,* 236–240.

Dikmen, S. S., Heaton, R. K., Grant, I., & Temkin, N. R. (1999). Test-retest reliability and practice effects of the expanded Halstead-Reitan neuropsychosocial test battery. *Journal of the International Neuropsychological Society, 5,* 346–356.

Dodrill, C. B. (1978). A neuropsychological battery for epilepsy. *Epilepsia, 19,* 611–623.

Dodrill, C. B. (1979). Sex differences on the Halstead-Reitan Neuropsychological Battery and on other neuropsychological measures. *Journal of Clinical Psychology, 35,* 236–241.

Dodrill, C. B., & Troupin, A. S. (1975). Effects of repeated administrations of a comprehensive neuropsychological battery among chronic epileptics. *Journal of Nervous and Mental Disease, 161,* 185–190.

Dufouil, C., Alperovitch, A., & Tzourio, C. (2003). Influence of education on the relationship between white matter lesions and cognition. *Neurology, 60,* 831–836.

Findeis, M. K., & Weight, D. K. (1994). *Meta-norms for two forms of neuropsychological test batteries for children.* Unpublished manuscript, Brigham Young University, Provo, Utah.

Finlayson, M. A., & Reitan, R. M. (1976). Handedness in relation to measures of motor and tactile-perceptual function in normal children. *Perceptual and Motor Skills, 43,* 475–481.

Finlayson, M. A. J., & Reitan, R. M. (1980). Effect of lateralized lesions on ipsilateral and contralateral motor functioning. *Journal of Clinical Neuropsychology, 2,* 237–243.

Fleishman, E. A., & Hempel, W. E. (1954). A factor analysis of dexterity tests. *Personnel Psychology, 7,* 15–32.

Fromm-Auch, D., & Yeudall, L. T. (1983). Normative data for the Halstead-Reitan neuropsychological tests. *Journal of Clinical Neuropsychology, 5,* 221–238.

Gill, D. M., Reddon, J. R., Stefanyk, W. O., & Hans, H. S. (1986). Finger tapping: Effects of trials and sessions. *Perceptual and Motor Skills, 62,* 674–678.

Goldstein, S. G., & Braun, L. S. (1974). Reversal of expected transfer as a function of increased age. *Perceptual and Motor Skills, 38,* 1139–1145.

Goldstein, G., & Watson, J. R. (1989). Test-retest reliability of the Halstead-Reitan battery and the WAIS in a neuropsychiatric population. *The Clinical Neuropsychologist, 3,* 265–273.

Greiffenstein, M. F., Baker, W. J., & Gola, T. (1996). Motor dysfunction profiles in traumatic brain injury and postconcussion syndrome. *Journal of the International Neuropsychological Society, 2,* 477–485.

Haaland, K. Y., & Delaney, H. D. (1981). Motor deficits after left or right hemisphere damage due to stroke or tumor. *Neuropsychologia, 19,* 17–27.

Haaland, K. Y., Temkin, N., Randahl, G., & Dikmen, S. (1994). Recovery of simple motor skills after head injury. *Journal of Clinical and Experimental Neuropsychology, 16,* 448–456.

Halstead, W. C. (1947). *Brain and intelligence.* Chicago: University of Chicago Press.

Harris, M., Cross, H., Van Nieuwkerk, R. (1981). The effects of state depression, induced depression and sex on the finger tapping and tactual performance tests. *Clinical Neuropsychology, 3,* 28–34.

Heaton, R. K., Chelune, G. J., & Lehman, R. A. W. (1978). Using neuropsychological and personality tests to assess the likelihood of patients employment. *Journal of Nervous and Mental Disease, 166,* 408–516.

Heaton, R. K., Grant, I., & Mathews, C. G. (1991). *Comprehensive norms for an expanded Halstead-Reitan Battery.* Odessa, Fla.: Psychological Assessment Resources.

Heaton, R. K., Miller, S. W., Taylor, M. J., & Grant, I. (2004). *Revised comprehensive norms for an expanded Halstead-Reitan Battery: Demographically adjusted neuropsychological norms for African American and Caucasian adults.* Lutz, FL: PAR.

Heaton, R. K., Smith, H. H., Lehman, R. A., & Vogt, A. T. (1978). Prospects for faking believable deficits on neuropsychological testing. *Journal of Consulting and Clinical Psychology, 46,* 892–900.

Hom, J., & Reitan, R. M. (1982). Effect of lateralized cerebral damage upon contralateral and ipsilateral sensorimotor performances. *Journal of Clinical Neuropsychology, 4,* 249–268.

Hom, J., & Reitan, R. M. (1990). Generalized cognitive function after stroke. *Journal of Clinical and Experimental Neuropsychology, 12,* 644–655.

Horton, A. M. (1999). Above-average intelligence and neuropsychological test score performance. *International Journal of Neuroscience, 99,* 221–231.

Johnson, S. C., & Prigatano, G. P. (2000). Functional MR imaging during finger tapping. *BNI Quarterly, 16,* 155–158.

Kennedy, J. E., Clement, P. F., & Curtiss, G. (2003). WAIS-III Processing Speed Index scores after TBI: The influence of working memory, psychomotor speed and perceptual processing. *The Clinical Neuropsychologist, 17,* 303–307.

Klonoff, H., & Low, M. (1974). Disordered brain function in young children and early adolescents: Neuropsychological and electroencephalographic correlates. In R. Reitan and L. A. Davidson (Eds.), *Clinical neuropsychology: Current status and applications.* Washington: V. H. Winston & Sons.

Larrabee, G. J. (2003). Detection of malingering using atypical performance patterns on standard neuropsychological tests. *The Clinical Neuropsychologist, 17,* 410–425.

Leckliter, I. N., & Matarazzo, J. D. (1989). The influence of age, education, IQ, gender, and alcohol abuse on Halstead-Reitan neuropsychological test battery performance. *Journal of Clinical Psychology, 45,* 484–512.

Lewis, R., & Kupke, T. (1992). Intermanual differences on skilled and unskilled motor tasks in nonlateralized brain dysfunction. *The Clinical Neuropsychologist, 6,* 374–382.

Massman, P. J., & Doody, R. S. (1996). Hemispheric asymmetry in Alzheimer's disease is apparent in motor functioning. *Journal of Clinical and Experimental Neuropsychology, 18,* 110–121.

Matarazzo, J. D., Wiens, A. N., Matarazzo, R. G., & Goldstein, S. G. (1974). Psychometric and clinical test-retest reliability of the Halstead Impairment Index in a sample of healthy, young, normal men. *Journal of Nervous and Mental Disease, 158,* 37–49.

McCurry, S. M., Gibbons, L. E., Uomoto, J. M., Thompson, M. L., Graves, A. B., Edland, S. D., Bowne, J., McCormick, W. C., & Larson, E. B. (2001). Neuropsychological test performance in a cognitively intact sample of older Japanese American adults. *Archives of Clinical Neuropsychology, 16,* 447–459.

Mitrushina, M. M., Boone, K. B., Razani, J. & D'Elia, L. F. (2005). *Handbook of normative data for neuropsychological assessment* (2nd ed.) New York: Oxford University Press.

Moehle, K. A., & Long, C. J. (1989). Models of aging and neuropsychological test performance decline with aging. *Journal of Gerontology, 44,* 176–177.

Morrison, M. W., Gregory, R. J., & Paul, J. J. (1979). Reliability of the finger tapping test and a note on sex differences. *Perceptual and Motor Skills, 48,* 139–142.

Muller, G., Weisbrod, S., & Klingberg, F. (1991). Finger tapping frequency and accuracy are decreased in early stage primary degenerative dementia. *Dementia, 2,* 169–172.

Nagasaki, H., Itoh, H., Maruyama, H., & Hashizume, K. (1988). Characteristic difficulty in rhythmic movement with aging and its relation to Parkinson's disease. *Experimental Aging Research, 14,* 171–176.

Ott, B. R., Ellias, S. A., & Lannon, M. C. (1995). Quantitative assessment of movement in Alzheimer's disease. *Journal of Geriatric Psychiatry and Neurology, 8,* 71–75.

Peters, M. (1990). Subclassification of non-pathological left-handers poses problems for theories of handedness. *Neuropsychologia, 28,* 279–289.

Prigatano, G. P., Altman, I. M., & O'Brien, K. P. (1990). Behavioral limitations that traumatic brain-injured patients tend to underestimate. *The Clinical Neuropsychologist, 4,* 163–176.

Prigatano, G. P., & Borgano, S. R. (2003). Qualitative features of finger movement during the Halstead Finger Oscillation Test following traumatic brain injury. *Journal of the International Neuropsychological Society, 9,* 128–133.

Prigatano, G., & Wong, J. L. (1997). Speed of finger tapping and goal attainment after unilateral cerebral vascular accident. *Archives of Physical Medicine and Rehabilitation, 78,* 847–852.

Provins, K. A., & Cunliffe, P. (1972). The reliability of some motor performance tests of handedness. *Neuropsychologia, 10,* 199–206.

Rabin, L. A., Barr, W. B., & Burton, L. A. (2005). Assessment practices of clinical neuropsychologists in the United States and Canada: A survey of INS, NAN, and APA Division 40 members. *Archives of Clinical Neuropsychology, 20,* 33–65.

Rapport, L. J., Farchione, T. J., Coleman, R. D., & Axelrod, B. N. (1998). Effects of coaching on malingered motor function profiles. *Journal of Clinical and Experimental Neuropsychology, 20,* 89–97.

Reitan, R. M. (1969). *Manual for administration of neuropsychological test batteries for adults and children.* Indianapolis, Ind.

Reitan, R. M., & Wolfson, D. (1985). *The Halstead-Reitan Neuropsychological Test Battery: Theory and interpretation*. Tucson, AZ: Neuropsychology Press.

Reitan, R. M., & Wolfson, D. (1994). Dissociation of motor impairment and higher-level brain deficits in strokes and cerebral neoplasms. *The Clinical Neuropsychologist, 8,* 193–208.

Reitan, R. M., & Wolfson, D. (1996). Relationships between specific and general tests of cerebral functioning. *The Clinical Neuropsychologist, 10,* 37–42.

Rosselli, M., Ardila, A., Bateman, J. R., & Guzman, M. (2001). Neuropsychological test scores, academic performance, and developmental disorders in Spanish-speaking children. *Developmental Neuropsychology, 20,* 355–373.

Roy, E. A., Clark, P., Aigbogun, S., & Quare-Storer, P. A. (1992). Ipsilesional disruptions to reciprocal finger tapping. *Archives of Clinical Neuropsychology, 7,* 213–219.

Ruff, R. M., & Parker, S. B. (1993). Gender- and age-specific changes in motor speed and eye-hand coordination in adults: Normative values for the Finger Tapping and Grooved Pegboard tests. *Perceptual and Motor Skills, 76,* 1219–1230.

Russell, E. W., & Starkey, R. (1993). *Halstead-Russell Neuropsychological Evaluation System—Revised (HRNES-R)*. Los Angeles: Western Psychological Services.

Salinsky, M. C., Storzbach, D., Dodrill, C. B., & Binder, L. M. (2001). Test-retest bias, reliability, and regression equations for neuropsychological measures repeated over a 12–16-week period. *Journal of the International Neuropsychological Society, 7,* 597–605.

Searight, H. R., Dunn, E. J., Grisso, T., Margolis, R. B., et al. (1989). The relation of the Halstead-Reitan neuropsychological battery to ratings of everyday functioning in a geriatric sample. *Neuropsychology, 3,* 135–145.

Schmidt, S. L., Oliveira, R. M., Krahe, T. E., & Filgueiras, C. C. (2000). The effect of hand preference and gender on finger tapping performance asymmetry by the use of an infra-red light measurement device. *Neuropsychologia, 38,* 529–534.

Shimoyama, I., Ninchoji, T., & Uemura, K. (1990). The Finger Tapping Test: A quantitative analysis. *Archives of Neurology, 47,* 681–684.

Sjogren, P., Thomsen, A., & Olsen, A. K. (2000). Impaired neuropsychological performance in chronic non-malignant pain patients receiving long-term oral opiod therapy. *Journal of Pain and Symptom Management, 19,* 100–108.

Snow, W. G. (1987). Standardization of test administration and scoring criteria: Some shortcomings of current practice with the Halstead-Reitan Test Battery. *The Clinical Neuropsychologist, 1,* 250–262.

Spreen, O., & Gaddes, W. H. (1969). Developmental norms for 15 neuropsychological tests age 6 to 15. *Cortex, 5,* 170–191.

Stanford, M. S., & Barratt, E. S. (1996). Verbal skills, finger tapping, and cognitive tempo define a second-order factor of temporal information processing. *Brain and Cognition, 31,* 35–45.

Thompson, L. L., Heaton, R. K., Mathews, C. G., & Grant, I. (1987). Comparison of preferred and nonpreferred hand performance on four neuropsychological motor tasks. *The Clinical Neuropsychologist, 1,* 324–334.

Trahan, D. E., Patterson, J., Quintana, J., & Biron, R. (1987). *The Finger Tapping Test: A re-examination of traditional hypotheses regarding normal adult performance*. Paper presented at the International Neuropsychological Society, Washington, D.C.

Triggs, W. J., Calvanio, R., Levine, M., Heaton, R. K., & Heilman, K. M. (2000). Predicting hand preference with performance on motor tasks. *Cortex, 36,* 679–689.

Trueblood, W., & Schmidt, M. (1993). Malingering and other validity considerations in the neuropsychological evaluation of mild head injury. *Journal of Clinical and Experimental Neuropsychology, 15,* 578–590.

Wefel, J. S., Hoyt, B. D., & Massman, P. J. (1999). Neuropsychological functioning in depressed versus nondepressed participants with Alzheimer's disease. *The Clinical Neuropsychologist, 13,* 249–257.

Welch, L. W., Cunningham, A. T., Eckardt, M. J., & Martin, P. R. (1997). Fine motor speed deficits in alcoholic Korsakoff's syndrome. *Alcoholism: Clinical and Experimental Research, 21,* 134–139.

Whitfield, K., & Newcomb, R. (1992). A normative sample using the Loong computerized tapping program. *Perceptual and Motor Skills, 74,* 861–862.

Yang, Y. K., Chiu, N. T., Chen, C. C., Chen, M., Yeh, T. L., & Lee, I. H. (2003). Correlation between fine motor activity and striatal dopamine D_2 receptor density in patients with schizophrenia and healthy controls. *Psychiatry Research: Neuroimaging, 123,* 191–197.

Ylikoski, R., Ylikoski, A., Erkinjuntti, T., Sulkava, R., Keskivaara, P., Raininko, R., & Tilvis, R. (1998). Differences in neuropsychological functioning associated with age, education, neurological status, and magnetic resonance imaging findings in neurologically healthy elderly individuals. *Applied Neuropsychology, 5,* 1–4.

Grip Strength

PURPOSE

The purpose of the Grip Strength test is to measure the strength or intensity of voluntary grip movements of each hand.

SOURCE

The Smedley Dynamometer can be ordered from the Stoelting Co., 1350 S. Kostner Avenue, Chicago, IL 60623 (http://www.stoeltingco.com), at a cost of $215 US, or from the Reitan Neuropsychology Laboratory (http://www.reitanlabs.com) at a cost of $245 US.

AGE RANGE

Norms are available for individuals aged 6 to 8 and 12 to 85 years.

DESCRIPTION

This test of hand strength (Reitan & Davison, 1974; Reitan & Wolfson, 1985) is frequently used to assess the integrity of motor function. It requires the person to hold the upper part of the dynamometer in the palm of the hand and squeeze the stirrup with the fingers as hard as he or she possibly can.

Figure 14–1 Instructions for Grip Strength.

> Ask the examine to stand, if able. The length of the dynamometer stirrup should be adjusted to the size of the subject's hand (see Instrument Manual). Demonstrate the use of the instrument to the subject. Indicate that the lower pointer will register the grip, so that the subject does not have to continue gripping while the scale is read. Then place the dynamometer in the subject's preferred hand (palm down) and instruct the subject to hold his or her arm down at the side and away from the body. The subject is then told to squeeze the dynamometer as hard as he or she can, taking as much time as needed to squeeze to the maximum. Allow two recorded trials with each hand, preferred and nonpreferred alternately, with pauses between each trial to avoid excessive fatigue. If either an increase or a decrease of more than 5 kg occurs on the second trial for either hand, wait a few moments and provide a third trial.

ADMINISTRATION

The procedure proposed by Reitan & Wolfson (1985), shown in Figure 14–1, is preferred, because a large normative base is available using this protocol.

ADMINISTRATION TIME

The time required is less than 5 min.

SCORING

According to Reitan & Wolfson (1985), two measurements within 5 kg of each other are recorded for each hand. The mean is calculated for each hand separately.

DEMOGRAPHIC VARIABLES

Age

Strength is related to age, increasing in childhood (Finlayson & Reitan, 1976) and declining with advancing age in adults (e.g., Bornstein, 1985; Christensen et al., 2001, 2004; Ernst, 1988; Heaton et al., 2004; MacDonald et al., 2004; Mitrushina et al., 2005). According to Heaton et al. (2004), about 5% to 7% of the variance in test scores of adults is accounted for by age. Longitudinal assessments of age-related changes in physical strength suggest that the decline in the older age groups is greater than is indicated by cross-sectional comparisons of different age groups. The underestimation of strength loss in cross-sectional estimates probably occurs because relatively fewer weak individuals are represented in older healthy samples (Clement, 1974).

Gender

As might be expected, males are stronger than females (e.g., Bornstein, 1985; Christensen et al., 2001, 2004; Ernst, 1988; Heaton et al., 2004; Mitrushina et al., 2005). In fact, gender is a strong predictor of grip strength, accounting for 55% to 60% of the variance in test scores (Heaton et al., 2004).

Education/IQ

Although some have reported a positive relationship between grip strength and education (Bornstein, 1985), others have reported minimal education effects (Christensen et al., 2004; Heaton et al., 2004; Mitrushina et al., 2005). IQ has little relationship with motor functioning (Anstey & Smith, 1999; Christensen et al., 2004; Seidenberg et al., 1983).

Ethnicity

Racial differences in grip strength have been reported. African American women have better grip strength than their Caucasian peers, perhaps due to differences in muscle mass (Rantanen et al., 1998).

Handedness

Performance tends to be better with the preferred than with the nonpreferred hand (e.g., Bornstein, 1985; Heaton et al., 2004).

Intermanual Differences

Age and education do not affect the magnitude of intermanual differences (Bornstein, 1986a; Ernst, 1988). The findings regarding gender differences in intermanual difference scores are inconsistent; some studies find gender-related differences (i.e., greater between-hand differences for males than for females; Bornstein, 1986a), and others do not (Ernst, 1988; Fromm-Auch & Yeudall, 1983; Mitrushina et al., 2005; Thompson et al; 1987). There is also evidence that right-handers show larger intermanual differences than left-handers do (Thompson et al., 1987).

NORMATIVE DATA

Adults

There are several normative studies of adults (e.g., Bornstein, 1985; Brennon et al., 2004; Ernst, 1988; Fromm-Auch & Yeudall, 1983; Koffler & Zehler, 1985). Because of the effects of age, ethnicity, and gender, we recommend the use of normative data provided by Heaton et al. (2004; see Table 14–10). Regression-based norms are provided separately for two ethnicity groups (Caucasians and African Americans) and are organized by age, gender, and education. The samples are large and cover a wide range in terms of age (20–85 years) and education (0–20 years); exclusion criteria are specified. T scores lower than 40 are classed as impaired. According to Heaton et al. (2004), the procedure used was the one specified by Reitan and Wolfson (1985).

Table 14-10 Characteristics of the Grip Strength Normative Sample Provided by Heaton et al. (2004)

Number	1482
Age (years)	20–85[a]
Geographic location	Various states in the United States and Manitoba, Canada
Sample type	Individuals recruited as part of multicenter studies
Education (years)	0–20[b]
Gender (%)	
Male	60.1
Female	39.9
Race/Ethnicity	
Caucasian	839
African American	643
Screening	No reported history of learning disability, neurological disorder, serious psychiatric disorder, or alcohol or drug abuse

[a]Age groups: 20–34, 35–39, 40–44, 45–49, 50–54, 55–59, 60–64, 65–69, 70–74, 75–79, and 80–89.
[b]Education groups: 7–8, 9–11, 12, 13–15, 16–17, and 18–20.

Therefore, it is assumed that the Smedley Dynamometer was used to test participants. However, the method for determining hand preference is not reported (Mitrushina et al., 2005), and the data were collected over a lengthy period (25 years).

Mitrushina et al. (2005) compiled data from five to nine studies, including 407 to 713 men and women aged 25 to 69 years. They noted that the integrity of their meta-norms was undermined by the lack of consistency in reporting hand preference.

Table 14–11 shows norms (Bornstein, 1985) for adults, ages 20 to 69 years. These are based on a sample of 365 individuals from the general population living in a large western Canadian city. They appear to agree reasonably well with those provided by Heaton et al. (2004) and Mitrushina et al. (2005). Hand preference was determined as the hand used for signing the consent form. Unfortunately, some cell sizes were quite small (e.g., $n = 13$). Although the health status and exclusion criteria were not reported in that paper, other reports (e.g., Bornstein, 1986b) with the same sample indicated that individuals with a history of neurological or psychiatric illness were excluded from the study.

For adults aged 53 to 90 years, Dixon (personal communication, April 5, 2005) provides normative data derived from a large sample of 457 typically aging, older, community-dwelling adults who participated in the Victoria Longitudinal Study (VLS), in Victoria, Canada. The sample was well-educated ($M = 15.23$ years; SD = 2.86), predominantly female (69.8%), Caucasian (98.2%), and considered English their native tongue (90.2%). Individuals with MMSE scores of 24 or less, moderate/severe visual or auditory impairment even with corrective aids, or a history of significant neurological or psychiatric disorder were excluded. Hand preference was self-reported, and the test was given with the participant standing

Table 14–11 Performance of Adults for Grip Strength (kilograms), by Education, Age, and Gender

Age Group (Years)	<Grade 12			≥Grade 12		
	N	M	SD	N	M	SD
Males, Preferred hand						
20–39	21	50.8	11.5	86	49.9	8.4
40–59	13	39.8	6.0	17	48.2	7.3
60–69	16	38.7	5.9	22	44.5	5.6
Males, Nonpreferred hand						
20–39	21	47.7	11.7	86	46.4	7.6
40–59	13	38.2	6.5	17	46.4	9.1
60–69	16	37.2	5.4	22	39.3	5.5
Females, Preferred hand						
20–39	13	32.7	8.7	50	31.0	5.4
40–59	22	27.7	5.9	43	29.8	5.8
60–69	22	25.6	5.3	34	25.0	4.9
Females, Nonpreferred hand						
20–39	13	31.2	8.0	50	28.7	5.0
40–59	22	24.9	6.7	43	26.9	5.4
60–69	22	24.0	6.0	34	22.8	4.8

Note: The sample consisted of 365 healthy individuals from the general population of a large Western Canadian city.

Source: From Bornstein, 1985. Reprinted with permission of John Wiley & Sons, Inc.

Table 14–12 Grip Strength (Mean and *SD*) by Age Range (Midpoint) and Gender

	53–60 (57)	55–65 (60)	60–75 (65)	65–75 (70)	70–80 (75)	75–85 (80)	80–90 (85)
N	92	180	172	145	135	112	58
F/M	71/21	138/42	121/51	93/52	88/47	74/38	39/19
Males							
Dominant hand	44.79 (8.79)	44.15 (7.93)	42.71 (6.58)	41.79 (6.35)	39.07 (6.27)	36.27 (5.08)	34.82 (4.36)
Nondominant hand	43.26 (7.19)	42.58 (7.00)	40.72 (7.32)	39.66 (6.82)	37.06 (6.40)	33.43 (4.79)	31.81 (4.57)
Discrepancy	5.08 (4.14)	4.46 (3.19)	4.16 (3.24)	3.66 (3.17)	3.31 (2.48)	3.70 (2.76)	3.90 (2.60)
Females							
Dominant hand	27.08 (5.20)	27.10 (5.02)	26.73 (4.63)	25.31 (5.26)	23.19 (5.61)	21.17 (4.30)	20.30 (3.76)
Non-dominant hand	25.86 (5.43)	25.34 (5.40)	24.29 (4.87)	22.94 (4.88)	21.38 (5.39)	19.84 (4.34)	19.22 (3.36)
Discrepancy	2.22 (1.62)	2.74 (1.84)	3.16 (2.28)	3.03 (2.49)	2.65 (1.85)	2.31 (1.50)	2.20 (1.54)

Note: Dominance self-reported; participant standing, alternating hands, average of two trials with Smedley dynamometer.

Source: R. Dixon, personal communication, April 5, 2005.

and alternating hands. The values shown in Table 14–12 reflect the average of two trials.

Children

A number of authors have provided norms for children. The meta-norms developed by Findeis and Weight (1994) are of limited value because they are given for combined groups of male and female children from middle- to upper-class homes.

Table 14–13 gives normative data for healthy male and female subjects aged 6 to 8 years (all right-handed as defined by scores on the Reitan-Klove Lateral dominance examination; Finlayson & Reitan, 1976); 12 to 15 years (the vast majority right-handed; C. Paniak, personal communication, April 14, 2004); and 15 to 20 years (79% right-handed; Yeudall et al., 1987). Note that cell size is relatively small for ages 6 to 8 (*n* = 10) and that norms for children aged 9 to 11 years are lacking.

None of the children studied by Finlayson and Reitan (1976) had significant medical, behavioral or academic diffi-

culties. The exclusion criteria for the sample studied by C. Paniak and colleagues included failure of one or more grades, enrollment in an English as a Second Language program, a history of hospitalization for brain injury or behavioral problems, or participation in a self-contained special education program. The sample had a WISC-III Vocabulary scaled score of about 10 (*SD* = 3). Individuals in the study by Yeudall et al. (1987) were excluded if there was any evidence of forensic involvements, head injury, neurological insult, prenatal or birth complications, psychiatric problems, or substance abuse.

RELIABILITY

Internal Consistency

Christensen et al. (2001) examined a sample of 838 older adults. Four trials were given to each hand. Across the eight trials, Chronbach's alpha was high (*r* = .82).

Table 14–13 Mean Performance (Mean and *SD*) of Children and Adolescents for Grip Strength (kilograms)

Age (Years)		Male			Female	
	n	Right Hand	Left Hand	*n*	Right Hand	Left Hand
6	10	10.40 (2.80)	9.45 (2.87)	10	9.05 (2.50)	7.90 (2.34)
7	10	11.45 (2.10)	11.10 (2.27)	10	9.30 (1.75)	8.80 (1.80)
8	10	12.25 (2.36)	11.40 (2.08)	10	11.55 (2.36)	10.15 (2.46)
12	38	26.88 (5.23)	25.41 (4.36)	56	24.17 (4.48)	21.97 (4.53)
13	39	30.54 (6.20)	28.64 (5.67)	57	25.73 (5.13)	23.95 (5.61)
14	46	35.71 (7.04)	33.23 (7.07)	70	27.96 (5.57)	25.73 (5.28)
15	29	38.31 (6.01)	35.78 (5.78)	23	25.50 (6.37)	23.83 (5.62)
15–20	32	43.58 (10.25)	40.46 (10.37)	30	30.20 (5.56)	28.07 (4.52)

Sources: Ages 6–8, Finlayson & Reitan (1976), all right-handed; Ages 12–15, C. Paniak, personal communication, April 10, 2004; the vast majority right-handed; Ages 15–20, Yeudall et al. (1988), mean age = 17.76, *SD* = 1.96; mean WAIS-R FSIQ = 111.75, *SD* = 10.16, 73% of females right-handed, 84% of males right-handed.

Test-Retest Reliability and Practice Effects

In adults and children, the performance of each hand is fairly reliable over test sessions, even with lengthy intervals between retest sessions (e.g., 30 months). Reliability coefficients ranging from .52 to .96, with most greater than .70, have been reported with both normal and neurologically impaired individuals (Anstey et al., 1997; Brown et al., 1989; Dikmen et al., 1999; Dodrill & Troupin, 1975; Dunn, 1978; Matarazzo et al., 1974; Provins & Cunliffe, 1972; Reddon et al., 1985; Thomas & Hageman, 2002). In head-injured individuals, however, performance may vary significantly from one session to the next (Burton et al., 2002).

The differences between hands are not highly reliable, and variations in performance do occur from time to time, perhaps influenced by variations in motivation (Provins & Cunliffe, 1972; Sappington, 1980).

Within a session, grip strength may deteriorate after an extended number of grip trials when brief (e.g., 15–30 s) intertrial intervals are used (Montazer & Thomas, 1992; Reddon et al., 1985). Performance drops significantly after two trials, with grip strength decreasing to about 80% with 10 trials and to about 40% in 100 trials. From trial 100 to 200, only an additional 10% drop occurs (Montazer & Thomas, 1992). However, with longer intertrial intervals (e.g., 120 s), performance improves across trials (at least over a series of four trials), with the greatest increase evident after the first trial (Dunwoody et al., 1996).

In healthy young adults, performance does improve somewhat with repeated practice over short intervals (about 1–2 kg over a retest interval of 3 weeks; Bornstein et al., 1987; about 5 kg over 10 weekly sessions, Reddon et al., 1985). Dikmen et al. (1999) reported slight declines in scores in a sample of 384 normal or neurologically stable individuals (aged 15–83 years, $M = 34.2$, $SD = 16.7$) who were retested about 9 months after initial testing. Table 14–14 provides information to determine whether there has been substantial change, taking practice into account. One first subtracts the mean T2 – T1 change (column 3) from the difference between the two testings for the individual and then compares the result with 1.64 times the standard deviation of the difference (column 4). The 1.64 comes from the normal distribution and is exceeded in the positive or negative direction only 10% of the time if indeed there is no real change in clinical condition.

VALIDITY

Relationships With Other Measures

Factor analysis of a variety of motor and sensory tasks in older, community-dwelling adults revealed a three-factor solution (MacDonald et al., 2004). Grip strength loaded on a sensorimotor factor, along with measures of close and distance vision, hearing in the speech frequency range, and peak expiratory flow. Measures of height, weight, and head circumference loaded on an anthrometric factor, whereas systolic and diastolic blood pressure indicators defined a biomedical factor.

Clinical Findings

Grip strength measures are included in neuropsychological examinations to assess gross and subtle motor impairment. Indeed, the task has proved useful in differentiating brain-damaged from normal people, and in detecting the laterality of brain lesion (Bornstein, 1986b; Dodrill, 1978; Finlayson & Reitan, 1980; Haaland & Delany, 1981; Hom & Reitan, 1982; Lewis & Kupke, 1990). Given the crossed nature of the motor system, right-hemisphere lesions tend to depress performance on the left hand, and left-hemisphere lesions tend to lower performance on the right hand. Dodrill (1978) reported that the dynamometer correctly identified the lateralization of brain lesions with higher accuracy than either the Finger Tapping Test or the Tactual Performance Test. The relative advantage of the dynamometer in making inferences regarding laterality of damage may lie, at least in part, in its relative simplicity and low demands on skill and adaptation, a function that may be compromised in brain-damaged individuals, particularly those with subcortical and/or bilateral disturbance (Haaland et al., 1994; Lewis & Kupke, 1990). Tests that require more skilled movement (e.g., tapping, Purdue pegboard) may place greater cognitive demands (e.g., in terms of speed, coordination, and pacing requirements), and patients may have more difficulty adapting to such tasks, particularly with the nonpreferred (less practiced) hand. In such cases, intermanual differences may reflect less a lateralized disturbance than a generalized reduction in cognitive efficiency (Lewis & Kupke, 1990). Grip strength has also proved useful in discriminating left-hemisphere speech from right-hemisphere speech in people with epilepsy (Strauss & Wada, 1988).

Table 14–14 Grip Strength Test-Retest Effects in 384 Normal or Neurologically Stable Individuals Assessed After Intervals of 2–16 months

| Measure | Time 1 | | Time 2 | | T2 – T1 | | T1, T2 |
	(1) Mean	SD	(2) Mean	SD	(3) M	(4) SD	r
Dominant	43.34	13.33	42.41	13.44	−.93	6.09	.90
Nondominant	40.60	12.89	39.65	13.19	−.96	5.67	.91

Note: Mean interval about 9 m, $SD = 3.0$.

Source: Adapted from Dikmen et al., 1999.

Haaland et al. (1994) found that grip strength was sensitive to recovery in the first year after head injury. Normal individuals showed no change, whereas head-injured patients showed improved performance from the 1-month to the 1-year evaluation. Burton et al. (2002) compared head-injured and healthy individuals and noted no differences between groups in mean level of grip strength. However, patients with traumatic head injuries were more variable in their right-hand performance, with scores fluctuating significantly from one week to the next. They suggested that single-occasion measures in such patients may not provide an accurate reflection of an individual's actual functioning.

Both cross-sectional and longitudinal studies (e.g., Christensen et al., 2000) indicate that grip strength declines with advancing age. Further, in old age, individuals with weaker grip tend to score lower on cognitive tests (e.g., slowed reaction times; Anstey et al., 2005). There is also evidence that changes in grip strength over a 3- to 4-year period correlate moderately with changes in cognitive functioning (e.g., information processing speed and memory); that is, they tend to move together longitudinally to some extent (Christensen et al., 2000, 2004). The decline appears be caused by a common factor or factors (e.g., vascular disease, decreased metabolic rate, programmed cell death, age-related myelin degeneration, dopaminergic depletion) that are responsible for age-related deterioration in cognitive and noncognitive processes (common cause hypothesis), in addition to more specific processes (Christensen et al., 2001, 2004). Of note, poor performance was predictive of cognitive decline in older adults over a 12-year period (MacDonald et al., 2004). Poor performance also predicted mortality over a period of 6 years, even after controlling for health (disease) and demographic factors (e.g., age, gender, education; Anstey et al., 2001). That is, grip strength is a reliable predictor of biological aging that is independent from health/disease processes.

Reduced grip strength has also been reported in a variety of other conditions, including autism (Hardan et al., 2003), multiple sclerosis (Paul et al., 1998), chemical exposure (Bowler et al., 1998; Dick et al., 2002), and pseudoseizures (Sackellares & Sackellares, 2001) and after unilateral posterior ventral pallidotomy in the treatment of Parkinson's disease (Cahn et al., 1998). Hemispherectomized children show impaired grip strength in the limb contralateral to the excised hemisphere (e.g., Holloway et al., 2000). However, no reliable association was found between side of lesion and lateralized motor deficits in one study of children with neonatal unilateral damage, perhaps a reflection of the milder nature of the damage (Glass et al., 1998).

As might be expected, pain is associated with decreased grip strength (Pienimaeki et al., 2002). However, perceived increases in level of fatigue as a consequence of cognitive work are not associated with decreases in strength (Paul et al., 1998). Depression may affect grip strength, with failure to demonstrate asymmetric grip strength observed in depressed adults and children (e.g., Crews & Harrison, 1994; Emerson et al., 2001; but see Crews et al., 1999). In addition, there is evidence that perceptions/beliefs of relevance and self-efficacy (e.g., competence) affect performance. Burkhalter & Wendt (2001) reported that, independent of gender and age, alienated youth and children with lower perceptions of physical competence are less able. Finally, Shapiro et al. (1996) reported that ambient sensory conditions (e.g., bright light, noise) can affect left-hand grip strength in older adults, although the extent of the declines do not appear to be sufficiently large to be clinically significant.

Intermanual Differences

The assumption is often made that a right-handed person should perform better on the dynamometer with the right hand, and that a left-handed person should perform better with the left hand (e.g., Reitan & Wolfson, 1985). In general, performance with the preferred hand is superior (about 10% stronger) to that with the nonpreferred hand (Bornstein, 1985, 1986a; Mitrushina et al., 2005; Triggs et al., 2000). However, there is considerable variability in the normal population, and the preferred hand is not necessarily the stronger one, especially when left-handed people are considered (Benton et al., 1962; Bohannon, 2003; Koffler & Zehler, 1985; Lewandowski et al., 1982; Satz et al., 1967; Smiljanic-Colanovic, 1974). Patterns indicating equal or better performance with the nonpreferred hand occur with considerable regularity in the normal population, and neurological involvement should not be inferred from an isolated lack of concordance. Even fairly large discrepancies between the hands on grip strength alone cannot be used to suggest unilateral impairment (Bornstein, 1986a; Koffler & Zehler, 1985; Thompson et al., 1987). Large-magnitude discrepancies (more than 1 SD from the mean) are not uncommon (about 25%) in the normal population. Greater confidence in the clinical judgment of impaired motor function with one hand or the other can be derived from consideration of the consistency of intermanual discrepancies across several motor tasks (Bornstein, 1986b; Thompson et al., 1987). Consistent deviant performances are quite rare in the normal population and therefore, in the absence of peripheral injury, are likely to indicate lateralized brain dysfunction (Bornstein, 1986b; Thompson et al., 1987).

Ecological and Predictive Validity

Impaired grip strength in older adults is related to reduced levels of daily function (e.g., Femia et al., 2001; Judge et al., 1996) and is predictive of functional decline over a 3-year window (Ishizaki et al., 2000). As noted earlier, poor performance is also predictive of cognitive decline (MacDonald et al., 2004) and mortality (Anstey et al., 2001) in older adults.

In stroke patients, grip strength can be used as a gross index of recovery of arm function and has some prognostic value. Sunderland et al. (1989) noted that the absence of measureable grip strength 1 month after stroke indicated that there would be poor outcome with regard to motor function. If there was detectable grip at 1 month, then the clinician could be reasonably certain that there would be at least rudimentary function 5 months later.

Malingering

A number of investigators (e.g., Greiffenstein et al., 1996; Heaton et al., 1978; Rapport et al., 1998) have reported that grip strength is sensitive to suboptimal performance. In addition, Greiffenstein et al. (1996) observed that compensation-seeking patients with postconcussion syndrome (PCS) demonstrated a nonphysiological profile (grip strength < finger tapping < grooved pegs), compared with a group of patients with proven traumatic brain injury, whose performance followed a gradient of increasing impairment corresponding to the sensory-motor complexity of these tasks. However, Rapport et al. (1998) found that the presence of nonphysiological configurations showed poor predictive accuracy among simulators (coached and uncoached) and controls. The authors also found that a significant proportion of normal individuals show poorer performance on grip strength compared with fine motor tasks and cautioned that the motor dysfunction profile does not appear to be a reliable or valid decision-making tool that can be used independently in the assessment of malingering.

COMMENT

The test is brief, is easy to give, and yields fairly reliable results. It is sensitive to a variety of disturbances, including aging. In fact, in older adults it may be viewed as a general indicator of the integrity of the central nervous system (e.g., Anstey & Smith, 1999).

Measurement of grip strength also provides information regarding everyday competence, given its importance for a variety of functional activities including dressing, picking up objects, and eating.

When establishing impairment, measurements can be compared with normative values or with values obtained from the presumably unimpaired side. However, large-magnitude discrepancies are relatively common in the normal population. Accordingly, judgments about impairments should not be made simply on the basis of between-side comparisons but should be supported by abnormal results on additional tests. Clinicians should also note that mild peripheral injury may impair grip strength long after subjective symptoms (e.g., pain, numbness) have subsided (Reitan, 2001). Therefore, inferences regarding lateralized deficits should be made with caution.

It should be noted that relatively little attention has been paid to the standardization of the procedure. For example, the amount of time between trials is left up to the individual examiner, despite evidence that the length of the intertrial in-

terval can have a significant influence on grip strength (e.g., Dunwoody et al., 1996). Intervals shorter than 1 min should not be used. Although some researchers (e.g., Reitan & Wolfson, 1985) do not provide a practice trial, familiarity with the task may reduce the likelihood of type 1 error; that is, reporting of "significant" results that may reflect the patient's learning how to use the equipment (Dunwoody et al., 1996). The number of trials given also varies, with some investigators giving two trials (Reitan & Wolfson, 1985) and others giving more (e.g., Salthouse et al., 1998). Further, scoring procedures differ among investigators. Some (e.g., Anstey et al., 1997; Glass et al., 1998) use the best trial for each hand, whereas others (e.g., Reitan & Wolfson, 1985) take the mean value of the trials given for each hand. Users should also note that the method of determination of hand preference is rarely reported, despite the fact that interpretation of normative data is based on assumptions of handedness.

Finally, it is worth pointing out that norms are lacking for certain age groups (e.g., 9–11 years) and that some of the reports (especially those for children) are quite dated (e.g., meta-norms provided by Findeis & Weight, 1994; Finlayson & Reitan, 1976). More recent norms (e.g., Paniak, personal communication, April 10, 2004) appear to establish a higher standard, perhaps reflecting changes in nutrition and cultural factors. Accordingly, further research is needed to improve the normative base.

REFERENCES

Anstey, K. J., Dear, K., Christensen, H., & Jorn, A. F. (2005). Biomarkers, health, lifestyle, and demographic variables as correlates of reaction time performance in early, middle, and late adulthood. *The Quarterly Journal of Experimental Psychology, 58A,* 5–21.

Anstey, K. J., Luszcz, M. A., Giles, L. C., & Andrews, G. R. (2001). Demographic, health, cognitive, and sensory variables as predictors of mortality in very old adults. *Psychology and Aging, 16,* 3–11.

Anstey, K. J., & Smith, G. A. (1999). Interrelationships among biological markers of aging, health, activity, acculturation, and cognitive performance in late adulthood. *Psychology and Aging, 14,* 605–618.

Anstey, K. J., Smith, G. A., & Lord, S. (1997). Test-retest reliability of a battery of sensory, motor and physiological measures of aging. *Perceptual and Motor Skills, 84,* 831–834.

Benton, A. L., Meyers, R., & Polder, G. J. (1962). Some aspects of handedness. *Psychiatrica et Neurologica Basel, 144,* 321–337.

Bohannon, R. W. (2003). Grip strength: A summary of studies comparing dominant and nondominant limb measurements. *Perceptual and Motor Skills, 96,* 728–730.

Bornstein, R. A. (1985). Normative data on selected neuropsychological measures from a nonclinical sample. *Journal of Clinical Psychology, 41,* 651–659.

Bornstein, R. A. (1986a). Normative data on intermanual differences on three tests of motor performance. *Journal of Clinical and Experimental Neuropsychology, 8,* 12–20.

Bornstein, R. A. (1986b). Consistency of intermanual discrepancies in normal and unilateral brain lesion patients. *Journal of Consulting and Clinical Psychology, 54,* 719–723.

Bornstein, R. A., Baker, G. B., & Douglas, A. B. (1987). Short-term retest reliability of the Halstead-Reitan Battery in a normal sample. *Journal of Nervous and Mental Disease, 175,* 229–232.

Bowler, R. M., Hartney, C., & Ngo, L. H. (1998). Amnestic disturbance and posttraumatic stress disorder in the aftermath of a chemical release. *Archives of Clinical Neuropsychology, 13,* 455–471.

Brennan, P., Bohannon, R., Pescatello, L., Marischke, L., Hasson, S., & Murphy, M. (2004). Grip strength norms for elderly women. *Perceptual and Motor Skills, 99,* 899–902.

Brown, S. J., Rourke, B. P., & Cicchetti, D. V. (1989). Reliability of tests and measures used in the neuropsychological assessment of children. *The Clinical Neuropsychologist, 3,* 353–368.

Burkhalter, N. A., & Wendt, J. C. (2001). Prediction of selected fitness indicators by gender, age, alienation, and perceived competence. *Journal of Teaching in Physical Education, 21,* 3–15.

Burton, C. L., Hultsch, D. F., Strauss, E., & Hunter, M. A. (2002). Intraindividual variability in physical and emotional functioning: Comparison of adults with traumatic brain injuries and healthy adults. *The Clinical Neuropsychologist, 16,* 264–279.

Cahn, D. A., Sullivan, E. V., Shear, P. K., Heit, G., Lim, K. O., Marsh, L., Lane, B., Wasserstein, P., & Silverberg, G. D. (1998). Neuropsychological motor functioning after unilateral anatomically guided posterior ventral pallidotomy: Preoperative performance and three-month follow-up. *Neuropsychiatry, Neuropsychology, & Behavioral Neurology, 11,* 136–145.

Christensen, H., Korten, A. E., Mackinnon, A. J., Jorn, A. F., Henderson, A. S., & Rodgers, B. (2000). Are changes in sensory disability, reaction time, and grip strength associated with changes in memory and crystallized intelligence? *Gerontology, 46,* 276–292.

Christensen, H., Mackinnon, A. J., Korten, A., & Jorm, A. F. (2001). The "common cause hypothesis" of cognitive aging: Evidence for not only a common factor but also specific associations of age with vision and grip strength in a cross-sectional analysis. *Psychology and Aging, 16,* 588–599.

Christensen, H., Mackinnon, A. J. Jorm, A. F., Korten, A., Jacomb, P., Hofer, S. M., & Henderson, S. (2004). The Canberra Longitudinal Study: Design, aims, methodology, outcomes and recent empirical investigations. *Aging, Neuropsychology and Cognition, 11,* 169–195.

Clement, F. J. (1974). Longitudinal and cross-sectional assessments of age changes in physical strength as related to sex, social class, and mental ability. *Journal of Gerontology, 29,* 423–429.

Crews W. D. Jr., & Harrison, D. W. (1994). Functional asymmetry in the motor performances of women: Neuropsychological effects of depression. *Perceptual and Motor Skills, 78,* 1315–1322.

Crews, W. D., Harrison, D. W., & Rhodes, R. D. (1999). Neuropsychological test performances of young depressed outpatient women: An examination of executive functions. *Archives of Clinical Neuropsychology, 14,* 517–529.

Dick, F., Semple, S., Osborne, A., Soutar, A., Seaton, A., Cherrie, J. W., Walker, L. G., & Haites, N. (2002). Organic solvent exposure, genes, and risk of neuropsychological impairment. *QJM: Monthly Journal of the Association of Physicians, 95,* 379–387.

Dikmen, S. S., Heaton, R. K., Grant, I., & Temkin, N. R. (1999). Test-retest reliability and practice effects of expanded Halstead-Reitan neuropsychological test battery. *Journal of the International Neuropsychological Society, 5,* 346–356.

Dodrill, C. B. (1978). The hand dynamometer as a neuropsychological measure. *Journal of Consulting and Clinical Psychology, 46,* 1432–1435.

Dodrill, C. B., & Troupin, A. S. (1975). Effects of repeated administrations of a comprehensive neuropsychological battery among chronic epileptics. *Journal of Nervous and Mental Disease, 161,* 185–190.

Dunn, J. M. (1978). Reliability of selected psychomotor measures with mentally retarded adult males. *Perceptual and Motor Skills, 46,* 295–301.

Dunwoody, L., Tittmar, H. G., & McClean, W. S. (1996). Grip strength and intertrial rest. *Perceptual & Motor Skills, 83,* 275–278.

Emerson, C. S., Harrison, D. W., Everhart, D. E., & Williamson, J. B. (2001). Grip strength asymmetry in depressed boys. *Neuropsychiatry, Neuropsychology, and Behavioral Neurology, 14,* 130–134.

Ernst, J. (1988). Language, grip strength, sensory-perceptual, and receptive skills in a normal elderly sample. *The Clinical Neuropsychologist, 2,* 30–40.

Femia, E. E., Zarit, S. H., & Johansson, B. (2001). The disablement process in very late life. *Journal of Gerontology Series B: Psychological Sciences and Social Sciences, 56,* P12–P23.

Findeis, M. K., & Weight, D. K. (1994). *Meta-norms for two forms of neuropsychological test batteries for children.* Unpublished manuscript, Brigham Young University, Provo, Utah.

Finlayson, M. A., & Reitan, R. M. (1976). Handedness in relation to measures of motor and tactile-perceptual functions in normal children. *Perceptual and Motor Skills, 43,* 475–481.

Finlayson, M. A., & Reitan, R. M. (1980). Effect of lateralized lesions on ipsilateral and contralateral motor functioning. *Journal of Clinical Neuropsychology, 2,* 237–243.

Fromm-Auch, D., & Yeudall, L. T. (1983). Normative data for the Halstead-Reitan Neuropsychological Tests. *Journal of Clinical Neuropsychology, 5,* 221–238.

Glass, P., Bulas, D. I., Wagner, A. E., Rajasingham, S. R., Civitello, L. A., & Coffman, C. E. (1998). Pattern of neuropsychological deficit at age five years following neonatal unilateral brain injury. *Brain and Language, 63,* 346–356.

Greiffenstein, M. F., Baker, W. J., & Gola, T. (1996). Motor dysfunction profiles in traumatic brain injury and postconcussion syndrome. *Journal of the International Neuropsychological Society, 2,* 477–485.

Haaland, K. Y., & Delaney, H. D. (1981). Motor deficits after left or right hemisphere damage due to stroke or tumor. *Neuropsychologia, 19,* 17–27.

Haaland, K. Y., Temkin, N., Randahl, G., & Dikmen, S. (1994). Recovery of simple motor skills after head injury. *Journal of Clinical and Experimental Neuropsychology, 16,* 448–456.

Hardan, A. Y., Kilpatrick, M., Keshavan, M. S., & Minshew, N. J. (2003). Motor performance and anatomic Magnetic Resonance Imaging (MRI) of the basal ganglia in autism. *Journal of Child Neurology, 18,* 317–324.

Heaton, R. K., Smith, H. H., Lehman, R. A., & Vogt, A. T. (1978). Prospects for faking believable deficits on neuropsychological testing. *Journal of Consulting and Clinical Psychology, 46,* 892–900.

Heaton, R. K., Miller, S. W., Taylor, M. J., & Grant, I. (2004). *Revised comprehensive norms for an expanded Halstead-Reitan Battery: Demographically adjusted neuropsychological norms for African American and Caucasian adults.* Lutz, FL: PAR.

Holloway, V., Gadian, D. G., Vargh-Khadem, F., Porter, D. A., Boyd, S. G., & Connelly, A. (2000). The reorganization of sensorimotor function in children after hemispherectomy. *Brain, 123,* 2432–2444.

Hom, J., & Reitan, R. M. (1982). Effect of lateralized cerebral damage upon contralateral and ipsilateral sensorimotor performances. *Journal of Clinical Neuropsychology, 4,* 249–268.

Ishizaki, T., Watanabe, S., Suzuki, T., Shibata, H., & Haga, H. (2000). Predictors of functional decline among nondisabled older Japanese living in a community during a 3-year follow-up. *Journal of the American Geriatrics Society, 48,* 1424–1429.

Judge, J. O., Schechtman, K., & Cress, E. (1996). The relationship between physical performance measures and independence in instrumental activities of daily living. *Journal of the American Geriatrics Society, 44,* 1332–1341.

Koffler, S. P., & Zehler, D. (1985). Normative data for the hand dynamometer. *Perceptual and Motor Skills, 61,* 589–590.

Lewandowski, L., Kobus, D. A., Church, K. L., & Van Orden, K. (1982). Neuropsychological implications of hand preference versus hand grip performance. *Perceptual and Motor Skills, 55,* 311–314.

Lewis, R., & Kupke, T. (1990). Intermanual differences on skilled and unskilled motor tasks in nonlateralized brain dysfunction. *The Clinical Neuropsychologist, 6,* 374–382.

MacDonald, S. W. S., Dixon, R. A., Cohen, A-L., & Hazlitt, J. E. (2004). Biological age and 12-year cognitive change in older adults: Findings from the Victoria Longitudinal Study. *Gerontology, 50,* 64–81.

Matarazzo, J. D., Wiens, A. N., Matarazzo, R. G., & Goldstein, S. (1974). Psychometric and clinical test-retest reliability of the Halstead Impairment Index in a sample of healthy, young, normal men. *Journal of Nervous and Mental Disease, 158,* 37–49.

Mitrushina, M. N., Boone, K. B., Razani, J. & d'Elia, L. F. (2005). *Handbook of normative data for neuropsychological assessment* (2nd ed.) New York: Oxford University Press.

Montazer, M. A., & Thomas, J. G. (1992). Grip strength as a function of 200 repetitive trials. *Perceptual and Motor Skills, 75,* 1320–1322.

Paul, R. H., Beatty, W. W., Schneider, R., Blanco, C. R., & Hames, K. A. (1998). Cognitive and physical fatigue in multiple sclerosis: Relations between self-report and objective performance. *Applied Neuropsychology, 5,* 143–148.

Pienimaeki, T., Tarvainen, T., Siira, P., Malmivaara, A., & Vanharanta, H. (2002). Associations between pain, grip strength, and manual tests in the treatment evaluation of chronic tennis elbow. *Clinical Journal of Pain, 18,* 164–170.

Provins, K. A., & Cunliffe, P. (1972). The reliability of some motor performance tests of handedness. *Neuropsychologia, 10,* 199–206.

Rantanen, T., Guralnik, J. M., Leveille, S., Izmirlian, G., Simonsick, E., Ling, S., & Fried, L. P. (1998). Racial differences in muscle strength in disabled older women. *Journal of Gerontology: Series A: Biological Sciences and Medical Sciences, 53A,* B355–B361.

Rapport, L. J., Farchione, T. J., Colemna, R. D., & Axelrod, B. N. (1998). Effects of coaching on malingered motor function profiles. *Journal of Clinical and Experimental Neuropsychology, 20,* 89–97.

Reddon, J. R., Stefanyk, W. O., Gill, D. M., & Renney, C. (1985). Hand dynamometer: Effects of trials and sessions. *Perceptual and Motor Skills, 61,* 1195–1198.

Reitan, R. M. (2001). Differentiating between peripheral and central lateralized neuropsychological deficits. *Journal of Forensic Neuropsychology, 2,* 21–27.

Reitan, R. M., & Davison, L. A. (1974). *Clinical Neuropsychology: Current Status and Applications.* Washington, DC: V. H. Winston.

Reitan, R. M.., & Wolfson, D. (1985). *The Halstead-Reitan Neuropsychological Test Battery: Theory and interpretation.* Tucson, AZ: Neuropsychology Press.

Sackellares, D. K., & Sackellares, J. C. (2001). Impaired motor function in patients with psychogenic pseudoseizures. *Epilepsia, 42,* 1600–1606.

Salthouse, T. A., Hambrick, D. Z., & McGurthy, K. E. (1998). Shared age-related influences on cognitive and noncognitive variables. *Psychology and Aging, 13,* 486–500.

Sappington, J. T. (1980). Measures of lateral dominance: Interrelationships and temporal stability. *Perceptual and Motor Skills, 50,* 783–790.

Satz, P., Achenbach, K., & Fennel, E. (1967). Correlations between assessed manual laterality and predicted speech laterality in a normal population. *Neuropsychologia, 5,* 295–310.

Seidenberg, M., Giorani, B., Berent, S., & Boll, T. J. (1983). IQ level and performance on the Halstead-Reitan Neuropsychological Test Battery for older children. *Journal of Consulting and Clinical Psychology, 51,* 406–413.

Shapiro, D. M., Crews, W. D., Harrison, D. W., & Everhart, D. E. (1996). Age differences in hemispheric activation to sensory condition. *International Journal of Neuroscience, 87,* 249–256.

Smiljanic-Colanovic, V. (1974). The measurement of different aspects and degrees of hand dominance. *Studiae Psychologica, 16,* 204–208.

Strauss, E., & Wada, J. (1988). Hand preference and proficiency and cerebral speech dominance determined by the carotid Amytal test. *Journal of Clinical and Experimental Neuropsychology, 10,* 169–174.

Sunderland, A., Tinson, D., Bradley, L., & Langton-Hewer, R. (1989). Arm function after stroke. An evaluation of grip strength as a measure of recovery and a prognostic indicator. *Journal of Neurology, Neurosurgery, and Psychiatry, 52,* 1267–1272.

Thomas, V. S., & Hageman, P. A. (2002). A preliminary study on the reliability of physical performance measures in older day-care center clients with dementia. *International Psychogeriatrics, 14,* 17–23.

Thompson, L. L., Heaton, R. K., Mathews, C. G., & Grant, I. (1987). Comparison of preferred and nonpreferred hand performance on four neuropsychological motor tasks. *The Clinical Neuropsychologist, 1,* 324–334.

Triggs, W. J., Calvanio, R., Levine, M., Heaton, R. K., & Heilman, K. M. (2000). Predicting hand preference with performance on motor tasks. *Cortex, 36,* 679–689.

Yeudall, L. T., Reddon, J. R., Gill, D. M., & Stafanyk, W. O. (1987). Normative data for the Halstead-Reitan neuropsychological tests stratified by age and sex. *Journal of Clinical Psychology, 43,* 346–367.

PURPOSE

The Grooved Pegboard task measures eye-hand coordination and motor speed.

SOURCE

The pegboard can be ordered from Lafayette Instrument Company, 3700 Sagamore Parkway, P.O. Box 5729, Lafayette, IN 47904, at a cost of $90 US, or from Psychological Assessment Resources (http://www.parinc.com) at a cost of $129 US.

AGE RANGE

Norms are available for ages 6 to 85 years.

DESCRIPTION

The Grooved Pegboard (Matthews & Klove, 1964) requires considerable manual precision and is included in neuropsychological examinations in order to assess motor impairment. It consists of a metal board with a matrix of 25 holes with randomly positioned slots (see Figure 14–2). Pegs have a ridge along one side and must be rotated to match the hole before they can be inserted. The patient's task is to insert metal pegs as quickly as possible into the slots in sequence, first with the dominant hand and then with the nondominant one. The patient continues until all pegs have been placed. The score is the time in seconds required to complete the array with each hand. According to the test manual, children aged 5 to 8 years are asked to fill only the first two rows of the pegboard, totalling 10 pegs. However, recent work (Rosselli et al., 2001) has used the full version with young children.

Figure 14–2 Grooved Pegboard. Reproduced with permission.

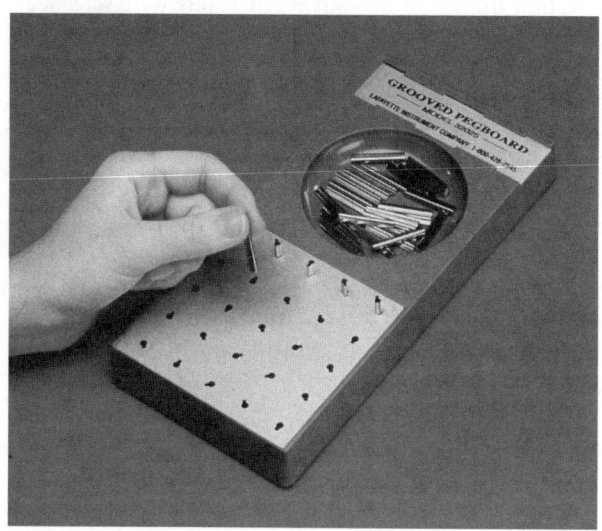

The test is also part of the Halstead-Russell Neuropsychological Evaluation System (HRNES; Russell and Starkey, 1993).

ADMINISTRATION

The instructions are provided in the test manual from the Lafayette Instrument Company. Briefly, the apparatus is placed with the peg tray oriented above the pegboard. The person is instructed to insert the pegs, matching the groove of the peg with the groove of the hole, filling the rows in a given direction as quickly as possible, without skipping any slots. Using the right hand, the patient is asked to work from left to right, and with the left hand, in the opposite direction. The dominant hand is tested first. The patient is warned that only one peg should be picked up at a time and that only one hand is to be used. If a peg is dropped, the examiner does not retrieve it; rather, one of the pegs correctly placed (usually, the first or second peg) is taken out and used again.

The examiner demonstrates one row before allowing the patient to begin. A practice trial is not given, and a trial may be discontinued after 5 min. In the HRNES (Russell and Starkey, 1993) version, the person continues until all pegs have been placed or until a time limit of 3 min has been reached. In both versions, the examiner begins timing after cueing the individual to begin.

ADMINISTRATION TIME

The time required is about 5 min.

SCORING

The score is computed for each hand separately and is the time required to place the pegs. Some researchers also record the number of pegs not placed and the number of pegs dropped; these errors may be considered clinically and are rarely seen in neurologically normal individuals (Heaton et al., 2004).

DEMOGRAPHIC EFFECTS

When each hand is considered separately, several trends emerge.

Age

Age has a strong impact on test scores, with performance improving (faster times) in childhood (Rosselli et al., 2001; Solan, 1987) and declining with advancing age (e.g., Bornstein, 1985; Concha et al., 1995; Mitrushina et al., 2005; Ruff & Parker, 1993; Selnes et al., 1991). According to Heaton et al. (2004), about 30% to 34% of the variance in test scores is accounted for by age.

Gender

Some have found significant gender differences in performance, with women outperforming men (Bornstein, 1985; Ruff & Parker, 1993; Schmidt et al., 2000), perhaps reflecting differences in finger size (Peters et al., 1990). However, others have noted that gender has little effect on test scores (Concha et al., 1995; Heaton et al., 2004; Mitrushina et al., 2005), accounting for less than 1% of the variance in test scores (Heaton et al., 2004). No gender effect has been found in children (Rosselli et al., 2001).

Hand Preference

Performance is faster with the dominant/preferred hand (Bryden et al., 1998; Heaton et al., 2004). Handedness (right, left) does not affect test scores (Ruff & Parker, 1993).

Education/IQ

Some have reported that better educated individuals perform faster (Ruff & Parker, 1993). However, others have found that education has little or only a small effect (Bornstein, 1985; Concha et al., 1995; Mitrushina et al., 2005; Selnes et al., 1991), accounting for about 3% to 6% of the variance test scores (Heaton et al., 2004).

Ethnicity

The impact of ethnicity has not been reported.

Intermanual Differences

Neither age, education, nor hand preference is related to intermanual differences scores on the Grooved Pegboard (Bornstein, 1986c; Ruff & Parker, 1993; Thompson et al., 1987); however, intermanual differences tend to be larger for females than for males (Rosselli et al., 2001; Thompson et al., 1987; but see Bornstein, 1986c).

NORMATIVE DATA

The use of simple cutoff scores is discouraged, because such a practice leads to a high rate of misclassification (Bornstein, 1986b). Normative data (ages 5 to 60+ years) provided by Dr. R. Trites (1977) are available in the manual; however, the sample is not well described, and the data are not stratified by gender.

Adults

Heaton et al. (2004) have developed normative data based on a large sample of Caucasians and African Americans (see Table 14–15). They provide norms separately for these two ethnicity groups, organized by age, gender and education.

Table 14–15 Characteristics of the Grooved Pegboard Normative Sample provided by Heaton et al. (2004)

Number	1482
Age (years)	20–85[a]
Geographic location	Various states in the United States and Manitoba, Canada
Sample type	Individuals recruited as part of multicenter studies
Education (years)	0–20[b]
Gender (%)	
Male	60.1
Female	39.9
Race/Ethnicity	
Caucasian	839
African American	643
Screening	No reported history of learning disability, neurological disorder, serious psychiatric disorder, or alcohol or drug abuse

[a]Age groups: 20–34, 35–39, 40–44, 45–49, 50–54, 55–59, 60–64, 65–69, 70–74, 75–79, and 80–89 years.
[b]Education groups: 7–8, 9–11, 12, 13–15, 16–17, and 18–20 years.

The data set covers a wide range in terms of age (20–85 years) and education (0–20 years), and exclusion criteria are specified. T scores lower than 40 are classed as impaired. According to Heaton et al. (2004), the procedure used was the one specified by the Lafayette Instrument Company. Unfortunately, the method for determining hand preference was not described.

Mitrushina et al. (2005) provide meta-norms, based on six studies and representing 2382 participants, aged 20 to 64 years. They noted that the integrity of the results is undermined by the lack of consistency in reporting of hand preference.

Table 14–16 provides data (Ruff and Parker, 1993) based on a sample of 357 individuals aged 16 to 70 years, ranging in education from 7 to 22 years. Participants were screened to exclude those with a positive history of psychiatric hospitalization, chronic polydrug abuse, or neurological disorders. Hand preference was evaluated using a lateral dominance examination. The data agree reasonably well with those provided by Mitrushina et al. (2005).

Children/Adolescents

Older normative data sets are available for children (Knights, 1970; Knights & Moule, 1968; Trites, 1977). However, use of these norms is not recommended, because they are quite dated and cell sizes are quite small.

Recently, Rosselli et al. (2001) used the 25-hole pegboard and provided data (see Table 14–17) on a sample of 290 Spanish-speaking children (141 boys, 149 girls), aged 6 to 11

Table 14–16 Mean Performance of Adults for Grooved Pegboard, by Education, Age, and Gender

Age group (Years)	≤Grade 12			>Grade 12		
	N	M	SD	N	M	SD
Females, Preferred hand						
16–39	30	62.8	8.9	60	57.8	6.2
40–54	14	63.1	4.4	30	63.3	7.4
55–70	15	78.6	11.7	29	75.3	11.3
Females, Nonpreferred hand						
16–39	29	66.8	10.7	60	65.2	10.3
40–54	14	69.6	6.5	30	70.8	8.9
55–70	13	84.3	15.3	29	82.0	12.5
Males, Preferred hand						
16–39	29	67.8	9.2	60	64.7	10.9
40–54	15	71.9	15.1	30	70.4	10.9
55–70	15	83.7	10.2	30	74.1	13.0
Males, Nonpreferred hand						
16–39	29	74.5	10.9	59	67.8	10.8
40–54	15	79.1	14.9	30	73.7	9.9
55–70	15	91.0	12.7	28	83.5	13.4

Note: Based on a sample of 357 healthy participants.

Source: From Ruff & Parker, 1993. © Perceptual and Motor Skills 1993. Reprinted with permission.

years, in Bogota, Colombia. None of the subjects was mentally retarded. Based on the Waterloo Handedness questionnaire, 268 children were right-handed, and 22 were left-handed. Rosselli et al. (2001) noted that the older the group,

Table 14–17 Grooved Pegboard (Time in Seconds) Normative Data for Spanish-Speaking Boys and Girls Aged 6–11 Years (25-Hole Pegboard), by Age

	6–7 years (*n* = 83)	8–9 years (*n* = 121)	10–11 years (*n* = 86)
Preferred hand	92.46 (17.80)	81.96 (13.79)	69.47 (10.47)
Nonpreferred hand	104.00 (21.44)	93.58 (17.67)	76.41 (12.22)

Source: Adapted from Rosselli et al., 2001.

the smaller the difference in performance between hands. The performance of older children was similar to that of adults aged 40 to 59 years (e.g., Bornstein, 1985; Ruff & Parker, 1993), suggesting that additional gains are made during adolescence.

In line with this proposal are the findings by Paniak (personal communication, April 10, 2004) for a sample of 358 adolescents living in a large western Canadian city (see Table 14–18). The exclusion criteria for this sample included failure of one or more grades, enrollment in an English as a Second Language program, a history of hospitalization for brain injury or behavioral problems, or participation in a self-contained special education program. The sample was largely right-handed and had a WISC-III Vocabulary scaled score of about 10 (*SD* = 3).

Table 14–18 Mean Performance (Seconds) on Grooved Pegboard in Adolescents

Age (Years)	Males			Females		
	N	Right Hand	Left Hand	N	Right Hand	Left Hand
12	38	64.61 (10.8)	70.03 (10.85)	56	66.05 (8.64)	71.61 (9.37)
13	39	61.82 (6.74)	67.33 (10.85)	57	62.93 (6.27)	70.60 (9.57)
14	46	64.00 (10.54)	70.09 (10.88)	70	62.43 (9.12)	67.30 (10.06)
15	29	62.21 (7.04)	63.34 (8.95)	23	64.78 (9.52)	67.48 (10.72)

Note: Based on a sample of 358 healthy adolescents in a large Western Canadian city.

Source: C. Paniak, H. Miller & D. Murphy (personal communication, April 10, 2004).

Table 14-19 Grooved Pegboard Test-Retest Effects in 121 Normal Individuals Assessed After Intervals of 2 to 16 Months

| Measure | Time 1 | | Time 2 | | T2–T1 | | T1, T2 |
	(1) Mean	SD	(2) Mean	SD	(3) M	(4) SD	r
Dominant	69.66	19.27	68.68	21.04	−.98	10.03	.86
Nondominant	75.80	21.56	73.70	19.69	−2.09	11.11	.86

Note: Based on a sample of 121 normal individuals (mean age = 43.6, *SD* = 19.6; mean education = 12.0, *SD* = 3.3) after retest intervals of about 2–16 months (mean = 5.4, *SD* = 2.5). One first subtracts the mean T2–T1 change (column 3) from the difference between the two testings for the individual and then compares it to 1.64 times the standard deviation of the difference (column 4). The 1.64 comes from the normal distribution and is exceeded in the positive or negative direction only 10% of the time if indeed there is no real change in clinical condition.

Source: Adapted from Dikmen et al., 1999.

Table 14-20 Grooved Pegboard Test-Retest Effects in 605 Healthy Males Assessed After Intervals of 2 to 24 Months

| Measure | Time 1 | | Time 2 | | T2–T1 | | T1, T2 |
	(1) Mean	SD	(2) Mean	SD	(3) M	(4) SD	r
Dominant	64.2	8.94	61.7	8.16	−2.50	7.01	.67
Nondominant	69.1	10.39	66.5	9.55	−2.61	7.37	.73

Note: Based on a sample of 605 healthy males, mostly Caucasian (mean age = 39.5, *SD* = 8.5; mean education = 16.4, *SD* = 2.3) after retest intervals of about 2–24 months (mean = 218 days, *SD* = 95).

Source: Adapted from Levine et al., 2004.

RELIABILITY

Test-Retest Reliability and Practice Effects

With retest intervals of about 4 to 24 months, reliability coefficients are marginal/high (.67 to .86) in normal individuals (aged 15 years and older; Dikmen et al., 1999; Levine et al., 2004; Ruff & Parker, 1993). No information is available for children.

When repeated trials are given within a session, performance improves particularly after the first trial (Schmidt et al., 2000). With two or more sessions (e.g., assessments 1 and 2 occurring within 1 week of each other, assessments 3 and 4 about 3 and 6 months later), performance improves steadily (McCaffrey et al., 1993; but see Bornstein et al., 1987).

Detecting Change

When individuals are retested after intervals of about 2 to 24 months, practice effects are evident (Dikmen et al., 1999; Levine et al., 2004; Ruff & Parker, 1993). Dikmen et al. (1999) examined a sample of 121 normal adults (age *M* = 43.6, *SD* = 19.6; education *M* = 12.0, *SD* = 3.3) after retest intervals of about 2 to 16 months (*M* = 5.4, *SD* = 2.5). Table 14–19 provides information to assess change, taking practice effects into

account (RCI-PE). Using values in Table 14–19, one first subtracts the mean T2 – T1 change (column 3) from the difference between the two testings for the individual and then compares the result with 1.64 times the standard deviation of the difference (column 4). The 1.64 comes from the normal distribution and is exceeded in the positive or negative direction only 10% of the time if indeed there is no real change in clinical condition.

Drawing from a database of 605 well-educated men (education *M* = 16.4, *SD* = 2.3), mostly Caucasian males (age *M* = 39.5, *SD* = 8.7), Levine and colleagues (2004) used both RCI-PE and simple linear regression approaches to derive estimates of change. The retest interval ranged from 4 to 24 months (*M* = 218 days, *SD* = 95). The length of retest interval did not contribute significantly to the regression equation. Table 14–20 shows the means, standard deviations of the change scores, and test-retest correlations for use in RCI equations. Table 14–21 shows the regression formulas used to estimate time 2 scores. The residual standard deviations for the regression formulas are also shown and can be used to establish the normal range for retest scores. For example, a 90% confidence interval can be created around the scores by multiplying the residual standard deviation by 1.645, which allows for 5% of people to fall outside of both the upper and lower extremes. Individuals whose scores exceed the extremes are considered to have significant changes.

Table 14–21 Regression Equations for Estimating Retest Scores

Measure	Regression Equation	Regression SD
Dominant	22.57 + (.609 × Time 1 score)	6.08
Nondominant	20.15 + (.671 × Time 1 score)	6.53

Note: Based on a sample of 605 healthy males, mostly Caucasian (mean age = 39.5, SD = 8.5; mean education = 16.4, SD = 2.3) after retest intervals of about 2–24 months (mean = 218 days, SD = 95).

Source: Adapted from Levine et al., 2004.

VALIDITY

Relationships With Other Measures

Pegboard time (dominant hand) shows a modest relation with tapping speed (−.35; Schear & Sato, 1989), and factor analytic findings indicate that the two tasks load differently (Baser & Ruff, 1987). Examination of relations among manual performance tasks in healthy individuals suggests that finger tapping and pegboard tasks are more closely related to one another than to grip strength (Corey et al., 2001).

In addition to requiring motor execution, the pegboard task also requires adequate vision. Schear and Sato (1989) found a moderately strong correlation (−.62) between near visual acuity and dominant-hand pegboard time.

Moderate/high associations have also been reported with measures of attention (e.g., reaction time $r = .31$; TMT-B $r = .46$; Schear & Sato, 1989; Strenge et al. 2002), perceptual speed (Digit Symbol $r = −.60$; Schear & Sato, 1989) and nonverbal reasoning (Block Design $r = −.34$; Object Assembly $r = −.45$; Schear & Sato, 1989; see also Haaland & Delaney, 1981).

There is little relation between pegboard scores (preferred hand) and grades in academic subjects (Rosselli et al., 2001), although Solan (1987) noted a moderate relation ($r = −.41$) with WRAT arithmetic.

Clinical Findings

There is evidence that pegboard-placing speed is reduced in a number of conditions, including stroke (Haaland & Delaney, 1981), tumor (Haaland & Delaney, 1981), autism (Hardan et al., 2003), nonverbal learning disabilities (Harnadek & Rourke, 1994), Williams syndrome (MacDonald & Roy, 1988), bipolar disorder (Wilder-Willis et al., 2001), end-stage heart disease (Putzke et al., 2000), toxic exposure (Bleecker et al., 1997; Mathiesen et al., 1999), substance abuse (withdrawn cocaine users; Smelson et al., 1999), and HIV-1 infection (Carey et al., 2004; Hestad et al., 1993). Various drug treatments (carbamazepine, phenytoin) also impair performance (Meador et al., 1991).

The test is also a sensitive, but not totally accurate, indicator of lateralized disturbances (Bornstein, 1986a; Haaland & Delaney, 1981). Left cerebral lesions tend to attenuate the more typical pattern of manual asymmetry; right lesions move the discrepancies in the opposite direction. However, ipsilateral impairment is also seen—perhaps a reflection of the significant sequencing, visual-spatial, and monitoring requirements of the tasks (Haaland & Delaney, 1981). Lewis & Kupke (1992) also suggested that difficulty adapting to a novel task, especially with the nonpreferred hand, may affect performance.

Typically, performances of the preferred and nonpreferred hands are compared on motor tasks to determine whether there is consistent evidence of poor performance with one hand relative to the other. In general, performance with the preferred hand is superior (by about 10%) to that with the nonpreferred hand (Mitrushina et al., 2005; Thompson et al., 1987). However, there is considerable variability in the normal population, and the preferred hand is not necessarily the faster one (Bornstein, 1986c; Corey et al., 2001), especially when left-handed people are considered (Corey et al., 2001; Thompson et al., 1987). Patterns indicating equal or better performance with the nonpreferred hand occur with considerable regularity in the normal population (about 25%), and neurological involvement should not be inferred from an isolated lack of concordance. Fairly large discrepancies between the hands on the Grooved Pegboard Test alone also cannot be used to suggest unilateral impairment, because discrepancies of large magnitude are not uncommon (about 20%) in the normal population (Bornstein, 1986a, 1986c; Thompson et al., 1987). In addition, intermanual discrepancies (even of large magnitude) are not perfect predictors of the side of lesion (Bornstein, 1986a). Greater confidence in the clinical judgment of impaired motor function with one or the other hand can be gained from consideration of the consistency of intermanual discrepancies across several motor tasks, because truly consistent, deviant performances are quite rare in the normal population (Bornstein, 1986a, 1986b; Thompson et al., 1987).

It is important to note that there may be reasons other than neurological impairment for an individual to perform poorly on this task. Deficits in tactile acuity at the fingertips can also translate into significant difficulties in tasks, such as the Grooved Pegboard, that require fine manipulations (Tremblay et al., 2002). Depression has also been associated with lower performance (Hinkin et al., 1992) as are some medications (e.g., Meador et al., 1991).

Ecological/Predictive Validity

Weak/modest associations have been noted between pegboard scores and daily functioning (complex activities of daily living) in patients with multiple sclerosis (Kessler et al., 1992) and after head injury (Farmer & Eakman, 1995). In those with HIV infection, poor performance may represent an early sign of a dementing process: Defective performance on the Grooved Pegboard was linked with an increased risk of becoming demented over a 30-month follow-up period (Stern et al., 2001).

Malingering

Individuals simulating head injury tend to suppress their performance on the Grooved Pegboard (Johnson & Lesniak-Karpiak, 1997; Rapport et al., 1998; but see Wong et al., 1998), although warning participants of the possibility of detection (Johnson & Lesniak-Karpiak, 1997) or coaching them on how to avoid detection (Rapport et al., 1998) may improve test scores.

Greiffenstein and colleagues (1996) examined the average performance of the dominant and nondominant hands on tests of motor functioning and reported that compensation-seeking patients with postconcussion syndrome (PCS) demonstrated a nonphysiological profile on grip strength, finger tapping, and Grooved Pegboard (grip strength < finger tapping < grooved pegs). However Rapport et al. (1998) found that the presence of nonphysiological configurations (grip strength < finger tapping < grooved pegs) showed poor predictive accuracy among simulators and controls.

COMMENT

The test is brief and easy to give. The availability of large normative reports is also an asset. Heaton et al (2004) appears not to have found problems with sample distribution for pegboard scores. However, Hamby et al. (1997) examined a sample of HIV-positive individuals and reported that the Grooved Pegboard test may not be well suited for identifying subtle deficits or making fine discriminations because of nonnormal sampling distributions (e.g., ceiling effects). They noted that such restrictions in range also make it difficult to apply simple conversions (e.g., to z scores and percentiles), identify changes over time, and investigate relationships among tests (because restricted ranges reduce the magnitude of correlations). For example, a dominant-hand Grooved Pegboard score of 74.1 s would receive a z score of $-.5$, using the mean and SD found in their sample. If the data were normally distributed, this would translate into a percentile score of 31%, within the average range. However, the actual percentile for that score, according to the sample distribution, is 13%, which might be interpreted as below average. That is, an individual's performance may be judged to be within normal limits when it actually indicates some degree of impairment. To deal with this problem, Hamby et al. (1997) recommended that norms for the test include true percentiles, not merely the mean and SD.

There is some variability among authors in terms of administration procedures. Most authors demonstrate the procedure, although some (e.g., Ruff & Parker, 1993; Selnes et al., 1991) allow the individual to practice before the actual test. The amount of time permitted for a trial also differs (5 min according to instructions provided by the Lafayette Instrument Company, 3 min according to Russell & Starkey, 1993). The number of trials (one or two) also varies (Mitrushina et al., 2005). Nonetheless, test-retest reliability is good. Note that, for young children, the best available norma-

tive data set (Rosselli et al., 2001) requires administration of the entire pegboard.

The Grooved Pegboard is a more cognitively demanding task than grip strength or finger tapping (Haaland & Delaney, 1981). In addition to motor dexterity, vision, speed, attention, and continuous monitoring of accuracy are also important components of task performance. Interpretation should take into account the possibility of peripheral limb injuries, as well as the performance on other related tasks (Bornstein, 1986a; Thompson et al., 1987). It is also worth bearing in mind that large-magnitude discrepancies between the hands and patterns indicating equal or better performance with the nonpreferred hand occur with considerable regularity in the normal population (Bornstein, 1986c; Thompson et al., 1987).

REFERENCES

Baser, C. N., & Ruff, R. M. (1987). Construct validity of the San Diego Neuropsychological Test Battery. *Archives of Clinical Neuropsychology, 2,* 13–32.

Bleecker, M. L., Lindgren, K. N., & Ford, D. P. (1997). Differential contribution of current and cumulative indices of lead dose to neuropsychological performance by age. *Neurology, 48,* 639–645.

Bornstein, R. A. (1985). Normative data on selected neuropsychological measures from a nonclinical sample. *Journal of Clinical Psychology, 41,* 651–658.

Bornstein, R. A. (1986a). Consistency of intermanual discrepancies in normal and unilateral brain lesion patients. *Journal of Consulting and Clinical Psychology, 54,* 719–723.

Bornstein, R. A. (1986b). Classification rates obtained with "standard" cut-off scores on selected neuropsychological measures. *Journal of Clinical and Experimental Neuropsychology, 8,* 413–420.

Bornstein, R. A. (1986c). Normative data on intermanual differences on three tests of motor performance. *Journal of Clinical and Experimental Neuropsychology, 8,* 12–20.

Bornstein, R. A., Baker, G. B., & Douglas, A. B. (1987). Short-term test-retest reliability of the Halstead-Reitan Battery in a normal sample. *The Journal of Nervous and Mental Disease, 175,* 229–232.

Bryden, P. J., Roy, E. A., & Bryden, M. P. (1998). Between task comparisons: Movement complexity affects the magnitude of manual asymmetries. *Brain and Cognition, 37,* 47–50.

Carey, C. L., Woods, S. P., Rippeth, J. D., Gonzalez, R., Moore, D. J., Marcotte, T. D., Grant, I., Heaton, R. K., & the HNRC Group. (2004). Initial validation of a screening battery for the detection of HIV-associated cognitive impairment. *The Clinical Neuropsychologist, 18,* 234–248.

Concha, M., Selnes, O. A., McArthur, J. C., Nance-Sproson, T., Updike, M. L., Royall W., Solomon, L., & Vlahov, D. (1995). Normative data for a brief neuropsychologic test battery in a cohort of injecting drug users. *International Journal of the Addictions, 30,* 823–841.

Corey, D. M., Hurley, M. M., & Foundas, A. L. (2001). Right and left handedness defined. *Neuropsychiatry, Neuropsychology, and Behavioral Neurology, 14,* 144–152.

Dikmen, S. S., Heaton, R. K., Grant, I., & Temkin, N. R. (1999). Test-retest reliability and practice effects of expanded Halstead-Reitan neuropsychological test battery. *Journal of the International Neuropsychological Society, 5,* 346–356.

Farmer, J. E., & Eakman, A. M. (1995). The relationship between neuropsychological functioning and instrumental activities of daily living following acquired brain injury. *Applied Neuropsychology, 2,* 107–115.

Greiffenstein, M. F., Baker, W. J., & Gola, T. (1996). Motor dysfunction profiles in traumatic brain injury and postconcussion syndrome. *Journal of the International Neuropsychological Society, 2,* 477–485.

Haaland, K. Y., & Delaney, H. D. (1981). Motor deficits after left or right hemisphere damage due to stroke or tumor. *Neuropsychologia, 19,* 17–27.

Hamby, S. L., Bardi, C. A., & Wilkins, J. W. (1997). Neuropsychological assessment of relatively intact individuals: Psychometric lessons from an HIV+ sample. *Archives of Clinical Neuropsychology, 12,* 545–556.

Hardan, A. Y., Kilpatrick, M., Keshavan, M. S., & Minshew, N. J. (2003). Motor performance and anatomic magnetic resonance imaging (MRI) of the basal ganglia in autism. *Journal of Child Neurology, 18,* 317–324.

Harnadek, M. C., & Rourke, B. P. (1994). Principal identifying features of nonverbal learning disabilities in children. *Journal of Learning Disabilities, 27,* 144–154.

Heaton, R. K., Miller, S. W., Taylor, M. J., & Grant, I. (2004). *Revised comprehensive norms for an expanded Halstead-Reitan Battery: Demographically adjusted neuropsychological norms for African American and Caucasian adults.* Lutz, FL: PAR.

Hestad, K., McArthur, J. H., Dal Pan, G. J., Selnes, O. A., et al., (1993). Regional brain atrophy in HIV-1 infection: Association with specific neuropsychological test performance. *Acta Neurological Scandinavica, 88,* 112–118.

Hinkin, C. H., van Gorp, W. G., Satz, P., Weisman, J. D., Thommes, J., & Buckingham, S. (1992). Depressed mood and its relationship to neuropsychological test performance in HIV-1 seropositive individuals. *Journal of Clinical and Experimental Neuropsychology, 14,* 289–297.

Johnson, J. L., & Lesniak-Karpiak, K. (1997). The effect of warning on malingering on memory and motor tasks in college samples. *Archives of Clinical Neuropsychology, 12,* 231–238.

Kessler, H. R., Cohen, R. A., Lauer, K., & Kausch, D. F. (1992). The relationship between disability and memory dysfunction in multiple sclerosis. *International Journal of Neuroscience, 62,* 17–34.

Knights, R. M. (1970). *Smoothed normative data on tests for evaluation of brain damage in children.* Unpublished manuscript. Carleton University, Ottawa, Ontario.

Knights, R. M., & Moule, A. D. (1968). Normative data on the Motor Steadiness Battery for children. *Perceptual and Motor Skills, 26,* 643–650.

Levine, A. J., Miller, E. N., Becker, J. T., Selnes, O. A., & Cohen, B. A. (2004). Normative data for determining significance of test-retest differences on eight common neuropsychological instruments. *The Clinical Neuropsychologist, 18,* 373–384.

Lewis, R., & Kupke, T. (1992). Intermanual differences on skilled and unskilled motor tasks in nonlateralized brain dysfunction. *The Clinical Neuropsychologist, 6,* 374–382.

MacDonald, G. W., & Roy, R. D. (1988). Williams Syndrome: A neuropsychological profile. *Journal of Clinical and Experimental Neuropsychology, 10,* 125–131.

Matthews, C. G., & Klove, K. (1964). *Instruction manual for the Adult Neuropsychology Test Battery.* Madison, Wisc.: University of Wisconsin Medical School.

Mathiesen, T., Ellingsen, D. G., & Kjuus, H. (1999). Neuropsychological effects associated with exposure to mercury vapor among former chloralkali workers. *Scandinavian Journal of Work, Environment and Health, 25,* 342–250.

McCaffrey, R. J., Ortega, A., & Haase, R. F. (1993). Effects of repeated neuropsychological assessments. *Archives of Clinical Neuropsychology, 8,* 519–524.

Meador, K. J., Loring, D. W., Allen, M. E., Zamini, E. Y., et al. (1991). Comparative cognitive effects of carbamazepine and phenytoin in healthy adults. *Neurology, 41,* 1537–1540.

Mitrushina, M. N., Boone, K. B., Razani, J. & d'Elia, L. F. (2005). *Handbook of normative data for neuropsychological assessment* (2nd ed.). New York: Oxford University Press.

Peters, M., Servos, P., & Day, R. (1990). Marked sex difference between right-handers and left-handers disappear when finger size is used as a covariate. *Journal of Applied Psychology, 75,* 87–90.

Putzke, J. D., Williams, M. A., Daniel, F. J., Foley, B. A., Kirklin, J. K., & Boll, T. J. (2000). Neuropsychological functioning among heart transplant candidates: A case control study. *Journal of Clinical and Experimental Neuropsychology, 22,* 95–103.

Rapport, L. J., Farchione, T. J., Coleman, R. D., & Axelrod, B. N. (1998). Effects of coaching on malingered motor function profiles. *Journal of Clinical and Experimental Neuropsychology, 20,* 89–97.

Rosselli, M., Ardila, A., Bateman, J. R., & Guzman, M. (2001). Neuropsychological test scores, academic performance, and developmental disorders in Spanish-speaking children. *Developmental Neuropsychology, 20,* 355–373.

Ruff, R. M., & Parker, S. B. (1993). Gender- and age-specific changes in motor speed and eye hand coordination in adults: Normative values for the Finger Tapping and Grooved Pegboard tests. *Perceptual and Motor Skills, 76,* 1219–1230.

Russell, E. W., & Starkey, R. I. (1993). *Halstead Russell Neuropsychological Evaluation System (HRNES).* Los Angeles: Western Psychological Services.

Schear, J. M., & Sato, S. D. (1989). Effects of visual acuity and visual motor speed and dexterity on cognitive test performance. *Archives of Clinical Neuropsychology 4,* 25–32.

Schmidt, S. L., Oliveira, R. M., Rocha, F. R.., & Abreu-Villaca, Y. (2000). Influences of handedness and gender on the Grooved Pegboard Test. *Brain and Cognition, 44,* 445–454.

Selnes, O. A., Jacobson, L., Machado, A. M., Becker, J. T., Wesch, J., Miller, E. N., Visscher, B., McArthur, J. C. (1991). Normative data for a brief neuropsychological screening battery. *Perceptual and Motor Skills, 71,* 539–550.

Smelson, D. A., Roy, A., Santana, S., & Engelhart, C. (1999). Neuropsychological deficits in withdrawn cocaine-dependent males. *American Journal of Drug and Alcohol Abuse, 25,* 377–381.

Solan, H. A. (1987). Perceptual norms in grades 4 and 5: A preliminary report. *Journal of the American Optometric Association, 58,* 979–982.

Stern, Y., McDermott, M. P., Albert, S., Palumbo, D., Selnes, O. A., McArthur, J., Sacktor, N., Schifitto, G., Kieburtz, K., Epstein, L., Marder, K. S., & Dana Consortium on the Therapy of HIV-Dementia and Related Cognitive Disorders. (2001). Factors associated with incident human immunodeficiency virus-dementia. *Archives of Neurology, 58,* 473–479.

Strenge, H., Niedenberger, U., & Seelhorst, U. (2002). Correlation between tests of attention and performance on Grooved and Purdue

Pegboards in normal subjects. *Perceptual and Motor Skills, 95,* 507–514.

Thompson, L. L., Heaton, K. R., Matthews, C. G., & Grant, I. (1987). Comparison of preferred and nonpreferred hand performance on four neuropsychological motor tasks. *The Clinical Neuropsychologist, 1,* 324–334.

Tremblay, F., Wong, K., Sanderson, R., & Cote, L. (2002). Tactile spatial acuity in elderly persons: Assessment with grating domes and relationship with manual dexterity. *Somatosensory and Motor Research, 20,* 127–132.

Trites, R. (1977). *Neuropsychological test manual.* Ottawa, Ontario: Royal Ottawa Hospital (available from Lafayette Instrument Company).

Wilder-Willis, K. E., Sax, K., Rosenberg, H. L., Fleck, D. E., Shear, P. K., & Strakowski, S. M. (2001). Persistent attentional dysfunction in remitted bipolar disorder. *Bipolar Disorders, 3,* 58–62.

Wong, J. L., Lerrner-Poppen, L., & Durham, J. (1998). Does warning reduce obvious malingering on memory and motor tasks in college samples? *International Journal of Rehabilitation and Health, 4,* 153–165.

Purdue Pegboard Test

PURPOSE

The purpose of this test is to measure unimanual and bimanual finger and hand dexterity.

SOURCE

The pegboard, manual, and record forms can be ordered from Lafayette Instrument Company, 3700 Sagamore Parkway, P.O. Box 5729, Lafayette, IN 47904, for $109 US, or from Psychological Assessment Resources (http://www.parinc.com) at a cost of $133 US.

AGE RANGE

Norms are available for individuals aged 5 to 89 years.

DESCRIPTION

The Purdue Pegboard was developed in the 1940s as a test of manipulative dexterity for use in personnel selection (Tiffin, 1968; Tiffin & Asher, 1948). In addition to this use, the Purdue Pegboard Test has been employed in neuropsychological assessment to assist in localizing cerebral lesions and deficits (Reddon et al., 1988). The board consists of two parallel rows of 25 holes each (see Figure 14–3). Pins (pegs) are located at the extreme right-hand and left-hand cups at the top of the board. Collars and washers occupy the two middle cups. In the first three subtests, the subject places as many pins as possible in the holes, first with the preferred hand, then with the nonpreferred hand, and finally with both hands, within a 30-s time period. To test the right hand, the subject must insert as many pins as possible in the holes, starting at the top of the right-hand row. The left-hand test uses the left row. Both hands then are used together to fill both rows top to bottom. In the fourth subtest, the subject uses both hands alternately to construct "assemblies," which consist of a pin, a washer, a collar, and another washer. The subject must complete as many assemblies as possible within 1 minute.

ADMINISTRATION

The instructions are described in the test manual. Briefly, the individual is required to take pins with the preferred (e.g., right) hand from the right-hand cup and place them as quickly

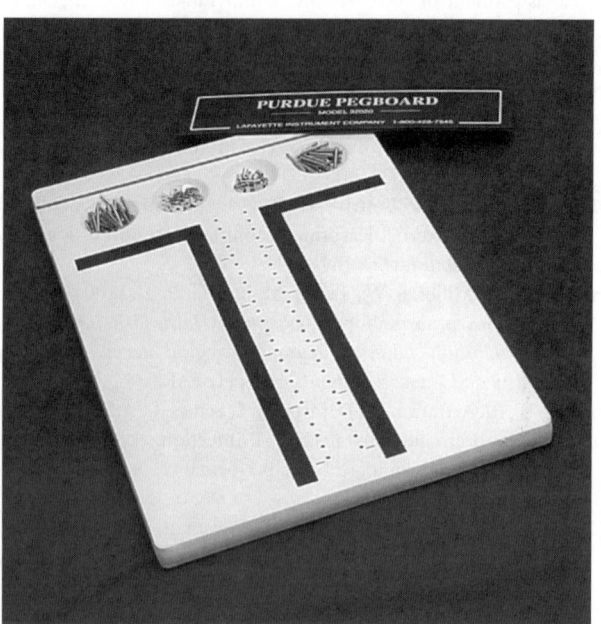

Figure 14–3 Purdue Pegboard. Reproduced with permission.

as possible in the right column of holes, during a 30-s period. The pins are allowed to remain in the holes and the procedure is repeated with the nonpreferred hand. The pins are then removed and the test is repeated with the individual using both hands simultaneously. Again the trial period is 30 s. The pins are then removed and the person is asked to form "assemblies." The person is asked to use continuous alternating movements of the right and left hands, one picking up a pin, one a washer, one a collar, and so on. The time allowed is 60 s. Demonstration and practice are provided before each subtest.

Examiners may repeat each task three times. If three-trial administration is desired, the right hand test is given three times before proceeding to the left hand test, and so on throughout the series of tests.

SCORING

Scores are derived for each part of the test. The scores for the pin (peg) placement subtests consist of the number of pins inserted in the time period for each hand. The score for the bimanual condition consists of the total number of pairs of pins inserted. The assembly score refers to the number of parts assembled (see *Source*).

DEMOGRAPHIC EFFECTS

Age

Performance improves during childhood and slows with advancing age (Agnew et al., 1988; Brito & Santos-Morales, 2002; DesRosiers et al., 1995; Gardner & Broman, 1979; Mathiowetz et al., 1986; McCurry et al., 2001; Wilson et al., 1982).

Gender

Females tend to perform better than males (e.g., Agnew et al., 1988; Brito & Santos-Morales, 2002; DesRosiers et al., 1995; Mathiowetz et al., 1986; Peters, 1990; Sattler & Engelhardt, 1982; Yeudall et al., 1986; but see Costa et al., 1963, who did not find sex-related differences). Gender differences in fine manual dexterity may be confounded by gender differences in finger size. Peters et al. (1990) reported that when measures of index finger and thumb thickness were used as covariates, gender differences in performance disappeared. Further, negative correlations between performance and finger size were observed in both men and women. The implication is that, for most men, the fingers are of a size that is relatively unsuitable for this task. With larger-sized pegs, men may no longer be at a disadvantage.

Education

Education appears to be unrelated to performance (Costa et al., 1963; McCurry et al., 2001; Yeudall et al., 1986).

Handedness

In general, performance is better with the preferred than with the nonpreferred hand (e.g., Brito & Santos-Morales, 2002; DesRosiers et al., 1995; Judge & Stirling, 2003; Triggs et al., 2000). There is evidence that left-handers perform more proficiently on the assembly component (Judge & Stirling, 2003).

Ethnicity/Socioeconomic Status

Ethnicity and social class had no impact on test performance of children residing in the greater Rio de Janeiro area (Brito & -Santo-Morales, 2002). Primary language spoken (English, Japanese) among Japanese adults (aged 65 years and older) also had no effect on peg placement scores (McCurry et al., 2001).

NORMATIVE DATA

Some normative data for various occupational groups are available in the test manual (see *Source*). Note, however, that the data are quite old; they are not stratified by age and information regarding hand preference is not provided.

Adults

Table 14–22 provides normative data for adults, stratified on the basis of age (15–40 years) and gender (Yeudall et al., 1986). Participants were excluded based on evidence from interview of forensic involvement, prenatal or birth complication, psychiatric disorders or substance abuse problems. Hand preference was determined by the hand used to write with. Administration was one trial per subtest.

Table 14–23 shows normative data (DesRosiers et al., 1995) based on a random sample of 360 individuals, stratified for age and gender, drawn from the electoral pool of a city in Quebec. All subjects were aged 60 to 89 years, lucid and independent in activities of daily living; all could see sufficiently well and had no impairment affecting upper limb functioning. Most (92%) were classed as right-handed based on the Edinburgh Handedness Inventory.

McCurry et al. (2001) presented data for the Purdue Peg placing trials based on a sample of Japanese American adults, aged 70 years and older, who were enrolled in a prospective study of aging and dementia in King County, Washington. None was classed as demented based on clinical and screening neuropsychological examinations. Hand preference was determined by asking subjects which hand they preferentially used. Accordingly, 94% of the participants were classed as right-handed (S. McCurry, personal communication May 11, 2004). Participants completed two 30-s trials for each hand. The data are provided in Table 14–24 and represent an important source of information for this understudied segment of the U.S. population.

Agnew et al. (1988) provide data (see Table 14–25) based on a sample of 212 healthy, well-educated, 40- to 85-year-olds, who were screened for cognitive impairment. Subtest scores consist of the average of three trials per subtest. Differences between dominant and nondominant hands were also calculated. The manual difference was greater for women than for men. There was a trend for this difference to become greater with increasing age, but the effect did not prove statistically significant.

Children

Gardner and Broman (1979) provide data (see Tables 14–26 and 14–27) for children, ages 5 years to 15 years 11 months. One trial was given per subtest. The 1334 school children (663 boys, 671 girls) were all in regular classes in a New Jersey suburb. They were primarily in the 95 to 110 IQ range and scored mainly in the middle range on national achievement tests. No children in special classes or children with a history of grade repetition were included in the study. Similar findings were reported for Brazilian children (Brito & Santo-Morales, 2002). These authors noted that the performance differences between hands were equivalent in boys and girls.

Table 14–22 Mean Performance of Young Adults for the Purdue Pegboard (One Trial Per Subtest)

	Age Groups				
	15–20	21–25	26–30	31–40	15–40
Females					
n	30	36	16	16	98
Preferred hand	16.69	16.64	17.25	15.94	16.64
SD	2.16	2.31	1.38	1.61	2.10
Nonpreferred hand	16.10	15.89	16.13	15.63	15.95
SD	1.57	1.79	1.50	1.89	1.68
Both hands	13.76	13.75	13.31	13.13	13.58
SD	1.41	1.54	1.45	1.31	1.45
Assemblies	41.83	42.47	40.44	41.44	41.77
	5.08	5.43	5.90	5.75	5.42
Males					
n	32	37	32	26	127
Preferred hand	15.56	15.44	16.22	15.35	15.65
SD	1.52	1.71	1.81	1.72	1.71
Nonpreferred hand	15.09	15.08	15.41	15.12	15.17
SD	1.42	1.98	2.08	1.77	1.82
Both hands	12.59	12.97	12.94	12.42	12.75
SD	1.56	1.18	1.29	1.65	1.42
Assemblies	40.25	38.89	39.13	37.50	39.01
SD	4.64	6.60	3.58	3.64	4.92

Note: Data were compiled from 225 healthy adults, largely right-handed (87.7%), with above average IQ, residing in a large city in Western Canada.

Source: Adapted from Yeudall et al. (1986).

Table 14–23 Performance(One Trial) on the Purdue Pegboard in Older Adults, by Age and Sex

	Males		Females	
	Mean	SD	Mean	SD
60–69 years				
Right	12.7	1.5	14.3	1.3
Left	12.7	1.5	13.7	1.3
Both	10.2	1.3	10.9	1.5
Assembly	27.6	5.1	30.6	5.3
70–79 years				
Right	11.2	1.9	12.7	1.8
Left	10.7	2.1	11.8	1.8
Both	8.2	2.0	9.7	1.7
Assembly	23.1	5.5	25.0	5.8
80 + years				
Right	10.1	2.0	11.5	1.8
Left	9.8	1.7	10.7	2.1
Both	7.4	1.6	8.3	1.9
Assembly	18.5	5.2	21.8	5.5

Note: Each age group contained 60 males and 60 females.

Source: Adapted from DesRosiers et al., 1995.

Mathiowetz et al. (1986) provided normative data, based on a three-trial administration, for 176 subjects aged 14 to 19 years. The adolescents had no history of neuromuscular or orthopedic dysfunction that would affect finger dexterity. Unfortunately, hand preference was not reported. The scores, shown in Table 14–28, are somewhat higher than those reported by Gardner and Broman (1979), perhaps reflecting the influence of practice afforded by additional trials.

Others (Tupper cited in Baron, 2004; Wilson et al. 1982) have modified the pegboard by shortening the board from 25 to 15 holes in each row so that it can be used with preschoolers. They compiled data for the peg placement portions only. Table 14–29 presents the data reported by Wilson et al. (1982). Participants completed one trial on each subtest.

RELIABILITY

Test-Retest Reliability and Practice Effects

The number of trials allowed per subtest affects reliability. For one-trial administrations over intervals of 1 to 2 weeks, correlation coefficients, ranging from .37 to .82, have been obtained for normal individuals (Buddenberg & Davis, 2000; DesRosiers et al., 1995; Reddon et al., 1988; Tiffin, 1968). Three-trial administrations yield higher reliabilities (.76 to .89)

Table 14–24 Purdue Peg-Placing Means, Standard Deviations, and Quartiles by Age and Gender for Japanese Americans (Two Trials per Subtest)

	Mean	SD	25th Percentile	Median	75th Percentile
Males 70–79 years					
Dominant hand (*n* = 52)	12.96	2.30	11	13	14.5
Nondominant hand (*n* = 52)	11.85	2.08	10	11.5	14.0
Females 70–79 years					
Dominant (*n* = 39)	14.17	1.55	13	13.5	15
Nondominant hand (*n* = 38)	13.31	2.14	12	13	14
Males 80–89 years					
Dominant hand (*n* = 17)	11.41	1.79	11	12	12.5
Nondominant hand (*n* = 17)	11.47	2.52	9.5	12.5	13.5
Females 80–89 years					
Dominant (*n* = 26)	13.08	2.34	11.5	12.5	14.5
Nondominant hand (*n* = 25)	11.28	1.49	11.0	11.5	12.5

Note: Age and gender but not education or language spoken significantly affected test scores.

Source: From McCurry et al., personal communication, May 10, 2004.

Table 14–25 Mean Performance of Adults for the Purdue Pegboard (Three Trials per Subtest)

	Age Groups				
	40–49	50–59	60–69	70–79	80–89
Males					
n	19	20	24	17	11
Preferred hand	14.6	14.4	13.6	13.0	10.8
SD	2.08	2.15	1.74	1.90	1.33
Nonpreferred hand	14.4	13.9	13.1	12.4	10.6
SD	2.35	2.19	1.56	1.48	1.84
Both hands	12.2	11.9	10.9	10.4	8.5
SD	2.43	2.22	1.46	1.27	1.21
Purdue Assembly	34.9	33.8	28.0	27.5	21.5
SD	7.66	9.66	5.06	5.06	4.81
Pref. minus nonpref.	0.16	0.23	0.44	0.59	0.18
SD	1.19	1.21	1.86	0.93	1.46
Females					
n	21	27	29	31	13
Preferred hand	15.9	15.0	14.6	13.8	12.9
SD	1.45	1.56	2.03	1.27	1.80
Nonpreferred hand	15.2	14.4	13.9	12.9	11.3
SD	1.48	1.69	1.78	1.52	2.05
Both hands	13.1	12.1	11.6	10.5	9.2
SD	1.56	1.30	1.87	1.19	1.92
Purdue Assembly	39.8	34.6	31.7	29.1	21.9
SD	4.54	8.21	6.83	4.85	4.54
Pref. minus nonpref.	0.73	0.63	0.71	0.94	1.56
SD	1.05	1.31	1.23	1.39	1.24

Source: Agnew et al., 1988. Reprinted with permission of Lawrence Erlbaum Associates, Inc.

Table 14-26 Performance of Children on Purdue Pegboard (One Trial per Subtest)

Age	n	Preferred Hand		Nonpreferred Hand		Both Hands		Assembly	
		M	SD	M	SD	M	SD	M	SD
Boys									
5:0–5:5	30	9.33	1.81	8.40	1.33	6.73	1.17	14.10	3.29
5:6–5:11	30	9.93	1.51	8.83	1.95	6.97	1.54	15.57	3.56
6:0–6:5	30	9.77	1.57	9.13	1.83	7.30	1.53	15.93	2.94
6:6–6:11	30	11.57	1.45	10.17	2.17	8.23	1.77	19.20	3.84
7:0–7:5	30	11.67	1.67	11.00	1.70	8.77	1.41	19.23	4.95
7:6–7:11	30	12.07	1.95	11.23	1.68	9.57	1.59	20.40	4.10
8:0–8:5	30	12.70	1.60	12.17	1.51	9.83	1.51	22.20	3.80
8:6–8:11	30	13.90	2.19	12.57	1.85	10.90	1.73	24.47	5.35
9:0–9:5	30	13.33	1.60	12.43	1.59	10.50	1.48	24.57	3.75
9:6–9:11	30	13.87	1.91	12.87	2.05	11.33	1.65	27.37	4.55
10:0–10:5	30	14.03	1.88	12.87	1.72	10.93	1.84	26.37	6.15
10:6–10:11	30	14.93	1.51	13.90	1.84	11.77	1.65	28.17	5.38
11:0–11:5	30	14.93	1.86	14.00	1.98	11.30	1.68	29.53	6.19
11:6–11:11	30	14.83	1.60	13.93	1.60	12.27	1.41	31.13	5.19
12:0–12:5	30	14.83	1.78	13.67	2.02	11.67	1.52	31.13	5.78
12:6–12:11	30	15.37	2.81	14.00	2.38	11.87	1.87	30.13	6.08
13:0–13:5	40	15.15	1.92	13.90	2.00	11.85	1.58	33.73	5.00
13:6–13:11	30	14.87	1.72	14.10	1.47	11.53	1.80	34.57	5.88
14:0–14:5	30	15.67	1.47	14.40	1.57	12.03	1.67	33.97	6.58
14:6–14:11	30	14.70	1.49	14.33	1.65	12.20	1.61	31.37	7.24
15:0–15:5	30	15.57	1.50	14.87	1.50	12.57	1.48	32.20	6.21
15:6–15:11	23	15.09	1.50	14.30	1.61	12.65	1.30	33.04	6.24
Girls									
5:0–5:5	30	10.00	1.53	8.50	1.36	6.97	1.25	14.70	2.55
5:6–5:11	30	9.30	1.73	9.13	1.59	6.77	1.28	14.37	4.02
6:0–6:5	30	11.43	1.33	10.23	1.52	8.53	1.46	18.03	3.54
6:6–6:11	30	11.87	1.68	10.47	1.38	8.67	1.79	20.63	4.27
7:0–7:5	30	12.03	1.65	10.47	2.08	8.83	1.80	19.77	4.49
7:6–7:11	30	12.47	1.53	11.50	1.80	9.50	1.70	20.20	4.61
8:0–8:5	30	13.07	1.78	12.03	1.40	10.10	1.81	21.93	4.31
8:6–8:11	30	13.77	1.63	12.30	1.26	10.43	1.59	24.50	5.83
9:0–9:5	30	13.37	1.79	11.83	2.12	9.83	1.62	24.97	6.81
9:6–9:11	30	14.40	1.52	13.03	1.67	11.60	1.65	29.07	6.01
10:0–10:5	30	15.13	1.48	13.20	1.35	11.33	1.42	27.90	5.10
10:6–10:11	30	15.47	1.59	13.63	1.33	12.27	1.46	31.70	6.02
11:0–11:5	30	14.90	1.79	14.00	2.00	11.67	1.63	32.77	5.50
11:6–11:11	30	15.70	1.84	13.83	1.88	12.00	1.82	33.47	7.24
12:0–12:5	30	15.57	1.65	14.20	1.73	12.00	1.23	34.57	5.20
12:6–12:11	30	15.40	1.96	14.07	1.66	12.03	1.65	34.70	7.52
13:0–13:5	40	15.55	1.69	14.15	1.64	12.03	1.44	34.85	5.57
13:6–13:11	32	15.38	1.58	14.09	1.44	12.13	1.31	37.40	5.34
14:0–14:5	30	16.33	1.73	14.93	1.78	12.63	1.61	36.43	6.76
14:6–14:11	30	16.03	1.77	14.83	1.66	12.40	1.94	34.17	6.62
15:0–15:5	28	16.68	1.49	14.89	1.40	12.89	1.64	36.89	7.75
15:6–15:11	31	16.42	1.84	15.29	2.04	12.77	1.45	37.35	8.24

Note: Data were derived from 1,334 normal schoolchildren.

Source: Adapted from Gardner & Broman (1979).

Table 14–27 Performance of Children on Purdue Pegboard: Percentiles

Age	n	10	20	30	40	50	60	70	80	90
Percentiles for Boys: Preferred Hand										
5:0–5:5	30	7.0	8.0	8.0	9.0	9.0	10.0	10.0	11.0	11.0
5:6–5:11	30	8.0	9.0	9.0	10.0	10.0	10.0	11.0	11.8	12.0
6:0–6:5	30	7.1	9.0	9.0	9.0	9.5	10.0	11.0	11.0	11.9
6:6–6.11	30	9.1	10.2	11.0	11.0	12.0	12.0	12.0	13.0	13.0
7:0–7:5	30	9.1	10.2	11.0	11.4	12.0	12.0	12.7	13.0	13.9
7:6–7:11	30	9.0	10.0	11.0	12.0	12.0	12.6	13.0	14.0	14.0
8:0–8:5	30	11.0	12.0	12.0	12.0	13.0	13.0	14.0	14.0	14.0
8:6–8:11	30	11.1	12.0	12.3	13.0	14.0	15.0	15.0	16.0	17.0
9:0–9:5	30	11.0	12.0	12.0	13.0	13.0	14.0	15.0	15.0	15.0
9:6–9:11	30	12.0	12.0	13.0	13.0	14.0	14.6	15.0	15.0	15.9
10:0–10:5	30	11.1	12.2	13.0	14.0	14.0	15.0	15.0	15.8	16.9
10:6–10:11	30	13.0	13.2	14.0	14.0	15.0	15.0	15.0	16.0	17.0
11:0–11:5	30	13.0	13.0	13.0	14.0	14.5	16.0	16.0	16.8	17.0
11:6–11:11	30	13.0	14.0	14.0	14.0	15.0	15.0	15.0	16.8	17.0
12:0–12:5	30	13.0	13.0	14.0	14.0	14.5	15.0	15.7	16.0	17.9
12:6–12:11	30	13.0	13.2	15.0	15.0	15.0	15.0	16.0	17.0.	18.9
13:0–13:5	40	12.1	14.0	14.0	15.0	15.0	15.0	16.0	16.8	18.0
13:6–13:11	30	13.0	13.0	14.0	14.4	15.0	15.0	16.0	16.0	17.0
14:0–14:5	30	14.0	14.0	14.3	15.0	16.0	16.0	17.0	17.0	17.9
14:6–14:11	30	13.0	13.0	14.0	14.4	15.0	15.0	15.0	16.0	16.9
15:0–15:5	30	14.0	14.0	14.0	15.0	15.5	16.0	16.7	17.0	18.0
15:6–15:11	23	13.0	14.0	14.0	15.0	15.0	15.0	16.0	17.0	17.0
Percentiles for Boys: Nonpreferred Hand										
5:0–5:5	30	6.1	7.0	8.0	8.0	8.5	9.0	9.0	9.0	10.0
5:6–5:11	30	6.1	8.0	8.0	8.0	9.0	9.6	10.0	10.0	11.0
6:0–6:5	30	6.0	8.0	9.0	9.0	9.0	10.0	10.0	10.0	12.0
6:6–6.11	30	7.1	8.2	9.0	10.0	10.3	11.0	11.7	12.0	13.0
7:0–7:5	30	9.0	10.0	10.0	11.0	11.0	11.0	12.0	12.0	12.9
7:6–7:11	30	9.1	10.0	10.0	11.0	11.0	11.0	12.0	13.0	13.9
8:0–8:5	30	10.0	11.0	11.0	12.0	12.5	13.0	13.7	13.0	15.9
8:6–8:11	30	10.1	11.0	11.0	12.0	12.0	13.0	13.7	14.0	15.9
9:0–9:5	30	10.0	11.0	11.3	12.0	13.0	13.0	13.7	14.0	14.0
9:6–9:11	30	10.0	11.2	12.0	12.0	12.0	13.0	14.0	15.0	16.0
10:0–10:5	30	10.1	12.0	12.0	13.0	13.0	13.6	14.0	14.0	15.0
10:6–10:11	30	11.0	12.2	13.0	13.0	14.0	14.0	15.0	15.8	17.0
11:0–11:5	30	12.0	13.0	13.0	13.0	13.5	14.0	15.0	15.8	16.9
11:6–11:11	30	11.1	13.0	13.0	14.0	14.0	14.0	15.0	15.0	16.0
12:0–12:5	30	12.0	13.0	13.0	13.0	14.0	14.0	15.0	15.0	16.0
12:6–12:11	30	11.0	12.2	13.0	13.4	14.0	14.0	15.0	16.0	16.9
13:0–13:5	40	11.0	11.2	13.0	14.0	14.0	15.0	15.0	16.0	16.0
13:6–13:11	30	12.0	13.0	13.0	14.0	14.0	14.0	15.0	15.8	16.0
14:0–14:5	30	12.1	13.0	14.0	14.0	14.5	15.0	15.7	16.0	16.0
14:6–14:11	30	11.2	13.2	14.0	14.0	14.5	15.0	15.0	15.8	16.0
15:0–15:5	30	13.0	14.0	14.3	15.0	15.0	15.0	16.0	16.0	16.9
15:6–15:11	23	12.0	13.0	13.0	14.0	15.0	15.0	15.0	16.0	16.6
Percentiles for Boys: Both Hands										
5:0–5:5	30	5.1	6.0	6.0	6.0	7.0	7.0	7.0	8.0	8.0
5:6–5:11	30	5.0	6.0	6.0	6.4	7.0	7.0	8.0	8.0	9.0
6:0–6:5	30	5.0	6.0	6.3	7.0	7.0	7.6	8.0	9.0	9.0
6:6–6.11	30	6.0	7.0	8.0	8.0	9.0	8.6	9.0	9.0	10.9
7:0–7:5	30	7.0	8.0	8.0	8.0	8.0	9.0	10.0	10.0	10.0
7:6–7:11	30	8.0	8.0	8.0	9.0	9.5	10.0	10.7	11.0	12.0
8:0–8:5	30	8.0	8.0	9.0	9.0	10.0	10.0	11.0	11.0	12.0
8:6–8:11	30	9.0	9.2	10.0	10.0	11.0	11.0	12.0	12.8	13.0

(continued)

Table 14–27 Performance of Children on Purdue Pegboard: Percentiles (*continued*)

Age	*n*	10	20	30	40	50	60	70	80	90
9:0–9:5	30	8.1	9.0	10.0	10.0	10.0	11.0	11.0	12.0	12.0
9:6–9:11	30	9.1	10.0	10.0	11.0	11.0	11.6	12.0	13.0	13.9
10:0–10:5	30	9.0	9.0	10.0	10.4	11.0	11.0	11.0	12.8	13.9
10:6–10:11	30	10.0	10.2	11.0	11.0	12.0	12.0	12.0	13.0	14.0
11:0–11:5	30	9.0	10.0	10.3	11.0	11.0	12.0	12.7	13.0	13.0
11:6–11:11	30	11.0	11.0	12.0	12.0	12.0	13.0	13.0	13.8	14.0
12:0–12:5	30	9.1	11.0	11.0	11.0	12.0	12.0	12.0	12.8	14.0
12:6–12:11	30	9.1	10.2	11.0	12.0	12.0	12.6	13.0	13.8	14.0
13:0–13:5	40	9.1	11.0	11.0	11.4	12.0	12.0	13.0	13.0	14.0
13:6–13:11	30	9.1	10.0	11.0	11.0	11.0	12.0	12.0	13.0	14.0
14:0–14:5	30	10.1	11.0	11.0	11.0	12.0	12.0	13.0	14.0	14.0
14:6–14:11	30	10.0	11.0	11.0	12.0	12.0	12.0	13.0	14.0	15.0
15:0–15:5	30	10.1	11.0	12.0	12.0	13.0	13.0	13.0	14.0	14.9
15:6–15:11	23	11.0	11.8	12.0	12.0	13.0	13.0	13.0	14.0	14.0

Percentiles for Boys: Assembly

Age	*n*	10	20	30	40	50	60	70	80	90
5:0–5:5	30	10.0	11.2	12.0	13.0	14.0	14.6	16.0	16.0	17.0
5:6–5:11	30	10.1	12.2	14.0	15.0	16.0	16.0	17.7	18.0	20.0
6:0–6:5	30	12.1	14.0	15.0	15.0	16.0	16.0	17.0	19.0	20.0
6:6–6.11	30	14.0	16.2	18.0	18.0	19.5	20.6	22.0	22.8	24.0
7:0–7:5	30	12.1	16.0	17.3	18.4	19.0	20.6	21.7	23.0	26.7
7:6–7:11	30	16.0	17.2	18.3	19.4	21.0	22.0	22.7	24.0	25.0
8:0–8:5	30	19.0	20.2	21.0	22.4	23.5	24.0	24.0	26.8	28.9
8:6–8:11	30	18.0	20.0	20.3	23.4	24.0	25.0	27.1	30.0	32.0
9:0–9:5	30	20.0	21.2	23.0	24.0	24.0	26.0	26.0	27.0	28.0
9:6–9:11	30	21.1	24.0	24.3	25.4	26.0	29.2	30.7	31.8	32.0
10:0–10:5	30	19.1	20.2	24.0	25.0	26.0	26.0	28.7	30.0	35.7
10:6–10:11	30	22.0	24.0	25.3	28.4	29.0	30.0	30.0	31.0	33.8
11:0–11:5	30	22.0	22.2	26.0	27.4	28.0	31.0	32.0	34.6	39.9
11:6–11:11	30	25.1	27.0	28.6	30.0	31.0	32.6	33.7	35.0	39.0
12:0–12:5	30	25.0	26.0	27.0	29.0	29.0	32.6	35.4	36.0	40.9
12:6–12:11	30	23.1	25.4	28.0	29.0	30.5	32.2	34.0	35.8	37.0
13:0–13:5	40	27.0	30.0	31.0	32.0	34.0	34.8	36.0	37.0	40.9
13:6–13:11	30	27.1	30.0	30.0	33.0	34.5	35.6	36.7	39.8	43.8
14:0–14:5	30	26.1	29.2	31.0	32.0	34.0	36.0	38.7	40.0	41.0
14:6–14:11	30	23.0	25.2	26.3	29.0	30.5	32.0	34.7	35.8	45.4
15:0–15:5	30	24.0	26.0	28.0	31.4	33.5	35.6	36.0	37.8	39.9
15:6–15:11	23	24.4	26.8	29.4	32.0	33.0	34.4	35.8	39.0	42.0

Percentiles for Girls: Preferred Hand

Age	*n*	10	20	30	40	50	60	70	80	90
5:0–5:5	30	8.0	8.2	9.3	10.0	10.0	10.6	11.0	11.0	12.0
5:6–5:11	30	7.0	8.0	8.0	9.0	9.5	10.0	11.0	11.0	11.0
6:0–6:5	30	9.1	10.2	11.0	11.0	11.5	10.0	12.0	12.0	13.0
6:6–6.11	30	10.1	11.0	11.0	11.0	11.0	12.0	3.0	14.0	14.0
7:0–7:5	30	10.0	11.0	11.0	12.0	12.0	12.0	13.0	13.0	14.9
7:6–7:11	30	10.1	11.0	12.0	12.0	13.0	13.0	13.0	14.0	14.0
8:0–8:5	30	11.0	12.0	12.0	12.4	13.0	13.0	14.0	14.8	15.9
8:6–8:11	30	12.0	12.0	13.0	13.0	14.0	14.0	14.7	15.0	16.9
9:0–9:5	30	10.1	12.0	13.0	13.0	13.0	14.0	14.0	15.0	16.0
9:6–9:11	30	12.0	13.0	14.0	14.0	14.0	15.0	15.0	16.0	16.9
10:0–10:5	30	13.0	14.0	14.0	15.0	15.0	15.0	16.0	16.0	17.9
10:6–10:11	30	13.1	14.0	14.8	15.0	15.5	16.0	16.0	16.8	17.9
11:0–11:5	30	12.0	13.2	14.0	15.0	15.0	15.0	15.7	16.8	17.0
11:6–11:11	30	14.0	14.0	15.0	15.0	16.0	16.0	17.0	17.0	18.0
12:0–12:5	30	14.0	14.0	14.0	15.0	15.0	16.0	17.0	17.0	17.9
12:6–12:11	30	12.1	13.2	15.0	15.0	16.0	16.0	16.0	17.0	18.0
13:0–13:5	40	14.0	14.0	15.0	15.0	16.0	16.0	16.0	17.0	18.0

(*continued*)

Table 14-27 Performance of Children on Purdue Pegboard: Percentiles (*continued*)

Age	n	10	20	30	40	50	60	70	80	90
13:6–13:11	30	13.3	14.0	14.0	15.0	15.0	15.0	16.0	17.0	18.0
14:0–14:5	30	14.1	15.0	15.0	16.0	16.0	16.0	17.0	17.8	19.0
14:6–14:11	30	14.0	14.0	15.0	15.0	16.0	16.6	17.0	17.0	18.9
15:0–15:5	30	15.0	15.0	16.0	16.0	17.0	17.0	18.7	18.0	19.0
15:6–15:11	23	14.0	15.0	15.6	16.0	16.0	17.0	17.4	18.0	19.0

Percentiles for Girls: Nonpreferred Hand

Age	n	10	20	30	40	50	60	70	80	90
5:0–5:5	30	7.0	7.0	8.0	8.0	9.0	9.0	9.0	10.0	10.0
5:6–5:11	30	7.0	7.2	8.0	8.4	9.0	10.0	10.0	11.0	11.0
6:0–6:5	30	8.0	8.2	9.3	10.0	10.0	11.0	11.0	11.8	12.0
6:6–6:11	30	9.0	9.2	10.0	10.0	10.0	11.0	11.0	12.0	12.0
7:0–7:5	30	8.0	9.0	10.0	10.0	11.0	11.0	11.0	12.0	13.0
7:6–7:11	30	9.0	10.0	10.3	11.0	11.0	12.0	13.0	13.0	14.0
8:0–8:5	30	10.0	11.0	11.0	12.0	12.0	12.0	12.7	13.0	14.0
8:6–8:11	30	11.0	11.0	12.0	12.0	12.0	12.6	13.0	13.8	14.0
9:0–9:5	30	9.0	10.0	11.0	11.0	11.5	12.6	13.0	14.0	14.9
9:6–9:11	30	11.0	11.0	12.0	12.0	13.0	13.6	14.0	14.8	15.0
10:0–10:5	30	11.0	12.0	13.0	13.0	13.0	13.6	14.0	14.8	15.0
10:6–10:11	30	11.2	13.0	13.0	13.4	14.0	14.0	14.0	14.8	15.0
11:0–11:5	30	10.2	12.4	14.0	14.0	14.0	15.0	15.0	15.0	16.8
11:6–11:11	30	11.0	12.0	13.0	14.0	14.0	14.0	15.0	15.0	16.0
12:0–12:5	30	12.0	13.0	13.3	14.0	14.0	14.0	15.0	16.0	16.9
12:6–12:11	30	12.0	13.0	13.0	13.0	14.0	14.0	15.0	15.0	16.9
13:0–13:5	40	12.1	13.0	13.0	13.4	14.0	14.0	15.0	16.0	16.0
13:6–13:11	30	12.0	13.0	14.0	14.0	14.0	15.0	15.0	15.0	16.0
14:0–14:5	30	13.0	13.0	14.0	15.0	15.0	15.0	15.7	16.0	17.0
14:6–14:11	30	13.0	13.2	14.0	14.0	15.0	15.0	16.0	16.8	17.0
15:0–15:5	30	12.9	14.0	14.0	14.6	15.0	15.4	16.0	16.0	17.0
15:6–15:11	23	13.0	13.0	14.0	14.0	15.0	16.0	16.4	17.8	18.0

Percentiles for Girls: Both Hands

Age	n	10	20	30	40	50	60	70	80	90
5:0–5:5	30	5.0	6.0	6.0	7.0	7.0	7.6	8.0	8.0	8.0
5:6–5:11	30	5.0	6.0	6.0	6.4	7.0	7.0	7.7	8.0	8.0
6:0–6:5	30	6.1	7.2	8.0	8.0	9.0	9.0	9.0	10.0	10.0
6:6–6:11	30	6.1	8.0	8.0	8.0	8.0	8.6	9.7	10.0	12.0
7:0–7:5	30	6.0	7.2	8.0	9.0	9.0	9.0	10.0	10.8	11.0
7:6–7:11	30	7.0	8.0	9.0	9.0	9.5	10.0	10.7	11.0	11.0
8:0–8:5	30	8.0	8.2	9.0	10.0	10.0	11.0	11.0	11.0	12.0
8:6–8:11	30	8.0	9.0	10.0	10.0	10.5	11.0	11.0	12.0	12.9
9:0–9:5	30	8.0	8.0	9.0	9.4	10.0	10.0	11.0	11.0	12.0
9:6–9:11	30	9.0	10.0	11.0	12.0	12.0	12.0	13.0	13.0	13.0
10:0–10:5	30	10.0	10.0	11.0	11.0	11.0	11.6	12.0	12.0	13.0
10:6–10:11	30	11.0	11.0	11.3	12.0	12.0	12.0	13.0	13.8	14.9
11:0–11:5	30	9.1	10.0	11.0	11.4	12.0	12.0	12.7	13.0	13.0
11:6–11:11	30	9.1	10.2	11.0	11.0	13.0	13.0	13.0	14.0	14.0
12:0–12:5	30	10.0	11.0	12.0	12.0	12.0	12.0	12.0	13.0	14.0
12:6–12:11	30	10.0	10.2	11.0	12.0	12.0	12.0	13.0	13.8	14.0
13:0–13:5	40	10.0	11.0	11.0	12.0	12.0	12.0	13.0	13.0	14.0
13:6–13:11	30	10.3	11.0	11.9	12.0	12.0	12.0	13.0	13.0	13.7
14:0–14:5	30	11.0	11.0	12.0	12.0	12.0	13.0	13.0	14.8	15.0
14:6–14:11	30	9.1	11.0	11.3	12.0	12.0	13.0	13.7	14.0	15.0
15:0–15:5	30	11.0	11.0	12.0	12.0	13.0	13.0	14.0	14.0	16.0
15:6–15:11	23	11.0	11.0	12.0	13.0	13.0	13.0	13.4	14.0	14.0

(*continued*)

Table 14–27 Performance of Children on Purdue Pegboard: Percentiles (*continued*)

Age	*n*	10	20	30	40	50	60	70	80	90
Percentiles for Girls: Assembly										
5:0–5:5	30	11.1	13.0	13.0	14.0	15.0	15.6	16.0	17.0	18.0
5:6–5:11	30	9.0	11.0	12.3	13.4	14.0	15.6	16.0	17.0	20.0
6:0–6:5	30	14.0	16.0	16.0	16.0	17.0	18.0	20.0	22.0	23.9
6:6–6:11	30	16.0	17.0	18.0	19.0	20.0	21.0	22.7	25.6	27.8
7:0–7:5	30	14.0	15.2	17.0	18.0	19.5	21.6	22.0	24.0	24.9
7:6–7:11	30	14.0	16.0	17.0	18.4	19.5	21.6	23.4	25.8	26.9
8:0–8:5	30	16.0	17.0	20.0	21.0	22.0	23.0	23.0	24.8	28.9
8:6–8:11	30	18.0	19.2	20.3	21.4	23.0	24.6	27.4	31.8	32.0
9:0–9:5	30	18.0	19.0	20.3	22.0	23.5	26.0	29.0	31.8	16.0
9:6–9:11	30	22.1	23.2	26.0	27.0	28.0	31.0	32.0	34.8	37.9
10:0–10:5	30	20.3	23.2	26.0	27.0	28.0	29.0	29.7	30.8	35.8
10:6–10:11	30	24.1	27.0	28.3	29.4	30.5	31.6	35.7	37.8	39.8
11:0–11:5	30	25.1	28.0	29.3	31.4	32.5	34.0	35.7	37.0	40.9
11:6–11:11	30	22.2	25.4	28.3	31.0	34.5	37.0	39.0	40.0	41.0
12:0–12:5	30	28.0	31.0	32.0	34.0	34.0	34.6	36.7	39.0	43.6
12:6–12:11	30	24.0	28.0	30.3	32.8	35.0	36.0	38.7	41.7	45.7
13:0–13:5	40	27.0	31.2	32.3	33.4	35.0	37.6	38.0	39.0	41.9
13:6–13:11	30	29.5	33.0	34.9	36.4	38.0	38.0	40.0	42.0	44.1
14:0–14:5	30	25.3	30.2	34.0	34.0	36.0	38.0	40.7	43.0	45.9
14:6–14:11	30	27.1	28.2	30.3	32.0	33.0	35.2	37.7	40.8	44.9
15:0–15:5	30	28.7	29.8	31.7	33.6	35.5	38.4	41.3	43.2	50.2
15:6–15:11	23	23.2	29.4	33.0	36.8	39.0	40.0	41.0	43.0	47.8

Note: Data were derived from 1,334 normal schoolchildren.

Source: Adapted from Gardner & Broman (1979).

Table 14–28 Performance (Sum of Three Trials) on the Purdue Pegboard in Adolescents, by Age and Gender

	Males			Females		
	N	Mean	SD	N	Mean	SD
14–15 years	26			28		
Right		49.5	4.0		51.6	4.8
Left		46.4	5.0		47.9	5.0
Both		39.5	5.1		40.3	3.6
Assembly		119.7	18.4		114.0	17.0
16–17 years	32			33		
Right		49.6	4.5		52.6	4.4
Left		47.8	4.9		49.4	5.2
Both		40.2	4.0		42.4	4.3
Assembly		119.8	18.2		122.4	18.2
18–19 years	29			28		
Right		49.5	5.4		54.8	5.8
Left		48.0	4.6		51.1	4.1
Both		40.4	4.3		44.3	4.9
Assembly		123.2	15.4		134.5	16.4

Notes: Based on a sample of 176 males and females, aged 14–19 years, with no history of neuromuscular or orthopedic dysfunction that could affect finger dexterity.

Source: Adapted from Mathiowetz et al., 1986.

after retest intervals of 1 week (.81 to .89; Buddenberg & Davis, 2000) and 6 months (.76 for peg-placing trials; Doyen & Carlier, 2002).

It is important to note that right-left difference scores or ratios tend not to be very reliable, with correlations ranging from .22 to .61 (Reddon et al., 1988; Sappington, 1980). Reddon et al. (1998) noted that, when normal right-handed adults were tested weekly over five occasions, the right-hand was greater than the left-hand score on the average 50% of the time in men (range, 0% to 100%) and in women, the right-hand score was greater than the left-hand score on the average 62.9% of the time (range 10% to 100%). Because changes in performance occur commonly in normal adults, considerable caution should be exercised in interpreting any changes in between-hand asymmetry.

There are practice effects, with scores improving on subsequent trials (DesRosiers et al., 1995; Feinstein et al., 1994; Reddon et al., 1988; Wilson et al., 1982). For example, Feinstein et al. (1994) examined the effects of practice in healthy volunteers tested at 2- to 4-week intervals over eight test sessions. Performance improved with time and was still discernible at the eighth session. Age also appears to interact with practice. The improvement was more marked for younger subjects, aged 25 to 33 years, who performed better than older subjects, aged 41 to 57 years, and who continued to improve for a greater length of time.

Table 14–29 Mean Performance on Purdue Pegboard in Children, by Age (One Trial per Hand)

Age (Years. Months)	No. of Males	No. of Females	Right Hand			Left Hand			Both Hands		
			M	SD	Range	M	SD	Range	M	SD	Range
2.6–2.11	10	10	4.70	1.08	3–7	4.05	1.15	2–7	2.95	1.28	0–5
3.0–3.5	10	14	5.54	1.62	3–9	5.13	1.42	2–8	3.63	1.53	0–6
3.6–3.11	10	15	6.80	1.26	4–9	6.00	1.38	3–8	4.20	1.23	2–7
4.0–4.5	23	17	8.08	1.49	4–11	6.68	1.25	4–9	5.23	1.44	2–8
4.6–4.11	27	19	9.07	1.58	6–13	8.20	1.56	4–11	6.07	1.20	4–9
5.0–5.5	15	16	10.16	1.77	7–14	9.19	2.02	6–14	6.81	1.76	4–10
5.6–5.11	10	10	9.90	1.59	7–13	9.00	1.26	6–11	6.35	1.69	3–9

Source: From Wilson et al., 1982. Reprinted with the kind permission of Psychology Press.

VALIDITY

Relationships With Other Measures

Factor-analytic studies (Fleishman & Ellison, 1962; Fleishman & Hempel, 1954) have shown that the Purdue Pegboard Test loads on a finger dexterity factor defined as "the ability to make rapid, skillful, controlled manipulative movements of small objects, where the fingers are primarily involved." However, the assembly test appears to measure something in addition to finger dexterity and also loads on a manual dexterity factor defined as "the ability to make skillful, controlled arm-hand manipulations of larger objects." Strenge et al. (2002) also highlighted the importance of attention as a key factor on the assembly and nondominant hand tasks.

The literature suggests that there is more than one type of dexterity. Factor analytic findings suggest that pegboard dexterity and finger tapping measure independent dimensions of manual proficiency (Fleishman & Hempel, 1954; Stanford & Barratt, 1996). However, when between-hand asymmetry is considered, Purdue peg-placement correlates highly (.78) in normal adults with finger tapping, a task that requires independent, precise finger movements, suggesting that both tasks depend at least in part on a common neural substrate; namely, asymmetry in the corticospinal system (Triggs et al., 2000). Laterality indices derived from the Purdue Pegboard Test also correlates moderately well (.52 to .68) with those from other manual dexterity tasks (e.g., Annett's peg-moving task; Doyen & Carlier, 2002). Correlations between hand preference and relative manual proficiency on the Purdue Pegboard Test are moderately high, about .70 (Triggs et al., 2000). However, left-handers have smaller mean between-hand discrepancy scores in Purdue performance (Judge & Stirling, 2003; Verdino & Dingman, 1998) and much greater variance in performance than right-handed individuals, suggesting that preference may not identify peg-placement proficiency within a left-handed group (Verdino & Dingman, 1998). Left-handers, however, perform more proficiently than right-handers on the assembly component, a task that requires timely coordination of both hands (Judge & Stirling, 2003).

This advantage seems to depend on a more proficient use of the nonpreferred hand in left-handers than in right-handers (Judge & Stirling, 2003).

Clinical Findings

Impairment has been noted in a variety of conditions. For example, Schmidt et al. (1993) reported that normal individuals without neuropsychiatric disorder or other disease, who showed MRI white matter hyperintensities (WMH), performed worse on the Assemblies subtest than did patients without WMH. Impaired peg placement (particularly on the bilateral condition) was observed in patients with Parkinson's disease (Brown et al., 1993; Pernat et al., 1996) with improvement noted after pallidotomy (Uitti et al., 1997). Impairment also occurs in progressive supranuclear palsy (Zakzanis et al., 1998), Huntington's (Brown et al., 1993), cerebellar disease (Brown et al., 1993) and schizophrenia (Flyckt et al., 1999; Roy et al., 2003). Occupational lead exposure also reduces performance on the various Purdue tasks (Stewart et al., 1999).

Further, the peg placement portion of the Purdue Pegboard Test may provide information of lateralizing significance in adults (Costa et al., 1983; Gardner & Broman, 1979; Rapin et al., 1966; Vaughan & Costa, 1962) as well as children (Braun et al., 2000). Right-hemisphere lesions tend to impair left-hand scores, whereas left-hemisphere lesions result in a right-sided decrement.

Ecological/Predictive Validity

Adequate fine motor dexterity is critical in the performance of almost all tasks of daily living. Therefore, faster performance on the Purdue Pegboard Test is associated with better social functioning in patients with schizophrenia (Lehoux et al., 2003) and with a good vocational outcome after TBI in children and adults (Asikainen et al., 1999; Nybo & Koskiniem, 1999). Perhaps the Purdue Pegboard Test taps not only motor dexterity but also the cognitive speed needed for good social or occupational functioning.

COMMENT

The task is brief and easy to administer. Users should note that administration rules vary among studies with respect to the number of trials (one, two, or three). The most reliable scores result from averaging subtest scores for the three-trial administration of the test. However, norms for such a version are not currently available for all segments of the population.

At a minimum, hand preference, age and gender need to be considered when evaluating test scores. Although normative reports provided here do present data stratified by age and gender, hand preference, and the method of determining handedness, is frequently not reported.

As noted earlier, reliability is better when three trials are given per subtest. Accordingly, clinicians who administer the one-trial test should exercise caution when interpreting changes in scores (Buddenberg & Davis, 2000). Further, right-left differences (or ratios) on the Purdue Pegboard Test are not very reliable. Therefore, asymmetries may have diagnostic value only if differences are also found on other tests (Reddon et al., 1988). In this context it is important to bear in mind that measures of lateral preference are imperfect indicators of performance asymmetry.

The Purdue Pegboard Test has proved useful in the assessment of motor deficits in both adults and children. It is perhaps not only because the task taps motor ability but also because it is demanding of cognitive speed and attentional control that it makes a useful predictor of functioning in daily life.

REFERENCES

Agnew, J., Bolla-Wilson, K., Kawas, C. H., & Bleeker, M. L. (1988). Purdue Pegboard age and sex norms for people 40 years old and older. *Developmental Neuropsychology, 4*, 29–35.

Asikainen, L., Nybo, T., Mueller, K., Sarna, S., & Kaste, M. (1999). Speed performance and long-term functional and vocational outcome in a group of young patients with moderate or severe traumatic brain injury. *European Journal of Neurology, 6*, 179–185.

Baron, I-S. (2004). *Neuropsychological evaluation of the child.* New York: Oxford University Press.

Braun, C. M. J., Archambault, M-A., Daigneault, S., & Larocque, C. (2000). Right body side performance decrement in congenitally dyslexic children and left body side performance decrement in congenitally hyperactive children. *Neuropsychiatry, Neuropsychology, and Behavioral Neurology, 13*, 89–100.

Brito, G. N. O., & Santos-Morales, T. R. (2002). Developmental norms for the Gardner Steadiness Test and the Purdue Pegboard: A study with children of a metropolitan school in Brazil. *Brazilian Journal of Medical and Biological Research, 35*, 931–949.

Brown, R. G., Jahanshahai, M., & Marsden, D. C. (1993). The execution of bimanual movements in patients with Parkinson's, Huntington's, and cerebellar disease. *Journal of Neurology, Neurosurgery and Psychiatry, 56*, 295–297.

Buddenberg, L. A., & Davis, C. (2000). Test-retest reliability of the Purdue Pegboard Test. *American Journal of Occupational Therapy, 54*, 555–558.

Costa, L. D., Vaughan, H. G., Levita, E., & Farber, N. (1963). Purdue Pegboard as a predictor of the presence and laterality of cerebral lesions. *Journal of Consulting Psychology, 27*, 133–137.

Costa, L. D., Scarola, L. M., & Rapin, I. (1983). Purdue Pegboard scores for normal grammar school children. *Perceptual and Motor Skills, 18*, 748.

DesRosiers, J., Hebert, R., Bravo, G., & Dutil, E. (1995). The Purdue Pegboard Test: Normative data for people aged 60 and over. *Disability and Rehabilitation, 17*, 217–224.

Doyen, A-L., & Carlier, M. (2002). Measuring handedness: A validation study of Bishop's reaching card test. *Laterality, 7*, 115–130.

Feinstein, A., Brown, R., & Ron, M. (1994). Effects of practice of serial tests of attention in healthy subjects. *Journal of Clinical and Experimental Neuropsychology, 16*, 436–447.

Fleishman, E. A., & Ellison, G. D. (1962). A factor analysis of fine manipulative tests. *Journal of Applied Psychology, 46*, 96–105.

Fleishman, E. A., & Hempel, W. E. Jr. (1954). A factor analysis of dexterity tests. *Personnel Psychology, 7*, 15–32.

Flyckt, L., Sydow, O., Bjerkenstedt, L., Edman, G., Rydin, E., & Wiesel, F-A. (1999). Neurological signs and psychomotor performance in patients with schizophrenia, their relatives and healthy controls. *Psychiatry Research, 86*, 113–129.

Gardner, R. A., & Broman, M. (1979). The Purdue Pegboard: Normative data on 1334 school children. *Journal of Clinical Child Psychology, 8*, 156–162.

Judge, J., & Stirling, J. (2003). Fine motor skill performance in left- and right-handers: Evidence of an advantage for left-handers. *Laterality, 8*, 297–306.

Lehoux, C., Everett, J., Laplante, L., Emond, C., Trepanier, J., Brassard, A., Rene, L., Cayer, M., Merette, C., Maziade, M., & Roy, M.A.. (2003). Fine motor dexterity is correlated to social functioning in schizophrenia. *Schizophrenia Research, 62*, 269–273.

Mathiowetz, V., Rogers, S. L., Dowe-Keval, M., Donahoe, L., & Rennels, C. (1986). The Purdue Pegboard: Norms for 14- to 19-year-olds. *The American Journal of Occupational Therapy, 40*, 174–179.

McCurry, S. M., Gibbons, L. E., Uomoto, J. M., Thompson, M. L., Graves, A. B., Edland, S. D., Bowne, J., McCormick, W. C., & Larson, E. B. (2001). Neuropsychological test performance in a cognitively intact sample of older Japanese American adults. *Archives of Clinical Neuropsychology, 16*, 447–459.

Nybo, T., & Koskiniem, M. (1999). Cognitive indicators of vocational outcome after severe traumatic brain injury (TBI) in childhood. *Brain Injury, 13*, 759–766.

Pernat, K., Kritikos, A., Phillips, J. G., Bradshaw, J. L., Iansek, R., Kempster, P., & Bradshaw, J. A. (1996). The association between clinical and quantitative indexes of Parkinsonian symptomatology. *Neuropsychiatry, Neuropsychology and Behavioral Neurology, 9*, 234–241.

Peters, M. (1990). Subclassification of non-pathological left-handers poses problems for theories of handedness. *Neuropsychologia, 28*, 279–289.

Peters, M., Servos, P., & Day, R. (1990). Marked sex differences on a fine motor skill task disappear when finger size is used as a covariate. *Journal of Applied Psychology, 75*, 87–90.

Rapin, I., Tourk, L. M., & Costa, L. D. (1966). Evaluation of the Purdue Pegboard as a screening test for brain damage. *Developmental Medicine and Child Neurology, 8*, 45–54.

Reddon, J. R., Gill, D. M., Gauk, S. E., & Maerz, M. D. (1988). Purdue Pegboard: Test-retest estimates. *Perceptual and Motor Skills, 66*, 503–506.

Roy, M-A., Lehoux, C., Emond, C., Laplante, L., Bouchard, R. H., Everett, J., Merette, C., & Maziade, M. (2003). A pilot neuropsychological study of Kraepelinian and non-Kraepelinian schizophrenia. *Schizophrenia Research, 62,* 155–163.

Sappington, T. J. (1980). Measures of lateral dominance: Interrelationships and temporal stability. *Perceptual and Motor Skills, 50,* 783–790.

Sattler, J. M., & Engelhardt, J. (1982). Sex differences on Purdue Pegboard norms for children. *Journal of Clinical Child Psychology, 11,* 72–73.

Schmidt, R., Fazekas, F., Offenbacher, H., Dusek, T., Zac, E., Reinhart, B., Grieshofer, P., Freidl, W., Eber, B., Schumacher, M., et al. (1993). Neuropsychologic correlations of MRI white matter hyperintensities: A study of 150 normal volunteers. *Neurology, 43,* 2490–2492.

Stanford, M. S., Barratt, E. S. (1996). Verbal skills, finger tapping, and cognitive tempo define a second-order factor of temporal information processing. *Brain and Cognition, 31,* 35–45.

Stewart, W. F., Schwartz, B. S., Simon, D., Bola, K. I., Todd, A. C., & Links, J. (1999). Neurobehavioral function and tibial and chelatable lead levels in 543 former organolead workers. *Neurology, 52,* 1610–1617.

Strenge, H., Niederberger, U., & Seelhorst, U. (2002). Correlation between tests of attention and performance on Grooved and Purdue Pegboards in normal subjects. *Perceptual and Motor Skills, 95,* 507–514.

Tiffin, J. (1968). *Purdue Pegboard: Examiner manual.* Chicago: Science Research Associates.

Tiffin, J., & Asher, E. J. (1948). The Purdue Pegboard: Norms and studies of reliability and validity. *Journal of Applied Psychology, 32,* 234–247.

Triggs, W. J., Calvanio, R., Levine, M., Heaton, R. K., & Heilman, K. M. (2000). Predicting hand preference with performance on motor tasks. *Cortex, 36,* 679–689.

Uitti, R. J., Wharen, R. E., Turk, M. F., Lucas, J. A., Finton, M. J., Graff-Radford, N. R., Boylan, K. B., Goerss, S. J., Kall, B. A., Adler, C. H., Caviness, J. N., & Atkinson, E. J. (1997). Unilateral pallidotomy for Parkinson's disease: Comparison of outcome in younger versus elderly patients. *Neurology, 49,* 1072–1077.

Vaughan, H. G., & Costa, L. D. (1962). Performance of patients with lateralized cerebral lesions: II. Sensory and motor tests. *Journal of Nervous and Mental Disease, 134,* 237–243.

Verdino, M., & Dingman, S. (1998). Two measures of laterality in handedness: The Edinburgh Handedness Inventory and the Purdue Pegboard test of manual dexterity. *Perceptual and Motor Skills, 86,* 476–478.

Wilson, B. C., Iacovello, J. M., Wilson, J. J., & Risucci, D. (1982). Purdue Pegboard performance of normal preschool children. *Journal of Clinical Neuropsychology, 4,* 19–26.

Yeudall, L. T., Fromm, D., Reddon, J. R., & Stefanyk, W. O. (1986). Normative data stratified by age and sex for 12 neuropsychological tests. *Journal of Clinical Psychology, 42,* 918–946.

Zakzanis, K. K., Leach, L., & Freedman, M. (1998). Structural and functional meta-analytic evidence for fronto-subcortical system deficit in progressive supranuclear palsy. *Brain and Cognition, 38,* 283–296.

15

Assessment of Mood, Personality, and Adaptive Functions

PSYCHOLOGICAL DISORDERS

The assessment of psychological disorders of the neurologically impaired patient has a long history, dating back to descriptions of the "frontal lobe syndrome" (the most publicized example being Phineas Gage, first reported by John Harlow in 1868); the "catastrophic reactions of patients" (Goldstein, 1948); and the search for the "epileptic personality" (Blumer & Benson, 1975). As one might expect, there are many ways in which neurological disorders and emotion can interact (Heilman et al., 2003). For example, central nervous system disturbance may interfere with the brain mechanisms that underlie emotion. Alternatively, patients with neurological disorders may develop emotional reactions to their disorder (e.g., patients may become depressed because they are disabled). Or, premorbid personality features and emotional states may enhance neurological symptoms (e.g., anxiety may aggravate tremor) and cognitive concerns (e.g., depression may exacerbate memory complaints). Abnormalities in postinjury personality may also predate the injury and be falsely attributed to the insult (Greiffenstein & Baker, 2001). Finally, emotional states may induce neurological symptoms (e.g., stress may cause headaches). Our selection covers a number of frequently used instruments (see Table 15–1).

Depression is a very common condition in the general population. For example, a recent survey identified a 6-month prevalence of depression of 17% in a European population (Tyee, 2000). The prevalence of depression after neurological disorders such as stroke or traumatic brain injury (TBI) is higher, about 20% to 40% at any point in time in the first year (Fleminger et al., 2003). Similar high rates have been reported among older adults (e.g., Lebowitz et al., 1997). Because depression is such a common condition, and because it lends itself to treatment, it should always be part of the assessment. The Beck Depression Inventory-II (BDI-II) is a very popular screening tool. It is brief, easy to administer, and easy to score, and its reliability and validity have been established across a broad spectrum of ages and populations. Note, however, that the level of cognitive status at which self-report data from the BDI-II becomes invalid remains to be determined.

When assessing depression among older adults, the GDS may be preferred. It too is brief and easy to administer and to score. In addition, cognitive status prerequisites have been developed: a cutoff of 20 on the MMSE has been recommended (Bedard et al., 2003).

The GDS deliberately omits items that may be inappropriate for elderly individuals (e.g., sexuality). It also contains no somatic items that might inflate scores. However, because of cultural differences in the expression of emotion, high scores may not signify depression, and low scores may not mean the absence of depression, because some individuals may endorse somatic items, purposely excluded from the GDS, rather than affective items as idioms of distress. In such cases, other tests (e.g., the BDI) may be preferred. Users should keep in mind that self-report inventories such as the BDI-II and GDS are subject to response bias (e.g., positive or negative impression management) and random responding. Neither the BDI-II nor the GDS includes scales to detect such patterns.

The TSI is a self-report measure concerning various aspects of a client's psychological state, including posttraumatic stress and dysphoric mood. Administration and scoring are relatively brief and straightforward. Of note, the TSI also includes validity scales designed to detect random or biased responding and therefore may be especially appropriate for assessing persons alleging trauma-related symptoms in forensic contexts.

Tests such as the MMPI-2 and PAI tap a broader range of symptomatology. The MMPI-2 boasts an extensive research base and has software that can provide a wealth of information. Reliability is best for the content scales; however, code-type stability is less than optimal. Evidence for convergent validity is generally considered better than for discriminant validity. The inclusion of various scales to assess test-taking attitude and profile validity is a significant strength. The availability of scales

Table 15–1 Some Measures of Mood and Personality

Measure	Age Range (Years)	Purpose	Some Key Processes	Administration Time (min)	Test-Retest	Validity Scales	Cognitive Levels Required
BDI-II	13–86	Self-report of depression	Somatic-affective; cognitive aspects	5–10	Adequate to high	No	Reading—NA MMSE—NA
BRIEF	5–18	Parent/teacher report of executive functioning	Behavioral regulation; emotional regulation; metacognition	10–15	Adequate to high	Negative impression; inconsistency	Grade 5 reading level is minimal
GDS	17+	Self-report of depression	Affective-behavioral aspects	5–10	High over short intervals	No	MMSE ≥20
MMPI-2	18–90	Self-report of personality and psychological disorders	General maladjustment and psychotic mentation; neurotic tendencies	45–50	Adequate for clinical scales; high for content and supplementary scales; but code-type stability can be poor	Inconsistency; positive impression; negative impression-cognitive/somatic symptoms, psychiatric symptoms	Grade 6 reading level is minimal but a few scales require at least grade 8 levels. May produce invalid results with loss of >20 IQ points or when WMS memory or attention/concentration indices <70.
PAI	18–89	Self-report of personality and psychological disorders	Neurotic spectrum, psychotic spectrum, behavior disorder, treatment attitude, interpersonal style; risk for suicide, violence/misbehavior	40–50	Adequate to high depending on the scale; high-point codes not as stable as overall profile configuration	Inconsistency; positive impression; negative impression	Grade 4 reading level is minimal; IQ/memory/attention—NA
TSI	18–88	Self-report of trauma symptomatoloty	Dysphoric mood; posttraumatic stress; sexual difficulties; self-dysfunction	20	NA	Defensiveness; overreporting; inconsistency	Grade 5–7 reading level required

Note: NA = Not Available

Table 15–2 Measures of Adaptive Function

Measure	Age Range	Purpose	Processes	Administration Time	Test-Retest Reliability	Interrater Reliability	Caution
IADL	Typically older adults	Informant rating of functional status	General functional status	10 min	High	High	Subject to ceiling and floor effects; may need more refined analysis of specific domains; no scales to evaluate reporting bias
SIB-R	Infancy to 90 years	Informant rating of functional status	Motor skills; social interaction and communication skills; personal living skills; community living skills; problem behaviors	60 min for Long Form; 15–20 min for Short Form and Early Development Form	High	Higher between parents than between parents and teachers	Most studies done with children; none with adults, the elderly in particular; no scales to evaluate reporting bias

(e.g., FBS) that are relevant to the neuropsychological/forensic context is particularly valuable.

Strengths of the PAI relative to the MMPI-2 include nonoverlapping scales that enhance discriminant validity, lower reading levels, fewer items, and four response options that allow for gradations of responses. In addition, the PAI includes a number of scales that may contribute information relevant to the neuropsychological context, such as indications about aggression, suicide potential, and attitudes toward treatment. Although the PAI also includes scales to evaluate test-taking attitude and profile validity, it is not known whether these are as effective as the MMPI-2 FBS in detecting the types of exaggeration (e.g., cognitive, somatic symptoms) often encountered in the neuropsychological setting.

For children and adolescents, we include the BRIEF, a rating scale for parents and teachers designed to evaluate executive functioning. The instrument is brief, has good psychometric properties, and, despite its recent publication, has generated a considerable literature. The inclusion of validity scales is also a strength.

It is important to bear in mind that the measures considered here provide information relevant to DSM-IV diagnoses. None, however, are diagnostic measures; rather, results from these measures should be used to inform the decision-making process with information derived from other sources (e.g., structured interviews).

ADAPTIVE FUNCTIONING

Two major categories of functional abilities are commonly distinguished: (a) activities of daily living, typically known as ADLs, which focus primarily on overlearned self-care activities such as feeding, bathing, toileting, and basic mobility; and (b) instrumental activities of daily living, commonly known as IADLs, which are viewed as involving fairly complex cognitive abilities and include activities such as managing medication, finances, and household duties. It is the IADLs that are of primary interest to neuropsychologists, because it is often the patient's inability to perform these activities that motivates caregivers to seek assessment in the first place. Further, poor performance on these complex tasks of daily living may guide decision making. For example, impairment in adaptive functioning is a defining diagnostic feature of dementia of the Alzheimer type (AD) and related dementing disorders, as well as mental retardation (American Psychiatric Association, 1994).

Both the Lawton and Brody IADL and the SIB-R (see Table 15-2) are proxy-based ratings of an individual's ability to carry out activities of daily living. The IADL is brief and provides a gross rating of an individual's everyday functioning. The SIB-R is more comprehensive. It also includes a measure of problem behaviors that may interfere with school, work, and community adjustment.

It is important to bear in mind that informant-based measures such as the Lawton and Brody IADL and the SIB-R

provide only one view of the patient's adaptive functioning. They have been criticized for being contaminated with reporter bias, and, in comparison to self-report, caregivers underestimate patients' abilities. Self-report measures, however, are considered problematic because individuals may lack insight into their own abilities. Performance-based measures such as the DAFS (Loewenstein et al., 1989), the Everyday Problems Test (Willis, 1993), SAILS (Mahurin et al., 1991), and the Daily Living tests of the NAB (see *Neuropsychological Assessment Battery*) offer another view of the patient's functioning, although they also have their limitations. They lack the environmental supports or distractions that affect the individual in everyday life. Self-ratings and informant ratings have the advantage in that they evaluate the individual's ability in his or her regular milieu and are also influenced by a longer time frame than is afforded in a single test session. Given the moderate associations among the different methods of assessment, the clinician should incorporate various approaches to gain a broader understanding of everyday competence.

REFERENCES

American Psychiatric Association. (1994). *Diagnostic and statistical manual of mental disorders—IV.* Washington, DC: American Psychiatric Association.

Bedard, M., Molloy, D. W., Squire, L., Minthorn-Biggs, M-B., Dubois, S., Lever, J. A., & O'Donnell, M. (2003). Validity of self-reports in dementia research: The Geriatric Depression Scale. *Clinical Gerontologist, 26,* 155–163.

Blumer, D., & Benson, D. F. (1975). Personality changes with frontal and temporal lobe lesions. In D. F. Benson & D. Blumer (Eds.). *Psychiatric aspects of neurological disease.* New York: Grune & Stratton.

Fleminger, S., Oliver, D. L., Williams, W. H., & Evans, J. (2003). The neuropsychiatry of depression after brain injury. *Neuropsychological Rehabilitation, 13,* 65–87.

Goldstein, K. (1948). *Language and language disturbances.* New York: Grune and Stratton.

Greiffenstein, M. F., & Baker, W. J. (2001). Comparison of premorbid and postinjury MMPI-2 profiles in late postconcussion claimants. *The Clinical Neuropsychologist, 15,* 162–170.

Heilman, K. M., Blonder, L. X., Bowers, D., & Valenstein, E. (2003). Emotional disorders associated with neurological diseases. In K. M. Heilman & E. Valenstein (Eds.). *Clinical neuropsychology* (4th ed.). New York: Oxford University Press.

Lawton, M. P., & Brody, E. M. (1969). Assessment of older people: Self-maintaining and instrumental activities of daily living. *Gerontologist, 9,* 179–185.

Lebowitz, B. D., Pearson, J. L., Schneider, L. S., Reynolds, C. F. 3rd, Alexopoulos, G. S., Bruce, M. L., Conwell, Y., Katz, I. R., Meyers, B. S., Morrison, M. F., Mossey, J., Niederehe, G., & Parmelee, P. (1997). Diagnosis and treatment of depression in late life: Consensus statement update. *Journal of the American Medical Association, 278,* 1186–1190.

Loewenstein, D. A., Amigo, A., Duara, R., Gutterman, A., et al. (1989). A new scale for the assessment of functional status in

Alzheimer's disease and related disorders. *Journal of Gerontology, 44,* 114–121.

Mahurin, R. K., DeBettignies, B. H., & Pirozzolo, F. J. (1991). The structured assessment of independent living skills: Preliminary report on a performance measure of functional abilities in dementia. *Journal of Gerontology, 46,* 58–66.

Tyee, A. (2000). Depression in Europe: Experience from the DEPRESS II survey. *European Neuropsychopharmacology, 10,* S445–S448.

Willis, S. L. (1993). *Test manual for the Everyday Problems Test for cognitively challenged elderly.* University Park, PA: The Pennsylvania State University.

Beck Depression Inventory—Second Edition (BDI-II)

PURPOSE

The purpose of the Beck Depression Inventory—Second Edition (BDI-II) is to measure the severity of self-reported depression in adolescents and adults.

SOURCE

The test (manual and 25 forms) can be ordered from Harcourt Assessment, 19500 Bulverde Rd, San Antonio, TX 78259 (http://www.harcourtassessment.com), at a cost of $77 US.

Other Versions

The test has also been translated into numerous languages including Arabic (Al-Musawi, 2001), Japanese (Kojima et al., 2002), Spanish (Novy et al., 2001; Penley et al., 2003) and Portuguese (Coelho et al., 2002). A computerized version is also available from the test publisher.

AGE RANGE

The test can be given to individuals aged 13 to 86 years.

DESCRIPTION

The BDI-II (Beck et al., 1996b) is a 21-item self-report instrument for measuring the presence and severity of depression in adults and adolescents. For this most recent version, some items were added (agitation, worthlessness, concentration difficulty, loss of energy) and others were dropped (weight loss, body image change, somatic preoccupation, work difficulty) or revised from the original (BDI, Beck et al., 1961) and the amended (BDI-IA, Beck et al., 1979; Beck & Steer, 1987) versions, so that the test corresponds more closely to the criteria for diagnosing major depressive disorders listed in the DSM-IV. Another important change is that the authors extended the required duration of symptoms in the BDI-II from 1 to 2 weeks, which corresponds to the DSM-IV criteria for assessing major depressive disorders.

Each of the 21 BDI-II items requires the respondent to endorse one of four options, scored 0 to 3, with increasing scores reflecting greater severity of a given depressive symptom. The statements refer to the following areas:

1. Sadness
2. Pessimism
3. Past failure
4. Loss of pleasure
5. Guilty feelings
6. Punishment feelings
7. Self-dislike
8. Self-criticalness
9. Suicidal thoughts or wishes
10. Crying
11. Agitation
12. Loss of interest
13. Indecisiveness
14. Worthlessness
15. Loss of energy
16. Changes in sleeping pattern
17. Irritability
18. Changes in appetite
19. Concentration difficulty
20. Tiredness or fatigue
21. Loss of interest in sex

A sample similar to that in the BDI-II follows:[1]

0 I do not feel unhappy.
1 I feel unhappy.
2 I am unhappy.
3 I am so unhappy that I can't stand it.

ADMINISTRATION

The test can be self-administered, or the examiner can present the items orally. The computerized version of the test provides equivalent results with respect to the standard form (Schulenberg & Yutrzenka, 2001).

Instructions are provided in the test manual. Briefly, the examiner informs the patient that the questionnaire consists of 21 groups of statements. After reading each group of statements carefully, the patient (examiner) indicates by circling the number (0, 1, 2, or 3) next to the one statement in each group that best describes the way the patient has been feeling in the *past two weeks,* including *today.*

ADMINISTRATION TIME

The time required is 5 to 10 min.

SCORING

Scores for each option range from 0 to 3, with higher scores indicating more severe symptoms. The total score is obtained by adding the highest score circled for each of the 21 items. The maximum score is 63. Interpretation is based on cut scores provided in the manual (see later discussion). However, alternate cut-scores exist for specific clinical populations (see *Validity*).

The BDI-II can be fractionated into two related but distinct dimensions of depression (see *Factor Analytic Findings*). The Cognitive subscale can be calculated (Kumar et al., 2002) by summing the ratings for the following eight symptoms: pessimism, past failure, guilty feelings, punishment feelings, self-dislike, self-criticalness, suicidal thoughts, and worthlessness (items 2, 3, 5–9, and 14). The Noncognitive subscale can be formed (Kumar et al., 2002) by summing the ratings for the 13 symptoms not included in the cognitive scale (items 1, 4, 10–13, and 15–21). A third scale, the BDI-FastScreen (BDI-FS; Beck et al., 2000), can also be calculated, by summing the ratings for the following seven symptoms: sadness, pessimism, past failure, loss of pleasure, self-dislike, self-criticalness, and suicidal thoughts.

Computer analysis and interpretation in combination with other Beck scales (Hopelessness, Anxiety, and Suicide Ideation Scales) is also available from the publisher. The warnings about computer interpretation apply (see *Chapter 4*).

DEMOGRAPHIC EFFECTS

Age

Some have reported little relationship between age and BDI-II scores in samples of outpatients or college students (Beck et al., 1996b; Kojima et al., 2002; Penley et al., 2003; Steer et al., 1997), geriatric inpatients (Steer et al., 2000), or adolescents (Krefetz et al., 2003; Kumar et al., 2002). However, others have found that depression is more likely with increasing age in adults (Glenn et al., 2001) and adolescents (Steer et al., 1998). Steer, Ball et al. (1999) reported that, in depressed outpatients, the severity of self-reported depression gradually increased from 18 to 38 years of age and then decreased to age 82 years. The quadratic age effect appeared to be largely due to one item: self-dislike.

Gender

Although some have reported no significant gender differences on the BDI-II (Beck et al., 1996a; Dozois et al., 1998; O'Hara et al., 1998; Penley et al., 2003; Schulenberg & Yutrzenka, 2001; Steer & Clark, 1997; Steer et al., 2000), a number of studies have found that females score higher than males (Arnau et al., 2001; Beck et al., 1996b; Coelho et al., 2002; Kojima et al., 2002; Kumar et al., 2002; Leigh & Anthony-Tolbert, 2001; Osman et al., 2004; Steer et al., 1997b, 1998b, 1999). Some (Krefetz et al., 2002) have found that the

effect size associated with gender is small ($r = .22$), with differences limited to one symptom—loss of energy (Steer et al., 1999) or difficulty with concentration (Steer et al., 1998). However, others have reported moderate (.34; Leigh & Anthony-Tolbert, 2001) to large (.63; Kumar et al., 2002) effect sizes.

Education

Scores are inversely related to education ($r = -.24$; Arnau et al., 2001).

Ethnicity, Socioeconomic Status (SES), and Acculturation

Researchers have not found significant differences in BDI-II scores between ethnic groups (e.g., Caucasian versus African Americans, Caucasian versus non-Caucasian; Beck et al., 1996a, 1996b; Buckley et al., 2001; Kumar et al., 2002; Steer et al., 1997, 1998b, 1999, 2000). SES correlates modestly with BDI-II scores ($r = -.20$ to $-.28$; Arnau et al., 2001; Penley et al., 2003). There is no unique effect for acculturation on scores after the effect of SES is taken into account (Penley et al., 2003).

NORMATIVE DATA

Standardization Sample

Cut-scores were developed by classifying 127 outpatients (see Table 15–3) from the University of Pennsylvania into four groups: single-episode or recurrent major depression (1) mildly depressed, (2) moderately depressed, or (3) severely depressed, and (4) nondepressed, according to clinical diagnoses based on the administration of the Structured Clinical Interview for DSM-III (SCID). Optimal cut-scores were derived through the use of receiver operating characteristic

Table 15–3 Characteristics of the BDI-II Sample Used to Determine Interpretive Guide

Number	127
Age	Not reported
Geographic location	Philadelphia (USA)
Sample type	Outpatients from the University of Pennsylvania Medical School's Department of Psychiatry
Education	Not reported
Gender	Not reported
Race/Ethnicity	Largely Caucasian
Screening	Diagnosed according to the outpatient version of the SCID for DSM-III-R

Table 15–4 Interpretation Guidelines for the BDI-II

Total Score	Range
0–13	Minimal
14–19	Mild
20–28	Moderate
29–63	Severe

Source: From Beck et al., 1996b.

(ROC) curves. The cut-score guidelines for total scores are provided in Table 15–4. It is important to note that the description of the clinical sample is sparse, with no information provided regarding demographic variables such as age, gender, and education.

RELIABILITY

Internal Consistency

Among university samples (including deaf persons), internal reliability coefficients for the BDI-II (including its various translations) have ranged from .84 to .93 (Al-Musawi, 2001; Beck et al., 1996b; Dozois et al., 1998; Leigh & Anthony-Tolbert, 2001; Schulenberg & Yutrzenka, 2001; Steer & Clark, 1997; Storch et al., 2004; Whisman et al., 2000). Among medical or psychiatric samples of adults and adolescents, internal reliability has also been found to be high (≥.88; Arnau et al., 2001; Beck et al., 1996a, 1996b; Buckley et al., 2001; Coelho et al., 2002; Grothe et al., 2005; Kojima et al., 2002; Krefetz et al., 2003; Kumar et al., 2002; Novy et al., 2001; Osman et al., 2004; Penley et al., 2003; Sprinkle et al., 2002; Steer et al., 1997, 1998b, 1999, 2000).

Cognitive, Noncognitive and combined cognitive/affective (BDI-FS) subscales of the BDI-II have been developed (see *Validity*). Cronbach's alpha is reported to range from .81 to .91 for these scales (Grothe et al., 2005; Kumar et al., 2002; Steer et al., 1999; Storch et al., 2004), suggesting excellent internal consistency.

Item-total correlations range from .35 to .68 (Beck et al., 1996b; Dozois et al., 1998; Grothe et al., 2005).

Test-Retest Reliability and Stability

Over short intervals (1 day to about 2 weeks), test-retest correlations are adequate (.74 to .75; Al-Musawi, 2001; Leigh & Anthony-Tolbert, 2001) to high (.93 to .96; Beck et al., 1996b; Sprinkle, 2002). Most authors have reported no significant change in scores in outpatients (Beck et al., 1996b) or in university students (Al-Musawi, 2001). Some have noted a significant change (about 1 point) that does not translate into a clinically meaningful difference (Schulenberg & Yutrzenka, 2001; Sprinkle et al., 2002) over similar intervals.

VALIDITY

Factor Analytic Findings

Research has established the BDI-II as a multifactorial test that taps into a higher-order general distress factor. Although the factor structure and item composition have varied somewhat across clinical samples (Arnau et al., 2001; Buckley et al., 2001; Norris et al., 2003; Osman et al., 2004) and university student samples (Al-Musawi, 2001), support has generally been found in both adolescents and adults of varying ages, males and females, Caucasians and African Americans, for two first-order correlated factors (Arnau et al., 2001; Beck et al., 1996b; Bedi et al., 2001; Dozois et al., 1998; Grothe et al., 2005; Kojima et al., 2002; Steer & Clark, 1997; Steer et al., 1998, 1999, 2000; Storch et al., 2004; Viljoen et al., 2003; Whisman et al., 2000) and, in some studies, a single second-order factor (Arnau et al., 2001; Grothe et al., 2005; Penley et al., 2003; Steer et al., 1998, 1999). The first factor, with loadings on items such as fatigue, loss of energy, changes in sleep and appetite, and crying, is considered to represent a Somatic-Affective dimension (items 1, 4, 10–13, and 15–21) that is related to loss and impairment. The second factor's salient symptoms include feelings of pessimism, guilt, punishment, self-dislike, self-criticism, suicidal thoughts, and worthlessness and is considered to reflect a Cognitive dimension (items 2, 3, 5–9, and 14) related to a negative theory of self and social environment.

Relationship With Earlier Versions

The BDI-II correlates well (.66 to .93) with the earlier version of the test (BDI-IA), although the revised version tends to yield slightly higher scores (about 2–3 points), with approximately one more symptom endorsed on average (Beck et al., 1996a, 1996b; Dozois et al., 1998; Wong et al., 2000). A table is provided in the test manual that allows conversion of test scores from one version to the other. Whether the BDI-II is a better discriminator of mood disorders than its predecessor is not known (Beck et al., 1996a).

Relationships With Other Tests

The BDI-II correlates highly with other depression-related instruments (e.g., SCID-I $r = .83$, Sprinkle et al., 2002; CES-D $r = .69$, Kojima et al., 2002; Reynolds Adolescent Depression Scale $r = .84$, Krefetz et al., 2002; MMPI-A, Beck Hopelessness Scale, Osman et al., 2004), providing strong evidence of convergent validity.

With regard to divergent validity, scores on the BDI-II show somewhat higher correlations with self-report measures of depression (e.g., Hamilton Psychiatric Rating Scale for Depression $r = .71$; Depression subscale of SCL-90 $r = .89$) compared with anxiety (e.g., Beck Anxiety Inventory $r =$ about .50 to .60, Beck et al., 1996b, Novy et al., 2001, Steer et al., 1999; State-Trait Anxiety Inventory $r = .41$ to .77, Al-Musawi, 2001,

Storch et al., 2004; anxiety subscale of SCL-90 $r = .71$, Steer et al., 1997). Factor analytic findings from an outpatient psychiatric sample suggest that the BDI-II and Beck Anxiety Inventory (BAI) assess both common and distinct symptom dimensions (Steer et al., 1999).

The BDI-II also correlates negatively ($r = -.10$ to $-.46$) with measures of happiness, ego strength, boldness (Al-Musawi, 2001), and independence (Steer & Clark, 1997), providing additional evidence of divergent validity. Al-Musawi (2001) noted an absence of significant correlations between the total and factor scores of the BDI-II and a measure of neuroticism. The implication is that the test does assess depression and is not just a measure of general psychopathology.

Clinical Findings

The test has utility in discriminating between individuals with and without an active depressed mood diagnosis. For example, Beck et al. (1996b) gave both the BDI-II and the SCID to a sample of 127 outpatients, 57 with major depression and 70 without; they noted that, for their sample, a score of 17 was optimal, yielding a 93% sensitivity rate and an 18% false-positive rate for identifying major depression. Similarly, Sprinkle et al. (2002) gave both the BDI-II and the major depressive episode portion of the SCID to a sample of 137 students (87 classed as depressed, 50 not depressed based on the SCID) who were receiving treatment at a university counseling center. In this sample, a BDI-II cut score of 16 yielded a sensitivity rate of 84% and a false-positive rate of 18% in identifying depressed mood. Among medical patients (about 70% Caucasian) presenting to a clinic, Arnau et al. (2001) reported that a cutoff score of 18 yielded the best balance between sensitivity (94%) and specificity (92%), with a positive predictive power of 54% and a negative predictive power of 99%. The low positive predictive power (ratio of the number of individuals screening positive who actually have the disorder to the total number of individuals who screen positive) reflects the very low base rate of depression in this sample (less than 10% with major depressive disorder). Therefore, in this setting, such a cutoff, although useful for screening purposes, lacks utility for diagnostic decision making. Another study of African Americans attending a clinic revealed a higher prevalence rate of depression (about 30%; Dutton et al., 2004). In this sample, a cutoff score of 14 proved optimal and yielded a sensitivity of 87.7%, a specificity of 83.9%, a positive predictive value of .70, and a negative predictive value of .94.

In adolescent samples, higher BDI-II values are needed to optimally identify depression, although clinical efficacy may be lower. Kumar et al. (2002) reported that, among adolescent inpatients (54 with major depressive disorder, 46 without), a cutoff score of 21 yielded maximal clinical efficiency, with a sensitivity of 85%, a specificity of 83%, a positive predictive power of .85, and a negative predictive power of .83. Krefetz et al. (2002) also evaluated adolescent inpatients with ($n = 57$) and without ($n = 43$) major depression and reported that a cut-score of 24 had the highest clinical efficiency, with a sensitivity

rate of 74%, a specificity rate of 70%, a positive predictive power of .76, and a negative predictive power of .67.

These studies illustrate that the clinical guidelines (cutoffs) provided in the test manual may not be the most clinically efficient ones for use in all samples to screen for the presence and characterize the severity of depression. In addition to levels of depression and sample characteristics (e.g., inpatient versus outpatient, adult versus youth) and the underlying prevalence of disorders, Beck et al. (1996b) cautioned users that the decision to use various cut-scores for the BDI-II needs to be based on the purpose of using the test, in light of the relative importance of sensitivity versus specificity to their specific question. If the purpose is to detect the maximum number of persons with depression, then the cut-score threshold must be lowered to minimize false negatives. If it is important to obtain as pure a group of persons with depression as possible, the cut-score must be raised to reduce the number of false positives.

As might be expected, in patients diagnosed with a major depressive disorder, BDI-II scores increase with increasing severity of disorder (Steer et al., 2001). Further, patients with mood disorders (e.g., major depression, dysthymia, bipolar disorders) tend to obtain higher BDI-II scores than patients with other conditions, including anxiety and adjustment disorders (Beck et al., 1996b). Similarly, patients with a major depressive disorder obtain higher scores than those with other conditions such as dysthymia, bipolar disorder, and impulse control disorders (Ball & Steer, 2003; Krefetz et al., 2002).

There is also evidence that the BDI-II is as effective as other self-report instruments (e.g., the Reynolds Adolescent Depression Scale, RADS) in differentiating patients with and without major depressive disorder. In adolescent inpatients, ROC analysis revealed that the areas under the curves were .78 for the BDI-II and .76 for the RADS (Krefetz et al., 2002).

The BDI-II can be fractionated into two related but distinct dimensions of depression (see *Scoring* and *Factor Analytic Findings*): the Cognitive subscale and the Noncognitive subscale. A third scale, the BDI-FS (Beck et al., 2000), can also be calculated (see *Scoring*). The total score and each of the subscales appears to be equally effective in differentiating adolescents with and without major depressive disorder (Kumar et al., 2002).

Somatic symptoms such as reduced energy, loss of interest, and sleep disturbance can be signs of physical illness, raising the concern that the BDI-II overidentifies depression in some samples (e.g., Buckley et al., 2001). There is evidence that, in medical patients, these symptoms tend to contribute to a general factor of depression (Arnau et al., 2001; Norris et al., 2003). In addition, in patients with medical disorders, disease severity is positively correlated with both cognitive and somatic-affective symptoms on the BDI-II (Penley et al., 2003). Further, Arnau et al. (2001) found that, in medical patients, cognitive and somatic-affective dimensions showed only small correlations with other measures of physical functioning and pain ($r = -.18$ to $-.24$). The implication is that the BDI-II physical symptoms, while sometimes reflecting physical illness, may also be accurate indices of depression in these patients.

Individuals with psychiatric disorders may also have comorbid attention-deficit/hyperactivity disorder (ADHD). Based on a study of adult psychiatric outpatients who were given the BDI-II and a symptom-report of attention deficit (CAARS-S:SV), Steer et al. (2003) concluded that ratings higher than 1 on the concentration item (no. 19) might be useful in determining whether follow-up evaluation of ADHD symptoms is warranted.

Depression is common in neurological samples. For example, Glenn et al. (2001) found that about 59% of outpatients with traumatic brain injury scored in the depressed range (BDI-II > 13). Scores tend to be higher in those with mild as opposed to moderate-severe injury (Findler et al., 2001; Glenn et al., 2001). A strong link has also been reported between postconcussion symptoms and BDI-II scores, even in the absence of neurological insult, suggesting that depression has a significant role in producing and/or maintaining such symptoms (Trahan et al., 2001).

COMMENT

The earlier version of the BDI proved to be one of the most frequently used tests by clinical psychologists or neuropsychologists, ranking about 10th in a list of 20 most commonly used tests (Camara et al., 2000). The BDI-II represents a substantial revision, with only 3 of the original 21 items unchanged. It appears to be a stronger instrument than the BDI-IA in terms of its factor structure, with two factors more clearly delineated (Dozois et al., 1998), and therefore it may assess conditions in different ways than its predecessor (Whisman et al., 2000). Given its brevity, ease of administration and scoring, congruence with the DSM-IV, and strong psychometric characteristics, the BDI-II will likely also prove very popular and of substantial clinical utility.

Paper-and-pencil and computer administrations appear to yield equivalent results. The BDI-II can be self-administered or given by an examiner. However, users should note that the equivalence of these two types of administration has not been empirically verified, and they may lead to different results.

Guidelines for interpretation of scores are provided by the test authors; however, the BDI-II standardization group is poorly described, and others have recommended different cutoff values (see *Validity*). The choice of the particular cutoff point depends in part on the purpose for using the test. If the purpose is to detect the maximum number of persons with depression, then the cut-score threshold must be lowered to minimize false negatives. If it is important to obtain as pure a group of persons with depression as possible, the cut-score must be raised to reduce the number of false positives.

The BDI-II is typically scored by summing its 21 cognitive, affective, and somatic symptoms; however, interpretation of the total score may obscure important individual differences (Bedi et al., 2001). For example, two individuals with the same total score may differ in terms of the relative severity and frequency of somatic-affective versus cognitive symptomatology. Therefore, calculation of separate scores for the somatic and cognitive dimensions may increase clinical utility with regard to diagnostic and therapeutic decisions and when tracking change (Bedi et al., 2001).

The BDI-II has been translated into many languages. There is evidence of psychometric comparability across the various versions, suggesting that the test is applicable to both western and non-western societies (e.g., Al-Musawi, 2001; Kojima et al., 2002; Novy et al., 2001). There is also some support for its use among ethnic minorities in the United States (e.g., Grothe et al., 2005; Penley et al., 2003). Further, its reliability and validity have been established across a broad spectrum of ages and clinical and nonclinical populations.

Internal reliability is high. The BDI-II has moderate to high test-retest reliability over short intervals, suggesting that it can be used effectively to measure change. However, its sensitivity to temporal fluctuations in the depressive experience and to treatment efficacy would benefit from study (Dozois et al., 1998).

The BDI-II shows strong evidence of convergent and divergent validity with other instruments (self-report and structured interview) and appears to be fairly sensitive to the presence and severity of depression, particularly in adult samples. Bear in mind that, although the BDI-II is a useful screening measure for depressive symptoms, it was not developed to specify a diagnosis. It does not contain an equal number of items for each of the DSM-IV depressive symptoms, and, although it contains items that correspond to those of the DSM-IV, it does not specify any criteria for use as a diagnostic tool (Osman et al., 2004).

Further, practitioners should keep in mind that self-report inventories are subject to response bias (Beck et al., 1996b; Hunt et al., 2003). Some individuals may magnify symptoms, and others may minimize them. Therefore, determination of the presence and severity of depression will require additional exploration. Attention to individual items is also important. In particular, patients admitting to suicide ideation and hopelessness (item 2) should be scrutinized closely for suicide potential (Beck et al., 1996b).

The BDI-II appears to tap the same noncognitive and cognitive dimensions in adolescents, young adults, and the elderly, providing support for its use in the evaluation of individuals across the age span. However, the level of mental status at which self-reported data from the BDI-II becomes invalid remains to be determined. A cutoff score of 20 on the MMSE has been recommended for another self-report measure, the Geriatric Depression Scale (GDS, Brink et al., 1982; Bedard et al., 2003). When assessing depression in older women, the GDS may be preferred, because its specific questions may be more relevant to that specific population (Jefferson et al., 2001).

Finally, users should note that depressed individuals often perceive themselves as being more disabled emotionally, cognitively, and physically than their nondepressed counterparts. Differential diagnosis and treatment of individuals with known health problems (e.g., head trauma) should take into consideration the potential role that depression can have in producing and maintaining such symptoms (Trahan et al., 2001).

NOTE

1. Simulated item similar to that in the Beck Depression Inventory-II. Copyright 1996 by Aaron T. Beck with permission of publisher, Harcourt Assessment, Inc. Reprinted with permission. All rights reserved.

REFERENCES

Al-Musawi, N. (2001). Psychometric properties of the Beck Depression Inventory-II with university students in Bahrain. *Journal of Personality Assessment, 77,* 568–579.

Arnau, R. C., Meagher, M. W., Norris, M. P., & Bramson, R. (2001). Psychometric evaluation of the Beck Depression Inventory-II with primary care medical patients. *Health Psychology, 20,* 112–119.

Beck, A. T., & Steer, R. A. (1987). *Beck Depression Inventory manual.* San Antonio, TX: Psychological Corporation.

Ball, R., & Steer, R. A. (2003). Mean Beck Depression Inventory-II scores of outpatients with dysthymic or recurrent-episode major depressive disorders. *Psychological Reports, 93,* 507–512.

Beck, A. T., Rush, A. J., Shaw, B. R., & Emery, G. (1979). *Cognitive therapy of depression.* New York: Guilford Press.

Beck, A. T., Steer, R. A., Ball, R., & Ranieri, W. F. (1996a). Comparison of Beck Depression Inventories-IA and -II in psychiatric outpatients. *Journal of Personality Assessment, 67,* 588–597.

Beck, A. T., Steer, R. A., & Brown, G. K. (1996b). *Beck Depression Inventory* (2nd ed.). San Antonio, TX: The Psychological Corporation.

Beck, A. T., Steer, R. A., & Brown, G. K. (2000). *Manual for the Beck Depression Inventory—FastScreen for Medical Patients.* San Antonio, Tex.: Psychological Corporation.

Beck, A. T., Ward, C. H., Mendelson, M., Mock, J., & Erbaugh, J. (1961). An inventory for measuring depression. *Archives of General Psychiatry, 4,* 561–571.

Bedard, M., Molloy, D. W., Squire, L., Minthorn-Biggs, M-B., Dubois, S., Lever, J. A., & O'Donnell, M. (2003). Validity of self-reports in dementia research: The Geriatric Depression Scale. *Clinical Gerontologist, 26,* 155–163.

Bedi, R. P., Koopman, R. F., & Thompson, J. (2001). The dimensionality of the Beck Depression Inventory-II and its relevance for tailoring the psychological treatment of women with depression. *Psychotherapy, 38,* 306–318.

Brink, T. L., Yesavage, J. A., Owen, L., Heersema, P. H., Adey, M., & Rose, T. L. (1982). Screening tests for geriatric depression. *Clinical Gerontologist, 1,* 37–43.

Buckley, T. C., Parker, J. D., & Heggie, J. (2001). A psychometric evaluation of the BDI-II in treatment-seeking substance abusers. *Journal of Substance Abuse Treatment, 20,* 197–204.

Camara, W. J., Nathan, J. S., & Puente, A. E. (2000). Psychological test usage: Implications in professional psychology. *Professional Psychology: Research and Practice, 31,* 141–154.

Coelho, R., Martins, A., & Barros, H. (2002). Clinical profiles relating gender and depressive symptoms among adolescents ascertained by the Beck Depression Inventory II. *European Psychiatry, 17,* 222–226.

Dozois, D. J. A., Dobson, K. S., & Ahnberg, J. L. (1998). A psychometric evaluation of the Beck Depression Inventory-II. *Psychological Assessment, 10,* 83–89.

Dutton, G. R., Grothe, K. B., Jones, G. N., Whitehead, D., Kendra, K., & Brantley, P.J.. (2004). Use of the Beck Depression Inventory-II with African American primary care patients. *General Hospital Psychiatry, 26,* 437–442.

Findler, M., Cantor, J., Haddad, L., Gordon, W., & Ashman, T. (2001). The reliability and validity of the SF-36 health survey questionnaire for use with individuals with traumatic brain injury. *Brain Injury, 15,* 715–723.

Glenn, M. B., O'Neil-Pirozzi, T., Goldstein, R., Burke, D., & Jacob, L. (2001). Depression amongst outpatients with traumatic brain injury. *Brain Injury, 15,* 811–818.

Grothe, K. B., Dutton, G. R., Jones, G. N., Bodenlos, J., Ancona, M., & Brantley, P. J. (2005). Validation of the Beck Depression Inventory-II in a low-income African American sample of medical outpatients. *Psychological Assessment, 17,* 110–114.

Hunt, M., Auriemma, J., & Cashara, A. C. (2003). Self-report bias and underreporting of depression on the BDI-II. *Journal of Personality Assessment, 80,* 26–30.

Jefferson, A. L., Powers, D. V., & Pope, M. (2001). Beck Depression Inventory-II (BDI-II) and the Geriatric Depression Scale (GDS) in older women. *Clinical Gerontologist, 22,* 3–12.

Kojima, M., Furukawa, T. A., Takahashi, H., Kawai, M., Nagaya, T., & Tokudome, S. (2002). Cross-cultural validation of the Beck Depression Inventory-II in Japan. *Psychiatry Research, 110,* 291–299.

Krefetz, D. G., Steer, R. A., Gulab, N. A., & Beck, A. T. (2002). Convergent validity of the Beck Depression Inventory-II with the Reynolds Adolescent Depression Scale in psychiatric inpatients. *Journal of Personality Assessment, 78,* 451–460.

Krefetz, D. G., Steer, R. A., & Kumar, G. (2003). Lack of age differences in the Beck Depression Inventory-II scores of clinically depressed adolescent outpatients. *Psychological Reports, 92,* 489–497.

Kumar, G., Steer, R. A., Teitelman, K. B., & Villacis, L. (2002). Effectiveness of Beck Depression Inventory-II subscales in screening for Major Depressive Disorders in adolescent psychiatric inpatients. *Assessment, 9,* 164–170.

Leigh, I. W., & Anthony-Tolbert, S. (2001). Reliability of the BDI-II with deaf persons. *Rehabilitation Psychology, 46,* 195–202.

Norris, M. P., Arnau, R. C., Bramson, R., & Meagher, M. W. (2003). The efficacy of somatic symptoms in assessing depression in older primary care patients. *Clinical Gerontologist, 27,* 43–57.

Novy, D. M., Stanley, M. A., Daza, P., & Averill, P. (2001). Psychometric comparability of English- and Spanish-language measures of anxiety and related affective symptoms. *Psychological Assessment, 13,* 347–355.

O'Hara, M., Sprinkle, S. D., & Ricci, N. A. (1998). Beck Depression Inventory-II: College population study. *Psychological Reports, 82,* 1395–1401.

Osman, A., Kopper, B. A., Barrios, F., Gutierrez, P. M., & Bagge, C. L. (2004). Reliability and validity of Beck Depression Inventory-II with adolescent psychiatric inpatients. *Psychological Assessment, 16,* 120–132.

Penley, J. A., Wiebe, J. S., & Nwosu, A. (2003). Psychometric properties of the Spanish Beck Depression Inventory-II in a medical sample. *Psychological Assessment,* 569–577.

Schulenberg, S. E., & Yutrzenka, B. A. (2001). Equivalence of computerized and conventional versions of the Beck Depression Inventory-II (BDI-II). *Current Psychology, 20,* 216–230.

Sprinkle, S. D., Lurie, D., Insko, S. L., Atkinson, G., Jones, G. L., Logan, A. R., & Bissada, N. M. (2002). Criterion validity, severity cut scores, and test-retest reliability of the Beck Depression Inventory-II in a university counselling center sample. *Journal of Counselling Psychology, 49*, 381–385.

Steer, R. A., Ball, R., Ranieri, W. F., & Beck, A. T. (1997). Further evidence for the construct validity of the Beck Depression Inventory-II with psychiatric outpatients. *Psychological Reports, 80*, 443–446.

Steer, R. A., Ball, R., Ranieri, W. F., & Beck, A. T. (1999). Dimensions of the Beck Depression Inventory-II in clinically depressed outpatients. *Journal of Clinical Psychology, 55*, 117–128.

Steer, R. A., Brown, G. K., Beck, A. T., & Sanderson, W. C. (2001). Mean Beck Depression Inventory-II scores by severity of major depressive disorder. *Psychological Reports, 88*, 1075–1076.

Steer, R. A., & Clark, D. A. (1997). Psychometric characteristics of the Beck Depression Inventory-II with college students. *Measurement and Evaluation in Counselling and Development, 30*, 128–136.

Steer, R. A., Clark, D. S., Beck, A. T., & Ranieri, W. F. (1999). Common and specific dimensions of self-reported anxiety and depression: The BDI-II versus the BDI-IA. *Behavior Research and Therapy, 37*, 183–190.

Steer, R. A., Kumar, G., Ranieri, W. F., & Beck, A. T. (1998). Use of the Beck Depression Inventory-II with adolescent psychiatric outpatients. *Journal of Psychopathology and Behavioral Assessment, 20*, 127–137.

Steer, R. A., Ranieri, W. F., & Kumar, G., & Beck, A. T. (2003). Beck Depression Inventory-II items associated with self-reported symptoms of ADHD in adult psychiatric outpatients. *Journal of Personality Assessment, 80*, 58–63.

Steer, R. A., Rismiller, D. J., & Beck, A. T. (2000). Use of the Beck Depression Inventory-II with depressed geriatric inpatients. *Behavior Research & Therapy, 38*, 311–318.

Storch, E. A., Roberti, J. W., & Roth, D. A. (2004). Factor structure, concurrent validity, and internal consistency of the Beck Depression Inventory–Second Edition in a sample of college students. *Depression and Anxiety, 19*, 187–189.

Trahan, D. E., Ross, C. E., & Trahan, S. L. (2001). Relationships among postconcussional-type symptoms, depression, and anxiety in neurologically normal young adults and victims of mild brain injury. *Archives of Clinical Neuropsychology, 16*, 435–445.

Viljoen, J. L., Iverson, G. L., Griffiths, S., & Woodward, T. S. (2003). Factor structure of the Beck Depression Inventory-II in a medical outpatient sample. *Journal of Clinical Psychology in Medical Settings, 10*, 289–291.

Whisman, M. A., Perez, J. E., & Ramel, W. (2000). Factor structure of the Beck Depression Inventory–Second Edition (BDI-II) in a student sample. *Journal of Clinical Psychology, 56*, 545–551.

Wong, J. L., Wetterneck, C., & Klein, A. (2000). Effects of depressed mood on verbal memory performance verus self-reports of cognitive difficulties. *International Journal of Rehabilitation and Health, 5*, 85–97.

Behavior Rating Inventory of Executive Function (BRIEF)

PURPOSE

The Behavior Rating Inventory of Executive Function (BRIEF) is a parent- and teacher-rated scale designed to measure executive functioning in children and adolescents.

SOURCE

The BRIEF and its preschool version (BRIEF-P) can be obtained from Psychological Assessment Resources, Inc. (http://www.parinc.com). An Introductory Kit (Professional Manual, 25 rating forms, and 25 scoring/summary forms) retails for $165 US for the BRIEF and $105 US for the BRIEF-P. A Combination Kit including both forms can be obtained for $259 US. Scoring and interpretive software is also available (BRIEF Software Portfolio, or BRIEF-SP) for $399 US. There is also a self-report version (BRIEF-SR) for adolescents, and an adult version including self-report and informant report versions (BRIEF-A).

AGE RANGE

The BRIEF can be administered to subjects aged 5 to 18 years. The BRIEF-P can be given to children aged 2 years 0 months to 5 years 11 months.

DESCRIPTION

Executive functions are not as amenable to paper-and-pencil assessment formats as are domain-specific functions such as language, memory, and visual-spatial skills (Gioia et al., 2000). In addition, because they are administered in a structured, novel, quiet, one-on-one testing environment, standard tests of executive functioning do not always allow executive deficits to emerge during administration. Therefore, clinicians and researchers in the field have developed specialised questionnaires completed by family members to assess executive functioning. The only executive functioning scale for use with children is the BRIEF (Gioia et al., 2000). Designed for assessing a broad range of childhood disorders, the BRIEF is intended as one component of a comprehensive evaluation (Gioia et al., 2002a).

The BRIEF is completed by raters who have observed a child in different settings (i.e., parents and teachers). It yields eight theoretically and empirically derived subscales, each of which reflects a specific aspect of executive functioning (Inhibit, Shift, Emotional Control, Initiate, Working Memory, Plan/Organize, Organization of Materials, and Monitor; see Table 15–5). These yield two broad composites, the Behavioral Regulation Index (BRI) and the Metacognition Index (MI), and an overall score, the Global Executive Composite (GEC; see Table 15–6). In addition, the BRIEF includes two scales designed to assess validity (Inconsistency and Negativity). Parent and Teacher forms both contain 86 items, 18 of which differ across forms.

Other versions, including a self-report version for adolescents (BRIEF-SR; Guy, Isquith & Gioia, 2004), an informant/self-report version for adults (BRIEF-A; Roth, Isquith & Gioia,

Table 15–5 Description of Executive Functions Underlying BRIEF Scales

Scale	Scale	Description	Examples of Deficit
BRI	Inhibit	The ability to resist or delay impulses, and/or to appropriately stop one's activity at the proper time	Acting without thinking Being easily distracted Inability to sit still
	Shift	The ability to alter problem-solving strategy, to think flexibly, and to switch or alternate attention	Perseveration
	Emotional Control	The ability to modulate emotional responses	Overblown emotional reaction to minor events General affective reactivity
MI	Initiate	The ability to start or to begin a task, or the ability to generate ideas or problem-solving strategies	Difficulty getting started with homework Need for prompts/cues to start a task, despite interest in the task
	Working Memory	The process of holding information in mind for the purposes of completing a task; necessary for following complex instructions, completing mental arithmetic, or performing multistep tasks	Difficulty remembering information for even a few minutes Forgetting when sent on simple errand
	Plan/Organize	The ability to anticipate future events, set goals, and develop steps ahead of time to complete multistep tasks; imagining or developing a goal and strategically determining how to reach it effectively	Lack of planning ability Tendency to start assignments at the last minute Not thinking ahead about possible problems or consequences of actions
		The ability to establish and maintain order within an activity or to carry out an activity in a systematic manner	Scattered approach to problem-solving Being overwhelmed by large tasks or assignments
	Organization of Materials	The ability to maintain order during play or work and with regard to personal belongings; keeping track of and organizing belongings	Difficulty organizing personal belongings Frequently losing personal belongings Messy or disorganized desk, closet, locker, or backpack
	Monitor	Self-monitoring; checking one's own actions during or immediately after finishing a task to assure goal attainment	Rushing through a task without checking work for mistakes Unawareness of effects of own behavior in social settings

2005), and preschool version (BRIEF-P; Gioia et al., 2003) are available but will not be reviewed here.

ADMINISTRATION TIME

Each form takes 10 to 15 min to complete.

Table 15–6 Clinical Scales and Composites of the BRIEF

Global Executive Composite (GEC)	
Behavioral Regulation Index (BRI)	**Metacognition Index (MI)**
Inhibit	Initiate
Shift	Working Memory
Emotional Control	Plan/Organize
	Organization of Materials
	Monitor

ADMINISTRATION

See the Professional Manual. Instructions for respondents are printed on the rating forms. In the manual, the authors also supply additional instructions to the respondents that emphasize the importance of completing all items.

Respondents are asked to rate the child's behavior on a 3-point scale ("Never," "Sometimes," and "Often"). Respondents with reading skills below a fifth-grade level should not be administered the BRIEF.

SCORING

Scores

T scores and percentiles can be derived for all scores.

Missing Responses

The BRIEF cannot be scored if the total number of missing responses is greater than 14, excluding any items that do not contribute to the subscales (i.e., items 73 to 86 on the Parent Form, 74 to 86 on the Teacher Form). T scores cannot be derived if more than two items are missing for an individual scale. The authors note that if only one or two responses are missing for a scale, a score of 1 should be assigned for those items.

Negativity Scale

The Negativity scale consists of nine items; the total score reflects the extent of negative bias on the part of the respondent, compared with the BRIEF clinical sample. A high Negativity score indicates that the respondent endorsed "Often" for most of the items on the Negativity scale. In the clinical sample, fewer than 3% of subjects scored higher than 7 on this scale; consequently, scores of 5 or more are considered elevated, and scores greater than 7 are considered either excessively negative, or, according to the authors, reflective of a child who "may have substantial executive dysfunction" (Professional Manual, p. 15). Specifically, because four of the nine Negativity items on the Parent Form are from the Shift scale, excessive cognitive rigidity should be evaluated as a possible explanation of elevations on the Negativity scale. Protocols should therefore be deemed invalid only after a careful review of items in the context of other test scores, history, and observations.

Inconsistency Scale

The Inconsistency scale consists of 10 item pairs that are similar in content. High scores on this scale indicate that the rater responded in an inconsistent manner within item pairs, compared with a large clinical sample. The manual notes that the calculation of the Inconsistency scale must be made carefully, because it is somewhat complex. For each pair, the absolute value of the difference between items is calculated. The Inconsistency scale is the sum of the absolute differences for each item pair. Based on this total, protocols are rated as Acceptable, Questionable, or Inconsistent (cumulative percentiles in the clinical sample of ≤98, 99 and <99). The authors recommend that protocols in the Questionable and Inconsistent range be reviewed carefully, to rule out actual differences caused by minor content variation across item pairs.

Index Score Interpretation

The manual notes that GEC scores should not be interpreted if the BRI and MI scores differ by 13 (Parent Form) or 19 (Teacher Form) T-score points.

DEMOGRAPHIC EFFECTS

Gender

Gender affects BRIEF ratings on parent and teacher forms on all scales except Shift and Organization of Materials on the Parent Form. Therefore, there are separate norms for gender, along with age.

Education/Socioeconomic Status (SES)

The manual indicates that there was a low, negative correlation between parental education and BRIEF ratings (accounting for 5% of the variance). SES was only mildly related to BRIEF scores in the standardization sample (i.e., ≤5% of the variance). However, children from low-SES families tended to be rated as having more executive problems.

IQ

Correlations with IQ differ across studies but suggest a modest relation to IQ in some samples (see *Validity*).

Ethnicity

Ethnicity is not related to BRIEF scores in the standardization sample (see manual).

NORMATIVE DATA

Standardization Sample

The BRIEF parent and teacher normative samples included individuals from schools in Maryland, along with a small number of cases from a research study ($n = 18$). Tables 15-7 and 15–8 show the sample characteristics for both scales.

A total of 1419 Parent Forms were completed by respondents in the normative sample. The Teacher Form was completed by 720 respondents. Corresponding ratings from parents and teachers were available for 296 children. Additional data were also collected to assess reliability and validity in clinical samples (Parent Form, 852 children; Teacher Form, 475 children). The mean level of education of parent respondents was 14.2 years.

Cases were weighted for ethnicity and gender according to the 1999 U.S. Census. T scores for the Parent Form were based on census-weighted data; Teacher Form scores were based on unweighted data. Although this did not appear to change the percentages significantly in most ethnicity classifications, subjects in the Hispanic category were underrepresented and, as a result, relatively highly weighted. Specifically, there were 42 Hispanic cases for the parent scale, representing 3.1% of the actual sample; this was weighted to reach 11.6% of the total sample (see Table 15–7).

Norms are organized along four age groupings in addition to gender (ages 5–7, 8–10, 11–13, and 14–18 years). The

Table 15–7 Characteristics of the BRIEF Normative Sample—Parent Version

Sample type	25 schools (12 elementary, 9 middle, and 4 high schools); 18 additional cases were obtained from a normal control group in a TBI study in Cleveland, Ohio	
N	1419[a]	
Age	5 to 18 years[b]	
Geographic location	State of Maryland, USA[c]	
Parental Education (years)	Mean, 14.2 (SD = 2.57)	
Gender (%)		
Boys	43	
Girls	57	
Race/Ethnicity (%)	Actual	Weighted
White	80.5	71.7
African American	11.9	12.2
Hispanic	3.1	11.6
Asian/Pacific Islander	3.8	3.8
Native American/Eskimo	0.5	0.7
Socioeconomic status (%)		
Upper	3.0	
Upper-middle	21.8	
Middle-middle	36.1	
Lower-middle	31.8	
Lower	6.2	
Unassigned	1.2	
Screening	Excluded if a history of special education or psychotropic medication use was present or >10% of items were missing	

[a]Norms were organized along four age groupings in addition to gender: ages 5–7, 8–10, 11–13, and 14–18 years.
[b]Only nine 18-year-olds were included.
[c]26.5%, 59%, and 14.5% of children were from urban, suburban, and rural settings, respectively.

Source: Adapted from Gioia et al., 2000.

Table 15–8 Characteristics of the BRIEF Normative Sample—Teacher Version

Sample type	25 schools (12 elementary, 9 middle, and 4 high schools); 18 additional cases were obtained from a normal control group in a TBI study in Cleveland, Ohio	
N	720[a]	
Age (years)	5 to 18 years[b]	
Geographic location	State of Maryland, USA[c]	
Parental education	Not specified	
Gender (%)		
Boys	44	
Girls	56	
Race/Ethnicity (%)	Actual	Weighted
White	72.1	71.7
African American	13.5	12.2
Hispanic	4.2	11.6
Asian/Pacific Islander	6.1	3.8
Native American/Eskimo	0.4	0.7
Socioeconomic status (%)		
Upper	7.4	
Upper-middle	20.0	
Middle-middle	28.0	
Lower-middle	21.0	
Lower	2.5	
Unassigned	21.0	
Screening	Excluded if a history of special education or psychotropic medication was present or >10% of items were missing	

[a]Norms were organized along four age groupings in addition to gender: ages 5–7, 8–10, 11–13, and 14–18 years.
[b]Only one 18-year-old was included.
[c]26.5%, 59% and 14.5% of children were from urban, suburban, and rural settings, respectively.

Source: Adapted from Gioia et al., 2000.

manual presents the actual age breakdown of the normative sample for the Parent and Teacher Forms, which indicates that cell numbers were not equivalent across age. For instance, although cell sizes were greater than 100 for each age from 6 to 14 years for the Parent Form, fewer than fifty 17-year-olds and only nine 18-year-olds were included in the normative sample. Overall, cell sizes were somewhat smaller on average for the Teacher Form (approximately 50 to 100 cases per age), but some ages included very few children. For example, there were twenty 5-year-olds, ten 16-year-olds, nineteen 17-year-olds, and only *one* 18-year-old. The unevenness in age representation was lessened somewhat by presenting norms by age groupings instead of absolute age, resulting in similar overall numbers across the four age bands. However, this means that there is an uneven representation of ages within some of these age groupings. Thus, because of the relative lack of older adolescents, younger adolescents are overrepresented in the 14–18

year age band. On average, numbers for the four age groupings by gender are larger for the Parent Form (144–262) than for the Teacher Form (29–224).

The majority of respondents in the normative sample for the Parent Form were mothers (i.e., 83%); no significant differences were found between mothers' and fathers' ratings. BRIEF data from the normative group are positively skewed, with the majority of cases at the lower end of the continuum (i.e., with few executive deficits).

RELIABILITY

Internal Consistency

Cronbach's alpha for the Parent and Teacher forms is high (r = .80 to .98). Reliabilities are very high for the GEC for both Parent and Teacher forms, in both standardization and clinical samples (r = .97 to .98). The other two composite indices

Table 15–9 Magnitude of Test-Retest Reliability Coefficients for the BRIEF for Three Groups

Magnitude of Coefficient	Parent Normative Sample	Parent Clinical Sample	Teacher Normative Sample
Very High (≥.90)	—	—	Inhibit Emotional Control *Behavior Regulation Index* *Metacognition Index* *Global Executive Composite*
High (.80 to .89)	Inhibit Initiate Working Memory Plan/Organize *Behavioral Regulation Index* *Metacognition Index* *Global Executive Composite*	Working Memory Plan/Organize Organization of Materials Monitor *Behavioral Regulation Index* *Metacognition Index* *Global Executive Composite*	Shift Initiate Working Memory Plan/Organize Organization of Materials Monitor
Adequate (.70 to .79)	Shift Emotional Control Organization of Materials Monitor	Inhibit Shift Emotional Control Initiate	—
Marginal (.60 to .69)	—	—	—
Low (≤.59)	—	—	—

Note: Index scores are shown in italics.

also have very high reliabilities in both normative and clinical samples for both forms (*r* = .94 to .98).

In the normative sample, the lowest reliabilities were for Initiate, Shift, and Monitor on the Parent Form (*r* = .81 to .83); the same general pattern was found in the clinical sample (*r* = .82 to .88). On the Teacher Form, scale reliabilities all exceeded .90 in the normative sample. In the clinical sample, Teacher Form reliability was lowest for Initiate (*r* = .84).

Test-Retest Reliability

Stability was evaluated in three different groups. For the Parent Form, 54 children from the normative sample and 40 children from the clinical sample were readministered the BRIEF after a 2- to 3-week interval. For the Teacher Form, 41 children were readministered the BRIEF after a 3.5-week interval. Table 15–9 shows the magnitude of correlations across groups. On average, Teacher Form stability was slightly higher than that of the Parent Form. Teacher Form stability was especially good for all the composites and for the Inhibit and Emotional Control scales (*r* > .90).

"Practice" Effects

The authors also examined the magnitude of T-score changes over time for the three test-retest groups. For the Parent and Teacher normative groups, T-score changes were minimal, on average (i.e., 1 point). Changes were larger in the clinical group (*M* = 3 points). Scales showing the largest changes included the Plan/Organize scale on the Parent Form, with a 3-point drop in the normative sample and a 7.5-point drop in the clinical sample. On the Teacher Form normative sample,

the greatest drop was for the Working Memory scale (3 points). Overall, these results indicate that the BRIEF is suitable for repeat assessments.

Interrater Reliability

Correlations between different raters (parents and teachers) are presented in the manual for 296 children. Overall, parent-teacher correlations are moderate at best (average *r* = .32), which is not unusual for parent-teacher rating agreement. In particular, the authors note that correlations were low for two scales, Initiate (*r* = .18) and Organization of Materials (*r* = .15). They also note that parents consistently rated children as having more difficulties on all scales than did teachers, a finding that is also fairly typical in the literature on parent-teacher agreement. Given these findings, parent and teacher ratings are likely to be measuring slightly different aspects of executive functioning and therefore are not interchangeable.

VALIDITY

Content Validity

The BRIEF appears to have been carefully constructed. According to the authors, scale structure was initially derived through literature review and consultation with colleagues and an expert panel, and then verified with factor analysis. Item content was based on review of interview notes of actual clinical cases, to generate items reflecting specific behaviors and characteristics. Common behavior rating scales were also reviewed to minimize redundancy with other scales (e.g., CBCL, TRF, BASC,

Conners Parent and Teacher Questionnaires, VABS). Other aspects of item derivation are described in the manual.

Factor Structure

The manual describes a two-factor solution for the normative and clinical samples that corresponds to the two composite scores: a metacognitive problem-solving factor composed of Initiate, Working Memory, Plan/Organize, and Organization of Materials, and a behavioral regulation factor comprised of Emotional Control, Shift, and Inhibit. This factor solution was obtained by specifying two factors a priori. In a pediatric epilepsy sample, the best fit for the Parent BRIEF was a two-component solution, using principal components analysis (Slick et al., submitted). The BRI and MCI were generally replicated, but Organization of Materials was found to load equivalently on both components.

Gioia and Isquith (2002) re-examined the item content of the Monitor scale and found that the scale actually reflected two distinct subcomponents instead of a single unitary dimension: task-monitoring (items 14, 21, 31, and 60 on the Parent Form) and self-monitoring (items 34, 42, 52, 63 on the Parent Form). They noted that these subcomponents were only moderately correlated with each other ($r = .47$) and that they loaded differently in exploratory factor analyses (i.e., task-monitoring with Metacognition, and self-monitoring with Behavioral Regulation). The factor structure of this revised 9-scale BRIEF (i.e., with the Monitor scale divided into two distinct domains) was therefore re-examined via confirmatory factor analysis in a large mixed clinical sample (Gioia et al., 2002b). A three-factor solution, thought to be most consistent with Barkley's (1997) model, was the best fit: a Behavioral Regulation factor comprising Inhibit and Self-Monitor, an Emotional Regulation factor defined by Emotional Control and Shift, and a Metacognition factor made up of Initiate, Working Memory, Plan/Organize, Organization of Materials, and Task-Monitor. This analysis did not support the view that executive functions as measured by the BRIEF consist of one unitary dimension. The authors noted that either the two-factor or the three-factor model could be used to interpret scores.

Correlations With Executive Functioning Tests

Generally, only modest (Anderson et al., 2002; Mahone et al., 2002a; Mangeot et al., 2002) or minimal (Slick et al., 2002; Vriezen & Pigott, 2002) correlations with clinical tests of executive functioning such as the WCST have been reported in various clinical populations. However, a small number of studies have reported some concordance between BRIEF scores and executive functioning tests. For example, Mangeot et al. (2002) observed that, of a number of executive functioning tests, only Consonant Trigrams was a consistent predictor of BRIEF composite scores in children with traumatic brain injury (TBI). Anderson et al. (2002) found that Contingency Naming, a measure of mental flexibility, was moderately related to

the BRIEF in a mixed clinical group. Moderate correlations between the BRIEF Working Memory and COWAT were also reported. Correlations with other tests, such as the Tower of London, were minimal.

Correlations With Behavior Rating Scales and Interviews

Because there exist no other rating scales of executive functioning designed for children, the authors examined correlations between BRIEF ratings and other rating scales measuring similar dimensions of behavior. Correlations with other behavior scales are described in the manual and in a number of recent publications describing clinical samples.

Good concordance has been reported between conceptually similar scales on the BRIEF and a commonly used measure of ADHD symptoms, the ADHD-RS-IV (DuPaul et al., 1998). The manual shows that, in 100 clinically referred children administered the parent forms of the BRIEF and ADHD-RS-IV, BRIEF scales reflecting attentional functioning (Metacognition Index, Working Memory, Plan/Organize, Initiate, Monitor) correlated highly with the ADHD-RS-IV Inattention scale ($r = .54$ to .67). At the same time, BRIEF scales reflecting behavioral disinhibition (Behavioral Inhibition Index, Inhibit, Shift, Emotional Control) correlated highly with the conceptually similar Hyperactivity-Impulsivity scale from the ADHD-RS-IV ($r = .56$ to .73). In our own studies on pediatric epilepsy (Slick et al., 2002), we found a high degree of association between BRIEF ratings and the ADHD-RS-IV ($r = .79$). Ratings of attention from the ADHD-IV were most highly correlated with the Working Memory, Initiate, and Plan/Organize scales from the BRIEF, whereas ratings of hyperactivity were most associated with the Inhibit Scale.

Correlations with the CBCL supporting BRIEF validity are presented in the manual for 200 children; correlations between scales were not as clear as with the ADHD-RS-IV, due to the multifactorial nature of some of the CBCL scales (e.g., CBCL Attention also includes items reflecting impulsivity and hyperactivity). However, principal factor analysis of the BRIEF and CBCL supported the validity of the Metacognition and Behavioral Regulation factors as separate from the Externalizing and Internalizing factors of the CBCL (see manual for details).

Correlations with BASC PRS (Reynolds & Kamphaus, 1998) reviewed in the manual are also supportive of the construct validity of the BRIEF scales. The Behavior Regulation Index was highly correlated with BASC Aggression and Hyperactivity, and Metacognition correlated highly with the BASC Attention scale (see manual for further details). Correlations with the Conners' scale (Conners, 1989) are also described; these instruments show the most overlap between the BRIEF Behavior Regulation Index scales and the Conners Restless-Disorganized, Conduct Disorder, and Hyperactive-Immature scales.

Other independent research studies have shown similar findings regarding the concordance of the Parent Form BRIEF and other child behavior rating scales (Mahone et al., 2002a; Mangeot et al., 2002), particularly scales that measure attention or hyperactivity such as CBCL Attention, DICA-IV ADHD Scale, and ADHD Rating Scale–IV (Mahone et al., 2002a). However, this is not always the case. For example, Mahone et al. (2002b) found that BRIEF ratings were selectively elevated in a group of children with myelomeningocele and hydrocephalus, whereas other scales of behavior (i.e., BASC scores) were in the normal range. This is consistent with the expected executive difficulties of this patient group (Mahone et al., 2002b) and suggests a limited sensitivity of broadband behavior scales to executive deficits.

Other studies have also found a significant relationship between BRIEF scores and measures of adaptive functioning. In children with autism, communication and social functioning on the Vineland were negatively related to BRIEF scales (Gilotty et al., 2002). BRIEF scores were related to adaptive functioning, behavioral adjustment, parent psychological distress, perceived family burden, and general family functioning in a long-term outcome study on childhood TBI (Mangeot et al., 2002). The authors of that study noted that shared method variance may partially account for the strong relationship between the BRIEF and other child behavior rating scales.

Correlations With IQ and Achievement

Low correlations with IQ have been reported in clinical groups such as ADHD and Tourette syndrome (<.28; Mahone et al., 2000a). In one study on TBI, verbal IQ had a moderate correlation with the Metacognition Index ($r = .30$; Vriezen & Pigott, 2002). In another study involving children with TBI, full-scale IQ significantly predicted the GEC and Metacognition Index, accounting for a small to medium amount of variance (Mangeot et al., 2002). The BRIEF is reportedly moderately related to math achievement as measured by the WIAT Math Composite (Mahone et al., 2002a), which may indicate a role for executive functioning in math skills.

Utility in ADHD Screening

The BRIEF is described as a measure that can assist in the diagnosis of ADHD. As noted earlier, the BRIEF Behavioral Inhibition index is highly related to measures of overactivity (ADHD-RS-IV Hyperactivity-Impulsivity Scale), and the BRIEF Metacognition Index is highly related to inattention symptoms (ADHD-RS-IV Inattention Scale). These findings also were replicated in a clinical study involving ADHD and Tourette syndrome (Mahone et al., 2000a). Gioia et al. (2000) noted that BRIEF profiles in ADHD indicate a broader range of deficits than are indicated in the DSM-IV, such as deficits in metacognition and modulation of emotions. This is consistent with recent theories of ADHD that propose a central problem with executive functioning rather than attention per se (Barkley, 1997).

ADHD subtypes have also been studied with regard to BRIEF profiles. The manual describes data for 53 children with ADHD, in which almost all Parent Form BRIEF subscales were elevated compared with controls. In addition, the Behavioral Regulation Index and its scales were higher in the ADHD-Combined type than in the ADHD-Inattentive type. A similar pattern was found for 121 children with ADHD on the Teacher Form. In a separate study, Gioia et al. (2000) reported that children with ADHD-Combined type showed high elevations across all scales; 89% had elevations on the Inhibit Scale that were greater than those of other clinical disorders including autism. In contrast, children with ADHD-Inattentive type showed elevations on metacognitive executive skills on the BRIEF.

In terms of the sensitivity and specificity of BRIEF composites to ADHD subtypes, the manual lists recommended cutoff values for the Working Memory and Inhibit scales to aid in the diagnosis of ADHD. For example, a T score of 70 on the Parent Form Working Memory scale identified 74% of children with ADHD-Inattentive but incorrectly identified 13% of controls. Similarly, a T score of 70 on the Parent Form Inhibit scale correctly identified 85% of children with ADHD-Combined, but also misidentified 13% of controls and 48% of ADHD-Inattentive subjects as ADHD-Combined.

On the Teacher Form, the recommended cutoff of 75 for the Working Memory scale identified 71% of children with ADHD-Inattentive, 72% of children with ADHD-Combined, and 15% of controls. A cutoff of 70 for the Teacher Form Inhibit scale yielded a 78% rate of correct identification of ADHD-Combined but misclassified 21% of controls. A higher cutoff of 80 correctly identified 69% of children with ADHD-Combined and misclassified 13% of controls. Other cutoffs with specific sensitivities and specificities are shown in Tables 54 through 57 in the Professional Manual.

BRIEF Profiles of Diagnostic Groups

The BRIEF manual presents Parent Form BRIEF profiles for a number of other diagnostic groups, including TBI, Tourette's syndrome, reading disorder, low birth weight, high-functioning autism, PDD, mental retardation, and frontal lesions. Teacher Form data are presented for high-functioning autism and PDD. Results are presented in terms of mean item raw score instead of T scores, which makes comparison with actual clinical protocols more difficult. Children with TBI described in the manual showed elevations across BRIEF scales; this was also true for children with extremely low birth weight, high-functioning autism, or PDD. Children with Tourette syndrome were no different than controls, but children with reading disorder showed deficits in Working Memory and Plan/Organize. Children with frontal lesions were rated as marginally more disinhibited than children with extrafrontal lesions, but both groups had BRIEF elevations compared with controls. Children with early-treated PKU had elevations on the Emotional Control scale.

Clinical profiles have also been described in several separate research studies, primarily with the Parent Form. Gioia et al. (2002a) reported that children with reading disorders showed elevations on metacognitive executive skills on the BRIEF, whereas children with autism showed high elevations across scales, along with particularly severe difficulties with Shifting, compared with other diagnostic groups. In children with severe epilepsy, Slick et al. (submitted) found that more than 50% of the sample had clinically significant elevations on the Working Memory scale, and 44% showed clinically significant impairments on Plan/Organize. Although executive profiles are not sufficiently specific to be used for diagnosis, they support the validity of the BRIEF in clinical groups.

With regard to TBI, the degree of executive dysfunction as measured by the BRIEF is related to the severity of injury in TBI (Mangeot et al., 2002). Interestingly, one long-term outcome study on childhood TBI reported that, although the BRIEF GEC was clinically elevated in 42% of children with severe TBI and 26% of children with moderate TBI, a full 21% of control children with orthopedic injuries also had clinically significant elevations, which underlines the fact that children who receive orthopedic injuries may have a higher incidence of executive functioning deficits than their normally functioning peers (Mangeot et al., 2002). See Gioia and Isquith (2004) for more on the use of the BRIEF in pediatric TBI.

In another study, BRIEF Parent ratings were not higher in TBI children with confirmed frontal pathology compared to those without such a classification (Vriezen & Pigott, 2002), although these authors noted that the diffuse nature of brain injury in TBI and the lack of sensitivity of imaging techniques may have confounded group assignment. In a larger study, children with frontal lesions were reported to have significant elevations on the BRIEF compared to children with early-treated PKU or hydrocephalus; more than 50% of the group with frontal lesions had clinically significant impairments in executive functions, as measured by the BRIEF, compared to less than 20% of the other clinical groups (Anderson et al., 2002). However, because the PKU and hydrocephalus groups had higher rates of executive impairments on the BRIEF compared with controls, the authors concluded that the BRIEF is also sensitive to the more subtle effects of diffuse brain dysfunction, in addition to the more focal effects of frontal lesions.

In one study examining BRIEF profiles in a psychiatric sample, adolescents with bipolar disorder showed elevations on all of the BRIEF subscales, consistent with the presumed executive dysfunction present in this disorder; adolescents with comorbid ADHD and bipolar disorder were disproportionally impaired according to BRIEF ratings (Shear et al., 2002).

COMMENT

The BRIEF is a well-designed, psychometrically sound instrument that, despite its recent publication, already boasts a substantial body of literature on its application in clinical contexts. This includes a number of studies on clinical groups, including children with ADHD, Tourette syndrome, reading disorders, TBI, autism, frontal lesions, PKU, hydrocephalus, epilepsy, and bipolar disorder (e.g., Gioia et al., 2002a;

Mahone et al., 2002a, 2002b; Shear et al., 2002; Slick et al., 2002; Vriezen & Pigott, 2002). These studies all appear to support the validity and clinical utility of the BRIEF. In addition, the manual is well written and thorough, and it includes detailed examination of psychometric properties in clinical groups, a feature that is sometimes overlooked in other tests and questionnaires. Its reliability is generally sound, and the composite scores, particularly those for the Teacher Form, are high enough for reliable diagnostic decision making.

In contrast to commonly used questionnaires designed for adults (e.g., MMPI-2, PAI), the inclusion of validity scales is often overlooked in childhood questionnaires. Although more research is needed on the BRIEF Inconsistency and Negativity scales, these scales are a clear asset for BRIEF users.

The BRIEF appears to be a useful tool in screening for ADHD. In addition, from a theoretical standpoint, the test is based on contemporary models of ADHD such as that of Barkley (1997), which proposes executive dysfunction as the core deficit, rather than inattention per se. Moreover, the BRIEF appears to be useful in the evaluation of other neurological and medical disorders. In some cases, it may be sensitive to deficits that are not detected by other broadband rating scales (e.g., Mahone et al., 2002b).

Limitations

The BRIEF has few limitations; however, some specific aspects deserve mention. First, to date, independent clinical studies on the BRIEF have examined the Parent Form only; similarly, most of the information from clinical samples provided in the manual involves the Parent Form. Given the relatively minimal overlap between parent and teacher ratings on the BRIEF, the significance of relying on one rater over another deserves more study, particularly for diagnostic decision making in conditions such as ADHD, which the BRIEF is intended to supplement. Of note is the fact that reliabilities for the Teacher version were uniformly good, whereas some test-retest reliabilities for some Parent Form subscales were only adequate (see Table 15–7). In addition, less case weighting was used in the Teacher form because of a closer approximation to U.S. Census data in the standardization sample.

Second, the BRIEF normative sample includes uneven numbers across age (the most extreme example being the inclusion of only *one* 18-year-old in the Teacher Form). This unevenness is lessened somewhat by the clustering of ages into four broad age bands, but equal representation across age should be sought in future revisions of the test. In particular, the upper age limit of 18 years is somewhat misleading, and there is a relatively small number of older adolescents overall. Case weighting, also used in many tests when the normative sample differs from Census composition, should be avoided if possible in future revisions. In some cases, case weighting is an attempt to compensate for inadequate sampling in the standardization sample. It is important to note that there were relatively few low SES children in the sample, and that low SES was associated with higher BRIEF ratings. More research on the test's appropriateness in specific populations (e.g., defined by ethnicity and/or SES) is needed.

More information on the utility and psychometric validity of the supraordinate GEC score would also be helpful, because factor analyses support a two- or three-dimension view of executive functions as measured by the BRIEF, not a unitary dimension (Gioia et al., 2002b).

The BRIEF Versus Tests of Executive Functioning

Overall, the BRIEF appears to measure aspects of executive functioning that are somewhat distinct from those measured by standard tests of executive functioning such as the WCST. Some have suggested that this lack of concordance indicates that the BRIEF may be more sensitive to executive deficits in daily life and that clinical tests simply lack ecological validity (Vriezen & Pigott, 2002). Known disadvantages of standard tests of executive function include a narrow focus, possible lack of sensitivity to subtler forms of executive deficits, the fact that many rely on novelty to assess skills, and use of paradigms based on tests validated in adults (Denckla, 2002; Silver, 2000).

Until there is further research on this question, the lack of strong overlap between the BRIEF and standard tests of executive functioning does not necessarily mean that one method is superior to the other. Rather, they may be tapping different aspects of behavior (e.g., the individual's capacity to function with or without support or distractions) and over different time intervals (e.g., questionnaires sample behavior over a longer time line than do standard clinical tests). Questionnaire formats also have their disadvantages (Denckla, 2002), including the need for competent language skills in the respondent and the possible distortion of responses due to emotional biases (i.e., positive and negative "halo effects"). In addition, clinical tests and questionnaires use different methodologies that have traditionally yielded only moderate correlations, at best, when used to assess other related domains such as attention (e.g., Barkley, 1991; Barkley, 1998). Clinical tests and BRIEF scores may therefore identify slightly different groups of children, with different manifestations of executive dysfunction in daily life. Until further research sheds light on the differential utility of these tests in clinical diagnosis, the best approach is a comprehensive assessment that includes both methods in the evaluation of executive functions in children.

REFERENCES

Anderson, V. A., Anderson, P., Northam, E., Jacobs, R., & Mikiewicz, O. (2002). Relationships between cognitive and behavioral measures of executive function in children with brain disease. *Child Neuropsychology, 8*(4), 231–240.

Barkley, R. A. (1991). The ecological validity of laboratory and analogue assessment methods of ADHD symptoms. *Journal of Abnormal Child Psychology, 19,* 149–178.

Barkley, R. A. (1997). *ADHD and the nature of self-control.* New York: Guildford.

Barkley, R. A. (1998). *Attention Deficit Hyperactivity Disorder: A handbook for diagnosis and treatment* (2nd ed.). New York: Guilford.

Conners, C. K. (1989). *Manual for Conners' Rating Scales.* North Tonawanda, NY: MultiHealth Systems.

Denckla, M. B. (2002). The Behavior Rating Inventory of Executive Function: Commentary. *Child Neuropsychology, 8*(4), 304–306.

DuPaul, G. J., Power, T. J., Anastopoulos, A. D., & Reid, R. (1998). *ADHD Rating Scale–IV: Checklists, norms, and clinical interpretation.* New York: Guilford.

Gilotty, L., Kenworthy, L., Sirian, L., Black, D. O., & Wagner, A. E. (2002). Adaptive skills and executive function in autism spectrum disorders. *Child Neuropsychology, 8*(4), 241–248.

Gioia, G. A., Espy, K. A., & Isquith, P. K. (2003). *Behavior Rating Inventory of Executive Function—Preschool Version.* Lutz, FL: Psychological Assessment Resources.

Gioia, G. A., & Isquith, P. K. (2002). Two faces of Monitor: Thy self and thy task [Abstract]. *Journal of the International Neuropsychological Society, 8,* 229.

Gioia, G. A., & Isquith, P. K. (2004). Ecological assessment of executive function in traumatic brain injury. *Developmental Neuropsychology, 25*(1&2), 135–158.

Gioia, G. A., Isquith, P. K., Guy, S. C., & Kenworthy, L. (2000). *Behavior Rating Inventory of Executive Function.* Lutz, FL: Psychological Assessment Resources.

Gioia, G. A., Isquith, P. K., Kenworthy, L., & Barton, R. M. (2002a). Profiles of everyday executive function in acquired and developmental disorders. *Child Neuropsychology, 8*(4), 121–137.

Gioia, G. A., Isquith, P. K., Retzlaff, P. D., & Espy, K. A. (2002b). Confirmatory factor analysis of the Behavior Rating Inventory of Executive Function (BRIEF) in a clinical sample. *Child Neuropsychology, 8*(4), 249–257.

Guy, S. C., Isquith, P. K., & Gioia, G. A. (2004). *Behavior Rating Inventory of Executive Function—Self-Report.* Lutz, FL: Psychological Assessment Resources.

Mahone, E. M., Cirino, P. T., Cutting, L. E., Cerrone, P. M., Hagelthorn, K. M., Hiemenz, J. R., Singer, H. S., & Denckla, M. B. (2002a). Validity of the Behavior Rating Inventory of Executive Function in children with ADHD and/or Tourette syndrome. *Archives of Clinical Neuropsychology, 17,* 643–662.

Mahone, E. M., Zabel, T. A., Levey, E., Verda, M., & Kinsman, S. (2002b). Parent and self-report ratings of executive function in adolescents with myelomeningocele and hydrocephalus. *Child Neuropsychology, 8*(4), 258–270.

Mangeot, S., Armstrong, K., Colvin, A. N., Yeates, K. O., & Taylor, H. G. (2002). Long-term executive function deficits in children with traumatic brain injuries: Assessment using the Behavior Rating Inventory of Executive Function (BRIEF). *Child Neuropsychology, 8*(4), 271–284.

Reynolds, C. R., & Kamphaus, R. W. (1998). *Behavior Assessment System for Children manual.* Circle Pines, MN: American Guidance Service.

Roth, R. R, Isquith, P. K., & Gioia, G. A. (2005). *Behavior Rating Inventory of Executive Function—Adult Version.* Lutz, FL: Psychological Assessment Resources.

Shear, P. K., DelBello, M. P., Rosenberg, H. L., & Strakowski, S. M. (2002). Parental reports of executive dysfunction in adolescents with bipolar disorder. *Child Neuropsychology, 8*(4), 285–295.

Silver, C. H. (2000). Ecological validity of neuropsychological assessment in childhood traumatic brain injury. *Journal of Head Trauma Rehabilitation, 15,* 973–988.

Slick, D. J., Lautzenhsier, A., Sherman, E. M. S., Eyrl, K., Connolly, M. B., & Steinbok, P. (Submitted). Component structure and profiles of Behavioral Rating Inventory of Executive Function (BRIEF) scales in children and adolescents with intractable epilepsy.

Slick, D. J., Sherman, E. M. S., Connolly, M. B., & Eyrl, K. (2002). Correlates of parent ratings of executive functions in children with intractable epilepsy. [Abstract]. *Journal of the International Neuropsychological Society, 8,* 320.

Vriezen, E. R., & Pigott, S. E. (2002). The relationship between parental report on the BRIEF and performance-based measures of executive function in children with moderate to severe traumatic brain injury. *Child Neuropsychology, 8*(4), 296–303.

Geriatric Depression Scale (GDS)

OTHER TEST NAME

Another test name for the Geriatric Depression Scale (GDS) is the Mood Assessment Scale.

PURPOSE

This test screens for depression in the elderly.

SOURCE

There is no commercial source for this test. The user can refer to the website http://www.stanford.edu/~yesavage/GDS.html to access the standard 30-item GDS and 15-item short-form (Brink et al., 1982; Yesavage et al., 1983). The questions are also provided in Figure 15–1. The test has been translated into more than 17 languages (refer to the GDS website for further details).

AGE RANGE

The test can be given to individuals aged 17 years and older.

DESCRIPTION

Depression is very common in the elderly. About 1% to 3% of community-dwelling older adults suffer from major depression, with the incidence rising to 10% to 15% in hospital and nursing home settings (Rinaldi et al., 2003). Research suggests that between 15% and 27% of older adults in the United States experience subsyndromal depression that does not meet criteria for a specific depressive syndrome (Lebowitz et al., 1997). Because depression is such a common condition in the elderly, and because it lends itself to treatment, it should always be part of the geriatric assessment. However, the detection of depression is difficult in this population, because symptoms often attributed to depression may be confused with problems associated with the aging process (e.g., slowness, insomnia, problems with memory and concentration).

The GDS was designed specifically to screen for depression among the geriatric population. Therefore, it taps affective and behavioral symptoms of depression and excludes those concerns that may be readily confused with somatic diseases or dementia. The GDS consists of 30 yes/no questions designed for ease of self-administration (see Figure 15–1). The directionality of answers scored for depression changes randomly. The purpose of the scale is partially disguised by the title "Mood Assessment Scale" at the top of the questionnaire. It is commonly used in primary care settings, geriatric clinics, and hospitals and in community studies. It is among the measures included in the recently proposed criteria for subsyndromal depression (Lavretsky & Kumar, 2002).

A 15-item short form has been developed (GDS-15) (Sheikh & Yesavage, 1986) as have 12- 10-, 5-, 4-, and 1-item versions (e.g., Cheng & Chan, 2004; D'Ath et al., 1994; Galaria et al., 2000; Gori et al., 1998; Hoyl et al., 1999; Sutcliffe et al., 2000). The 15- and 5-item short forms appear more commonly in the literature and are also shown in Figure 15–1.

ADMINISTRATION

The examiner asks the patient to complete a simple questionnaire (see Figure 15–1) referring to changes in mood, and to answer these questions by circling yes or no, whichever appropriately describes his or her feelings at that time. Alternatively, the questions can be read to the patient if there is any concern about his or her ability to read or comprehend written material.

ADMINISTRATION TIME

About 5 to 10 min is required for the long form and 5 to 7 min for the GDS-15.

SCORING

One point is given for each of the answers marked in bold in Figure 15–1. Scores may range from 0 (no depression) to 30 (severe depression). Dr. Yesavage recommends that, if a patient misses a few items, scores may be prorated according to the ratio of endorsed responses to endorsable responses (see website for further information). For example, if the patient scored 4 of 12 or ⅓ positive on the items completed, add ⅓ each for the 3 missing items, or 1 point, for a total of 5. For information on cutoff values, see *Normative Data*.

Figure 15–1 Geriatric Depression Scale: *Items comprising the 5-item GDS,   **Items comprising the 15-item GDS. *Source:* From Brink et al., 1982; Yesavage, 1983.

MOOD ASSESSMENT SCALE

1. Are you basically satisfied with your life?	Yes/**No***	**
2. Have you dropped many of your activities and interests?	**Yes**/ No	**
3. Do you feel that your life is empty?	**Yes**/No	**
4. Do you often get bored?	**Yes**/ No*	**
5. Are you hopeful about the future?	Yes/ **No**	
6. Are you bothered by thoughts that you can't get out of your head?	**Yes**/ No	
7. Are you in good spirits most of the time?	Yes/ **No**	**
8. Are you afraid that something bad is going to happen to you?	**Yes**/ No	**
9. Do you feel happy most of the time?	Yes/ **No**	**
10. Do you often feel helpless?	**Yes**/ No*	**
11. Do you often get restless and fidgety?	**Yes**/ No	
12. Do you prefer to stay home rather than go out and doing new things?	**Yes**/No*	**
13. Do you frequently worry about the future?	**Yes**/ No	
14. Do you feel that you have more problems with memory than most?	**Yes**/ No	**
15. Do you think it is wonderful to be alive now?	Yes/ **No**	**
16. Do you often feel downhearted and blue?	**Yes**/ No	
17. Do you feel pretty worthless the way you are now?	**Yes**/ No*	**
18. Do you worry a lot about the past?	**Yes**/ No	
19. Do you find life very exciting?	Yes/ **No**	
20. Is it hard for you to get started on new projects?	**Yes**/ No	
21. Do you feel full of energy?	Yes/ **No**	**
22. Do you feel that your situation is hopeless?	**Yes**/ No	**
23. Do you think that most people are better off than you are?	**Yes**/ No	**
24. Do you frequently get upset by little things?	**Yes**/ No	
25. Do you frequently feel like crying?	**Yes**/ No	
26. Do you have trouble concentrating?	**Yes**/ No	
27. Do you enjoy getting up in the mornings?	Yes/ **No**	
28. Do you prefer to avoid social gatherings?	**Yes**/ No	
29. Is it easy for you to make decisions?	Yes/ **No**	
30. Is your mind as clear as it used to be?	Yes/ **No**	

DEMOGRAPHIC EFFECTS

Age

Age does not appear to have a strong influence on test performance. Some authors have reported small but positive associations with increasing age on the 30-item test (Colenda & Smith, 1993; Knight et al., 2004; Monopoli & Vaccaro, 1998), and others have not (e.g., Dunn & Sacco, 1989; Ingram, 1996; Parmelee et al., 1989; Rule et al., 1990; Tamkin et al., 1985). Similarly, some have noted age effects on the 15-item form (Chou & Chi, 2005; Ferraro & Chelminski, 1996; Jang et al., 2001; Knight et al., 2004) but others have not (D'Ath et al., 1994; Ingram, 1996; Steiner et al., 1996).

Gender

Some researchers have found no effect (D'Ath et al., 1994; Steiner et al., 1996) or only small effects (Parmelee et al., 1989) of gender. However, there may be a risk of increased false-negative results in men compared to women. Allen-Burge et al.

(1994) reported that the GDS was twice as likely to classify depressed men as nondepressed using a cutoff of 11 and that one quarter to one half of the depressed men were missed by the GDS.

Education/IQ

Lower education is linked to higher scores on the 30-item test (Colenda & Smith, 1993; Monopoli & Vaccaro, 1998) and on the 15-item version (Jang et al., 2001), although Ferraro and Chelminski (1996) found only a small positive correlation ($r = .18$) in young adults. Premorbid IQ as measured by the NART appears to be unrelated to GDS scores (Knight et al., 2004).

Race/Ethnicity

A number of studies have found that older African Americans are less likely than their Caucasian counterparts to self-report depression, and, therefore, GDS scores underestimate depression in this group (see Stiles & McGarrahan, 1998 for review; see *Validity*).

NORMATIVE DATA

The norms were developed from small groups of normal and depressed elderly (Brink et al., 1982; Yesavage et al., 1983; Table 15–10). Table 15–11 provides cutoff scores for the 30-item and 15-item versions of the GDS (Brink et al., 1982; Yesavage et al., 1983, 1986; Sheik & Yesavage, 1986).

Rule et al. (1990) noted that, on the full GDS, mean performance in healthy individuals aged 17 to 55 years (5.83,

Table 15–10 Characteristics of the GDS Sample Used to Determine Interpretive Guide

Number	30-item: 20 normal elders, 51 elders receiving treatment for depression
Age (years)	>55
Geographic location	California, USA
Sample type	Normal subjects—elderly individuals recruited at local senior centers and housing projects Depressed subjects—elderly patients and outpatients in Veterans Administration, county, and private treatment settings
Education	Not reported
Gender	Not reported
Race/Ethnicity	Not reported
Screening	Diagnosed as mild or severe according to Research Diagnostic criteria for major affective disorder elicited during clinical interview.

Source: From Brink et al., 1982, and Yesavage et al., 1983.

Table 15–11 Cutoff Scores for the 30- and 15-item GDS

	Normal	Mild	Moderate	Severe
GDS-30	0–9	10–19	—	20–30
GDS-15	0–4	5–8	8–11	12–15

Note: The distinction between mild and severe depression is based on Research Diagnostic Criteria (Spitzer et al., 1978).

Sources: Brink et al., 1982; Yesavage et al., 1983; Sheik et al., 1986.

$SD = 4.52$) was similar to that seen in normal individuals aged 65 and older. Furthermore, fewer than 5% of young adults aged 17 to 20 enrolled in university obtained scores of 6 or greater on the 15-item short form (Ferraro & Chelminski, 1996). These findings attest to the wide applicability of the GDS.

RELIABILITY

Internal Consistency

The item-total correlations of the GDS range from .32 to .83, with a mean of .56 (Yesavage et al., 1983). In general, longer versions of the test have increased score reliability (Kieffer & Reese, 2002). For the 30-item GDS, internal consistency (alpha) is high, with values ranging from .82 to .94 (Chattat et al., 2001; Fernandez-San Martin et al., 2002; Knight et al., 2004; Lyons et al., 1989; Mui, 2003; Mui & Shibusawa, 2003; Parmelee et al., 1989; Rule et al., 1990; Yesavage et al., 1983). Split-half reliability ranges from .78 to .94 (Mui & Shibusawa, 2003; Yesavage et al., 1983). Abraham (1991) reported an internal consistency between .69 and .88 over 18 occasions during a 39-week period in frail, multiply impaired nursing home patients, aged 71 to 97 years, attesting to the longitudinal internal reliability of the GDS.

In community-dwelling older individuals, the 15-item short form (GDS-15) shows Cronbach's alpha values of .71 to .84 (Iglesias, 2004; Jang et al., 2001; Knight et al., 2004; Mui, 2003; Steiner et al., 1996) and split-half reliability of .73 (Jang et al., 2001). However, Cronbach's alpha has been found to range from .46 to .80 for the GDS-15 in samples of older medical inpatients and outpatients, raising concerns about the interpretation of the final score in this setting (Chattat et al., 2001; Incalzi et al., 2003). Internal consistency declines with increasing severity of Alzheimer's disease (AD), suggesting that it should not be used in the later stages of the disease (Muller-Thomsen et al., 2005; see also *Clinical Findings*).

Internal consistency of the 5-item version is low ($r = .49$), a not surprising finding given the reduction in the number of items (Chattat et al., 2001).

Test-Retest Reliability and Assessment of Change

Over intervals of 1 week to 2 months, test-retest correlations for the GDS-30 are high ($r = .80$ to .98; Ingram, 1996; Parmelee et al., 1989; Laprise & Vezina, 1998; Lyons et al., 1989; Yesavage et al., 1983). After intervals of about 6 months, correlations are lower, although still reasonable (>.70) for those with MMSE scores greater than 24; however, correlations deteriorate significantly (<.70) for cognitively impaired individuals (Bedard et al., 2003).

Test-retest reliability of the short forms (GDS-15, GDS-5) is high (.84 to .85) after an interval of about 7 to 14 days in cognitively intact older individuals (Mui et al., 2001; Rinaldi et al., 2003). Parmelee et al. (1989) reported that 1-year reliabilities were high (.86) in cognitively intact as well as impaired individuals; however, others have reported lower values after intervals of about 8 weeks in independent, community-dwelling individuals ($r = .67$, Ingram, 1996).

There is evidence that the GDS-15 is able to measure changes in depressive symptomatology. Vinkers et al. (2004) reported that the GDS-15 was able to detect change in depressive symptoms after a negative life event, loss of a partner. Scores in their subjects showed a gain of about 1.2 points, whereas scores in controls were unaltered. Based on these findings, the authors suggested that an increase of 2 points or more of the GDS-15 score is clinically relevant.

Alternate Form Reliability: Written Versus Oral Administration

The GDS was designed for self-administration, via written format. However, the test authors recommend that the examiner read the items if the client needs assistance. Although written and oral administrations yield adequate correlations for cognitively intact individuals ($r = .77$; Cannon et al., 2002), in general, high-functioning individuals endorse significantly more items on the written than on the oral administration (see also O'Neill et al., 1992). In addition, the correlation between oral and written versions is low ($r = .38$) for cognitively impaired individuals (those scoring below the cutoff of 123/144 on the Mattis DRS; Cannon et al., 2002). Individual item analysis reveals good consistency for high-functioning but not for low-functioning individuals (average kappa = .59 and .28, respectively). Such lack of agreement in test scores renders GDS results invalid in cognitively impaired individuals (Cannon et al., 2002). See *Validity* for further discussion.

VALIDITY

Factor Analytic Findings

Several studies have applied principal component analysis to the GDS long form (e.g., Abraham et al., 1994; Parmelee et al., 1989; Salamero & Marcs, 1992; Sheikh et al., 1991) but with little agreement. Sheikh et al. (1991) found five distinct factors, whereas Abraham et al. (1994) found a six-factor solution. Two other studies concluded that the GDS was basically unidimensional and strongly recommended the use of the single composite score (Parmelee et al., 1989; Salamero & Marcos, 1992).

The test and its various short forms have been translated into a number of languages. There is evidence, however, that the structure may not replicate across cultures (Jang et al., 2001), suggesting that the concept of depression may differ across cultures. Jang et al. (2001) used the GDS-15 and found a three-factor solution for the Korean version; however, in a U.S. sample, four factors were extracted.

Relationships With Other Tests

Test scores from the GDS correlate moderately well with other self-report measures such as the BDI (.73 to .90; Hyer & Blount, 1984; Laprise & Vezina, 1998; Scogin, 1987), the Zung scale (.59 to .89; Brink et al., 1982; Dunn & Sacco, 1989; Gilleard et al., 1981; Hickie & Snowden, 1987; Rule et al., 1989; Yesavage et al., 1983, 1986) and the Hamilton scale (.33 to .83; Brink et al., 1982; Clayton et al., 1997; Lyons et al., 1989; Salamero & Moarcos, 1982; Yesavage et al., 1983, 1986), providing support for the convergent validity of the GDS.

A number of studies have also compared scores from the GDS with cognitive screening tests (Blessed, MMSE) and found low correlations (e.g., Feher et al., 1992; Parmelee et al., 1991; Rapp et al., 1988), providing support for the divergent validity of the GDS.

Clinical Findings

The GDS has been extensively validated against a variety of criteria, including Research Diagnostic Criteria, DSM-III-R, structured interview (e.g., Dunn & Sacco, 1989; Gilley & Wilson, 1997; Laprise & Vezina, 1998; Lesher, 1986; Norris et al., 1987; Rapp et al., 1988; Yesavage et al., 1983), checklists (Dunn & Sacco, 1989; Parmelee et al., 1989), and consensual clinical diagnoses (Parmelee et al., 1989), with depressed individuals scoring significantly higher than nondepressed subjects on the GDS. The test is also sensitive to severity of depression in the elderly (Parmelee et al., 1989; Yesavage et al., 1983) and appears to be as useful as other measures (e.g., BDI) in identifying depression (Laprise and Vezina, 1998; Scogin, 1987; Tamkin et al., 1985). Nonresponse rates of items on the BDI-II and GDS appear to be quantitatively equivalent (Jefferson et al., 2001). Further, the GDS appears comparable to the Beck Depression Inventory in detecting change in mood (Scogin, 1987).

In their initial validation studies, the authors of the GDS set a score of 11 as the cutoff for depression on the scale (Brink et al., 1982; Yesavage et al., 1983). This score provided a sensitivity/specificity ratio of 84%/95%, which they believed would offer the best balance of false positives and false negatives. They also reported that a cutoff value of 14, while lowering the sensitivity to 80%, raised the specificity to 100%. Since the initial validation studies, numerous other studies have examined the sensitivity and specificity of the GDS in diverse populations, with a wide range of results and no clear consensus (for review, see Stiles & McGarrahan, 1998). For example, a cut-score of 12 on the GDS has been recommended to detect depression in older adults (Lavretsky & Kumar, 2002). Such a cut-score has been found to have sensitivities ranging from 83% to 89% and specificities from 68% to 80% for major depression in primary care settings (Watson & Pignone, 2003). The average age of participant in these studies was close to 70 years. However, such a cutoff performs poorly in other samples. For example, Watson & Pignone (2003) reported that, in healthy retirees aged about 80 years, a cutoff of 12 resulted in a sensitivity of 60% for major depression and a specificity of 93%. The positive predictive value, which takes into account the prevalence of the disorder with a positive screening test, was only 55%, which is no better than chance. The negative predictive value (probability that an individual with a negative screening test is truly free of the disorder) was 95%. Using optimal cutoff points based on ROC analysis, a score of 9 or more on the GDS captured 80% of the major depression cases (specificity was 85%). When used to detect minor depression, the GDS lost accuracy, with a sensitivity of 33% using a cut-score of 12 (Watson et al., 2004) and 70% using a cutpoint of 10 (Lyness et al., 1999).

Cultural factors also affect sensitivity and specificity. For example, Robison et al.s (2002) noted that the optimal cutpoint (based on ROC analyses) for Hispanic primary care patients (aged 50 years and older) was 13 on the 30-item GDS and resulted in a sensitivity of 81% and a specificity of 65%. The authors noted that the GDS displayed sensitivity and specificity rates similar to those of the 10-item CES-D but was lengthier to administer. The GDS-15 displayed a poorer combination of sensitivity (73%) and specificity (71%). In their review, Mui et al. (2001) concluded that neither the long nor the short form of the GDS was adequate for cross-cultural use.

These studies illustrate that the conventional guidelines may not be the most clinically efficient ones for use in all samples to screen for the presence of depression. In addition to level of depression, state of health (e.g., patient versus community sample), ethnicity/cultural factors, and the underlying prevalence of disorders may also affect sensitivity and specificity. The purpose of the assessment also affects the cut-point (e.g., is the purpose to rule in or rule out depression). The lower the cutoff, the higher the sensitivity and the lower the specificity. The higher the cutoff, the lower the sensitivity and the higher the specificity.

It is important to bear in mind that cognitive impairment can render test scores invalid (Brink, 1984; Burke et al., 1989; Burke et al., 1991; Cannon et al., 2002; de Craen et al., 2003; Feher et al., 1992; Ferrario et al., 1990; Gilley & Wilson, 1997; Montorio & Izal, 1996; Nussbaum & Sauer, 1993; but see Burke et al., 1992; Parmelee et al., 1989). For example, Bedard et al. (2003) found that, compared with individuals with MMSE scores of 29 to 30, those with scores of 18 or less answered fewer items and tended to display a positive response set bias. They suggested that the GDS score should not be interpreted once MMSE scores decline below 20. In general, cognitive impairment tends to suppress GDS scores such that there is underidentification of the level of depressive symptomatology (Gilley & Wilson, 1997). Obviously, use of the GDS or other self-

report measures with persons who have impaired insight is not recommended (e.g., Feher et al., 1992; Ott & Fogel, 1992).

The GDS correlates substantially with physical health and functional status, underscoring the important relation between health and depression (Jongenelis et al., 2004; Parmelee et al., 1989; Steiner et al., 1996). In addition, there is evidence that patients with mild cognitive impairment and depression are at increased risk, compared to those without depression, for development of AD, raising the question of a common neurobiological basis for both disorders (Modrego & Ferrandez, 2004). Further, cerebrovascular disease may be a factor in the pathogenesis of some forms of late-life depression. MRI studies of older adults suggest a relationship between hyperintensities in the deep white matter and depressive symptoms on the GDS, especially of impaired motivation, concentration, and decision making; this relationship is especially strong in individuals carrying the APOE-4 allele (Nebes et al., 2001).

Finally, it should be noted that the GDS, although designed for use with the elderly, may also prove useful in other age groups and diagnostic categories where core symptoms may be confused with depression. For example, Zalsman et al. (2001) found the GDS-15 useful for the detection of depression in adolescents diagnosed with anorexia nervosa. In this group, weight loss is a core symptom of the disorder, even in the absence of depression.

Long Versus Short Forms

The 15-item version correlates highly ($r = .66$ to .92) with the full GDS (e.g., Alden et al., 1989; Chattat et al., 2001; Ingram, 1996; Knight et al., 2004; Lesher & Berryhill, 1994; Sheikh & Yesavage, 1986) and with other measures such as the BDI ($r = .84$; Ferraro & Chelminski, 1996; Zalsman et al., 2001), the Zung Self-Rating Depression Scale (Iglesias, 2004) and CESD ($r = .68$, Knight et al., 2004), providing some support for its concurrent validity. Evaluation of diagnostic validity suggests that the short form has sensitivity and specificity similar to those of the long form (Lesher & Berryhill, 1994) and may be better than other tools (e.g., Minimum Data Set) in identifying depression (Heiser, 2004). However, classification congruence between the short and long forms of the GDS in community-dwelling older adults can be poor. Ingram (1996) reported that, among 15 of 73 individuals categorized as depressed by the GDS, 9 (60%) were classed as not depressed by the short form.

The correlation of the GDS-5 with the complete GDS is respectable ($r = .82$; Chattat et al., 2001). The GDS-5 appears to be as effective as the GDS-15 for the screening of depression in cognitively intact older adult patients (Chattat et al., 2001; Rinaldi et al., 2003; Wall et al., 1999). For example, Rinaldi et al. (2003) reported that, in a geriatric setting, a cutoff of 2 on the GDS-5 had a sensitivity of .94 (.92 for a cutoff of >5 on the GDS-15 version), a specificity of .81 (.83 for the GDS-15), a positive predictive value of 0.81 (.83 for the GDS-15), and a negative predictive value of 0.94 (.92 for the GDS-15). The various short forms appear to be good screening instruments for depression, but usually at the expense of specificity and positive predictive power (Almeida & Almeida, 1999; Chattat et al., 2001; Lesher & Berryhill, 1994).

In the presence of cognitive deficits, the full GDS may be particularly burdensome for both patient and examiner, and some have suggested that the completion rates and reliability of the scale may be improved with the use of one of the short forms. Unfortunately, although some have found satisfactory sensitivity and specificity rates with short forms in cognitively impaired older adults (e.g., 4 items, Cheng & Chan, 2004; 10 and 15 item, Shah et al., 1996; 4 and 15 items, Valeria et al. 2001; 15 items, Wall et al., 1999), others have found inadequate sensitivity rates (e.g., 15 items, Burke et al., 1992; 4 items, Shah et al., 1996). Discrepancies most likely relate to differences in item sets and different prevalence and severity rates of depressive symptomatology, as well as the severity of cognitive impairment. Bedard et al. (2003) suggested caution in interpreting GDS scores on both long and short forms in individuals with MMSE scores lower than 20. (See also *Response Biases*.)

Response Biases

It is important to note that the GDS is dichotomously scored, and blind application of cutoff scores neglects the possibility that the patient may have responded to items in a random fashion or may have put forth incomplete effort. In fact, scores falling in the "mild" range (11–20), do not differ significantly from chance responding ($p < .05$; Woodard & Axelrod, 1999). Demented individuals may be more likely to produce a random or pseudorandom response pattern. In one sample of cognitively impaired individuals, almost half of the GDS scores were in the chance range, raising questions about the accuracy of their responses and overall test-taking approach. Woodard and Axelrod (1999) cautioned that verification of depressive symptomatology in such cases requires referral to external data (e.g., behavioral observations, reports from caregiver).

COMMENT

The GDS is a fairly brief, easy to administer task developed specifically for older populations. A strength of the GDS is that it deliberately omits items dealing with guilt, sexuality, and suicide, which the authors considered inappropriate for elderly subjects. It also contains no somatic items that might inflate scores. Rather, it includes items dealing with perceived locus of control, making this test more suitable for subjects in hospital or long-term care. The yes/no format makes fewer demands on the cognitive skills of the patient and leads to better completion rates than point-scales such as the BDI in clinical populations with mild cognitive impairment (Dunn & Sacco, 1989; Norris et al., 1987). Completion rates of the GDS are also higher than multiple-choice measures such as the Zung Self Rating Depression Scale (Dunn & Sacco, 1989).

The GDS can be given in written or oral format. The oral format is available if patients are unable to read or complete the scale independently. However, in answering questions, clients may make lengthy and vague responses, rendering scoring difficult. Standardization of the oral administration procedure and detailed scoring criteria are needed to ensure that the test is used in a reliable manner (Wong et al., 2002). Further, the written administration results in greater item endorsement, suggesting that this format is preferred to elicit the greatest degree of openness in self-report (Cannon et al., 2002). Obviously, the test cannot be used if comprehension or awareness of deficits is seriously impaired (Feher et al., 1994). The test also should not be used to screen for depression in those with moderate cognitive impairment (e.g., MMSE scores <20), regardless of the method of administration. In such cases, close informants should be consulted about depressive symptoms.

It is important to note that the description of the original normative sample is sparse and that it consists of very few individuals, with an unknown age range. Subsequent studies have suggested that age has little impact on test scores, supporting its use over a wide spectrum of ages. However, the impacts of gender and race/ethnicity are less clear. The question of whether separate cutoffs are needed for certain groups (e.g., males versus females, African Americans versus Caucasians) requires additional research.

The GDS has been shown to have high internal consistency and is stable over time in older adults (Stiles & McGarrahan, 1998). Validity has also been demonstrated by comparing the results of the GDS with clinical diagnoses and with other scales that purport to measure depression. There is also evidence of divergent validity. Factorial studies have produced mixed results; in the absence of consistent findings, the scale should be used as a single-factor instrument (Miu et al., 2001; Stiles & McGarrahan, 1998).

In general, research shows that the utility of the English version of the GDS is satisfactory, with sensitivity and specificity scores typically exceeding 80% in community-dwelling persons and physically impaired patients (see Stiles & McGarrahan, 1998, for a review). A conventional cut-score of 11 or 12 has been recommended to screen for the presence of depression. However, depending on factors such as the prevalence of the disorder and the relative importance of sensitivity and specificity, the cut-point may have to be altered to improve recognition of clinically significant depression. For example, to detect major depression in healthy community-dwelling elderly, a score of 9 may be optimal (Watson et al., 2004). By contrast, to identify suicidal ideation in geriatric patients, a cut-off of 15 may be most effective (Uncapher and Sandberg, 1998). However, it should be noted that there are no items on the test that specifically address suicidal ideation.

The simplicity, reliability, and validity of the GDS have encouraged its translation into numerous languages and its use in various cultures. Studies that evaluate the utility of the instrument in different cultural groups are, however, inconclusive (Mui et al., 2001). Because of cultural differences in the expression of emotion, high scores may not signify depression (Jang et al., 2001). Similarly, low scores may not mean absence of depression, because individuals from some ethnic groups may endorse somatic items, which are purposely excluded from the GDS, rather than affective items as idioms of distress (Robison et al., 2002). In such cases, the GDS should be used with considerable caution (Stiles & McGarrahan, 1998), and other measures (e.g., BDI, CES-D) may be preferred (see also Mui et al., 2001). Additional research is needed to evaluate the cultural sensitivity of the various screening instruments.

It is also important to bear in mind that recommended cut-off scores of 11 or greater actually fall in the range of random responding. Reporting the presence of depressive symptomatology based on blind interpretation of a score that simply exceeds the cutoff yet falls in the range of random responding can be extremely misleading if other information is not taken into account (Woodard & Axelrod, 1999). Although scores that exceed chance can be interpreted with greater confidence, scores in the chance range require greater consideration to assess response validity (Woodard & Axelrod, 1999). It is extremely important to use the GDS as a screening rather than a diagnostic tool, in view of the potential for errors in classification (Woodard & Axelrod, 1999; Yesavage et al., 1983).

Various brief versions have been proposed as time-saving alternatives. The 15-item version is popular and appears to be sensitive to change. However, the extent to which the GDS-15 is representative of or as reliable as the long form is questionable (Mui et al., 2001). In addition, diagnostic accuracy is reduced with this form, at least in some populations (e.g., Hispanic; Robison et al., 2002), including cognitively impaired individuals. The 4 or 5-item versions may be a better screening instruments than the GDS-15 (Cheng & Chan, 2004; Rinaldi et al., 2003). However, additional studies are needed that compare these short forms with different screening instruments in the same sample. Therefore, at this time, it is still advisable to use the long form whenever possible (Stiles & McGarrahan, 1998).

REFERENCES

Abraham, I. L. (1991). The Geriatric Depression Scale and Hopelessness Index: Longitudinal psychometric data on frail nursing home residents. *Perceptual and Motor Skills, 72,* 875–880.

Abraham, I. L., Wofford, A. B., Lichtenberg, P. A., & Holroyd, S. (1994). Factor structure of the Geriatric Depression Scale in a cohort of depressed nursing-home residents. *International Journal of Geriatric Psychiatry, 9,* 611–617.

Alden, D., Austin, C. N., & Sturgeon, R. (1989). A correlation between the Geriatric Depression Scale long and short form. *Journal of Gerontology, 44,* 124–125.

Allen-Burge, R., Storandt, M., Kinscherf, D. A., & Rubin, E. H. (1994). Sex differences in the sensitivity of two self-report depression scales in older depressed inpatients. *Psychology and Aging, 9,* 443–445.

Almeida, O. P., & Almeida, S. A. (1999). Short versions of the Geriatric Depression Scale: A study of their validity for the diagnosis of a major depressive episode according to ICD-10 and DSM-IV. *International Journal of Geriatric Psychiatry, 14,* 858–865.

Bedard, M., Molloy, D. W., Squire, L., Minthorn-Biggs, M-B., Dubois, S., Lever, J. A., & O'Donnell, M. (2003). Validity of self-reports in dementia research: The Geriatric Depression Scale. *Clinical Gerontologist, 26,* 155–163.

Brink, T. L. (1984). Limitations of the GDS in cases of pseudodementia. *Clinical Gerontology, 2,* 60–61.

Brink, T. L., Yesavage, J. A., Lum, O., Heersema, P. H., Adey, M., & Rose, T. S. (1982). Screening tests for geriatric depression. *Clinical Gerontologist, 1,* 37–43.

Burke, W. J., Houston, M. J., Boust, S. J., & Roccaforte, W. H. (1989). Use of the Geriatric Depression Scale in dementia of the Alzheimer type. *Journal of the American Geriatrics Society, 37,* 856–860.

Burke, W. J., Nitcher, R. L., Roccaforte, W. H., & Wengel, S. P. (1992). A prospective evaluation of the Geriatric Depression Scale in an outpatient geriatric assessment center. *Journal of the American Geriatrics Society, 40,* 1227–1230.

Burke, W. J., Roccaforte, W. H., & Wengel, S. P. (1991). The short form of the Geriatric Depression Scale: A comparison with the 30-item form. *Journal of Geriatric Psychiatry and Neurology, 4,* 173–178.

Cannon, B. J., Thaler, T., & Roos, S. (2002). Oral verus written administration of the Geriatric Depression Scale. *Aging and Mental Health, 6,* 418–422.

Chattat, R., Ellena, L., Cucinotta, D., Savorani, G., & Mucciarelli, G. (2001). A study of the validity of different short versions of the Geriatric Depression Scale. *Archives of Gerontology and Geriatrics Supplement, 7,* 81–86.

Cheng, S-T., & Chan, A.C.M. (2004). A brief version of the Geriatric Depression Scale for the Chinese. *Psychological Assessment, 16,* 182–186.

Chou, K-L., & Chi, I. (2005). Prevalence and correlates of depression in Chinese oldest-old. *International Journal of Geriatric Psychiatry, 20,* 41–50.

Clayton, A. H., Holroyd, S., & Sheldon-Keller, A. (1997). Geriatric Depression Scale vs. Hamilton Rating Scale for Depression in a sample of anxiety patients. *Clinical Gerontologist, 17,* 3–13.

Colenda, C., & Smith, S. (1993). Multivariate modelling of anxiety and depression in community-dwelling elderly persons. *American Journal of Geriatric Psychiatry, 1,* 327–338.

D'Ath, P., Katona, P., & Mullan, E. (1994). Screening detection and management of depression in elderly primary care attenders: The acceptability and performance of the 15 item Geriatric Depression Scale (GDS 15) and the development of short version. *Family Practice, 1,* 260–266.

De Craen, A., Heeren, T. J., & Gussekloo, J. (2003). Accuracy of the 15-item Geriatric Depression Scale (GDS-15) in a community sample of the oldest old. *International Journal of Geriatric Psychiatry, 18,* 63–66.

Dunn, V. K., & Sacco, W. P. (1989). Psychometric evaluation of the Geriatric Depression Scale and the Zung Self-Rating Depression Scale using an elderly community sample. *Psychology and Aging, 4,* 125–126.

Feher, E. P., Larrabee, G. J., & Crook, T. H. (1992). Factors attenuating the validity of the Geriatric Depression Scale in a dementia population. *Journal of the American Geriatrics Society, 40,* 906–909.

Fernandez-San Martin, M. I., Andrade, C., Molina, J., Munoz, P. E., Carretero, B., Rodriguez, M., & Silva, A. (2002). Validation of the Spanish version of the Geriatric Depression Scale (GDS) in primary care. *International Journal of Geriatric Psychiatry, 17,* 279–287.

Ferrario, E., Cappa, G., Bertone, O., Poli, L., & Fabris, F. (1990). Geriatric Depression Scale and assessment of cognitive-behavioural disturbances in the elderly: A preliminary report on an Italian sample. *Clinical Gerontologist, 10,* 67–73.

Ferraro, F. R., & Chelminski, I. (1996). Preliminary normative data on the Geriatric Depression Scale–Short Form (GDS-SF) in a young adult sample. *Journal of Clinical Psychology, 52,* 443–447.

Galaria, I. I., Casten, R. J., & Rovner, B. W. (2000). Development of a shorter version of the Geriatric Depression Scale for visually impaired older patients. *International Psychogeriatrics, 12,* 435–443.

Gilleard, C. J., Willmott, M., & Vaddadi, K. S. (1981). Self-report measures of mood and morale in elderly depressives. *British Journal of Psychiatry, 138,* 230–235.

Gilley, D. W., & Wilson, R. S. (1997). Criterion-related validity of the Geriatric Depression Scale in Alzheimer's disease. *Journal of Clinical & Experimental Neuropsychology, 19,* 489–499.

Gori, C., Appollonio, I., Riva, G. P., Spiga, D., Ferrari, A., Trabucchi, M., & Frattola, L. (1998). Using a single question to screen for depression in the nursing home. *Archives of Gerontology and Geriatrics Supplement, 6,* 235–240.

Heiser, D. (2004). Depression identification in the long-term care setting: The GDS vs. the MDS. *Clinical Gerontologist, 27,* 3–18.

Hickie, C., & Snowdon, J. (1987). Depression scales for the elderly: GDS, Gilleard, Zung. *Clinical Gerontologist, 6,* 51–53.

Hoyl, M. T., Alessi, C. A., Harker, J. O., Josephson, K. R., Pietruszka, F. M., Koelfgen, M., Mervis, J. R., Fitten, L. J., & Rubenstein, L. Z. (1999). Development and testing of a five-items version of the Geriatric Screening Scale. *Journal of the American Geriatric Society, 47,* 873–878.

Hyer, L., & Blount, J. (1984). Concurrent and discriminant validities of the GDS with older psychiatric patients. *Psychological Reports, 54,* 611–616.

Iglesias, G. H. (2004). Geriatric Depression Scale short form and Zung Self-Rating Depression Scale: A study of homebound elders. *Clinical Gerontologist, 27,* 55–66.

Incalzi, R. A., Cesari, M., Pedone, C., & Carbonin, P. (2003). Construct validity of the 15-item Geriatric Depression Scale in older medical inpatients. *Journal of Geriatric Psychiatry and Neurology, 16,* 23–28.

Ingram, F. (1996). The short Geriatric Depression Scale: A comparison with the standard form in independent older adults. *Clinical Gerontologist, 16,* 49–56.

Jang, Y., Small, B. J., & Haley, W. E. (2001). Cross-cultural comparability of the Geriatric Depression Scale: Comparison between older Koreans and older Americans. *Aging and Mental Health, 5,* 31–37.

Jefferson, A. L., Powers, D. V., & Pope, M. (2001). Beck Depression Inventory-II (BDI-II) and the Geriatric Depression Scale (GDS) in older women. *Clinical Gerontologist, 22,* 3–12.

Jongenelis, K., Pot, A. M., Eisses, A. M. H. et al. (2004). Prevalence and risk indicators of depression in elderly nursing home patients: The AGED study. *Journal of Affective Disorders, 83,* 135–142.

Kieffer, K. M., & Reese, R. J. (2002). A reliability generalization study of the Geriatric Depression Scale. *Educational and Psychological Measurement, 62,* 969–994.

Knight, R. G., McMahon, J., Green, T. J., & Skeaf, C. M. (2004). Some normative and psychometric data for the Geriatric Depression Scale and the Cognitive Failures Questionnaire from a sample of healthy older persons. *New Zealand Journal of Psychology, 33,* 163–170.

Laprise, R., & Vezina, J. (1998). Diagnostic performance of the Geriatric Depression Scale and the Beck Depression Inventory with nursing home residents. *Canadian Journal on Aging, 17,* 401–413.

Lavretsky, H., & Kumar, A. (2002). Clinically significant non-major depression: Old concepts, new insights. *American Journal Geriatric Psychiatry, 10,* 239–255.

Lebowitz, B. D., Pearson, J. L., Schneider, L. S., Reynolds, C. F. 3rd, Alexopoulos, G. S., Bruce, M. L., Conwell, Y., Katz, I. R., Meyers, B. S., Morrison, M. F., Mossey, J., Niederehe, G., & Parmelee, P. (1997). Diagnosis and treatment of depression in late life: Consensus statement update. *Journal of the American Medical Association, 278,* 1186–1190.

Lesher, E. L. (1986). Validation of the Geriatric Depression Scale among nursing home residents. *Clinical Gerontologist, 4,* 21–28.

Lesher, E. L., & Berryhill, J. S. (1994). Validation of the Geriatric Depression Scale–Short Form among inpatients. *Journal of Clinical Psychology, 50,* 256–260.

Lyons, J. S., Strain, J. J., Hammer, J. S., Ackerman, A. D., & Fulop, G. (1989). Reliability, validity, and temporal stability of the Geriatric Depression Scale in hospitalized patients. *International Journal of Psychiatry in Medicine, 19,* 203–209.

Lyness, J. M., King, D. A., Cox, C., Yoediono, Z., & Caine, E. D. (1999). The importance of subsyndromal depression in older primary care patients: Prevalence and associated functional disability. *Journal of the American Geriatric Society, 47,* 647–652.

Modrego, P. J., & Ferrandez, J. (2004). Depression in patients with mild cognitive impairment increases the risk of developing dementia of Alzheimer type. *Archives of Neurology, 61,* 1290–1293.

Monopoli, J., & Vaccaro, F. (1998). Depression, hypochondriasis and demographic variables in a non-institutionalized elderly sample. *Clinical Gerontologist, 19,* 75–78.

Montorio, I., & Izal, M. (1996). The Geriatric Depression Scale: A review of its development and utility. *International Psychogeriatrics, 8,* 103–112.

Mui, A. C., & Shibusawa, T. (2003). Japanese American elders and the Geriatric Depression Scale. *The Clinical Gerontologist, 26,* 91–104.

Mui, A. C., Burnette, D., & Chen, L. M. (2001). Cross-cultural assessment of geriatric depression: A review of the CES-D and the GDS. *Journal of Mental Health and Aging, 7,* 137–164.

Muller-Thomsen, T., Arlt, S., Mann, U., Mass, R., Ganzer, S. (2005). Detecting depression in Alzheimer's disease: Evaluation of four different scales. *Archives of Clinical Neuropsychology, 20,* 271–276.

Nebes, R. D., Vora, I. J., Meltzer, C. C., Fukui, M. B., Williams, R. L., Kamboh, M. I., Saxton, J., Houck, P. R., DeKosky, S. T., & Reynolds, C. F. (2001). Relationship of deep white matter hyperintensities and apoliprotein E genotype to depressive symptoms in older adults without clinical depression. *American Journal of Psychiatry, 158,* 878–884.

Norris, J. T., Gallagher, D., Wilson, A., & Winograd, C. H. (1987). Assessment of depression in geriatric medical outpatients: The validity of two screening measures. *Journal of the American Geriatrics Society, 35,* 989–995.

Nussbaum, P. D., & Sauer. L. (1993). Self-report of depression in elderly with and without progressive cognitive deterioration. *Clinical Gerontologist, 13,* 69–79.

O'Neill, D., Rice, I., Blake, P., & Walsh, J. B. (1992). The Geriatric Depression Scale: Rater-administered or self-administered? *International Journal of Geriatric Psychiatry, 7,* 511–515.

Ott, B. R., & Fogel, B. S. (1992). Measurement of depression in dementia: Self vs. clinician rating. *International Journal of Geriatric Psychiatry, 7,* 899–904.

Parmelee, P. A., Lawton, M. P., & Katz, I. R. (1989). Psychometric properties of the Geriatric Depression Scale among the institutionalized aged. *Psychological Assessment, 1,* 331–338.

Rapp, S. R., Parisi, S. A., Walsh, D. A., & Wallace, C. E. (1988). Detecting depression in elderly medical inpatients. *Journal of Consulting and Clinical Psychology, 56,* 509–513.

Rinaldi, P., Mecocci, P., Benedetti, C., Ercolani, S., Bregnocchi, M., Menculini, G., Catani, M., Senin, U., & Cherubini, A. (2003). Validation of the five-item Geriatric Depression Scale in elderly subjects in three different settings. *Journal of the American Geriatric Society, 51,* 694–698.

Robison, J., Gruman, C., Gaztambide, S., & Blank, K. (2002). Screening for depression in middle-aged and older Puerto Rican primary care patients. *Journal of Gerontology, 57A,* M308–M314.

Rule, B. G., Harvey, H. Z., & Dobbs, A. R. (1989). Reliability of the Geriatric Depression Scale for younger adults. *Clinical Gerontologist, 9,* 37–43.

Salamero, M., & Marcus, T. (1992). Factor study of the Geriatric Depression Scale. *Acta Psychiatrica Scandinavica, 86,* 282–286.

Scogin, F. (1987). The concurrent validity of the Geriatric Depression Scale with depressed older adults. *Clinical Gerontologist, 7,* 23–31.

Shah, A., Phongsathorn, V., Bielawska, C., & Katona, C. (1996). Screening for depression among geriatric inpatients with short versions of the Geriatric Depression Scale. *International Journal of Geriatric Psychiatry, 11,* 915–918.

Sheikh, J. I., & Yesavage, J. A. (1986). Geriatric Depression Scale (GDS): Recent evidence and development of a shorter version. *Clinical Gerontologist, 5,* 165–173.

Shiekh, J. J., Yesavage, J. A., & Brooke, J. O. (1991). Proposed factor structure of the Geriatric Depression Scale. *International Psychogeriatrics, 3,* 23–28.

Steiner, A., Raube, K., Stuck, A. E., Aronow, H. U., Draper, D., Rubenstein, L. Z., & Beck, J. C. (1996). Measuring psychosocial aspects of well-being in older community residents: Performance of four short scales. *The Gerontologist, 36,* 54–62.

Stiles, P. G., & McGarrahan, J. F. (1998). The Geriatric Depression Scale: A comprehensive review. *Journal of Clinical Geropsychology, 4,* 89–110.

Sutcliffe, C., Cordingly, L., Burns, A., Mozley, C., Bagley, H., Uxley, P., & Challis, D. (2000). A new version of the Geriatric Depression Scale for nursing and residential home populations: The Geriatric Depression Scale (Residential) (GDS-12R). *International Psychogeriatrics, 12,* 173–181.

Tamkin, A. S., Carson, M. F., Nixon, D. H., & Hyer, L. A. (1985). A comparison among some measures of depression in alcoholics. *IRCS Medical Science: Psychology & Psychiatry, 13,* 231.

Uncapher, H., & Sandberg, D. A. (1998). Using the Geriatric Depression Scale to detect suicidal ideation in inpatient older adults. *Journal of Clinical Geropsychology, 4,* 349–358.

Valeria, I., Villa, M. L., & Appolonio, I. (2001). Screening and quantification of depression in mild-to-moderate dementia through the GDS short forms. *Clinical Gerontologist, 24,* 115–125.

Vinkers, D. J., Gussekloo, J., Stek, M. L., Westendorp, R. G. J., & van der Mast, R. C. (2004). The 15-item Geriatric Depression Scale (GDS-15) detects changes in depressive symptoms after a major life event. The Leiden 85-Plus Study. *International Journal of Geriatric Psychiatry, 19,* 80–84.

Wall, J. R., Lichtenberg, P. A., MacNeill, S. E., Walsh, P., & Deshpande, S. A. (1999). Depression detection in geriatric rehabilitation: Geriatric Depression Scale short form vs. long form. *Clinical Gerontologist, 20,* 13–21.

Watson, L. C., Lewis, C. L., Kistler, C., Amick, H. R., & Boustani, M. (2004). Can we trust depression screening instruments in healthy "old–old" adults? *International Journal of Geriatric Psychiatry, 19,* 278–285.

Watson, L. C., & Pignone, M. P. (2003). Screening accuracy for late-life depression in primary care: A systematic review. *Journal of Family Practice, 52,* 956–964.

Wong, M. T. P., Ho, T. P., Ho, M. Y., Yu, C. S., Wong, Y. H., & Lee, S. Y. (2002). Development and inter-rater reliability of a standardized verbal instruction manual for the Chinese Geriatric Depression Scale–short form. *International Journal of Geriatric Psychiatry, 17,* 459–463.

Woodard, J. L., & Axelrod, B. N. (1999). Interpretative guidelines for neuropsychiatric measures with dichotomously scored items. *International Journal of Geriatric Psychiatry, 14,* 385–388.

Yesavage, J. A., Brink, T. L., Rose, T. L., & Adey, M. (1986). The Geriatric Depression Rating Scale: Comparison with other self-report and psychiatric rating scales. In L. W. Poon (Ed.), *Handbook of clinical memory assessment of older adults* (pp. 153–167). Washington, DC: American Psychological Association.

Yesavage, J. A., Brink, T. L., Rose, T. L., Lum, O., Huang, V., Adey, M. B., & Leirer, V. O. (1983). Development and validation of a geriatric depression rating scale: A preliminary report. *Journal of Psychiatric Research, 17,* 37–49.

Zalsman, G., Weizman, A., Carel, C. A., & Aizenberg, D. (2001). Geriatric Depression Scale (GDS-15): A sensitive and convenient instrument for measuring depression in young anorexic patients. *Journal of Nervous and Mental Disease, 189,* 338–339.

Instrumental Activities of Daily Living (IADL)

PURPOSE

The Instrumental Activities of Daily Living (IADL) is a caregiver/informant-based rating scale designed to measure functional status.

SOURCE

There is no commercial source. Users can refer to Figure 15–2.

AGE RANGE

The test was designed for use with older individuals.

DESCRIPTION

Interest in the ability to live independently has increased for a number of reasons, including the growing numbers of older adults who require nursing home placement or family support, the rapidly escalating financial burden of such arrangements, and the psychosocial implications for the individual and his or her family and friends. Two major categories of functional abilities are commonly distinguished: (a) activities of daily living, commonly known as ADLs, which focus primarily on overlearned self-care activities such as feeding, bathing, toileting, and basic mobility, and (b) instrumental activities of daily living, commonly known as IADLs, which

Figure 15–2 Instrumental Activities of Daily Living. Note for the MAI version (Lawton et al., 1982; Lawton, 1988), a ninth item is added: Can do own handyman work. Also, each item is rated on a three-point scale: 3, can do without help; 2, can do with some help; 1, completely unable to do. *Sources:* Lawton & Brody, 1969.

For each item listed below, please circle one number which best describes the person's abilities.

1. Ability to use telephone.
   1. Operates telephone on own initiative—looks up and dials numbers etc.
   2. Dials a few well-known numbers
   3. Answers telephone but does not dial
   4. Does not telephone at all

2. Shopping
   1. Takes care of all shopping needs independently
   2. Shops independently for small purchases
   3. Needs to be accompanied on any shopping trip
   4. Completely unable to shop

3. Food Preparation
   1. Plans, prepares and serves adequate meals independently
   2. Prepares adequate meals if supplied with ingredients
   3. Heats and serves prepared meals OR prepares meals but does not maintain adequate diet
   4. Needs to have meals prepared and served

4. Housekeeping
   1. Maintains house alone or with occasional assistance (e.g., heavy work-domestic assistance)
   2. Performs light daily tasks such as dishwashing, bed making
   3. Performs light daily tasks but cannot maintain acceptable level of cleanliness
   4. Needs help with all home maintenance tasks
   5. Does not participate in any housekeeping tasks

5. Laundry
   1. Does personal laundry completely
   2. Launders small items, rinses socks, stockings, etc.
   3. All laundry must be done by others

6. Mode of Transportation
   1. Travels independently on public transportation or drives own car
   2. Arranges own travel via taxi, but does not otherwise use public transportation
   3. Travels on public transportation when assisted or accompanied by another
   4. Travel limited to taxi or automobile with assistance of another
   5. Does not travel at all

7. Responsibility for own medications
   1. Is responsible for taking medication in correct dosages at correct time
   2. Takes responsibility if medication is prepared in advance in separate dosages
   3. Is not capable of dispensing own medication

8. Ability to handle finances
   1. Manages financial matters independently (budgets, writes checks, pays rent, bills, goes to bank), collects and keeps track of income.
   2. Manages day-to-day purchases, but needs help with banking, major purchases, etc.
   3. Incapable of handling money.

Table 15–12 Characteristics of the IADL Normative Sample (MAI Version)

Number	253
Age (years)	Mean = 76.0
Geographic location	Five census tracts in Philadelphia
Sample type	Sample of Social Security recipients recruited to represent three living arrangement groups of each gender (live-alones, marital pairs alone, residence with a younger family member)
Education (years)	Mean = 9.2
Gender (%)	
Men	43
Women	57
Race/Ethnicity	94% Caucasian
Screening	Not reported

are viewed as involving fairly complex cognitive abilities and include activities such as managing medication, managing finances, using transportation, using the telephone, maintaining one's household (housekeeping), meal preparation, and nutrition. It is the IADLs that are of primary interest to neuropsychologists, because loss of competence in complex tasks of daily living is a defining diagnostic feature of Alzheimer's disease (AD) and related dementing disorders (American Psychiatric Association, 1994). Decline is often noted in IADLs before declines in self-maintenance tasks (ADLs; e.g., Juva et al., 1994; Njegovan et al., 2001). This is not surprising, given that IADLS rely on complex cognitive processes that may be affected early in the course of the disorder (Willis et al., 1998). Indeed, it is a person's inability to perform these demanding everyday tasks (e.g., taking medication, managing financial affairs, driving) that frequently motivates the family to seek assessment (Willis et al., 1998).

The IADL, developed by Lawton and Brody (1969), has been used extensively in gerontological research. It is a Likert-type evaluation of the rater's perception of the client's everyday competence in eight domains (telephone usage, food preparation, housekeeping, laundry, mode of transportation, shopping, ability to handle finances, and responsibility for own medications (see Figure 15–2).

These items were also incorporated into the Philadelphia Geriatric Multilevel Assessment Instrument (MAI; Lawton et al., 1982). However, these items ask whether the person can (as opposed to does) perform a task; this avoids the problems associated with sex-role or situation-limited aspects of some of the tasks (e.g., cooking). A ninth item, "Can do own handyman work" is also included. In addition, each item is rated on a 3-point scale (3 = can do without help; 2 = can do with some help; 1 = completely unable to do).

A self-rated version (Lawton & Brody, 1988) has also been developed. This version uses similar items as the informant version. Each item is rated on the same 3-point scale as the IADL. We focus mainly on the informant version here, because much of the literature pertains to this form.

ADMINISTRATION

A respondent who is familiar with the patient reads each item and rates each item. Some of the items depend on gender. In fact, cooking meals, housekeeping, and washing clothes are traditionally seen as feminine roles, particularly in the older generations. Lawton and Brody (1969) recommended that these items be excluded when evaluating men.

ADMINISTRATION TIME

About 10 min is needed to complete the form.

SCORING

Authors differ in their scoring of the IADL. For example, according to Lawton and Brody (1969), item scores of 1 reflect complete independence in performing the task, and scores of 0 reflect partial or complete dependence. By contrast, others (e.g., Bertrand et al., 2001; Boyle et al., 2002) employ a greater range of scores to increase sensitivity, with scores of 0 used to reflect complete independence and higher scores (e.g., 1 or 2) used to reflect partial or complete dependence. Users should note the disparity in response scales for individual items. If the examiner sums the scores of individual items, a misleading summary score may be produced, because greater weight is assigned to those items with a greater number of points. For example, the ability to handle transportation needs is rated on a 5-point Likert scale, whereas responsibility for medication is rated on a 3-point scale. As a consequence, the ability to handle transportation is given more weight than the ability to handle medications. To address this disparity, items can be transformed so that each is equally weighted (e.g., Bertrand & Willis, 1999), or simple binary coding (0, 1) can be used. Alternatively, users can refer to the 9-item MAI version (Lawton et al., 1982), in which scores for each item range from 1 (complete dependence) to 3 (complete independence) (see *Description*).

DEMOGRAPHIC EFFECTS

Age

Age has a significant relation with adaptive functioning (e.g., Ford et al., 1996; Lechowski et al., 2003). Being of younger age tends to elicit higher competence ratings from caregivers (Bertrand et al., 2001; Ford et al., 1996). The latter may reflect, at least in part, a subtle type of ageism, with caregivers expecting less of older individuals simply because of their age.

Education

Adults with lower levels of education tend to be rated as less competent (Farias et al., 2003).

Gender

Being a female tends to elicit higher competence rating from caregivers (Bertrand et al., 2001).

Ethnicity

No differences have been noted between African American and Caucasian patients with dementia (Ford et al., 1996).

NORMATIVE DATA

Tabert et al. (2002) scored the IADL items dichotomously (0 = no difficulty, 1 = any difficulty), with the range of the sum of scores being 0 to 8. Normal controls ($N = 46$; 54% women; age $M = 63.8$, $SD = 9.7$; education $M = 16.5$, $SD = 2.7$) self-reported no deficits. Self- and informant-reported deficits of individuals with very mild cognitive impairment ($N = 48$; 42% women; age $M = 63.2$, $SD = 9.9$; education $M = 16.7$, $SD = 2.4$) also elicited very few deficits (self-report $M = 0.4$, $SD = 0.9$; informant report $M = 0.3$, $SD = 0.7$).

Lawton et al. (1982) tested a sample of independently living older people with the MAI 9-item version (see Table 15–12). They reported a mean score of 24.51 ($SD = 3.66$).

RELIABILITY

Internal Consistency

This is reported to be high (.93) in patients in the early stages of dementia (Farias et al., 2003).

Test-Retest Reliability and Practice Effects

One-month retest reliability of the standard form was high (>.90) in a sample of patients with probable AD (Green et al., 1993). Retest reliability of the OARS/MAI form after a 3-week interval was adequate (.73; Lawton et al., 1982).

Interrater Reliability

At a given assessment, the items show high reliability for the standard informant-rating form (≥.85; Green et al., 1993; Hokoishi et al., 2001; Lawton & Brody, 1969) as well as for the MAI form (.91; Lawton et al., 1982). At different points in time, however, raters may disagree on whether to rate a particular item (food preparation, housekeeping, laundry) for male patients and for those who were mildly demented when first seen (Green et al., 1993).

VALIDITY

Relationships With Other Measures

The scale shows moderate to high correlations with other measures of functioning. For example, Lawton and Brody (1969) tested a group of older adults and reported correlations of .61 with physical self-maintenance, .48 with a mental status questionnaire, and .36 with a rating of behavior and adjustment. Bertrand & Willis (1999) reported a correlation of .47 between AD patient and caregiver IADL ratings, and of .25 between caregiver ratings and a test of everyday problem-solving. Farias et al. (2003) found a correlation of .66 with a behaviorally-based measure of daily living skills (the DAFS) in a sample of individuals diagnosed with AD.

Clinical Findings

Research has shown that there are declines in functional competence with increasing age (e.g., Lechowski et al., 2003). There are a number of other characteristics of adults that make them vulnerable to functioning at lower levels of competence as they age. Education emerges as a significant risk factor (Cho et al., 2001; Farias et al., 2003); adults with lower levels of education tend to show lower levels of functional competence and may become particularly vulnerable in old age, when their level of functioning becomes even further diminished by age-related changes in performance.

Other factors—physical, emotional/social, and cognitive—may also affect the ability to function independently in one's environment. Common medical conditions (e.g., urinary incontinence, falls; Cho et al., 2001) and measures of sensory deficits (e.g., visual impairment) and motor disabilities (e.g., fine motor speed, apraxia) have been reported to be determinants of functional capacity (Barberger-Gateau et al. 1999b; Boyle et al., 2002; Farias et al., 2003). Emotional factors, such as feelings of depression, may also affect functional status in mild-to-moderately demented individuals (Cho et al., 2001; Monini et al., 1998; Pearson et al., 1989; but see Farias et al., 2003).

With respect to cognitive functioning, overall intellectual status (e.g., MMSE, DRS) has been found to be a strong predictor of functional ability (e.g., Barberger-Gateau et al., 1992; Bertrand et al., 2001; Cahn et al., 1998; Cho et al., 2001; Ford et al., 1996; Green et al., 1993; Juva et al., 1994; Lechowski et al., 2003; Shay et al., 1991). Lower functioning and increasing severity of disorder generate lower caregiver ratings.

In addition to overall cognitive status, a number of specific cognitive abilities are predictive of everyday functioning. For example, numerous studies have found that executive dysfunction is a significant predictor of functional disturbance for community-dwelling older individuals (Cahn-Weiner et al., 2002) and for individuals with a variety of neurological disorders (e.g., AD, VAD, PD; Back-Madruga et al., 2002; Bertrand et al., 2001; Boyle et al., 2003, 2004; Cahn et al., 1998; Farias et al., 2003). Other cognitive abilities, such as attention (Boyle et al., 2002), speed (Barberger-Gateau et al., 1999a), memory (Farias et al., 2003), and confrontation naming (Farias et al., 2003) have also been found to correlate with IADL scores.

Barberger-Gateau et al. (1992) reported that four IADL items (telephone, transportation, medication, and finances) are correlated with cognitive impairment independent of age, gender, and education. A summary score based on these four items (items rated 0 = fully independent, 1 = dependent) had a sensitivity of .62 and a specificity of .80 for the diagnosis of cognitive impairment at a cutoff score > 0. Accordingly, they suggested that independence in these four items may serve as a useful screen to rule out cognitive impairment in elderly community dwellers. Loss of independence in any one of these items signals the need for more thorough assessment to determine whether the failure might be related to physical or cognitive impairment.

To date, a few studies of everyday competence in cognitively impaired individuals have examined change across multiple measurements (Bertrand et al., 2001; Green et al., 1993; Schmeidler et al., 1998). Green et al. (1993) evaluated patients with AD every 6 months over a 30-month period. IADL scores changed an average of 2 points annually, and change scores were smaller for patients with severe dementia (see also Schmeidler et al., 1998). Further, IADL change was highly dependent on baseline scores. Ratings changed rapidly for patients who were initially classed as highly functional, but there was a steady decrease in the amount of change as baseline increased (i.e., less functional rating). Bertrand et al. (2001) assessed caregivers and a community-dwelling sample of patients with AD over an 18-month period, involving four 6-month data points. Although patients self-reported a constant, linear rate of decline in everyday competence, caregivers reported a nonlinear rate of decline, with the rate slowing over time. Furthermore, patients rated their level of everyday competence higher than their caregivers did, and they perceived their rate of decline as less precipitous than their caregivers rated it.

Among community-dwelling elderly (aged 70 years and older) who were followed for a 3-year period, decline tended to be minimal, translating into loss of one self-reported IADL every 2 years (Royall et al., 2004). However, deterioration in executive functioning appeared to be linked to declines in self-reported functional status (Royall et al., 2004). The association appeared to be independent of factors such as initial level of performance, age, and comorbid disease.

The IADL has been used to evaluate the efficacy of various drugs (e.g., Cutler et al., 1993; Feldman et al., 2003). It has also been used in the assessment of younger adults (e.g., Schifitto et al., 2001).

Predictive Validity

Functional impairments (particularly on those items requiring high-level cognitive skills, such as managing finances or medications) are present a few years before a diagnosis of dementia is made—that is, in the pre-clinical phase (Barberger-Gateau et al., 1999a, 1999b; Bidzan & Bidzan, 2002). The implication is that their presence may signify an increased risk of subsequent dementia. However, one study monitored individuals with mild cognitive impairment over a 2-year period and did not find informant-reported functional deficits to be greater in those who did or did not convert to a diagnosis of AD (Tabert et al., 2002). Other scales (Pfeffer Functional Activity Questionnaire) that evaluate more complex cognitive

competencies (e.g., assembling tax or business records, playing games of skill, keeping track of current events) and the discrepancy between self and other ratings proved more useful (Tabert et al., 2002).

COMMENT

Measures of functional ability are important for diagnostic purposes, to monitor disease progression, to guide treatment decisions, and to assess their efficacy. Measures such as the IADL have been criticized for being contaminated with reporter bias. In comparison to performance-based measures, patients tend to overestimate their ability to perform tasks, whereas caregivers underestimate patients' abilities (Bertrand et al., 2001). Self-report measures are considered to be particularly problematic, because individuals in the early stages of dementing disorders often lack insight into their abilities. That is, the very mechanisms that give rise to functional impairment may be associated with misidentification of such difficulty in self-report. While not ruling out the value of self-report, these findings suggest that caregiver ratings or performance-based measures may be needed to identify critical information. It is important to bear in mind, however, that performance-based measures of everyday tasks (e.g., DAFS, Loewenstein et al., 1989; Everyday Problems Test, Willis, 1993; SAILS, Mahurin et al., 1991) do not necessarily represent the gold standard. Performance measures and self or informant ratings may be assessing somewhat different dimensions of behavior (Bertrand et al., 2001). Performance-based measures may assess the potential or capacity of the individual but are devoid of information on the environmental support or distractions that may allow (or hinder) an individual in carrying out the task in real life. On the other hand, self- or caregiver ratings may evaluate the application of everyday competence in one's regular milieu (Bertrand et al., 2001). Another advantage of ratings is that they are influenced by a longer time frame than is afforded in a single test session. Given the moderate correlations among the different methods of assessment, it seem prudent to incorporate various approaches in order to gain a broader understanding of everyday competence behaviors.

The IADL is easy to administer. However, there are problems of standardization with the test. Different versions are available (e.g., versions with 8 or 9 items), as well as different scoring procedures, and these variations may lead to different results. Further, Lawton & Brody (1969) recommended deleting three gender-linked items (food preparation, laundry, housekeeping), although some authors give all items regardless of gender. In longitudinal assessment, clinicians/researchers need to document at the baseline assessment the data on which the decision to rate was made, so that it can be referred to at subsequent assessments (Green et al., 1993).

The IADL is highly reliable over the short term. However, it is subject to ceiling and floor effects, limiting its sensitivity to change over the long term. The use of a dichotomous scoring system also leads to a loss of sensitivity to change, and more fine-grained ratings may be preferable (Demers et al., 2000).

Numerous factors are related to IADL performance, including age, education, and motor and sensory ability. In addition, a major risk factor for poor functional ability is cognitive disturbance. A number of specific sources of cognitive difficulty have been identified, with the presence of prominent executive dysfunction appearing to place the individual at increased risk. This finding is not surprising, because high-level skills such as self-regulation, organization, and planning are required for tasks such as shopping and handling finances.

Users should also note that, although the test is brief and provides a gross rating of an individual's everyday functioning, other tests (e.g., SIB-R, Vineland) may be needed to provide a more refined analysis of specific domains of functioning (e.g., personal living skills, financial abilities) and the particular aspects of tasks that are problematic.

REFERENCES

American Psychiatric Association (1994). *Diagnostic and statistical manual of mental disorders–IV.* Washington, DC: American Psychiatric Association.

Back-Madruga, C., Boone, K. B., Briere, J., Cummings, J., McPherson, S., Fairbanks, L., & Thompson, E. (2002). Functional ability in executive variant Alzheimer's disease and typical Alzheimer's disease. *The Clinical Neuropsychologist, 16,* 331–340.

Barberger-Gateau, P., Commenges, D., Gagnon, M., Letenneur, Sauvel, C., & Dartigues, J-F. (1992). Instrumental activities of daily living as a screening tool for cognitive impairment and dementia in elderly community dwellers. *Journal of the American Geriatric Society, 40,* 1129–1134.

Barberger-Gateau, P., Fabrigoule, C., Helmer, C., Rouch, I., & Dartigues, J-F. (1999a). Functional impairment in instrumental activities of daily living: An early clinical sign of dementia. *Journal of the American Geriatrics Society, 47,* 456–462.

Barberger-Gateau, P., Fabrigoule, C., Rouch, I., Letenneur, L., & Dartigues, J-F. (1999b). Neuropsychological correlates of self-reported performance in instrumental activities of daily living and prediction of dementia. *Journal of Gerontology: Psychological Sciences, 54B,* P293–P303.

Bertrand, R. M., & Willis, S. L. (1999). Everyday problem solving in Alzheimer's patients: A comparison of subjective and objective assessments. *Aging & Mental Health, 3,* 281–293.

Bertrand, R. M., Willis, S. L., & Sayer, A. (2001). An evaluation of change over time in everyday cognitive competence among Alzheimer's patients. *Aging, Neuropsychology, and Cognition, 8,* 192–212.

Bidzan, L., & Bidzan, M. (2002). The predictive value of MMSE, ADAS-Cog, IADL and PSMS as instruments for the diagnosis of pre-clinical phase of dementia of Alzheimer type. *Archives of Psychiatry and Psychotherapy, 4,* 27–33.

Boyle, P. A., Cohen, R. A., Paul, R., Moser, D., & Gordon, N. (2002). Cognitive and motor impairments predict functional declines in patients with vascular dementia. *International Journal of Geriatric Psychiatry, 17,* 164–169.

Boyle, P. A., Paul, R., Moser, D. et al. (2003). Cognitive and neurologic predictors of functional impairment in vascular dementia. *American Journal of Geriatric Psychiatry, 11,* 103–106.

Boyle, P. A., Paul, R. H., Moser, D. J., & Cohen, R. A. (2004). Executive impairments predict functional declines in vascular dementia. *The Clinical Neuropsychologist, 18,* 75–82.

Cahn, D. A., Sullivan, E. V., Shear, P. K., Pfefferbaum, A., Heit, G., & Silverberg, G. (1998). Differential contributions of cognitive and motor component processes to physical and instrumental activities of daily living in Parkinson's disease. *Archives of Clinical Neuropsychology, 13,* 575–583.

Cahn-Weiner, D. A., Boyle, P. A., & Malloy, P. F. (2002). Tests of executive function predict instrumental activities of daily living in community-dwelling older individuals. *Applied Neuropsychology, 9,* 187–191.

Cho, C., Cho, H., Cho, K., Choi, K., Oh, H., & Bae, C. (2001). Factors associated with functional dependence in Alzheimer's disease. *Journal of Clinical Geropsychology, 7,* 79–89.

Cutler, N. R., Fakouhi, T. D., Smith, W. T., Hendrie, H. C., Matsuo, F., Sramek, J. J., & Herting, R.L. (1993). Evaluation of multiple doses of milacemide in the treatment of senile dementia of the Alzheimer's type. *Journal of Geriatric Psychiatry and Neurology, 6,* 115–119.

Demers, L., Oremus, M., Perrault, A., Champoux, N., & Wolfson, C. (2000). Review of outcome measurement instruments in Alzheimer's disease drug trials: Psychometric properties of functional and quality of life scales. *Journal of Geriatric Psychiatry and Neurology, 13,* 170–180.

Green, C. R., Mohs, R. C., Schmeider, J., Aryan, M., & Davis, K. L. (1993). Functional decline in Alzheimer's disease: A longitudinal study. *Journal of the American Geriatric Society, 41,* 654–661.

Farias, S. T., Harrell, E., Neumann, C., & Houtz, A. (2003). The relationship between neuropsychological performance and daily functioning in individuals with Alzheimer's disease: Ecological validity of neuropsychological tests. *Archives of Clinical Neuropsychology, 18,* 655–672.

Feldman, H., Gauthier, S., Hecker, J., Vellas, B., Emir, B., Mastey, V., Subbiah, P., & Donepezil MSAD Study Investigators Group. (2003). Efficacy of Donepezil on maintenance of activities of daily living in patients with moderate to severe Alzheimer's disease and the effect on caregiver burden. *Journal of the American Geriatrics Society, 51,* 737–744.

Ford, G. R., Haley, W. E., Thrower, S. L., West, C. A. C., & Harrell, L. E. (1996). Utility of Mini-Mental State Exam scores in predicting functional impairment among White and African American dementia patients. *Journal of Gerontology: Medical Sciences, 51A,* M185–M188.

Hokoishi, K., Ikeda, M., Nomura, M., Torikawa, S., Fujimoto, N., Fukuhara, R., Komori, K., & Tanabe, H. (2001). Interrater reliability of the Physical Self-Maintenance Scale and the Instrumental Activities of Daily Living Scale in a variety of health professional representatives. *Aging and Mental Health, 5,* 38–40.

Juva, K., Sulkava, R., Erkinjuntti, T., Ylikoski, R., Valvanne, J., & Tilvis, R. (1994). Staging the severity of dementia: Comparison of clinical (CDR, DSM-III-R), functional (ADL, IADL) and cognitive (MMSE) scales. *Acta Neurolica Scandinavica, 90,* 293–298.

Lawton, M. P., & Brody, E. M. (1969). Assessment of older people: Self-maintaining and instrumental activities of daily living. *Gerontologist, 9,* 179–185.

Lawton, M. P., & Brody, E. M. (1988). Instrumental Activities of Daily Living (IADL) scale—Self-rated version. *Psychopharmacology Bulletin, 24,* 789–791.

Lawton, M. P., Moss, M., Fulcomer, M., & Kleban, M. H. (1982). A research and service oriented multilevel assessment instrument. *Journal of Gerontology, 37,* 91–99.

Lechowski, L., Dfieudonne, B., Tortar, D., Teillet, L., Robert, P. H., Beroit, M., et al. (2003). Role of behavioural disturbance in the loss of autonomy for activities of daily living in Alzheimer patients. *International Journal of Geriatric Psychiatry, 18,* 977–982.

Loewenstein, D. A., Amigo, A., Duara, R., Gutterman, A., et al. (1989). A new scale for the assessment of functional status in Alzheimer's disease and related disorders. *Journal of Gerontology, 44,* 114–121.

Mahurin, R. K., DeBettignies, B. H., & Pirozzolo, F. J. (1991). The structured assessment of independent living skills: Preliminary report on a performance measure of functional abilities in dementia. *Journal of Gerontology, 46,* 58–66.

Monini, P., Tognetti, A., Sergio, G., & Bartorelli, L. (1998). Depressive disorder in Alzheimer's disease patients: Different aspects in the early and late stages. *Archives of Gerontology and Geriatrics Supplement, 6,* 343–346.

Njegovan, V., Man-Son-Hing, M., Mitchell, S. L., & Molnar, F. J. (2001). The hierarchy of functional loss associated with cognitive decline in older persons. *Journal of Gerontology: Medical Sciences, 56A,* M638–M643.

Pearson, J. L., Teri, L., Reifler, B. V., & Raskind, M. A. (1989). Functional status and cognitive impairment in Alzheimer's patients with and without depression. *Journal of the American Geriatric Society, 37,* 1117–1121.

Royall, D. R., Palmer, R., Chiodo, L. K., & Polk, M. J. (2004). Declining executive control in normal aging predicts change in functional status: The Freedom House Study. *Journal of the American Geriatric Society, 52,* 346–352.

Schifitto, G., Kieburtz, K., McDermott, M. P., McArthur, J., Marder, K., Sacktor, N., Palumbo, D., Selnes, O., Stem, Y., Epstein, L., & Albert, S. (2001). Clinical trials in HIV-associated cognitive impairment. *Neurology, 56,* 415–418.

Schmeidler, J., Mohs, R. C., & Aryan. M. (1998). Relationship of disease severity to decline on specific cognitive and functional measures in Alzheimer disease. *Alzheimer Disease and Associated Disorders, 12,* 146–151.

Shay, K. A., Duke, L. W., Conboy, T., Harrell, L. E., Callaway, R., & Folks, D. G. (1991). The clinical validity of the Mattis Dementia Rating Scale in staging Alzheimer's dementia. *Journal of Geriatric Psychiatry and Neurology 4,* 18–25.

Tabert, M. H., Albert, S. M., Borukhova-Milov, B. A., Camacho, M. S., Peltion, G., Liu, X., Stern, Y., & Devanand, D. P. (2002). Functional deficits in patients with mild cognitive impairment. *Neurology, 58,* 758–764.

Willis, S. L. (1993). *Test manual for the Everyday Problems Test for cognitively challenged elderly.* University Park, PA: The Pennsylvania State University.

Willis, S. L., Allen-Burge, R., Dolan, M. M., Bertrand, R. M., Yesavage, J., & Taylor, J. L. (1998). Everyday problem solving among individuals with Alzheimer's disease. *The Gerontologist, 38,* 569–577.

Minnesota Multiphasic Personality Inventory-2 (MMPI-2)

PURPOSE

The Minnesota Multiphasic Personality Inventory-2 (MMPI-2) is a self-report test that assesses personality functioning and psychological disorders.

SOURCE

The MMPI-2 is available from National Computer Systems (NCS), P.O. Box 1416, Minneapolis, MN 55343 (http://www.pearsonassessments.com). The MMPI-2 Hand Scoring Kit (includes manual, 2 test booklets, 50 answer sheets, profile forms, and answer keys) costs $680 US. The test can be given in several formats: paper-and-pencil, audiocassette, and computer. It can also be given in English, Spanish, Hmong, and French. In addition to hand-scoring, there are a number of other scoring options, including MICROTEST Q™ Assessment System software, mail-in service, and optical scanning; each provides a basic one-page report as well as more extensive interpretive reports, with costs ranging from about $9 to $30 US per report.

AGE RANGE

The test is intended for use with individuals aged 18 to 90 years.

DESCRIPTION

This self-report test ranks as one of the most popular measures among neuropsychologists (Camara et al. 2000; Rabin et al., 2005). The original version, the MMPI, was published by Hathaway and McKinley in 1940. The scales were developed by means of an empirical approach: Items were selected for each scale on the basis of their ability to discriminate between clinical and normal groups. As a result, these scales tend to be heterogeneous in nature. Table 15–13 summarizes the standard validity and clinical scales included in the MMPI. Clinical scales are often simply known by their number (e.g., "scale 8").

Because of concerns regarding the adequacy of the normative base and item content, the test was revised and restandardized by Butcher et al. (1989). The revision eliminates duplicate, nonworking, objectionable, or outmoded items and rewords 14% of the items in more modern, simplified language, eliminating potential sexist wording and grammatical ambiguities (Graham, 2000; Butcher et al., 2001). The MMPI-2 consists of 567 true/false questions. The patient marks his or her answers on the standard answer sheet, which is then scored by overlay scoring keys or by computer entry for a variety of scales. The revision uses the same (slightly revised) validity and clinical scales and the critical item list of the original MMPI but adds a myriad of new validity or response-style indicators (see *Malingering* for details), as well as new scales (see Table 15–14). Information derived from these other scales (e.g., Content, Supplementary, Restructured Clinical [RC]) may reinforce that provided by the clinical scales, but it may also elaborate and refine inferences or even suggest opposing interpretive hypotheses (Nichols, 2001).

Table 15–13 Summary of MMPI Validity and Clinical Scales

Validity Scales

L—Lie	Assesses attempt to present oneself in favorable light by denying minor weaknesses
F—Infrequency	Detects atypical ways of responding
K—Correction	Detects attempt to deny or exaggerate problems

Clinical Scales

(1) HS—Hypochondriasis	Measures tendency to deny good health and admit a variety of physical symptoms
(2) D—Depression	Measures symptoms of depression
(3) Hy—Hysteria	Measures somatic complaints and a tendency to deny psychological or social problems
(4) PD—Psychopathic Deviate	Measures alienation, rebellion
(5) Mf—Masculinity-Feminity	Measures patterns of interest and attitudes that tend to follow gender stereotypes
(6) Pa—Paranoia	Measures ideas of being misunderstood, persecuted, treated unfairly
(7) Pt—Psychasthenia	Measures tendency to be anxious, worry, obsess, ruminate
(8) Sc—Schizophrenia	Measures disturbed thinking, mood, and behavior
(9) Ma—Hypomania	Measures activity/energy level, excitability
(10) Si—Social Introversion	Measures introversion, tendency to withdraw from social contact and responsibilities

Interpreting the MMPI-2 scales involves three aspects: (a) evaluating the acceptability/validity of the protocol, (b) examining the clinical scales to generate possible descriptors of the person's personality and emotional status that are based on the results of studies of normal individuals and psychiatric patients, and (c) examining the scores on the content, supplementary, and RC scales (and noting critical items) to elaborate, refine, or refute interpretive hypotheses.

High scores on the clinical scales are usually expressed in a 1-, 2-, or 3-point "high-point code," listing scale elevations above a T score of 65. Butcher et al. (2001) recommend that code-type interpretation be limited to those cases in which scales in the code-type have T scores greater than 64. Definition refers to the differences in scores between the scales in the code-type and those not in the code-type. The T-score differences between the lowest scale in the code-type and the next highest clinical scale should be considered. For example, for a 2-point code-type, the difference between the second- and third-highest scales is examined. For a 3-point code-type, the difference between the third- and fourth-highest scales is evaluated. Because scales are not perfectly reliable (see *Reliability*), only code-types in which there is a relatively large difference between the lowest scale in the code-type and the next highest scale should be interpreted; small differences between scores (<5 T-score points) should not be interpreted. In cases where sufficient definition does not exist, interpretation should be based primarily on individual scales (Butcher et al., 2001). For interpretive possibilities of MMPI-2 code-types, the reader is referred to other authors (e.g., Archer et al., 1995; Gass, 2000; Graham, 2000; Greene, 2000).

ADMINISTRATION

Instructions are printed on the front of the reusable booklet. Briefly, the patient is instructed to read each statement and to decide whether it is true or false as applied to himself or herself. The patient is then asked to mark his or her answer on the answer sheet and is encouraged to answer all items. The test can also be given by personal computer, using software available from the source. Computer administration has been shown to be equivalent to booklet administration (Finger & Ones, 1999, cited in Butcher et al., 2001).

Although breaks are permitted, allowing the client to complete the MMPI-2 at home is not recommended, because norms were generated under carefully controlled conditions, circumstances during test-taking that may affect validity cannot be observed, and responses may be influenced by others at home (and indeed someone else may have completed the instrument; Butcher & Pope, 1992).

A grade 6 reading ability is considered minimal (see *Source*). Although the average reading difficulty of items corresponds roughly to the fifth grade, a few subscales (e.g., Hypomania [Ma]) require proficiency above grade 8 (Paolo et al., 1991). For poor readers, tape-recorded versions are available. However, it is possible that the audiotaped format is more demanding of memory or attention than the printed version (Mittenberg et al., 1996).

Within the context of the neuropsychological examination, many clinicians avoid routine administration of the MMPI-2 because of its length and significant demands on attention and comprehension. Mittenberg et al. (1996) suggested that the MMPI-2 tends to produce invalid scores in those with a loss of 20 or more IQ points below premorbid estimates or when WMS-R Memory or Attention/Concentration indices fall below 70.

ADMINISTRATION TIME

Approximately 1 to 2 hours is required for test administration.

SCORING

Hand-scoring is possible with the use of various scoring keys; however, given the large number of scales that are routinely scored, computer scoring systems are preferred to reduce time

Table 15–14 MMPI-2 Scales

Validity Scales	VRIN—Variable Response Inconsistency
	TRIN—True Response Inconsistency
	F—Infrequency
	F_B—Back F
	F_p—Infrequency—Psychopathology
	L—Lie
	K—Correction
	S—Superlative Self-Presentation
	? Cannot Say
Superlative Self-Presentation Subscales	S1—Beliefs in Human Goodness
	S2—Serenity
	S3—Contentment with Life
	S4—Patience and Denial of Irritability and Anger
	S5—Denial of Moral Flaws
Clinical Scales	1—HS
	2—D
	3—HY
	4—Pd
	5—Mf
	6—PA
	7—Pt
	8—Sc
	9—MA
	0—Si
RC (Restructured Clinical) Scales	RCd—dem—Demoralization
	RC1—som—Somatic Complaints
	RC2—lpe—Low Positive Emotions
	RC3—cyn—Cynicism
	RC4—abs—Antisocial Behavior
	RC6—per—Ideas of Persecution
	RC7—dne—Dysfunctional Negative Emotions
	RC8—abx—Aberrant Experiences
	RC9—hpm—Hypomanic Activation
Clinical Subscales	Harris-Lingoes Subscales
	Social Introversion Subscales
Content Scales	ANX—Anxiety
	FRS—Fears
	OBS—Obsessiveness
	DEP—Depression
	HEA—Heath Concerns
	BIZ—Bizarre Mentation
	ANG—Anger
	CYN—Cynicism
	ASP—Antisocial Practices
	TPA—Type A
	LSE—Low Self-Esteem
	SOD—Social Discomfort
	FAM—Family Problems
	WRK—Work Interference
	TRT—Negative Treatment Indicators
Content Components Scales	Fears Subscales
	Depression Subscales
	Health Concerns Subscales
	Bizarre Mentation Subscales
	Anger Subscales
	Cynicism Subscales

(continued)

Table 15–14 MMPI-2 Scales (*continued*)

	Antisocial Practices Subscales
	Type A Subscales
	Low Self-Esteem Subscales
	Social Discomfort Subscales
	Family Problems Subscales
	Negative Treatment Indicators
Supplementary Scales	Personality Psychopathology Five Scales (Psy-5)
	AGGR—Aggressiveness
	PSYC—Psychoticism
	DISC—Disconstraint
	NEGE—Negative Emotionality/ Neuroticism
	INTR—Introversion/ Low Positive Emotionality
	Broad Personality Characteristics
	A—Anxiety
	R—Repression
	Es—Ego Strength
	Do—Dominance
	Re—Social Responsibility
	Generalized Emotional Distress
	Mt—College Maladjustment
	PK—Post-Traumatic Stress Disorder—Keane
	MDS—Marital Distress
	Behavioral Dyscontrol
	Ho—Hostility
	O-H—Overcontrolled Hostility
	MAC-R—MacAndrew—Revised
	AAS—Addiction Admission
	APS—Addiction Potential
	Gender Role
	GM—Gender Role—Masculine
	GF—Gender Role—Feminine
Special Indices/ Scores	Welsch Code
	F-K Dissimulation Index
	Percent True
	Percent False
	Average Profile Elevation
	Megargee Classification
	P-A-I-N Classification
	Behavioral Dimensions
	Possible Problem Areas
	Gass Head Injury Items

and errors (see *Source*; Nichols, 2001). However, even computer scoring can result in scoring errors. For example, if demographic data are omitted when entering raw data, the program may interpret the data based on default options (e.g., 18-year-old with 12 years of education; Lees-Haley, 2001).

Scores for clinical and content scales are transformed into uniform T scores that have a mean of 50 and standard deviation of 10. Uniform T scores mean that the percentile equivalent for any given T score is identical across all of the scales.

Each scale produces the sum of answers relevant to that scale. Raw scores are then transferred to a profile sheet, which also provides corrections for some scales that are affected by a concealing attitude or by an attempt to appear in a favorable light (K-Scale). Corrected scores are plotted on the profile sheet, which directly translates into T scores. In general, T scores of 65 or greater are considered high, and T scores below 40 are considered low.

DEMOGRAPHIC EFFECTS

Age

Age contributes little to most MMPI-2 scales (Graham, 2000).

Gender

Differences in raw scores are found between men and women (Graham, 2000). Accordingly, separate norms are provided for men and women.

Education/Socioeconomic Status (SES)

According to the test authors (Butcher et al., 2001), there is no substantial association between education and other SES in-dictors and scores on the MMPI-2 scales.

NORMATIVE DATA

Standardization Sample

Norms were developed from a sample of 2600 community-dwelling individuals (see Table 15–15) recruited by ads, direc-tories, and mailing lists (Butcher et al., 2001). Unlike the original MMPI, participants in the restandardization project were not disqualified for being under the care of a physician or mental health professional (Nichols, 2001). About 300 subjects were removed from a larger sample of 2900 subjects because of an excess of omitted items or excessively high

Table 15–15 Characteristics of the MMPI-2 Standardization Sample

Number	2600
Age (years)	18–90; in comparison to 1990 U.S. Census data, there is an underrepre-sentation of young (18–19) and old (70+) individuals
Geographic location	Seven US states: California, Minnesota, North Carolina, Ohio, Pennsylvania, Virginia, and Washington
Sample type	Individuals drawn from directories, advertising lists, and, in one site, by advertisement and special appeals
Education	In comparison to 1990 U.S. Census data, there is an excess of individuals with college and postgraduate education
Gender	
Men	1,138
Women	1,462
Race/Ethnicity	In comparison to 1990 U.S. Census data, proportions are comparable for blacks and whites; however Hispanic and Asian American groups are underrepresented whereas Native Americans are somewhat overrepresented in the normative sample
Screening	Individuals dropped from sample because of excessive item omissions or an excessively high F or F_B

scores (≥ 20) on either the F or the F_B scale. In comparison to the 1990 U.S. Census data, there was some underrepresenta-tion of Hispanics and Asian Americans, as well as subjects at the extremes of the age distribution (see Table 15–15). There was also an excess of college-educated individuals. However, a study by Schinka and LaLone (1997) found that differences on standard validity, clinical, content, and supplementary scales were nonexistent between the full restandardization sample and a census-matched subsample.

RELIABILITY

Internal Consistency

The internal consistency of the clinical scales is quite variable, ranging from .34 (Pa) to .85 (Pt, Sc) in males and .37 (Mf) to .87 (Pt) in females. This finding is not surprising, because Hathaway and McKinley constructed the clinical scales with the explicit expectation that they would not all be homoge-neous in content (Butcher et al., 2001). Coefficient alphas are adequate (>.70) for the content scales but variable for the sup-plementary scales (.34 for scale O-H to .89 for scale A in males; .24 for scale O-H to .90 for scale A in females).

Test-Retest Reliability and Stability

For a 1-week interval, test-retest coefficients of the clinical scales ranged from .67 (Pa) to .93 (Si) for a sample of 82 men, and from .54 (Sc) to .92 (Si) for a sample of 82 men and 111 women in the normative sample (Butcher et al., 2001). Similar findings were reported by Wetter and Deitsch (1996) in a sample of undergraduate students with a 2-week interval between testings. The average reliability coefficient for the clinical scales was about .75 (Wetter & Deitch, 1996). Group means on retesting were quite similar, within about 1 or 2 points. Test-retest coefficients are typically high (>.80) for the content and supplementary scales (Butcher et al., 2001). Code-type stability, however, tends to be poor (Graham, 2000; Senior & Douglas, 2001). For example, Senior and Douglas (2001) found a high rate of instability (30%) in their forensic psychiatric sample (test-retest interval not reported). Graham (2000) reported that, with a 1-week retest interval, about 49% of the normative sample obtained the same 1-point code-type, 26% had the same 2-point code-type, and 15% had the same 3-point code-type.

Standard Errors of Measurement (SEM)

The error of measurement of T scores on the clinical scales ranges from 2.74 (Si) to 5.74 (Pa) for males and from 2.76 (Si) to 6.82 (Sc) for females. The SEMs for the content and supple-mentary scales are slightly smaller (Butcher et al., 2001). This information is important to determine whether scale scores are significantly different from one another or have changed significantly over time.

VALIDITY

Relations Within Test

Factor-analytic findings of the MMPI-2 in the normative sample suggest two major dimensions. One major factor seems related to general maladjustment and psychotic mentation, with scales F, 7, and 8 loading highly on this factor (Graham, 2000; Nichols, 2001). The second factor represents neurotic tendencies, with highest loading from scales L, 2, 3, and 9 (Graham, 2000; Nichols, 2001). The factor structure tends to be somewhat different for men and women, suggesting that certain MMPI-2 patterns have somewhat different interpretive meanings for each gender (Graham, 2000).

Relations With Other Tests

Scores on the standard clinical scales have shown moderate convergence with scores on a variety of self-report inventories (including the original MMPI), rating scales, and clinical judgments (Graham, 2000; Miller & Paniak, 1995; Nichols, 2001). However, the degree of congruence between the MMPI and MMPI-2 with regard to 2-point code-type match is modest in neurologically impaired patients. Miller and Paniak (1995) found that only 50% of their sample had similar 2-point code-types on both versions. Therefore, caution must be exercised when drawing inferences about the MMPI-2 from MMPI research (Miller & Paniak, 1995).

Evidence for convergent validity of the clinical scales is generally considered better than that for divergent validity. That is, the item overlap between MMPI-2 clinical scales and the resulting enhanced correlations among them reduces their specificity and thereby compromises their discriminant validity (Nichols, 2001). In fact, Senior and Douglas (2001) raised significant concerns with regard to the efficacy of traditional code-type analysis and the accuracy of the MMPI-2 to discriminate between diagnostic classes. They advocated an hypothesis-testing approach in which interpretations are checked against other scale and subscale elevations.

In this context, it is important to emphasize that the content of the clinical scales tends to be heterogeneous in nature, and some items on a scale may not be rationally related to the construct that they are supposed to be measuring. Therefore, the examinee's ability to directly communicate his or her distress is reduced (Palav et al., 2001). The content scales may provide an avenue for the client to identify distressing concerns and to verify interpretation of the clinical scale (e.g., elevation of D is interpreted as reflecting depression-related symptoms only if DEP is also elevated). Indeed, there is evidence that the content scales add incremental validity beyond the clinical scales to the prediction of self-reported psychopathology in college students (Ben Porath et al., 1993), psychiatric inpatients (Archer et al., 1996), and head-injured patients (Palav et al., 2001). The incremental contributions made by the supplementary scales appeared relatively limited, at least in an inpatient population (Archer et al., 1997).

Neuropsychological Studies

Diagnosis of "organicity," although attempted by some authors, is not a question that can or should be answered by the MMPI or MMPI-2. Nor is the MMPI-2 sensitive to the general location of brain lesions (right versus left, anterior versus posterior; Gass, 2000; King et al., 2002).

Central nervous system impairment is likely to produce elevations on scales 1, 2, 3, 7, and 8 (for review, see Gass, 2000), consistent with the notion that such patients present with symptoms such as depression, dissatisfaction with life, anxiety, and cognitive and somatic concerns. For example, patients with multiple sclerosis (MS) tend to show elevations on scales 1, 3, and 8 (Nelson et al., 2003), and patients with amnesic disorders display elevations on scales 2 and 8 (Bachna et al., 1998). In those with end-stage pulmonary disease, elevations are noted on scales 1 and 3 (Crews et al., 2003), whereas patients with intractable seizures tend to show elevations on scales 1, 2, 3, and 8 (King et al., 2002 reported elevations on these scales and on scale 7; Nelson et al., 2004).

There is some evidence that head-injured individuals show more pathology than those diagnosed with stroke or dementia (Golden & Golden, 2003) and that patients with mild head injury demonstrate greater symptomatology on the MMPI-2 than do patients with moderate-to-severe head injury (Hoffman et al., 1999; Miller & Donders, 2001; Youngjohn et al., 1997). Litigation after head injury is also associated with increased reporting of psychopathology (Hoffman et al., 1999; Youngjohn et al., 1997). Of note, Greiffenstein and Baker (2001) compared premorbid and postinjury MMPI-2 profiles in patients with mild cranial/cervical injuries (those with persistent postconcussion symptoms). Although all claimants attributed major personality change to their injuries, their premorbid MMPI-2 profiles were all abnormal and indicated somatoform psychopathology. The postaccident profiles showed persistent somatization trends, along with increased defensiveness and a general decline in global psychopathology. The implication is that in these patients, reports of posttraumatic change reflected at least a response bias that minimized preinjury adjustment problems. Greiffenstein and Baker (2001) noted that a somatoform MMPI-2 profile is the most frequently encountered pattern in late postconcussion cases and that such a profile most likely represents premorbid personality trends.

Two sets of decision rules have been developed to distinguish those with epileptic seizures from those with psychogenic nonepileptic seizures (PNES; Derry & McLachlan, 1996; Wilkus et al., 1984). However, Cragar et al. (2003) found that the two sets of decision rules yielded sensitivities of 68% and 48% and specificities of 55% and 58%. Positive predictive values were unacceptably low for predicting the presence of the condition. Therefore, use of these rules can result in a large number of false-positive diagnoses of PNES.

Emotional distress on the MMPI-2 is associated with cognitive complaints (Gass & Apple, 1997). Whether distress as measured by the MMPI-2 adversely affects objectively measured cognition is less clear. Some have found MMPI-2 indices of psychological disturbance to be related to performance on measures of list learning, attention, and psychomotor speed (Gass, 1996; Solbakk et al., 2000), although the effect on test scores tended to be relatively modest (Ross et al., 2003; Sherman et al., 2000) or not reliable (Binder et al., 1998; Rohling et al., 2002; Ruttan & Heinrichs, 2003). The reason for the discrepancy is not certain but may relate to the level and type of distress present in the particular sample as well as the severity, etiology, and chronicity of the neurological disturbances. Typically, in these studies, patients who display suboptimal effort are excluded from study.

Findings on the MMPI-2 are often used to determine whether a person is employable (Rabin et al., 2005). However, Fox and Lees-Haley (2001) found no meaningful association between MMPI-2 scores (including scores on the WRK scale) and employment status among claimants in litigation. The results suggested that the MMPI-2 is not an effective indicator of work disability in litigating patients.

Neurocorrections

One concern with the MMPI-2 is that scale elevations may be caused by valid neurological disturbance, rather than reflecting a patient's emotional state. Gass (1991; Gass & Wald, 1997) identified a list of items that might affect the clinical profile and constructed a correction factor to be used with individuals who have a neurological condition. The 14 items are listed in Table 15–16. Each of the items distinguished patients with head injury from the MMPI-2 normative sample, was endorsed by at least 25% of the head injury sample, comprised a unitary factor separate from a set of psychiatric symptoms, and showed face validity as representing physical and cognitive symptoms. Gass

Table 15–16 MMPI-2 Gass Correction Factor for Closed Head Injury

Item No.	Scoring	Scales
31	T	2, 3, 4, 7, 8, 0
101	T	1, 3
106	F	8, 9, 0
147	T	2, 7, 8
149	T	1
165	F	2, 7, 8
170	T	2, 7, 8
172	T	3
175	T	1, 2, 3, 7
179	F	1, 3, 8
180	T	F, 8
247	T	1, 8
295	F	8
325	T	7, 8

(2000) recommended that the MMPI-2 profiles of patients with closed head injury be scored twice—once in the standard manner and again after elimination of any correction items endorsed in the scored direction. He suggested that interpretation of code-types be based on the corrected protocol. Others have developed different correction factors (e.g., Alfano et al., 1990, 1992, 1993) for head-injured individuals, although the correction factor for head-injured individuals developed by Gass (1991) appears to provide better sensitivity and specificity (Glassmire et al., 2003; but see Dunn & Lees-Haley, 1995). Others have proposed correction factors for stroke cases (Gass, 1992), patients with seizures (Derry et al., 1997; Nelson et al., 2004) and patients with MS (Nelson et al., 2003).

Based on the available literature, Gass (2000) recommended that the standard application of the correction factor for head injury should be limited to the MMPI-2 protocols of individuals who have clear evidence of bona fide brain injury and no premorbid history of psychopathology or drug addiction. Rayls et al. (2000) noted that correction-factor item endorsement frequencies typically return to normal levels 3 to 6 months after mild head trauma. Therefore, endorsement of items after this period most likely reflects psychological factors (Rayls et al., 2000), including depression (Brulot et al., 1997) and litigation status (Hoffman et al., 1999). In short, Gass (2000) argued that the correction should not be applied in cases in which symptoms persist beyond 6 months.

Some, however, oppose the use of a correction factor, because they believe that it removes important information from the profile that has neurological relevance (e.g., Cripe, 1996; Glassmire et al., 2003); that it threatens the psychometric properties of the MMPI-2 and invalidates the empirical procedure used for scale construction (Edwards et al., 2003); or that the factor/scales relate more to psychological distress than to neurological compromise (e.g., Brulot et al. 1997; Derry et al., 1997; Glassmire et al., 2003; but see Rayls et al., 1997). Glassmire and colleagues (2003) cautioned that items on correction factors (e.g., Gass, 1991; Alfano et al., 1993), although sensitive to head injury, are not specific to head injury; rather, they may be endorsed equally commonly in psychiatric patients (see also Dunn & Lees-Haley, 1995; Edwards et al., 2003). That is, an item might be endorsed because of the head injury itself, a premorbid psychiatric condition, an emotional response to the injury, and/or nonspecific generalized distress. Currently, there is no way to determine which of these reasons underlie the item endorsement. Glassmire et al. (2003) recommended that the correction factor should not be used if there is any indication of a comorbid psychiatric condition (e.g., premorbid psychopathology or a significant emotional reaction to the head injury).

Short Forms

The length of the MMPI-2 (567 items) can be prohibitive. The original validity scales (L, F, K) and the clinical scales are scored from the first 370 items, but it is desirable to have the entire test completed so that all the validity indicators, content

Table 15–17 Descriptive Data on MMPI-2 Feigning Indexes

Scale	Items	Development	Detection Strategy	r with F
F	60	Normative	Rare symptoms	—
F_B	40	Normative	Rare symptoms	.86/.59[a]
F_p	27	Discriminant	Rare symptoms	.75/.57[a]
Ds	58	Discriminant	Erroneous stereotypes	.84/.61[a]
Dsr	32	Discriminant	Erroneous stereotypes	—
LW	107	Content	Symptom severity	.84/.67[a]
O-S	253	Rational	Obvious vs. subtle	.81/.58[a]
FBS	43	Rational-discriminant	Erroneous sterotypes	.21[b]

Note: Normative = uncharacteristic responses based on norms; discriminant = empirically derived items that differentiate between feigning and honest responding; content = nominated by clinical psychologists as representing a specific content area of psychological concerns; rational = heuristic division of items (obvious and subtle); rational-discriminant = rational selection of items taking into account differences between criterion groups; F = Infrequency; F_B = Back Infrequency; F_p = Infrequency—Psychopathology; Ds = Dissimulation; Dsr-Dissimulation—Revised; LW = Lachar-Wrobel; O-S = T-score difference of Obvious–Subtle; FBS = Fake Bad Scale.
[a]Derived from Greene (2000), p. 66. First correlations are based on 50,966 patients (Caldwell, 1998), whereas second correlations are based on the normative sample (Butcher et al., 1989).
[b]Derived from Guez et al. (2005).

Source: From Rogers et al., 2003, p. 161. Reprinted with the permission of Sage Publications, Inc.

scales, and supplementary scales can be scored (Butcher et al., 2001). A shortened version consisting of the first 180 items has been proposed (MMPI-2-180; Dahlstrom & Archer, 2000). However, when cases are examined individually, this short form is unreliable for predicting clinical code-types, identifying the high-point scales, or predicting the scores on most of the basic scales (Gass & Gonzales, 2003; Gass & Luis, 2001a). However, the MMPI-2-180 might be useful as a means of salvaging information from an unfinished administration, in order to estimate whether a full-scale score would fall above or below 65T. This information might alert the clinician to particular problem areas, although such an inference would have to be treated with considerable caution (Gass & Gonzales, 2003). In the absence of psychometric studies dealing with the MMPI-2-180, Gass and Gonzales (2003) advised against routine use of this short form.

Malingering

Numerous studies have reported elevations on MMPI-2 scales 1, 2, 3, 7, and 8 in individuals likely malingering neurocognitive disturbances (e.g., Berry et al., 1995; Boone & Lu, 1999; Larrabee, 1998, 2003a; Millis et al., 1995). Such individuals tend to score higher on scales 1, 3, and 7 than persons in other clinical groups, including those with depression, chronic pain, nonlitigating severe closed head injury, MS, and spinal cord injury (Larrabee, 2003a). One implication is that clinicians need to carefully evaluate the credibility of cognitive scores produced by patients with such elevations through a variety of techniques (Boone & Lu, 1999).

A major advantage of the MMPI-2 is its measurement of test-taking attitude and profile validity (see Table 15–14). Detection of incomplete effort on the MMPI-2 has focused on the identification of persons using scales composed of items with low normative endorsement rates (rare symptoms), an evaluation of symptom severity (the endorsement of an unexpectedly high number of critical items), a comparison of obvious and subtle symptoms (the endorsement of more obvious than subtle symptoms), and the use of erroneous stereotypes (see Table 15–17). These scales include the Infrequency (F) scale, the Fback (F_B), F-psychopathology (F_p), the Infrequency minus Correction (F − K), and Gough's Dissimulation Index. For a more complete listing and description, see Lees-Haley et al. (2002), Meyers et al. (2002), and Rogers et al. (2003). Table 15–18 shows the item composition of two of these scales, F_p and FBS.

Although these scales, particularly F and F_p, have proved useful in distinguishing persons feigning various types of psychiatric disorders from true patients and normal controls[1] (Rogers et al., 2003), their use in forensic neuropsychological settings has produced mixed results (Ross et al., 2004), perhaps because persons feigning head injury tend to endorse high rates of somatic rather than psychiatric symptoms.[2] Larrabee (1998) has astutely observed that only one F-scale item occurs on scales 1 or 3, making it less likely that an individual enhancing somatic concerns (e.g., pain, malaise) would be identified by an F-scale elevation. To this end, recent studies in the detection of malingered head injury have focused on the Fake Bad Scale (FBS) developed by Lees-Haley et al. (1991) to detect invalid response style in personal injury cases. In contrast to F and its cousins (e.g., F_p, F_B), the FBS appears to detect somatic ("acts hurt") rather than psychiatric ("acts crazy") malingering (Greiffenstein et al., 2002; Larrabee, 2003a, 2003b).

Lees-Haley et al. (1991) developed the FBS scale using unpublished frequency counts of malingerers' MMPI test results and observations of personal injury malingerers. The items incorporated both social desirability ("faking good") and symptom exaggeration ("faking bad") with a focus of (a) appearing honest; (b) appearing psychologically normal except

Table 15–18 Items comprising the FBS and F_p Indices.

Scale		Items[a]	Suggested Cutoff Values[b]	
FBS	True	11, 18, 28, 30, 31, 39, 40, 44, 59, 111, 252, 274, 325, 339, 464, 469, 505, 506	Lees-Haley et al. (1991)	≥20
			Lees-Haley (1992)	≥24 men
				≥26 women
			Greiffenstein et al. (2002)	≥20 mild HI
				≥24 moderate/severe HI
	False	12, 41, 57, 58, 81, 110, 117, 152, 164, 176, 224, 227, 248, 249, 250, 255, 264, 284, 362, 373, 374, 419, 433, 496, 561		
F_p	True	66, 114, 162, 193, 216, 228, 252, 270, 282, 291, 294, 322, 323, 336, 371, 387, 478, 555	Millis et al. (1995)	$T \geq 93$
			Arbisi & Ben-Porath (1997)	$T \geq 90$
			Lees-Haley et al. (2002)	≥5 items
			Rogers et al. (2003)	$T \geq 98$
	False[c]	*51, 77,* 90, *93, 102,* 126, 192, 276, 501		

Note: HI = head injury.
[a]The examiner adds one point for each item marked in the scored direction (true or false)
[b]Suggested cutoffs vary depending on the sample. See Lees-Haley et al. (2001), Meyers et al. (2002), and Rogers et al. (2004) for a more complete listing of these and other scales.
[c]Gass and Luis (2001b) recommend dropping items 51, 77, 93, and 102 because they load on the L scale and are associated with defensiveness, not with symptom exaggeration. They found that removing these four items improved the scale's correlation with other measures of symptom magnification.

for the influence of the alleged cause of injury; (c) avoiding admitting preexisting psychopathology; (d) attempting to minimize the impact of previously disclosed preexisting complaints; (e) minimizing or hiding preinjury antisocial or illegal behavior; and (f) presenting a degree of injury or disability within perceived limits of plausibility (Larrabee, 2005). The 43 items in this scale and scored direction are shown in Table 15–18. Most of the FBS items occur on scales 1 and 3. In their initial study, they used a cutoff score of 20 and reported 96% accurate classification for suspected malingerers, 93% for patients believed to be suffering from bona fide injuries, and 74% for various simulator groups. Other studies have suggested different cutoffs, such as 20 or greater for mild head injury claimants seen more than 1 year after injury and 24 or greater for those with moderate/severe head injuries (Greiffenstein et al., 2002); 21 (Larrabee, 2003b, 2003c); and 24 for men and 26 for women (Lees-Haley, 1992). See Table 15–18 for a list of suggested cutoffs.

Butcher et al. (2003; Arbisi & Butcher, 2004) have questioned the merit of this scale, arguing that the FBS contains a high number of physical symptoms and therefore is unacceptably prone to false-positive errors (but see others, such as Greve & Bianchini, 2004; Lees-Haley & Fox, 2004). However, a number of authors have found the FBS to be particularly useful in patients claiming personal injury (e.g., Greiffenstein et al., 2002; Iverson et al., 2002; Larrabee, 2003b; Meyers et al., 2002; Miller & Donders, 2001). Indeed, the FBS has proved more sensitive to symptom exaggeration than other validity scales, including F, F_B, F_p, and the recently developed Meyers'

Weighting Validity Index (Meyers et al., 2002) in simulation (Dearth et al., 2005) and personal injury settings (Greiffenstein et al., 2002, 2004; Larrabee, 1998, 2003a, 2003b; Millis et al., 1995; Tsushima & Tsushima, 2001). For example, Ross et al. (2004) examined head-injured patients (litigants with suspect performance versus nonlitigants with moderate/severe head injuries) and found that a cutoff score of 21 on the FBS had a sensitivity of 90% and a specificity of 90%. Positive predictive values ranged from 50% when the base rate of suboptimal effort was 10% to 79% when the base rate was 30%. Therefore, the use of the FBS is not advised when the base rate of suboptimal effort is 10% or less (see also Larrabee, 2003b). Further, these authors noted that traditional MMPI-2 indices (F and F-K) added no predictive power over the FBS alone in detecting suboptimal effort in cases of mild head injury. Although the utility of the FBS is clearest in the context of exaggerated neurotrauma claims, it also extends to other psychological changes, such as inauthentic pain report (Guez et al., 2005; Larrabee 2003d). Further, Greiffenstein et al. (2004) used a known groups comparison (litigants with implausible symptoms versus nonlitigants exposed to severe stressors) and found the FBS better than the F-family scales (F, F_p, and F-K) at detecting improbable psychological trauma claims. They found that cut-scores of 30 or greater had a 100% probability of symptom magnification.

There is also evidence (Larrabee, 2003b; Slick et al., 1996) that FBS, but not scales such as F_p, correlates with symptom validity tests such as the VSVT and the PDRT. However, it is important to bear in mind that validity indices (e.g., F, FBS) derived from the MMPI-2 show only moderate convergent validity with scores from symptom validity tests (e.g., Greiffenstein et al., 1995; Larrabee, 2003b, 2003d; Slick et al., 1996; Temple et al., 2003). This should not be surprising, because the tests differ considerably in task demand (self report versus actual performance) and domain (e.g., psychiatric versus somatic versus memory complaints). Therefore, pathologically elevated F-family or FBS scales do not necessarily imply malingering of neurobehavioral deficits, nor does the absence of pathological elevations imply compliance on neuropsychological measures (Greiffenstein et al., 1995).

Nonetheless, there is evidence that the FBS is more effective at detecting suspect effort than indicators derived from conventional tests. Larrabee (2005) reported that the FBS was the single most sensitive measure for discriminating definite malingerers from those with moderate-severe TBI, when compared with indices derived from the Benton Visual Form Discrimination, Finger Tapping, Reliable Digit Span, and WCST FMS.

If the clinician is reviewing an MMPI-2 profile and there is no computed FBS or True-False answer sheet, the FBS can be estimated with a regression equation developed by Larrabee (2003b), shown in Table 15–19. He recommended that, pending

Table 15–19 Regression Equation to Predict MMPI-2 FBS from T Scores of Validity and Standard Scales

$$FBS = -.028(L) + 0.051(F) - 0.032(K) + 0.127(Hs) + 0.106(D)$$
$$+ 0.169(Hy) - 0.176(Pd) +$$
$$0.017(MF) + 0.083(Pa) + 0.049(Pt)$$
$$- 0.002(Sc) - 0.004(Ma) - 0.015(Si) - 4.886$$
$$R^2 = .788, SEE = 3.667$$

Source: Adapted from Larrabee, 2003b.

independent replication, a conservative confidence interval employing the standard error of estimate of 3.667 should be used along with measures of effort independent of the MMPI-2. If only the first 370 items have been given, then the full FBS can be prorated by multiplying the short FBS score by 1.3 (*SEE* = .003; Fox's FBS Short Form; Lees-Haley, personal communication, July 8, 2004).

It is also useful for clinicians to know which raw scores on other validity scales are rare in the general population or in patients with psychiatric problems. These cutoffs are shown in Table 15–20 and are based on the MMPI-2 normative sample of 2600 community controls, Caldwell's clinical sample of 50,966 psychiatric patients (Lees-Haley et al., 2002), and the patient sample included in a meta-analysis of 65 MMPI-2 feigning studies (Rogers et al., 2003). The 98th percentile is used as the standard. Conceivably, a percentage of the clinical samples may be undetected cases of malingering; however, their inclusion in these normative estimates is likely to decrease the number of false positives found with these cutscores (Rogers et al., 2003).

Clinicians should note that response stability on the MMPI-2 may be a useful marker of suboptimal effort for some disorders. Wetter and Deitch (1996) found that individuals attempting to feign postconcussion symptoms on the MMPI-2 showed increased inconsistency across serial testings (spaced 2 weeks apart). By contrast, participants feigning posttraumatic stress disorder showed relatively high levels of reliability.

Graham (2000) suggested that the content scales may be more susceptible to distortion (faking) than the clinical scales because of their greater face validity. A similar possibility was raised for the recently introduced RC scales, because they contain more obvious item content than the heterogeneous clinical scales. However, findings from simulation studies suggest

Table 15–20 Raw Scores Corresponding to the 98% Rank (2 Standard Deviations Above the Mean) for Normal and Clinical Groups on the MMPI-2

Scale	MMPI-2 Normative	Caldwell Clinical Data Set	Cut Scores from Patient Sample in Rogers et al. (2003)
F	12	24	Men: 22 Women: 20
F_B[a]	9	20	Men: 18 Women: 19
F minus K	3	15	18
Fp	4	7	Men: 8 Women: 9
Obvious-Subtle T-Difference	135	240	256
Dissimulation Scale	24	35	Men: 32 Women: 34

[a]Rogers et al. (2003) noted that F_B cut scores should not be used because many bona fide patients have moderate elevations and considerable variation on F_B. That is, the scale appears confounded by genuine psychopathology as genuine patients' attention may falter during the latter part of the administration. They also found extreme endorsement levels by presumptively genuine patients with PTSD and recommend not using O-S with any patients with histories of PTSD. They also noted that O-S was unlikely to be clinically useful except in rare cases of extreme endorsement levels.

Source: From Lees-Haley et al., 2002, and Rogers et al., 2003.

that the clinical scales are not less susceptible to distortion than the content or RC scales and that, if overreporting is suspected, MMPI-2 users should exercise equal caution when interpreting the three sets of scales (content, RC, and clinical; Sellbom et al., 2005).

COMMENT

Strengths of the MMPI-2 include its extensive research base with a wide variety of populations and a large contemporary normative standardization sample. Users should bear in mind, however, that certain groups, particularly those with low education and those at the ends of the age distribution, tend to be underrepresented. Therefore, although the norms may be appropriate for some clients (e.g., private psychotherapy), they may overly pathologize individuals with very limited education (Nichols, 2001), as well as the very young or very old.

The test is also easy to administer and includes a variety of administration formats. However, the audiotape version may be more demanding of attention and memory than the printed version. The influence of administration format in a neuropsychological setting requires additional study (Mittenberg et al., 1996). Another strength is the scoring software, which provides a wealth of information.

Reliability (internal and test-retest) is best for the content scales, with values falling in the acceptable range or better. Code-type stability, however, appears less than optimal. Evidence for the convergent validity of the MMPI-2 is generally considered better than for its discriminant validity (Nichols, 2001). The availability of various scales to assess test-taking attitude and profile validity (e.g., underreporting or overreporting of symptoms) is also a significant strength. However, the validity of traditional code-type interpretations in the neuropsychological/forensic context has been seriously questioned (Lees-Haley, 2001; Senior & Douglas, 2001).

Correction factors have been proposed for use with patients with neurological disturbance, including head injury (e.g., Gass, 1991). However, clinicians should bear in mind that the correction factors, although sensitive to neurological injury, are not specific to such injury and may merely reflect general psychological distress. As a general guide, the correction is not appropriate for routine application in the majority of individuals who are seeking compensation for persisting symptoms after mild head injury (i.e., >6 months after injury), because head injury symptoms are likely to have resolved, or in those with a comorbid psychiatric condition (Brulot et al., 1997; Dunn & Lees-Haley, 1995; Gass, 2000; Glassmire et al., 2003). In such cases, symptoms may well relate to psychological factors (including premorbid psychopathology and motivational issues), and correction would probably distort the accuracy of profile interpretation (Gass, 2000; Greiffenstein & Baker, 2001). Clinicians should also bear in mind that excessive elevations on somatically oriented scales may well preexist personal injuries (Greiffenstein & Baker, 2001).

In other conditions (e.g., epilepsy, MS), "pathological" endorsement may reflect understandable physical symptoms and experiences of the neurological disorder, and correction procedures may have some utility. Therefore, further evaluation of the content of items derived from correction scales (e.g., via additional interview) may provide some insight into the nature of complaints (i.e., their physical and/or emotional basis) and the impact of the condition on patient's lives (Nelson et al., 2003, 2004).

It is important to note the independence of exaggeration of cognitive, somatic, and psychiatric symptomatology (e.g., Greiffenstein et al., 1995, 2002; McCaffrey et al., 2003; Slick et al., 1996; Temple et al., 2003). Some individuals may feign one type (e.g., cognitive disturbance) but not another (e.g., psychiatric disorder); others may show a different pattern. There appear to be at least two different types of malingering on the MMPI-2: (a) malingered psychopathology characterized by elevations on scales F, 6, and 8, and (b) malingered injury/illness with elevations on FBS and scales 1, 2, 3, 7, and 8 (Larrabee, 2003a). Therefore, reliance on the F-family, as opposed to FBS, may be most appropriate in the exaggeration of psychotic syndromes—a not very common condition in a personal injury population. Although the value of the FBS to detect suboptimal effort has been questioned (e.g., Butcher et al., 2003), the available evidence suggests that it provides unique information over and above traditional MMPI-2 validity indices in personal injury cases, including exaggerated pain, posttraumatic anxiety, and neurological problems. Its utility in a forensic setting is most evident in the context of exaggerated neurotrauma. However, here its use should be limited to compensation-seeking patients with mild head injury where the base rate of malingering exceeds 10% (Larrabee, 2003b; Ross et al., 2004), which includes most forensic/medicolegal settings. At very high levels of endorsement, FBS scores are associated with high positive predictive power. FBS scores of 30 or more are unlikely to result in false positives in patients with chronic pain or head-injury who have cognitive and somatic complaints (Meyers et al., 2002; Larrabee, 2003a, 2003b). However, FBS cutoffs of 21 to 29 do result in cases of false-positive identification (Larrabee, 2003a). Therefore, the presence of additional indicators of suboptimal performance (e.g., from clinical history, SVTs) should be sought to reduce the potential of false-positive findings (Larrabee, 2003b, 2003c). At the very least, elevated FBS scores should alert the clinician to examine premorbid or comorbid difficulties that may contribute to the maintenance of symptoms in patients with mild head injuries (Miller & Donders, 2001).

NOTES

1. Rogers et al. (2003) recommend Fp as the primary MMPI-2 scale for the assessment of feigning.

2. Greiffenstein et al. (2004) suggest other possible reasons for the insensitivity of F-family scales to feigned non-psychotic problems: namely, (a) that their validity in detecting feigned mental disorder relies largely on role-playing college simulators who tend to

engage in extreme item endorsement, and (b) the F-family was never designed for use in a litigating population.

REFERENCES

Alfano, D. P., Finlayson, M. A. J., Stearns, G. M., & Neilson, P. M. (1990). The MMPI and neurologic dysfunction: Profile configuration and analysis. *The Clinical Neuropsychologist, 4*, 69–79.

Alfano, D. P., Neilson, P. M., Paniak, C. E., & Finlayson, M. A. J. (1992). The MMPI and closed head injury. *The Clinical Neuropsychologist, 6*, 134–142.

Alfano, D. P., Paniak, C. E., & Finlayson, M. A. J. (1993). The neurocorrected MMPI for closed head injury. *Neuropsychiatry, Neuropsychology, and Behavioral Neurology, 6*, 111–116.

Arbisi, P. A., & Ben-Porath, Y. S. (1997). Characteristics of the MMPI-2 F_p scale as a function of diagnosis in an inpatient sample of veterans. *Psychological Assessment, 9*, 102–105.

Arbisi, P. A., & Butcher, J. N. (2004). Failure of the FBS to predict malingering of somatic symptoms: Response to critiques by Greve and Binachini and Less Haley and Fox. *Archives of Clinical Neuropsychology, 19*, 341–345.

Archer, R. P., Aiduk, R., Griffin, R., & Elkins, D. E. (1996). Incremental validity of the MMPI-2 Content Scales in a psychiatric sample. *Assessment, 3*, 79–90.

Archer, R. P., Elkins, D. E., Aiduk, R., & Griffin, R. (1997). The incremental validity of MMPI–2 supplementary scales. *Assessment, 4*, 193–205.

Archer, R. P., Griffin, R., & Aiduk, R. (1995). MMPI-2 clinical correlates for the common codes. *Journal of Personality Assessment, 65*, 391–407.

Bachna, K., Sieggreen, M. A., Cermak, L., Penk, W., & O'Connor, M. (1998). MMPI/MMPI-2: Comparisons of amnesic patients. *Archives of Clinical Neuropsychology, 13*, 535–542.

Ben Porath, Y. S., McCully, E., Almagor, M. (1993). Incremental validity of the MMPI-2 Content Scales in the assessment of personality and psychopathology by self-report. *Journal of Personal Assessment, 61*, 557–575.

Berry, D. T. R., Wetter, M. W., Baer, R. A., Youngjohn, J. R., Gass, C. S., Lamb, D. G., Franzen, M. D., MacInnes, W. D., & Bucholz, D. (1995). Overreporting of closed-head injury symptoms on the MMPI-2. *Psychological Assessment, 7*, 517–523.

Binder, L. M., Kinderman, S. S., Heaton, R. K., & Salinsky, M. C. (1998). Neuropsychologic impairment in patients with nonepileptic seizures. *Archives of Clinical Neuropsychology, 13*, 513–522.

Boone, K. B., & Lu, P. H. (1999). Impact of somatoform symptomatology on credibility of cognitive performance. *The Clinical Neuropsychologist, 13*, 414–419.

Brulot, M. M., Strauss, E. H., & Spellacy, F. J. (1997). The validity of MMPI-2 correction factors for use with patients with suspected head injury. *The Clinical Neuropsychologist, 11*, 391–401.

Butcher, J. N., Arbisi, P. A., Atlis, M. M., & McNulty, J. L. (2003). The construct validity of Lees-Haley Fake Bad Scale: Does this scale measure somatic malingering and feigned emotional distress? *Archives of Clinical Neuropsychology, 18*, 473–485.

Butcher, J. N., Dahlstrom, W. G., Graham, J. R., Tellegen, A. M., & Kaemmer, B. (1989). *MMPI-2, Minnesota Multiphasic Personality Inventory–2: Manual for administration and scoring.* Minneapolis, MN: University of Minnesota Press.

Butcher, J. N., Graham, J. R., Ben Porath, Y. S., Tellegen, A., Dahlstrom, W. G., & Kaemmer, B. (2001). *Manual for administration, scoring, and administration* (revised ed.). Minneapolis: University of Minnesota Press.

Butcher, J. N., & Pope, K. S. (1992). The research base, psychometric properties, and clinical uses of the MMPI-2 and MMPI-A. *Canadian Psychology, 33*, 61–78.

Camara, W. J., Nathan, J. S., & Puente, A. E. (2000). Psychological test usage: Implications in professional psychology. *Professional Psychology: Research and Practice, 31*, 141–154.

Cragar, D. E., Schmitt, F. A., Berry, D. T. R., Cibula, J. E., Dearth, C. M. S., & Fakhoury, T. A. (2003). A comparison of MMPI-2 decision rules in the diagnosis of nonepileptic seizures. *Journal of Clinical and Experimental Neuropsychology, 25*, 793–804.

Crews, W. D., Jefferson, A. L., Broshel, D. K., Rhodes, R. D., Williamson, J., Brazil, A. M., Barth, J. T., & Robbins, M. K. (2003). Neuropsychological dysfunction in patients with end-stage pulmonary disease: Lung transplant evaluation. *Archives of Clinical Neuropsychology, 18*, 353–362.

Cripe, L. I. (1996). The MMPI in neuropsychological assessment: A murky measure. *Applied Neuropsychology, 3*, 97–103.

Dahlstrom, W. G., & Archer, R. P. (2000). A shortened version of the MMPI-2. *Assessment, 7*, 131–137.

Dearth, C. S., Berry, D. T. R., Vickery, C. D., Vagnini, V. L., Baser, R. E., Orey, S. A., & Cragar, D. E. (2005). Detection of feigned head injury symptoms on the MMPI-2 in head injured patients and community controls. *Archives of Clinical Neuropsychology, 20*, 95–110.

Derry, P. A., Harnadek, M. C. S., McLachlan, R. S., & Sontrob, J. (1997). Influence of seizure content on interpreting psychopathology on the MMPI-2 in patients with epilepsy. *Journal of Clinical and Experimental Neuropsychology, 19*, 396–404.

Derry, P. A., & McLachlan, R. S. (1996). The MMPI-2 as an adjunct to the diagnosis of pseudoseizures. *Seizure, 5*, 35–40.

Dunn, J. T. & Lees-Haley, P. R. (1995). The MMPI-2 correction factor for closed-head-injury: A caveat for forensic cases. *Assessment, 2*, 47–51.

Edwards, D. W., Dahmen, B. A., Wanlass, R. L., Holmquist, L. A., Wicks, J. J., Davis, C., & Morrison, T. L. (2003). Personality assessment in neuropsychology: The nonspecificity of MMPI-2 neurocorrection methods. *Assessment, 10*, 222–227.

Fox, D. D., & Lees-Haley, P. R. (2001). MMPI-2 scores do not correlate with employment status. *Journal of Forensic Neuropsychology, 2*, 53–56.

Gass, C. S. (1991). MMPI-2 interpretation and closed head injury: A correction factor. *Psychological Assessment, 3*, 27–31.

Gass, C. S. (1992). MMPI-2 interpretation of patients with cerebrovascular disease: A correction factor. *Archives of Clinical Neuropsychology, 7*, 17–27.

Gass, C. S. (1996). MMPI-2 variables in attention and memory test performance. *Psychological Assessment, 8*, 135–138.

Gass, C. S. (2000). Assessment of emotional functioning with the MMPI-2. In G. Groth-Marnat (Ed.), *Neuropsychological assessment in clinical practice.* New York: John Wiley & Sons.

Gass, C. S., & Apple, C. (1997). Cognitive complaints in closed-head injury: Relationship to memory test performance and emotional disturbance. *Journal of Clinical and Experimental Neuropsychology, 19*, 290–299.

Gass, C. S., & Gonzales, C. (2003). MMPI-2 short form proposal: CAUTION. *Archives of Clinical Neuropsychology, 18*, 521–527.

Gass, C. S., & Luis, C. A. (2001a). MMPI-2 short form: Psychometric characteristics in a neuropsychological setting. *Assessment, 8*, 213–219.

Gass, C. S., & Luis, C. A. (2001b). MMPI-2 Scale F(p) and symptom feigning: Scale refinement. *Assessment, 8,* 425–429.

Gass, C. S., & Wald, H. S. (1997). MMPI-2 interpretation and closed-head trauma: Cross-validation of a correction factor. *Archives of Clinical Neuropsychology, 12,* 199–205.

Glassmire, D. M., Kinney, D. L., Greene, R. L., Stolberg, R. A., Berry, D. T. R., & Cripe, L. (2003). Sensitivity and specificity of MMPI-2 neurologic correction factors: Receiver operating characteristic analysis. *Assessment, 10,* 299–309.

Golden, Z., & Golden, C. J. (2003). The differential impacts of Alzheimer's dementia, head injury, and stroke on personality function. *International Journal of Neuroscience, 113,* 869–878.

Graham, J. R. (2000). *MMPI-2: Assessing personality and psychopathology* (3rd ed.). New York: Oxford University Press.

Greene, R. L. (2000). *The MMPI-2/MMPI: An interpretative manual* (2nd ed.). Odessa, FL: Psychological Assessment Resources.

Greiffenstein, M. F., & Baker, W. J. (2001). Comparison of premorbid and postinjury MMPI-2 profiles in late postconcussion claimants. *The Clinical Neuropsychologist, 15,* 162–170.

Greiffenstein, M. F., Baker, W. J., Gola, T., Donders, J., & Miller, L. (2002). The Fake Bad Scale in atypical and severe closed head injury litigants. *Journal of Clinical Psychology, 58,* 1591–1600.

Greiffenstein, M. F., Baker, W. J., Axelrod, B., Peck, E. A., & Gervais, R. (2004). The Fake Bad Scale and MMPI-2–family in detection of implausible psychological trauma claims. *The Clinical Neuropsychologist, 18,* 573–591.

Greiffenstein, M. F., Gola, T., & Baker, W. J. (1995). MMPI-2 validity scales versus domain specific measures of detection of factitious traumatic brain injury. *The Clinical Neuropsychologist, 9,* 230–240.

Greve, K. W., & Bianchini, K. J. (2004). Response to Butcher et al., The construct validity of the Lees-Haley Fake-Bad Scale. *Archives of Clinical Neuropsychology, 19,* 337–339.

Guez, M., Brannstrom, R., Nyberg, L., Toolanen, G., & Hildingsson, C. (2005). Neuropsychological functioning and MMPI-2 profiles in chronic neck pain: A comparison of whiplash and non-traumatic groups. *Journal of Clinical and Experimental Neuropsychology, 27,* 151–163.

Hathaway, S. R., or McKinley, J. C. (1940). A Multiphasic Personality Schedule (Minnesota): I. Construction of the schedule. *Journal of Psychology, 10,* 249–254.

Hoffman, R. G., Scott, J. G., Emick, M. A., & Adams, R. L. (1999). The MMPI-2 and closed head injury: Effects of litigation and head injury severity. *Journal of Forensic Neuropsychology, 1,* 3–13.

Iverson, G. L., Henrichs, T. F., Barton, E. A., & Allen, S. (2002). Specificity of the MMPI-2 Fake Bad Scale as a marker for personal injury malingering. *Psychological Reports, 90,* 131–136.

King, T. Z., Fennell, E. B., Bauer, R., Crosson, B., Dede, D., Riley, J. L., Robinson, M. E., Uthman, B., Gilmore, R., & Roper, S. N. (2002). MMPI-2 profiles of patients with intractable epilepsy. *Archives of Clinical Neuropsychology, 17,* 583–593.

Larrabee, G. J. (1998). Somatic malingering on the MMPI and MMPI-2 in personal injury litigants. *The Clinical Neuropsychologist, 12,* 179–188.

Larrabee, G. J. (2003a). Exaggerated MMPI-2 symptom report in personal injury litigants with malingered neurocognitive deficit. *Archives of Clinical Neuropsychology, 18,* 673–686.

Larrabee, G. J. (2003b). Detection of symptom exaggeration with the MMPI-2 in litigants with malingered neurocognitive deficit. *The Clinical Neuropsychologist, 17,* 54–68.

Larrabee, G. J. (2003c). Detection of malingering using atypical performance patterns on standard neuropsychological tests. *The Clinical Neuropsychologist, 17,* 410–425.

Larrabee, G. J. (2003d). Exaggerated pain report in litigants with malingered neurocognitive dysfunction. *The Clinical Neuropsychologist, 17,* 395–410.

Larrabee, G. J. (2005). Assessment of malingering. In G. J. Larrabee (Ed.) *Forensic Neuropsychology: A scientific approach.* New York: Oxford University Press.

Lees-Haley, P. R. (1992). Efficacy of the MMPI-2 validity scales and MCMI-II modifier scales for detection of spurious PTSD claims: F, F-K, Fake-Bad scale, ego strength, subtle-obvious subscales, Dis, and Deb. *Journal of Clinical Psychology, 48,* 681–689.

Lees-Haley, P. R.. (2001). Commentary on misconceptions and misuse of the MMPI-2 in assessing personal injury claimants. *Neurorehabilitation, 16,* 301–302.

Lees-Haley, P. R., English, L. T., & Glenn, W. G. (1991). A Fake-Bad-Scale for personal injury claimants. *Psychological Reports, 68,* 203–210.

Lees-Haley, P. R., & Fox, D. D. (2004). Commentary on Butcher, Arbisi, Atlis, & McNulty (2003) on the Fake Bad Scale. *Archives of Clinical Neuropsychology, 19,* 333–336.

Lees-Haley, P. R., Iverson, G. L., Lange, R. T., Fox, D. D., & Allen L. M. III. (2002). Malingering in forensic neuropsychology: Daubert and the MMPI-2. *Journal of Forensic Neuropsychology, 3,* 167–203.

McCaffrey, R. J., O'Bryant, S. E., Ashendorf, L., & Fisher, J. M. (2003). Correlations among the TOMM, Rey-15, and MMPI-2 validity scales in a sample of TBI litigants. *Journal of Forensic Neuropsychology, 3,* 45–53.

Meyers, J. E., Millis, S. R., & Volkert, K. (2002). A validity index for the MMPI-2. *Archives of Clinical Neuropsychology, 17,* 157–169.

Miller, H. B., & Paniak, C. E. (1995). MMPI and MMPI-2 profile and code type congruence in a brain-injured sample. *Journal of Clinical and Experimental Neuropsychology, 17,* 58–64.

Miller, L. J., & Donders, J. (2001). Subjective symptomatology after traumatic head injury. *Brain Injury, 15,* 297–304.

Millis, S. R., Putnam, S. H., & Adams, K. M. (1995). *Neuropsychological malingering and the MMPI-2: Old and new indicators.* Paper presented at the 30th Annual Symposium on the use of the MMPI, MMPI-2, and MMPI-A. St. Petersburg, Fla.

Mittenberg, W., Tremont, G., & Rayls, K. R. (1996). Impact of cognitive function on MMPI-2 validity in neurologically impaired patients. *Assessment, 3,* 157–163.

Nelson, L. D., Elder, J. T., Groot, J., Tehrani, P., & Grant, A. C. (2004). Personality testing and epilepsy: Comparison of two MMPI-2 correction procedures. *Epilepsy and Behavior, 5,* 911–918.

Nelson, L. D., Elder, J. T., Tehrani, P., & Groot, J. (2003). Measuring personality and emotional functioning in multiple sclerosis: A cautionary note. *Archives of Clinical Neuropsychology, 18,* 419–429.

Nichols, D. S. (2001). *Essentials of MMPI-2 assessment.* New York: John Wiley & Sons.

Palav, A., Ortega, A., & McCaffrey, R. J. (2001). Incremental validity of the MMPI-2 Content Scales: A preliminary study with brain-injured patients. *Journal of Head Trauma Rehabilitation, 16,* 275–283.

Paolo, A. M., Ryan, J. J., & Smith, A. J. (1991). Reading difficulty of the MMPI-2 subscales. *Journal of Clinical Psychology, 47,* 529–533.

Rabin, L. A., Barr, W. B., & Burton, L. A. (2005). Assessment practices of clinical neuropsychologists in the United States and Canada: A survey of INS, NAN, and APA Division 40 members. *Archives of Clinical Neuropsychology, 20,* 33–65.

Rayls, K. R., Mittenberg, W., Burns, W. J., & Theroux, S. (2000). Prospective study of the MMPI-2 correction factor after mild head injury. *The Clinical Neuropsychologist, 14,* 546–550.

Rayls, K., Mittenberg, W. B., Williams, J., & Theroux, S. (1997). Longitudinal analysis of the MMPI-2 neurocorrection factor in mild head trauma [Abstract]. *Archives of Clinical Neuropsychology, 12,* 390–291.

Rohling, M. L., Green, P., Allen, L. M., & Iverson, G. L. (2002). Depressive symptoms and neurocognitive test scores in patients passing symptom validity tests. *Archives of Clinical Neuropsychology, 17,* 205–222.

Rogers, R., Sewell, K. W., Martin, M. A., & Vitacco, M. J. (2003). Detection of feigned mental disorders: A meta-analysis of the MMPI-2 and malingering. *Assessment, 10,* 160–177.

Ross, S. R., Millis, S. R., Krukowski, R. A., Putnam, S. H., & Adams, K. M. (2004). Detecting incomplete effort on the MMPI-2: An examination of the Fake-Bad Scale in mild head injury. *Journal of Clinical and Experimental Neuropsychology, 26,* 115–134.

Ross, S. R., Putnam, S. H., Gass, C. S., Bailey, D. E., & Adams, K. M. (2003). MMPI-2 indices of psychological disturbance and attention and memory test performance in head injury. *Archives of Clinical Neuropsychology, 18,* 905–916.

Ruttan, L. A., & Heinrichs, R. W. (2003). Depression and neurocognitive functioning in mild traumatic brain injury patients referred for assessment. *Journal of Clinical and Experimental Neuropsychology, 25,* 407–419.

Schinka, J. A., & LaLone, L. (1997). MMPI-2 norms: Comparisons with a census-matched subsample. *Psychological Assessment, 9,* 307–311.

Sellbom, M., Ben Porath, Y., Graham, J. R., Arbisi, P. A., & Bagby, R. M. (2005). Susceptibility of the MMPI-2 Clinical, Restructured Clinical (RC), and Content scales to overreporting and underreporting. *Assessment, 12,* 79–85.

Senior, G., & Douglas, L. (2001). Misconceptions and misuse of the MMPI-2 in assessing personal injury claimants. *Neurorehabilitation, 16,* 203–213.

Sherman, E. M. S., Strauss, E., Slick, D. J., & Spellacy, F. (2000). Effect of depression on neuropsychological functioning in head injury: Measurable but minimal. *Brain Injury, 14,* 621–632.

Slick, D. J., Hopp, G., Strauss, E., & Spellacy, F. J. (1996). Victoria Symptom Validity Test: Efficiency for detecting feigned memory impairment and relationship to neuropsychological tests and MMPI-2 validity scales. *Journal of Clinical and Experimental Neuropsychology, 18,* 911–922.

Solbakk, A-K., Reinvang, I., & Nielsen, C. S. (2000). ERP indices of resource allocation difficulties in mild head injury. *Journal of Clinical and Experimental Neuropsychology, 22,* 743–760.

Temple, R. O., McBride, A. M., Horner, M. D., & Taylor, R. M. (2003). Personality characteristics of patients showing suboptimal effort. *The Clinical Neuropsychologist, 17,* 402–409.

Tsushima, W. T., & Tsushima, V. G. (2001). Comparison of the Fake Bad Scale and other MMPI-2 validity scales with personal injury litigants. *Assessment, 8,* 205–212.

Wetter, M. W., & Deitsch, S. E. (1996). Faking specific disorders and response consistency on the MMPI-2. *Psychological Assessment, 8,* 39–47.

Wilkus, R. J., Dodrill, C. B., & Thompson, P. M. (1984). Intensive EEG monitoring and psychological studies of patients with pseudoepileptic seizures. *Epilepsia, 25,* 200–207.

Youngjohn, J. R., Davis, D., & Wolf, I. (1997) Head injury and the MMPI-2: Paradoxical severity effects and the influence of litigation. *Psychological Assessment, 9,* 177–184.

Personality Assessment Inventory (PAI)

PURPOSE

The Personality Assessment Inventory (PAI) is a self-report test that assesses personality functioning and psychological disorders.

SOURCE

The PAI is available from Psychological Assessment Resources (http://www.parinc.com). The PAI Comprehensive Kit (including a manual, 2 test booklets, 2 administration folios, 25 answer sheets, profile forms, and critical items) costs $239 US. The test can be given in several formats: paper-and-pencil, audiocassette, and computer. It is available in English or Spanish. Hand-scoring is possible. However, two other scoring options, mail-in service and computer software, also provide interpretive reports. The PAI software costs $695 US. A separate screener, the Personality Assessment Screener, consisting of 22 items, is available for $83 US.

AGE RANGE

The test is intended for use with individuals 18 to 89 years of age.

DESCRIPTION

This self-report multiple-scale inventory (Morey, 1991) has been gaining in popularity (Edens et al., 2001) and ranks fourth in terms of objective instruments in doctoral-level clinical training programs approved by the American Psychiatric Association (Belter & Piotrowski, 2001). It consists of 344 items that constitute four sets of nonoverlapping scales: 4 validity scales, 11 clinical scales covering major categories of pathology corresponding to DSM nosology (neurotic spectrum—SOM, ANX, ARD, DEP; psychotic spectrum—MAN, PAR, SCZ; behavior disorder or impulse control problems—BOR, ANT, ALC, DRG), 5 treatment scales measuring constructs relevent to treatment, and 2 interpersonal scales (see Table 15–21; Morey, 2003). In contrast to the MMPI-2, the clinical scales were developed to measure particular constructs that are represented by the names of the individual scales, with content validity and discriminative validity playing important roles in the development of the PAI (Morey, 2003).

To ensure adequate depth of coverage, the scales were designed to include items that address the multidimensionality and full range of severity of the construct. As a consequence,

Table 15–21 Summary of PAI Scales and Subscales

Validity Scales	Inconsistency (ICN)	Consists of pairs of highly correlated items
	Infrequency (INF)	Items with very high or low endorsement rates
	Negative Impression (NIM)	Suggests an exaggerated unfavourable impression
	Positive Impression (PIM)	Suggests an enhanced positive impression
Clinical Scales	Somatic Complaints (SOM) 　Conversion 　Somatization 　Health Concerns	Focuses on preoccupation with health matters and somatic complaints
	Anxiety (ANX) 　Cognitive 　Affective 　Physiological	Focuses on phenomenology and observable signs of anxiety
	Anxiety-Related Disorders (ARD) 　Obsessive-Compulsive 　Phobias 　Traumatic Stress	Focuses on symptoms related to specific disorders—especially phobias, traumatic stress, and obsessive-compulsive symptoms
	Depression (DEP) 　Cognitive 　Affective 　Physiological	Focuses on symptoms of depressive disorders
	Mania (MAN) 　Activity Level 　Grandiosity 　Irritability	Focuses on symptoms of mania and hypomania
	Paranoia (PAR) 　Hypervigilence 　Persecution 　Resentment	Focuses on symptoms of paranoid disorders
	Schizophrenia (SCZ) 　Psychotic Experiences 　Social Detachment 　Thought Disorder	Focuses on symptoms relevant to schizophrenic disorders
	Borderline Features (BOR) 　Affective Instability 　Identity Problems 　Negative Relationships 　Self-Harm	Focuses on attributes suggestive of borderline personality functioning
	Antisocial Features (ANT) 　Antisocial Behaviors 　Egocentricity 　Stimulus Seeking	Focuses on history of illegal acts, egocentrism, lack of empathy, instability, excitement-seeking
	Alcohol Problems (ALC)	Focuses on problems associated with alcohol use
	Drug Problems (DRG)	Focuses on problems associated with drug use
Treatment Scales	Aggression (AGG) 　Aggressive Attitude 　Verbal Aggression 　Physical Aggression	Focuses on behaviors/attitudes related to anger, assertiveness
	Suicidal Ideation (SUI)	Focuses on suicidal ideation
	Stress (STR)	Measures impact of recent stressors in major life areas
	Nonsupport (NON)	Measures a lack of perceived social support
	Treatment Rejection (RXR)	Focuses on attitudes indicating a lack of interest in making personal/psychological changes
Interpersonal Scales	Dominance (DOM)	Assesses dominance/submissive style
	Warmth (WRM)	Assesses whether person is interested in supportive/empathetic relationships

most of the clinical scales are arrayed as a collection of sub-scales, each of which taps an important component of the superordinate construct (e.g., Depression: affective, cognitive, and physiological components). In addition, test items are answered on a graded four-alternative scale, with the anchors being *totally false, slightly true, mainly true, and very true.*

Generally, the beginning point in the interpretation is a determination of the validity of the profile. This is followed by an examination of the individual scales (those with scores of 70 T or greater), their component parts, and a consideration of particular combinations of scales (Morey, 2003). The simplest approach to configurational analysis involves describing the profile by its two-point code. However, other approaches are also provided. The PAI software (Morey, 2000) includes an empirical comparison of the respondent's profile to the average profile of various diagnostic groups (e.g., major depression). In addition, Morey (1991, 1996) has developed a series of diagnostic rules that are incorporated into the PAI interpretive computer program (Morey, 2000) and are designed to aid in diagnosis. These diagnostic rules are a combination of empirically based algorithms and conceptually derived rules based on DSM-IV criteria for psychopathology (Morey, 2003; Morey et al., 1998). Twenty-seven critical items have also been identified and are intended to indicate potential crisis situations. Positive responses to any of these items suggest the need for follow-up.

The ordering of PAI items allows a sampling of item content on almost all scales and subscales within the first 160 items (Morey, 2003). From these items, estimates of scores for 20 of the 22 full scales can be obtained. Scores for the ICN and STR full scales cannot be obtained from this short form. Morey (1991) warned that the short form may be useful in certain research and screening applications, or in unusual clinical circumstances, but should not be used when important clinical decisions must be made. The PAS (see *Source*) is a very rapid, broadband screening instrument consisting of a subset of 22 PAI items.

ADMINISTRATION

Instructions are printed on the front of the booklet. Briefly, the patient is instructed to read each statement and to decide whether it is totally false, slightly true, mainly true, or very true as applied to himself or herself. The test can also be given by personal computer, with software available from the source. An audiotape is available from the test publisher for those patients who cannot read, although Morey (2003) noted that such a departure from standard administration may affect test results.

A fourth-grade reading level is required. The level of IQ or memory ability required to ensure test validity is not known.

ADMINISTRATION TIME

Approximately 40 to 50 min is required.

SCORING

If 18 or more items were left unanswered, the client should be asked to review and complete those items if possible; in general, scores on a scale or subscale should not be interpreted if more than 20% of the items on that scale were left unanswered (Morey, 2003). Hand-scoring is possible with the use of an answer sheet; however, computer scoring is preferred, because it is faster, is less susceptible to error, automatically computes a variety of supplemental indices, and provides an interpretive report.

Scores for scales are transformed into linear T scores that have a mean of 50 and standard deviation of 10. For example, a T score of 40 corresponds to the 16th percentile, whereas a T score of 70 is equivalent to the 96th percentile. Typically, T scores of 70 or greater merit attention, because they represent pronounced deviations from the typical responses of adults living in the community. The PAI T scores are referenced against a representative sample of American adults living in the community. Reference to various comparison groups (e.g., clinical sample, individuals with PIM elevations) is also possible. Such comparisons can be made by referring to the test manual (Morey, 1991) and by using the Interpretive Explorer component of the PAI scoring and interpretation software (Morey, 2000). The hand-scoring profile form also includes a reference line that lies two standard deviations above the mean of the clinical standardization sample. Morey (2003) recommended that if profile elevations suggest problems of clinical significance, the clinician should also evaluate the profile in the context of specific contextual referents. If such problems are not present, the initial comparison should focus on the community norms.

DEMOGRAPHIC EFFECTS

Age

Age has an impact on PAI scores, especially at the extremes (Morey, 1991). The youngest age group (18–29 years) shows mean scores on the ANX, PAR, BOR, and ANT scales that are 5 to 7 T scores above the mean for the entire sample. Older adults (60 years and older) generally obtain T scores that are below the mean for the entire sample.

Gender

In general, differences between males and females in scale means for the full scales are less than 4 T-score units—a difference that is equivalent to the standard error of measurement (*SEM*) for these scales (Morey, 1991). Differences for the subscales are similarly small, although exceptions occur on ANT and ALC scales, for which the gender difference is greater than 5 T-score units, corresponding to the higher incidence of antisocial personality disorder and alcoholism reported in males (Morey, 1991).

Education

Education has significant effects across the scales (Morey, 1991). Those with the fewest years of education (4–11 years) have T scores that are 4 to 5 units above the sample means, whereas those with the most years of education (≥16) have T-scores slightly below the mean.

Ethnicity

According to Morey (1991), differences in PAI scores attributable to race appear to be small and are generally equivalent to or less than the *SEM*. The major exception occurs on the PAR scale, where blacks and other races have T scores that are about 7 T-score units higher than those of Caucasians. Fantoni-Salvador and Rogers (1997) also noted that PAI scales did not appear to be influenced by ethnic background in Hispanic patients.

NORMATIVE DATA

Standardization Sample

Norms were developed from a U.S. 1995 Census-matched sample of 1000 community-dwelling individuals, stratified according to age, race, and gender (see Table 15–22). Data were also gathered from samples of college students ($N = 1051$) and clinical subjects ($N = 1246$), the latter drawn from a wide variety of clinical facilities, including outpatient psychiatric settings (35%), inpatient psychiatric settings (25%), medical settings (2%), substance abuse programs (15%), and correctional settings (12%; Morey, 1991). A large database of profiles obtained from individuals applying for public safety positions is also available (Roberts et al., 2000). Data for additional diagnostic

Table 15–22 Characteristics of the PAI Normative Standardization Sample

Number	1000 adults selected from an initial sample of 1462 adults residing in the United States
Age (years)	18–89 conforming to 1995 US census data
Geographic location	12 states in the United States representing both rural and urban areas
Sample type	Individuals drawn from directories and special appeals to community groups
Education (years)	Mean = 13.7
Gender (%)	
Men	48
Women	52
Race/Ethnicity	In comparison to 1995 U.S. Census data, proportions are comparable for blacks, whites, and other
Screening	No more than 33 items could be left blank

or evaluation groups are also presented in the interpretive guide (Morey, 1996).

RELIABILITY

Internal Consistency

The internal consistency of the clinical scales is quite high, with median alphas for the full scales of .81, .86 and .82 for the normative, clinical, and college samples, respectively (Morey, 2001). Similar findings have been reported by others in clinical (Boone, 1998; Schinka, 1995) and nonclinical (Costa & McCrae, 1992) samples. Internal consistency estimates for ICN and INF tend to be low (<.60), but these scales do not measure theoretical constructs but rather the care with which the test was completed (Morey, 1991). Internal consistency of the subscales is lower and ranges from .42 to .89 (Boone, 1998; Morey, 1991; Schinka, 1995). This is perhaps to be expected given their shorter item length. Mean interitem correlations for the PAI scales and subscales is typically about .20, indicating that the items tap reasonably independent content (Morey, 1991). There is very little variability in internal consistency as a function of race, gender, or age (Morey, 1991).

Test-Retest Reliability and Practice Effects

Normal individuals from the community and college samples were retested after intervals of about 24 to 28 days. Test-retest coefficients of the clinical scales were generally adequate/high, ranging from .68 (DOM) to .92 (DRG; Morey, 1991). Only ICN and INF showed low consistency (<.50; Morey, 1991). Boyle and Lennon (1994) found the median test-retest reliability (across all scales) to be .73 using a similar retest interval with a sample of 70 nonpsychiatric adults.

Mean scores show little change over time (about 2 to 3 T-score points), and profiles show substantial stability in configuration over time ($r = .83$; Morey, 1991). In general, however, high-point codes are not as stable as the reliability of the overall profile configuration, nor are they as stable as the T-score values of the scales themselves. For this reason, Morey (1991) suggested that the use of high-point codes should be considered only as a first step in profile interpretation; in general, the consideration of total profile configuration in interpretation is preferable.

Standard Errors of Measurement

The *SEM* of T scores on the clinical scales ranges from 2.8 (ANT) to 4.6 (DRG). This information is important to determine whether scale scores are significantly different from one another or have changed significantly over time. For example, changes in T scores that are 2 *SEM*s or more in magnitude can serve as a threshold for detecting statistically reliable change in a given client (Morey, 2003).

VALIDITY

Relations Within the Test

The pattern of correlations between scales is generally consistent with expectation (Morey, 1991). For example, NIM and PIM display a moderate inverse relationship, and NIM is positively related with clinical scales, especially with scales involving the reporting of subjective distress.

Factor-analytic findings of the PAI in normal and clinical samples suggest four major dimensions (Morey, 1991). The first factor seems related to general maladjustment and affective disruption, with scales DEP, ANX, ARD, SCZ, and BOR loading highly on this factor. The second factor represents acting-out behavior, with highest loading from scales ANT, ALC, and DRG. The third factor is defined by loadings on MAN, ANT, and DOM and appears to involve egocentricity and exploitativeness in interpersonal relationships. The fourth factor was defined by high positive loadings on INF and ICN in the clinical group, suggesting a dimension of profile validity/carelessness. In the normal group, this factor is defined by high negative loadings on WRM and positive loadings on NON, SCZ, and PAR. For this group, the meaning of this factor seems to involve a social detachment and touchiness/sensitivity in social relationships. Similar factor-analytic findings have been found by others in nonclinical samples (Deisinger, 1995) and clinical samples (Schinka, 1995; but see Boyle & Lennon, 1994; Boyle et al., 1994; see also Conger & Conger, 1996, who attempted to clarify the controversy). Morey (1991) noted that, although the factor structure seems to converge with a number of relevant distinctions, a large amount of variance (more than 25%) remains unaccounted for and appears to be unique to each of the scales. Accordingly, the factor scores should not be emphasized at the expense of these unique sources of variance.

Ten of the clinical scales were designed to have a subscale structure. Therefore, two identical elevations on a particular scale may be interpreted differently depending on the configuration of the subscales. Jackson and Trull (2001) were unable to replicate the four-factor model of the BOR items in a nonclinical sample. Therefore, caution is needed in interpreting PAI-BOR subscale scores in similar populations. Rather, their results revealed a different six-factor structure.

Computer modeling (of random responding, item response set) and simulation studies (to assess performance of subjects attempting to manage their impression) provide support for the notion that the PAI validity scales have some utility in capturing invalid profiles (Morey, 1991).

Relations With Other Measures

The convergent and discriminant validity of the PAI has received some support from evaluations of mean profiles of relevant clinical groups (Morey, 1991, 2003), correlations of the scales with other markers (e.g., MMPI, BDI, NEO-PI, Rorschach) of similar constructs (e.g., Costa & McCrae, 1992;

Hays, 1997; Klonsky, 2004; Morey, 1991, 2003; Parker et al., 1999; Rogers et al., 1998b; Wang et al., 1997; Young & Schinka, 2001), and evaluations of diagnostic accuracy with reference to clinical judgments/structured diagnostic interviews (e.g., Bell-Pringle et al., 1997; Fantoni-Salvador & Rogers, 1997; Klonsky, 2004). However, Edens et al. (2001) raised some concerns with regard to the ability of the PAI psychotic spectrum scales to identify specific patient groups. In addition, the ability of the PAI to evaluate substance abuse problems is mixed (Edens et al., 2001). Item content has been noted to be face valid, rendering ALC and DRG scales very susceptible to dissimulation (Fals-Stewart, 1996; but see Morey, 2003, for some strategies to detect substance abuse underreporting). Even when the profile appears valid, the DRG and ALC scales may not discriminate well between past and present psychoactive substance use (Fals-Stewart, 1996).

Predictive Validity

Research suggests that the PAI may be useful in assessing risk. For example, investigations have supported the utility of the SUI scale as a marker of suicide risk (Edens et al., 2001; Rogers et al., 1998b; Wang et al., 1997). Further, the PAI has several scales and indices (e.g., AGG, ANT) that are relevant to the assessment of violence potential. A number of studies have reported positive evidence regarding the relation between these scales and various types of violence and misbehavior among offender populations (Caperton et al., 2004; Douglas et al., 2001; Wang et al., 1997; see Edens et al., 2001, and Duellman & Bowers, 2004, for review). However, the obtained correlations tended to be relatively small, suggesting that use of specific cut-scores (e.g., $T \geq 70$) might result in significant errors (both false positive and false negative).

Neuropsychological Studies

Few studies have been published bearing on the utility of the PAI in the neuropsychological context. Roselli et al. (2001) noted abnormality in PAI profiles among chronic cocaine abusers, pointing to a Borderline/Antisocial personality, frequently associated with features of mania. Mild cognitive deficits were observed in these individuals; however, neuropsychological test performance showed no robust association with personality profile, suggesting that neuropsychological test performance is independent from personality traits in this sample.

Validity of Self-Report

Clients may alter their responses to present themselves in a particular light (e.g., feign psychopathology or underreport symptoms), and the PAI contains several scales and indices that assess symptom exaggeration or fabrication.

There are several indicators of negative distortion (see Table 15–23). The NIM scale is composed of nine items, collectively designed to measure an exaggerated unfavorable impression of the self and present circumstances, and contains

Table 15–23 PAI Indicators of Distortion

Indicator	Composition	Suggested Cutoff for Suspicion
NIM	Items of low endorsement frequency	≥73T
MAL	Eight configural features from PAI	≥3
RDF	Weighted combination of PAI scores	>0
PIM	Items of low endorsement frequency	≥57T
DEF	Eight configural features from PAI	≥6
CDF	Weighted combination of PAI scores	>160

Source: Adapted from Morey, 2003.

extremely bizarre and unlikely symptoms (Morey, 1991). Generally, NIM scores lower than 8 (73 T) suggest little distortion in the negative direction on the clinical scales, with the likelihood of distortion increasing with higher scores (Rogers et al., 1998a; Morey, 2003). The effectiveness of NIM is mixed (see Edens et al., 2001, and Morey, 2003, for review), seeming to work best with efforts to simulate severe, but not milder, forms of mental disorder. The Malingering Index (MAL) is derived from eight scoring criteria drawn from various PAI scales and subscales that tend to be observed more frequently in the profiles of persons simulating severe mental disorders than in actual clinical patients. MAL is scored by determining the number of positive features, with scores ranging from 0 to 8. Scores of 3 or more raise suspicion, whereas scores of 5 or greater are considered highly specific for malingering (Morey, 2003; Rogers et al., 1998). The sensitivity of MAL appears to decline when milder forms of psychopathology (e.g., depression, posttraumatic stress disorder) are being simulated (e.g., Calhoun et al., 2000; see Morey, 2003, for review). The Rogers Discriminant Function (RDF) involves a weighted combination of PAI scales that best discriminated overreporters of psychopathology from respondents answering honestly (Rogers et al., 1996). Scores greater than 0 suggest malingering, whereas scores less than 0 suggest that no effort at negative distortion was made. Results in simulation studies have been promising; however, the results have been less promising in forensic contexts (Rogers et al., 1998; see Edens et al., 2001, and Morey, 2003, for review). A similar discriminant function has been developed by Cashel et al., 1995 (CDF) but with mixed results in detecting distortion (Morey, 2003; also see later discussion).

Morey (2003) indicated that the correlations among the various negative distortion indicators (NIM, MAL, RDF) are low to moderate and suggested that patterns of performance may shed light on the relative contributions of covert and overt influences on the profile. For example, he suggested that the NIM scale is relatively highly saturated with influences of psychopathology. Accordingly, if all three indicators are markedly elevated (e.g., 90 T or greater), overt exaggeration is likely. If NIM is elevated, RDF is average, and MAL falls somewhere in between, the pattern suggests that covert factors are likely responsible for the distortion. If NIM > MAL > RDF with RDF still moderately elevated, it suggests a mixture of

covert and overt influences. Research is required to examine the validity of these interpretive guidelines.

The MMPI-2 also offers a number of indicators of overreporting. Blanchard et al. (2003) compared the effectiveness of the MMPI-2 and the PAI in college students attempting to feign a mental disorder (e.g., insanity, depression) in a psychiatric or forensic setting. The MMPI-2 indicators of overreporting included F, F_B, F_p, Ds, Ds-R, FBS, F-K, and O-S. Four scales or scale combinations were used with the PAI: NIM, MAL, RDF, and CDF. The best single predictor was the F-K index, followed closely by F_p, and the performance of MAL from the PAI was only slightly poorer. The MMPI-2 set of indicators was consistently better as a set. However, each inventory offered incremental validity over the other (see also Bagby et al., 2002).

It is important to note that, to date, studies have focused on the detection of exaggeration of psychiatric symptomatology. The relative efficacy of the various PAI indicators in detecting the kinds of exaggeration typically encountered in the neuropsychological context (i.e., overreporting of somatic and/or cognitive disturbances) remains to be evaluated. Duncan and Ausborn (2002) reported a strong correlation of .73 between the MMPI-2 F and PAI NIM scales in a criminal pretrial forensic population. In addition, NIM showed a modest correlation (−.34) with the Reliable Digit Span score from the WAIS-R. These findings suggest that NIM, like F, may be sensitive to exaggeration of psychiatric symptomatology and that other tools (e.g., MMPI-2 FBS) may be more useful in the detection of exaggeration of somatic and cognitive symptoms.

The PAI also provides several positive distortion indicators. The PIM scale was developed to evaluate underreporting and defensiveness. For the most part, PIM items offer the individual an opportunity to admit minor personal fault. Low scores (<44 T) are strongly indicative of honest responding. Scores of 18 or above (between 57 T and 68 T) raise the suspicion index; high scores on PIM, at or above 68 T, suggest extreme caution in interpretation of the PAI (see Morey, 2003, for a review). In addition to PIM, two configural indices have been developed: the Defensiveness Index (DEF; Morey, 1996) and the Cashel Discriminant Function (CDF; Cashel et al., 1995). DEF is a composite score of eight different configural features from the PAI profile. Scores of 6 or greater suggest that the person is overtly defensive, although the sensitivity of this cut-score appears to be limited in coached dissimulators (Morey, 2003). The CDF was developed in response to poor classification of defensive students and offenders using either PIM or DEF. It involves multiplying the T scores for six PAI scales (BOR, PIM, MAN, RXR, ALC, STR) by weights and then summing these products to create a function score. Morey and Lanier (1998) found the CDF to correlate positively with PIM ($r = .23$) and DEF ($r = .40$); however, it also correlated positively with indices of overreporting ($r = .30$ to .41 for NIM, MAL, and RDF), leading the researchers to suggest that CDF may serve as a general indicator of impression management, in either direction. However, Bagby et al. (2002) found that CDF was ineffective in detecting fake-bad responding using a simulation paradigm. Morey (2003) suggested that low scores on the Cashel function (<135) indicate honest responding, scores between 145 and 160 suggest some efforts at impression management, and scores greater than 160 indicate distortion.

Morey (2003) noted that correlations among the three positive distortion indicators are low to modest, suggesting that they have somewhat different properties. He suggested that PIM is relatively influenced by true adjustment status. Accordingly, if all three indicators are markedly elevated, the client is effortfully attempting to present a favorable impression. If PIM is elevated, the CDF is average, and DEF falls in between, covert factors such as lack of insight may be distorting the profile. If PIM > DEF > CDF, with CDF still elevated, a mixture of overt and covert influences is likely. If CDF > DEF > PIM, overt positive dissimulation is suggested. If neither DEF nor PIM is elevated, then there is overt negative profile distortion. Research is required to verify these various proposals.

In addition to altering response style to overreport or underreport symptoms, clients may adopt a particular response set (e.g., all-true, all-false) or respond randomly. As a consequence, tests such as the MMPI-2 and the PAI include scales to detect the presence of random responding (e.g., MMPI-2: F, F_B, VRIN; PAI: ICN, INF). Back random responding (BRR; i.e., changing from initial content-based responding somewhere within the instrument and continuing throughout the remaining test items) results in clinically meaningful changes on PAI scales, especially on the STR scale (Clark et al., 2003). However, PAI validity scales (ICN, INF) perform poorly in identifying the presence of low to moderate levels of BRR. Moreover, MMPI-2 Clinical and Content scales are less susceptible to the effects of BRR, and MMPI-2 validity indices are better at detecting its presence. In addition, if BRR is detected on the PAI, the entire test must be discarded, because there is no way to distinguish between BRR and all-random responding (Clark et al., 2003). This is unfortunate, because the PAI has a built-in short form available that is based on responses to the first 160 items and includes abbreviated versions of most (20 of 22) PAI full scales (Morey, 1991).

Based on this concern, Morey and Hopwood (2004) developed a new strategy to identify BRR that relies on the high correlation of short- and long-form full-scale T scores. They recommended that a short/full difference in T scores greater than 5 on both the SUI and ALC scales, in the absence of elevations on ICN or INF, should be used to detect BRR from nonrandom responding. In such circumstances, the clinician should interpret T scores derived from the 160-item short form, because the full instrument is likely to contain significant distortion. T-score transformation for the short-form scales can be found in Appendix F-1 of the PAI manual (Morey, 1991).

COMMENT

The PAI is simple to administer and score. Identified psychometric strengths of the PAI, relative to the MMPI-2, include nonoverlapping scales that enhance discriminant validity (Rogers et al., 1993), lower reading levels (grade 4; Cashel et al., 1995), fewer items (Lepage & Mogge, 2001), extensive response set features (Edens et al., 2000), and four response options for each item, which allows for gradation of responses (Rogers et al., 1993). The availability of different normative referents is also an asset. Reliability of the instrument is generally very good. On the basis of their *SEM*s, however, greater confidence can be placed in the interpretation of the PAI full scales than in the subscales.

The PAI is based on current notions of psychopathology, taps a broad range of symptomatology, and therefore is relevant in a variety of clinical contexts, including inpatient, outpatient, and criminal settings. Bear in mind that the PAI assesses patterns of psychopathology that are related to DSM-IV diagnoses. However, the PAI does not evaluate formally the DSM-IV inclusion and exclusion criteria. Therefore, it is not a diagnostic measure (Rogers, 2003); rather, its results should be used to inform diagnostic information derived from other sources (e.g., structured interviews).

Historically, multiscale inventories such as the PAI were referred to as "objective tests." However, this term is a misnomer: Although the scoring is objective, the interpretation is not (Rogers, 2003). The availability of a variety of interpretations offered in the computerized report is an asset; however, Rogers (2003) warned against "cherry picking"—an extreme form of confirmatory bias. It is also important to bear in mind that almost none of the published research has attempted to examine the diagnostic utility of interpretive strategies or decision rules other than the clinical cutoffs associated with full-scale scores, which might provide incremental validity beyond the full-scale scores in isolation (Edens et al., 2001).

The PAI may provide important data about patients who abuse alcohol and drugs; however, the instrument should be used with considerable caution when assessing individuals suspected of having such problems who are in situations where they may be motivated to deny it (Fals-Stewart & Lucent, 1997). Further, the ways in which the PAI may help the clinician understand the patient in a neuropsychological setting (e.g., provide a sense of specific problems and motivations, suggest or rule out various disorders), select appropriate treatment, and anticipate the course of therapy remains to be determined. Of note, the PAI includes a number of features that may contribute information that is highly relevant to the neuropsychological context, such as indications about substance use, aggression, suicide potential, and attitudes toward treatment.

The PAI includes a number of indicators to detect distorting influences. There is some evidence that the PAI is less successful than the MMPI-2 in detecting exaggeration of psychiatric disturbance (Blanchard et al., 2003). However, administration of both inventories may enhance detection of feigning psychiatric disorder (Blanchard et al., 2003). Whether the PAI is as effective as other tools (e.g., MMPI-2 FBS) to detect manipulation in the neuropsychological context (e.g., personal injury) remains to be determined.

REFERENCES

Bagby, R., Nicholson, R. A., Bacchiochi, J. R., Ryder, A. G., & Bury, A. S. (2002). The predictive capacity of the MMPI-2 and PAI validity scales and indexes to detect coached and uncoached feigning. *Journal of Personality Assessment, 78,* 69–86.

Bell-Pringle, V. J., Pate, J. L., & Brown, R. C. (1997). Assessment of borderline personality disorder using the MMPI-2 and the Personality Assessment Inventory. *Assessment, 2,* 131–139.

Belter, R. W., & Piotrowski, C. (2001). Current status of doctoral-level training in psychological testing. *Journal of Clinical Psychology, 57,* 717–726.

Blanchard, D. D., McGrath, R. E., Pogge, D. L., & Khadivi, A. (2003). A comparison of the PAI and MMPI-2 as predictors of faking bad in college students. *Journal of Personality Assessment, 80,* 197–205.

Boone, D. (1998). Internal consistency reliability of the Personality Assessment Inventory with psychiatric inpatients. *Journal of Clinical Psychology, 54,* 839–843.

Boyle, G. J., & Lennon, T. J. (1994). Examination of the reliability and validity of the Personality Assessment Inventory. *Journal of Psychopathology and Behavioral Assessment, 16,* 173–187.

Boyle, G. J., Ward, J., & Lennon, T. J. (1994). Personality Assessment Inventory: A confirmatory factor analysis. *Perceptual and Motor Skills, 79,* 1441–1442.

Calhoun, P. S., Earnst, K. S., Tucker, D. D., Kirby, A. C., & Beckham, J. C. (2000). Feigning combat-related posttraumatic stress disorder on the Personality Assessment Inventory. *Journal of Personality Assessment, 75,* 338–350.

Caperton, J. D., Edens, J. F., & Johnson, J. K. (2004). Predicting sex offender institutional adjustment and treatment compliance using the Personality Assessment Inventory. *Psychological Assessment, 16,* 187–191.

Cashel, M. L., Rogers, R., Sewell, K., & Martin-Cannici, C. (1995). The Personality Assessment Inventory (PAI) and the detection of defensiveness. *Assessment, 2,* 333–342.

Clark, M. E., Gironda, R. J., & Young, R. W. (2003). Detection of back random responding: Effectiveness of MMPI-2 and Personality Assessment Inventory validity indices. *Psychological Assessment, 15,* 223–234.

Conger, A. J., & Conger, J. C. (1996). Did too, did not! Controversies in the construct validation of the PAI. *Journal of Psychopathology and Behavioral Assessment, 18,* 205–212.

Costa, P. T., & McCrae, R. R. (1992). Normal personality assessment in clinical practice: The NEO Personality Inventory. *Psychological Assessment, 4,* 5–13.

Deisinger, J. A. (1995). Exploring the factor structure of the Personality Assessment Inventory. *Assessment, 2,* 173–179.

Douglas, K. S., Hart, S. D., & Kropp, P. R. (2001). Validity of the Personality Assessment Inventory for forensic assessments. *International Journal of Offender Therapy and Comparative Criminology, 45,* 183–197.

Duellman, R. M., & Bowers, T. G. (2004). Use of the Personality Assessment Inventory (PAI) in forensic and correctional settings: Evidence for concurrent validity. *International Journal of Forensic Psychology, 1,* 42–57.

Duncan, S. A., & Ausborn, D. L. (2002). The use of reliable digits to detect malingering in a criminal forensic pretrial population. *Assessment, 9,* 56–61.

Edens, J. F., Cruise, K. R., & Buffington-Vollum, J. K. (2001). Forensic and correctional applications of the Personality Assessment Inventory. *Behavioral Sciences and the Law, 19,* 519–543.

Edens, J. F., Hart, S. D., Johnson, D. W., Johnson, J. K., & Olver, M. E. (2000). Use of the Personality Assessment Inventory to assess psychopathy offender populations. *Psychological Assessment, 12,* 132–139.

Fals-Stewart, W. (1996). The ability of individuals with psychoactive substance use disorders to escape early detection by the Personality Assessment Inventory. *Psychological Assessment, 8,* 60–68.

Fals-Stewart, W., & Lucente, S. (1997). Identifying positive dissimulation by substance-abusing individuals on the Personality Assessment Inventory: A cross-validation study. *Journal of Personality Assessment, 68,* 455–469.

Fantoni-Salvador, P., & Rogers, R. (1997). Spanish versions of the MMPI-2 and PAI: An investigation of concurrent validity with Hispanic patients. *Assessment, 4,* 29–39.

Hays, J. R. (1997). Note on concurrent validation of the Personality Assessment Inventory in law enforcement. *Psychological Reports, 81,* 244–246.

Jackson, K. M., & Trull, T. J. (2001). The factor structure of the Personality Assessment Inventory-Borderline features (PAI-BOR) scale in a nonclinical sample. *Journal of Personality Disorders, 15,* 536–545.

Klonsky, E. D. (2004). Performance of Personality Assessment Inventory and Rorschach indices of schizophrenia in a public psychiatric hospital. *Psychological Services, 1,* 107–110.

Lepage, J. P., Mogge, N. L., & Sharpe, W. R. (2001). Validity rates of the MMPI-2 and PAI in a rural inpatient psychiatric facility. *Assessment, 8,* 67–74.

Morey, L. C. (1991). *The Personality Assessment Inventory.* Odessa, FL: Psychological Assessment Inventory.

Morey, L. C. (1996). *An interpretive guide to the Personality Assessment Inventory.* Odessa, FL: PAR.

Morey, L. C. (2000). *PAI software portfolio manual.* Odessa, FL: PAR.

Morey, L. C. (2003). *Essentials of PAI assessment.* New York: John Wiley & Sons.

Morey, L. C., Goldin, J. N., & White, T. (1998). *PAI-SP manual.* Odessa, FL: PAR.

Morey, L. C., & Hopwood, C. J. (2004). Efficacy of a strategy for detecting back random responding on the Personality Assessment Inventory. *Psychological Assessment, 16,* 197–200.

Morey, L. C., & Lanier, V. W. (1998). Operating characteristics for six response distortion indicators for the Personality Assessment Inventory. *Assessment, 5,* 203–214.

Parker, J. D., Daleiden, E. L., & Simpson, C. A. (1999). Personality Assessment Inventory substance-use scales: Convergent and discriminant relations with the Addiction Severity Index in a residential chemical dependence treatment setting. *Psychological Assessment, 11,* 507–513.

Roberts, M. D., Thompson, J. A., & Johnson, M. (2000). *PAI law enforcement, corrections, and public safety selection report module.* Odessa, Fla.: PAR.

Rogers, R. (2003). Forensic use and abuse of psychological tests: Multiscale inventories. *Journal of Psychiatric Practice, 9,* 316–320.

Rogers, R., Ornduff, S. R., & Sewell, K. W. (1993). Feigning specific disorders: A study of the Personality Assessment Inventory (PAI). *Journal of Personality Assessment, 60,* 554–560.

Rogers, R., Sewell, K. T., Morey, L. C., & Ustad, K. (1996). Detection of feigned mental disorders on the Personality Assessment Inventory: A discriminant analysis. *Journal of Personality Assessment, 67,* 629–640.

Rogers, R., Sewell, K. W., Cruise, K. R., Wang, E. W., & Ustad, K. L. (1998a). The PAI and feigning: A cautionary note on its use in forensic-correctional settings. *Assessment, 5,* 399–405.

Rogers, R., Ustad, K. L., & Salekin, R. T. (1998b). Convergent validity of the Personality Assessment Inventory: A study of emergency referrals in a correctional setting. *Assessment, 5*, 3–12.

Rosselli, M., Ardila, A., Lubomski, M., Murray, S., & King, K. (2001). Personality profile and neuropsychological test performance in chronic cocaine. *International Journal of Neuroscience, 110*, 55–72.

Schinka, J. A. (1995). Personality Assessment Inventory scale characteristics and factor structure in the assessment of alcohol dependency. *Journal of Personality Assessment, 64*, 101–111.

Wang, E. W., Rogers, R., Giles, C. L., Diamond, P. M., Herrington-Wang, L. E., & Taylor, E. R. (1997). A pilot study of the Personality Assessment Inventory (PAI) in corrections: Assessment of malingering, suicide risk, and aggression in male inmates. *Behavioral Sciences and the Law, 15*, 469–482.

Young, M. S., & Schinka, J. A. (2001). Research validity scales for the NEO-PI-R: Additional evidence for reliability and validity. *Journal of Personality Assessment, 76*, 412–420.

Scales of Independent Behavior—Revised (SIB-R)

PURPOSE

The Scales of Independent Behavior—Revised (SIB-R) assesses adaptive and problem behaviors.

SOURCE

The SIB-R is available from Riverside Publishing (http://www.riverpub.com). The complete kit (interview book, manual, 15 full-scale response booklets, 5 short-form response booklets, and 5 early development form response booklets) costs $229 US. SIB-R scoring and reporting software costs $287.50 US.

AGE RANGE

The test covers a wide age range, from early infancy to 90 years.

DESCRIPTION

This measure (Bruininks et al., 1996) is designed to assess functional independence and adaptive functioning in school, home, employment, and community settings. The items sample skills from early life to adulthood, varying from profound to mild disabilities. The SIB-R has several different forms—the Full Scale, the Short Form, and the Early Development Form—along with a Problem Behavior Scale.

The SIB-R Full Scale is a broad measure of adaptive behavior comprising 14 subscales organized into four adaptive behavior clusters (Motor, Social Interaction and Communication, Personal Living, and Community Living; see Table 15–24). These clusters form the primary interpretive level. Each cluster contains from two to five subscales, and each subscale has up to 20 items, for a total of 259 items. The respondent rates the patient on each item (e.g., "Plans and prepares meals regularly for self and family") using a 4-point scale:

0 Never or rarely—even if asked
1 Does but not well or about 1/4 of the time—may need to be asked
2 Does fairly well or about 3/4 of the time—may need to be asked
3 Does very well always or almost always—without being asked.

The performance rating is based on the underlying requirement that the patient does (or could do) all parts of the task without help or supervision.

The SIB-R also summarizes an individual's overall performance across the various clusters/domains. This overall score (SIB-R Broad Independence Score) can be directly compared to the WJ-R Broad Cognitive Ability Scale, allowing users to determine whether any strength or discrepancy exists between adaptive and cognitive skills.

The Short Form contains 40 items from all 14 subscales of the SIB-R Full Scale. The Early Development Form was designed primarily for use with children from early infancy through age 6 years or with older individuals with severe disabilities whose developmental levels are below 8 years of age. It contains 40 items sampled from the Full Scale. Both the Short Form and the Early Development Form can be used as either separate assessments or screeners.

The Problem Behavior Scale provides a general summary of eight problem behaviors organized into three broad maladaptive behavior indices (Internalized, Externalized, and Asocial; see Table 15–24) and a total maladaptive score. Each problem behavior is rated according to its frequency of occurrence and severity. The five ratings on the frequency scale are

1 Less than once a month
2 1 to 3 times a month
3 1 to 6 times a week
4 1 to 10 times a day
5 1 or more times an hour.

The five ratings on the severity scale are

0 Not serious; not a problem
1 Slightly serious; a mild problem
2 Moderately serious; a moderate problem
3 Very serious; a severe problem
4 Extremely serious; a critical problem

Results from an individual's adaptive behavior and problem behavior assessments can be weighted and combined (70% adaptive behavior, 30% problem behavior) to produce a Support Score. This score is used to help determine the overall intensity of resources needed to improve and/or maintain the individual's functional independence. The structure of the Full SIB-R is shown in Figure 15–3.

Table 15–24 Summary of SIB-R Clusters and Subscales

Broad Independence	Clusters	Subscales	Sample Skills
	Motor Skills	Gross Motor	Balance, coordination, strength, endurance
		Fine Motor	Eye-hand coordination
	Social Interaction and Communication Skills	Social Interaction	Interactions include entertaining, making plans
		Language Comprehension	Tasks range from simple recognition of one's name to searching for information
		Language Expression	Tasks range from simple repetition to delivering formal reports
	Personal Living Skills	Eating and Meal Preparation	Tasks range from simple eating to meal preparation
		Toileting	Tasks range from staying dry to using appropriate bathroom facilities outside the home
		Dressing	Tasks range from simple removal of clothes to selection and maintenance of clothes
		Personal Self-Care	Tasks range from simple use of a toothbrush to seeking professional assistance to treat illness
		Domestic Skills	Tasks range from clearing dishes to complex home repairs
	Community Living Skills	Time and Punctuality	Tasks range from assessing concept of time to ability to keep appointments
		Money and Value	Tasks range from selecting particular coins to consumer decisions involving investments and use of credit
		Work Skills	Tasks range from indicating when a chore is finished to completing job resumes
		Home/Community Orientation	Tasks assess concept of space at home and more complex travel skill in the community
Problem Behaviors	Internalized	Hurtful to Self	e.g., hitting self
		Unusual or Repetitive Habits	e.g., rocking
		Withdrawal or Inattentive Behavior	e.g., keeping away from other people
	Externalized	Hurtful to Others	e.g., biting
		Destructive to Property	e.g., throwing
		Disruptive Behavior	e.g., picking fights
	Asocial	Socially Offensive Behavior	e.g., talking too loudly
		Uncooperative Behavior	e.g., breaking laws

ADMINISTRATION

The test can be given as an interview, with the examiner asking questions and recording the respondent's answers in the SIB-R response booklet. Although the SIB-R can be given to the patient directly, the authors advise caution in using such self-report information if there is any reason to question the accuracy of responses. There are suggested starting points to minimize testing time. To use the starting point, the examiner needs to estimate the age level at which the individual is functioning developmentally. Basal and Ceiling rules are included in each Response Booklet but differ depending on the form (Full, Short, and Early Development).

In the checklist administration procedure, the respondent reads each item and records answers directly in the Response Booklet. This format does not rely on basal or ceiling rules; every item is responded to and scored in the adaptive behavior subscales.

For the Problem Behavior Scale, the respondent indicates whether the individual currently exhibits any type of problem behavior within each category, provides open-ended descriptions of the single most serious behavior within each category, and rates its frequency and severity. The respondent also

Figure 15–3 Structure of the SIB-R. *Source:* Reproduced with permission of Riverside Publishing.

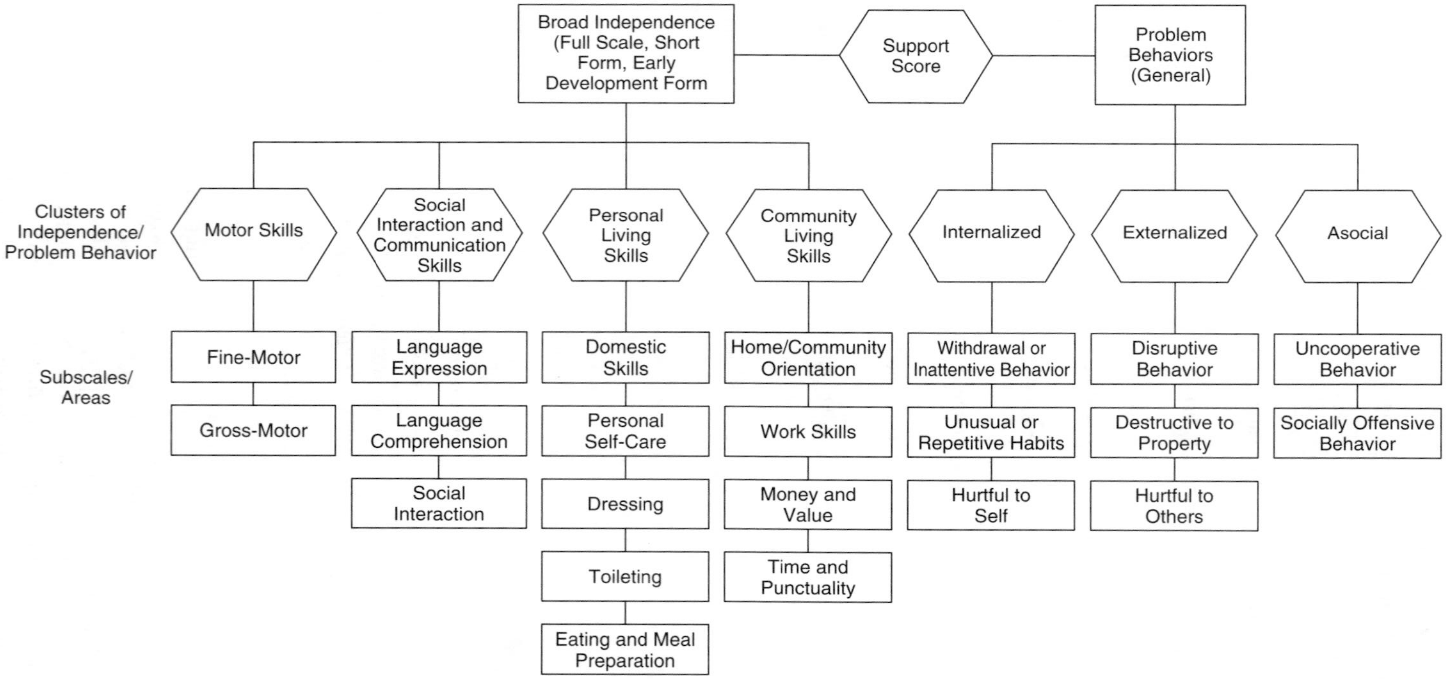

describes how the problem behavior is usually managed by others.

ADMINISTRATION TIME

About 1 hour is required for the Full Scale. Administration time is about 15 to 20 min for the Short Form or the Early Development Form.

SCORING

For the Full Scale, the sum of adaptive behavior item scores (each rated 0, 1, 2, or 3) becomes the raw score for each subscale. The age-equivalent of each subscale can be obtained directly from tables in the Response Booklet. Clusters of related subscales provide the primary basis for normative interpretations. Briefly, each raw score for each subscale has a corresponding W score, which is a special transformation of the Rasch ability scale. The W scores for each cluster are averaged to obtain the cluster W score. These are then summed to form the Broad Independence W score. Relative Mastery Indices (RMIs), reflecting relative quality of performance), standard scores (SSs, with a mean of 100 and an *SD* of 1; range, 0 to 200), percentile ranks (PRs), and adaptive behavior skill levels (with age-level tasks ranging from limited to advanced) are then determined for each cluster and the Broad Independence Score. Standard scores can also be converted by means of a table (H in the manual) into T scores, stanines, and normal curve equivalents.

For the Short Form, raw adaptive behavior item scores range from 0 to 120. Raw scores on the Early Development Form range from 0 to 120.

The ratings of problem behaviors are used to derive four maladaptive indices: an Internalized Maladaptive Index (IMI), an Asocial Maladaptive Index (AMI), an Externalized Maladaptive Index (EMI), and a General Maladaptive Index (GMI). The GMI is an aggregate of all problem behaviors. The Maladaptive Behavior Indices range from about +5 to −70, with an average of 0, and have a mean of 0 for normal individuals of any age, with negative scores indicating greater problem behaviors.

The Support Score ranges from 0 (pervasive) to 100 (infrequent or none), with higher scores reflecting increased functional independence.

An individual's adaptive behavior and problem behavior can also be displayed in profiles. Computer scoring is available and is recommended to reduce time and error.

DEMOGRAPHIC EFFECTS

Age

As might be expected, age has a significant relation to adaptive functioning (Bruininks et al., 1996). There is a progressive increase in scores until about age 39 years, with scores declining slightly from 40 to 90 years. Problem behaviors become less common with increasing age, but the correlations with age are very small.

Gender

Gender has little impact on scores (Bruininks et al., 1996).

Race

Race has little relation to the Broad Independence Score (Bruininks et al., 1996).

NORMATIVE DATA

Standardization Sample

Norms for the original SIB ($N = 1764$) were gathered in the 1980s to reflect the characteristics of the 1980 U.S. Census. In gathering additional data for the SIB-R, a supplemental sample of 418 individuals was chosen so that the total norm group ($N = 2182$) would conform to 1990 U.S. Census data in terms of gender; race (white, black, native American, Asian); Hispanic origin; occupational status (not in labor force, employed, unemployed); occupational level (white-collar, blue-collar, service, farm); geographical region (Northeast, North Central, South, West); and type of community (urban, rural; see Table 15–25). However, there are disparities between the

Table 15–25 Characteristics of the SIB-R Normative Standardization Sample

Number	2182 (1764 from original SIB sample + 418 from supplemental sample)
Age	3 months to 90 years[a]
Geographic location	United States
Sample type	Representative of U.S. population based on 1990 U.S. Census data with respect to gender, race, occupation, region, and degree of urbanization
Education	Not reported
Gender (%)	
Males	48.6
Females	51.4
Race/Ethnicity (%)	
Caucasian	83.9
Black	12.3
Native or Asian	3.5
Hispanic	8.5
Screening	Norming sample did not include students with severe disabilities unless they were in regular education programs. Individuals who had participated in an English-speaking environment for <1 year were also exluded

[a]Age groups 3–11 mo, $n = 140$; 1yr, $n = 145$; 2yr, $n = 128$; 3yr, $n = 125$; 4 yr, $n = 132$; 5 yr, $n = 109$; 6 yr, $n = 166$; 7–8 yr, $n = 187$; 9–10 yr, $n = 192$; 11–12 yr, $n = 104$; 13–14 yr, $n = 174$; 15-16 yr, $n = 115$; 17–19 yr, $n = 100$; 20–39 yr, $n = 211$; 40–59 yr, $n = 83$; 60–90 yr, $n = 71$. SIB-R age-based norm tables are accessed by month from age 2 through age 18, and by year from age 19+.

normative group and the census data. Specifically, there is a preponderance of individuals from the Midwest and a relative shortage of people from the Northeast. Note too that, although sample sizes are adequate for children and adolescents, there are only 83 individuals aged 40 to 59 years and 71 people aged 60 to 90 years.

Of the SIB-R norm group, 325 individuals (aged 2 to 90 years) were also given the WJ-R Broad Cognitive Ability Cluster (Early Development Scale).

RELIABILITY

Internal Consistency

The internal consistency of the subscales is generally quite high, most in the high .70s to low .90s. A few subscales (e.g., Toileting, Money and Value) show a truncation in the coefficients at some age levels, because most individuals have (or have not yet) developed such skills.

Median reliabilities (high .80s and .90s) are higher for the cluster scores than the subscales, with 15 of the 20 coefficients at .90 or higher. The median coefficient for the Broad Independence Score for the entire standardization sample is .98 (Bruininks et al., 1996). Similar values were obtained in a group of individuals with disabilities (Bruininks et al., 1996). The manual does not report reliability coefficients for the Problem Behavior Scale.

Standard Error of Measurement (SEM)

SEMs are expressed in W scale units, which are given in Rasch analysis, not in the more common standard score distribution with $M = 100$ and $SD = 15$ (Sattler, 2002). The size of the SEM differs according to the test region in which an individual receives a score: people who receive scores near the bottom or top of the test have measures that are subject to larger error than people whose scores fall near the middle.

Test-Retest Reliability

An elementary school age sample ($N = 31$, age 6–13 years) was used to assess the test-retest reliability characteristics of SIB-R Full Scale scores. The two tests were completed by the same respondent within a 4-week period. Test-retest correlations for the Short Form and Full Scale Broad Independence scores were .97 and .98, respectively. The cluster reliabilities were between .96 and .98. Subtest reliabilities were all high (>.80; Bruininks et al., 1996). Test-retest correlations for the four Maladaptive Behavior Indices ranged from .80 to .83. The Support Score produced a coefficient of .96. Bruininks et al. (1996) noted that reliability was also acceptable (>.70) for the Maladaptive Behavior Indices in other samples, including students with behavior disorders. Test-retest reliability of the Early Development Form after intervals of 7 to 14 days was reported to be high (>.97).

Interrater Reliability

Bruininks et al. (1996) reported that the SIB-R is quite consistent between parents for the same child, with most correlations in the .80s. Correlations between parents tend to be somewhat higher than those found between parents and teachers (especially in children without disabilities; r about .64; Bruininks et al., 1996).

VALIDITY

Relations Within Test

SIB-R subscales intercorrelate highly. Not surprisingly, subscale correlations with the clusters of which they are members are always higher than subscale correlations with other clusters. Correlations between the subscales and Broad Independence Scores are also quite high (Bruininks et al., 1996). The intercorrelations among the four cluster scores are high; the correlations between the Motor Skills cluster and each of the other three clusters are generally lower than the intercorrelations among the other three clusters, except in those younger than 5 years of age (Bruininks et al., 1996).

Relations With Other Measures

As might be expected given the developmental nature of adaptive behaviors, the relationship between age and SIB-R adaptive behavior skills is curvilinear, increasing rapidly in early ages, increasing more slowly in adolescence, and gradually declining in later life.

Analyses were conducted to assess the relationship between the original SIB, based on 1985 norms using the original Rasch item calibration, and the SIB-R, which used the same individuals but was based on the 1994 norms and Rasch calibration. These analyses revealed high correlations (most in the .90s) between the SIB and SIB-R (Bruininks et al., 1996). Evidence of convergent and divergent validity based on correlations with other measures (e.g., Vineland) is available for the older version (SIB; Middleton et al., 1990) and shows that both tests measure similar traits (correlation between total scores = .83). However, measures between more discrete traits exhibit lower correlations, with the most valid scales being Personal Living Skills, Communication Skills, and Community Living Skills.

Adaptive ability, assessed by the SIB-R, and cognitive ability, assessed by the WJ-R, tend to be highly correlated in individuals without disabilities ($r = .82$ between SIB-R Broad Independence and WJ-R Broad Cognitive Ability W scores; Bruininks et al., 1996). However, they do show different patterns of growth. Bruininks et al. (1996) noted that, among young children (aged 3–4 years), correlations between adaptive behavior and cognitive ability are quite low, typically in the .20s. Among 5- to 12-year-olds, correlations are relatively high, typically in the .70s. Among adolescents and adults without disabilities, where variance is more limited because most adults have mastered most adaptive behavior skills, correlations between adaptive and cognitive domains are again quite low, typically in the teens. Bruininks et al. (1996) noted that both adaptive behavior skills and cognitive ability are age dependent. They proposed that, if age were partialled out, the correlation between adaptive behavior and cognitive ability of individuals without disabilities would be quite low.

In samples with disabilities, correlations between the original SIB and the Original WJ are high (median correlation of about .85; Bruininks et al., 1996). According to the test authors, about 50% to 65% of the variance in adaptive behavior scores for subjects with disabilities is explained by cognitive abilities scores.

The SIB-R Maladaptive Behavior Indices

The problem behavior section of the SIB did not change in the revised version. The SIB-R Maladaptive Behavior Indices correlate in the expected manner with other measures of problem behaviors (Bruininks et al., 1996; McIntyre et al., 2002). The indices tend to assess more outwardly aggressive behaviors, rather than withdrawal and attention behavior problems. Maladaptive behaviors are predictive of family stress and tendency toward out-of-home placement (McIntyre et al., 2002).

Clinical Findings

Bruininks et al. (1996) reported that individuals with disabilities score lower on the SIB and show more problem behaviors than same-aged individuals without such disabilities. In addition, more severe limitations are found among individuals with more severe disabilities. Given the high correlation between the SIB and the SIB-R, similar findings are expected for the revised version.

SIB-R Early Development Form

Children with disabilities obtain significantly lower adaptive behavior scores and show more maladaptive behaviors than do children without such disabilities (Bruininks et al., 1996). Correlations between this form and a similar measure (Early Screening Profiles) are quite high (>.70; Bruininks et al., 1996).

COMMENT

The SIB-R provides a comprehensive rating of an individual's everyday functioning, tapping basic self-care activities (e.g., toileting) as well as instrumental activities of daily living (e.g., managing finances, using transportation). The latter involve fairly complex cognitive abilities and are of primary interest to neuropsychologists, because it is a person's ability to perform these very demanding everyday tasks that frequently motivates families/caregivers to seek assessment. Further, poor performance on these instrumental activities may guide diagnostic decision making. For example, the SIB-R includes coverage of those adaptive skills recommended in the assessment process for defining mental retardation. Similarly, loss of competence in complex tasks of daily living is a defining feature of Alzheimer's disease and related dementing disorders (American Psychiatric

Association, 1994). In short, because lack of or loss of these skills has important implications for patients, families, and health care and legal professionals, the SIB-R may provide valuable information for diagnostic and placement purposes.

One advantage of the SIB-R is that overall cluster and subscale performances can be evaluated, enabling a refined analysis of specific domains of functioning. It also includes a broad measure for assessing problem behaviors that may interfere with school, work, and community adjustment. It is important to note, however, that the SIB-R provides a proxy-report of a patient's functional abilities. Although it does provide an indication of an individual's everyday competence in his or her regular milieu, it is not a direct measure of the patient's functioning. In fact, the authors do not report the results of studies bearing on the relations between informant report and adaptive behaviors directly observed by examiners (Zlomke, 2001). Therefore, the SIB-R should be viewed as one approach to understanding an individual's functional capacity that should be supplemented by other methods of assessment (e.g., performance-based measures of everyday problem-solving)—with the realization that each method may be assessing somewhat different dimensions of behavior (see *Introduction to Assessment of Mood, Personality, and Adaptive Functions*).

The SIB-R can be given to the respondent by an examiner, or the respondent can complete a checklist. Whether the two forms yield identical findings is not reported. Further, the method of administration used with the standardization sample is not clearly described.

The norms cover a broad age range; however, sample size for adults, especially in the older age range, are less than optimal, and screening procedures for the adult sample are not described. In addition, the norm sample does not match U.S. Census data with regard to region.

Reliability of the instrument is excellent, although additional test-retest reliability studies are needed over the entire age range covered by the scale (Sattler, 2002). Further, its sensitivity to change remains to be determined.

There is some evidence of construct validity; however, it is limited and derives largely from the test authors. Importantly, the efficacy of the SIB-R subscales and cluster scores in describing actual competencies (degree of congruence between reported and directly observed behaviors; see earlier discussion) and in predicting real-life adjustment needs to be determined. The translation of overall adaptive and maladaptive scores into a taxonomy of support needs appears to be useful for making decisions regarding planning and treatment services. However, research is required to assess the validity of such decisions.

Users should note that most studies to date have focused on children and young adults, and the utility of the SIB-R in characterizing functional capacities of older adults requires study. Further, whether characteristics on the SIB-R (both adaptive behavior and problem behavior) vary as a function of type of disorder is not known.

The SIB-R can be used together with the WJ-R to provide a comprehensive assessment of adaptive and cognitive ability. However, the WJ-R has recently been revised (WJ-III), making it more difficult to compare adaptive behavior to cognitive behavior.

REFERENCES

American Psychiatric Association (1994). *Diagnostic and statistical manual of mental disorders–IV.* Washington, DC: American Psychiatric Association.

Bruininks, R. H., Woodcock, R. W., Weatherman, R. F., & Hill, B. K. (1996). SIB-R: Scales of Independent Behavior-Revised. Itasca, IL: Riverside Publishing Company.

McIntyre, L. L., Blacher, J., & Baker, B. L. (2002). Behavior/mental health problems in young adults with intellectual disability: The impact on families. *Journal of Intellectual Disability Research, 46,* 239–249.

Middleton, H. A., Keene, R. G., & Brown, G. W. (2000). Convergent and discriminant validities of the Scales of Independent Behavior and the Revised Vineland Adaptive Behavior Scales. *American Journal on Mental Retardation, 94,* 669–673.

Sattler, J. (2002). *Assessment of children: Behavioral and clinical application.* San Diego: Jerome Sattler.

Zlomke, L. (2001). Review of the Scales of Independent Behavior-Revised. In Plake, B. S., & Impara, J. C. (Eds.). *The fourteenth mental measurements yearbook.* Lincoln, NE: Buros Institute of Mental Measurements.

Trauma Symptom Inventory (TSI)

PURPOSE

The Trauma Symptom Inventory (TSI) assesses acute and chronic traumatic symptomatology.

SOURCE

The test (manual, 10 item booklets, 25 hand-scorable answer sheets, and 25 each of male and female profile forms) can be ordered from PAR (http://www.parinc.com) at a cost of $182 US. An alternate 86-item version (TSI-A) is also available for $182 US. It is identical to the TSI but does not contain the Sexual Concerns scale, the Dysfunctional Sexual Behavior scale, or two Critical Items with sexual content. A computer scoring program can be purchased at a cost of $265 US.

AGE RANGE

The test can be given to individuals aged 18 years and older.

DESCRIPTION

Psychological trauma is very common. About 1% to 7% of the general population suffers from posttraumatic stress disorder (PTSD), whereas Vietnam veterans, firefighters, rape victims, and others exposed to extremely stressful events can have incidences of PTSD as high as 20% to 40% (Briere, 1995). The TSI was designed to assess psychological sequelae of potentially traumatic events, including physical violence, sexual assault, combat, automobile accidents, and natural disasters. It consists of 100 items (e.g., nightmares or bad dreams, irritability) that tap four broad areas of distress: dysphoric mood, posttraumatic stress, sexual difficulties, and self-dysfunction. Respondents rate each symptom item according to its frequency of occurrence over the preceding 6 months, using a 4-point scale ranging from 0 (*never*) to 3 (*often*). The items are organized into 10 clinical scales (see Table 15–26). In contrast to other trauma measures, the TSI also contains three validity scales (see Table 15–26). Twelve critical items have also been identi-fied, covering issues such as self-mutilation, potential for suicide, and potential for violence against others. These items are intended to indicate possible problems that need follow-up.

Interpretation begins with an assessment of the validity scales, followed by an examination of TSI scales that are clinically significant (T scores $\geq$ 65). The three TSI scales most relevant to posttraumatic stress disorder are IE, DA, AA (Briere & Elliot, 1998). Beyond specific scale configurations, TSI profiles can be interpreted according to which of two general factors (trauma symptoms—primarily scales AA, D, IE, DA, DIS, TRB, and ISR; self-dysfunction—primarily scales DSB, TRB, ISR, SC, AI) are elevated. Profiles that involve multiple elevations in "trauma" symptoms are more likely to reflect intrusive, avoidant, and dysphoric symptoms, whereas elevations in "self-dysfunction" are indicative of difficulties in identity, affect regulation, and dysfunctional behavior. Briere (1995) suggests that a patient with trauma symptom elevations tends to present more as a classic/uncomplicated trauma victim, often in response to a relatively recent trauma. A respondent with relatively low trauma symptomatology but with multiple self-difficulties would be seen as someone more likely to have the identity and affect regulation difficulties often associated with dysfunctional personality traits; and a person with both trauma and self-disturbance indicators would be most likely to present as a complex trauma victim—chronically distressed, overwhelmed by intrusive symptoms and potentially more likely to act out painful internal states because of lower self-resources.

ADMINISTRATION

The test can be given individually or in a group-testing format. The respondent completes the questionnaire on the answer sheet. A fifth- to seventh-grade reading level is required (Briere, 1995).

ADMINISTRATION TIME

About 20 min is required to complete the TSI.

Table 15–26 Brief Description of TSI Validity and Clinical Scales

	Scale	Description
Validity	Response Level (RL)	Items with very high endorsement rates; high scores reflect tendency toward defensiveness
	Atypical Response (ATR)	Items not commonly endorsed; high scores suggest psychosis, extreme distress, or overendorsement
	Inconsistency Response (INC)	Assesses consistency of response; high scores suggest inconsistent responses to TSI items
Clinical Scales	Anxious Arousal (AA)	Measures symptoms of anxiety, especially hyperarousal (e.g., jumpiness)
	Depression (D)	Measures mood state (e.g., sadness) and depressive cognitive distortions (e.g., hopelessness)
	Anger/ Irritability (AI)	Measures angry or irritable affect, cognitions, and behavior
	Intrusive Experiences (IE)	Measures intrusive symptoms such as flashbacks, nightmares, intrusive thoughts
	Defensive Avoidance (DA)	Measures posttraumatic avoidance, both cognitive (e.g., pushing painful thoughts out of mind) and behavioral (e.g., avoidance of stimuli associated with trauma)
	Dissociation (DIS)	Measures symptoms such as depersonalization, derealization, out-of-body experiences, and psychic numbing
	Sexual Concerns (SC)	Measures self-reported sexual distress (e.g., dissatisfaction, dysfunction, unwanted thoughts and feelings)
	Dysfunctional Sexual Behavior (DSB)	Measures behavior that is dysfunctional because it is indiscriminant, has potential for self-harm or is used to achieve nonsexual goals
	Impaired Self-Reference (ISR)	Measures problems such as identity confusion, self-other disturbance, and lack of self-support
	Tension Reduction Behavior (TRB)	Measures tendency to turn to external methods to reduce distress, such as self-mutilation, angry outbursts, suicide threats

SCORING

Each item on the scoring sheet is identified by scale. The raw score for each scale consists of the total for that scale. The two exceptions are RL and INC. For the RL scale, the number of RL items endorsed with a zero is recorded. For the INC scale, the absolute values of the differences between specific items pairs are summed. The raw scores for each scale are then transferred onto an age-based profile form that lists the corresponding T score. T scores have a mean of 50 and a standard deviation of 10. For all TSI scales, T scores of 65 or higher are considered clinically significant. Profile forms are provided separately for males and females.

DEMOGRAPHIC EFFECTS

Age

Younger respondents tend to score higher than older ones (Briere, 1995).

Gender

In general, females score higher than males (Briere, 1995).

Education

Effects of education are not reported.

Race/Ethnicity

Ethnicity has a small effect on some of the scales (particularly validity scales), accounting for about 2% of the variance in TSI raw scores (Briere, 1995).

NORMATIVE DATA

Standardization Sample

The norms (see Table 15–27) were developed from a stratified random sample based on geographical location of registered owners of automobiles and/or individuals with listed telephones. The sample is generally comparable to 1990 U.S. Census data, although it overrepresents, to some extent, Caucasian, married individuals, and more educated individuals.

Table 15–27 Characteristics of the TSI Sample Used to Determine Interpretive Guide

Number	836
Age (years)	Mean = 47.3, SD = 16.2; range = 18–88
Geographic location	United States
Sample type	Mail-out standardization sample of general population. Random sample based on geographical region of registered owners of automobiles and/or with listed telephones. Subjects completed mail-out TSI surveys.
Education	66% had at least some college or trade school
Gender(%)	
Male	50.8
Female	49.2
Race/Ethnicity(%)	
Caucasian	77.5
African American	10.3
Hispanic	6.1
Asian	2.9
Native American	2.3
Screening	Not reported

Normative data derived from the 836 respondents in the standardization sample are based on combinations of age (18–54 years, 55 years and older) and gender groupings. Because African American and Hispanic respondents in the standardization sample scored an average of 3 to 5 points above Caucasians on the validity scales, Briere (1995) recommends that the examiner adjust cutoff scores to obtain a valid profile for these two groups.

Additional normative data from a sample of 3659 female and male Navy recruits are provided in the test manual (Appendix B) for potential use when the respondent is a member of the U.S. Armed Forces.

RELIABILITY

Internal Consistency

Reliability coefficients for the clinical scales range from .74 to .91 (M = .86 in the standardization sample, .84 in a university sample, .87 in a clinical sample, and .85 in a Navy recruit sample), indicating relatively high internal consistency (Briere, 1995). Similar findings were reported by Purves & Erwin (2004) in a university sample and by Merrill (2001) among female U.S Navy recruits.

Test-Retest Reliability

This is not reported.

VALIDITY

Factor-Analytic Findings

Scales are moderately intercorrelated (Briere, 1995). Exploratory factor analyses within the standardization sample and a clinical sample yielded two factors, designated "Generalized Trauma and Distress" and "Self-Dysfunction" (Briere, 1995). Confirmatory factor analysis suggested that a three-factor model fit the underlying structure of the TSI. The first factor, Trauma, had loadings from intrusive experiences (IE), defensive avoidance (DA), dissociation (DIS), and impaired self-reference (ISR). The second factor, Self, had loadings from ISR, sexual concerns (SC), dysfunctional sexual behavior (DSB), tension-reduction behavior (TRB), and anger/irritability (AI). AI, depression (D), and anxious arousal (AA) contributed to the third factor, Dysphoria. However, Gebhart-Eaglemont (2001) argued that this model is ill-conceived and that the Trauma and Dysphoria components are highly correlated (r = .95), indicating that they constitute one factor.

Relations With Other Measures

Validity was examined by correlating TSI scales with indices from other measures thought to measure similar constructs

(Briere, 1995; Briere & Elliott, 1998). For example, with regard to the validity scales, ATR and RL correlated in the expected manner with PAI and MMPI-2 impression management scales (PAI: PIM, NIM; MMPI-2: F, K, L; Briere, 1995). Similarly, TSI scales showed reasonable convergent validity with those scales from other measures (e.g., the Brief Symptom Inventory, Impact of Event Scale) that overlapped in content. Those scales not similar in content were less strongly correlated with one another (Briere, 1995; Briere & Elliot, 1998).

The TSI also shows incremental validity, providing additional information regarding victimization (particularly in females) beyond that tapped by two other trauma scales (IES, SCL) and a more generic measure of psychological symptoms (BSI; Briere, 1995; Briere & Elliott, 1998).

Clinical Findings

Validity of the TSI was also demonstrated by examining mean differences between traumatized and nontraumatized groups (e.g., Briere, 1995; Elliott et al., 2004; Merrill, 2001; Runtz & Roche, 1999). For example, in psychiatric patients, those reporting a history of child abuse or adult assault tended to have higher TSI raw scores than did those not reporting victimization (Briere, 1995). Similarly, female university students with a history of childhood maltreatment (physical abuse, sexual abuse) had higher TSI scores than did nonmaltreated women. In addition, indicators of greater severity of abuse were predictive of higher symptom scores (Runtz & Roche, 1999). Further, those who had experienced multiple traumatic events were more distressed than those who had experienced fewer events (Green et al., 2000).

Briere (1995) also provided data showing that the TSI has some ability to detect PTSD status in the general population and to identify psychiatric inpatients with and without a diagnosis of Borderline Personality Disorder. However, its ability to differentiate among disorders (e.g., PTSD, Borderline Personality Disorder), however, is not known (Gebhart-Eaglemont, 2001).

Malingering

Little is known about the utility of the ATR scale in distinguishing honest respondents from those exaggerating or fabricating trauma-related symptomatology. Based on score distributions in the standardization sample, Briere (1995) suggested that a score of T > 90 should be used as a cutoff for considering a TSI profile as valid, and that scores greater than T 65 should be considered questionable. Using an analog design, Edens et al. (1998) found that a T-score cutoff of 61 and below produced good sensitivity (81%) and specificity (92%) in a university sample. Application of a cutoff of T 65 in clinical samples generally resulted in low false-positive rates, suggesting that relatively few genuinely symptomatic individuals would be misclassified as malingering. Using a simulation paradigm with university students, Guriel et al. (2004) recently reported that coaching (provision of symptom-specific information and/or strategies for avoiding detection) has little impact on the success of avoiding detection.

A recent study, however, suggested caution in the use of ATR to detect fabrication or enhancement of posttraumatic stress disorder (PTSD). Elhai et al. (2005) compared students simulating PTSD with clinically diagnosed PTSD outpatients. The T-score cutoff of 61 correctly classified only 61% of simulators and patients (PPP = .66, NPP = .54). Elhai et al. (2005) noted that the MMPI-2 Fake Bad Scales have a better record of detecting simulated PTSD.

COMMENT

The TSI is a self-report measure that provides the clinician with information about various aspects of a patient's psychological state, including posttraumatic stress, dysphoric mood, and self-functioning. Administration is straightforward; however, because the individual TSI scales cannot be used in isolation (all 100 items must be administered together), other measures (e.g., Impact of Event Scale) may be more useful in situations where time constraints might make the TSI less appropriate, such as screening (Briere & Elliot, 1998).

The normative base is reasonably large, allowing the clinician to estimate the importance of a TSI score in terms of its frequency in the general population. Internal reliability is good. However, information on test-retest reliability is lacking, as is its sensitivity to change in psychological state.

The incorporation of clinical items indicating potential risks is an asset. Further, the inclusion of validity scales to examine underreporting or overreporting is a particularly positive feature that distinguishes the TSI from essentially all other standardized measures of trauma-related symptomatology. The TSI therefore may be especially appropriate for assessing persons alleging trauma-related symptomatology in forensic contexts (Edens et al., 1998). However, the available data on the utility of the ATR are mixed, and additional study is needed in a forensic setting (e.g., personal injury). At present, the ATR should not be used alone to evaluate trama-related symptomatology. Other measures (e.g., MMPI-2) should be included when assessing symptom accuracy.

The TSI exhibits reasonable convergent and incremental validity. Evidence of divergent validity appears weaker, suggesting that the instrument should not be used as the sole basis in diagnostic evaluations. Other tools (e.g., MMPI-2, PAI), in conjunction with the TSI and the interview, are needed to provide information useful for differential diagnosis. Another possible weakness relates to indications of gender-specificity of the TSI items, suggesting that it performs better with females (Fernandez, 2001; Gebhart-Eaglemont, 2001). Further, although the TSI appears sensitive to potential trauma history, to date most of the studies derive from Briere and his students. Additional research regarding the reliability and validity of the TSI by other researchers is needed.

REFERENCES

Briere. J. (1995). *Trauma symptom inventory: Professional manual.* Odessa, FL: PAR.

Briere, J., & Elliott, D. M. (1998). Clinical utility of the Impact of Event Scale: Psychometrics in the general population. *Assessment, 5,* 171–180.

Edens, J. F., Otto, R. K, & Dwyer, T. J. (1998). Susceptibility of the Trauma Symptom Inventory to malingering. *Journal of Personality Assessment, 71,* 379–392.

Elhai, J. D., Gray, M. D., Naifeh, J. A., Butcher, J. L., Davis, J. L., Falsetti, S. A., & Best, C. L. (2005). Utility of the Trauma Symptom Inventory's Atypical Response Scale in detecting malingered post-traumatic stress disorder. *Assessment, 12,* 210–219.

Elliott, D. M., Mok, D. S., & Briere, J. (2004). Adult sexual assault: Prevalence, symptomatology, and sex differences in the general population. *Journal of Traumatic Stress, 17,* 203–211.

Fernandez, E. (2001). Review of the Trauma Symptom Inventory. In B. S. Plake & J. C. Impara (Eds.). *The fourteenth mental measurements yearbook.* Lincoln, NE: Buros Institute of Mental Measurements.

Gebhart-Eaglemont, J. E. (2001). Review of the Trauma Symptom Inventory. In B. S. Plake & J. C. Impara (Eds.). *The fourteenth mental measurements yearbook.* Lincoln, NE: Buros Institute of Mental Measurements.

Green, B. L., Goodman, L. A., Krupnick, J. L., Corcoran, C. B., Petty, R. M., Stockton, P., & Stern, N. M. (2000). Outcomes of single versus multiple trauma exposure in a screening sample. *Journal of Traumatic Stress, 13,* 271–286.

Guriel, J., Yanez, T., Fremouw, W., Shreve-Neiger, A., Ware, L., Filcheck, H., Farr, C. (2004). Impact of coaching on malingered posttraumatic stress symptoms on the M-FAST and the TSI. *Journal of Forensic Psychology Practice, 4,* 37–56.

Merrill, L. L. (2001). Trauma symptomatology among female U.S. Navy recruits. *Military Medicine, 166,* 621–624.

Purves, D. G., of Erwin, P. G. (2004). Posttraumatic stress and self-disclosure. *Journal of Psychology: Interdisciplinary and Applied, 138,* 23–33.

Runtz, M. G., & Roche, D. N. (1999). Validation of the Trauma Symptom Inventory in a Canadian sample of university women. *Child Maltreatment: Journal of the American Professional Society on the Abuse of Children, 4,* 69–80.

16

Assessment of Response Bias
and Suboptimal Performance

DEFINITION AND CRITERIA

Neuropsychologists are frequently asked to evaluate the nature and severity of deficits in examinees about whom secondary gain is an issue, such as those involved in personal injury litigation, those pursuing long-term disability or worker's compensation awards, or those who are defendants in criminal injury proceedings. Increasingly, neuropsychological opinion is sought regarding whether cognitive deficits are legitimate or feigned; that is, whether the examinee is exaggerating or fabricating deficits. This trend has been driven in part by the increased awareness among clinicians of the frequency with which suboptimal performance (SOP: instances of an examinee not performing to the best of his or her ability as directed on tests) may be encountered in various settings. For example, a recent survey of neuropsychologists in active practice found that as many as 30% of individuals who present for evaluation in the context of personal injury litigation or worker's compensation may be feigning impairments (Mittenberg et al., 2002). Higher rates (about 40%) reportedly obtain among litigants with mild traumatic brain injury (TBI; Larrabee, 2005; Mittenberg et al., 2002). The increased attention to SOP has also been driven by a heightened awareness among those who request and scrutinize neuropsychological assessments of the frequency of this behavior and the increasing variety and utility of detection methods. This has led in turn to increasing requests by referring parties for clinicians to explicitly address SOP and also to increasing stringent evidentiary standards being applied to measures for detecting SOP in the medical-legal arenas where they are most commonly used. It should be noted that the term SOP encompasses *any* instance of less than maximal performance on testing, including those that may arise in the context of somatization, conversion, factitious disorder, or other forms of poor motivation and opposition that are not directly related to secondary gain. Malingering is only one of a number of explanations for SOP and is *not* a synonym for it.

Various definitions and criteria for the diagnosis of malingering have been published, most notably those of the *Diagnostic and Statistical Manual of Mental Disorders—Fourth Edition* (DSM-IV; American Psychiatric Association, 1994). According to this definition, malingering is "the intentional production of false or grossly exaggerated physical or psychological symptoms, motivated by external incentives such as avoiding military duty, avoiding work, obtaining financial compensation, evading criminal prosecution, or obtaining drugs." With respect to diagnostic criteria, the DSM-IV indicates that malingering should be strongly suspected if any combination of the following pertains: (a) medicolegal context of presentation; (b) marked discrepancy between the person's claimed stress or disability and the objective findings; (c) lack of cooperation during the diagnostic evaluation and in complying with the prescribed treatment regimen; and (d) the presence of Antisocial Personality Disorder. A number of authors have noted problems with the DSM-IV criteria, including the lack of relevance to the neuropsychological (as opposed to the psychiatric) context, the difficulty in assessing examinees' internal states, the possibility that conscious and unconscious motivations may contribute to an examinee's behavior and that fabricated or exaggerated deficits may coexist with real impairments.

These limitations have prompted researchers and clinicians to offer alternative definitions and criteria for malingering. Building on the work of Greiffenstein et al. (1994), Slick et al. (1999) presented a set of diagnostic criteria that define psychometric, behavioral, and collateral data indicative of possible, probable, and definite malingering of cognitive dysfunction, for use in clinical practice and for defining populations for clinical research. Their definition of malingering of neurocognitive dysfunction (MND) and criteria are shown in Table 16–1. Although these criteria have not been universally accepted, they are being used increasingly by researchers and have therefore assumed a prominent role in the literature concerning psychometric properties of commonly used measures of SOP.

I. *Definitions*

 A. *Malingering of Neurocognitive Dysfunction (MND)* is the volitional exaggeration or fabrication of cognitive dysfunction for the purpose of obtaining substantial material gain, or avoiding or escaping formal duty or responsibility. Substantial material gain includes money, goods, or services of nontrivial value (e.g., financial compensation for personal injury). Formal duties are actions that people are legally obligated to perform (e.g., prison, military, or public service, or child support payments or other financial obligations). Formal responsibilities are those that involve accountability or liability in legal proceedings (e.g., competency to stand trial).

 B. *Definite MND* is indicated by the presence of clear and compelling evidence of volitional exaggeration or fabrication of cognitive dysfunction and the absence of plausible alternative explanations. The specific diagnostic criteria necessary for Definite MND are listed below.

  1. Presence of a substantial external incentive [Criterion A]
  2. Definite negative response bias [Criterion B1]
  3. Behaviors meeting necessary criteria from group B are not fully accounted for by psychiatric, neurological, or developmental factors [Criterion D]

 C. *Probable MND* is indicated by the presence of evidence strongly suggesting volitional exaggeration or fabrication of cognitive dysfunction and the absence of plausible alternative explanations. The specific diagnostic criteria necessary for Probable MND are listed below.

  1. Presence of a substantial external incentive [Criterion A]
  2. Two or more types of evidence from neuropsychological testing, excluding definite negative response bias [two or more of Criteria B2–B6]

  Or

  One type of evidence from neuropsychological testing, excluding definite negative response bias, and one or more types of evidence from Self-Report [one of Criteria B2–B6 and one or more of Criteria C1–C5]
  3. Behaviors meeting necessary criteria from groups B or C are not fully accounted for by psychiatric, neurological, or developmental factors [Criterion D]

 D. *Possible MND* is indicated by the presence of evidence suggesting volitional exaggeration or fabrication of cognitive dysfunction and the absence of plausible alternative explanations. Alternatively, possible MND is indicated by the presence of criteria necessary for Definite or Probable MND except that other primary etiologies can not be ruled out. The specific diagnostic criteria for Possible MND are listed below.

  1. Presence of a substantial external incentive [Criterion A]
  2. Evidence from Self-Report [one or more of Criteria C1–C5]
  3. Behaviors meeting necessary criteria from groups B or C are not fully accounted for by psychiatric, neurological, or developmental factors [Criterion D]

  Or

  Criteria for Definite or Probable MND are met except for Criterion D (i.e., primary psychiatric, neurological, or developmental etiologies cannot be ruled out). In such cases, the alternate etiologies that cannot be ruled out should be specified.

II. *Criteria*

 A. *Presence of a substantial external incentive*
 At least one clearly identifiable and substantial external incentive for exaggeration or fabrication of symptoms (see definition) is present at the time of examination (e.g., personal injury settlement, disability pension, evasion of criminal prosecution, or release from military service).

 B. *Evidence from neuropsychological tests*
 Evidence of exaggeration or fabrication of cognitive dysfunction on neuropsychological tests, as demonstrated by at least one of the following.

  1. *Definite response bias.* Below chance performance ($p < .05$) on one or more forced-choice measures of cognitive function.
  2. *Probable response bias.* Performance on one or more *well-validated* psychometric tests or indices designed to measure exaggeration or fabrication of cognitive deficits is consistent with feigning.
  3. *Discrepancy between test data and known patterns of brain functioning.* A pattern of neuropsychological test performance that is markedly discrepant from currently accepted models of normal and abnormal central nervous system (CNS) function. The discrepancy must be consistent with an attempt to exaggerate or fabricate neuropsychological dysfunction (e.g., a patient performs in the severely impaired range on verbal attention measures but in the average range on memory testing; a patient misses items on recognition testing that were consistently provided on previous free-recall trials, or misses many easy items when significantly harder items from the same test are passed).
  4. *Discrepancy between test data and observed behavior.* Performance on two or more neuropsychological tests within a domain are discrepant with observed level of cognitive function in a way that suggests exaggeration or fabrication of dysfunction (e.g., a well-educated patient who presents with no significant visual-perceptual deficits or language disturbance in conversational speech performs in the severely impaired range on verbal fluency and confrontation naming tests).
  5. *Discrepancy between test data and reliable collateral reports.* Performance on two or more neuropsychological tests within a domain are discrepant with day-to-day level of cognitive function described by at least one reliable collateral informant in a way that suggests exaggeration or fabrication of dysfunction (e.g., a patient handles all family finances but is unable to perform simple math problems in testing).
  6. *Discrepancy between test data and documented background history.* Improbably poor performance on two or more standardized tests of cognitive function

(continued)

within a specific domain (e.g., memory) that is inconsistent with documented neurological or psychiatric history (e.g., a patient with no documented LOC or PTA, multiple negative neurological investigations, and no other history of CNS trauma or disease consistently obtains verbal memory scores in the severely impaired range after a motor vehicle accident).

C. *Evidence from Self-Report*

The following are indicators of possible malingering of cognitive deficits but are not sufficient for the diagnosis. However, presence of one or more of these criteria provides additional evidence in support of a diagnosis of malingering. These criteria involve significant inconsistencies or discrepancies in the patient's self-reported symptoms that suggest a deliberate attempt to exaggerate or fabricate cognitive deficits.

1. *Self-reported history is discrepant with documented history.* Reported history is markedly discrepant with documented medical or psychosocial history and suggests attempts to exaggerate injury severity or deny premorbid neuropsychological dysfunction (e.g., exaggerated severity of physical injury or length of LOC/PTA; exaggerated premorbid educational or occupational achievement; denial of previous head injury or previous psychiatric history).

2. *Self-reported symptoms are discrepant with known patterns of brain functioning.* Reported or endorsed symptoms are improbable in number, pattern, or severity or markedly inconsistent with expectations for the type or severity of documented injury or pathology (e.g., claims of extended retrograde amnesia without loss of memory for the accident, or claims of loss of autobiographical information after mild head trauma without LOC).

3. *Self-reported symptoms are discrepant with behavioral observations.* Reported symptoms are markedly inconsistent with observed behavior (e.g., a patient complains of severe episodic memory deficits yet has little difficulty remembering names, events, or appointments; a patient complains of severe cognitive deficits yet has little difficulty driving independently and arrives on time for an appointment in an unfamiliar area; a patient complains of severely slowed mentation and concentration problems yet easily follows complex conversation).

4. *Self-reported symptoms are discrepant with information obtained from collateral informants.* Reported symptoms, history, or observed behavior is inconsistent with information obtained from other informants judged to be adequately reliable. The discrepancy must be consistent with an attempt to exaggerate injury severity or deny premorbid neuropsychological dysfunction (e.g., a patient reports severe memory impairment and/or behaves as if severely memory-impaired, but spouse reports that the patient has minimal memory dysfunction at home).

5. *Evidence of exaggerated or fabricated psychological dysfunction.* Self-reported symptoms of psychological dysfunction are substantially contradicted by behavioral observation and/or reliable collateral information. *Well-validated* validity scales or indices on self-report measures of psychological adjustment (e.g., MMPI-2) are strongly suggestive of exaggerated or fabricated distress or dysfunction.

D. *Behaviors meeting necessary criteria from groups B or C are not fully accounted for by psychiatric, neurological, or developmental factors*

Behaviors meeting necessary criteria from groups B and C are the product of an informed, rational, and volitional effort aimed at least in part toward acquiring or achieving external incentives as defined in Criterion A. As such, behaviors meeting criteria from groups B or C cannot be fully accounted for by psychiatric, developmental, or neurological disorders that result in significantly diminished capacity to appreciate laws or mores against malingering, or inability to conform behavior to such standards (i.e., psychological need to "play the sick role," or in response to command hallucinations).

III. *Additional Considerations*

A. *Informed consent* In the process of obtaining informed consent prior to examination, clinicians should ensure that patients understand that a consistent high level of effort is required and that any evidence of poor or inconsistent effort, or exaggeration or fabrication of dysfunction, may be noted in resulting reports or other professional communications.

B. *Differential diagnoses* If criteria for definite, probable, or possible malingering are met by a patient who is unable to appreciate the implications and consequences of his or her behavior (i.e., failure to meet Criterion D) but is instead responding to directions or pressure from others, the term "MND by proxy" may be considered. In cases where psychiatric, developmental, or neurological disorders are the primary cause of feigned cognitive deficits, then a diagnosis of "feigned cognitive deficits secondary to [specify psychiatric/developmental/neurological disorder]" may be considered.

C. *Ruling out malingering* No psychological test has perfect negative predictive power. Therefore, one cannot automatically conclude that patients are not malingering if they obtain "passing" scores on measures designed to detect exaggerated or fabricated deficits. Patients who attempt to malinger may exaggerate or fabricate symptoms from a variety of different domains (e.g., anxiety, mood, memory, language) and present with varying degrees of sophistication. Similarly, failure to meet the proposed criteria for malingering does not constitute conclusive evidence that a patient is not malingering.

D. *Reliability, validity, and standardized administration of diagnostic measures* In order to meet Criteria B2–B6, tests or indices should have adequate reliability and validity, test data should be obtained through standardized procedures under adequate testing conditions, and norms referenced should be applicable to the patient. Forced-choice measures are unique in that they may be excepted from the requirement that

(*continued*)

Table 16–1 Proposed Definition and Criteria for Possible, Probable, and Definite Malingering of Neurocognitive Dysfunction *(continued)*

scores be norm referenced (i.e., raw scores can be "standardized" by referencing random response distributions). Clinicians need to be well aware of the positive and negative predictive power of any signs, symptoms, or test scores that inform the diagnostic process. Although psychometric data are relied upon heavily for a diagnosis of malingering, current psychometric methods and instruments are in a relatively early stage of development. Most current measures or indices of exaggeration or fabrication are experimental and lack adequate normative data. Therefore, scores from such instruments should be interpreted with due caution. Test developers and publishers are strongly encouraged to ensure that their products meet established standards for reliability and validity.

E. *Individual differences* Clinicians must be cognizant of cultural differences, level of acculturation, and demand characteristics of the examination and how these factors may influence patient performance.

F. *Prior patient behavior* A documented or self-reported prior history of malingering, functional findings on medical examination, or sociopathic behavior may support a diagnosis of malingering, but these are neither necessary nor sufficient for diagnosis. Similarly, although uncooperativeness, resistance, or refusal may be associated with malingering, these behaviors are not evidence of exaggeration or fabrication.

G. *Clinical judgment* Many of the malingering criteria require some degree of expert clinical judgment. Expert clinical judgment is (a) an opinion about the nature and causes of specific behaviors in the absence of definitive data, (b) based on an objective evaluation of all obtainable data relevant to the particular case, and (c) supported by the weight of empirical research relevant to the behaviors in question.

H. *Self-reported symptoms* The scope of this paper does not permit a review or listing of all the things to consider when evaluating patient self-report in the context of documented history. However, clinicians should not rush to judgment about intent when self-reports are not congruent with other data. Special care should be taken to distinguish deliberate from nondeliberate misattribution or exaggeration of deficits. Patients may become highly sensitized (particularly in medical-legal settings) to *any* cognitive failings, and it is possible to falsely attribute preexisting symptoms to an

accident, report a higher than actual level of premorbid function, catastrophize or overreport current symptoms, or have difficulty reporting symptoms precisely, without intending to deceive. Clinicians should be cognizant of the literature on base rates of neuropsychological symptoms in the general population. An inability to provide an accurate history or accurately gauge current level of cognitive function may be symptomatic of legitimate brain dysfunction. The task of judging the veracity of reported symptoms is most difficult when significant injuries are documented. Often, there are no objective data on day-to-day functioning that can be compared to reported symptoms for evaluating veracity.

IV. *Malingered Neurocognitive Dysfunction Criteria Checklist*

☐ A.   Clear and substantial external incentive

☐ B1. Definite response bias
☐ B2. Probable response bias
☐ B3. Discrepancy between known patterns of brain function/dysfunction and test data
☐ B4. Discrepancy between observed behavior and test data
☐ B5. Discrepancy between reliable collateral reports and test data
☐ B6. Discrepancy between history and test data

☐ C1. Self-reported history is discrepant with documented history
☐ C2. Self-reported symptoms are discrepant with known patterns of brain functioning
☐ C3. Self-reported symptoms are discrepant with behavioral observations
☐ C4. Self-reported symptoms are discrepant with information obtained from collateral informants
☐ C5. Evidence of exaggerated or fabricated psychological dysfunction on standardized measures

☐ D.   Behaviors satisfying Criteria B and/or C were volitional and directed at least in part toward acquiring or achieving external incentives as defined in Criteria A

☐ E.   The patient adequately understood the purpose of the examination and the possible negative consequences of exaggerating or fabricating cognitive deficits

☐ F.   Test results contributing to Criteria B are sufficiently reliable and valid

Source: From Slick et al., 1999, pp. 552–555. Reprinted with the kind permission of Psychology Press.

METHODS OF DETECTION

In concert with the increased use of neuropsychological data and opinions in the medical-legal arena, interest in methods of detecting SOP has burgeoned over the past decade. There are essentially two types of methods for detecting SOP. The first encompasses those indices derived from conventional measures. The second includes measures that have been developed specifically to detect SOP. Both methods rely on the

detection of inconsistency; that is, performance within and across test sessions that is inconsistent with patterns expected of healthy individuals or of individuals with particular types of neurological damage.

Caveat

When selecting which measures of SOP to use in clinical practice, clinicians should ensure that validity has been adequately established. Ideally, any measure used clinically can be referenced to a reasonably large and representative clinical sample of a type similar to that seen in practice but without any significant influence of secondary gain (e.g., nonlitigating patients with mild TBI). This, at the very least, provides an indication of the rarity of scores in the "invalid" range among examinees with bona fide injuries, thereby providing an estimate of the likelihood that such scores may in fact be false positives. Unfortunately, data from large, directly applicable, nonlitigating clinical samples are not yet available for most measures, and specificity remains inadequately characterized. Complimenting specificity data should be information on sensitivity. However, much of the research and normative data available for measures of SOP are derived from analog samples of convenience (i.e., college students instructed to malinger) rather than true clinical cases of malingering. Such analog samples often do not match the demographics and experiences of those seen clinically, and such subjects probably are not as highly motivated to feign dysfunction in a believable manner. As a consequence, simulation studies tend to overestimate a test's sensitivity when used in clinical practice (Vickery et al., 2001). Even when known-group (e.g., examinees identified using well-defined criteria such as those of Slick et al., 1999) or differential prevalence designs (e.g., litigating versus nonlitigating examinees) are used, problems may arise, because findings may be based on examinees with extreme performance patterns and symptoms and therefore may not be adequately sensitive to more subtle response distortions (Lezak et al., 2004). Therefore, sensitivity, like specificity, remains inadequately characterized for many measures.

Sensitivity and specificity concern the performance of the measure in the validity studies, where participants' actual status is known or assumed. Where sensitivity and specificity are reasonably well characterized, these validity data need to be translated into more clinically relevant indexes, such as positive and negative predictive power, that reflect real-world assessment settings in which the clinician uses the results of a test to predict actual motivational status (see Chapter 1; see also Boone et al., 2002; Kaye & Koehler, 2003; Lindeboom, 1989; Millis & Volinsky, 2001; Mossman, 2000a, 2000b, 2003; Mossman & Hart, 1996; Streiner, 2003). Positive and negative predictive power values refer to probabilities that an examinee's

score does or does not reflect the condition of interest (e.g., malingering). For example, if specificity at a particular cutoff score is 85%, then the false-positive rate at that cutoff is 15% (100% − 85%). However, predictive accuracy varies as a function of the base rate of the condition.

Estimates of base rates of malingering or other types of SOP vary widely, depending on the clinical context (e.g., compensation versus noncompensation). A figure of 15% can be considered a lower bound for the base rate of suspect effort in a general clinical setting (Boone et al., 2002). The 30% figure cited earlier (Mittenberg et al., 2002) can be viewed as an estimate of the base rate in practice settings where a mixture of nonlitigating and medical-legal referrals is seen. A 45% base rate might refer to practices that specialize in compensation-seeking referrals (Boone et al., 2002). In general, cut-scores are chosen that minimize false positives while still maintaining adequate sensitivity for detecting SOP. The use of a positive predictive value ≥80% with a base rate of ≤30% has been recommended as meeting the criteria of scientific evidence established in *Daubert v. Merrell Dow Pharmaceuticals* (Vallabhajosula & van Gorp, 2001). This standard means that, using a particular cut-score, 8 of 10 individuals who receive a suspect-effort result are truly displaying SOP (and 2 of the 10 are false positives who have been incorrectly identified as displaying noncredible performance). It is important to bear in mind that this standard is arbitrary and that a different standard may be appropriate in specific settings or circumstances.

In general, as the base rate increases, positive predictive accuracy increases and negative predictive accuracy decreases. The indexes of predictive accuracy indicate how much a test improves on random selection as a means of selecting individuals with a particular condition (Boone et al., 2002). Table 16–2 presents values of positive and negative predictive accuracy (PPP and NPP) for three hypothetical tests (A, B, and C) at base-rate assumptions of 15%, 30%, and 45%. An assumed base rate of 15% for suboptimal effort (or 85% for normal effort) means that, even with random selection from a large group of test-takers, one would choose a cooperative individual 85% of the time. The NPP values are quite high, although theoretically these values cannot be less than 85%, which is the assumed base rate for normal effort. The cutoff for identifying SOP on all tasks (PPP) improves selection

Table 16–2 Cutoffs for Suspect Performance on Three Tests and Indices of Sensitivity, Specificity, and Predictive Power at Three Base Rates of Suboptimal Performance

Test	Cutoff Value	Sensitivity (%)	Specificity (%)	15% PPP (%)	15% NPP (%)	30% PPP (%)	30% NPP (%)	45% PPP (%)	45% NPP (%)
A	20	68.2	95.0	70.7	94.4	85.4	87.5	91.8	78.5
B	22	62.4	88.9	49.8	93.0	70.6	84.6	82.1	74.3
C	14	88.2	95.3	76.9	97.9	89.0	95.0	93.9	90.8

Source: Adapted from Boone et al., 2002.

accuracy beyond that expected on the basis of random selection (which would produce a "hit" for suspect effort only 15% of the time). However, the 15% base-rate PPP column demonstrates that in no task does accuracy exceed 80%. In test A, PPP is about 70%, meaning that with this cutoff score, about 3 of every 10 people would be incorrectly identified as displaying SOP. In test B, the situation is worse, with 5 of 10 honest people being incorrectly labeled as suspect. In settings where the base rate of SOP is higher, PPP values increase, although at a base rate of 30% only tests A and C would meet adequate scientific criteria (PPP ≥ 80%). When the base rate is assumed to be 45%, PPP is high for all tasks.

By focusing more on predictive power (particularly with associated confidence intervals) than on sensitivity and specificity or a simple binary positive-negative test score interpretation, clinicians adopt a more sophisticated approach to data analysis that is likely to serve them far better in increasingly sophisticated and demanding legal settings. In an excellent and highly recommended technical overview of *Daubert* and methods for determining the probative value of SOP measures, Mossman (2003) proposed a considerably more sophisticated (and technically more demanding) approach than that of Vallabhajosula & van Gorp (2001). One of the more important highlights of Mossman's approach is an emphasis on the fact that predictive power is an estimate like any other psychological measure, and as such it is associated with measurement error that should be quantified (i.e., in the form of a confidence interval) and considered when such values are interpreted in clinical and legal settings. Given the amount of research activity in this area, findings reported here should be viewed as tentative, and clinicians are advised to keep abreast of current developments in the field.

CONVENTIONAL MEASURES

The indices of SOP that have been derived from conventional neuropsychological tests can be subdivided into two groups based on complexity: simple cutoffs and atypical patterns of performance (see Table 16–3). The reader is referred to the *Malingering* sections in the various test write-ups in this volume for more complete descriptions and evaluations of these and other indicators.

Cutoffs

The simplest indices represent application of cutoff scores to level of performance. These indices take advantage of low floors that may be found on some conventional tests. That is, tests for which the clinical floor (i.e., lowest scores) seen in examinees with bona fide injuries and/or impairments is well above the lowest score that can be obtained on the test (Digit Span is an example; see Iverson & Tulsky, 2003). Malingerers may be unaware that a test has a clinical floor, and if they also typically perceive the test to be more difficult

than it actually is, or as more likely to be affected by brain injury than it actually is, there is potential for derivation of a useful SOP cutoff. These cutoff scores are developed by comparing score distributions of control or clinical samples of interest (e.g., TBI) with score distributions of suspected or analog malingerers. Despite the appeal of simplicity of clinical application, the sensitivity of these measures tends to be low. Studies have demonstrated that suspected or analog malingerers do not often perform at a level consistent with severe or profound deficits (i.e., below the cutoff). In addition, although specificity appears moderately high for some tasks (e.g., WAIS-III Digit Span, RAVLT Recognition, WMS-III Faces I) in some groups (e.g., patients with mild head injury), it is modest for others (e.g., RMT), increasing the risk of false-positive errors. Therefore, performance on these tasks may suggest concerns about a person's motivation but should not be used in isolation.

New Indices

A more sophisticated approach than the simple cutoff method is based on the identification of atypical within- or across-test patterns of performance. Here, new indices are derived by combining existing indices within a test (e.g., Reliable Digit Span, discrepancies in recognition-recall on the RAVLT or the Rey-O; combination of existing indices in the WCST or the RAVLT EI). The development of these measures has typically been informed by assumptions about the naiveté in the lay population regarding the relative difficulties of different tasks and common patterns of performance seen in neurological conditions (e.g., recognition is usually better than recall).

In a related vein, new indices of within-test performance may be derived based on item analyses. For example, analysis may reveal that particular items on a test are infrequently missed by persons with bona fide injuries or impairments, and that multiple errors across a number of these infrequently missed items are extremely rare (e.g., SPM, Category Test, Rey-O, WMS-III Logical Memory Delayed Recognition). Naïve persons are probably not aware of such normative trends and therefore may be identified by a high "infrequent error" count. This type of index is conceptually similar to certain validity scales on personality tests with which most clinicians are already familiar (e.g., F scale on the MMPI-2).

The advantage of these new indices is that they are often associated with greater separation of group distributions. Specificity tends to be higher, so these measures are less likely to generate false-positive errors than simple cutoffs are. However, sensitivity is typically limited. Therefore, scores that fall in the range of biased responding may be considered as "red flags," but the examiner should not rely on these indices alone, because doing so would result in an unacceptable high number of false-negative decisions. Rather, the examiner should also use specialized techniques (e.g., symptom validity tests) to detect SOP.

Table 16–3 Subtypes and Examples of Indices Derived from Conventional Tests

Subtype	Rationale	Examples	Comment
Cutoffs	Level of performance	WAIS-III—Digit Span WCST—FMS TOVA omissions TMT—time, errors CVLT-II—FC RMT RAVLT Recognition Rey-O Recognition WMS-III Auditory Recognition Delayed Index; Word List II Recognition; Faces I Token Test Judgment of Line Orientation Smell Identification Test Finger Tapping Brief—Inconsistency and Negativity MMPI-2—F Scale PAI—NIM TSI—ATR	Sensitivity varies depending on the measure; for most measures, sensitivity is limited; risk of false positives varies depending on the measure but can be high
Derivation of new indices	Pattern of performance	IVA subscales Standard Progressive Matrices—Rate of decay; Rare errors WAIS-III Vocabulary Minus Digit Span; Reliable Digit Span Category Test—Rare errors; inconsistency across test sessions WCST—Formulas combining various scores RMT—Longest run of incorrect responses; rare errors RAVLT—Abnormal serial position effects; discrepancies between recall and recognition; inconsistency in recall; EI index; combined indices of recognition memory Rey-O—Test trial configurations (Memory Error Patterns); rare recognition errors; combination scores (Copy and Recognition) WMS-III—Rarely Missed Index MMPI-2—FBS PAI—MAL, RDF, CDF	Sensitivity varies but tends to be low; less prone to false positives than simple cutoffs

Importance of Indices From Conventional Tests

The value of indices developed from conventional tests is that they do "double duty," providing evidence regarding both performance and the validity of results (see also Meyers & Volbrecht, 2003). One can argue that such measures should be investigated for all existing tests that are widely used, and that all new conventional measures or revisions of existing measures should be constructed with "built-in" or intrinsic indices of SOP that are evaluated as part of the norming process. In addition to being cost-efficient, use of these indicators is important for other reasons.

First, because individuals can have variable or inconsistent motivation across the course of an assessment, these indicators complement specialized tools (e.g., symptom validity tests) that are typically given at a few points in time, serving as useful additional validity checks. Second, the literature suggests that these intrinsic indicators, although somewhat correlated with one another, may provide relatively independent information regarding performance validity. This is probably due in part to interindividual variability; some examinees may feign or exaggerate a memory problem, whereas others may exaggerate cognitive slowing or reading difficulties. These different SOP profiles may be better detected by techniques intrinsic to various conventional neuropsychological measures than by standard symptom validity tests, which, with few exceptions, are presented as tests of memory (see later discussion). In addition, analog studies have demonstrated that special tests (e.g., symptom validity tests) do not have perfect sensitivity and therefore will always miss some malingerers. Further, given the ready availability of the neuropsychological literature to the general public (as well as to lawyers), claimants may recognize standard forced-choice procedures and evade detection by them. Finally, as Bernard et al (1993) pointed out, development of validity checks in neuropsychological instruments allows the clinician to make inferences about the vulnerability of the other tests used in the examination. Considering these issues, whenever an examination is done in the context of incentives to malinger or SOP is otherwise possible, clinicians should make use of all well-validated indices of SOP derived from the conventional measures that they employ.

It is important to bear in mind, however, that most SOP indices have been developed for use with young adults and for the purpose of assessing the performance of individuals with traumatic head injury (who are predominantly young adult males). Their use with persons outside this age range (e.g., the very young or very old) or with those complaining of other conditions (e.g., chronic pain, depression, stress-related disorders) has received relatively less study and should be undertaken with due caution. More generally, all psychometric measures of SOP are inherently limited in that, whereas they may reliably detect underperformance, they cannot be used in isolation to diagnose malingering. Such a diagnosis requires integration of multiple types of information beyond test scores and full consideration of exclusionary conditions or factors (Slick, et al., 1999).

SPECIALLY DESIGNED TESTS

A number of tests have been devised specifically to detect SOP (see Table 16–4). These are generally of two types. One type relies on the production of errors that are atypical for persons with bona fide cognitive deficits (e.g., incorrect recall of character sets, reading wrong letters, counting dots incorrectly). These typically employ tasks that are designed to appear face-valid as measures of cognitive ability but are very easy, so that, presumably, patients with even significant neuropsychological deficits can perform perfectly or almost perfectly (Larrabee, 2005), although this assumption of course requires validation. The Rey 15-Item test is one of the most frequently used measures of this type (Slick et al., 2004), despite the fact that it is sensitive to genuine cognitive impairment and not sufficiently sensitive to SOP. Low cost, ready availability, and ease of administration probably account for its popularity. The test should not be used in isolation, and if it is administered, it should be given early in the examination, before the client is exposed to more difficult tests that would reveal the simplicity of the measure by comparison (Iverson & Franzen, 1996). If poor scores in the SOP range occur on the task, clinicians

should first consider the possibility that these reflect bona fide cognitive deficits; low scores can occur in those with low IQ or severe neurological or psychiatric disorders (e.g., Greiffenstein et al., 1994, 1996).

Because individuals may be selective in which domains they choose to feign or enhance complaints (e.g., memory, counting, reading), tests such as the b-test and Dot Counting are available to capture these differing approaches to symptom magnification. Although specificity tends to be high for these tasks, they lack adequate sensitivity. Therefore, positive findings suggest SOP, but use of these tasks in isolation will result in high rates of false negatives. It is also important to note that, although they have good specificity, in practices where base rates of malingering are less than 30%, the risk of false-positive results is high with these tests. Therefore, the clinician is encouraged to supplement these tasks with others, particularly forced-choice procedures.

Symptom Validity Tests

The second type of task consists of forced-choice tests and relies on a probabilistic analysis of patient performance (Pankratz, 1979). The technique is most often used to evaluate complaints about memory, but it can be used with other symptoms (e.g., sensory) as well. Most tests use a two-choice response format. For example, in two-choice recognition tests, the probability of responding correctly on all items by chance alone (i.e., guessing) is 50%. Overall performance should therefore approximate 50% correct in the most severe cases of memory impairment. Assuming random responses to a given number of two-choice items, confidence intervals for chance-level performance can be calculated. Scores within the confidence interval about chance-level performance are assumed to reflect either severe impairment or possibly exaggeration of deficits. High or low scores that are outside this large confidence interval are highly unlikely to occur by chance alone. Such scores are assumed to be the product of purposeful selection of correct or incorrect answers (in either case depending on intact memory), with the latter being suggestive of exaggerated or faked memory deficits. Because studies have shown that individuals suspected of feigning mild to moderate head injury (the type of case most likely to be seen in litigation) often perform above chance levels, reliance on probability-derived cutoffs results in very conservative decisions. By evaluating nonlitigants with significant cognitive deficits (including profound memory impairment), investigators have also provided empirically based cutoff scores to improve the sensitivity of these measures while maintaining adequate floors.

There is evidence to suggest that these special techniques, particularly forced-choice symptom validity tests, achieve the best hit rates for detection of SOP (e.g., Greiffenstein et al., 1994; Strauss et al., 2002; Vickery et al., 2001; Williamson et al., 2003), although, in the case of forced-choice measures, this is always the case when normative cutoffs rather than below-chance cutoffs are employed. Considering the tests shown in Table 16–4, the TOMM appears to be more useful

Table 16–4 Some Characteristics of Symptom Validity Tests

Measure	Age Range	Administration Time (min)	Comment	Caution
b-test	17+	15	Relatively unaffected by demographic variables. Impact of mild learning disabilities minimal; unknown if contaminated by more severe learning disorders. Moderate sensitivity, high specificity	Contraindicated in those with significant visual or motor impairments, moderate to severe dementia, stroke, or acute psychosis; in practices where base rate of malingering is less than 30%, risk of false positives is high
Dot Counting	17+	10	Relatively unaffected by demographic variables or emotional disorder. Moderate sensitivity, high specificity.	Contraindicated in those with stroke, mental retardation, MMSE <24; in practices where base rate of malingering is less than 30%, risk of false positives is high
Rey 15-Item	11+	5	Performance is related to age, educational and intellectual status. Modest sensitivity; specificity variable	Ineffective in detecting malingering and overly sensitive to real impairment; contraindicated in those with cognitive impairment or psychiatric disorder and in young children
TOMM	5+	15	Age, low education, cultural factors, depression, anxiety, and pain have little impact on scores; performance is relatively insensitive to cognitive impairment; specificity is high, but other computerized tasks (VSVT, WMT) show higher sensitivity	Contraindicated in those with moderate-to-severe dementia or moderate mental retardation
21-Item Test	Adults	5	Age and education do not affect forced-choice performance. Poor sensitivity, high specificity; other forced-choice tasks more effective	Because of low sensitivity, need to use more than this task; if used, give early on in examination
VSVT	18+	15–20	Age, education, profound memory impairment, depression, and sophistication with symptoms of head injury have little impact on accuracy; more sensitive than the TOMM and compares favorably with the WMT	Requires familiarity with Arabic numerals; accuracy scores more effective than latency scores
WMT	7+	20	Age, education, IQ, significant cognitive impairment, psychiatric disorder, and pain do not affect accuracy on effort trials; sophistication with symptoms of head injury does not affect performance; coaching on how to avoid detection improved performance, but such individuals can still be detected; more sensitive than tests such as the TOMM and has better face validity than the TOMM and VSVT; unique in that test measures both effort and memory	Computer format requires grade 3 reading level

than tests such as the Rey 15-Item and the 21-Item tests; however, it may be redundant when used with other symptom validity tests such as the WMT and the VSVT, which have better sensitivity (Gervais et al., 2004; Tan et al., 2002), at least when the TOMM is administered face-to-face by an examiner. It is possible that computer administration of tasks, as is usually the case for the VSVT and the WMT, increases their sensitivity. That is, it may be less threatening to give wrong responses when tested by a computer than when tested by an experimenter (Bolan et al., 2002). Alternatively, people may be disinclined to feign nonverbal (picture) as opposed to verbal (word) memory deficits. Nonetheless, the TOMM may be the instrument of choice when one is faced with clients who are from another culture (e.g., from a non-English-speaking country), who have significant reading disorders (e.g., less than a grade 3 reading level), or who are young children (e.g., younger than 10–11 years of age).

Good measures of motivational status should be relatively insensitive to actual impairment. The available evidence suggests that tests such as the TOMM, VSVT, and WMT are relatively easy, even for individuals with significant neurological impairment (e.g., patients with moderate to severe head injury). Additional evidence that these tests tap effort rather than ability comes from the finding that a variety of factors, such as age, low education, depression, anxiety, and pain typically do not affect scores on these tests. Therefore, low scores should not be attributed to these conditions.

It is important to recognize that symptom validity tests, like all measures of SOP, are at best capable only of indicating that factors other than, or perhaps in addition to, cognitive impairment may be influencing a client's performance. To rule out false positives, clinicians must consider not only scores on the various symptom validity tasks but also performance on the other tests, as well as clinical data, to ensure that the pattern makes neuropsychological sense (see the criteria listed in Slick et al., 1999, and reproduced in Table 16–1). It is also important to bear in mind that scores that fall in the normal range on these tests do not rule out a motivational defect. For example, the individual may have been feigning symptoms that he or she perceives to be unrelated to performance on these tests (e.g., motor or sensory deficit).

MULTIPLE MEASURES

As noted earlier, one can have greater confidence in diagnostic decisions concerning SOP when multiple measures are employed in the context of a logical and comprehensive diagnostic framework. Such an approach is supported on a statistical basis, particularly with regard to increasing specificity. For example, Larrabee (2003) examined litigants with definite evidence of malingering and patients with moderate or severe TBI on five tests: Benton Form Discrimination, Finger Tapping, Reliable Digit Span, WCST FMS, and the Lees-Haley FBS from the MMPI-2. The sensitivity and specificity of the individual tests at specific cutting scores ranged from .40 (sensitivity for Finger Tapping) to .935 (specificity for Finger Tapping and Reliable Digit Span). Evaluation of all possible pair-wise combinations of scores exceeding cutoff (e.g., FBS and FMS, FT and RDS) resulted in a sensitivity of .875 and a specificity of .889. Evaluation of all possible three-way combinations (i.e., three test failures) resulted in a sensitivity of .54 (higher than the individual sensitivities of Visual Form Discrimination, Finger Tapping, Reliable Digit Span, and FMS), and a specificity of 100% (i.e., no false positives), a value better than that achieved by any single test.

Similar results were reported by Vickery et al. (2004), who used a simulation design in which healthy controls and persons with moderate/severe TBI completed three symptom validity tests (Digit Memory, Letter Memory, and the TOMM) under standard as well as malingering instructions. Sensitivity dropped with increasingly stringent criteria (i.e., increasing numbers of tests failed) whereas specificity increased. Perfect specificity was achieved at three or more test failures, the same result as that reported by Larrabee (2003). Subjects with three or more test failures had 100% positive predictive accuracy regardless of the base rate (15%, 40%, or 50%). Inspection of PPP and NPP data at various base rates (see Table 16–5) indicates that, in low-base-rate environments (15%), NPP is usually high and PPP is lower. Therefore, in low base-rate settings, a more conservative threshold for predicting malingering may be appropriate, such as requiring that three or more indicators be failed. In contrast, in settings where the base rate is high (e.g., 50%), use of conservative criteria to predict malingering, such as failure on three or more indicators,

Table 16–5 Classification Rate Data Requiring Failure of Increasing Numbers of Symptom Validity Tests for Identifying Malingering by Base Rate

No. of Tests Failed	Sensitivity	Specificity	Hit Rate	15%		40%		50%	
				PPP	NPP	PPP	NPP	PPP	NPP
≥1	89.1	93.5	91.5	70.8	98.0	90.1	92.8	93.2	89.6
≥2	65.2	97.8	79.9	84.0	94.1	95.2	80.8	96.7	73.8
≥3	32.6	100.0	63.6	100.0	89.4	100.0	69.0	100.0	59.4

Note: PPP = Positive Predictive Power; NPP = Negative Predictive Power.

Source: From Vickery et al., 2004, with permission from Elsevier.

would result in high PPP (100%) but unacceptably low NPP (59.4% in the Vickery et al. [2004] study). Vickery et al. (2004) suggested that more liberal criteria may be appropriate in high-base-rate settings.

The finding of improved specificity when data from multiple measures are aggregated reflects the rarity of multiple test scores in the suboptimal range in truly impaired patients. That is, although an examinee may on rare occasion obtain a "failing" score on one SOP measure, he or she is not likely to obtain scores on two or more measures in this range (Larrabee, 2005). Specificity is typically set at .90 to minimize false positives. Using the Slick et al. (1999) criteria for probable response bias, the probability of a false-positive score for two indicators exceeding the cutoff, each with a specificity of .90 and with little correlation between the two tests in a nonlitigating clinical sample, is $1/10 \times 1/10$, or .01 (Larrabee, 2005). Therefore, administration of several independent and well-validated techniques serves to substantially increase diagnostic accuracy (Boone & Lu, 2003; Larrabee, 2005).

MULTIPLE ASSESSMENTS

Individuals seen in medical-legal contexts often undergo repeated evaluations during the course of their litigation. Cullum et al. (1991) argued that to "produce consistent (but exaggerated or feigned) results, the patient would have to replicate the same levels of inadequate effort across multiple tests and time periods." This may be difficult to achieve, particularly on lengthy test batteries. They suggested that assessment of response consistency across serial evaluations might prove to be an especially powerful technique to detect invalid results. There is some evidence that this is the case.

For example, Reitan and Wolfson (1995, 1996, 1997) compared the test results of two groups of head-injured adults, one group involved in litigation and the other not. Every patient was tested twice, about 1 year apart, on subtests of the Wechsler Intelligence Scale and components from the Halstead-Reitan Battery. Litigants tended to demonstrate more inconsistent scores on retesting than those not in litigation.

Demakis (1999) used an analog design and examined performance on a number of standard neuropsychological tasks. Participants were tested on two occasions spaced about 3 weeks apart. Simulators demonstrated a less consistent recall pattern than did controls across the five CVLT learning trials (i.e., they recalled different words on successive trials).

Strauss et al. (2002) used an analog design in which half of the participants (composed of three groups: naïve healthy people, professionals working with head-injured people, and nonlitigating head-injured people) were asked to try their best, and the remainder were asked to feign believable injury. Participants were assessed with the Reliable Digit Span task, the VSVT, and a computerized Dot Counting Test on three separate occasions spaced about 2 weeks apart. Regardless of an individual's experience, forced-choice tests achieved the best hit rate on a single test session. In addition, inconsistency of response on the forced-choice task across test sessions contributed uniquely to prediction accuracy. The authors recommended that clinicians consider changes of 3 or more points up or down on the overall easy items of the VSVT as increasing the index of suspicion. This suggestion was based on the observation that none of the head-injured controls obtained deviations of 3 or more points on easy items. An important finding here is that any inconsistency across assessments that might be associated with head injury (e.g., Bleiberg et al., 1997; Burton et al., 2002; Stuss et al., 1994, 1999) appears to differ from that seen on such simple tasks in the context of SOP. Finally, it is worth noting that an assessment of within-test consistency has been incorporated into one of the symptom validity tasks, the WMT. Similar indices are also available for the CVLT-II, although no data concerning their value for the detection of SOP have been reported.

MANAGEMENT OF CLIENTS

Neuropsychologists identified from the literature as expert in handling financial compensation or personal injury litigation were recently surveyed regarding their assessment practices (Slick et al., 2004). These experts reported that they always give at least one symptom validity test, although the precise measure varied from one expert to another. They also indicated that they supported their diagnostic impressions from multiple sources of evidence, including indices derived from standard neuropsychological tests. These practices are consistent with guidelines recently proposed by the NAN Policy and Planning Committee (Bush et al., 2005).

Opinion is divided on whether to warn clients before testing that SOP, exaggeration, or faked impairments may be detected by the tests given during the neuropsychological examination. More than half of experts surveyed by Slick et al. (2004) never gave any type of warning before the testing. More than a third gave some type of warning. This division of opinion is reflected in the literature. Some authors have expressed concern that warning individuals about the presence of specific measures to detect SOP may reduce the sensitivity of various measures (e.g., Suhr & Gunstad, 2000; Youngjohn et al., 1999). Increasingly, this issue is being recognized as a problem, because almost 50% of lawyers believe that they should provide their clients with specific information about psychological tests, including information about validity measures (Wetter & Corrigan, 1995). Youngjohn et al. (1999) cautioned that the validity of forensic neuropsychological evaluations will be further jeopardized if psychologists also engage in this practice. They recommend that examinees be asked if there is anything limiting their ability to answer all questions accurately to the best of their knowledge, or if there is anything besides their injury limiting their ability to put forth their best effort on performance tests. Thereafter, the issue of symptom validity should not be emphasized or re-emphasized during the course of the evaluation. On the other hand, a recent NAN position paper recommended that examiners "inform the examinee at the outset of the evaluation that good effort and honesty will be required (the examiner may inform the examinee that such factors will be directly assessed)" (Bush et al., 2005, p. 424).

There is evidence that order of test administration can affect detection rates. Guilmette et al. (1996) gave a number-recognition symptom validity task (Hiscock Forced-Choice procedure), either at the beginning or at the end of a battery of neuropsychological tests, to simulators and disability claimants. For both groups, poorer performance was obtained on the earlier administration. The authors recommended that the symptom validity tests should be given at the very beginning of the session, before the patient is exposed to more difficult clinical tests, which may serve by comparison to "unmask" the low difficulty level of symptom validity measures. Despite this evidence, only half of the experts surveyed by Slick et al. (2004) reported that they always give measures specifically designed to detect suboptimal effort at the beginning of the assessment; the remainder reported that they give such measures at any time during the course of an assessment, as the need arises.

Once suspicion is raised, more than half of the experts surveyed by Slick et al. (2004) altered their assessment routine, at least on some occasions, by encouraging good effort or by administering additional symptom validity tests. A minority directly confronted or warned clients, terminated the examination earlier than planned, or contacted the referring attorney immediately.

COMMUNICATION OF FINDINGS

Communication of positive findings concerning SOP can be difficult, given the pejorative overtones associated with the term "malingering," the substantial consequences that such a diagnosis can have for an individual, the difficulty in confirming its presence, and the complex motivations that underlie a person's behavior. Virtually all experts surveyed by Slick et al. (2004) stated that they always gave some opinion in their report regarding indicators of invalidity. However, the majority rarely used the term "malingering." Most stated that the test results are invalid, inconsistent with the severity of the injury, or indicative of exaggeration. For example, an examiner might state the following: "Results from the neuropsychological examination raise the concern that Ms. Jones may be exaggerating her memory complaints. Her scores on a number of forced-choice recognition tests were significantly lower than expected. Although such low scores can occur in severely demented individuals, they are rarely, if ever, obtained by normal people or by individuals suffering from mild brain injury." Or the examiner might state that "the results are not consistent with any known diagnosis" or that "the results are not consistent with the presenting complaint."

There is relatively little research on the coexistence of legitimate neuropsychological dysfunction and SOP and whether it is possible to tease apart exaggerated from real impairment.

A number of authors (e.g., Boone & Lu, 2003; Larrabee, 2005) recommend that it may be possible to reach conclusions in such cases, based on published outcome data in patient groups sharing similar injury severity characteristics (e.g., Belanger et al., 2005; Dikmen et al., 1995; Rohling et al., 2003; Vanderploeg et al., 2005).

Finally, it is important to note that instances have been reported of individuals searching the Internet and other sources for information about malingering and about how to evade detection. Accordingly, as a precaution to reduce the opportunity to use such previously learned information, the client should not see the names of tests during the administration. Further, Green (2003) advised that the nature of the task (e.g., number recognition) but not the name of the task should be identified in the body of the report. The name of the task can, however, be listed in the appendix.

REFERENCES

American Psychiatric Association. (1994). *Diagnostic and statistical manual of mental disorders* (4th ed.). Washington, DC: Author.

Belanger, H. G., Curtiss, G., Demery, J. A., Lebowitz, B. K., & Vanderploeg, R. D. (2005). Factors moderating neuropsychological outcomes following mild traumatic brain injury: A meta-analysis. *Journal of the International Neuropsychological Society, 11,* 215–227.

Bernard, L. C., Houston, W., & Natoli, L. (1993). Malingering on neuropsychological memory tests: Potential objective indicators. *Journal of Clinical Psychology, 49,* 45–53.

Bleiberg, J., Garmoe, W. S., Halpern, E. L., Reeves, D. L., & Nadler, J. D. (1997). Consistency of within-day and across-day performance after mild brain injury. *Neuropsychiatry, Neuropsychology, and Behavioral Neurology, 10,* 247–253.

Bolan, B., Foster, J. K., Schmand, B., & Bolan, S. (2002). A comparison of three tests to detect feigned amnesia: The effects of feedback and the measurement of response latency. *Journal of Clinical and Experimental Neuropsychology, 24,* 154–167.

Boone, K. B., & Lu, P. H. (2003). Noncredible cognitive performance in the context of severe brain injury. *The Clinical Neuropsychologist, 17,* 244–254.

Boone, K., Lu, P., & Hertzberg, D. (2002). *The Dot Counting Test.* Los Angeles: Western Psychological Services.

Burton, C. L., Hultsch, D. F., Strauss, E., & Hunter, M. A. (2002) Intraindividual variability in physical and emotional functioning: Comparison of adults with traumatic brain injuries and healthy adults. *The Clinical Neuropsychologist, 16,* 264–279.

Bush, S. S., Ruff, R. R., Troster, A. I., Barth, J. T., Koffler, S. P., Pliskin, N. H., Reynolds, C. R., & Silver, C. H. (2005). Symptom validity assessment: Practice issues and medical necessity. NAN Policy & Planning Committee. *Archives of Clinical Neuropsychology, 20,* 419–426.

Cullum, C., Heaton, R., & Grant, I. (1991). Psychogenic factors influencing neuropsychological performance: Somatoform disorders, factitious disorders, and malingering. In H. O. Doerr & A. S. Carling (Eds.), *Forensic neuropsychology: Legal and scientific bases* (pp. 141–171). New York: Guilford Press.

Demakis, G. J. (1999). Serial malingering on verbal and nonverbal fluency and memory measures: An analog investigation. *Archives of Clinical Neuropsychology, 14,* 401–410.

Dikmen, S. S., Machamer, J. E., Winn, H. R., & Temkin, N. R. (1995). Neuropsychological outcome at 1-year post head injury. *Neuropsychology, 9,* 80–90.

Gervais, R. O., Rohling, M. L., Green, P., & Ford, W. (2004). A comparison of WMT, CARB, and TOMM failure rates in non-head injury disability claimants. *Archives of Clinical Neuropsychology, 19,* 475–487.

Green, P. (2003). *Green's Word Memory Test for Microsoft Windows.* Edmonton, Alberta: Green's Publishing.

Greiffenstein, M. F., Baker, W. J., & Gola, T. (1994). Validation of malingered amnesia measures with a large clinical sample. *Psychological Assessment, 6,* 218–224.

Greiffenstein, M. F., Baker, W. J., & Gola, T. (1996). Comparison of multiple scoring methods for Rey's malingered amnesia measures. *Archives of Clinical Neuropsychology, 11,* 283–293.

Guilmette, T. J., Whelihan, W. M., Hart, K. J., Sparadeo, F. R., & Buongiorno, G. (1996). Order effects in the administration of a forced-choice procedure for detection of malingering in disability claimants' evaluation. *Perceptual and Motor Skills, 83,* 1007–1016.

Iverson, G. L., & Franzen, M. D. (1996). Using multiple object memory procedures to detect simulated malingering. *Journal of Clinical and Experimental Neuropsychology, 8,* 1–14.

Iverson, G. L., & Tulsky, D. S. (2003). Detecting malingering on the WAIS-III: Ususual Digit Span performance patterns in the normal population and in clinical groups. *Archives of Clinical Neuropsychology, 18,* 1–9.

Kaye, D. H., & Koehler, J. J. (2003). The misquantification of probative value. *Law and Human Behavior, 27*(6), 645–659.

Larrabee, G. J. (2003). Detection of malingering using atypical performance patterns on standard neuropsychological tests. *The Clinical Neuropsychologist, 17,* 410–425.

Larrabee, G. J. (2005). Assessment of malingering. In G. J. Larrabee (Ed.), *Forensic neuropsychology: A scientific approach.* New York: Oxford University Press.

Lezak, M. D., Howieson, D. B., & Loring, D. W. (2004). *Neuropsychological assessment* (4th ed.). New York: Oxford University Press.

Lindeboom, J. (1989). Who needs cutting points? *Journal of Clinical Psychology, 45,* 679–683.

Meyers, J. E., & Volbrecht, M. E. (2003). A validation of multiple malingering detection methods in a large clinical sample. *Archives of Clinical Neuropsychology, 18,* 261–276.

Millis, S. R. & Volinsky, C. T. (2001). Assessment of response bias in mild head injury: Beyond malingering tests. *Journal of Clinical and Experimental Neuropsychology, 23,* 809–828.

Mittenberg, W., Patton, C., Canyock, E. M., & Condit, D. C. (2002). Base rates of malingering and symptom exaggeration. *Journal of Clinical and Experimental Neuropsychology, 24,* 1094–1102.

Mossman, D. (2000a). The meaning of malingering data: Further applications of Bayes' theorem. *Behavioral Sciences and the Law, 18*(6), 761–779.

Mossman, D. (2000b). Interpreting clinical evidence of malingering: A Bayesian perspective. *Journal of the American Academy of Psychiatry and the Law, 28*(3), 293–302.

Mossman, D. (2003). Daubert, cognitive malingering, and test accuracy. *Law and Human Behaviour, 27,* 229–249.

Mossman, D., & Hart, K. J. (1996). Presenting evidence of malingering to courts: Insights from decision theory. *Behavioral Sciences & the Law, 14*(3), 271–291.

Pankratz, L. (1979). Symptom validity testing and symptom retraining: Procedures for the assessment and treatment of functional sensory deficits. *Journal of Consulting and Clinical Psychology, 47,* 409–410.

Reitan, R. M., & Wolfson, D. (1995). Consistency of response on retesting among head-injured subjects in litigation versus head-injured subjects not in litigation. *Applied Neuropsychology, 2,* 67–71.

Reitan, R. M., & Wolfson, D. (1996). The question of validity of neuropsychological test scores among head-injured litigants: Development of a Dissimulation Index. *Archives of Clinical Neuropsychology, 11,* 573–580.

Reitan, R. M., & Wolfson, D. (1997). Consistency of neuropsychological test scores of head-injured subjects involved in litigation compared with head-injured subjects not involved in litigation: Development of the Retest Consistency Index. *The Clinical Psychologist, 11,* 69–76.

Rohling, M. L., Meyers, J. E., & Millis, S. R. (2003). Neuropsychological impairment following traumatic brain injury: A dose-response analysis. *The Clinical Neuropsychologist, 17,* 289–302.

Slick, D. J., Sherman, E. M. S., & Iverson, G. L. (1999). Diagnostic criteria for malingered neurocognitive dysfunction: Proposed standards for clinical practice and research. *The Clinical Neuropsychologist, 13,* 545–561.

Slick, D. J., Tan, J. E., Strauss, E. H., & Hultsch, D. F. (2004). Detecting malingering: A survey of experts' practices. *Archives of Clinical Neuropsychology, 19,* 465–473.

Strauss, E., Slick, D. J., Levy-Bencheton, J., Hunter, M., MacDonald, S. W. S., & Hultsch, D. F. (2002). Intraindividual variability as an indicator of malingering in head injury. *Archives of Clinical Neuropsychology, 17,* 423–444.

Streiner, D. L. (2003). Diagnosing tests: Using and misusing diagnostic and screening tests. *Journal of Personality Assessment, 81,* 209–219.

Stuss, D. T., Murphy, K. J., & Binns, M. A. (1999). The frontal lobes and performance variability: Evidence from reaction time. *Journal of the International Neuropsychological Society, 5,* 123.

Stuss, D. T., Pogue, J., Buckle, L., & Bonndar, J. (1994). Characterization of stability of performance in patients with traumatic brain injury: Variability and consistency on reaction time tests. *Neuropsychology, 8,* 316–324.

Suhr, J. A., & Gunstad, J. (2000). The effects of coaching on the sensitivity and specificity of malingering measures. *Archives of Clinical Neuropsychology, 15,* 415–424.

Tan, J. E., Slick, D. J., Strauss, E., & Hultsch, D. F. (2002). How'd they do it? Malingering strategies on symptom validity tests. *The Clinical Neuropsychologist, 16,* 495–505.

Vallabhajosula, B., & van Gorp, W. G. (2001). Post-Daubert admissibility of scientific evidence on malingering of cognitive deficits. *Journal of the American Academy of Psychiatry Law, 29,* 207–221.

Vanderploeg, R. D., Curtiss, G., & Belanger, H. (2005). Long-term neuropsychological outcomes following mild traumatic brain injury. *Journal of the International Neuropsychological Society, 11,* 228–236.

Vickery, C. D., Berry, D. T. R., Dearth, C. S., Vagnini, V. L., Baser, R. E., Cragar, D. E., & Orey, S. A. (2004). Head injury and the ability to feign neuropsychological deficits. *Archives of Clinical Neuropsychology, 19,* 37–48.

Vickery, C. D., Berry, D. T. R., Inman, T. H., Harris, M. J., & Orey, S. A. (2001). Detection of inadequate effort on neuropsychological testing: A meta-analytic review of selected procedures. *Archives of Clinical Neuropsychology, 16,* 45–73.

Wetter, M. W., & Corrigan, S. K. (1995). Providing information to clients about psychological tests: A survey of attorneys' and law students' attitudes. *Professional Psychology: Research and Practice, 26*, 474–477.

Wetter, M. W., & Deitsch, S. E. (1996). Faking specific disorders and temporal response consistency on the MMPI-2. *Psychological Assessment, 8*, 39–47.

Williamson, D. J. G., Green, P., Allen, L., & Rohling, M. L. (2003). Evaluating effort with the Word Memory Test and Category Test—or not: Inconsistencies in a compensation-seeking sample. *Journal of Forensic Neuropsychology, 3*, 19–44.

Youngjohn, J. R., Lees-Haley, P. R., & Binder, L. M. (1999). Comment: Warning malingerers produces more sophisticated malingering. *Archives of Clinical Neuropsychology, 14*, 511–516.

The b Test

PURPOSE

The b Test is a letter-recognition task that is designed to detect suspect test-taking effort.

SOURCE

The b Test is available from Western Psychological Services (http://www.wpspublish.com). The kit (including the manual, 10 stimulus booklets, 1 set of scoring templates, and 50 record forms) costs $128 US.

AGE RANGE

The test is intended for use with individuals aged 17 years and older.

DESCRIPTION

The b Test (Boone et al., 2000, 2002) is a recently developed task that assesses an overlearned skill, the ability to detect "b"s from distractors—an ability that is fairly resistant to acquired brain injury. Because individuals who feign or exaggerate cognitive deficits may not be aware of this relative preservation, they may be tempted to display their "impairment" and thereby be flagged as having given suspect effort. Anecdotally, Boone assessed several malingerers who stated that they had become dyslexic (i.e., seeing letters upside down and backward) after an equivocal head injury, a complaint not reported in cooperative head-injured patients. This experience led to the development of this measure.

The test consists of a 15-page stimulus booklet, each page of which contains an array of lowercase "b"s interspersed among other letters such as "d"s and "q"s and same letters rotated at a diagonal angle or with double stems. In each successive presentation, the array becomes progressively smaller, to make the task appear harder while actually maintaining a trivial level of difficulty. The client is asked to circle all the "b"s that appear on each page, working as quickly as possible. The error totals along with the time required to complete the task are needed to calculate the Effort Index score (E-score), which is the primary measure of test-taking effort.

ADMINISTRATION

Instructions are found in the test manual. Briefly, the patient is instructed to circle all the letter "b"s on the pages as quickly as possible. The patient is also informed that the test may become more difficult with each subsequent page.

The authors caution that the test should not be given to those subjects who have significant visual or motor impairments, moderate to severe dementia, or acute psychosis and/or substance intoxication.

ADMINISTRATION TIME

Approximately 15 min is required.

SCORING

Scoring the b Test involves recording the total response time and counting symbols that the client circled ("d" errors, non-"b"s) as well as certain symbols ("b"s) that the client may not have circled. The error and time scores are used to compute the E-score, which is the primary score required for interpretation. In the equation used to calculate the E-score, commission errors are given added weight to reflect their importance as signs of suspect effort.

The client's performance can be evaluated against that of normal-effort (cooperative) respondents and respondents whose effort is known to be suspect. Data on a number of normal-effort groups are provided, including a non-neurological group and patients with a variety of neurological and psychiatric conditions (depression, schizophrenia, head injury, stroke, learning disability; see Table 16–6). The examiner selects a normal-effort group whose clinical status best matches the presenting complaint of the client. The authors indicate that the combined normal-effort comparison should be used only if the examinee's presenting complaint does not match well with any of the specific normal-effort comparison groups.

A table is provided (Table 5 in the test manual) that presents recommended cutoffs and the associated values for four indices of classification accuracy: sensitivity, specificity, positive predictive accuracy (PPA), and negative predictive accuracy (NPA). PPA and NPA are calculated using three hypothetical base rates: 15%, 30%, and 45%. If the E-score is less than the specified

Table 16–6 Normal-Effort Comparison Groups for the b Test

Normal-Effort Group	Description	N (Gender)	Mean Age in Years (Range)	Mean Education in Years (Range)
Nonclinical	No psychiatric disorder, substance abuse, or neurological disorders	26 (8 M, 18 F)	73.1 (52–84)	14.5 (10–21)
Depression	Met DSM-III-R criteria for Major Depression	38 (18 M, 20 F)	60.9 (51–81)	14.3 (10–21)
Schizophrenia	Met DSM-III-R criteria for Schizophrenia	28 (18 M, 10 F)	35.3 (22–56)	13.1 (6–21)
Head Injury	Head trauma with brain lesion documented with CT or MRI	20 (14 M, 6F)	34.6 (18–56)	12.9 (10–17)
Stroke	CVA with brain lesion documented with CT or MRI	18 (10 M, 8 F)	63.2 (35–81)	15.9 (12–22)
Learning Disability	LD documented by cognitive testing; receiving special services	31 (14 M, 17 F)	31.0 (19–72)	15.6 (13–18)
Normal-Effort Groups Combined	All of above	161 (82 M, 79 F)	49.8 (18–84)	14.4 (6–22)

cutoff, the client's performance is considered to fall within the range of normal effort. The recommended cutoffs were chosen to minimize false positives while maintaining adequate sensitivity for suspect effort. Appendix A in the test manual includes tables showing other cutoff scores with associated values of sensitivity, specificity, PPA, and NPA. These tables allow the examiner to opt for different cutoff scores in order to maximize sensitivity or specificity in various situations. As the cutoff score is raised, specificity and PPA increase, and sensitivity and NPA decrease. This occurs because a higher cutoff reduces the likelihood of false-positive errors.

Although the E-score is the primary score used to interpret performance, clinicians can also examine the component scores (commission errors, "d" errors, omission errors, total time) to evaluate whether a client chose inaccurate or slowed responding as the method of symptom fabrication. Appendix B in the test manual provides sensitivity and specificity values for b Test component scores.

DEMOGRAPHIC VARIABLES

Age

Boone et al. (2002) reported that age did not affect test scores.

Gender

Gender has no effect on E-scores (Boone et al., 2002).

Education

Education does affect E-scores, although the amount of variance accounted for by education is reported to be small ($R^2 = .03$; Boone et al., 2002).

Ethnicity

Effects of ethnicity are not reported.

NORMATIVE DATA

Standardization Sample

As noted earlier (see *Scoring*), performance is evaluated relative to a suspect-effort group and a normal-effort group that corresponds most closely to the complaint of the client. As shown in Table 16–6, 161 individuals were included in the normal-effort group. None were involved in litigation or seeking disability payments. The suspect-effort group consisted of 91 individuals, 88 of whom were in personal injury litigation or seeking disability benefits associated with alleged medical or psychiatric disorders (37% head injury; 27% stress/chronic pain). One was diagnosed with a factitious disorder, and two were inmates in a county jail seeking to obtain more lenient sentences.

Boone et al. (2002) found that only 3.3% of the suspect-effort participants produced E-scores of 50 or less, whereas 32.3% of all the normal-effort participants produced such scores. Accordingly, based on their analysis of suspect- and normal-effort groups, they suggested that an E-score of 50 or less is very likely to represent a credible, normal-effort performance. Only 6.8% of the normal-effort participants produced E-scores of 160 or greater. By contrast, 58.2% of the suspect-effort individuals produced such scores. Accordingly, E-scores of 160 or greater are typically associated with suspect effort.

The test authors found that "d" errors are highly suggestive of suspect effort. Only 2.5% of the normal-effort participants committed three or more such errors.

RELIABILITY

Boone et al. (2002) did not provide data on reliability, arguing that test-taking effort is not a stable trait or skill; rather "it is a capacity that responds to the external contingencies of the assessment setting. When the test-taking situation itself introduces a variable effect on the construct being measured, traditional reliability statistics have little meaning" (p. 23). They argued that the best evidence for the reliability of an effort test is that the test can discriminate among groups whose effort statuses have been established by other means, and that it can do so consistently across groups representing different problems and clinical states.

VALIDITY

Relations With Other Measures

The test shows modest to moderate correlations with other measures of effort (e.g., Dot Counting $r = .60$, Rey 15-Item $r = -.42$; Digit Span $r = -.57$, Complex Figure $r = .37$, Warrington Recognition Memory $r = -.18$; Nelson et al., 2003). The elapsed time variables from the Dot Counting and b Test were highly correlated, sharing about 42% of the variance. This finding suggests that these two scores may provide some, but not total, redundancy of information regarding effort.

Clinical Findings

In support of the validity of the task, Boone et al. (2002) found that it was able to discriminate a suspect-effort group (91 personal injury claimants) from seven normal-effort groups (see Table 16–6). In order to be included in the suspect-effort group, clients had to show noncredible performance on two other tasks and behavioral features consistent with suspect effort (e.g., implausible self-reported symptoms). None of the individuals in the normal-effort groups was involved in litigation or seeking compensation. The suspect group made more errors and took significantly longer to complete the task than did the normal-effort groups. Data from this study were used to calculate sensitivity, specificity, PPA, and NPA over a range of possible cutoff scores (see *Scoring*). The primary criterion for selecting the cutoff score was to obtain a specificity of at least 85%. The recommended cutoff scores

yielded sensitivities of about 70% for all comparison groups except Schizophrenia and Stroke, for which sensitivity was low, 56%.

Boone et al. (2002) reported that the b Test performed best when used with the Head Injury comparison group. The recommended cutoff score of 90 had a sensitivity of 76.9% and a specificity of 90% in detecting suspect effort. Positive predictive values were 57.6% with a base rate of suboptimal effort of 15%, 76.7% with a base rate of 30%, and 86.3% with a base rate of 45%. Therefore, the use of the b Test appears limited when the base rate of suboptimal effort is about 30% or less, because the likelihood of a false-positive error is high (more than 2 of 10 claimants would be incorrectly labeled as malingering).

The b Test appears to be less useful in patients with schizophrenia or stroke than in other clinical groups. The recommended cutoffs had to be set substantially higher than the other groups to avoid false positives, suggesting that the cognitive impairments associated with these two conditions may affect test performance independent of effort. The authors recommend that the test findings be interpreted cautiously when assessing such patients.

COMMENT

Because malingerers may be selective as to which domains they choose to feign impairment (e.g., memory, mental speed, reading), it is important to have tests such as the b Test available that capture these differing approaches to symptom magnification. Other strengths of the test include the availability of different normal-effort reference groups and the provision of sensitivity, specificity, and predictive accuracy scores corresponding to different base rates of suspect effort.

Boone et al. (2002) do not provide information on reliability, arguing that tests of effort are "state" measures, reflecting behavioral responses to environmental contingencies. This does not mean that information on reliability would not be interesting or useful, particularly if one could isolate those factors that predicted repeated good or bad performance, or variability. One might, for example, expect that some factors underlying symptom validity performance are in fact stable "traits" (e.g., sociopathy or its opposite) that would, all things being equal, promote reliably bad or good scores, although admitting that environmental contingencies might outweigh those tendencies (e.g., contingencies for getting caught malingering).

One would also be interested in knowing how reliable the test is among a clinical group of interest (e.g., nonlitigants with head injury or severe memory impairment). Although test-retest reliability need not be demonstrated among litigants, it would be important to know that persons with legitimate injuries reliably produce good scores.

The b Test is based on the notion that certain skills are highly resistant to the effects of brain injury and other diseases. Although the authors present data showing that the task is minimally affected by the presence of neurological, psychiatric, or learning disabilities, users should note that cognitive impairments can affect test performance (at least in the case of schizophrenia or stroke). Boone et al. (2002) also reported that the test could distinguish individuals with suspect effort from those with bona fide learning disabilities. It is important to bear in mind that the learning-disabled subjects comprised a highly educated group of university students (mean education, 13–18 years). Whether the task will prove equally effective with a more diverse group of learning-disabled individuals remains to be determined. At present, the instrument should be used with considerable caution when assessing individuals with possible learning disorders and lower educational achievement.

The b Test appears to be most effective in the assessment of the effects of head injury. Clinicians should note, however, that its utility appears most evident in settings where the base rate of malingering exceeds 30%; that is, practices that specialize primarily in medical-legal evaluations. In clinical settings with base rates of 30% and lower, the risk of false positives may be unacceptably high.

Data provided by the test authors suggest that the b Test is a useful addition to complement other measures of motivational status. The task is moderately but not highly correlated with other measures of effort, suggesting that it provides relatively independent information. Additional studies by other investigators are needed to confirm these initial findings. Finally, users should bear in mind that determination of motivational status should not be based solely on the results of any single test, but rather must rely on a comprehensive assessment in which the clinician evaluates multiple aspects of the patient's performance, history, and behavior (Slick et al., 1999).

REFERENCES

Boone, K., Lu, P., Herzberg, D. S. (2002). *The b Test*. Los Angeles: Western Psychological Services.

Boone, K. B., Lu, P., Sherman, D., Palmer, B., Back, C., Warner-Chacon, K., & Berman, N. G. (2000). Validation of a new technique to detect malingering of cognitive symptoms: The b Test. *Archives of Clinical Neuropsychology, 15,* 227–241.

Nelson, N. W., Boone, K., Dueck, A., Wagener, L., Lu, P., & Grills, C. (2003). Relationships between eight measures of suspect effort. *The Clinical Neuropsychologist, 17,* 263–272.

Slick, D. J., Sherman, E. M. S., & Iverson, G. L. (1999). Diagnostic criteria for malingered neurocognitive dysfunction: Proposed standards for clinical practice and research. *The Clinical Neuropsychologist, 13,* 545–561.

The Dot Counting Test (DCT)

PURPOSE

The Dot Counting Test (DCT) is designed to detect suspect test-taking effort.

SOURCE

Users may refer to the description that follows to reproduce the task. A version has recently been standardized by Boone et al. (2002a) and is available through Western Psychological Services (http://www.wpspublish.com). The kit includes the manual, stimulus booklet, and 50 record forms and costs $108 US.

AGE RANGE

The test is intended for use with individuals aged 17 years and older.

DESCRIPTION

Original Version

The DCT was developed as two separate tasks by Andre Rey (1941; described in Frederick, 2002) and adapted by Lezak (1983; Lezak et al., 2004) to detect suboptimal effort; the tasks are currently used in tandem. Each task requires that the client count the number of dots appearing on six cards. The first part (Ungrouped) consists of six 3×5 inch cards on which are printed dots randomly arranged. Card 1 has 7 dots; card 2, 11; card 3, 15; card 4, 19; card 5, 23; and card 6, 27 (see Figure 16–1). The cards are shown to the client one at a time in the following order: 2, 4, 3, 5, 6, 1. The time required to count the number of dots is expected to increase gradually with increasing number of dots. More than one pronounced deviation from this pattern raises the concern of suspect effort. The second part of the task (Grouped) consists of six cards containing dots arrayed in a nonrandom pattern: (1) two four-dot squares, (2) two five-dot squares and two separate dots, (3) four four-dot diamonds, (4) four five-dot squares, (5) four six-dot rectangles, and (6) four five-dot squares and two four-dot squares (see Figure 16–1). The order of presentation is the same as in the first part: 2, 4, 3, 5, 6, 1. Because the dots can be grouped and patients can apply simple heuristics (i.e., addition or basic multiplication of sets), the time taken to count the dots should be much less than for the ungrouped items, which must be counted individually.

Figure 16–1 Example of DCT ungrouped and grouped items.

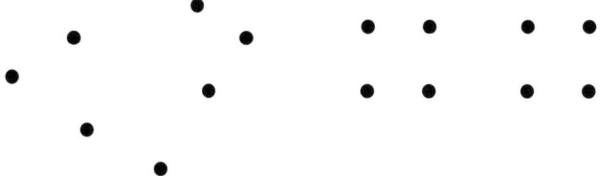

Accordingly, performance can be evaluated in terms of the difference between the time required to perform each task, with deviations from expectation (little difference between grouped and ungrouped conditions, grouped longer than ungrouped) raising the index of suspicion.

Boone et al.

The version offered by Boone et al. (2002a) is similar to the original, but the cards are enlarged to 5 × 7 inches to facilitate ease of handling, and the dots were limited to 1/16 inch. Further, both accuracy (errors) and speed (counting time) are considered in the Effort Index score (E-score), which is the primary measure on this version of the DCT.

ADMINISTRATION

The client is asked to count and tell the number of dots appearing on each card as quickly as possible. The examiner presents each card individually and records the latency and response for each card. The examiner does not inform the client that there are some trials with grouped dots and some with ungrouped dots.

ADMINISTRATION TIME

Approximately 10 min is required.

SCORING

Original Version

Scoring of the original DCT involves recording the response time for each item. Some investigators also record errors.

Boone et al.

For the version developed by Boone et al. (2002a), both time and errors are recorded for each card, and these are used to compute the E-score. It consists of the sum of the total number of counting errors, the mean ungrouped time (first set of cards) and the mean grouped time (second set of cards).

In the Boone et al. version, the client's performance can be evaluated against that of normal-effort (cooperative) respondents and respondents whose effort is known to be suspect (based on other cognitive and behavioral criteria). A number of normal-effort groups are provided, including a non-neurological group and patients with a variety of neurological and psychiatric conditions (depression, schizophrenia, head injury, stroke, learning disability, mild dementia; see Table 16–7). The examiner selects a normal-effort group whose clinical status best matches the presenting complaint of the client. The authors indicate that the combined normal-effort comparison should be used only if the examinee's presenting complaint does not match well with any of the specific normal-effort comparison groups.

Table 16–7 Normal-Effort Comparison Groups for the Dot Counting Test

Normal-Effort Group	Description	N (Gender)	Mean Age in Years (Range)	Mean Education in Years (Range)
Nonclinical	No psychiatric disorder, substance abuse, or neurological disorder; age >45 yr	51 (16 M, 35 F)	65.3 (46–80)	15.3 (12–20)
Depression	Met DSM-III-R criteria for Major Depression; age >45 yr	64 (30 M, 34 F)	59.8 (50–85)	15.1 (11–20)
Schizophrenia	Met DSM-III-R criteria for Schizophrenia	28 (18 M, 10 F)	35.3 (22–56)	13.1 (6–21)
Head Injury	Head trauma with brain lesion documented with CT or MRI	20 (14 M, 6 F)	34.6 (18–56)	12.9 (10–17)
Stroke	CVA with brain lesion documented with CT or MRI	18 (10 M, 8 F)	61.2 (35–81)	15.9 (12–22)
Learning Disability	LD documented by cognitive testing; receiving special services	31 (14 M, 17 F)	31.0 (19–72)	15.6 (13–18)
Mild Dementia	Met DSM-III-R criteria for AD; MMSE score >21	16 (10 M, 6 F)	75.4 (54–88)	12.7 (8–18)
Normal-Effort Groups Combined	All of above	228 (112 M, 116 F)	52.8 (18–88)	14.6 (6–22)

A table is provided (Table 5 in the test manual) that presents recommended cutoffs and the associated values for four indexes of classification accuracy: sensitivity, specificity, positive predictive accuracy (PPA), and negative predictive accuracy (NPA). PPA and NPA are calculated using three hypothetical base rates: 15% (general clinical assessment setting), 30% (practices in which a mixture of clinical and medical-legal referrals is seen), and 45% (practices that specialize in medical-legal evaluations). If the E-score is less than the specified cutoff, the client's performance is considered to fall in the range of normal effort. The recommended cutoff points were chosen to minimize false positives while maintaining adequate sensitivity for suspect effort. Appendix A in the test manual includes tables showing other cutoff scores with associated values of sensitivity, specificity, PPA, and NPA. These tables allow the examiner to opt for different cutoff scores in order to maximize sensitivity or specificity in various situations. As the cutoff score is raised, specificity and PPA increase, and sensitivity and NPA decrease. This occurs because a higher cutoff reduces the likelihood of false-positive errors.

DEMOGRAPHIC EFFECTS

Age

Age is related to performance (Arnett & Franzen, 1997; Back et al., 1996); however, the impact appears to be minimal. Boone et al. (2002a) reported that correlations with age are less than .20.

Gender

Gender has no effect on E-scores (Boone et al., 2002a).

Education

Education does affect E-scores, although the amount of variance accounted for by education is reported to be small ($R^2 = .04$; Boone et al., 2002a).

Ethnicity

The effect of ethnicity is not reported.

NORMATIVE DATA

Original Version

Lezak et al. (2004) provided percentile norms for the time (in seconds) taken to count ungrouped and grouped dots on each card. The data appear quite dated because they are based on work published more than 60 years ago (Rey, 1941). Others have described different cutoffs. For example, Paul et al. (1992) recommended the following cutoff points: (a) longer than 130 s total time on grouped dots, (b) longer than 180 s total time for ungrouped dots, (c) less than three correct responses on grouped-dot cards, (d) less than one correct response on ungrouped-dot cards, and (e) more than four trend reversals (instances in which the respondent fails to show the expected pattern of requiring more time to count larger arrays of dots). However, the sensitivity of these cutoffs is poor (Boone et al., 2002a; Rose et al., 1998).

Boone et al.

As noted earlier, performance is evaluated relative to a suspect-effort group and a normal-effort group that corresponds closest to the complaint of the client. A total of 228 individuals were included in the normal-effort group (see Table 16–7). None was involved in litigation or seeking disability payments. The suspect-effort group consisted of 99 individuals, 85 of whom were in personal injury litigation or seeking disability benefits associated with alleged medical or psychiatric disorders. All were suspected of noncredible effort based on other behavioral and cognitive criteria. Data from this study were used to calculate sensitivity, specificity, PPA, and NPA over a range of possible cutoff scores (see *Scoring*). The primary criterion for selecting the cutoff score was to obtain a specificity of at least 90% (achieved for all but the stroke group). The recommended cutoff scores achieved a PPA of at least 80% (except for stroke cases), using a base rate assumption of 30% for suspect effort.

Boone et al. (2002a) found that only 3.5% of all the suspect-effort participants produced E-scores of 9 or less, whereas 50.8% of all the normal-effort participants produced such scores. Accordingly, based on their analysis of suspect- and normal-effort groups, they suggested that an E-score of 9 or less is very likely to represent a credible, normal-effort performance. Fewer than 10% of the normal effort participants produced E-scores of 22 or greater, but 55.3% of the suspect-effort individuals produced such scores. Therefore, E-scores of 22 or greater are typically associated with suspect effort.

Boone et al. (2002b) also noted other indicators of suspect effort on the DCT: longer than 7 s mean grouped-dot counting time, more than three errors, and a ratio of ungrouped-to grouped-dot counting time of less than 1.5. Sensitivities of these indicators are low, suggesting that these findings are relatively uncommon even in those with verified suspect effort; however, specificities tend to be high, meaning that these signs are almost never present in those who exert normal effort.

RELIABILITY

Boone et al. (2002a) did not provide data on reliability, arguing that test-taking effort is not a stable trait or skill; rather "it is a capacity that responds to the external contingencies of the assessment setting. When the test-taking situation itself introduces a variable effect on the construct being measured, traditional reliability statistics have little meaning" (p. 23). They argued that the best evidence for the reliability of an effort test is that the test can discriminate among groups whose effort statuses have been established by other means, and that it can do so consistently across groups representing different problems and clinical states. Our view is that test-retest reliability need not be demonstrated among litigants; however, it would be important to know that persons with legitimate injuries reliably produce good scores.

VALIDITY

Relations Within the Test

Total errors correlate modestly with grouped-dot counting time ($r = .25$) and with the ratio of ungrouped- to grouped-dot counting time ($r = -.34$); however, the amount of shared variance among scores does not exceed 12%, suggesting that speed and accuracy of dot-counting performance are separable constructs (Boone et al., 2002a). Of note, Binks et al. (1997) found that dot-counting accuracy appeared to be more important than the time scores in detecting suboptimal effort.

Relations With Other Measures

The DCT shows moderately high correlations with other measures assessing feigning of cognitive symptoms (e.g., b Test $r = .60$, Rey 15-Item $r = -.56$; Complex Figure $r = .69$, Warrington Recognition Memory $r = .41$, Nelson et al., 2003; PDRT $r = -.41$, Youngjohn et al., 1995), suggesting that the task provides somewhat independent information regarding effort in this arena. However, the association between the DCT (E-score) and Digit Span (age-corrected scaled score) is high ($r = -.75$; 56% shared variance), indicating that these two measures may provide somewhat redundant information. One implication is that it may not be appropriate to use scores from these two tests as additive evidence of suspect effort (Nelson et al., 2003).

Correlations are small between validity indicators on measures of psychopathology (e.g., MMPI-2, MCMI) and scores on the DCT (Boone et al., 1995; Youngjohn et al., 1995). Therefore, the DCT may be sensitive to exaggeration of neuropsychological impairment but not of psychopathology.

Clinical Findings

The efficacy of the test in detecting noncredible cognitive symptoms is mixed. For example, Boone et al. (2002a, 2002b) found that the task was able to discriminate a suspect-effort group (86 personal injury claimants) from groups displaying normal effort. Using cut-scores based on ungrouped-dot counting time, grouped-dot counting time, and number of errors, sensitivity was about 70% in this sample, and

specificity was about 90% in a variety of clinical groups. Other researchers (e.g., Beetar & Williams, 1995; Binks et al., 1997; Erdal, 2004; Martin et al., 1996; Strauss et al., 2002) have also found that simulators (even those with considerable knowledge or expertise regarding the effects of head injuries) suppress their performance, taking longer to respond and being less accurate than nonsimulators. Simulators are also more inconsistent than controls, showing greater variability in performance from one test session to another (Strauss et al., 2002).

However, some authors (Greiffenstein et al., 1994; Hayes et al., 1997; Hiscock et al., 1994; Rose et al., 1998) have reported that the DCT does not reliably distinguish probable or simulating malingerers from compliant patients. In addition, there is evidence that other tests (e.g., forced-choice recognition) are more sensitive than the DCT to suspect effort (Hiscock et al., 1994; Martin et al., 1996; Rose et al., 1998; Strauss et al., 2002; see also Vickery et al., 2001 for a recent meta-analytic review of various procedures). The DCT appears to be as effective (or ineffective) as the Rey 15-Item Test in differentiating honest from dissimulating groups of respondents (Vickery et al., 2001).

Some studies have shown DCT performance to be preserved in the context of actual memory impairment (e.g., substance abuse, Arnett & Franzen, 1997; Wernicke-Korsakoff syndrome, Pachana et al., 1998). However, cognitive status does affect performance, and the task should not be used with patients who have more extensive cognitive impairments (e.g., stroke, mental retardation, MMSE scores ≤24), because their cognitive problems may well interfere with accurate assessment of effort (Back et al., 1996; Boone et al., 2002a; Hayes et al., 1996). Psychiatric disturbance (e.g., depression, psychosis) appears to have little impact on test scores (Back et al., Boone et al., 2002a, 2002b; Lee et al., 2000).

COMMENT

Overall, the test appears to display moderate sensitivity and high specificity. Positive findings imply suspect effort, but use of the task in isolation may result in an unacceptable number of false negatives. Therefore, the clinician is encouraged to supplement this task with others, particularly forced-choice procedures.

The DCT taps somewhat different sources of information regarding effort than other tasks used to detect feigning of cognitive symptoms. However, the association between the DCT (E-score) and Digit Span (age-corrected scaled score) is high, suggesting that these two measures may provide somewhat redundant sources of information regarding effort (Nelson et al., 2003).

The task appears to be relatively unaffected by age or educational level. It also is minimally affected by emotional disorder, suggesting that it is appropriate for use with patients with psychiatric disorders. It is also not affected by true memory impairment. However, users should bear in mind that the DCT is not impervious to cognitive impairment.

The availability of DCT data on various clinical groups allows the clinician to tailor cutoffs to the individual case. When the DCT was used in the context of evaluation of traumatic head injury, the recommended cutoff E-score of 20 had a sensitivity of 68.2% and a specificity of 95% in detecting suspect effort (Boone et al., 2002a). The PPV was reported to be 70.7% when the base rate of suboptimal effort is 15%, 85.4% when it was 30%, and 91.8% when it was 45%. Therefore, the efficacy of the task appears limited when the base rate of suboptimal effort is less than about 30%, because the risk of a false-positive finding is high (i.e., about 2 in 10 claimants will be incorrectly labeled as malingering using a 30% figure). Users should also note that the cutoffs recommended by Boone et al. (2002a) are estimates that require independent confirmation.

Boone et al. (2002a, 2002b) suggested that individuals in different settings may take different approaches to feigning. For example, prison inmates may slow their performance on both tasks, whereas civil litigants may slow grouped time to approximate ungrouped time and commit errors (Boone et al., 2002a, b). Additional studies are needed to confirm these preliminary findings.

REFERENCES

Arnett, P. A., & Franzen, M. D. (1997). Performance of substance abusers with memory deficits on measures of malingering. *Archives of Clinical Neuropsychology, 12*, 513–518.

Back, C., Boone, K. B., Edwards, C., Burgoyne, K., & Silver, B. (1996). The performance of schizophrenics on three cognitive tests of malingering, Rey 15-Item Memory test, Rey Dot Counting, and Hiscock Forced-Choice Method. *Assessment, 3*, 449–458.

Beetar, J. T., & Williams, J. M. (1995). Malingering response styles on the Memory Assessment Scales and symptom validity tests. *Archives of Clinical Neuropsychology, 10*, 57–72.

Binks, P. G., Gouvier, W. D., & Waters, W. F. (1997). Malingering detection with the Dot Counting Test. *Archives of Clinical Neuropsychology, 12*, 41–46.

Boone, K., Lu, P., Herzberg, D. S. (2002a). *The Dot Counting Test.* Los Angeles: Western Psychological Services.

Boone, K. B., Lu, P., Back, C., King, C., Lee, A., Philpott, L., Shamieh, E., & Warner-Chacon, K. (2002b). Sensitivity and specificity of the Rey Dot Counting Test in patients with suspect effort and various clinical samples. *Archives of Clinical Neuropsychology, 17*, 625–642.

Boone, K. B., Sadovnik, I., Ghaffarian, S., Lee, A., Freeman, D., & Berman, N. G. (1995). Rey 15-Item Memory and Dot Counting scores in a "stress" claim worker's compensation population: Relationship to personality (MCMI) scores. *Journal of Clinical Psychology, 5*, 457–463.

Erdal, K. (2004). The effects of motivation, coaching, and knowledge of neuropsychology on the simulated malingering of head injury. *Archives of Clinical Neuropsychology, 19*, 73–88.

Frederick, R. I. (2002). A review of Rey's strategies for detecting malingered neuropsychological impairment. *Journal of Forensic Neuropsychology, 2*, 1–25.

Greiffenstein, M., Baker, W., & Gola, T. (1994). Validation of malingered amnesia measures with a large clinical sample. *Psychological Assessment, 6*, 218–224.

Hayes, J. S., Hale, D. B., & Gouvier, W. D. (1997). Do tests predict malingering in defendants with mental retardation? *The Journal of Psychology, 131*, 575–576.

Hiscock, C. K., Branham, J. D., & Hiscock, M. (1994). Detection of feigned cognitive impairment: The two-alternative forced-choice method compared with selected conventional tests. *Journal of Psychopathology and Behavioral Assessment, 16*, 95–110.

Lee, A., Boone, K. B., Lesser, I., Wohl, M., Wilkins, S., & Parks, C. (2000). Performance of older depressed patients on two cognitive malingering tests: False positive rates for the Rey 15-Item Memorization and Dot Counting tests. *The Clinical Neuropsychologist, 14*, 303–308.

Lezak, M. D. (1983). *Neuropsychological assessment.* New York: Oxford University Press.

Lezak, M. D., Howieson, D. B., & Loring, D. W. (2004). *Neuropsychological assessment* (4th ed.). New York: Oxford University Press.

Martin, R. C., Hayes, J. S., & Gouvier, W. D. (1996). Differential vulnerability between postconcussion self-report and objective malingering tests in identifying mild head injury. *Journal of Clinical and Experimental Neuropsychology, 18*, 265–275.

Nelson, N. W., Boone, K., Dueck, A., Wagener, L., Lu, P., & Grills, C. (2003). Relationships between eight measures of suspect effort. *The Clinical Neuropsychologist, 17*, 263–272.

Pachana, N. A., Boone, K. B., & Ganzell, S. (1998). False positive errors on selected tests of malingering. *American Journal of Forensic Psychology, 16*, 17–25.

Paul, D., Franzen, M. D., Cohen, S. H., & Fremouw, W. (1992). An investigation into the reliability and validity of two tests used in the detection of simulation. *International Journal of Clinical Neuropsychology, 14*, 1–9.

Rey, A. (1941). L' examen psychologique dans les cas d'encephalopathie traumatique. *Archives de Psychologie, 28*, 286–340.

Rose, F. E., Hall, S., & Szalda-Petree, A. D. (1998). A comparison of four tests of malingering and the effects of coaching. *Archives of Clinical Neuropsychology, 13*, 349–363.

Strauss, E., Slick, D. J., Levy-Bencheton, J., Hunter, M., MacDonald, S. W. S., & Hultsch, D. F. (2002). Intraindividual variability as an indicator of malingering in head injury. *Archives of Clinical Neuropsychology, 17*, 423–444.

Vickery, C. D., Berry, D. T. R., Inman, T. H., Harris, M. J., & Orey, S. A. (2001). Detection of inadequate effort on neuropsychological testing: A meta-analytic review of selected procedures. *Archives of Clinical Neuropsychology, 16*, 45–73.

Youngjohn, J. R., Burrows, L., & Erdal, K. (1995). Brain damage or compensation neurosis? The controversial post-concussion syndrome. *The Clinical Neuropsychologist, 9*, 112–123.

Rey Fifteen-Item Test (FIT)

OTHER TEST NAMES

The Rey Fifteen-Item Test (FIT) is also called the Fifteen-Item Memory Test, Rey's Memory Test, or Rey's 3×5 Test.

PURPOSE

This test is used to assess exaggeration or feigning of memory complaints.

SOURCE

The test can be made using the description provided here.

AGE RANGE

The task can be used with people aged about 11 years and older.

DESCRIPTION

Andre Rey developed an interest in detecting malingering partly in response to accusations by insurance companies that most, if not all, claimants were probably only feigning impairment (Frederick, 2002). The FIT (Rey, 1964) is probably the best known of Rey's procedures (Frederick, 2002). Lezak (1983) adapted the task. Currently, it is one of the most commonly used symptom validity tasks (Slick et al., 2004). It consists of 15 items that are arranged in three columns by five rows (see Figure 16–2). Patients are shown a card (21.5 cm in width and 28 cm in height) containing the 15 items for 10 s and are then asked to draw the items from memory. In the instructions, the number "15" is stressed to make the test appear difficult (Lezak et al., 2004). In reality, because this is primarily a test of immediate memory and attention and because of item redundancy (i.e., ABC, 123, abc, and so on), the FIT is actually rather easy and patients need recall only three or four ideas to recall most of the items. Malingerers are thought to misjudge the difficulty of the task and thus to perform more poorly than all but those patients with severe intellectual impairment. In their discussion of the FIT, Lezak et al. (2004) suggested that anyone who is not significantly impaired can recall at least three of the five character sets, or 9 of the 15 items.

Figure 16–2 Rey's Fifteen-Item Test.

Figure 16–3 Rey FIT Recognition Simuli. *Source:* From Boone et al., 2002. Reprinted with the kind permission of Psychology Press.

Other Variants

A number of authors have suggested various modifications of the FIT to increase the sensitivity of the test (see *Validity*). For example, Paul et al. (1992) developed a 16-item version of the FIT consisting of four rows and four items (ABCD, 1234, abcd, I II III IIII). Griffin et al. (1997) redesigned the figures, increasing the internal logic and pattern redundancy. Boone et al. (2002) included a recognition trial after the recall trial. The client is requested to recognize the 15 stimuli out of 15 targets and 15 foils (see Figure 16–3).

ADMINISTRATION

The client is provided with a blank sheet of paper. The instructions for the standard FIT (Goldberg & Miller, 1986) are shown in Figure 16–4. Other researchers have emphasized different aspects of the instructions. For example, Arnett et al. (1995) emphasize that it is a "difficult" memory task and that the client must "draw as many of the designs as you can remember and arrange them in the same way as they were on the card."

ADMINISTRATION TIME

About 5 min is required for the test.

SCORING

A number of scores can be computed. Typically, examiners record the total number of items recalled correctly, regardless

Figure 16–4 Instructions for Rey's Fifteen-Item Test. *Source:* From Goldberg & Miller, 1986.

*I am going to show you a card with **15** (emphasized) things on it to remember. When I take the card away, I want you to write down as many of the 15 things as you can remember. The stimulus card is removed after a 10-s exposure.*

of their spatial location. The range is 0 to 15. One can also record the number of correct rows in proper sequence; that is, the number of rows that are in the correct place in the 3 × 5 matrix and that contain all of the correct items arranged in the correct order. The range is 0 to 5. One can also sum the number of symbols correctly placed within a row. For example, ACB would receive a score of 1. The range of scores is 0 to 15. Analysis of type of error (e.g., rotations, distortions, perseverations) may also be of some use (e.g., Erdal, 2004; Greiffenstein et al. 1996; Griffen et al. 1996; also see *Validity*).

DEMOGRAPHIC EFFECTS

Age

Modest associations have been reported between number correct and age. For example, Schretlen et al. (1991) found that, in adults, the number of items recalled was inversely related to age ($r = -.25$). Others have also reported that scores on the FIT decline with advancing age (e.g., Boone et al., 2002; Griffin et al., 1997; Philpott & Boone, 1994), although the amount of shared variance tends to be small (<10%). In children, test performance correlates highly with age ($r = .61$ to .72), with scores improving with increasing age (Constantinou & McCaffrey, 2003).

IQ/Education

Intellectual level is also related (.38 to .81) to performance on the test (e.g., Goldberg & Miller, 1986; Griffin et al., 1997; Schretlen et al., 1991; but see Back et al., 1996, who failed to find a relation between MMSE and FIT scores in schizophrenic patients). Level of education affects scores in adults (e.g., Back et al., 1996; Boone et al., 2002) and children (Constantinou & McCaffrey, 2003), with scores increasing with higher levels of education. Therefore, the FIT may be inappropriate for individuals with less than average IQ/education.

Gender

No differences between males and females have been reported (Constantinou & McCaffrey, 2003).

NORMATIVE DATA

Adults

For the standard FIT, cutoff scores of 7 items correct or fewer (Lee et al., 1992), 8 items or fewer (Bernard & Fowler, 1990; Schretlen et al., 1991), 9 items or fewer (Greiffenstein et al., 1996; Lezak et al., 2004; Taylor et al., 2003), and 11 items (Hiscock et al., 1994) have been suggested to determine suboptimal effort in adults (see *Validity*). Adjusting the cutoff score higher tends to increase the FIT's sensitivity but at the expense of its specificity (Lee et al., 1992; Schretlen et al., 1991).

Although most researchers focus on the total number of items recalled, some have suggested more complex scoring schemes involving appraisals of item placement and accuracy of reproductions. For example, examiners can use a cutoff of fewer than two rows in proper location (Arnett et al., 1995) or fewer than nine symbols accurately placed within rows (Greiffenstein et al., 1996).

The five rows that comprise the FIT differ in degree of difficulty. In nonlitigating brain-damaged individuals, recall of the three capital letters is best, followed by arabic numerals, lowercase letters, geometric figures, and Roman numerals (Morgan, 1991). The most frequent qualitative error is misordering of geometric shapes (Morgan, 1991). In honest responders, perseverations/repetitions of correct stimuli and errors in the correct placement of rows appear to be relatively common; however, other types of errors (e.g., dyslexic errors, such as d for b; gestalt error, such as >3 items in a row; embellishments or confabulatory errors) are rare (Griffin et al., 1996; Lee et al., 2000). It is important to bear in mind, however, that some of these errors (e.g., confabulations) may occur commonly in the context of low IQ or a diagnosis of dementia (Hays et al., 2000).

If the recognition trial is also given, Boone et al (2002) suggest a combination cutoff score (total FIT score + [recognition score − false positives]) of less than 20 to indicate "failed" performance.

Children

Mean scores for 67 children (44 girls, 23 boys), aged 5 to 12 years, living in upstate New York were provided for the FIT by Constantinou and McCaffrey (2003). The data are shown in Table 16–8. These authors also provided similar data from a second site (Cyprus). Although the sample is very small, the data suggest that errorless levels are reached by about age 11 years.

RELIABILITY

Test-Retest Reliability

Information regarding test-retest reliability is not available for the standard protocol. However, Paul et al. (1992) devised a

Table 16–8 Mean Scores of Children in the United States on the FIT

Age	*n*	Mean	SD
5	7	3.57	2.44
6	10	8.90	5.61
7	14	9.79	2.69
8	14	12.78	3.09
9	13	12.85	1.95
10	1	12	—
11	1	15	—
12	7	14.14	1.46

Source: Adapted from Constantinou & McCaffrey, 2003.

16-item version of the FIT (described earlier) and gave the task to community volunteers. On retesting after a 2-week interval, community dwellers achieved a reliability coefficient of .48 (due to the fact that normal subjects typically obtain perfect scores on both tests), which rose to .88 under simulation conditions.

Interrater Reliability

Goldberg and Miller (1986) reported that independent raters showed 95% agreement for items correct and 97% agreement for rows correct scores.

VALIDITY

Relations With Other Measures

The FIT shows modest to moderate correlations (.19 to .78) with other cognitive measures of effort (e.g., b Test, Dot Counting, TOMM, Warrington Recognition Memory Test; McCaffrey et al., 2003; Nelson et al., 2003), with shared variances tending to be less than 50% (Nelson et al., 2003). Therefore, the FIT may provide some nonredundant information regarding motivational status. There appears to be little relationship between various MMPI-2 validity scales (e.g., F, F-K) and scores on cognitive tasks such as the FIT (Greiffenstein et al., 1995; McCaffrey et al., 2003). The implication is that the FIT is measuring a different construct than the traditional MMPI-2 validity scales.

Clinical Findings

Ideally, a test designed to detect malingered memory defects should be sensitive to faking but insensitive to genuine memory disturbance. However, the FIT appears to fall far short of this ideal. In general, honest responders achieve higher scores on the test than dissimulating responders, but the sensitivity of the FIT in identifying deception is weak and lower than that of other tests (e.g., Digit Memory Test, TOMM; Shum et al., 2004; Vickery et al., 2001; Vallabhajosula & van Gorp, 2001).

Further, patients with focal memory disturbance, as well as those with more extensive cognitive impairment, may perform poorly on the task. For example, Schretlen et al. (1991) gave the test to 76 subjects faking various mental disorders; 148 patients with amnesia, dementia, severe mental illness, or other neuropsychiatric disorder; and 80 normal controls. They reported that 27% of the patients scored in the "malingering" range, and only 15% of those instructed to fake impairment were detected as malingerers with the FIT. Similarly, Morgan (1991) examined 60 nonlitigating subjects with mild-to-severe memory impairment and found that 12 of them "failed" the FIT when a criterion of three rows or nine items was used. Goldberg and Miller (1986) gave the task to 50 adult psychiatric inpatients of average intelligence ($M = 101.1$, $SD = 12.5$) and 16 retarded adults (WAIS-R IQ range, 40–69,

$M = 63.4$, $SD = 7.54$). They found that all of the psychiatric patients recalled at least 9 of the 15 items, and more than 37% of the retarded subjects recalled fewer than 9 items. Nine of the 16 retarded adults failed to recall at least three of the five rows (see also Hayes et al., 1997).

Philpott and Boone (1994) gave the FIT to patients with probable dementia of the Alzheimer type (AD) who varied with respect to level of cognitive impairment (from mild to severe according to scores on the MMSE) and to healthy adults, aged 46 to 80 years. They found that performance on the FIT varied with severity of dementia. Only 2 of the 49 patients with AD obtained a FIT score greater than 9. Even patients with mild cognitive decline exhibited a high rate of "failure" on this test. Finally, Back et al. (1996) reported that in a sample of 30 patients with schizophrenia, 13% obtained a score less than 9.

Adjusting the cutoff score to 7 has been recommended to improve diagnostic efficiency (Lee et al., 1992). Lee et al. (1992) gave the FIT to inpatients with 100 temporal lobe epilepsy, 56 nonlitigating outpatients, and 16 outpatients who were in litigation and whose optimal performance could not be assumed. They found that a score of 7 items recalled was at or below the 5th percentile for each reference group except the outpatient group in litigation. However, concerns have also been raised about the merits of this cutoff. For example, Millis and Kler (1995) gave the FIT to seven individuals who were claiming to have severe cognitive deficits as a result of closed head injuries but who were judged to be malingerers because of significantly below-chance performance on the Recognition Memory Test, a forced-choice memory measure. A reference group of seven patients with acute moderate-to-severe traumatic brain injury was also given the FIT. The brain-injured subjects recalled significantly more items on the FIT than the malingering subjects did. Using a cutoff score of 7, the FIT was able to detect only about half of the malingerers but did not misclassify any brain-injured subjects. Guilmette et al. (1994) also used this modified cutoff score and found that the FIT was overly sensitive to genuine memory impairment and not sensitive enough to identify individuals feigning brain damage. Using a cutoff of 7 or fewer items correct, 40% of nonlitigating patients with moderate-to-severe brain damage and 20% of depressed psychiatric inpatients would have been classified as possible malingerers. In contrast, only 5% of a group of normal subjects asked to feign believable deficits fell in the "malingering" range.

Others have recommended different adjustments to improve the utility of the test. Arnett et al. (1995) compared the performance of a mixed sample of neurological patients (predominantly patients with traumatic brain-injury and intracerebral hemorrhage) to normal individuals instructed to simulate impairment on several quantitative and qualitative variables derived from the FIT. They found that a cutoff of less than two rows in proper location provided the best discrimination of groups (in comparison to cutoffs of less than three rows correct, fewer than nine items correct, and less than rows correct), producing sensitivity of 47% and a specificity of 97%. The same cutoff applied to a replication study yielded a sensitivity of 64% and a specificity of 96%. Note, however, that their group of brain-damaged patients was not ideal, because they suffered moderate-to-severe damage. Patients with minor traumatic brain injury would provide a more appropriate comparison. Nonetheless, the finding that patients with documented evidence of cerebral damage can achieve two or more correct rows on the FIT suggests that performance below this cutoff in the context of minor head injury should be considered as suspect.

Griffin et al. (1996) recommended altering the administration by requesting that subjects record the 15 items "just as they appear on the card." They suggested, based on a study of psychiatrically disabled subjects and normal nonmalingerers, as well as possible malingerers, that both quantitative and qualitative analysis should be used. Although omissions were most common, possible malingerers made significantly more gestalt (failure to reproduce the 3×5 configuration), row sequence, dyslexic (character reversal), and embellishment errors than did nonmalingerers. Simulators also produced significantly more errors than honest responders on a redesigned version of the Rey test (Griffin et al., 1997). Note, however that these errors (e.g., gestalt errors, wrong item) are uncommon even among simulators or probable malingerers (Griffin et al., 1996). The fact that some of these errors (e.g., embellishments/confabulations) occur commonly in the context of low IQ or dementia (Hays et al., 2000) indicates that it is important to rule out these conditions before accepting them as pathognomic signs of suspect effort.

Greiffenstein et al. (1996) examined the utility of some other scoring modifications. In 60 patients with severe traumatic brain injury and 90 litigating postconcussion patients who were probably malingering, hit rates (64% sensitivity, 72% specificity) with Rey's original scoring method (≤9 items) could be improved somewhat (69% sensitivity, 77% specificity) with a spatial scoring system in which the correct within-row reproductions are computed. Note that the specificity levels are quite low, with a false-positive error rate of about 33%. A 15-word forced-choice recognition memory test proved to be more effective than the FIT.

More recently, Boone et al. (2002) suggested yet another approach to improve the efficacy of the test. They developed a recognition trial to follow the recall trial in which the patient is asked to circle the 15 stimuli (out of 15 targets and 15 foils) recognized from the original stimulus page. Boone et al. suggested that sensitivity is increased by 50% relative to recall alone when the recognition trial is added (to >70%), with no appreciable loss in specificity (>90%). Note that patients with mental retardation and dementia were excluded from the study, which probably enhanced specificity values. With a base rate of suspect effort of 28%, a combined score (computed as recall correct plus recognition correct minus false-positive recognitions) of 20 or less yielded a positive predictive value (PPV) of 77.8% and a negative predictive value (NPV) of 89.5%.

Depression appears to have relatively little impact on test scores, at least when outpatients are evaluated. Lee et al. (2000) assessed a sample of older adult outpatients with major depression and found that about 5% failed the FIT using the cutoffs of less than 9 total items and less than 9 spatial score (number of items accurately placed within a row). By contrast, as noted earlier, Guilmette et al. (1994) used a cutoff score of 7 items and found that 20% of depressed psychiatric inpatients would have been classified as possible malingerers.

Performance on the FIT (recall/recognition) does not appear to be contaminated by mild learning disorders. Boone et al. (2002) found that learning-disabled college students performed well on the tasks. However, it remains to be determined whether performance is contaminated by more severe learning disorders (e.g., those found in non-university students).

There is considerable evidence that forced-choice recognition tasks are more useful than the standard FIT (Greiffenstein et al., 1996; Hiscock et al., 1994; Vallabhajosula & van Gorp, 2001; Vickery et al., 2001). For example, Guilmette et al. (1994) found that a version of the Hiscock and Hiscock (1989) forced-choice procedure was superior to the FIT as a malingering detection procedure within neuropsychological assessment (see the *Victoria Symptom Validity Test* for an adaptation of Hiscock and Hiscock's procedure). Using a cutoff of 90% or less correct as suggesting malingering on the Hiscock and Hiscock forced-choice procedure, all of the brain-damaged subjects and all but 15% of the simulators were correctly classified.

Iverson and Franzen (1996) evaluated students, psychiatric patients, and a mixed group of memory-impaired patients on a number of tasks, including the 16-item version of the FIT. The 16-item version was not effective in classifying individuals instructed to malinger (22.5%), although forced-choice procedures had relatively high rates of correct classification. Greiffenstein et al. (1994) tested a sample of 106 postconcussion patients with and without overt signs of malingering (e.g., improbable poor performance on two or more neuropsychological measures, contradiction between collateral sources and symptom history) on a battery of neuropsychological tests (e.g., RAVLT, WMS, WMS-R) and a number of malingered amnesia measures, including the FIT. Probable malingerers could not be differentiated from seriously brain-injured patients on free-recall measures from the Wechsler scales and the RAVLT. In contrast, probable malingerers performed poorly on the malingering measures, including the FIT, although the Portland Digit Recognition Test achieved a better hit rate. Greiffenstein et al. (1995) noted, however, that malingered amnesia measures, including the FIT, were generally more sensitive to noncompliance than were MMPI-2 measures.

COMMENT

A recent survey addressing practices of expert neuropsychologists in handling financial compensation or personal injury litigation cases revealed the FIT to be one of the most frequently used measures (Slick et al., 2004). Low cost, ready availability, and ease of administration probably account for its popularity.

The available evidence suggests that the FIT may provide complementary information to that of other measures of motivational status. On the other hand, it appears to be sensitive to genuine cognitive dysfunction (including dementia, amnesia, and visual-spatial problems) and insufficiently sensitive to malingering (e.g., Arnott et al., 1995; Beetar & Williams, 1994; Greiffenstein et al., 1996; Guilmette et al., 1994; Iverson & Franzen, 1996; Morgan, 1991; Schretlen et al., 1991; Vickery et al., 2001). One potential approach to improve sensitivity is to include the recognition trial in the administration (Boone et al., 2002). However, it should be noted that the FIT, even with the addition of the recognition trial, does not meet the Daubert standard for admissibility of scientific evidence based on its failure to achieve a criterion of PPV of 80% or higher using a base rate of suspect effort of 30% (Vallabhajosula & van Gorp, 2001).

The FIT should not be used in isolation. If clinicians choose to use the FIT in combination with other measures, its greatest utility may be in detecting blatant malingering strategies after mild brain injury (Millis & Kler, 1995; Palmer et al., 1995). In such cases, the test should be given at the very beginning of the evaluation, before the patient is exposed to more difficult tests and subsequently understands the simplicity of the procedure (Iverson & Franzen, 1996). The use of the test in patients with severe cerebral dysfunction is not recommended. In fact, if poor scores occur on the standard FIT, clinicians should first consider the possibility of low IQ and/or severe neurological disturbance before drawing conclusions about the validity of malingering scores (e.g., Greiffenstein et al., 1994, 1996; Hayes et al., 1997). We, like others, prefer forced-choice procedures (e.g., Greiffenstein et al., 1994; Guilmette et al., 1994; Iverson & Franzen, 1996; Millis & Kler, 1995; Vickery et al., 2001).

It is worth noting that the motivation that an individual has can affect the magnitude of his or her dissimulation on the FIT. Erdal (2004) used a simulation paradigm and reported that people who are motivated to gain compensation malinger more flagrantly than do those who are motivated to avoid blame.

Most research on suboptimal effort has examined adults while ignoring the possibility that children may not put forth optimal effort. The FIT should not be used with young children whose experience with geometric shapes, letters, and numbers is limited (Constantinou & McCaffrey, 2003). Whether it is useful in assessing motivational status in older children requires study. Further, although the impact of mild learning disorders on task performance appears to be minimal, it is not known whether the task is contaminated by language processing deficits found in more severe forms of learning disability.

REFERENCES

Arnett, P. A., Hemmeke, T. A., & Schwartz, L. (1995). Quantitative and qualitative performance on Rey's 15-Item Test in neurological patients and dissimulators. *The Clinical Neuropsychologist, 9,* 17–26.

Back, C., Boone, K. B., Parks, C., Burgoyne, K., & Silver, B. (1996). The performance of schizophrenics on three cognitive tests of malingering, Rey 15-Item Memory Test, Rey Dot Counting, and Hiscock forced-choice method. *Assessment, 3,* 449–457.

Beetar, J. T., & Williams, J. M. (1994). Malingering response styles on the Memory Assessment Scales and symptom validity tests. *Archives of Clinical Neuropsychology, 10,* 57–72.

Bernard, L. C., & Fowler, W. (1990). Assessing the validity of memory complaints: Performance of brain-damaged and normal individuals on Rey's task to detect malingering. *Journal of Clinical Psychology, 46,* 432–436.

Boone, K. B., Salazar, X., Lu, P., Warner-Chacon, K., & Razani, J. (2002). The Rey 15-Item Recognition Trial: A technique to enhance sensitivity of the Rey 15-Item Memorization Test. *Journal of Clinical and Experimental Neuropsychology, 24,* 561–573.

Constantinou, M., & McCaffrey, R. J. (2003). Using the TOMM for evaluating children's effort to perform optimally on neuropsychological measures. *Child Neuropsychology, 9,* 81–90.

Erdal, K. (2004). The effects of motivation, coaching, and knowledge of neuropsychology on the simulated malingering of head injury. *Archives of Clinical Neuropsychology, 19,* 73–88.

Frederick, R. I. (2002). A review of Rey's strategies for detecting malingered neuropsychological impairment. *Journal of Forensic Neuropsychology, 2,* 1–25.

Goldberg, J. O., & Miller, H. R. (1986). Performance of psychiatric inpatients and intellectually deficient individuals on a task that assesses the validity of memory complaints. *Journal of Clinical Psychology, 42,* 792–795.

Greiffenstein, M., Baker, W. J., & Gola, T. (1994). Validation of malingered amnesia measures with a large clinical sample. *Psychological Assessment, 6,* 218–224.

Greiffenstein, M. F., Baker, W. J., & Gola, T. (1996). Comparison of multiple scoring methods for Rey's malingered amnesia measures. *Archives of Clinical Neuropsychology, 11,* 283–293.

Greiffenstein, M. F., Gola, T., & Baker, W. J. (1995). MMPI-2 validity scales versus domain specific measures in detection of factitious traumatic brain injury. *The Clinical Neuropsychologist, 9,* 230–240.

Griffin, G. A., Glassmire, D. M., Henderson, E. A., & McCann, C. (1997). Rey II: Redesigning the Rey Screening Test of malingering. *Journal of Clinical Psychology, 53,* 757–766.

Griffin, G. A. E., Normington, J., & Glassmire, D. (1996). Qualitative dimensions in scoring the Rey Visual Memory Test of malingering. *Psychological Assessment, 8,* 383–387.

Guilmette, T. J., Hart, K. J., Giuliano, A. J., & Leininger, B. E. (1994). Detecting simulated memory impairment: Comparison of the Rey Fifteen-Item Test and the Hiscock Forced-Choice Procedure. *The Clinical Neuropsychologist, 8,* 283–294.

Hays, J. R., Emmons, J., & Stallings, G. (2000). Dementia and mental retardation on the Rey 15-Item Visual Memory Test. *Psychological Reports, 86,* 179–182.

Hayes, J. S., Hale, D. B., & Gouvier, W. D. (1997). Do tests predict malingering in defendants with mental retardation? *The Journal of Psychology, 131,* 575–576.

Hiscock, M., & Hiscock, C. K. (1989). Refining the forced choice method for the detection of malingering. *Journal of Clinical and Experimental Neuropsychology, 11,* 967–974.

Hiscock, C., Branham, J., & Hiscock, M. (1994). Detection of feigned cognitive impairment: The two-alternative forced-choice method compared with selected conventional tests. *Journal of Psychopathology and Behavioral Assessment, 16,* 95–109.

Iverson, G. L., & Franzen, M. D. (1996). Using multiple object memory procedures to detect simulated malingering. *Journal of Clinical and Experimental Neuropsychology, 8*, 1–14.

Lee, A., Boone, K. B., Lesser, I., Wohl, M., Wilkins, S., & Parks, C. (2000). Performance of older depressed patients on two cognitive malingering tests: False positive rates for the Rey 15-Item Memorization and Dot Counting tests. *The Clinical Neuropsychologist, 14*, 303–308.

Lee, G. P., Loring, D. W., & Martin, R. C. (1992). Rey's 15-Item Visual Memory Test for the detection of malingering: Normative observations on patients with neurological disorders. *Psychological Assessment, 4*, 43–46.

Lezak, M. D. (1983). *Neuropsychological assessment* (2nd ed.). New York: Oxford University Press.

Lezak, M. D., Howieson, D. B., & Loring, D. W. (2004). *Neuropsychological assessment* (4th ed.). New York: Oxford University Press.

McCaffrey, R. J., O'Bryant, S. E., Ashendorf, L., & Fisher, J. M. (2003). Correlations among the TOMM, Rey-15, and MMPI-2 validity scales in a sample of TBI litigants. *Journal of Forensic Neuropsychology, 3*, 45–53.

Millis, S. R., & Kler, S. (1995). Limitations of the Rey Fifteen-Item test in the detection of malingering. *The Clinical Neuropsychologist, 9*, 241–244.

Morgan, S. F. (1991). Effect of true memory impairment on a test of memory complaint validity. *Archives of Clinical Neuropsychology, 6*, 327–334.

Nelson, N. W., Boone, K., Dueck, A., Wagener, L., Lu, P., & Grills, C. (2003). Relationships between eight measures of suspect effort. *The Clinical Neuropsychologist, 17*, 263–272.

Palmer, B. W., Boone, K. B., Allman, L., & Castro, D. B. (1995). Co-occurrence of brain lesions and cognitive deficit exaggeration. *The Clinical Neuropsychologist, 9*, 68–73.

Paul, D. S., Franzen, M. D., Cohen, S. H., & Fremouw, W. (1992). An investigation into the reliability and validity of two tests used in the detection of dissimulation. *International Journal of Clinical Neuropsychology, 14*, 1–9.

Philpott, L. M., & Boone, K. B. (1994). *The effects of cognitive impairment and age on two malingering tests: An investigation of the Rey Memory Test and Rey Dot Counting Test in Alzheimer's patients and normal middle aged/older adults.* Paper presented to the International Neuropsychological Society, Cincinnati, Ohio.

Rey, A. (1964). *L'examen clinique en psychologie.* Paris: Presses Universitaires de France.

Schretlen, D., Brandt, J., Krafft, L., & Van Gorp, W. (1991). Some caveats using the Rey 15-Item Memory Test to detect malingered amnesia. *Psychological Assessment, 3*, 667–672.

Shum, D. H. K., O'Gorman, J. G. O., & Alpar, A. (2004). Effects of incentive and preparation time on performance and classification accuracy on standard and memory-specific memory tests. *Archives of Clinical Neuropsychology, 19*, 817–823.

Slick, D. J., Tan, J. E., Strauss, E. H., & Hultsch, D. F. (2004). Detecting malingering: A survey of experts' practices. *Archives of Clinical Neuropsychology, 19*, 465–473.

Taylor, L. A., Kreutzer, J. S., & West, D. D. (2003). Evaluation of malingering cut-off scores for the Rey 15-Item Test: A brain injury case study series. *Brain Injury, 17*, 295–308.

Vallabhajosula, B., & van Gorp, W. G. (2001). Post-Daubert admissibility of scientific evidence on malingering of cognitive deficits. *Journal of the American Academy of Psychiatry and the Law, 29*, 207–215.

Vickery, C. D., Berry, D. T. R., Inman, T. H., Harris, M. J., & Orey, S. A. (2001). Detection of inadequate effort on neuropsychological testing: A meta-analytic review of selected procedures. *Archives of Clinical Neuropsychology, 16*, 45–73.

Test of Memory Malingering (TOMM)

PURPOSE

The Test of Memory Malingering (TOMM) is used to assess exaggeration or feigning of memory impairment.

SOURCE

The complete kit (including two stimulus booklets, 25 score sheets, and a manual) can be ordered from Multi Health Systems (MHS), Inc., 908 Niagara Falls Blvd, North Tonawanda, NY 14120-2060 (http://www.mhs.com), at a cost of $131 US. Software is available that administers, scores, and reports the results of the TOMM. The software manual and three uses costs $45 US.

AGE RANGE

The test can be used with individuals aged 5 years and older.

DESCRIPTION

The TOMM (Tombaugh, 1996) is the symptom validity test (SVT) most commonly used by neuropsychologists who are expert in handling personal injury cases (Slick et al., 2004). It is similar to the Recognition Memory Test—Faces (Warrington, 1984) in that it involves recognition of pictorial stimuli. Visual stimuli were chosen because the literature suggests that recognition memory for pictures is remarkably robust in older adults and in various neurologically impaired populations.

The TOMM consists of two learning trials and a retention trial. On each learning trial, the patient is shown 50 line drawings (target pictures) of common objects, for 3 s each, at 1-s intervals. The patient is then shown 50 recognition panels, one at a time. Each panel contains one of the previously presented target pictures and a new picture. On this forced-choice recognition task, the patient is required to select the previously shown target picture. Explicit feedback on response correctness is given on each item. The same 50 pictures are used on each trial. However, they are presented in a different order during the second learning trial. There is an optional retention trial that is administered about 15 min after Trial 2. This is similar to the previous trials except that the target pictures are not readministered. Tombaugh (1996) suggested that the two learning trials are usually sufficient to assess malingering. However, use of the retention trial helps corroborate results.

ADMINISTRATION

See *Source.* Briefly, the patient is told that the examiner will test the patient's ability to remember 50 pictures of common objects. The examiner then presents the test stimuli, records responses on the record sheet for the two-choice recognition test, and provides feedback regarding the correctness of the response.

The computerized version appears to give equivalent results to the standard booklet version, at least in a simulation paradigm (Rees et al., 1998). However, differences may arise in the context of clinical evaluations, with the computerized version yielding a higher sensitivity to suboptimal effort (see *Validity* and *Comment*). The computerized version may also be preferred in order to avoid challenges based on imprecise administrative procedures (Tombaugh, 2002).

ADMINISTRATION TIME

About 15 min is required for the test.

SCORING

One point is given for each correct answer provided by the patient on the recognition and retention trials. Therefore, the maximum score on each trial is 50.

DEMOGRAPHIC EFFECTS

Age

Some have reported that age has little impact on test scores (Tombaugh, 1996, 1997); others have noted moderately strong relationships for Trial 2 ($r = -.40$) and the Retention trial ($r = -.50$) in older adults (Teichner & Wagner, 2004). In children, age has no significant association with Trial 2 scores (Constantinou and McCaffrey, 2003; Donders, 2005).

Education/IQ

Education has little relation to performance in adults (Gervais et al., 2004; Teichner & Wagner, 2004; Tombaugh, 1996) or children (Constantinou & McCaffrey, 2003). For example, Gervais et al. (2004) reported a correlation of .06 between the TOMM and years of education. Therefore, limited educational attainment probably cannot account for failure on the TOMM. The influence of IQ is not reported, although moderate to severe cognitive deficit appears to have an impact (see *Validity*).

Gender

Gender has no impact on test scores (Constantinou & McCaffrey, 2003; Donders, 2005; Rees et al., 1998).

Ethnicity/Culture

No differences were found between children living in New York and in Cyprus (Constantinou and McCaffrey, 2003). Similarly, Donders (2005) reported no impact of ethnicity in a pediatric sample in the United States.

NORMATIVE DATA

Standardization Samples

The test was developed on samples of community-dwelling individuals, ranging in age from 16 to 84 years, and on a sample of patients referred for neuropsychological evaluation (see Table 16–9). Tombaugh (1996, 1997) reported that performance on Trial 2 was very high for nonmalingerers regardless of neurological dysfunction (except in the case of dementia). More than 95% of adults living in the community obtained a score of 49 or 50 on the second trial. Moreover, scores for different clinical samples showed that most nondemented individuals obtained a perfect score on Trial 2. In contrast, simulators tended to score below 45 on Trial 2 or the Retention trial. Accordingly, Tombaugh (see *Source*) recommends that any score lower than 45 on Trial 2 or on the Retention Trial should raise concern that the individual is not putting forth maximum effort. Others (Powell et al., 2004; Teichner & Wagner, 2004) have also reported that nondemented adults obtain high scores on the TOMM, with a cutoff point of 5 or more errors on Trial 2 or the Retention trial yielding a high rate of correct classification.

Tombaugh (see *Source*) recommends that, rather than using the score of 45 as a rigid cutoff, it should be viewed as a guideline, with the likelihood of malingering increasing as the score deviates further from the performance of specific clinical samples (see Tables 3-5 and 3-7 in source).

Typically, the number of correct responses is evaluated. However, the computerized version also allows examination of response latencies. Rees et al. (1998) found that response latencies are longer (on average by about 1–2 s) for simulators.

Children

Constantinou and McCaffrey (2003) provided normative data for a sample of 67 children (44 girls, 23 boys) living in upstate New York. These data are shown in Table 16–10. Similar values were obtained for a group of children living in Cyprus. Of note, 9 children (4 Cypriot, 5 U.S.) had a significant medical or psychiatric history. Nonetheless, they all performed above the cutoff of 45 on Trial 2.

RELIABILITY

Internal Consistency

According to Tombaugh (personal communication, November, 1996), coefficient alphas ($n = 40$) were high for each trial (Trial 1 = .94, Trial 2 = .95, Retention Trial = .94).

Table 16–9 Characteristics of the TOMM Standardization Sample

Number	Experiment 1: 475 community-dwelling adults Experiment 2: 70 community-dwelling adults Experiment 3: 135 inpatients and outpatients at the Boston VA diagnosed with a variety of disorders including amnesia, MS, PD, aphasia, dementia, head injury; 23 head-injured individuals involved in a study in Ottawa, Canada, were also included
Age (years)	Experiment 1: 16–84. $M = 54.8$, $SD = 20.2$ Experiment 2: 17–73, $M = 37.8$, $SD = 14.2$ Experiment 3: 19–90, $M = 56.2$, $SD = 18.8$
Geographic location	Experiments 1 and 2: Ottawa, Canada Experiment 3: Boston and Ottawa
Sample type	Experiment 1 and 2: Community-dwelling individuals participating in studies of aging on memory; recruited at shopping centers, social organizations, work, psychology classes, word of mouth Experiment 3: 138 consecutive patients referred for neuropsychological examination at Boston VA (3 excluded because of severe dementia); 23 head-injured participants in a study for PhD thesis
Education (years)	Experiment 1: 8–21, $M = 13.1$, $SD = 3.2$ Experiment 2: 7–20, $M = 12.7$, $SD = 1.9$ Experiment 3: 4–21, $M = 12.7$, $SD = 2.8$
Gender	Experiment 1: 223 M, 252 F Experiment 2: 44 M, 26 F Experiment 3: NA
Race/Ethnicity	Not reported
Screening	Experiments 1 and 2: Any person with a self-reported history of neurological disease, psychiatric illness, head injury, or stroke was excluded Experiment 3: Not involved in litigation or compensation hearings

Note: In the initial validation study (Experiment 1, Tombaugh, 1997), normal individuals were shown the target and three distractors in the test phase. Explicit feedback on the correctness of each response was not given. In Experiment 2 and the subsequent clinical validation studies, the TOMM was made a two-choice, rather than a four-choice, recognition test to facilitate evaluation of below-chance performance. In addition, trial-by-trial feedback was given, allowing individuals to more accurately track their performance and adjust it accordingly. Further, the effects of visual neglect and homonomous hemianopsia were minimized by placing the pictures vertically on the page.

Test-Retest Reliability

No information is available.

VALIDITY

Clinical Findings

A test designed to detect malingered memory defects should be sensitive to deception but insensitive to genuine memory impairment. The available evidence suggests that the TOMM shows considerable promise in this regard.

The test gives the impression of being more difficult than it really is, supporting its potential usefulness in the detection of poor effort (Rees et al., 1998; Tombaugh, 1997). When it is given in the context of other legitimate neuropsychological tests, individuals do not identify its true intent (Rees et al., 1998). That is, it does have face validity as a measure of memory. In addition, performance appears to be relatively insensitive to neurological impairment, although profound cognitive impairment appears to affect performance. Using a criterion

cutoff score of 45 on Trial 2, Tombaugh's studies (Rees et al., 1998; Tombaugh, 1996, 1997) revealed specificity rates greater than 90% when considering cognitively impaired (from a variety of neurological conditions), aphasic, and non-compensation-seeking TBI patients. However, correct classification of demented patients as not malingering was poor. About 27% of

Table 16–10 Mean Scores and SDs of Children in the United States on the TOMM

Age	n	Trial 1	SD	Trial 2	SD
5	7	44.57	3.15	49.71	0.48
6	10	45.60	3.50	49.90	0.32
7	14	43.28	4.87	49.92	0.27
8	14	46.21	3.07	49.93	0.27
9	13	48.08	1.93	49.92	0.28
10	1	50.00	—	50.00	—
11	1	48.00	—	50.00	—
12	7	47.57	2.29	50.00	—

Source: Adapted from Constantinou & McCaffrey, 2003.

patients diagnosed with dementia obtained scores lower than 45 on Trial 2. Similarly, Teicher and Wagner (2004) reported that older adults (including those with mild cognitive impairment) perform almost perfectly on Trial 2 and on the Retention trial; however, misclassification rates were high (>70%) for patients with dementia.

Colby (2001) suggested that false-positive errors are reduced (without a substantial decline in sensitivity) in individuals with and without dementia when a cutoff of more than 14 errors on Trial 2 and Retention combined (or >13 errors if only Trial 2 is given) is used and dementia cannot be ruled out. Weinborn et al. (2003) provided support for the use of these cutoffs among patients with mild mental retardation.

Performance on the TOMM is unrelated to length of coma (Donders, 2005) and only modestly related to measures of learning and memory. Tombaugh (1996) reported that TOMM scores show correlations ranging from .20 to .35 with free-recall measures of visual and verbal learning (Visual Reproduction from the WMS-R, CVLT, and Word-List subtest from the LAMB). Similarly, Hill et al. (2003) examined the relation between measures of declarative memory and the TOMM in patients with and without temporal lobe dysfunction. They reported that temporal lobe dysfunction might affect Retention Trial performance, but not to a degree that TOMM performance fell below the cutoff criteria for malingering. In short, persons who score in the impaired range on standardized tests of learning and retention generally perform well on the TOMM.

Further, the TOMM appears to be moderately sensitive to motivational defects. For example, Tombaugh (see *Source*) gave a battery of neuropsychological tests, including the TOMM, to a group of 27 undergraduate students who were asked to simulate symptoms after head injury and 22 controls. Simulating participants demonstrated lower scores than controls. On Trial 2 in particular, all controls achieved a score of 49 or greater (100% specificity), whereas 93% of the simulators scored lower than 49 (93% sensitivity). Analysis of debriefing questionnaires revealed that participants did not distinguish the TOMM from other tests as a measure of malingering. In a subsequent study, the performance of litigating TBI patients ($n = 11$) was contrasted with that of a nonlitigating control group ($n = 17$), a group of cognitively intact normal subjects ($n = 11$), and a group of patients with focal neuropsychological impairment recruited from a neurological unit ($n = 12$). On Trial 1, TBI patients "not-at-risk" for malingering performed slightly lower than either normal subjects or patients with focal impairment, but they performed at comparable levels on the other two trials. This was in marked contrast to the substantially lower performance of the "at-risk" TBI group. On all three trials, the scores from the "at-risk" TBI group were significantly lower than those from the other groups, which did not differ from one another.

Clients who inflate cognitive concerns may also exaggerate psychological distress (Hill et al., 2003). However, Tombaugh (2002) warned that the TOMM is not an appropriate test to evaluate whether a person is faking a psychiatric disorder. In

support of this proposal, there is evidence that the MMPI-2 validity scales measure a different construct than tests of the validity of cognitive complaints. McCaffrey et al. (2003) found that MMPI-2 validity scales did not correlate with any trial on the TOMM, with the exception of the F_B scale, which was negatively correlated ($r = -.34$) with TOMM Trial 1.

Nonetheless, the task may have some utility in detecting motivational disorders in forensic psychiatric settings. Individuals suspected of feigning incompetence to stand trial (e.g., those facing murder charges) tend to produce low scores on the TOMM (Heinze & Purisch, 2001; Weinborn et al., 2003). Using the cutoffs described in the test manual, specificity tends to be high (90% or higher), although sensitivity is lower (about 60% to 67%) in these settings.

Tombaugh (1996, 2002) cautioned that interpretation of the TOMM involves many factors and that patients may fail one type of symptom validity test more than another because of the relevance of the test material to their presenting complaints. For example, Moore and Donders (2004) examined TBI referrals to a rehabilitation facility and found that the TOMM and the Forced Choice trial of the CVLT-II were equally sensitive to invalid test performance. There was strong but not perfect agreement between the two instruments, suggesting that clinicians should not rely solely on the results of a single measure. McCaffrey et al (2003) noted that, although scores on the TOMM and on the Rey 15-Item test were moderately correlated with one another (.89 to .78), the TOMM identified more than twice as many litigants (27%) as possible malingerers than the Rey 15-Item Test did (11%).

Although the TOMM appears to be more efficient than the Rey at detecting suboptimal effort, other tests appear to be more powerful indicators. Tan et al (2002) used a simulation paradigm to compare the efficacy of the TOMM; the Word Memory Test (WMT), a word-recognition task; and the Victoria Symptom Validity Test (VSVT), a digit recognition task. Although all tasks differentiated groups, the TOMM proved least effective. Using suggested cutoffs from the test manuals, the TOMM misclassified 4% of the controls as suspect, whereas both the VSVT and the WMT correctly classified all controls into their group. All simulators were accurately identified by the WMT; 12% were not identified by the VSVT, and 20% were not identified by the TOMM.

Similar findings were recently reported by Gervais et al. (2004). They gave 519 disability claimants the TOMM and two other SVTs, one based on digit recognition (Computerized Assessment of Response Bias, CARB) and one employing verbal recognition memory (WMT). Of the total sample, 35% failed one or more of the SVTs. More importantly, the rates of failure varied widely from one SVT to another. More than twice as many people failed the WMT than the TOMM. CARB failure rates were intermediate between those of the other two tests but closer to the TOMM. Notably, only one individual failed the TOMM but passed the WMT. Therefore, tests of recognition memory using pictorial stimuli, digits, or verbal stimuli resulted in highly different failure rates. The lower failure rate on the TOMM may suggest a general disinclination to feign nonverbal memory impairments in favor of verbal memory deficits. However, scores lower than 45 on the TOMM were highly specific, correctly identifying suboptimal effort in almost 100% of the cases in which failure on the WMT and/or CARB was used as the external criterion.

Financial compensation-seeking and a prior psychiatric history increase the risk of invalid test performance on the TOMM (Moore & Donders, 2004). Individuals with long-standing emotional difficulties may be more likely to make misattribution errors, associated with underestimation of their premorbid problems and selective augmentation of cognitive and somatic symptoms due to the perception that dysfunction as the result of physical trauma is more socially acceptable (Moore & Donders, 2004).

Of note, depression (even of a severe form; Ashendorff et al., 2004; Rees et al., 2001) and anxiety (Ashendorff et al., 2004) do not adversely affect performance on the TOMM. Even cognitive impairment associated with psychosis generally does not impair TOMM performance to a level that would produce a false-positive finding (Duncan, 2005). Colby's (2001) cutoffs may help to reduce the risk of false-positive assessments further in cases of severe psychotic mental illness (Weinborn et al., 2003). The experience of pain (e.g., low, high) within the assessment also appears to be unrelated to test scores (Etherton et al., 2005; Gervais et al., 2004).

Much of the literature on suboptimal effort has focused on adults. There is evidence that the TOMM also has potential for identifying children who do not put forth maximal effort. Constantinou and McCaffrey (2003) found that the performance of children in both the United States and Cyprus was comparable to that of adults (with scores > 45 on Trial 2). Similarly, Donders (2005) reported that 97% of a pediatric sample (more than half of whom had sustained a TBI) exceeded the adult cutoff for sufficient effort on the second trial. Therefore, unusual findings may not be attributed to factors such as age or cultural background.

COMMENT

The TOMM appears to be more useful than the Rey 15-Item Test to detect exaggeration of cognitive difficulties. It has also been suggested that the TOMM possesses sufficient validity to meet the Daubert criteria for admissibility of scientific evidence in the courtroom (Vallabhajosula & van Gorp, 2001; Tombaugh, 2002). Specificity is high, resulting in few false positives when dementia or mental retardation can be ruled out. In the context of mild dementia, residual psychosis, or mild mental retardation, the use of Colby's (2001) cutoffs is recommended. The test is not recommended for use if moderate mental retardation or moderate/severe forms of dementia cannot be ruled out.

Financial incentives and premorbid psychiatric maladjustment are important risk factors with regard to invalid performance. Users should note that a variety of factors such as age, low education, depression, anxiety, and pain do not

negatively affect TOMM performance. Therefore, low scores should not be attributed to these conditions. However, sensitivity is lower than that of other tests such as the VSVT, the WMT, and the CARB, resulting in a high rate of false-negative classifications.

There is some evidence that the TOMM is redundant when used with other SVTs (e.g., WMT, VSVT) to detect response bias (Gervais et al., 2004; Tan et al., 2002). Further, it is more often perceived as a measure of malingering than other tests (WMT, VSVT), at least when administered face-to-face by an examiner (Tan et al., 2002; but see Tombaugh, 1997). It is possible that computerized administration increases the sensitivity of the task. Bolan et al. (2002) proposed that it may be less threatening to give wrong responses when tested by a computer (e.g., as is typically done for the WMT and VSVT) than when tested by an experimenter (as is commonly done for the TOMM). Alternatively, people may be disinclined to feign nonverbal (picture recognition) as opposed to verbal (word recognition) memory deficits.

Nonetheless, the TOMM may be a useful measure of the extent of the motivational defect, with task failure associated with more blatant forms of exaggeration (Gervais et al., 2004). It may also be of value when assessing clients from other cultures (Tombaugh, 2002) and therefore has a broader range of application than other tasks such as the Rey 15-Item, VSVT, and WMT. Recall that Tombaugh (1996) found that even patients with aphasic disturbances achieve high scores on the TOMM. In addition, Constantinou and McCaffrey (2003) examined children in Cyprus and the United States and found that TOMM performance was unaffected by differences in cultural background.

A recent simulation study suggested that the test is relatively insensitive to different coaching paradigms (symptom-coached, test-coached; Powell et al., 2004). However, the test publisher has noted instances of individuals searching the Internet for information about malingering and how to respond to specific commonly used tests such as the TOMM in order to evade detection. Accordingly, as a precaution, the publisher recommends that the respondent not see the name of the test at any time during the administration, thereby reducing the opportunity to use any previously learned information.

REFERENCES

Ashendorf, L., Constantinou, M., & McCaffrey, R. J. (2004). The effect of depression and anxiety on the TOMM in community-dwelling older adults. *Archives of Clinical Neuropsychology, 19*, 125–130.

Bolan, B., Foster, J. K., Schmand, B., & Bolan, S. (2002). A comparison of three tests to detect feigned amnesia: The effects of feedback and the measurement of response latency. *Journal of Clinical and Experimental Neuropsychology, 24*, 154–167.

Colby, F. (2001). Using the binomial distribution to assess effort: Forced-choice testing in neuropsychological settings. *Neurorehabilitation, 16*, 253–265.

Constantinou, M., & McCaffrey, R. J. (2003). Using the TOMM for evaluating children's effort to perform optimally on neuropsychological measures. *Child Neuropsychology, 9*, 81–90.

Donders, J. (2005). Performance on the Test of Memory Malingering in a mixed pediatric sample. *Child Neuropsychology, 11*, 221–227.

Duncan, A. (2005). The impact of cognitive and psychiatric impairment or psychotic disorders on the Test of Memory Malingering (TOMM). *Assessment, 12*, 123–129.

Etherton, J. L., Bianchini, K. J., Greve, K. W., & Ciota, M. A. (2005). Test of Memory Malingering performance is unaffected by laboratory-induced pain: Implications for clinical cue. *Archives of Clinical Neuropsychology, 20*, 375–384.

Gervais, R. O., Rohling, M. L., Green, P., & Ford, W. (2004). A comparison of WMT, CARB, and TOMM failure rates in non-head injury disability claimants. *Archives of Clinical Neuropsychology, 19*, 475–487.

Heinze, M., & Purisch, A. D. (2001). Beneath the mask: Use of psychological tests to detect and subtype malingering in criminal defendants. *Journal of Forensic Psychology Practice, 1*, 23–52.

Hill, S. K., Ryan, L. M., Kennedy, C. H., & Malamut, B. L. (2003). The relationship between measures of declarative memory and the Test of Memory Malingering in patients with and without temporal lobe dysfunction. *Journal of Forensic Neuropsychology, 3*, 1–18.

McCaffrey, R. J., O'Bryant, S. E., Ashendorf, L., & Fisher, J. M. (2003). Correlations among the TOMM, Rey-15, and MMPI-2 validity scales in a sample of TBI litigants. *Journal of Forensic Neuropsychology, 3*, 45–53.

Moore, B. A., & Donders, J. (2004). Predictors of invalid neuropsychological test performance after traumatic brain injury. *Brain Injury, 18*, 975–984.

Powell, M. R., Gfeller, J. D., Hendricks, B. L., & Sharland, M. (2004). Detecting symptom- and test-coached simulators with the Test of Memory Malingering. *Archives of Clinical Neuropsychology, 19*, 693–702.

Rees, L. M., Tombaugh, T. N., & Boulay, L. (2001). Depression and the Test of Memory Malingering. *Archives of Clinical Neuropsychology, 16*, 501–506.

Rees, L. M., Tombaugh, T. N., Gansler, D. A., & Moczynski, N. P. (1998). Five validation experiments of the the Test of Memory Malingering (TOMM). *Psychological Assessment, 10*, 10–20.

Slick, D. J., Tan, J. E., Strauss, E. H., & Hultsch, D. F. (2004). Detecting malingering: A survey of experts' practices. *Archives of Clinical Neuropsychology, 19*, 465–473.

Tan, J. E., Slick, D. J., Strauss, E., & Hultsch, D. F. (2002). How'd they do it? Malingering strategies on symptom validity tests. *The Clinical Neuropsychologist, 16*, 495–505.

Teicher, G., & Wagner, M. T. (2004). The Test of Memory Malingering (TOMM): Normative data from cognitively intact, cognitively impaired, and elderly patients with dementia. *Archives of Clinical Neuropsychology, 19*, 455–464.

Tombaugh, T. N. (1996). *Test of Memory Malingering (TOMM)*. North Tonawanda, NY: Multi Health Systems.

Tombaugh, T. (1997). The Test of Memory Malingering (TOMM): Normative data from cognitively intact and cognitively impaired individuals. *Psychological Assessment, 9*, 260–268.

Tombaugh, T. (2002). The Test of Memory Malingering (TOMM) in forensic neuropsychology. *Journal of Forensic Neuropsychology, 2*, 69–96.

Vallabhajosula, B., & van Gorp, W. G. (2001). Post-Daubert admissibility of scientific evidence on malingering of cognitive deficits. *Journal of the American Academy of Psychiatry and the Law, 29*, 207–215.

Warrington, E. (1984). *Recognition Memory Test*. Windsor, England: NFER-Nelson.

Weinborn, M., Orr, T., Woods, S. P., Canover, E., & Feix, J. (2003). A validation of the Test of Memory Malingering in a forensic psychiatric setting. *Journal of Clinical and Experimental Neuropsychology, 25*, 979–990.

21-Item Test

PURPOSE

The 21-Item Test is designed to identify exaggeration or feigning of memory impairment.

SOURCE

The manual and test protocols can be ordered from Grant Iverson, Ph.D., Department of Psychiatry, 2255 Wesbrook Mall, University of British Columbia, Vancouver, B.C., Canada V6T 2A1, at a cost of $23 US or $28 Cdn.

AGE RANGE

The test is used with adults.

DESCRIPTION

The 21-Item Test was designed as a rapid screen for nonoptimal effort (Iverson et al., 1991). The test is a refinement of the symptom validity paradigm that was popularized by Pankratz (1983; Pankratz et al., 1975). It is composed of a target list of 21 nouns that are read to the client (see Figure 16–5). The word lists contain 7 rhyming word pairs, 7 semantically similar word pairs, and 7 semantically unrelated word pairs. After presentation of the list, the client is instructed to freely recall

Figure 16–5 Target words on the 21-Item Test. *Source:* Copyright Grant Iverson & Michael Franzen. Reproduced with permission of the authors.

1. Hat	8. Snow	15. Wood
2. House	9. Road	16. Chart
3. Table	10. Plane	17. Stone
4. Door	11. Boys	18. Hand
5. Dish	12. Ball	19. Nose
6. Clock	13. Station	20. City
7. Oil	14. Arms	21. Sugar

as many words as possible. A second list of 21 nouns is used as foils in a recognition task. Immediately after the free-recall trial, the client is given the two-alternative forced-choice recognition task and is instructed to select the word that was previously presented from the target list.

ADMINISTRATION

The client is told that the examiner will present a list of words and that the client is to remember as many as possible. The examiner then reads the list of words at a rate of one word per 1.5 s (taking about 30 to 33 s to read the entire list). Immediately after the last word is read, the client is asked to recall all the words heard. After the client has recalled the last word, the examiner reads a list of word pairs, and the client is asked to choose the word that was on the original list. On both the free-recall and forced-choice trials, the examiner records the client's responses on the answer form.

ADMINISTRATION TIME

The entire test takes about 5 min to administer and score.

SCORING

The primary score derived from the test is the total number of correct responses on the forced-choice task. Additional scores include the total number of correct responses on free recall that are subsequently missed on forced choice (inconsistency score), and the greatest number of consecutive misses on the forced-choice task.

DEMOGRAPHIC EFFECTS

Age

Iverson et al. (1994) found a moderate negative relationship between free-recall scores and age ($r = -.38$) among nonmalingering individuals. Similar findings were also reported by Arnett and Franzen (1997). Age showed no relation with forced-choice performance in nonmalingering subjects (Iverson et al., 1994).

Education

Iverson et al. (1994) reported that education was not related to free-recall performance. By contrast, Arnett and Franzen (1997) noted that, in a substance abusing population, education was correlated significantly (value not reported) with the number correct on the free-recall score. Education was not correlated with forced-choice performance in nonmalingering subjects (Iverson et al., 1994).

Gender

Gender effects are not reported.

Ethnicity

Effects of ethnicity are not reported.

NORMATIVE DATA

A cutoff score of 9 on the forced-choice component is recommended, because it appears to approximate a lower limit of performance for actual memory-impaired individuals (Iverson & Franzen, 1996; see also Gontkovsky & Souheaver, 2000). Random responding on the forced-choice component of the test results in a score between 7 and 14. Therefore, if a person obtains a score of 6 or less, it can be presumed that he or she was deliberately choosing incorrect answers.

Two additional scores on the 21-Item Test have shown promise as indicators of biased responding. The inconsistency score represents the number of words recalled on free recall that are subsequently missed on forced-choice recognition. This finding is rare in control samples and in patients giving full effort. Iverson (1998) recommended an inconsistency cutoff score of 3 as an indicator of response bias. The second significant score is the greatest number of consecutive misses. A large number of consecutive misses on the forced-choice task is both clinically unlikely and statistically improbable. Five consecutive misses on the forced-choice component rarely occurs among individuals who are trying their best. The probability of missing 5 consecutive responses, assuming a random response strategy, is .03.

Iverson (1998) provided an interpretation scheme to be used with patients who have mild head injuries or other forms of mild brain impairment. The scheme is provided in Table 16–11 and is reported to be based on samples of patients seen for neuropsychological evaluation of significant neurological or psychiatric disturbance.

RELIABILITY

Internal Consistency

Coefficient alpha in simulators feigning head injury is marginal to good (.65 to .81; Inman et al., 1998).

Test-Retest Reliability

No information is available.

Table 16–11 Interpretation of 21 Item Test performance

Score	Suspicious	Highly Suspicious	Biased
Forced Choice	12	9–11	8 or less
Inconsistency		3–4	5 or more
Greatest Consecutive Misses		5–6	7 or more

Source: Adapted from Iverson, 1998.

VALIDITY

Clinical Findings

Iverson and his colleagues (Iverson & Franzen, 1996; Iverson et al., 1991, 1994) showed that controls perform better than simulators on the task. For example, Iverson & Franzen (1996) gave the 21-Item Test along with several measures (Personal History/Orientation Questionnaire, Modification of Rey's 15-Item Test, Digit Span, WMS-R Logical Memory with Forced-Choice Supplement) to 20 undergraduates and 20 psychiatric inpatients. The tests were given twice in a repeated-measures, counterbalanced design. In one condition subjects were instructed to try their best, and in the other condition they were instructed to malinger memory impairment. Malingering subjects performed worse on both free-recall and forced-choice recognition than controls or memory-impaired participants. The forced-choice procedure was, however, more sensitive to the effects of dissimulation. Applying a cut-score of 9, which eliminated false positives on the forced-choice component, resulted in a correct classification rate of 100% for normal control and memory-impaired subjects, 22.5% for experimental malingerers, and 69% overall. A cutoff score of 13 resulted in a much higher classification rate but also some false-positive classifications. Subjects' performances were also compared with chance. On the forced-choice component, individuals employing a random response strategy would score between 7 and 15 correct 95% of the time. Subjects scoring 6 or less are performing below chance, clearly indicating that they are providing nonoptimal effort. No control or memory-impaired subjects in these three studies performed below chance, whereas 10% to 60% of the experimental malingerers scored in this range (Iverson & Franzen, 1993).

It is worth noting that sophisticated individuals (e.g., individuals with training in psychology) may easily avoid detection on this task and perform above the recommended cutoff (Franzen & Martin, 1996). However, these same individuals are easily detected by other techniques (e.g., evaluation of Digit Span, Logical Memory recognition scores).

A recent meta-analytic review (Vickery et al., 2001) of a variety of procedures to detect feigning/exaggeration suggested that the 21-Item Test shows high specificity (100%) but poor sensitivity (22%). Other tests (e.g., Hiscock & Hiscock digit recognition procedure, Portland Digit Recognition Test, forced-choice test of nonverbal ability, Letter Memory Test) are more effective in distinguishing honest and dissimulating responders (Frederick et al., 1994; Inman et al., 1998; Rose et al., 1998; see Vickery et al., 2001 for review). The low sensitivity of the 21-Item Test suggests that some modification of the cut-score may need to be considered (Vickery et al., 2001).

Arnett and Franzen (1997) found the free-recall measure to be sensitive to actual memory impairment in a substance-abusing group. They noted a correlation of .52 between the WMS-R Delayed Memory Index and the free-recall index of the 21-Item test.

COMMENT

The 21-Item Test recognition scores shows high specificity but low sensitivity, suggesting that use of this measure as a single screen would result in an unacceptable number of false-negative decisions (Vickery et al., 2001). Therefore, the clinician should use more than this one procedure. Given its brevity and high specificity, the 21-Item Test may be best used at the very beginning of a neuropsychological examination, as a rapid screen as part of a battery of tasks for less than optimal effort. The test likely will prove less sensitive to exaggeration if it is used reactively; that is, if it is used midway through the evaluation, after suspicions of biased effort have been raised. The client will have been exposed to a variety of difficult neuropsychological measures, so that the 21-Item Test will appear relatively simple and straightforward. Users should bear in mind that individuals who have some working knowledge of normal memory can easily avoid detection on this task. The free-recall score appears to be sensitive to true memory impairment and therefore should not be used to infer malingering.

The word lists contain rhyming word pairs, semantically similar word pairs, and semantically unrelated word pairs. The pairing was done to determine whether any of these variables would have discriminating value (Iverson, 1998). To date, there has been no research to support the discriminating value of these variables.

REFERENCES

Arnett, P. A., & Franzen, M. D. (1997). Performance of substance abusers with memory deficits on measures of malingering. *Archives of Clinical Neurospychology, 12,* 513–518.

Franzen, M. D., & Martin, N. (1996). Do people with knowledge fake better? *Applied Neuropsychology, 3,* 82–85.

Frederick, R. I., Sarfaty, S. D., Johnston, J. D., & Powel, J. (1994). Validation of a detector of response bias on a forced-choice test of nonverbal ability. *Neuropsychology, 8,* 118–125.

Gontkovsky, S. T., & Souheaver, G. T. (2000). Are brain-damaged patients inappropriately labelled as malingering using the 21-Item Test and the WMS-R Logical Memory Forced Choice Recognition Test? *Psychological Reports, 87,* 512–514.

Inman, T. H., Vickery, C. D., Lamb, D. G., Edwards, C. L., & Smith, G. T. (1998). Development and initial validation of a new procedure for evaluating adequacy of effort given during neuropsychological testing: The Letter Memory Test. *Psychological Assessment, 10,* 128–139.

Iverson, G. L. (1998). *21-Item Test research manual.* Vancouver, B.C.: Author.

Iverson, G. L., & Franzen, M. D. (1993). A brief assessment instrument designed to detect malingered memory deficits. *The Behavior Therapist,* May, 134–135.

Iverson, G. L., & Franzen, M. D. (1994). The Recognition Memory Test, Digit Span, and Knox Cube Test as markers of malingered memory impairment. *Assessment, 1,* 323–334.

Iverson, G. L., & Franzen, M. D. (1996). Using multiple objective memory procedures to detect simulated malingering. *Journal of Clinical and Experimental Neuropsychology, 18,* 38–51.

Iverson, G. L., Franzen, M. D., & McCracken, L. M. (1991). Evaluation of an objective assessment technique for the detection of malingered memory deficits. *Law and Human Behavior, 15,* 667–676.

Iverson, G. L., Wilhelm, K., & Franzen, M. D. (1992). *Objective assessment of simulated memory deficits: Additional scoring criteria for the 21 Item Test.* Paper presented to the National Academy of Neuropsychology, Pittsburgh, Penn.

Iverson, G. L., Franzen, M. D., & McCracken, L. M. (1994). Application of a forced-choice memory procedure designed to detect experimental malingering. *Archives of Clinical Neuropsychology, 9,* 437–450.

Pankratz, L. (1983). A new technique for the assessment and modification of feigned memory deficit. *Perceptual and Motor Skills, 57,* 367–372.

Pankratz, L., Fausti, S. A., & Peed, S. (1975). A forced-choice technique to evaluate deafness in the hysterical or malingering patient. *Journal of Consulting and Clinical Psychology, 433,* 421–422.

Rose, F. E., Hall, S., Szalda-Petree, A. D., & Bach, P. J. (1998). A comparison of four tests of malingering and the effects of coaching. *Archives of Clinical Neuropsychology, 13,* 349–363.

Vickery, C. D., Berry, D. T. R., Inman, T. H., Harris, M. J., & Orey, S. A. (2001). Detection of inadequate effort on neuropsychological testing: A meta-analytic review of selected procedures. *Archives of Clinical Neuropsychology, 16,* 45–73.

Victoria Symptom Validity Test (VSVT)

PURPOSE

The Victoria Symptom Validity Test (VSVT) is used to assess exaggeration or feigning of memory complaints.

SOURCE

The computerized version of this test (including disk for unlimited use and manual) can be ordered from Psychological Assessment Resources, Inc., P.O. Box 998, Odessa, FL 33556 (http://www.parinc.com). The cost is $499 US. A flip-card version can be made, using the description provided here, if a computer is not available.

AGE RANGE

The test has been used with individuals aged 18 years and older.

DESCRIPTION

Hiscock and Hiscock (1989) developed a two-alternative forced-choice recognition task in order to assess memory complaints. In their task, a five-digit number is presented on a card for a 5-s study period, followed after a brief delay by another card containing the correct choice and a foil. The correct answers can always be distinguished from foils by recognizing the first or last digit. In order to increase the face validity of the task, the period between study and recognition is overtly increased to 10 and then 15 s. Malingering subjects are cued to perform poorly by being told that the test is difficult for those with memory problems and that the level of difficulty increases with retention interval. Because all items have two response possibilities, overall error rates should be approximately 50% under conditions of random responding. That is, scores in this range would result from either (a) severe disturbances in attention and/or memory or (2) symptom exaggeration. Error rates that depart from 50% are less likely to have occurred by chance alone, with an associated probability that is easily calculated. Performance below chance at a low probability (e.g., $p < .05$) is indicative of deliberate choice of incorrect answers (i.e., malingering).

Protocols in which the number of correct items is above chance are considered valid.

Slick et al. (1994, 1996, 1997) modified the task in a number of ways. First, the administration time of the original task was quite lengthy, about 30 to 40 min. The number of items was therefore reduced from 72 to 48, halving the administration time. Second, item difficulty was manipulated, making items appear more difficult than in fact they are. *Easy* items are those in which the foil and the study number share no common digits (e.g., 34092 and 56187), so that recognition of the first, last, or any other digit or pattern of digits from the study number will facilitate a correct choice. *Hard* items are those in which the foil is identical to the study number with the exception of a transposition of the second and third or third and fourth digits (e.g., 46923 and 46293). To choose correctly on hard items, the order of the middle digits must be remembered; recognition of the first or last digit of the study number will not aid in making a correct choice. Like the increase in retention intervals, the difference in actual difficulty between easy and hard items is assumed to be small. Third, response time is also recorded. Below-chance performance at $p < .05$ is labeled as unequivocally invalid/malingered, and performance significantly above chance at $p < .05$ is labeled as unequivocally valid. A third category, labeled "questionable," consists of scores that fall within the remaining 90% confidence interval of chance performance. More recent data based on patients with bona fide severe memory disorders has resulted in additional guidelines (see *Normative Data*).

The VSVT includes a total of 48 items, presented in three blocks of 16 items each. In each block, a five-digit number is presented at the center of a computer monitor, followed by a blank screen retention interval, after which the previously shown study number and a five-digit foil are displayed, one to each side of center screen. Subjects respond by striking one of two keys (left or right shift) on the keyboard. Side of correct choices and foils are counterbalanced and pseudorandomized. The retention interval is 5 s in the first block and increases to 10 and then 15 s in the second and third blocks, respectively. All three sections contain an equal number (eight each) of easy and difficult items. Within sections, the order of easy and difficult items and the screen location (left or right) of foils is pseudorandomized.

ADMINISTRATION

Test presentation is controlled by the computer program. The examiner should ensure that the patient is properly oriented to the monitor and keyboard. The examiner may input responses for clients who are unable to use both hands for the keyboard. Clients should be familiar with reading Arabic numerals.

ADMINISTRATION TIME

About 15 to 20 min is required for the test.

SCORING

Test scoring is provided by the computer program. Results are printed for the test as a whole (i.e., out of 48), as well as for each section. The following summary information is provided.

1. The number of correct trials for each block and item difficulty level, along with the maximum number of correct items (e.g., 6/8).
2. Z scores derived from a binomial probability curve centered at chance-level performance (50% correct). A z score of 0 indicates exact chance-level performance, with half of the items passed. Z scores are translated directly to p values, indicating the likelihood of a patient's obtaining a particular score by chance alone (i.e., responding randomly). High positive scores ($z > 1.65$) indicate better than chance performance, and low negative scores ($z < -1.65$) represent worse than chance performance.
3. Bias is a measure of the tendency to use one hand more than the other. Scores can range from −1 (using only the left hand) to +1 (using only the right hand). High scores (<.6) raise the question of a perceptual (e.g., visual field defect), motoric defect, or some other unusual response set.
4. Mean response latency (and standard deviation) to easy and hard items in milliseconds.

DEMOGRAPHIC EFFECTS

Age

In adults (ages 18 years and older), age has no (Grote et al., 2000; Slick et al., 1997; Strauss et al., 2002) or little (Loring et al., 2005) impact on accuracy.

Education

Years of education do not influence accuracy scores on the VSVT (Slick et al., 1997; Strauss et al., 2002).

Gender

Similarly, gender has no impact on test scores (Slick et al., 1997; Strauss et al., 2002).

Ethnicity

Effects of ethnicity are not reported.

NORMATIVE DATA

Interpretation of the computer-generated VSVT scores has been based largely on binomial probability theory (Slick et al., 1996, 1997). This approach provides an indicator of the validity of the respondent's performance relative to what would be predicted on the basis of chance alone (i.e., if a respondent had endorsed items in a completely random manner). Scores for the total, easy, and hard items can be evaluated with reference to Table 16–12. These are the guidelines used in the computer-generated report. It is important to note that cutoff scores do not make allowances for differing base-rate conditions. Accordingly, a classification confidence matrix is available in the test manual so that scores on hard items can be evaluated with respect to various base-rate conditions.

The binomial probability scores answer the question: how likely is this score to occur by chance alone? An alternative method of determining the likelihood of malingering is to evaluate normative data obtained from healthy individuals and from persons with genuine cognitive impairment. In this way, the clinical rarity of a (litigating) client's scores can be evaluated. If the individual performed more poorly than the majority of nonlitigants with injuries or conditions of similar

Table 16–12 Classification of Client Performance by Scores on the VSVT Derived From Probabilistic Analysis

	Valid (Above Chance)	Questionable (At Chance)	Invalid/Malingering (Below Chance)
Total correct	≥30	18–29	≤17
Easy	≥16	8–15	≤7
Hard	≥16	8–15	≤7

Table 16–13 Classification of Client Performance by Scores on the VSVT Derived from Nonlitigating Patients With Memory Impairment

	Compliant	Questionably Compliant	Probably Noncompliant	Noncompliant
Easy	21–24	16–20	8–15	0–7
Hard	21–24	16–20	8–15	0–7

or greater severity than those of the client, malingering must be considered.

Slick et al. (1996) found that no healthy individual or non-compensation-seeking patient obtained a score of 15 or less on the hard items. Subsequent studies (Doss et al., 1999; Grote et al., 2000; Slick et al., 2003) have cross-validated and extended the initial findings of Slick and his colleagues. By evaluating nonlitigants with significant cognitive deficits (including profound memory impairment), they have provided empirically based cutoff scores to improve the sensitivity of the measure. For example, Slick et al. (2003) tested six nonlitigating patients with significant memory impairment (e.g., due to aneurysm of the ACA, Korsakoff's disease). All obtained perfect scores on the easy items and near-perfect scores (≥22) on the hard items. Doss et al. (1999) noted that one of their patients with a diagnosis of probable dementia was able to obtain scores well above chance on the VSVT (easy items, 23/24; hard items, 20/24) despite extremely low scores on traditional memory tasks. Grote et al. (2000) found that 28 (93%) of 30 non-compensation-seeking patients with intractable epilepsy had VSVT hard scores of 21 or greater, compared with only 19 (36%) of 53 compensation-seeking patients. Recently, Loring et al. (2005) reported that 86 of 97 (89%) non-litigating patients with intractable epilepsy obtained scores of at least 21/24 on the hard VSVT items. Based on these clinical data, we agree with Grote et al. (2000) that scores between 16 and 20 correct on the easy or hard items should not be thought of as "valid" but instead as a level of performance that is rarely seen among non-compensation-seeking patients with documented brain damage. Based on review of the published research, Table 16–13 provides some "qualitative" labels for various VSVT score ranges, with the caveat that users must consider them as hypotheses to be confirmed or disconfirmed when integrated with other data.

There are a number of other measures from the VSVT that may prove useful. Slick et al. (1996) noted that steep drops in scores across retention intervals were unusual in bona fide brain-damaged individuals. Further, it is rare for any non-compensation-seeking patient to obtain scores of 0 to 5 (where 8 is the highest possible score) on any of the six blocks of scores referred to in the VSVT printout (Grote et al., 2000).

Slick et al. (1996) suggested that average response times in excess of 4 s in patients who do not appear to be confused or disoriented may be indicative of motivational problems. Based on an examination of non-compensation-seeking and compensation-seeking patients, Grote et al. (2000) suggested

alternative criteria: 3 s for the easy items and 4 s for hard items.

Standard deviation scores for response latencies are provided on the computer printout. Compensation-seeking patients tend to be more variable in their response latencies than non-compensation-seeking clients. Grote et al. (2000) recommended a cutoff for the standard deviation score of 1.9 s or less.

RELIABILITY

Internal Consistency

Slick (1996) reported that alphas for the 24 easy items, the 24 hard items, and the entire set of 48 items were .82, .87, and .89, respectively.

Test-Retest Reliability

The VSVT was administered twice to 31 healthy participants and 27 compensation-seeking patients (Slick et al., 1997). The median retest interval was 14 days for controls and 31 days for compensation-seeking patients (range = 1–550 days). Test-retest correlations for selected measures from the VSVT were low (.53 to .54 for latency measures) among the control sample, most likely a reflection of restriction of range. Among the compensation-seeking group, correlations were higher (.56 easy RT to .84 total items correct). All of the control participants obtained the same classification at retest (valid) as they did at first testing. Among the compensation-seeking patients, 86% obtained the same classification at retest. Overall, these findings suggest that the VSVT exhibits adequate reliability and suggests that changes in classification across test-retest intervals most likely reflect the VSVT's sensitivity to changes in effort or performance exhibited by patients and not error variance (Thompson, 2002).

VALIDITY

Clinical Findings

The VSVT appears to be sensitive to motivational defects (for a discussion of the original Hiscock and Hiscock procedure [1989], see Binder, 1990; Guilmette et al., 1993, 1994). Analog malingerers and compensation-seeking individuals obtain lower scores on this task (especially on the hard items) than do honest respondents and non-compensation-seeking people (Doss et al., 1999; Grote et al., 2000; Slick et al., 1994, 1996; Strauss et al., 1999, 2002; Tan et al., 2002). For example, Slick et al. (1994, 1996) gave the task to healthy adults ($n = 43$), normal individuals instructed to simulate postconcussion symptoms ($n = 42$), compensation-seeking patients ($n = 121$), and patients not seeking compensation ($n = 26$). They found that simulating participants demonstrated lower scores on hard items. Adoption of the three-category classification system (below chance, above chance, and questionable) showed excellent specificity, producing zero false-positive classifications, and reasonable sensitivity. All control and non-compensation-seeking participants performed above chance. About 83% of individuals simulating impairment fell within the questionable or invalid range. Approximately 83% of the compensation-seeking patients achieved above-chance scores. Further, individuals who produced invalid protocols took about twice as long to respond as those who produced valid protocols, suggesting that response time may be a useful adjunct to measures of symptom validity. Although slowing of response (and inconsistency of response) tends to occur more commonly among those with suspect performance, the diagnostic utility of the accuracy score on the hard items appears to be greater (e.g., Grote et al., 2000; Strauss et al., 1999, 2002).

There is evidence that malingerers (even those with considerable experience with regard to head injury) tend to be more inconsistent across serial testings. Using an analog design, Strauss et al. (1999, 2002) found that simulators fluctuated more than controls in terms of their accuracy (on hard items) and response latency. Successful feigning of the same level of performance across different test sessions appears to require higher levels of self-monitoring or more sophisticated knowledge of human behavior than most malingerers possess. Therefore, evaluation of response consistency across test occasions may increase the accuracy of detection. Clinicians should consider changes of three or more points up or down on the easy items as increasing the index of suspicion.

In addition, the available data indicate that severe cognitive impairment has minimal impact on the VSVT (Berry, personal communication, July 1995; Doss et al., 1999; Grote et al., 2000; Slick et al., 2003). For example, Berry et al. (personal communication, July 1995) found a low false-positive rate when the VSVT was given to a group of 30 moderately to severely head-injured adults (mean number of days of unconsciousness = 21, $SD = 29$) who were not seeking compensation at the time of assessment. Twenty-nine (97%) of the patients obtained scores in the valid range, and only one patient (3%) obtained a score in the questionable range. These data demonstrate that scores in the questionable range are unlikely in patients who do not have obvious, grossly impaired function (e.g., severe attentional disturbance or impaired consciousness). Slick et al. (2003) examined six non-litigating patients with severe memory impairment whose scores on conventional memory tasks were generally below the first percentile. Despite their obvious impairment on these tasks, they obtained perfect scores on

the easy items (24/24) and near-perfect scores (≥ 22) on the hard items.

Depression has little impact on VSVT performance (Slick et al., 1996; see also Guilmette et al., 1994, with regard to an abbreviated version of the Hiscock and Hiscock procedure). Similarly, expertise with head injury (e.g., head-injured individuals, professionals working with head-injured individuals) does not affect the test's sensitivity (Strauss et al., 2002).

Divergent validity has also been demonstrated by small correlations between the VSVT and scores on tests designed to measure dissimilar constructs. Slick et al. (1996) reported that no memory test (e.g., RAVLT, Rey Figure) shared more than 5% of its variance with easy- or hard-item scores from the VSVT, indicating that the VSVT is largely unaffected by level of cognitive function. The implication is that low scores probably reflect some degree of exaggeration. Response times to easy and hard items, however, showed considerably less divergent validity, being moderately correlated (.32 to .53) with Digit Span and measures with heavy processing-speed components (e.g., Stroop, Trails), suggesting caution in the interpretation of response times.

The question arises regarding the effectiveness of the VSVT relative to other procedures. Tan et al. (2002) used a simulation paradigm to compare the efficacy of the VSVT, the TOMM, and Word Memory Test (WMT). The VSVT compared favorably with the WMT and was better than the TOMM in detecting feigned impairment associated with head injury. However, use of the TOMM delayed recognition score in combination with the VSVT or WMT significantly improved prediction. There is also evidence that the task shows superior classification accuracy, compared with other procedures such as the Rey 15-Item Test, the 21-Item Test, and the Portland Digit Recognition (PDRT) tests (Vickery et al., 2001). The VSVT (hard items) has also proved to be a better predictor of instructional set (respond honestly, feign head injury) than Dot Counting, Reliable Digit Span, or Vocabulary minus Digit Span measures (Strauss et al., 1999, 2002), consistent with other research showing that forced-choice recognition tasks achieve the best hit rate in the detection of noncompliance (e.g., Greiffenstein et al., 1994; Rose et al., 1998).

In terms of face validity, the WMT fares best, with about one third of the individuals perceiving it to be a legitimate measure of memory, followed by about one quarter who perceived the VSVT in this way (Tan et al., 2002). Fewer than 10% of subjects perceived the TOMM as a legitimate measure of cognitive function as opposed to malingering (Tan et al., 2002).

Correlations between MMPI-2 validity scales and VSVT scores are in the small-to-medium range (Slick et al., 1996). For Easy Items Correct score and the MMPI-2 F scale T score, $r = -.29$, indicating that higher F-scale scores were associated with lower VSVT Easy Correct scores. Of note, easy and difficult item correlations with the Lees-Haley FBS scale were higher (.42 and .43, respectively), consistent with the notion that the FBS scale has greater utility than F-scale scores in the context of exaggerated neurotrauma claims (see *Minnesota Multiphasic Personality Inventory–2*). However, when participant classifications from the two tests are compared, a low rate of agreement is found between the MMPI-2 and the VSVT. This is perhaps not surprising, because the tests differ considerably in task (self-report versus actual performance) and in domain (memory versus personality assessment; see also Greiffenstein et al., 1995, with regard to a number of other malingered amnesia measures and the MMPI-2).

COMMENT

The available data suggest that subnormal VSVT scores obtained by litigants should be considered as an indicator of possible malingering. Age, education, depression, and sophistication regarding the effects of head injury have little impact on test scores. Even the presence of profound cognitive/memory impairment affects VSVT performance minimally. In addition, the VSVT includes a left-right preference score that could alert clinicians to one of the few conditions that might cause spurious false-positive results on the VSVT (e.g., left neglect). The VSVT also demonstrates adequate reliability and appears sensitive to changes in patient effort and performance. The fact that the VSVT is administered by computer probably enhances its reliability by minimizing any error variance that might be associated with minor variations with which different clinicians administer the test. Accordingly, based on its ease of use, short administration time, and other positive characteristics, Thompson (2002) concluded that the VSVT most likely meets Daubert standards for the admissibility of scientific evidence presented in the courtroom. In their initial studies, the test authors relied on binomial probability theory for guidelines for VSVT interpretation. This resulted in quite conservative cutoff values for suspect performance. More recent studies have suggested some empirically based cutoff scores for the VSVT that may serve to enhance its sensitivity.

We, like others (Doss et al., 1999), view performance on the easy items as a baseline indicator of general effort and attention to the task. That is, if a patient obtains an almost perfect score on the easy items, there seems to be less likelihood that a low score on the hard items can be attributed to poor effort or an attention deficit.

Although the VSVT procedure is useful, several issues should be noted. First, the placement of the VSVT in the test battery could influence performance. The work of Guilmette et al. (1996) suggests that more failures occur when it is placed at the beginning of the test battery, before clients have had experience with more demanding memory measures. Second, the task is commonly used with adults. Although the basic Hiscock and Hiscock procedure was initially validated on a young child, research is needed to develop norms for children. Third, although the VSVT is easy to administer, it has generated relatively little research (Hartman, 2002)—and much that exists is from the test authors. Fourth, perfect

performance does not definitively rule out fabrication or exaggeration of symptomatology (Guilmette et al., 1993, 1994). Further, Slick et al. (1996) cautioned that symptom validity tests such as the VSVT are at best capable only of indicating that factors other than, or perhaps in addition to, certain forms of cognitive impairment may be influencing client performance (see also Palmer et al., 1995). Even in cases where financial or other incentives exist and the patient's performance is suspect, the patient may be legitimately impaired and/or acting without conscious intent (see Slick et al., 1999). For example, patients with impaired judgment (perhaps reflecting executive dysfunction) may exhibit chance-level performance. If suspect performance is detected, the use of multiple measures is recommended to clarify whether poor performance is intentional and to evaluate alternative explanations for suspect scores.

REFERENCES

Binder, L. M. (1990). Malingering following minor head trauma. *The Clinical Neuropsychologist, 4*, 25–36.

Doss, R. C., Chelune, G. J., & Naugle, R. I. (1999). Victoria Symptom Validity Test: Compensation-seeking vs. non-compensation-seeking patients in a general clinical setting. *Journal of Forensic Neuropsychology, 14*, 5–20.

Greiffenstein, M. F., Baker, W. J., & Gola, T. (1994). Validation of malingered amnesia measures with a large clinical sample. *Psychological Assessment, 6*, 218–224.

Greiffenstein, M. F., Gola, T., & Baker, W. J. (1995). MMPI-2 validity scales versus domain specific measures in detection of factitious traumatic brain injury. *The Clinical Neuropsychologist, 9*, 230–240.

Grote, C. L., Kooker, E. K., Garron, D. C., Nyenhuis, D. L., Smith, C. A., & Mattingly, M. L. (2000). Performance of compensation seeking and non-compensation seeking samples on the Victoria Symptom Validity Test: Cross validation and extension of a standardization study. *Journal of Clinical and Experimental Neuropsychology, 22*, 709–719.

Guilmette, T. J., Hart, K. J., & Giuliano, A. J. (1993). Malingering detection: The use of a forced-choice method in identifying organic versus simulated memory impairment. *The Clinical Neuropsychologist, 7*, 59–69.

Guilmette, T. J., Hart, K. J., Giuliano, A. J., & Leininger, B. E. (1994). Detecting simulated memory impairment: Comparison of the Rey Fifteen-Item Test and the Hiscock Forced-Choice Procedure. *The Clinical Neuropsychologist, 8*, 283–294.

Hartman, D. E. (2002). The unexamined lie is a lie worth fibbing: Neuropsychological malingering and the Word Memory Test. *Archives of Clinical Neuropsychology, 17*, 709–714.

Hiscock, M., & Hiscock, C. K. (1989). Refining the forced choice method for the detection of malingering. *Journal of Clinical and Experimental Neuropsychology, 11*, 967–974.

Loring, D. W., Lee, G. P., & Meador, K. J. (2005). Victoria Symptom Validity Test performance in non-litigating epilepsy surgery candidates. *Journal of Clinical and Experimental Neuropsychology, 27*, 610–617.

Palmer, B. W., Brauer Boone, K., Allman, L., & Castro, D. B. (1995). Co-occurrence of brain lesions and cognitive deficit exaggeration. *The Clinical Neuropsychologist, 9*, 68–73.

Rose, F. E., Hall, S., & Szalda-Petree, A. D. (1998). A comparison of four tests of malingering and the effects of coaching. *Archives of Clinical Neuropsychology, 13,* 349–363.

Slick, D. (1996). *The Victoria Symptom Validity Test: A new clinical measure of response bias.* Ph.D. dissertation, University of Victoria, British Columbia, Canada.

Slick, D., Hopp, G., Strauss, E., Hunter, M., & Pinch, D. (1994). Detecting dissimulation: Profiles of simulated malingerers, traumatic brain-injury patients, and normal controls on a revised version of Hiscock and Hiscock's forced choice memory test. *Journal of Clinical and Experimental Neuropsychology, 16,* 472–481.

Slick, D., Hopp, G., Strauss, E., & Spellacy, F. (1996). Victoria Symptom Validity Test: Efficiency for detecting feigned memory impairment and relationship to neuropsychological tests and MMPI-2 validity scales. *Journal of Clinical and Experimental Neuropsychology, 18,* 911–922.

Slick, D., Hopp, G., Strauss, E., & Thompson, G. B. (1997). *Victoria Symptom Validity Test.* Odessa, Fla.: Psychological Assessment Resources.

Slick, D. J., Sherman, E. M. S., & Iverson, G. L. (1999). Diagnostic criteria for malingered neurocognitive dysfunction: Proposed standard for clinical practice. *The Clinical Neuropsychologist, 13,* 545–561.

Slick, D. J., Tan, J. E., Strauss, E., Mateer, C. A., Harnadek, M., & Sherman, E. M. S. (2003). Victoria Symptom Validity Test scores of patients with profound impairment: Nonlitigant case studies. *The Clinical Neuropsychologist, 17,* 390–394.

Strauss, E., Hultsch, D. F., Hunter, M., Slick, D. J., Patry, B., & Levy-Bencheton, J. (1999). Using intraindividual variability to detect malingering in cognitive performance. *The Clinical Neuropsychologist, 14,* 420–432.

Strauss, E., Slick, D. J., Levy-Bencheton, J., Hunter, M., MacDonald, S. W. S., & Hultsch, D. F. (2002). Intraindividual variability as an indicator of malingering in head injury. *Archives of Clinical Neuropsychology, 17,* 423–444.

Tan, J. E., Slick, D. J., Strauss, E., & Hultsch, D. F. (2002). How'd they do it? Malingering strategies on symptom validity tests. *The Clinical Neuropsychologist, 16,* 495–505.

Thompson, G. B. III. (2002). The Victoria Symptom Validity Test: An enhanced test of symptom validity. *Journal of Forensic Neuropsychology, 2,* 43–67.

Vickery, C. D., Berry, D. T. R., Inman, T. H., Harris, M. J., & Orey, S. A. (2001). Detection of inadequate effort on neuropsychological testing: A meta-analytic review of selected procedures. *Archives of Clinical Neuropsychology, 16,* 45–73.

Word Memory Test (WMT)

PURPOSE

The Word Memory Test (WMT) assesses exaggeration or feigning of memory complaints.

SOURCE

Green's Word Memory Test for Windows (Green, 2003) can be ordered from Paul Green, 1-866-INFO-WMT (1-866-463-6968) or (1-780-484-5550), or from http://www.word memorytest.com. Contact Paul Green (paulgreen@shaw.ca) for pricing information. The license fee includes the compact disc and test manual in any available language (English, Spanish, French, German, Dutch, and Turkish), 1 year unlimited use, free updates, upgrades, membership in the WMT USER Internet group, and support). There is an additional license fee after 1 year. The oral version is not sold separately but comes free with the purchase of the WMT Windows version.

AGE RANGE

The test can be used with individuals aged 7 years and older.

DESCRIPTION

A variety of forced symptom validity formats are used to detect exaggerated cognitive problems, including digit recognition (e.g., CARB, Allen et al., 1997; PDRT, Binder & Willis, 1991; VSVT, Slick et al., 1997), picture recognition (TOMM, Tombaugh, 1996; RMT, Warrington, 1984), and word recognition (WMT, Green et al., 1997). The WMT is a commonly used measure (Slick et al., 2004) that evaluates the immediate and delayed recognition of 20 semantically linked word pairs (e.g., pig—bacon). The list is presented twice (either shown on the computer screen or read aloud by the examiner); this is followed by an immediate recognition (IR) trial in which the client must select each of the original words from 40 new pairs (e.g., "pig" from the pair cow—pig). Feedback regarding correctness is given to assist motivated patients in learning for later subtests. Without advance warning, a second similar recognition subtest is administered after a 30-min delay (DR), and the client is required to select each of the 40 words on the original list from pairs that incorporate new foils (e.g., feed—pig). The IR and DR scores, as well as the consistency of response (Cons) between the two trials, are the primary measures of motivational status. The conventional definition of WMT failure is IR or DR or Cons below the cutoff value.

The effort measures are followed by a series of memory tests of gradually increasing difficulty, intended to be sensitive to verbal memory impairment. After the DR trial, the client is presented with a multiple-choice (MC) task in which he or she is shown the first word from each pair and is asked to select the matching word from a list of eight options. A paired-associate (PA) subtest can also be given. Here, the tester says the first word from each pair and the client must supply the word that was paired with it. This is followed by a delayed free recall subtest (DFR), in which the client is asked to recall all of the words from the list in any order while the tester records responses on the computer or on a sheet of paper. After a further delay of 20 min, free recall of the word list can be tested again (LDFR).

The IR and DR subtests serve a dual function as effort measures and also as additional learning trials, because all of the words from the list are presented and feedback is given on correctness of responses. The MC and PA trials provide further exposure to the 20 first words from the pairs, again serving a dual purpose as tests of memory and as learning trials, before the free recall trials. Therefore, the WMT generates three effort scores (IR, DR, Cons) and four memory scores (MC, PA, DFR, LDFR).

Although the recognition subtests (IR, DR) are very easy, the MC and PA subtests are more difficult, and the DR subtests are even more difficult. Green (2003) proposed that the differing levels of subtest difficulty produce a characteristic gradient of scores in those who are making full effort and that deviations from this pattern increase the index of suspicion. The free-recall scores are interpreted as a measure of memory only when poor or inconsistent effort has been ruled out.

ADMINISTRATION

The WMT can be given orally or partially unattended with the client working on a computer. The WMT requires at least a grade 3 reading level (Green & Faro, 2003). When taking the computerized WMT, people are given assistance with reading and understanding the task instructions if needed. If there is a question about reading problems, the examiner can ask the person to say each word aloud as it appears (Green, 2003). If there is an error, the examiner corrects the word immediately. If the person is expected to have difficulty on the computerized task (e.g., reading difficulty, blindness), the oral version can be given.

APPROXIMATE TIME FOR ADMINISTRATION

About 20 min is required for the test (excluding the delays).

SCORING

Test scoring is provided by the computer program. Multiple measures can be derived from the task, including the following:

1. The number correct on IR and DR trials
2. A measure of response consistency between IR and DR
3. The number correct on the MC, PA and DR trials

The computer printout shows the patient's results graphically (e.g., a graph plots percentage correct for each subtest, a z-score graph plots the person's scores in terms of the number of standard deviations above or below the mean from a reference group) and as a list of raw scores on all measures. Tables are provided so that the person's scores can be compared with the mean scores obtained from each of a number of reference groups, including patients with moderate to severe brain injury, neurological patients, patients with normal verbal memory, patients with impaired verbal memory, and bright normal controls.

DEMOGRAPHIC EFFECTS

Effort Trials

Age.   The scores on the effort tasks (IR, DR) are unrelated to age in adults (Green, 2003; Green et al., 2002). Although Green and Flaro (2003) reported no impact of age in individuals aged 7 to 18 years, Courtney et al. (2003) reported moderately strong relationships (.54 to .58) between age and effort measures.

Education, IQ, and Reading Level.   The scores on the effort tasks (IR, DR) are unrelated to intelligence and education in adults (Green, 2003; Green et al., 2002). They also appear to be unrelated to intellectual level in children (Courtney et al., 2003; Green & Flaro, 2003). However, reading level is correlated with WMT effort scores (.23 to .62) (Courtney et al., 2003; Green & Flaro, 2003) and with memory scores (.40 to .61; Green & Flaro, 2003).

Gender.   Gender has no impact on effort measures (Courtney et al., 2003; Green et al., 2002).

Memory Trials

Age.   Age has a significant effect on the memory trials, with scores improving with increasing age in childhood (Green & Flaro, 2003). In individuals aged 15 to 68 years, age had a significant effect for PA, but not for MC, FR, or LDFR (Green, 2003). Note however, that there were only 11 individuals older than 60 years of age.

Education, IQ, and Reading Level.   Education has only a weak relation ($r = .10$) with the delayed recall scores (Gervais et al., 2004). Reading level is correlated with memory scores (.40 to .61). Memory scores increase with increasing verbal IQ (Green, 2003).

Gender.   There are gender differences on memory measures, with women scoring higher than men on both FR and LDFR.

NORMATIVE DATA

Standardization Sample

When the WMT was devised by Paul Green, it was given to every outpatient referred to him for neuropsychological assessment. Over several years, the WMT was given to more than 1000 consecutive adults in this series, all involved in compensation or disability claims. This is the central data set from which much of the WMT research has evolved (Green et al., 2002).

The adult cutoffs were initially set at the 2nd percentile relative to 157 patients with moderate to severe head injury or other neurological disorders, after excluding 10% of individuals in whom there was strong independent evidence of poor effort (e.g., worse than chance scores on other tests; Green & Flaro, 2003). Adults were classed as a "pass" if IR, DR, and Cons were all above 82.5%. If not, the person was classed as failing the WMT effort test.

Norms for children are based on data from 130 children, between the ages of 7 and 18 years, with a variety of clinical disorders (e.g., schizophrenia, FAS, ADHD; Green & Flaro, 2003). The median score on the IR and DR subtests was at or above 97.5% in all child diagnostic groups. After excluding 5 children in whom there was evidence of poor effort (e.g., initially failed the WMT, but passed it when given an incentive; Green & Faro, 2003), cutoff scores at the 5th percentile were derived. These are 82.5% for IR and DR and 75% for Cons. The values for IR and DR are the same as the adult cutoffs, below which effort should be considered inadequate. Courtney et al. (2003), however, found that performance varied as a function of age in children, with only those 11 years of age and older producing results similar to those of adults. Accordingly, they recommended against the use of adult-based norms with children younger than about 11 years of age.

Green (2003, submitted) recently revised these cutoffs (see Table 16–14). He reported that normal adult controls obtain perfect scores on the WMT (Iverson et al., 1999) and that nearly perfect scores are obtained from adults and children with neurological diseases or mental retardation. Accordingly, he recommended that scores less than 91% correct on the effort subtests should raise the concern of low effort—with rare exceptions, such as people with dementia who need care 24 hours per day or children younger than 7 years of age with less than a grade 3 reading level.

Green (2003) indicated that, although MC and PA can be affected by actual neurological impairment, they are fairly easy even for those with severe brain injuries. He suggested that scores less than 70% correct on MC or less than 60% on PA should be considered suspicious, except in individuals with dementia or profound amnesia. Discrepancies (inconsistencies) in the expected gradient of performance across subtests also raise the concern of suspect effort. More precise interpretation of a person's WMT test results can be done by selecting appropriate comparison groups available through the scoring program and by referring to the test manual.

Table 16–14 Guidelines for WMT Interpretation

Clear Pass	Clear Fail	Caution
IR, DR, Cons >90% correct	Any of one of IR, DR, Cons ≤ 82.5% correct	Any of one of IR, DR, Cons 83%–90% correct

Source: Adapted from Green, 2003.

RELIABILITY

Internal Consistency

Green (2003) reported that, in 1207 consecutive outpatients, correlations were high between IR and DR ($r = .88$), MC and PA ($r = .90$) and FR and LDFR ($r = .86$).

Test-Retest Reliability

Green (2003) reported that 33 individuals were seen for retesting after 1 year or more. At any given time, WMT effort measures were found to correlate highly with one another (IR and DR $r = .87$ on initial testing and .94 on retesting). However, because effort can fluctuate markedly from one test occasion to another, correlations were modest ($r = .43$ for IR and $r = .33$ for DR).

VALIDITY

Clinical Findings

The WMT effort scores appear sensitive to motivational defects. Patients with moderate to severe head injuries performed better on these measures than did those with mild head injuries (Green, submitted; Green & Faro, 2003; Green et al., 1999, 2002). This is explained by lower effort, on average, in the mild group. Further, simulators (e.g., Dunn et al., 2003; Iverson et al., 1999; Tan et al., 2002) and compensation-seeking individuals (e.g., Gervais et al., 2001; Green et al., 2002) suppress their performance on this task. They are less accurate, and their response latencies are longer and more variable than those of honest responders (Dunn et al., 2003). In addition, low scores on the WMT are associated with a general suppression of test scores, in particular learning and memory tests (Gervais et al., 2001, 2004; Green & Faro, 2003; Green et al., 2001, 2002), but other domains (e.g., smell identification, Green et al., 2003; mood, Rohling et al., 2002; see Green, submitted, for a recent review) are also affected. Therefore, failure on the WMT effort components suggests invalid results on other tests as well (Green et al., 2002). Neuropsychological test scores tend to be progressively reduced to a degree corresponding with the level of effort indicated by the WMT (Green, submitted). There is also an association between failure on the WMT effort measures and a general over-reporting of symptoms (Gervais et al., 2001).

Good effort measures should be as insensitive as possible to actual impairment. The available evidence suggests that WMT effort trials are very easy, even for adults with significant neurological impairment (e.g., moderate to severe head injury, multiple sclerosis, tumor, ADHD, Conduct Disorder; Green & Faro, 2003; Green et al., 1999, 2001, 2002; Williamson et al., 2003b). For example, Green et al. (2002) reported that patients with moderate to severe brain injury (mean GCS of 9) who showed impairment on actual measures of memory scored above 95% (38/40) correct on the IR and DR portions of the WMT. IR/DR consistency was about 93%. In healthy volunteers, the mean score on these effort measures was similar (see also Tan et al., 2002). Moreover, within the brain-injured group, WMT effort measures were unrelated to measures of head injury severity, including GCS scores, duration of posttraumatic amnesia, and duration of loss of consciousness. In children, the effort trials also appear to be unaffected by a variety of disorders, including schizophrenia, FAS, and ADHD (Green & Faro, 2003).

Another sign that the WMT effort scores measure effort rather than ability is that they appear to be unrelated to age in children and adults (Green & Faro, 2003; but see Courtney et al., 2003, who found performance affected in those younger than 10 years of age). Further, having a specific reading disability does not, in itself, imply difficulty with the WMT, as long as the individual's reading level is above grade 2 (Green & Faro, 2003). Limited educational or intellectual attainment does not affect performance on the IR and DR trials (Gervais et al., 2004; Green & Faro, 2003). In fact, Green and Faro (2003) reported that even those children with low IQs (VIQ <75) performed well on the effort portion. Their mean IR score was 95% ($SD = 4.5$), their mean DR score was 98.2% ($SD = 2.4$), and their mean Cons score was 93.5% ($SD = 5.5$) Pain at the time of the assessment also did not affect test performance (Gervais et al., 2004).

The effect of mood disorder on WMT performance in nonlitigants has been the subject of some study. Patients who put forth poor effort appear more likely to produce elevated complaints of subjective distress, as indexed by the MMPI-2 (Williamson et al., 2003b). Rohling et al (2002) found that, after removal of litigating/disability cases with failing scores on effort tests (either WMT or CARB), there was no association between self-reported symptoms of depression and scores on conventional neuropsychological tests. They argued that, if depression did not affect scores on relatively difficult neuropsychological tests, it should not explain failure on effort tests.

The WMT effort measures correlate strongly with one another (>.80; Green et al., 1997). They also show moderate relations with scores from other SVTs (e.g., $r > .60$ with the CARB; >.6 with the Amsterdam Short Term Memory Test (ASTM), >.6 with the 21-Item Test, and >.68 with TOMM Trial 2; Green, submitted; Green et al., 1997). In addition, there is agreement in classification (pass-fail) between the WMT and other symptom validity tests (e.g., CARB shows 85% agreement; Green et al., 1997). However, symptom validity tests vary considerably in their sensitivity to response bias. Recently, Gervais et al. (2004) compared the WMT, CARB, and TOMM in 519 claimants referred for disability or personal injury–related assessments. The WMT proved more sensitive than the other two tasks. More than twice as many people failed the WMT than failed the TOMM, with the CARB occupying an intermediate position. Similarly, Tan et al. (2002) compared the VSVT, TOMM, and WMT in a simulation paradigm. Using the conventional cut scores, the WMT proved to be most efficient, classifying all controls and all malingerers accurately. The TOMM proved least efficient, and the efficacy of the VSVT approached that of the WMT. In terms of face validity, the WMT fared best, with about one third of the participants perceiving it to be a legitimate measure of memory, followed by about one quarter for the VSVT and 10% for the TOMM.

Sophisticated simulators (psychologists, patients asked to simulate impairment) perform poorly on the task (Green et al., 2002). Coaching of individuals on how to avoid detection improves performance, although such individuals still perform worse than controls (Dunn et al., 2003).

The use of the WMT memory tasks to measure memory has been subjected to less study. The memory measures (MC, PA, DFR) correlate highly with one another ($r > .80$) and show moderately strong correlations with independent verbal memory measures (e.g., CVLT Total $r = .67$), providing support for the validity of WMT measures (Green et al., 1997). Although WMT effort scores show strong ceiling effects, WMT memory scores appear to be normally distributed and are affected by neurological compromise (Green et al., 2002).

COMMENT

Hartman (2002) suggested a number of criteria to evaluate the efficacy of SVTs. They should

> Measure willingness to exert basic effort and be insensitive to cognitive dysfunction (sensitive and specific)
>
> Appear to the patient to be a realistic measure of the cognitive facet under study (face validity)
>
> Measure abilities likely to be exaggerated by patients claiming brain damage
>
> Have a strong normative basis underlying test results to satisfy scientific and Daubert concerns
>
> Be based on validation studies that include normal subjects, patient populations, and individuals who are suspected and/or verified malingerers in actual forensic or disability assessment conditions
>
> Be difficult to fake or coach
>
> Be relatively easy to administer
>
> Be supported by continuing research.

The WMT clearly meets all of these criteria, and it is unique among SVTs in that it measures effort as well as memory (Lynch, 2004). Unlike many of the other symptom validity techniques, validation of the WMT has been based primarily on claimants rather than simulators. It has a large database derived from clinical forensic settings. It can be used with a wide age range, children to adults. Further, the effort measures are quite insensitive to differences in ability levels and can be used even with individuals of limited verbal intelligence. Pain also does not explain patient failure on the effort portions (Green et al., 2002), although the impact of significant emotional distress requires additional study.

Of note, findings from the author of the WMT and his collaborators have generated important questions with regard to the effect of effort in the interpretation of neuropsychological test data (Hartman, 2002). For example, Green and his colleagues (Green, submitted; Green et al., 2001, 2002) have suggested that about half of the variance in neuropsychological test results can be accounted for by motivation; that effort has a much larger effect on neuropsychological test scores than age, education, severity of brain injury, or neurological disease;

and that compensation-driven effort may account for findings often attributed to disease or injury.

Clearly, the WMT is an important tool, especially in financial compensation cases (e.g., neurological trauma, pain, fibromyalgia, emotional disorder; e.g., Gervais et al., 2001; Rohling et al., 2002). However, use of the WMT (or other similar measures) in other settings (including research ones) is also recommended in order to rule out possible contaminating effects of suboptimal effort (e.g., Green et al., 2001; Williamson et al., 2003a). For example, Williamson et al. (2003a) reported that the majority of patients with psychogenic seizures obtained WMT scores in the invalid range.

It is important that clinicians do not misinterpret WMT scores. To rule out false positives, clinicians must consider not only the scores on the effort measures but also performance on the other subtests (as well as other test and clinical data), to ensure that the pattern of results makes neuropsychological sense.

The task can be given either orally or by computer. However, users should note that studies comparing the equivalence of both procedures are not yet available. The WMT may be easier to feign when it is administered by a computer than by a person. Users should also bear in mind that the computerized version of the WMT requires some basic reading skills and is not appropriate for those with less than a grade 3 reading level. Accordingly, it is important to measure word identification skills, so as not to be misled regarding the meaning of low test scores. The effort portion of the computerized version can be used with children (with at least a grade 3 reading level), although norms for the memory subtests are needed.

Green has argued that consideration of the gradient of scores across both effort and memory tasks has diagnostic utility. Research is needed on the reliability and incremental validity of scores contained within the entire profile. Finally, much of the current literature on the WMT derives from Green and his colleagues. Additional studies from other investigators would be useful.

REFERENCES

Allen, L. M., Condor, R. L., Green, P., & Cox, D. R. (1997). *CARB 97 manual for computerized assessment of response bias.* Durham, NC: CogniSyst.

Binder, L. M., & Willis, S. C. (1991). Assessment of motivation after financially compensable minor head trauma. *Psychological Assessment: A Journal of Consulting and Clinical Psychology, 3,* 175–181.

Courtney, J. C., Dinkins, J. P., Allen, L. M., & Kuroski, K. (2003). Age related effects in children taking the Computerized Assessment of Response Bias and Word Memory Test. *Child Neuropsychology, 9,* 109–116.

Dunn, T. D., Shear, P. K., Howe, S., & Ris, M. D. (2003). Detecting neuropsychological malingering: Effects of coaching information. *Archives of Clinical Neuropsychology, 18,* 121–134.

Gervais, R. O., Russell, A. S., Green, P., Allen, L. M., Ferrari, R., & Pieschl, S. D. (2001). Effort testing in fibromyalgia patients with disability incentives. *Journal of Rheumatology, 28,* 1892–1899.

Gervais, R. O., Rohling, M. L., Green, P., & Ford, W. (2004). A comparison of WMT, CARB, and TOMM failure rates in non-head injury disability claimants. *Archives of Clinical Neuropsychology, 19,* 475–487.

Green, P. (2003). *Green's Word Memory Test for Microsoft Windows.* Edmonton, Alberta: Green's Publishing Inc.

Green, P. (Submitted). The pervasive influence of effort on neuropsychological tests.

Green, P., Allen, L. M., & Astner, K. (1997). *The Word Memory Test: A user's guide to the oral and computer-administered forms, US version 1.1.* Durham, NC: CogniSyst.

Green, P., & Faro, L. (2003). Word Memory Test performance in children. *Child Neuropsychology, 9,* 189–207.

Green, P., Iverson, G., & Allen, L. (1999). Detecting malingering in head injury litigation with the Word Memory Test. *Brain Injury, 13,* 813–819.

Green, P., Lees-Haley, P., & Allen, L. (2002). The Word Memory Test and the validity of neuropsychological test scores. *Forensic Neuropsychology, 2,* 97–124.

Green, P., Rohling, M. L., Iverson, G. L., & Gervais, R. O. (2003). Relationships between olfactory discrimination and head injury severity. *Brain Injury, 17,* 479–496.

Green, P., Rohling, M. L., Lees-Haley, P. R., & Allen, L. M. (2001). Effort has a greater effect on test scores than severe brain injury in compensation claimants. *Brain Injury, 15,* 1045–1060.

Hartman, D. E. (2002). The unexamined lie is a lie worth fibbing: Neuropsychological malingering and the Word Memory Test. *Archives of Clinical Neuropsychology, 17,* 709–714.

Iverson, G., Green, P., & Gervais, R. (1999). Using the word memory test to detect biased responding in head injury litigation. *Journal of Cognitive Rehabilitation, 17,* 4–8.

Lynch, W. J. (2004). Determination of effort level, exaggeration, and malingering in neurocognitive assessment. *Journal of Head Trauma Rehabilitation, 19,* 277–283.

Rohling, M. L., Green, P., Allen, L. M., & Iverson, G. L. (2002). Depressive symptoms and neurocognitive test scores in patients passing symptom validity tests. *Archives of Clinical Neuropsychology, 17,* 205–222.

Slick, D., Hopp, G., Strauss, E., & Thompson, G. B. (1997). *Victoria Symptom Validity Test.* Odessa, FL: Psychological Assessment Resources.

Slick, D. J., Tan, J. E., Strauss, E. H., & Hultsch, D. F. (2004). Detecting malingering: A survey of experts' practices. *Archives of Clinical Neuropsychology, 19,* 465–471.

Tan, J. E., Slick, D. J., Strauss, E., & Hultsch, D. F. (2002). How'd they do it? Malingering strategies on symptom validity tests. *The Clinical Neuropsychologist, 16,* 495–505.

Tombaugh, T. (1996). *Test of Memory Malingering (TOMM).* North Tonawanda, NY: Multi-Health Systems.

Warrington, E. K. (1984). *Recognition Memory Test manual.* Windsor, England: NFER-Nelson.

Williamson, D. J., Drane, D. L., Stroup, E. S., Miller, J. W., & Holmes. M. D. (2003a). *Most patients with psychogenic seizures do not exert valid effort on neurocognitive testing.* Poster presented to the Annual Meeting of the American Epilepsy Society, Boston, MA.

Williamson, D. J. G., Green, P., Allen, L., & Rohling, M. L. (2003b). Evaluating effort with the Word Memory Test and Category Test—or not: Inconsistencies in a compensation-seeking sample. *Journal of Forensic Neuropsychology, 3,* 19–44.

Test Index

Note: page numbers followed by *f* and *t* indicate figures and tables.

Adjusting-Paced Serial Addition Test
  (Adjusting-PSAT)
  description of, 594
  practice effects on, 597
  source of, 583*t*
Advanced Progressive Matrices. *See* Raven's
  Progressive Matrices
  description of, 229–231
  normative data, 232
  reliability of, 233
American National Adult Reading Test
  (AMNART)
  dementia effects on performance, 197
  Mayo's Older Americans Normative Studies
    scaled scores, 195, 195*t*
  WAIS-R predictions from, 194–195
Auditory Consonant Trigrams. *See also*
    Brown-Peterson Task
  administration of, 705
  children's version, 705, 707*f*, 709*f*,
    709–710
  description of, 704
  instructions for, 709*f*
  normative data, 709–710
  reliability of, 711
  scoring of, 706*f*–707*f*
  validity of, 711
Autobiographical Memory Interview (AMI),
    681*t*, 687–690

b Test
  administration of, 1158
  age range for, 1158
  characteristics of, 1153*t*
  description of, 1158
  head injury assessments, 1161
  normal-effort comparison groups, 1159*t*
  normative data, 1159–1160
  purpose of, 1158
  reliability of, 1160
  scoring of, 1158–1159
  source of, 1158
  standardization sample for, 1159–1160

summary of, 1160–1161
validity of, 1160
Balloons Test, 964*t*, 965–967
Bayley Scales of Infant Development (BSID)
  Bayley Scales of Infant Development—Second
    Edition vs., 115–116, 126
  norms, 129
  overview of, 114
Bayley Scales of Infant Development—Second
    Edition (BSID-II)
  administration of, 116–118, 117*t*–118*t*
  age range for, 114
  basals for, 116
  Behavior Rating Scale
    description of, 115, 115*t*
    percentiles for, 121
    scores, 119, 119*t*
  BSID vs., 115–116, 126
  ceiling for, 116
  change assessments, 125
  characteristics of, 102*t*
  clinical studies using, 127–128
  cognitive tests correlated with, 127
  content of
    description of, 115
    validity of, 126
  corrected age vs. chronological age, 129–130
  demographic effects
    age, 120
    education, 120
    ethnicity, 120–121
    socioeconomic status, 120–121
  description of, 101, 114–116
  as developmental test, 114
  factor structure, 126
  intelligence quotient and, correlations
    between, 126–127
  interpretation of, 130
  item sets, 115
  limitations of, 128
  manipulatives used in, 116
  Mental Developmental Index, 124*t*, 127
  Mental Scale

description of, 115, 115*t*, 119*t*
  intercorrelations, 126
  reliability of, 122
Motor Scale
  description of, 115, 115*t*
  intercorrelations, 126
  reliability of, 122
normative data
  ability levels, 122
  cutoff points, 129
  demographically adjusted norms, 121–122
  extrapolated standard scores, 122, 123*t*–124*t*
  limitations of, 128–129
  standardization sample, 121
in premature infants, 129
in profoundly impaired children, 130
psychometric issues associated with, 128
Psychomotor Development Index, 124*t*
purpose of, 114
reliability of, 122, 125*t*, 125–126
scoring of
  corrected age vs. chronological age, 129–130
  domain scores, 119
  guidelines for, 117*t*–118*t*
  scores, 118–119, 128
in severely impaired children, 130
source of, 114
start points for, 116, 129
structure of, 114–115
testing time for, 118
translations, 116
in treatment studies, 128
validity of, 126
WPPSI-III vs., 346
Beck Depression Inventory—Second Edition
    (BDI-II)
  administration of, 1084, 1088
  in adolescents, 1087
  age range for, 1084
  attention-deficit/hyperactivity disorder, 1088
  characteristics of, 1081*t*
  clinical findings, 1087–1088
  Cognitive subscale, 1085

Beck Depression Inventory (*continued*)
  demographic effects, 1085
  depression-related tests correlated with,
      1086–1087
  description of, 1080, 1084
  early version of, 1086, 1088
  factor analytic findings, 1086
  major depressive disorder evaluations, 1087
  Noncognitive subscale, 1085
  normative data, 1085–1086
  purpose of, 1084
  reliability of, 1086, 1088
  scoring of, 1085, 1088
  source of, 1084
  standardization sample for, 1085–1086
  summary of, 1088–1089
  translated versions of, 1088
  validity of, 1086–1088
Beery Developmental Test of Visual Motor
      Integration (VMI), 832
Behavior Rating Inventory of Executive Function
      (BRIEF)
  adaptive functioning and, 1096
  ADHD, 1096
  ADHD-RS-IV and, 1095
  administration of, 1091
  age range for, 1090
  behavior rating scales correlated with, 1095
  characteristics of, 1081*t*
  demographic effects, 1092
  description of, 1083, 1090–1091
  executive functioning tests and, 1095, 1098
  factor structure of, 1095
  Inconsistency scale, 1092
  limitations of, 1097–1098
  Negativity scale, 1092
  normative data, 1092–1093, 1093*t*, 1097
  practice effects, 1094
  purpose of, 1090
  reliability of, 1093–1094, 1094*t*
  scales, 1091*t*
  scoring of, 1091–1092
  source of, 1090
  standardization sample for, 1092–1093
  summary of, 1097–1098
  in traumatic brain injury patients, 1096–1097
  validity of, 1094–1097
  versions of, 1090–1091
Behavioral Assessment of the Dysexecutive
      Syndrome (BADS)
  administration of, 410
  age range for, 408
  characteristics of, 402*t*
  conditions that affect, 412–413
  demographic effects, 410
  description of, 408–410
  Dysexecutive Questionnaire, 409*t*, 412–414
  neuropsychological tests correlated with, 412
  normative data, 410–411, 411*t*, 414
  purpose of, 408
  reliability of, 411–412, 412*t*, 414
  scoring of, 410
  source of, 408
  standardization sample, 410–411
  subtests of, 409*t*, 410
  summary of, 414
Bells Cancellation Test, 964*t*, 968–971

Benton Visual Retention Test (BVRT-5)
  administration of, 691–692, 692*t*
  age range for, 691
  ceiling effects of, 699
  characteristics of, 681*t*
  in children, 694–695
  clinical studies of, 697–698
  dementia effects, 697–698
  demographic effects, 693
  drawing administration of, 691–692
  limitations of, 698
  malingering detection, 698
  multiple-choice administration of, 691–692
  normative data, 693–695, 694*t*–695*t*
  practice effects on, 696
  purpose of, 691
  reliability of, 695–697
  scoring of, 692–693
  source of, 691
  summary of, 698–699
  validity of, 697–698
Biber Cognitive Estimation Test (BCET)
  administration of, 439*f*
  characteristics of, 403*t*
  conditions that affect, 442
  description of, 439
  general cognitive status effects on, 442
  items on, 439*f*, 440*t*
  normative data, 441
  scoring of, 440
Bolter Validity Index, 433
Boston Diagnostic Aphasia Examination (BDAE)
  administration of, 893
  age range for, 893
  in Alzheimer's disease, 898–899
  aphasia evaluations, 898
  characteristics of, 892*t*
  clinical studies of, 898–899
  demographic effects, 895
  description of, 891, 893
  Language Competency Index, 895*f*
  neuroanatomic correlates, 898
  normative data, 896, 897*t*
  Parietal Lobe Battery, 898
  purpose of, 892
  reliability of, 896
  scoring of, 893–895
  source of, 892
  Spatial-Quantitative Battery, 895*t*
  Speech Characteristics Profile, 896
  standardization sample for, 896
  subtests, 894*t*
  summary of, 899
  validity of, 896–899
  versions of, 892
Boston Naming Test—2 (BNT-2)
  administration of, 902–903
  age range for, 901
  in Alzheimer's disease patients, 911
  Canadian norms, 907
  characteristics of, 892*t*
  in children, 907–908
  demographic effects, 904–905, 912
  description of, 901–902
  head injury effects on, 912
  language versions, 901
  long form

  administration of, 902
  normative data, 905–909
  Mack SF4, 902–903, 903*f*
  MOAANS norms, 907*t*
  neurological conditions that affect, 911
  non-normality of, 7
  normative data, 905–910, 906*t*
  practice effects, 910–911
  premorbid indicators as score estimators for,
      908–909
  purpose of, 901
  reliability of, 910–911
  scoring of, 903–904, 912
  short form
      administration of, 901–903
      normative data, 909–910
      validity of, 912
  source of, 901
  Spot-the-Word test and, relations between,
      274, 278*t*
  summary of, 912
  validity of, 911–912
  verbal intelligence effects on performance, 904
Brief Test of Attention (BTA)
  administration of, 550
  age range for, 547
  attention tests correlated with, 552
  characteristics of, 548*t*
  in children, 553
  clinical studies of, 552
  demographic effects, 550
  description of, 547, 550
  discontinuing of, 550–551
  neuropsychological tests correlated with, 552
  normative data, 551, 551*t*, 553
  PASAT and, 552
  practice effects on, 552
  purpose of, 547
  reliability of, 551–552
  scoring of, 550
  source of, 547
  summary of, 552–553
  validity of, 552
Brief Visuospatial Memory Test—Revised
      (BVMT-R)
  administration of, 701–702
  age range for, 701
  characteristics of, 681*t*
  clinical studies of, 704
  demographic effects, 702
  description of, 701
  limitations of, 704
  normative data, 702–703, 703*t*
  practice effects, 703
  purpose of, 701
  reliability of, 703
  scores and scoring of, 701–702, 702*t*
  source of, 701
  standardization sample for, 702–703,
      703*t*
  summary of, 704
  validity of, 703–704
Brixton Spatial Anticipation Test
  clinical studies of, 464–465
  demographic effects, 461
  description of, 460
  normative data, 462

scoring of, 461
summary of, 465
Brown-Peterson Task
  age range for, 704, 705*t*
  Auditory Consonant Trigrams
    administration of, 705
    children's version, 705, 707*f*, 709*f*, 709–710
    description of, 704
    instructions for, 709*f*
    normative data, 709–710
    reliability of, 711
    scoring of, 706*f*–707*f*
    validity of, 711
  characteristics of, 681*t*
  clinical studies of, 711–712
  demographic effects, 708–709
  description of, 705
  practice effects, 711
  purpose of, 704
  reliability of, 711
  source of, 704
  summary of, 712
Buschke Selective Reminding Test (SRT)
  administration of, 714, 717*f*
  in adolescents, 714
  advantages of, 727
  age range for, 713
  alternate forms, 714, 716*f*
  characteristics of, 681*t*
  for children
    alternate forms, 714, 716*f*
    demographic effects, 716, 721
    description of, 714, 716*f*–717*f*
    normative data, 722–724
    scoring sheets for, 719*f*–720*f*
    word lists, 717*f*
  clinical studies of, 726–727
  dementia evaluations, 726–727
  demographic effects, 716, 721
  description of, 713–714
  items for, 715*f*
  in multiple sclerosis patients, 727
  normative data, 721–724
  purpose of, 713
  reliability of, 724
  scoring of, 714, 718*f*–721*f*
  short form, 722–724
  source of, 713
  summary of, 727
  validity of, 724, 726–727
  Verbal Selective Reminding Test, 721*t*
  versions of, 713–714

California Verbal Learning Test—Children's
    Version (CVLT-C)
  administration of, 737
  age range for, 735
  cancer applications of, 744
  characteristics of, 681*t*
  Children's Category Test, 739
  clinical studies of, 743–744
  cluster analysis of, 742
  CMS and, 752
  contrast variables for, 737, 738*f*, 739–740
  demographic effects, 738
  description of, 680
  factor analysis of, 741–742

head injury evaluations, 743–744
  intelligence quotient and, 743
  learning strategy variables, 735–736
  neuropsychological tests and, correlation
      between, 742–743
  normative data, 738–740, 739*t*
  overview of, 735
  paradigm for, 735, 736*t*
  practice effects, 741
  psychometric properties of, 744–745
  purpose of, 735
  reliability of, 740–741
  scoring of, 737, 745
  source of, 735
  Spanish version of, 737, 737*t*, 740
  standardization sample, 738–739
  summary of, 744–745
  validity of, 741–744
California Verbal Learning Test-II (CVLT-II)
  administration of, 730
  age range for, 730
  characteristics of, 681*t*
  clinical studies of, 733–734
  CVLT vs., 733
  demographic effects, 731
  description of, 680, 730
  factor analysis of, 733
  malingering evaluations, 734
  normative data, 731–732, 734
  practice effects, 732
  purpose of, 730
  reliability of, 732–733
  scoring of, 730–731
  Short Form, 730
  source of, 730
  standardization sample, 731–732
  summary of, 734
  validity of, 733–734
  WRAML2 and, 887
Cambridge Contextual Reading Test (CCRT),
      190–191
Cambridge Neuropsychological Test Automated
      Batteries (CANTAB)
  administration of, 416
  age range for, 415
  Alzheimer's disease affected by, 421
  characteristics of, 402*t*
  clinical studies, 421–422
  conditions that affect, 422
  demographic effects, 416
  description of, 415–416
  normative data, 416, 418–419, 420*t*, 422
  practice effects on, 419
  purpose of, 415
  reliability of, 419
  scoring of, 416
  source of, 415
  standardization sample, 416
  summary of, 422–423
  tasks of, 416, 417*t*–418*t*, 419*f*
  validity of, 419, 421–422
Category Test (CT)
  administration of, 425, 427
  adult version of, 426*f*, 428
  age range for, 424
  characteristics of, 402*t*
  children's version of, 426*f*, 429–431, 430*t*, 739

clinical studies of, 432–433
  demographic effects, 427–428
  description of, 425
  factor-analytic findings, 432
  intermediate version of, 426*f*, 429–431
  malingering issues, 433
  manual version of, 425–427, 426*f*
  neurological conditions that affect, 432–433
  neuropsychological measures correlated
      with, 432
  normative data, 428–431
  practice effects, 431–432
  purpose of, 424
  reliability of, 431–432
  scoring of, 427
  short forms, 425
  source of, 424
  summary of, 433–434
  validity of, 432–433
  WCST vs., 433–434
CCC. *See* Auditory Consonant Trigrams (Brown-
      Peterson Task)
Childrens' Category Test. *See* Category Test
Children's Color Trails Test (CCTT), 554–557
Children's Memory Scale (CMS)
  academic achievement and, 752–753
  administration of, 747–748
  age range for, 746
  characteristics of, 682*t*
  clinical studies of, 753
  CVLT-C and, 752
  demographic effects, 749
  description of, 746–747, 753–754
  executive functioning and, 753
  factor structure of, 754
  General Memory Index, 753
  intellectual ability and, 752
  language skills and, 753
  limitations of, 754
  normative data, 749, 749*t*
  primary index scores for, 747*t*–748*t*
  purpose of, 746
  reliability of, 749–751, 750*t*, 754
  scoring of, 747*t*–748*t*, 748–749
  source of, 746
  structure of, 747*f*
  subtest intercorrelations, 751
  summary of, 753–755
  validity of, 751–753
  WMS-III and, 751–752
  WRAML and, 752
  WRAML2 and, 752
Children's Paced Auditory Serial Addition Test
      (CHIPASAT)
  administration of, 586, 587*f*
  age range for, 582, 584
  characteristics of, 548*t*, 585*t*
  computerized, 583*t*, 585*t*
  mathematical ability correlated with
      performance on, 603–604
  normative data, 597, 601*t*–602*t*
  protocol for, 591*f*–592*f*
  source of, 583*t*
Clock Drawing Test (CDT)
  administration of, 972, 973*t*, 974*f*, 975
  characteristics of, 964*t*
  in children, 975–977, 976*t*, 979, 981

Clock Drawing Test (*continued*)
  dementia evaluations, 978–979
  demographic effects, 975–976
  depression effects on, 979
  description of, 972
  evaluative criteria, 975t–976t
  hemianopsia effects on, 979
  neuroanatomical correlates of, 979–980
  normative data, 976–977
  purpose of, 972
  reliability of, 977
  scoring of, 974f, 975, 977–978
  source of, 972
  summary of, 980–981
  validity of, 977–980
Cognitive Assessment System (CAS)
  achievement correlated with, 142
  administration of, 135, 137
  age range for, 133
  age-related changes and, 138
  Attention subtests, 136t
  Basic Battery, 135
  characteristics of, 102t
  clinical studies of, 142
  concerns regarding, 143
  demographic effects, 138
  description of, 101, 133–135
  ethnicity and, 138
  Expressive Attention subtest, 136t
  factor structure, 140–141, 143
  Figure Memory subtest, 136t
  forms of, 135
  gender differences, 138
  intelligence quotient and, 141–142
  Matching Numbers subtest, 136t
  materials used in, 135
  neuropsychological tests correlated with, 141
  Nonverbal Matrices subtest, 136t
  normative data for, 138
  Number Detection subtest, 136t
  PASS processes, 133, 134t
  Planned Codes subtest, 136t
  Planned Connections subtest, 136t
  Planning subtests, 136t
  purpose of, 133
  Receptive Attention subtest, 136t
  reliability of, 138–139, 140t
  scoring of, 137–138
  Sentence Questions subtest, 137t
  Sentence Repetition subtest, 136t
  Simultaneous subtests, 136t
  source of, 133
  Speech Rate subtest, 137t
  Standard Battery, 135
  Successive subtests, 136t–137t
  summary of, 142–143
  uses of, 133–135
  validity of, 139–142
  Visual-Spatial Relations subtest, 136t
Cognitive Estimation Test (CET)
  administration of, 439
  age range for, 437
  characteristics of, 403t
  conditions that affect, 442
  demographic effects, 440
  description of, 437, 439
  general knowledge effects on, 441

  intelligence levels and, 441
  normative data, 440–441
  purpose of, 437
  reliability of, 441
  scoring of, 438f, 439–440
  source of, 437
  summary of, 442
  validity of, 441–442
Color Trails Test (CTT), 554–557
Colored Progressive Matrices (Raven's
    Progressive Matrices)
  description of, 229–230
  example of, 230f
  normative data, 232, 232t
  reliability of, 233
Comprehensive Trail Making Test (CTMT)
  administration of, 558–559
  age range for, 557
  characteristics of, 548t
  clinical studies of, 561
  demographic effects, 559
  description of, 557–558
  neuropsychological tests correlated with, 561
  normative data, 559, 560t
  practice effects, 560
  purpose of, 557
  reliability of, 559–560
  scoring of, 559
  source of, 557
  summary of, 561
  trials, 558, 558f, 558t
  validity of, 561
Conners' Continuous Performance Test
    (CPT-II)
  administration of, 563
  age range for, 562
  attention deficit hyperactivity disorder
      evaluations, 569–571
  characteristics of, 548t
  commission errors, 573
  confidence indices, 563
  confidence intervals from, 563
  demographic effects, 566–567
  demographically corrected norms, 568–569
  diagnostic utility of, 562–563, 570, 573
  group differences for, 570–571
  normative data, 567–569, 573–574
  overview of, 562
  previous versions of, 562, 562t
  psychometric properties of, 574
  purpose of, 562
  reliability of, 569–570
  repeat assessment of, 565–566
  scoring of, 563–566, 564t
  source of, 562
  standardization sample for, 567–568
  summary of, 572–574
  validity of, 570–572
Controlled Oral Word Association Test
    (COWA), 274, 278t, 936. *See also* Verbal
    Fluency Test
CVLT (California Verbal Learning Test), 733

Delis-Kaplan Executive Function System
    (D-KEFS)
  administration of, 445
  advantages of, 449

  age range for, 443
  characteristics of, 403t
  clinical studies, 448
  conditions that affect, 448
  demographic effects, 445
  description of, 443–445
  Design Fluency Test, 456
  frontal lobe lesions effect on, 448–449
  normative data, 446, 446t
  purpose of, 443
  reliability of, 446
  scoring of, 445
  source of, 443
  standardization sample, 446
  summary of, 449
  tests, 444t
  WCST and, correlation between, 448
Dementia Rating Scale (DRS), 104
Dementia Rating Scale—2 (DRS-2)
  administration of, 144–145
  age range for, 144
  Alzheimer's disease differentiation, 155
  bias in, 156
  characteristics of, 102t
  clinical studies of, 155–156
  demographic effects, 145
  depression effects on, 155–156
  description of, 144
  Mayo's African American Normative Studies
      scaled scores, 146–147, 151t–155t
  Mayo's Older Americans Normative Studies
      scaled scores, 146, 146t–150t
  MMSE score conversion, 156t, 183t
  normative data, 145–147, 146t–148t
  purpose of, 144
  reliability of
    alternate form, 150
    internal, 148–149
    practice effects on, 149–150
    test-retest, 149–150
  scoring of, 145
  screening uses of, 157
  source of, 144
  subscales of, 145t
  subtests of, 145t
  summary of, 157
  validity of
    construct, 151–155
    ecological, 156
  versions of, 156
Design Fluency Test
  administration of, 450, 451f–452f
  characteristics of, 403t
  in children, 453
  clinical studies of, 454–455
  criticisms of, 455
  demographic effects, 453
  description of, 450
  D-KEFS, 456
  NEPSY, 456
  normative data, 453
  practice effects on, 453–454
  purpose of, 450
  reliability of, 453–454
  scoring of, 450, 452
  summary of, 455
  validity of, 454

Dichotic Learning—Words
  administration of, 916, 917f–918f
  age range for, 916
  characteristics of, 892t
  demographic effects, 916–917
  description of, 916
  dyslexia effects, 919
  Fused Dichotic Words Test vs., 920
  lateralized deficits and, 920
  malingering, 920
  normative data, 917
  purpose of, 916
  reliability of, 917
  right ear advantage, 916, 919
  source of, 916
  summary of, 920
  validity of, 917, 919–920
Doors and People Test (DPT)
  administration of, 756
  age range for, 755
  characteristics of, 682t
  clinical studies of, 759
  demographic effects, 757
  description of, 755–756
  NART and, 757
  normative data, 757–758, 758t
  purpose of, 755
  reliability of, 758
  scoring of, 756
  source of, 755
  standardization sample, 757
  summary of, 759
  verbal recall evaluations, 755t, 756
  verbal recognition evaluations, 755t, 756
  visual recall evaluations, 755, 755t
  visual recognition evaluations, 755, 755t
Dot Counting Test (DCT)
  administration of, 1162
  age range for, 1161
  characteristics of, 1153t
  demographic effects, 1163
  description of, 1161–1162
  normal-effort comparison groups, 1162t
  normative data, 1163
  purpose of, 1161
  reliability of, 1163–1164
  scoring of, 1162–1163
  source of, 1161
  summary of, 1164–1165
  validity of, 1164
Dysexecutive Questionnaire (DEX), 409t,
    412–414. See also Behavioral Assessment
    of the Dysexecutive Syndrome

Excluded Letter Fluency task, 500
Expressive One-Word Picture Vocabulary Test—
    Third Edition (EOWPVT3)
  administration of, 923
  age range for, 922
  characteristics of, 892t
  clinical studies of, 926–927
  demographic effects, 923–924
  description of, 923
  language tests correlated with, 926
  normative data, 924t, 924–925
  purpose of, 922
  reliability of, 925

  scoring of, 923–925
  source of, 922
  standardization sample for, 924, 925t
  summary of, 927
  verbal intelligence assessments using, 927
Expressive Vocabulary Test (EVT)
  administration of, 929
  age range for, 928
  characteristics of, 892t
  clinical studies of, 931–932
  demographic effects, 929–930
  items on, 929f
  language impairment evaluations,
    931–932
  language tests correlated with, 931
  overview of, 928–929
  PPVT-III vs., 932–933
  practice effects, 931
  purpose of, 928
  receptive-expressive discrepancies, 932
  reliability of, 930–931
  scoring of, 929
  source of, 928
  structure of, 929
  summary of, 932–933
  validity of, 931–932

Facial Recognition Test (FRT)
  administration of, 983
  age range for, 983
  characteristics of, 964t
  clinical findings of, 987–988
  conditions that affect, 988
  demographic effects, 985
  description of, 983–984
  Long Form, 987–989
  normative data, 985–987
  purpose of, 983
  reliability of, 986–987
  scoring of, 984
  source of, 983
  standardization sample for, 985–986
  summary of, 988–989
  validity of, 987–988
  vision effects, 988
Fake Bad Scale, 1120–1121, 1121t
Finger Localization, 1012t, 1013–1017
Finger Tapping (FTT)
  administration of, 1043–1044
  in adolescents, 1046–1047
  age range for, 1043
  characteristics of, 1042t
  in children, 1046–1047
  conditions that affect, 1048
  demographic effects, 1044–1045
  intermanual differences, 1044–1045
  malingering detection, 1049
  normative data, 1045–1047
  purpose of, 1043
  reliability of, 1047
  scoring of, 1044
  source of, 1043
  summary of, 1049–1050
  tapping speed, 1048
  validity of, 1047–1049
  WAIS-R and, 1048
Five-Point Test

administration of, 456–458
  in adolescents, 458–459
  age range for, 456
  characteristics of, 403t
  in children, 458–459
  clinical studies of, 459
  demographic effects, 458
  description of, 456
  normative data, 458–459
  purpose of, 456
  scoring of, 458
  source of, 456
  summary of, 459
  validity of, 459
Four Word Short-Term Memory Test
  administration of, 705
  description of, 705
  illustration of, 708f
  instructions for, 709f
  normative data, 710
Fused Dichotic Words Test, 920

General Ability Index (GAI)
  Wechsler Adult Intelligence Scale—III, 286, 287t
  Wechsler Intelligence Scale for Children—
    Fourth Edition, 312, 316t, 319t
Geriatric Depression Scale (GDS)
  administration of, 1099, 1104
  age range for, 1099
  brief versions of, 1105
  characteristics of, 1081t
  clinical findings, 1102–1103
  cognitive impairment effects on, 1103
  cultural factors that affect, 1103
  demographic effects, 1100–1101
  description of, 1080, 1099
  factor analytic findings, 1102
  long form, 1103–1104
  normative data, 1101, 1104
  physical health status and, 1103
  purpose of, 1099
  reliability of, 1101–1102, 1104
  response biases, 1104
  scoring of, 1099, 1100f
  self-administration of, 1102
  short form, 1103–1104
  source of, 1099
  summary of, 1104–1105
  translated versions of, 1104–1105
  validity of, 1102–1104
Golden Version (Stroop Test)
  administration of, 479
  in adults, 481, 484
  in children, 484, 490
  description of, 477–478
  normative data, 481, 484, 485t–490t, 490
  scoring of, 479
  standardization sample, 481
Gray Oral Reading Tests—Fourth Edition
    (GORT-4)
  administration of, 365–366, 369
  age range for, 365
  alternate forms reliability, 368, 370
  basals for, 366
  ceilings for, 366, 370
  clinical studies of, 369
  demographic effects, 366–367

Gray Oral Reading Tests (*continued*)
    description of, 365
    floor effects, 370
    intelligence quotient and, 369
    normative data, 367
    overview of, 364*t*
    purpose of, 365
    reading tests correlated with, 368–369
    reliability of, 367–368, 368*t*
    scoring of, 366, 366*t*
    source of, 365
    summary of, 369–370
    validity of, 368–369
Grip Strength
    administration of, 1053
    age range for, 1052
    characteristics of, 1042*t*
    in children, 1055
    demographic effects, 1053, 1055*t*
    depression effects on, 1057
    gender-based findings, 1055*t*
    instructions for, 1053, 1053*f*
    malingering detection using, 1058
    neurological conditions that affect, 1056–1057
    normative data, 1053–1055, 1054*t*–1055*t*
    pain effects, 1057
    practice effects, 1056
    purpose of, 1052
    reliability of, 1055–1056
    source of, 1052
    summary of, 1058
    validity of, 1056–1058
Gronwall Version of Paced Auditory Serial
        Addition Test
    administration of, 584
    characteristics of, 583*t*, 585*t*
    form for, 587*f*
    instructions for, 586*f*
    normative data for, 595*t*–596*t*, 595–596
Grooved Pegboard
    administration of, 1061, 1066
    in adolescents, 1062–1063
    characteristics of, 1042*t*
    in children, 1062–1063
    conditions that affect, 1065
    demographic effects, 1061–1062
    description of, 1061
    malingering on, 1066
    normative data, 1062*t*–1063*t*, 1062–1063
    practice effects, 1064
    purpose of, 1061
    reliability of, 1064
    source of, 1061
    summary of, 1066
    validity of, 1065–1066

Halstead-Reitan Category Test. *See also*
        Category Test
    children's version of, 426*f*, 429–431, 430*t*
    description of, 425–427, 426*f*
    manual version of, 425–427, 426*f*
Halstead-Russell Neuropsychological Evaluation
        System
    description of, 428
Hayling and Brixton Tests. *See also* Brixton
        Spatial Anticipation Test
    administration of, 460–461

age range for, 460
    characteristics of, 403*t*
    clinical studies of, 464
    correlations between, 463–464
    demographic effects, 461
    description of, 460
    normative data, 461–462
    purpose of, 460
    reliability of, 462–463
    scoring of, 461
    source of, 460
    standardization sample, 461–462
    summary of, 465
Homophone Meaning Generation Test, 500
Hooper Visual Organization Test (VOT)
    administration of, 991
    age range for, 990
    characteristics of, 964*t*
    in children, 993
    clinical studies of, 994–995
    conditions that affect, 994–995
    description of, 990
    normative data, 991–993
    object naming, 994
    psychiatric disorders that affect, 995
    purpose of, 990
    reliability of, 993–994
    scoring of, 991
    short form, 995
    source of, 990
    standardization sample for, 991–992
    summary of, 995–996
    validity of, 994–996
Hopkins Verbal Learning Test—Revised
        (HVLT-R)
    administration of, 760
    for African Americans, 763*t*–765*t*
    age range for, 760
    in Alzheimer's disease, 766–767
    assessment of change, 765–766
    characteristics of, 682*t*
    clinical studies of, 766–768
    dementia screenings, 767
    demographic effects, 760–761
    diagnostic validity of, 768
    normative data, 761*t*–762*t*, 761–762
    practice effects, 765–766
    purpose of, 760
    reliability of, 762, 765–766
    scoring of, 760
    source of, 760
    standardization sample, 761, 761*t*
    summary of, 768
    validity of, 766–768
    verbal memory and, 766

Information-Memory-Concentration test, 151
Instrumental Activities of Daily Living (IADL)
    administration of, 1109, 1111
    age range for, 1107
    characteristics of, 1082*t*
    cognitive status and, 1110
    demographic effects, 1109–1110
    description of, 1083, 1107, 1109
    factors that affect, 1112
    geriatric uses of, 1107, 1109
    limitations of, 1111

normative data, 1109*t*, 1110
    purpose of, 1107
    reliability of, 1110
    scoring of, 1109
    source of, 1107, 1108*f*
    summary of, 1111–1112
    validity of, 1110–1111
Integrated Visual and Auditory Continuous
        Performance Test (IVA + Plus)
    administration of, 576–577
    age range for, 576
    attention deficit hyperactivity disorder
        detection by, 580–581
    attention tests correlated with, 580
    characteristics of, 548*t*
    clinical studies of, 580
    demographic effects, 577–578
    factor structure for, 580
    limitations of, 581–582
    malingering, 580, 581*t*
    normative data, 579, 579*t*
    overview of, 576
    parameters for, 576
    purpose of, 575
    reliability of, 579
    scores and scoring of, 576–577, 577*t*–578*t*
    source of, 575
    standardization sample for, 579
    summary of, 580–582
    validity of, 579–580

Judgment of Line Orientation (JLO)
    administration of, 998
    age range for, 997
    characteristics of, 964*t*
    in children, 1003
    clinical studies of, 1002–1003
    demographic effects, 998–999
    description of, 997–998
    malingering detection, 1004
    MOAANS norms for, 1001*t*
    MOANS norms for, 1000*t*
    neurological conditions that affect, 1003
    normative data, 999*t*, 999–1001
    purpose of, 997
    reliability of, 1001–1002
    scoring of, 998
    short forms, 998, 1001, 1002*t*, 1003–1004
    source of, 997
    standardization sample for, 999, 999*t*
    summary of, 1004
    validity of, 1002–1004
    visual acuity and, 1003

Kaplan Baycrest Neurocognitive Assessment
        (KBNA)
    administration of, 161
    age effects on, 161
    age range for, 159
    characteristics of, 102*t*
    clinical studies of, 163
    demographic effects, 161–162
    description of, 103–104, 159, 161
    education effects on, 161
    indices, 161, 161*t*
    normative data, 162, 162*t*
    purpose of, 159

reliability of, 162, 163t
scoring of, 161
source of, 159
subtests of, 159, 160t, 164t
summary of, 163–164
validity of, 162–163
Kaufman Brief Intelligence Test (K-BIT)
administration of, 165
advantages of, 101
age effects on, 165
age range for, 164
characteristics of, 102t
clinical studies of, 167
cognitive tests correlated with, 167
demographic effects, 165
description of, 164–165
intelligence quotient tests correlated with,
166–167
Matrices subtest of, 164–165
nonverbal intelligence measures, 167
normative data, 165, 166t, 167
practice effects on, 166
purpose of, 164
reliability of, 165–166
scoring of, 165
source of, 164
standardization sample for, 165
summary of, 167–168
validity of, 166–167
verbal intelligence measures, 167
Vocabulary subtest of, 164

Levin Version of Paced Auditory Serial
Addition Test
administration of, 584–586
characteristics of, 583t, 585t
form for, 588f–589f
normative data, 596–597, 597t, 600t
Milwaukee Card Sorting Test, 527

Mini-Mental State Examination (MMSE).
See also 3MS
administration of, 169, 176
age effects, 176, 178t–179t
age range for, 168
Alzheimer's disease and, 183–184
characteristics of, 102t
children's version
illustration of, 175f
normative data for, 177, 179
cutoff points, 185
Dementia Rating Scale-2 and, correlation
between, 151, 156t, 183t
demographic effects of, 176–177
description of, 104, 168–169
education effects, 176, 178t–179t
ethnicity effects on, 177
factor-analytic studies of, 183
gender effects, 176
item sensitivity, 184
Modified. See 3MS
Modified Mini-Mental State Examination,
169, 170f–174f
normative data for, 177, 178t–179t
purpose of, 168
race effects on, 177
RBMT and, 847

reliability of, 180–181, 182t
scoring of, 176
source of, 168
summary of, 185–186
validity of, 182–185
Minnesota Multiphasic Personality Inventory—2
(MMPI-2)
administration of, 1114, 1123
characteristics of, 1081t
convergent validity of, 1118
correction factors for, 1119, 1119t, 1123
demographic effects, 1116–1117
description of, 1080, 1113–1114
emotional distress during, 1119
factor-analytic findings, 1118
Fake Bad Scale, 1120–1121, 1121t
feigning indexes, 1120t, 1123
head injury effects, 1118
malingering detection using, 1120t, 1120–1123
neurocorrections, 1119, 1119t
neurological conditions that affect, 1118–1119
normative data, 1117
PAI vs., 1083
purpose of, 1113
reading level necessary for, 1114
reliability of, 1117, 1123
response stability on, 1122
scales, 1114t–1116t
scoring of, 1114, 1116
in seizure patients, 1118
short forms, 1119–1120
source of, 1113
standardization sample for, 1117
strengths of, 1123
summary of, 1123
validity of, 1114t, 1118–1123
VSVT and, 1182
MMSE. See Mini-Mental State Examination
Multilingual Aphasia Examination (MAE)
age range for, 933
clinical studies of, 938–939
demographic effects, 935
description of, 891, 933–934
factor structure of, 938
head injuries effect on, 938–939
limitations of, 939
MOANS norms, 936–937, 937t
normative data, 935–937
purpose of, 933
reliability of, 937
scoring of, 934–935, 935t
source of, 933
Spanish version of, 934, 939
standardization sample for, 935–936
subtests, 933, 934t
summary of, 939
Token Test, 938
validity of, 937–939

National Adult Reading Test (NART)
age range for, 190
clinical observations to supplement, 198
contraindicated groups for, 198
dementia effects on performance, 197
demographic effects, 194
description of, 190–192
development of, 107

DPT scores and, 758
limitations of, 198
neurological conditions that affect, 197
neurological decline and, 107
premorbid intelligence estimates using,
196–198
psychiatric disorders that affect, 197–198
purpose of, 189
reliability of, 196
scores of, 107
scoring of, 192–193
short, 192–193
source of, 189–190
structure of, 107–108
summary of, 198
TEA and, correlation between, 634
validity of, 196–198
versions of, 190t
Wechsler intelligence scores predicted
from, 194
National Adult Reading Test-2 (NART-2)
administration of, 191–192
description of, 190
reliability of, 196
NEPS, 201
NEPSY
achievement tests and, 212
administration of, 202, 204
advantages of, 214–215
age effects on, 204
age range for, 201
ceiling effects on, 216
characteristics of, 102t
for children, 104
clinical studies of, 213–214
clinical utility of, 215
Core domains of, 202, 205t
demographic effects, 204, 206
description of, 201–202
Design Fluency Test, 456
ethnicity effects on, 204, 206
factor structure of, 211
flexibility of, 216
floor effects on, 216
gender effects on, 204
intelligence quotient and, 206, 211–212
limitations of, 215
materials used in, 202, 204
neuropsychological tests correlated with,
212–213
normative data for, 206–208
psychometric properties of, 215
purpose of, 201
reliability of, 208–211
scores and scoring of
conversion of, 207–208
description of, 204
interpretation of, 215–216
sensitivity of, 215
source of, 201
standardization sample for, 206, 206t
structure of, 201–202
subtests, 202t–204t, 211–213, 216
summary of, 214–217
theoretical orientation of, 201
validity of, 211–214
visual assessment using, 217

NEUROPSI, 500
Neuropsychological Assessment Battery (NAB)
  administration of, 219t, 221, 226t
  age range for, 218
  characteristics of, 102t
  clinical studies of, 227
  demographic effects, 222
  description of, 104, 218–221
  ecological validity of, 227
  factor-analytic findings, 227
  familiarity with, 228
  malingering on, 227
  normative data, 222–223, 228
  organization of, 218, 219t
  purpose of, 218
  reliability of, 223–225, 224t, 228
  scores and scoring of, 218–222, 222t
  Screening Module of, 218, 219t, 226, 228
  source of, 218
  standardization sample for, 222–223
  subtests of, 218, 220t
  summary of, 227–228
  validity of, 225–228
North American Adult Reading Test 35
    (NAART35), 193
North American Adult Reading Test (NAART)
  demographic effects, 194
  description of, 190
  instructions for, 193f
  reliability of, 196
  scoring sheet for, 191f
  WAIS-R predictions from, 193–195

Paced Auditory Serial Addition Test (PASAT)
  PASAT-50, 589f–590f
  PASAT-100, 589f–590f
  PASAT-200, 589f–590f
  administration of, 584, 586, 593
  age range for, 582, 584
  anxiety effects, 605–606
  attention tests correlated with, 601, 603
  auditory version of, 601, 607
  BTA and, 552
  ceiling effects, 601
  characteristics of, 548t
  Children's. See Children's Paced Auditory
    Serial Addition Test (CHIPASAT)
  chunking scoring of, 593, 594f, 597
  clinical studies of, 604–606
  computer-derived scoring of, 593–594
  computerized, 585t, 607
  conditions that affect performance on,
    604–605
  demographic effects, 594–595
  description of, 584
  dyad scoring of, 593, 594f, 597
  fast speech responses required by, 607
  fatigue effects, 606
  Gronwall Version
    administration of, 584
    characteristics of, 583t, 585t
    form for, 587f
    instructions for, 586f
    normative data for, 595t–596t, 595–596
  head injury effects on, 604
  intelligence quotient and, 603
  Levin Version

  administration of, 584–586
  characteristics of, 583t, 585t
  form for, 588f–589f
  normative data, 596–597, 597t, 600t
  limitations of, 606
  malingering detection using, 606
  mathematical ability correlated with
    performance on, 603–604
  modalities, 606–607
  mood effects, 605–606
  in multiple sclerosis patients, 604–605
  neuroanatomic correlates of, 605
  normative data, 595–597
  postconcussion syndrome identified using, 604
  practice effects on, 597–598, 601
  processing speed estimations, 607
  purpose of, 582
  reliability of, 597–598, 601
  scoring of, 593–594, 594f, 607
  short forms, 597, 600t
  source of, 582, 583t
  summary of, 606–607
  versions of, 583t, 584, 601, 606
  visual version of, 601
Paced Visual Serial Addition Test (PVSAT), 583t
Peabody Picture Vocabulary Test—Revised
    (PPVT-R)
  in children, 942
  PPVT-III vs., 941, 945, 949–950
Peabody Picture Vocabulary Test—Third Edition
    (PPVT-III)
  administration of, 941–942
  age range for, 940
  autism assessments, 950–951
  background of, 940
  characteristics of, 892t
  clinical studies of, 948–949
  demographic effects, 942–944
  ethnicity effects, 942–944
  EVT vs., 932–933
  language tests correlated with, 946
  mental retardation assessments, 949
  non-language domains correlated with,
    946–947
  normative data, 944, 944t
  overview of, 940–941
  PPVT-R vs., 941, 945, 949–950
  practice effects, 945
  in premorbid estimation, 948
  purposes of, 940–941
  receptive-expressive discrepancies, 946
  reliability of, 944–945
  scoring of, 942
  source of, 940
  standardization sample for, 944, 944t
  summary of, 949–951
  validity of, 945–949
Personality Assessment Inventory (PAI)
  administration of, 1128, 1132
  age range for, 1126
  characteristics of, 1081t
  demographic effects, 1128–1129
  description of, 1080, 1126, 1128
  distortion indicators, 1130–1132, 1131t
  factor-analytic findings, 1130
  MMPI-2 vs., 1083
  neuropsychological studies of, 1130

  overreporting on, 1131
  purpose of, 1126
  reliability of, 1129
  scales, 1127t
  self-report validity, 1130–1132
  source of, 1126
  subscales, 1127t
  substance abuse evaluations, 1132
  summary of, 1132
  validity of, 1130–1132
Philadelphia Geriatric Multilevel Assessment
    Instrument, 1109
Phonemic fluency (Verbal Fluency Test)
  administration of, 502f
  in adolescents, 512–513
  in children, 512–513
  demographic effects, 503
  description of, 499–500
  normative data, 506, 508
  semantic fluency vs., 512
Primary Mental Abilities test, 521
Purdue Pegboard Test
  administration of, 1068
  characteristics of, 1042t
  in children, 1069–1070, 1072t–1076t
  demographic effects, 1069
  description of, 1068
  factor-analytic studies of, 1077
  neurological conditions that affect, 1077
  normative data, 1069–1070, 1070t
  practice effects, 1076
  purpose of, 1068
  reliability of, 1070, 1076, 1078
  scoring of, 1068–1069
  source of, 1068
  summary of, 1078
  validity of, 1077

Raven's Progressive Matrices
  administration of, 231
  Advanced Progressive Matrices
    description of, 229–231
    normative data, 232
    reliability of, 233
  age effects on, 231
  age range for, 229
  Alzheimer's disease and, 234
  characteristics of, 102t
  Colored Progressive Matrices
    description of, 229–230
    example of, 230f
    normative data, 232, 232t
    reliability of, 233
  demographic effects, 231
  description of, 229–231
  gender effects on, 231
  indications for, 103
  neurological conditions that affect, 234
  purpose of, 229
  scoring of, 231
  source of, 229
  Standard Progressive Matrices
    description of, 229–230
    example of, 229f
    malingering detection, 234–235
    normative data, 231–232
    reliability of, 233

summary of, 235–236
validity of, 233–235
visual field defects and, 234
Recognition Memory Test (RMT)
administration of, 769
age range for, 769
characteristics of, 682t
clinical studies of, 772–773
dementia diagnosis using, 774
demographic effects, 770
description of, 769
evaluation of amnesia, 772–773
laterality of disturbance and, 773
limitations of, 774
malingering detection using, 774
normative data, 770, 770t
perceptual abilities' effect on, 773
practice effects, 772
psychiatric disorders' effect on, 773
purpose of, 769
reliability of, 771–772
scoring of, 769–770
source of, 769
standardization sample, 770
summary of, 774–775
validity of, 772–775
Repeatable Battery for the Assessment of
    Neuropsychological Status (RBANS)
administration of, 238
age effects, 239
age range for, 237
Alzheimer's disease effects on, 254
assessments of change, 244–246
characteristics of, 102t
clinical studies of, 252, 254, 256–257
demographic effects, 239
demographically adjusted normative data
    for, 243
description of, 104, 237–238
education effects, 239
ethnicity effects, 239
gender effects, 239
indices of, 238t
limitations of, 257
neurological conditions that affect, 252, 254
normative data, 239–244, 240t–244t
Parkinson's disease effects on, 254, 256
psychiatric screenings, 256
purpose of, 237
reliability of, 244–248
scoring of
    description of, 238–239
    score conversions, 242t–249t
source of, 237
subtests of, 238t, 240t–244t
summary of, 257
validity of, 249–257
Rey Auditory Verbal Learning Test (RAVLT)
administration of, 779, 784f
in adults, 786–794
age range for, 776
alternate forms, 779, 780f–782f
ceiling effects, 806–807
characteristics of, 682t
in children, 794–796
clinical studies of, 801, 804–805
conditions that affect, 801, 804

demographic effects, 779, 782–783
description of, 776–779, 777f
malingering detection using, 805–806
mental stress effects, 804–805
metanorms, 786t
MOANS scaled scores, 788t–792t
MOANS summary scores, 784t
normative data, 783, 785–794, 806
practice effects, 797–800
purpose of, 776
reliability of, 796–800
scoring of, 777f–778f, 779
source of, 776
summary of, 806–807
validity of, 800–806
WHO/UCLA version of, 783f
within-test relations, 800
Rey Fifteen-Item Memory Test (FIT)
administration of, 1166
in Alzheimer's disease, 1169
characteristics of, 1153t
in children, 1167
demographic effects, 1167
description of, 1152, 1166
efficacy of, 1169
instructions for, 1166f
purpose of, 1166
reliability of, 1167–1168
scoring of, 1166–1167
summary of, 1169–1170
validity of, 1168–1169
variants of, 1166
Rey-Osterrieth Complex Figure Test (ROCF)
administration of, 813, 820, 820f
age range for, 811
alternate figures for, 811, 814f–819f, 836
Beery Developmental Test of Visual Motor
    Integration and, 832
central nervous system disorders' effect on,
    832–833
clinical studies of, 832–834
conditions that affect, 832–834
demographic effects, 826
description of, 811
developmental patterns, 832
factor analysis of, 831
history of, 811
malingering detection using, 834–835
memory ability and, 831
normative data, 827t–829t, 827–829
practice effects, 830
psychiatric disorders' effect on, 833–834
purpose of, 811
reliability of, 829–831, 830t
in schizophrenia, 833
scores and scoring of
    accuracy of, 821, 836
    Bennett-Levy Scoring System, 825
    Boston Qualitative Scoring System,
        824–826, 825t
    Bylsma Scoring System, 825
    Chiulli Scoring System, 825
    description of, 811, 820
    Developmental Scoring System, 821,
        824t, 826
    Hamby Scoring System, 825
    quality of, 821

Rapport Scoring System, 825
Rey Complex Figure Organizational
    Strategy Score, 821, 823
Savage Scoring System, 825
systems for, 820–821
Taylor criteria, 821, 822f–823f
source of, 811
summary of, 835–836
three-minute recall, 813, 820
traumatic brain injury effects, 834
validity of, 831–835
visuomotor ability and, 831
Right-Left Orientation (RLO), 1012t, 1017–1020
Rivermead Assessment of Somatosensory
    Performance (RASP), 1012t, 1020–1023
Rivermead Behavioural Memory Test—
    Children's Version (RBMT-C)
for children, 844–845
description of, 841
scoring of, 843
standardization sample for, 844–845
tasks, 842t
Rivermead Behavioural Memory Test—E
    (RBMT-E)
conditions that affect performance on, 848
description of, 841
scoring of, 843
summary of, 849
tasks, 842t
Rivermead Behavioural Memory Test—Second
    Edition (RBMT-II)
administration of, 842
age range for, 841
Alzheimer's disease effects, 847
characteristics of, 683t
in children, 849
clinical studies of, 847–848
demographic effects, 843
description of, 841
disorders that affect, 847
expressive language disorders' effect on, 848
factor analytic findings, 847
MMSE and, 847
modifications for mobility-impaired
    individuals, 849
mood disorders that affect, 848
normative data, 843–844, 844t–845t
purpose of, 841
reliability of, 845–847
scoring of, 842–843
source of, 841
standardization sample for, 843–844
summary of, 848–849
Ruff 2 & 7 Selective Attention Test (2 & 7 Test)
administration of, 610–611
age range for, 610
attention tests correlated with, 614
characteristics of, 548t
clinical studies of, 614
demographic effects, 612
description of, 610
diagnostic utility of, 614–615, 615t
factor structure of, 614
limitations of, 615–616
neuropsychological tests correlated with, 614
normative data, 612, 612t–613t
practice effects on, 613–614

Ruff 2 & 7 (*continued*)
  psychometric properties of, 615
  purpose of, 610
  reliability of, 612–614, 613*t*
  scoring of, 611*t*, 611–612
  source of, 610
  standardization sample for, 612
  summary of, 615–616
  validity of, 614–615, 615*t*
Ruff Figural Fluency Test (RFFT)
  administration of, 466
  age range for, 466
  characteristics of, 403*t*–404*t*
  clinical studies of, 469
  demographic effects, 467
  description of, 456, 459, 466
  factor-analytic findings, 469
  neurological conditions that affect, 469
  normative data, 467, 470
  phonemic fluency and, 469
  practice effects on, 468
  purpose of, 466
  reliability of, 467–468, 470
  scoring of, 466
  source of, 466
  summary of, 470
Ruff-Light Trail Learning Test (RULIT)
  administration of, 851
  age range for, 851
  characteristics of, 683*t*
  clinical studies of, 853–854
  components of, 851–852, 852*t*
  demographic effects, 852
  factor analytic findings, 853
  neuropsychological tests correlated with, 853
  normative data, 852–854
  purpose of, 851
  reliability of, 853–854
  scoring of, 851–852, 852*t*
  source of, 851
  standardization sample for, 852–853, 853*t*
  stimulus card, 851, 851*f*
  summary of, 854

Scales of Independent Behavior—Revised (SIB-R)
  administration of, 1135, 1137
  advantages of, 1139
  age range for, 1134
  characteristics of, 1082*t*
  clusters, 1135*t*
  demographic effects, 1137
  description of, 1083, 1134
  Full Scale, 1134
  Maladaptive Behavior Indices, 1139
  normative data, 1137–1139
  Problem Behavior Scale, 1134–1135
  purpose of, 1134
  reliability of, 1138–1139
  scoring of, 1137
  Short Form, 1134
  source of, 1134
  standardization sample for, 1137–1138
  structure of, 1136*f*
  subscales, 1135*t*
  summary of, 1139–1140
  validity of, 1138–1139
  WJ-R and, 1138

Self-Ordered Pointing Test (SOPT)
  administration of, 472
  age range for, 471
  characteristics of, 404*t*
  in children, 473
  clinical studies of, 475–476
  demographic effects, 473
  description of, 471
  executive function measures and, 475
  frontal lobe lesions effect on, 475–476
  normative data, 473
  purpose of, 471
  reliability of, 474, 476
  scoring of, 472–473, 474*f*
  source of, 471
  summary of, 476
Semantic fluency (Verbal Fluency Test)
  administration of, 502*f*
  dementia detection using, 519
  description of, 500–501
  normative data, 508–510
  phonemic fluency vs., 512
  summary of, 521
  validity of, 521
Sentence Repetition Test
  administration of, 857
  age range for, 854
  characteristics of, 683*t*
  clinical studies of, 858–859
  demographic effects, 857
  description of, 854, 857
  forms, 854, 855*f*–856*f*
  instructions for, 857*f*
  normative data, 858
  purpose of, 854
  reliability of, 858
  scoring of, 857
  source of, 854
  summary of, 859
  validity of, 858–859
Smell Identification Test (SIT)
  administration of, 1024
  age range for, 1023
  in Alzheimer's disease patients, 1027
  characteristics of, 1012*t*
  clinical studies of, 1027
  demographic effects, 1024
  description of, 1023–1024
  lexical functioning and, 1027
  malingering detection using, 1028
  neuroanatomical correlates of, 1026–1027
  normative data, 1024–1025
  purpose of, 1023
  reliability of, 1026, 1028
  scoring of, 1024
  short forms, 1028
  source of, 1023
  standardization sample for, 1024–1025
  summary of, 1028–1029
  validity of, 1026–1028
Speed and Capacity of Language Processing Test (SCOLP)
  administration of, 273
  age range for, 272
  description of, 272–273
  normative data, 273–274
  purpose of, 272

  scoring of, 273
  source of, 272
  Speed of Comprehension Test
    demographic effects, 273
    description of, 272–273
    neurological conditions that affect, 277
    normative data, 274
    reliability of, 274–275
    scaled scores for, 275*t*
    validity of, 276
  Spot-the-Word test
    Boston Naming test and, 274, 278*t*
    Controlled Oral Word Association test and, 274, 278*t*
    demographic effects, 273
    description of, 108, 272–273
    neurological conditions that affect, 277
    normative data, 274
    reliability of, 275–276
    validity of, 276–278
  standardization sample for, 273–274
  summary of, 278–279
Standard Progressive Matrices (Raven's Progressive Matrices)
  description of, 229–230
  example of, 229*f*
  malingering detection, 234–235
  normative data, 231–232
  reliability of, 233
Stanford-Binet Intelligence Scales—Fifth Edition (SB5)
  Abbreviated Battery IQ, 265
  ability-achievement discrepancies, 260, 267
  achievement and, correlation between, 266
  administration of, 260, 262*f*, 266–267
  age effects, 262
  age range for, 258
  characteristics of, 102*t*
  clinical studies of, 266
  components of, 259*f*
  demographic effects, 262
  description of, 101
  format of, 266–267
  Full-Scale IQ (FSIQ)
    demographics used to estimate scores in, 105
    description of, 259–260
    premorbid estimations and, 104
  history of, 258*f*
  intelligence tests correlated with, 265–266
  Nonverbal IQ, 259*f*, 267
  normative data, 262–263, 263*t*
  overview of, 258–259
  purpose of, 258
  reliability of, 263–264, 264*t*
  SB-IV and, correlation between, 265
  scoring of, 260
  source of, 258
  standardization sample for, 262–263
  structure of, 259–260
  subtests of, 261*t*
  summary of, 266–267
  validity of, 264–266
  Verbal IQ, 259*f*
Stroop Test
  age range for, 477
  characteristics of, 404*t*

clinical studies of, 493–494
Comalli Version, 478
demographic effects, 479, 481
depression effects on, 494
description of, 477–478
error analysis of, 496
Golden Version
    administration of, 479
    in adults, 481, 484
    in children, 484, 490
    description of, 477–478
    normative data, 481, 484, 485t–490t, 490
    scoring of, 479
    standardization sample, 481
interference, 493, 496
malingering and, 495
neuroanatomical correlates, 494–495
practice effects, 490
purpose of, 477
reading effects on, 495
reliability of, 490, 492
source of, 477
summary of, 495–496
tests correlated with, 492–493
time-of-day effects, 495–496
versions of, 477–478, 495–496
Victoria
    administration of, 479
    advantages of, 478
    description of, 477–478
    normative data, 481, 482t–483t
    scoring of, 479, 480f
visual function and, 495–496
working memory effects, 492
Symbol Digit Modalities Test (SDMT)
    age range for, 617
    alternate forms of, 617, 621f–622f
    attention tests correlated with, 624–625
    change assessments, 622–623
    characteristics of, 548t, 618t
    clinical studies of, 625
    demographic effects, 618
    description of, 617
    in Huntington's disease patients, 625
    incidental recall version of, 617
    malingering, 626
    in multiple sclerosis patients, 625
    normative data, 618–620, 626
    practice effects, 622
    purpose of, 617
    reliability of, 620, 622–623
    scoring of, 617
    source of, 617
    standardization sample for, 618t, 618–620
    summary of, 626
    traumatic brain injury effects, 625
    validity of, 623–626

Tactual Performance Test (TPT)
    administration of, 1031–1032, 1032f
    in adolescents, 1034
    characteristics of, 1012t
    in children, 1034
    clinical studies of, 1037–1038
    criticisms of, 1038–1039
    demographic effects, 1033–1034
    description of, 1031

instructions for, 1032f
metanorms, 1034t–1035t
neurological conditions that affect, 1037–1038
normative data, 1034–1036
practice effects, 1036–1037
purpose of, 1031
reliability of, 1036–1037, 1039
scoring of, 1032–1033
source of, 1031
summary of, 1038–1039
validity of, 1037–1038
Test of Everyday Attention for Children
    (TEA-Ch)
    achievement and, 643
    administration of, 638–640
    age range for, 638
    in attention deficit hyperactivity disorder
        patients, 643
    attention tests correlated with, 642–643
    ceiling effects, 644
    characteristics of, 549t
    clinical studies of, 643
    demographic effects, 640
    description of, 638
    floor effects, 644
    intelligence quotient and, 642
    normative data, 640–641, 641t
    practice effects on, 641–642
    purpose of, 638
    reliability of, 641–642, 644
    scoring of, 640
    source of, 638
    in special populations, 640
    standardization sample for, 640, 641t
    subtests of, 639t
    summary of, 643–644
    validity of, 642–644
Test of Everyday Attention (TEA)
    administration of, 629–630
    advantages of, 629
    attention measures correlated with, 633
    ceiling effects, 636
    characteristics of, 549t
    clinical studies of, 634–635
    closed head injury effects on performance, 634
    demographic effects, 630–631
    description of, 628–629
    floor effects, 636
    Hong Kong version of, 634
    NART and, correlation between, 634
    normative data, 631–632
    practice effects, 633
    psychometric limitations of, 636
    reliability of, 632–633, 633t
    scoring of, 630
    standardization sample for, 631, 631t
    stroke effects on performance, 634
    subtests, 629
    summary of, 636–637
    in traumatic brain injury patients, 634, 635t
    validity of, 633–635
Test of Memory Malingering (TOMM)
    administration of, 1172
    age range for, 1171
    characteristics of, 1153t
    in children, 1172

clinical findings of, 1173–1174
demographic effects, 1172
description of, 1152, 1154, 1171–1172
learning trials, 1171
mood disorders' effect on, 1175
motivational defects effect on, 1174–1175
normative data, 1172
psychological distress and, 1174
purpose of, 1171
reliability of, 1172–1173
scoring of, 1172
source of, 1171
standardization sample for, 1172
summary of, 1175
validity of, 1173–1175
Test of Nonverbal Intelligence—3 (TONI-3)
    achievement and, correlation between, 271
    administration of, 269
    age range for, 268
    characteristics of, 102t
    clinical studies of, 271
    demographic effects, 269
    description of, 268
    ethnicity effects, 269
    floor effects on, 271
    indications for, 103
    intelligence quotient tests correlated with,
        270–271
    limitations of, 271
    normative data, 269
    psychometric properties of, 271–272
    purpose of, 268
    reliability of, 269–270
    scoring of, 269
    source of, 268
    summary of, 271–272
    validity of, 270–271
Test of Variables of Attention (T.O.V.A.)
    administration of, 646
    advantages of, 652
    age range for, 645
    in attention deficit hyperactivity disorder
        patients, 651
    attention rating scales correlated with,
        650–651
    characteristics of, 549t
    clinical studies of, 651–652
    demographic effects, 647
    description of, 645
    factor structure, 649–650
    normative data, 647t–648t, 647–648
    psychometric properties of, 652–653
    purpose of, 645
    rating scales, 645
    reliability of, 648–649
    scoring of, 646
    source of, 645
    standardization sample for, 647–648
    validity of, 649–652
3MS. See also Mini-Mental State Examination
    (MMSE)
    children's version of, 179–180
    description of, 169
    illustration of, 170f–174f
    modifications to, 185
    normative data for, 177
    reliability of, 182

Token Test (TT)
  administration of, 954
  advantages of, 960
  age range for, 953
  in Alzheimer's disease, 959
  aphasia evaluations, 959
  in children, 957
  clinical studies of, 959
  demographic effects, 954, 956–957
  description of, 891, 953–954
  head injury evaluations, 959
  limitations of, 960
  malingering detection using, 960
  MOANS norms, 937t
  NCCEA subtest, 955f–956f
  normative data, 957, 958t
  practice effects, 957
  purpose of, 953
  reliability of, 957
  scoring of, 954
  source of, 953
  summary of, 960
  validity of, 957, 959–960
  Western Aphasia Battery and, 957
Trail Making Test (TMT)
  administration of, 655
  in adolescents, 658, 661
  age range for, 655
  characteristics of, 549t
  in children, 663
  demographic effects, 657–658
  description of, 655
  instructions for, 656f–657f
  malingering detection using, 670
  neuroanatomical correlates, 670
  neurocognitive deficits and, 669–670
  in non-neurological procedures, 670
  normative data, 658–663, 659t–661t
  oral, 657f, 658, 663, 667, 671–672
  practice effects, 666–667
  purpose of, 655
  reliability of, 663, 665–667
  scoring of, 657
  source of, 655
  summary of, 672
  validity of, 668–672
Trauma Symptom Inventory (TSI)
  administration of, 1140
  age range for, 1140
  characteristics of, 1081t
  demographic effects, 1142
  description of, 1080, 1140
  factor-analytic findings, 1142
  malingering detection by, 1143
  normative data, 1142
  posttraumatic stress disorder detected by,
      1140, 1143
  purpose of, 1140
  reliability of, 1142
  scoring of, 1141
  source of, 1140
  standardization sample for, 1142
  summary of, 1143
  validity of, 1141t, 1142–1143
2 & 7 Test. See Ruff 2 & 7 Test
21-Item Test, 1153t, 1176–1178

Verbal Fluency Test
  administration of, 501, 502f–503f
  in adolescents, 512–514
  age range for, 500
  category fluency, 513–514
  characteristics of, 404t
  in children, 512–514
  clinical studies of, 519–520
  clustering/switching scores, 520
  cognitive measures correlated with, 517–518
  demographic effects, 503–505
  depression effects on, 519
  description of, 500–501
  error-based performance evaluations, 502
  fluency tasks correlated with, 517
  frontal lobe lesions effect on, 518
  language versions of, 500
  neuroanatomical correlates, 518
  normative data, 506–514
  performance of, 522
  phonemic fluency
    administration of, 502f
    in adolescents, 512–513
    in children, 512–513
    demographic effects, 503
    description of, 499–500
    normative data, 506, 508
    semantic fluency vs., 512
  practice effects, 514–517
  purpose of, 499
  reliability of, 514–517
  schizophrenia effects on, 519–520
  scoring of, 502–503
  semantic fluency
    administration of, 502f
    dementia detection using, 519
    description of, 500–501
    normative data, 508–510
    phonemic fluency vs., 512
    summary of, 521
    validity of, 521
  source of, 499–500
  summary of, 521–522
  traumatic brain injury effects on, 519
  validity of, 517–521
  written word fluency
    administration of, 503f
    description of, 501–502, 510
    validity of, 521
Victoria Stroop Test (VST)
  administration of, 479
  advantages of, 478
  description of, 477–478
  normative data, 481, 482t–483t
  scoring of, 479, 480f
Victoria Symptom Validity Test (VSVT)
  administration of, 1180
  characteristics of, 1153t
  clinical findings, 1181–1183
  cognitive impairment effects on, 1182
  demographic effects, 1180
  depression effects on, 1182
  description of, 1179–1180
  MMPI-2 and, 1182–1183
  normative data, 1180–1181
  purpose of, 1179

  reliability of, 1181
  scoring of, 1180
  source of, 1179
  summary of, 1183
  validity of, 1181–1183
Visual Object and Space Perception Battery
    (VOSP)
  administration of, 1006
  age range for, 1006
  British norms for, 1011
  characteristics of, 964t
  demographic effects, 1006–1008
  factor analytic findings, 1010–1011
  normative data, 1008–1009, 1009t
  practice effects, 1009–1010
  purpose of, 1006
  reliability of, 1009–1010
  source of, 1006
  standardization sample for, 1008–1009
  summary of, 1010–1011
  tasks, 1007t
  validity of, 1010

Warrington Recognition Memory Test. See
    Recognition Memory Test (RMT)
Wechsler Abbreviated Scale of Intelligence
    (WASI)
  administration of, 280
  characteristics of, 103t
  demographic effects, 280
  description of, 101, 279–280
  history of, 311f
  Kaufman Brief Intelligence Test and,
      correlation between, 166
  normative data, 281
  purpose of, 279
  reliability of, 281
  scoring of, 280
  summary of, 282–283
  validity of, 281–282
  WIAT and, 282
Wechsler Adult Intelligence Scale—Revised
    (WAIS-R)
  Finger Tapping and, 1048
  Freedom from Distractibility factor, 603
  Kaufman Brief Intelligence Test and,
      correlation between, 166
  National Adult Reading Test standardized
      for, 190
  scores
    North American Adult Reading Test 35
        equations for predicting, 193
    North American Adult Reading Test
        equations for predicting, 193–195
Wechsler Adult Intelligence Scale—III
    (WAIS-III)
  administration of, 285–286, 288
  age range for, 283
  basals, 289
  Canadian norms, 294, 307
  assessment of change, 296–298
  clinical findings, 300
  data reporting, 307
  demographic effects, 289, 291
  description of, 101, 283–285
  Digit Symbol, 301

discrepancies, 302
education effects and, 289, 291
ethnicity effects, 293–294, 305–306
factor-analytic findings, 299–300
Full-Scale IQ, 286*t*, 298, 305
gender effects, 293
General Ability Index, 286, 287*t*
history of, 311*f*
Incidental Learning scores, 301
interpretation of, 301
Letter-Number Sequencing task, 285
malingering, 303, 305
Matrix Reasoning subtest of, 101
normative data, 291, 293–294, 305
Oklahoma Premorbid Intelligence Estimate
    and, 109
practice effects on, 295–296, 306
premorbid estimation of intellectual ability,
    302–303
profile analysis, 301–302
purpose of, 283
reliability of, 294–298
Reliable Digit Span score, 305
revisions, 306–307
scores and scoring of, 109*t*, 288–289
short forms, 285–286, 305
socioeconomic status effects and, 289, 291
source of, 283
standardization sample for, 291, 293–294
strengths of, 305
structure of, 284*t*
subtests of, 284, 284*t*, 300
summary of, 305–307
traumatic brain injury effects, 300
validity of, 298–305
Vocabulary and Block Design, 285
WAIS-R vs., 283–284, 298
WISC-III vs., 298
WISC-IV vs., 298
WMS-III and, relationship between, 873
Wechsler Individual Achievement Test (WIAT)
    changes to, 371
    NEPSY and, correlation between, 212
    WASI and, 282
    WIAT-III vs., 379
Wechsler Individual Achievement Test—Second
        Edition (WIAT-III)
    ability-achievement discrepancy analysis, 371,
        376*t*, 382
    administration of, 371, 373
    with adolescents, 382
    with adults, 382
    age bands, 373, 375
    age range for, 371
    ceiling effects, 381
    clinical groups assessed using, 380–381
    floor effects, 381–382
    intelligence tests correlated with, 378–379
    language assessments, 383
    limitations of, 381
    normative data, 375–376, 381
    overview of, 364*t*, 371
    Parent Report, 383
    practice effects, 377–378
    preschooler evaluations, 381–382
    purpose of, 370

Qualitative Observations checklist, 375*f*
Reading Comprehension subtest, 383
reliability of, 376–378
school grades correlated with, 379–380
school-age children evaluations, 382
scoring of, 373, 375
source of, 370
subtests, 372*t*–373*t*
summary of, 381–383
supplemental scores, 382–383
usability of, 381
validity of, 378–381
WIAT vs., 371, 374*t*–375*t*, 379
WJ-R correlations with, 379
Wechsler Intelligence Scale for Children—Third
        Edition (WISC-III)
    Cognitive Assessment System and, correlation
        between, 141
    Full-Scale IQ, 270
    Kaufman Brief Intelligence Test and, correla-
        tion between, 166
    NEPSY and, correlation between, 212
    SB5 and, correlation between, 265
    WAIS-III vs., 298
    WISC-IV vs., 313*t*, 335–336
    WPPSI-III vs., 344
Wechsler Intelligence Scale for Children—Fourth
        Edition (WISC-IV)
    ability-achievement comparisons, 317,
        319*t*–322*t*
    ability-memory comparisons, 317, 323*t*–331*t*
    achievement and, 335
    administration of, 314
    age range for, 311
    characteristics of, 103*t*
    clinical studies of, 335–336
    CMS, 323*t*–330*t*
    demographic effects, 317–318
    description of, 101, 311–314
    factor structure, 334–335
    Full-Scale IQ
        CMS composite scores predicted from,
            323*t*–326*t*
        description of, 314, 317
    General Ability Index
        description of, 312, 316*t*, 319*t*
        WIAT-II subtests and, differences between,
            320*t*–322*t*
    index scores on, 311, 311*t*
    limitations of, 336
    memory function and, 335
    normative data, 319, 322, 331
    Perceptual Reasoning Index, 311, 311*t*
    practice effects on, 332
    process scores, 312, 314*t*
    Processing Speed Index
        CMS composite scores predicted from,
            329*t*–330*t*
        description of, 311, 311*t*
        intercorrelations, 333–334, 334*t*
    purpose of, 310
    reliability of, 331–332
    score conversions, 319, 322, 331
    scoring of, 314, 317
    sensitivity of, 336
    source of, 310

structure of, 312
subtests of
    description of, 312, 313*t*
    intercorrelations among, 333–334, 334*t*
    specificity, 334
summary of, 336
validity of, 332–336
Verbal Comprehension Index
    CMS composite scores predicted from,
        327*t*–328*t*
    description of, 311*t*, 311–312
    intercorrelations, 333–334, 334*t*
    WAIS-III vs., 298, 335
    WIAT-II and, 312
    WISC-III vs., 313*t*, 335–336
Working Memory Index
    description of, 311, 311*t*
    intercorrelations, 334
    limitations of, 336
    WPPSI-III vs., 335
Wechsler Intelligence Scale for Children—
        Revised (WISC-R), 166
Wechsler Intelligence Scales, 311*f*. *See also specific
        scales*
Wechsler Memory Scale—Revised (WMS-R), 759
Wechsler Memory Scale—Third Edition
        (WMS-III)
    Abbreviated, 860
    ability-memory discrepancies, 865
    administration of, 862–863
    advantages of, 878
    age range for, 860
    aging effects, 874–875
    Auditory Recognition Delayed Index, 878
    ceiling effects, 878
    characteristics of, 683*t*
    clinical studies of, 874
    CMS and, correlation between, 751–752
    demographic effects, 863
    description of, 860, 862
    discrepancy data, 864–868
    factor structure of, 871, 873
    floor effects, 878
    laterality of disturbance effects, 874
    malingering detection using, 876–877
    memory indices, 873–874
    neurological disorders that affect, 874
    normative data, 864–868
    practice effects, 868–869
    premorbid memory functioning predictions,
        876
    prorated versions of, 862
    purpose of, 860
    regression equations, 872*t*
    reliability of, 868–870, 869*t*–870*t*
    Reliable Change Index, 869, 872*t*, 876–877
    scoring of, 863
    short forms, 860, 862
    source of, 860
    standardization sample for, 864
    subtests of
        description of, 860*t*–861*t*, 860–862
        Digital Span, 861*t*, 875–876, 878
        discrepancy data for, 865, 868
        Faces, 861*t*, 875, 877
        Family Pictures, 861*t*, 875

Wechsler Memory Scale (*continued*)
    intercorrelations among, 870–871
      scores, 869*t*
      Spatial Span, 861*t*, 875–876, 878
      summary of, 878
      Word Lists, 861*t*, 876
    summary of, 877–878
    validity of, 870–877
    verbal memory deficits assessed using, 874
    WAIS-III and, relationship between, 873
    Working Memory Index, 878
Wechsler Preschool and Primary Scale of
        Intelligence—Revised (WPPSI-R)
    SB5 and, correlation between, 265
    WPPSI-III vs., 338*t*, 343, 346
Wechsler Preschool and Primary Scale of
        Intelligence—Third Edition (WPPSI-III)
    ability-achievement comparisons, 341
    achievement correlations, 344
    administration of, 339
    age bands, 345–346
    age range for, 337
    breadth of, 345–346
    BSID-II vs., 346
    Carroll-Horn-Cattell theory and, 338
    ceiling effects, 346
    characteristics of, 103*t*
    clinical studies of, 344–345
    demographic effects, 341–342
    description of, 101, 337–339
    factor structure, 345
    floor effects, 346
    Full-Scale IQ, 339, 346
    interpretation of, 341
    limitations of, 345
    normative data, 342
    purpose of, 337
    reliability of, 342, 343*t*
    score conversions, 342
    scoring of, 339–341
    source of, 337
    standardization sample for, 342
    structure of, 338*f*
    subtests
      description of, 338–339, 340*t*
      intercorrelations among, 343
      specificity of, 343–344
      substitution of, 346
    summary of, 345–346
    validity of, 343–345
    WISC-III vs., 344
    WISC-IV vs., 335, 344
    WPPSI-R vs., 338*t*, 343, 346
Wechsler Test of Adult Reading (WTAR), 108,
      347–351
Western Aphasia Battery (WAB), 957
Wide Range Achievement Test—3 (WRAT-3)
    achievement tests correlated with, 387
    administration of, 384–385
    age range for, 384
    ceiling effects, 389
    clinical studies of, 387–388
    cross-cultural use of, 389
    demographic effects, 385
    description of, 384
    floor effects, 389
    as "hold" test, 388

intelligence quotient and, 387
literacy measurements, 388
normative data, 385, 386*t*
overview of, 364*t*
premorbid intelligence estimations using, 388
psychometric issues, 389
purpose of, 384
reading subtest of, 108
reliability of, 385–386
scoring of, 385
source of, 384
summary of, 389
Wide Range Assessment of Memory and
      Learning (WRAML)
    characteristics of, 683*t*
    CMS and, 752
Wide Range Assessment of Memory and
      Learning—Second Edition (WRAML2)
    achievement and, 888
    age range for, 881
    clinical studies of, 888
    CMS and, 752
    demographic effects, 883
    description of, 881–882
    floor effects, 889
    intellectual ability and, 888
    limitations of, 889
    memory scales correlated with, 887
    normative data, 883, 885*t*
    practice effects, 885
    purpose of, 881
    reliability of, 883–885, 886*t*
    scoring of, 882–883
    source of, 881
    standardization sample for, 883, 885*t*
    structure of, 881–882, 882*f*
    subtests, 884*t*, 887
    summary of, 888–889
    validity of, 885, 887–888
Wisconsin Card Sorting Test (WCST)
    administration of, 527–528
    age range for, 526
    aging-related declines and, 536
    Brixton Spatial Anticipation Test based on, 460
    Category Test vs., 433–434
    characteristics of, 404*t*
    in children, 530–531, 531*t*–532*t*, 533, 537
    clinical studies of, 536–537
    computer-administered versions of, 527, 539
    conceptual processing measurements, 535
    Delis-Kaplan Executive Function System
      and, 448
    demographic effects, 529
    description of, 526–528
    executive function measures correlated with,
      535–536
    Failure to Maintain Set scores, 8
    frontal lobe dysfunction effects on, 536, 539
    malingering detection using, 538
    modified version of, 527
    mood disorders' effect on, 537
    neuropsychological tests correlated with, 535
    non-normality of, 7
    normative data, 529–531, 530*t*–531*t*
    practice effects, 532
    purpose of, 526
    reliability of, 531–534, 539

schizophrenia effects on, 536–537
scoring of, 528–529
short form, 527, 537–538
source of, 526
standardization sample for, 529–530, 530*t*
summary of, 539
traumatic brain injury effects on, 536, 538
validity of, 534–538
Wisconsin Card Sorting Test-64 (WCST-64), 531,
    537, 539
Woodcock-Johnson—Revised (WJ-R)
    SIB-R and, 1138
    WIAT-III correlations with, 379
    WJ III ACH vs., 392
    WJ III COG vs., 353, 359
Woodcock-Johnson III Tests of Achievement
      (WJ III ACH)
    ability-achievement discrepancies, 267
    administration of, 392, 394, 399
    advantages of, 399
    background of, 391
    Cattell-Horn-Carroll theory and, 391
    characteristics of, 103*t*
    clusters, 392*t*, 399–400
    demographic effects, 396
    intelligence quotient and, 399
    normative data, 396, 399
    overview of, 364*t*
    practice effects, 397–398
    psychometric properties of, 399
    purpose of, 390
    Relative Proficiency Index, 395
    reliability of, 396–398, 398*t*
    scoring of, 394–396
    source of, 390–391
    standardization sample for, 396
    structure of, 391, 391*t*
    subtests, 391–392, 393*t*–394*t*
    summary of, 399–400
    theoretical principles of, 391–392
    validity of, 398–399
    WJ-R vs., 392
Woodcock-Johnson III Tests of Cognitive
      Abilities (WJ III COG)
    achievement and, 359–360
    administration of, 353, 355, 361
    advantages of, 361
    background of, 351
    Carroll-Horn-Cattell theory and, 311,
      351, 352*f*
    categories of, 352*t*
    clinical studies of, 360
    demographic effects, 356–357
    description of, 101
    disadvantages of, 361–362
    factor structure of, 359
    normative data, 357, 361
    practice effects, 357
    purpose of, 351
    reliability of, 357–359
    SB5 and, correlation between, 265–266
    scoring of, 355–356
    semantic fluency tasks, 500
    source of, 351
    standardization sample for, 357
    structure of, 351, 353
    subtests of, 352*t*–355*t*, 361

summary of, 360–362
theoretical principles of, 351, 353
validity of, 359–360
WJ-R vs., 353, 359
Word Fluency Test. *See* Verbal Fluency Test
Word Memory Test (WMT)
    administration of, 1185, 1188
    characteristics of, 1153*t*

demographic effects, 1185
description of, 1184–1185
efficacy criteria for, 1187
mood disorder effects on, 1187
normative data, 1185–1186
purpose of, 1184
reliability of, 1186
scoring of, 1185

source of, 1184
standardization sample for, 1185–1186
summary of, 1187–1188
validity of, 1186–1187
Written word fluency (Verbal Fluency Test)
    administration of, 503*f*
    description of, 501–502, 510
    validity of, 521

Subject Index

Note: page numbers followed by *f* and *t* indicate figures and tables.

Ability-achievement discrepancy
  description of, 363
  Stanford-Binet Intelligence Scales—Fifth
    Edition, 260, 267
  Wechsler Individual Achievement Test—
    Second Edition, 371, 376t, 382
  Wechsler Intelligence Scale for Children—
    Fourth Edition, 317, 319t–322t
  Wechsler Preschool and Primary Scale of
    Intelligence—Third Edition, 341
  WJ III ACH, 267
Acculturation. *See also* Ethnicity, Race
  Boston Naming Test—2 and, 905
  Multilingual Aphasia Examination and, 935
  Token Test and, 956–957
Achievement
  Behavior Rating Inventory of Executive
    Function correlated with, 1096
  Children's Memory Scale and, 752–753
  Cognitive Assessment System and, 142
  Expressive One-Word Picture Vocabulary
    Test—Third Edition and, 926
  Expressive Vocabulary Test and, 931
  Peabody Picture Vocabulary Test—Third
    Edition and, 948
  Stanford-Binet Intelligence Scales—Fifth
    Edition scores and, 266
  Test of Everyday Attention for Children and, 643
  Wechsler Intelligence Scale for Children—
    Fourth Edition and, 335
  Wechsler Preschool and Primary Scale of
    Intelligence—Third Edition and, 344
  Wide Range Assessment of Memory and
    Learning—Second Edition and, 885
  Woodcock-Johnson III Tests of Cognitive
    Abilities and, 359–360
Achievement tests
  clinical uses of, 363
  scoring considerations for, 365
Activities of daily living, 1083, 1107, 1134
Adaptive functioning
  description of, 1083
  tests of, 1082t

ADHD. *See* Attention Deficit Hyperactivity
    Disorder
Adolescents. *See also* Children
  Beck Depression Inventory—Second Edition
    and, 1087
  Brown-Peterson Task and, 704
  Buschke Selective Reminding Test and, 714
  Category Test and, 424
  Comprehensive Trail Making Test and, 557
  Dementia Rating Scale—2 and, 156
  Finger Tapping and, 1046–1047
  Five-Point Test and, 458–459
  Grooved Pegboard and, 1062–1063
  Rivermead Behavioural Memory Test—
    Children's Version and, 844–845
  Symbol digit Modalities Test and, 617
  Tactual Performance Test and, 1034
  Token Test and, 959
  Trail Making Test and, 658, 661
  Verbal Fluency and, 512–517
  Wechsler Adult Intelligence Scale and,
    285, 296
Age
  Beck Depression Inventory—Second Edition
    and, 1085
  Benton Visual Retention Test and, 693
  Boston Diagnostic Aphasia Examination
    and, 895
  Boston Naming Test—2 and, 904
  Brief Test of Attention and, 550
  Brief Visuospatial Memory Test—Revised
    and, 702
  Brixton Spatial Anticipation Test and, 465
  Brown-Peterson Task and, 708–709
  Buschke Selective Reminding Test and, 716
  California Verbal Learning Test—Children's
    Version (CVLT-C) and, 738
  California Verbal Learning Test-II and, 731
  Cambridge Neuropsychological Test
    Automated Batteries and, 416
  Category Test and, 427
  Clock Drawing Test and, 975–976
  Cognitive Estimation Test and, 440

Conners' Continuous Performance Test
    and, 566
Delis-Kaplan Executive Function System
    and, 445
Design Fluency Test and, 453
Dichotic Learning—Words and, 916–917
Expressive One-Word Picture Vocabulary
    Test—Third Edition and, 923
Expressive Vocabulary Test and, 929
Finger Localization and, 1015
Finger Tapping and, 1044
Five-Point Test and, 458
Geriatric Depression Scale and, 1100
Grip Strength and, 1053
Grooved Pegboard and, 1061
Hayling and Brixton Tests and, 461
Hooper Visual Organization Test and, 991
Hopkins Verbal Learning Test—Revised
    and, 760
Instrumental Activities of Daily Living and, 1109
Integrated Visual and Auditory Continuous
    Performance Test and, 577–578
Judgment of Line Orientation and, 998
Kaplan Baycrest Neurocognitive Assessment
    and, 161
Kaufman Brief Intelligence Test and, 165
MMSE and, 176, 178t–179t
Multilingual Aphasia Examination and, 935
Paced Auditory Serial Addition Test and,
    594–595
Peabody Picture Vocabulary Test—Third
    Edition (PPVT-III) and, 942
Personality Assessment Inventory and, 1128
Purdue Pegboard Test and, 1069
Recognition Memory Test and, 770
Repeatable Battery for the Assessment of
    Neuropsychological Status and, 239
Rey Auditory Verbal Learning Test and, 782
Rey Fifteen-Item Memory Test and, 1167
Rey-Osterrieth Complex Figure Test and, 826
Right-Left Orientation and, 1018
Rivermead Behavioural Memory Test—Second
    Edition (RBMT-II) and, 843

Ruff 2 & 7 Selective Attention Test and, 612
Ruff Figural Fluency Test and, 467
Scales of Independent Behavior—Revised
    and, 1137
Self-Ordered Pointing Test and, 473
Sentence Repetition Test and, 858
Smell Identification Test and, 1024
Stanford-Binet Intelligence Scales—Fifth
    Edition and, 262
Stroop Test and, 479, 481
Tactual Performance Test and, 1033
Test of Everyday Attention for Children
    and, 640
Test of Memory Malingering and, 1172
Test of Nonverbal Intelligence—3 and, 269
Test of Variables of Attention and, 647
Token Test and, 954, 956–957
Trail Making Test and, 658
21-Item Test and, 1177
Verbal Fluency Test and, 503–504
Visual Object and Space Perception Battery
    and, 1006–1007
Wechsler Adult Intelligence Scale—III and,
    289
Wechsler Memory Scale—Third Edition and,
    863, 874–875
Wechsler Test of Adult Reading and, 348
Wide Range Achievement Test—3 and, 385
Wide Range Assessment of Memory and
    Learning—Second Edition and, 883
Wisconsin Card Sorting Test and, 529, 536
Woodcock-Johnson III Tests of Achievement
    and, 396
Woodcock-Johnson III Tests of Cognitive
    Abilities and, 356
Word Memory Test and, 1185
Age bands, 48
Age range, 47
Aging, 422, 448, 464–465, 475, 493, 536, 670, 711,
    804, 874, 988, 1027, 1057
Alcohol use, 297, 350, 412, 422, 442, 464, 469,
    493, 536, 651, 669, 669, 698, 711, 753, 833,
    848, 888, 988, 1027, 1038, 1048, 1186
Alternate form reliability
    of Benton Visual Retention Test, 696–697
    of Boston Diagnostic Aphasia Examination, 896
    of Brief Test of Attention, 552
    of Brief Visuospatial Memory Test—Revised,
        703
    of Buschke Selective Reminding Test, 724
    of California Verbal Learning Test-II, 732–733,
        733t
    of Children's Color Trails Test, 556
    definition of, 12
    of Delis-Kaplan Executive Function System,
        446, 449
    of Dementia Rating Scale-2, 150
    of Geriatric Depression Scale, 1102
    of Gray Oral Reading Tests—Fourth Edition,
        368, 370
    of Hopkins Verbal Learning Test—Revised
        (HVLT-R), 762, 765
    of Multilingual Aphasia Examination, 937
    of Peabody Picture Vocabulary Test—Third
        Edition, 945
    of Repeatable Battery for the Assessment of
        Neuropsychological Status, 246–248

of Rey Auditory Verbal Learning Test, 797
of Rey-Osterrieth Complex Figure Test,
    830–831
of Rivermead Behavioural Memory Test—
    Children's Version, 846
of Rivermead Behavioural Memory Test—
    Second Edition, 845
of Ruff-Light Trail Learning Test, 853
of Sentence Repetition Test, 858
for speed tests, 10
of Stroop Test, 492
of Symbol Digit Modalities Test, 623
of Test of Everyday Attention for Children, 642
of Test of Nonverbal Intelligence—3, 269–272
of Trail Making Test, 667
of Verbal Fluency Test, 516–517
of Wide Range Achievement Test—3, 386
of Wisconsin Card Sorting Test, 534
of Woodcock-Johnson III Tests of
    Achievement, 398
Alzheimer's disease. See also Dementia
    anomia in, 911
    Autobiographical Memory Interview in
        patients with, 689–690
    Benton Visual Retention Test for detection of,
        698
    Biber Cognitive Estimation Test and, 442
    Boston Diagnostic Aphasia Examination in
        patients with, 898–899
    Boston Naming Test—2 in patients with, 911
    Brief Visuospatial Memory Test—Revised
        and, 704
    CANTAB and, 421
    Clock Drawing Test for evaluation of, 978–979
    Cognitive Estimation Test and, 442
    Dementia Rating Scale-2 for, 153–155
    description of, 155
    Dichotic Listening and, 919
    D-KEFS and, 448
    Doors and People Test and, 759
    Facial Recognition Test and, 988
    Hayling and Brixton Test and, 464
    Hopkins Verbal Learning Test—Revised
        (HVLT-R) performance and, 766–767
    Judgement of Line Orientation Test and, 1003
    MMSE and, 183–184
    National Adult Reading Test performance
        and, 197
    Raven's Progressive Matrices and, 234
    Recognition Memory Test and, 773
    Repeatable Battery for the Assessment of
        Neuropsychological Status performance
        and, 254
    Rey Auditory Verbal Learning Test and,
        804–805
    Rey Fifteen-Item Memory Test in patients
        with, 1168
    Rey Osterrieth Complex Figure Test and, 832
    Rivermead Behavioural Memory Test—Second
        Edition and, 845–847
    Ruff Figural Fluency and, 469
    screening for, 155, 183–185
    Smell Identification Test in patients with, 1027
    Token Test in patients with, 959
    Wechsler Adult Intelligence Scale—III and,
        297, 301
    Wechsler Memory Scale-III and, 874

Wechsler Test of Adult Reading and, 350
Wide Range Achievement Test—3 and, 388
Wide Range Assessment of Memory and
    Learning—2 and, 888
American Psychological Association, 75
Anoxia, 911
Anterior communicating artery aneurysm, 442,
    801, 832, 919, 1181
Anxiety, 81, 605, 734, 804, 834, 848, 1086. See also
    Posttraumatic stress disorder, Depression,
    Psychiatric Disorder
Aphasia
    Boston Diagnostic Aphasia Examination
        evaluations, 895
    Dichotic Listening Test, 926
    Facial Recognition Test, 987
    Multilingual Aphasia Examination, 938
    Raven's Progressive Matrices, 234
    Right-Left Orientation Test, 1019
    Sentence Repetition, 859
    Test of Memory Malingering, 1173
    Token Test evaluations, 959
    Verbal Fluency, 519
Apperceptive agnosia, 963
Area under the normal curve, 4
Assessment of Reliable Change. See Reliable
    Change Index
Attention
    deficits in, 547
    description of, 546
    models of, 546
    processes involved in, 546
    working memory and, 546
Attention deficit hyperactivity disorder
    Beck Depression Inventory-II, 1088
    Behavior Rating Inventory of Executive
        Function for screening of, 1096
    Behavioral Assessment of the Dysexecutive
        Syndrome, 412–413
    Brief Test of Attention, 556
    Brown-Peterson Task, 711
    California Verbal Learning Test—Children's
        Version, 744
    CANTAB, 422
    Clock Drawing Test, 979
    Cognitive Assessment System, 143
    Conners' Continuous Performance Test
        detection of, 569–571
    Gray Oral Reading Test-4, 369
    Hayling and Brixton Tests, 464
    Integrated Visual and Auditory Continuous
        Performance Test detection of, 580
    NEPSY, 213
    psychiatric disorders concomitantly presenting
        with, 1088
    Self-Ordered Pointing Test, 476
    Smell Indetification Test, 1027
    Stanford Binet Intelligence Scale—Fifth
        Edition, 266
    Stroop Test, 493
    Test of Everyday Attention for Children, 643
    Test of Nonverbal Intelligence-3, 271
    Test of Variables of Attention (T.O.V.A.), 651
    Wechsler Individual Achievement Test-II, 380
    Wechsler Intelligence Scale for Children-IV,
        336
    Wechsler Memory Scale-III, 874

Attention deficit hyperactivity disorder (*continued*)
  Wechsler Preschool and Primary Scale of
    Intelligence-III, 336
  Wisconsin Card Sorting Test, 536–537
  Woodcock Johnson III Tests of Cognitive
    Abilities, 360
  Word Memory Test, 1186
Attention tests
  characteristics of, 548*t*–549*t*
  description of, 547
  in neuropsychological batteries, 547
Autism, 422, 442, 533, 536, 537, 651, 926, 959,
  994, 1057, 1065

Background history, 88
Baserates
  estimating of, 22–23
  predictive power and, 22
  of impairment, 28, 300, 875
Bayesian statistics, 23
Behavioral observations
  during interview, 56
  in report, 89
Bias
  in Dementia Rating Scale-2, 156
  in test-retest situations, 11*t*
Bilingual patients, 82–83
Bipolar Disorder, 257, 494, 1065, 1097.
    See also Depression
Body orientation tests, 1012–1013
Boston "process" approach, 76

Cancer, 744
Carroll-Horn-Catell *Gf-Gc* theory
  description of, 98, 99*f*
  WJ III ACH and, 391
  WJ III COG and, 311, 351, 352*f*
Ceiling effects, 8
Cerebellar disease, 1027, 1048,1077
Cerebro-vascular accident, 183, 561, 634–635,
    744, 833, 847, 848, 859, 911, 920, 967, 970,
    980, 989, 995, 1022, 1049, 1057, 1065,
    1103, 1118, 1159, 1162, 1164
Change. *See also* Reliable Change Index
  assessments of, 24
  clinically significant, 27
  reference group change score distributions, 25
  Reliable Change Index, 25–26
  standardized regression-based (SRB) change
    scores, 26–27
Chemical exposure. *See* Toxic exposure
Children. *See also* Adolescents
  Bayley Scales of Infant Development and, 114
  Bells Cancellation Test and, 970
  Benton Visual Retention Test and, 694–695
  Boston Naming Test—2 and, 907–908, 912
  Behavior Rating Inventory of Executive
    Function, 1090
  Brief Test of Attention and, 553
  Brown Peterson Task and, 704
  Buschke Selective Reminding Test and, 713
  California Verbal Learning Test—Children's
    Version and, 735
  CANTAB and, 415
  Category Test and, 424
  Children's Memory Scale and, 746
  Clock Drawing Test in, 975–977, 976*t*, 979, 981

Cognitive Assessment System and, 133
Color Trails Test and, 555
Conners' Continuous Performance Test-II
  and, 562
cooperation by, 82
Design Fluency Test and, 450
D-KEFS and, 443
Expressive One-Word Picture Vocabulary
  Test-3 and, 933
Expressive Vocabulary Test and, 928
Facial Recognition Test and, 986, 988
Finger Localization and, 1015–1016
Finger Tapping and, 1046–1047
Five-Point Test and, 456, 458–459
Golden Stroop Test and, 484, 490
Gray Oral Reading Test—Fourth Edition
  and, 365
Grip Strength and, 1055
Grooved Pegboard and, 1062–1063
history-taking questionnaire for, 67*f*–73*f*
Hooper Visual Organization Test and, 993
Integrated Visual and Auditory Continuous
    Performance Test (IVA + Plus) and, 575
Judgment of Line Orientation and, 1003
Kaufman Brief Intelligence Test and, 164
MMSE for, 175*f*, 177
Multilingual Aphasia Examination and, 936
NEPSY and, 201
neuropsychological assessment of, 81–82
Paced Audtiory Serial Addition Test and, 582
Peabody Picture Vocabulary Test—III and, 940
premorbid estimations and, 109–111
profile forms for, 35*f*–40*f*
Purdue Pegboard Test and, 1069–1070,
    1072*t*–1076*t*
Raven's Progressive Matrices and, 229
reinforcements for, 81
Rey Auditory Verbal Learning Test and,
    794–796
Rey Fifteen-Item Memory Test and, 1167
Rey Osterrieth Complex Figure Test and, 811
Right-Left Orientation Test and, 1017
Rivermead Behavioural Memory Test—
    Children's Version (RBMT-C) and,
    844–845
Ruff figural Fluency Test and, 466
Scales of Independent Behavior and, 1134
Self-Ordered Pointing Test and, 473
Sentence Repetition Test and, 854
Smell Identification Test and, 1025
Stanford Binet—Fifth Edition and, 258
Stroop Test and, 484, 492
Symbol Digit Modalities Test and, 620
Tactual Performance Test and, 1034
testing of, 81–82
Test of Everyday Attention for Children
  and, 638
Test of Memory Malingering and, 117, 1175
Test of Nonverbal Intelligence and, 268
Test of Variables of Attention (T.O.V.A.)
  and, 645
Token Test and, 957, 959
Trail Making Test and, 663
Verbal Fluency and, 512–515
Victoria Symptom Validity Test and, 1183
Wechsler Abbreviated Scale of Intelligence
  and, 279

Wechsler Individual Achievement Test—II
  and, 370
Wechsler Intelligence Scale for Children-IV
  and, 310
Wechsler Preschool and Primary Scale of
  Intelligence-III and, 337
Wide Range Achievement Test—3 and, 384
Wide Range Assessment of Memory and
  Learning 2 and, 881
Wisconsin Card Sorting Test in, 530–531,
    531*t*–532*t*, 533, 537
Word Memory Test and, 1186
Woodcock-Johnson III Tests of Cognitive
  Abilities and, 351
Woodcock-Johnson Tests of Achievement
  and, 390
Chronic Fatigue Syndrome, 605, 711, 804
Circadian arousal, 82
Classification accuracy statistics, 21–24
Cochlear Implants, 926, 949
Coefficient alpha, 9, 25, 9*t. See also* Internal
  Reliability
Cognitive abilities
  Carroll-Horn-Catell *Gf-Gc* model of,
    98, 99*f*
  description of, 98
Cognitive tests, 120
Computer(s)
  reports generated using, 94–95
  scores generated using, 94–95
  test administration using, 77–78
Concurrent validity, 18, 233
Concussion, 252, 494, 604, 614–615, 652, 1182.
    See also Head Injury, Traumatic Brain
    Injury
Condition of interest
  cutoff scores for, 23
  definition of, 20
  prevalence of, 22
  test accuracy for, 21
Conduct Disorder, 464, 1186
Confidence intervals, 16
Confidentiality, of report, 87
Consolidation, memory, 678, 684
Construct validity
  of Dementia Rating Scale-2, 151–155
  description of, 17–18
  of executive function tests, 405–406
  of Kaplan Baycrest Neurocognitive
    Assessment, 162–163
  of MMSE, 182–183
  of National Adult Reading Test, 196–198
  of Paced Auditory Serial Addition Test, 601
  of Raven's Progressive Matrices, 233
  of Scales of Independent Behavior—Revised,
    1139
  of Speed and Capacity of Language Processing
    Test
    Speed of Comprehension Test, 276
  of Spot-the-Word test, 276–278
  of Wechsler Abbreviated Scale of Intelligence,
    281–282
Content validity
  of Behavior Rating Inventory of Executive
    Function, 1094–1095
  of Children's Memory Scale, 751
  of Comprehensive Trail Making Test, 561

of Expressive One-Word Picture Vocabulary Test—Third Edition, 925
of Expressive Vocabulary Test, 931
of Gray Oral Reading Tests—Fourth Edition, 368
of Neuropsychological Assessment Battery, 225–226
of Peabody Picture Vocabulary Test—Third Edition, 945
of Ruff 2 & 7 Selective Attention Test, 614
of Stanford-Binet Intelligence Scales—Fifth Edition, 264–265
of Test of Everyday Attention, 633
of Test of Nonverbal Intelligence—3, 270
of Wechsler Individual Achievement Test—Second Edition, 378
of Wechsler Intelligence Scale for Children—Fourth Edition, 332–333
of Wechsler Preschool and Primary Scale of Intelligence—Third Edition, 343
of Wide Range Achievement Test—3, 386–387
of Wide Range Assessment of Memory and Learning—Second Edition, 885
of Woodcock-Johnson III Tests of Achievement, 398
of Woodcock-Johnson III Tests of Cognitive Abilities, 359
Continuous performance tests, 562
Convergent validity
description of, 18
of Minnesota Multiphasic Personality Inventory—2, 1118
of Personality Assessment Inventory, 1130
of Repeatable Battery for the Assessment of Neuropsychological Status, 250, 252
of Speed and Capacity of Language Processing Test, Spot-the-Word test, 277
of Wechsler Abbreviated Scale of Intelligence, 282
of Wechsler Adult Intelligence Scale—III, 298–299
Criminal offenders, 834, 1165
Cronbach's α, 9, 9t, 25. See also Internal reliability
Culture, 49
Cutoff scores
determining of, 23–24
predictive power and, 24, 1150,1154

Daubert v. Merrell Dow Pharmaceuticals, 94
Dementia. See also Alzheimer's disease
Beck Depression Inventory-II and, 1088
Benton Visual Retention Test in patients with, 697–698
Boston Diagnostic Aphasia Examination in patients with, 898–899
Brown-Peterson Task and, 711
Buschke Selective Reminding Test evaluations, 726–727
Clock Drawing Test for evaluation of, 978–979
Cognitive Estimation Test and, 442
Dementia Rating Scale-2 and, 144–159
Design Fluency Test and, 454–455
Dot Counting Test and, 1162
Finger Tapping Test and, 1048
Geriatric Depression Scale and, 1103
Hooper Visual Organization Test and, 995

Hopkins Verbal Learning Test—Revised (HVLT-R) evaluations, 767
Instrumental Activities of Daily Living and, 1060
Kaplan Baycrest Neurocognitive Assessment and, 163
Minnesota Multiphasic Personality Inventory-2 and, 1118
Mini-Mental State Examination and, 168
National Adult Reading Test performance and, 197
Neuropsychological Assessment Battery and, 227
Raven's Progressive Matrices and, 234
Recognition Memory Test for diagnosis of, 774
Repeatable Battery for the Assessment of Neuropsychological Status and, 254
Rey Fifteen-Item Memory Test and, 1168
Right-Left Orientation in patients with, 1019
Smell Identification Test and, 1027–1028
Speed and Capacity of Language Processing Test (SCOLP) and, 277
Stroop interference and, 493
Test of Everyday Attention and, 634
Test of Memory Malingering and, 1174
Trail Making Test and, 670
Verbal Fluency Test for detection of, 519
Victoria Symptom Validity Test and, 1181
Visual Object and Space Perception Battery and, 1010
Demographically corrected norms
description of, 46–47, 50–51
for minority groups, 51
practical considerations for, 51–52
Demographics, premorbid estimation using, 105–107
Depression. See also Mood disorders
Beck Depression Inventory-II and, 1090
Boston Naming Test-2 and, 912
B Test in, 1159
Buschke Selective Relinding Test and, 727
California Verbal Learning Test-II and, 734
CANTAB and, 422
Category Test and, 433
Clock Drawing Test and, 979
Dementia Rating Scale-2 and, 155–156
Design Fluency Test and, 455
Dichotic Listening and, 920
Dot Counting Test and, 1162
in elderly, 1099
Grip Strength and, 1057
Grooved Pegboard Test and, 1065
Judgement of Line Orientation and, 1003
National Adult Reading Test and, 197
prevalence of, 1080
Recognition Memory Test and, 773
Rey Auditory Verbal Learning Test and, 804
Rey Fifteen-Item Memory Test and, 1169
Rey Osterrieth Complex Figure and, 834
Rivermead Behavioral Memory Test-II and, 848
Ruff 2 & 7 Test and, 614
Stroop Test and, 494
Test of Memory Malingering and, 1175
tests for assessing, 1080, 1081t, 1083
Trail Making Test and, 670
Verbal Fluency Test and, 519

Victoria Symptom Validity Test and, 1182
Wisconsin Card Sorting Test performance and, 537
Word Memory Test and, 1187
Developmental growth curves, 47–48
Diabetes, 804
Diagnosis threat, 834
Diagnostic tests, 20
Disabled patients, 82
Distribution(s)
near-uniform, 8
skewed, 7f, 8
third moment of a, 8
truncated, 8, 52
uniform, 8
Divergent validity, 18
of Personality Assessment Inventory, 1130
of Speed and Capacity of Language Processing Test, Spot-the-Word test, 277
of Victoria Symptom Validity Test, 1182
of Wechsler Abbreviated Scale of Intelligence, 282
of Wechsler Adult Intelligence Scale—III, 298–299
Down Syndrome, 127, 1027
Driving, 93
Drug Abuse, 476, 536, 635, 669, 697, 832, 847, 1065, 1130, 1164, 1178
Dyslexia. See Learning Disorders

Eating disorders, 465, 1103
Ecological validity
of Behavioral Assessment of the Dysexecutive Syndrome, 413
of Benton Visual Retention Test, 698
of Boston Diagnostic Aphasia Examination, 899
of Brief Test of Attention, 552
of Buschke Selective Reminding Test, 727
of California Verbal Learning Test—Children's Version, 744
of Cognitive Estimation Test, 442
of Dementia Rating Scale-2, 156
of Expressive One-Word Picture Vocabulary Test—Third Edition, 926
of Grip Strength, 1057–1058
of Grooved Pegboard, 1065
of Hayling Test, 464
of Hooper Visual Organization Test, 995
of MMSE, 184–185
of Neuropsychological Assessment Battery, 227
of Paced Auditory Serial Addition Test, 606
of Purdue Pegboard Test, 1077
of Rey Auditory Verbal Learning Test, 805
of Rey-Osterrieth Complex Figure Test, 834
of Rivermead Behavioural Memory Test—Second Edition, 848
of Ruff 2 & 7 Selective Attention Test, 614
of Smell Identification Test, 1027–1028
of Tactual Performance Test, 1038
of Test of Everyday Attention, 635
of Trail Making Test, 671
of Verbal Fluency Test, 520–521
of Wechsler Memory Scale—Third Edition, 876
of Wisconsin Card Sorting Test, 537

Education effects
    Autobiographical Memory Interview
      and, 688
    Behavior Rating Inventory of Executive
      Function and, 1092
    Bells Cancellation Test and, 970
    Benton Visual Retention Test and, 693
    Boston Diagnostic Aphasia Examination
      and, 895
    Boston Naming Test—2 and, 904
    Brief Visuospatial Memory Test—Revised
      and, 702
    Buschke Selective Reminding Test and, 716
    California Verbal Learning Test—Children's
      Version (CVLT-C) and, 738
    California Verbal Learning Test-II and, 731
    Category Test and, 427
    Cognitive Estimation Test and, 440
    Design Fluency Test and, 453
    Expressive Vocabulary Test and, 930
    Finger Tapping and, 1044
    Five-Point Test and, 458
    Geriatric Depression Scale and, 1101
    Grip Strength and, 1053
    Grooved Pegboard and, 1062
    Hayling and Brixton Tests and, 461
    Hooper Visual Organization Test and, 991
    Hopkins Verbal Learning Test—Revised
      and, 760
    Instrumental Activities of Daily Living and,
      1109
    Integrated Visual and Auditory Continuous
      Performance Test and, 578
    Judgment of Line Orientation and, 999
    Kaplan Baycrest Neurocognitive Assessment
      and, 161
    Minnesota Multiphasic Personality
      Inventory—2 and, 1117
    MMSE and, 176, 178t–179t
    Multilingual Aphasia Examination and, 935
    Paced Auditory Serial Addition Test and, 595
    Peabody Picture Vocabulary Test—
      Edition (PPVT-III) and, 942
    Personality Assessment Inventory and, 1129
    Purdue Pegboard Test and, 1069
    Recognition Memory Test and, 770
    Repeatable Battery for the Assessment of Neu-
      ropsychological Status and, 239
    Rey Auditory Verbal Learning Test and, 783
    Rey Fifteen-Item Memory Test and, 1167
    Rey-Osterrieth Complex Figure Test and, 826
    Right-Left Orientation and, 1018
    Rivermead Behavioural Memory Test—Second
      Edition (RBMT-II) and, 843
    Ruff 2 & 7 Selective Attention Test and, 612
    Ruff Figural Fluency Test and, 467
    Self-Ordered Pointing Test and, 473
    Sentence Repetition Test and, 858
    Stroop Test and, 481
    Tactual Performance Test and, 1033
    Test of Memory Malingering and, 1172
    Token Test and, 956
    Trail Making Test and, 658
    21-Item Test and, 1177
    Verbal Fluency Test and, 504
    Visual Object and Space Perception Battery
      and, 1008
    Wechsler Adult Intelligence Scale—III and,
      289, 291
    Wechsler Intelligence Scale for Children—
      Fourth Edition and, 318
    Wechsler Memory Scale—Third Edition and,
      863
    Wechsler Preschool and Primary Scale of
      Intelligence—Third Edition and, 342
    Wide Range Achievement Test—3 and, 385
    Wide Range Assessment of Memory and
      Learning—Second Edition and, 883
    Wisconsin Card Sorting Test and, 529
    Woodcock-Johnson III Tests of Achievement
      and, 396
    Woodcock-Johnson III Tests of Cognitive
      Abilities and, 356–357
    Word Memory Test and, 1185
Educational records, 56t
Education-corrected norms, 49
Employment records, 56t
Encephalitis, 690, 711, 919
Encoding, 678
English as a second language patients, 82–83
Epilepsy, 297, 448, 459, 469, 493, 571–572, 704,
    744, 753, 773, 832–833, 848, 920, 938,
    1027, 1038, 1057, 1118, 1181
Episodic memory
    characteristics of, 679–680, 684
    tests of, 680
Equivalent form reliability, 225. See also
    Alternate form reliability
Error
    measurement of, 9
    reliability coefficients and, 9, 9t
    in test-retest situations, 11t
    types of, 15–17, 25
Estimated prevalence value, 6
Estimated true scores, 14–16
Ethical Principles of Psychologists, 90
Ethnically adjusted norms, 49–50
Ethnicity effects. See also Race, Acculturation
    Beck Depression Inventory—Second Edition
      and, 1085
    Bells Cancellation Test and, 970
    Benton Visual Retention Test and, 693
    Boston Diagnostic Aphasia Examination and,
      895
    Boston Naming Test—2 and, 905
    Brief Test of Attention and, 550
    Buschke Selective Reminding Test and, 716
    Conners' Continuous Performance Test and,
      567
    description of, 49
    Expressive One-Word Picture Vocabulary
      Test—Third Edition and, 924
    Expressive Vocabulary Test and, 930
    Finger Tapping and, 1044
    Geriatric Depression Scale and, 1101
    Gray Oral Reading Tests—Fourth Edition and,
      366–367
    Grip Strength and, 1053
    Hooper Visual Organization Test and, 991
    Hopkins Verbal Learning Test—Revised
      and, 761
    Judgment of Line Orientation and, 999
    MMSE and, 176
    Multilingual Aphasia Examination and, 935
    Paced Auditory Serial Addition Test and, 595
    Peabody Picture Vocabulary Test—Third
      Edition (PPVT-III) and, 942–944
    Personality Assessment Inventory and, 1129
    Purdue Pegboard Test and, 1069
    Repeatable Battery for the Assessment of
      Neuropsychological Status and, 239
    Rey Auditory Verbal Learning Test and, 783
    Rey-Osterrieth Complex Figure Test and, 826
    Right-Left Orientation and, 1018–1019
    Rivermead Behavioural Memory Test—Second
      Edition (RBMT-II) and, 843
    Smell Identification Test and, 1024
    Stanford-Binet Intelligence Scales—Fifth
      Edition and, 262
    Stroop Test and, 481
    Tactual Performance Test and, 1033
    Test of Everyday Attention for Children
      and, 640
    Test of Nonverbal Intelligence—3 and, 269
    Test of Variables of Attention and, 647
    Token Test and, 956–957
    Trail Making Test and, 658
    Verbal Fluency Test and, 504
    Visual Object and Space Perception Battery
      and, 1008
    Wechsler Adult Intelligence Scale—III and,
      293–294, 305–306
    Wechsler Intelligence Scale for Children—
      Fourth Edition and, 317–318
    Wechsler Memory Scale—Third Edition
      and, 863
    Wechsler Preschool and Primary Scale of
      Intelligence—Third Edition and, 341–342
    Wechsler Test of Adult Reading and, 348
    Wide Range Achievement Test—3 and, 385
    Wide Range Assessment of Memory and
      Learning—Second Edition and, 883
    Woodcock-Johnson III Tests of Achievement
      and, 396
    Woodcock-Johnson III Tests of Cognitive
      Abilities and, 356
Exclusionary criteria, 52
Executive function
    assessment recommendations, 407, 407t
    definition of, 401
    frontal lobe processes and, 401, 405
    importance of, 401
    intelligence and, 406–407
    processes involved in, 406
Executive function tests
    behavioral ratings, 407
    characteristics of, 402t–404t
    construct validity issues for, 405–406
    test-retest reliability of, 406
Explicit memory
    definition of, 679
    episodic memory, 679–680, 684
    semantic memory, 684
Extrapolations, 9
Extreme test scores, 6

Face validity, 18
Fatigue, 537, 605
Feedback
    during neuropsychological assessment, 79
    of results, 95

Finger gnosis, 1017
Fixed battery approach, 75–76
Flexible battery approach, 75–76
Floor effects, 8
Flynn effect, 45–46
Forensic assessment reports, 93–94
Fragile X syndrome, 668
Freidrich's ataxia, 493
Frontal lobe dysfunction, 421–422, 433, 442, 448, 454–455, 459, 464, 469, 475, 494–495, 518, 519, 521, 537, 670, 684, 690, 711, 733, 744, 980, 1027, 1038, 1097
Frye standard, 94

Gaussian distribution, 3
Gender effects
    Beck Depression Inventory—Second Edition and, 1085
    Behavior Rating Inventory of Executive Function and, 1092
    Benton Visual Retention Test and, 693
    Boston Diagnostic Aphasia Examination and, 895
    Boston Naming Test—2 and, 904
    Brief Test of Attention and, 550
    Buschke Selective Reminding Test and, 716
    California Verbal Learning Test—Children's Version (CVLT-C) and, 738
    California Verbal Learning Test-II and, 731
    Cambridge Neuropsychological Test Automated Batteries and, 416
    Clock Drawing Test and, 976
    Cognitive Estimation Test and, 440
    Conners' Continuous Performance Test and, 566–567
    Design Fluency Test and, 453
    Dichotic Learning—Words and, 917
    Expressive One-Word Picture Vocabulary Test—Third Edition and, 923
    Finger Tapping and, 1044
    Five-Point Test and, 458
    Geriatric Depression Scale and, 1100–1101
    Grip Strength and, 1053
    Grooved Pegboard and, 1062
    Hayling and Brixton Tests and, 461
    Hopkins Verbal Learning Test—Revised and, 760–761
    Instrumental Activities of Daily Living and, 1110
    Integrated Visual and Auditory Continuous Performance Test and, 578
    Judgment of Line Orientation and, 999
    Minnesota Multiphasic Personality Inventory—2 and, 1117
    MMSE and, 176
    Multilingual Aphasia Examination and, 935
    Paced Auditory Serial Addition Test and, 595
    Personality Assessment Inventory and, 1128
    Purdue Pegboard Test and, 1069
    Repeatable Battery for the Assessment of Neuropsychological Status and, 239
    Rey Auditory Verbal Learning Test and, 782–783
    Rey-Osterrieth Complex Figure Test and, 826
    Rivermead Behavioural Memory Test—Second Edition (RBMT-II) and, 843
    Self-Ordered Pointing Test and, 473

    Sentence Repetition Test and, 858
    Smell Identification Test and, 1024
    Stroop Test and, 481
    Tactual Performance Test and, 1033
    Test of Everyday Attention for Children and, 640
    Test of Nonverbal Intelligence—3 and, 269
    Test of Variables of Attention and, 647
    Trail Making Test and, 658
    Verbal Fluency Test and, 504
    Visual Object and Space Perception Battery and, 1007
    Wechsler Adult Intelligence Scale—III and, 293
    Wechsler Intelligence Scale for Children—Fourth Edition and, 317
    Wechsler Memory Scale—Third Edition and, 863
    Wide Range Assessment of Memory and Learning—Second Edition and, 883
    Wisconsin Card Sorting Test and, 529
    Woodcock-Johnson III Tests of Cognitive Abilities and, 356
Generalizability coefficients, 12–13
Generalizability theory, 12–13
Geographic region, 905
Gerstmann syndrome, 1019

Head injury. See Traumatic brain injury, Concussion
Hemianopsia. See Visual field defect
Hemispherectomy, 959, 1057
History taking
    description of, 55
    information obtained, 55
    interview. See Interview
    neuropsychological report section, 87–88
    questionnaires used in
        for adults, 57f–66f
        for children, 67f–73f
HIV-AIDS, 614, 669, 704, 767, 804, 1027, 1065
Hormone replacement therapy, 848
Huntington's disease, 155, 183, 254, 301, 350, 421, 448, 475, 493, 519–520, 552, 625, 697, 804, 832, 874, 1010, 1027
Hydrocephalus, 744, 1097
Hyperbilirubinemia, 959
Hyperexia, 919
Hypoglycemia, 605

Implicit memory, 679
Informed consent
    description of, 78
    flowchart for, 79f
    sample, 80f
Informing interview, 95
Instrumental activities of daily living, 1083, 1107, 1134
Intelligence
    Cognitive Estimation Test and, 441
    executive function and, 406–407
    models of, 98, 100
Intelligence quotient (IQ)
    Behavior Rating Inventory of Executive Function correlated with, 1096

    Benton Visual Retention Test and, 693
    Boston Naming Test—2 and, 904
    Brief Visuospatial Memory Test—Revised and, 702
    Buschke Selective Reminding Test and, 716
    California Verbal Learning Test—Children's Version and, 743
    California Verbal Learning Test-II and, 731
    Cambridge Neuropsychological Test Automated Batteries and, 416
    Children's Memory Scale and, 752
    classification of, 91t
    Conners' Continuous Performance Test and, 567
    Expressive One-Word Picture Vocabulary Test—Third Edition and, 924
    Expressive One-Word Picture Vocabulary Test—Third Edition and, 926
    Expressive Vocabulary Test and, 931
    Finger Tapping and, 1044
    Geriatric Depression Scale and, 1101
    Gray Oral Reading Tests—Fourth Edition and, 369
    Hayling and Brixton Tests and, 461
    Hooper Visual Organization Test and, 991
    Hopkins Verbal Learning Test—Revised and, 760
    Integrated Visual and Auditory Continuous Performance Test and, 578
    Judgment of Line Orientation and, 999
    MMSE and, 176
    NEPSY and, 206, 211–212
    Paced Auditory Serial Addition Test and, 595, 603
    Peabody Picture Vocabulary Test—Third Edition and, 942, 947–948, 951
    premorbid estimation of. See Premorbid estimation
    Recognition Memory Test and, 770
    Rey Auditory Verbal Learning Test and, 783
    Rey Fifteen-Item Memory Test and, 1167
    Rey-Osterrieth Complex Figure Test and, 826
    Right-Left Orientation and, 1018
    Rivermead Behavioural Memory Test—Second Edition (RBMT-II) and, 843
    Ruff 2 & 7 Selective Attention Test and, 612
    Ruff Figural Fluency Test and, 467
    screening methods, 101, 103–104
    Sentence Repetition Test and, 858
    Stroop Test and, 481
    Tactual Performance Test and, 1033
    Test of Everyday Attention for Children and, 640
    Test of Memory Malingering and, 1172
    Test of Variables of Attention and, 647
    Token Test and, 956
    Trail Making Test and, 658
    Verbal Fluency Test and, 505
    Visual Object and Space Perception Battery and, 1008
    Wide Range Assessment of Memory and Learning—Second Edition and, 883
    Wisconsin Card Sorting Test and, 529
    Word Memory Test and, 1185
Intelligence tests. See also Intelligence Quotient (IQ)
    acceptance of, 98

Intelligence tests (*continued*)
   content of, 100
   educational achievement and, 100
   nonverbal, 103
   overview of, 98, 100
   reliability of, 100
   scores from, 100
   selection of, 100–101, 102*t*–103*t*
Intermediate position, 75
Internal reliability
   acceptable level of, 13
   of Beck Depression Inventory—Second
      Edition, 1086
   of Behavior Rating Inventory of Executive
      Function, 1093–1094
   of Behavioral Assessment of the Dysexecutive
      Syndrome, 411
   of Benton Visual Retention Test, 695–696
   of Boston Diagnostic Aphasia Examination,
      896
   of Boston Naming Test—2, 910
   of Brief Test of Attention, 551
   of Brixon Tests, 463
   of Brown-Peterson Task, 711
   of California Verbal Learning Test—Children's
      Version, 740
   of California Verbal Learning Test-II, 732
   of Cambridge Neuropsychological Test
      Automated Batteries, 419
   of Category Test, 431
   of Children's Memory Scale, 749, 750*t*
   of Cognitive Assessment System, 139
   of Cognitive Estimation Test, 441
   of Comprehensive Trail Making Test, 559
   definition of, 9
   of Delis-Kaplan Executive Function System,
      446, 447*t*
   of Dementia Rating Scale-2, 148–149
   of Expressive One-Word Picture Vocabulary
      Test—Third Edition, 925
   of Expressive Vocabulary Test, 930
   of Geriatric Depression Scale, 1101
   of Gray Oral Reading Tests—Fourth Edition,
      367
   of Grip Strength, 1055
   of Hayling Tests, 462–463
   of Hooper Visual Organization Test, 993
   importance of, 13
   of Instrumental Activities of Daily Living,
      1110
   of Judgment of Line Orientation, 1001–1002
   of Kaplan Baycrest Neurocognitive
      Assessment, 162
   of Kaufman Brief Intelligence Test, 165
   of Minnesota Multiphasic Personality
      Inventory—2, 1117
   of MMSE, 180
   of NEPSY, 208, 208*t*–209*t*
   of Neuropsychological Assessment Battery,
      223, 228
   of Paced Auditory Serial Addition Test, 597
   of Peabody Picture Vocabulary Test—Third
      Edition, 944
   of Personality Assessment Inventory, 1129
   of Recognition Memory Test, 771
   of Repeatable Battery for the Assessment of
      Neuropsychological Status, 244

   of Rey Auditory Verbal Learning Test, 796
   of Rey-Osterrieth Complex Figure Test, 829
   of Rivermead Behavioural Memory Test—
      Second Edition, 845
   of Scales of Independent Behavior—Revised,
      1138
   speed tests and, 10–11
   of Stanford-Binet Intelligence Scales—Fifth
      Edition, 263
   of Symbol Digit Modalities Test, 620
   of Tactual Performance Test, 1036, 1039
   of Test of Everyday Attention, 632
   of Test of Everyday Attention for Children, 641
   of Test of Nonverbal Intelligence—3, 269
   of Test of Variables of Attention, 648
   of Token Test, 957
   of Verbal Fluency Test, 514
   of Victoria Symptom Validity Test, 1181
   of Visual Object and Space Perception Battery,
      1009
   of Wechsler Abbreviated Scale of Intelligence,
      281
   of Wechsler Adult Intelligence Scale—III,
      294–295
   of Wechsler Individual Achievement Test—
      Second Edition, 376–377
   of Wechsler Intelligence Scale for Children—
      Fourth Edition, 331
   of Wechsler Memory Scale—Third Edition,
      868
   of Wechsler Preschool and Primary Scale of
      Intelligence—Third Edition, 342
   of Wechsler Test of Adult Reading, 348
   of Wide Range Achievement Test—3, 385
   of Wide Range Assessment of Memory and
      Learning—Second Edition, 883–884
   of Woodcock-Johnson III Tests of
      Achievement, 396–397
   of Woodcock-Johnson III Tests of Cognitive
      Abilities, 357
Internal-consistency reliability, 25. *See also*
      Internal reliability
Interpolation, 9
Interpreter, 83
Interrater reliability
   acceptable level of, 13
   of Autobiographical Memory Interview, 688
   of Behavior Rating Inventory of Executive
      Function, 1094
   of Behavioral Assessment of the Dysexecutive
      Syndrome, 411
   of Benton Visual Retention Test, 697
   of Boston Diagnostic Aphasia Examination,
      896
   of Brixon Tests, 463
   of Children's Memory Scale, 751
   of Clock Drawing Test, 977
   of Cognitive Estimation Test, 441
   of Comprehensive Trail Making Test, 560
   of Delis-Kaplan Executive Function
      System, 446
   description of, 12
   of Doors and People Test, 759
   of Expressive One-Word Picture Vocabulary
      Test—Third Edition, 925
   of Gray Oral Reading Tests—Fourth Edition,
      368

   of Hayling Tests, 463
   of Instrumental Activities of Daily Living,
      1110
   of Kaplan Baycrest Neurocognitive
      Assessment, 162
   of MMSE, 181
   of National Adult Reading Test, 196
   of NEPSY, 210–211
   of Neuropsychological Assessment Battery, 225
   of Peabody Picture Vocabulary Test—Third
      Edition, 945
   of Repeatable Battery for the Assessment of
      Neuropsychological Status, 248
   of Rey Fifteen-Item Memory Test, 1168
   of Rey-Osterrieth Complex Figure Test, 830
   of Rivermead Assessment of Somatosensory
      Performance, 1022
   of Ruff Figural Fluency Test, 468, 470
   of Stanford-Binet Intelligence Scales—Fifth
      Edition, 264
   of Test of Nonverbal Intelligence—3, 270
   of Trail Making Test, 667
   of Verbal Fluency Test, 517
   of Wechsler Abbreviated Scale of Intelligence,
      281
   of Wechsler Adult Intelligence Scale—III, 298
   of Wechsler Individual Achievement Test—
      Second Edition, 378
   of Wechsler Intelligence Scale for Children—
      Fourth Edition, 332
   of Wechsler Memory Scale—Third Edition,
      870
   of Wechsler Preschool and Primary Scale of
      Intelligence—Third Edition, 342
   of Wisconsin Card Sorting Test, 534
   of Woodcock-Johnson III Tests of
      Achievement, 398
   of Woodcock-Johnson III Tests of Cognitive
      Abilities, 359
Interview
   behavioral observations during, 56
   description of, 55
   framing of questions in, 56
   information obtained in, 55
   informing, 95
   length of, 56
   note-taking during, 56
   questionnaire used in
      for adults, 57*f*–66*f*
      for children, 67*f*–73*f*
   review of records, 56, 56*t*
   structure of, 55
   symptom report/response styles, 66, 73
Item analysis, 44

Klinefelter's syndrome, 464
Korsakoff's syndrome, 350, 442, 536, 678,
      689, 711, 712, 804, 833, 874, 1027, 1048,
      1164, 1181
Kuder-Richardson reliability coefficient, 9, 9*t*

Landau-Kleffner syndrome, 919
Language, 504–505
Language tests, 891, 892*t*
Laplace-Gauss distribution, 3
Laterality, 759, 769, 833, 848, 874, 917–920, 1003,
      1038, 1047–1048, 1056–1057, 1065, 1077

Learning disorders, 360, 369, 380, 382, 387, 464, 533, 571, 643, 698, 744, 804, 833, 858, 888, 919, 926, 931, 939, 949, 959, 1019, 1038, 1065, 1159, 1162, 1169, 1187
Legal records, 56t
Long-term memory, 678–679
Lupus, 605
Lurian principles, 201
    And NEPSY, 201–202

Major depressive disorder. *See* Depression, Psychiatric disorders
Malaria, 652, 919
Malingering. *See also* Suboptimal performance
    base rates of, 1149
    Benton Visual Retention Test detection of, 698
    California Verbal Learning Test-II detection of, 734
    Category Test and, 433
    client management, 1155–1156
    communication of findings about, 1156
    definition of, 1145
    Dichotic Learning—Words and, 920
    DSM-IV diagnostic criteria for, 1145, 1146t–1148t
    Finger Tapping detection of, 1049
    Grip Strength for detection of, 1058
    Grooved Pegboard and, 1066
    indicators of, 1147t
    Integrated Visual and Auditory Continuous Performance Test detection of, 580, 581t
    Minnesota Multiphasic Personality Inventory—2 detection of, 1120t, 1120–1123
    multiple assessments, 1155
    of neurocognitive dysfunction, 1145, 1146t
    Neuropsychological Assessment Battery and, 227
    Paced Auditory Serial Addition Test detection of, 606
    Raven's Progressive Matrices and, 234–235
    Recognition Memory Test detection of, 774
    Rey Auditory Verbal Learning Test detection of, 805–806
    Rey-Osterrieth Complex Figure Test detection of, 834–835
    Slick criteria for, 1145, 1146t
    Smell Identification Test detection of, 1028
    Stroop Test and, 495
    Test of Variables of Attention and, 652
    Token Test detection of, 960
    Trail Making Test in, 671
    Trauma Symptom Inventory detection of, 1143
    Wechsler Adult Intelligence Scale—III and, 303, 305
    Wechsler Memory Scale—Third Edition detection of, 876–877
    Wisconsin Card Sorting Test for detection of, 538
Mayo's Older African American Normative Studies scaled scores
    Boston Naming Test-2, 907t
    Dementia Rating Scale-2 (DRS-2), 146–147, 151t–155t
    Judgement of Line Orientation, 938t
    MAE Token Test, 938t
    Rey Auditory Verbal Learning Test, 795t–800t

Stroop norms, 491t–492t
Trail Making Test, 662t–663t
Verbal Fluency, 509t, 511t–512t
Mayo's Older Americans Normative Studies
    AMNART, 195t
    Boston Naming Test, 906t
    Dementia Rating Scale-2, 146t–151t
    Judgement of Line Orientation, 1000t
    MAE Token Test, 937t
    Rey Auditory Verbal Learning Test, 788t–795t
    Stroop, 485t–490t
    Verbal Fluency, 507t, 510t
Measurement error
    confidence intervals, 16
    description of, 9
    standard error of estimation, 16–17
    standard error of measurement. *See* Standard error of measurement
    standard error of prediction, 17
    true scores, 14–16
Medical records, 56t
Memory
    acquisition, 684
    consolidation of, 678, 684
    definition of, 678
    episodic, 679–680, 684
    explicit, 679
    implicit, 679
    long-term, 678–679
    neural correlates of, 684–686
    recognition, 680, 684–685
    semantic, 684
    tests for assessing, 681t–683t
    working, 678–679
Memory tests
    characteristics of, 681t–683t
    practice effects on, 686
    reliability of, 686
Meningitis, 960
Menopause, 697
Mental health records, 56t
Mental retardation, 155, 156, 266, 271, 282, 336, 804, 921, 931, 849, 1164, 1186
Military records, 56t
Minority groups. *See also* Ethnicity
    demographically based norms for, 51
    norms for, 50
Mood disorders. *See also* Anxiety, Depression, Psychiatric Disorders
    Rivermead Behavioural Memory Test—Second Edition and, 848
    Test of Memory Malingering and, 1175
    Wisconsin Card Sorting Test performance and, 537
    Word Memory Test and, 1187
Motor function tests, 1042t, 1042–1043
Multimodality
    definition of, 8
    example of, 7f
Multiple sclerosis
    Autobiographical Memory Inventory with, 689–690
    Behavioral Assessment of the Dysexecutive Syndrome with, 412
    Benton Visual Retention Test-5 with, 697
    Brown-Peterson Task with, 711

Boston Naming Test-2 with, 911
Buschke Selective Reminding Test in patients with, 727
Dichotic Listening with, 919–920
Facial Recognition Test with, 988
Finger Tapping Test with, 1048
Grip Strength with, 1057
Paced Auditory Serial Addition Test in patients with, 604–605
Symbol Digit Modalities Test in patients with, 625
Tactual Performance Test with, 1038
Wisconsin Card Sorting Test with, 536
Word Memory Test with, 1186
Myelomeningocele, 744

NCCEA, 955f
Near-uniform distribution, 8
Negative predictive power, 21–22, 494, 571, 580, 615, 670, 767, 835, 877, 932, 1049, 1087, 1103, 1149–1150, 1154, 1163
Neuropsychological assessment
    anxiety reduction, 81
    of children, 81–82
    comfort during, 81
    description of, 3
    of English as a second language patients, 82–83
    environment for, 81
    feedback during, 79
    informed consent for, 78, 79f–80f
    older adults and, 82
    patient cooperation/effort during, 81
    patient preparation for, 78–79
    rules for, 78–79, 81
    special-needs patients and, 82
    stress reduction, 81
    third-party presence during, 79, 81
Neuropsychological batteries, 103–104
Neuropsychological report. *See* Report
Neuropsychological tests
    Flynn effect, 45–46
    imprecision of, 28
    precision of, 9
    selection of, 75–76
    standards for, 3
    translation of, 83
    variability among, 3
Non-normality
    causative factors, 8
    ceiling effects, 8
    floor effects, 8
    near-uniform distribution, 8
    overview of, 7–8
    percentile derivations and, 8–9
    skew, 8
    truncated distributions, 8
    uniform distribution, 8
Normal curve
    area under, 4
    characteristics of, 3–4
    definition of, 3
    illustration of, 4f
    test construction and, 6–7
    Z scores, 4, 5t, 6f
Normal distribution. *See* Normal curve
Normal variation, 27–28

Normative data
    dataset size, 44–45
    date of norming, 45–46
    demographically adjusted, 46–47, 50–51
    education-corrected, 49
    ethnically adjusted, 49–50
    geographical location considerations, 52–53
    lifespan of, 45
    for minority groups, 50
    older, 46
    older adults and, 52
    population-based, 47
    in report, 92
    selection of, 44
    size of, 44–45
    stratified general population, 47
    types of, 46–47
    within-group, 50

Obsessive-compulsive disorder, 422, 459, 536, 635
Object perception disorders, 963
Obtained scores, 14, 17
Occupation, 693
Oklahoma Premorbid Intelligence Estimate
    calculation worksheet for, 304f
    description of, 108–109, 302–303
    subtests, 109, 302–303
    WAIS-III intelligence quotient and,
        correlations between, 109
Older adults
    circadian arousal considerations for, 82
    neuropsychological assessment of, 82
    norms for, 52
    testing of, 82
Olfactory function tests, 1012–1013

Pain, 66, 305, 605, 1048, 1057
Parental intelligence, 111
Parietal lobe dysfunction, 698, 980, 995, 1019
Parkinson's disease, 155, 183, 234, 254, 256, 350,
        421–422, 442, 464, 475, 493, 519–520,
        536, 537, 711, 804, 832, 874, 888, 911, 919,
        988, 995, 1003, 1027–1028, 1038, 1057,
        1077, 1175, 1188
Pearson, Karl, 3
Pearson correlations
    advantages of, 12
    description of, 12
Percentile-rank reporting, 91
Percentiles
    definition of, 4
    interpretation of, 4
    non-normality effects on, 8–9
    scores converted to, 4, 5t
    Z scores and, nonlinear relation between, 4
Personality disorders, 422, 834, 1130, 1143
Persistent postconcussive syndrome. See
        Postconcussion syndrome
Phenylketonuria (PKU), 128, 476, 744, 1097
Population-based norms, 47
Positive predictive power, 21–22, 494, 571, 580,
        615, 670, 767, 805, 835, 877, 932, 1049,
        1087, 1103, 1149–1150, 1154, 1159, 1163
Postconcussive symptoms, 73, 652, 699, 1118
Postconcussion syndrome
    Grip Srength in, 1058
    Paced Auditory Serial Addition Test and, 604

Posttraumatic stress disorder, 727, 804, 834, 848,
        1140, 1143. See also Anxiety
Practice effects, 11. See also under individual tests
Predictive power
    baserates and, 22, 1149
    cutoff scores and, 24, 1150
    in multiple test context, 24
    negative, 21–22, 1149–1150
    positive, 21, 1149–1150
Predictive validity, 18
    of Clock Drawing Test and, 980
    of Grip Strength and, 1057–1058
    of Grooved Pegboard, 1065
    of Instrumental Activities of Daily Living,
        1111
    of Personality Assessment Inventory, 1130
    of Purdue Pegboard Test, 1077
    of Rivermead Behavioural Memory Test—
        Second Edition, 848
    of Tactual Performance Test, 1038
    of Trail Making Test, 671
    of Wisconsin Card Sorting Test, 537
Prematurity, 127
Premorbid estimation of intelligence
    in children, 109–111
    current performation for, 107–109
    demographics for, 105–109
    description of, 104
    methods of, 104–105
    National Adult Reading Test for, 107–108,
        197–198
    Oklahoma Premorbid Intelligence Estimate
        for. See Oklahoma Premorbid Intelligence
        Estimate
    self-report for, 104
    sociodemographic variables for, 111
    Wechsler Adult Intelligence Scale—III,
        302–303
    Wide Range Achievement Test—3 for, 388
    WTAR for, 108, 302
Process approach, 76
Profile forms
    for adults, 29f–34f
    for children, 35f–40f
Progressive Supranuclear Palsy, 1077
Psychiatric disorders, 197, 256, 422, 571, 635,
        804, 833, 926, 988, 995, 1164, 1174, 1175.
        See also Depression, Schizophrenia,
        Anxiety
Psychological disorders
    description of, 1080
    history of, 1080
Psychometrist, 77

Questionnaires, history taking
    for adults, 57f–66f
    for children, 67f–73f

Race, 49. See also Ethnicity
    MMSE and, 176
    Repeatable Battery for the Assessment of
        Neuropsychological Status and, 239
Race-norming, 50
Reading ability, 768, 1081
Reason for referral, 87
Receiver operating characteristics analyses
        (ROC), 23–24

Recognition memory, 680, 684–685
Reference group change score distributions, 25
Referral, reason for, 87
Regression-based change scores (SRB scores).
        See also Change
    limits of, 27
    standardized, 26–27
Reliability. See also Alternate form reliability;
        Internal reliability; Interrater reliability;
        Test-retest reliability
    acceptable level of, 13
    of b Test, 1160
    of Balloon Test, 966–967
    of Beck Depression Inventory—Second
        Edition, 1086, 1088
    of Behavior Rating Inventory of Executive
        Function, 1093–1094, 1094t
    of Behavioral Assessment of the Dysexecutive
        Syndrome, 411–412, 412t
    of Bells Cancellation Test, 970
    of Benton Visual Retention Test, 695–697
    of Boston Diagnostic Aphasia Examination,
        896
    of Boston Naming Test—2, 910–911
    of Brief Test of Attention, 551–552
    of Brief Visuospatial Memory Test—Revised,
        703
    of Brown-Peterson Task, 711
    of Buschke Selective Reminding Test, 724
    of California Verbal Learning Test—Children's
        Version, 740–741
    of California Verbal Learning Test-II, 732–733
    of Cambridge Neuropsychological Test
        Automated Batteries, 419
    of Category Test, 431–432
    of Children's Memory Scale, 749–751,
        750t, 754
    of Clock Drawing Test, 977
    Color Trails Test in, 555–556
    of Comprehensive Trail Making Test, 559–560
    of Conners' Continuous Performance Test,
        569–570
    definition of, 9
    of Delis-Kaplan Executive Function System,
        446, 447t
    of Design Fluency Test, 453–454
    of Dichotic Learning—Words, 917
    of Doors and People Test, 758
    of Dot Counting Test, 1163–1164
    evaluation of, 13
    of Expressive One-Word Picture Vocabulary
        Test—Third Edition, 925
    of Expressive Vocabulary Test, 930–931
    of Facial Recognition Test, 986–987
    factors that affect, 9
    of Finger Localization, 1016
    of Finger Tapping, 1047
    of Geriatric Depression Scale, 1101–1102
    Gray Oral Reading Tests—Fourth Edition and,
        367–368, 368t
    of Grip Strength, 1055–1056
    of Grooved Pegboard, 1064
    of Hayling and Brixton Tests, 462–463
    of Hooper Visual Organization Test, 993–994
    of Hopkins Verbal Learning Test—Revised
        (HVLT-R), 762, 765–766
    of Instrumental Activities of Daily Living, 1110

of Integrated Visual and Auditory Continuous Performance Test, 579
of intelligence quotient tests (IQ), 100
of Judgment of Line Orientation, 1001–1002
of Kaplan Baycrest Neurocognitive Assessment, 162, 163t
of Kaufman Brief Intelligence Test, 165–166
limits of, 14
of Minnesota Multiphasic Personality Inventory—2, 1117
of MMSE, 180–181, 182t
of Multilingual Aphasia Examination, 937
of National Adult Reading Test, 196
of National Adult Reading Test-2, 196
of North American Adult Reading Test, 196
of Paced Auditory Serial Addition Test, 597–598, 601
of Peabody Picture Vocabulary Test—Third Edition, 944–945
of Personality Assessment Inventory, 1129
of Recognition Memory Test, 771–772
of Repeatable Battery for the Assessment of Neuropsychological Status, 244–248
of Rey Auditory Verbal Learning Test, 796–800
of Rey Fifteen-Item Memory Test, 1167–1168
of Rey-Osterrieth Complex Figure Test, 829–831, 830t
of Right-Left Orientation, 1019
of Rivermead Assessment of Somatosensory Performance, 1022
of Rivermead Behavioural Memory Test— Second Edition, 845–847
of Ruff 2 & 7 Selective Attention Test, 612–614
of Ruff Figural Fluency Test, 467–468
of Ruff-Light Trail Learning Test, 853
of Scales of Independent Behavior—Revised, 1138
of Self-Ordered Pointing Test, 474, 476
of Sentence Repetition Test, 858
of Smell Identification Test, 1026
of Speed and Capacity of Language Processing Test
   Speed of Comprehension Test, 274–275
of Spot-the-Word test, 275–276
of Stanford-Binet Intelligence Scales—Fifth Edition, 263–264
of Stroop Test, 490–492
of Symbol Digit Modalities Test, 620, 622–623
of Tactual Performance Test, 1036–1037
of Test of Everyday Attention, 632–633
of Test of Everyday Attention for Children, 641–642, 644
of Test of Memory Malingering, 1172–1173
of Test of Variables of Attention, 648–649
of 3MS, 182
of Token Test, 957
of Trail Making Test, 663, 665–667
of Trauma Symptom Inventory, 1142
true scores and, 15t
of 21-Item Test, 1177
of Victoria Symptom Validity Test, 1181
of Visual Object and Space Perception Battery, 1009–1010
of Wechsler Abbreviated Scale of Intelligence, 281
of Wechsler Adult Intelligence Scale—III, 294–298

of Wechsler Individual Achievement Test— Second Edition, 376–378
of Wechsler Intelligence Scale for Children— Fourth Edition, 331–332
of Wechsler Memory Scale—Third Edition, 868–870, 869t–870t
of Wechsler Preschool and Primary Scale of Intelligence—Third Edition, 342–343
of Wechsler Test of Adult Reading, 348–349
of Wide Range Achievement Test—3, 385
of Wide Range Assessment of Memory and Learning—Second Edition, 883–885, 886t
of Wisconsin Card Sorting Test, 531–534
of Woodcock-Johnson III Tests of Achievement (WJ III ACH), 396–398, 398t
of Woodcock-Johnson III Tests of Cognitive Abilities, 357–359
of Word Memory Test, 1186
Reliability coefficients
   adequacy of, 13–14
   error variance and, 9, 9t
   factors that affect, 9
   generalizability, 12–13
   Kuder-Richardson, 9, 9t
   limits of, 14
   magnitude of, 14t
   split-half, 9, 9t
Reliable Change Index, 25–26
   in Bayley Scales of Infant Development, 2, 125
   in Boston Naming Test, 910–911
   in Buschke Selective Reminding Test, 724
   in Category Test, 431
   in Conners' Continuous Performance Test II, 565
   in Dementia Rating Scale-2, 150
   in Finger Tapping Test, 1047
   in Geriatric Depression Scale, 1101–1102
   in Grip Strength, 1056
   in Grooved Pegboard, 1064
   in Hopkins Verbal Learning Test-Revised, 765–766
   in Mini-Mental State Examination, 181
   in Personality Assessment Inventory, 1129
   in Recognition Memory Test, 772
   in Repeatable Battery for the Assessment of Neuropsychological Status, 244–257
   in Rey Auditory Verbal Learning Test, 800, 804t
   in Rey Osterrieth Complex Figure, 830
   in Ruff Figural Fluency Test, 468
   in Symbol Digit Modalities Test, 622–623
   in Tactual Performance Test, 1036–1037
   in Test of Variables of Attention, 649
   in Trail Making Test, 666–668
   in Verbal Fluency, 515–517
   in Visual Object and Space Perception Battery, 1010
   in Wechsler Adult Intelligence Scale-III, 296–298
   in Wechsler Memory Scale-III, 868–870, 871t–872t
   in Wisconsin Card Sorting Test, 531–534
Report
   appendices, 93
   behavioral observations in, 89
   computer-generated, 94–95
   confidentiality of, 87
   content of, 87, 87t

current complaints and concerns, 88
description of, 86
forensic assessment, 93–94
history-taking information in, 87–88
informant information, 88–89
irrelevant information omitted from, 87
length of, 86–87
normative dataset used, 92
opinions in, 92
percentile-rank reporting, 91
privacy issues for, 87
reason for referral, 87
recipients of, 93
recommendations in, 92–93
review of relevant previous reports, 88
style of, 86
summary of, 92
test results in, 89–90
test scores, 90–93
wording of, 86
Response biases, 66

Sample
   of convenience, 53
   standardized, 53
Schizophrenia
   Autobiographical Memory Interview in patients with, 688–690
   B Test and, 1159
   Behavioral Assessment of the Dysexecutive Syndrome and, 413
   Benton Visual Retention Test-5 and, 698
   Boston Naming Test-2 and, 912
   Buschke Selective Reminding Test and, 727
   CANTAB and, 422
   Category Test and, 433
   Clock Drawing Test and, 979,
   Cognitive Estimation Test and, 442
   Conners' Continuous Performance Test and, 572
   Dichotic Listening Test and, 920
   Dot Counting Test and, 1162
   Hayling and Brixton Test and, 464–465
   National Adult Reading Test, 197
   Paced Auditory Serial Addition Test and, 605
   Purdue Pegboard and, 1077
   Repeatable Battery for the Assessment of Neuropsychological Status, 250, 256
   Rivermead Behavioral Memory Test and, 847
   Ruff 2 & 7 Test and, 614
   Rey-Osterrieth Complex Figure Test and, 833–834
   Sentence Repetition Test and, 859
   Smell Identification Test and, 1027
   Stroop Test and, 493
   Trail Making Test and, 670
   Wechsler Adult Intelligence Scale-III and, 297
   Wechsler Test of Adult Reading and, 388
   Wisconsin Card Sorting Test performance and, 536
   Word Memory Test and, 1186
Screening tests
   accuracy of, 20t, 21
   description of, 20
   efficiency of, 21
Self-knowledge, 688
Self-report, 104

SEM. See Standard error of measurement
Semantic memory, 684
Sensitivity, 21, 185, 215, 305, 380, 382, 387, 433, 469, 494, 538, 570–571, 759, 767, 773, 805, 876–877, 932, 947, 974, 977, 1087, 1102, 1121, 1149, 1169, 1174, 1178, 1182, 1186
Sibling intelligence, 111
Sickle Cell disease, 652
Skew, 8
Sleep deprivation, 476, 711
Sleep disorders, 652
Smoking, 1024
Sociodemographic factors
    older norms interaction with, 46
    premorbid estimations based on, 111
Socioeconomic status
    Boston Diagnostic Aphasia Examination and, 895
    parental education and, 120
    Wechsler Adult Intelligence Scale—III and, 289, 291
Somatosensory function tests, 1012–1013
Spatial neglect tests, 964
Spatial processing, 963
Special-needs patients, 82
Specific language disorders, 804
Specificity, 21, 185, 216, 300, 305, 334, 343, 380, 433, 469, 494, 570–571, 580, 615, 651, 669–676, 759, 767, 773, 805, 876–877, 974, 977, 1087, 1102, 1121, 1149, 1169, 1173, 1178
Speed tests, 10–11
Split-half reliability coefficient, 9, 9*t*
Standard error for individual predicted scores, 26
Standard error of estimation, 16–17
Standard error of measurement
    of California Verbal Learning Test—Children's Version, 740
    of Children's Memory Scale, 749
    of Conners' Continuous Performance Test, 569
    description of, 15–17
    of Expressive One-Word Picture Vocabulary Test—Third Edition, 925
    of Expressive Vocabulary Test, 930
    of Gray Oral Reading Tests—Fourth Edition, 367
    of Kaufman Brief Intelligence Test, 165–166
    of Minnesota Multiphasic Personality Inventory—2, 1117
    of NEPSY, 208
    of Neuropsychological Assessment Battery, 225
    of Peabody Picture Vocabulary Test—Third Edition, 944
    of Personality Assessment Inventory, 1129
    of Repeatable Battery for the Assessment of Neuropsychological Status, 244
    of Ruff 2 & 7 Selective Attention Test, 613
    of Scales of Independent Behavior—Revised, 1138
    of Stanford-Binet Intelligence Scales—Fifth Edition, 263
    of Test of Nonverbal Intelligence—3, 269
    of Test of Variables of Attention, 648
    of Wechsler Adult Intelligence Scale—III, 295
    of Wechsler Individual Achievement Test—Second Edition, 377

of Wechsler Intelligence Scale for Children—Fourth Edition, 331
    of Wechsler Memory Scale—Third Edition, 868
    of Wechsler Preschool and Primary Scale of Intelligence—Third Edition, 342
    of Wide Range Achievement Test—3, 386
    of Wide Range Assessment of Memory and Learning—Second Edition, 884–885
    of Woodcock-Johnson III Tests of Achievement, 397
    of Woodcock-Johnson III Tests of Cognitive Abilities, 357–358
Standard error of the difference, 25
Standard error of prediction, 17
Standard regression-based change (SRB) scores. *See* Change
Standardized sample, 53
Standardized scores
    interpretation of, 6
    linear transformation of, 4, 5*t*
    non-normality of
        causative factors, 8
        ceiling effects, 8
        floor effects, 8
        near-uniform distribution, 8
        overview of, 7–8
        percentile derivations and, 8–9
        skew, 8
        truncated distributions, 8
        uniform distribution, 8
    normalizing of, 9
Standards for Educational and Psychological Testing
    description of, 3
    validity as described by, 17
Stratified general population norms, 47
Stress, 81
Stroke. *See* Cerebro-Vascular Accidents
Suboptimal performance. *See also* Malingering
    client management, 1155–1156
    communication of findings about, 1156
    description of, 1145
    measures for detection of
        conventional, 1150–1152
        cutoffs, 1150, 1151*t*
        description of, 1148
        indices from conventional tests, 1151–1152
        multiple measures, 1154–1155
        new indices, 1150, 1151*t*
        selection of tests, 1148–1150
        specially designed tests, 1152–1154
        symptom validity tests, 1152–1154
    multiple assessments, 1155
    risk factors for, 1175
Substance abuse treatment records, 56*t*
Symbolic play
    Bayley Scales of Infant Development—Second Edition and, 128
    description of, 128
Symptom report/response styles, 66, 73

Temporal lobe dysfunction, 421–422, 454, 459, 469, 475, 518, 519, 536, 684–685, 689, 726, 759, 772, 773, 801, 832, 847, 988, 1027

T scores
    classification of, 91*t*
    conversion of, 5*t*
    description of, 4
Test(s)
    Flynn effect, 45–46
    imprecision of, 28
    order of, 78
    precision of, 9
    selection of, 75–76
    standards for, 3
    timing of, 76–77
    translation of, 83
    variability among, 3
Test administration
    computer-based, 77–78
    note-taking during, 77
    order of, 78
    by psychometrist, 77
    in report, 93
    time required for, 77
    timing of, 76–77
Test data
    graphical representations of, 28, 40
    profile forms for, 29*f*–40*f*
Test scores
    extreme, 6
    normalizing of, 9
    practice effects and, 11
    prior exposure effects on, 11–12
    in report, 90–93
    standardization of, 6
    variability in, 11
Test-retest reliability
    of Balloon Test, 966–967
    of Beck Depression Inventory—Second Edition, 1086
    of Behavior Rating Inventory of Executive Function, 1094
    of Behavioral Assessment of the Dysexecutive Syndrome, 411
    of Bells Cancellation Test, 970
    of Benton Visual Retention Test, 696
    of Boston Diagnostic Aphasia Examination, 896
    of Boston Naming Test—2, 910–911
    of Brief Test of Attention, 551–552
    of Brief Visuospatial Memory Test—Revised, 703
    of Brixton Tests, 463
    of Brown-Peterson Task, 711
    of Buschke Selective Reminding Test, 724
    of California Verbal Learning Test—Children's Version, 740–741, 743*t*
    of California Verbal Learning Test-II, 732
    of Cambridge Neuropsychological Test Automated Batteries, 419, 421*t*
    of Category Test, 431
    of Children's Color Trails Test, 555–556
    of Children's Memory Scale, 749–751, 750*t*, 754
    of Clock Drawing Test, 977
    of Cognitive Assessment System, 139, 140*t*
    of Cognitive Estimation Test, 441
    of Color Trails Test, 555–556
    of Comprehensive Trail Making Test, 560
    of Conners' Continuous Performance Test, 569–570

of Delis-Kaplan Executive Function System, 446, 447*t*
of Dementia Rating Scale-2, 149–150
description of, 11
of Design Fluency Test, 453–454
of Doors and People Test, 759
of Expressive One-Word Picture Vocabulary Test—Third Edition, 925
of Expressive Vocabulary Test, 930
of Facial Recognition Test, 987
of Finger Localization, 1016
of Finger Tapping, 1047
of Geriatric Depression Scale, 1101–1102
of Gray Oral Reading Tests—Fourth Edition, 367–368, 368*t*
of Grip Strength, 1056
of Grooved Pegboard, 1064
of Hayling Tests, 463
of Hooper Visual Organization Test, 994
of Hopkins Verbal Learning Test—Revised (HVLT-R), 762, 766*t*
of Instrumental Activities of Daily Living, 1110
of Integrated Visual and Auditory Continuous Performance Test, 579, 579*t*
of Judgment of Line Orientation, 1002
of Kaplan Baycrest Neurocognitive Assessment, 162, 163*t*
of Kaufman Brief Intelligence Test, 166
of Minnesota Multiphasic Personality Inventory—2, 1117
of MMSE, 181
of National Adult Reading Test, 196
of NEPSY, 208–209, 210*t*
of Neuropsychological Assessment Battery, 223, 225, 228
of Paced Auditory Serial Addition Test, 597
of Peabody Picture Vocabulary Test—Third Edition, 944–945
of Personality Assessment Inventory, 1129
practice effects, 11
prior exposure effects, 11–12
of Purdue Pegboard Test, 1070, 1076
of Recognition Memory Test, 772, 774
of Repeatable Battery for the Assessment of Neuropsychological Status, 244–246
of Rey Auditory Verbal Learning Test, 797
of Rey Fifteen-Item Memory Test, 1167–1168
of Rey-Osterrieth Complex Figure Test, 829–830
of Right-Left Orientation, 1019
of Rivermead Assessment of Somatosensory Performance, 1022
of Rivermead Behavioural Memory Test—Second Edition, 845
of Ruff 2 & 7 Selective Attention Test, 613, 613*t*
of Ruff Figural Fluency Test, 467–468, 470
of Scales of Independent Behavior—Revised, 1138
of Self-Ordered Pointing Test, 474
of Sentence Repetition Test, 858
for speed tests, 10–11
of Stanford-Binet Intelligence Scales—Fifth Edition, 263
of Stroop Test, 490–492
of Symbol Digit Modalities Test, 620, 622
of Tactual Performance Test, 1036–1037

of Test of Everyday Attention, 632, 633*t*
of Test of Everyday Attention for Children, 641
of Test of Nonverbal Intelligence—3, 269
of Test of Variables of Attention, 648–649
of Token Test, 957
of Trail Making Test, 663, 665–666
of Verbal Fluency Test, 514
of Victoria Symptom Validity Test, 1181
of Visual Object and Space Perception Battery, 1009–1010
of Wechsler Abbreviated Scale of Intelligence, 281
of Wechsler Adult Intelligence Scale—III, 295
of Wechsler Individual Achievement Test—Second Edition, 377, 378*t*
of Wechsler Intelligence Scale for Children—Fourth Edition, 331–332
of Wechsler Memory Scale—Third Edition, 868–870
of Wechsler Preschool and Primary Scale of Intelligence—Third Edition, 342
of Wechsler Test of Adult Reading, 348–349
of Wide Range Achievement Test—3, 386
of Wide Range Assessment of Memory and Learning—Second Edition, 885
of Wisconsin Card Sorting Test, 531–534
of Woodcock-Johnson III Tests of Achievement, 397
of Woodcock-Johnson III Tests of Cognitive Abilities, 358, 358*t*
Third moment of a distribution, 8
Time of day effects, 495, 668, 768, 1003
Toxic exposure, 669, 804, 912, 919, 949, 1057, 1065, 1077
Traumatic brain injury. *See also* Head injury
Assessment of response bias and, 1145
Beck Depression Inventory and, 1088
Behavior Rating Inventory of Executive Function (BRIEF) and, 1096–1097
Behavioral Assessment of the Dysexecutive Syndrome and, 412–414
Benton Visual Retention Test-5 and, 697–698
Boston Naming Test—2 and, 912
Brown-Peterson Test and, 712
b Test assessments of, 1161
Buschke Selective Reminding Test and 726–727
California Verbal Learning Test—Children's Version evaluation of, 743–744
Category Test and, 433
Cognitive Estimation Test and, 442
Design Fluency and, 445
Dichotic Listening and, 919–920
Dot Counting Test and, 1162
Facial Recognition Test and, 988
Finger Tapping Test and, 1048
Grip Strength and, 1057
Kaplan Baycrest Neurocognitive Assessment and, 163
Kaufman Brief Intelligence Test and, 167
MAE and, 938–939
Minnesota Multiphasic Personality Inventory—2 and, 1118
National Adult Reading Test and, 197
Neuropsychological Assessment Battery and, 227
PASAT and, 604

Peabody Picture Vocabulary Test-III and, 949,
Recognition Memory Test and, 773
report writing and, 88
Rey Auditory Verbal Learning Test and, 804–805
Rey Fifteen-Item Test and, 1168–1169
Rey-Osterrieth Complex Figure Test and, 833–834
Rivermead Behavioral Memory Test-II and, 847–848
Ruff figural Fluency Test and, 469
Ruff 2 & 7 Test and, 614
Self-Ordered Pointing Test and, 476
Sentence Repetition Test and, 859
Smell Identification Test and 1027–1028
Stroop Test and, 493
Symbol Digit Modalities Test and, 625
TEA performance and, 634, 635*t*
Test of Everday Attention-Ch and, 643
Test of Memory Malingering and, 1174
Tactual Performance Test and, 1038
Token Test evaluations, 959
Trail Making Test and, 669–671
Verbal fluency and, 519
Victoria Symptom Validity Test and, 1182
Wechsler Abbreviated Scale of Intelligence, 281
Wechsler Adult Intelligence Scale—III scores, 297, 299, 300, 303
Wechsler Intelligence Scale for Children—IV and, 336
Wechsler Memory Scale-II and, 874
Wechsler Test of Adult Reading and, 350
Wide Range Achievement Test-3 and, 388
Wide Range Assessment of Memory and Learning-2 and, 888
Wisconsin Card Sorting Test performance and, 536, 537, 538
Word Memory Test and, 1186
Tripartite model of validity, 18
True scores
in clinical practice, 15
definition of, 14
estimated, 14–16
obtained scores vs., 17
reliability and, 15*t*
Truncated distributions, 8, 52
Turner's Syndrome, 833, 1003

Uniform distribution, 8

Validity. *See also* Construct validity; Content validity; Convergent validity; Divergent validity; Ecological validity; Predictive validity
of Autobiographical Memory Interview, 688
of b Test, 1160
of Balloon Test, 967
of Beck Depression Inventory—Second Edition, 1086–1088
of Behavior Rating Inventory of Executive Function, 1094–1097
of Behavioral Assessment of the Dysexecutive Syndrome, 412–414
of Bells Cancellation Test, 970–971
of Benton Visual Retention Test, 697–698
of Boston Diagnostic Aphasia Examination, 896–899

Validity (*continued*)
  of Brief Visuospatial Memory Test—Revised, 703–704
  of Brixton Tests, 463–465
  of Brown-Peterson Task, 711–712
  of Buschke Selective Reminding Test, 724, 726–727
  of California Verbal Learning Test—Children's Version, 741–744
  of Cambridge Neuropsychological Test Automated Batteries, 419, 421–422
  of Category Test, 432–433
  of Children's Color Trails Test, 556
  of Children's Memory Scale, 751–753
  of Clock Drawing Test, 977–980
  of Cognitive Assessment System, 139–142
  of Cognitive Estimation Test, 441–442
  of Comprehensive Trail Making Test, 561
  concurrent, 18, 233
  of Conners' Continuous Performance Test, 570–572
  content-related, 19t
  criterion-related, 19t
  definition of, 18
  of Delis-Kaplan Executive Function System, 446–447
  description of, 17–18
  of Design Fluency Test, 454–455
  of Dichotic Learning—Words, 917, 919–920
  divergent, 18
  of Doors and People Test, 759, 760
  of Dot Counting Test, 1164
  evaluation of, 18–19
  of Expressive One-Word Picture Vocabulary Test—Third Edition, 925–927
  of Expressive Vocabulary Test, 931–932
  of Facial Recognition Test, 987–988
  of Finger Localization, 1016–1017
  of Finger Tapping, 1047–1049
  of Five-Point Test, 459
  of forensic reports, 94
  of Geriatric Depression Scale, 1102–1104
  of Gray Oral Reading Tests—Fourth Edition, 368–369
  of Grip Strength, 1056–1058
  of Grooved Pegboard, 1065–1066
  of Hayling Tests, 463–465
  of Hooper Visual Organization Test, 994–996
  of Hopkins Verbal Learning Test—Revised (HVLT-R), 766–768
  of Instrumental Activities of Daily Living, 1110–1111
  of Judgment of Line Orientation, 1002–1004
  of Kaplan Baycrest Neurocognitive Assessment, 162–163

  of Kaufman Brief Intelligence Test, 166–167
  Messick's model of, 18, 18t
  of Minnesota Multiphasic Personality Inventory—2, 1118–1123
  models of, 18
  of Multilingual Aphasia Examination, 937–939
  of National Adult Reading Test, 196–198
  of NEPSY, 211–214
  of Neuropsychological Assessment Battery, 225–228
  of Personality Assessment Inventory, 1130–1132
  of Purdue Pegboard Test, 1077
  of Raven's Progressive Matrices, 233–235
  of Recognition Memory Test, 772–775
  of Repeatable Battery for the Assessment of Neuropsychological Status, 249–257
  report description of, 90
  of Rey Auditory Verbal Learning Test, 800–806
  of Rey Fifteen-Item Memory Test, 1168–1169
  of Rey-Osterrieth Complex Figure Test, 831–835
  of Right-Left Orientation, 1019–1020
  of Rivermead Assessment of Somatosensory Performance, 1022–1023
  of Ruff 2 & 7 Selective Attention Test, 614–615
  of Scales of Independent Behavior—Revised, 1138–1139
  of Self-Ordered Pointing Test, 474–476
  of Sentence Repetition Test, 858–859
  of Smell Identification Test, 1026–1028
  of Speed and Capacity of Language Processing Test
    Speed of Comprehension Test, 276
    Spot-the-Word test, 276–278
  Standards for Educational and Psychological Testing description of, 17
  of Stanford-Binet Intelligence Scales—Fifth Edition, 264–266
  of Stroop Test, 492–495
  subtypes of, 18
  of Symbol Digit Modalities Test, 623–626
  of Tactual Performance Test, 1037–1038
  of Test of Everyday Attention, 633–635
  of Test of Everyday Attention for Children, 642–644
  of Test of Memory Malingering, 1173–1175
  of Test of Nonverbal Intelligence—3, 270–271
  of Test of Variables of Attention, 649–652
  test-centric assessment of, 18

  of Token Test, 957, 959–960
  of Trail Making Test, 668–672
  of Trauma Symptom Inventory, 1141t, 1142–1143
  of 21-Item Test, 1178
  of Verbal Fluency Test, 517–521
  of Visual Object and Space Perception Battery, 1010
  of Wechsler Abbreviated Scale of Intelligence, 281–282
  of Wechsler Adult Intelligence Scale—III, 298–305
  of Wechsler Individual Achievement Test—Second Edition, 378–381
  of Wechsler Intelligence Scale for Children—Fourth Edition, 332–336
  of Wechsler Memory Scale—Third Edition, 870–877
  of Wechsler Preschool and Primary Scale of Intelligence—Third Edition, 343–345
  of Wechsler Test of Adult Reading, 349–350
  of Wide Range Achievement Test—3, 386–388
  of Wide Range Assessment of Memory and Learning—Second Edition, 885, 887–888
  of Wisconsin Card Sorting Test, 534–538
  of Woodcock-Johnson III Tests of Achievement, 398–399
  of Woodcock-Johnson III Tests of Cognitive Abilities, 359–360
  of Word Memory Test, 1186–1187
Validity coefficient, 19–20
Vascular dementia, 155,183, 767, 832, 1027
Velo-cardio-facial syndrome, 1010
Visual field defect, 234, 979, 966, 988
Visual neglect, 234, 834, 979, 970, 964–966, 987, 1003
Visual perception tests, 963–965
Visual-spatial disorders, 964

White matter hyperintensities, 1077, 1103
Williams Syndrome, 988, 1065
Within-group norming, 50
Word reading tests
  description of, 107
Working memory
  description of, 678–679
  neural correlates of, 684–685

Z scores
  classification of, 91t
  conversion of, 5t
  description of, 4
  estimated prevalence value of, 6
  linear transformation of, 4, 5t
  percentiles and, nonlinear relation between, 4